MW00846021

Fundamental and Advanced Fetal Imaging Ultrasound and MRI

Second Edition

EDITORS

Beth M. Kline-Fath, MD

Professor of Radiology
Chief of Fetal and Neonatal Imaging
Department of Radiology
College of Medicine, University of Cincinnati
Cincinnati Children's Hospital Medical Center
Cincinnati, Ohio

Dorothy I. Bulas, MD

Professor of Pediatrics and Radiology
George Washington University
Chief
Division of Diagnostic Imaging and Radiology
Director of Fetal Imaging
Prenatal Pediatrics Institute
Children's National Hospital
Washington, District of Columbia

Wesley Lee, MD

Professor of Obstetrics and Gynecology
Director, Division of Women's and Fetal Imaging
Department of Obstetrics and Gynecology
Baylor College of Medicine
Medical Staff, Texas Children's Pavilion for Women
Houston, Texas

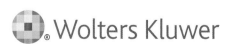

Philadelphia • Baltimore • New York • London
Buenos Aires • Hong Kong • Sydney • Tokyo

Executive Editor: Sharon Zinner
Development Editor: Eric McDermott
Editorial Coordinator: Ashley Pfeiffer
Senior Production Project Manager: David Saltzberg
Design Coordinator: Holly Reid McLaughlin
Prepress Vendor: S4Carlisle Publishing Services

Copyright © 2021 Wolters Kluwer Health

All rights reserved. This book is protected by copyright. No part of this book may be reproduced or transmitted in any form or by any means, including as photocopies or scanned-in or other electronic copies, or utilized by any information storage and retrieval system without written permission from the copyright owner, except for brief quotations embodied in critical articles and reviews. Materials appearing in this book prepared by individuals as part of their official duties as U.S. government employees are not covered by the above-mentioned copyright. To request permission, please contact Wolters Kluwer Health at Two Commerce Square, 2001 Market Street, Philadelphia, PA 19103, via email at permissions@lww.com, or via our website at shop.lww.com (products and services).

9 8 7 6 5 4 3 2 1

Printed in China

Library of Congress Cataloging-in-Publication Data

ISBN-13: 978-1-975117-00-9

ISBN-10: 1-975117-00-X

Library of Congress Control Number: 2020932318

Care has been taken to confirm the accuracy of the information presented and to describe generally accepted practices. However, the authors, editors, and publisher are not responsible for errors or omissions or for any consequences from application of the information in this book and make no warranty, expressed or implied, with respect to the currency, completeness, or accuracy of the contents of the publication. Application of this information in a particular situation remains the professional responsibility of the practitioner; the clinical treatments described and recommended may not be considered absolute and universal recommendations.

The authors, editors, and publisher have exerted every effort to ensure that drug selection and dosage set forth in this text are in accordance with the current recommendations and practice at the time of publication. However, in view of ongoing research, changes in government regulations, and the constant flow of information relating to drug therapy and drug reactions, the reader is urged to check the package insert for each drug for any change in indications and dosage and for added warnings and precautions. This is particularly important when the recommended agent is a new or infrequently employed drug.

Some drugs and medical devices presented in this publication have Food and Drug Administration (FDA) clearance for limited use in restricted research settings. It is the responsibility of the health care provider to ascertain the FDA status of each drug or device planned for use in his or her clinical practice.

shop.lww.com

CCS0420

To my husband, Tom, without whose love and support, this book would not have been possible. To my daughters, Kelsey and Abby, and new sons, Matt and John, I will always love you more. To my parents, thank you for your love and for teaching me to always reach for more. And to my family, especially my nieces Natasha and Naomi, it is through your lives that I understood the importance of this field.
BMKF

To my husband, Neal, whose incredible support and encouragement remain key to whatever I accomplish. To my sons, Mark and Adam, and their growing families, for the love and joy they bring to my life. And finally to my parents Romuald and Benigna, as well as my sister Barbara, who have been the inspiration to explore the fascinating field of fetal medicine.
DIB

To my wife, Pam, who has been a constant inspiration throughout my career. To those among us who value the pursuit of academic medicine and to others who will serve in the future.
WL

Jacques S. Abramowicz, MD, FACOG, FAIUM
Professor
Department of Obstetrics and Gynecology
University of Chicago
Director of Ultrasound Quality Assurance
Department of Obstetrics and Gynecology
University of Chicago Medical Center
Chicago, Illinois

Nickie Andescavage, MD
Assistant Professor
Department of Pediatrics
George Washington University School of Medicine
Attending, Neonatal-Perinatal Medicine/Director,
    Neonatal Transport
Department of Neonatology
Children's National Hospital
Washington, District of Columbia

Fred E. Avni, MD, PhD
Professor in Radiology
Faculty of Medicine
Free University of Brussels (ULB)
Senior Consultant in Pediatric and Fetal Imaging
Department of Imaging
Delta Hospital (CHIREC)
Brussels, Belgium

Richard A. Barth, MD
Professor and Associate Chair of Radiology
Department of Radiology
Stanford University School of Medicine
Radiologist in Chief
Department of Radiology
Lucile Packard Children's Hospital at Stanford
Stanford, California

Michael A. Belfort, MBBCH, MD, PhD
Ernst W. Bertner Chairman and Professor
FB McGuyer Family Endowed Chair in Fetal Surgery
Department of Obstetrics and Gynecology
Baylor College of Medicine
Obstetrician and Gynecologist-In-Chief
Texas Chlldren's Hospital
Medical Director, Texas Children's Fetal Center
Houston, Texas

Krista Lynn Birkemeier, MD
Clinical Associate Professor of Practice
Department of Medical Education
Texas A&M College of Medicine
Bryan, Texas
Staff Radiologist
Department of Radiology
Baylor Scott & White, McLane Children's Medical Center
Temple, Texas

Dorothy I. Bulas, MD
Professor of Pediatrics and Radiology
Division of Diagnostic Imaging and Radiology
George Washington University
Chief, Director of Fetal Imaging
Division of Diagnostic Imaging and Radiology
Children's National Hospital
Washington, District of Columbia

Maria A. Calvo-Garcia, MD
Associate Professor of Radiology
Department of Radiology
College of Medicine, University of Cincinnati
Cincinnati Children's Hospital Medical Center
Cincinnati, Ohio

Christopher Ian Cassady, MD
Professor
Departments of Radiology, Obstetrics &
    Gynecology, and Pediatrics
Baylor College of Medicine
EB Singleton Department of Radiology
Texas Children's Hospital and Fetal Center
Houston, Texas

Teresa Chapman, MD, MA
Professor
Department of Radiology
University of Washington
Radiologist
Department of Radiology
Seattle Children's Hospital
Seattle, Washington

Sarah B. Clauss, MD
Associate Professor
Department of Pediatrics
George Washington University
Washington, District of Columbia
Pediatric Cardiologist
Department of Cardiology
Children's National Medical Center
Washington, District of Columbia

Gregory DeVore, MD
Clinical Professor
David Geffen School of Medicine, UCLA
Pasadena, California

Mary T. Donofrio, MD
Professor
Department of Pediatric Cardiology
George Washington University School of Medicine and
    Health Sciences
Director, Fetal Heart Program
Department of Cardiology
Children's National Hospital
Washington, District of Columbia

Judy A. Estroff, MD
Associate Professor
Department of Radiology
Harvard Medical School
Division Chief, Fetal-Neonatal Imaging
Department of Radiology
Boston Children's Hospital
Boston, Massachusetts

Karin A. Fox, MD, MEd, FACOG
Associate Professor
Department of Obstetrics and Gynecology
Clinical Director, Placenta Accreta Spectrum Care Team
Medical Director of Maternal Transport, Kangaroo Crew
Baylor College of Medicine
Texas Children's Pavilion for Women
Houston, Texas

Henry L. Galan, MD
Professor
Department of Obstetrics & Gynecology
University of Colorado School of Medicine
Colorado Fetal Care Center
Children's Hospital of Colorado
Aurora, Colorado

Luis F. Goncalves, MD
Professor
Department of Radiology and Child Health
University of Arizona Medical College
Director of Fetal Imaging
Department of Radiology
Phoenix Children's Hospital
Phoenix, Arizona

Mourina Habli, MD
Associate Professor
Department of Pediatric Surgery
University of Cincinnati
Trihealth Fetal care Center
Director
Obstetrics and Gynecology Department
Good Samaritan Hospital
Cincinnati, Ohio

Sonia S. Hassan, MD
Associate Vice President
Office of Women's Health
Wayne State University
Detroit, Michigan

Edgar Hernandez-Andrade, MD
Professor
Division of Maternal-Fetal Medicine
Department of Obstetrics and Gynecology
Wayne State University School of Medicine
Detroit, Michigan
Head (Coordinator)
Maternal-Fetal Imaging Unit
Perinatology Research Branch
Division of Obstetrics and Maternal-Fetal Medicine
Division of Intramural Research
Eunice Kennedy Shriver National Institute of Child Health and Human Development, National Institutes of Health
U. S. Department of Health and Human Services
Hutzel Women's Hospital
Detroit, Michigan

Adam K. Hiett, MD, RDMS
Clinical Professor
Department of Obstetrics/Gynecology
Wright State University, Boonshoft School of Medicine
Maternal-Fetal Medicine
Miami Valley Hospital
Dayton, Ohio

Robert J. Hopkin, MD
Associate Professor
Department of Pediatrics
University of Cincinnati
Associate Professor
Division of Human Genetics
Cincinnati Children's Hospital
Cincinnati, Ohio

Sarah Mayes Huguenard, MS, CGC
Instructor
Department of Molecular and Human Genetics
Baylor College of Medicine
Houston, Texas

Jon Hyett, MBBS, BSc, MD, MRCOG, FRANZCOG
Clinical Professor
Departments of Obstetrics, Gynaecology and Neonatology
University of Sydney
Head, High Risk Obstetrics
RPA Women and Basics
Camperdown, New South Wales, Australia

Jiri D. Sonek, MD
Clinical Professor
Department of Maternal-Fetal Medicine
Wright State University
Fairborn, Ohio
Medical Director
Department of Maternal-Fetal Medicine, Ultrasound, and Genetics
Miami Valley Hospital
Dayton, Ohio

Cristiano D. Jodicke, MD
Maternal-Fetal Medicine Specialist
Department of Obstetrics and Gynecology
Winnie Palmer Hospital for Women and Babies
Orlando, Florida

Jennifer H. Johnston, MD
Assistant Professor
Department of Diagnostic and Interventional Imaging
McGovern Medical School
Staff, Department of Radiology
Children's Memorial Hermann Hospital
Houston, Texas

Beth M. Kline-Fath, MD, FAIUM
Professor of Radiology
Chief of Fetal and Neonatal Imaging
Department of Radiology
College of Medicine, Univeristy of Cincinnati
Cincinnati Children's Hospital Medical Center
Cincinnati, Ohio

Anita Krishnan, MD
Pediatric Cardiologist
Department of Cardiology
George Washington University
Children's National Medical Center
Washington, District of Columbia

Wesley Lee, MD
Professor of Obstetrics and Gynecology
Director, Division of Women's and Fetal Imaging
Department of Obstetrics and Gynecology
Baylor College of Medicine
Medical Staff, Texas Children's Pavilion for Women
Houston, Texas

Catherine Limperopoulos, PhD
Professor
Department of Neurology, Radiology, and Pediatrics
George Washington University School of Medicine
Director, Advanced Pediatric Brain Imaging Research
Director, Center for the Developing Brain
Vice Chair of Research, Diagnostic Imaging & Radiology
Co-Director of Research, Division of Neonatology
Department of Diagnostic Imaging & Radiology
Children's National Hospital
Washington, District of Columbia

Leann E. Linam, MD
Associate Professor
Department of Radiology and Pediatrics
Emory University
Physician Lead for Ultrasound
Department of Radiology
Children's Healthcare of Atlanta-Egleston Hospital
Atlanta, Georgia

Anderson J. Lo, DO
Fellow, Maternal-Fetal Medicine
Perinatology Research Branch
Division of Obstetrics and Maternal-Fetal Medicine
Division of Intramural Research
Eunice Kennedy Shriver National Institute of Child Health and
    Human Development, National Institutes of Health
    U. S. Department of Health and Human Services
Hutzel Women's Hospital
Fellow, Maternal-Fetal Medicine
Division of Maternal-Fetal Medicine
Department of Obstetrics and Gynecology
Wayne State University School of Medicine
Detroit, Michigan

Jorge Lopes, PhD
Assistant Professor
Department of Arts and Design
Pontifícia Universidade Católica (PUC-Rio)
Rio de Janeiro-RJ
Brazil

Davide Marini
Staff Cardiologist
The Labatt Family Heart Centre
The Hospital for Sick Children
Assistant Professor
University of Toronto
Toronto, Ontario, Canada

Juan S. Martin-Saavedra, MD
Post-Doctoral Research Fellow
Department of Radiology
The Children's Hospital of Philadelphia
Philadelphia, Pennsylvania

Dev Maulik, MD, PhD
Professor and Chair
Department of Obstetrics and Gynecology
Senior Associate Dean, Women's Health
UMKC School of Medicine
Chair, Department of Obstetrics and Gynecology
Truman Medical Center
Chair, Department of Maternal Fetal Medicine
Children's Mercy Hospital
Kansas City, Missouri

Amy R. Mehollin-Ray, MD
Associate Professor
Departments of Radiology and Obstetrics and Gynecology
Baylor College of Medicine
Chief, Division of Fetal Radiology, E.B. Singleton
Department of Pediatric Radiology
Houston, Texas

Mariana Laura Meyers, MD
Associate Professor
Department of Radiology
University of Colorado School of Medicine
Director of Fetal MRI
Department of Pediatric Radiology
Children's Hospital Colorado
Aurora, Colorado

David Michael Mirsky, MD
Associate Professor
Department of Radiology
University of Colorado School of Medicine
Pediatric Neuroradiologist
Department of Radiology
Children's Hospital Colorado
Aurora, Colorado

Usha D. Nagaraj, MD
Assistant Professor
Department of Radiology
University of Cincinnati College of Medicine
Assistant Professor
Department of Clinical Radiology and Pediatrics
Cincinnati Children's Hospital Medical Center
Cincinnati, Ohio

Salma A. Nassef, MS, CGC
Associate Program Director
Genetic Counseling Program
School of Health Professions
Baylor College of Medicine
Assistant Professor
Board Certified Genetic Counselor
Department of Molecular and Human Genetics
Houston, Texas

Ahmed A. Nassr, MD, PhD
Assistant Professor
Department of Obstetrics and Gynecology
Baylor College of Medicine
Texas Children's Fetal Center
Houston, Texas

Kypros H. Nicolaides, FRCOG
Professor of Fetal Medicine
Department of Women & Children's Health
King's College London
Director of Fetal Medicine Research Institute
King's College Hospital
London, UK

David Perry, MBChB, FRANZCR
Department of Radiology
National Women's and Starship Children's Health
University of Auckland
Auckland, New Zealand

Rupa Radhakrishnan, MBBS, MS
Assistant Professor
Department of Radiology and Imaging Sciences
Indiana University School of Medicine
Neuroradiologist
Department of Radiology and Imaging Sciences
Riley Hospital for Children at Indiana University Health
Indianapolis, Indiana

Shane Reeves, MD
Associate Professor
Department of OB/GYN
University of Colorado School of Medicine
Director of Prenatal Diagnosis and Genetics
Department of OB/GYN
University of Colorado Hospital
Aurora, Colorado

Gerson Ribeiro
Fellowship
Department of Arts and Design
Pontifícia Universidade Católica (PUC-Rio)
Rio de Janeiro-RJ
Brazil

Timothy P. L. Roberts, PhD
Professor
Department of Radiology
University of Pennsylvania
Vice-chair Research and Oberkircher Family Chair in
  Pediatric Radiology
Department of Radiology
Children's Hospital of Philadelphia
Philadelphia, Pennsylvania

Ashley James Robinson, BSc, MB ChB, FRCR, FRCPC
Associate Professor
Department of Radiology
Weill Cornell Medical College
New York, New York
Vice-Chair
Diagnostic Imaging
Sidra Medicine
Doha, Qatar

Roberto Romero, MD, D.Med.Sci.
Chief
Perinatology Research Branch
Division of Obstetrics and Maternal-Fetal Medicine
Division of Intramural Research
Eunice Kennedy Shriver National Institute of Child Health and
  Human Development, National Institutes of Health, U.S.
  Department of Health and Human Services
Hutzel Women's Hospital
Detroit, Michigan

Eva Ilse Rubio, MD
Associate Professor
Department of Radiology
The George Washington University
Vice Chief
Division of Diagnostic Imaging and Radiology
Children's National Hospital
Washington, District of Columbia

Stephanie L. Santoro, MD
Assistant Professor
Department of Pediatrics
Harvard Medical School
Clinical Geneticist
Department of Pediatrics
Massachusetts General Hospital
Hospital or Institution
Boston, Massachusetts

Gary M. Satou, MD, FASE, FAHA
Director, Pediatric Echocardiography
Co-Director, Fetal Cardiology Program
UCLA Mattel Children's Hospital, Ronald Reagan UCLA
  Medical Center & UCLA Health
Clinical Professor, Pediatrics, David Geffen School of Medicine
  at UCLA
UCLA Children's Heart Center
Los Angeles, California

David N. Schidlow, MD, MMus
Cardiac Imaging, Pediatric and Fetal Cardiology
Department of Cardiology
Boston Children's Hospital
Assistant Professor of Pediatrics
Harvard Medical School
Boston, Massachusetts

William T. Schnettler, MD, FACOG
Department of Maternal-Fetal Medicine
Cincinnati Children's Hospital Medical Center
Director
Center for Maternal Cardiac and Critical Care
Department of Obstetrics and Gynecology
Good Samaritan Hospital
Cincinnati, Ohio

Mike T. M. Seed, MBBS, MRCHPCH, FRCR
Associate Professor
Department of Paediatrics and Medical Imaging
University of Toronto
Division Head, Cardiology
Departments of Pediatrics and Diagnostic Imaging
The Hospital for Sick Children
Toronto, Ontario, Canada

Neeta Jain Sethi, MD
Advanced Cardiac Imaging Fellow
Division of Cardiology
Children's National Hospital
Washington, District of Columbia

Alireza A. Shamshirsaz, MD
Associate Professor
Department of Maternal Fetal Medicine
Baylor College of Medicine
Fetal Surgeon
Department of Obstetrics and Gynecology
Texas Children's Pavilion for Women
Houston, Texas

Paul Singh, MD
Clinical Instructor
Division of Maternal-Fetal Medicine
Department of Obstetrics and Gynecology
Kansas City, Missouri

Mark Sklansky, MD
Professor and Chief
Division of Pediatric Cardiology
Department of Pediatrics
David Geffen School of Medicine at UCLA
UCLA Mattel Children's Hospital
Los Angeles, California

Eleazar E. Soto Torres, MD
Assistant Professor
Division of Maternal-Fetal Medicine
Obstetrics, Gynecology and Reproductive Sciences
McGovern Medical School
The University of Texas Health Science
   Center at Houston
Houston, Texas
Head
Maternal-Fetal Imaging Unit
The University of Texas Health Science Center at Houston
Houston, Texas

Dan Tirosh, MD
Senior Physician, Clinical Lecturer
Ultrasound Unit
Department of Obstetrics and Gynecology
Soroka University Medical Center and the Faculty of
   Health Sciences
Ben-Gurion University of the Negev
Beer Sheva, Israel

Ignatia B. Van den Veyver, MD
Professor
Department of Obstetrics and Gynecology and
   Molecular and Human Genetics
Baylor College of Medicine
Director of Clinical Prenatal Genetics
Department of Obstetrics and Gynecology and
   Molecular and Human Genetics
Texas Children's Hospital Pavilion for Women
Houston, Texas

Teresa Victoria, MD, PhD
Associate Professor
Department of Radiology
Children's Hospital of Philadelphia
Philadelphia, Pennsylvania

Heron Werner Jr, MD
Department of Fetal Medicine
Clínica de Diagnóstico por Imagem (CDPI)
Rio de Janeiro-RJ
Brazil

Lami Yeo, MD, FACOG, FAIUM
Professor
Division of Maternal-Fetal Medicine
Department of Obstetrics and Gynecology
Wayne State University School of Medicine
Director of Fetal Cardiology
Perinatology Research Branch
Division of Obstetrics and Maternal-Fetal Medicine
Division of Intramural Research
Eunice Kennedy Shriver National Institute of Child Health and
   Human Development, National Institutes of Health, U.S.
   Department of Health and Human Services
Hutzel Women's Hospital
Detroit, Michigan

Prenatal ultrasound (US) ushered in an exciting new age in fetal assessment and represented the proverbial great leap forward. The systematic investigation of both fetal behavior and anatomy became a reality. Subsequent technologic advances have ensued at a relentless pace. Pulse and color Doppler facilitated the near complete interrogation of the fetal vasculature while three-dimensional (3D) and four-dimensional (4D) US provided enhanced realism and novel perspectives of fetal structure.

Fetal magnetic resonance imaging (MRI) is equally transformational. Structural details have been dramatically enhanced, providing a previously unachievable fingerprint of fetal tissues. Techniques such as bright blood imaging for cardiac detail, diffusion, spectroscopy, and other functional modalities promise to transform our understanding of intrauterine life.

Evidence now clearly shows that these two modalities are deeply complementary and that their simultaneous deployment is critical for optimal fetal assessment for many important fetal disorders. Utilizing US and MRI together, our knowledge of fetal pathophysiology, including genetic disorders, has increased immensely. With the information gained from both US and fetal MRI, improved counseling, directed prenatal intervention, and guided postnatal care continue to evolve.

In this second edition, the specialties of radiology and obstetrics again converge to provide an updated reference on the complex field of fetal imaging. The first part of the book is dedicated to normal prenatal US and MRI. US evaluation in the first and second trimesters, growth, Doppler, basic cardiac anatomy, and 3D/4D US techniques are reviewed. MRI chapters include a how-to technical section and provide normal examples of the entire fetal anatomy, with emphasis on the fetal brain. Additional information with regard to US and MRI safety is provided, with discussion of 3 Tesla fetal MRI and 3D printing techniques reviewed. Advanced fetal brain and cardiac MR techniques are also detailed. The second part of the book reviews the major fetal pathologies by organ system, updated to changes and new advances in the field. The incidence, pathogenesis, etiology, and diagnosis with US and MRI, as well as prognosis and management for fetal pathologies are examined. Color diagrams, tables, and, most importantly, images utilizing both US and MRI provide the reader with an enhanced understanding of the anomalies. There is a new section dedicated to placenta accreta spectrum and diagnostic fetal imaging necessary for surgical intervention. The appendix and biometry tables are updated. These tables contain restructured normal MR values, including essential measurements of the fetal brain at different gestational ages.

A unique feature of this book is that a diverse group of fetal subspecialists again graciously helped author chapters, including cardiologists, geneticists, and Doppler specialists. International experts, including Kypros Nicolaides, Heron Werner, and Fred Avni, provided a global perspective of this discipline.

Our goal for the second edition of *Fundamental and Advanced Fetal Imaging* was to improve on the prior edition by including new and the most up-to-date and encompassing reference for fetal imaging. We hope all fetologists, including radiologists and obstetricians, as well as pediatric specialists such as surgeons, geneticists, counselors, neurologists, urologists, and neurosurgeons, will turn to this reference for basic and advanced imaging information. This book should also serve as an excellent resource for the resident and medical student.

Understanding normal development and pathologies in the fetus is essential for optimal prenatal and postnatal care. We hope you find this book illuminating and that it will continue to contribute to fetal research, therapeutic techniques, perinatal care, and counseling.

Beth M. Kline-Fath
Dorothy I. Bulas
Wesley Lee

ACKNOWLEDGMENTS

First and foremost, we would like to thank all the authors from so many different specialties who have generously shared their expertise, research, and images.

We cannot thank them enough for their hard work and leadership in this growing field of fetology.

We thank the sonographers, obstetricians, radiologists, and fetal specialists who have worked together to improve the care of the fetus.

We thank the fellows, residents, and students in training who have asked compelling questions and pushed us to search for better answers.

We would like to thank Glenn Minano for his creative assistance with regard to the artwork presented in this book.

We would like to thank the staff of Wolters Kluwer Health, including Sharon Zinner, Eric McDermott, Samson Premkumar, and Ashley Pfeiffer for their assistance in making this second edition happen.

BMKF, DIB, WL

I would like to thank Dorothy Bulas and Wesley Lee for their constant support and enthusiasm about this project. To those who encouraged and directed my medical career, I would like to express gratitude to Ben Felson, Hugh Hawkins, Alan Chambers, John Egelhoff, and Lane Donnelly. For those who taught me the importance of teamwork to improve fetal and neonatal care at Cincinnati Children's Hospital Medical Center, I would like to thank Constance Bitters, Kristina Stenger, Maria Calvo-Garcia, Bill Polzin, Foong-Yen Lim, Tim Crombleholme, and all of my fetal coworkers and fellows, many of whom have gone to other institutions to continue work in this innovative field. Finally, I would like to thank all families who entrust the care of their unborn; it is their lives that inspire me to learn more to improve fetal care.

BMKF

Working on this second edition was even more rewarding than the first. The field continues to grow exponentially and it is exciting to see how many brilliant and caring experts from multiple specialties have turned their focus to this fascinating discipline. It was a joy to work with Beth Kline Fath and Wes Lee, amazing experts whose hard work and tenaciousness have resulted in such a strong second edition.

I must thank all those in my department who do such great work that has allowed me the time to spend on this project. I am grateful to all the colleagues in our fetal center at Children's National who have shared my enthusiasm for caring for the fetus. Their collaboration has been a source of inspiration through the years. Lastly, I want to thank all the families I have had the privilege to work with. It is their stories that move me to continue to work in this field.

DIB

CONTENTS

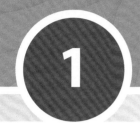

Bioeffects and Safety of Ultrasound for the Clinician

Jacques S. Abramowicz

Diagnostic ultrasound (DUS) in clinical medicine, in general, and in obstetrics, in particular, is convenient, painless, relatively inexpensive, and results are available immediately. The almost universal belief is that it does not pose any risk to the pregnant patient or her fetus. Ultrasound, however, is a form of energy and, as such, has effects in any scanned biological tissues (bioeffects). The two major physical mechanisms responsible for these effects are nonthermal (mechanical) or thermal. The issue of whether any of these bioeffects may be harmful is as old as medical DUS[1-3] and continues to be discussed currently.[4-8]

This chapter presents very basic notions of acoustics and physics as they relate to ultrasound and its effects. Mechanisms for bioeffects are described. Literature on bioeffects and the safety of ultrasound are briefly reviewed as are statements of various ultrasound organizations. It also affords a practical approach to the ultrasound end users to limit the potential risks to the fetus of exposure to DUS.

BASIC PHYSICS OF ULTRASOUND

A detailed description of ultrasound physics can be found in various publications.[9-12] However, certain basic properties of ultrasound are very important when trying to understand safety and bioeffects. Equally important are tissue characteristics, such as attenuation coefficient. A basic knowledge of instrument controls ("knobology") is also essential not only for appropriate clinical usage but it is also imperative to avoid potential harm, since many of the controls that are in the hands of the examiner will alter the acoustic output and, hence, the energy applied to the tissues.

The Ultrasound Wave

Sound is a mechanical vibratory form of energy with alternating positive and negative components of the wave. Megapascal (MPa) is the unit for pressure. Ultrasound instrumentation can generate peak pressures of 5 MPa and above. Atmospheric pressure is 0.1 MPa. Frequency is the number of cycles/second, measured in hertz (Hz). DUS is, generally, 2 to 10 million hertz (megahertz, MHz). The higher the frequency, the better the resolution but the lower the penetration.

DUS is pulsed, that is, pulses of acoustic energy separated by "silent" gaps. The number of pulses occurring in 1 second is the pulse repetition frequency (PRF) and is controlled by the instrument in B-mode. In Doppler mode, it can be altered by the end user. Average intensity of a beam is expressed by the beam power (in mW), divided by the cross-sectional area of the beam (in cm^2) and is, therefore, expressed in mW/cm^2. Since DUS is a pulsed

wave, there are pulses of energy intermingled with "silent" periods where no energy is emitted. Depending on the time and location of the measurement, several parameters can be described in relation to time or space, thus defining several types of intensity. Spatial peak–temporal average intensity (I_{SPTA}) is the most practical, and commonly referred to.

The maximal permitted value varies by clinical application. This had been determined in 1976 by the U.S. Food and Drug Administration (FDA) to be 46 mW/cm^2 for fetal application,[13] but was modified in 1986 to 94 mW/cm^2.[14] The most recent definition dates from 1992 and is 720 mW/cm^2.[15] Thus, for fetal imaging, the I_{SPTA} has been allowed to increase by a factor of almost 16-fold from 1976 and almost 8-fold from 1986 to 1992. It is important to keep in mind that all epidemiological information available regarding possible fetal effects predates 1992.[16]

Instrument Outputs

Some publications of various instrument outputs are available.[17-19] These are generally quickly outdated, since manufacturers introduce new commercial machines to the market (or modify existing ones) at a rate too fast for immediate objective evaluation. Over the years, output of instruments has increased.[18,20] From a clinical standpoint, there is no easy way to verify the actual output of the instrument in use. In addition, each transducer generates a specific output, further complicated by the different modes that may be applied. When comparing modes, the I_{SPTA} increases from a low 34 mW/cm^2, average in B-mode to M-mode to color Doppler to spectral Doppler where it can reach 1,180 mW/cm^2, but the temporal averaged intensity in Doppler mode can reach 10 W/cm^2.[21] Therefore, caution should be exercised when applying Doppler mode, particularly in the first trimester. Color Doppler displays higher intensities than does B-mode but is still much lower than spectral Doppler, mainly due to the mode of operation—sequences of pulses, scanned through the region of interest (or "box"). Most measurements are available in manufacturers' manuals. These have been derived in laboratory conditions, and real-life conditions may be different.[22] Furthermore, various machine controls can alter the output when modified by the end user. For example, the degree of temperature elevation is proportional to the product of the amplitude of the sound wave by the pulse length and the PRF. Hence, any increase in one of them can add to the risk of elevating the temperature, a potential mechanism for bioeffects (see section "Thermal Effects" below). The three important parameters under end user control are the scanning (or operating) mode, including transducer choice, the system setup and output control, and the dwell time.

1. Scanning mode: As mentioned earlier, B-mode carries the lowest risk, and spectral Doppler carries the highest, with M-mode and color Doppler in between. In spectral Doppler, the beam needs to be held in a relatively constant position over the vessel of interest, which may lead to further increase in temporal average intensity.
2. System setup: Starting or default output power and, particularly, mode (B-mode, Doppler, etc.) control changes. A subtler element is fine-tuning performed by the examiner to optimize the image and influence output but with no visible effect (except if one follows thermal index [TI] and/or mechanical index [MI] displays, see below). It is very important that each clinician knows how controls on his/her machine alter the output. Controls that regularize output in B-mode include focal depth, increasing frame rate, and limiting the field of view, for instance, by high-resolution magnification or certain zooms. In Doppler mode, changing sample volume and/or velocity range (all done to optimize received signals) changes output. A very important control in every mode is receiver gain. While it has similar effects to the controls on the displayed or recorded image, it has none on the output of the outgoing beam and is, therefore, completely safe to manipulate.
3. Dwell time is directly under the control of the examiner. Directly related with dwell time is examiner experience: knowledge of anatomy, bioeffects, instrument controls, and scanning techniques. It can be safely assumed that the more experienced the examiner, the less scanning time will be needed to obtain the needed diagnostic images.

ULTRASOUND BIOEFFECTS

When the ultrasound wave penetrates tissues, two major effects occur: The alternance of positive and negative pressure may cause a direct effect (mechanical effect) and an indirect effect, when the acoustic energy is transformed into heat (thermal effect).

Mechanical Effects

These are interactions between the ultrasound wave and the tissue that do not cause a significant degree of temperature increase ($<1°C$; hence, the term nonthermal, often used to design them). These include acoustic cavitation as well as radiation torque and force, and acoustic streaming secondary to propagation of the ultrasound waves. Cavitation, which necessitates the presence of bubbles in the path of the ultrasound beam, seems to be the major factor in mechanical effects.[23-25] Two types of cavitation can be demonstrated: stable and inertial (previously defined as transient). In stable cavitation, bubbles acquire small backward and forward movements with possible resulting microstreaming. Inertial cavitation indicates expansion and reduction in bubble volume, also secondary to alternating positive and negative pressures generated by the ultrasound wave. Expansion in growth is less with each cycle until collapse occurs with production of very high pressure (hundreds of atmospheres) and very elevated temperature (thousands of degrees), but on such a small area (<100 nm) and for such a brief time (few tens of nanoseconds) that it will not be felt and is very hard to measure (adiabatic reaction—occurring without the gain or loss of heat) but can produce

microstreaming or even release of free radicals.[26] Biological effects of ultrasound in animals such as local intestinal,[27] renal,[28] and pulmonary[29] hemorrhages have been attributed to mechanical effects, although cavitation could not always be implicated. Furthermore, since gas bubbles are not present in fetal lungs or bowels (where effects have been described in neonates or adult animals), the risk, in the human fetus, from mechanical effect secondary to cavitation appears to be minimal unless ultrasound contrast agents, a source of cavitation nuclei, are injected into the body before the ultrasound examination. There is, for now, no clear clinical indication for the use of ultrasound contrast agents in fetal ultrasound, and, to date, no studies have specifically investigated the interaction of ultrasound and microbubble contrast agents in fetal tissues *in vivo*.

In addition, fetal stimulation caused by pulsed ultrasound insonation has been described, with no apparent relation to cavitation.[30] This effect may be secondary to radiation forces associated with ultrasound exposures. These forces were suspected at the earliest stages of ultrasound research[31] and are known to possibly stimulate auditory,[32] sensory,[33] and cardiac tissues.[34] The pressure generated by the ultrasound have been alleged to be capable of causing acoustic damage,[35] but no harmful effects of DUS, secondary to nonthermal mechanisms, have been reported in human fetuses.[36]

Thermal Effects

During the entire gestation, temperature of the human embryo/fetus is higher than maternal core body temperature,[37] generally exceeding maternal temperature by 0.5°C and gradually rises until the final trimester (near term). Teratogenesis secondary to temperature elevation has been demonstrated in many animal studies, as well as in several controlled human studies.[38] While elevated maternal temperature in early gestation has been associated with an increased incidence of congenital anomalies,[39] the majority of these studies do not involve ultrasound-induced temperature elevation. A 1.5°C temperature elevation above the normal value has been suggested as a universal threshold after which teratological effects are suspected to occur.[40] There is, however, some evidence that any positive temperature differential for any period of time has some effect. In other words, a thermal threshold for hyperthermia-induced birth defects may not exist.[41] Gestational age is a vital factor: Milder exposure during the preimplantation period can have consequences similar to more severe exposures during embryonic and fetal development and can result in prenatal death and abortion or a wide range of structural and functional defects.

In experimental animals, the most common defects thought to result from heat teratogenesis are of the neural tube, microcephaly, microphthalmia and cataract,[40] as well as defects of craniofacial development including clefts,[42] skeleton,[43] the body wall, teeth, and heart.[44] In humans, hyperthermia *in utero* (due to maternal influenza, for instance) has been described as a risk factor for congenital anomalies and subsequent childhood psychological/behavioral disturbances[45] and, more particularly, schizophrenia.[46] Most of these defects have been found in human epidemiological studies following maternal fever or hyperthermia during pregnancy, but none of these investigations have involved ultrasound-induced hyperthermia effects. Yet, there are experimental data on the effects of hyperthermia and measurements of *in vivo* temperature induced by pulsed ultrasound, but not in human beings.[47,48] These data have been widely reviewed.[49,50] Can DUS induce a sufficient rise in fetal temperature to be harmful?[51–53] For prolonged exposures, temperature elevations of up to 5°C have been obtained.[53] Temperature change in insonated tissues depends on the balance between heat production and heat loss. A particular tissue property that strongly influences the amount of heat transported is local perfusion, which very clearly diminishes the risk, if present. In early pregnancy, under 6 weeks' gestation, there appears to be minimal maternal–fetal circulation, that is, minimal fetal perfusion, which may potentially reduce heat dispersion.[54] Only at about weeks 10 to 11 does the embryonic circulation actually link up with the maternal circulation.[55] In addition, at about weeks 4 to 5, the gestational sac is about 2.5 cm in diameter, and by week 8 it is around 8 cm in diameter. This may allow whole-body fetal scanning (and, possibly, temperature increase), a concept that is generally ignored in the literature dealing with thermal effects of ultrasound. The issue of transducer heating, which may be particularly relevant in the first trimester, specifically if performing endovaginal scanning, is also often ignored.[56] Contrariwise, motions (even very small) of the examiner's hand as well as the patient's breathing and body movements (in the case of obstetrical ultrasound, both the mother and the fetus) tend to spread through the region being heated. However, for spectral (pulsed) Doppler studies, it is necessary to have the transducer as steady as possible. As described earlier, the intensity (I_{SPTA}) and acoustic power associated with Doppler ultrasound are the highest of all the general-use categories. Ziskin[57] reported a total of 121,000 patient examinations, obstetrical and general, including 15,973 Doppler ultrasound examinations. In this report, there was no information concerning the reason for each examination. The average duration of the Doppler examination was 27 minutes (and the longest 4 hours!). Although this is an older report, this shows the extent of Doppler use in clinical medicine and the need for precaution.

There is a mathematical/physical relation between certain beam characteristics and temperature elevation. The elevation is proportional to the product of the wave amplitude, length of the pulse, and PRF. Hence, manipulating any of these via instrument controls will alter the *in situ* conditions. A temperature increase of 1°C can be reached easily in routine scanning. Computer-generated estimates of elevation of up to 1.5°C were obtained in the first trimester and up to 4°C in the second and third trimesters, particularly with the use of pulsed Doppler.[58]

A standardized method of providing the end user a parameter related to acoustic output and expressing potential for bioeffects was clearly needed—hence, the origin of the Output Display Standard (ODS), based on the two most likely interactions of ultrasound with tissues, namely, thermal and nonthermal or mechanical.[38]

THE OUTPUT DISPLAY STANDARD

In 1992, the FDA, under pressure from ultrasound clinical users as well as from manufacturers, allowed an increase in the power output of instruments. The general opinion was that higher outputs would generate better images, and thus improve diagnostic accuracy. To reflect the two major potential biological consequences of ultrasound (see sections "Mechanical Effects" and "Thermal Effects" above), the American Institute of Ultrasound in Medicine (AIUM), the National Electrical Manufacturers' Association (NEMA), and the FDA (with representatives from the Canadian Health Protection Branch, the National Council on Radiation Protection and Measurements, and 14 other medical organizations) developed a standard related to the potential for the two most plausible ultrasound bioeffects. The full name was the Standard for Real-Time Display of Thermal and Mechanical Indices on Diagnostic Ultrasound Equipment, generally known as the ODS.[15] To be allowed to increase instruments' output for fetal use, the manufacturers were requested to display, on screen and in real time, two types of indices with the intent of making the user aware of the potential for bioeffects. These indices are the TI, to provide some indication of potential temperature increase, and the MI, to provide indication of potential for nonthermal (i.e., mechanical) effects.[15,59] The TI is the ratio of total instantaneous acoustic power to the acoustic power estimated to be required to increase tissue temperature by a maximum of 1°C. It is an estimate of the maximal temperature rise at a given exposure and does not represent an actual or assumed temperature increase. It certainly bears some correlation with temperature rise in degrees Celsius, but in no way does it allow an estimate of what that temperature change actually is in the tissue.[59] There are three variants: thermal index for soft tissue (TIS), to be used mostly in early pregnancy when ossification is low; thermal index for bones (TIB), to be used when the ultrasound beam impinges on bone at or near the beam focus, such as late second and third trimesters of pregnancy, because bone is the tissue that absorbs most of the acoustic energy, and hence a higher risk of temperature increase in the vicinity of that bone; and thermal index for transcranial studies (TIC) when the transducer is essentially against bone, mostly for examinations in adult patients, but also in neonatal scanning, which is an area that has been largely ignored. These indices were required to be displayed if equal to or over 0.4. The MI represents the potential for nonthermal damage in tissues, or rather the risk of cavitation, but is not based on actual *in situ* measurements. It is a theoretical formulation of the ratio of the pressure to the square root of the ultrasound frequency (hence, the higher the frequency, the lesser risk of mechanical effect). Both the TI and MI can and should be followed as an indication of change in output during the clinical examination, with higher values indicating the potential for higher thermal and nonthermal effects than do lower values. As a consequence, for fetal imaging, the output, as expressed by the I_{SPTA}, was allowed to go from a previous value of 92 to 720 mW/cm². It takes only one pulse to induce cavitation, and about a minute to raise temperature to its peak. Dwell time, however, is not taken into account in the calculation of the ODS.

This document was the first attempt to provide the ultrasound practitioner with semiquantitative safety-related information. The end users are able to see how manipulation of certain instrument controls during an ultrasound examination may cause alterations in the output and, thus, on the exposure, assuming they follow changes in the thermal and mechanical indices. A clear requirement in the ODS original document was training of the end user in bioeffects and the significance of the indices, as a major part in their implementation. Attempts have been made to educate the end users,[60] but, unfortunately, this aspect of the ODS does not seem to have succeeded as end users' knowledge of bioeffects, safety, and output indices is found lacking.[61,62] In a questionnaire that was distributed to ultrasound end users (82% were obstetricians) attending review courses and hospital grand rounds, in the United States, only 17.7% gave the correct answer of the definition of the TI, and only 3.8% described MI properly. Almost 80% of end users did not know where to find the acoustic indices during a clinical examination (the correct answer being: on the monitor in real time).[63] Similar results were recorded in surveys performed in Europe, Asia, or the Middle East,[64–66] indicating that clinical end users worldwide show poor knowledge regarding safety issues of ultrasound during pregnancy. Knowledge of residents in obstetrics and gynecology and maternal–fetal medicine fellows was also found to be grossly lacking.[67] Furthermore, identical results were obtained when surveying sonographers, with no difference in depth (or lack thereof) of knowledge based on years of experience.[68]

Compliance with the ALARA (as low as reasonably achievable) principle by practitioners seeking credentialing for nuchal translucency (NT) measurement between 11 and 14 weeks' gestation was evaluated. Only 5% of the providers used the correct TI type (TIB) at lower than 0.5 for all submitted images, 6% at lower than 0.7, and 12% at 1.0 or lower. A TI higher than 1.0 was used by 19.5% of the providers. Proficiency in NT measurement and educational background (physician or sonographer) did not influence compliance with ALARA. The authors concluded that clinicians seeking credentialing in NT do not demonstrate compliance with the recommended use of the TIB in monitoring acoustic output.[69]

A further concern is that several assumptions were made when calculating the TI and MI, which prompts some questions on the clinical value of these indices. Maybe the most significant (from a clinical aspect) is the choice of the tissue phantom used in the calculations of the ODS. In National Council on Radiation Protection and Measurements (NCRP) report number 140,[38] there is an entire chapter (Chapter 9) listing conditions where both indices may be inaccurate, for example, long fluid path (full bladder, amniotic fluid, ascites, or hydrocephalus) or path through increased amounts of soft tissue such as obese patients.

Because of the possible errors inherent in the calculation of the TI and MI, various attempts have been made to find a better quantification of the potential risk.[70,71] These have not been adopted by the clinical community.

BRIEF REVIEW OF HISTORICAL RESEARCH

In the late 19th century, the French engineer Paul Langevin designed an ultrasound machine, using Pierre Curie's principle of the piezoelectric effect.[72] During World War I, he attempted to use this instrument to detect submarines through echo location (hence the later coined term SONAR: SOund Navigation And Ranging). He also demonstrated that the waves produced by his machine could kill small fish in an insonated water bath and could cause pain when hands were plunged into the water bath in the path of the beam. Experimental findings cannot always be extrapolated to human clinical situations but are helpful in understanding the mechanism of processes. Historical details can be found in various publications.[7,73–77]

Initially, cell suspensions and cell and tissue cultures were employed, and many reports described clear effects of the ultrasound waves on these, mostly secondary to cavitational and other nonthermal mechanisms. Plants were another extensively studied organism for effects of ultrasound,[78] particularly the Elodea leaf, since internal gas channels are present.[79] Insects have been exposed to ultrasound with significant effects, such as death of eggs and larvae as well as abnormal development, presumably secondary to the presence of gas-filled channels.[80] In addition, alterations at the chromosomal and even DNA levels have been described.[81]

Animal Research

Multiple studies have been performed with ultrasound on a wide variety of species (such as mice, rats, cats, and monkeys) with a wide assortment of effects, with ultrasound levels generally higher than those in human clinical medicine and too numerous to mention in detail. But it should be noted that some similar effects have also been demonstrated with acoustic fields much closer to clinically pertinent ones, in particular lung and intestinal hemorrhage.[82] Several major clinical end points for bioeffects that could have direct relevance to human studies include fetal growth and birth weight, effects on brain and central nervous system (CNS) function, and change in hematological function. Decreased birth weight after prenatal exposure to ultrasound has been reported in some species but not convincingly in others. Therefore, clear species differences seem to exist,[83] making it difficult to generalize, and even more difficult to extrapolate to humans.

Two specific studies merit somewhat detailed description: Ang et al.[84] and Schneider et al.[85] Neurons of the cerebral neocortex in mammals, including humans, are generated during fetal life in the brain proliferative zones and then migrate to their final destinations by following an inside-to-outside sequence. Ang et al.[84] evaluated in mice the effect of ultrasound waves on neuronal positioning within the embryonic cerebral cortex. A small, but statistically significant, number of neurons failed to acquire their proper position and remained scattered within inappropriate cortical layers and/or in the subjacent white matter when exposed to ultrasound for a total of 30 minutes or longer during the period of their migration. The magnitude of dispersion systematically increased with duration of exposure to ultrasound (although not linearly, with some extended exposure yielding less effect than did lower ones). It is unclear whether a relatively small misplacement in a relatively small number of cells that retain their origin cell class is of any clinical significance. It is also important to note that there are several major differences between the experimental setup and the clinical use of ultrasound in humans.[86] The most noticeable difference was the length of exposure of up to 7 hours in the setup of Ang et al. Moreover, scans were performed over a small period of several days. The experimental setup was such that embryos received whole-brain exposure to the beam, which is rare in humans, although quite possible in the earliest stages of gestation. In addition, brains of mice are much smaller than are those in humans and develop over days. This should not completely deter from the study, but encourages caution.

In another study, chick brains were exposed, in ovo, on day 19 of a 21-day incubation period to B-mode (5 or 10 minutes), or to pulsed Doppler (1, 2, 3, 4, or 5 minutes) ultrasound.[85] After hatching, learning and memory function were assessed at day 2 post-hatch. B-mode exposure did not affect memory function. However, significant memory impairment occurred following 4 and 5 minutes of pulsed Doppler exposure. Short-, intermediate-, and long-term memory was equally impaired, suggesting an inability to learn. Chicks were also unable to learn with a second training session. In this study, exposure to pulsed Doppler ultrasound adversely affected cognitive function in chicks. Although some methodological issues exist and extrapolation to humans is unwarranted, these findings justify further investigations and caution in applying pulsed Doppler to human fetuses in the first trimester.

Human Research and Epidemiology

In 2016, the AIUM reapproved the following statement:

Based on the epidemiological data available and on current knowledge of interactive mechanisms, there is insufficient justification to warrant a conclusion of a causal relationship between diagnostic ultrasound and recognized adverse effects in humans. Some studies have reported effects of exposure to diagnostic ultrasound during pregnancy, such as low birth weight, delayed speech, dyslexia, and non–right-handedness. Other studies have not demonstrated such effects. The epidemiological evidence is based on exposure conditions prior to 1992, the year in which acoustic limits of ultrasound machines were substantially increased for fetal/obstetrical applications.[87]

Laboratory animal experiments under similar diagnostic exposure levels have shown some effects from ultrasound, under certain conditions. Effects have also been reported in humans, but a definitive statement regarding risk should, ideally, include direct analysis of the effects in human populations. Several epidemiological studies have been published.[88,89] In humans, prenatal exposure to DUS has been implicated as a possible etiology for intrauterine growth restriction and low birth weight, delayed speech, dyslexia, neurological and mental development or behavioral issues, and, more recently, non–right-handedness. Occasional studies did report an association between DUS and some specific abnormalities such as lower birth weight,[90] delayed speech,[91] dyslexia,[92] and non–right-handedness.[93,94] With the exception of low birth weight, these findings have never been duplicated, and the majority of studies have been negative for any association. Furthermore, the difference was small and was not detectable at 8 years of age.[90] In a large study (originally 10,000 pregnancies exposed to ultrasound matched with 500 controls) with a 6-year follow-up, Lyons et al.[95] did not find differences in birth weight (nor increased congenital malformations, chromosomal abnormalities, infant neoplasms, speech or hearing impairment, or developmental problems). A second major potential effect extensively evaluated is delayed speech. A study of over 1,100 children exposed to ultrasound *in utero* and over 1,000 controls found no significant differences in delayed speech, limited vocabulary, or stuttering.[96] Dyslexia (and other neurological problems) is another widely studied subject. Long-term follow-up studies were conducted in over 2,100 children with various tests for dyslexia such as spelling and reading. No statistically significant differences were found between ultrasound-exposed children and controls for reading, spelling, arithmetic, or overall performance as reported by teachers. Specific dyslexia tests showed similar rates of occurrence among scanned children and controls in reading, spelling, and intelligence scores, and no discrepancy between intelligence and reading or spelling.[97–99]

The first report of a possible link between prenatal exposure to ultrasound and subsequent non–right-handedness in children who were exposed to ultrasound *in utero* was published in 1993 by Salvesen et al.,[100] but according to the authors, "only barely significant at the 5% level." In a later analysis of the data, they described that the association was restricted to males. Salvesen then published a meta-analysis of these two studies and of previously unreported results.[101] No difference was found in general, but a small increase in non–right-handedness was present when analyzing boys separately. No valid mechanistic explanation is given in the studies to explain the findings. Therefore, although there may be a small increase in the incidence of non–right-handedness in male infants, there is not enough evidence to infer a direct effect on brain structure or function or even that non–right-handedness is an adverse effect. A more recent and intriguing study showed that fetuses self-touched their faces more often with the left hand than with the right, as observed by ultrasound, in correlation to stress levels of the mother.[102] Furthermore, laterality is, mostly, genetically determined,[103] and the role of ultrasound, if any, cannot be determined without specific studies, none having been published.

Other end points that have been considered but not found to be associated with ultrasound exposure include congenital malformations, hearing problems, and malignancies.[98,104] There have been several publications (most with flawed methods or analysis) attempting to link exposure to ultrasound with the development of autism spectrum disorder (ASD)[105] or worsening of symptoms.[106] Etiology of ASD is multifactorial, including genetic components and exposure to infection, toxins, or other environmental factors, particularly unfavorable perinatal/neonatal conditions. There certainly has been an increase in the frequency of diagnosis of ASD over the past 20 years with a parallel increase in the use of obstetrical DUS with prenatal ultrasound exposure. Hence, some blame ultrasound as the main etiology for the autism "epidemics."[107,108] CNS alterations have been described in ASD and certain similar changes have been described in animals after exposure to ultrasound.[84] However, analysis of *in utero* exposure in humans has failed to demonstrate harmful effects in neonates or children, particularly in school performance, attention disorders, or behavioral changes. There is no independently confirmed, peer-reviewed, published evidence that a cause–effect relation exists between *in utero* exposure to clinical ultrasound and development of ASD in childhood.[109]

CLINICAL EXPOSIMETRY

There is, unfortunately, no way to perform actual sonographic exposure measurements in the human fetus. Acoustic output, as expressed by MI and TI, was recorded in several prospective observational studies investigating first-trimester ultrasound,[110,111] Doppler studies,[112] and 3D/4D studies.[113] First-trimester ultrasound was associated with very low TI values (with a mean of 0.2 ± 0.1).[111] The TI was significantly higher in the pulsed wave Doppler (mean 1.5 ± 0.5, range 0.9 to 2.8) and color flow imaging studies (mean 0.8 ± 0.1, range 0.6 to 1.2) as compared to B-mode ultrasound (mean 0.3 ± 0.1, range 0.1 to 0.7; $P < 0.01$).[112] In the same study, TI was above 1.5 in 43% of the Doppler studies. Figure 1.1 shows a TI of 2 when performing a spectral Doppler study. Mean TI during the 3D (0.27 ± 0.1) and 4D examinations (0.24 ± 0.1) was comparable to the TI during the B-mode scanning (0.28 ± 0.1; $P = 0.343$).[113] The ever-increasing use of 3D/4D ultrasound begs the question of whether this modality exposes the fetus to higher levels of acoustic energy. Since the process begins with acquisition of multiple 2D images through sweeps across the organ of interest, computer reconstructions and offline (or on the ultrasound machine after the patient's scan is completed) manipulations of the volumes obtained, this results in no additional exposure of the fetus to ultrasound. Some studies have evaluated volume acquisitions for subsequent interpretation (unpublished data) and suggest that this new scanning method has the potential to

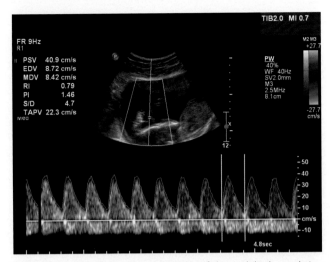

FIGURE 1.1: Color and spectral Doppler of the umbilical vessels in a third-trimester fetus. The spectral Doppler was active when the image was frozen. Note the TI of 2. EDV, end-diastolic velocity; FR, frame rate; MDV, minimum diastolic velocity; PI, pulsatility index; PSV, peak systolic velocity; PW, Power; RI, resistive index; S/D, systolic/diastolic ratio; TAPV, time-averaged peak velocity; WF, wall filter.

decrease scanning time, thereby decreasing exposure. On the other hand, continuous scanning, such as might occur with 4D ultrasonography to observe fetal movements over time, could potentially generate high exposure levels. The potential risks may increase with unnecessary prolonged exposure, or when less than optimally trained users operate the device.

Adequate diagnostic information may be obtained with low output levels (as documented by values of the TI), with increase in the gain. This is post-processing and has no effect on the emitted acoustic energy. This has been reported in the literature, specifically for Doppler, the mode with the highest output, both in early and later pregnancy.[114,115] It should be noted that, under pressure from Bioeffects and Safety Committees of various professional organizations (AIUM, European Federation of Ultrasound in Medicine and Biology [EFSUMB], International Society for Ultrasound in Obstetrics and Gynecology [ISUOG], and World Federation for Ultrasound in Medicine and Biology [WFUMB]), several manufacturers have changed their default settings, specifically for pulsed Doppler in fetal mode, from very high (as it was originally, presumably in an attempt to obtain better images) to very low, with the end user capable of raising the output, if desired. Since acoustic output is high in Doppler, special precaution is recommended, particularly in early gestation.[4]

RECOMMENDATIONS

Many national and international organizations or societies have issued official statements regarding the epidemiology, bioeffects, and safety of ultrasound, as well as the nonmedical usage of ultrasound such as the AIUM,[116] ISUOG,[117] WFUMB,[118] British Medical Ultrasound Society (BMUS),[119] and European Committee of Medical Ultrasound Safety (ECMUS).[120] They all state, in one way or another, that ultrasound appears safe if performed for clinical indications by appropriately trained personal, but that prudence is recommended because of the possibility of yet unknown deleterious effects. The sonographer and sonologist are interested in knowing how to keep the examination safe.

A general recommendation is that DUS should be used only when indicated, and minimal exposure should be used to obtain the diagnostic images. Furthermore, exposure time should be kept as short as possible. Precautions are, naturally, of particular importance in early gestation,[121] and, particularly for Doppler exposure.[122] Several published recommendations are available.[119,123-126] The most rigorous is the BMUS with strict time recommendations, based on value of the TI: "For equipment for which the safety indices are displayed over their full range of values, the TI should always be less than 0.7 and the MI should always be less than 0.3 . . . Frequent exposure of the same subject is to be avoided."[126] An easy rule to remember is if the TI is below 1, examination of the fetus is safe, as long as it lasts less than 1 hour (with TI <0.7, there is no time limit, as long as ALARA is respected).[7,8]

REFERENCES

1. Wood WR, Loomis AL. The physical and biological effects of high frequency sound waves of great intensity. *Phil Mag.* 1927;4:414.
2. Neuweiler W, Renfer HR. The effect of ultra-sound on the ovary. *Gynaecologia.* 1950;129:280–283.
3. Donald I. Approaches to determining foetal hazard from ultrasound. *Br J Radiol.* 1971;44:563.
4. ter Haar GR, Abramowicz JS, Akiyama I, et al. Do we need to restrict the use of Doppler ultrasound in the first trimester of pregnancy? *Ultrasound Med Biol.* 2013;39:374–380. doi:10.1016/j.ultrasmedbio.2012.11.024.
5. Pooh RK, Maeda K, Kurjak A, et al. 3D/4D sonography—any safety problem. *J Perinat Med.* 2016;44:125–129. doi:10.1515/jpm-2015-0225.
6. Harris GR, Church CC, Dalecki D, et al. Comparison of thermal safety practice guidelines for diagnostic ultrasound exposures. *Ultrasound Med Biol.* 2016;42:345–357. doi:10.1016/j.ultrasmedbio.2015.09.016.
7. Abramowicz J. Ultrasound bioeffects and safety: what the practitioner should know. In: Fleischer A, Abramowicz J, Gonçalves L, et al, eds. *Fleischer's Sonography in Obstetrics and Gynecology: Textbook and Teaching Cases.* New York, NY: McGraw Hill; 2018:2–23.
8. Van den Hof MC. Obstetric ultrasound biological effects and safety. *J Obstet Gynaecol Can.* 2018;40:627–632. doi:10.1016/j.jogc.2017.11.023.
9. Ziskin MC. Fundamental physics of ultrasound and its propagation in tissue. *Radiographics.* 1993;13:705–709.
10. Lawrence JP. Physics and instrumentation of ultrasound. *Crit Care Med.* 2007;35:S314–S322.
11. O'Brien WD Jr. Ultrasound-biophysics mechanisms. *Prog Biophys Mol Biol.* 2007;93:212–255.
12. Kremkau F. *Sonography Principles and Instruments.* 9 ed. St. Louis, MO: Saunders; 2016.
13. U.S. Food and Drug Administration. *501(k) Guide for Measuring and Reporting Acoustic Output of Diagnostic Ultrasound Medical Devices.* Rockville, MD: Center for Devices and Radiological Health; 1985.
14. U.S. Food and Drug Administration. *Diagnostic Ultrasound Guidance Update.* Rockville, MD: Center for Devices and Radiological Health; 1987.
15. American Institute of Ultrasound in Medicine, The National Electrical Manufacturers' Association. *Standard for Real-Time Display of Thermal and Mechanical Acoustic Output Indices on Diagnostic Ultrasound Devices.* Laurel, MD: American Institute of Ultrasound in Medicine;1992.
16. Abramowicz JS, Fowlkes JB, Stratmeyer ME, et al. Bioeffects and safety of fetal ultrasound exposure: why do we need epidemiology? In: Sheiner E, ed. *Textbook of Epidemiology in Perinatology.* New York, NY: Nova Science Publishers, Inc.; 2010.
17. Carson PL, Fischella PR, Oughton TV. Ultrasonic power and intensities produced by diagnostic ultrasound equipment. *Ultrasound Med Biol.* 1978;3:341–350.
18. Duck FA, Henderson J. Acoustic output of modern instruments: is it increasing? In: Barnett SB, Kossoff G, eds. *Safety of Diagnostic Ultrasound.* New York, NY: The Parthenon Publishing Group; 1998:15–25.
19. Cibull SL, Harris GR, Nell DM. Trends in diagnostic ultrasound acoustic output from data reported to the US Food and Drug Administration for device indications that include fetal applications. *J Ultrasound Med.* 2013;32:1921–1932. doi:10.7863/ultra.32.11.1921.
20. Shaw A, Martin K. The acoustic output of diagnostic ultrasound scanners. In: ter Haar G, ed. *The Safe Use of Ultrasound in Medical Diagnosis.* 3rd ed. London, England: The British Institute of Radiology; 2012.
21. Duck FA. Acoustic dose and acoustic dose-rate. *Ultrasound Med Biol.* 2009; 35:1679–1685.
22. Jago JR, Henderson J, Whittingham TA, et al. How reliable are manufacturer's reported acoustic output data? *Ultrasound Med Biol.* 1995;21:135–136.
23. Carstensen EL. Acoustic cavitation and the safety of diagnostic ultrasound. *Ultrasound Med Biol.* 1987;13:597–606.

24. Holland CK, Deng CX, Apfel RE, et al. Direct evidence of cavitation in vivo from diagnostic ultrasound. *Ultrasound Med Biol.* 1996;22:917–925.

25. Kimmel E. Cavitation bioeffects. *Crit Rev Biomed Eng.* 2006;34:105–161.

26. Kondo T, Kodaira T, Kano E. Free radical formation induced by ultrasound and its effects on strand breaks in DNA of cultured FM3A cells. *Free Radic Res Commun.* 1993;19(suppl 1):S193–S200.

27. Dalecki D, Raeman CH, Child SZ, et al. Intestinal hemorrhage from exposure to pulsed ultrasound. *Ultrasound Med Biol.* 1995;21:1067–1072.

28. Wible JH Jr, Galen KP, Wojdyla JK, et al. Microbubbles induce renal hemorrhage when exposed to diagnostic ultrasound in anesthetized rats. *Ultrasound Med Biol.* 2002;28:1535–1546.

29. Dalecki D, Child SZ, Raeman CH, et al. Ultrasonically induced lung hemorrhage in young swine. *Ultrasound Med Biol.* 1997;23:777–781.

30. Fatemi M, Ogburn PL Jr, Greenleaf JF. Fetal stimulation by pulsed diagnostic ultrasound. *J Ultrasound Med.* 2001;20:883–889.

31. Harvey EN, Harvey EB, Loomis RW. Further observations on the effect of high frequency sound waves on living matter. *Biol Bull.* 1928;55:459–469.

32. Siddiqi TA, Plessinger MA, Meyer RA, et al. Bioeffects of diagnostic ultrasound on auditory function in the neonatal lamb. *Ultrasound Med Biol.* 1990;16:621–625.

33. Dalecki D, Child SZ, Raeman CH, et al. Tactile perception of ultrasound. *J Acoust Soc Am.* 1995;97:3165–3170.

34. Dalecki D, Raeman CH, Child SZ, et al. Effects of pulsed ultrasound on the frog heart: III. The radiation force mechanism. *Ultrasound Med Biol.* 1997;23:275–285.

35. Fatemi M, Alizad A, Greenleaf JF. Characteristics of the audio sound generated by ultrasound imaging systems. *J Acoust Soc Am.* 2005;117:1448–1455.

36. Abramowicz JS, Kremkau FW, Merz E. Obstetrical ultrasound: can the fetus hear the wave and feel the heat? [in German]. *Ultraschall Med.* 2012;33:215–217. doi:10.1055/s-0032-1312759.

37. Asakura H. Fetal and neonatal thermoregulation. *J Nippon Med Sch.* 2004;71:360–370.

38. National Council on Radiation Protection and Measurements. *Report No. 140: Exposure Criteria for Medical Diagnostic Ultrasound: II. Criteria Based on All Known Mechanisms.* Bethesda, MD: National Council on Radiation Protection and Measurements; 2002.

39. Shaw GM, Todoroff K, Velie EM, et al. Maternal illness, including fever and medication use as risk factors for neural tube defects. *Teratology.* 1998;57:1–7.

40. Edwards MJ, Saunders RD, Shiota K. Effects of heat on embryos and foetuses. *Int J Hyperthermia.* 2003;19:295–324.

41. Miller MW, Brayman AA, Abramowicz JS. Obstetric ultrasonography: a biophysical consideration of patient safety—the "rules" have changed. *Am J Obstet Gynecol.* 1998;179:241–254.

42. Toneto AD, Lopes RA, Oliveira PT, et al. Effect of hyperthermia on rat fetus palate epithelium. *Braz Dent J.* 1994;5:99–103.

43. Martinez-Frias ML, Garcia Mazario MJ, Caldas CF, et al. High maternal fever during gestation and severe congenital limb disruptions. *Am J Med Genet.* 2001;98:201–203.

44. Tikkanen J, Heinonen OP. Maternal hyperthermia during pregnancy and cardiovascular malformations in the offspring. *Eur J Epidemiol.* 1991;7:628–635.

45. Dombrowski SC, Martin RP, Huttunen MO. Association between maternal fever and psychological/behavior outcomes: a hypothesis. *Birth Defects Res A Clin Mol Teratol.* 2003;67:905–910.

46. Edwards MJ. Hyperthermia in utero due to maternal influenza is an environmental risk factor for schizophrenia. *Congenit Anom (Kyoto).* 2007;47:84–89. doi:10.1111/j.1741-4520.2007.00151.x.

47. Duggan PM, Liggins GC, Barnett SB. Ultrasonic heating of the brain of the fetal sheep in utero. *Ultrasound Med Biol.* 1995;21:553–560.

48. Horder MM, Barnett SB, Vella GJ, et al. Ultrasound-induced temperature increase in guinea-pig fetal brain in utero: third-trimester gestation. *Ultrasound Med Biol.* 1998;24:1501–1510.

49. Miller MW, Nyborg WL, Dewey WC, et al. Hyperthermic teratogenicity, thermal dose and diagnostic ultrasound during pregnancy: implications of new standards on tissue heating. *Int J Hyperthermia.* 2002;18:361–384.

50. WFUMB. WFUMB symposium on safety of ultrasound in medicine recommendations on the safe use of ultrasound. *Ultrasound Med Biol.* 1998;24:xv–xvi.

51. Abramowicz JS. Ultrasound in obstetrics and gynecology: is this hot technology too hot? *J Ultrasound Med.* 2002;21:1327–1333.

52. Barnett SB. Can diagnostic ultrasound heat tissue and cause biological effects. In: Barnett SB, Kossoff G, eds. *Safety of Diagnostic Ultrasound.* Carnforth, England: Parthenon Publishing; 1998:30–31.

53. Miller MW, Ziskin MC. Biological consequences of hyperthermia. *Ultrasound Med Biol.* 1989;15:707–722.

54. Jauniaux E, Gulbis B, Burton GJ. The human first trimester gestational sac limits rather than facilitates oxygen transfer to the foetus—a review. *Placenta.* 2003;24(suppl A):S86–S93.

55. Makikallio K, Tekay A, Jouppila P. Uteroplacental hemodynamics during early human pregnancy: a longitudinal study. *Gynecol Obstet Invest.* 2004;58:49–54.

56. Calvert J, Duck F, Clift S, et al. Surface heating by transvaginal transducers. *Ultrasound Obstet Gynecol.* 2007;29:427–432.

57. Ziskin MC. Intrauterine effects of ultrasound: human epidemiology. *Teratology.* 1999;59:252–260.

58. Bly SH, Vlahovich S, Mabee PR, et al. Computed estimates of maximum temperature elevations in fetal tissues during transabdominal pulsed Doppler examinations. *Ultrasound Med Biol.* 1992;18:389–397.

59. Abbott JG. Rationale and derivation of MI and TI—a review. *Ultrasound Med Biol.* 1999;25:431–441.

60. European Federation of Societies for Ultrasound in Medicine and Biology. Thermal and mechanical indices: EFSUMB safety tutorial. *Eur J Ultrasound.* 1996;4:144–150.

61. Marsal K. The output display standard: has it missed its target? *Ultrasound Obstet Gynecol.* 2005;25:211–214. doi:10.1002/uog.1864.

62. Sheiner E, Abramowicz JS. Clinical end users worldwide show poor knowledge regarding safety issues of ultrasound during pregnancy. *J Ultrasound Med.* 2008;27:499–501.

63. Sheiner E, Shoham-Vardi I, Abramowicz JS. What do clinical users know regarding safety of ultrasound during pregnancy? *J Ultrasound Med.* 2007;26:319–325; quiz 326–327.

64. Piscaglia F, Tewelde AG, Righini R, et al. Knowledge of the bio-effects of ultrasound among physicians performing clinical ultrasonography: results of a survey conducted by the Italian Society for Ultrasound in Medicine and Biology (SIUMB). *J Ultrasound.* 2009;12:6–11.

65. Akhtar W, Arain MA, Ali A, et al. Ultrasound biosafety during pregnancy: what do operators know in the developing world?: national survey findings from Pakistan. *J Ultrasound Med.* 2011;30:981–985.

66. Sharon N, Shoham-Vardi I, Aricha-Tamir B, et al. What do ultrasound performers in Israel know regarding safety of ultrasound, in comparison to the end users in the United States? [in Hebrew]. *Harefuah.* 2012;151:146–149, 190.

67. Houston LE, Allsworth J, Macones GA. Ultrasound is safe... right?: resident and maternal-fetal medicine fellow knowledge regarding obstetric ultrasound safety. *J Ultrasound Med.* 2011;30:21–27.

68. Bagley J, Thomas K, DiGiacinto D. Safety practices of sonographers and their knowledge of the biologic effects of sonography. *J Diagn Med Sonogr.* 2011;27:252–261.

69. Bromley B, Spitz J, Fuchs K, et al. Do clinical practitioners seeking credentialing for nuchal translucency measurement demonstrate compliance with biosafety recommendations? Experience of the Nuchal Translucency Quality Review Program. *J Ultrasound Med.* 2014;33:1209–1214. doi:10.7863/ultra.33.7.1209.

70. Bigelow TA, Church CC, Sandstrom K, et al. The thermal index: its strengths, weaknesses, and proposed improvements. *J Ultrasound Med.* 2011;30:714–734.

71. Ziskin MC. The thermal dose index. *J Ultrasound Med.* 2010;29:1475–1479.

72. Langevin P. *Procédés et appareils d' émission et de reception des ondes élastiques sous-marines à l'aide des ultrasons.* French Patent No. 505 703. 1920.

73. Nyborg WL. Biological effects of ultrasound: development of safety guidelines. Part I: Personal histories. *Ultrasound Med Biol.* 2000;26:911–964.

74. Nyborg WL. History of the American Institute of Ultrasound in Medicine's efforts to keep ultrasound safe. *J Ultrasound Med.* 2003;22:1293–1300.

75. Sikov MR. Effect of ultrasound on development. Part 2: Studies in mammalian species and overview. *J Ultrasound Med.* 1986;5:651–661.

76. Sikov MR. Effect of ultrasound on development. Part 1: Introduction and studies in inframammalian species. Report of the bioeffects committee of the American Institute of Ultrasound in Medicine. *J Ultrasound Med.* 1986;5:577–583.

77. Suhr D, Brummer F, Irmer U, et al. Bioeffects of diagnostic ultrasound in vitro. *Ultrasonics.* 1996;34:559–561.

78. Miller DL. The botanical effects of ultrasound: a review. *Environ Exp Bot.* 1983;23:1–27.

79. Carstensen EL, Child SZ, Crane C, et al. Lysis of cells in Elodea leaves by pulsed and continuous wave ultrasound. *Ultrasound Med Biol.* 1990;16:167–173.

80. Child SZ, Carstensen EL, Lam SK. Effects of ultrasound on Drosophila: III. Exposure of larvae to low-temporal-average-intensity, pulsed irradiation. *Ultrasound Med Biol.* 1981;7:167–173.

81. Barnett SB, Miller MW, Cox C, et al. Increased sister chromatid exchanges in Chinese hamster ovary cells exposed to high intensity pulsed ultrasound. *Ultrasound Med Biol.* 1988;14:397–403.

82. Dalecki D. Mechanical bioeffects of ultrasound. *Ann Rev Biomed Eng.* 2004;6:229–248.

83. O'Brien WD Jr, Januzik SJ, Dunn F. Ultrasound biologic effects: a suggestion of strain specificity. *J Ultrasound Med.* 1982;1:367–370.

84. Ang ESBC, Gluncic V, Duque A, et al. Prenatal exposure to ultrasound waves impacts neuronal migration in mice. *Proc Natl Acad Sci U S A.* 2006;103:12903–12910.

85. Schneider-Kolsky ME, Ayobi Z, Lombardo P, et al. Ultrasound exposure of the foetal chick brain: effects on learning and memory. *Int J Dev Neurosci.* 2009;27:677–683. doi:10.1016/j.ijdevneu.2009.07.007.

86. Abramowicz JS. Prenatal exposure to ultrasound waves: is there a risk? *Ultrasound Obstet Gynecol.* 2007;29:363–367.

87. American Institute of Ultrasound in Medicine. AIUM official statement: conclusions regarding epidemiology for obstetric ultrasound. https://www.aium .org/officialStatements/16. Published 2010. Reaffirmed 2016. Accessed June 1, 2019.

88. Salvesen KA. Epidemiological prenatal ultrasound studies. *Prog Biophys Mol Biol.* 2007;93:295–300.

89. Ziskin MC, Petitti DB. Epidemiology of human exposure to ultrasound: a critical review. *Ultrasound Med Biol.* 1988;14:91–96.

90. Newnham JP, Doherty DA, Kendall GE, et al. Effects of repeated prenatal ultrasound examinations on childhood outcome up to 8 years of age: follow-up of a randomised controlled trial. *Lancet.* 2004;364:2038–2044.

91. Campbell JD, Elford RW, Brant RF. Case-control study of prenatal ultrasonography exposure in children with delayed speech. *CMAJ.* 1993;149:1435–1440.

92. Stark CR, Orleans M, Haverkamp AD, et al. Short- and long-term risks after exposure to diagnostic ultrasound in utero. *Obstet Gynecol* 1984;63:194–200.

93. Kieler H, Cnattingius S, Haglund B, et al. Sinistrality—a side-effect of prenatal sonography: a comparative study of young men. *Epidemiology.* 2001;12:618–623.

94. Salvesen KA. Ultrasound in pregnancy and non-right handedness: meta-analysis of randomized trials. *Ultrasound Obstet Gynecol.* 2011;38:267–271. doi:10.1002/uog.9055.

95. Lyons EA, Dyke C, Toms M, et al. In utero exposure to diagnostic ultrasound: a 6-year follow-up. *Radiology.* 1988;166:687–690. doi:10.1148/radiology.166.3.3277240.

96. Salvesen KA, Vatten LJ, Bakketeig LS, et al. Routine ultrasonography in utero and speech development. *Ultrasound Obstet Gynecol.* 1994;4:101–103. doi:10.1046/j.1469-0705.1994.04020101.x.

97. Eik-Nes SH, Okland O, Aure JC, et al. Ultrasound screening in pregnancy: a randomised controlled trial. *Lancet.* 1984;1:1347.

98. Salvesen KA, Eik-Nes SH. Ultrasound during pregnancy and birthweight, childhood malignancies and neurological development. *Ultrasound Med Biol.* 1999;25:1025–1031.

99. Salvesen KA, Vatten LJ, Jacobsen G, et al. Routine ultrasonography in utero and subsequent vision and hearing at primary school age. *Ultrasound Obstet Gynecol* 1992;2:243–244, 245–247.

100. Salvesen KA, Vatten LJ, Eik-Nes SH, et al. Routine ultrasonography in utero and subsequent handedness and neurological development. *BMJ.* 1993;307:159–164.

101. Salvesen KA, Eik-Nes SH. Ultrasound during pregnancy and subsequent childhood non-right handedness: a meta-analysis. *Ultrasound Obstet Gynecol.* 1999;13:241–246.

102. Reissland N, Aydin E, Francis B, et al. Laterality of foetal self-touch in relation to maternal stress. *Laterality.* 2015;20:82–94. doi:10.1080/1357650X.2014.920339.

103. Hepper PG. The developmental origins of laterality: fetal handedness. *Dev Psychobiol.* 2013;55:588–595. doi:10.1002/dev.21119.

104. Harbarger CF, Weinberger PM, Borders JC, et al. Prenatal ultrasound exposure and association with postnatal hearing outcomes. *J Otolaryngol Head Neck Surg.* 2013;42:3. doi:10.1186/1916-0216-42-3.

105. Rosman NP, Vassar R, Doros G, et al. Association of prenatal ultrasonography and autism spectrum disorder. *JAMA Pediatr.* 2018;172:336–344. doi:10.1001/jamapediatrics.2017.5634.

106. Webb SJ, Garrison MM, Bernier R, et al. Severity of ASD symptoms and their correlation with the presence of copy number variations and exposure to first trimester ultrasound. *Autism Res.* 2017;10:472–484. doi:10.1002/aur.1690.

107. Rodgers C. Questions about prenatal ultrasound and the alarming increase in autism. *Midwifery Today Int Midwife.* 2006:16–19, 66–67.

108. Williams EL, Casanova MF. Potential teratogenic effects of ultrasound on corticogenesis: implications for autism. *Med Hypotheses.* 2010;75:53–58. doi:10.1016/j.mehy.2010.01.027.

109. Abramowicz JS. Ultrasound and autism: association, link, or coincidence? *J Ultrasound Med.* 2012;31(8):1261-1269. Review. PMID: 22837291

110. Sheiner E, Abramowicz JS. Acoustic output as measured by thermal and mechanical indices during fetal nuchal translucency ultrasound examinations. *Fetal Diagn Ther.* 2009;25:8–10.

111. Sheiner E, Shoham-Vardi I, Hussey MJ, et al. First-trimester sonography: is the fetus exposed to high levels of acoustic energy? *J Clin Ultrasound.* 2007;35:245–249.

112. Sheiner E, Shoham-Vardi I, Pombar X, et al. An increased thermal index can be achieved when performing Doppler studies in obstetric sonography. *J Ultrasound Med.* 2007;26:71–76.

113. Sheiner E, Hackmon R, Shoham-Vardi I, et al. A comparison between acoustic output indices in 2D and 3D/4D ultrasound in obstetrics. *Ultrasound Obstet Gynecol.* 2007;29:326–328.

114. Sande RK, Matre K, Eide GE, et al. Ultrasound safety in early pregnancy: reduced energy setting does not compromise obstetric Doppler measurements. *Ultrasound Obstet Gynecol.* 2012;39:438–443. doi:10.1002/uog.10148.

115. Sande RK, Matre K, Eide GE, et al. The effects of reducing the thermal index for bone from 1.0 to 0.5 and 0.1 on common obstetric pulsed wave Doppler measurements in the second half of pregnancy. *Acta Obstet Gynecol Scand.* 2013;92:790–796. doi:10.1111/aogs.12114.

116. AIUM. As low as reasonably achievable (ALARA) principle. https://www.aium.org/officialStatements/39. Published 2014. Accessed January 6, 2019.

117. Abramowicz JS, Kossoff G, Marsal K, et al. Safety statement, 2000 (reconfirmed 2003). International Society of Ultrasound in Obstetrics and Gynecology (ISUOG). *Ultrasound Obstet Gynecol.* 2003;21:100. doi:10.1002/uog.36.

118. WFUMB. WFUMB clinical safety statement for diagnostic ultrasound. https://wfumb.info/2019/04/15/echoes-2-2-2-2-2-2-2-2-2-2-2-2-2-2-2-2-2-2-2-2-2-2-2/. Accessed June 1, 2019.

119. British Medical Ultrasound Society. Guidelines for the safe use of diagnostic ultrasound equipment. http://www.bmus.org/ultras-safety/us-safety03.asp. Published 2009. Accessed August 10, 2016.

120. Clinical safety statement for diagnostic ultrasound–2008. *Ultraschall Med.* 2008;29:552. doi:10.1055/s-0028-1098034.

121. Lees C, Abramowicz JS, Brezinka C, et al; Royal College of Obstetricians and Gynaecologists. Ultrasound from conception to 10^{+0} weeks gestation (scientific impact paper 49). https://www.rcog.org.uk/globalassets/documents/guidelines/scientific-impact-papers/sip-49.pdf. Published 2015. Accessed January 6, 2019.

122. Abramowicz JS. Fetal Doppler: how to keep it safe? *Clin Obstet Gynecol.* 2010;53:842–850. doi:10.1097/GRF.0b013e3181fbae34.

123. Safety Group of the British Medical Ultrasound Society. Guidelines for the safe use of diagnostic ultrasound equipment. *Ultrasound.* 2010;18:52–59.

124. Maulik D. The use of Doppler in early pregnancy. In: Abramowicz JS, ed. *First-Trimester Ultrasound—A Comprehensive Guide.* New York, NY: Springer; 2015.

125. Nelson TR, Fowlkes JB, Abramowicz JS, et al. Ultrasound biosafety considerations for the practicing sonographer and sonologist. *J Ultrasound Med.* 2009;28:139–150.

126. ter Haar G. Guidelines and recommendations for the safe use of diagnostic ultrasound: the user's responsibilities. In: ter Haar G, ed. *The Safe Use of Ultrasound in Medical Diagnosis.* 3rd ed. London, England: British Institute of Radiology; 2012:142–157.

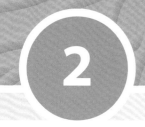

First-Trimester Evaluation

Jiri D. Sonek • Adam K. Hiett • Kypros H. Nicolaides

In the past 30 years, ultrasound examination in the first trimester (11^{+0} to 13^{+6} weeks) has evolved from just an assessment of fetal viability and gestational age to become a central component of an integrated clinic for the diagnosis of fetal abnormalities and assessment of risk for a wide range of pregnancy complications. This chapter reviews the accumulated data on the role of the first-trimester scan in pregnancy care.

SCREENING FOR FETAL ANEUPLOIDIES

Aneuploidies are major causes of perinatal death and childhood handicap. Consequently, detection of chromosomal disorders constitutes the most frequent indication for prenatal screening and diagnostic testing. However, invasive testing, by amniocentesis or chorionic villus sampling (CVS), is associated with a risk of miscarriage. Therefore, these tests are carried out mainly in pregnancies considered to be at high risk for aneuploidies.[1]

In the past 45 years, prenatal screening for aneuploidies has focused on trisomy 21. The first method of screening for trisomy 21 in the general population of pregnant women was introduced in the 1970s. It was based just on maternal age and yielded a detection rate (DR) of 30% for a false-positive rate (FPR) of 5%. In the 1980s and the 1990s, second-trimester maternal serum biochemical markers were added to maternal age, which increased the DR to 60% to 70% for an FPR of 5%. In the past 25 years, screening in the first trimester (11^{+0} to 13^{+6} weeks) has been shown to improve detection of trisomy 21 even further. A combination of maternal age, maternal history, fetal nuchal translucency (NT) thickness, and maternal serum levels of free beta-hCG (beta-human chorionic gonadotropin) and PAPP-A (pregnancy-associated plasma protein A; combined screening) can achieve a DR of 90% and an FPR of 5%.[2] Studies in the past 15 years have shown that this performance can be improved by the addition of ultrasound assessment of the nasal bone and Doppler evaluation of flow in the ductus venosus (DV), hepatic artery (HA), and across the tricuspid valve.

It was quickly noted that in the process of screening for trisomy 21, it was possible to also make an early diagnosis of trisomies 18 and 13, which are the second and third most common chromosomal abnormalities. The relative prevalence of trisomy 21 at 11 to 13 weeks' gestation is 1:3 for trisomy 18 and 1:7 for trisomy 21.[3,4] Since all three trisomies have some risk factors, such as increased maternal age, increased fetal NT, and decreased serum PAPP-A, in common, screening using solely the algorithm for trisomy 21 can detect about 70% to 75% of cases of trisomies 18 and 13, at an FPR of 4% to 5%.[5,6] However, using specific algorithms for each trisomy, which incorporate not only their similarities but also their differences in maternal serum biomarker pattern (low level of free beta-hCG in both trisomies 18 and 13 and high levels in trisomy 21) and increased fetal heart rate in trisomy 13, further improves their performance. The resultant DR for trisomies 18 and 13 is about 95% at the same overall FPR of about 4% to 5%.[5,6]

In addition to trisomies 21, 18, and 13, invasive testing in the screen positive group from the combined test can lead to detection of many other clinically significant aneuploidies.[7] However, the biomarker profile for many of the rare aneuploidies and chromosomal imbalance syndromes is not clearly defined, and it is uncertain whether their incidence in the screen positive group for trisomy 21 is higher than that in the screen negative group. The only exceptions are monosomy X, which is associated with large fetal NT, and triploidy where serum-free beta-hCG is very high and NT is increased if it is diandric in origin and both serum-free beta-hCG and PAPP-A are low if it is digynic in origin.[2,8–10]

In the past 5 years, studies have reported on clinical validation and implementation of screening for aneuploides by analysis of cell-free (cf) DNA in maternal blood.[11] The quality of this approach is high when screening for trisomy 21 with a DR of greater than 99% and an FPR less than 0.1%; performance in screening for trisomies 18 and 13 and for Turner syndrome is also high but less so than for trisomy 21.[12] Several proof of principle studies have examined the potential value of cfDNA testing in the detection of triploidy, trisomies other than those affecting chromosomes 21, 18, and 13, and chromosomal deletions and duplications with varying results.[13–15]

Unfortunately, cfDNA analysis is inconclusive in at least 2% of the cases. Most commonly, this is due to a low fetal fraction in maternal blood (<4%). There is a strong association between low fetal fraction and maternal weight.[16] Consequently, the performance of this test is diminished in obese populations. Low fetal fraction is also more common in pregnancies affected by trisomy 18 or 13.[17] Even though this is not the case in pregnancies with trisomy 21, a recommendation has been made to offer invasive testing in those instances where the cfDNA analysis is inconclusive.[18] This recommendation could be challenged depending on the fact that the vast majority of fetuses with trisomies 18 and 13 are detectable by a detailed ultrasound examination.[19]

In the long term, it is likely that cfDNA testing will replace classical first-trimester combined screening as the primary test for detection of trisomy 21. The practical advantages of this test include simplicity of the screening process for the clinician (obtaining a blood sample) and high efficiency. However, the current high cost of the test and the fact that at least 2% of the test results are inconclusive still limit its use.[20]

Finally, an important aspect of cfDNA testing needs to be kept in mind: As with any other screening test, the positive predictive value changes with the prevalence of disease in the population. Overall, assuming an age-independent trisomy 21 prevalence of approximately 1:500, the positive predictive value is about 66%. However, this falls under 50% in a population younger than 30 years of age. This reality underscores the fact that cfDNA analysis is truly just a screening test. The diagnosis of a chromosomal defect can be made only by invasive testing, which needs to be always offered to clarify an abnormal cfDNA test result.[21]

It is also noteworthy that even though cfDNA technology performs very well in screening for the common aneuploidies, it has very limited application in screening for other chromosomal defects and has no benefit in detection of fetal structural

9

anomalies. By comparison, first-trimester screening, which includes a fetal ultrasound evaluation with NT measurement and additional markers (see section Clinical Implementation, page 13), casts a much wider net in diagnosing fetal defects. An approach that combines the two approaches provides the best results (see section Clinical Implementation of Cell-Free DNA Testing in Maternal Blood, page 14).

Nuchal Translucency Thickness

NT is the sonographic appearance of a collection of fluid under the skin behind the fetal neck in the first trimester of pregnancy.[22] The term translucency is used, irrespective of whether it is septated or not and whether it is confined to the neck or envelops the whole fetus. The incidence of chromosomal and other abnormalities is related to the size, rather than to the appearance of NT.[23] During the second trimester, the translucency usually changes into normally appearing subcutaneous tissue even if it had been thickened in the first trimester. In a few cases, it evolves into either nuchal edema, which is referred to as increased nuchal fold thickness, or into a cystic septated structure, which in the second trimester is referred to as cystic hygromas. The latter can be accompanied by generalized hydrops.

Measurement of Nuchal Translucency Thickness

NT measurement is best done when the fetal crown-rump length (CRL) is 45 to 84 mm. This corresponds to the approximate gestational age of 11^{+0} to 13^{+6} weeks. The lower limit is selected to allow the sonographic diagnosis of many major fetal abnormalities, which would have otherwise been missed. The upper limit has been chosen due to the increasing difficulty of obtaining an accurate NT measurement due to fetal position and the somewhat reduced effectiveness of screening with advancing gestational age. In addition, this limit provides women with affected fetuses the option of an earlier and safer form of termination. Fetal NT can be measured by either transabdominal or transvaginal sonography, and the results are similar. When measuring the NT, the magnification of the image should be such that the fetal head and upper thorax occupy the whole screen. A midsagittal section with the fetus in a neutral position must be obtained (Fig. 2.1). The widest part of translucency must always be measured, and care must be taken

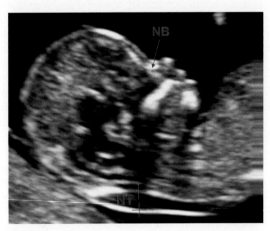

FIGURE 2.1: US of a fetus at 12 weeks' gestation illustrating the measurement of nuchal translucency (NT) thickness and assessment of the nasal bone (NB).

to distinguish between fetal skin and amnion. Measurements should be taken with the inner border of the horizontal line of the calipers placed on the two echogenic lines that define the NT thickness—the crossbar of the calipers should be such that it is hardly visible as it merges with the white lines of the border and does not protrude into the nuchal fluid. During the scan, more than one measurement must be taken, and the largest one that meets all the above-mentioned criteria is used for risk calculation. Accreditation and ongoing quality assurance have been shown to be critical in maintaining the high performance of this screening test. A number of accrediting organizations exist around the world, with the Fetal Medicine Foundation (FMF) being available in most countries.

Implications of Increased Nuchal Translucency Thickness

The measurement of fetal NT thickness provides effective and early screening for trisomy 21 and other major aneuploidies.[24–26] Furthermore, high NT is associated with fetal death, cardiac defects, and a wide range of other fetal malformations and genetic syndromes.[27–31] The heterogeneity of conditions associated with thickened NT suggests that there may not be a single underlying mechanism for the increase in the amount of fluid beneath the skin of the fetal neck. Possible mechanisms include cardiac dysfunction in association with abnormalities of the heart and great arteries, venous congestion in the head and neck, altered composition of the extracellular matrix, failure of lymphatic drainage due to abnormal or delayed development of the lymphatic system or impaired fetal movements, fetal anemia or hypoproteinemia, and congenital infection.

In normal fetuses, NT thickness increases with fetal CRL. The median and 95th percentiles of NT at a CRL of 45 mm are 1.2 and 2.1 mm, and the respective values at CRL of 84 mm are 1.9 and 2.7 mm. The 99th percentile does not change significantly with CRL, and it is about 3.5 mm. Increased NT refers to a measurement above the 95th percentile.

The prevalence of fetal abnormalities and adverse pregnancy outcome increases exponentially with NT thickness (Table 2.1). However, the parents can be reassured that the chances of delivering a baby with no major abnormalities are more than 90% if the fetal NT is between the 95th and 99th percentiles, about 70% for NT of 3.5 to 4.4 mm, 50% for NT 4.5 to 5.4 mm, 30% for NT of 5.5 to 6.4 mm, and 15% for NT of 6.5 mm or more.[27]

Management of Pregnancies with Increased Nuchal Translucency Thickness

In pregnancies with fetal NT below the 99th percentile (3.5 mm), the decision by the parents in favor of or against fetal karyotyping will depend on the patient-specific risk for chromosomal defects, which is derived from the combination of maternal age and history, sonographic findings, and serum-free beta-hCG and PAPP-A with or without additional markers such as nasal bone and blood flow through the DV or across the tricuspid valve. If the risk assessment places the patient in a low-risk category or if the fetal karyotype is shown to be normal, a detailed fetal scan in the mid-second trimester is still useful to check fetal growth and look for fetal abnormalities that were not identified at the time of the first-trimester screen.

A fetal NT measurement above 3.5 mm is found in about 1% of pregnancies. The risk of major chromosomal abnormalities is very high and increases from about 20% for NT of 4.0 mm to

TABLE 2.1   **Relation between Nuchal Translucency Thickness and Prevalence of Chromosomal Defects, Miscarriage or Fetal Death, and Major Fetal Abnormalities**

NUCHAL TRANSLUCENCY	CHROMOSOMAL DEFECTS (%)	FETAL DEATH (%)	MAJOR FETAL ABNORMALITIES (%)	ALIVE AND WELL[a] (%)
<95th centile	0.2	1.3	1.6	97
95th–99th centiles	3.7	1.3	2.5	93
3.5–4.4 mm	21.1	2.7	10.0	70
4.5–5.4 mm	33.3	3.4	18.5	50
5.5–6.4 mm	50.5	10.1	24.2	30
>6.5 mm	64.5	19.0	46.2	15

[a]Estimated prevalence of delivery of a healthy baby with no major abnormalities.

33% for NT of 5.0 mm, 50% for NT of 6.0 mm, and 65% for NT of 6.5 mm or more. Consequently, the first line of management of such pregnancies should be to offer fetal karyotyping by CVS. In the chromosomally normal group, a detailed scan, including fetal echocardiography, should be attempted at the time of the first-trimester screening ultrasound and again at about 16 weeks' gestation. The latter serves to evaluate the appearance of the NT over time and to look for fetal defects at still a relatively early gestational age. If this scan demonstrates resolution of the NT, that is, a normal nuchal fold thickness measurement and absence of any major abnormalities, the parents can be reassured that the prognosis is likely to be good and the chances of delivering a baby with no major abnormalities is more than 95%. Nonetheless, a detailed scan at 20 to 22 weeks' gestation still is useful to check for major abnormalities, especially congenital heart defects, and for more subtle defects that may be seen in certain genetic syndromes. If none of these is found, the parents can be counseled that the risk of delivering a baby with a serious abnormality or neurodevelopmental delay is essentially no higher than in the general population.

Persistence of unexplained increased NT or evolution to nuchal edema with or without associated hydrops fetalis at either the 16 weeks' or at the 20 to 22 weeks' scan further increases the risk of either congenital infection or a genetic syndrome being present. Maternal blood should be tested for toxoplasmosis, cytomegalovirus, and parvovirus B19. Serial ultrasounds approximately every 4 weeks are useful to look at the evolution of the edema and associated changes in fetal anatomy. In addition, consideration should be given to DNA testing for certain genetic conditions, such as spinal muscular atrophy, even if there is no family history of these conditions. In pregnancies with unexplained nuchal edema at the 20 to 22 weeks' scan, the parents should be counseled that there is up to a 10% risk of evolution to hydrops and perinatal death or a live birth with a genetic syndrome, such as Noonan syndrome. The risk of neurodevelopmental delay is estimated at 3% to 5%.

Additional Ultrasound Markers

At the time of the first-trimester screen, fetuses with trisomy 21 have an increased prevalence of nasal bone absence (60%), reversed atrial contraction (a-wave) in the DV (66%), tricuspid

regurgitation (55%), and increased peak systolic velocity (PSV) in the HA (80%). By contrast, these are seen in 2.5%, 3.0%, 1.0%, and 5.0% of euploid fetuses, respectively.[32–41]

Absent or Hypoplastic Nasal Bone

At the time of first-trimester combined screening, the nasal bone is assessed for its presence or absence, not its length. The sonographic technique is similar to the one employed for NT measurements: A midsagittal view of the fetal profile should be obtained, and the magnification of the image should be such that the head and upper thorax occupy the whole screen. However, care must be taken so the angle of insonation is such that the face of the ultrasound transducer is the nasal bridge. The ultrasound probe is then gently tilted from one side of the nose to the other. The facial landmarks that help establish that the view is in midsagittal plane are the following: The skin over the tip of the nose and the nasal bridge is seen as two short echogenic lines, one in front of the other, and the hard palate is rectangular in shape. In addition, this view should include a translucent diencephalon, which is located approximately at the center of the fetal brain.

When the nasal bone is present, this view should demonstrate three distinct echogenic lines in the region of the fetal nose. As mentioned earlier, two are in tandem and represent the nasal bridge and the tip of the nose. The third line, which lies beneath the nasal bridge and is distinct from it, is the nasal bone. These two lines run in parallel and are, therefore, referred to as the "equal sign." By definition, the nasal bone is considered present if the bottom line is more echogenic than the overlying skin line. Usually, if the nasal bone is present, the bottom line will also be thicker than the skin line (Fig. 2.1). Absence of the nasal bone is diagnosed if the echogenicity of the bottom line is the same as or less than the overlying skin or if no bottom line is be identified, that is, the "equal sign" is absent.

Abnormal Flow across the Ductus Venosus

The DV is a short fetal vessel that connects the hepatic portion of the umbilical vein (UV) to the inferior vena cava. It delivers oxygenated blood to the heart and, through intracardiac shunting, preferentially to the fetal brain. About 20% of oxygenated blood is thus delivered directly to the heart, bypassing the liver. It enters the right atrium and is shunted across the foramen ovale into the left atrium. It than passes through the left heart into the aorta and

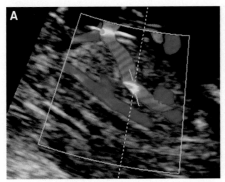
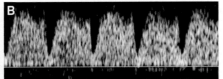
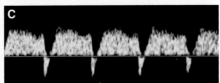

FIGURE 2.2: Midsagittal view of the fetal trunk demonstrating insonation of the ductus venosus **(A)** of a fetus at 12 weeks with normal waveform **(B)** and reversed a-wave **(C)**.

is delivered to the neck vessels, which supply the fetal brain. The DV usually closes within a few minutes of birth.

Due to proximity of its insertion to the right atrium, blood flow through the DV is affected by the changes in pressure in the right heart, which occur during the cardiac cycle. Blood flow in the DV has a characteristic waveform with high velocity during ventricular systole (S-wave) and diastole (D-wave). The flow decreases during an a-wave but usually remains in the forward direction. Increased impedance to flow in the fetal DV at 11 to 13 weeks' gestation is associated fetal aneuploidies, cardiac defects, and other adverse pregnancy outcomes.[36,42–46] The reason for this finding is not entirely clear, but it may represent decreased compliance of the right heart, which results in increased pressure during the right atrial contraction. In most studies examining DV flow, look at the appearance of the a-wave as a *categorical* variable: It is classified as normal when forward flow is observed during atrial contraction and abnormal when flow stops (a-wave is absent) or if it is reversed. DV flow can also be measured using the pulsatility index for veins (PIV). This is the preferred alternative for estimation of patient-specific risk because it is a continuous variable and removes some of the subjectivity that is associated with assessing DV flow based solely on the appearance of the a-wave.[47]

Assessment of DV flow begins by obtaining a right ventral longitudinal view of the fetal trunk. Magnification of the image should be such that the fetal thorax and abdomen occupy the whole screen (Fig. 2.2). The Doppler examination should be during fetal quiescence, and color flow mapping must be used to differentiate between the UV, DV, and fetal heart. The pulsed Doppler sample gate should be small (0.5 to 1.0 mm) to avoid

contamination from the adjacent veins. It must be placed in the yellowish aliasing area at an insonation angle of less than 30° with respect to the longitudinal axis of the DV. The filter should be set at a low frequency (50 to 70 Hz) to allow visualization of the whole waveform and the sweep speed should be high (2 to 3 cm/s) so that the waveforms are widely spread. The DV PIV is measured by the ultrasound machine after the waveform is traced manually. *As always, adhering to the As Low As Reasonably Achievable (ALARA) principle is highly recommended. The time that the fetus is exposed to Doppler should be minimized and the lowest possible power output to obtain diagnostic information should be used.*[48]

Tricuspid Regurgitation

Tricuspid regurgitation at 11 to 13 weeks' gestation has increased prevalence in fetal aneuploidies and major cardiac defects.[37–39,49] The exact reason for this is yet to be determined. However, there are essentially two possible anatomical causes of tricuspid regurgitation. One is dilatation of the tricuspid valve annulus that leads to an incomplete valve closure and the other one is congenital malformation of the valve itself. The first mechanism is likely at play in fetuses with aneuploidy but normal cardiac structure. In fetuses that have a cardiac defect, with or without fetal aneuploidy, abnormality of the structure of the valve is also a likely contributing factor.

In the assessment of tricuspid flow, an apical four-chamber view of the fetal heart should be obtained, and the magnification of the image should be such that the fetal thorax occupies most of the screen. The pulsed Doppler sample should be large (2.0 to 3.0 mm) and positioned across the tricuspid valve. The insonation angle to the direction of flow should be less than 30° with respect

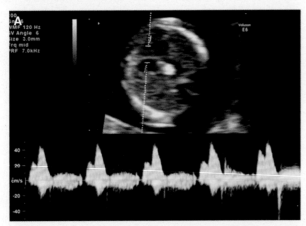
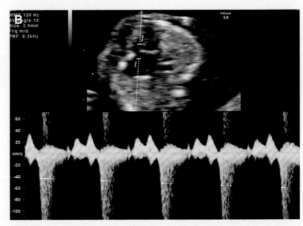

FIGURE 2.3: Transverse view of the fetal heart demonstrating Doppler assessment of flow across the tricuspid valve of a fetus at 12 weeks with normal waveform **(A)** and tricuspid regurgitation **(B)**.

to the interventricular septum, and the sweep speed should be high (2 to 3 cm/s) so that the waveforms are widely spread (Fig. 2.3). The tricuspid valve could be insufficient in one or more of its three cusps; therefore, the sample gate should be placed across the valve several times, in an attempt to interrogate the entire valve. In order for the diagnosis of tricuspid regurgitation to be made, the regurgitant stream has to last at least half of the systole and the velocity must be over 60 cm/s. The latter criterion is needed so that contamination by aortic or pulmonary arterial blood flow, which at this point in gestation has a maximum velocity of approximately 50 cm/s, is not erroneously interpreted as tricuspid regurgitation. *As always, adhering to the ALARA principle is highly recommended. The time that the fetus is exposed to Doppler should be minimized and the lowest possible power output to obtain diagnostic information should be used.*[48]

Increased Blood Velocity in the Hepatic Artery

In fetal life, the liver has a number of critical functions, which include both metabolic and hemopoietic activities. Normally, more than 90% of the blood supply to the liver is provided by the umbilical and portal veins and less than 10% comes directly from the HA. The HA branches from the celiac trunk, which originates from the descending aorta. At 11 to 13^{+6} weeks' gestation, HAs in fetuses affected by trisomy 21 have an increased PSV and decreased pulsatility index (PI).[40,41]

Landmarks for the assessment of the HA flow are similar to those used for DV evaluation. A right ventral midsagittal view of the fetal trunk is obtained, and the magnification of the image should be such that the fetal thorax and abdomen occupy the whole screen. The Doppler examination should be performed during fetal quiescence and color flow mapping is used to demonstrate the hepatic portion of the UV, DV, descending aorta, and HA (Fig. 2.4). Initially, the size of the pulsed Doppler gate must be set at 2.0 mm and is placed so that it includes both the DV and the adjacent upper part of the HA. This ensures that the HA, rather than celiac trunk, is sampled. After these vascular structures are identified, the size of the gate should be reduced to 1.0 mm, so that only the HA is being sampled. The insonation angle must be less than 30° with respect to the longitudinal axis of the HA. The filter should be set at a high frequency (120 Hz) to avoid contamination from adjacent veins and the sweep speed should be high (2 to 3 cm/s) so that the waveforms are widely spread. The pulsed wave pulse repetition frequency should be adjusted to optimize the PSV measurement. When three similar consecutive waveforms are obtained, they are traced manually and the software in the ultrasound equipment is used to measure the PSV and PI. *As always, adhering to the ALARA principle is highly recommended. The time that the fetus is exposed to Doppler should be minimized and the lowest possible power output to obtain diagnostic information should be used.*[48]

Clinical Implementation

If each of the additional ultrasound markers is added to the standard first-trimester combined screening, the DR of trisomy 21 increases from 93% to 96% and the FPR decreases to less than 3%. This improvement in screening can be achieved if this is done in every patient examined or using a contingent approach. Using the latter algorithm, the first step is performing standard combined screening using maternal age, fetal NT, and serum-free beta-hCG and PAPP-A in each patient (Fig. 2.5).[50] Patients are then stratified according to this initial risk assessment. Those with a risk of 1 in 50 or more are offered invasive testing. Those with a risk of less than 1 in 1,000 are offered no further testing except for a second-trimester detailed ultrasound. Patients who

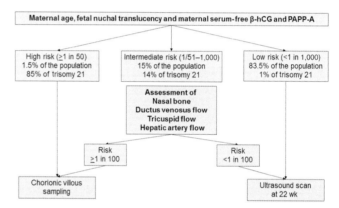

FIGURE 2.5: Two-stage screening for fetal aneuploidies. In the first stage, all patients have screening by a combination of maternal age, fetal nuchal translucency thickness, and maternal serum-free beta-human chorionic gonadotropin *(beta-hCG)* and pregnancy-associated plasma protein A *(PAPP-A)*, and according to the results they are classified into high-risk, intermediate-risk, and low-risk groups. In the intermediate-risk group, second-stage screening is carried out by one or more sonographic markers, including nasal bone, blood flow in the ductus venosus, hepatic artery, or across the tricuspid valve, and on the basis of the results they are then classified as high-risk or low-risk groups.

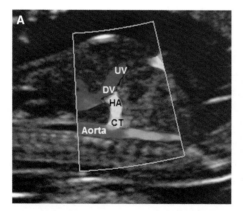
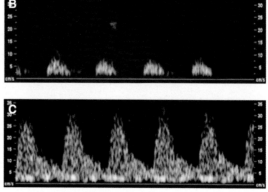

FIGURE 2.4: A: Right ventral midsagittal view of a fetus at 12 weeks demonstrating the umbilical vein *(UV),* ductus venosus *(DV),* descending aorta, hepatic artery *(HA),* and celiac trunk *(CT).* The peak systolic velocity in the waveform from the fetus with trisomy 21 **(C)** is much higher than that in a euploid fetus **(B).**

fall in the intermediate-risk category (1 in 51 to 1 in 1,000), which constitutes 15% to 20% of the total population, undergo second-stage screening using nasal bone, DV, or tricuspid blood flow evaluations. The results are then used to modify the risk based on the initial combined screen. If the adjusted risk is 1 in 100 or more, the patient is offered invasive testing. Those with a lesser risk are reassured and only a second-trimester detailed ultrasound is recommended. Using the contingent approach results in reducing the need for more specialized services, which are then needed in only 15% to 20% of the population.

Screening in Twins

The first step in screening for trisomies in twins is to determine their chorionicity. This is easily performed by ultrasound at 11 to 13⁺⁶ weeks' gestation (Fig. 2.6).[51] The ultrasound appearance of the dividing membrane becomes more similar between monochorionic and dichorionic twins as the pregnancy progresses: The membrane in dichorionic twins thins out as the chorion laeve atrophies during the course of the pregnancy and assumes an appearance similar to that of monochorionic twins. Since all monochorionic twins are monozygotic, a single risk assessment is calculated for both fetuses. This is done by averaging the two NT measurements. In dichorionic twins, each fetus is assigned its individual risk based on the NT measurements in that fetus.[52,53] The latter approach is accurate in most but not all dichorionic twins as approximately 10% of these gestations are monozygotic. Measurement of serum-free beta-hCG and PAPP-A is also useful in screening for trisomies in twins. However, these levels need to be adjusted since normal ranges are different in twins compared to those in singletons. Furthermore, the levels are lower in monochorionic than in dichorionic pregnancies.[54–56]

In twins, the DR of trisomy 21 by the combined test is about 90% but at a higher FPR than in singletons (6% vs. 5%).[52] In monochorionic twins, the FPR is even higher, at about 9%. This is due to the fact that increased NT measurement may be an early sign of not only aneuploidy but also of twin-to-twin transfusion syndrome, a condition that is specific to monochorionic pregnancies.[52]

Clinical Implementation of Cell-Free DNA Testing in Maternal Blood

The performance of screening for trisomies 21, 18, and 13 by cfDNA analysis of maternal blood is superior to that of the combined test.[11] However, the test is expensive, and it is therefore unlikely that it would be used for routine screening of the whole population in the near future. Employing cfDNA testing on contingent basis after first-trimester combined screening has a number of advantages. We suggest that at the present time, offering first-trimester combined screen as the first step and offering cfDNA testing on contingent basis may be the best approach.[7,57] Similarly to the contingent approach described earlier for the use of additional ultrasound markers, the population is divided into three groups: high risk, intermediate risk, and low risk. In this model, invasive testing is offered to all patients who fall into the high-risk (e.g., risk ≥ 1:10) group and that cfDNA testing is offered to those in the intermediate-risk (e.g., 1:11 to 1:1,000) group. Invasive testing is offered to those who have a positive cfDNA screening result (Fig. 2.7). Those who have negative cfDNA results or those who fall into the low-risk (e.g., <1:1,100) group are recommended a detailed ultrasound in the mid-second trimester.

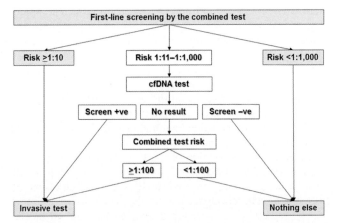

FIGURE 2.7: First-line screening by the combined test is carried out in all pregnancies. In those with a risk for trisomies 21, 18, or 13 greater than or equal to 1:10, invasive testing is performed, and in those with a risk less than 1:1,000, there is no further testing. In women with risk between 1:11 and 1:1,000 cell-free (cf) DNA testing is carried out. In those with a positive cfDNA result, invasive testing is performed, and in those with a negative result, there is no further testing. In the group of women with no result from cfDNA testing, the results of the combined test are considered, and invasive testing is carried out for those with a risk for trisomies 21, 18, or 13 greater than or equal to 1:100.

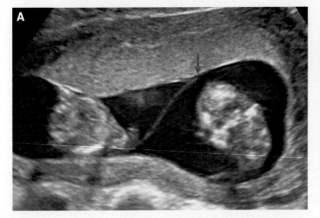
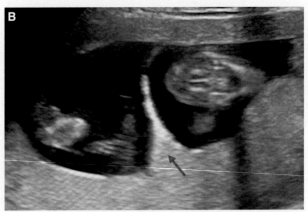

FIGURE 2.6: US illustrating the difference in the junction of the intertwin membrane (shown by the *red arrow*) with the placenta in monochorionic **(A)** and dichorionic twins **(B)** at 12 weeks' gestation.

Such a strategy retains the advantages of the first-trimester scan such as establishing a very accurate gestational age, the diagnosis of over 50% major defects, and assessment of risk for pregnancy complications such as preeclampsia (PE; see section Preeclampsia, page 23). At the same time, it would detect about 98% of fetuses with trisomies 21, 18, and 13, at an overall invasive testing rate of less than 1%. The intermediate-risk group requiring cfDNA testing constitutes about 25% of the population. However, if the measurement of DV PIV is added to the first-line use of combined screening, this proportion can be reduced to about 10%, without affecting the overall performance of screening.[57]

In the future, detection of other chromosomal abnormalities and rare syndromes may also be improved using cfDNA technology.[58,59] In the context of screening, however, it will take considerable time for the true detection and FPRs to be determined. Given the inherently low prevalence of most of these disorders, it will be difficult to achieve high positive predictive values using screening based solely on cfDNA. Thus, introduction of screening for more uncommon disorders has not thus far gained wide acceptance.[60] Microdeletion 22q11.2 may be one possible exception as the prevalence of this chromosomal abnormality is up to 1 in 1,000.[61] Given the wide spectrum of anomalies associated with this disorder and the follow-up examinations that are needed after an abnormal test result, the appropriateness of antenatal screening in the general obstetrical population is difficult to determine.[62] The prevalence of the other currently detectable diseases is certainly too low for general screening programs. However, the tests can be useful in individual cases. For example, they may be useful in the setting of a strongly positive family history, such as a previously affected offspring, or if the level of suspicion is sufficiently raised by the presence of specific ultrasound markers.

DIAGNOSIS OF MAJOR FETAL DEFECTS

It is no longer acceptable to consider an ultrasound examination of the fetus between 11 and 13[+6] weeks just as an opportunity to establish gestational age and perhaps measure the NT. It requires the operator to evaluate the fetal anatomy in as much detail as possible. This is reflected in the current guidelines issued by ISUOG and AIUM.[48,63] In addition to the structures enumerated in Table 2.2, both recommend careful evaluation of the adnexa and the uterus and location of the pregnancy, including cervical, cesarean scar, and extrauterine locations. This approach allows for major fetal anomalies to be diagnosed at an early point in pregnancy, which gives the parents more time to consider their options, including an earlier and safer pregnancy termination.

The ability to diagnose major fetal abnormalities depends on a number of factors. As with all fetal evaluations, maternal factors such as habitus, fetal position, quality of ultrasound equipment, time allotted for the examination, and the level of expertise of the sonographer/sonologist all play a role. Aside from these factors, anomalies can be divided into roughly three categories with respect to ease of first-trimester diagnosis.[64] One group consists of anomalies that are relatively easy to identify. Anomalies such as body stalk anomaly, alobar holoprosencephaly, omphalocele, and gastroschisis should be evident on ultrasound even to a relatively inexperienced sonographer. Megacystis, which in the first trimester is associated with either a development of serious renal problems or may serve as a marker for aneuploidy, is also relatively easy to identify. Anencephaly also falls into this category. However, the sonographer

TABLE 2.2	Suggested Anatomical Assessment at Time of 11-to-13[+6]-Week Scan	
ORGAN/ANATOMICAL AREA	**PRESENT AND/OR NORMAL?**
Head	Present Cranial bones Midline falx Choroid-plexus-filled ventricles
Neck	Normal appearance Nuchal translucency thickness (if accepted after informed consent and trained/certified operator available)
Face	Eyes with lens Nasal bone Normal profile/mandible Intact lips
Spine	Vertebrae (longitudinal and axial) Intact overlying skin
Chest	Symmetrical lung fields No effusions or masses
Heart	Cardiac regular activity Four symmetrical chambers
Abdomen	Stomach present in left upper quadrant Bladder Kidneys
Abdominal wall	Normal cord insertion No umbilical defects
Extremities	Four limbs each with three segments Hand and feet with normal orientation
Placenta	Size and texture
Cord	Three-vessel cord

From Salomon LJ, Alfirevic Z, Bilardo CM, et al. ISUOG Practice Guidelines: performance of first-trimester fetal ultrasound scan. *Ultrasound Obstet Gynecol.* 2013;41(1):102–113. doi:10.1002/uog.12342. Copyright © 2013 ISUOG. Reprinted by permission of John Wiley & Sons, Inc.

must be aware of the fact that this condition has a very different appearance in the first trimester as compared to later gestation. At the other end of the spectrum, there are anomalies that become evident on ultrasound only during the second or third trimester of pregnancy and are, therefore, not detectable in the first trimester. These include microcephaly, agenesis of the corpus callosum, semilobar holoprosencephaly, hypoplasia of the cerebellum or vermis, congenital pulmonary airway malformations, and bowel obstruction. A third group includes abnormalities that are either potentially detectable but require extremely detailed investigation or those that are often associated with ultrasound markers that increase the level of suspicion of their presence. Examples of such associations are thickened NT in fetuses with major cardiac defects, lethal skeletal dysplasia, or diaphragmatic hernia or abnormal posterior brain in the presence of an open spine defect.

Several studies reported the diagnosis of a wide range of fetal abnormalities during the first-trimester scan. A randomized study of 35,792 pregnancies where a routine anomaly scan was performed at either 12 or 18 weeks' gestation using a checklist (skull, neck and brain, face, chest, heart, diaphragm, abdominal wall, stomach, kidneys, bladder, spine, and limbs), reported that the rate of prenatal detection of major abnormalities was not significantly different between the two groups (38% vs. 47%).[65] In our center, we evaluated the DR of fetal anomalies at the time of first-trimester screening for aneuploidy in 45,191 pregnancies.[64] Results from ultrasound examinations at 20 to 23 weeks' gestation and neonatal examinations were available. Chromosomally abnormal cases were excluded from the analysis. Fetal abnormalities were observed in 488 (1.1%) cases and 213 (43.6%) of these were detected at 11 to 13 weeks. The early scan detected all cases of exencephaly/anencephaly sequence, alobar holoprosencephaly, exomphalos, gastroschisis, megacystis, and body stalk anomaly, 77% of absent hand or foot, 50% of diaphragmatic hernias, 50% of lethal skeletal dysplasias, 60% of polydactyly, 34% of major cardiac defects, 5% of facial clefts, and 14% of open neural tube defects.

Suggested Protocol for First-Trimester Anomaly Scan

The ultrasound examination is usually performed transabdominally, using 3 to 7.5 MHz curvilinear transducers, but in about 1% of cases when there are technical difficulties to obtain adequate views, a transvaginal scan (3 to 9 MHz transducer) should also be carried out. The time allocated for the ultrasound examination of the fetus should be about 20 minutes. The goal is to obtain at minimum the following views: Transverse section of the head to demonstrate the skull, midline echo, and the choroid plexuses; a midsagittal view of the face to demonstrate the nasal bone and maxilla; sagittal section of the spine to look for kyphoscoliosis; a transverse section of the thorax to demonstrate the four-chamber view of the heart and record blood flow across the tricuspid valve; transverse and sagittal sections of the trunk to demonstrate the stomach, bladder, and abdominal cord insertion; and extremities (all the long bones, hands, and feet).

Acrania and Anencephaly

The ossification of the skull and the development of the two cerebral hemispheres are usually evident at 11 weeks' gestation. The underlying defect in development of anencephaly is absence of the cranial vault (acrania) and overlying muscles and skin. In the first trimester, neural tissue is still present above the base of the skull. However, it is disordered, and normal hemispheres are absent. This condition is termed exencephaly and exposes the neural tissues to the caustic effects of the amniotic fluid. By the mid-second trimester, this interaction leads to essentially complete resorption of brain tissue. The result is the typical appearance of anencephaly that is seen later in pregnancy and at birth, and that is a complete absence of recognizable neural tissue above the level of ocular orbits.

The sonographer must be aware of the fact that the first-trimester appearance of anencephaly differs from what is seen later on. The diagnosis of anencephaly may be missed in the first trimester unless the correct views are obtained. The ultrasonographic hallmarks of the exencephaly/anencephaly sequence between 11 and 13[+6] weeks' gestation are the lack of ossified calvarium and lack of normal intracranial anatomy. Even though these findings are best demonstrated on the axial view of the fetal head, they can also be readily seen in a longitudinal section (Fig. 2.8).[66]

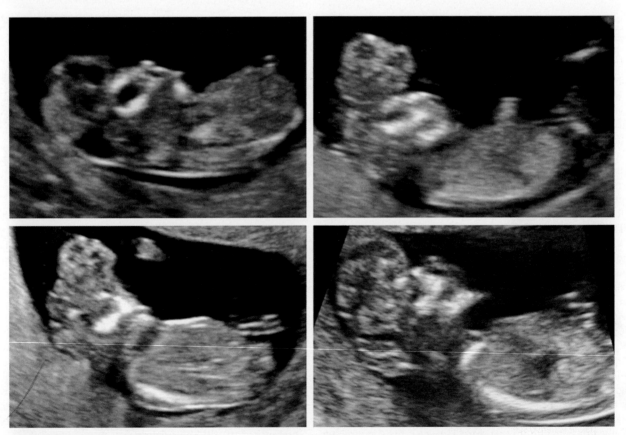

FIGURE 2.8: Acrania with varying degrees of distortion and disruption of the brain at 11 to 13 weeks' gestation.

Holoprosencephaly

Holoprosencephaly, with a birth prevalence of about 1 in 10,000, is characterized by a spectrum of cerebral abnormalities resulting from incomplete cleavage of the forebrain. In a normal pregnancy, it is already possible to clearly visualize falx cerebri and the butterfly appearance of the cerebral hemispheres at 11 weeks' gestation. At this point, the bulk of the hemispheres is composed of the choroid plexuses of the lateral ventricles (Fig. 2.9). In the standard transverse view of the fetal head, alobar or semilobar holoprosencephaly is characterized by a single dilated midline ventricle replacing the two lateral ventricles (fusion of the anterior horns of the lateral ventricles) or partial segmentation of the ventricles and the absence of the butterfly sign.[67] The alobar and semilobar types are often associated with facial defects, such as hypotelorism, cyclopia, midline facial cleft, nasal hypoplasia, or proboscis. In about 65% of cases diagnosed in the first trimester, there is an underlying aneuploidy, mainly trisomy 13.[68]

Cleft Lip and Palate

Cleft lip and cleft palate (CLP) are strongly associated with chromosomal and syndromic disorders, which make their early diagnosis important.[69] There are several markers that improve the rate of CLP detection in the first trimester. Sepulveda et al. described the "retronasal triangle" to facilitate this diagnosis[70] (Fig. 2.10). Chaoui et al. reported on a so-called maxillary gap to identify fetuses with CLP. Approximately 80% of affected fetuses were noted to have this finding[71] (Fig. 2.11). Hoopman et al. used a line tangentially applied to the ventral edge of the mandible and maxilla (so-called maxillomandibular line [MML]) in screening for CLP (Fig. 2.12). The distance of the line from the frontal bone (frontal space distance) was found to be above the 99th or below the first percentile in 35 of 36 affected fetuses.[72]

Open Neural Tube Defects

In almost all cases of open neural tube defects, there is an associated Arnold–Chiari malformation. In the second trimester of pregnancy, the ultrasound manifestations of the Arnold–Chiari malformation include an easily recognizable banana sign, which is often accompanied by the lemon sign.[73]

Intracranial findings associated with open neural tube defects in the first trimester are much subtler. However, it is now recognized that caudal displacement of the brain is associated with the presence of an open neural tube defect already at 11 to 13 weeks' gestation. This can be evaluated in the same midsagittal view of the fetal face as for measurement

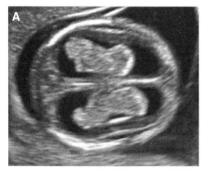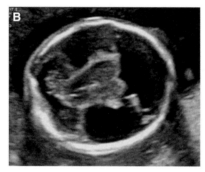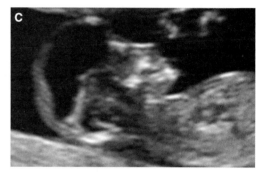

FIGURE 2.9: Cross-sectional view of the fetal brain at 12 weeks demonstrating the normal butterfly appearance of the lateral ventricles with the choroid plexuses **(A)** and alobar holoprosencephaly with fusion of the anterior horns of the lateral ventricles **(B)**. **C:** Sagittal view of the fetal brain demonstrating alobar holoprosencephaly.

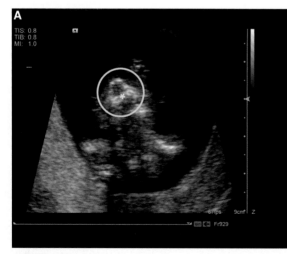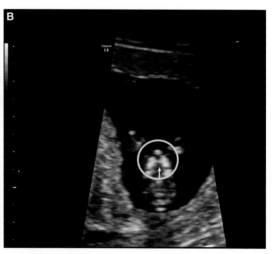

FIGURE 2.10: Retronasal triangle *(circle)*. **A:** Normal retronasal triangle: two frontal processes of the maxilla and the hard palate *(asterisk)* seen in a coronal view of the central portion of the face. **B:** Retronasal triangle view in a fetus with a cleft palate: two frontal processes of the maxilla are present, but the hard palate is absent *(arrow)*.

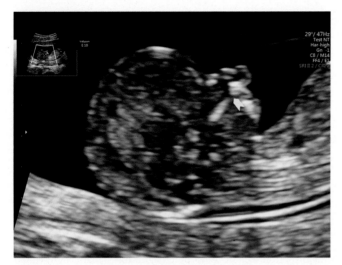

FIGURE 2.11: Maxillary gap *(chevron)* in a fetus with bilateral cleft lip and palate.

of fetal NT and assessment of the nasal bone.[74,75] In this view, the posterior and lower portion of the brain that is located between the sphenoid bone and the occipital bone (OB) is divided into two main sections. One section starts at the sphenoid bone and extends to the first echogenic line that is encountered as one proceeds posteriorly. This section is the brain stem (BS) and the echogenic line is the interface between the posterior edge of the BS and the floor of the fourth ventricle. The second section begins at the echogenic line and extends to the inner edge of the OB. This section includes the fourth ventricle and its roof (developing cerebellar vermis) and the cisterna magna (Fig. 2.13). The two sections can be measured individually in the anteroposterior direction and their relationship is established by calculating the ratio of the measurements (BS/BSOB). As the posterior fossa structures that are displaced caudally, the measurement of the BSOB distance decreases and the BS/BSOB increases. Ratio of 1.0 or greater has been associated with high risk for open neural tube defects.

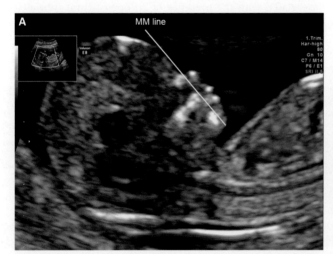

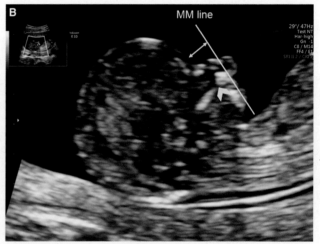

FIGURE 2.12: Mandibulomaxillary line (MML). **A:** MML in a normal fetus. In this case, the line is apposed to the forehead and the frontal space measurement is 0 (in normal fetuses, the line is usually located close to the forehead). **B:** Increased frontal space measurement *(double arrow)* in a fetus with bilateral cleft lip and palate. *Chevron,* maxillary gap.

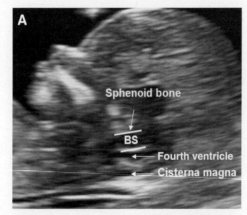

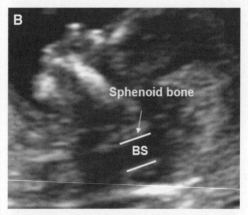

FIGURE 2.13: Midsagittal view of the fetal brain in a normal **(A)** and a spina bifida **(B)** fetus at 12 weeks demonstrating the measurement of brain stem *(BS)* diameter. In open spina bifida, the brain stem diameter is increased.

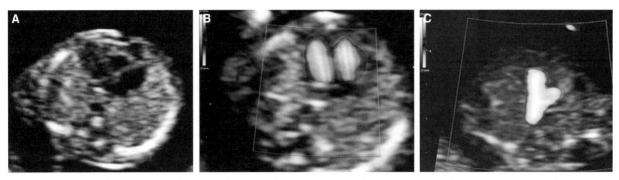

FIGURE 2.14: Four-chamber view of the fetal heart at 12 weeks' gestation **(A)**, color flow imaging of an apical four-chamber view demonstrating equal diastolic flows from right and left atrium into right and left ventricle **(B)**, and color flow imaging showing the V-sign formed by the ductal arch and aortic arch **(C)**.

Major Cardiac Defects

Abnormalities of the heart and great arteries are the most common congenital defects. They account for about 20% of all stillbirths and 30% of neonatal deaths that are attributable to congenital anomalies.[76] Although most major cardiac defects are amenable to prenatal diagnosis by specialist fetal echocardiography, routine ultrasound screening in pregnancy fails to identify the majority of affected fetuses.[77–79] Consequently, effective population-based prenatal diagnosis necessitates improved methods of identifying the high-risk group for referral to specialists.

The traditional method of screening for cardiac defects, which relies on family history of cardiac defects, maternal history of diabetes mellitus, and maternal exposure to teratogens, identifies only about 10% of affected fetuses.[80] A major improvement in screening came with the realization that an increase in fetal NT thickness increases the risk of cardiac defects. It was noted that risk of congenital heart disease (CHD) also is increased in fetuses with abnormal flow in the DV and across the tricuspid valve.[29,31,43,81–84] Reversed a-wave in the DV or tricuspid regurgitation are observed in about 2% and 1% of normal fetuses, respectively. However, it is found in about 30% of fetuses with CHD. If specialist fetal echocardiography is performed in cases with NT above the 99th percentile, and those with reversed a-wave in the DV or tricuspid regurgitation, irrespective of NT, specialized service would be required in only about 4% of the population, but it would detect about 50% of major CHDs.

Some studies evaluated the use of DV PIV in screening for cardiac defects. Timmerman et al. observed that in the group of euploid fetuses with a cardiac defect and increased NT, the DV PIV was above the 95th percentile in about three-quarters of the cases.[85] In a study that was performed in a low-risk population, the detection and FPR was 38% and 5%, respectively.[86]

Informative evaluation of patients who are identified as being at high risk for cardiac defects in the first trimester can begin much earlier than 20 weeks' gestation. First-trimester fetal echocardiography is technically more difficult than at 20 weeks, because the heart is much smaller and the fetus is usually more mobile. However, it is still possible to demonstrate the four-chamber view, outflow tracts, ductus arteriosus, and the aortic arch (Fig. 2.14). Overall, an adequate assessment of the fetal heart can be performed in about 45% and 90% of the cases at 11 and 13 weeks' gestation, respectively.[87] In many instances,

a scan as early as at 13 weeks' gestation can effectively reassure the parents that there is no suggestion of a major cardiac defect. Similarly, in many cases with a major cardiac defect, the early scan can raise a suspicion that a defect is present, and often leads to the correct diagnosis even at this gestational age. A systematic review based on 10 studies (1,243 patients) to determine the accuracy of first-trimester ultrasound in detecting congenital heart disease was published in 2006. The pooled sensitivity was 85% and specificity was 99%.[88]

However, an echocardiogram done later in gestation is still important, especially in those cases where the fetal heart appears to be normal during the early evaluation.

Diaphragmatic Hernia

Even though it can be part of a syndrome, this is usually a sporadic defect with a birth prevalence of about 1 in 4,000. In up to 30% of affected fetuses, there are associated chromosomal abnormalities, mainly trisomy 18, or other anomalies. Increased NT thickness is present in about 40% of fetuses with diaphragmatic hernia, including more than 80% of those that result in neonatal death owing to pulmonary hypoplasia and in about 20% of those that survive (Fig. 2.15).[89] The reason for the association between NT measurement and survival is unclear. It may be that the diaphragmatic hernia in those that have an increased NT exerts a greater amount of intrathoracic pressure perhaps due to its greater size. Another explanation may be that

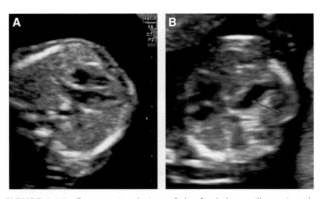

FIGURE 2.15: Cross-sectional view of the fetal thorax illustrating the normal position of the heart and lungs **(A)**, and intrathoracic herniation of the stomach (*arrow* in **B**) in a case of diaphragmatic hernia.

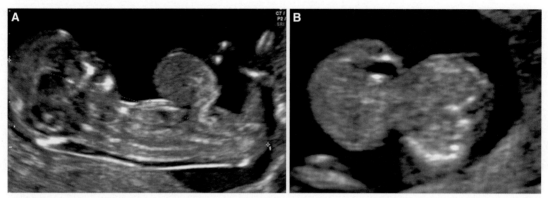

FIGURE 2.16: Sagittal **(A)** and transverse **(B)** views of the fetal abdomen at the level of the umbilicus illustrating cases of exomphalos containing the liver at 12 weeks' gestation.

in those that have a normal NT measurement, herniation of abdominal organs does not occur until later in pregnancy.

Ventral Wall Defects

Omphalocele

An omphalocele is a midline anterior abdominal wall defect where the herniated visceral organs are covered by a membrane and the umbilical cord insertion at the apex of the sac (Fig. 2.16). First-trimester diagnosis of an omphalocele is complicated by the fact that physiological exomphalos (midgut herniation) is part of normal embryonic and very early fetal development. All fetuses at 8 to 10 weeks' gestation demonstrate herniation of the midgut, which is visualized as a hyperechogenic mass in the base of the umbilical cord. In some fetuses, it persists until 11 weeks' gestation or beyond, but retraction into the abdominal cavity is normally completed by 12 weeks. Occasionally, a delay in retraction of physiological exomphalos occurs. In these cases, there may be an increased risk of congenital bowel defects such as malrotations.

At 11 to 13 weeks, omphalocele is observed in about 1:1,000 fetuses, and in 55% of cases there is an associated chromosomal abnormality, usually trisomy 18.[68] Omphaloceles are variable in content and size. In most cases, they include bowel only but additional intra-abdominal organs such as the liver can be involved. Giant omphaloceles are more difficult to surgically correct, but they have a lesser association with aneuploidy.

Gastroschisis

This is a sporadic defect with a birth prevalence of about 1 in 4,000. Its incidence has significantly increased over the past two decades, particularly in younger gravidas. It is rarely associated with chromosomal abnormalities. Evisceration of the intestine occurs through a small abdominal wall defect, which is usually located to the right of an intact umbilical cord insertion. Early in pregnancy, it is only the loops of the intestine that protrude and lie uncovered in the amniotic fluid (Fig. 2.17). Prenatal diagnosis by ultrasound is based on the demonstration of the normally located umbilical cord insertion and the herniated loops of intestine, which are free floating.

Megacystis

The fetal bladder can be visualized by sonography in about 95% of fetuses at 11 weeks of gestation and in all cases by 13 weeks. At this point in gestation, the length of fetal bladder in a sagittal section is normally less than 7 mm. Fetal megacystis is defined being 7 mm or more in length. It is found in about 1 in 1,500 of pregnancies. This finding is associated with an increased risk for chromosomal defects, mainly trisomies 13 and 18. These are seen in approximately 30% of fetuses with megacystis (Fig. 2.18).[68,90,91] In chromosomally normal fetuses, mild to moderate megacystis, that is, 7 to 15 mm, usually resolves spontaneously and is not associated with a significant increase in long-term sequelae. However, in fetuses with bladder length of greater than 15 mm

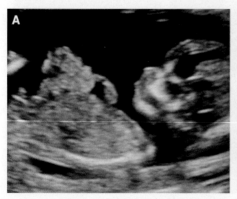
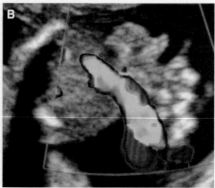

FIGURE 2.17: Sagittal **(A)** and transverse **(B)** views of the fetal abdomen at the level of the umbilicus illustrating cases of gastroschisis at 12 weeks' gestation.

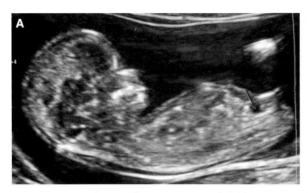 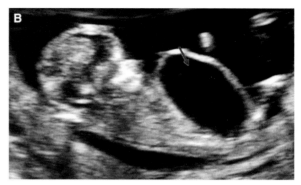

FIGURE 2.18: Midsagittal illustrating a normal bladder *(arrow)* in a fetus at 12 weeks' gestation **(A)** and one with megacystis *(arrow)* **(B)**.

(severe megacystis), there is usually progression to severe obstructive uropathy. The presence of smooth muscle in the bladder and autonomic innervation develop only after 13 weeks' gestation; prior to this point, the bladder wall consists of epithelium and connective tissue with no contractile elements. It is likely that in most cases, the etiology of mild megacystis is simply a delay in development of the muscular element rather than an underlying urethral obstruction.

Skeletal Dysplasias

In the first trimester, it is possible to identify and evaluate each of the three segments of the limbs (proximal, middle, and distal) and their movements. The diagnosis of any but the most severe types of skeletal dysplasias is difficult in the first trimester. However, a careful evaluation of the limbs can raise the suspicion of polydactyly, clenched hands, clubfoot, and severe dysplasias such as thanatophoric dysplasia, osteogenesis imperfecta, achondrogenesis, and asphyxiating thoracic dystrophy. Many skeletal dysplasias also have an association with increased NT thickness. In the cases associated with a narrow chest, the cause of increased NT may be venous congestion in the head and neck due to superior mediastinal compression. An additional or alternative mechanism for the increased NT may be altered composition of the extracellular matrix found in association with some of the skeletal dysplasias, such as osteogenesis imperfecta.

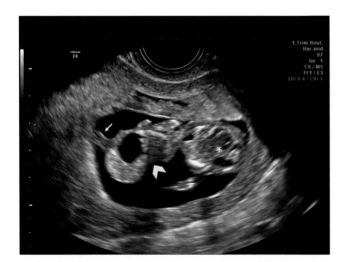

FIGURE 2.19: Fetus with a body stalk defect. *Arrow,* short umbilical cord; *asterisk,* head; *chevron,* major disruption of the chest and abdomen.

Body Stalk Anomaly

This lethal sporadic anomaly has a birth prevalence of 1 in 15,000. The ultrasound features include major abdominal wall defect, severe kyphoscoliosis, and short umbilical cord with a single artery.[92] Half of the fetal body is seen in the amniotic cavity and the other half in the celomic cavity, suggesting that early amnion rupture before obliteration of the celomic cavity is a possible cause of the syndrome (Fig. 2.19). A defect of somatic clefting is also a plausible contributing factor.[93] The fetal NT is increased in about 85% of the cases, but the karyotype is usually normal. The increase in NT thickness is most likely due to the severe limitation of fetal movement that is associated with this condition.

Cesarean Scar Pregnancy

A cesarean scar pregnancy (CSP) is the result of the embryo implanting in or near an existing cesarean scar. The total cesarean section rate in the United States has doubled since 1980 and is increasing worldwide. According to the Centers for Disease Control, of the 3,945,875 births registered in the United States in 2016, 1,258,581 were delivered by cesarean section for a total cesarean rate of 31.9%.[94] This resulted in an increase in the incidence of CSP, a condition that is associated with a number of serious complications. The true incidence of CSP is unknown; however, in the United States, the current estimates range from 1 in 1,800 to 1 in 2,500 pregnancies.[95]

The implantation process in the cesarean scar is different from that in the rest of the uterus. The cesarean scar is poorly vascularized due to scar healing and resulting fibrosis. Low oxygen tension in the region of the scar stimulates the invasiveness of the implanting cytotrophoblasts. Therefore, the placental villi tend to invade deeply into the thin residual myometrial layer (placenta accreta spectrum), which can lead to scar rupture, preterm birth, hemorrhage, and maternal death.[96] Many ongoing CSP pregnancies require peripartum hysterectomy at delivery and have significant surgical morbidities.[97]

In 2012, Timor-Tritsch compiled seven published sonographic criteria for the diagnosis of CSP.[98] All seven criteria had to be present:

1. Visualization of an empty uterine cavity and a positive pregnancy test
2. Detection of the placenta and/or a gestational sac embedded in the hysterotomy scar
3. In early gestations (<8 weeks' gestation), a triangular gestational sac that fills the niche of the scar; at greater than

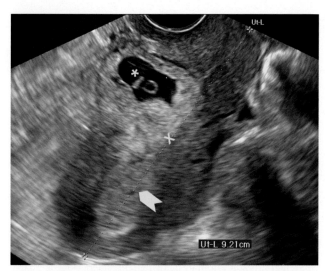

FIGURE 2.20: Cesarean scar pregnancy, which includes an embryo and a yolk sac. *Asterisk*, middle of the gestational sac; *chevron*, empty fundus; ✕, midpoint of the uterine length.

8 postmenstrual weeks this shape may become rounded or even oval.

4. A thin (1 to 3 mm) or absent myometrial layer between the gestational sac and the bladder
5. A closed and empty cervical canal
6. The presence of embryonic/fetal pole and/or yolk sac with or without heart activity
7. The presence of a prominent and at times rich vascular pattern at or in the area of a cesarean scar

The primary sonographic characteristic of CSP, which is most commonly described in published reports, is the location of the gestational sac: It is at the level of the cervico-isthmic junction, that is, in the region of the cesarean scar (Figs. 2.20 and 2.21). Early in gestation (5 to 10 weeks), an objective method of establishing its location is to look at the location of the center of

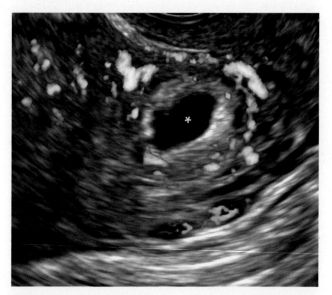

FIGURE 2.21: Magnified view of a cesarean scar pregnancy. Color Doppler demonstrates increased peripheral blood perfusion. *Asterisk*, middle of the gestational sac.

the gestational sac relative to the midpoint of the uterus along its longitudinal axis.[99] First, the length of the uterus (from the external cervical os to the top of the fundus) is established. The relative location of the center of the gestational sac to the midpoint the uterus (half of the total measured length) is then established (Fig. 2.20). Most CSPs are located between the midpoint of the uterus and the external cervical os, while most intrauterine pregnancies are located above the midpoint and closer to the uterine fundus. Using this approach as a marker of CSP early in the first trimester has a sensitivity of 93.0% and specificity of 98.9%.

There is a growing consensus that women with a history of cesarean delivery should be evaluated with transvaginal sonography in the first trimester to screen for CSP.[100] Early diagnosis of CSP allows for comprehensive counseling, including a discussion regarding the various management options. These include expectant management and interventions that interrupt the pregnancy. The latter include injecting the gestational sac with potassium chloride or methotrexate, administration of systemic methotrexate, uterine artery embolization followed by ultrasound-guided dilation and curettage (D&C), intrauterine Foley balloon placement, and hysteroscopic or laparoscopic resection.[101,102] Early diagnosis and treatment reduce the known complications of CSP such as uterine rupture and severe hemorrhage.

Women who choose expectant management require close monitoring. A meta-analysis of 17 published studies reviewed the outcome of 69 cases of CSP managed expectantly.[103] This included 52 pregnancies with and 17 without embryonic cardiac. In CSPs with embryonic cardiac activity, 13% experienced an uncomplicated miscarriage. Uterine rupture during the first or second trimester of pregnancy occurred in approximately 10% of cases. Forty of these cases continued into the third trimester. Of these women, 39% experienced severe bleeding, 60% underwent a hysterectomy at delivery, and 75% of the cases had either a surgical or pathological diagnosis of abnormally invasive placenta. In women with a CSP without embryonic cardiac activity, 69% ended in an uncomplicated miscarriage. Uterine rupture during the first trimester of pregnancy occurred in 13% of these cases. None of these pregnancies resulted in a hysterectomy.

An early diagnosis of CSP is extremely important and treatment must be individualized to the patient's desires after a detailed counseling regarding risks and benefits of various approaches.

ASSESSMENT OF RISK FOR PREGNANCY COMPLICATIONS

The current approach to prenatal care, which involves office visits at 16, 24, 28, 30, 32, 34, and 36 weeks' gestation and then weekly until delivery, was established 90 years ago.[104,105] The high concentration of visits in the third trimester implies that, firstly, most complications occur at this late stage of pregnancy and, secondly, that most major adverse outcomes are unpredictable during the first or even the second trimester.

In the past 20 years, it has become apparent that an integrated first hospital visit at 11 to 13 weeks combining data from maternal characteristics and history with findings of biophysical and biochemical tests can define the patient-specific risk for a wide spectrum of pregnancy complications, including miscarriage and stillbirth, PE, preterm birth, gestational diabetes, fetal

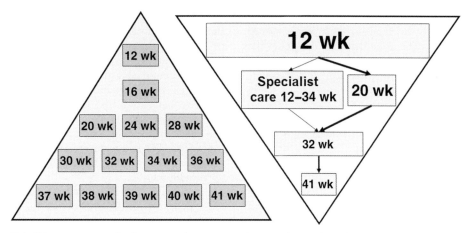

FIGURE 2.22: Pyramid of gestational ages according to the traditional model of prenatal care established in the 1920s *(left)* and according to the proposed new model of inverted pyramid *(right)*.

growth restriction, and macrosomia.[106] Early estimation of patient-specific risks for these pregnancy complications would improve pregnancy outcome by changing prenatal care from a series of routine visits to a more individualized patient- and disease-specific approach in terms of both the schedule and the content of such visits. Each visit would have a predefined objective in each patient. The intensity and type of care would be based on likelihood ratios estimated from the initial assessment at 11 to 13 weeks' gestation.

At 11 to 13 weeks, the great majority of women would be classified as being at low risk for pregnancy complications. The number of routine medical visits in the low-risk group could potentially be reduced to as few as three. After the initial first-trimester assessment, the subsequent visit at 20 to 22 weeks would include an ultrasound to reevaluate fetal anatomy and growth and reassess risk for such complications as PE and preterm delivery. Another visit during the third trimester would assess maternal and fetal well-being and determine the best time and method of delivery. The small proportion of women who constitute the high-risk group would require close surveillance in specialist clinics. This would include more frequent visits and increased number of investigations that would be supervised by clinicians who specialize in pregnancy-related complications. The risk would be reassessed during each of these visits. In some cases, the risk would potentially be lowered, and the intensity of their care could be reduced.

Future research will inevitably expand the number of conditions that can be identified in early pregnancy and define genetic markers of disease that will improve the accuracy of the *a priori* risk based on maternal characteristics and medical history. Similarly, new biophysical and biochemical markers that may replace some of the current ones and modify the value of others will be described. With the passage of time, it will become necessary to reevaluate and improve the timing and content of each visit and the likelihood ratios for each test. Early identification of high-risk groups will also stimulate further research that will define the best protocol for their follow-up and development of strategies for the prevention of disorders of pregnancy or mitigation of their adverse consequences. A new approach to prenatal care is represented in the so-called inverted pyramid of antenatal care (Fig. 2.22). This approach proposes to use the results of a comprehensive assessment at 11 to 13 weeks to change the current prenatal care paradigm on a large scale and in a systematic manner.[106]

Preterm Birth

Preterm birth is the leading cause of perinatal death and handicap in children, and the vast majority of mortality and morbidity is due to early delivery before 34 weeks. The rates of delivery at this point depend on the population, but, overall, occur in about 2% of singleton pregnancies. In two-thirds of the cases, this is due to spontaneous onset of labor or preterm premature rupture of membranes, and it is indicated in the other one-third, mainly because of PE.[107]

The patient-specific risk for spontaneous delivery before 34 weeks can be determined at 11 to 13 weeks using an algorithm, which combines maternal characteristics and obstetrical history with the sonographic measurement of cervical length using transvaginal ultrasound.[108,109] When measuring cervical length,

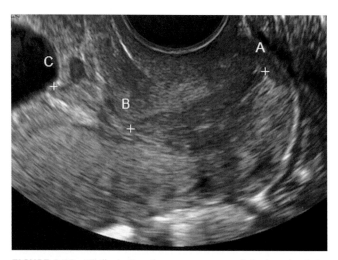

FIGURE 2.23: US illustrating the measurement of the length of the endocervix (A to B) and the isthmus (B to C).

it is important to distinguish between the true cervix and the uterine isthmus. True cervix is characterized by the presence of the endocervical canal, which is bordered by the somewhat hypoechoic endocervical mucosa (Fig. 2.23). Making this distinction is especially important in the first trimester when juxtaposition of the anterior and posterior portions of the lower uterine segments is especially common.

Effective early identification of the high-risk group for subsequent spontaneous early delivery could potentially improve outcome by directing such patients to specialist clinics for regular monitoring of cervical length, and stimulating research for identification of potentially useful biomarkers and the investigation of the potential role of earlier intervention with such measures as prophylactic use of vaginal progesterone or cervical cerclage.

Preeclampsia

PE is a major cause of maternal and perinatal morbidity and mortality. Both the degree of impaired placentation and the incidence of adverse fetal and maternal short-term and long-term sequelae are inversely related to the gestational age at onset of the disease. Consequently, in screening for PE, the condition should be subdivided according to gestational age at delivery. Traditional approach to screening for PE is to identify risk factors from maternal demographic characteristics and medical history.[110,111] More recently, algorithms that use a combination of these factors and maternal biophysical and serum markers have been developed.[112–114] All available screening algorithms

have higher DRs for PE at early gestational ages compared to those that occur at term.

The first trimester appears to be an ideal time for screening for PE for two main reasons. First, reduction of risk for PE using low-dose aspirin can be achieved only if its use is started early in pregnancy (<16 weeks' gestation). Second, it has now been shown that a first-trimester screening algorithm developed by the FMF, which combines maternal characteristics, maternal mean arterial pressure, uterine artery pulsatility index (UtA-PI), and maternal serum biochemical test (placental growth factor [PlGF]) can efficiently select patients at risk for developing PE.

A nonintervention, multicenter screening study using the FMF algorithm demonstrated that the incidence of early PE (<32 weeks' gestation), preterm PE (<37 weeks' gestation), and term PE (≥37 weeks' gestation) was 0.2%, 0.8%, and 2.1%, respectively. The FMF algorithm predicted 90% of early PE, 75% of preterm PE and 41% of term PE, at screen positive rate (SPR) of 10% (Table 2.3).[115] This compared favorably to screening using maternal characteristics and obstetrical history alone where only 53% of early PE, 45% of preterm PE, and 34% of term PE were predicted at a 10% SPR.[115] Using National Institute for Health and Care Excellence (NICE) guidelines, which are similar to the US Preventative Services Task Force (USPSTF guidelines), the SPR was 12% and the DRs for the three types of PE ranged from 32% to 46%, with the highest DR being for early PE. Implementation of current American College of Obstetricians and Gynecologists (ACOG) guidelines results in an extremely high (66%) SPR for DRs of 89% to 91%.[115]

TABLE 2.3	**Detection Rate with 95% Confidence Interval, at Screen Positive Rate of 10%, of Preeclampsia with Delivery at <32, <37 and ≥37 Weeks' Gestation in Screening by Maternal Factors, Biomarkers, and Their Combination**		
METHOD OF SCREENING	**PE < 32 wk**	**PE < 37 wk**	**PE ≥ 37 wk**
Maternal factors	52.6 (43.6–61.4)	44.8 (40.5–49.2)	33.5 (31.0–36.2)
Maternal factors plus			
MAP	61.2 (52.1–69.6)	50.5 (46.1–54.9)	38.2 (35.6–40.9)
UtA-PI	69.8 (61.0–77.4)	58.4 (54.0–62.7)	35.2 (32.6–37.8)
PAPP-A	55.2 (46.1–63.9)	48.5 (44.1–52.9)	35.2 (32.7–37.9)
PlGF	72.4 (63.7–79.3)	60.6 (56.3–64.9)	34.5 (32.0–37.2)
MAP, UtA-PI	82.8 (74.9–88.6)	68.4 (64.1–72.3)	41.4 (38.8–44.2)
MAP, PAPP-A	65.5 (56.5–73.5)	55.8 (51.4–60.1)	39.1 (36.4–41.8)
MAP, PlGF	79.3 (71.1–85.7)	66.1 (61.8–70.2)	39.3 (36.7–42.0)
UtA-PI, PAPP-A	69.8 (61.0–77.4)	59.2 (54.8–63.5)	36.3 (33.7–39.0)
UtA-PI, PlGF	81.0 (73.0–87.1)	66.9 (62.7–70.9)	36.9 (34.3–39.6)
PlGF, PAPP-A	74.1 (65.5–81.2)	63.5 (59.2–67.6)	35.7 (33.1–38.4)
MAP, UtA-PI, PAPP-A	82.8 (74.9–88.6)	68.2 (63.9–72.1)	40.6 (37.9–43.3)
MAP, PAPP-A, PlGF	81.0 (73.0–87.1)	67.3 (63.1–71.3)	39.3 (36.7–42.0)
MAP, UtA-PI, PlGF	89.7 (82.8–94.0)	74.8 (70.8–78.5)	41.0 (38.3–43.7)
UtA-PI, PAPP-A, PlGF	81.0 (73.0–87.1)	68.2 (63.9–72.1)	36.9 (34.3–39.6)
MAP, UtA-PI, PAPP-A, PlGF	89.7 (82.8–94.0)	74.8 (70.8–78.5)	41.3 (38.7–44.1)

MAP, mean arterial pressure; PAPP-A, pregnancy-associated plasma protein A; PE, preeclampsia; PlGF, placental growth factor; UtA-PI, uterine artery pulsatility index.
From Tan MY, Syngelaki A, Poon LC, et al. Screening for pre-eclampsia by maternal factors and biomarkers at 11–13 weeks' gestation. *Ultrasound Obstet Gynecol.* 2018;52(2): 186–195. doi:10.1002/uog.19112. Copyright © 2018 Crown. Ultrasound in Obstetrics & Gynecology © 2018 ISUOG. Reprinted by permission of John Wiley & Sons, Inc.

Using the FMF algorithm and a fixed risk cutoff, it has been shown that in screening for PE, the DR and SPR are influenced by the characteristics of the study population, which define the *prior* risk. Both the DR and the SPR are higher in nulliparous than in parous women and in black than in white women (Table 2.4). In all groups, the risk of being affected was increased considerably if the screen result was positive and was considerably decreased if the screen result was negative.[115] In a white population, for risk cutoff of 1 in 100 and 1 in 150 for the respective SPRs are about 10% and 16%, the DRs for early PE are 88% and 94% and DRs for preterm PE are 69% and 81% (Table 2.5). It would therefore be reasonable use a risk cutoff of 1:150 in screening for PE in a predominantly white population to use a risk cutoff of 1 in 150 to define the high-risk group. This approach increases the number of women placed on prophylactic aspirin only by 6%, but the DR of early PE increases by 12%.

The fact that prophylactic use of low-dose aspirin is associated with a reduction in preterm PE assuming that it is started early (<16 weeks' gestation) was initially demonstrated in two meta-analyses.[116,117] A more recent meta-analysis suggests that aspirin reduces the risk of preterm PE by 67%, only if the daily dose of the drug is greater than or equal to 100 mg *and* the gestational age at onset of therapy is less than or equal to 16 weeks.[118] In addition, aspirin at a daily dose of greater than or equal to 100 mg initiated at less than or equal to 16 weeks may decrease the risk of placental abruption or antepartum hemorrhage. This effect is not seen if the same dose is started after 16 weeks' gestation.[119]

The effectiveness of combining the FMF algorithm and aspirin prophylaxis in reducing the rate of preterm PE was prospectively investigated in a recently published trial (so-called ASPRE [Aspirin versus Placebo in Pregnancies at High Risk for Preterm Preeclampsia] trial). The FMF algorithm was used at 11 to 13[+6]

weeks' gestation to identify women at an increased risk (>1:100) for PE. Subjects with an increased risk were randomized into either a placebo group or a group that received 150 mg of aspirin nightly starting shortly after a positive screen until 36 weeks' gestation. A reduction in early PE with delivery at less than 32 weeks' gestation was 90% and reduction in preterm PE with delivery at less than 37 weeks' gestation was 60%. No appreciable change in term PE was noted.[120]

Secondary analyses of the ASPRE trial further delineated benefits of aspirin prophylaxis and factors that affect its efficacy. It was shown that the use of aspirin prophylaxis reduces the length of stay in the neonatal intensive unit by about 70%. This was mainly due to a decrease in the rate of births due to PE at less than 32 weeks' gestation.[121] Not surprisingly, it was also shown that improved compliance (≥90%) results in increased reduction of preterm PE (75% vs. 60% overall).[122] Finally, evaluation of aspirin effect in subgroups defined according to maternal characteristics, obstetrical history, and history of preexisting medical conditions showed no heterogeneity, with the exception of those with chronic hypertension. In this study, it appeared that aspirin prophylaxis may not be useful in this group.[123]

The FMF algorithm can be relatively easily implemented into practice. Recording maternal characteristics and medical history, measurement of blood pressure, and hospital attendance are an integral part of routine early antenatal care in most countries. Many countries also consider an ultrasound at 11 to 13[+6] weeks' gestation an integral part of prenatal evaluation. Measurement of serum PlGF and quality assurance for such measurement can be put in place. This process already exists for many other maternal serum markers. Measurement of UtA-PI can be performed at the time of a first-trimester ultrasound examination using the same ultrasound equipment. Briefly, the steps to measure

TABLE 2.4 **Performance of Screening for Preterm PE by an Algorithm Combining Maternal Factors, MAP, UtA-PI, and PlGF at a Risk Cutoff of 1 in 100**

GROUP	n	PREVALENCE n/N (%)	SCREEN +VE RATE n/N (%)	FALSE +VE RATE (%)	DETECTION RATE % (95% CI)	RISK OF BEING AFFECTED GIVEN RESULT	
						SCREEN +VE (%)[a]	SCREEN -VE (%)[b]
All pregnancies	61,174	493 (0.81)	8,970 (14.7)	8,576 (14.1)	394 (79.9, 76.2–83.2)	394/8,970 (4.4)	99/52,204 (0.2)
Nulliparous	29,075	271 (0.93)	5,579 (19.2)	3,177 (10.9)	214 (79.0, 73.7–83.4)	214/5,579 (3.8)	57/23,496 (0.2)
No previous PE	30,253	146 (0.48)	2,337 (7.7)	2,230 (7.4)	107 (73.3, 65.6–79.8)	107/2,337 (4.6)	39/27,916 (0.1)
Previous PE	1,846	76 (4.12)	1,054 (57.1)	981 (53.1)	73 (96.1, 89.0–98.7)	73/1,054 (6.9)	3/792 (0.4)
Black race	10,108	183 (1.81)	3,433 (34.0)	3,264 (32.9)	169 (92.3, 87.6–95.4)	169/3,433 (4.9)	14/6,675 (0.2)
Nulliparous	3,742	72 (1.92)	1,691 (45.2)	1,624 (43.4)	67 (93.1, 84.8–97.0)	67/1,691 (4.0)	5/2,051 (0.2)
No previous PE	5,873	75 (1.28)	1,347 (22.9)	1,281 (21.8)	66 (88.0, 78.7–93.6)	66/1,347 (4.9)	9/4,526 (0.2)
Previous PE	493	36 (7.30)	395 (80.1)	359 (72.8)	36 (100, 90.4–100)	36/395 (9.1)	0/98 (0.0)
White race	44,684	256 (0.57)	4,647 (10.4)	4,470 (10.1)	177 (69.1, 63.2–74.5)	177/4,647 (3.8)	79/40,037 (0.2)
Nulliparous	22,256	164 (0.74)	3,293 (14.8)	3,177 (14.3)	116 (70.7, 63.4–77.2)	116/3,293 (3.5)	48/18,963 (0.3)
No previous PE	21,225	63 (0.30)	782 (3.7)	748 (3.5)	34 (54.0, 41.8–65.7)	34/782 (4.3)	29/20,443 (0.1)
Previous PE	1,203	29 (2.41)	572 (47.5)	545 (45.3)	27 (93.1, 78.0–98.1)	27/572 (4.7)	2/631 (0.3)

[a]Same as positive predictive value.
[b]Same as 1−negative predictive value.
MAP, mean arterial pressure; PE, preeclampsia; PlGF, placental growth factor; UtA-PI, uterine artery pulsatility index.
From Tan MY, Syngelaki A, Poon LC, et al. Screening for pre-eclampsia by maternal factors and biomarkers at 11–13 weeks' gestation. *Ultrasound Obstet Gynecol.* 2018;52(2): 186–195. doi:10.1002/uog.19112. Copyright © 2018 Crown. Ultrasound in Obstetrics & Gynecology © 2018 ISUOG. Reprinted by permission of John Wiley & Sons, Inc.

TABLE 2.5	Performance of Screening for Early and Preterm PE by an Algorithm Combining Maternal Factors, MAP, UtA-PI, and PlGF at Different Risk Cutoffs in White and Black Women					
	WHITE RACE			**BLACK RACE**		
RISK CUTOFF	**SPR** n/44,684 (%)	**DR PE < 32 wk** n/48 (%)	**DR PE < 37 wk** n/256 (%, 95% CI)	**SPR** n/10,108 (%)	**DR PE < 32 wk** n/56 (%)	**DR PE < 37 wk** n/183 (%, 95% CI)
1 in 20	674 (1.5)	20 (41.7, 28.9–55.7)	80 (31.3, 25.9–37.2)	1,011 (10.0)	50 (89.3, 78.5–95.0)	134 (73.2, 66.4–79.1)
1 in 50	2,129 (4.8)	35 (72.9, 59.0–83.4)	143 (55.9, 49.7–61.8)	2,126 (21.0)	53 (94.6, 85.4–98.2)	155 (84.7, 78.8–89.2)
1 in 70	3,110 (7.0)	39 (81.3, 68.1–89.8)	165 (64.5, 58.4–70.1)	2,693 (26.6)	55 (98.2, 90.6–99.7)	161 (88.0, 82.5–91.9)
1 in 100	4,647 (10.4)	42 (87.5, 75.3–94.1)	177 (69.1, 63.2–74.5)	3,433 (34.0)	56 (100, 93.6–100)	169 (92.3, 87.6–95.4)
1 in 150	6,960 (15.6)	45 (93.8, 83.2–97.9)	206 (80.5, 75.2–84.9)	4,383 (43.4)	56 (100, 93.6–100)	175 (95.6, 91.6–97.8)
1 in 200	9,016 (20.2)	45 (93.8, 83.2–97.9)	213 (83.2, 78.1–87.3)	5,098 (50.4)	56 (100, 93.6–100)	180 (98.4, 95.3–99.4)
1 in 250	10,858 (24.3)	45 (93.8, 83.2–97.9)	218 (85.2, 80.3–89.0)	5,610 (55.5)	56 (100, 93.6–100)	180 (98.4, 95.3–99.4)

DR, detection rate; MAP, mean arterial pressure; PE, preeclampsia; PlGF, placental growth factor; SPR, screen positive rate; UtA-PI, uterine artery pulsatility index.
From Tan MY, Syngelaki A, Poon LC, et al. Screening for pre-eclampsia by maternal factors and biomarkers at 11–13 weeks' gestation. *Ultrasound Obstet Gynecol.* 2018;52(2): 186–195. doi:10.1002/uog.19112. Copyright © 2018 Crown. Ultrasound in Obstetrics & Gynecology © 2018 ISUOG. Reprinted by permission of John Wiley & Sons, Inc.

UtA-PI at 11 to 13^{+6} weeks' gestation are as follows. A sagittal section of the uterus is obtained, and the cervical canal and internal cervical os are identified. The transducer should be gently tilted from side to side, and color flow mapping is used to identify each uterine artery along the side of the cervix and uterus at the level of the internal os (Fig. 2.24). Pulsed wave Doppler is used with the sampling gate set at 2 mm to obtain the waveform. The angle of insonation must be less than 30°. When three similar consecutive waveforms are obtained, the UtA-PI should be measured, and the mean PI of the left and right arteries calculated. There is a need for additional training to perform the UtA-PI in a standardized manner, but this can be accomplished

online. Generally, this measurement adds only 2 to 3 minutes to the examination.

In summary, the performance of screening for PE by a combination of maternal factors, MAP, UtA-PI, and PlGF is by far superior to the traditional methods of screening based on maternal factors alone. Screening at 11 to 13^{+6} weeks' gestation identifies a group of pregnancies that would benefit from prophylactic use of aspirin. This benefit is predominantly seen in reduction of preterm PE. Screening for preterm PE should be universal rather than selective, and in countries with a predominantly White population, it would be reasonable to use a risk cutoff of 1 in 150 to define the high-risk group for treatment with aspirin. There are various levels of complexity and implications in terms of general applicability and costs for the various components of the combined test. The choice of which biomarkers should be used in a particular setting will ultimately depend not only on the basis of performance but also on the feasibility of implementation and health economic considerations.

In conclusion, the first-trimester scan has evolved recently into one of the milestones of prenatal care. As shown in this chapter, the aims of the 11 to 13^{+6} weeks scan include not only the confirmation of the viability of the pregnancy and the accurate dating of the gestation based on the CRL measurement but, especially screening for aneuploidies and complications of various pregnancies, early diagnosis of major fetal abnormalities, and the detection of multiple pregnancies with reliable identification of chorionicity. Even in the age of cfDNA testing, the versatility of this evaluation is unmatched by other methods.

REFERENCES

1. Tabor A, Alfirevic Z. Update on procedure-related risks for prenatal diagnosis techniques. *Fetal Diagn Ther.* 2010;27:1–7.
2. Nicolaides KH. Screening for fetal aneuploidies at 11 to 13 weeks. *Prenat Diagn.* 2011;31:7–15.
3. Snijders RJM, Holzgreve W, Cuckle H, et al. Maternal age-specific risks for trisomies at 9–14 weeks' gestation. *Prenat Diagn.* 1994;14:543–552.
4. Snijders RJM, Sebire NJ, Nicolaides KH. Maternal age and gestational age-specific risks for chromosomal defects. *Fetal Diagn Ther.* 1995;10:356–367.

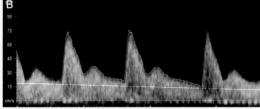

FIGURE 2.24: Parasagittal view of the cervix with color flow imaging to illustrate the uterine arteries **(A)** and characteristic waveform at 12 weeks' gestation **(B)**.

5. Kagan KO, Wright D, Valencia C, et al. Screening for trisomies 21, 18 and 13 by maternal age, fetal nuchal translucency, fetal heart rate, free beta-hCG and pregnancy-associated plasma protein-A. *Hum Reprod.* 2008;23:1968–1975.
6. Wright D, Syngelaki A, Bradbury I, et al. First trimester screening for trisomies 21, 18 and 13 by ultrasound and biochemical testing. *Fetal Diagn Ther.* 2014;35(2):118–126.
7. Syngelaki A, Pergament E, Homfray T, et al. Replacing the combined test by cell-free DNA testing in screening for trisomies 21, 18 and 13: impact on the diagnosis of other aneuploidies. *Fetal Diagn Ther.* 2014;35:174–184.
8. Kagan KO, Anderson JM, Anwandter G, et al. Screening for triploidy by the risk algorithms for trisomies 21, 18 and 13 at 11 weeks to 13 weeks and 6 days of gestation. *Prenat Diagn.* 2008;28:1209–1213.
9. Sebire NJ, Snijders RJ, Brown R, et al. Detection of sex chromosome abnormalities by nuchal translucency screening at 10–14 weeks. *Prenat Diagn.* 1998;18:581–584.
10. Spencer K, Tul N, Nicolaides KH. Maternal serum free beta-hCG and PAPP-A in fetal sex chromosome defects in the first trimester. *Prenat Diagn.* 2000;20:390–394.
11. Gil MM, Akolekar R, Quezada MS, et al. Analysis of cell-free DNA in maternal blood in screening for aneuploidies: meta-analysis. *Fetal Diagn Ther.* 2014;35:156–173.
12. Gil MM, Accurti V, Santacruz B, et al. Analysis of cellfree DNA in maternal blood in screening for aneuploidies: updated meta-analysis. *Ultrasound Obstet Gynecol.* 2017;50:302–314. doi:10.1002/uog.17484.
13. Nicolaides KH, Syngelaki A, Gil MM, et al. Prenatal detection of fetal triploidy from cell-free DNA testing in maternal blood. *Fetal Diagn Ther.* 2014;35:212–217.
14. Guex N, Iseli C, Syngelaki A, et al. A robust 2nd generation genome-wide test for fetal aneuploidy based on shotgun sequencing cell-free DNA in maternal blood. *Prenat Diagn.* 2013;33:707–710.
15. Srinivasan A, Bianchi DW, Huang H, et al. Noninvasive detection of fetal sub-chromosome abnormalities via deep sequencing of maternal plasma. *Am J Hum Genet.* 2013;92:167–176.
16. Ashoor G, Syngelaki A, Poon LCY, et al. Fetal fraction in maternal plasma cell-free DNA at 11–13 weeks' gestation: relation to maternal and fetal characteristics. *Ultrasound Obstet Gynecol.* 2013;41:26–32. doi:10.1002/uog.12331.
17. Revello R, Sarno L, Ispas A, et al. Screening for trisomies by cell-free DNA testing of maternal blood: consequences of a failed result. *Ultrasound Obstet Gynecol.* 2016;47:698–704. doi:10.1002/uog.15851.
18. ACOG. Committee Opinion No. 640: cell-free DNA screening for fetal aneuploidy. *Obstet Gynecol.* 2015;126:e31–e37. doi:10.1097/ AOG.0000000000001051.
19. Wagner P, Sonek J, Hoopmann M, et al. First-trimester screening for trisomies 18 and 13, triploidy and Turner syndrome by detailed early anomaly scan. *Ultrasound Obstet Gynecol.* 2016;48:446–451. doi:10.1002/uog.15829.
20. Grati FR, Kagan KO. Rate of no result in cell-free DNA testing and its influence on test performance metrics. *Ultrasound Obstet Gynecol.* 2017;50:134–137. doi:10.1002/uog.17330.
21. Salomon LJ, Alfirevic Z, Audibert F, et al. ISUOG updated consensus statement on the impact of cfDNA aneuploidy testing on screening policies and prenatal ultrasound practice. *Ultrasound Obstet Gynecol.* 2017;49:815–816. doi:10.1002/uog.17483.
22. Nicolaides KH, Azar G, Byrne D, et al. Fetal nuchal translucency: ultrasound screening for chromosomal defects in first trimester of pregnancy. *BMJ.* 1992;304:867–889.
23. Molina FS, Avgidou K, Kagan KO, et al. Cystic hygromas, nuchal edema, and nuchal translucency at 11–14 weeks of gestation. *Obstet Gynecol.* 2006;107:678–683.
24. Snijders RJ, Noble P, Sebire N, et al; Fetal Medicine Foundation First Trimester Screening Group. UK multicentre project on assessment of risk of trisomy 21 by maternal age and fetal nuchal-translucency thickness at 10–14 weeks of gestation. *Lancet.* 1998;352:343–346.
25. Wald NJ, Rodeck C, Hackshaw AK, et al; SURUSS Research Group. First and second trimester antenatal screening for Down's syndrome: the results of the Serum, Urine and Ultrasound Screening Study (SURUSS). *Health Technol Assess.* 2003;7:1–88.
26. Malone FD, Canick JA, Ball RH, et al; for the First- and Second-Trimester Evaluation of Risk (FASTER) Research Consortium. First-trimester or second-trimester screening, or both, for Down's syndrome. *N Engl J Med.* 2005;353:2001–2011.
27. Souka AP, Snidjers RJM, Novakov A, et al. Defects and syndromes in chromosomally normal fetuses with increased nuchal translucency thickness at 10–14 weeks of gestation. *Ultrasound Obstet Gynecol.* 1998;11:391–400.
28. Souka AP, Von Kaisenberg CS, Hyett JA, et al. Increased nuchal translucency with normal karyotype. *Am J Obstet Gynecol.* 2005;192:1005–1021.
29. Hyett J, Perdu M, Sharland G, et al. Using fetal nuchal translucency to screen for major congenital cardiac defects at 10–14 weeks of gestation: population based cohort study. *BMJ.* 1999;318:81–85.
30. Hyett J, Moscoso G, Papapanagiotou G, et al. Abnormalities of the heart and great arteries in chromosomally normal fetuses with increased nuchal translucency thickness at 11–13 weeks of gestation. *Ultrasound Obstet Gynecol.* 1996;7:245–250.
31. Atzei A, Gajewska K, Huggon IC, et al. Relationship between nuchal translucency thickness and prevalence of major cardiac defects in fetuses with normal karyotype. *Ultrasound Obstet Gynecol.* 2005;26:154–157.
32. Cicero S, Curcio P, Papageorghiou A, et al. Absence of nasal bone in fetuses with trisomy 21 at 11–14 weeks of gestation: an observational study. *Lancet.* 2001;358:1665–1667.
33. Cicero S, Avgidou K, Rembouskos G, et al. Nasal bone in first-trimester screening for trisomy 21. *Am J Obstet Gynecol.* 2006;195:109–114.
34. Kagan KO, Cicero S, Staboulidou I, et al. Fetal nasal bone in screening for trisomies 21, 18 and 13 and Turner syndrome at 11–13 weeks of gestation. *Ultrasound Obstet Gynecol.* 2009;33:259–264.
35. Matias A, Gomes C, Flack N, et al. Screening for chromosomal abnormalities at 10–14 weeks: the role of ductus venosus blood flow. *Ultrasound Obstet Gynecol.* 1998;12:380–384.
36. Maiz N, Valencia C, Kagan KO, et al. Ductus venosus Doppler in screening for trisomies 21, 18 and 13 and Turner syndrome at 11–13 weeks of gestation. *Ultrasound Obstet Gynecol.* 2009;33:512–517.
37. Huggon IC, DeFigueiredo DB, Allan LD. Tricuspid regurgitation in the diagnosis of chromosomal anomalies in the fetus at 11–14 weeks of gestation. *Heart.* 2003;89:1071–1073.
38. Faiola S, Tsoi E, Huggon IC, et al. Likelihood ratio for trisomy 21 in fetuses with tricuspid regurgitation at the 11 to 13 +6-week scan. *Ultrasound Obstet Gynecol.* 2005;26:22–27.
39. Kagan KO, Valencia C, Livanos P, et al. Tricuspid regurgitation in screening for trisomies 21, 18 and 13 and Turner syndrome at 11+0 to 13+6 weeks of gestation. *Ultrasound Obstet Gynecol.* 2009;33:18–22.
40. Bilardo CM, Timmerman E, Robles de Medina PG, et al. Low-resistance hepatic artery flow in first trimester fetuses: an ominous sign. *Ultrasound Obstet Gynecol.* 2011;37(4):438–443. doi:10.1002/uog.7766.
41. Zvanca M, Gielchinsky Y, Abdeljawad F, et al. Hepatic artery Doppler in trisomy 21 and euploid fetuses at 11–13 weeks. *Prenat Diagn.* 2011;31:22–27.
42. Maiz N, Nicolaides KH. Ductus venosus in the first trimester: contribution to screening of chromosomal, cardiac defects and monochorionic twin complications. *Fetal Diagn Ther.* 2010;28:65–71.
43. Matias A, Huggon I, Areias JC, et al. Cardiac defects in chromosomally normal fetuses with abnormal ductus venosus blood flow at 10–14 weeks. *Ultrasound Obstet Gynecol.* 1999;14:307–310.
44. Maiz N, Kagan KO, Milovanovic Z, et al. Learning curve for Doppler assessment of ductus venosus flow at 11+0 to 13+6 weeks. *Ultrasound Obstet Gynecol.* 2008;31:503–506.
45. Maiz N, Valencia C, Emmanuel EE, et al. Screening for adverse pregnancy outcome by ductus venosus Doppler at 11–13+6 weeks of gestation. *Obstet Gynecol.* 2008;112:598–605.
46. Borrell A, Borobio V, Bestwick JP, et al. Ductus venosus pulsatility index as an antenatal screening marker for Down's syndrome: use with the Combined and Integrated tests. *J Med Screen.* 2009;16:112–118.
47. Maiz N, Wright D, Ferreira AF, et al. A mixture model of ductus venosus pulsatility index in screening for aneuploidies at 11–13 weeks' gestation. *Fetal Diagn Ther.* 2012;31:221–229.
48. ISUOG Practice Guidelines: performance of first-trimester fetal ultrasound scan. *Ultrasound Obstet Gynecol.* 2013;41:102–113. doi:10.1002/uog.12342.
49. Falcon O, Faiola S, Huggon I, et al. Fetal tricuspid regurgitation at the 11+0 to 13+6-week scan: association with chromosomal defects and reproducibility of the method. *Ultrasound Obstet Gynecol.* 2006;27:609–612.
50. Nicolaides KH, Spencer K, Avgidou K, et al. Multicenter study of first-trimester screening for trisomy 21 in 75 821 pregnancies: results and estimation of the potential impact of individual risk-orientated two-stage first-trimester screening. *Ultrasound Obstet Gynecol.* 2005;25:221–226.
51. Sepulveda W, Sebire NJ, Hughes K, et al. The lambda sign at 10–14 weeks of gestation as a predictor of chorionicity in twin pregnancies. *Ultrasound Obstet Gynecol.* 1996;7:421–423.
52. Sebire NJ, Snijders RJ, Hughes K, et al. Screening for trisomy 21 in twin pregnancies by maternal age and fetal nuchal translucency thickness at 10–14 weeks of gestation. *Br J Obstet Gynaecol.* 1996;103:999–1003.
53. Vandecruys H, Faiola S, Auer M, et al. Screening for trisomy 21 in monochorionic twins by measurement of fetal nuchal translucency thickness. *Ultrasound Obstet Gynecol.* 2005;25:551–553.
54. Spencer K, Nicolaides KH. First trimester prenatal diagnosis of trisomy 21 in discordant twins using fetal nuchal translucency thickness and maternal serum free beta-hCG and PAPP-A. *Prenat Diagn.* 2000;20:683–684.
55. Spencer K, Nicolaides KH. Screening for trisomy 21 in twins using first trimester ultrasound and maternal serum biochemistry in a one-stop clinic: a review of three years' experience. *BJOG.* 2003;110:276–280.
56. Madsen H, Ball S, Wright D, et al. A re-assessment of biochemical marker distributions in T21 affected and unaffected twin pregnancies in the first trimester. *Ultrasound Obstet Gynecol.* 2011;37:38–47.
57. Nicolaides KH, Syngelaki A, Poon LC, et al. First-trimester contingent screening for trisomies 21, 18 and 13 by biomarkers and maternal blood cell-free DNA testing. *Fetal Diagn Ther.* 2014;35:185–192.
58. Everett TR, Chitty LS. Cell-free fetal DNA: the new tool in fetal medicine. *Ultrasound Obstet Gynecol.* 2015;45:499–507. doi:10.1002/uog.14746.
59. Wapner RJ, Babiarz JE, Levy B, et al. Expanding the scope of noninvasive prenatal testing: detection of fetal microdeletion syndromes. *Am J Obstet Gynecol.* 2015;212(3):332.e1–e9. doi:10.1016/j. ajog.2014.11.041.

60. Gammon BL, Kraft SA, Michie M, et al. "I think we've got too many tests!": prenatal providers' reflections on ethical and clinical challenges in the practice integration of cell-free DNA screening. *Ethics Med Public Health.* 2016;2:334–342. doi:10.1016/j.jemep.2016.07.006.

61. Grati FR, Molina Gomes D, Ferreira JCPB, et al. Prevalence of recurrent pathogenic microdeletions and microduplications in over 9500 pregnancies. *Prenat Diagn.* 2015;35:801–809. doi:10.1002/pd.4613.

62. Dugoff L, Mennuti MT, McDonald McGinn DM. The benefits and limitations of cell-free DNA screening for 22q11.2 deletion syndrome. *Prenat Diagn.* 2017;37:53–60. doi:10.1002/pd.4864.

63. AIUM-ACR-ACOG-SMFM-SRU Practice parameter for the performance of standard diagnostic obstetric ultrasound examinations. *J Ultrasound Med.* 2018;37:E13–E24.

64. Syngelaki A, Chelemen T, Dagklis T, et al. Challenges in the diagnosis of fetal non-chromosomal abnormalities at 11–13 weeks. *Prenat Diagn.* 2011;31:90–102.

65. Saltvedt S, Almström H, Kublickas M, et al. Detection of malformations in chromosomally normal fetuses by routine ultrasound at 12 or 18 weeks of gestation—a randomised controlled trial in 39,572 pregnancies. *BJOG.* 2006;113:664–674.

66. Johnson SP, Sebire NJ, Snijders RJM, et al. Ultrasound screening for anencephaly at 10–14 weeks of gestation. *Ultrasound Obstet Gynecol.* 1997;9:14–16.

67. Sepulveda W, Dezerega V, Be C. First-trimester sonographic diagnosis of holoprosencephaly: value of the "butterfly" sign. *J Ultrasound Med.* 2004;23: 761–765.

68. Kagan KO, Staboulidou I, Syngelaki A, et al. The 11–13-week scan: diagnosis and outcome of holoprosencephaly, exomphalos and megacystis. *Ultrasound Obstet Gynecol.* 2010;36:10–14.

69. Maarse W, Rozendaal AM, Pajkrt E, et al. A systematic review of associated structural and chromosomal defects in oral clefts: when is prenatal genetic analysis indicated? *J Med Genet.* 2012;49:490–498. doi:10.1136/jmedgenet-2012-101013.

70. Sepulveda W, Wong AE, Martinez-Ten P, et al. Retronasal triangle: a sonographic landmark for the screening of cleft palate in the first trimester. *Ultrasound Obstet Gynecol.* 2010;35:7–13. doi:10.1002/uog.7484.

71. Chaoui R, Orosz G, Heling KS, et al. Maxillary gap at 11–13 weeks' gestation: marker of cleft lip and palate. *Ultrasound Obstet Gynecol.* 2015;46:665–669. doi:10.1002/uog.15675.

72. Hoopmann M, Sonek J, Esser T, et al. Frontal space distance in facial clefts and retrognathia at 11–13 weeks' gestation. *Ultrasound Obstet Gynecol.* 2016; 48:171–176.

73. Nicolaides KH, Campbell S, Gabbe SG, et al. Ultrasound screening for spina bifida: cranial and cerebellar signs. *Lancet.* 1986;2:72–74.

74. Chaoui R, Benoit B, Mitkowska-Wozniak H, et al. Assessment of intracranial translucency (IT) in the detection of spina bifida at the 11–13-week scan. *Ultrasound Obstet Gynecol.* 2009;34:249–252.

75. Lachmann R, Chaoui R, Moratalla J, et al. Posterior brain in fetuses with spina bifida at 11–13 weeks. *Prenat Diagn.* 2011;31:103–106.

76. Office for National Statistics. *Mortality Statistics, Childhood, Infancy and Perinatal.* Newport, England: Office for National Statistics; 2007. Series DH3, 40.

77. Bull C. Current and potential impact of fetal diagnosis on prevalence and spectrum of serious congenital heart disease at term in the UK. *Lancet.* 1999;35:1242–1247.

78. Bricker L, Garcia J, Henderson J, et al. Ultrasound screening in pregnancy: a systematic review of the clinical effectiveness, cost-effectiveness and women's views. *Health Technol Assess.* 2000;4:1–193.

79. Tegnander E, Williams W, Johansen OJ, et al. Prenatal detection of heart defects in a non-selected population of 30,149 fetuses-detection rates and outcome. *Ultrasound Obstet Gynecol.* 2006;27:252–265.

80. Allan LD. Echocardiographic detection of congenital heart disease in the fetus: present and future. *Br Heart J.* 1995;74:103–106.

81. Maiz N, Plasencia W, Dagklis T, et al. Ductus venosus Doppler in fetuses with cardiac defects and increased nuchal translucency thickness. *Ultrasound Obstet Gynecol.* 2008;31:256–260.

82. Martinez JM, Comas M, Borrell A, et al. Abnormal first-trimester ductus venosus blood flow: a marker of cardiac defects in fetuses with normal karyotype and nuchal translucency. *Ultrasound Obstet Gynecol.* 2010;35:267–272.

83. Chelemen T, Syngelaki A, Maiz M, et al. Contribution of ductus venosus Doppler in first trimester screening for major cardiac defects. *Fetal Diagn Ther.* 2011;29:127–134.

84. Pereira S, Ganapathy R, Syngelaki A, et al. Contribution of fetal tricuspid regurgitation in first trimester screening for major cardiac defects. *Obstet Gynecol.* 2011;117:1384–1391.

85. Timmerman E, Clur SA, Pajkrt E, et al. First-trimester measurement of the ductus venosus pulsatility index and the prediction of congenital heart defects. *Ultrasound Obstet Gynecol.* 2010;36(6):668–675.

86. Borrell A, Grande M, Bennasar M, et al. First-trimester detection of major cardiac defects with the use of ductus venosus blood flow. *Ultrasound Obstet Gynecol.* 2013;42(1):51–57.

87. Persico N, Moratalla J, Lombardi CM, et al. Fetal echocardiography at 11–13 weeks by transabdominal high frequency ultrasound. *Ultrasound Obstet Gynecol.* 2011;37:296–301.

88. Rasiah SV, Publicover M, Ewer AK, et al. A systematic review of the accuracy of first-trimester ultrasound examination for detecting major congenital heart disease. *Ultrasound Obstet Gynecol.* 2006;28:110–116.

89. Sebire NJ, Snijders RJM, Davenport M, et al. Fetal nuchal translucency thickness at 10–14 weeks of gestation and congenital diaphragmatic hernia. *Obstet Gynecol.* 1997;90:943–947.

90. Sebire NJ, von Kaisenberg C, Rubio C, et al. Fetal megacystis at 10–14 weeks of gestation. *Ultrasound Obstet Gynecol.* 1996;8:387–390.

91. Liao AW, Sebire NJ, Geerts L, et al. Megacystis at 10–14 weeks of gestation: chromosomal defects and outcome according to bladder length. *Ultrasound Obstet Gynecol.* 2003;21:338–341.

92. Daskalakis G, Sebire NJ, Jurkovic D, et al. Body stalk anomaly at 10–14 weeks of gestation. *Ultrasound Obstet Gynecol.* 1997;10:416–418.

93. Paul C, Zosmer N, Jurkovic D, et al. A case of body stalk anomaly at 10 weeks of gestation. *Ultrasound Obstet Gynecol.* 2001;17:157–159.

94. Martin JA, Hamilton BE, Osterman MJK, et al. Births: final data for 2016. *Natl Vital Stat Rep.* 2018;67(1):1–55.

95. Timor-Tritsch IE, Monteagudo A, Bennett TA, et al. A new minimally invasive treatment for cesarean scar pregnancy and cervical pregnancy. *Am J Obstet Gynecol.* 2016;215(3):351.e1–e8.

96. Timor-Tritsch IE, Khatib N, Monteagudo A, et al. Cesarean scar pregnancies: experience of 60 cases. *J Ultrasound Med.* 2015;34(4):601–610.

97. Timor-Tritsch IE, Monteagudo A, Cali G, et al. Cesarean scar pregnancy and early placenta accreta share common histology. *Ultrasound Obstet Gynecol.* 2014;43(4):383–395.

98. Timor-Tritsch IE, Monteagudo A, Santos R, et al. The diagnosis, treatment, and follow-up of cesarean scar pregnancy. *Am J Obstet Gynecol.* 2012;207(1):44. e1–e13.

99. Timor-Tritsch IE, Monteagudo A, Cali G, et al. Easy sonographic differential diagnosis between intrauterine pregnancy and cesarean delivery scar pregnancy in the early first trimester. *Am J Obstet Gynecol.* 2016;215(2):225.e1–e7.

100. Timor-Tritsch IE, D'Antonio F, Cali G, et al. Early first trimester transvaginal ultrasound is indicated in pregnancies after a previous cesarean delivery: should it be mandatory? *Ultrasound Obstet Gynecol.* 2019;54:156–163. doi:10.1002/uog.20225.

101. Michaels AY, Washburn EE, Pocius KD, et al. Outcome of cesarean scar pregnancies diagnosed sonographically in the first trimester. *J Ultrasound Med.* 2015;34(4):595–599.

102. Timor-Tritsch IE, Cali G, Monteagudo A, et al. Foley balloon catheter to prevent or manage bleeding during treatment for cervical and Cesarean scar pregnancy. *Ultrasound Obstet Gynecol.* 2015;46(1):118–123.

103. Calì G, Timor-Tritsch IE, Palacios-Jaraquemada J, et al. Outcome of Cesarean scar pregnancy managed expectantly: systematic review and meta-analysis. *Ultrasound Obstet Gynecol.* 2018;51(2):169–175.

104. Ballantyne JW. A plea for a pro-maternity hospital. *Br Med J.* 1901;1(2101): 813–814.

105. Ministry of Health Report. *1929 Memorandum on Antenatal Clinics: Their Conduct and Scope.* London, England: His Majesty's Stationery Office; 1930.

106. Nicolaides KH. Turning the pyramid of prenatal care. *Fetal Diagn Ther.* 2011;29:183–196.

107. Celik E, To M, Gajewska K, et al; for the Fetal Medicine Foundation Second Trimester Screening Group. Cervical length and obstetric history predict spontaneous preterm birth: development and validation of a model to provide individualized risk assessment. *Ultrasound Obstet Gynecol.* 2008;31:549–554.

108. Beta J, Ventura W, Akolekar R, et al. Prediction of spontaneous preterm delivery from maternal factors and placental perfusion and function at 11–13 weeks. *Prenat Diagn.* 2011;31:75–83.

109. Greco E, Lange A, Ushakov F, et al. Prediction of spontaneous preterm delivery from endocervical length at 11–13 weeks. *Prenat Diagn.* 2011;31:84–89.

110. National Collaborating Centre for Women's and Children's Health. *Hypertension in Pregnancy: The Management of Hypertensive Disorders During Pregnancy.* London, England: RCOG Press, 2010.

111. Committee opinion No. 638: First-trimester risk assessment for early-onset preeclampsia. *Obstet Gynecol.* 2015;126:e25–e27.

112. Akolekar R, Syngelaki A, Sarquis R, et al. Prediction of preeclampsia from biophysical and biochemical markers at 11–13 weeks. *Prenat Diagn.* 2011;31: 66–74.

113. Akolekar R, Syngelaki A, Poon L, et al. Competing risks model in early screening for preeclampsia by biophysical and biochemical markers. *Fetal Diagn Ther.* 2013;33:8–15.

114. Wright D, Syngelaki A, Akolekar R, et al. Competing risks model in screening for preeclampsia by maternal characteristics and medical history. *Am J Obstet Gynecol.* 2015;213:62.e1–e10.

115. Tan MY, Syngelaki A, Poon LC, et al. Screening for pre-eclampsia by maternal factors and biomarkers at 11-13 weeks' gestation. *Ultrasound Obstet Gynecol.* 2018;52:186–195. doi:10.1002/uog.19112.

116. Bujold E, Roberge S, Lacasse Y, et al. Prevention of preeclampsia and intrauterine growth restriction with aspirin started in early pregnancy: a meta-analysis. *Obstet Gynecol.* 2010;116:402–414.

117. Roberge S, Villa P, Nicolaides K, et al. Early administration of low dose aspirin for the prevention of preterm and term pre-eclampsia: a systematic review and meta-analysis. *Fetal Diagn Ther.* 2012;31:141–146.
118. Roberge S, Bujold E, Nicolaides KH. Aspirin for the prevention of preterm and term preeclampsia: systematic review and meta-analysis. *Am J Obstet Gynecol.* 2018;218:287–293.e1.
119. Roberge S, Bujold E, Nicolaides KH. Meta-analysis on the effect of aspirin use for prevention of preeclampsia on placental abruption and antepartum hemorrhage. *Am J Obstet Gynecol.* 2018;218:483–489.
120. Rolnik DL, Wright D, Poon LC, et al. Aspirin versus placebo in pregnancies at high risk for preterm preeclampsia. *N Engl J Med.* 2017;377:613–622.
121. Wright D, Rolnik DL, Syngelaki A, et al. Aspirin for evidence-based preeclampsia prevention trial: effect of aspirin on length of stay in the neonatal intensive care unit. *Am J Obstet Gynecol.* 2018;218:612.e1–e6.
122. Wright D, Poon LC, Rolnik DL, et al. Aspirin for evidence-based preeclampsia prevention trial: influence of compliance on beneficial effect of aspirin in prevention of preterm preeclampsia. *Am J Obstet Gynecol.* 2017;217:685.e1–e5.
123. Poon LC, Wright D, Rolnik DL, et al. Aspirin for evidence-based preeclampsia prevention trial: effect of aspirin in prevention of preterm preeclampsia in subgroups of women according to their characteristics and medical and obstetrical history. *Am J Obstet Gynecol.* 2017;217:585.e1–e5.

3 Normal Fetal Ultrasound Survey

Jiri D. Sonek • Adam K. Hiett • Jon Hyett

Prenatal ultrasound represents one of the most important advances in modern obstetrics. Prior to the advent of this technology, the contents of the uterus were essentially a black box. Ultrasound has evolved significantly since Donald et al. first demonstrated its potential value. It provides an effective means of evaluating the fetus from both a structural and a functional perspective. As a consequence, obstetrics has evolved from a discipline that deals almost exclusively with maternal health concerns to one that also focuses on the health and development of the fetus.[1,2]

A complete obstetric ultrasound includes evaluation of the uterus, the adnexa, and the intrauterine contents.[3–7] In this chapter, we focus on examination of the fetus. Examinations of the umbilical cord, placenta, and amniotic fluid are discussed in Chapter 13.1, and assessment of the uterine cervix is discussed in Chapter 14.

The obstetric ultrasound is a comprehensive exam with different components of the exam emphasized at various stages of fetal development. While examination at 8 weeks' gestation is not currently considered the optimal gestational age for fetal ultrasound assessment, it does provide an opportunity to assess viability and intrauterine location of the pregnancy, to reliably determine chorionicity in the case of a multiple gestation, and to date the pregnancy with a great degree of accuracy. The 12-week scan is a relatively recent addition, but is now accepted as a point for routine assessment and is rapidly gaining recognition as one of the most important points for fetal evaluation. Most fetal chromosomal and severe structural abnormalities can be detected even at this early stage of development. Recognition of a problem at this point in pregnancy allows the parents ample time for counseling with a wide range of options regarding termination or continuation of pregnancy.[8–12] More recently, the 12-week scan has also been shown to be valuable in the prediction of obstetric complications such as preeclampsia and growth restriction, allowing obstetricians to take preventive action at a point early in gestation, potentially reducing the risk of adverse pregnancy outcome.[13] Discussion regarding utility of ultrasound evaluation at this point in pregnancy, including up-to-date references, is detailed in Chapter 2.

For many years, the 20-week scan has been the cornerstone of obstetric imaging. Systematic examination at this stage identifies a high proportion of major structural anomalies. At this gestation, the fetus is already relatively large, and the formation of major fetal structures except for the brain has been completed. Therefore, more anomalies can be detected at this point than at 12 weeks, and those that are suspected at an earlier gestational age can now be confirmed and better defined. Still, some important abnormalities such as neuronal migration defects will remain undetectable until the late third trimester or until after birth. Finally, most data regarding the value of cervical assessment also pertain to the 20-week gestational age window.

Even though a complete structural survey can be performed at ≥28 weeks' gestation, scans at this stage are limited by bone shadowing from the calvarium, ribs, spine, and limbs. However, investigation at this point in gestation provides invaluable information regarding fetal well-being and placental function. In addition to the evaluation of fetal growth and amniotic fluid volume, Doppler ultrasound can be employed to evaluate placental and fetal hemodynamics, and to look for changes indicative of placental insufficiency and fetal hypoxia. This information is helpful in determining timing and mode of delivery of growth-restricted fetuses as well as whether antepartum fetal testing is appropriate. This approach is also useful in identifying late onset growth restriction and the failing placenta at term.[14–23]

Obstetric ultrasound has its limitations, a fact that both clinicians and patients need to recognize. Anomalies may be missed for a variety of reasons. In early pregnancy, structures may be too small for examination, the embryological development process may be incomplete, or secondary pathological change may have not yet occurred. As noted earlier, development of some structures, such as the central nervous system, continues throughout the pregnancy and even into infancy; therefore, anomalies may not be evident at the time of a routine 20-week ultrasound examination. Other important abnormalities, such as autism, are functional rather than structural and therefore cannot be detected by ultrasound.[24]

The exact prognosis associated with a particular anomaly finding might be unclear. For example, with certain ultrasound findings most fetuses might have a normal outcome, yet a small proportion may be severely incapacitated. Clinicians who report ultrasound findings have to be able to define risks as clearly as possible, recognize the inherent uncertainties, and have the skill to communicate them effectively to the patient.[25]

The quality of the ultrasound image may be affected by a number of maternal and fetal factors, including maternal obesity and fetal position. Increased maternal body mass index (BMI) has become a notable impediment to the performance of obstetric ultrasound. Ultrasound does not penetrate adipose tissue well, leading to decreased image quality and prolonged examination time. The increased study length and physical stress is a major health issue for sonographers.[26,27] Nonetheless, it also needs to be kept in mind that increased maternal BMI is associated with an increased risk of a number of fetal anomalies such as neural tube defects, cardiac defects, and facial clefts.[28] It therefore becomes important to attempt to maximize the diagnostic potential of the ultrasound examination, while minimizing risks to staff. This can be accomplished by defining a maximum time limit for an exam and termination of an exam at a point where it is determined that optimal images are not obtainable. Difficulties relating to fetal position are relatively easier to deal with by alteration of the angle of insonation, manipulation of the fetus, combined transabdominal and transvaginal imaging, or simply waiting until the fetus spontaneously changes its position. Despite these difficulties, we need to remember that image interpretation is fundamentally dependent on image quality, and sonographers

TABLE 3.1 Summary of Recommendations for Diagnostic Ultrasound Parameters and Indices

In the low-megahertz frequency range, there have been no independently confirmed adverse biological effects in mammalian tissues exposed *in vivo* under experimental ultrasound conditions, as follows:

1. Thermal mechanisms
   a. No effects have been observed for an unfocused beam having free-field spatial-peak temporal-average (SPTA) intensities[a] below 100 mW/cm², or a focused[b] beam having intensities below 1 W/cm², or thermal index values of <2.
   b. For fetal exposures, no effects have been reported for a temperature increase above the normal physiological temperature, ΔT, when $\Delta T < 4.5 - (\log_{10} t/0.6)$, where t is exposure time ranging from 1 to 250 min, including off time for pulsed exposure.[30]
   c. For postnatal exposures producing temperature increases of 6°C or less, no effects have been reported when $\Delta T < 6 - (\log_{10} t/0.6)$, including off time for pulsed exposure. For example, for temperature increases of 6.0°C and 2.0°C, the corresponding limits for the exposure durations t are 1 and 250 min.[31]
   d. For postnatal exposures producing temperature increases of 6°C or more, no effects have been reported when $\Delta T < 6 - (\log_{10} t/0.3)$, including off time for pulsed exposure. For example, for a temperature increase of 9.6°C, the corresponding limit for the exposure duration is 5 s (=0.083 min).[31]
2. Nonthermal mechanisms
   a. In tissues that contain well-defined gas bodies, e.g., lung, no effects have been observed for in situ peak rarefactional pressures below approximately 0.4 MPa or mechanical index values approximately <0.4.
   b. In tissues that do not contain well-defined gas bodies, no effects have been reported for peak rarefactional pressures below approximately 4.0 MPa or mechanical index values approximately <4.0.[29]

[a]Free-field SPTA intensity for continuous wave and pulsed exposures.
[b]Quarter-power (−6 dB) beam width smaller than four wavelengths or 4 mm, whichever is less at the exposure frequency.
Modified from American Institute of Ultrasound in Medicine. AIUM Statement on Mammalian *In Vivo* Ultrasonic Biological Effects. http://www.aium.org/. With permission. Accessed November 8, 2008.

should be encouraged to be single-minded in their pursuit of excellence.

Sound waves transmit energy, which has the potential to heat and disrupt tissue.[29–44] While diagnostic grayscale imaging delivers a low amount of energy, other forms of ultrasound such as pulse wave and color Doppler ultrasound focus higher levels of energy on small areas of tissue. The limited data available suggest that the application of diagnostic ultrasound to human pregnancy is safe and that the value of the information gained through examination easily outweighs any risk to the fetus. All ultrasound machines report power output as the thermal index (TI), a measure of the potential increase in temperature that ultrasound causes in tissue, and the mechanical index (MI), a measure of the potential for tissue cavitation (Table 3.1).[29–32] Ultrasound technology should always be applied according to the "as low as reasonably achievable" (ALARA) principle, which states that one should perform the shortest exam with the lowest amount of ultrasound energy required to successfully complete a diagnostic examination. The Bioeffects Committee of the American Institute of Ultrasound in Medicine, comprising 35 experts in various fields pertaining to ultrasound safety, has defined acceptable limits for diagnostic investigation. Selected safety recommendations are included in Table 3.2.[33,34]

Effective prenatal diagnosis relies on a high standard of imaging. Several national and international bodies have described standards for imaging in the first, second, and third trimester of pregnancy. These include organizations such as the American College of Obstetricians and Gynecologists (ACOG), American Institute of Ultrasound in Medicine (AIUM), Australasian Society of Ultrasound in Medicine (ASUM), National Health Service (NHS) in the United Kingdom, and the International Society of Ultrasound in Obstetrics and Gynecology (ISUOG)

(Table 3.3).[3–7] Guidelines typically describe the essential components of an obstetric ultrasound examination. However, many experts in the field advocate the use of additional views to improve diagnostic performance. In the United States, Current Procedural Terminology (CPT) codes are used to determine the

TABLE 3.2 Selected Safety Recommendations for Diagnostic Ultrasound

- Ultrasound exposures that elevate fetal temperature by 4°C above normal for 5 min or more have the potential to induce severe developmental defects
- Apply the ALARA principle if the tissues to be exposed contain stabilized gas bodies (lung) and the MI exceeds 0.4
- There is no epidemiological support for a causal relationship between diagnostic ultrasound during pregnancy and adverse biological effects to the fetus observed for outputs under a spatial-peak temporal-average intensity of 94 mW/cm²
- The temperature of the fetus should not safely rise more than 0.5°C above its normal temperature
- When MI is above 0.5 or the TI is above 1.0, the NCRP recommends that the risks of ultrasound be weighed against the benefits

ALARA, as low as reasonably achievable; MI, mechanical index; NCRP, National Council on Radiation Protection and Measurements.
From Fowlkes JB, Bioeffects Committee of the American Institute of Ultrasound in Medicine. American Institute of Ultrasound in Medicine consensus report on potential bioeffects of diagnostic ultrasound. *J Ultrasound Med*. 2008;27(4):503–515. National Council on Radiation Protection and Measurements. Exposure Criteria for Medical Ultrasound, II: Criteria Based on All Known Mechanisms. Bethesda, MD: National Council on Radiation Protection and Measurements; 2002. NRCP report 140.

TABLE 3.3	Summary of Recommendations Regarding Evaluation of Fetal Anatomy on Prenatal Ultrasound			
	ISUOG	**AIUM AND ACOG**	**ASUM**	**NHS (UK)**
Head and Neck				
Skull bones, calvarium	X		X	X (shape)
Biparietal diameter (measure)	X	X	X	
Head circumference (measure)	X	X	X	X
Nuchal fold	X	X (measure if increased age)	X	X (measure if increased)
Brain				
Cavum septum pellucidum	X	X	X	X
Cerebral ventricles, choroid plexus	X	X	X	X (measure)
Cerebellum	X	X	X	X (measure)
Cisterna magna	X	X	X	
Midline falx	X	X	X	
Face				
Orbits	X		X	
Nose	X (if tech feas)		X	
Lips	X (upper)	X (upper)	X	X (coronal)
Mouth	X			
Jaw			X	
Profile	X (if tech feas)		X	
Chest				
Heart				
Cardiac activity	X	X	X	
Four-chamber view	X	X	X	X
Outflow tracts	X (if tech feas)	X (if tech feas)	X	X
Lungs	X			X
Diaphragm	X		X (right/left)	
Abdomen and Pelvis				
Stomach	X (presence, situs)	X (presence, size, situs)	X (presence, situs)	X
Abdominal wall			X	X
Abdominal circumference (measure)	X	X	X	X
Umbilical cord insertion	X	X	X	
Umbilical cord vessel number	X	X	X	
Bowel	X			X
Kidneys	X	X	X	X
Renal pelvis (measure if increased)	X			X
Bladder	X	X	X	X
Spine				
Vertebrae	X	X	X	X
Skin covering			X	X
Limbs				
Upper extremity	X	X	X	X
Metacarpals (right and left)	X		X	X
Lower extremity	X	X	X	X
Femur length	X (measure)	X (measure)	X	X (measure)
Metatarsals (right and left)	X		X	X

	ISUOG	AIUM AND ACOG	ASUM	NHS (UK)
TABLE 3.3 Summary of Recommendations Regarding Evaluation of Fetal Anatomy on Prenatal Ultrasound (*continued*)				
Uterus, Cervix, and Adnexa				
Cervical length		X (if tech feas)	X	
Adnexa	X (if tech feas)	X (if tech feas)	X	
Amniotic fluid volume (subj or meas)	X	X	X	X
Placental position	X	X	X	X

ACOG, American College of Obstetricians and Gynecologists; AIUM, American Institute of Ultrasound in Medicine; ASUM, Australasian Society of Ultrasound in Medicine; ISUOG, International Society of Ultrasound in Obstetrics and Gynecology; NHS, National Health Service, UK.
From Salomon LJ, Alfirevic Z, Berghella V, et al. Practice guidelines for performance of the routine midtrimester fetal ultrasound scan (ISUOG). *Ultrasound Obstet Gynecol.* 2011;37:116–126; American Institute of Ultrasound in Medicine. AIUM practice guideline for the performance of obstetric ultrasound examinations. *J Ultrasound Med.* 2010;29:157–166; American College of Obstetricians and Gynecologists. ACOG Practice Bulletin No. 101: ultrasonography in pregnancy. *Obstet Gynecol.* 2009;113:451–461; Australasian Society for Ultrasound in Medicine. Guidelines, policies and statements—D2: Guidelines for the midtrimester obstetric scan. https://www.asum.com.au/files/public/SoP/curver/Obs-Gynae/Guidelines-for-the-Performance-of-Second-Mid-Trimester-Ultrasound.pdf. Accessed October 12, 2018; National Collaborating Centre for Women's and Children's Health. *Antenatal Care: Routine Care for the Healthy Pregnant Woman.* 2nd ed. London, England: RCOG Press; 2008.

level of service and billing. They delineate the specific structures that need to be evaluated to fulfill criteria for that level of service. For example, in the second and third trimesters of pregnancy, two codes 76805 (basic ultrasound) and 76811 (detailed ultrasound) are most commonly used.[45,46]

The detailed obstetric examination includes all the components of the basic examination with the addition of examinations of the face, chest, cardiac outflow tracts, limbs, placenta, umbilical cord, and a more detailed examination of the brain anatomy as well as "other fetal structures as clinically indicated." The justification for performing a detailed rather than basic ultrasound can be based on maternal or family history of congenital anomalies, an abnormality or a marker that is detected on basic ultrasound (either at the time when the basic ultrasound is performed or as a referral from a center with only a basic examination capability), or if the ultrasound is significantly compromised by maternal habitus (BMI > 30). However, most persons experienced in performing obstetric ultrasounds would consider the "detailed scan" as a minimum standard for each initial ultrasound examination. In addition to describing the basic components of an obstetrical ultrasound examination in this chapter, we also present extended views that improve the quality of the examination and the detection of pregnancy-related problems. This chapter deals with normal fetal anatomy; however, frequent references to anomalies are made to underscore the pertinence of a good anatomic evaluation. Each image used in this chapter was obtained using two-dimensional (2D) ultrasound. Three-dimensional (3D) ultrasound can be a useful adjunct to 2D ultrasound in select circumstances and will be discussed in Chapter 7. All stated gestational ages are according to last menstrual period (LMP) dating.

EARLY FIRST-TRIMESTER SCAN (5 TO 10 WEEKS' GESTATION)

The embryonic stage, ending at 10 weeks' gestation, is a time of very rapid change in the small, developing conceptus.[47] Ultrasound before 11 weeks' gestation is not typically regarded as a

routine part of pregnancy assessment. When performed, the examination is generally limited to determination of the location and number of gestations present, determination of chorionicity in cases of multiple gestations, assessment for viability, and estimation of gestational age.[48] Although the anatomy of embryo is not typically examined in detail, a variety of severe congenital anomalies (e.g., severe amniotic band syndrome, body-stalk anomalies, and conjoined twins) may be identified even at this point. A finding that is commonly seen in the early first trimester and that deserves special mention is physiological herniation of the midgut into the root of the abdominal cord insertion (Fig. 3.1).[49] This finding is considered normal until the early portion 12th week of gestation and should not be mistaken for an omphalocele.

Most examinations at this stage are performed for a specific clinical indication such as pain or vaginal bleeding associated with a positive pregnancy test. Systematic evaluation is needed to accurately distinguish between a viable intrauterine pregnancy, a miscarriage, or an ectopic pregnancy. Ultrasound findings are frequently best interpreted in combination with quantitative

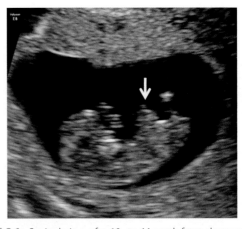

FIGURE 3.1: Sagittal view of a 10- to 11-week fetus demonstrating a physiological midgut herniation *(arrow)*.

maternal serum hCG (human chorionic gonadotropin) with or without progesterone levels. Serial examinations may be needed to reach a diagnosis. The transvaginal approach should be used in all circumstances where a viable intrauterine pregnancy is not obvious on transabdominal assessment. The uterus and adjacent structures should be assessed in both longitudinal and axial sections, taking care to pass completely from side to side and from fundus to cervix to determine the number and location of gestational sacs and embryos. In the early first trimester, the transvaginal approach is ideal to detect any adnexal pathology or free fluid.

Using transvaginal ultrasound, the presence of an intrauterine gestational sac can be consistently demonstrated by the completion of the fifth week of gestation. At this early stage, the gestational age is being estimated by determination of the mean sac diameter (MSD): the average of the sac length, width, and depth. The yolk sac becomes visible within the gestational sac by the midportion of the sixth gestational week, corresponding to an MSD of approximately 10 mm. An embryonic pole with a heartbeat is generally detected by the middle of the seventh gestational week (MSD of ~18 mm). When an embryonic pole becomes identifiable, the best method of establishing the gestational age is measurement of the crown-rump length (CRL). Prior to the completion of the seventh gestational week, the anatomy of the embryonic pole is difficult to clearly delineate. At this stage, the CRL is defined as the longest dimension of the embryonic pole (Fig. 3.2). Beginning with the eighth week of gestation, the embryonic head and torso become identifiable. At this point, the CRL is defined as measurement between the top of the fetal head and the fetal rump along its longitudinal axis (Fig. 3.3).[50] Whereas some investigators advocate using the average of three CRL measurements to establish gestational age, most use the single best measurement. In the 11th week of gestation, the fetus begins to flex and extend its body to a degree that may significantly affect CRL; therefore, CRL measurements need to be carefully standardized from this point on (Fig. 3.4).[51,52]

The accuracy of CRL measurement decreases with gestational age. Between 7 and 11[+6] weeks' gestation measurements should be within 4 days of dates by LMP. At 12 to 13[+6] weeks, an error of ±7 days is considered to be acceptable.[53,54]

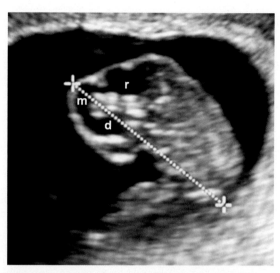

FIGURE 3.3: Sagittal view of an 8-week gestation. *Calipers*, crown-rump length measurement; *d*, diencephalon; *m*, mesencephalon; *r*, rhombencephalon.

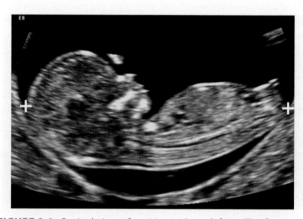

FIGURE 3.4: Sagittal view of an 11- to 12-week fetus. The fetus is in a neutral position and occupies the majority of the image. *Calipers*, crown-rump length measurement.

LATE FIRST-TRIMESTER SCAN (11[+1] TO 13[+6] WEEKS' GESTATION)

The late first-trimester scan is generally considered to be the first scheduled point for routine ultrasound assessment in pregnancy. It provides the same information as the early first-trimester scan with a number of additional benefits. Since it includes highly accurate estimation of gestational age, routine implementation of the late first-trimester scan would lead to a significant reduction in postterm pregnancies. During this time frame, the fetus reaches a size and stage of development sufficient to allow for the performance of an informative anatomic survey.[10,11,55] A number of markers, the most important of which is the nuchal translucency measurement, can be employed to provide an accurate risk assessment for aneuploidy. It should also be stressed that an increased translucency and the presence of other markers, most notably tricuspid valve regurgitation and an abnormal ductus venosus (DV) Doppler waveform, increase the risk of structural abnormalities even in chromosomally normal fetuses.[56]

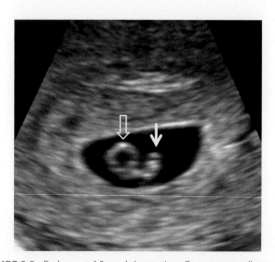

FIGURE 3.2: Embryo at 6.5 weeks' gestation. *Open arrow*, yolk sac; *solid arrow*, embryo.

Optimal timing of the first-trimester scan involves some compromise. Nuchal translucency assessment is easier to perform and more sensitive at an earlier gestation (11 to 12 weeks), whereas anatomy is best assessed at a slightly later gestation (12 to 13 weeks).[8] The examination may be performed transabdominally, and if necessary transvaginally, but a combination of the two approaches often yields the best results. Regardless of the approach used, the fetus needs to be assessed in all planes: longitudinal, axial, and coronal.

The midsagittal section of the fetus is very important, as this allows accurate measurement of CRL and, when adequately magnified, nuchal translucency (Fig. 3.5). Nuchal translucency measurement is typically increased in fetuses affected by chromosomal abnormality. Measurement according to standardized methodology allows individualized levels of risk for trisomy 21, 18, and 13 to be calculated. Another marker for aneuploidy, the fetal nasal bone, can be examined in the same section. Absence of the nasal bone is associated with an increased risk of trisomy 21.[57] Similarly, the intracranial anatomy of the posterior fossa can be examined and used to screen for spina bifida in this view.[12] The methodology for assessment of these features as well as the overall utility of the 11 to 13[+6] week scan is discussed in detail in Chapter 2.

Fetal anatomy is most readily assessed with a transverse sweep, running from head to toe. In this section, the intracranial anatomy essentially consists of the lateral ventricles and a very thin layer of brain parenchyma. The lateral ventricles are essentially filled by choroid plexi, which are seen as paired echogenic structures, one within each hemisphere ("butterfly view"). The midline falx is visible as an echogenic line running anteroposteriorly in the midline bisecting the "butterfly" (Fig. 3.6). The posterior fossa contains the developing cerebellum. Since the cerebellar vermis is not yet fused, a large midline communication is seen between the developing fourth ventricle and the cisterna magna (CM) (Fig. 3.7). The posterior fossa undergoes rapid change during the late first trimester, and by 13 to 14 weeks the cerebellum begins to assume a shape resembling that seen in the mid-second trimester (Fig. 3.8).

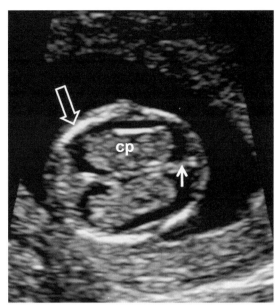

FIGURE 3.6: Axial view of the fetal head at 12 weeks' gestation. *cp*, choroid plexus; *open arrow*, ossified portion of calvarium; *solid arrow*, falx cerebri.

Occasionally, the third ventricle can be detected in a midcoronal section of the head (Fig. 3.9).

After 11 weeks' gestation, the calvarium should be ossified and is seen as an echogenic ring around the intracranial structures (see Fig. 3.6). Absence of an ossified calvarium in association with abnormal intracranial anatomy is consistent with exencephaly/anencephaly sequence. As the transducer is moved caudally, the orbits can be identified. However, these are often better seen in a coronal section of the face (Fig. 3.10). The face, specifically lips and nose, is best examined in sagittal section (see Fig. 3.5). In this view, an upper lip seen extending beyond the tip of the nose raises the possibility of cleft lip and palate.

In an axial section at the superior aspect of the thorax, clavicles can be seen even early in gestation (Fig. 3.11). The four-chamber view and outflow tracts can be assessed using both grayscale and color Doppler ultrasound imaging (Figs. 3.12 to 3.14). The stomach should be visible in the upper abdomen, and the integrity of the diaphragm can be assessed in sagittal or coronal sections (Figs. 3.15 and 3.16). Returning to an axial section, the anterior abdominal wall and cord insertion are evaluated (Fig. 3.17). The kidneys are generally difficult to see owing to their small size and echogenicity, which is similar to that of the small bowel. Both axial and coronal views are often required in order to identify them with confidence (Figs. 3.18 and 3.19). Color Doppler ultrasound may be used to look for the renal arteries. However, it should be kept in mind that since the vessels are very small, only small adjustments of the transducer can affect their visualization (Fig. 3.20).[58,59]

The bladder should be visible in all cases from 12 weeks' onward. It is best assessed in the midsagittal section. A standardized longitudinal measurement of the bladder in the first trimester should be performed in this view if it appears to be enlarged.[60] The same section provides information regarding fetal gender by qualitative evaluation or measurement of the angle between the genital tubercle and the fetal longitudinal axis.

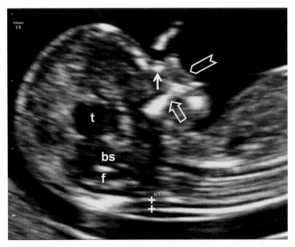

FIGURE 3.5: Sagittal view of a 12- to 13-week fetus. The fetal head and upper torso occupy the majority of the image, and the fetus is in a neutral position. *bs*, brain stem; *calipers*, nuchal translucency measurement; *chevron*, upper lip; *f*, fourth ventricle; *open arrow*, maxilla; *solid arrow*, nasal bone; *t*, thalamus.

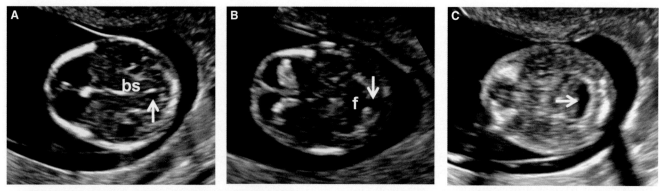

FIGURE 3.7: Transverse views of a fetal head at 12 weeks' gestation demonstrating hindbrain appearance at various levels in descending order. **A:** *Arrow*, developing aqueduct of Sylvius; *bs*, brain stem. **B:** *Arrow*, open communication with cisterna magna; *f*, fourth ventricle. **C:** *Arrow*, cisterna magna.

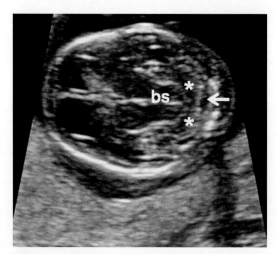

FIGURE 3.8: Transverse views of a fetal head at 13.5 weeks' gestation demonstrating progressive development of the cerebellum. Compare with Figure 3.7. *Arrow*, cisterna magna; *asterisks*, cerebellar hemispheres; *bs*, brain stem.

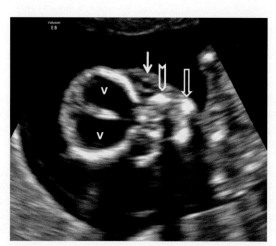

FIGURE 3.10: Coronal view of the fetal face. *Chevron*, maxilla; *open arrow*, body of the mandible; *solid arrow*, ocular orbit with a lens within it; *v*, lateral ventricles.

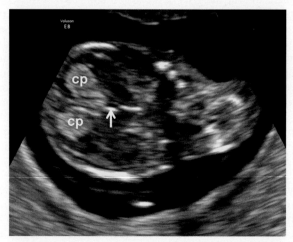

FIGURE 3.9: Midcoronal view of the head at 12 to 13 weeks' gestation. *Arrow*, third ventricle; *cp*, choroid plexus.

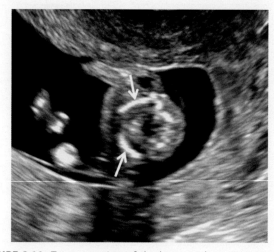

FIGURE 3.11: Transverse view of the lower neck at 12 to 13 weeks' gestation. *Solid arrows*, clavicles.

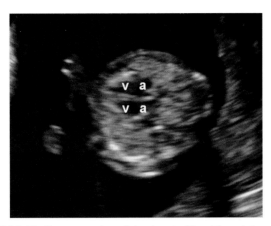

FIGURE 3.12: Transverse view of the chest at 12 to 13 weeks' gestation containing a four-chamber heart view. *a*, atria; *v*, ventricles.

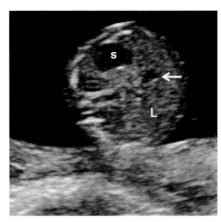

FIGURE 3.15: Transverse view of the abdomen at 13 weeks' gestation at the level of the abdominal circumference. *Arrow*, portal sinus; *L*, liver; *s*, stomach.

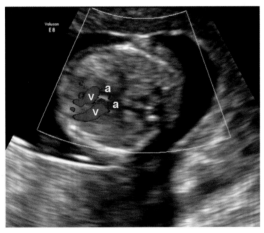

FIGURE 3.13: Transverse view of the chest at 12 to 13 weeks' gestation containing a four-chamber heart view in diastole with the ventricles *(v)* highlighted using color Doppler. *a*, atria.

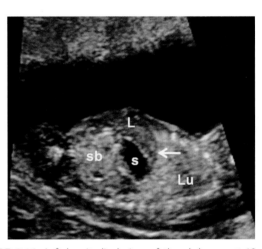

FIGURE 3.16: Left longitudinal view of the abdomen at 12 weeks' gestation demonstrating the left lung *(Lu)*, intact diaphragm *(arrow)*, left lobe of the liver *(L)*, stomach *(s)*, and small bowel *(sb)*. Note the difference in echogenicities between the various organs.

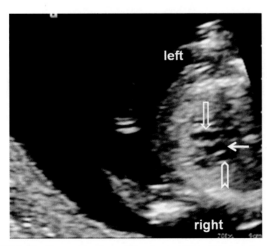

FIGURE 3.14: Transverse view of the chest at 12 to 13 weeks' gestation at the level of the three-vessel view. *Chevron*, superior vena cava; *open arrow*, pulmonary artery; *solid arrow*, aorta.

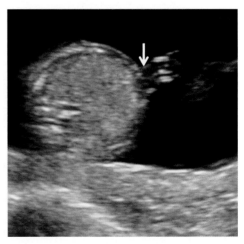

FIGURE 3.17: Transverse view of the abdomen at 13 weeks' gestation at the level of abdominal cord insertion *(arrow)*.

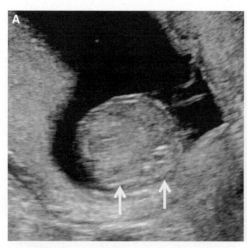 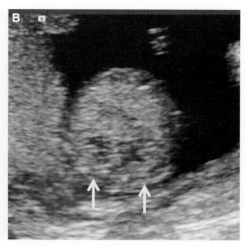

FIGURE 3.18: Transverse view of the abdomen at the level of the kidneys *(arrows)* at 12 weeks' gestation **(A)** and at 13 weeks' gestation **(B)**.

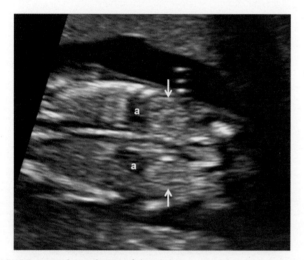

FIGURE 3.19: Coronal view of the abdomen at 12 weeks' gestation at the level of the kidneys *(arrows)*. Note the relatively prominent adrenal glands *(a)*, which need to be kept in mind in order not to mistake them for the kidneys.

A small angle, which is essentially parallel to the longitudinal axis of the fetus, indicates a female gender, whereas an angle measuring 30° or more suggests a male gender (Figs. 3.21 and 3.22). Using this method, the accuracy of sex determination is only 70% at 11 weeks' gestation but increases to nearly 100% at 13 to 14 weeks' gestation.[61]

A skeletal survey is best performed by utilizing both axial and transverse sections. Both hands are commonly held in front of the chest or fetal face, and the legs are generally flexed at the hip at this gestation. The number of fingers is relatively easy to assess in the first trimester as all fingers, including the thumb, lie in approximately the same ultrasound plane (Fig. 3.23). Fetal feet can also be identified, though evaluating the number of toes may be difficult because of their small size (Fig. 3.24). There is a tendency of the ankles to turn inward, making the diagnosis of clubfoot in the first trimester challenging. Both the femur and the humerus can be identified and measured (Figs. 3.25 and 3.26).

Color Doppler ultrasound may be used to help define the cord insertion and the number of arteries in the cord

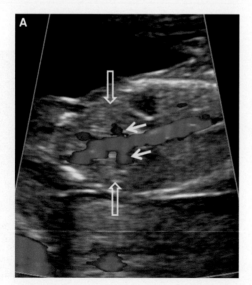 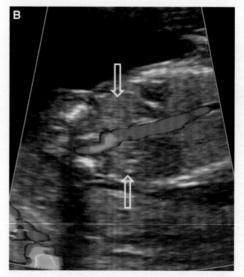

FIGURE 3.20: Coronal view of the abdomen at the level of the kidneys *(open arrows)* in a 12- to 13-week fetus. Color Doppler is used to demonstrate the renal arteries *(solid arrows)* in **(A)**, which can become nondetectable with only a slight adjustment of the transducer, as in **(B)**.

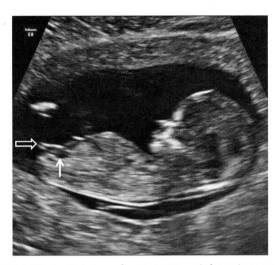

FIGURE 3.21: Sagittal view of a 12- to 13-week fetus demonstrating the presence of a small urinary bladder *(solid arrow)*. The genital tubercle *(open arrow)* points in a direction parallel to the longitudinal axis of the fetus, indicating female gender.

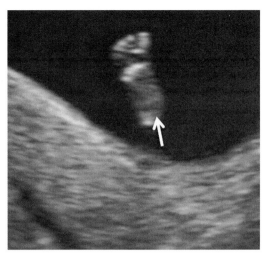

FIGURE 3.24: Fetal foot *(arrow)* with all five toes visible (12 to 13 weeks' gestation).

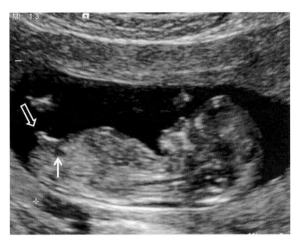

FIGURE 3.22: Sagittal view of a 12- to 13-week fetus demonstrating the presence of a small urinary bladder *(solid arrow)*. The genital tubercle *(open arrow)* up from the fetal longitudinal axis (>30°).

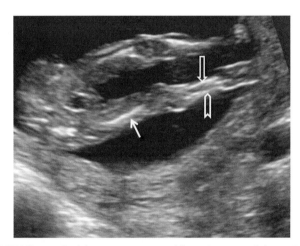

FIGURE 3.25: Both lower extremities visible at 13 to 14 weeks' gestation. *Chevron*, fibula; *open arrow*, tibia; *solid arrow*, femur.

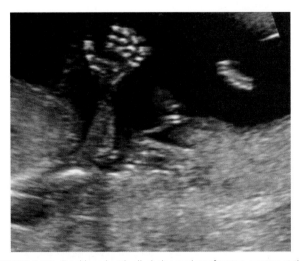

FIGURE 3.23: Fetal hand with all phalangeal ossification centers visible (13 to 14 weeks' gestation).

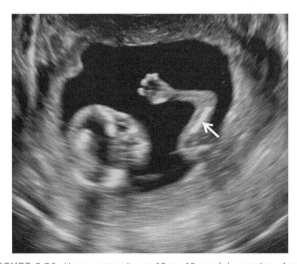

FIGURE 3.26: Upper extremity at 12 to 13 weeks' gestation. *Arrow*, humerus.

(Fig. 3.27). It can also be used to localize the DV in a right parasagittal section, allowing pulse wave assessment of this vessel for aneuploidy and cardiac screening. The hepatic artery peak systolic velocity may be evaluated in the same section to aid in aneuploidy risk assessment (Fig. 3.28).[8] Doppler examination involves higher power levels and consequently should generally be avoided during the embryonic period (≤10 weeks' menstrual gestational age) unless the benefits clearly outweigh the risks. When using Doppler during the 11 to 13[+6] week scan, power indices should be reduced to a minimum, and the region of interest should be interrogated for the minimum time necessary. Often, the region of interest can be effectively identified using grayscale prior to employing Doppler, resulting in reduced energy exposure to the fetus. Please see Chapter 2 for a detailed discussion regarding the utility of ultrasound evaluation between 11 and 13 weeks 6 days as well as up-to-date references.

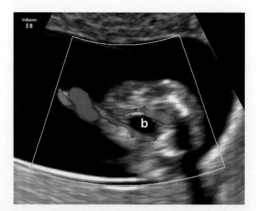

FIGURE 3.27: Transverse/oblique section of the lower abdomen and the pelvis showing the urinary bladder *(b)* with two umbilical arteries coursing around it in a 12- to 13-week fetus.

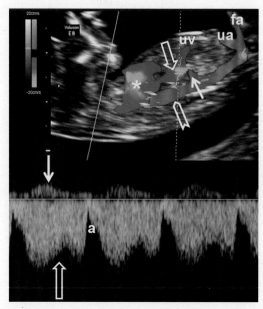

FIGURE 3.28: Right parasagittal section of a fetus at 12 to 13 weeks' gestation with color and pulsed Doppler. *Asterisk,* heart; *chevron,* aorta; *fa,* femoral artery; *open arrows,* ductus venosus and its corresponding waveform; *solid arrows,* hepatic artery and its corresponding waveform; *ua,* umbilical artery; *uv,* umbilical vein.

ASSESSING FETAL ANATOMY DURING THE SECOND AND THIRD TRIMESTERS

Standard assessment of the fetus is quite complex. It is best to develop a systematic approach to the examination. A complete examination of the uterine contents in pregnancy includes much more than evaluation of the fetal anatomy; the remaining issues will be discussed in later chapters. The issue of fetal biometry is discussed in this chapter only to illustrate the proper technique rather than clinical applicability.

Fetal anatomy is best assessed at 20 to 24 weeks' gestation. At this point, the pregnant uterus is out of the pelvis and is located well within the maternal abdomen. The fetus usually presents itself in a better axis for examination. The fetus is also larger and more developed, making the detection of anomalies easier.[62–75] In some jurisdictions, the anomaly scan is performed earlier (e.g., at 18 to 20 weeks' gestation) in view of the legal restrictions related to interruption of pregnancy if there are abnormal findings. However, it should be pointed out that there is a statistically significant difference in being able to complete the fetal anatomic survey if it is performed at 18 to 18[+6] (in 76% of cases) versus 20 to 22[+6] weeks' gestation (in 90% of cases).[76]

The approach to the anatomical survey is essentially the same in both the second and the third trimesters. However, fetal position, reduction in amniotic fluid volume, and increased bony ossification often make the third-trimester examination more challenging. It is, however, good practice to briefly check fetal anatomy at the third-trimester scan, even if a more comprehensive survey has previously been done at 20 to 24 weeks. Some anomalies may be more readily detectable with the fetus in a different position and others (e.g., duodenal atresia, X-linked aqueductal stenosis, certain skeletal dysplasias, and fetal tumors) generally only become apparent after the mid-second-trimester examination. The exact timing of the examination may also depend on maternal habitus. Increased BMI can significantly compromise the ultrasound examination and may require a change in the usual strategy. One reasonable approach to evaluating a fetus in an obese patient is to perform a thorough examination at 12 weeks' gestation using the transvaginal route and delay the anomaly scan until 22 to 24 weeks' gestation to increase the likelihood of successfully completing the structural examination.

Immediately after starting the scan, the fetal heart is checked, establishing viability and providing some reassurance to the mother. The uterus should then be scanned in cross section, from left to right and from top to bottom, determining the number of fetuses that are present and defining the lie of the fetus. Placental site and cervical length can then be assessed, although true cervical assessment requires a transvaginal approach, which is best performed at the end of the examination.

Standard fetal biometry includes the following measurements: biparietal diameter (BPD), head circumference (HC), abdominal circumference (AC), and femur diaphysis length (FDL).[77–82] Other measurements that are commonly performed as a part of a routine examination in some centers are the humerus diaphysis length (HDL) and the transcerebellar diameter (TCD).[83,84] The correct manner in which each of these measurements should be obtained is described in the individual sections later. Additional fetal biometry is performed if clinically appropriate. Standard measurements of essentially all fetal structures have been published.

Calvarium

The shape, measurements, and integrity of the calvarium are best assessed utilizing axial and sagittal views. In the axial section, the contour of the fetal head is normally oval in shape. In order to assess the symmetry of the two halves of the brain, regardless of the level of the axial view, care should be taken to keep the falx cerebri truly in the midline. The BPD is assessed using an axial image of the head at a level where standard anatomic landmarks are visible: the globular and slightly hypoechoic paired structures representing the thalami in the midportion of the head with a slit-like hypoechoic structure representing the third ventricle located between them, the cavum septi pellucidi (CSP) in front of the thalami, and the lateral ventricles, with the frontal horns seen anteriorly and the atria (trigones) seen posteriorly. Care should be taken with caliper placement as the authors of some charts measure from the outer aspect of the calvarium in the near field to the inner aspect of the calvarium in the far field, while others use an outer–outer approach. The HC is measured by tracing around the outside of the calvarium in the same axial section as the BPD. In addition to measuring the BPD and HC, the occipito-frontal diameter (OFD) can be measured and expressed in ratio to the BPD (BPD/OFD) as the cephalic index (CI) (Fig. 3.29). This ratio is valuable in describing the shape of the head. The normal range for CI is 0.74 to 0.83. A CI, which is below 0.74, connotes a relatively flat head (dolichocephaly), while a CI above 0.83 describes a relatively round head (brachycephaly).[85] Dolichocephaly is not uncommon and is often seen in fetuses that are in a persistently breech presentation or in association with chronic oligohydramnios. Dolichocephaly has been reported in fetuses with sagittal synostosis. Brachycephaly may also be a normal variant but has been described in association with trisomy 21. It can also be seen in conditions where the skull is poorly ossified such as certain types of osteogenesis imperfecta and hypophosphatasia. In these conditions, the skull is also easily compressible, which can be demonstrated by applying gentle pressure with the ultrasound transducer.

The shape of the skull may be abnormal in association with a number of specific fetal anomalies. In the mid-second trimester, bifrontal scalloping occurs in greater than 95% of open neural tube defects resulting in a "lemon"-shaped calvarium seen in the axial section.[86,87] The occipital portion of the skull is typically flattened in trisomy 18, while the frontal and parietal portions of the skull gently slope toward one another anteriorly, creating a "strawberry" shape in axial view. Premature closure of multiple cranial sutures restricts expansion of the skull, particularly with advancing gestation, resulting in a "cloverleaf" appearance. The sagittal section offers the best view of the fetal forehead. Abnormalities such as frontal bossing, which are part of a number of skeletal dysplasias or a sloping forehead present in conditions such as microcephaly, are best visualized in this fashion.

The calvarium should be systematically examined to ensure that it is intact. The most common defects are a cephalocele or an encephalocele. These are generally located in the occipital portion of the calvarium, but can be seen less frequently in the area of the nasal root anteriorly or parietally. Disruption of the skull can also occur at more unusual sites, especially when it is caused by amniotic bands. The calvarium will be completely absent in anencephaly.

Intracranial Anatomy

Intracranial anatomy is complex and gestational age–dependent owing to rapid embryological and later fetal development.[88] The sections most commonly employed to look at the fetal anatomy are axial ones. This is because of the fact that they are the easiest to obtain and are very familiar to operators who are involved in fetal scanning.

The half of the brain that is closest to the transducer is much more difficult to image clearly when compared with the distal half. This is due to ossification of the skull, which casts an acoustic shadow over the proximal portion of the fetal brain. With advancing gestation, increasing calcification of the calvarium limits resolution. Images can often be improved by rotating the probe so the brain is imaged through the suture lines and fontanelles, using techniques similar to those applied during neonatal examination. Employing the transvaginal route to image a fetus that is cephalic in presentation can facilitate a detailed examination of the intracranial anatomy.

The general symmetry of the fetal brain is first assessed using standard axial views. The presence and position of the falx cerebri should be noted. The falx cerebri is seen as an echogenic line running in the anteroposterior direction. It is a structure that is usually very easy to visualize, and if absent, the possibility of a severe structural defect such as alobar holoprosencephaly should be entertained. The cerebral cortex is a hypoechoic structure, which is fairly thin and difficult to visualize at early gestations. The proportion of the cranial cavity that it fills progressively increases as the gestation advances. The structures that are easiest to identify because of their well-delineated boundaries and greatest differences in echogenicity from the surrounding cortex are the lateral ventricles and the CSP. Routine examination of the intracranial anatomy should always include identification of these structures.

Each lateral ventricle is divided into five parts: the frontal horn, the body of the lateral ventricle, the occipital horn, the

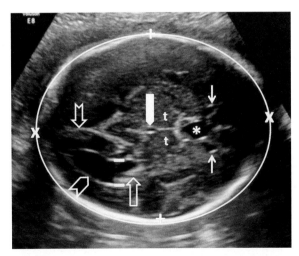

FIGURE 3.29: Axial view of the fetal head at the biparietal diameter (BPD) level. Please note the difference in anatomic detail between the proximal and distal half of the brain. *Asterisk*, cavum septi pellucidi; *calipers*, BPD measurement; *chevron*, lateral ventricle (occipital horn); *notched arrow*, lateral ventricle (occipital horn); *open arrow*, lateral ventricle (atrium containing echogenic choroid plexus); *t*, thalamus; *thick solid arrow*, third ventricle; *thin solid arrows*, lateral ventricle (frontal horns) *two (-) signs*, lateral atrial diameter measurement of the lateral ventricle.

inferior (temporal) horn, and the atrium (trigone). The atrium is the point of confluence between the occipital horn, inferior horn, and the body of the lateral ventricle and is the largest, most easily identifiable portion of the lateral ventricle. In axial section at the level of the thalami, the atrium can be measured. This is normally done at the level of the posterior margin of the choroid plexus using a magnified image so that calipers can be accurately placed on the inner margins of the ventricular walls (Fig. 3.29). Enlargement of the lateral ventricle (ventriculomegaly) will be recognized by measurement at this point. At 20 weeks' gestation, the upper limit of normal is considered to be 10 mm, although recently some authors have suggested that even measurements up to 12 mm are very unlikely to be associated with significant pathology.[89–92] The ventricles become less prominent with advancing gestation, although a threshold of measurement less than 10 mm is typically also used in the third trimester.

It needs to be kept in mind that the shape of the lateral ventricle is 3D complex; unless it is enlarged, it is difficult to visualize in its entirety in a single ultrasound plane. The atrium is located medially. The body and the anterior horn of the lateral ventricle radiate anteriorly, superiorly, and laterally from the atrium. The occipital horns project posteriorly. The temporal horn extends from the atrium in an inferior and anterior direction. Additionally, the bodies of the lateral ventricle and their continuation, the frontal horns, are domed in shape in the sagittal section; therefore, their appearance differs significantly when viewed in various axial planes. The inferior (temporal) horns run through the area of the temporal lobe and are difficult to identify unless they are enlarged. The shape of the ventricles is best assessed using the combination of longitudinal and coronal views (Figs. 3.30 to 3.33). The atrium contains a globular and echogenic structure, the glomus of the choroid plexus. In the majority of cases, the glomus is homogeneous in its ultrasound appearance. However, occasionally echolucent structures of varying complexity and size called choroid plexus cysts (CPCs) are present.[93–95] They can develop in any portion of the choroid plexus, but those that are ≥3 mm tend to be located in the glomus.

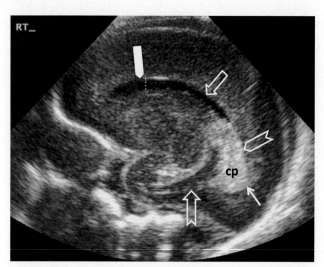

FIGURE 3.30: Sagittal view of the lateral ventricle at 24 weeks' gestation. Note that this is a neonatal image to show the anatomy in its entirety. *Chevron*, trigone; *cp*, choroid plexus; *notched arrow*, inferior (temporal) horn; *open arrow*, body of the lateral ventricle; *thick solid arrow*, frontal horn; *thin solid arrow*, portion of the occipital horn.

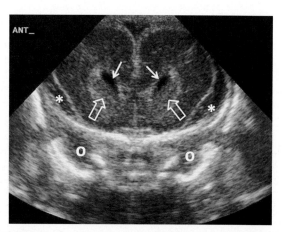

FIGURE 3.31: Anterior coronal view of the brain at 24 weeks' gestation. Please note the increased amount of extra-axial fluid, which is normal early in gestation. Note that this is a neonatal image to show the anatomy in its entirety. *Asterisks*, extra-axial fluid; *o*, orbit; *open arrows*, caudate nuclei; *solid arrows*, frontal horns of the lateral ventricles.

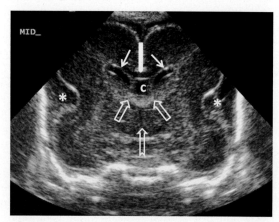

FIGURE 3.32: Midcoronal view of the brain at 24 weeks' gestation. Please note the increased echogenicity of the roof of the third ventricle extending into the foramina of Monro. This represents the choroid plexus. Note that this is a neonatal image to show the anatomy in its entirety. *Asterisks*, operculization of the insula; *c*, cavum septi pellucidi; *notched arrow*, third ventricle; *open arrows*, location of the foramina of Monro; *thick solid arrow*, corpus callosum; *thin solid arrows*, bodies of the lateral ventricles.

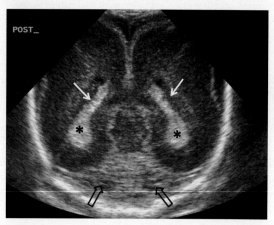

FIGURE 3.33: Posterior coronal view of the brain at 24 weeks' gestation. Note that this is a neonatal image to show the anatomy in its entirety. *Asterisks*, choroid plexi; *black arrows*, section through a portion of the cerebellum; *white arrows*, trigones.

Unilateral or bilateral CPCs are a common finding affecting 1% to 4% of euploid fetuses but have also been associated with aneuploidy, particularly trisomy 18. They invariably resolve spontaneously and do not represent a true pathological entity. When found in isolation, risk for aneuploidy is not increased, but it is worth reviewing the results of first-trimester screening, and in particular of first-trimester biochemistry (both free β-hCG [beta human chorionic gonadotropin] and PAPP-A [pregnancy-associated plasma protein A] are low in trisomy 18), to check there are no common themes through different modalities of screening. The choroid plexus does not extend into the anterior horn of the lateral ventricle; therefore, cystic structures seen anterior to the caudothalamic notch will have a different underlying etiology.

The CSP and its posterior extension, the cavum septi vergae (CSV), are seen as a continuous hypoechoic structure located in the midline. It represents a space between the two septi pellucidi, which is filled with cerebrospinal fluid (CSF). Not infrequently, the cavum septi pellucidi et vergae (CSPV) contains septations, especially in its posterior portion (Fig. 3.34). The CSPV begins to close in the third trimester, a process that is completed in infancy.

There is no direct communication between the ventricular system and CSPV; it is diffusion across the thin septi pellucidi that allows CSF to enter this space. This space begins to close in late gestation, a process that is completed during infancy. It is bounded by the corpus callosum anteriorly and superiorly, the fornix posteriorly, and the anterior commissure inferiorly. In a midsagittal section, the CSPV is arched in shape. Therefore, in the standard axial section at the level of the BPD, usually it is only the CSP that is visible. In this section, the CSP appears as a hypoechoic roughly rectangular structure located anteriorly to the thalami. As a normal variant, the CSV can be unusually large and visible in this section. Since the CSPV is arched in shape, it may appear to be separate from the cavum septi pellucid, simulating a cyst (Fig. 3.35). Examination of the CSPV in the sagittal section will help to elucidate the diagnosis (see Fig. 3.34). A cystic midline structure that is

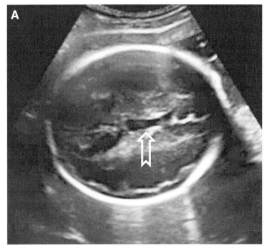

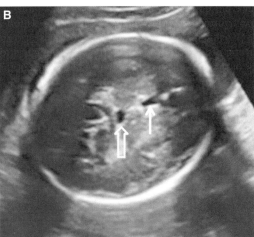

FIGURE 3.35: Axial view of a fetal head at 32 weeks. **A:** Section through the cavum septum pellucidi et vergae at a point when continuity between the two is evident *(arrow)*. **B:** Axial view in a plane slightly caudal to **(A)**, where the cavum septi pellucidi *(solid arrow)* and cavum septi vergae *(open arrow)* are seen as two separate structures. The latter should not be mistaken for a cyst.

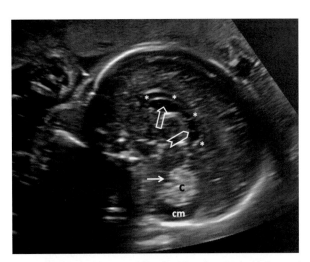

FIGURE 3.34: Sagittal view of the fetal head at 24 weeks' gestation. Please note the septations in the cavum septi vergae seen as echogenic lines running anteroposteriorly. *Asterisks,* corpus callosum; *c,* cerebellum; *chevron,* cavum septi vergae; *cm,* cisterna magna; *open arrow,* cavum septi pellucidi; *solid arrow,* fourth ventricle.

occasionally seen located posteriorly and inferiorly to the CSV is the cavum veli interpositi (Fig. 3.36). This is a normal variant and is part of the leptomeningeal space between the roof of the third ventricle and the body of the fornices. The size of this structure normally does not exceed 1 cm. It can be difficult to distinguish from an arachnoid cyst located at the quadrigeminal cistern.[96,97]

The importance of positively identifying the CSPV lies in the fact that it can be absent in association with midline defects. It should be remembered that the anterior pillars of the fornices lie in the same general area as the CSP. They are hypoechoic and have a generally rectangular shape in the axial plane. This can lead to a false impression that the CSP is present, consequently missing the diagnosis of anomalies that can be associated with absent CSPV such as agenesis of corpus callosum, septo-optic dysplasia, lobar holoprosencephaly, and neuronal migration defects. However, unlike the CSP, a thin echogenic line can be seen between the two fornices, which helps to differentiate between the two entities (Fig. 3.37).[98] In the sagittal view, visualization of the pericallosal artery helps to confirm the

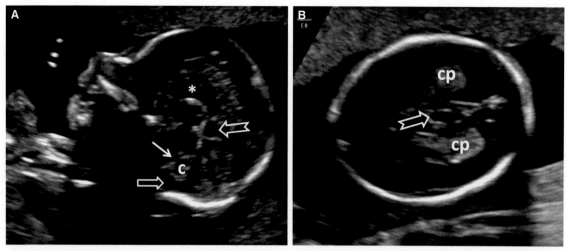

FIGURE 3.36: A: Sagittal section of a fetal head at 22 weeks' gestation with a cavum veli interpositi *(notched arrow)* located posteriorly and inferiorly to CSPV *(asterisk)*. *c*, cerebellum; *open arrow*, cisterna magna; *solid arrow*, fourth ventricle. **B:** Axial view of the same fetus. *Arrow*, cavum veli interpositi; *cp*, choroid plexus.

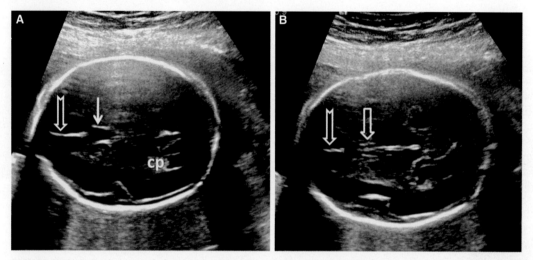

FIGURE 3.37: A: Axial section of a fetal head at 22 weeks' gestation at the level of the cavum septi pellucidi *(solid arrow)*. *cp*, choroid plexus; *notched arrow*, falx cerebri. **B:** Axial view of the same fetus in slightly more caudal section. Note the two juxtaposed pillars of the fornix *(open arrow)* with a midline echogenic division. *Notched arrow*, falx cerebri.

presence of the corpus callosum (Fig. 3.38). Since the corpus callosum is a structure that completes its formation relatively late in pregnancy, the CSPV should not be expected to be visible prior to 18 to 19 weeks' gestation.

The third ventricle is located inferiorly to the CSP, between the paired thalami. This slit-like structure is filled with CSF and is hypoechoic in its ultrasound appearance (see Fig. 3.29). It is normally small (<3 mm diameter) and may be difficult to visualize. Enlargement of the third ventricle is typically only seen in association with enlargement of the lateral ventricles.

Examination of the cerebral cortex focuses on ruling out any space-occupying lesions, either cystic or solid in nature. Cortical maturation continues throughout pregnancy, as the brain develops gyri and loses its smooth appearance (Fig. 3.39). The process of cortical maturation can be most easily observed in the insula. Even though operculization of the insula begins at approximately 14 weeks' gestation, on ultrasound, this process does not become evident until approximately 19 weeks' gestation. It begins as infolding of the cerebral cortex at the lateral edge of

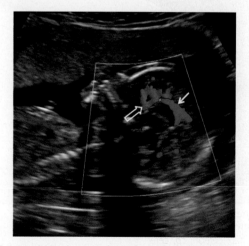

FIGURE 3.38: Sagittal view of the fetal head at 22 weeks. Anterior cerebral *(open arrow)* and pericallosal *(solid arrow)* arteries with some of their branches are demonstrated using color Doppler.

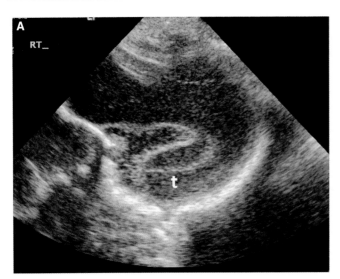
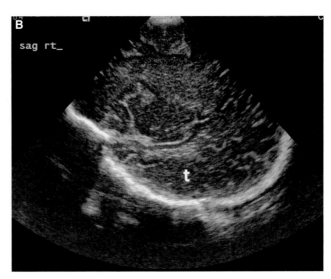

FIGURE 3.39: Parasagittal section of the fetal head with the temporal lobe *(t)* visible. Please note the difference in the texture of the surface of the cortex, with absent sulci and gyri at 22 weeks' gestation **(A)** and well-developed pattern of sulci and gyri at term **(B)**.

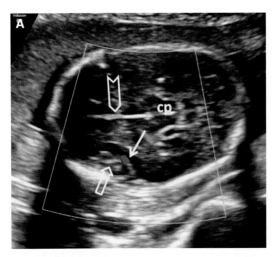

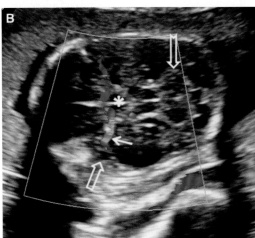

FIGURE 3.40: A: Axial section of a fetal head at 20 weeks' gestation demonstrating the insula at an early stage of operculization *(open arrow)* with the middle cerebral artery (color Doppler) at its base *(solid arrow)*. *Chevron,* falx cerebri; *cp,* cerebral peduncles. **B:** Slightly more caudal section of the same fetus demonstrating the course of the middle cerebral artery *(solid arrow)* to the base of the insula *(open arrow)* with color Doppler. *Asterisk,* center of the circle of Willis; *notched arrow,* cerebellum.

the cerebrum located initially in the anterior half of the distance between the occiput and the forehead. It first appears as a heterogeneous depression, which is increased in echogenicity. Prominent pulsations can be seen at the bottom of the depression, which represents the Sylvian segment of the middle cerebral artery (Fig. 3.40). As operculization progresses, the depression is roofed over by the temporal lobe. By the completion of the process at the beginning of the third trimester, it remains as only a slit-like structure, representing the Sylvian fissure (Fig. 3.41). Absence of normal operculization raises the possibility of a neuronal migration defect such as lissencephaly.

Posterior Fossa

Another axial section routinely employed to evaluate the intracranial anatomy is the suboccipitobregmatic view: Starting with the BPD view, the posterior aspect of the probe is rotated caudally until the posterior fossa becomes visible. Even though this view is primarily designed to evaluate the posterior fossa and

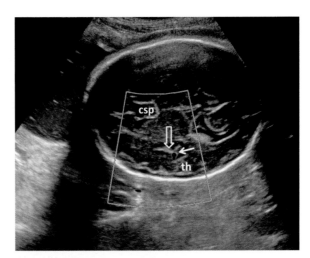

FIGURE 3.41: Axial view of a fetal head in the third trimester after the completion of insular operculization. *csp,* cavum septi pellucidi; *open arrow,* Sylvian fissure; *solid arrow,* color Doppler of the middle cerebral artery; *th,* temporal horn.

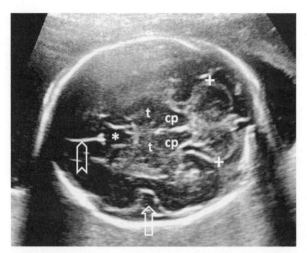

FIGURE 3.42: Suboccipitobregmatic view of the head. *Asterisk*, cavum septi pellucidi; *calipers*, transcerebellar diameter; *cp*, cerebral peduncles; *chevron*, falx cerebri; *open arrow*, insula; *t*, thalami.

the back of the fetal head, it also offers a good view of the CSP, thalami, and the midbrain as well as their anatomic relationship (Fig. 3.42). Sagittal views of the posterior fossa are also very informative. Coronal sections add very little information to the axial ones, but depending on the position of the fetus, this approach may provide the clearest view.

Routine examination of the posterior fossa is critical to detect not only anomalies that originate in the posterior fossa but also changes that are indicative of problems in the spine. In addition to the bifrontal scalloping of the cranium described earlier, open spine defects are accompanied by the Chiari Type II malformation (herniation of the cerebellar tonsils through the foramen magnum and downward displacement of the cerebellar vermis). In the axial view, this defect translates into flattening of the cerebellar hemispheres with an anterior bend (so-called banana sign) and obliteration of the CM.[86,87,99–101] Finally, since most cephaloceles and encephaloceles are located in the occipital region of the skull, examination of the posterior fossa must also include a careful evaluation of the calvarium in that region.[102]

The formation of the cerebellar hemispheres and the connecting vermis continues throughout the first half of the pregnancy. Since the vermis is not fully developed until mid-gestation,

vermian defects, especially small ones, are difficult to diagnose prior to 18 to 20 weeks' gestation. Using axial planes, the mid-second-trimester cerebellum is seen as a dumbbell-shaped structure consisting of two hemispheres connected by the vermis. The shape of the cerebellar hemispheres becomes somewhat flattened on its anterior surface. As gestation advances, the vermis increases in echogenicity in relation to the hemispheres, and the caudal part of the vermis becomes notched (cerebellar tonsils). The hemispheres develop gyri through the third trimester, which are visible on ultrasound, and the cerebellar tonsils become more elongated. An axial view of the inferior aspect of the cerebellum at this point in pregnancy may reveal a fluid-filled space between the tonsils, which may lead to the erroneous diagnosis of a defect in the vermis. The TCD is measured in an axial section using the suboccipitobregmatic view. Care must be taken so that the cerebellar hemispheres are symmetrical, and the measurement is done at a point where the distance between the lateral edges of the two hemispheres is the greatest.[103,104]

Every attempt should be made to visualize both cerebellar hemispheres to allow a comparison of their size and echotexture. There are conditions that may affect only one of the cerebellar hemispheres such as unilateral hypoplasia, hemorrhage, or infarction. If a cerebellar defect or ventriculomegaly is suspected, the fourth ventricle should be evaluated. It is seen as a hypoechoic structure between the cerebral peduncles and the cerebellum (Fig. 3.43). Isolated enlargement of the fourth ventricle is unlikely to occur and is of limited clinical significance.

The CM is a CSF-filled structure that is located behind the cerebellum. If it appears to be exceptionally large, it can be objectively assessed by measurement of its anteroposterior diameter in an axial section of the posterior fossa (Fig. 3.44). Even though the normal CM diameter is below 10 mm, isolated CM enlargement (mega-CM) is considered to be a normal variant. Nonetheless, a large CM should lead to a detailed evaluation of the fetal anatomy overall and the cerebellar vermis specifically, as this finding has a weak association with trisomy 13 and 21 and vermian defects. Septations within the CM are a common finding and occasionally they can simulate a small cyst. These are due to subarachnoid trabeculae and represent a normal finding.[105–107]

With the exception of the above-described Chiari Type II malformation, most defects affecting the posterior fossa are cystic in nature (Dandy–Walker malformation, Blake pouch, arachnoid cysts, and dysgenesis of the cerebellar vermis). These diagnoses

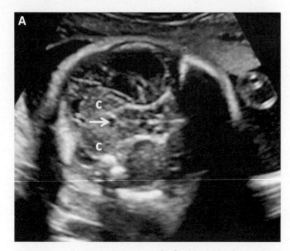

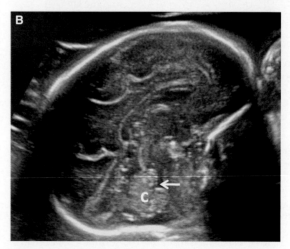

FIGURE 3.43: A: Axial section of a fetal head in the mid-second trimester weeks demonstrating the fourth ventricle (*arrow*). *c*, cerebellar hemispheres. **B:** Sagittal section of a fetal head in the early third trimester. *Arrow*, fourth ventricle; *c*, cerebellum.

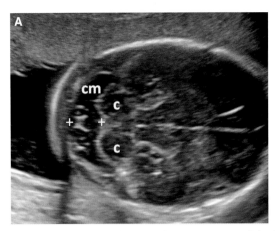
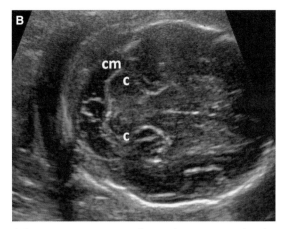

FIGURE 3.44: A, B: Suboccipitobregmatic views of the head demonstrating a variety of normal septations within the cisterna magna *(cm)*. Note the formation of a cyst-like structure in **(B)**. *c*, cerebellar hemispheres; *calipers*, cisterna magna measurement.

can be difficult to tease out and depend on findings in axial, mid-sagittal, and coronal sections. The posterior fossa anomalies are one area where fetal magnetic resonance imaging may be especially helpful in arriving at the correct diagnosis.

Finally, the suboccipitobregmatic view is also used as a standardized view for nuchal fold measurement. Thickened (>6 mm) nuchal fold is associated with an increased risk of trisomy 21.

Spine

Assessment of the central nervous system is not complete without detailed examination of the fetal spine. This involves evaluation of the vertebrae and the contents of the spinal canal. Open spinal defects also disrupt the skin, so careful examination of the cutaneous covering of the spine is also important. The vertebral column should be evaluated in at least two of the three planes: coronal, axial, and longitudinal (midsagittal). The vertebrae have three ossification centers visible prenatally: vertebral body anteriorly and one in each of the vertebral arches (laminae) posteriorly. In the axial section, the three ossification centers are in a triangular arrangement. The vertebral body ossification center is round and is located in the midline. The paired laminar ossification centers are slightly offset from the midline. They are linear in shape and form a roof over the spinal canal (Fig. 3.45).[108,109] In the presence of an open spine defect, this arrangement is disrupted, and the laminar ossification centers are displaced laterally, forming the shape of the letter U or V in the axial view of the spine. Often, axial views are best for assessing the integrity of the skin. Both individual vertebrae and their skin covering should be evaluated by sliding the transducer along the entire length of the spine.

The whole length of the vertebral column can be seen in both a coronal and in a sagittal section, and the ossification centers should be spaced evenly in these views. In the coronal view, the two lateral points of ossification can be visualized cleanly, and by moving the probe anteriorly, ossification of the vertebral body can be brought into view. As the spine is curved, it is common to be able to visualize the vertebral bodies at some levels and the arches at other levels in the same view (Fig. 3.46). In longitudinal section, the line of ossification of vertebral bodies is seen anteriorly and, if there is a slight oblique cut, one set of posterior ossification sites will be visualized. In the anteroposterior axis, the spine is curved, being convex in the thoracic region and concave in the lumbosacral region. The sacral portion of the

spine usually has a more persistent curvature, with the tip of the spine pointing posteriorly (Fig. 3.47). This sacral upswing may be absent in the presence of an open spine defect and in the presence of caudal regression syndrome.

Overcurvature of the thoracic spine, kyphosis, or lateral curvature of the spine, scoliosis, can be detected by careful assessment of at least two of the three standard planes. Abnormal curvature may be due to the presence of a hemivertebra, which is a feature of a number of genetic syndromes such as vertebral defects, anal atresia, cardiac defects, trachea-esophageal fistula, renal anomalies, and limb abnormalities (VACTERL); therefore, other anomalies known to be associated with this syndrome should be actively sought.

The spinal cord can be delineated within the spinal canal using ultrasound on most exams (Fig. 3.48). However, the presence of multiple vertebral ossification centers does obscure it to a variable degree, especially later in gestation. The ultrasound appearance of the spinal cord is fairly uniform with slightly decreasing size moving cranial to caudal. The conus medullaris can be identified as the place where the spinal cord comes to its end point (Fig. 3.49). Measuring the distance between the tip of the conus medullaris to the tip of the spine is potentially useful in diagnosing tethered cord, and therefore spina bifida occulta.[110] Fetal hair can occasionally be seen on ultrasound, especially in the third trimester.[111] It can also form a prominent echogenic line behind the fetal back generally following the outline of the spine, which may be a confusing finding for those who are not aware of this possibility (Fig. 3.50).

Face

The face is a large and complex structure. As such, it needs to be examined at multiple levels and in multiple planes.[112] At a minimum, complete examination requires axial sections to evaluate the orbits and maxilla, a midsagittal section that identifies the nasal bone and demonstrates the profile, and a coronal section demonstrating the lips. The face should be investigated for right–left symmetry and defects of fusion. Since the formation of the face involves fusion in the midline, many of the defects are located close to the midline. Also, since the cleavage of the prosencephalon is intimately associated with formation of the facial structures, in cases where holoprosencephaly is suspected, normal facial structures also need to be evaluated carefully.

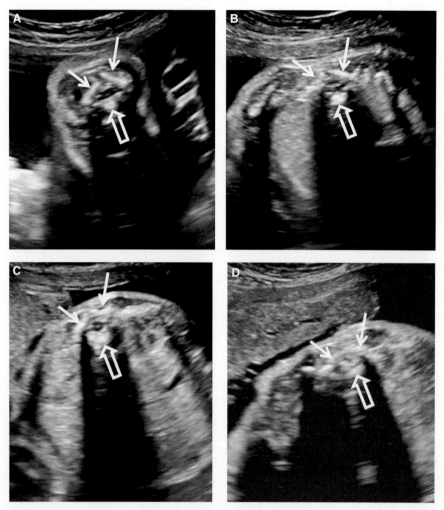

FIGURE 3.45: A transverse view of vertebrae at various levels of the vertebral column: cervical **(A)**; thoracic **(B)**; lumbar **(C)**; sacral **(D)**. The three ossification centers (*solid arrows*, vertebral arches; *open arrow*, vertebral body) are seen. Note the differences in their appearance depending on the level.

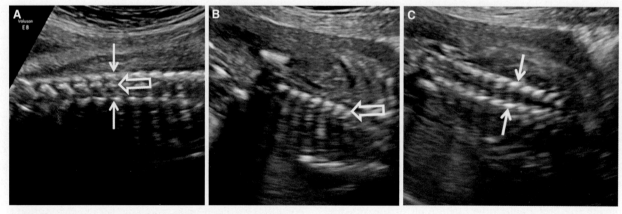

FIGURE 3.46: Coronal views of the vertebral column. **A:** Section demonstrating all three types of ossification centers in the same view. *Open arrow*, vertebral body ossification; *solid arrows*, vertebral arch ossifications. **B:** Section demonstrating vertebral body ossification centers *(open arrow)* only. **C:** Section demonstrating vertebral arch ossification centers *(solid arrows)* only.

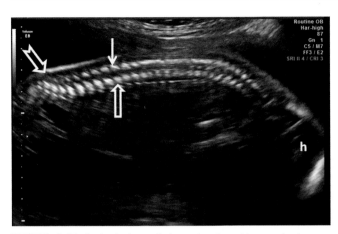

FIGURE 3.47: Sagittal view of the spine in mid-second trimester demonstrating its normal curvature. Note the sacral upswing *(notched arrow)*. *h*, head; *open arrow*, vertebral body ossification center; *solid arrow*, vertebral arch ossification center.

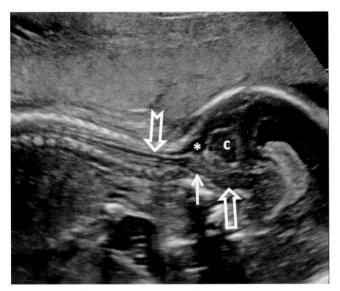

FIGURE 3.48: Sagittal view of the cervical spinal cord *(notched arrow)* in late second trimester. *Asterisk*, cisterna magna; *c*, cerebellum; *open arrow*, pons; *solid arrow*, medulla oblongata.

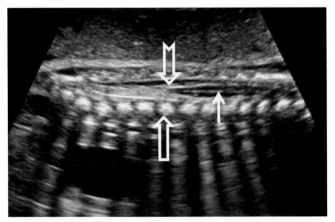

FIGURE 3.49: Sagittal view of the lumbar spinal cord *(solid arrow)* ending in the conus medullaris *(notched arrow)* in late second trimester. *Open arrow*, vertebral body ossification center.

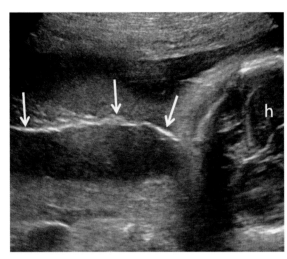

FIGURE 3.50: Superficial coronal view along the fetal back in the third trimester. A thin line of hair along the fetal back *(arrows)* is seen. *h*, fetal head.

The orbits should be assessed in an axial section. This is best achieved by moving the probe caudally from the standard axial section of the head and brain. The orbits are round bony structures, each containing a hypoechoic bulbus oculi. Although gestational charts for intraorbital and extraorbital diameter are available, these measurements are not routinely made. However, visually, the interorbital distance should be approximately one-third of the extraorbital distance (Fig. 3.51). A number of fetal syndromes are associated with decreased (hypotelorism) or increased (hypertelorism) interorbital distance.[113,114] Visualization of the lens of the eye will rule out anophthalmia or aphakia. This can be done in both the axial and the coronal sections. In the coronal view, the lens is a round hypoechoic structure with a thin echogenic border (Fig. 3.52). Congenital cataracts can be demonstrated as an additional thick echogenic ring within the lens oculi. In the axial view, an echogenic linear structure, the hyaloid artery, can be visualized running from the midposterior aspect of the lens to the back of the ocular orbit (Fig. 3.53). This vessel is easily visualized in the mid-second trimester but starts

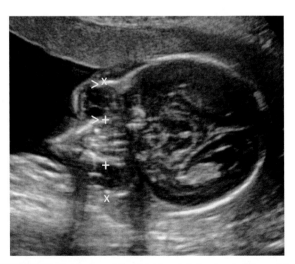

FIGURE 3.51: Axial view of the fetal head at the level of the orbits in mid-second trimester. The distance between two orbits is designated by + (interocular diameter), external ocular diameter by ✕, and the ocular diameter by >.

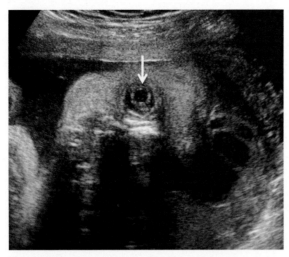

FIGURE 3.52: Coronal view of the eye demonstrating a normal lens *(arrow)* in the third trimester.

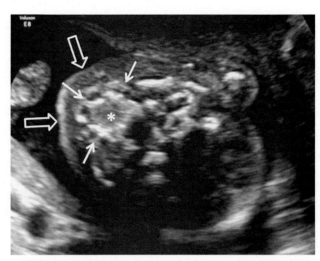

FIGURE 3.54: Axial view of the fetal head at the level of the maxilla *(asterisk)* and the upper lip *(open arrows)*. Multiple hypoechoic structures within the alveolar ridge are dental alveoli, with the two large ones in front being the incisors. *Solid arrows,* external border of the alveolar ridge.

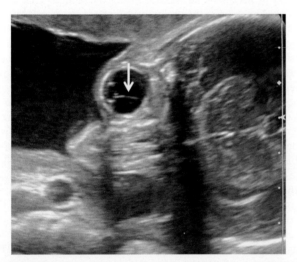

FIGURE 3.53: Axial view of the fetal head at the level of the orbits late second trimester. The echogenic line *(arrow)* extending from the posterior aspect of the lens to the posterior border of bulbus oculi is the hyaline artery, the future hyaline (Cloquet) canal.

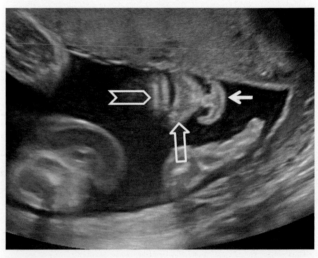

FIGURE 3.55: Coronal view of the upper lip *(open arrow)* with both the tip of the nose *(solid arrow)* and the lower lip *(chevron)* visible.

to become obliterated at about 28 weeks' gestation, eventually becoming the hyaloid (Cloquet) canal.

Moving the probe caudally, the maxilla, alveolar ridge, and upper lip can also be examined in transverse section (Fig. 3.54). These structures should be examined to ensure continuity over the midline. The presence of a defect would be indicative of the presence of a cleft lip and/or palate, which is by far the most common facial anomaly (approximately 1:700 pregnancies). The lips should also be examined in a coronal section (Fig. 3.55), taking care not to identify the natural depression of the philtrum as an anomaly (Fig. 3.56). Any cleft in the lip or palate will effectively be filled by amniotic fluid and will therefore be hypoechoic. Fetal small parts or a loop of umbilical cord positioned in front of the lips may create a false impression of a defect (Fig. 3.57). Therefore, if a facial cleft is suspected, it needs to be confirmed in a number of different views.

The front of the maxilla can be evaluated in the coronal view as well. In this view, generally only the two alveolar processes, the

incisors, are seen. The alveolar processes with a thin bony division between them and bones on each side create the so-called three-line view (Fig. 3.58). However, an axial examination of the maxilla allows for the entire alveolar ridge to be visualized (see Fig. 3.54).

Isolated cleft palate involves the posterior aspect of the palate. This can vary from just a bifid uvula or a defect in the soft palate to a defect that involves the palatine portion of the maxilla. The usual views to detect cleft palate in association with a cleft lip are not useful. Isolated cleft palate is extremely difficult to diagnose, especially if it just involves the soft palate. Evaluation of fluid flow through the nasal cavity and the nasopharynx using color Doppler ultrasound can aid in making the diagnosis of an isolated cleft palate as fluid will be noted to flow directly between the nasal and oral cavities in the presence of a large defect (Fig. 3.59).

The fetal mandible can be seen in the axial plane (Fig. 3.60). Its contour in severe micrognathia tends to be less domed than seen in normal cases.

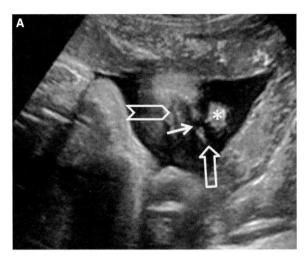

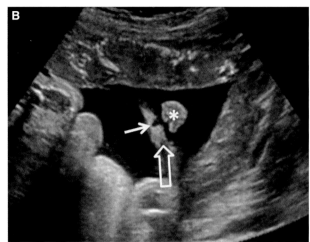

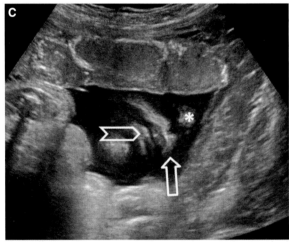

FIGURE 3.56: Coronal view of the upper lip in a fetus with a deep philtrum. **A, B:** Sections through the philtrum simulate a midline defect *(solid arrow)*. **C:** A deeper section through the face demonstrates an intact upper lip. *Asterisk,* tip of the nose; *chevron,* lower lip; *open arrow,* upper lip.

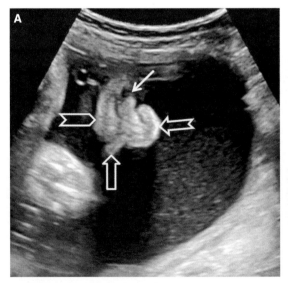

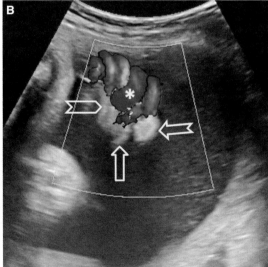

FIGURE 3.57: A: Coronal view of the upper lip with an apparent deep defect *(solid arrow)*. **B:** Color Doppler demonstrating that the false impression of a defect is being created by a loop of umbilical cord *(asterisk)*. *Chevron,* lower lip; *notched arrow,* tip of the nose; *open arrow,* upper lip.

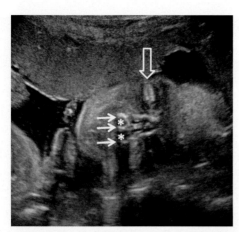

FIGURE 3.58: Coronal view of the front of the maxilla in the early third trimester demonstrating the two hypoechoic alveoli of the incisors *(asterisks)* with the surrounding bone creating the so-called "three-line view" *(solid arrows). Open arrow,* eyelids.

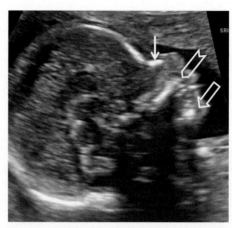

FIGURE 3.61: Sagittal view of the fetal profile. *Chevron,* front of the maxilla; *open arrow,* mandibular mentum; *solid arrow,* nasal bone.

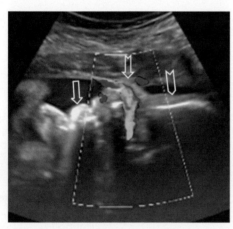

FIGURE 3.59: Sagittal view of the fetal face demonstrating normal flow of amniotic fluid across the upper palate with color Doppler. *Chevron,* forehead; *notched arrow,* tip of the nose; *open arrow,* chin.

The fetal profile is best evaluated in a sagittal section (Fig. 3.61). The evaluation is done subjectively by visually evaluating the contour of the profile. The nasal bone can be simply evaluated for its presence or absence, or it can be measured. Delayed ossification (absence of the nasal bone) and hypoplasia of the nasal bone are strong markers for trisomy 21. Prenasal skin and the prefrontal space ratio evaluation and measurements are useful markers for Down syndrome, although they are not currently included in the routine anomaly scan in most departments.[115-117] The portion of the mandible, which is seen in the midline, is the mentum. Its position relative to the front of the maxilla provides a subjective assessment for the presence of micrognathia. A parasagittal section can be used to assess the ear (Fig. 3.62). This is not routinely done, but can be of value in defining risk for aneuploidy and may be significant in identifying a number of genetic syndromes.[118] As the ear is a small, complex and irregular structure, 3D ultrasound may be a useful adjunct to evaluation.

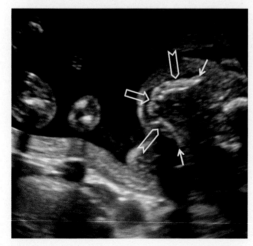

FIGURE 3.60: Axial view of the fetal head at the level of the mandible in the mid-second trimester. Note the small hypoechoic structures representing dental alveoli within the mandibular alveolar ridge. Note also its normal domed appearance. *Chevrons,* bodies of the mandible; *open arrow,* chin; *solid arrows,* portions of the mandibular rami.

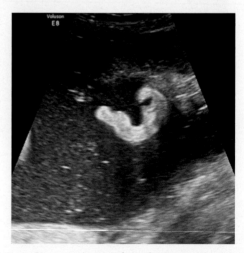

FIGURE 3.62: Parasagittal view of the fetal external ear in the third trimester.

Neck

Examination typically centers on the identification of any abnormal fluid accumulation (nuchal edema or cystic hygroma) in the posterior aspect of the neck. In a transverse section, normal anatomy includes the cervical vertebrae, muscles, vessels, pharynx, upper trachea, and fetal thyroid, which can be identified as a slightly echogenic paired organ in the lower anterior aspect of the neck (Fig. 3.63). The thyroid becomes more obvious when enlarged, and a fetal goiter can be readily apparent. Any protrusion in the skin line, either anteriorly or posteriorly, should raise the suspicion of fetal abnormality. Cervical meningomyeloceles are a rare but well-recognized subgroup of neural tube defects, and cervical teratomas (epignathus; with mixed cystic and solid components), and lymphatic malformations can be found both anteriorly and posteriorly.

Nuchal fold measurement at 16 to 20 weeks is performed in the suboccipitobregmatic view (see Fig. 3.41). Increased thickness (≥6 mm) is associated with trisomic aneuploidy.[119] A septated cystic lesion (cystic hygroma) is more commonly associated with monosomy X (Turner syndrome). Assessment of nuchal fold thickness at 20 weeks has value in screening for aneuploidy, but the efficacy of the test at this gestation is significantly lower than that performed at 11 to 13[+6] weeks.

Thorax

Examination of the thorax may be split into three parts: the thoracic cage and mediastinum, the lungs, and the heart. Most information about thoracic anatomy can be obtained using transverse sections. The thoracic cage is comprised of the thoracic vertebrae posteriorly, the ribs laterally, and the sternum anteriorly. The ribs can be examined in both transverse and parasagittal sections. They will normally wrap around the lateral wall of the abdomen and remain visible in the part of the chest. Ribs may be shortened, fractured, or have areas of focal echogenicity in a variety of skeletal dysplasias, and this can affect the size of the chest. The circumference of the lower portion of the thorax should be similar to the AC. If there is concern that the chest may be small, then axial sections of the thorax and abdomen can be compared directly. Gestational age–adjusted ranges for measurement of the anteroposterior and transverse diameters

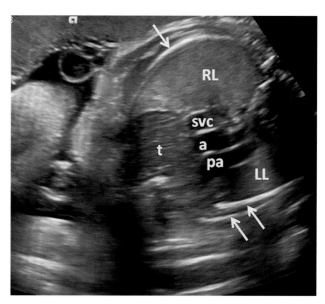

FIGURE 3.64: Axial view of the thoracic cavity demonstrating the presence of the thymus *(t)* at the level of the three-vessel view. *a*, aorta; *LL*, left lung; *pa*, pulmonary artery; *RL*, right lung; *solid arrows*, ribs; *svc*, superior vena cava.

and the thoracic circumference are also available.[120] The fetus with a small chest will also look abnormal in sagittal section, with an apparent "step" between the thorax and the abdomen at the level of the diaphragm.

The fetal thymus can be identified within the thoracic inlet, located anteriorly to the great vessels within the mediastinum (Fig. 3.64). Its echogenicity is similar to or slightly less than that of the lung. Occasionally, it is seen to extend to the level of the heart and may lead to the erroneous diagnosis of an anterior intrathoracic mass. In fetuses with cardiac abnormalities that are associated with 22q11 deletion, the identification of the thymus provides some reassurance, as it may be absent in this chromosomal abnormality. Lesions of the anterior mediastinum are exceptionally rare. Generally, these are echogenic in nature, and teratomas are most common.

The trachea lies to the right and slightly anterior to the spine. It is relatively small and difficult to visualize on ultrasound. It is best seen in the upper thorax at the level used to demonstrate the cardiac three-vessels and trachea view (Fig. 3.80). The trachea bifurcates into right and left mainstem bronchi between the lower portion of the fourth and the seventh thoracic vertebrae. A dilated and distended trachea is more easily seen as in congenital high airway obstructive sequence (CHAOS). The whole lower airway below the level of obstruction becomes visible in coronal or sagittal section, while the lungs are large and hyperechoic, the diaphragms depressed, and the heart and mediastinum compressed.

The esophagus runs posteriorly and to the left of the trachea. It is normally collapsed and free of fluid, and consequently difficult to identify on ultrasound. It is most easily seen in sagittal or coronal section as two or more parallel, echogenic lines.[121,122] Occasionally, if the esophagus is insonated during fetal swallowing, it has hypoechoic content (Fig. 3.65). In esophageal atresia, the proximal esophagus (the "esophageal pouch") may be seen as a dilated tubular structure in the upper chest.

The lungs fill the major part of each hemithorax. Abnormalities of the lung are rare, and the process of examination is relatively straightforward. The lungs are homogeneous with a moderately

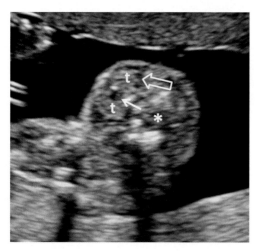

FIGURE 3.63: Transverse view of the neck demonstrating the trachea *(solid arrow)*, thyroid *(t)*, and the neck vessels *(open arrow). Asterisk*, spine.

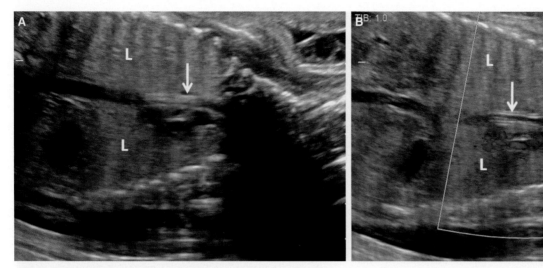

FIGURE 3.65: Coronal view of the esophagus *(arrow)* in late second trimester. Note the presence of echogenic dots around the periphery of the chest representing cross sections of the ribs and their acoustic shadows within the proximal lung. **A:** The esophagus is at rest consisting of three solid lines. **B:** The esophagus of the same fetus containing hypoechoic fluid during swallowing. *L*, lungs.

hyperechoic appearance on ultrasound (see Figs. 3.64 and 3.65). The periphery of the lungs should be inspected carefully to identify a pleural effusion as a hypoechoic layer surrounding the lung. Lesions of the lung can be either cystic or solid in appearance and of variable echogenicity. Furthermore, lesions within the thorax may be extrathoracic in origin such as a diaphragmatic hernia. Displacement of the heart may be the first indication of the presence of a lung abnormality. It can be displaced to one side or the other depending on the location and size of the lesion. It can also be displaced with congenital agenesis of the lung. As the pregnancy progresses beyond the mid-second trimester, the shadowing by the fetal ribs increases due to their ossification. The resultant alternating areas of echogenicity and acoustic shadows located within the thorax may give the false impression of a mass (see Fig. 3.65). Therefore, if a mass is suspected, it should be evaluated in multiple sections to rule out an artifact.

Heart

Cardiac defects are very common, affecting approximately 1% of infants. However, they are also commonly missed on prenatal ultrasound.[72] The two main reasons for this are the fact that the range of cardiac abnormalities is wide and that the 3D anatomy of the heart is very complex. However, over 90% of cardiac defects are detectable, so it is important to develop an effective screening strategy that will alert clinicians to the risk of an abnormality. The basic components of this strategy include the four-chamber view, outflow tracts, and three-vessel view in the mid-second trimester. Not only do cardiac anomalies have a high association with neonatal and childhood morbidity and mortality, but they are also markers for chromosomal and genetic anomalies. Therefore, the importance of a careful cardiac cannot be overstated.[123-125]

The cardiac examination begins outside the chest by checking situs. First, fetal position is assessed to define the left and right sides of the fetus. The abdomen is then examined in axial sections to define the position of the stomach and of the great vessels. The stomach should normally be on the left side of the abdomen, and the aorta should be anterior to the spine and slightly to the left of the midline (see section on Abdomen and Pelvis in this chapter). The vena cava normally is more anterior

and to the right of the aorta. Once abdominal situs is established, the examination moves to the chest. In axial section, the apex of the heart should lie to the left side of the midline. The heart occupies one-third of the surface area of the chest, and the axis of the ventricular septum should be at 45° (±7°) to the anteroposterior axis of the thorax (Fig. 3.66).[126] An abnormal position of the heart may arise as a result of an abnormal space-occupying lesion in the left or right chest. The cardiac axis can also be displaced in the setting of certain cardiac malformations (e.g., tetralogy of Fallot and truncus arteriosus) and is a useful screening tool for cardiac defects.

Once situs and basic relationships are established, heart rate and rhythm are evaluated. Primary detection of rhythm anomalies is done by qualitative observation of cardiac motion. Detailed analysis of cardiac rhythm requires measurement of heart rate, the time intervals in the cardiac cycle, and, in particular, the relationship between atrial and ventricular contractions.

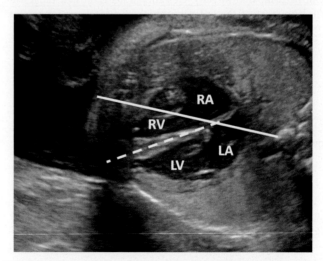

FIGURE 3.66: Axial view of the thoracic cavity at the level of the four-chamber view of the heart in diastole. The cardiac axis is formed by the anteroposterior axis of the thorax *(solid line)* and the longitudinal axis of the ventricular septum *(dashed line)* and is within normal limits. *LA*, left atrium; *LV*, left ventricle; *RA*, right atrium; *RV*, right ventricle.

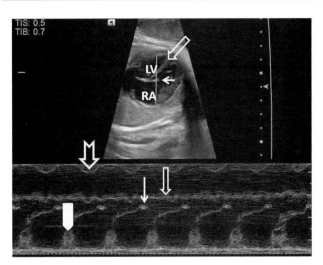

FIGURE 3.67: Axial view of the four-chamber heart with an M-mode through the left ventricle (*LV, notched arrow* on M-mode) and the right atrium (*RA, thick solid arrow* on M-mode). The cursor also includes the ventricular septum (*open arrow* on both grayscale and M-mode) and the medial leaflet of the tricuspid valve (*thin solid arrow* on both grayscale and M-mode).

The exact rate can be determined using either pulse wave Doppler or M-mode ultrasound, both of which document movement over time (Fig. 3.67). When using M-mode ultrasound, the sampling line is placed across both ventricle and atrium to display the temporal relationship of ventricular and atrial motion on one image. The timing and frequency of atrial and ventricular contractions may be used to classify the specific form of arrhythmia present. Premature atrial or ventricular contractions are a common benign finding and, in the absence of a cardiac structural defect, are of no clinical significance.

Before discussing issues regarding the circulation, it is appropriate to briefly review some of the specialized aspects of fetal circulatory anatomy. The fetal circulation is oxygenated by the placenta and therefore has several anatomical differences compared with the postnatal circulation. The fetal cardiovascular system is designed in such a way that the most highly oxygenated blood is delivered to the myocardium and brain. This is achieved in the fetus by both the preferential streaming of oxygenated blood and the presence of intracardiac and extracardiac shunts. The fetal circulation runs in parallel and is shunt dependent. The three vascular structures most important in the fetal circulation are the DV, foramen ovale (FO), and ductus arteriosus (DA). Briefly, during fetal life, DV delivers highly oxygenated blood from the umbilical vein directly into the inferior vena cava (IVC). The IVC also contains poorly oxygenated blood from the lower abdomen and pelvis. The blood coming from the DV is preferentially streamed across the FO into the left atrium owing to anatomic adaptations in the right atrium and a differential in flow velocity between the blood coming from the DV and the rest of the blood in the IVC. The oxygenated blood then empties into the left ventricle to be expelled into the aorta. In this way, the most oxygen-rich blood is delivered to the coronary arteries and the upper portion of the body, including the brain. Most of the deoxygenated blood from the IVC joins the deoxygenated blood returning via the superior vena cava (SVC) in the right atrium and is preferentially directed into the right ventricle and subsequently the pulmonary artery. The majority of this blood reenters the systemic circulation through the DA, which enters the aorta below the isthmus and mixes with more oxygenated blood coming from the left ventricle. In this way, the organs of the lower part of the body, which have a lower oxygen demand than the brain and the heart, receive blood with lower oxygen content. Also, the relatively deoxygenated blood is pumped to the placenta for re-oxygenation via the umbilical arteries, which originate from the internal iliac arteries.

Comprehensive evaluation of anatomy is best performed in a sequential fashion. Because of the 3D complexity of the anatomy of the heart and its arterial and venous connections, many views and transducer positions have been developed to assist in their examination. To complicate matters even further, optimal positions of the transducer are also greatly influenced by the position of the fetus, which changes during the examination as the fetus moves. Optimization of views requires frequent adjustment of the position of the transducer and the angle of insonation. It is important to recognize that even a slight alteration in angle or level at which the heart or great vessels are insonated leads to a significant change in their appearance. An added degree of difficulty is added by the fact that multiple cardiac structures lie in close proximity to each other. The operator should frequently return to a familiar and easily obtainable view such as the four-chamber, which acts as a point of reference. In the following section, we present the views that produce the highest yield and efficiency.

The four chambers of the heart can be seen in an axial section through the lower portion of the thorax. Normally, the heart is primarily located in the left hemithorax but does extend slightly to the right side. A line drawn along the anteroposterior axis transects the heart close to its crux. The entire left ventricle and a portion of the right ventricle will be located in the left hemithorax, whereas the entire right atrium and portion of the left atrium will be on the right (see Fig. 3.66). A careful search for a thoracic mass needs to be performed for cases in which the heart's location significantly deviates from this relationship. A small amount of pericardial fluid is usually present (Fig. 3.68). The amount of fluid is considered increased if the measurement between the wall of the heart and the pericardial sac exceeds 2 mm.

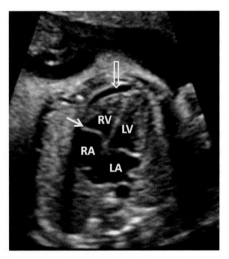

FIGURE 3.68: Axial view of the four-chamber heart demonstrates a prominent layer of pericardial fluid (*open arrow*) and apical displacement of the tricuspid valve (*solid arrow*). Compare the location of this valve to that of the mitral valve. *LA*, left atrium; *LV*, left ventricle; *RA*, right atrium; *RV*, right ventricle.

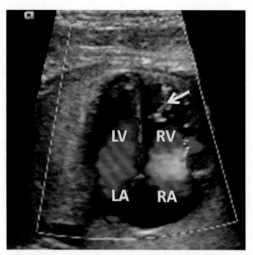

FIGURE 3.69: Axial and apical view of the four-chamber heart during early diastole with color Doppler demonstrating inflow of blood. Please note the moderator band *(arrow)* in the right ventricle *(RV)*. *LA*, left atrium; *LV*, left ventricle; *RA*, right atrium.

In the four-chamber view, two atria and two ventricles with a septum at midcavity are present. There are two atrioventricular valves; the tricuspid valve opens in to the right ventricle and the mitral valve opens in the left ventricle. The crux is the center of the heart where the atrial septum meets the ventricular septum and at which the atrioventricular valves also insert.[127,128]

The two ventricles are approximately equal in size. The right ventricle lies anteriorly, just behind the anterior chest wall, and the left ventricle is located behind it. The right ventricle can be identified morphologically by the fact that the tricuspid valve inserts into the interventricular septum (IVS) at a slightly lower level than the mitral valve and has a septal attachment, whereas the mitral valve has only a free wall attachment. The right ventricle is more coarsely trabeculated than the left and contains a thick band of tissue called the moderated band, which is located close to its apex (Fig. 13.69). While the right ventricle extends toward the apex, the left ventricle makes the apex of the heart

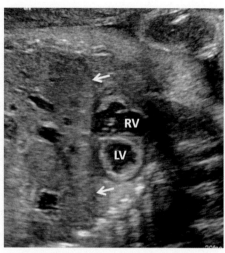

FIGURE 3.71: Short axis of the heart demonstrating the differences between the ventricular shapes. Note the rounded appearance of the left ventricle *(LV)* and the more flattened appearance of the right ventricle *(RV)*, which appears to "wrap" around the left one. Also note the echogenic projections into the right ventricular lumen representing trabeculations and chordae tendineae/papillary muscles. *Arrows*, domes of the diaphragm.

(Fig. 3.70). In the short axis view, the shapes of the two ventricles also differ: The right ventricle appears to slightly wrap around the more rounded left ventricular lumen (Fig. 3.71). The two atrioventricular valves should be visualized and seen to open and close through the cardiac cycle. Color flow and pulse wave Doppler can be used to demonstrate filling of the ventricular chambers and to look for valvular regurgitation (Fig. 3.72).

A common finding is an intracardiac echogenic focus, which is usually located in the left ventricle. As an isolated finding, it is of no consequence, though it is considered to be a weak marker for trisomy 21. It is thought to represent an area of calcification in a papillary muscle, though it may be caused by reflection from a papillary muscle surface during diastole (Fig. 3.73).[94,95,129,130]

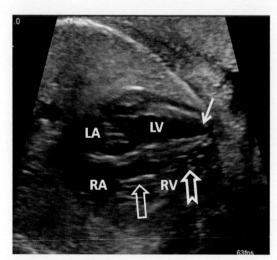

FIGURE 3.70: Axial view of the four-chamber heart. Please note that the tip of the left ventricle *(LV)* forms the apex of the heart *(solid arrow)* and the more "full" appearance of the right ventricular *(RV)* lumen due to chordae tendineae/papillary muscles *(open arrow)* and trabeculations *(notched arrow)*. *LA*, left atrium; *RA*, right atrium.

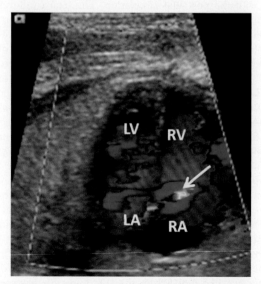

FIGURE 3.72: Apical view of the four-chamber heart at the time of valve closure. There is an area of turbulent flow *(arrow)* across the tricuspid valve, which is often seen at the time of valve closure and should not be mistaken for regurgitation. *LA*, left atrium; *LV*, left ventricle; *RA*, right atrium; *RV*, right ventricle.

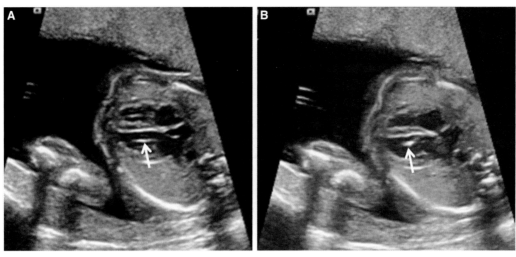

FIGURE 3.73: Axial view of the four-chamber heart. **A:** Appearance of the papillary muscle *(arrow)* when it is stretched during ventricular systole. **B:** Papillary muscle in the same patient presenting as an intracardiac echogenic focus *(arrow)* when it is relaxed during ventricular diastole.

The IVS separates the two ventricular cavities. It has muscular (basal) and membranous (inlet) parts. A number of different views should be employed to assure its integrity from the apex to the crux as ventricular septal defects (VSDs) are relatively common but often difficult to detect. The septum is best examined with the ultrasound beam perpendicular to the longitudinal axis. In this view, the entire septum, including both muscular and membranous portions, can be seen, and large defects can be visualized. Color Doppler ultrasound is a valuable adjunct for smaller muscular VSDs, which may be identified owing to the presence of flow across the septum. However, generally, this method is limited to the detection of muscular septal defects. Color Doppler evaluation of the subaortic portion of the septum is compromised by its proximity to the outflows and valves, rendering it less helpful due to "color bleed." Demonstration of bidirectional flow on Doppler helps to identify a VSD as outflow tracts will contain unidirectional flow only. The septum can also be insonated apically, that is, with the direction of the ultrasound beam parallel to the longitudinal axis of the septum. In this view, the membranous portion of the septum, which is close to the crux cordis, is not well imaged. This portion of the IVS is particularly thin, creating a "drop out," giving the erroneous impression of a VSD (Fig. 3.74). However, an echogenic dot (so-called "flashlight" sign) is often seen at the margin of a true VSD. This may in fact be the initial indication of its presence.

The two atria are also approximately the same in size and are of similar appearance. The atria are separated by the interatrial septum (IAS), which is significantly thinner than the IVS. The IAS contains a prominent conduit (FO) that lets oxygenated blood to stream into the left atrium from the right. A flap valve, which is associated with FO, is seen fluttering in the left atrium, reflecting the right to left direction of blood flow. Occasionally, it assumes the shape of an aneurysm, which is considered a benign variant (Fig. 3.75). Atrial septal defects are very difficult to detect prenatally as the majority are ostium secundum defects involving the FO. Ostium primum atrial septal defects are located close to the atrioventricular valves and are considered to be part of an atrioventricular septal (atrioventricular canal) defect spectrum.

The objective of imaging the left and right ventricular outflow tracts is to determine their size and relationship to each other,

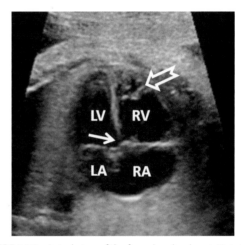

FIGURE 3.74: Apical view of the four-chamber heart. Note the "fall-out" in the membranous portion of the ventricular septum *(solid arrow)*. *LA*, left atrium; *LV*, left ventricle; *notched arrow*, moderator band; *RA*, right atrium; *RV*, right ventricle.

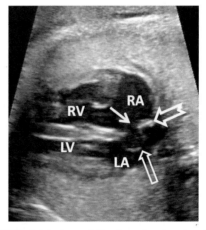

FIGURE 3.75: Axial view of the four-chamber heart showing the foramen ovale *(solid arrow)* with a foramen flap forming a small aneurysm *(open arrow)*. Most of the time, foramen ovale flap aneurysm is of limited clinical significance. *LA*, left atrium; *LV*, left ventricle; *notched arrow*, atrial septum; *RA*, right atrium; *RV*, right ventricle.

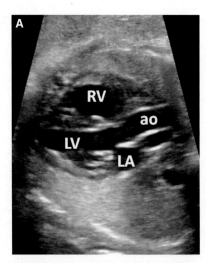 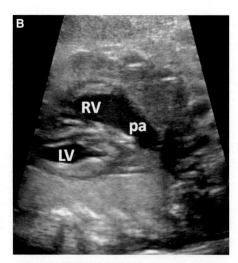

FIGURE 3.76: Axial views of the outflow tracts. **A:** Aortic outflow *(ao)* tract exiting from the left ventricle *(LV)*. *LA*, left atrium. **B:** Pulmonary artery outflow *(pa)* exiting from the right ventricle *(RV)*.

and to their respective ventricles (Fig. 3.76).[131,132] These views are necessary for identification of a number of cardiac anomalies not detectable using the four-chamber view alone. Evaluation of the left and then right outflow tract involves moving the probe progressively cranially in an axial section from the four-chamber view. The left ventricular outflow tract appears first, and this view can be improved by tilting the probe slightly toward the left shoulder of the fetus. As one continues to move cranially in axial section, the right ventricular outflow tract becomes apparent. The left ventricular outflow tract courses from left to right as it exits the left ventricle. The continuity of the IVS with the anterior wall of the aorta is more clearly seen in this view. An interruption in the IVS in this region is indicative of a perimembranous or outlet VSD. An overriding aorta is frequently found in association with an outlet VSD. The pulmonary trunk normally runs posteriorly, directly toward the spine, so the two vessels effectively cross one another at the level of their origin. Absence of this crossing suggests the presence of transposition of the great vessels. The pulmonary trunk divides into the right and left pulmonary arteries, a finding which is useful to differentiate between the two great arteries. An additional major vessel, which originates from the point of bifurcation of the pulmonary trunk or from the left pulmonary artery, is the DA. It is a fetal vessel, which connects the pulmonary circulation with the descending thoracic aorta. Color Doppler ultrasound is useful to define the direction of flow through the great arteries as they leave the heart.

Moving the probe further cranially into the upper mediastinum allows the outflow tracts to be imaged in the three-vessel view. This view includes from left to right: the main pulmonary trunk, a transverse section of the aorta and of the SVC. The lumen of the aorta and pulmonary trunk are similar in size, though the pulmonary artery tends to be slightly larger, and the SVC is the smallest. The DA is usually, but not always, seen in this view coursing posteriorly toward the descending aorta (Figs. 3.77 and 3.78). The DA is usually a fairly straight vessel, but occasionally a highly tortuous DA is found (Fig. 3.79). This is of no apparent clinical significance.

The tracheal view is obtained by moving the probe further cranially. This view also includes the aorta, the pulmonary artery, and the DA (Fig. 3.80). However, they are seen more along their long axis running anteroposteriorly from right to left. The cross section of the trachea is also seen in this section located anteriorly

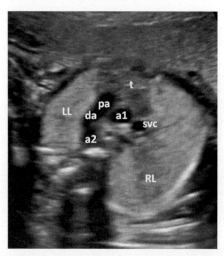

FIGURE 3.77: Axial section of the chest at the level of the three-vessel view with the ductus arteriosus *(da)* visible. *a1*, ascending thoracic aorta; *a2*, descending thoracic aorta; *LL*, left lung; *pa*, pulmonary artery; *RL*, right lung; *svc*, superior vena cava; *t*, thymus.

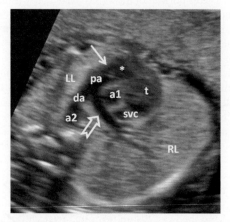

FIGURE 3.78: Modified (oblique) axial section of the chest at a similar level to Figure 3.16, demonstrating the right branch *(notched arrow)* of the pulmonary artery *(pa)* and ductus arteriosus *(da)*. *a1*, ascending thoracic aorta; *a2*, descending thoracic aorta; *asterisk*, upper portion of the right ventricle; *da*, ductus arteriosus; *LL*, left lung; *RL*, right lung; *solid arrow*, pulmonary valve; *svc*, superior vena cava; *t*, thymus.

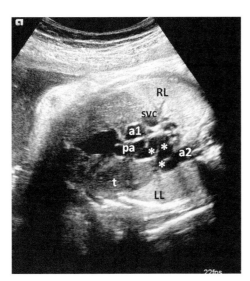

FIGURE 3.79: Axial section of the chest at the level of the three-vessel view. The convoluted vessel *(asterisks)* is an unusually tortuous ductus arteriosus. *a1,* ascending thoracic aorta; *a2,* descending thoracic aorta; *LL,* left lung; *pa,* pulmonary artery; *RL,* right lung; *svc,* superior vena cava; *t,* thymus.

FIGURE 3.80: Tracheal view with the entry of the azygos *(solid arrow)* vein visible. *a1,* ascending thoracic aorta; *a2,* descending thoracic aorta; *da,* ductus arteriosus; *notched arrow,* trachea; *pa,* pulmonary artery; *svc,* superior vena cava.

to the vertebral body and to the right of both the pulmonary artery and the aorta.

In addition to the axial views described earlier, the course of the great arteries can also be defined using longitudinal views of the chest (aortic and ductal arch views). Since the two lie close to each other, it is important to be able to differentiate them on the basis of their morphology. The ductal arch is formed by the DA as it travels from its origin at the pulmonary artery to the point of entry into the descending aorta. Its distinguishing features include a relatively flat shape ("hockey stick") and the fact that it does not give off any branches. The aortic arch, on the other hand, is more rounded (like a candy cane) and gives off branch vessels from its superior aspect (brachiocephalic, left common carotid, and left subclavian arteries) (Fig. 3.81).

Short axis views are defined as the views at right angles to the longitudinal axis of the IVS. The two views that are most

helpful are a cross section of the ventricles and a cross section at the level of the aortic valve. The easiest method for obtaining short axis views is to first obtain the four-chamber view and then rotate the transducer at right angles to the longitudinal axis of the heart.

As mentioned earlier, the short axis view of the ventricles is useful for defining right and left ventricular morphology (see Fig. 3.71). Also, sweeping the entire ventricular septum in this view while employing color Doppler ultrasound is helpful for the detection of VSDs.

A short axis view at the level of the aortic valve is very informative. However, it needs to be kept in mind that the components of this view change depending on even slight adjustments in angulation of the transducer. Nonetheless, the aortic valve ring should always be seen in a transverse section and should be located in the center of the image. The structures of

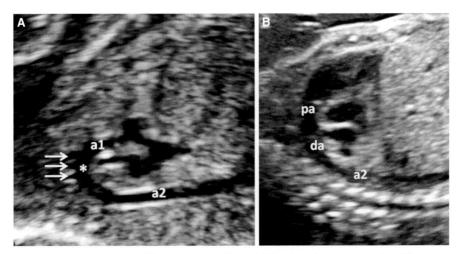

FIGURE 3.81: Axial views of the aortic **(A)** and ductal **(B)** arches demonstrating the difference in shape between the two. *Asterisk,* aortic arch; *a1,* ascending thoracic aorta; *a2,* descending thoracic aorta; *da,* ductus arteriosus; *pa,* pulmonary artery; *solid arrows,* three branches of the aortic arch.

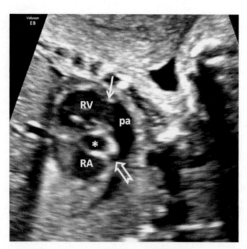

FIGURE 3.82: Short axis view at the level of the aortic valve. *Asterisk,* aortic valve annulus; *notched arrow,* right pulmonary artery; *pa,* pulmonary artery; *RA,* right atrium; *RV,* right ventricle; *solid arrow,* pulmonary valve annulus.

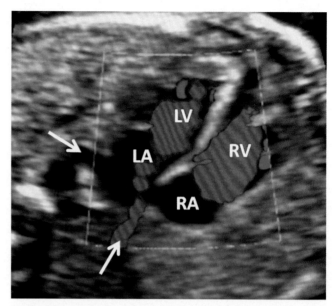

FIGURE 3.84: Axial view of the four-chamber heart with right and left pulmonary veins *(arrows)* visible entering the left atrium *(LA)* during diastole. Color Doppler is used to improve the ease of visualization. *LV,* left ventricle; *RA,* right atrium; *RV,* right ventricle.

the right heart are organized radially around the aortic valve: The upper portion of the right ventricle and the longitudinal view of the right outflow tract are located anteriorly; the right pulmonary artery wraps around the aortic root; the superior portion of the right atrium is located to the right of the aortic root and posteriorly to the right ventricle (Fig. 3.82). Since both the aortic and the pulmonary valves are seen in the same view, comparison of their relative size can be readily performed.

The venous connections of the heart also should be examined. The SVC and IVC are relatively large and are readily identifiable using grayscale ultrasound. The SVC can be seen on axial views of the chest (see Figs. 3.1, 3.77 to 3.80). Of note is that the azygos vein can be identified at its point of entry into the posterior aspect of the SVC in this view (see Fig. 3.80). Significant enlargement of this vessel indicates an interruption of IVC. In the longitudinal view, both the SVC and the IVC can be identified as they enter the right atrium. The DV can frequently be seen entering the IVC anteriorly just before its entry into the right atrium (Fig. 3.83).

The pulmonary veins are much smaller than the IVC and SVC; therefore, they are much more difficult to visualize with grayscale imaging. Color Doppler ultrasound (with a low pulse repetition frequency [PFR] setting) is very helpful. Normally, there are four pulmonary veins that enter the left atrium. Usually, it is the left and right lower veins that are seen on the four-chamber view, and it is reasonable to expect to be able to identify connection of only these two. The pulmonary veins may become confluent behind the left atrium without being connected, and it is important to demonstrate flow into the atria, not merely flow behind the atria (Fig. 3.84). In a total anomalous pulmonary venous drainage, the pulmonary veins cannot be seen connecting to the left atrium.

Diaphragm

The diaphragm forms the division between the abdomen and the chest. It is identified and examined most easily utilizing sweeping longitudinal and coronal views (Figs. 3.85 and 3.86). The diaphragm is a thin, hypoechoic, membrane-like structure that may be difficult to clearly visualize on ultrasound. If not directly visualized, the presence of the diaphragm may be implied by a clearly defined interface between the lungs and the intra-abdominal contents. If this border appears blurred, detailed examination of the diaphragm is indicated, and the relative levels of the intra-abdominal organs with respect to the heart should be determined. There should be no abdominal structures visible in a transverse view of the chest at the level of the four-chamber heart.

The coronal view offers the additional advantage of viewing both domes of the diaphragm at the same time. This is an important view for establishing that they are at approximately the same level. In some fetal disorders, such as eventration, both domes are present, but one is significantly higher than the other. Flattening or even inversion of the diaphragm may be seen in association with congenital upper airway obstruction.

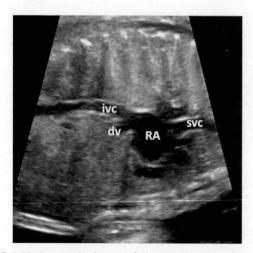

FIGURE 3.83: Longitudinal view of the superior and inferior venae cavae *(svc* and *ivc,* respectively) entering the right atrium *(RA).* Note the entry of the ductus venosus *(dv)* into the anterior aspect of the IVC.

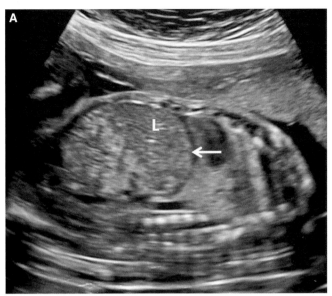
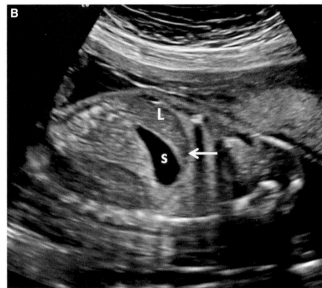

FIGURE 3.85: Longitudinal views of the right **(A)** and left **(B)** domes of the diaphragm *(arrows)*. *L*, liver; *s*, stomach.

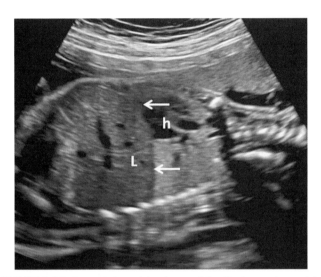

FIGURE 3.86: Coronal view of the dome of the diaphragm *(arrows)*. *h*, heart; *L*, liver.

Abdomen and Pelvis

During the morphology scan, the abdomen and pelvis are traditionally examined in four main axial planes. The landmarks used to assess the upper abdomen and to obtain the proper level for an AC measurement are the stomach, a portion of the umbilical vein, the portal sinus, and a portion of the right portal vein (RPV) (the so-called J sign). A true axial section is verified by ensuring that a single rib is visible through its length rather than a number of ribs cut in cross section. The adrenal glands are often seen in this section (Fig. 3.87). However, visualization of any portion of the kidneys indicates an improper plane for AC measurement. Moving caudally, the next axial section is taken at the level of the renal pelves. The kidneys are best visualized with the fetal back being closest to the transducer, and the probe should be manipulated to achieve this whenever possible. The next axial section is at the level of the umbilical cord, and is used to document the integrity of the anterior abdominal wall. Defects at the umbilicus

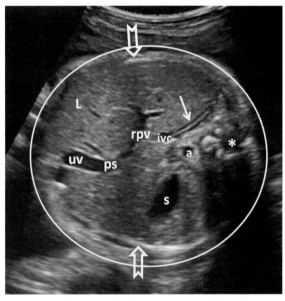

FIGURE 3.87: Axial view of the upper abdomen in the late second trimester at the level of the abdominal circumference *(circle)*. *a*, aorta; *asterisk*, vertebra; *ivc*, inferior vena cava; *L*, liver; *notched arrows*, ribs along their longitudinal axis; *ps*, portal sinus; *rpv*, right portal vein; *s*, stomach; *solid arrow*, adrenal; *uv*, hepatic portion of the umbilical vein.

can be subtle, so care needs to be taken to visualize this clearly. Finally, an axial section of the pelvis, showing the bladder and, with color Doppler ultrasound, the umbilical arteries around its lateral margins, should be recorded. In real time, these views can be linked by sweeping the probe through the abdomen and the pelvis. This allows the sonographer to identify any cystic or solid masses within the abdomen and to determine whether the bowel is abnormally echogenic. Some intra-abdominal anomalies, such as duodenal atresia or obstruction of the bowel, are not readily visualized at the time of the 20-week scan. Assessment of intra-abdominal anatomy during any third-trimester scan is therefore worthwhile.

In an axial section of the upper abdomen, the liver fills the right upper abdominal quadrant, and the stomach is seen on the left. The liver is homogeneous and slightly less echogenic than the lung. There are three interconnected vessels coursing through the liver, which are large enough to be easily visualized using grayscale ultrasound only: the intrahepatic portion of the umbilical vein, the RPV, and the portal sinus located between the two. The umbilical vein enters the abdomen at the abdominal cord insertion and courses a short distance through the falciform ligament to the anterior and inferior edge of the liver. It then courses obliquely in a posterior and caudal direction along the inferior aspect of the liver (Fig. 3.88). It changes into the portal sinus after the junction with the inferior left portal vein (LPV). The portal sinus ends at the point of origin of the RPV. The portal sinus and the RPV form a J-like shape in the axial section. Additional branches originate from the portal sinus (superior LPV, extrahepatic portal vein, and the DV), all of which are difficult to see without the aid of color Doppler ultrasound (Fig. 3.89). The DV originates at the point where the portal sinus takes a sharp bend toward the right. It travels in a posterior and cephalad direction without giving off any branches until it joins the IVC. The course that it takes is more directly cephalad than is the direction of the hepatic portion of the umbilical vein.[133]

Detailed analysis of hepatic vasculature is not part of the routine 20-week scan. Despite this, it is important to have a good understanding of hepatic vasculature (Figs. 3.88 to 3.90), as identification and assessment of the DV is necessary for assessment of cardiovascular compensation and then decompensation in the severely growth-restricted fetus. Pulse wave Doppler evaluation of the DV normally shows forward flow throughout the cardiac cycle. In the later stage of intrauterine growth restriction, as the myocardium becomes hypoxic and dysfunctional, resistance to atrial filling increases and reversal of the DV a-wave is seen. Additionally, this investigation can lead to the rare diagnosis of congenital absence of the DV, a condition that has an increased risk of poor perinatal outcome.

Moving the probe a fraction caudally from the axial section of the upper abdomen brings another elongated cystic structure

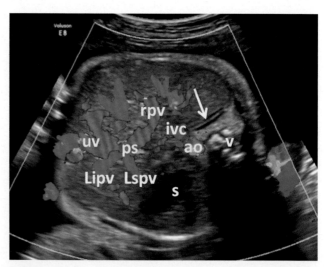

FIGURE 3.89: Anatomy of the hepatic portion of the umbilical vein and portal circulation in an axial section. Additional portions of the hepatic circulation are also seen. *ao*, aorta; *ivc*, inferior vena cava; *Lipv*, left inferior portal vein; *Lspv*, left superior portal vein; *ps*, portal sinus; *rpv*, right portal vein; *s*, stomach; *solid arrow*, adrenal; *uv*, umbilical vein; *v*, vertebra.

that runs along the inferior surface of the liver into view. The gallbladder is pear-like in shape, with the stem pointing toward the hepatic hilum (porta hepatis).[134] It is usually located between the right and the left hepatic lobes, and is located to the right of the intrahepatic portion of the umbilical vein and portal sinus (Fig. 3.91). On grayscale, the appearance of the vascular structures and the gallbladder can be fairly similar. However, color Doppler ultrasound can be used to distinguish between them by identifying flow in the vessels.

Congenital persistence of the right umbilical vein will lead to the intrahepatic portion of the umbilical vein being located to the right of the gallbladder (Fig. 3.92). This is not an uncommon finding (1:500 to 1:1,000) and is of no clinical significance when isolated. However, it does increase the risk of extrahepatic abnormalities such as cardiac and renal defects being present. As a normal variant, the gallbladder may also contain septations or have an unusual shape such as the "Phrygian cap"

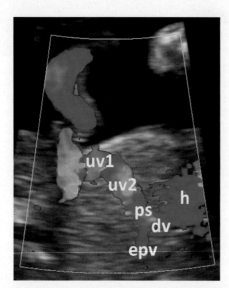

FIGURE 3.88: Anatomy of the hepatic portion of the umbilical vein and portal circulation in a longitudinal view. *dv*, ductus venosus; *epv*, extrahepatic portal vein; *h*, heart; *ps*, portal sinus; *uv1*, intra-abdominal portion of the umbilical vein; *uv2*, intrahepatic portion of the umbilical vein.

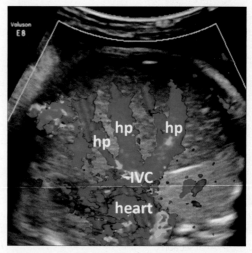

FIGURE 3.90: Color Doppler demonstrating the three hepatic veins *(hp)* in an axial oblique view of the liver. *IVC*, inferior vena cava.

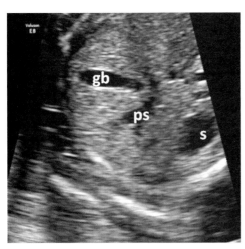

FIGURE 3.91: Axial section of the upper abdomen demonstrating a gallbladder *(gb)* in its normal location to the right of the portal sinus *(ps)*. *s,* stomach.

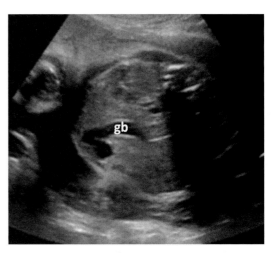

FIGURE 3.93: Axial section of the upper abdomen demonstrating a Phrygian cap gallbladder *(gb)*.

gallbladder (Fig. 3.93). The gallbladder is congenitally absent in 1:1,000 infants. Nonvisualization on prenatal ultrasound is usually a transient finding due to variable and intermittent emptying of biliary contents. However, a persistently absent gallbladder may be indicative of congenital hepatic problems, such as biliary atresia. Occasionally, in the third trimester, the gallbladder contains echogenic structures, which are consistent with sludge or gallstones (Fig. 3.94). These generally resolve in the neonatal period and are of limited clinical significance. Occasionally, a calcification can be seen at the periphery of the liver (Fig. 3.95). As an isolated finding, these are usually of no clinical significance.

The fetal stomach is normally located in the left upper quadrant of the abdomen. Its normal ultrasound appearance is that of an elongated cystic structure with uniformly hypoechoic contents (see Figs. 3.85, 3.87, 3.91, 3.92, and 3.94). However, the contents occasionally include structures with increased echogenicity,

which usually represent swallowed intra-amniotic debris such as blood (Fig. 3.96). Small echogenic foci may be seen associated with the gastric wall (Fig. 3.97). These are of unclear etiology and have been shown not to be associated with an increase in adverse fetal outcome.

The stomach varies in size depending on fetal swallowing and gastric emptying. Nonvisualization or enlargement of the stomach is typically transient, and serial examination may help in elucidating any abnormality. If obstruction is suspected, then assessment of the amniotic fluid index (AFI) may also be helpful to determine whether there is concurrent polyhydramnios. Obstruction may not become apparent until the fetus is swallowing more actively in the late second or third trimester.[135,136]

The spleen is located in the left upper quadrant of the abdomen along the periphery of the stomach. In the axial section, it is roughly oval in shape (Fig. 3.98). The spleen has echogenicity similar to the liver and, as such, is often difficult to clearly delineate

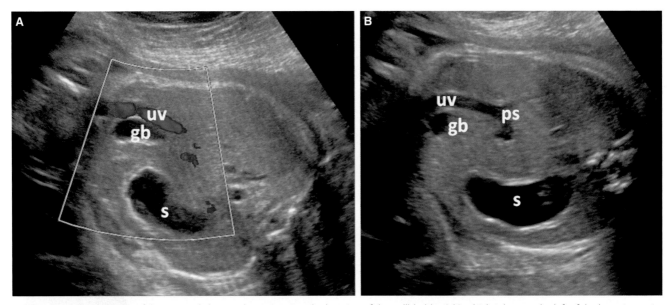

FIGURE 3.92: Axial section of the upper abdomen demonstrating the location of the gallbladder *(gb)*, which is here to the left of the hepatic portion of the umbilical vein *(uv)*. **(A and B)** The direction of the curvature of the portal sinus *(ps)* is to the left **(B)** rather than in its usual direction. These findings are indicative of persistent right umbilical vein. *s,* stomach.

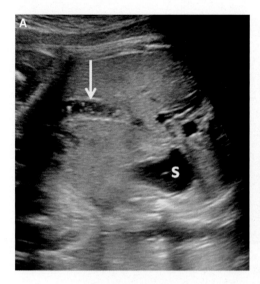

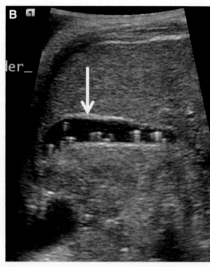

FIGURE 3.94: A and B: Axial sections of the upper abdomen demonstrating a gallbladder *(arrows)* with multiple small luminal echogenicities, which are suggestive of either gallstones or sludge **(B, magnified view)**. *s*, stomach.

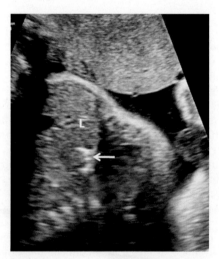

FIGURE 3.95: Sagittal view of the liver *(L)* of a fetus in the late second trimester. An isolated calcification of the liver capsule *(arrow)* is seen.

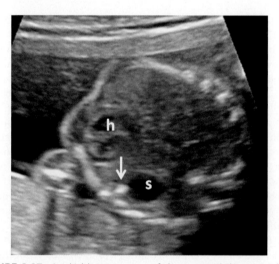

FIGURE 3.97: Axial/oblique section of the upper abdomen and the lower chest demonstrating a perigastric echogenic focus *(arrow)*. *h*, heart; *s*, stomach.

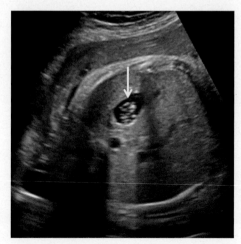

FIGURE 3.96: Axial section of the upper abdomen demonstrating a stomach *(arrow)* filled with echogenic debris.

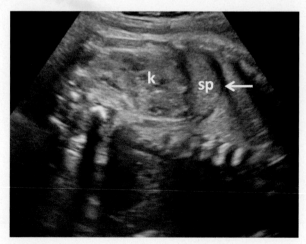

FIGURE 3.98: Longitudinal view of the left side of a fetus in the late second trimester. *Arrow*, diaphragm; *k*, kidney; *sp*, spleen.

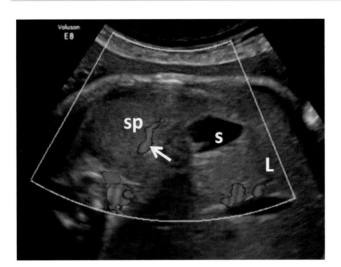

FIGURE 3.99: Axial view of the upper portion of the abdomen in a fetus in the late second trimester. Please note the similarity in echogenicity of the spleen *(sp)* and the liver *(L). Arrow,* splenic artery; *s,* stomach.

(Fig. 3.99). It is not routinely evaluated at 20 weeks' gestation, but an attempt to image it should be made in circumstances where polysplenia or asplenia is suspected.[137]

The fetal adrenals are also imaged within the upper abdomen, and can be often seen in the AC view (Fig. 3.100; see Figs. 3.87 and 3.89).[138] As such, it is often visualized during the 20-week anomaly scan, though a formal assessment is normally done only if a mass is discovered in this area. The adrenal gland is draped as a pyramidal structure over the upper pole of the kidney. Therefore, an axial view of the cephalic tip of the kidney can result in an image of the adrenal with a highly echogenic center. This is an artifact resulting from the anatomic relationship of the two organs and not an adrenal hemorrhage. A longitudinal view of the kidney and adrenal resolves this question: The interface

between the two organs can be visualized in this section, and the appearance of the adrenal can be evaluated independently of the kidney (Fig. 3.101).

Moving caudally, the kidneys are also imaged in axial section. They are in a posterior, retroperitoneal location next to the spine. Their visualization may be compromised by several factors, including the decreased penetration of ultrasound if scanning from the anterior aspect of the fetus, and one or the other kidney being obscured by the spine if scanning from the lateral aspect of the fetus. Similar to the first trimester, kidneys in the mid-second trimester are homogeneous and only slightly more

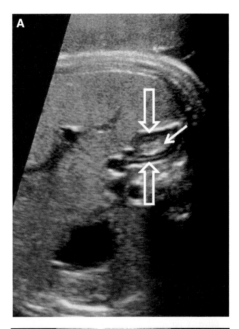

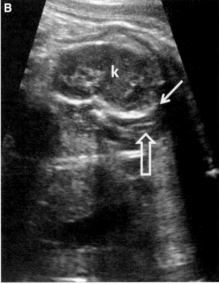

FIGURE 3.101: A: Axial view of the upper portion of the abdomen of the same fetus as in Figure 3.100. However, the section is slightly more caudal in location and includes the renal capsule over the superior pole of the kidney *(solid arrow),* which is surrounded by normal adrenal parenchyma *(open arrows).* This should not be mistaken for an adrenal hemorrhage. **B:** Longitudinal view of the same region depicting the anatomic relationship of the renal capsule *(solid arrow)* and the adrenal *(open arrow)* that produces the artifact presented in **(A).** Note that the adrenal gland is partially obscured by rib shadowing. *k,* kidney.

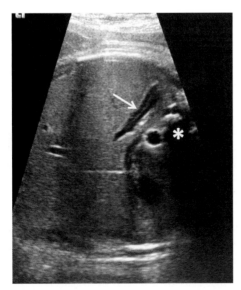

FIGURE 3.100: Axial view of the upper portion of the abdomen in a fetus in the early third trimester demonstrating the normal adrenal gland *(arrow)* appearance. The thin echogenic line located in the middle of the adrenal is a normal finding. *Asterisk,* vertebra.

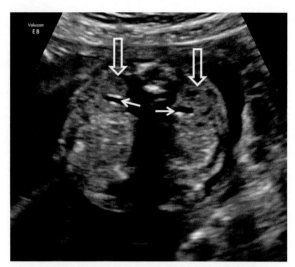

FIGURE 3.102: Axial view of the abdomen at the level of the renal pelves *(solid arrows)* in a midtrimester fetus. Please note that the echogenicity of the kidneys *(open arrows)* is very similar to that of the surrounding structures.

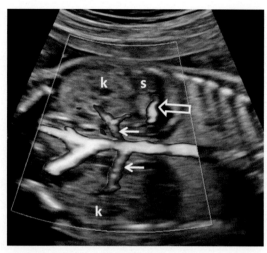

FIGURE 3.104: Coronal view of both kidneys *(k)* in a midtrimester fetus demonstrating the presence of renal vessels *(solid arrows)* bilaterally with color Doppler. *Open arrow*, splenic artery; *s*, spleen.

echogenic than neighboring structures, making them difficult to delineate (Fig. 3.102). In addition to scanning the kidneys with the ultrasound probe being pointed toward the fetal back, employing coronal and longitudinal views may be very helpful in establishing the presence of the kidneys (Fig. 3.103). Similarly, color Doppler ultrasound can be used to help define the renal vessels, which also helps in distinguishing renal presence versus absence (Fig. 3.104). The renal cortex becomes less echogenic in the third trimester, and the capsule is more sharply delineated, making them easier to see (Fig. 3.105). The surface of the kidney is often undulating in contour, consistent with fetal lobulations (Fig. 3.106).[139,140]

The renal hilum is located on the medial side of the kidney. The renal pelvis is located at the hilum and can be identified on ultrasound as a small, slit-like structure with anechoic content (see Figs. 3.102 and 3.105). Although the kidneys are not normally measured during the course of the 20-week anomaly scan, charts of measurements of the kidney throughout the

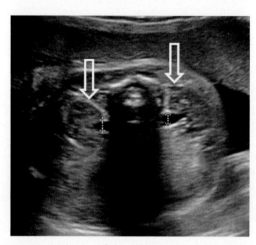

FIGURE 3.105: Axial view of the abdomen at the level of the renal pelves *(calipers)* in a third-trimester fetus. The renal parenchyma is now more hypoechoic as compared with Figure 3.102, and the renal capsule *(arrows)* is better defined and increased in echogenicity.

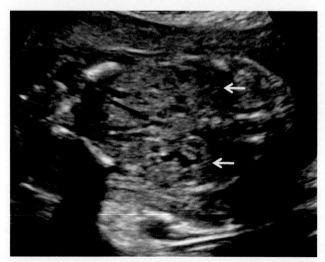

FIGURE 3.103: Coronal view of both kidneys in a midtrimester fetus *(arrows,* upper renal poles). The echogenicity of the kidneys is very similar to that of the surrounding structures.

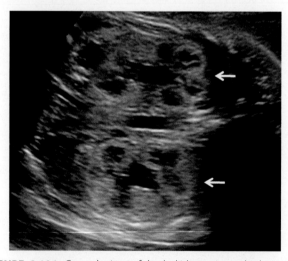

FIGURE 3.106: Coronal view of both kidneys in a third-trimester fetus. The hypoechoic structures within the renal parenchyma are renal pyramids with the surrounding cortical projections that are more echogenic. Also note the slightly undulating contour of the surface of the kidneys, consistent with fetal lobulations. *Arrows*, upper renal poles.

gestation are available. The renal pelvis is typically assessed in AP diameter and is commonly measured, as mild pyelectasis (measurement ≥4 mm) is recognized as a potential marker for trisomy 21 (see Fig. 3.105). This is, however, a weak marker of limited value within the context of modern screening strategies. However, pyelectasis, especially if associated with caliectasis, requires follow-up later in pregnancy and after delivery, as in some cases these can become clinically significant. A wide variety of renal abnormalities may be seen during the 20-week scan, or become apparent at later gestations. It is important to ensure that both kidneys are properly assessed and to remember that it is not uncommon for a fetus with one renal anomaly to have another problem affecting the contralateral kidney.[141-143]

Each kidney should be evaluated along its entire length in either a longitudinal or coronal section. Occasionally, isolated renal cysts may be present. These are generally not clinically significant but rarely may be an early sign of autosomal dominant polycystic kidney disease. It is important to include a sweep through the entire length of the kidney, as the cysts may be isolated. Large cysts are readily defined and are hypoechoic. Highly echogenic kidneys should undergo careful evaluation and follow-up. This finding may be due to perinatal type of polycystic kidney disease, which is a serious problem with a grave prognosis. In these circumstances, the kidneys are enlarged and diffusely echogenic, and the normal internal anatomy is absent. However, occasionally the renal parenchyma will be noted as highly echogenic, but the anatomy is otherwise normal as is the renal size (Fig. 3.107). The prognosis in these cases is generally good, but the risk of poor renal function later in childhood is increased.

The renal pyramids become better delineated as the pregnancy progresses. They are seen as hypoechoic structures surrounded by echogenic cortical projections, containing the straight tubules of the nephrons (see Fig. 3.106). Understanding that this represents normal architecture, especially in the third trimester, helps to prevent the incorrect diagnosis of renal cysts from being made.

Renal agenesis may be unilateral or bilateral. Unilateral renal agenesis does not normally complicate the postnatal period, and the amniotic fluid volume around the fetus is typically normal. The contralateral kidney is often enlarged, which appears to be a compensatory change. It is important to remember that an empty renal fossa does not necessarily mean that the kidney is absent; it may be present in an ectopic location, most commonly in the pelvis. Therefore, the finding of an empty renal fossa should always first lead to a careful search for a kidney in an unusual location. Fetuses with bilateral renal agenesis develop anhydramnios by mid-gestation. The absence of fluid around the fetus reduces the quality of imaging and makes the decision whether or not kidneys are absent that much more difficult. In the presence of anhydramnios, it is especially important to employ all views of the fetal abdomen (axial, longitudinal, and coronal) as well as undertake a detailed search for the kidneys in ectopic locations. This should also include an attempt to identify renal arteries using color Doppler ultrasound. This is best accomplished by scanning through the aorta and IVC in a coronal section.

Ureters are not normally visible during a prenatal scan. An obstructed, dilated ureter appears as a convoluted hypoechoic tubular structure; therefore, a cross section of a significantly dilated ureter will often have the appearance of multiple anechoic cysts. Common causes of pelvic and ureteral dilatation include vesicoureteral reflux and ureteral obstruction. Both of these problems can also be associated with renal duplication. Therefore, abnormal ureteral findings should always lead to a careful examination of the renal hilum (looking for a duplicated collecting system) and the urinary bladder (looking for a ureterocele), both of which can be seen in renal duplication.[142-145] A hypoechoic structure extending from the lower portion of the kidney to the pelvis is frequently noted in longitudinal views. This represents the psoas muscle and should not be mistaken for a prominent ureter (Fig. 3.108).

Defects of the anterior abdominal wall can occur anywhere along the midline but are most common at the level of the umbilicus. Therefore, the abdominal cord insertion should be clearly imaged. Although this is typically done in a transverse section, it may also be achieved with a midsagittal view (Fig. 3.109). Herniation of abdominal contents into the root of the umbilical cord beyond 12 weeks' gestation is never normal and constitutes an omphalocele. While an omphalocele has a membranous covering, and the umbilical cord is noted to insert

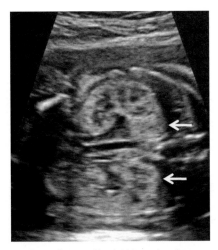

FIGURE 3.107: Coronal view of both kidneys in a late second-trimester fetus. The echogenicity of the renal parenchyma is increased. However, the normal renal architecture, including the hypoechoic pyramids, is preserved, and the kidneys are not enlarged. *Arrows*, upper renal poles.

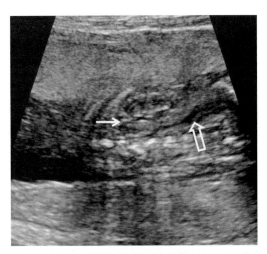

FIGURE 3.108: Longitudinal and slightly oblique view of the right kidney. The psoas muscle *(open arrow)* is clearly visible and should not be mistaken for a dilated ureter. *Solid arrow*, upper renal pole.

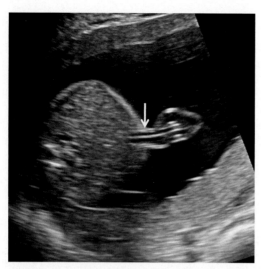

FIGURE 3.109: An axial view of the fetal abdomen at the level of the abdominal cord insertion *(arrow)*.

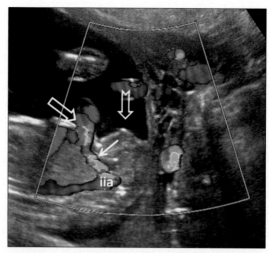

FIGURE 3.111: A longitudinal view of the umbilical cord insertion *(open arrow)* and the course of the intra-abdominal portion of the umbilical artery *(solid arrow)* to the point of its origin from the internal iliac artery *(iia)*. This is a female fetus *(notched arrow)*.

directly into this membranous sac, gastroschisis is an open abdominal wall defect located immediately to the right of an otherwise normal abdominal cord insertion. This diagnosis is also made in a transverse section, but in contrast to an omphalocele, the protruding bowel in a gastroschisis does not have a covering membrane and is free-floating in the amniotic fluid.

The umbilical cord normally contains a single vein, which carries oxygenated blood to the fetus and two arteries, which return deoxygenated blood to the placenta. These vessels are encased in Wharton jelly up to the point where the cord meets the anterior abdominal wall. A detailed discussion regarding the umbilical cord is included in Chapter 13.1. The umbilical vessels separate within the fetal abdomen. The umbilical vein first courses along the anterior abdominal wall in a cephalad direction and then enters the liver, following a course as described earlier. Between the umbilical cord insertion and the liver, the size of the umbilical vein is variable. If it is excessively large, it is termed a varix. This finding has been associated with other fetal anomalies and poor perinatal outcome. From the umbilical cord insertion, the direction of umbilical arteries is in the posterior and inferior direction around the bladder (Fig. 3.110). They originate from the internal

iliac arteries (Fig. 3.111). Following delivery, the segments of the umbilical arteries that bridge the distance between the dome of the bladder and the cord insertion become obliterated and become the medial umbilical ligaments. The remaining portions of the umbilical arteries stay patent and become the superior vesical arteries.

The bowel can be examined as the transducer is swept in transverse section from the upper abdomen, through the level of the umbilicus to the pelvis. The appearance of fetal bowel changes with gestation. In the first and early second trimester, the bowel is fairly uniform in appearance, and individual bowel loops are difficult to identify. The overall echogenicity is normally slightly greater and more heterogeneous than that of the liver parenchyma (Fig. 3.112). In the latter half of the second trimester and the third trimester, a variable amount of fluid may be visualized within some of the small bowel loops, and the differentiation between the small and large bowels becomes possible (Figs. 3.113 and 3.114). Under normal circumstances, the amount of fluid

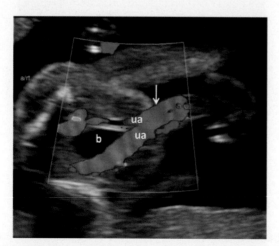

FIGURE 3.110: An axial/oblique view of the fetal lower abdomen and pelvis demonstrating the two umbilical arteries *(ua)* coursing from the abdominal cord insertion *(arrow)* around the bladder *(b)*.

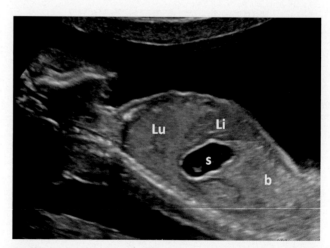

FIGURE 3.112: A longitudinal view of the torso and abdomen in the mid-second trimester demonstrating the differences in echogenicity of the lung *(Lu)*, liver *(Li)*, and the bowel *(b)*. Note the homogeneous appearance of the bowel. *s*, stomach.

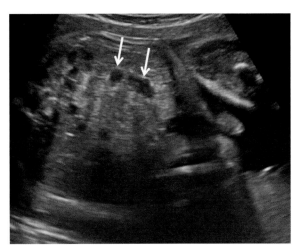

FIGURE 3.113: Transverse/oblique view of the fetal abdomen in the third trimester. Note the multiple hypoechoic spaces *(arrows)* representing fluid-filled small bowel loops. This is a normal finding in the third trimester.

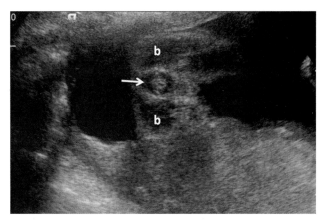

FIGURE 3.115: Transverse view of the anus *(arrow)*. The anal sphincter is hypoechoic, forming a ring around the anus, known as the "target sign." *b,* buttocks.

within the small bowel is relatively small. However, small bowel dilatation, defined as a diameter >6 mm,[146] may be indicative of bowel pathology such as jejunal or ileal atresia. The bowel may be abnormally echogenic, appearing as bright as bone, during the 20-week scan. This is most commonly due to a benign cause such as intra-amniotic bleeding, where the fetus has swallowed blood-stained amniotic fluid. However, it can also be associated with fetal aneuploidy, fetal hypoxia, intrauterine growth restriction, cystic fibrosis, meconium ileus, and fetal infection. The colon is identifiable on prenatal ultrasound consistently from 24 weeks onward. Its diameter is variable but tends to be significantly greater than the small bowel. The contents have greater echogenicity than those of the small bowel. The dilated large bowel may be associated with obstruction or neurological diseases affecting the bowel wall. Significantly increased echogenicity of the large colon contents may be associated with disease processes such as cystic fibrosis. Occasionally, the rectum is seen to have anechoic contents, which is a normal finding. The anus and the

anal sphincter can be identified readily as a hypoechoic ring with an echogenic center on careful examination of the posterior fetal pelvis (Fig. 3.115).[146-149]

The urinary bladder is visualized as an anechoic cystic structure within the fetal pelvis (Fig. 3.116; see Fig. 3.110). The size of the bladder is highly variable and dependent on the amount of fetal urine production and output at any point in time. After emptying, the bladder may be difficult to visualize, but this is normally a transient issue. Sustained absence of the urinary bladder throughout the examination is never a normal finding. If the bladder proves difficult to visualize, color Doppler ultrasound can be used to locate the intra-abdominal portions of the umbilical arteries, and therefore the location where the bladder should be seen (see Fig. 3.110). Persistent absence of a urinary bladder in association with a normal amniotic fluid volume is indicative of rare but serious fetal anomalies such as bladder or cloacal exstrophy. At the other extreme, a large bladder may be observed when there is outflow obstruction. There are a number of potential causes, but in male fetuses a "key hole" appearance with dilatation of the proximal portion of the urethra is indicative of the presence of posterior urethral valves. When an anomaly of the urinary tract is suspected, assessment of the amniotic fluid volume provides valuable information about its functional effect.

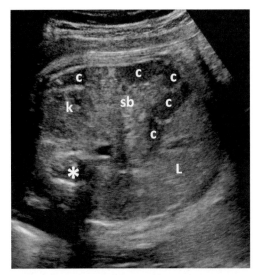

FIGURE 3.114: Transverse/oblique view of the fetal abdomen in the third trimester with the colon *(c)* clearly visible separately from the rest of the abdominal structures. *Asterisk,* vertebra; *k,* kidney; *L,* liver; *sb,* small bowel.

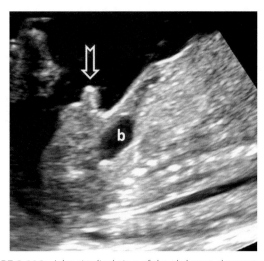

FIGURE 3.116: A longitudinal view of the abdomen demonstrating a normal size bladder *(b)*. This is a male fetus *(arrow)*.

External Genitalia

The gender of the fetus can be determined with a high degree of accuracy by using transverse and midsagittal planes. Accurate definition of fetal gender is important in a number of genetic conditions. It may help define the need for invasive testing in pregnancies at risk of X-linked dominant conditions. Alternatively, it may direct need for therapeutic intervention, for example, steroid therapy to prevent virilization in female fetuses at risk of congenital adrenal hyperplasia.

At the 20-week anomaly scan, the diagnosis of a male depends on demonstration of the penis and scrotum. The penis appears to be short compared with infancy, but this is normal (Fig. 3.117). Charts of penile length have been published if there are concerns about length. Anechoic fluid within the scrotum representing hydroceles is fairly common, and in the absence of hydrops fetalis or ascites, it is not associated with any specific fetal and neonatal problems. One or both testes appear within the scrotum at variable times during the third trimester (Fig. 3.118). Both the penis and the scrotum may also be visualized in the same view in a

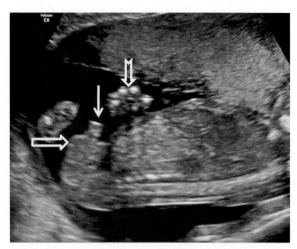

FIGURE 3.119: A sagittal view of external male genitalia in mid-second trimester. *Notched arrow,* transverse view of fingers; *open arrow,* scrotum; *solid arrow,* penis.

sagittal section of the genital area (Fig. 3.119). The fetal urethra is not identifiable under normal circumstances. However, in the presence of posterior urethral valves, the proximal urethra can be very dilated. Also, in the rare instance of a megalourethra, the urethra may be dilated and contain anechoic fluid along its entire length.

The diagnosis of female gender should not be reliant on merely being unable to demonstrate the presence of the penis/scrotum. In transverse section, the swelling of the labial folds can be visualized (Fig. 3.120). The clitoris is best identified in a sagittal section (Fig. 3.121). The labia minora, and later in pregnancy the labia majora, are seen as two elongated somewhat hypoechoic structures with an echogenic line dividing the two (Figs. 3.122 and 3.123). The latter represents the interface between the two labia. The echogenicity of the labia majora is the same as of the fetal skin and, therefore, greater than that of the labia minora.

Identification of fetal gender is made more difficult by several factors such as early gestational age, positioning of the fetal legs close together, umbilical cord coursing between the legs, maternal habitus, and fetal position. In both sagittal and transverse views, care should be taken to ensure the structures visualized represent

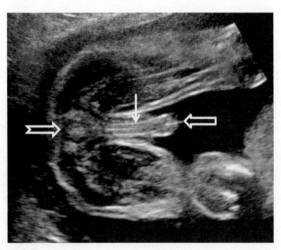

FIGURE 3.117: A transverse view of external male genitalia in mid-second trimester. *Notched arrow,* anus; *open arrow,* penis; *solid arrow,* corpus cavernosum.

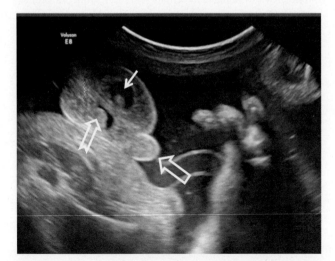

FIGURE 3.118: A coronal/oblique view of external male genitalia in mid-third trimester. *Notched arrow,* testis; *Open arrow,* penis; *solid arrow,* small hydrocele.

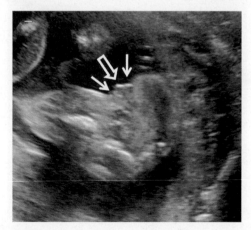

FIGURE 3.120: A transverse view of external female genitalia in mid-second trimester. *Open arrow,* confluence of labia minora; *solid arrows,* labia majora.

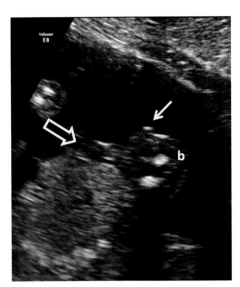

FIGURE 3.121: A sagittal view of external female genitalia in mid-second trimester. *b*, buttock; *open arrow*, abdominal cord insertion; *solid arrow*, clitoris.

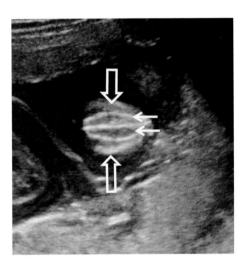

FIGURE 3.122: A transverse view of external female genitalia in early third trimester with prominent labia minora. *Open arrows*, labia majora; *solid arrows*, labia minora.

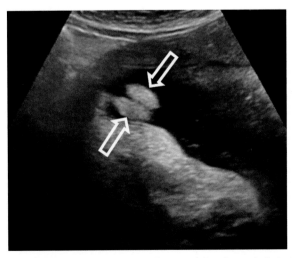

FIGURE 3.123: A transverse view of external female genitalia in late third trimester with only labia majora *(arrows)* visible.

male anatomy and not the rare case of ambiguous genitalia. If the labia majora are especially prominent in the third trimester, they may be erroneously identified as the scrotum. If the labia minora are particularly prominent, especially in the presence of clitoromegaly, the appearance of the external genitalia may be ambiguous. Erroneous assignment of female gender may occur in the presence of severe hypospadias.

Extremities

Careful, systematic sequential examination of the extremities is important as anomalies may affect one or more limbs and be seen at any level. These anomalies are frequently isolated. However, a wide range of fetal problems, including aneuploidy and genetic syndromes, are associated with limb defects. Therefore, a limb anomaly should lead to a careful examination of the rest of the fetal anatomy.[150]

Starting proximally, both humeri and femora should be examined to make sure they are of an appropriate length, are straight with normal mineralization, and have no evidence of fractures (Fig. 3.124). Both the femur and the humerus are measured in exactly the same fashion: The bone is insonated along its longitudinal axis with the ends of the bone being as sharply delineated as possible, and it is measured from one end to the other. In the second trimester, shortening of the humerus has a slightly better predictive value than shortening of the femur when screening for trisomy 21. Moving distally, the forearm or lower leg should contain two long bones, which are also assessed for mineralization and fractures. They are not routinely measured unless an anomaly is suspected. Identification of both bones in the forearm is important, as radial hypoplasia or aplasia is part of the phenotype of a number of syndromes. At the elbow, the ulna is located medially to the radius. Their relative position at the level of the wrist depends on the degree of rotation of the forearm (Fig. 3.125). Many skeletal dysplasias will be defined on the basis of shortening or fracture of long bones, and the pattern of shortening is often important in reaching a firm diagnosis. Unilateral limb deficiencies are rare but can be detected at 20 weeks' gestation. These can involve any portion of the limb; therefore, it is important to always attempt to evaluate each limb in its entirety (Fig. 3.126).

In the presence of normal amniotic fluid volume, the limbs should move freely at each of the joints. Freedom of movement is implied by documentation that the hip, knee, elbow, ankle, and wrist joints are held in normal anatomical positions. Abnormal angulation of the ankle joint (ankle clubbing, talipes equinovarus) is common, with a prevalence of 1 in 100 live births. The most useful view for ruling out this diagnosis is a coronal section of the ankle. The ankle normally extends straight along the same axis as the lower leg (Fig. 3.127). However, in the presence of ankle clubbing, the ankle deviates medially. The longitudinal view is also useful to evaluate the relationship between the lower leg and the ankle. Slight angulation of the ankle is common, especially in the third trimester due to intrauterine crowding (Fig. 3.128). Two findings help to differentiate positional angulation of the ankles from true clubbing. Firstly, the angulation of the ankle due to positional changes is not as severe as with true clubbing. Secondly, a clubbed ankle stays in a fixed position and never straightens out. Unilateral ankle clubbing is generally an isolated defect. However, bilateral clubbing can be seen in association with chromosomal or genetic conditions.

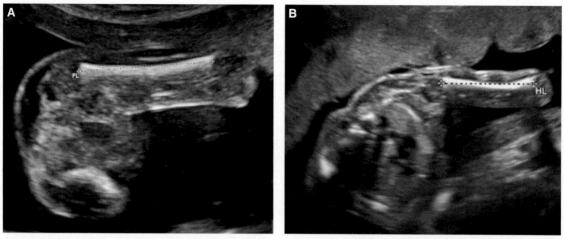

FIGURE 3.124: Longitudinal views of femur (*FL* in **A**) and humerus (*HL* in **B**). *Calipers* denote their measurements.

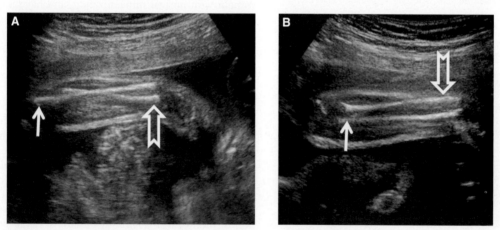

FIGURE 3.125: Views of ulna *(solid arrow)* and radius *(notched arrow)*. **A:** The bones are crossed during pronation. **B:** The bones are parallel in a supine position.

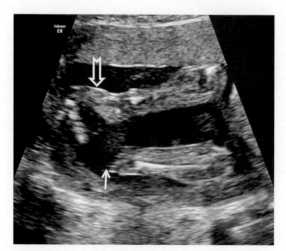

FIGURE 3.126: Longitudinal view of both forearms with a normal left hand *(notched arrow)* and a completely absent right hand *(solid arrow)*.

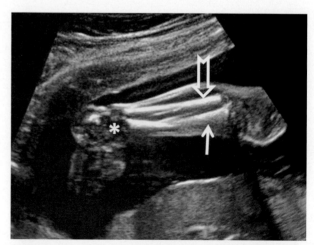

FIGURE 3.127: Coronal view of the lower leg and the ankle *(asterisk)*. The edges of the ankle are a fairly straight continuation of the lower leg, ruling out ankle clubbing. *Notched arrow*, fibula; *solid arrow*, tibia.

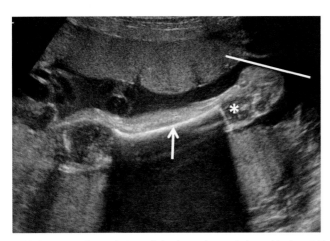

FIGURE 3.128: Coronal view of the lower leg and the ankle *(asterisk)*. Please note that the ankle is straight but the foot is turned in (*solid line* is parallel to the sole of the foot). This is related to fetal position rather than clubbing. *Arrow,* tibia.

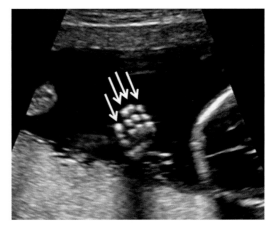

FIGURE 3.130: Image of four fingers *(arrows)* with all three phalangeal ossification centers visible in each digit.

The wrist is very flexible and may be seen in a variety of positions. The position of the fingers is also variable. In a resting position, the fingers often form a fist, but the hand can be stimulated to open, showing all four fingers and thumb (Fig. 3.129). Unlike in the first trimester, in the second and third trimesters the thumb is visible in a different plane from the rest of the fingers (Fig. 3.130). The most consistently reliable method for counting the fingers is in a transverse section that lines up the proximal phalanges or their respective metacarpals in a row (Fig. 3.131). Polydactyly is more common in some ethnic groups, such as African Americans. It may be seen in isolation and may affect both hands and feet. Both abnormal number of fingers or abnormal position of fingers (e.g., camptodactyly or clinodactyly) are associated with an increased risk of an underlying fetal syndrome. Fingers also can be missing, often due to the amniotic band syndrome. However, certain rare syndromes such as ectrodactyly–ectodermal dysplasia–cleft syndrome are associated with missing fingers as well.

The foot is best imaged with a superficial transverse section showing the heel, sole, and toes (Fig. 3.132). The position of the big toe with respect to the other toes can be evaluated for a "sandal gap" anomaly, which has a weak association with trisomy 21. The length of the foot can also be assessed in the same view. This is

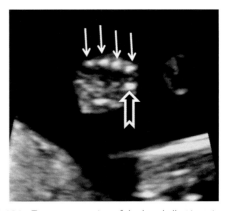

FIGURE 3.131: Transverse section of the hand allowing visualization of the phalanges of all four fingers *(solid arrows)* and the thumb *(notched arrow)* in the same view.

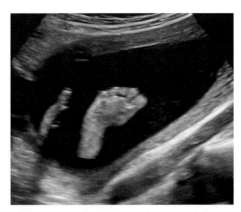

FIGURE 3.132: Superficial transverse section of the foot with all five toes evident.

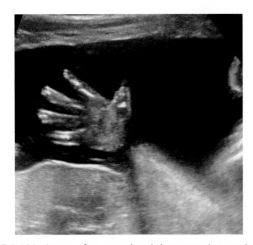

FIGURE 3.129: Image of an open hand demonstrating portions of all five fingers.

especially useful in assessment of skeletal dysplasias, where the femur is short but the foot length is typically preserved; therefore, the femur to foot length ratio will be significantly decreased (0.9). A normal ratio will be preserved in a fetus with a constitutionally short femur.

The phalangeal and/or metatarsal ossification centers can occasionally be counted in a transverse section (Fig. 3.133).

However, the interfaces between the toes can often be seen as thin echogenic lines and can be mistaken for phalanges (Fig. 3.134). Therefore, toes should also be counted in coronal section (Fig. 3.135). This view has the advantage of presenting the phalanges and/or metatarsals as discrete echogenic points that are easier to define individually. Essentially the same differential diagnosis applies to lower extremity polydactyly or missing toes as to their upper extremity counterparts.

The lower extremities should be visually evaluated for the presence of fluid accumulation since certain syndromes, such as congenital (hereditary) lymphedema, are associated with this finding.

Miscellaneous Bony Structures

There are a number of other bony structures that can be evaluated and/or measured, although this is not normally done as a routine. Extended, specialized examinations are generally performed as needed, based on recognized family history or on other abnormalities that are identified. For example, the fetal clavicles can be readily examined and measured as early as the first trimester (Fig. 3.136; see Fig. 3.11). This evaluation is helpful in those individuals who are at risk for cleidocranial dysplasia. Fetal scapulae are also readily identifiable, and may be of value in defining skeletal dysplasia, where the scapulae may be dysplastic (Fig. 3.137). Defining the anatomy of less commonly examined structures during routine exams helps to familiarize the operator with their typical appearance, experience that is very valuable in the event that they need to be assessed to clarify a diagnosis.

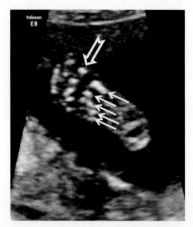

FIGURE 3.133: Transverse section of the foot with five metatarsals *(solid arrows)* and the row of their corresponding digits *(notched arrow)*.

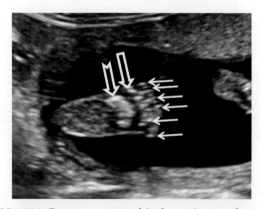

FIGURE 3.134: Transverse section of the foot with a row of metatarsals *(notched arrow)* and a row of digits *(open arrow)* visible. Note the echogenic skin *(solid arrows)* on the surface of the toes, which can often be even more prominent than presented here.

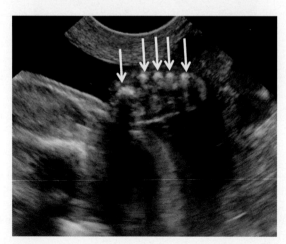

FIGURE 3.135: Coronal section of the foot with all five metatarsals or digits easily identified as separate echogenic dots *(arrows)*.

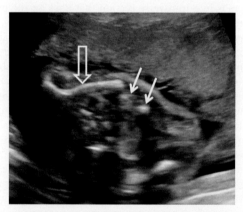

FIGURE 3.136: Axial view of the clavicle *(open arrow)* in the late second trimester. *Solid arrows,* upper portion of the manubrium.

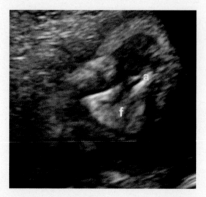

FIGURE 3.137: Coronal/oblique section of the fetal back in late second trimester demonstrating the scapula. *a,* acromion and spina scapulae; *f,* fossa infraspinata.

CONCLUSION

The list of complications that can affect pregnancy outcome is long and varied. Many of these issues can be assessed by a high-quality ultrasound performed by qualified personnel. The effectiveness of ultrasound is improved by taking a systematic approach to the examination. It cannot be overstated that thorough understanding of normal fetal anatomy is the first step toward fetal anomaly detection.[151] It is critical for individual ultrasound centers to perform ongoing audit, which includes a periodic review of image quality for each sonographer and to collect data related to pregnancy outcome. A detailed image review needs to be performed in each case where a fetal anomaly went unrecognized on prenatal ultrasound. If deficiencies are noted on the review, appropriate and prompt changes need to be made to improve techniques and methods of assessment.

REFERENCES

1. Donald I, MacVicar J, Brown TG. Investigation of abdominal masses by pulsed ultrasound. *Lancet.* 1958;1:1188–1195.
2. Donald I, Abdulla U. Ultrasonics in obstetrics and gynaecology. *Br J Radiol.* 1967;40:604–611.
3. Salomon LJ, Alfirevic Z, Berghella V, et al. Practice guidelines for performance of the routine midtrimester fetal ultrasound scan (ISUOG). *Ultrasound Obstet Gynecol.* 2011;37:116–126.
4. American Institute of Ultrasound in Medicine. AIUM-ACR-ACOG-SMFM-SRU Practice Parameter for the Performance of Standard Diagnostic Obstetric Ultrasound Examinations. *J Ultrasound Med.* 2018;37:E13-E24. doi: 10.1002/jum.14831. Epub 2018 Oct 11.
5. American College of Obstetricians and Gynecologists. ACOG Practice Bulletin No. 101: ultrasonography in pregnancy. *Obstet Gynecol.* 2009;113:451–461.
6. Australasian Society for Ultrasound in Medicine. Guidelines, policies and statements—D2: Guidelines for the mid trimester obstetric scan. https://www.asum.com.au/files/public/SoP/curver/Obs-Gynae/Guidelines-for-the-Performance-of-Second-Mid-Trimester-Ultrasound.pdf. Accessed October 23, 2018.
7. National Collaborating Centre for Women's and Children's Health. *Antenatal Care: Routine Care for the Healthy Pregnant Woman.* 2nd ed. London, England: RCOG Press; 2008.
8. Nicolaides KH. Screening for fetal aneuploidy at 11 to 13 weeks. *Prenat Diagn.* 2011;31:7–15.
9. Sonek JD. First trimester ultrasonography in screening and detection of fetal anomalies. *Am J Med Genet C Semin Med Genet.* 2007;145:45–61.
10. Souka AP, Pilalis A, Kavalakis Y, et al. Assessment of fetal anatomy at the 11–14-week ultrasound examination. *Ultrasound Obstet Gynecol.* 2004;24:730–734.
11. Becker R, Wegner RD. Detailed screening for fetal anomalies and cardiac defects at the 11–13 week scan. *Ultrasound Obstet Gynecol.* 2006;27:613–618.
12. Lanchmann R, Chaoui R, Moratalla J, et al. Posterior brain in fetuses with open spina bifida at 11–13 weeks. *Prenat Diagn.* 2011;31:103–106.
13. Poon LCY, Kametas NA, Chelemen T, et al. Maternal risk factors for hypertensive disorders in pregnancy: a multivariate approach. *J Hum Hypertens.* 2010;24:104–110.
14. Brenner WE, Edelman DA, Hendricks CH. A standard of fetal growth for the United States of America. *Am J Obstet Gynecol.* 1976;126:555–564.
15. Campbell S, Thoms A. Ultrasound measurement of fetal head to abdomen circumference ratio in the assessment of growth retardation. *Br J Obstet Gynaecol.* 1977;84:165–174.
16. Hadlock FP, Harrist RB, Martinez-Poyer J. In utero analysis of fetal growth: a sonographic weight standard. *Radiology.* 1991;181:129–133.
17. Robson SC, Gallivan S, Walkinshaw SA, et al. Ultrasonic estimation of fetal weight: use of targeted formulas in small for gestational age fetuses. *Obstet Gynecol.* 1993;82:359–364.
18. David C, Gabrielli S, Pilu G, et al. The head-to-abdomen circumference ratio: a reappraisal. *Ultrasound Obstet Gynecol.* 1995;5:256–259.
19. Gardosi J, Chang A, Kalyan B, et al. Customised antenatal growth charts. *Lancet.* 1992;339:283–287.
20. Clausson B, Gardosi J, Francis A, et al. Perinatal outcome in SGA births defined by customised versus population-based birthweight standards. *Br J Obstet Gynecol.* 2001;108:830–834.
21. Smith-Bindman R, Chu PW, Ecker JL, et al. US evaluation of fetal growth: prediction of neonatal outcomes. *Radiology.* 2002;223:153–161.
22. Nyberg DA, Abuhamad A, Ville Y. Ultrasound assessment of abnormal fetal growth. *Semin Perinatol.* 2004;28:3–22.
23. Bricker L, Neilson JP, Dowswell T. Routine ultrasound in late pregnancy (after 24 weeks' gestation). *Cochrane Database Syst Rev.* 2008;(8):CD001451.
24. Prayer D, Kasparian F, Krampl E, et al. MRI of normal brain development. *Eur J Radiol.* 2006;57:199–216.
25. Eurenius K, Axelsson O, Gallstedt-Fransson I, et al. Perception of information, expectations and experiences among women and their partners attending a second-trimester routine ultrasound scan. *Ultrasound Obstet Gynecol.* 1997;9:86–90.
26. Pike I, Russo A, Berkowitz J, et al. The prevalence of musculoskeletal disorders among diagnostic medical sonographers. *J Diagn Med Sonogr.* 1997;13:219–227.
27. Magnavita N, Bevilacqua L, Mirk P, et al. Work-related musculoskeletal complaints in sonologists. *J Occup Environ Med.* 1999;41:981–988.
28. Stothard KJ, Tennant PW, Bell R, et al. Maternal overweight and obesity and the risk of congenital anomalies: a systematic review and meta-analysis. *JAMA.* 2009;301:636–650.
29. Church CC, Carstensen EL, Nyborg WL, et al. The risk of exposure to diagnostic ultrasound in postnatal subjects: nonthermal mechanisms. *J Ultrasound Med.* 2008;27:565–592.
30. Miller MW, Nyborg WL, Dewey WC, et al. Hyperthermic teratogenicity, thermal dose and diagnostic ultrasound during pregnancy: implications of new standards on tissue heating. *Int J Hyperthermia.* 2002;18:361–384.
31. O'Brien WD Jr, Deng CX, Harris GR, et al. The risk of exposure to diagnostic ultrasound in postnatal subjects: thermal effects. *J Ultrasound Med.* 2008;27:517–535.
32. American Institute of Ultrasound in Medicine. AIUM statement on mammalian biological effects of ultrasonic in vivo. http://www.aium.org/. Revised March, 2015. Accessed December 13, 2018.
33. Fowlkes JB; Bioeffects Committee of the American Institute of Ultrasound in Medicine. American Institute of Ultrasound in Medicine consensus report on potential bioeffects of diagnostic ultrasound. *J Ultrasound Med.* 2008;27:503–515.
34. National Council on Radiation Protection and Measurements. *Exposure Criteria for Medical Ultrasound, II: Criteria Based on All Known Mechanisms.* Bethesda, MD: National Council on Radiation Protection and Measurements; 2002. NCRP report 140.
35. Cavicchi TJ, O'Brien WD. Heat generated by ultrasound in an absorbing medium. *J Acoust Soc Am.* 1984;76:1244–1245.
36. Barnett SB, Rott HD, ter Haar GR, et al. The sensitivity of biological tissue to ultrasound. *Ultrasound Med Biol.* 1997;23:805–812.
37. Hershkovitz R, Sheiner E, Mazor M. Ultrasound in obstetrics: a review of safety. *Eur J Obstet Gynecol Reprod Biol.* 2002;101:15–18.
38. Stark CR, Orleans M, Haverkamp AD, et al. Short- and long-term risks after exposure to diagnostic ultrasound in utero. *Obstet Gynecol.* 1984;63:194–200.
39. Lyons EA, Dyke C, Toms M, et al. In utero exposure to diagnostic ultrasound: a 6-year follow-up. *Radiology.* 1988;166:687–690.
40. Tarantal AF, Hendrickx AG. Evaluation of the bioeffects of prenatal ultrasound exposure in the cynomolgus macaque (*Macaca fascicularis*), II: growth and behavior during the first year. *Teratology.* 1989;39:149–162.
41. Kossoff G. Contentious issues in safety of diagnostic ultrasound. *Ultrasound Obstet Gynecol.* 1997;10:151–155.
42. Rott HD. Clinical safety statement for diagnostic ultrasound: European Committee for Medical Ultrasound Safety, Tours, France, March 1998. *Eur J Ultrasound.* 1998;8:67–68.
43. Zhu J, Lin J, Zhu Z, et al. Effects of diagnostic levels of color Doppler ultrasound energy on the cell cycle of newborn rats. *J Ultrasound Med.* 1999;18:257–260.
44. Ang ES, Gluncic V, Duque A, et al. Prenatal exposure to ultrasound waves impacts neuronal migration in mice. *Proc Natl Acad Sci U S A.* 2006;103:12903–12910.
45. Wax J, Minkoff H, Johnson A, et al. Consensus report on the detailed fetal anatomic ultrasound examination: indications, components, and qualifications. *J Ultrasound Med.* 2014;33(2):189–195. doi:10.7863/ultra.33.2.189.
46. Wax JR, Benacerraf BR, Copel J, et al. Consensus report on the 76811 scan: modification. *J Ultrasound Med.* 2015;34(10):1915. doi:10.7863/ultra.15.09006.
47. Warren WB, Timor-Tritsch I, Peisner DB, et al. Dating the early pregnancy by sequential appearance of embryonic structures. *Am J Obstet Gynecol.* 1989;161:747–753.
48. Sepulveda W, Sebire NJ, Hughes K, et al. The lambda sign at 10–14 weeks of gestation as a predictor of chorionicity in twin pregnancies. *Ultrasound Obstet Gynecol.* 1996;7:421–423.
49. Bowerman RA. Sonography of fetal midgut herniation: normal size criteria and correlation with crown-rump length. *J Ultrasound Med.* 1993;5:251–254.
50. Robinson HP, Fleming JEE. A critical evaluation of sonar "crown-rump length" measurements. *Br J Obstet Gynecol.* 1975;82:702–710.
51. Chalouhi GE, Bernard JP, Ville Y, et al. A comparison of first trimester measurements for prediction of delivery date. *J Matern Fetal Neonatal Med.* 2011;24:51–57.
52. Salomon LJ, Bernard M, Amarsy R, et al. The impact of crown-rump length measurement error on combined Down syndrome screening: a simulation study. *Ultrasound Obstet Gynecol.* 2009;33:506–511.
53. Hadlock FP, Shah YP, Kanon DJ, et al. Fetal crown-rump length: reevaluation of relation to menstrual age (5–18 weeks) with high resolution real-time US. *Radiology.* 1992;182:501–505.
54. Robinson HP. Gestational age determination: first trimester. In: Chervenak FA, Isaacson GC, Campbell S, eds. *Ultrasound in Obstetrics and Gynecology.* Boston, MA: Little, Brown and Company; 1993:295–304.

55. Blaas HG, Eik-Nes SH, Kiserud T, et al. Early development of the abdominal wall, stomach and heart from 7 to 12 weeks of gestation: a longitudinal ultrasound study. *Ultrasound Obstet Gynecol.* 1995;6:240–249.
56. Souka AP, Von Kaisenberg CS, Hyett JA, et al. Increased nuchal translucency with normal karyotype. *Am J Obstet Gynecol.* 2005;192:1005–1021.
57. Sonek J, Nicolaides KH. Additional first trimester ultrasound markers. *Clin Lab Med.* 2010;30:573–592.
58. Rosati P, Guariglia L. Transvaginal sonographic assessment of the fetal urinary tract in early pregnancy. *Ultrasound Obstet Gynecol.* 1996;7:95–100.
59. Haak MC, Twisk JW, Van Vugt JM. How successful is fetal echocardiographic examination in the first trimester of pregnancy? *Ultrasound Obstet Gynecol.* 2002;20:9–13.
60. Liao AW, Sebire NJ, Geerts L, et al. Megacystis at 10–14 weeks of gestation: chromosomal defects and outcome according to bladder length. *Ultrasound Obstet Gynecol.* 2003;21:338–341.
61. Efrat Z, Akinfenwa O, Nicolaides KH. First-trimester determination of fetal gender by ultrasound. *Ultrasound Obstet Gynecol.* 1999;13:305–307.
62. Saari-Kemppainen A, Karjalainen O, Ylostalo P, et al. Ultrasound screening and perinatal mortality: controlled trial of systematic one-stage screening in pregnancy: the Helsinki Ultrasound Trial. *Lancet.* 1990;336:387–391.
63. Chitty LS, Hunt GH, Moore J, et al. Effectiveness of routine ultrasonography in detecting fetal structural abnormalities in a low risk population. *BMJ.* 1991;303:1165–1169.
64. Brocks V, Bang J. Routine examination by ultrasound for the detection of fetal malformations in a low risk population. *Fetal Diagn Ther.* 1991;6:37–45.
65. Levi S, Hyjazi Y, Schaapst JP, et al. Sensitivity and specificity of routine antenatal screening for congenital anomalies by ultrasound: the Belgian Multicentric Study. *Ultrasound Obstet Gynecol.* 1991;1:102–110.
66. Shirley IM, Bottomley F, Robinson VP. Routine radiographer screening for fetal abnormalities by ultrasound in an unselected low risk population. *Br J Radiol.* 1992;65:564–569.
67. Luck CA. Value of routine ultrasound scanning at 19 weeks: a four year study of 8849 deliveries. *BMJ.* 1992;304:1474–1478.
68. Roberts AB, Hampton E, Wilson N. Ultrasound detection of fetal structural abnormalities in Auckland 1988–1989. *N Z Med J.* 1993;106:441–443.
69. Romero R. Routine obstetric ultrasound. *Ultrasound Obstet Gynecol.* 1993;3:303–307.
70. Vintzileos AM, Campbell WA, Rodis JF, et al. The use of second trimester genetic sonogram in guiding clinical management of patients at increased risk for fetal trisomy 21. *Obstet Gynecol.* 1996;87:948–952.
71. VanDorsten JP, Hulsey TC, Newman RB, et al. Fetal anomaly detection by second-trimester ultrasonography in a tertiary center. *Am J Obstet Gynecol.* 1998;178:742–749.
72. Grandjean H, Larroque D, Levi S. The performance of routine ultrasonographic screening of pregnancies in the Eurofetus Study. *Am J Obstet Gynecol.* 1999;181:446–454.
73. Vintzileos AM, Ananth CV, Smulian JC, et al. Routine second-trimester ultrasonography in the United States: a cost-benefit analysis. *Am J Obstet Gynecol.* 2000;182:655–660.
74. Filly RA. Obstetrical sonography: the best way to terrify a pregnant woman. *J Ultrasound Med.* 2000;19:1–5.
75. Timor-Tritsch IE. As technology evolves, so should its application: shortcomings of the "18-week anatomy scan." *J Ultrasound Med.* 2006;25:423–428.
76. Schwarzler P, Senat MV, Holden D, et al. Feasibility of the second-trimester fetal ultrasound examination in an unselected population at 18, 20 or 22 weeks of pregnancy: a randomized trial. *Ultrasound Obstet Gynecol.* 1999;14:92–97.
77. Hadlock FP, Deter RL, Harrist RB, et al. Fetal biparietal diameter: rational choice of plane of section for sonographic measurement. *AJR Am J Roentgenol.* 1982;138:871–874.
78. Shepard M, Filly RA. A standardized plane for biparietal diameter measurement. *J Ultrasound Med.* 1982;1:145–150.
79. Hadlock FP, Harrist RB, Deter RJ, et al. Fetal head circumference: relation to menstrual age. *AJR Am J Roentgenol.* 1982;138:649–653.
80. Hadlock FP, Deter RL, Harrist RB, et al. Fetal abdominal circumference as a predictor of gestational age. *AJR Am J Roentgenol.* 1982;139:367–370.
81. Queenan JT, O'Brien GD, Campbell S. Ultrasound measurement of fetal limb bones. *Am J Obstet Gynecol.* 1980;138:297–302.
82. Hadlock FP, Harrist RB, Deter RJ, et al. Fetal femur length as a predictor of menstrual age: sonographically measured. *AJR Am J Roentgenol.* 1982;138:875–878.
83. Jeanty P, Rodesch F, Delbeke D, et al. Estimation of gestational age form measurements of fetal long bones. *J Ultrasound Med.* 1984;3:75–79.
84. Smith PA, Johansson D, Tzannatos C, et al. Prenatal measurement of the fetal cerebellum and cisterna cerebellomedullaris by ultrasound. *Prenat Diagn.* 1986;6:133–141.
85. Hadlock FP, Deter RL, Carpenter RLL, et al. The effect of head shape on the accuracy of BPD on estimating fetal gestational age. *AJR Am J Roentgenol.* 1981;137:83–85.
86. Nicolaides KH, Campbell S, Gabbe SG, et al. Ultrasound screening for spina bifida: cranial and cerebellar signs. *Lancet.* 1986;2:72–74.

87. Van den Hof MC, Nicolaides KH, Campbell S, et al. Evaluation of the lemon and banana signs in one hundred thirty fetuses with open spina bifida. *Am J Obstet Gynecol.* 1990;162:322–327.
88. Nyberg DA. Recommendations for obstetric sonography in the evaluation of the fetal cranium. *Radiology.* 1989;172:309–311.
89. Cardoza JD, Goldstein RB, Filly RA. Exclusion of fetal ventriculomegaly with a single measurement: the width of the lateral ventricular atrium. *Radiology.* 1988;169:711–714.
90. Alagappan R, Browning PD, Laorr A, et al. Distal lateral ventricular atrium: re-evaluation of normal range. *Radiology.* 1994;193:405–408.
91. Farell TA, Hertzberg BS, Kliewer MA, et al. Fetal lateral ventricles: reassessment of normal values for atrial diameter at US. *Radiology.* 1994;193:409–411.
92. Pilu G, Falco P, Gabrielli S, et al. The clinical significance of fetal isolated cerebral borderline ventriculomegaly: report of 31 cases and review of the literature. *Ultrasound Obstet Gynecol.* 1999;14:320–326.
93. Ghidini A, Strobelt N, Locatelli A, et al. Isolated fetal choroid plexus cysts: role of ultrasonography in establishment of the risk of trisomy 18. *Am J Obstet Gynecol.* 2000;182:972–977.
94. Filly RA, Benacerraf BR, Nyberg DA, et al. Choroid plexus cyst and echogenic intracardiac focus in women at low risk for chromosomal anomalies. *J Ultrasound Med.* 2004;23:447–449.
95. Doubilet PM, Copel JA, Benson CB, et al. Choroid plexus cyst and echogenic intracardiac focus in women at low risk for chromosomal anomalies: the obligation to inform the mother. *J Ultrasound Med.* 2004;23:883–885.
96. D'Addario V, Pinto A, Rossi AC, et al. Cavum veli interpositi cyst: prenatal diagnosis and postnatal outcome. *Ultrasound Obstet Gynecol.* 2009;34:52–54.
97. Bannister CM, Russell SA, Rimmer S, et al. Fetal arachnoid cysts: their site, progress, prognosis and differential diagnosis. *Eur J Pediatr Surg.* 1999;9(suppl 1):27–28.
98. Callen PW, Callen AL, Glenn OA, et al. Columns of the fornix, not be mistaken for the cavum septi pellucidi on prenatal sonography. *J Ultrasound Med.* 2008;27:25–31.
99. Ulm B, Ulm MR, Deutinger J, et al. Dandy-Walker malformation diagnosed before 21 weeks of gestation: associated malformations and chromosomal abnormalities. *Ultrasound Obstet Gynecol.* 1997;10:167–170.
100. Bernard JP, Moscoso G, Renier D, et al. Cystic malformations of the posterior fossa. *Prenat Diagn.* 2001;21:1064–1069.
101. Boddaert N, Klein O, Ferguson N, et al. Intellectual prognosis of the Dandy-Walker malformation in children: the importance of vermian lobulation. *Neuroradiology.* 2003;45:320–324.
102. Bannister CM, Russell SA, Rimmer S, et al. Can prognostic indicators be identified in a fetus with an encephalocele? *Eur J Pediatr Surg.* 2000;10(suppl 1):20–23.
103. McLeary RD, Kuhns LR, Barr M Jr. Ultrasonography of the fetal cerebellum. *Radiology.* 1984;151:439–442.
104. Serthatlioglu S, Kocakoc E, Kiris A, et al. Sonographic measurement of the fetal cerebellum, cisterna magna, and cavum septum pellucidum in normal fetuses in the second and third trimesters of pregnancy. *J Clin Ultrasound.* 2003;31:194–200.
105. Mahony BS, Callen PW, Filly RA, et al. The fetal cisterna magna. *Radiology.* 1984;153:773–776.
106. Knutzon R, McGahan JP, Salamat MS, et al. Fetal cisterna magna septa: a normal anatomic finding. *Radiology.* 1991;180:799–801.
107. Laing FC, Frates MC, Brown DL, et al. Sonography of the fetal posterior fossa: false appearance of mega-cisterna magna and Dandy-Walker variant. *Radiology.* 1994;192:247–251.
108. Filly RA, Simpson GF, Linkowski G. Fetal spine morphology and maturation during the second trimester. *J Ultrasound Med.* 1987;6:631–636.
109. Gray DL, Crane JP, Rudolff MA. Prenatal diagnosis of neural tube defects: origin of midtrimester vertebral ossification centers as determined by sonographic water-bath studies. *J Ultrasound Med.* 1988;7:421–427.
110. Hoopman M, Able H, Yazdi B, et al. Prenatal evaluation of the position of the fetal conus medullaris. *Ultrasound Obstet Gynecol.* 2011;38:548–552.
111. Petrikovsky BM, Vintzileos AM, Rodis JF. Sonographic appearance of occipital fetal hair. *J Clin Ultrasound.* 1989;17:425–427.
112. Bowerman RA. Ultrasound of the fetal face. *Ultrasound Q.* 1993;11:211–258.
113. Mayden KL, Tortora M, Berkowitz RL, et al. Orbital diameters: a new parameter for prenatal diagnosis and dating. *Am J Obstet Gynecol.* 1982;144:289–297.
114. Jeanty P, Cantraine F, Cousaert E, et al. The binocular distance: a new way to estimate gestational age. *J Ultrasound Med.* 1984;3:241–243.
115. Sonek JD, Cicero S, Neiger R, et al. Nasal bone assessment in prenatal screening for trisomy 21. *Am J Obstet Gynecol.* 2006;195:1219–1230.
116. Persico N, Borenstein M, Molina F, et al. Prenasal thickness in trisomy 21 fetuses at 16–24 weeks of gestation. *Ultrasound Obstet Gynecol.* 2008;32(6):751–754.
117. Sonek J, Molina F, Hiett AK, et al. Prefrontal space ratio: comparison between trisomy 21 anneuploid fetuses in the second trimester. *Ultrasound Obstet Gynecol.* 2012;40:293–296.
118. Bimholz JC, The fetal external ear. *Radiology.* 1983;147:819–821.
119. Benacerraf BR, Frigoletto FD Jr. Soft tissue nuchal fold in the second trimester fetus: standards for normal measurements compared with those in Down syndrome. *Am J Obstet Gynecol.* 1987;157:1146–1149.

120. Fong K, Ohlsson A, Zaley A. Fetal thoracic circumference: a prospective cross-sectional study with real-time ultrasound. *Am J Obstet Gynecol.* 1988;158:1154–1160.
121. Cooper C, Mahony BS, Bowie JD, et al. Ultrasound evaluation of the normal fetal upper airway and esophagus. *J Ultrasound Med.* 1985;4:343–346.
122. Avni EF, Rypens F, Milaire J. Fetal esophagus: normal sonographic appearance. *J Ultrasound Med.* 1994;13:175–180.
123. Hess LW, Hess DB, McCaul JF, et al. Fetal echocardiography. *Obstet Gynecol Clin North Am.* 1990;17:41–79.
124. Bromley B, Estroff A, Sandets SP. Fetal echocardiography: accuracy and limitations in a population at high and low risk for heart defects. *Am J Obstet Gynecol.* 1992;166:1473–1481.
125. Abuhamad A. *A Practical Guide to Fetal Echocardiography.* Philadelphia, PA: Lippincott-Raven; 1997.
126. Comstock CH. Normal fetal heart axis and position. *Obstet Gynecol.* 1987;70:255–259.
127. McGahan JP. Sonography of the fetal heart: findings on the four-chamber view. *AJR Am J Roentgenol.* 1991;156:547–553.
128. Brown DL, Cartier MS, Emerson DS, et al. The peripheral hypoechoic rim of the fetal heart. *J Ultrasound Med.* 1989;8:603–608.
129. Levy DW, Mintz MC. The left ventricular echogenic focus: a normal finding. *AJR Am J Roentgenol.* 1988;150:85–86.
130. Petrikovsky BM, Challenger M, Wyse LJ. Natural history of echogenic foci within the ventricle of the fetal heart. *Ultrasound Obstet Gynecol.* 1995;5:92–94.
131. DeVore GR. The aortic and pulmonary outflow tract screening examination in the human fetus. *J Ultrasound Med.* 1992;11:345–348.
132. DeVore GR. Color Doppler examination of the outflow tracts of the fetal heart: a technique for identification of cardiovascular malformation. *Ultrasound Obstet Gynecol.* 1994;4:463–471.
133. Mavrides E, Moscoso G, Carvalho JS, et al. The anatomy of the umbilical, portal and hepatic venous systems in the human fetus at 14–19 weeks of gestation. *Ultrasound Obstet Gynecol.* 2001;18:598–604.
134. Hata K, Aoki S, Hata T, et al. Ultrasound identification of the human fetal gall bladder in utero. *Gynecol Obstet Invest.* 1987;23:79–83.
135. Pretorius DH, Gosink BB, Clautice-Engle T, et al. Sonographic evaluation of the fetal stomach: significance of non-visualization. *AJR Am J Roentgenol.* 1988;151:987–989.
136. Millener PB, Anderson NG, Chisholm RJ. Prognostic significance of non-visualization of the fetal stomach by sonography. *AJR Am J Roentgenol.* 1993;160:827–830.
137. Schmidt W, Yarkoni S, Jeanty P, et al. Sonographic measurements of the fetal spleen: clinical implications. *J Ultrasound Med.* 1985;4:667–672.
138. Rosenberg R, Bowie JD, Andreotti RF, et al. Sonographic evaluation of the fetal adrenal glands. *AJR Am J Roentgenol.* 1982;139:1145–1147.
139. Lawson TL, Foley WD, Berland LL, et al. Ultrasonic evaluation of fetal kidneys: analysis of normal size and frequency of visualization as related to stage of pregnancy. *Radiology.* 1981;138:153–156.
140. Bowie JD, Rosenberg R, Andreotti RF, et al. The changing sonographic appearance of the fetal kidneys during pregnancy. *J Ultrasound Med.* 1983;2:505–507.
141. Grannum P, Bracken M, Silverman R, et al. Assessment of fetal kidney size in normal gestation by comparison of ratio of kidney circumference to abdominal circumference. *Am J Obstet Gynecol.* 1980;136:249–254.
142. Cohen HL, Cooper J, Eisenberg P, et al. Normal length of fetal kidneys: sonographic study in 397 obstetric patients. *AJR Am J Roentgenol.* 1991;157:545–548.
143. Anderson N, Clautice-Engle T, Allan R, et al. Detection of obstructive uropathy in the fetus: predictive value of sonographic measurements of renal pelvic diameter at various gestational ages. *AJR Am J Roentgenol.* 1995;164:719–723.
144. Corteville JE, Gray DL, Crane JP. Congenital hydronephrosis: correlation of fetal ultrasonographic findings with infant outcome. *Am J Obstet Gynecol.* 1991;165:384–388.
145. Mandell J, Blyth BR, Peters CA, et al. Structural genitourinary defects detected in utero. *Radiology.* 1991;178:193–196.
146. Parulekar SG. Sonography of normal fetal bowel. *J Ultrasound Med.* 1991;10:211–220.
147. Nyberg DA, Mack LA, Pattern RM, et al. Fetal bowel: normal sonographic findings. *J Ultrasound Med.* 1987;6:3–6.
148. Vincoff S, Callen PW, Smith-Bindman R, et al. Effect of ultrasound transducer frequency on the appearance of the fetal bowel. *J Ultrasound Med.* 1999;18:799–803.
149. Fakhry J, Reiser M, Shapiro LR, et al. Increased echogenicity in the lower fetal abdomen: a common normal variant in the second trimester. *J Ultrasound Med.* 1986;5:489–492.
150. Mahony BS, Filly RA. High-resolution sonographic assessment of the fetal extremities. *J Ultrasound Med.* 1984;3:489–498.
151. Bowerman RA. *Atlas of Normal Fetal Ultrasonographic Anatomy.* 2nd ed. Chicago, IL: Year Book Medical Publishers; 1992.

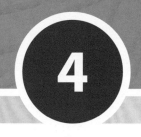

4 Fetal Growth and Doppler Ultrasound

Henry L. Galan • Shane Reeves

INTRODUCTION

Fetal growth restriction (FGR) is a common complication of pregnancy. There is a lack of consensus regarding optimal terminology, diagnostic criteria, and management options. The American College of Obstetrics and Gynecology (ACOG) and the Society for Maternal-Fetal Medicine (SMFM) define FGR as a fetus that measures less than the 10th percentile for the estimated fetal weight (EFW) on a standardized growth curve.[1] However, this does not optimally differentiate between a fetus that is constitutionally small and fulfilling its growth potential and a fetus that is not fulfilling its potential because of an underlying pathological condition. Pathologically, FGR has been associated with a variety of adverse perinatal outcomes including increased risk of intrauterine demise, neonatal morbidity and mortality, as well as the long-term sequelae of neurodevelopmental delay, cardiovascular disease, and diabetes.[2–4] Many experts have tried to refine the definition of FGR, and a Delphi survey of specialists incorporates EFW, abdominal circumference (AC), and Doppler ultrasound findings of the fetus.[5] The purpose of this chapter is to review the topic of FGR with a focus on methods for determining gestational age (GA), definitions of fetal undergrowth, and diagnostic biometric and surveillance tools. An algorithm for management and for timing the delivery of the FGR fetus is provided.

ESTABLISHMENT OF GESTATIONAL AGE

The *menstrual age* is defined as the age of a pregnancy when compared with the first day of the last menstrual period (LMP). This is the most commonly used method to determine the due date in clinical practice. The *conceptional age* is the true fetal age of the pregnancy, as it estimates the GA when compared with the day of conception. The difficulty with using the conceptional age is that it is truly known only in cases of assisted reproduction such as *in vitro* fertilization (IVF). Even in these cases, it is common in clinical practice to refer to the menstrual age by calculating backward 14 days from the day of conception and using this as a guide to determine the menstrual age. In this chapter, the GA of the pregnancy will be synonymous with the menstrual age, and the GA will be used throughout the remainder of the chapter.

Knowledge of the GA is important, as risk assessment, diagnosis, and interventions depend upon knowing the exact duration of the pregnancy. In the first trimester, for example, screening for aneuploidy through ultrasound assessment of the nuchal translucency is performed in a narrow window between 10 weeks 4 days and 13 weeks 6 days.[6] Chorionic villus sampling can be performed after 10 weeks, and performing this procedure earlier than this increases the risk of limb reduction defects.[7] Amniocentesis can be performed after 15 weeks, but prior to this GA, it increases the number of newborns with talipes equinovarus.[8] Therefore, if the precise GA is not known, there could be an increased risk of pregnancy complications from the diagnostic procedures. In addition, once a due date is established, the fetus will be compared with other fetuses at the same GA to determine whether the fetus is measuring too large or too small. This is particularly important in identifying pregnancies at risk for poor perinatal outcome because of FGR. If the GA is incorrect, then accurate classification of fetal growth is impossible. Similarly, management of preterm labor depends upon accurate determination of GA, as administration of tocolytics would be inappropriate after a certain GA. Finally, planning induction of labor or timed cesarean delivery is critically dependent upon accurate knowledge of the GA so as not to incur iatrogenic prematurity or stillbirth from a post-dates pregnancy. Virtually all clinical decisions depend upon accurate determination of GA.

The due date is commonly calculated by adding 280 days to the first day of the LMP. This assumes a normal menstrual cycle of 28 days, with ovulation occurring on the 14th day. Many women may not remember the first day of their LMP. Even in women with reliable recall, the LMP could be misleading as it is common for women to have cycle lengths that vary between 21 and 35 days. One study showed that up to 20% of women will have early or late ovulation,[9] increasing the probability of an inaccurate GA determination. For all of these reasons, determination of the due date using the LMP alone is fraught with inaccuracy.

FIRST-TRIMESTER ULTRASOUND

In the first trimester, the first ultrasonographic sign of pregnancy is the identification of the gestational sac. This is a fluid-filled structure containing mostly chorionic fluid. In the early days of ultrasonography, this could not reliably be seen until approximately 6 weeks' Gestational Age. However, with high-resolution, real-time sonography and transvaginal imaging, the sac can be seen as early as during the fourth or fifth week of gestation. Menstrual age can be estimated by measuring the size of the gestational sac. The mean sac diameter (MSD) is the average of the measurement of the gestational sac in three orthogonal planes. This measurement is obtained from the interface of the chorionic fluid and the sac wall. The sac wall is not included in the measurement (Fig. 4.1). The gestational sac can be seen with measurements as small as 2 to 3 mm, and the MSD increases approximately 1 mm per day in early gestation.[10] Table 1 in Appendix A1 shows the relationship between MSD, menstrual age, and human chorionic gonadotropin level.

The gestational sac can often be confused with a pseudo-sac seen in ectopic pregnancy. To distinguish a true gestational sac, one must identify a double sac sign. This is a finding that is created by visualization of the two layers of the decidua parietalis. The deep layer of the decidua parietalis and early villi is more echogenic, and this can be seen as separated from the less echogenic layer of the superficial layer. Also, the intradecidual sign can be seen, where the sac is imbedded in the decidua rather than between two layers of the endometrium (Fig. 4.2).

As the first trimester advances, the reliability of the MSD in predicting menstrual age decreases. Between 2 and 14 mm, the MSD is quite precise in determination of age, but after an MSD of 14 mm, an embryo can be seen at which time the MSD should not be used. Once an embryo is seen, the measurement of the

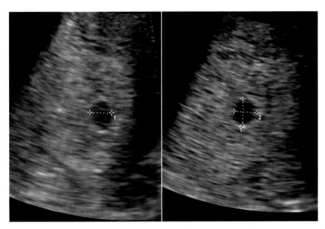

FIGURE 4.1: Mean sac diameter (MSD). The gestational sac is measured in three planes with the calipers placed at the interface between the wall of the sac and the embryonic fluid. Notice that the sac wall is not incorporated in the measurement. The MSD is the average of the three measurements.

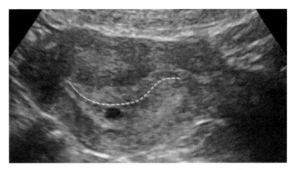

FIGURE 4.2: Characteristics of a gestational sac. In this image, the gestational sac is seen eccentrically located in the endometrial cavity. It is displaced inferiorly such that it is located in the decidua rather than the endometrial canal *(line)*. The sac also has a hypoechoic rim around a hyperechoic sac wall.

crown rump length (CRL) can be obtained, and this is now more accurate in obtaining the true estimation of GA. The CRL is not the true measurement of the length of the fetus, as fetuses in early gestation have flexion. In truth, the CRL is the measurement of the longest straight line from the head of the fetus to the caudal end. Figure 4.3 depicts measurements of the CRL at different GAs. When obtaining the CRL, the sonologist should obtain at least three measurements and average the values to obtain the GA (see Table 1 in Appendix A1).

The accuracy of GA determination based on CRL is best in the middle of the first trimester. As the pregnancy advances, the CRL loses precision in GA determination.[11] When examining pregnancies conceived through IVF, where the precise GA is known, from 7 to 11 weeks, the 95% confidence interval shows that the CRL is within 3 days of true GA. From 11 to 13 weeks, the 95% confidence interval CI is within 5 days.[12] Hadlock et al.[13] showed that the variability in the CRL remained fairly constant from 2 mm to 12 cm, where the 95% confidence interval for GA was 8%. Therefore, if a pregnancy measured 8 weeks 0 days, the true GA was 8 weeks 0 days ± 0.64 weeks. If the pregnancy measured 12 weeks, the true GA was 12 ± 0.96 weeks. Variation in fetal growth in the late second and third trimesters is an expectation in any given population reflecting individual genetic determinants of growth, but deviation in fetal CRL size may be a

predictor of growth pathology. Using pregnancies resulting from assisted reproductive technology, the FASTER trial showed that fetuses that measured small in the first trimester had a higher risk of being small for gestational age (SGA) at birth.[14] Alternatively, fetuses measuring larger than expected by CRL in the first trimester also may be at risk for macrosomia at birth.[15] Therefore, CRL is a useful tool not only for gestational dating but it may also predict patients at risk for developing abnormalities in fetal growth as pregnancy advances. Other measurements can be obtained in the first trimester that can help in the determination of GA. First-trimester biparietal diameter (BPD) and AC have been investigated by multiple authors. Two independent authors evaluated first-trimester measurement of BPD and compared this with the CRL between 7 and 13 weeks. Both showed that the CRL was superior to BPD in determining menstrual age.[16,17] This has come into question in a more recent analysis evaluating BPD and CRL in pregnancies conceived through IVF. In this study, the two measurements were similar in ability to predict GA, but the BPD had the advantage of having lower random measurement error.[18] Another recent analysis showed similar findings when evaluating first-trimester BPD, CRL, and AC. This analysis showed that both CRL and BPD were accurate in determining when a pregnancy will actually deliver, and both were superior to the fetal AC.[19] Given the precision and ease of obtaining a first-trimester CRL with high-resolution abdominal and vaginal ultrasonography, most practitioners utilize this measurement as the primary means of determining GA. However, in the event that CRL cannot be obtained because of fetal position, uterine anomalies, or maternal

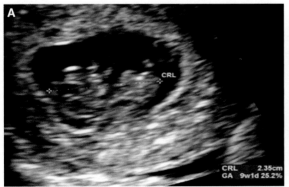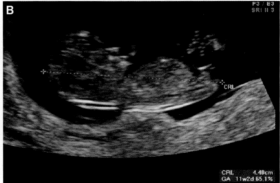

FIGURE 4.3: Crown rump length (CRL). **A:** The CRL is measured in a sagittal plane through the fetus. The image contains the head and body. Calipers are placed from the tip of the head to the edge of the caudal end. **B:** The CRL at later gestational ages allows for a clearer distinction of the fetal edges.

body habitus, first-trimester use of the BPD could be an alternative measurement in determining GA.

First-trimester ultrasound is the most accurate method of determining GA. The measurement of the gestational MSD between 2 and 14 mm, followed by CRL determination once a fetal pole is seen, will appropriately assign an estimated due date. Biological variability in the first trimester is present, but it is much smaller than later in gestation. Once a due date is determined from a precise first-trimester ultrasound, this due date should not be changed later in gestation. If a future ultrasound shows significant deviation from the due date established by first-trimester ultrasound, this identifies a fetus with abnormal growth. As detailed later in this chapter, these fetuses may be at risk for poor perinatal outcome and should have further evaluation.

SECOND- AND THIRD-TRIMESTER BIOMETRY

In order to calculate a second- or third-trimester GA, multiple structures should be evaluated with rigorous criteria, and those criteria are discussed here.

Biparietal Diameter

The BPD was originally defined as the widest distance between the parietal eminences. However, this measurement is often more cephalad in location when compared with the thalami.[20] Since standardization is the goal, the BPD is measured when certain landmarks are identified. The BPD can be measured in any plane that traverses the third ventricle and the thalami. By convention, the BPD is measured in a plane similar to the head circumference (HC), but since it is a single line that crosses through the thalamus, it can be measured in any plane. For the BPD to be accurate, the third ventricle and thalamus need to be identified and located centrally in the image. The calvarial walls should be symmetric, and the midline of the fetal brain should be equidistant from the parietal bones to ensure that an oblique measurement is not obtained as this will falsely increase the distance. The calipers are then placed on the outer edge of the proximal calvaria and measured to the inner edge of the distal calvaria (Fig. 4.4). With this

measurement, the BPD is compared with a dataset to determine the percentile of the value, which can help identify normal and abnormal growth (see Table 10 in Appendix A1).

Head Circumference

Unlike the BPD, the HC requires a specific plane for proper acquisition. To appropriately obtain the measurement, the proper plane needs to parallel the base of the skull, the transducer must be perpendicular to the parietal bones, and the image must transect the third ventricle and thalami. To ensure the correct plane of measurement, the cavum septum pellucidum (CSP) must be visualized as a boxlike structure in the anterior portion of the fetal brain. The thalamus needs to be visualized around the third ventricle, and the cerebellum should not be in the image. If the cerebellum is seen, the image was obtained in an oblique plane, and this will increase the overall circumference measurement. Once the appropriate plane is obtained with identification of the appropriate structures, the HC is measured as an ellipse around the perimeter of the fetal skull. The HC does not include the skin edge; rather, an accurate HC traces around the calvarial margins. Ideally, the entire calvarium is visualized (Fig. 4.5). Often, images of the head shape appear abnormal, as in cases of breech presentation or fetal head molding. The fetal head is called dolichocephalic when transverse diameter appears flattened with the anteroposterior (AP) diameter elongated. Conversely, the head is called brachycephalic when it appears more rounded than long. In both of these instances, the BPD may appear abnormal, but the overall size of the fetal head is within a normal range. The HC will not be altered by the relative shape of the head, and this provides an advantage over the BPD in determining whether a fetus has abnormal growth. Tables 7 and 10 in Appendix A1 show normal values for HC.

Abdominal Circumference

The AC is similar to the HC in that it requires a precise plane of obtainment in order to be accurate. Inclusive in the AC is the fetal liver, an organ that can be affected by pathological growth in that it will be small in instances of growth restriction because of

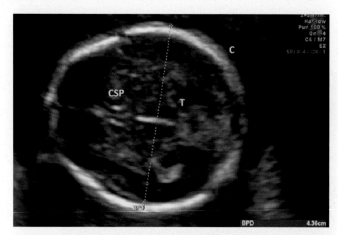

FIGURE 4.4: Biparietal diameter (BPD). The BPD is taken in an axial plane with the midline perpendicular to the transducer. The thalamus (T) is seen in the center, and the cavum septum pellucidum (CSP) is noted in the front of the image. The calipers are placed from the outer edge of the proximal calvarium (C) to the inside edge of the distal calvarium.

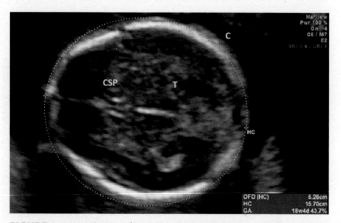

FIGURE 4.5: Head circumference (HC). The HC is taken in an axial plane. In the image, the landmarks of the thalamus (T) and cavum septum pellucidum (CSP) are visible. The midline is noted to be equidistant from both calvarial (C) edges. The HC is measured as the perimeter around the bone.

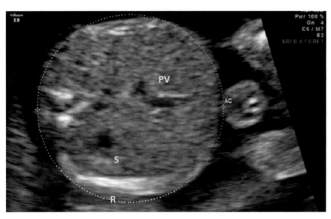

FIGURE 4.6: Abdominal circumference (AC). The AC is taken in an axial plain through the section of the abdomen containing the fetal liver. In this image, the liver is the proximal structure in the fetal abdomen. The portal vein (PV) can be seen curving away from the stomach (S). The PV makes a "C" shape, indicating that the image is taken appropriately. In addition, the three bright spots on the left side of the image mark the spine. The rib (R) is seen at the bottom of the image of the abdomen. There is only one rib seen, indicating that the plane is not oblique to the fetal lie.

glycogenolysis and large in instances of fetal macrosomia secondary to excessive glycogen storage. The appropriate AC incorporates the stomach, ribs, spine, and portal vein. The location of the confluence of the left portal vein and the right portal vein will create a "C-shape" in the fetal liver on ultrasound imaging, indicating an appropriate plane of obtainment. If the "C" is not seen in the fetal liver, either the transducer is too cephalad in the fetal abdomen or oblique to the correct plane. There should be one or two ribs seen in the image, but if the ribs are seen in cross-section with multiple segments visualized, the measurement will be falsely elevated. Figure 4.6 shows an appropriate image of the AC, including the stomach, portal vein, spine, and ribs. Tables 6 and 10 in Appendix A1 show measurements of the AC as GA progresses.

Femur Length

The femur is measured by aligning the transducer to the long axis of the femoral diaphysis. To measure the femur length (FL) correctly, the shaft should be aligned horizontally on the image. If the femur is not horizontal, shadowing from the edges of the bone will shorten the true length. Of note, ultrasound will detect only the ossified region of the femur, including the diaphysis and metaphysis. The cartilaginous regions are not well seen by ultrasound imaging. Once the entire length of the ossified bone is horizontal on the image, the calipers are placed on the central part of the femoral head and extended to the distal condyle. The calipers should be at the edge of the ossified site, between the bright bone and the dark cartilage. The correct measurement also does not incorporate the distal femoral point, as this is nonstandard and will incorrectly lengthen the measurement. Figure 4.7 depicts the proper measurement of the FL, and Tables 8 and 10 in Appendix A1 show the predicted GA for measured FL.

ACCURACY IN MEASUREMENTS

Biparietal Diameter Accuracy

The BPD has been well studied in its accuracy in determining GA. Between 14 and 21 weeks, Hadlock et al.[21] investigated 1,770 chromosomally normal fetuses, and they showed that the 95%

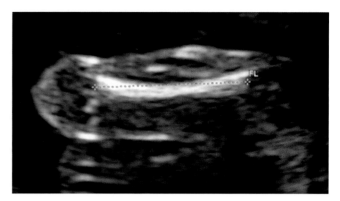

FIGURE 4.7: Femur length (FL). The FL is measured with the longest portion of the bone perpendicular to the transducer. If the femur is not horizontal, shadowing from the ossified bone may shorten the length. The calipers are placed in the center of the femur and measured to the end of the bright edges, ensuring not to include the femoral tip.

confidence interval for measuring the BPD was within 1 week of the known GA. Other authors showed findings similar in accuracy between 14 and 20 weeks when looking at pregnancies dated either by known dates of conception or first-trimester CRL.[22,23] In all of these studies, two standard deviations (SDs) for the accuracy of BPD in determining GA ranged between 0.92 and 1.02 weeks for GAs between 14 and 20 weeks. As GA advances, the variability in BPD measurement increases, diminishing the accuracy of GA determination. Benson and Doubilet[24] looked at pregnancies dated by early CRL, and they showed that the variability (±2 SD) in determining GA increased from 2.1 weeks at 20 to 26 weeks to 4.1 weeks from 32 to 42 weeks (Table 4.1). Similar to early CRL, BPD measurements are most accurate the earlier the study is performed; and as pregnancy progresses, deviation from normal will be more of a measure of abnormal growth rather than assigning GA.

As mentioned previously, the BPD can be significantly affected by the fetal head shape. In cases of breech presentation, uterine anomalies, fibroids, and multiple gestations, the fetal calvarium can be compressed so that the BPD is shortened or elongated relative to the true GA. The cephalic index (CI) is a ratio that assesses dolichocephaly and brachycephaly, and it is calculated from the

TABLE 4.1	Variability in Predicting Gestational Age in the Second Half of Pregnancy		
PARAMETER	20–26 wk	26–32 wk	32–42 wk
BPD	2.1	3.8	4.1
HC	1.9	3.4	3.8
AC	3.7	3.0	4.5
FL	2.5	3.1	3.5

The variability is expressed as ±2 SD. AC, abdominal circumference; BPD, biparietal diameter; FL, femur length; HC, head circumference.
Adapted from Benson CB, Doubilet PM. Sonographic prediction of gestational age: accuracy of second and third trimester fetal measurements. AJR. 1991;157:1275–1277. Copyright © 1991 American Roentgen Ray Society.

BPD and the fronto-occipital diameter (FOD). This measurement is from the outside of the anterior portion of the fetal skull to the outside of the posterior calvarium. The CI is calculated as follows:

$$CI = (BPD/FOD) \times 100$$

Hadlock et al. demonstrated that the CI remained relatively stable from 14 to 40 weeks, with a mean value of 78.3 and an SD of 4.4. In this study, CI measurements that were greater than 1 SD from the mean had BPD measurements that were inaccurate in determining GA. In such instances, the HC is a better measure as it is not as dependent upon head shape.[25]

Head Circumference Accuracy

The HC is not dependent upon fetal head shape, and its measurement has also been shown to be an accurate predictor of GA. In fact, at less than 20 weeks, the HC may be more predictive of GA than is BPD, as shown by Law and MacRae.[26] Like the BPD, this measurement is accurate to within 1 week (±2 SD) of the GA when the precise due date is known. Like other measures in pregnancy, the best prediction of GA occurs with earlier measurement with error in accuracy increasing as GA advances.[21,23] In the third trimester, the inaccuracies of HC parallel that of BPD in GA determination with a margin of error of ±3.8 weeks (2 SD) after 32 weeks.[24]

Abdominal Circumference Accuracy

The AC is the most difficult measure to obtain of all of the biometric assessments. Also, the AC contains the liver, which is subject to acute and subacute changes in metabolism by the fetus. In pathological states, it has been theorized that the liver size may shrink because of metabolic demands from nutrient deficiency. In instances of glucose excess, such as diabetes, the fetal liver should increase in size as glucose is stored in this organ. For these reasons, the AC would be expected to have the highest level of variability when predicting GA. This was observed by Benson and Doubilet[24] in their analysis, where they saw that the AC had the highest variability in predicting GA when compared with the other measures.

Femur Length Accuracy

With the ease of measuring the FL, this biometric parameter has been well studied in determining GA. Similar to other measures, the earlier the measurement is obtained, the more accurate the FL is in determining GA. As shown by Benson and Doubilet,[24] the FL has variability similar to that of other bony measures (e.g., BPD, HC) in the late second and third trimesters.

ASSIGNING THE ESTIMATED DATE OF CONFINEMENT

With the various methods of determining the fetal GA, an accurate assignment of the due date (estimated date of confinement [EDC]) is critical in assessing fetal growth. Determining the EDC has significant implications in pregnancy management, especially when considering the fetus where there is a suspected abnormality in fetal growth. As mentioned previously, the EDC is often determined by adding 280 days to the first day of the LMP. However, if there is a discrepancy between an ultrasound-determined EDC and the one determined by the LMP, this needs to be resolved in order to properly identify pregnancies with fetal growth abnormalities. ACOG, SMFM, and the American Institute for Ultrasound in Medicine (AIUM) have provided guidelines estimating the EDC and for changing the EDC when an ultrasound-determined GA differs from the one provided by the LMP[27] (Table 4.2). As biologic variability for growth is least early in pregnancy, an EDC established in the first trimester should serve as the final EDC and not changed due to a discrepancy in GA obtained by an ultrasound performed later in pregnancy.

OTHER BIOMETRIC PARAMETERS

Multiple other structures have been investigated for determining GA. These include measurements of the binocular distance, clavicular length, ulna, tibia, radius, and foot. Similar to the other measurements, earlier assessment is most accurate. One structure that shows promise in accuracy is the transcerebellar diameter (TCD). This measurement can be obtained during evaluation of the posterior fossa. The best image is obtained by having the transducer perpendicular to the parietal bones, in a plane slightly

---

TABLE 4.2	Recommendations Changing the Estimated Date of Confinement	
GA BY MEASUREMENT	**METHOD TO DETERMINE GA**	**DIFFERENCE BETWEEN GA MEASUREMENT AND LMP EDC THAT PROMPTS CHANGE OF EDC**
≤8w6d	CRL	More than 5 d
9w0d–13w6d	CRL	More than 7 d
14w0d–15w6d	BPD, HC, AC, FL	More than 7 d
16w0d–21w6d	BPD, HC, AC, FL	More than 10 d
22w0d–27w6d	BPD, HC, AC, FL	More than 14 d
28w0d and beyond	BPD, HC, AC, FL	More than 21 d

Third-trimester measurements should warrant caution in changing the estimated date of confinement due to the risk of mismanaging a fetus with growth restriction. AC, abdominal circumference; BPD, biparietal diameter; CRL, crown rump length; d, days; EDC, estimated date of confinement; FL, femur length; GA, gestational age; HC, head circumference; LMP, last menstrual period; w, weeks.

diagonal to that used for the BPD. The optimal image has the CSP seen anteriorly and the cerebellum seen posteriorly. The calipers are placed on the outer edge of the cerebellum and measured to the opposite side (Fig. 4.8). Table 19 in Appendix A1 shows the measurements of the cerebellar length as GA advances.

The accuracy in GA determination for the TCD is quite high. Chavez et al. studied the TCD in the second and third trimesters in singleton, nonanomalous, well-dated pregnancies. Between 17 and 21 weeks, the TCD predicted GA accurately within 4 days. In fact, as pregnancy advanced, the TCD maintained a higher accuracy than did any other biometric parameters. Between 29 and 36 weeks, the predicted age was within 5 days of the actual age, and at greater than 37 weeks, it was within 9 days.[28] However, measurement of the TCD may be challenging late in pregnancy. Fetal positioning and calcification of the skull can make visualization of cerebellar landmarks difficult. Unlike the BPD, HC, AC, and FL, the TCD is particularly important in determining GA at extremes of fetal growth. When evaluating pregnancies with good dating criteria, even in fetuses with growth restriction (estimated weight <10th percentile) and macrosomia (estimated weight >90th percentile), the TCD maintained accuracy in predicting GA.[29] Of note, like other measurements, chromosomally abnormal fetuses can have a TCD smaller than predicted,[30] which could further complicate assessment of GA. Despite this finding, clinicians are often challenged with patients presenting late in pregnancy with an uncertain GA. The TCD can be a measurement that will help in determining whether a fetus is measuring SGA or large for gestational age (LGA), as it seems to be less subject to variability when compared with other biometric parameters.

Although other long bone measurements do not provide any clear additional benefit for dating a pregnancy or for EFW calculation, in certain circumstances, they may be beneficial relative to bony abnormalities. Measurements for the humerus, radius, ulna, tibia, and fibula are captured in Table 13 in Appendix A1. The fetal foot length can be measured throughout gestation, beginning as early as the end of the first trimester. The literature on newborn and fetal foot length has been summarized elsewhere,[31] and

the foot length percentiles across gestation are shown in Table 15 in Appendix A1. In FGR, Meirowitz and colleagues showed that 60% of fetuses have foot length measurements that are less than the 10th percentile. Thus, the foot length may not be sufficiently spared to provide clinical utility.[32]

ESTIMATION OF FETAL WEIGHT

Up until this point, this chapter has focused on GA determination using ultrasound biometric parameters. This is crucial in determining the true due date and assigning an appropriate age to the pregnancy. Once the due date from early measurement has been established, it should not be altered later in pregnancy. In cases of deviation from the predicted GA, the fetus is demonstrating growth abnormalities—either in the case of excess fetal growth called LGA or inhibited growth called FGR. GA is not the only issue in assessing normal progression of a pregnancy; fetal weight is another key element in determining the status of growth.

Formulae

Shortly after the application of ultrasound to modern obstetrics, measurements of the fetus were evaluated in predicting birth weight (BW). One of the first publications showed that the AC alone was predictive of newborn weight with a moderate degree of accuracy if the AC was measured within 48 hours of delivery.[33] With this observation, multiple other investigators started adding additional biometric parameters in an attempt to improve accuracy. Several authors added the BPD as the first measurement, and regression analysis was used to create standardized formulae for estimating fetal weight. Warsof et al.[34] found that the addition of the BPD could improve accuracy with an SD of 106 g per kg if performed within 48 hours of delivery. Other investigators followed and generated other equations using the BPD and AC to estimate fetal weight.[35–38] Over time, FL was added to the equations in an attempt to improve prediction as the prior measurements did not take long bone growth into consideration. In addition, BPD was recognized as being influenced by head shape, so HC was added to the equation in some instances, and replaced the BPD in others.[39–43] Table 4.3 shows some of the most commonly used equations in calculating an EFW.

Accuracy of Specific Formulae

Numerous formulae exist for the estimation of fetal weight. Since none of the formulae has perfect accuracy, institutions may choose a particular formula as a standard or in specific scenarios. When looking at accuracy, investigators will assess bias (the systematic overprediction or underprediction of weight) and precision (random error). Systematic bias is often defined as the mean percentage error (MPE), where percentage error = 100 × (BW − EFW)/BW, and the MPE is the mean of percent errors in a given population. Random error is the SD of the MPE. This method has been used to compare the accuracies of different formulae, and it is one tool that can help determine which formula may be best. Of note, if an estimate of weight is calculated and the fetus progresses beyond 1 week from the measures, the EFW would be expected to be incorrect because of ongoing fetal growth. In addition, maternal body habitus has a significant effect on accuracy, where the MPE in women with a body mass index (BMI) greater than 30 is almost double that in women with a BMI less than 25.[44]

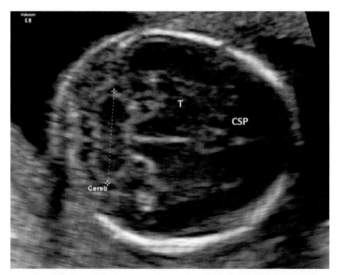

FIGURE 4.8: Cerebellar measurement. The cerebellum *(Cereb)* is measured from an axial plane in the fetal head. The plane is in the correct location when the cavum septum pellucidum *(CSP)* is located anteriorly with the thalamus *(T)* seen in the midline. The midline is equidistant from both calvarial edges.

TABLE 4.3	Common Formulae for Fetal Growth	
PARAMETERS	**REFERENCES**	**FORMULA**
AC, BPD	Thurnau et al.[33]	$BW = (BPD \times AC \times 9.337) - 229$
	Shepard et al.[36]	$\mathrm{Log_{10}}\ BW = 0.166(BPD) + 0.046(AC) - 0.002546(AC)(BPD) - 1.7492$
	Hadlock et al.[35]	$\mathrm{Log_{10}}\ BW = 1.1134 + 0.05845(AC) - 0.000604(AC)^2 - 0.007365(BPD)^2 + 0.000595(BPD)(AC) + 0.1694(BPD)$
	Vintzileos et al.[34]	$\mathrm{Log_{10}}\ BW = 1.879 + 0.084(BPD) + 0.026(AC)$
	Warsof et al.[32]	$\mathrm{Log_{10}}\ BW = 0.144(BPD) + 0.032(AC) - 0.000111(BPD)^2(AC) - 1.599$
AC, HC	Weiner et al.[37]	$\mathrm{Log_{10}}\ BW = 1.6575 + 0.04035(HC) + 0.01285(AC)$
AC, FL, BPD	Hadlock et al.[35]	$\mathrm{Log_{10}}\ BW = 1.182 + 0.0273(HC) + 0.07057(AC) - 0.00063(AC)^2 - 0.0002184(HC)(AC)$
	Combs et al.[40]	$BW = 0.23718(AC)^2(FL) + 0.03312(HC)^3$
	Hadlock et al.[38]	$\mathrm{Log_{10}}\ BW = 1.326 - 0.00326(AC)(FL) + 0.0107(HC) + 0.0438(AC) + 0.158(FL)$
	Weiner et al.[37]	$\mathrm{Log_{10}}\ BW = 1.6961 + 0.02253(HC) + 0.01645(AC) + 0.06439(FL)$
	Ott et al.[39]	$\mathrm{Log_{10}}\ BW = -2.0661 + 0.04355(HC) + 0.05394(AC) - 0.0008582(HC)(AC) + 1.2594(FL/AC)$
AC, FL, BPD, HC	Hadlock et al.[38]	$\mathrm{Log_{10}}\ BW = 1.3596 + 0.0064(HC) + 0.0424(AC) + 0.174(FL) + 0.00061(BPD)(AC) - 0.00386(AC)(FL)$
AD, FL, BPD	Rose and McCallum[41]	$\mathrm{Ln}\ BW = 0.143(BPD + AD + FL) + 4.198$

AC, abdominal circumference; BPD, biparietal diameter; BW, birth weight; FL, femur length; HC, head circumference.
From Burd I, Srinivas S, Pare E, et al. Is sonographic assessment of fetal weight influenced by formula selection? *J Ultrasound Med*. 2009;28(8):1019–1024. Copyright © 2016 by the American Institute of Ultrasound in Medicine. Reprinted by permission of John Wiley & Sons, Inc.

Therefore, appropriate comparisons can be made only if the EFW is made close to the time of delivery in a population where visualization of the fetus is possible.

Multiple factors can play a part in EFW accuracy, but how important is the specific formula used? When looking at each formula, using the same measurements from an individual fetus can provide considerable differences in values. Anderson et al. evaluated 12 different formulae for accuracy in population data from 1991 and 2000. They compared intraobserver and interobserver variability, and also looked at different formulae in the accuracy of predicting BW. They found that observer error (that obtained from multiple measures or from multiple sonologists on the same fetus) provided far less error than the use of different formulae. In fact, only six formulae were able to provide an MPE within 7%.[45] Edwards et al.[46] found that Hadlock[35] and Shepard[18] provided more accurate results than did other formulae. A systematic review of articles comparing EFW formulae was performed in an attempt to determine accuracy. In this analysis, the formulae by Hadlock et al. using BPD, HC, AC, and FL[35,38] seemed to provide the most consistent MPEs when used on various populations with the same amount of precision as in the case of other formulae. However, all formulae presented a fairly wide MPE and SD, and the authors conclude that no particular formula is ideal.[47] Other authors found that between 2,500 and 3,999 g, the Schild et al.[48] formula, is the most accurate in determining

weight ($EFW = -4,035.275 + 1.143\ BPD^{(3)} + 1,159.878\ AC^{(1)}/^{(2)} + 10.079\ FL^{(3)} - 81.277 \times FL^{(2)}$). However, in this study, most formulae performed similarly, and the MPE was still around 7% for the best ones.[49] A recent analysis looking at 18 different formulae showed that the formulae by Hadlock and Ott were the most accurate in predicting BW in all fetuses.[50] These studies have consistent findings, and Hadlock's formula may be more accurate than were others in determining fetal weight, but most formulae are similar and even the best do not have an MPE less than 5%. Further studies may help identify the optimal formula given a specific population.

Accuracy at Extremes of Measurement

EFW accuracy can be affected by multiple factors, and one of the most significant factors influencing inaccuracies is the fetus demonstrating abnormal growth. In the EFW formulae, FL, BPD, and HC are all measures of bony structures. The AC is the only measurement incorporating soft tissue, as it encompasses the outer perimeter of the abdomen, which includes the liver and subcutaneous tissue. Investigators have argued that formulae based on bone structures may be less accurate with abnormal growth. In growth restriction, nutrient deficiency may lead to a more pronounced decline in muscle and fat cell growth compared with bone growth. In macrosomia, subcutaneous tissues would be expected to be increased, and the current formulae could be particularly inaccurate owing to the lack of accounting for this tissue development.

Multiple studies have been published addressing the issue of accuracy in EFW determination at extremes of newborn weight. Dudley showed that regardless of EFW formula, all methods showed wide variation in accuracy when the BW was less than 1,500 g. In addition, for macrosomic newborns, the formulae were also more inaccurate, with a tendency to underestimate weight.[47] Ben-Haroush et al. studied 840 pregnancies that were induced for various reasons and had an ultrasound EFW from 1 to 3 days prior to delivery. In this cohort, ultrasound EFW underestimated suspected macrosomic fetuses by a mean of 110 g and overestimated suspected growth-restricted fetuses by 113 g.[51] The same group also looked at 26 different formulae and found that models that incorporated 3 or 4 biometric indices were more accurate than were those that only used 1 to 2. All models confirmed previous findings that the accuracy decreased at the extremes of newborn weight, where they overestimated low BW and underestimated large BW.[52] Regardless of the formula used, inaccuracy in EFW calculation exists when fetuses are small or large.

EFW is crucial in pregnancy management, where pregnancies identified as growth restricted will have increased surveillance and earlier delivery. Pregnancies identified as macrosomic will have changes in delivery planning in regard to route and timing. Clearly, improving accuracy at extremes of fetal weight will better guide the clinician in the management of a specific pregnancy. As mentioned, certain EFW models may be superior to others given a small or large fetus. In one study, when evaluating pregnancies with BW less than 2,500 g, Hadlock's formulae (Log_{10} EFW = 1.3596 − 0.00386 AC × FL + 0.0064 HC + 0.00061 BPD × AC + 0.0424 AC + 0.174 FL) and (Log_{10} EFW = 1.335 − 0.0034 AC × FL + 0.0316 BPD + 0.0457 AC + 0.1623 FL)[40] were the most accurate when compared with 11 other formulae in predicting EFW.[49] In a different study, for fetuses expected to be less than the 10th percentile, investigators found that symmetric (all measures small) versus asymmetric (AC and FL smaller than head measurements) growth restriction also affected accuracy in EFW. For symmetrically grown fetuses, Hadlock formulae incorporating three or more measures were the most accurate in determining weight. However, in asymmetric fetuses, the Hadlock formula with only two measures that excluded FL was more accurate.[53] Studies investigating small fetuses show that Hadlock's formulae have the highest degree of accuracy, but in the macrosomic fetus, other formulae could provide more appropriate EFWs. When comparing 36 commonly used formulae for EFW on 350 singleton fetuses with BW greater than 4,000 g, Hoopmann et al. showed that Hart's formula (e^7.6377445039 + 0.0002951035 × maternal weight + 0.0003949464 × HC + 0.0005241529 × AC + 0.0048698624 × FL [g, mm])[54] had the lowest MPE and the highest detection rate for macrosomic fetuses. This method also showed that 96% of fetuses fell within 10% of the EFW.[55]

Certain formulae may be more accurate than are others at the extremes of fetal weight, but it may be that customizing a calculation provides the most accuracy. In a Chinese study of 1,034 patients, comparing 25 existing models failed to demonstrate a superior formula for EFW calculation. In this group, they created a regional-specific EFW model that could be used on the whole population. When the model predicted fetuses greater than the 90th percentile or less than the 10th percentile, two different formulae were used: one for small fetuses and one for large fetuses. Using this method, they were able to more accurately predict fetal weight in growth-restricted and macrosomic fetuses.[56] Estimates of fetal soft-tissue mass have been attempted to be measured through three-dimensional (3D) fractional thigh volume, which is an attractive addition to EFW formulae for the accurate prediction of weight in fetuses at the extremes of GA.[57] In one study, it showed superiority over conventional formulae for predicting actual BW in diabetic pregnancies,[58] and in another study, it showed superiority over Hadlock's curve in accuracy of predicting BW.[59]

Accuracy Conclusions

The literature has yet to declare a clear superior formula in the prediction of fetal and newborn weight. Factors affecting EFW include maternal body habitus, formula used, individual variability of the measures taken, and extremes of fetal weight. Although new models incorporating 3D technology have promise because they can evaluate fetal soft-tissue mass, their clinical utility has not yet been adequately studied, and they have not yet entered into common practice. It seems that formulae involving three to four measures are more accurate than those involving one to two except in asymmetrically growth-restricted fetuses. It is recommended that each institution use a consistent formula for assigning an EFW rather than altering the formula for each patient. Universal application would lead to less confusion and more uniform care.

GROWTH CURVES

A growth curve is a graphic model of data that identifies the normal range of growth given a specific GA. Outliers are classified as too large or too small. Usually, a fetus measuring greater than the 90th percentile is defined as LGA, while a fetus measuring less than the 10th percentile is defined as SGA. SGA was originally defined in 1967 by neonatologists to categorize a newborn with a BW of less than the 10th percentile.[60] Over time, SGA was adopted by obstetricians to broadly classify the undergrown fetus regardless of etiology. The correct classification of fetuses as large or small is needed to accurately identify those fetuses that are at risk for poor perinatal outcome. An ideal standard would therefore allow a clinician to appropriately identify a pregnancy as high risk, and a good growth curve is the screening tool that would inform a clinician that increased surveillance is necessary.

Population-Specific Growth Curves

Normal neonatal BW differs depending upon the population studied. Race and ethnicity are key factors in determining normal weight, where black infants have lower mean BWs than do white infants.[61,62] Chinese neonates are lighter than are newborns in the United States,[63] and Asian newborns are smaller than are European newborns.[64] It is not surprising that newborns of different races and different locations across the globe have different BWs, but even when looking at BW ranges in Europe, regional differences exist. Knowing that differences exist is one thing, but does a BW in one region portend a different prognosis than does the same BW in another region? One study by Graafmans and coworkers tried to answer this question. They compared the modal BWs in specific countries, and they investigated their relationship to country-specific mortality curves. They found that shifts in the modal BW values paralleled the shift in the perinatal mortality curve. For example, Scotland has a modal BW of 3,446 g, with the lowest perinatal mortality found at 3,888 g. Norway has a heavier modal BW of 3,622 g, and the perinatal mortality nadirs at 4,305 g.[65] This shows that perinatal outcome related to BW is regionally specific, and each population has an "ideal birth weight." Many countries and institutions have created locally derived BW standards, and the curves generated from the data sources identify newborns at risk for poor outcome based on the individualized regional population. This seems to be a good strategy to identify those pregnancies that should be truly classified as high risk.

Fetal versus Neonatal Growth Curves

Neonatal BW standards vary by population, and European standards have been created identifying different normal weights depending upon the country of birth.[66] In the United States, many BW curves have been created, with one of the first standards defined by Lula Lubchencko in Denver.[67] The use of this BW curve to the general population came into question as this standard reported the BWs of newborns born at moderately high altitude, a known factor leading to smaller newborn size. This again emphasizes the importance of regional standards.

Questions began to arise about the validity of using a BW growth standard for *in utero* fetal weight standards as investigators realized that preterm birth was a pathological condition. In fact, at preterm GAs, the normal population is one in which the mother is still pregnant. As ultrasound technology improved, it was possible to estimate fetal weight using mathematical modeling by measuring certain fetal characteristics as described previously in this chapter. In 1991, Ott and coworkers compared BW percentile at various GAs as determined by an ultrasound-derived EFW curve versus a standard BW curve. When using the ultrasound fetal weight curve as the standard, they showed that the number of fetuses classified as FGR (<10th percentile) decreased as GA advanced. If the BW curve was used to classify a newborn's weight, the number of babies identified as FGR remained static. This caused the authors to draw the conclusion that growth restriction and preterm birth are related.[68] Hadlock et al.[69] created the most commonly used fetal growth curve, which was based on cross-sectional analysis of ultrasound data. By comparing EFW curves and newborn BW curves, the questions to be answered are as follows: (a) How do these curves differ, and (b) which growth standard better identifies fetuses at risk for adverse perinatal outcome?

To address the first question, Bernstein and colleagues created a regional ultrasound-derived EFW curve based on 1,331 normal pregnancies. They compared this curve with the same region's BW data from 9,553 births at various GAs. The estimates for the 10th percentile at each GA were different for all ages except 37 and 38 weeks. In preterm gestations, less than 2% of EFWs fall below the 10th percentile on the BW standard. Conversely, more than 26% of ultrasound EFWs were greater than the 90th percentile on the BW standard.[70] In a French population, Salomon et al. compared an EFW standard with a BW standard created from 18,989 singleton, nonanomalous fetuses and neonates. The growth curves were significantly different, showing that the 50th percentile on the BW standard matched the 10th percentile on the estimated weight standard from 28 to 32 weeks' gestation.[71] These two studies showed that a BW standard will underestimate the number of FGR fetuses and overestimate the number of LGA fetuses when compared with a growth curve created by EFW.

If a growth curve derived from EFW differs from that derived from BW, which curve is better at predicting adverse pregnancy and neonatal outcome? A Canadian study compared the outcomes of 37,377 nonanomalous pregnancies between 25 and 40 weeks classified as FGR on either a BW curve or Hadlock's curve.[69] This study showed that infants classified as FGR from a fetal weight standard were more likely to have preterm birth than those that were appropriately grown; however, if a fetus was classified as FGR on the BW standard, there was no association with preterm birth. The fetal standard identified 90 fetuses that eventually experienced a perinatal death compared with 57 fetuses identified employing the BW standard.[72] By classifying a fetus as FGR on a fetal weight standard, the ability to predict adverse pregnancy outcome is improved over that of using a BW standard. Like pregnancy outcomes, neonatal outcomes have also been investigated. Zaw et al. compared the outcomes of 1,267 newborns at less than 34 weeks and classified them as FGR using either a Canadian BW curve or Hadlock's curve. In this study, babies classified as FGR on the fetal weight standard were more likely to have the neonatal outcomes of respiratory distress syndrome (RDS), bronchopulmonary dysplasia, intraventricular hemorrhage, and retinopathy of prematurity. If the BW curve was used, newborns classified as FGR were more likely to have neonatal mortality, retinopathy of prematurity, and necrotizing enterocolitis.[73] The differences in predictive ability likely hinge on the fact that newborns identified as FGR on the BW curve are the smallest infants using either schema.

Using a fetal standard on ongoing pregnancies will better identify fetuses at risk for pregnancy and perinatal morbidity, whereas using a BW standard will better identify those fetuses destined for neonatal mortality. It is the obligation of the obstetrician to identify a diseased state, where fetuses classified as high risk are at an increased probability of developing poor outcome. Mortality is only one factor when considering poor outcome; therefore, the authors suggest using a fetal weight standard, such as that created by Hadlock et al.[69] when determining the percentile of a given EFW.

Fetal Growth Curves Based on Race or Nationality

As previously mentioned, regional differences in BW correlate with neonatal outcomes, and race has been associated with suboptimal fetal growth.[74,75] The World Health Organization (WHO) created a fetal growth curve looking at 10 different countries throughout the world. They showed that EFW growth varied depending upon the country of origin.[76] A large study by the National Institute of Child Health and Human Development (NICHD) established fetal growth standards for non-Hispanic white, non-Hispanic black, Hispanic, and Asian or Pacific Islander singleton fetuses in the United States. The study showed that EFW differed significantly by race/ethnicity at greater than 20 weeks, and specific growth curves based on race would identify differing amounts of growth abnormalities compared to a universal growth curve.[75] Showing that different populations have different distributions of EFW makes intuitive sense, but does it better predict poor outcome? A recent study by Blue et al. compared Hadlock's fetal growth standard to the NICHD race-specific standards to see which one better predicted neonatal morbidity. Despite its publication being more than 25 years ago, and despite the fact that it was created on a small, white population, Hadlock's standard was better at predicting neonatal morbidity in all races than were the race-specific NICHD fetal growth curves.[77] The INTERGROWTH-21st Century Project created an *in utero* growth curve based on normal pregnancies in eight countries using multiple races and nationalities.[78] When applied to an American population and compared to Hadlock's curve, both curves were comparable in predicting neonatal outcomes, but Hadlock's curve had a higher sensitivity for predicting low BW.[79] At this point, Hadlock's fetal growth standard has been the most-studied growth standard in regard to fetal outcome, and it should not be abandoned in favor of race-specific growth curves.

Alternative Approaches for Growth Assessment

Population growth curves can be generated using databases on either BW or EFW, but many have advocated that designing a regionally specific population curve is still not sensitive enough to appropriately identify those fetuses truly at risk for poor outcome. A baby born at 39 weeks weighing 3,000 g to parents both under 65 inches tall may not be at the same risk as a baby born at the same weight to parents who are above 70 inches tall. This has led some investigators to generate an individualized growth chart to more accurately identify the fetus at high risk.

Gardosi and coworkers have proposed a novel method for a customised growth curve. This group observed that multiple factors influence a neonatal BW, including maternal height, weight in early pregnancy, parity, and ethnic group.[80] Paternal height was also a minor variable that contributes to the infant's weight.[81] This group developed a software program to calculate a fetus' "term optimal weight" using coefficients of adjustment for each of the aforementioned variables. These coefficients were generated from multivariate analysis of large, well-dated BW databases of term infants. The confidence interval for the optimal BW was determined by the coefficient of variation for the mean term BW of the population database. A growth curve for each GA is then created using a log polynomial equation described by Hadlock.[82] This novel approach allows for the generation of a growth curve that takes into consideration normal term BW and normal preterm EFW, while adjusting for factors specific to the parents of a fetus.

Using this methodology, Clausson and coworkers compared perinatal outcomes of infants identified as FGR on a Swedish BW standard versus the individualized growth curve. Infants identified as appropriately grown for their customised standard but less than the 10th percentile on the BW standard were not at risk for poor outcome. Conversely, infants identified as appropriately grown by BW standards but less than the 10th percentile on the customized curve had an increased odds ratio of having a poor outcome.[83] The customised growth curve had a better ability to predict perinatal outcomes such as stillbirth, neonatal death, and Apgar scores less than 4 at 5 minutes.[82] The findings from this study were confirmed in French, Spanish, and US populations.[84–86] In addition, the methodology has been used to generate customized growth standards for multiple gestations. When comparing a growth curve customized for twins to a customized curve for singletons, the curve for twins was more accurate in predicting fetal demise.[87] From multiple studies, the individualized growth curve is superior to BW standards at identifying fetuses at risk for poor perinatal outcome.

The concept of an customised growth chart that takes into consideration maternal characteristics, paternal factors, and fetal number and sex is an attractive one. However, few data are available comparing this model directly to a fetal growth curve. A large study by Hutcheon and colleagues compared the customised curve to a BW curve and Hadlock's curve. When looking at 782,303 infants, compared with the BW standard, both the customised standard and the fetal standard identified more fetuses as less than the 10th percentile at preterm gestations. However, they identified a statistically similar number of patients as FGR when compared with each other. In addition, the study confirmed that the BW standard was inferior in predicting which fetuses will have stillbirth or neonatal death; however, the customised curve was similar to the fetal standard in predicting these outcomes.[88] This study suggests that the true benefit of an customised curve rests on establishing an *in utero* standard, and the effect of maternal and paternal characteristics is minimal. Further study is needed to confirm these findings; and until data are available, the use of a fetal growth curve, such as that provided by Hadlock et al.,[69] seems to provide as much accuracy as the customised curve in identifying fetuses that are at high risk of poor perinatal outcome.

Some authors have described other methods of assessing individualized growth assessment, and this is beyond the scope of this chapter. A good review article addressing these assessment tools can be found by Deter et al.[89]

MAGNETIC RESONANCE IMAGING

Ultrasound is the gold standard method for assessing fetal growth, but some authors have started using magnetic resonance imaging (MRI) as an adjunctive imaging modality in the assessment of at-risk fetuses. MRI has the advantage of a larger field of view, it is not affected by maternal body habitus or fetal position, and it has multiplanar and modal capabilities. One attractive feature of MRI is the ability to measure volume in 3D planes. In one of the first studies, Baker et al. measured fetal liver and placental and brain volumes in 32 fetuses to see whether there was any association with newborn weight below the 10th percentile. Interestingly, the liver volume was less than the 2.5th percentile in 10 of 11 fetuses who ultimately weighed less than the 10th percentile at birth. The placenta and brain did not show any reduction in measured volume compared with normally grown newborns.[90] Duncan et al. compared MRI with ultrasound in 74 fetuses, roughly half of which were growth restricted at birth. In this analysis, ultrasound fetal weight was superior to MRI in identifying fetuses that were measuring SGA. In contrast to the prior study, asymmetric FGR fetuses (head size preserved) had reduced brain volume on MRI, suggesting that cerebral growth is still affected by growth restriction.[91] This was not confirmed by another group in 2012. In this study, MRI was performed on 20 growth-restricted fetuses and 19 normal fetuses. There was a significant reduction in whole-body volume and of all internal organs in growth-restricted fetuses except the fetal brain. In fact, with a brain:liver volume ratio above 3.0, there was a 3.3-fold increased risk of perinatal mortality.[92] All three of these studies were small, and their assessments should be confirmed with larger analysis. However, the results parallel those seen by ultrasound in that fetuses that demonstrate growth abnormalities will have reduction in size of the fetal liver, which is incorporated in the ultrasonographic measurement of the AC. MRI is a relatively new technology in pregnancy assessment, and future studies could be performed to assess whether there is any benefit with assessment of fetal body composition, the macrosomic fetus, fetal brain perfusion, and the obese mother, all of which have limitations by current ultrasound technology.

USE OF DOPPLER VELOCIMETRY IN FETAL GROWTH RESTRICTION

Doppler Physics

The Doppler Effect, described by Johann Christian Doppler in 1842, shows that when energy is reflected from a moving boundary, the frequency of the reflected energy varies in relation to the velocity and direction of the moving boundary. In ultrasonography, Doppler velocimetry depends upon the ability of an ultrasound beam to be changed in frequency when encountering a moving object (e.g., red blood cells [RBCs]). The change in frequency ("frequency shift") is directly proportional to the speed with which the RBCs are moving within a particular vessel and it is also dependent on the cosine of the angle that the ultrasound beam makes with the direction of blood flow, also referred to as the angle of insonation (Fig. 4.9). After some cosmetic manipulation by ultrasound programming, a flow velocity waveform is generated with the velocity in centimeter per second (reflecting the Doppler frequency shift) on the y-axis and time on the x-axis. For arterial waveforms, there is a clear systolic and diastolic component, while venous waveforms are typically steady and without pulsations (exceptions are centrally located veins such as the hepatic veins [HV], ductus venosus [DV], inferior vena cava [IVC], and pulmonary veins). Two general characteristics of vascular

flow can be determined from the flow velocity waveforms. One of these is resistance or impedance to blood flow, and the second is the velocity of the blood moving through the vessel. To get the true velocity of the RBCs within a blood vessel, one needs to reduce the angle of insonation to 0°, as shown in Figure 4.10. Ultrasound machines that have pulsed-wave Doppler capabilities generally have the ability to have the operator angle correct the Doppler signal. Several indices of resistance have been described, and the more commonly used indices are shown in Figure 4.11. The systolic/diastolic ratio (S/D ratio) is the most commonly used clinically in the United States, although all three correlate very highly and are used throughout the literature.

One of the characteristics of these resistance indices is angle independence. Changing the angle of insonation between the ultrasound Doppler beam and blood flow direction will produce a different appearing waveform. However, the waveforms will still be proportionate in nature. Thus, regardless of the index of resistance used, the same value will be obtained (e.g., the S/D ratios will be the same; Fig. 4.12). This is an advantage in the interrogation of vessels given that one cannot always obtain the same angle

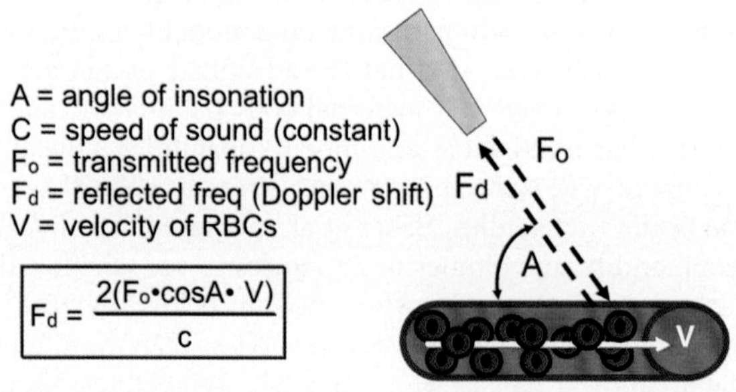

A = angle of insonation
C = speed of sound (constant)
F_o = transmitted frequency
F_d = reflected freq (Doppler shift)
V = velocity of RBCs

$$F_d = \frac{2(F_o \cdot \cos A \cdot V)}{c}$$

FIGURE 4.9: Relationship between the pulsed-wave Doppler signals transmitted (F_o) and received (F_d) by the transducer and the velocity of the red blood cells (RBCs). This relationship is defined in the above formula. The Doppler (frequency) shift is directly proportional to the speed with which the RBCs are moving within a particular vessel, and it is also dependent on the cosine of the angle the Doppler beam makes with the blood vessel (as defined in the equation).

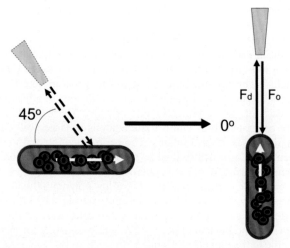

FIGURE 4.10: Example of angle correction with elimination of the angle between the Doppler beam and the interrogated vessel. This brings the angle of insonation to 0°, whereby the reflected Doppler signal (F_d) represents the actual speed of the blood. F_d, reflected frequency or Doppler shift; F_o, transmitted frequency.

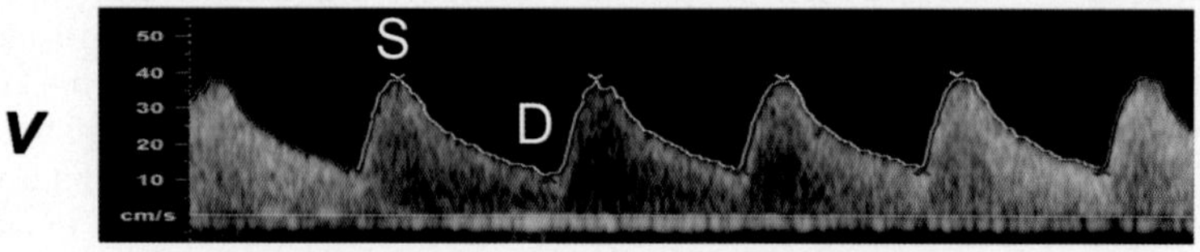

Index	Calculation
Systolic to diastolic (S/D) ratio	$\dfrac{\underline{\text{Systolic peak velocity}}}{\text{Diastolic peak velocity}}$
Resistance index (RI)	$\dfrac{\underline{\text{Systolic – end-diastolic peak velocity}}}{\text{Systolic peak velocity}}$
Pulsatility index (PI)	$\dfrac{\underline{\text{Systolic – end-diastolic peak velocity}}}{\text{Time-averaged maximum velocity}}$

FIGURE 4.11: Commonly used indices of resistance to assess blood flow velocity.

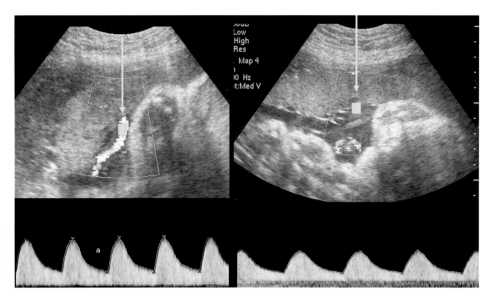

FIGURE 4.12: Two ultrasound images with color Doppler depicting different angles of insonation with flow velocity waveforms that are different in appearance, but proportionate in nature.

of insonation for any given vessel, especially when dealing with the uncontrollable and variable position of the fetus. A technical pearl to keep in mind is that the best waveform attainable is one in which the angle of insonation is closest to 0°. Obtaining the best possible waveform can be particularly useful when trying to determine whether there is low or absent end-diastolic flow (AEDF) in the umbilical artery. Also in this setting, a low wall filter setting is beneficial. In clinical practice, an angle less than 30° is generally acceptable for Doppler measurement.

Umbilical Artery Doppler Ultrasound

The fetal vessel most commonly interrogated with color and pulsed-wave Doppler ultrasound is the umbilical artery, which was first reported in 1977 by Fitzgerald and Drumm.[93] There is a GA-related increase in diastolic flow velocity in the umbilical artery both in human and in sheep pregnancies. This corresponds to the decreasing resistance to blood flow resulting from growth of placental vessels that branch from the umbilical arteries. Figure 4.13 depicts the progressive increase in diastolic flow

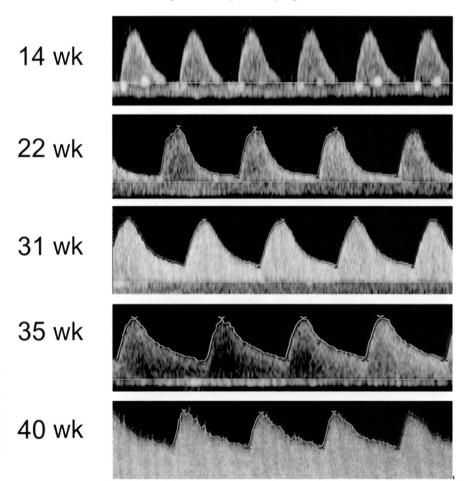

FIGURE 4.13: Umbilical artery flow velocity waveforms showing an increase in diastolic flow with advancing gestational age. This increase in diastolic flow is a result of the processes of placental branching angiogenesis at the end of the first trimester and beginning of the second, and nonbranching angiogenesis that starts at the end of the second and into the third trimesters.

velocity across gestation in normal pregnancy. Assessment of the flow velocity waveform in the umbilical artery has been described numerous times in the clinical setting of FGR. The abnormal flow velocity waveform in the umbilical artery of FGR fetuses was first described by Trudinger et al.[94] in 1985. In this study, 85% of 43 infants less than the 10th percentile BW had S/D ratios greater than the 95th percentile for GA, and this was secondary to a decrease in diastolic velocity in turn due to high resistance to blood flow downstream in the placenta. The degree of resistance in the umbilical artery, and thus in the smaller downstream placental arterial vasculature to which it is connected, can be determined by analysis of the flow velocity waveform. The three common resistance indices used for arterial flow are shown in Figure 4.11. Figure 4.14 shows an initially normal flow velocity waveform that becomes progressively abnormal in an FGR fetus. In FGR pregnancies with increased umbilical artery resistance indices, approximately 30% of the placental villous vessels are abnormal.[95] As the FGR placental disease worsens, the velocity waveforms may show AEDF and then reversed end-diastolic flow (REDF). At this stage, 60% to 70% of the villous vessels will be abnormal.[96,97] In addition, there is a rate of 50% to 80% of intrauterine hypoxia by the time AEDF is apparent.[98–100] From a clinical standpoint, AEDF in the umbilical artery is associated with an 80-fold increase in perinatal mortality.[101]

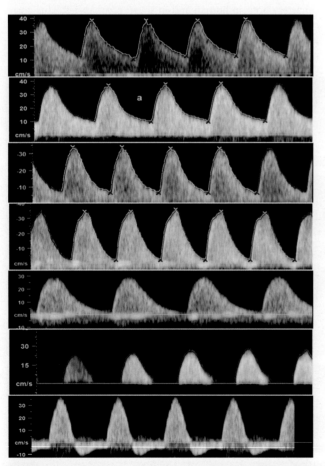

FIGURE 4.14: Multiple sequential umbilical artery flow velocity waveforms depicting a progressive increase in resistance over time in a fetal growth restriction fetus with advancing placental disease. Note that the end-diastolic flow progresses from normal in the first waveform to abnormal with absent end-diastolic flow and then to reversed end-diastolic flow.

Middle Cerebral Artery Doppler Ultrasound

The middle cerebral artery (MCA) is another commonly interrogated fetal vessel in the setting of FGR. The MCA is easy to visualize by obtaining a suboccipitobregmatic axial plane through the fetus and applying color Doppler ultrasound. This will allow the circle of Willis to be visualized with six cerebral vessels extending from the circle of Willis. These vessels are paired and named the anterior, middle, and posterior cerebral arteries. The MCA tends to be the easiest to visualize given the lateral orientation of the vessel and the fact that the vessel carries approximately 80% of the cerebral blood flow. In normal circumstances, the flow velocity waveform in the MCA reflects the normally high impedance of the cerebral circulation in comparison with the normal umbilical artery waveform. Several studies in humans and in animal models have shown that an increase in diastolic flow velocity in the MCA is consistent with a chronic hypoxemic state in the fetus (Fig. 4.15). In addition, there is a redistribution of blood flow from nonvital organ systems and the torso of the fetus toward the fetal heart, brain, and adrenal glands.[102–105]

Clinically, the MCA Doppler ultrasound in FGR management is useful primarily in two ways. The first is a combination of the MCA PI and the umbilical artery pulsatility index (PI) in the form of a ratio. This was first reported as the cerebroplacental ratio (CPR = MCA PI/Umb art PI) by Arbeille et al.[106] and subsequently by others.[102,107] CPR values less than 1.0 or 1.08 have been reported as abnormal. Bahado-Singh et al. reported that the CPR correlates well with BWs less than the fifth percentile with and without neonatal complications compared with the umbilical artery alone. They also showed that among 123 FGR fetuses, those with an abnormal CPR were born 5 weeks earlier, weigh 850 g less, and had a significantly greater number of neonatal complications. Importantly, this manuscript also identifies that the CPR beyond 34 weeks loses its predictive ability and thus clinical utility. This is because the umbilical artery waveform may not become abnormal in FGR pregnancies beyond 34 weeks. Their observation supports prior studies that report that the umbilical artery Doppler ultrasound may not become abnormal in the late (>34 week) FGR fetuses (Fig. 4.16).[107] A larger study by Akelekar et al. showed similar findings. When looking at the CPR in pregnancies between 35 and 37 weeks, there was a higher sensitivity for detecting abnormal perinatal outcome in FGR fetuses (60%), but this came with a false-positive rate of 34%.[108] A second area where the MCA Doppler velocimetry alone has begun to show some potential clinical utility is in the late FGR fetus. FGR fetuses with a normal umbilical artery, but a reduced MCA PI, show higher rates of neurological behavioral problems and a higher rate of nonreassuring fetal heart rate (FHR) pattern in labor, often leading to an emergency cesarean section.[109–111] Thus, although the late-onset FGR (>34 weeks) fetus may not develop abnormal umbilical artery Doppler velocimetry, the fetus may still develop an abnormal MCA Doppler waveform and still identify a pregnancy at risk for adverse outcome. This occurs in up to 40% of FGR pregnancies (98–100). In clinical practice, use of the CPR to identify pregnancies at greater risk for adverse outcomes can be used for counseling purposes. However, insufficient data are available to use CPR as a trigger for delivery. A reduction in the MCA peak systolic velocity, an index used clinically to assess for fetal anemia, has been associated with fetal polycythemia in FGR; however, the clinical utility of this measurement is yet to be determined.

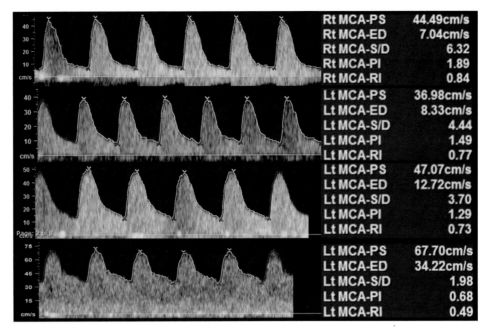

Rt MCA-PS	44.49cm/s
Rt MCA-ED	7.04cm/s
Rt MCA-S/D	6.32
Rt MCA-PI	1.89
Rt MCA-RI	0.84
Lt MCA-PS	36.98cm/s
Lt MCA-ED	8.33cm/s
Lt MCA-S/D	4.44
Lt MCA-PI	1.49
Lt MCA-RI	0.77
Lt MCA-PS	47.07cm/s
Lt MCA-ED	12.72cm/s
Lt MCA-S/D	3.70
Lt MCA-PI	1.29
Lt MCA-RI	0.73
Lt MCA-PS	67.70cm/s
Lt MCA-ED	34.22cm/s
Lt MCA-S/D	1.98
Lt MCA-PI	0.68
Lt MCA-RI	0.49

FIGURE 4.15: Normal and abnormal middle cerebral artery flow velocity waveforms in a fetal growth restriction (FGR) fetus. There is a progressive increase in the diastolic flow velocity, resulting in a progression from a normal waveform with a high resistance to flow to an abnormal waveform with very low resistance. The abnormal waveforms with increase in diastolic flow velocity are consistent with chronic hypoxemia of FGR.

Venous Vessel Doppler Ultrasound

The precardiac venous vessels have been studied extensively in FGR. These "venous structures" are a general reference to the DV, HV, and the IVC. The anatomical relationship of these venous structures to one another and the liver are elegantly described and illustrated in the 16-week human fetus microdissections by Mavrides et al.[112] Figure 4.17 depicts the vasculature of the fetal hepatic and portal circulations. The umbilical vein is a conduit vessel that delivers nutrient- and oxygen-rich blood from the placenta to the fetus. After entering the abdominal wall, the umbilical vein courses anteriorly through the falciform ligament entering the liver and becoming the portal sinus. On ultrasound, this portal sinus is depicted as the characteristic hypoechoic vascular structure with an L or hockey-stick appearance (Fig. 4.18) and has a typical steady venous flow velocity waveform Doppler pattern. The portal sinus delivers blood to the left lobe of the liver via the inferior and superior portal veins and venules, and terminates in the right lobe of the liver, where this fresh blood coalesces with flows from the portal circulation. Ultrasound resolution is sufficiently

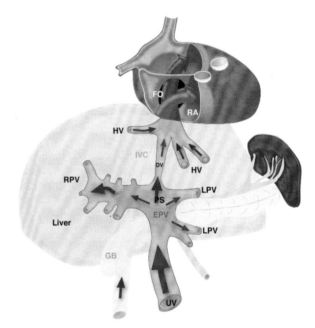

FIGURE 4.17: Schematic representation of the fetal umbilical, portal, and hepatic venous circulations. The *arrows* indicate the direction of blood flow. The *red color* reflects the more oxygenated blood and the *blue color* the lesser oxygenated blood. *DV*, ductus venosus; *EPV*, extrahepatic portal vein; *FO*, foramen ovale; *GB*, gall bladder; *HV*, hepatic veins; *IVC*, inferior vena cava; *LPV*, left portal vein; *PS*, portal sinus; *RA*, right atrium; *RPV*, right portal vein; *UV*, umbilical vein. (From Mavrides E, Moscoso G, Carvalho JS, et al. The anatomy of the umbilical, portal and hepatic venous systems in the human fetus at 14–19 weeks of gestation. *Ultrasound Obstet Gynecol.* 2001;18(6):598–604. Copyright © 2001 International Society of Ultrasound in Obstetrics and Gynecology. Reprinted by permission of John Wiley & Sons, Inc..)

FIGURE 4.16: The cerebroplacental ratio *(CPR)* is shown across gestation in 123 fetal growth restriction fetuses. Note that the CPR loses its ability to identify morbidity in fetuses less than the 10th percentile after 34 weeks *(box).* (Reprinted from Bahado-Singh RO, Kovanci E, Jeffres A, et al. The Doppler cerebroplacental ratio and perinatal outcome in intrauterine growth restriction. *Am J Obstet Gynecol.* 1999;180(3):750–756. Copyright © 1999 Elsevier. With permission.)

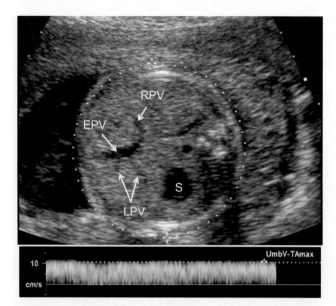

FIGURE 4.18: Axial ultrasound image of the fetal abdomen showing the portal sinus vasculature with the characteristic "hockey-stick" appearance. Also shown is a steady, nonpulsatile Doppler flow velocity waveform characteristic of the portal and umbilical venous vessels. *EPV*, extrahepatic portal vein; *LPV*, left portal vein; *RPV*, right portal vein; *S*, stomach.

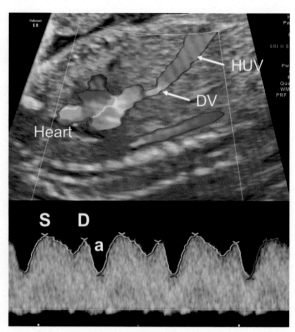

FIGURE 4.19: Longitudinal ultrasound image of the fetus with color Doppler showing the hepatic portion of the umbilical vein (*HUV*; also termed extrahepatic portal vein), the ductus venosus *(DV)*, and fetal heart. Note the aliasing of the DV that allows for easy identification of the DV. Also shown is the triphasic flow velocity waveform of the ductus venosus obtained by pulsed-wave *(PW)* Doppler. *a*, atrial contraction; *D*, early diastole; *S*, systole. (Courtesy of Simona Ivanov, RDMS, and Henry L. Galan, MD.)

high that even the echolucent lines representing the left portal veins can be seen (see Fig. 4.18). At the approximate bend of the L-shaped portal sinus, about 50% of the blood delivered by the umbilical veins is shunted through the cone-shaped DV vessel, allowing this fresh blood to bypass the highly metabolic liver and stream toward the fetal heart. These vessels coalesce into an area just beneath the diaphragm that has been described as the subdiaphragmatic vestibulum, where the process of differential streaming is initiated. Preferential streaming directs the more nutrient- and oxygen-rich blood across the foramen ovale into the left atrium and left ventricle. This results in the fetal heart (via coronary vessels) and the fetal brain through the aorta receiving this oxygen-rich blood.

The central venous vessels (DV, HV, and IVC) have characteristic triphasic pulsed-wave Doppler waveforms that reflect the normal central venous pressure changes, while the peripheral venous vessels (umbilical vein and portal sinus) have steady-flow velocity waveforms. The normal triphasic flow velocity waveforms of the central venous vessels have three components, which are shown in Figure 4.19. The highest pressure gradient between the venous vessels and the right atrium occurs during ventricular systole, resulting in the highest blood flow velocity. This is the first peak of forward flow. The second phase of forward flow occurs during early diastole when the atrioventricular (AV) valves open with passive early filling of the ventricles. The nadir of flow velocities occurs with atrial contraction during late diastole, at which time the foramen ovale flap and crista dividens meet. One advantage of venous Doppler ultrasound interrogation is that it provides assessment of cardiac forward function. The forward function is complex and is determined by afterload, compliance, and contractility. The DV waveform normally has forward flow throughout the cardiac cycles, whereas the IVC and HV waveforms have reverse or absent flow at the atrial kick. The complex triphasic waveform has been described by multiple venous Doppler indices, none of which has been shown to have a clear advantage (Table 4.4). Hecher et al.[113] and Rizzo et al.[114] performed fetal

blood sampling in fetuses who had reversal of flow in the DV or greatly reversed flow in the IVC and showed that this is consistent with an acidemic state in the fetus. The utility of umbilical artery and venous Doppler ultrasound in FGR management is discussed further later.

Uterine Artery Doppler Assessment

The uterine arteries that emanate from the maternal hypogastric arteries bilaterally have a variable and at times tortuous course along the lateral aspects of the uterus before terminating in the much smaller caliber spiral arteries embedded in the myometrium. In the nonpregnant state and early pregnancy period, the spiral arteries are characterized by a high vascular impedance state. Under normal circumstances, in the first trimester of pregnancy, placental cytotrophoblast cells differentiate into invasive and noninvasive cytotrophoblast cells.[115] These specialized trophoblast cells penetrate and cross the decidualized endometrium, invading the maternal and spiral radial arteries. This results in physiological remodeling of arterial musculature, transforming these normally high-resistance vessels into low-resistance vessels. If the trophoblast invasion remains confined to the decidualized endometrial portion of the myometrium, maternal spiral and radial arteries fail to undergo the physiological transformation into low-resistance vessels. Blood flow impedance in these small-caliber vessels can be detected upstream in the larger caliber uterine artery vessels through the use of color and pulsed-wave Doppler velocimetry. The normal flow velocity waveform in the uterine artery after vascular remodeling is characterized by a smooth gentle peak systolic component, absence of an early or protodiastolic notch, and high end-diastolic flow velocity that results in

TABLE 4.4	Formulae for the Doppler Indices Commonly Used for the Central Venous Vessels
INDEX	**CALCULATION**
Ductus venosus (DV) preload index	$\dfrac{\text{systolic} - \text{diastolic peak velocity}}{\text{systolic peak velocity}}$
Inferior vena cava (IVC) preload index	$\dfrac{\text{peak velocity during atrial contraction}}{\text{systolic peak velocity}}$
IVC and DV pulsatility index for veins (PIV)	$\dfrac{\text{systolic} - \text{diastolic peak velocity}}{\text{time} - \text{averaged maximum velocity}}$
IVC and DV peak velocity index for veins (PVIV)	$\dfrac{\text{systolic} - \text{atrial contraction peak velocity}}{\text{diastolic peak velocity}}$
Percentage reverse flow	$\dfrac{\text{systolic time averaged velocity}}{\text{diastolic time averaged velocity}} \times 100$

low-resistance indices. Normal and abnormal flow velocity waveforms in the uterine artery are shown in Figure 4.20. The low-resistance transformation in the small-caliber vessels is generally expected by 22 to 24 weeks. Many studies and reviews have illustrated that failure to achieve low resistance in these vessels is associated with an increased risk for adverse pregnancy outcomes, including the development of preeclampsia, FGR, placental abruption, and other adverse pregnancy outcomes.[116] While the evidence that uterine artery Doppler ultrasound abnormalities are associated with and predictive of adverse pregnancy outcomes is strong, the benefit and application of uterine artery Doppler assessment in pregnancy as a screening tool, either for routine use in low- or high-risk pregnancies, remain controversial and is currently not recommended.[117]

Cardiac Doppler Ultrasound

The fetal heart is probably the most challenging organ to interrogate in the fetus as blood that flows into, through, and out of the heart is affected by several factors including preload, afterload, heart rate, and compliance. Several investigators have reported on cardiac Doppler flow changes and function in FGR, and some of these have been conducted in a longitudinal manner. In addition to functional cardiac status, numerous sites in the fetal heart have

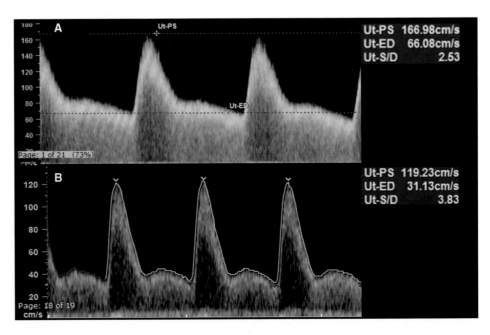

FIGURE 4.20: Normal **(A)** and abnormal **(B)** flow velocity waveforms in the uterine artery. Note the softer peak, absence of early diastolic notching, higher end-diastolic flow, and lower systolic/diastolic ratio (S/D ratio) in the normal uterine artery waveform in **A** compared with that of the abnormal waveform in **B**.

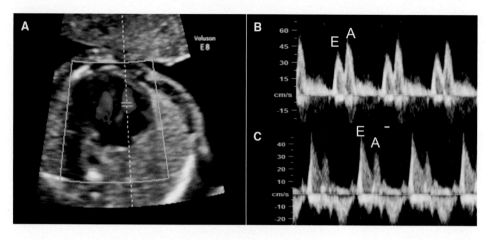

FIGURE 4.21: A: Four-chamber view of the heart showing the location of the Doppler sample volume at the distal point of the opening of the atrioventricular *(AV)* valve. **B:** The characteristic M shape of the flow velocity waveform with the E and A components through the valve. Reversal of the E/A waveform is seen in extrauterine life and can be seen in FGR **(C)**. (Courtesy of Lisa Howley, MD.)

been interrogated by real-time, color, and Doppler ultrasound. These include, but are not limited to, E/A ratios, DV, aortic isthmus, myocardial performance indices, cardiac outflow tracts, the right and left diastolic function, and coronary arteries.[113,118–124] The more commonly interrogated sites in the fetal heart are the aortic and pulmonary outflow tracts, DV, and atrioventricular (AV) valves. Because flow indices at the level of the heart are quantitative in nature, it is important to be cognizant of the angle of insonation and try to maintain it less than 20° since at greater angles than this, the measurements are less reliable.

The AV valve Doppler flow investigation is best obtained in a four- or five-chamber view, with the sample volumes placed just distal to the opening of the AV valves within the ventricular chamber. The Doppler beam should be nearly parallel to the flow of blood in order to obtain the best and most consistent waveforms possible. The waveform should have a characteristic "M" configuration from which the E/A ratio, which expresses the diastolic ventricular function, can be calculated. This M configuration is similar in the tricuspid and mitral valves, which suggests similar diastolic function in the two ventricles.[125] The E component of the ratio (initial peak velocity) represents early and fast ventricular filling, while the A component (second peak velocity) represents peak velocity with atrial contraction (Fig. 4.21). Under normal circumstances *in utero*, the E peak velocity is less than the A peak velocity. Because the ratio is related to preload and cardiac compliance, the ratio increases with advancing GA.[126] Postnatally, the E/A ratio reverses and assumes the adult pattern of the E peak velocity being greater than the A peak velocity. In FGR, diastolic function can be damaged by insufficient ventricular filling and can appear either as a lower E/A ratio or as a significant reduction of the atrial peak in the flow velocity waveform.[113,123,127,128]

Normally, the contributions of the right and left ventricles to the combined fetal cardiac output (CCO) are 60% and 40%, respectively. Approximately, 40% of the CCO is delivered to the low-resistance vascular bed of the placenta. In FGR, there are several mechanisms involved in affecting the flows through the fetal heart. These include (1) increase in afterload secondary to increases in placental blood flow resistance, (2) reduced blood flow volume, (3) reduction in diastolic function due to inadequate ventricular filling via the AV valves, and (4) progressive enlargement of the cardiac structures such as the AV valves and the outflow tract vessels. The net result is a decrease in CCO with an approximate 10% shift from the right ventricle to the left, resulting in a decrease in the right-to-left cardiac output ratio.[129] There is also a decrease in the peak velocities in both the aortic and the pulmonary outflow tracts.[121] In addition, the reduction of peak velocity in the pulmonary outflow tract is seen with more

frequency (95% of FGR cases) than in the aortic tract (57% of FGR cases), which is understandable given that it is the right side of the heart (via the ductus arteriosus) that is most affected by the increase in afterload. The reduction in ventricular peak velocities is considered to be a relatively late cardiovascular finding in the decompensating FGR fetus.[119] The ventricle damage that is seen in FGR because of inadequate filling of the ventricles is reflected in the AV valves where either a decrease in the E/A ratio or an isolated atrial peak systolic waveform may be seen.[113,123,127,128]

A less commonly discussed cardiac vascular structure in the setting of FGR is the coronary artery. In 1998, Baschat et al.[130] reported that fetal coronary artery blood flow could be visualized in normal fetuses at 32 weeks and beyond. Coronary artery blood flow identification requires close attention to color Doppler ultrasound setting, as described by these authors, including (1) adjustment of color Doppler velocity scale between 27 and 48 cm per second, depending on the depth of insonation and the transducer used, (2) reduction in size of the color Doppler box and gate as much as possible to optimize both temporal and spatial resolution, (3) setting the color filter to a high degree of motion discrimination, (4) setting the color amplification gain to eliminate color background noise on the screen, and (5) selection of a persistence setting from a range of 0 (no averaging of frames) to 3. They also verify the identification of coronary vessels by color Doppler ultrasound, with pulsed-wave Doppler flow showing the typical flow velocity waveform.[130] In a follow-up study, these authors also showed that coronary artery blood flow could be visualized at an earlier GA in FGR fetuses (e.g., <32 weeks) with abnormal arterial and venous Doppler findings, and that these fetuses with absent/reversed end-diastolic velocity (A/REDV) and centralization of blood flow are at high risk for hypoxemia, acidemia, and adverse outcome.[131] The authors speculated that the visualization of coronary blood flow less than 32 weeks represents another example of the "sparing" effects seen in FGR. While interrogation of coronary vessels was seen in conjunction with venous Doppler abnormalities, further investigation is needed to show whether there is additional benefit to interrogating the coronary vessels.

SURVEILLANCE OF THE FETAL GROWTH RESTRICTION FETUS

The FGR fetus is at increased risk for progressive placental dysfunction, deterioration of acid–base balance, and stillbirth. As such, fetal surveillance in this condition is warranted. Several tools are available to assess the status of the FGR fetus, and these are listed in Table 4.5.

TABLE 4.5   Surveillance Tools in Fetal Growth Restriction

Maternal monitoring of fetal activity

Amniotic fluid volume (AFV)

Nonstress testing

Biophysical profile

Modified biophysical profile (NST + AFV assessment)

Doppler velocimetry

Interval growth

NST, nonstress test.

Fetal Movement

Several methods have been described for maternal assessment of fetal movement. A simple technique involves having the patient lie on her side and record any fetal movement one or two times per day. The fetus should move 10 times within a 2-hour period, although most pregnant patients will feel their fetuses achieve the target movements in the first 5 to 10 minutes of maternal monitoring. Failure to achieve 10 movements in a 2-hour period warrants further fetal evaluation with nonstress testing (NST). In a 1975 study, Matthews[132] showed the predictive value of fetal activity counts in 50 FGR fetuses who subsequently demonstrated distress in labor.

Amniotic Fluid Volume

Assessment of amniotic fluid volume is important as the amniotic fluid is a reflection of fetal renal perfusion and an indirect measure of fetal vascular status.

Amniotic fluid assessment by ultrasound can be determined by one of the three general methods: amniotic fluid index (AFI) absolute value of less than 5 cm, AFI of less than the fifth percentile for GA, or deepest vertical pocket (DVP) or maximal vertical pocket (MVP). A nomogram for amniotic fluid across gestation is shown in Table 4 in Appendix A1. There are limitations to the use of ultrasound to assess the amniotic fluid volume. Ultrasound sources of error when estimating the amniotic fluid volume include excess abdominal pressure by the sonographer, multiple loops of cord, umbilical, or placental cysts, and particulate variation in the amniotic fluid (e.g., meconium). Controversy exists regarding the best cutoffs to use to define oligohydramnios and polyhydramnios. Assessment by ultrasound is only an indirect measurement of amniotic fluid volume, and previous studies of amniotic fluid volume determination comparing ultrasound with intra-amniotic dye tests have shown the limited accuracy of ultrasound at both extremes of amniotic fluid volumes.[133] Although there is no consensus regarding the best ultrasound method to predict adverse neonatal outcome, the single MVP has higher specificity than does AFI and reduces the likelihood of intervention without a demonstrable benefit and without increased risk of adverse effects for the fetus.[133–135]

While low amniotic fluid (anhydramnios or oligohydramnios) itself is a poor screening tool for FGR, it may be the first sign of a growth-restricted fetus. Up to 96% of fetuses with fluid pockets less than 1 cm in depth may be FGR.[136] A gradual reduction in amniotic fluid volume is due to redistribution of blood flow favoring the fetal heart, brain, and adrenal glands, and away from the lungs, digestive tract, kidneys, and torso, has been well described with hypoxia in lambs.[137] This "brain-sparing" effect has been described in human FGR pregnancies, and the reduction in renal blood flow is felt to account for the oligohydramnios.[138,139] The relationship of oligohydramnios and progressive worsening of both arterial and venous Doppler velocimetry findings has been previously described.[140] The large PORTO trial on FGR demonstrated that low AFI is most valuable clinically when the FGR fetus is less than the third percentile.[141]

Antepartum Testing

The NST and the biophysical profile (BPP) are the two most commonly used standard surveillance tools in high-risk pregnancies. The NST is a method of FHR analysis that uses Doppler technology to record and trace the FHR concomitantly with contraction monitoring. NST reactivity is defined as two accelerations (15 bpm above baseline for 15 seconds' duration) within a 20-minute window, and this must occur within 40 minutes of monitoring. In fetuses less than 32 weeks, reactivity has been defined as accelerations greater than 10 bpm above baseline for greater than 10 seconds. Antepartum testing with the NST is combined with amniotic fluid assessment, and when the testing is normal, it identifies a fetus with a normal fetal acid–base status and low risk of stillbirth.[142,143] While 80% of fetuses beyond 32 weeks have a reactive NST, the rate of reactivity is lower in FGR fetuses. Studies have shown that there is delay in central nervous system (CNS) maturation, including a delay in the normal decline of FHR with advancing gestation, decreased short- and long-term variability, and delay in reactivity, especially in early FGR.[144,145] Thus, additional testing with the BPP or prolonged monitoring is commonly required for FGR fetuses especially for those that are early in gestation (<30 weeks).

While CNS maturation is delayed, centrally regulated responses to hypoxia remain preserved.[146] Because of delay in reactivity in FGR fetuses and because FGR is seen early in pregnancy before reactivity is expected, the four-point BPP is commonly used. A BPP score of 4 or less is strongly associated with a pH less than 7.20. Further, a BPP score of 2 or less has 100% sensitivity for prediction of acidemia. With progressive fetal hypoxemia and acidemia, the FGR fetus will show a progressive loss of fetal breathing motions, body movements, and tone, and eventually cessation of all activity.[147–149] If the decrease in activity is acute, amniotic fluid volume may not be decreased. In contrast, if activity reduces gradually, the amniotic fluid volume may decrease. Given that reactivity is not generally expected in early FGR (<30 weeks), the four-component BPP without FHR assessment (e.g., the 8-point BPP) makes clinical sense. However, while reactivity is not necessarily anticipated, monitoring the fetus with the FHR tracing will allow for assessment of FHR decelerations that would likely be missed in a BPP unless the fetus were acidemic. A BPP score of 4 or less, recurrent decelerations, or nonreactive FHR tracing by computerized cardiac monitoring is associated with an increased rate of fetal hypoxemia, acidemia, cord compression from oligohydramnios, and increased perinatal mortality.[100,142,143,150] The frequency of fetal monitoring using these techniques is dependent on the GA of the fetus and the severity of the FGR condition. This is further elucidated in an algorithm for FGR management in Figure 4.22. Monitoring of the FGR fetus with pulsed-wave

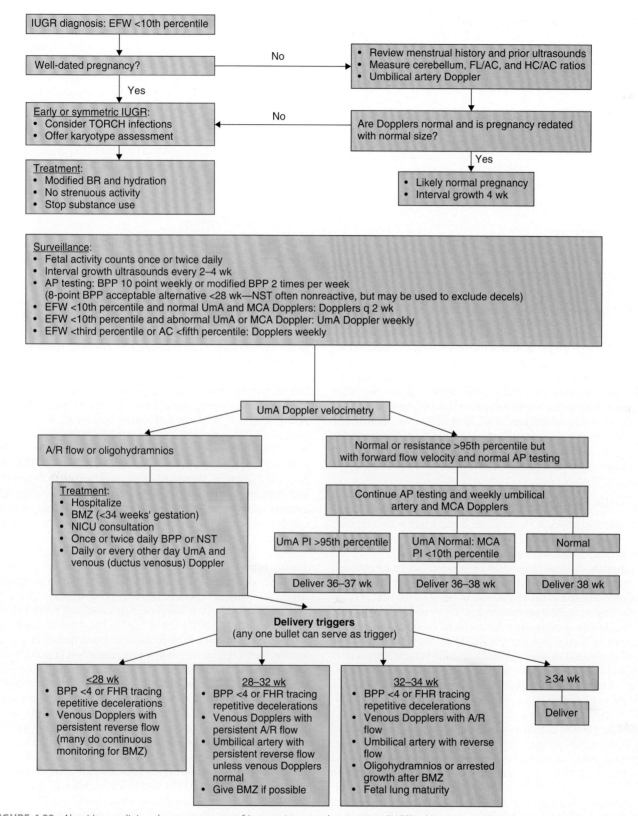

FIGURE 4.22: Algorithm outlining the management of intrauterine growth restriction (IUGR) taking into account the gestational dating, possible etiologies, and potential treatments, as well as providing a guideline for fetal surveillance (antepartum testing and Doppler studies) and timing of delivery. *AC*, abdominal circumference; *AP*, antepartum; *A/R*, absent/reverse; *BMZ*, betamethasone; *BPP*, biophysical profile; *BR*, bed rest; *EFW*, estimated fetal weight; *FL*, femur length; *FHR*, fetal heart rate; *HC*, head circumference; *MCA*, middle cerebral artery; *NICU*, neonatal intensive care unit; *NST*, nonstress test; *PI*, pulsatility index; *UmA*, umbilical artery.

Doppler velocimetry has been used effectively for three decades to assess the status of the FGR fetus. Use of Doppler ultrasound as a trigger for delivery is discussed further later. Interval growth of the fetus reflects the ongoing ability of the placenta to provide adequate nutrition to the fetus over time. Interval growth assessment is discussed earlier in the chapter, but, in general, the timing of these ultrasounds should not occur any more frequently than every 2 to 3 weeks. In practical terms, the frequency of interval growth prior to 34 weeks impacts pregnancy management less than do other parameters of fetal assessment.

MANAGEMENT AND DELIVERY OF PRETERM AND TERM FETAL GROWTH RESTRICTION FETUSES

Timing delivery of the FGR fetus requires close consideration of a variety of key factors listed in Table 4.6, which are discussed further in this section. These determinants represent different aspects of the FGR pregnancy. While any one determinant might serve as a trigger for delivery, in general, they are used in combination to assess the overall health and developmental status of the pregnancy.

The etiology of FGR for a given fetus is important to establish when the diagnosis of FGR is first assigned. While this is not always possible, efforts should be made as this not only allows for appropriate counseling of the patient but may also have a significant impact on the timing of delivery. For example, a fetus affected by aneuploidy or a congenital viral infection may not have its outcome affected by delaying delivery until term gestation. Furthermore, if a lethal condition is present, maternal preference and her safety take precedence in regard to the timing of delivery. In counseling patients with a new diagnosis of FGR, it is important to share that 70% of fetuses less than the 10th percentile will be small for normal reasons and not at risk for FGR complications; this is referred to as "constitutional" smallness.[141,151] This will help alleviate some of the patient's anxiety and give her hope that the pregnancy may still be normal. Often, the obstetrical provider will note that there are individuals of short stature in the family, which may account for the small constitutional size of the fetus. In contrast, 30% of fetuses less than the 10th percentile will be at risk for adverse perinatal outcomes and require surveillance. The risk of adverse outcomes has been shown to be highest in newborns

with BWs less than the third percentile.[141,151] Once poor pregnancy dating, aneuploidy (either with fetal karyotype or cell-free fDNA testing), structural abnormalities (e.g., gastroschisis), and congenital infection (cytomegalovirus [CMV], toxoplasmosis, herpes simplex virus, rubella, etc.) have been determined to be unlikely or excluded, the majority of the remaining cases will be due to constitutional smallness or placental insufficiency. Placental insufficiency may be due to a primary placental problem (circumvallate placenta, velamentous cord insertion, etc.), substance abuse, or chronic maternal disease, which may impact placentation, uterine blood flow, and placental perfusion. Table 4.7 depicts the typical phenotype of the FGR fetus due to placental insufficiency. Even with the use of this phenotype, distinguishing between placental insufficiency and small constitutional size can be challenging, and at times, the two may overlap. As such, fetuses that are constitutionally small should still be considered at risk and will require additional surveillance. Testing for the abovementioned congenital infections is generally not performed unless there is ultrasound evidence for infections (e.g., periventricular or hepatic calcifications).

The use of these delivery determinants, either alone or in combination, as an indication for delivery is largely dependent on the GA of the fetus. While fetuses weighing less than 500 g may survive, achieving an EFW of at least 500 g is generally considered to be a threshold for intervening on fetal behalf. While fetal weight is important, work by several groups has demonstrated that GA is a more important determinant of survival and intact survival. Beyond 27 weeks, survival and intact survival first exceed 50%; however, a BW less than 550 g is associated with a very high risk of neonatal death.[141,151–153] In 604 FGR fetuses between 24 and 32 weeks, Baschat et al. assessed the relationship between a variety of perinatal variables (Doppler studies, GA, BW, acid–base status, and Apgar scores) and major neonatal complications,

TABLE 4.6 Determinants of Delivery in the Fetal Growth Restriction Fetus

Etiology

Gestational age

Biophysical assessment (NST/BPP)

Umbilical artery Doppler velocimetry

Maternal comorbidity

Low amniotic fluid volume (anhydramnios/oligohydramnios)

Interval growth

BPP, biophysical profile; IUGR, intrauterine growth restriction; NST, nonstress test.

TABLE 4.7 Phenotype of the Fetus with Uteroplacental Insufficiency

Biometry: symmetric

Anatomical abnormalities: absent

Evidence of brain-sparing effect:
  Head circumference size maintained
  Cerebellum size maintained
  MCA Doppler index reduced

Amniotic fluid: reduced

Fetal Doppler velocimetry:
  Umbilical artery with elevated indices, absent or reversed end-diastolic flow
  Precordial venous Dopplers showing elevated indices or absent/reversed flow in the a-wave

Biophysical assessment:
  Nonstress test: nonreactive or with late decelerations
  Biophysical profile score: ≤4

Maternal comorbidity: Preeclampsia or chronic medical disease

MCA, middle cerebral artery.

survival, and intact survival. They found that GA was the most significant determinant of survival until 26 6/7 weeks and intact survival until 29 2/7 weeks. Beyond these cutoffs, DV Doppler assessment and cord artery pH predicted survival, and only DV Doppler assessment predicted intact survival.[152] Mari et al. similarly showed in 41 FGR fetuses delivered less than 32 weeks that GA is a critical factor in survival. Perinatal mortality decreased by 48% for each additional week gained, and 94% of deaths occurred when the delivery was less than 29 weeks.[154] The importance of both fetal size and GA further emphasized their inverse relationship with neonatal morbidities underscored by the work of McIntire and colleagues. These investigators demonstrated a decrease in RDS in more than 12,000 preterm infants with increasing GA and BW when stratified by these variables.[155] For example, the incidence of RDS at 35 to 36 weeks at less than the 10th percentile BW was approximately 5%, and the incidence decreased with increasing BW percentiles. These studies collectively suggest delaying delivery of the FGR fetus shows no signs of acidemia is further supported by the TRUFFLE (Trial of Umbilical and Fetal Flow in Europe) study that showed a mean GA at delivery of 30.2 weeks and mortality rate of 2% in each of the three groups of FGR fetuses studied.[156]

There is little argument that over the past 25 years, the use of color and spectral Doppler velocimetry has increased our understanding of the pathophysiology of FGR. Resultant studies have led to the use of Doppler ultrasound as a primary tool for assessing the vascular status and managing the FGR fetus. Initial Doppler studies were focused on the umbilical and cerebral circulations, and subsequently the venous circulations. As discussed previously, absent or reverse flow in the umbilical artery is associated with high rates of intrauterine hypoxemia (50% to 80%) and increased risk of perinatal mortality (80-fold). A 2017 Cochrane database systematic review of 19 studies and over 10,667 women demonstrated that the use of umbilical artery Doppler ultrasound reduces the rate of perinatal deaths (relative risk [RR] = 0.71; 95% confidence interval [CI], 0.52 to 0.98). It also reduced the rate of inductions of labor (RR = 0.89; 95% CI, 0.80 to 0.99) and cesarean sections (RR = 0.90; 95% CI, 0.84 to 0.97).[157]

In 1997, the ACOG reported that use of umbilical artery Doppler ultrasound in conjunction with standard antepartum testing (e.g., NST) reduced mortality.[158] In the 1990s, interrogation of the fetal venous structures gained significant attention. Fetal Doppler studies by investigators, such as those by Hecher et al.[113] and Rizzo et al.,[114] demonstrated that venous backflow during the atrial contraction in precordial venous structures is reflective of fetal metabolic acidemia. Subsequent studies were published to address longitudinal Doppler changes and biophysical testing in FGR fetuses in order to better understand the progressive nature of the FGR pathologic process. Several of these studies depicted how venous Doppler changes (especially the DV) precede BPP and FHR tracing abnormalities. Baschat and colleagues[147] showed that 70% of fetuses demonstrate Doppler abnormalities in the DV and other vessels prior to an abnormal BPP defined as less than 6/10 (Fig. 4.23). Ferrazzi et al.[119] similarly showed that as FGR fetuses decompensate, there is a fairly consistent pattern to which vessels show abnormal Doppler flow. These are depicted as early and late Doppler changes in Figure 4.24. Work by Hecher and colleagues in the FGR fetus with deteriorating condition very nicely demonstrated the close relationship between the DV and short-term variability.[140] This may be the first clear link between an abnormal Doppler flow in a vessel and the FHR parameter of short-term variability that reflects the balance between the parasympathetic and sympathetic nervous system in the fetus. More specifically, they showed a clear inverse relationship, namely, as the DV Doppler index became abnormal, so did the short-term variability (Fig. 4.25). This could suggest that as the DV becomes abnormal, so does the autonomic nervous system.

These last three studies collectively suggest that before a fetus becomes acidotic as indicated by an abnormal biophysical test, the majority of fetuses (50% to 70%) will demonstrate Doppler abnormalities, particularly the DV. These types of data have led several groups to propose that abnormal venous Doppler assessment, and the DV in particular, be considered as triggers for delivery of the FGR fetus, which became realized as the TRUFFLE study.[156] The TRUFFLE study was a randomized clinical trial (RCT) comparing maternal and fetal outcomes among fetuses randomized to delivery based on computerized FHR monitoring (cardiotocography and short-term variability [CTG/ STV]), DV S/a ratio elevated greater than the 95th percentile (DV p95) and DV with either absent or reversed (A/R) a-wave. Another publication from the previously mentioned PORTO trial of 1,100 FGR fetuses

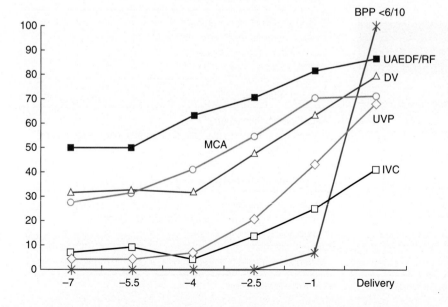

FIGURE 4.23: The percentage of abnormal Doppler findings in individual vessels and the incidence of a biophysical profile score below 6 in the week prior to delivery. *BPP,* biophysical profile; *DV,* abnormal ductus venosus flow; *IVC,* abnormal inferior vena cava flow; *MCA,* abnormal middle cerebral artery flow; *UAEDF/RF,* umbilical artery absent or reversed end-diastolic flow; *UVP,* umbilical vein pulsations. Deterioration of Doppler findings precedes the decline in biophysical profile score. (From Baschat AA, Gembruch U, Harman CR. The sequence of changes in Doppler and biophysical parameters as severe fetal growth restriction worsens. *Ultrasound Obstet Gynecol.* 2001;18(6): 571–577. Copyright © 2001 International Society of Ultrasound in Obstetrics and Gynecology. Modified by permission of John Wiley & Sons, Inc.)

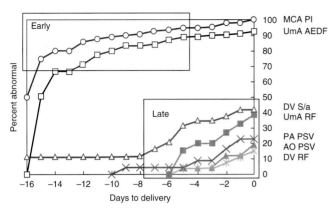

FIGURE 4.24: Temporal sequence of Doppler changes prior to delivery in decompensating fetal growth restriction fetuses. Fourteen days prior to delivery, the umbilical artery pulsatility index *(PI)* was abnormal in 100% of cases (not shown graphically). Early and late Doppler changes are depicted. *AO PSV*, aortic peak systolic velocity; *DV RF*, ductus venosus reversed a-wave; *DV S/a*, ductus vensosus S/a ratio; *MCA PI*, middle cerebral artery pulsatility index; *PA PSV*, pulmonary artery peak systolic velocity; *UmA AEDF*, umbilical artery absent end-diastolic flow; *UmA RF*, umbilical artery reverse end-diastolic flow.

demonstrated that the DV abnormality was seen in only 11% of the 1,100 FGR cases and that there was no specific or dominant sequence of abnormal Doppler changes seen in these 1,100 cases. However, this study was different in several ways from the TRUF-FLE study including that the PORTO trial did not categorize the severity of umbilical artery Doppler findings A/REDF changes are more severe Doppler findings and it is likely in this subgroup of fetuses where DV Doppler changes are likely to occur. Further, the type of FGR fetuses included were likely very different given that the mean GA for delivery in the PORTO trial was 37 weeks while that of the TRUFFLE study was 30 weeks.

Like other determinants of delivery listed in Table 4.6, Doppler triggers and timing of delivery need to be reconciled with the GA of the fetus, given that GA, at least until 29 weeks, is the strongest predictor of intact survival.[147,154] The timing of the delivery of the FGR fetus is best answered in RCTs. There is one reported RCT addressing FGR fetuses less than 36 weeks and one RCT for delivery beyond 36 weeks, and each of these have some long-term follow-up studies on the original study cohort. The Growth Restriction Intervention Trial (GRIT) had 548 study subjects, of which 196 were between 24 and 30 weeks, and 352 between 30 and 36 weeks. In this trial, patients were enrolled when physicians were unsure about delivery timing, and they were then randomized to a delivery-now or delayed-delivery group. The interval of time between randomization and delivery was 0.9 and 4.9 days, respectively. The cesarean delivery rates were 91% and 79%, respectively. There was no difference in mortality.[159] In a 2-year follow-up study, the GRIT study group reported similar neurological outcomes between groups for GA at delivery greater than 31 weeks. In contrast, they found a slightly higher rate of disability less than 31 weeks in the delivery-now group (14% vs. 5%). Clinically significant differences between immediate and deferred delivery were not found.[160] A 6- to 13-year follow-up report on one-half of the original cohort did not show the higher disability rate findings of the 2-year follow-up study. This long-term report showed similar cognitive, language, behavior, and motor ability between groups.[161] Although there were some limitations to the GRIT trial, such as the small difference in the interval of delivery between groups (0.9 to 4.9 days) and the possibility that the delivery-now group may not have had sufficient benefit from steroids (range of delivery from time of randomization 0.4 to 1.3 days), this study may suggest that the timing of delivery may not make a difference in early-onset FGR fetuses. The neurological injury in FGR may already be set by the time the usual triggers for delivery are used.

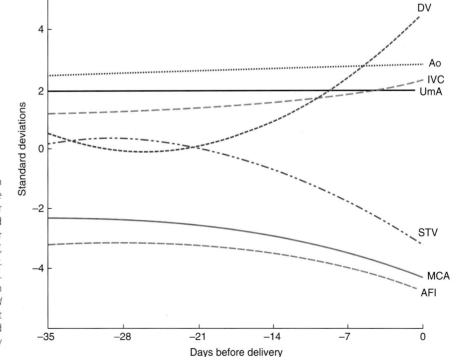

FIGURE 4.25: Trends over time of variables in relation to time before delivery and reference ranges (±2 SD; for fetuses delivered before or at 32 weeks of gestation). *AFI*, amniotic fluid index; *Ao*, aorta; *DV*, ductus venosus; *IVC*, inferior vena cava; *MCA*, middle cerebral artery; *STV*, short-term variation; *UmA*, umbilical artery. (From Hecher K, Bilardo CM, Stigter RH, et al. Monitoring of fetuses with intrauterine growth restriction: a longitudinal study. *Ultrasound Obstet Gynecol.* 2001;18(6):564–570. Copyright © 2001 International Society of Ultrasound in Obstetrics and Gynecology. Modified by permission of John Wiley & Sons, Inc.)

The TRUFFLE study represents the only RCT for early severe FGR assessing the utility of DV in determining the timing of delivery. In this study, the authors randomized patients with singleton FGR pregnancies between 26 and 32 weeks' GA to three timing delivery plans: abnormal cardiotocograph, early DV changes (PI of DV >95th percentile), or late DV changes (a-wave at or below the baseline). The primary endpoint assessed among the three treatment arms described previously was survival without cerebral palsy (CP) or neurosensory impairment, or Bayley III score of less than 85 at 2 years of age. Overall, the proportion of infants surviving without neuroimpairment did not differ between the groups. However, more infants in the delivery for late DV changes group had improved developmental outcomes at 2 years of age (95% vs. 85%). Overall, there was no difference among the groups for the rates of fetal death (2%), neonatal death (5%), or survival at 2 years (92%). Because the overall rates of survival were no different, some critics have stated that the DV should not be used in making delivery timing decisions. However, the survival rate in the study was much higher than predicted, thus affecting the power of the study. Arguably, if the survival of the fetus is the same regardless of the use of the DV, but if those fetuses that are delivered have a better neurological outcome at age 2, the DV may be a tool that can be used to identify a population of fetuses that should be delivered.

Available literature on fetal Doppler interrogation and its application to fetuses beyond 34 weeks is limited for two primary reasons: (1) the overwhelming majority of fetal vascular Doppler studies have been performed on fetuses less than 34 weeks of gestation, and (2) umbilical artery Doppler interrogation has been found to be less reliable after 34 weeks. The uteroplacental insufficiency seen in FGR fetuses diagnosed late in gestation (>34 weeks' gestation) is depicted by more mild placental dysfunction in which the elevated umbilical artery Doppler indices are often not seen. Other studies further show that the cerebroplacental Doppler ratio loses its predictive accuracy after 34 weeks' gestation.[102,107] Curiously, more recent data suggest that the only sign of placental dysfunction and nutrient and oxygen transfer insufficiency may be MCA Doppler changes characterized by an elevated diastolic flow velocity (e.g., brain-sparing effect), and these fetuses may still be at risk.[109–111]

As mentioned previously, amniotic fluid is an important component in the evaluation of the FGR fetus and is an integral part of the standard antepartum testing modalities (e.g., modified BPP and BPP). In addition, anhydramnios and oligohydramnios may also serve as triggers for delivery. There are no randomized trials of delivery on the basis of low amniotic fluid volume in FGR pregnancies. However, data have shown that the combination of FGR and oligohydramnios is associated with fetal hypoxia, abnormal Doppler studies and biophysical testing, and increased rates of fetal distress in labor and perinatal mortality.[162,163] This has led to expert opinion and committee consensus that delivery should occur as early as 34 weeks and probably not later than 37 weeks gestation when FGR is complicated by oligohydramnios.[133]

Timing delivery of the FGR fetus beyond 34 to 36 weeks has generally been based on the concern for stillbirth risk at a time when prematurity complications wane. In a study of 76 fetal demises with postmortem validated examinations and 582 controls, Froen et al.[164] found that 52% of the fetal death cases were growth restricted. Vergani et al.[165] assessed independent predictors of adverse neonatal outcomes in 481 FGR fetuses and, using a scoring model, determined that beyond 37.5 weeks, GA no longer had an independent impact on outcome. A more recent report demonstrates a progressive increase in the risk of stillbirth beyond 37 weeks (Table 4.8).[166] The only RCT for timing the delivery of the late FGR fetus (beyond 36 weeks) is the Disproportionate Intrauterine Growth Intervention Trial at Term (DIGITAT). Boers et al. reported the initial results of this trial that included 650 study subjects who were randomized after 36 weeks of gestation to induction of labor ($n = 321$) or expectant management ($n = 329$). Compared with the expectant management group, the induction of labor group delivered, on average, 10 days earlier, weighed 130 g less, and had similar composite adverse neonatal outcomes. Maternal outcomes showed no differences for spontaneous or operative vaginal delivery or for cesarean section rate. Preeclampsia was significantly more common in the expectant management group (7.9% vs. 3.7%).[167,168] A follow-up subanalysis of this study using a more sensitive analytic technique for neonatal morbidities (MAIN: Morbidity Index for Newborns) showed that while neonatal intensive care unit (NICU) admissions were higher in the induction of labor group, the percentage of adverse outcomes was similar between the two groups.[168] In a 2-year neurodevelopmental follow-up study, induction of labor and expectant management had similar developmental and behavioral outcomes.[169] Drawing clinical strategies about timing delivery of the late preterm/early term FGR fetus from the DIGITAT trial is limited by an absence of Doppler interrogation of these fetuses. Umbilical artery Doppler assessment was performed in the trial, and only 10% of cases were affected, which has been a previously described

TABLE 4.8	Risk of Stillbirth beyond 37 Weeks' Gestation		
GESTATIONAL AGE (wk)	ONGOING SGA PREGNANCIES	SGA STILLBIRTHS ($n = 20$)	STILLBIRTH RISK/10,000 ONGOING SGA PREGNANCIES (95% CI)
37–37 6/7	3,333	7	21 (13.0–32.1)
38–38 6/7	2,776	3	11 (5.5–19.7)
39–39 6/7	1,953	5	26 (17.0–38.1)
>40	832	5	60 (45.9–77.2)

SGA, small for gestational age.
Adapted from Trudell AS, Cahill AG, Methodius G, et al. Risk of stillbirth after 37 weeks in pregnancies complicated by small-for-gestational-age fetuses. *Am J Obstet Gynecol.* 2013;208(5):376.e1–376.e7. Copyright © 2013 Elsevier. With permission.

finding in late FGR. However, the MCA Doppler flow may be the only abnormal Doppler finding in late FGR, and it is suggestive of fetal hypoxemia, and these were not reported. This type of information may help distinguish between the constitutionally small fetus at or near term that may benefit from delivery at 39 weeks versus the pathologically small fetus that may benefit from earlier delivery. As such, the guidelines provided by the ACOG that recommends delivery of the otherwise uncomplicated (absence of maternal comorbidity, normal umbilical artery Doppler ultrasound, and amniotic fluid) late FGR fetus between 38 0/7 and 39 6/7 weeks is reasonable, at least until other studies show benefit of earlier delivery.[170]

Figure 4.22 depicts an algorithm for the management of FGR that is intended to serve as a guideline. The guideline begins with the most common definition used clinically for diagnosis of FGR: an EFW of less than the 10th percentile for gestation. Ascertainment of pregnancy dating remains a cornerstone for the correct diagnosis, something that at times is not possible when patients present late in gestation for prenatal care. A surveillance approach is outlined using BPPs, NST, and Doppler velocimetry tools. As previously discussed in this chapter, the BPP may be used prior to 28 weeks as a primary tool for fetal surveillance since the FHR tracing may not show reactivity; however, an FHR tracing may still be used to see whether variable or late decelerations are present. As mentioned previously, the umbilical artery Doppler flow may not become abnormal in late-onset FGR, whereas the MCA Doppler flow may become abnormal. Thus, the algorithm incorporates the use of Doppler ultrasound in both types of vessels to evaluate near-term or term FGR. Once absent or reversed umbilical artery diastolic flow or oligohydramnios is present, hospitalization is suggested for further evaluation and surveillance. In some cases, FGR may precede the development of preeclampsia in the mother. The triggers for delivery are divided into GA epochs based on the knowledge that FGR fetuses have less morbidity and mortality at certain GAs. The recent publication on multivessel fetal Doppler assessment from the PORTO trial showed that the interval of a Doppler abnormality to the time of delivery can be roughly predicted by the specific abnormality seen. For example, reverse flow in the umbilical artery has a very short interval to delivery (mean of 5 days), while an abnormal umbilical artery PI is nearly 40 days.[171] An abnormal MCA carried a mean interval to delivery of 30 days, while the DV interval was about 37 days. While this is useful for counseling, in reality, there are many variables that can shorten or lengthen the interval to delivery that need to be taken into account. Beyond 34 weeks, delivery is recommended for persistent oligohydramnios or anhydramnios, absence of interval growth, or for absent end-diastolic velocity in the umbilical artery. For an FGR fetus with isolated oligohydramnios beyond 34 weeks, timing the delivery can be individualized, and the ACOG has recommended delivery anytime between 34 0/7 and 37 6/7 weeks.[170] Finally, when delivery is anticipated prior to 34 weeks, the following should be considered: (1) betamethasone administration to reduce complications of prematurity and improve outcomes,[172-175] (2) magnesium sulfate administration for neuroprotection based on published protocols,[176-178] and (3) delivery at a facility that has NICU capabilities.[1]

Doppler Abnormalities and Long-Term Neurological Outcome

There are few studies relating neurodevelopment to antenatal surveillance parameters including Doppler studies. A 2004 study consisting primarily of preterm growth-restricted pregnancies and that evaluated developmental outcomes for 2 years reported that GA at delivery, BW, and reversal of umbilical artery end-diastolic velocity were the main determinants of motor and neurosensory morbidity. Fetal deterioration of venous Doppler flow or biophysical parameters did not have an impact on neurodevelopment.[160] Furthermore, a relatively more recent study assessed the long-term (6 to 13 years of age) impact on neurological outcomes that were reported for the GRIT study. This was an RCT of immediate versus delayed delivery of FGR fetuses with the majority born less than 34 weeks. Cognitive development was identical in both groups. In short, these findings are concerning in that they suggest that the intrauterine environment has a significant impact on neurodevelopment before delivery criteria arise and, accordingly, it suggests that any neurological injury may already be set by the time delivery is required and that it may not be mitigated by any specific delivery criteria.[161] There are few data on long-term neurological outcomes and delivery timing in late FGR fetuses. A 2-year follow-up study from patients enrolled in the DIGITAT trial concluded that in term FGR fetuses, neither a policy of labor induction nor one of expectant management has an effect on developmental or behavioral outcomes.[169] This study did not report on Doppler findings. As previously mentioned, changes in the MCA Doppler flow may be the only Doppler changes noted in late FGR fetuses, and these may be associated with neurological sequelae.[110,111] Currently, there is insufficient evidence to warrant early delivery of the FGR fetus less than 36 weeks for the sole purpose of reducing neurological injury.

Doppler Velocimetry Reference Ranges

Longitudinal reference ranges for Doppler velocimetry flow velocities and indices for the uterine arteries, umbilical arteries, MCA, and DV are shown in Appendix A1 in Tables 38 to 46.

REFERENCES

1. ACOG Practice Bulletin No. 204: Fetal growth restriction. *Obstet Gynecol.* 2019;133(2):e97–e109.
2. Barker DJ. Adult consequences of fetal growth restriction. *Clin Obstet Gynecol.* 2006;49(2):270–283.
3. Pallotto EK, Kilbride HW. Perinatal outcome and later implications of intrauterine growth restriction. *Clin Obstet Gynecol.* 2006;49(2):257–269.
4. Resnik R. Intrauterine growth restriction. *Obstet Gynecol.* 2002;99(3):490–496.
5. Gordijn SJ, Beune IM, Thilaganathan B, et al. Consensus definition of fetal growth restriction: a Delphi procedure. *Ultrasound Obstet Gynecol.* 2016;48(3):333–339.
6. Bulletins ACoP. ACOG Practice Bulletin No. 77: screening for fetal chromosomal abnormalities. *Obstet Gynecol.* 2007;109(1):217–227.
7. Firth HV, Boyd PA, Chamberlain P, et al. Severe limb abnormalities after chorion villus sampling at 56–66 days' gestation. *Lancet.* 1991;337(8744):762–763.
8. Sundberg K, Bang J, Smidt-Jensen S, et al. Randomised study of risk of fetal loss related to early amniocentesis versus chorionic villus sampling. *Lancet.* 1997;350(9079):697–703.
9. Matsumoto S, Nogami Y, Ohkuri S. Statistical studies on menstruation: a criticism on the definition of normal menstruation. *J Med Sci.* 1962;11:294.
10. Batzer FR, Weiner S, Corson SL, et al. Landmarks during the first forty-two days of gestation demonstrated by the beta-subunit of human chorionic gonadotropin and ultrasound. *Am J Obstet Gynecol.* 1983;146(8):973–979.
11. MacGregor SN, Tamura RK, Sabbagha RE, et al. Underestimation of gestational age by conventional crown-rump length dating curves. *Obstet Gynecol.* 1987;70(3 pt 1):344–348.
12. Daya S. Accuracy of gestational age estimation by means of fetal crown-rump length measurement. *Am J Obstet Gynecol.* 1993;168(3 pt 1):903–908.
13. Hadlock FP, Shah YP, Kanon DJ, et al. Fetal crown-rump length: reevaluation of relation to menstrual age (5–18 weeks) with high-resolution real-time US. *Radiology.* 1992;182(2):501–505.
14. Bukowski R, Smith GC, Malone FD, et al. Fetal growth in early pregnancy and risk of delivering low birth weight infant: prospective cohort study. *BMJ.* 2007;334(7598):836.
15. Hackmon R, Le Scale KB, Horani J, et al. Is severe macrosomia manifested at 11–14 weeks of gestation? *Ultrasound Obstet Gynecol.* 2008;32(6):740–743.

16. Selbing A. Gestational age and ultrasonic measurement of gestational sac, crown-rump length and biparietal diameter during first 15 weeks of pregnancy. *Acta Obstet Gynecol Scand.* 1982;61(3):233–235.

17. Silva PD, Mahairas G, Schaper AM, et al. Early crown-rump length. A good predictor of gestational age. *J Reprod Med.* 1990;35(6):641–644.

18. Wu FS, Hwu YM, Lee RK, et al. First trimester ultrasound estimation of gestational age in pregnancies conceived after in vitro fertilization. *Eur J Obstet Gynecol Reprod Biol.* 2012;160(2):151–155.

19. Chalouhi GE, Bernard JP, Benoist G, et al. A comparison of first trimester measurements for prediction of delivery date. *J Matern Fetal Neonatal Med.* 2011;24(1):51–57.

20. Shepard M, Filly RA. A standardized plane for biparietal diameter measurement. *J Ultrasound Med.* 1982;1(4):145–150.

21. Hadlock FP, Harrist RB, Martinez-Poyer J. How accurate is second trimester fetal dating? *J Ultrasound Med.* 1991;10(10):557–561.

22. Persson PH, Weldner BM. Reliability of ultrasound fetometry in estimating gestational age in the second trimester. *Acta Obstet Gynecol Scand.* 1986;65(5):481–483.

23. Rossavik IK, Fishburne JI. Conceptional age, menstrual age, and ultrasound age: a second-trimester comparison of pregnancies of known conception date with pregnancies dated from the last menstrual period. *Obstet Gynecol.* 1989;73(2):243–249.

24. Benson CB, Doubilet PM. Sonographic prediction of gestational age: accuracy of second- and third-trimester fetal measurements. *AJR Am J Roentgenol.* 1991;157(6):1275–1277.

25. Hadlock FP, Deter RL, Carpenter RJ, et al. Estimating fetal age: effect of head shape on BPD. *AJR Am J Roentgenol.* 1981;137(1):83–85.

26. Law RG, MacRae KD. Head circumference as an index of fetal age. *J Ultrasound Med.* 1982;1(7):281–288.

27. Committee Opinion No 700. Methods for estimating the due date. *Obstet Gynecol.* 2017;129(5):e150–e154.

28. Chavez MR, Ananth CV, Smulian JC, et al. Fetal transcerebellar diameter measurement with particular emphasis in the third trimester: a reliable predictor of gestational age. *Am J Obstet Gynecol.* 2004;191(3):979–984.

29. Chavez MR, Ananth CV, Smulian JC, et al. Fetal transcerebellar diameter measurement for prediction of gestational age at the extremes of fetal growth. *J Ultrasound Med.* 2007;26(9):1167–1171; quiz 1173–1164.

30. Vinkesteijn AS, Jansen CL, Los FJ, et al. Fetal transcerebellar diameter and chromosomal abnormalities. *Ultrasound Obstet Gynecol.* 2001;17(6):502–505.

31. Gottlieb AG, Galan HL. Nontraditional sonographic pearls in estimating gestational age. *Semin Perinatol.* 2008;32(3):154–160.

32. Meirowitz NB, Ananth CV, Smulian JC, et al. Foot length in fetuses with abnormal growth. *J Ultrasound Med.* 2000;19(3):201–205.

33. Campbell S, Wilkin D. Ultrasonic measurement of fetal abdomen circumference in the estimation of fetal weight. *Br J Obstet Gynaecol.* 1975;82(9):689–697.

34. Warsof SL, Gohari P, Berkowitz RL, et al. The estimation of fetal weight by computer-assisted analysis. *Am J Obstet Gynecol.* 1977;128(8):881–892.

35. Hadlock FP, Harrist RB, Carpenter RJ, et al. Sonographic estimation of fetal weight. The value of femur length in addition to head and abdomen measurements. *Radiology.* 1984;150(2):535–540.

36. Shepard MJ, Richards VA, Berkowitz RL, et al. An evaluation of two equations for predicting fetal weight by ultrasound. *Am J Obstet Gynecol.* 1982;142(1):47–54.

37. Thurnau GR, Tamura RK, Sabbagha R, et al. A simple estimated fetal weight equation based on real-time ultrasound measurements of fetuses less than thirty-four weeks' gestation. *Am J Obstet Gynecol.* 1983;145(5):557–561.

38. Vintzileos AM, Campbell WA, Rodis JF, et al. Fetal weight estimation formulas with head, abdominal, femur, and thigh circumference measurements. *Am J Obstet Gynecol.* 1987;157(2):410–414.

39. Combs CA, Jaekle RK, Rosenn B, et al. Sonographic estimation of fetal weight based on a model of fetal volume. *Obstet Gynecol.* 1993;82(3):365–370.

40. Hadlock FP, Harrist RB, Sharman RS, et al. Estimation of fetal weight with the use of head, body, and femur measurements—a prospective study. *Am J Obstet Gynecol.* 1985;151(3):333–337.

41. Ott WJ, Doyle S, Flamm S. Accurate ultrasonic estimation of fetal weight. Effect of head shape, growth patterns, and amniotic fluid volume. *Am J Perinatol.* 1986;3(3):193–197.

42. Rose BI, McCallum WD. A simplified method for estimating fetal weight using ultrasound measurements. *Obstet Gynecol.* 1987;69(4):671–675.

43. Weiner CP, Sabbagha RE, Vaisrub N, et al. Ultrasonic fetal weight prediction: role of head circumference and femur length. *Obstet Gynecol.* 1985;65(6):812–817.

44. Gandhi M, Ferrara L, Belogolovkin V, et al. Effect of increased body mass index on the accuracy of estimated fetal weight by sonography in twins. *J Ultrasound Med.* 2009;28(3):301–308.

45. Anderson NG, Jolley IJ, Wells JE. Sonographic estimation of fetal weight: comparison of bias, precision and consistency using 12 different formulae. *Ultrasound Obstet Gynecol.* 2007;30(2):173–179.

46. Edwards A, Goff J, Baker L. Accuracy and modifying factors of the sonographic estimation of fetal weight in a high-risk population. *Aust N Z J Obstet Gynaecol.* 2001;41(2):187–190.

47. Dudley NJ. A systematic review of the ultrasound estimation of fetal weight. *Ultrasound Obstet Gynecol.* 2005;25(1):80–89.

48. Schild RL, Sachs C, Fimmers R, et al. Sex-specific fetal weight prediction by ultrasound. *Ultrasound Obstet Gynecol.* 2004;23(1):30–35.

49. Siemer J, Egger N, Hart N, et al. Fetal weight estimation by ultrasound: comparison of 11 different formulae and examiners with differing skill levels. *Ultraschall Med.* 2008;29(2):159–164.

50. Esinler D, Bircan O, Esin S, et al. Finding the best formula to predict the fetal weight: comparison of 18 formulas. *Gynecol Obstet Invest.* 2015;80(2):78–84.

51. Ben-Haroush A, Yogev Y, Bar J, et al. Accuracy of sonographically estimated fetal weight in 840 women with different pregnancy complications prior to induction of labor. *Ultrasound Obstet Gynecol.* 2004;23(2):172–176.

52. Melamed N, Yogev Y, Meizner I, et al. Sonographic fetal weight estimation: which model should be used? *J Ultrasound Med.* 2009;28(5):617–629.

53. Proctor LK, Rushworth V, Shah PS, et al. Incorporation of femur length leads to underestimation of fetal weight in asymmetric preterm growth restriction. *Ultrasound Obstet Gynecol.* 2010;35(4):442–448.

54. Hart NC, Hilbert A, Meurer B, et al. Macrosomia: a new formula for optimized fetal weight estimation. *Ultrasound Obstet Gynecol.* 2010;35(1):42–47.

55. Hoopmann M, Abele H, Wagner N, et al. Performance of 36 different weight estimation formulae in fetuses with macrosomia. *Fetal Diagn Ther.* 2010;27(4):204–213.

56. Chen P, Yu J, Li X, et al. Weight estimation for low birth weight fetuses and macrosomic fetuses in Chinese population. *Arch Gynecol Obstet.* 2011;284(3):599–606.

57. Lee W, Balasubramaniam M, Deter RL, et al. New fetal weight estimation models using fractional limb volume. *Ultrasound Obstet Gynecol.* 2009;34(5):556–565.

58. Pagani G, Palai N, Zatti S, et al. Fetal weight estimation in gestational diabetic pregnancies: comparison between conventional and three-dimensional fractional thigh volume methods using gestation-adjusted projection. *Ultrasound Obstet Gynecol.* 2014;43(1):72–76.

59. Lee W, Deter R, Sangi-Haghpeykar H, et al. Prospective validation of fetal weight estimation using fractional limb volume. *Ultrasound Obstet Gynecol.* 2013;41(2):198–203.

60. Battaglia FC, Lubchenco LO. A practical classification of newborn infants by weight and gestational age. *J Pediatr.* 1967;71(2):159–163.

61. Goldenberg RL, Cliver SP, Cutter GR, et al. Black-white differences in newborn anthropometric measurements. *Obstet Gynecol.* 1991;78(5 pt 1):782–788.

62. Hulsey TC, Levkoff AH, Alexander GR, et al. Differences in black and white infant birth weights: the role of maternal demographic factors and medical complications of pregnancy. *South Med J.* 1991;84(4):443–446.

63. Yip R, Li Z, Chong WH. Race and birth weight: the Chinese example. *Pediatrics.* 1991;87(5):688–693.

64. Alvear J, Brooke OG. Fetal growth in different racial groups. *Arch Dis Child.* 1978;53(1):27–32.

65. Graafmans WC, Richardus JH, Borsboom GJ, et al. Birth weight and perinatal mortality: a comparison of "optimal" birth weight in seven Western European countries. *Epidemiology.* 2002;13(5):569–574.

66. Hemming K, Hutton JL, Glinianaia SV, et al. Differences between European birth-weight standards: impact on classification of "small for gestational age." *Dev Med Child Neurol.* 2006;48(11):906–912.

67. Lubchenco LO. Classification of high risk infants by birth weight and gestational age: an overview. *Major Probl Clin Pediatr.* 1976;14:1–279.

68. Ott WJ. Intrauterine growth retardation and preterm delivery. *Am J Obstet Gynecol.* 1993;168(6 Pt 1):1710–1715; discussion 1715–1717.

69. Hadlock FP, Harrist RB, Martinez-Poyer J. In utero analysis of fetal growth: a sonographic weight standard. *Radiology.* 1991;181(1):129–133.

70. Bernstein IM, Mohs G, Rucquoi M, et al. Case for hybrid "fetal growth curves": a population-based estimation of normal fetal size across gestational age. *J Matern Fetal Med.* 1996;5(3):124–127.

71. Salomon LJ, Bernard JP, Ville Y. Estimation of fetal weight: reference range at 20–36 weeks' gestation and comparison with actual birth-weight reference range. *Ultrasound Obstet Gynecol.* 2007;29(5):550–555.

72. Lackman F, Capewell V, Richardson B, et al. The risks of spontaneous preterm delivery and perinatal mortality in relation to size at birth according to fetal versus neonatal growth standards. *Am J Obstet Gynecol.* 2001;184(5):946–953.

73. Zaw W, Gagnon R, da Silva O. The risks of adverse neonatal outcome among preterm small for gestational age infants according to neonatal versus fetal growth standards. *Pediatrics.* 2003;111(6 pt 1):1273–1277.

74. Norris T, Tuffnell D, Wright J, et al. Modelling foetal growth in a bi-ethnic sample: results from the Born in Bradford (BiB) birth cohort. *Ann Hum Biol.* 2014;41(6):481–487.

75. Buck Louis GM, Grewal J, Albert PS, et al. Racial/ethnic standards for fetal growth: the NICHD Fetal Growth Studies. *Am J Obstet Gynecol.* 2015;213(4):449.e1–449.e41.

76. Kiserud T, Piaggio G, Carroli G, et al. The World Health Organization fetal growth charts: a multinational longitudinal study of ultrasound biometric measurements and estimated fetal weight. *PLoS Med.* 2017;14(1):e1002220.

77. Blue NR, Beddow ME, Savabi M, et al. Comparing the Hadlock fetal growth standard to the Eunice Kennedy Shriver National Institute of Child Health and Human Development racial/ethnic standard for the prediction of neonatal morbidity and small for gestational age. *Am J Obstet Gynecol.* 2018;219(5):474.e1–474.e12.

78. Papageorghiou AT, Ohuma EO, Altman DG, et al. International standards for fetal growth based on serial ultrasound measurements: the Fetal Growth Longitudinal Study of the INTERGROWTH-21st Project. *Lancet.* 2014;384(9946):869–879.

79. Nwabuobi C, Odibo L, Camisasca-Lopina H, et al. Comparing INTERGROWTH-21st Century and Hadlock growth standards to predict small for gestational age and short-term neonatal outcomes. *J Matern Fetal Neonatal Med.* 2019:1–7.

80. Gardosi J, Mongelli M, Wilcox M, et al. An adjustable fetal weight standard. *Ultrasound Obstet Gynecol.* 1995;6(3):168–174.

81. Wilcox MA, Newton CS, Johnson IR. Paternal influences on birthweight. *Acta Obstet Gynecol Scand.* 1995;74(1):15–18.
82. Gardosi J. Customized fetal growth standards: rationale and clinical application. *Semin Perinatol.* 2004;28(1):33–40.
83. Clausson B, Gardosi J, Francis A, et al. Perinatal outcome in SGA births defined by customised versus population-based birthweight standards. *BJOG.* 2001;108(8):830–834.
84. Ego A, Subtil D, Grange G, et al. Customized versus population-based birth weight standards for identifying growth restricted infants: a French multicenter study. *Am J Obstet Gynecol.* 2006;194(4):1042–1049.
85. Figueras F, Figueras J, Meler E, et al. Customised birthweight standards accurately predict perinatal morbidity. *Arch Dis Child Fetal Neonatal Ed.* 2007;92(4):F277–F280.
86. Odibo AO, Francis A, Cahill AG, et al. Association between pregnancy complications and small-for-gestational-age birth weight defined by customized fetal growth standard versus a population-based standard. *J Matern Fetal Neonatal Med.* 2011;24(3):411–417.
87. Odibo AO, Cahill AG, Goetzinger KR, et al. Customized growth charts for twin gestations to optimize identification of small-for-gestational age fetuses at risk of intrauterine fetal death. *Ultrasound Obstet Gynecol.* 2013;41(6):637–642.
88. Hutcheon JA, Zhang X, Cnattingius S, et al. Customised birthweight percentiles: does adjusting for maternal characteristics matter? *BJOG.* 2008;115(11):1397–1404.
89. Deter RL, Lee W, Yeo L, et al. Individualized growth assessment: conceptual framework and practical implementation for the evaluation of fetal growth and neonatal growth outcome. *Am J Obstet Gynecol.* 2018;218(2s):S656–S678.
90. Baker PN, Johnson IR, Gowland PA, et al. Measurement of fetal liver, brain and placental volumes with echo-planar magnetic resonance imaging. *Br J Obstet Gynaecol.* 1995;102(1):35–39.
91. Duncan KR, Issa B, Moore R, et al. A comparison of fetal organ measurements by echo-planar magnetic resonance imaging and ultrasound. *BJOG.* 2005;112(1):43–49.
92. Damodaram MS, Story L, Eixarch E, et al. Foetal volumetry using magnetic resonance imaging in intrauterine growth restriction. *Early Hum Dev.* 2012;88 Suppl 1:S35–S40.
93. FitzGerald DE, Drumm JE. Non-invasive measurement of human fetal circulation using ultrasound: a new method. *Br Med J.* 1977;2(6100):1450–1451.
94. Trudinger BJ, Giles WB, Cook CM. Uteroplacental blood flow velocity-time waveforms in normal and complicated pregnancy. *Br J Obstet Gynaecol.* 1985;92(1):39–45.
95. Giles WB, Trudinger BJ, Baird PJ. Fetal umbilical artery flow velocity waveforms and placental resistance: pathological correlation. *Br J Obstet Gynaecol.* 1985;92(1):31–38.
96. Kingdom JC, Burrell SJ, Kaufmann P. Pathology and clinical implications of abnormal umbilical artery Doppler waveforms. *Ultrasound Obstet Gynecol.* 1997;9(4):271–286.
97. Morrow RJ, Adamson SL, Bull SB, et al. Effect of placental embolization on the umbilical arterial velocity waveform in fetal sheep. *Am J Obstet Gynecol.* 1989;161(4):1055–1060.
98. Bilardo CM, Nicolaides KH, Campbell S. Doppler measurements of fetal and uteroplacental circulations: relationship with umbilical venous blood gases measured at cordocentesis. *Am J Obstet Gynecol.* 1990;162(1):115–120.
99. Nicolaides KH, Bilardo CM, Soothill PW, et al. Absence of end diastolic frequencies in umbilical artery: a sign of fetal hypoxia and acidosis. *BMJ.* 1988;297(6655):1026–1027.
100. Pardi G, Cetin I, Marconi AM, et al. Diagnostic value of blood sampling in fetuses with growth retardation. *N Engl J Med.* 1993;328(10):692–696.
101. Thornton JG, Lilford RJ. Do we need randomised trials of antenatal tests of fetal wellbeing? *Br J Obstet Gynaecol.* 1993;100(3):197–200.
102. Gramellini D, Folli MC, Raboni S, et al. Cerebral-umbilical Doppler ratio as a predictor of adverse perinatal outcome. *Obstet Gynecol.* 1992;79(3):416–420.
103. Gudmundsson S, Tulzer G, Huhta JC, et al. Venous Doppler in the fetus with absent end-diastolic flow in the umbilical artery. *Ultrasound Obstet Gynecol.* 1996;7(4):262–267.
104. Mari G, Deter RL. Middle cerebral artery flow velocity waveforms in normal and small-for-gestational-age fetuses. *Am J Obstet Gynecol.* 1992;166(4):1262–1270.
105. Wladimiroff JW, Tonge HM, Stewart PA. Doppler ultrasound assessment of cerebral blood flow in the human fetus. *Br J Obstet Gynaecol.* 1986;93(5):471–475.
106. Arbeille P, Roncin A, Berson M, et al. Exploration of the fetal cerebral blood flow by duplex Doppler-linear array system in normal and pathological pregnancies. *Ultrasound Med Biol.* 1987;13(6):329–337.
107. Bahado-Singh RO, Kovanci E, Jeffres A, et al. The Doppler cerebroplacental ratio and perinatal outcome in intrauterine growth restriction. *Am J Obstet Gynecol.* 1999;180(3 Pt 1):750–756.
108. Akolekar R, Ciobanu A, Zingler E, et al. Routine assessment of cerebroplacental ratio at 35–37 weeks' gestation in the prediction of adverse perinatal outcome. *Am J Obstet Gynecol.* 2019;221(1):65.e1–65.e18.
109. Cruz-Martinez R, Figueras F, Hernandez-Andrade E, et al. Fetal brain Doppler to predict cesarean delivery for nonreassuring fetal status in term small-for-gestational-age fetuses. *Obstet Gynecol.* 2011;117(3):618–626.
110. Eixarch E, Meler E, Iraola A, et al. Neurodevelopmental outcome in 2-year-old infants who were small-for-gestational age term fetuses with cerebral blood flow redistribution. *Ultrasound Obstet Gynecol.* 2008;32(7):894–899.
111. Oros D, Figueras F, Cruz-Martinez R, et al. Middle versus anterior cerebral artery Doppler for the prediction of perinatal outcome and neonatal neurobehavior in term small-for-gestational-age fetuses with normal umbilical artery Doppler. *Ultrasound Obstet Gynecol.* 2010;35(4):456–461.
112. Mavrides E, Moscoso G, Carvalho JS, et al. The anatomy of the umbilical, portal and hepatic venous systems in the human fetus at 14–19 weeks of gestation. *Ultrasound Obstet Gynecol.* 2001;18(6):598–604.
113. Hecher K, Snijders R, Campbell S, et al. Fetal venous, intracardiac, and arterial blood flow measurements in intrauterine growth retardation: relationship with fetal blood gases. *Am J Obstet Gynecol.* 1995;173(1):10–15.
114. Rizzo G, Capponi A, Arduini D, et al. The value of fetal arterial, cardiac and venous flows in predicting pH and blood gases measured in umbilical blood at cordocentesis in growth retarded fetuses. *Br J Obstet Gynaecol.* 1995;102(12):963–969.
115. Zhou Y, Fisher SJ, Janatpour M, et al. Human cytotrophoblasts adopt a vascular phenotype as they differentiate. A strategy for successful endovascular invasion? *J Clin Invest.* 1997;99(9):2139–2151.
116. Lovgren TR, Dugoff L, Galan HL. Uterine artery Doppler and prediction of preeclampsia. *Clin Obstet Gynecol.* 2010;53(4):888–898.
117. Berkley E, Chauhan SP, Abuhamad A. Doppler assessment of the fetus with intrauterine growth restriction. *Am J Obstet Gynecol.* 2012;206(4):300–308.
118. Benavides-Serralde A, Scheier M, Cruz-Martinez R, et al. Changes in central and peripheral circulation in intrauterine growth-restricted fetuses at different stages of umbilical artery flow deterioration: new fetal cardiac and brain parameters. *Gynecol Obstet Invest.* 2011;71(4):274–280.
119. Ferrazzi E, Bozzo M, Rigano S, et al. Temporal sequence of abnormal Doppler changes in the peripheral and central circulatory systems of the severely growth-restricted fetus. *Ultrasound Obstet Gynecol.* 2002;19(2):140–146.
120. Figueras F, Puerto B, Martinez JM, et al. Cardiac function monitoring of fetuses with growth restriction. *Eur J Obstet Gynecol Reprod Biol.* 2003;110(2):159–163.
121. Groenenberg IA, Wladimiroff JW, Hop WC. Fetal cardiac and peripheral arterial flow velocity waveforms in intrauterine growth retardation. *Circulation.* 1989;80(6):1711–1717.
122. Mari G, Hanif F, Kruger M. Sequence of cardiovascular changes in IUGR in pregnancies with and without preeclampsia. *Prenat Diagn.* 2008;28(5):377–383.
123. Reed KL, Anderson CF, Shenker L. Changes in intracardiac Doppler blood flow velocities in fetuses with absent umbilical artery diastolic flow. *Am J Obstet Gynecol.* 1987;157(3):774–779.
124. Baschat AA, Muench MV, Gembruch U. Coronary artery blood flow velocities in various fetal conditions. *Ultrasound Obstet Gynecol.* 2003;21(5):426–429.
125. Kenny JF, Plappert T, Doubilet P, et al. Changes in intracardiac blood flow velocities and right and left ventricular stroke volumes with gestational age in the normal human fetus: a prospective Doppler echocardiographic study. *Circulation.* 1986;74(6):1208–1216.
126. Stoddard MF, Pearson AC, Kern MJ, et al. Influence of alteration in preload on the pattern of left ventricular diastolic filling as assessed by Doppler echocardiography in humans. *Circulation.* 1989;79(6):1226–1236.
127. Rizzo G, Arduini D, Romanini C. Doppler echocardiographic assessment of fetal cardiac function. *Ultrasound Obstet Gynecol.* 1992;2(6):434–445.
128. Forouzan I, Graham E, Morgan MA. Reduction of right atrial peak systolic velocity in growth-restricted discordant twins. *Am J Obstet Gynecol.* 1996;175(4 Pt 1):1033–1035.
129. al-Ghazali W, Chita SK, Chapman MG, et al. Evidence of redistribution of cardiac output in asymmetrical growth retardation. *Br J Obstet Gynaecol.* 1989;96(6):697–704.
130. Baschat AA, Gembruch U, Harman CR. Coronary blood flow in fetuses with intrauterine growth restriction. *J Perinat Med.* 1998;26(3):143–156.
131. Baschat AA, Gembruch U, Gortner L, et al. Coronary artery blood flow visualization signifies hemodynamic deterioration in growth-restricted fetuses. *Ultrasound Obstet Gynecol.* 2000;16(5):425–431.
132. Mathews DD. Maternal assessment of fetal activity in small-for-dates infants. *Obstet Gynecol.* 1975;45(5):488–493.
133. Chauhan SP, Doherty DD, Magann EF, et al. Amniotic fluid index vs single deepest pocket technique during modified biophysical profile: a randomized clinical trial. *Am J Obstet Gynecol.* 2004;191(2):661–667; discussion 667–668.
134. Nabhan AF, Abdelmoula YA. Amniotic fluid index versus single deepest vertical pocket as a screening test for preventing adverse pregnancy outcome. *Cochrane Database Syst Rev.* 2008(3):CD006593.
135. Spong CY, Mercer BM, D'Alton M, et al. Timing of indicated late-preterm and early-term birth. *Obstet Gynecol.* 2011;118(2 Pt 1):323–333.
136. Manning FA, Hill LM, Platt LD. Qualitative amniotic fluid volume determination by ultrasound: antepartum detection of intrauterine growth retardation. *Am J Obstet Gynecol.* 1981;139(3):254–258.
137. Peeters LL, Sheldon RE, Jones MD Jr, et al. Blood flow to fetal organs as a function of arterial oxygen content. *Am J Obstet Gynecol.* 1979;135(5):637–646.
138. Arabin B, Bergmann PL, Saling E. Simultaneous assessment of blood flow velocity waveforms in uteroplacental vessels, the umbilical artery, the fetal aorta and the fetal common carotid artery. *Fetal Ther.* 1987;2(1):17–26.
139. Veille JC, Kanaan C. Duplex Doppler ultrasonographic evaluation of the fetal renal artery in normal and abnormal fetuses. *Am J Obstet Gynecol.* 1989;161(6 Pt 1):1502–1507.
140. Hecher K, Bilardo CM, Stigter RH, et al. Monitoring of fetuses with intrauterine growth restriction: a longitudinal study. *Ultrasound Obstet Gynecol.* 2001;18(6):564–570.

141. Unterscheider J, Daly S, Geary MP, et al. Optimizing the definition of intrauterine growth restriction: the multicenter prospective PORTO Study. *Am J Obstet Gynecol.* 2013;208(4):290.e1–290.e6.

142. Nageotte MP, Towers CV, Asrat T, et al. Perinatal outcome with the modified biophysical profile. *Am J Obstet Gynecol.* 1994;170(6):1672–1676.

143. Baschat AA, Galan HL, Bhide A, et al. Doppler and biophysical assessment in growth restricted fetuses: distribution of test results. *Ultrasound Obstet Gynecol.* 2006;27(1):41–47.

144. Arduini D, Rizzo G, Caforio L, et al. Behavioural state transitions in healthy and growth retarded fetuses. *Early Hum Dev.* 1989;19(3):155–165.

145. Henson G, Dawes GS, Redman CW. Characterization of the reduced heart rate variation in growth-retarded fetuses. *Br J Obstet Gynaecol.* 1984;91(8):751–755.

146. Pillai M, James D. Continuation of normal neurobehavioural development in fetuses with absent umbilical arterial end diastolic velocities. *Br J Obstet Gynaecol.* 1991;98(3):277–281.

147. Baschat AA, Gembruch U, Harman CR. The sequence of changes in Doppler and biophysical parameters as severe fetal growth restriction worsens. *Ultrasound Obstet Gynecol.* 2001;18(6):571–577.

148. Ribbert LS, Nicolaides KH, Visser GH. Prediction of fetal acidaemia in intrauterine growth retardation: comparison of quantified fetal activity with biophysical profile score. *Br J Obstet Gynaecol.* 1993;100(7):653–656.

149. Visser GH, Dawes GS, Redman CW. Numerical analysis of the normal human antenatal fetal heart rate. *Br J Obstet Gynaecol.* 1981;88(8):792–802.

150. Vintzileos AM, Fleming AD, Scorza WE, et al. Relationship between fetal biophysical activities and umbilical cord blood gas values. *Am J Obstet Gynecol.* 1991;165(3):707–713.

151. Ott WJ. The diagnosis of altered fetal growth. *Obstet Gynecol Clin North Am.* 1988;15(2):237–263.

152. Baschat AA, Cosmi E, Bilardo CM, et al. Predictors of neonatal outcome in early-onset placental dysfunction. *Obstet Gynecol.* 2007;109(2 Pt 1):253–261.

153. Garite TJ, Clark R, Thorp JA. Intrauterine growth restriction increases morbidity and mortality among premature neonates. *Am J Obstet Gynecol.* 2004;191(2):481–487.

154. Mari G, Hanif F, Treadwell MC, et al. Gestational age at delivery and Doppler waveforms in very preterm intrauterine growth-restricted fetuses as predictors of perinatal mortality. *J Ultrasound Med.* 2007;26(5):555–559; quiz 560–552.

155. McIntire DD, Bloom SL, Casey BM, et al. Birth weight in relation to morbidity and mortality among newborn infants. *N Engl J Med.* 1999;340(16):1234–1238.

156. Lees CC, Marlow N, van Wassenaer-Leemhuis A, et al. 2 year neurodevelopmental and intermediate perinatal outcomes in infants with very preterm fetal growth restriction (TRUFFLE): a randomised trial. *Lancet.* 2015;385 (9983):2162–2172.

157. Alfirevic Z, Stampalija T, Gyte GM. Fetal and umbilical Doppler ultrasound in high-risk pregnancies. *Cochrane Database Syst Rev.* 2010(1):CD007529.

158. ACOG Committee Opinion. Utility of antepartum umbilical artery Doppler velocimetry in intrauterine growth restriction. Number 188, October 1997 (replaces no. 116, November 1992). Committee on Obstetric Practice. American College of Obstetricians and Gynecologists. *Int J Gynaecol Obstet.* 1997;59(3):269–270.

159. The GRIT Study Group. A randomised trial of timed delivery for the compromised preterm fetus: short term outcomes and Bayesian interpretation. *BJOG.* 2003;110(1):27–32.

160. Thornton JG, Hornbuckle J, Vail A, et al. Infant wellbeing at 2 years of age in the Growth Restriction Intervention Trial (GRIT): multicentred randomised controlled trial. *Lancet.* 2004;364(9433):513–520.

161. Walker DM, Marlow N, Upstone L, et al. The growth restriction intervention trial: long-term outcomes in a randomized trial of timing of delivery in fetal growth restriction. *Am J Obstet Gynecol.* 2011;204(1):34.e1–34.e9.

162. Groome LJ, Owen J, Neely CL, et al. Oligohydramnios: antepartum fetal urine production and intrapartum fetal distress. *Am J Obstet Gynecol.* 1991;165(4 Pt 1):1077–1080.

163. Peipert JF, Donnenfeld AE. Oligohydramnios: a review. *Obstet Gynecol Surv.* 1991;46(6):325–339.

164. Froen JF, Gardosi JO, Thurmann A, et al. Restricted fetal growth in sudden intrauterine unexplained death. *Acta Obstet Gynecol Scand.* 2004;83(9):801–807.

165. Vergani P, Roncaglia N, Ghidini A, et al. Can adverse neonatal outcome be predicted in late preterm or term fetal growth restriction? *Ultrasound Obstet Gynecol.* 2010;36(2):166–170.

166. Trudell AS, Cahill AG, Tuuli MG, et al. Risk of stillbirth after 37 weeks in pregnancies complicated by small-for-gestational-age fetuses. *Am J Obstet Gynecol.* 2013;208(5):376.e1–376.e7.

167. Boers KE, Vijgen SM, Bijlenga D, et al. Induction versus expectant monitoring for intrauterine growth restriction at term: randomised equivalence trial (DIGITAT). *BMJ.* 2010;341:c7087.

168. Boers KE, van Wyk L, van der Post JA, et al. Neonatal morbidity after induction vs expectant monitoring in intrauterine growth restriction at term: a subanalysis of the DIGITAT RCT. *Am J Obstet Gynecol.* 2012;206(4):344.e1–344.e7.

169. van Wyk L, Boers KE, van der Post JA, et al. Effects on (neuro)developmental and behavioral outcome at 2 years of age of induced labor compared with expectant management in intrauterine growth-restricted infants: long-term outcomes of the DIGITAT trial. *Am J Obstet Gynecol.* 2012;206(5):406.e1–406.e7.

170. ACOG Committee Opinion No. 560: medically indicated late-preterm and early-term deliveries. *Obstet Gynecol.* 2013;121(4):908–910.

171. Unterscheider J, Daly S, Geary MP, et al. Predictable progressive Doppler deterioration in IUGR: does it really exist? *Am J Obstet Gynecol.* 2013;209(6):539.e1–539.e7.

172. Effect of corticosteroids for fetal maturation on perinatal outcomes. *NIH Consens Statement.* 1994;12(2):1–24.

173. Antenatal corticosteroids revisited: repeat courses. *NIH Consens Statement.* 2000;17(2):1–18.

174. Roberts D, Dalziel S. Antenatal corticosteroids for accelerating fetal lung maturation for women at risk of preterm birth. *Cochrane Database Syst Rev.* 2006;3:CD004454.

175. Bernstein IM, Horbar JD, Badger GJ, et al. Morbidity and mortality among very-low-birth-weight neonates with intrauterine growth restriction. The Vermont Oxford Network. *Am J Obstet Gynecol.* 2000;182(1 Pt 1):198–206.

176. Committee Opinion No. 455: magnesium sulfate before anticipated preterm birth for neuroprotection. *Obstet Gynecol.* 2010;115(3):669–671.

177. Marret S, Marpeau L, Zupan-Simunek V, et al. Magnesium sulphate given before very-preterm birth to protect infant brain: the randomised controlled PREMAG trial. *BJOG.* 2007;114(3):310–318.

178. Rouse DJ, Hirtz DG, Thom E, et al. A randomized, controlled trial of magnesium sulfate for the prevention of cerebral palsy. *N Engl J Med.* 2008;359(9):895–905.

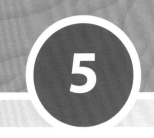

5 The Normal Fetal Echocardiogram

Anita Krishnan • Mary T. Donofrio

INTRODUCTION

Structural cardiac disease is the most commonly diagnosed congenital malformation. The incidence of congenital heart disease (CHD) has been estimated to be between 6 and 12 per 1,000 live births,[1-4] or approximately 1% of the general population. It is likely that the incidence prenatally is much higher, given that some pregnancies affected by CHD are terminated and other fetuses may die *in utero*. One study from Belgium[5] reported a CHD incidence of 8.3% in chromosomally normal infants born at 26 weeks of gestation.

INDICATIONS FOR REFERRAL

There are many fetal, maternal, and familial factors that can increase the risk of CHD in the fetus above that of the general population (Table 5.1). It is often these fetuses that are referred for additional cardiac evaluation beyond the routine mid-gestation obstetric ultrasound. All of these indications for referral increase the chance or likelihood of identifying CHD somewhat above that of the general population, but with varying effects on relative risk.

Maternal Factors

Diabetes Mellitus

Pregestational diabetes mellitus (DM) is found in approximately 1% of all pregnant women and, in the fetuses of these women, approximately 3% to 5% show CHD, which is significantly higher than that in the general population.[6] There are conflicting data regarding whether strict glycemic control prior to pregnancy affects the incidence of CHD.[7,8] As the fetal heart is fully formed within the first trimester of pregnancy, and gestational DM usually does not develop until the third trimester, it is not considered to be a reason for routine fetal cardiac evaluation. However, some fetuses may develop ventricular hypertrophy in the setting of poor glycemic control. Gestational diabetes, acquired late in pregnancy, is not thought to carry a risk of CHD[9]; however, there may be women with pregestational diabetes not uncovered until pregnancy whose fetuses are at risk for CHD.

Autoimmune Disease

Maternal autoimmune disease such as systemic lupus erythematosus (SLE) and Sjögren syndrome have been shown to be associated with congenital complete heart block (CHB) in the fetus, especially in those women demonstrating the autoantibodies anti-Ro/SSA and/or anti-La/SSB, and even in the setting of a mother who demonstrates no clinical symptoms of autoimmune disease. The incidence of CHB can be as low as 1% in those with no previously affected fetuses, but rises to nearly 20% in those with a previously affected child. The American Heart Association recommends screening between 16 and 28 weeks' gestation.[10] This includes structural and functional assessment, as well as measurement of the mechanical PR interval to evaluate for first- or second-degree heart block.[11] The mechanical PR interval (Fig. 5.1) measures the time for the electrical signal to travel from the atria to the ventricle. It has been hypothesized that prolongation of this measurement may represent an early marker of inflammation of the conduction system, although multiple studies have shown reversal to normal sinus rhythm with no intervention. The types of structural disease and arrhythmias associated with anti-SSA antibodies include ventricular arrhythmias,[11,12] sinus bradycardia,[13,14] junctional ectopic tachycardia,[15] structural cardiac disease,[16,17] valve regurgitation,[18,19] and aortic root dilation.[20,21] A recent multicenter study provided data that home Doppler monitor can be used to detect early signs of heart block and could be an adjunct to echocardiography.[22]

Medication Exposure

Fetal exposure to many different maternal medications has been shown to increase the risk of CHD in the fetus. This is dependent on the potential teratogenicity of the substance, when during gestation the fetus is exposed, and how likely it is to cross the placenta in significant quantities. Maternal medications that have been shown to lead to an increased risk of CHD in the fetus include anticonvulsants such as carbamazepine,[23] lithium (although more recent literature has suggested that the relative risk is not as high as initially thought),[24,25] retinoic acid[26] antihypertensives such as angiotensin-converting enzyme (ACE) inhibitors,[27] selective serotonin reuptake inhibitors,[28] and nonsteroidal anti-inflammatory drugs.[29]

Metabolic Diseases

Uncontrolled phenylketonuria may lead to an increased risk of CHD in the fetus.[30,31] Phenylketonuria, with elevated phenylalanine level greater than 10 mg/dL, may carry up to 12% to 14% risk of CHD for the fetus.

Viral Infections

Maternal rubella,[32] parvovirus, or other infections, including coxsackievirus,[33] adenovirus, and cytomegalovirus, can have adverse effects on fetal myocardial function. HIV is not associated with structural CHD[34]; however, fetuses of HIV-infected women may have alterations of left ventricular function. Parvovirus infection is a common cause of nonimmune hydrops fetalis in the fetus. It can cause direct myocardial damage, with reports of conduction system disease,[35] or fetal anemia with secondary congestive heart failure. Cardiovascular changes can include chamber dilation, ventricular thickening, and valvular regurgitation.

Assisted Reproductive Technology

An increasingly common indication for fetal echocardiography is the use of assisted reproductive technologies such as *in vitro* fertilization (IVF), which may or may not be combined with intracytoplasmic sperm injection (ICSI). It is difficult to accurately assess the increase in risk imposed by IVF and/or ICSI on the development of CHD in the fetus, as its use is often

TABLE 5.1   Indications for Fetal Echocardiography

	ABSOLUTE RISK, % LIVE BIRTHS	RELATIVE RISK OR LIKELIHOOD RATIO (CI)	COR/LOE	TIMING/ FREQUENCY OF EVALUATION	COMMENTS
Maternal factors					
Pregestational DM (pre-conception metabolic control may affect risk) or DM identified in the first trimester	3–5	≈5	I/A	18–22 wk repeat evaluation in third trimester if HbA$_{1c}$ >6% may be considered	DM is associated with a higher relative risk of certain specific cardiac defects, including 6.22 for heterotaxy, 4.72 for truncus arteriosus, 2.85 for d-TGA, and 18.24 for single-ventricle defects Poorly controlled DM is associated with ventricular hypertrophy in the third trimester
Gestational DM with HbA$_{1c}$ <6%	<1	1	III/B		If HbA$_{1c}$ >6%, fetal echocardiography in the third trimester may be considered to assess for ventricular hypertrophy
Phenylketonuria (pre-conception metabolic control may affect risk)	12–14	10–15	I/A	18–22 wk	Only if periconception phenylalanine level >10 mg/dL
Lupus or Sjögren only if SSA/SSB autoantibody positive Note: increased risk with maternal hypothyroidism or maternal vitamin D deficiency	1–5	Unknown	IIa/B	16 wk, then weekly or every other week to 28 wk	Recent studies have suggested that high SSA values (≥50 U/mL) correlate with increased fetal risk Concern for late myocardial involvement may justify additional assessments in the third trimester
With prior affected child with CHB or neonatal lupus, risk increased	11–19		I/B	16 wk, then at least weekly to 28 wk	
Medication exposures					
Teratogens Anticonvulsants Lithium ACE inhibitors Retinoic acids Vitamin A (>10,000 IU retinol/d) SSRIs	1–2 1.8 <2 2.9 8–20 1.8 1–2	1.1–1.8 1.2–1.72	IIb/A IIb/B IIa/B I/B IIb/B IIb/A (for paroxetine) III/A (for others)	18–22 wk 18–22 wk 18–22 wk 18–22 wk 18–22 wk 18–22 wk	Unless otherwise specified, exposure in the first trimester of pregnancy. For a more detailed review, see elsewhere 3.3 (95% CI, 1.3–8.8) for RVOT lesions only
Vitamin K antagonists (i.e., Coumadin) NSAIDs	<1 1%–2% for structural CHD 5%–50% for ductal constriction	1 1.8 (1.32–2.62)	III/B IIb/B (first-trimester exposure) I/A (third-trimester exposure)	Not indicated 18–22 wk Up to daily during exposure	Detailed anatomical survey should be performed Recommendation for exclusion of ductal constriction only

TABLE 5.1   Indications for Fetal Echocardiography (*continued*)

	ABSOLUTE RISK, % LIVE BIRTHS	RELATIVE RISK OR LIKELIHOOD RATIO (CI)	COR/LOE	TIMING/ FREQUENCY OF EVALUATION	COMMENTS
Maternal infection	1–2	1.8 (1.4–2.4)	I/C (rubella) III/C (other viruses with only seroconversion) I/C (if pericarditis/myocarditis suspected)	18–22 wk	Certain infections, specifically maternal rubella, have been associated with a higher incidence of specific cardiac malformations. Parvovirus, Coxsackie virus, adenovirus, and cytomegalovirus have been implicated in fetal myocarditis
Use of assisted reproduction technology	1.1–3.3		IIa/A	18–22 wk	Both IVF alone and IVF with ICSI seem to carry similar risk
Family history					
Maternal structural cardiac disease	3–7 (all) 10–14 (AVSD) 13–18 (AS) <3 (TOF, d-TGA)	≈5	I/B	18–22 wk	
Paternal structural cardiac disease	2–3, although may be slightly higher		I/B	18–22 wk	A single study reported a 7.5% recurrence when fetal echocardiography was used in addition to postnatal evaluation; this study included small VSDs and ASDs that were not detectable on fetal echocardiography
Sibling with structural disease	3%, 8% for HLHS	≈4	I/B	18–22 wk	For most lesions, <50% concordance has been observed, although exact concordance may be in the range of 20%–35% for the majority of cardiac malformations
Second-degree relative with structural cardiac disease	<2	1.39 (1.25–1.54)	IIb/B	18–22 wk	Studies have established heritability for left-sided obstructive lesions; and some now advocate screening for all first- and second-degree relatives of affected individuals
Third-degree relatives with structural cardiac disease	≈1	1.18 (1.05–1.32)	III/B	18–22 wk	
First- or second-degree relative with disease, disorder, or syndrome with Mendelian inheritance associated with structural cardiac disease	Up to 50		I/C	18–22 wk	There is little value to fetal echocardiography in detecting disease with postnatal onset of cardiovascular manifestations such as hypertrophic cardiomyopathy, Marfan or Ehlers–Danlos syndromes

(continued)

TABLE 5.1   Indications for Fetal Echocardiography (*continued*)

	ABSOLUTE RISK, % LIVE BIRTHS	RELATIVE RISK OR LIKELIHOOD RATIO (CI)	COR/LOE	TIMING/ FREQUENCY OF EVALUATION	COMMENTS
Fetal factors					
Suspected cardiac abnormality on obstetric ultrasound	>40		I/B	At detection	Repeat fetal echocardiography if abnormality is found or if progressive disease is suspected
Rhythm abnormalities:					
Tachycardia	1% for associated CHD		I/C	At detection	Fetal echocardiography to ascertain the mechanism of tachycardia and to guide therapy
Bradycardia/CHB	50–55		I/C	At detection	Fetal echocardiography to ascertain mechanism of bradycardia, and if persistent, monitoring to assess heart rate, rhythm and cardiac function
Irregular rhythm	0.3% with CHD; 2% with arrhythmia	(0–0.7)	I/C (frequent) IIa/C (persistent > 1–2 wk)	At detection 1–2 wk after detection	Baseline fetal echocardiography, and if persistent, weekly heart rate monitoring until resolved to assess for tachycardia
Noncardiac abnormality	20–45		I/B	At detection	Risk depends on organ systems affected
Known or suspected chromosomal abnormality	Varies, may be as high as 90		I/C	12–14 wk and/or 18–22 wk	See section Extracardiac Assessment of the Fetus with CHD for specific risks for aneuploidies and deletion syndromes
Increased NT, mm					
3.0–3.4	3		IIa/A I/A (if abnormal ductus venosus flow)	18–22 wk	
≥3.5	6	24	I/A	12–14 wk and/or 18–22 wk	
>6	24		I/B		
>8.5	>60		I/B		
Abnormality of umbilical cord, placenta, or intra-abdominal venous anatomy	3.9	>2	IIb/C	18–22 wk	Significant bias may be present in estimate

	ABSOLUTE RISK, % LIVE BIRTHS	RELATIVE RISK OR LIKELIHOOD RATIO (CI)	COR/LOE	TIMING/ FREQUENCY OF EVALUATION	COMMENTS
Monochorionic twinning	2–10	9.18 (5.5–15.3)	I/A	12–14 wk and 18–22 wk; additional evaluation based on clinical findings	Estimated at 2%–2.5%; 11% when pregnancy complicated by TTTS
Hydrops fetalis	15–25		I/B	At diagnosis	Can be extended to the evaluation of the at-risk fetus and to the fetus with effusions in the absence of hydrops (isolated pericardial or pleural effusion, ascites)

TABLE 5.1   Indications for Fetal Echocardiography (*continued*)

ACE, angiotensin-converting enzyme; AS, aortic stenosis; ASD, atrial septal defect; AVSD, atrioventricular septal defect; CHB, complete heart block; CHD, congenital heart disease; CI, confidence interval; COR, classification of recommendation; DM, diabetes mellitus; d-TGA, dextro-transposition of the great arteries; HbA$_{1c}$, hemoglobin A$_{1c}$; HLHS, hypoplastic left heart syndrome; ICSI, intracytoplasmic sperm injection; IVF, *in vitro* fertilization; LOE, level of evidence; NSAID, nonsteroidal anti-inflammatory drug; NT, nuchal translucency; RVOT, right ventricular outflow tract; SSRI, selective serotonin reuptake inhibitor; TOF, tetralogy of Fallot; TTTS, twin–twin transfusion syndrome; and VSD, ventricular septal defect.

Reprinted with permission from Donofrio MT, Moon-Grady AJ, Hornberger LK, et al. Diagnosis and treatment of fetal cardiac disease. *Circulation*. 2014;129(21):2183–2242. Copyright ©2014 American Heart Association, Inc.

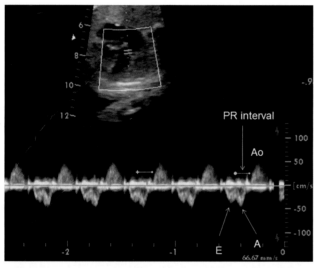

FIGURE 5.1: The mechanical PR or AV interval corresponds to the electrocardiogram (ECG) measurement of the *PR* interval, the time for the electrical impulse to travel from atrium to ventricle. A pulsed-wave Doppler is placed to simultaneously sample mitral inflow and aortic outflow in the four-chamber view. The mitral inflow during diastole consists of two phases, *E* or passive filling and *A* or active atrial contraction. *Ao* indicates aortic outflow during ventricular systole. The PR interval is measured from the beginning of the mitral A wave to the beginning of the aortic ejection phase. Normative data for 2 and 3 standard deviations exist in the literature.

more common in mothers of advanced parental age and also leads to an increased risk of monozygous twins, both of which can slightly increase the incidence of CHD. Regardless, the risk of CHD in infants conceived through such assisted reproductive technologies is considered increased and is an indication for fetal echocardiography.[36–38]

Family History

Another common indication for fetal cardiac evaluation is a family history of CHD. The incidence of recurrence in subsequent family members can vary depending on what the relationship of the fetus to the proband is, and what the nature of the CHD is. The highest risk of recurrence occurs when CHD is present in the mother of the fetus,[39] and fetal echocardiography is indicated in all such cases. The increase in risk overall is 3% to 7%, but is lesion dependent, with the most pronounced increase for lesions of atrioventricular septal defect[40] (10% to 14%) and aortic stenosis (13% to 18%). There is also an increased risk of CHD in the fetuses of affected fathers; although the risk of 2% to 3% is not as significant, fetal echocardiography remains reasonable. The recurrence risk for siblings is approximately 3%, although higher for hypoplastic left heart syndrome.[41–44] The risk to the fetus increases as the number of previously affected siblings increases, and it is not unusual for multiple fetuses of the same parents to be affected with heterotaxy syndrome or aortic valve stenosis.[45] Although fewer data are available for the incidence of recurrence in second-degree relatives of affected patients, the risk is thought to be somewhat above that of the general population, but not significant enough to require routine screening in these fetuses.[39,46]

Fetal Factors

Multiple factors relating to the fetus itself can be indications for fetal echocardiography.

Suspected Fetal Cardiac Disease

The indication for fetal echocardiography yielding the greatest likelihood of CHD is an abnormal four-chamber view on obstetrical ultrasound. The detection rate of the four-chamber view for significant CHD in the fetus is only 40%. When outflow tract views are included in the obstetrical screening examination, this number increases to over 50% in low risk populations.[47,48]

Suspected Fetal Arrhythmia

All fetuses thought to have an abnormal cardiac rhythm, whether it be tachycardia, bradycardia, or an irregular rhythm with the exception of isolated premature atrial contractions, should have a fetal echocardiogram to better assess the specific rhythm abnormality and to diagnose any associated structural heart disease. This can help both in guiding therapy and in evaluating for the underlying cause of the arrhythmia.

Chromosomal Abnormalities

Previously diagnosed or suspected chromosomal abnormalities that are associated with CHD are a common indication for referral for fetal echocardiography. The incidence of detecting CHD varies with the specific chromosomal abnormality in the fetus.[44] Commonly referred chromosomal abnormalities include trisomy 21, 18, or 13, DiGeorge syndrome, and Turner syndrome.

Extracardiac Abnormalities

Even in a genetically normal fetus, extracardiac abnormalities may warrant an echocardiogram. Some abnormalities that are highly associated with CHD in the affected fetus include omphalocele, congenital diaphragmatic hernia, genitourinary abnormalities, and central nervous system abnormalities.[49–54]

Increased Nuchal Translucency

An increased nuchal translucency (NT) found in fetuses between 11 and 14 weeks' gestational age has been shown to increase the risk of aneuploidy and other congenital anomalies, including CHD.[55,56] The risk of CHD in the fetus rises with increasing NT, even in the absence of known aneuploidy or other genetic abnormality.[57]

Vascular Malformations

Vascular abnormalities in the fetus that are indications for fetal cardiac evaluation include a single umbilical artery or absence of the ductus venosus. Single umbilical artery is associated with CHD of various types, and in association with renal and vertebral anomalies in the VACTERL (vertebral defects, anal atresia, cardiac defects, tracheo-esophageal fistula, renal anomalies, and limb abnormalities) syndrome.

Twin Pregnancy

Monochorionic twin gestation carries an overall risk of 2% for CHD.[58] A second indication for fetal echocardiography is to evaluate the heart in fetuses with twin–twin transfusion syndrome. If twin–twin transfusion syndrome is present, structural cardiac anomalies including pulmonary valve stenosis have been described.

Fetal Hydrops

Fetal echocardiography is indicated to rule out structural cardiac disease, arrhythmia, tumor, or vascular anomalies in fetuses with hydrops fetalis. In addition, scoring systems based on heart size, function, and umbilical Doppler parameters have been created and shown to correlate with outcome.[59]

FETAL ECHOCARDIOGRAPHY

Timing and Technical Considerations

Timing of fetal echocardiography can vary depending on the indication for referral. The major cardiac structures are present by 9 weeks, and the developmental sequence has been delineated in anatomical specimens using advanced imaging techniques.[60]

During pregnancy, Doppler assessment of cardiac function can be performed in the early first trimester, even before fetal cardiac development is complete.[61] A complete fetal echocardiogram, with the exception of pulmonary vein assessment, is possible at 12 to 16 weeks, with a high level of sensitivity for major CHD.[62] However, in general, screening echocardiography for maternal risk factors such as family history or pregestational DM occurs between 18 and 22 weeks' gestational age. Follow-up examinations should be performed whenever the initial cardiac evaluation occurs earlier in gestation and/or if any abnormalities are suspected. Once CHD is diagnosed, interval follow-up occurs throughout pregnancy.

Imaging of the fetal heart is limited by the small size of the fetal heart, the rapid heart rate, and the depth of imaging in all cases, and can be additionally compromised by factors such as maternal body habitus and fetal positioning. To optimize imaging, the highest frequency transducer (usually between 4 and 12 MHz) that sufficiently penetrates the maternal abdomen should be used. This may become more difficult later in gestation as the need for increased depth penetration necessitates using a lower frequency transducer. The ultrasound system used should be able to perform two-dimensional (2D) imaging, M-mode, color Doppler, and pulsed-wave Doppler.

Evaluation of the Normal Fetal Heart

Fetal Visceral Situs

The initial step in evaluating the fetal heart is to determine the visceral situs of the fetus, or the laterality of the organs. The normal arrangement of the visceral organs is described as situs solitus, with morphological right atrium, major hepatic lobe, inferior vena cava, trilobed lung, and short eparterial bronchus on the right side. Situs inversus refers to a reversal in laterality, when these anatomical findings occur on the left side of the fetus. In situs ambiguous, the laterality cannot be determined, and does not fit easily into the solitus or inversus description. Visceral/atrial situs ambiguous is commonly associated with significant CHD, most notably heterotaxy[63] (see Chapter 24.2).

The first step in determining fetal visceral situs is to determine the exact position of the fetus within the maternal abdomen. By sweeping from maternal foot to head, and from maternal right to left, the exact position of the fetus can be determined. A transverse view of the fetal abdomen and thorax should be obtained, and it can confirm that the fetal heart is pointing to the left side of the chest, as well as to the stomach and descending aorta. Typically, the inferior vena cava can be seen on the right side, and the atria into which the inferior vena cava enters is the morphological right atrium. The inferior vena cava can be interrupted, with azygous continuation to the superior vena cava.

Fetal Cardiac Axis

A transverse view of the chest at the level of the four-chamber view of the heart is found to determine the cardiac axis. A normal cardiac axis lies at approximately 45° from the midline, with the apex of the heart pointing leftward[63] (Fig. 5.2). Abnormal cardiac axis, either significantly more or less, can indicate either structural heart disease or other abnormality within the thorax of the fetus such as congenital cystic malformation of the lung or congenital diaphragmatic hernia.

Fetal Cardiac Size

The fetal heart occupies approximately one-third of the area in the thorax. This can be evaluated by tracing the circumference of both the heart and the thorax, and comparing either the area or the circumference. The cardiothoracic area ratio remains

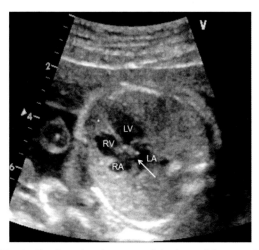

FIGURE 5.2: The four-chamber view of the heart delineates the right atrium (*RA*), left atrium (*LA*), right ventricle (*RV*), and left ventricle (*LV*). The *asterisk* indicates the moderator band characteristic of a morphologic right ventricle. The foramen ovale, indicated with an *arrow*, bows into the left atrium. Note that a line drawn through the apex of the left ventricle is at a 45° angle with the midline, which is a normal cardiac axis. The heart lies in the left chest, with the apex pointing leftward, and occupies less than one-third of the area of the thorax.

consistent throughout gestation and should range between 0.25 and 0.35. Greater ratios may indicate cardiomegaly in the fetus[64] and are associated with hydrops fetalis, volume overload lesions such as arteriovenous malformations or sacrococcygeal teratoma, fetal anemia, or myocardial injury from structural heart disease, valvular regurgitation, or arrhythmia.

Fetal Cardiac Position

The position of the heart within the fetal chest is referred to as cardiac position. The normal position is described as levocardia, with the heart located in the left chest (see Fig. 5.2). In dextrocardia, the heart is located in the right chest, and in mesocardia, the heart is located in the midline. The determination of cardiac position is independent of the cardiac axis. For example, with a left-sided congenital diaphragmatic hernia, the heart is positioned in the right chest, but the apex is still pointing leftward. This is known as dextroposition of the heart.

Evaluation of the Fetal Cardiac Chambers

As ultrasound uses 2D images to evaluate the 3D anatomy of the heart, multiple views of all of the fetal cardiac chambers should be obtained.

The Right Atrium

The normal right atrium is located anterior and to the right of the left atrium. Typically, the right atrium receives desaturated blood from the inferior vena cava, superior vena cava, and coronary sinus (Fig. 5.3). At times, the inferior vena cava can be interrupted, but if it enters directly into an atrium, it is typically the morphological right atrium. The right atrial body is smooth posteriorly and trabeculated anteriorly, with a broad-based right atrial appendage.[65] The Eustachian valve, which is located over the opening of the inferior vena cava, directs the highly oxygenated blood from the maternal circulation and, subsequently, the ductus venosus (Fig. 5.4), across the foramen ovale to the left side of the heart, so that the most oxygenated blood supplies the head vessels of the aorta.[66]

The atrial septum separates the right and left atria, which is formed by the septum primum and septum secundum. The fossa ovalis is on the right atrial side, and flow across the fossa ovalis is

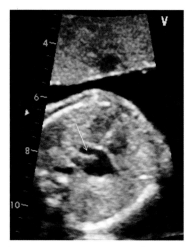

FIGURE 5.3: The coronary sinus is a normal structure located in the posterior–inferior aspect of the heart. Care should be taken not to mistake this normal structure for a *primum* atrial septal defect. An enlarged coronary sinus, highlighted by the *arrow*, can be associated with a left superior vena cava, anomalous pulmonary venous connection to the coronary sinus, or with elevated right-sided pressure.

typically right to left (Fig. 5.5). The septum primum forms the valve of the foramen ovale, and is located within the left atrium. Atrial septal defects are classified by where they lie within the atrial septum.

The Left Atrium

The normal left atrium is located posteriorly within the chest cavity and is smooth walled. It should receive all four pulmonary veins in the normal heart and is smooth walled throughout. The left atrial appendage is narrow and fingerlike.[58] It contains the septum primum or the flap valve of the foramen ovale (see Fig. 5.2).

The Right Ventricle

Located behind the sternum, the right ventricle is the most anterior chamber in the normal heart. It is coarsely trabeculated in contrast to the smooth trabeculations of the left ventricle. It is crescent shaped as opposed to elliptical like the left ventricle. Although the left ventricle is designed to handle the demands of the systemic circulation after birth, *in utero* it is the right ventricle

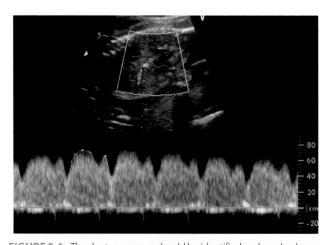

FIGURE 5.4: The ductus venosus should be identified and a pulsed-wave Doppler performed in a fetal echocardiogram. Here, a normal Doppler flow pattern is seen, with continuous flow entering the fetal heart. Ductus venosus tissue restricts the volume of highly oxygenated maternal blood returning to the fetal heart. Absence of the ductus venosus can cause right heart volume overload. Reversed flow in the ductus venosus is abnormal and can indicate right ventricular diastolic dysfunction or early atrial contraction/arrhythmia, where the atrium contracts against a closed valve.

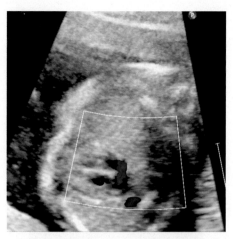

FIGURE 5.5: Unrestricted foramen ovale flow is seen crossing from right to left (normal) in this fetus. Restriction of the atrial septum can be seen in congenital heart disease and also as an isolated finding, and careful attention should be paid to the size and direction of the foramen flow. The foramen ovale typically constitutes less than one-third of the atrial septum.

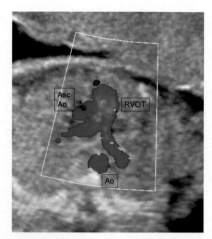

FIGURE 5.6: The branch pulmonary arteries are seen in the right ventricular outflow tract *(RVOT)* view in the transverse imaging plane. *Asc Ao,* Ascending aorta; *Ao,* aorta.

that pumps against high resistance of the pulmonary circulation. It contains a moderator band (see Fig. 5.2).

Tricuspid Valve

The atrioventricular valve is defined by its ventricle, with the tricuspid valve directing blood into the right ventricle. The tricuspid valve should be slightly more apically displaced within the heart than the mitral valve. The tricuspid valve is comprised of three leaflets—the anterior, posterior, and septal leaflets—which are anchored by the chordae tendineae to the three papillary muscles within the body of the right ventricle. Chordae tendineae from the tricuspid valve attach directly to the septal wall in the right ventricle, a feature that is not found in the left ventricle.

The Left Ventricle

The left ventricle is smooth walled, and located posterior and leftward of the right ventricle. It is elliptical or bullet shaped and should form the apex of the heart. It does not have a moderator band and has two distinct papillary muscles that should be clearly separated (the anterolateral and posteromedial papillary muscles).

Mitral Valve

The mitral valve is the atrioventricular valve associated with the morphological left ventricle. The mitral valve has two leaflets—the anterior and posterior—that attach to the anterolateral and posteromedial papillary muscles, which then insert into the free wall of the left ventricle, without the septal attachments apparent in the morphologic right ventricle.

The Pulmonary Valve, Conus, and Pulmonary Arteries

The subpulmonic conus separates the pulmonary valve anteriorly from the tricuspid valve and the body of the right ventricle.[65] The main pulmonary artery arises from the right ventricle and crosses the aorta, with the pulmonary valve located anterior and leftward of the aortic valve. The pulmonary valve has three leaflets. The main pulmonary artery then divides into the right and left branch pulmonary arteries (Fig. 5.6) and the ductus arteriosus, which subsequently joins the descending aorta.

The Aortic Valve and Aorta

The aortic semilunar valve has three leaflets, the right and left coronary cusps, and the posterior or noncoronary cusp. The ascending aorta arises from the left ventricle and is crossed by the pulmonary artery so that the aortic valve is posterior and rightward of the

pulmonary valve. The valve is in fibrous continuity with the mitral valve. The ascending aorta curves posteriorly into the aortic arch and gives rise to the three main head vessels—the innominate artery, which divides into the right subclavian and right common carotid artery, the left common carotid artery, and the left subclavian artery. The descending thoracic aorta lies posterior to the left atrium and becomes the abdominal aorta at the level of the diaphragm.[65] Arch sidedness is typically leftward, which means that the arch crosses to the left of the trachea. A right aortic arch is common in conotruncal abnormalities, but can occur as an isolated finding or in association with a vascular ring (Fig. 5.7). Arch sidedness is delineated in the trachea view, described later. A right aortic arch carries an increased risk of 22q microdeletion syndrome.[67]

Standard Imaging Planes

Depending on the source, the standard imaging views may carry different names. For the purposes of this discussion, the imaging planes described by the American Institute of Ultrasound in

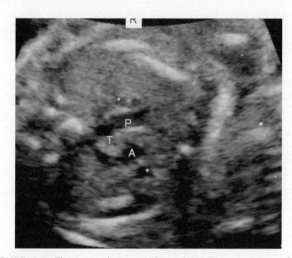

FIGURE 5.7: Three-vessel view with trachea *(T)* is seen in a fetus diagnosed with right aortic arch and a left-sided superior vena cava *(*)*. In this fetus, the pulmonary artery *(P)* is seen to the left of the trachea. The ascending aorta *(A)* is seen crossing right of the trachea, and a left-sided ductus is seen posterior to the trachea. This provides the substrate for a vascular ring at birth that can cause compression of the trachea and esophagus. If symptoms of emesis or respiratory difficulties are noted, this type of lesion would need surgical repair. A right aortic arch can also be associated with 22q microdeletion syndrome.

Medicine are used.[68] These guidelines were recently updated in 2020, but with no significant changes to the imaging planes.

Transverse Views

The transverse scanning planes consist of the four-chamber view, the left and right arterial outflow tract views, and the three-vessel and trachea view.

Four-Chamber View: A four-chamber view of the heart can be obtained by imaging transversely through the fetal chest

(Fig. 5.8). In the normal four-chamber view, the apex of the heart should be pointing leftward at approximately 45° (see Fig. 5.2). The descending aorta should be visualized to the left and anterior to the fetal spine. The atria should be approximately equal in size, and the ventricles should be approximately equal in size and contractility (although this can vary by gestational age). The ventricular septum should appear intact, and the foramen ovale (see Fig. 5.5) should be visible within the atrial septum. In addition, the anatomical right atrium and ventricle should be rightward, and the anatomical left atrium and ventricle should

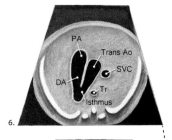

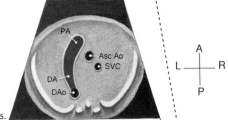

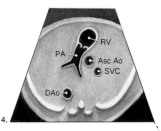

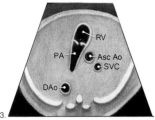

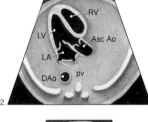

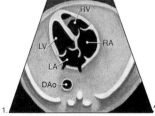

Representative Scan Planes

1. Four Chamber View
2. Left Ventricular Outflow Tract
3. Right Ventricular Outflow Tract
4. Three Vessel View with Main PA Bifurcation
5. Three Vessel View with Ductal Arch
6. Three Vessels and Trachea View

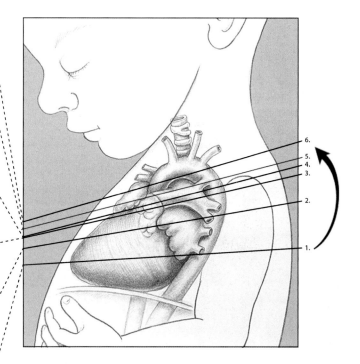

FIGURE 5.8: Representative scan planes for fetal echocardiography include an evaluation of the 4-chamber view (1), left and right arterial outflow tracts (2 and 3, respectively), two variants of the 3-vessel view, one demonstrating the main pulmonary artery bifurcation (4) with another more superior plane that demonstrates the ductal arch (5), and the 3-vessel and trachea view (6). Not all views may be seen from a single cephalic transducer sweep without some minor adjustments in the position and orientation of the transducer due to anatomic variations and the fetal lie. *Asc Ao*, ascending aorta; *DAo*, descending aorta; *LA*, left atrium; *LV*, left ventricle; *PA*, pulmonary artery; *RA*, right atrium; *RV*, right ventricle; *Tr*, trachea. (From American Institute of Ultrasound in Medicine. AIUM practice guideline for the performance of fetal echocardiography. *J Ultrasound Med.* 2013;32(6):1067–1082. Copyright © 2016 by the American Institute of Ultrasound in Medicine. Reprinted by permission of John Wiley & Sons, Inc.)

be leftward, as described later. It can be challenging to assess the pulmonary venous return to the left atrium as only a small amount of blood is directed to the lungs during fetal life. Often, the transverse, four-chamber view of the fetal heart yields the most helpful images of the pulmonary veins entering the left atrium (Fig. 5.9). Ideally, at least one left and one right pulmonary vein should be visualized.

Outflow Tract Views: Following initial determination of situs and evaluation of the four-chamber fetal heart from the transverse view, the transducer can be tipped anteriorly within the fetus (toward the fetal head) to obtain the "five-chamber view" of the fetal heart, which includes the left ventricular outflow tract (see Fig. 5.9). The membranous ventricular septum and much of the muscular portion of the ventricular septum can also be assessed in this view. Moving the transducer cranially will bring in the right ventricular outflow tract view (see Fig. 5.6), and then moving it again cranially will define the three-vessel view with trachea.

Three-Vessel and Trachea View: In the three-vessel and trachea view (Fig. 5.10), the aorta, main pulmonary artery, and superior vena cava are visualized. This angulation of the three-vessel view shows the relationship of the arch to the trachea. Relative size can be evaluated as can arch sidedness. A right aortic arch, suggested by an aorta positioned rightward of the trachea, warrants further evaluation for associated structural heart disease. From the three-vessel view, tilting the transducer cranially can yield a transverse view of the ductus arteriosus with the ductus joining the descending aorta leftward of the spine.

Sagittal Views

The sagittal views consist of the bicaval, the aortic arch, and the ductal arch views.

Bicaval Sagittal View: From a sagittal view of the fetus (parallel to the fetal spine), the systemic venous anatomy can be assessed (Fig. 5.11). The bicaval view (Fig. 5.12) can be obtained by tilting the probe rightward in the fetus from the midline sagittal plane. The superior and inferior vena cava can be seen entering the right atrium posteriorly. A portion of the atrial septum and left atrium can be visualized. The superior vena cava is seen anterior to the

right pulmonary artery. At the junction of the inferior vena cava and right atrium, the Eustachian valve can sometimes be appreciated.[63]

Aortic Arch View: From a sagittal view of the fetus (parallel to the fetal spine), the aortic and ductal arches can be assessed. In the left sagittal plane, a view of the aortic arch can be obtained (Fig. 5.13). The aortic arch arises from the middle of the chest and curves in a "candy-cane" appearance posteriorly. The three head vessels can be seen arising from the aortic arch and heading superiorly toward the neck and head of the fetus. The right pulmonary artery is seen in cross section posterior to the ascending aorta. The aortic isthmus can be visualized distal to the left subclavian artery, before the insertion of the ductus arteriosus. This is the narrowest aspect of the aortic arch, and most aortic coarctations are located just distal to this part of the arch.

Ductal Arch View: By sweeping further leftward with a slight change of angulation, the ductal arch can be imaged (Figs. 5.14 and 5.15). The ductal arch arises more anteriorly within the chest and has a more acute curvature, previously described as having a "hockey stick" appearance. The ductal arch connects to the descending aorta distal to the aortic isthmus.

Short-Axis Views

Oblique, or short-axis, views of the fetal heart can be obtained (Fig. 5.16). The short-axis view of the fetal heart can assist in evaluation of the right ventricular outflow tract (Fig. 5.17) and can be obtained by orienting the transducer from right fetal hip to left fetal shoulder. The right ventricle is visualized anteriorly, as is the main pulmonary artery as it crosses over the aorta, which is viewed in cross section. The main pulmonary artery then divides into the right pulmonary artery and the ductus arteriosus. Both the atrium and the foramen ovale can also be visualized from this plane.

By adjusting the transducer from apical to basal within the fetal heart, multiple short-axis views can be obtained. With these views, the ventricular chamber size, ventricular wall thickness, ventricular septum, and systolic function can be assessed (Fig. 5.18). The left ventricle should appear posterior, circular, and smooth walled, while the right ventricle is more trabeculated, crescent shaped, and anterior.

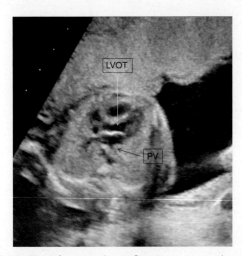

FIGURE 5.9: The left ventricular outflow tract view in the transverse imaging plane. The *PV* indicates a left pulmonary vein entering the left atrium. Note the normal unobstructed left ventricular outflow tract (*LVOT*).

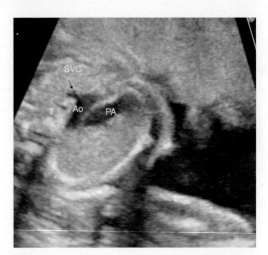

FIGURE 5.10: The three-vessel view shows the relative size of the main pulmonary artery and aorta, and their position relative to the trachea. This figure highlights a typical left arch in which both the aorta and pulmonary artery cross to the left of the trachea. *Ao*, aorta; *PA*, pulmonary artery; *SVC*, superior vena cava; *T*, trachea.

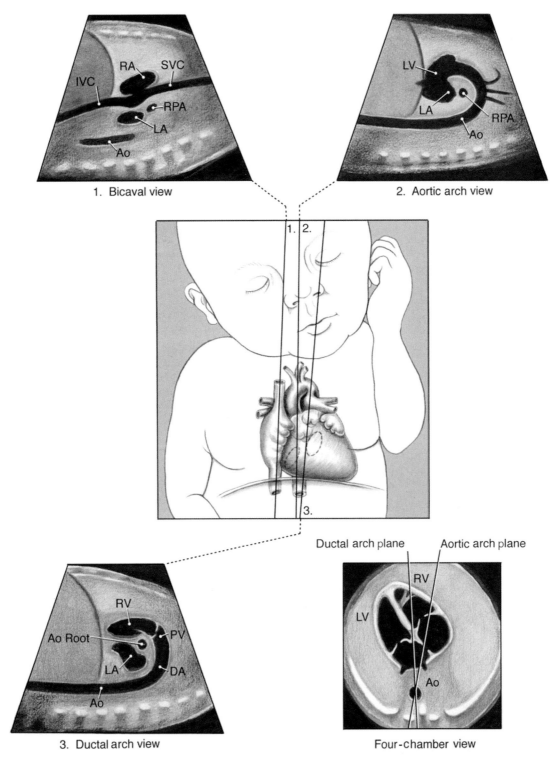

1. Bicaval view

2. Aortic arch view

3. Ductal arch view

Four-chamber view

FIGURE 5.11: The standard sagittal imaging planes. *Ao,* aorta; *Ao Root,* aortic root; *DA,* ductus arteriosus; *IVC,* inferior vena cava; *LA,* left atrium; *LV,* left ventricle; *PV,* pulmonary valve; *RA,* right atrium; *RPA,* right pulmonary artery; *RV,* right ventricle; *SVC,* superior vena cava. (From American Institute of Ultrasound in Medicine. AIUM practice guideline for the performance of fetal echocardiography. *J Ultrasound Med.* 2013;32(6):1067–1082. Copyright © 2016 by the American Institute of Ultrasound in Medicine. Reprinted by permission of John Wiley & Sons, Inc.)

CARDIAC BIOMETRY

Quantitative assessment of cardiac structure and function is valuable in both structurally normal and abnormal hearts. Normative values and Z-score equations are available for all valves and chambers of the heart, at all periods during gestation.[69–71] Measurement of atrioventricular and semilunar valves, ventricular length, and subsequent comparison of left- and right-sided structures can give significant insight into underlying structural cardiac disease. For example, a small pulmonary valve

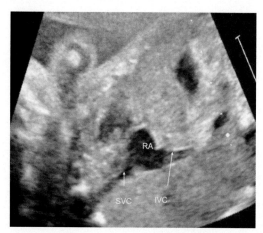

FIGURE 5.12: The bicaval sagittal view illustrates the inferior and superior vena cava (*SVC*) entering the right atrium (*RA*). A portion of the atrial septum is seen. The inferior vena cava (*IVC*) can be interrupted in certain types of congenital heart disease, specifically the heterotaxy syndromes. Anomalous pulmonary venous drainage to the superior or inferior vena cava can cause dilation of these vessels.

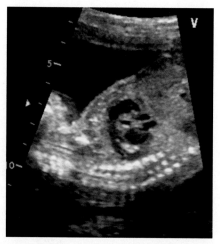

FIGURE 5.14: The ductal arch is seen in its entirety. Typically, the peak systolic velocity in the ductus arteriosus is less than 2 m/s, and diastolic velocity is 0.35 m/s. Restriction of the ductus can be caused by maternal ingestion of nonsteroidal anti-inflammatory medications. It is imperative to image the entire ductus, particularly where it enters the aortic isthmus, as restriction may occur primarily in this area.

annulus may be the first indication of tetralogy of Fallot in a fetal heart with a relatively normal four-chamber view with a questionable ventricular septal defect, while a small aortic valve may be the first indication of coarctation of the aorta. Both by qualitative assessment and by established normative values, the right-sided atrioventricular and semilunar valves should be slightly larger than their left-sided counterparts, while the right and left ventricles should be approximately equal in length and width.[69–71] However, in late gestation, the right ventricular width can be noticeably larger than the left.

COLOR DOPPLER EVALUATION

The fetal heart is a moving, beating organ, and full assessment of it should include evaluation of blood flow. Color Doppler can be useful in the assessment of atrioventricular and semilunar valve stenosis or regurgitation, anatomy and flow through the ductal and aortic arches, drainage of the systemic and pulmonary veins, as well as in the evaluation of septal defects,[72,73] and is now recommended as part of a comprehensive fetal echocardiographic examination.[74]

Technical Considerations

A high frame rate improves the quality of 2D imaging of the fetal heart. Once color Doppler imaging commences, the frame rate

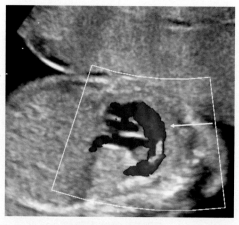

FIGURE 5.15: Color imaging of the ductal arch is helpful in evaluating for critical congenital heart disease. Reversed color flow in the ductus arteriosus is abnormal and can indicate ductal-dependent pulmonary blood flow arrow points to the ductal arch.

decreases, and a balance must be reached between optimizing frame rate and allowing for adequate color Doppler assessment. The narrower the width of the color box, the higher the frame rate, yielding improved quality of images. The quality of color Doppler

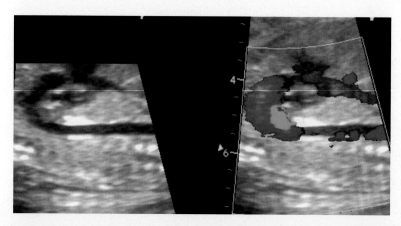

FIGURE 5.13: The aortic arch is seen in black and white, and color imaging. It typically has a candy-cane appearance, although this is altered in diseases like transposition of the great arteries. The head vessels are usually equally spaced. Color imaging of the arches is helpful in ruling out critical congenital heart disease, in which there will be reversed flow in one of the arches, but can obfuscate finer details about the size of the distal ductus and aortic isthmus. Relying on only color imaging may cause the clinician to miss milder disease.

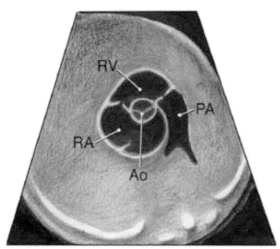

1. High Short Axis View - Great Arteries

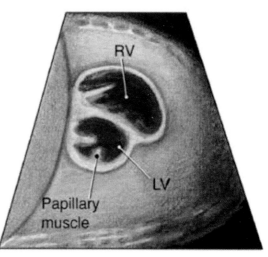

2. Low Short Axis View - Ventricles

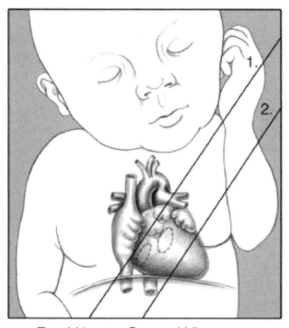

Fetal Heart - Coronal View

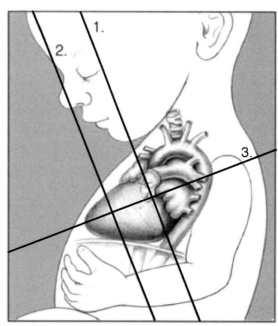

Fetal Heart - Sagittal View

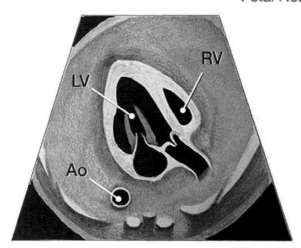

3. Long Axis View

FIGURE 5.16: High short-axis view (1), low short-axis view (2), and long-axis view (3) of the fetal heart. *Ao,* aortic valve; *LV,* left ventricle; *PA,* pulmonary artery; *RA,* right atrium; *RV,* right ventricle. (From American Institute of Ultrasound in Medicine. AIUM practice guideline for the performance of fetal echocardiography. *J Ultrasound Med.* 2013;32(6):1067–1082. Copyright © 2016 by the American Institute of Ultrasound in Medicine. Reprinted by permission of John Wiley & Sons, Inc.)

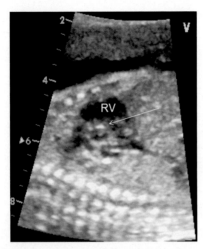

FIGURE 5.17: In the "high" short-axis view, the aortic valve in cross section is indicated with an *arrow*. The right ventricular outflow tract crosses anteriorly. This view is helpful in evaluating for diseases like tetralogy of Fallot, in which there is small and anteriorly deviated right ventricular outflow tract. *RV*, right ventricle.

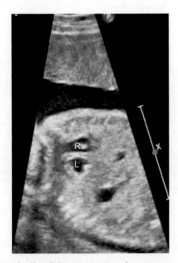

FIGURE 5.18: In the "low" short-axis view, the two ventricles are seen in cross section. This view can be used to obtain the shortening fraction, a measure of function. R, right ventricle; L, left ventricle.

imaging can also be affected by the velocity scale. For the majority of the fetal cardiac evaluation, a relatively high-velocity scale can be used (>40 cm/s). This allows for adequate imaging across the atrioventricular and semilunar valves as well as the great vessels, without color aliasing that would be apparent at a lower scale. Lower velocity scales are more appropriate for low-velocity vessels such as the pulmonary and systemic veins. Doppler interrogation of the heart with the probe angled parallel to the blood flow will optimize color imaging. All standard views, including the four-chamber view, outflow tracts, three-vessel view with trachea, and arch, should be acquired with 2D and color. 2D images allow assessment of anatomical features, and color adds physiological information.

OTHER CARDIAC EVALUATIONS

Pulsed-Wave Doppler Evaluation

Less commonly used in obstetrical fetal heart ultrasound screening, but important to the full fetal echocardiogram, is pulsed-wave Doppler, which is discussed in more detail in

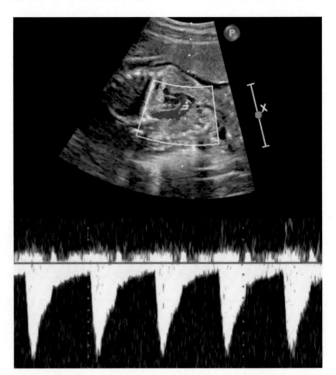

FIGURE 5.19: A pulsed-wave Doppler tracing in the aortic isthmus.

Chapter 6. Normative data for peak velocities and typical blood flow patterns are available for all of the cardiac valves and great vessels, and should be applied in the comprehensive evaluation of the fetal heart. An example of a pulsed-wave Doppler tracing in the aortic isthmus is seen in Figure 5.19.

Fetal Rhythm Assessment

Suspected fetal arrhythmias are a common indication for referral for fetal echocardiography. In addition to a comprehensive assessment of the structure of the fetal heart, an assessment of fetal rhythm should be performed. M-mode or pulsed-wave Doppler imaging allows assessment of the mechanical measure of fetal cardiac rhythm.

M-Mode Echocardiography

M-mode imaging allows for the visual representation of the movement of a structure over time. To evaluate the rhythm of the heart, the sample line is placed through the right atrium and either ventricle. The M-mode images show the change in wall motion over time, so that the relationship between atrial and ventricular contractions can be assessed, and the fetal heart rate and rhythm can be measured.[75]

Pulsed-Wave Doppler

Another method of assessing mechanical atrial and ventricular systole as a means of fetal rhythm assessment is through pulsed-wave Doppler. This can be evaluated by simultaneous Doppler of the left ventricular inflow and outflow and/or the superior vena cava and ascending aorta so that the fetal rhythm can be more accurately assessed.[76,77] In this way, the relationship between atrial and ventricular contractions can be more clearly visualized than when using 2D ultrasound alone. In women with anti-SSA antibodies, the mechanical PR interval can be measured and followed up over the duration of pregnancy using simultaneous left ventricular inflow and outflow Dopplers.

Fetal Cardiac Functional Assessment

In addition to an assessment of fetal cardiac structure and rhythm, an assessment of function of the fetal heart is also an integral part of a comprehensive fetal cardiac evaluation. Persistent arrhythmias, cardiomyopathies, maternal infections, and structural heart disease are some of the factors that can affect fetal cardiac function. A qualitative assessment of fetal cardiac function is part of the basic cardiac evaluation. Cardiomegaly can indicate impaired fetal cardiac function or altered loading conditions.[78] Quantitatively, the shortening fraction of the left ventricle can be evaluated from 2D or M-mode imaging (shortening fraction [%] = [end diastolic diameter-end systolic diameter]/end diastolic diameter).[79] The Tei index is a global additional assessment of cardiac function, calculated from the inflow–outflow Doppler of the mitral and aortic valve.[80] Additional measures for evaluating fetal cardiac function use pulsed-wave Doppler, and are discussed in more detail in Chapter 6.

LIMITATIONS OF FETAL ECHOCARDIOGRAPHY

There are limitations to fetal echocardiography due to the small size of the fetal heart, the rapid fetal heart rate, and the fact that imaging occurs through the maternal abdomen and uterus. In addition, factors such as maternal body habitus and fetal position may worsen already suboptimal imaging. Fortunately, major structural heart disease can usually be identified with a complete fetal echo, and most of the lesions less consistently diagnosed prenatally often have little impact on neonatal well-being or hemodynamic stability. These include small ventricular or atrial septal defects, minor valve abnormalities, and partial pulmonary venous drainage abnormalities.[81] Imaging with the four-chamber view alone cannot detect major malformations such as tetralogy of Fallot or transposition of the great arteries, making the outflow views essential in accurately diagnosing cardiac defects. Because of the nature of fetal cardiac circulation, persistence of a patent foramen ovale and patent ductus arteriosus cannot be predicted. In addition, some cardiac anomalies develop later in gestation or progress throughout gestation, and may not be apparent at the routine mid-gestation evaluation. These include fetal arrhythmias, cardiomyopathies, rhabdomyomas, and some obstructive lesions.[82–84] Certain conditions, such as coarctation and anomalous pulmonary venous return, are challenging but possible to detect prenatally by experienced clinicians. Coarctation often becomes more severe when ductal tissue in the aortic isthmus constricts after birth. Prenatally, a small aorta relative to the pulmonary outflow may be seen in the three-vessel view with the trachea,[85] and bidirectional or low-velocity flow may be seen in the aortic isthmus. In total anomalous pulmonary venous connection, an additional venous structure entering either the superior vena cava or crossing below the diaphragm may be noted.

REFERENCES

1. Ferencz C, Rubin JD, McCarter RJ, et al. Congenital heart disease: prevalence at livebirth. The Baltimore-Washington Infant Study. *Am J Epidemiol.* 1985;121(1):31–36.
2. Hoffman JI. Congenital heart disease: incidence and inheritance. *Pediatr Clin North Am.* 1990;37(1):25–43.
3. Tegnander E, Williams W, Johansen OJ, et al. Prenatal detection of heart defects in a non-selected population of 30,149 fetuses—detection rates and outcome. *Ultrasound Obstet Gynecol.* 2006;27(3):252–265.
4. Wren C, Richmond S, Donaldson L. Temporal variability in birth prevalence of cardiovascular malformations. *Heart.* 2000;83(4):414–419.
5. Moons P, Sluysmans T, De Wolf D, et al. Congenital heart disease in 111 225 births in Belgium: birth prevalence, treatment and survival in the 21st century. *Acta Paediatr.* 2009;98(3):472–477.
6. Moore T. *Maternal-Fetal Medicine: Principles and Practice.* Philadelphia, PA: WB Saunders; 1999.
7. Miller E, Hare JW, Cloherty JP, et al. Elevated maternal hemoglobin A1c in early pregnancy and major congenital anomalies in infants of diabetic mothers. *N Engl J Med.* 1981;304(22):1331–1334.
8. Lisowski LA, Verheijen PM, Copel JA, et al. Congenital heart disease in pregnancies complicated by maternal diabetes mellitus: an international clinical collaboration, literature review, and meta-analysis. *Herz.* 2010;35(1):19–26.
9. Hagay Z, Reece A. *Reece and Hobbins: Medicine of the Fetus and Mother.* Philadelphia, PA: Lippincott Williams & Wilkins; 1999.
10. Donofrio MT, Moon-Grady AJ, Hornberger LK, et al. Diagnosis and treatment of fetal cardiac disease: a scientific statement from the American Heart Association. *Circulation.* 2014 May 27;129(21):2183–2242.
11. Friedman DM, Kim MY, Copel JA, et al. Utility of cardiac monitoring in fetuses at risk for congenital heart block: the PR Interval and Dexamethasone Evaluation (PRIDE) prospective study. *Circulation.* 2008;117(4):485–493.
12. Hornberger LK, Al Rajaa N. Spectrum of cardiac involvement in neonatal lupus. *Scand J Immunol.* 2010;72(3):189–197.
13. Chockalingam P, Jaeggi ET, Rammeloo LA, et al. Persistent fetal sinus bradycardia associated with maternal anti-SSA/Ro and anti-SSB/La antibodies. *J Rheumatol.* 2011;38(12):2682–2685.
14. Askanase AD, Friedman DM, Copel J, et al. Spectrum and progression of conduction abnormalities in infants born to mothers with anti-SSA/Ro-SSB/La antibodies. *Lupus.* 2002;11(3):145–151.
15. Zhao H, Cuneo BF, Strasburger JF, et al. Electrophysiological characteristics of fetal atrioventricular block. *J Am Coll Cardiol.* 2008;51(1):77–84.
16. Costedoat-Chalumeau N, Amoura Z, Lupoglazoff JM, et al. Outcome of pregnancies in patients with anti-SSA/Ro antibodies: a study of 165 pregnancies, with special focus on electrocardiographic variations in the children and comparison with a control group. *Arthritis Rheum.* 2004;50(10):3187–3194.
17. Eronen M. Long-term outcome of children with complete heart block diagnosed after the newborn period. *Pediatr Cardiol.* 2001;22(2):133–137.
18. Cuneo BF, Fruitman D, Benson DW, et al. Spontaneous rupture of atrioventricular valve tensor apparatus as late manifestation of anti-Ro/SSA antibody-mediated cardiac disease. *Am J Cardiol.* 2011;107(5):761–766.
19. Krishnan AN, Sable CA, Donofrio MT. Spectrum of fetal echocardiographic findings in fetuses of women with clinical or serologic evidence of systemic lupus erythematosus. *J Matern Fetal Neonatal Med.* 2008;21(11):776–782.
20. Radbill AE, Brown DW, Lacro RV, et al. Ascending aortic dilation in patients with congenital complete heart block. *Heart Rhythm.* 2008;5(12):1704–1708.
21. Davey DL, Bratton SL, Bradley J, et al. Relation of maternal anti-Ro/La antibodies to aortic dilation in patients with congenital complete heart block. *Am J Cardiol.* 2011;108(4):561–564.
22. Cuneo BF, Sonesson SE, Levasseur S, et al. Home monitoring for fetal heart rhythm during anti-Ro pregnancies. *J Am Coll Cardiol.* 2018;72(16):1940–1951.
23. Matalon S, Schechtman S, Goldzweig G, et al. The teratogenic effect of carbamazepine: a meta-analysis of 1255 exposures. *Reprod Toxicol.* 2002;16(1):9–17.
24. Jenkins KJ, Correa A, Feinstein JA, et al. Noninherited risk factors and congenital cardiovascular defects: current knowledge: a scientific statement from the American Heart Association Council on Cardiovascular Disease in the Young: endorsed by the American Academy of Pediatrics. *Circulation.* 2007;115(23):2995–3014.
25. Warner JP. Evidence-based psychopharmacology 3. Assessing evidence of harm: what are the teratogenic effects of lithium carbonate? *J Psychopharmacol.* 2000;14(1):77–80.
26. Lammer EJ, Chen DT, Hoar RM, et al. Retinoic acid embryopathy. *N Engl J Med.* 1985;313(14):837–841.
27. Cooper WO, Hernandez-Diaz S, Arbogast PG, et al. Major congenital malformations after first-trimester exposure to ACE inhibitors. *N Engl J Med.* 2006;354(23):2443–2451.
28. Louik C, Lin AE, Werler MM, et al. First-trimester use of selective serotonin-reuptake inhibitors and the risk of birth defects. *N Engl J Med.* 2007;356(26):2675–2683.
29. Moise KJ Jr, Huhta JC, Sharif DS, et al. Indomethacin in the treatment of premature labor: effects on the fetal ductus arteriosus. *N Engl J Med.* 1988;319(6):327–331.
30. Platt LD, Koch R, Hanley WB, et al. The international study of pregnancy outcome in women with maternal phenylketonuria: report of a 12-year study. *Am J Obstet Gynecol.* 2000;182(2):326–333.
31. Levy HL, Waisbren SE. Effects of untreated maternal phenylketonuria and hyperphenylalaninemia on the fetus. *N Engl J Med.* 1983;309(21):1269–1274.
32. Botto LD, Lynberg MC, Erickson JD. Congenital heart defects, maternal febrile illness, and multivitamin use: a population-based study. *Epidemiology.* 2001;12(5):485–490.
33. Ornoy A, Tenenbaum A. Pregnancy outcome following infections by Coxsackie, echo, measles, mumps, hepatitis, polio and encephalitis viruses. *Reprod Toxicol.* 2006;21(4):446–457.

34. Hornberger LK, Lipshultz SE, Easley KA, et al. Cardiac structure and function in fetuses of mothers infected with HIV: the prospective PCHIV multicenter study. *Am Heart J.* 2000;140(4):575–584.
35. Fishman SG, Pelaez LM, Baergen RN, et al. Parvovirus-mediated fetal cardiomyopathy with atrioventricular nodal disease. *Pediatr Cardiol.* 2011;32(1):84–86.
36. Bahtiyar MO, Campbell K, Dulay AT, et al. Is the rate of congenital heart defects detected by fetal echocardiography among pregnancies conceived by in vitro fertilization really increased?: a case-historical control study. *J Ultrasound Med.* 2010;29(6):917–922.
37. Tararbit K, Houyel L, Bonnet D, et al. Risk of congenital heart defects associated with assisted reproductive technologies: a population-based evaluation. *Eur Heart J.* 2010;32(4):500–508.
38. Reefhuis J, Honein MA, Schieve LA, et al. Assisted reproductive technology and major structural birth defects in the United States. *Hum Reprod.* 2009;24(2):360–366.
39. Oyen N, Poulsen G, Boyd HA, et al. Recurrence of congenital heart defects in families. *Circulation.* 2009;120(4):295–301.
40. Emanuel R, Somerville J, Inns A, et al. Evidence of congenital heart disease in the offspring of parents with atrioventricular defects. *Br Heart J.* 1983;49(2):144–147.
41. Nora JJ, Nora AH. Genetic epidemiology of congenital heart diseases. *Prog Med Genet.* 1983;5:91–137.
42. Hinton RB Jr, Martin LJ, Tabangin ME, et al. Hypoplastic left heart syndrome is heritable. *J Am Coll Cardiol.* 2007;50(16):1590–1595.
43. Pradat P. Recurrence risk for major congenital heart defects in Sweden: a registry study. *Genet Epidemiol.* 1994;11(2):131–140.
44. Pierpont ME, Basson CT, Benson DW Jr, et al. Genetic basis for congenital heart defects: current knowledge: a scientific statement from the American Heart Association Congenital Cardiac Defects Committee, Council on Cardiovascular Disease in the Young: endorsed by the American Academy of Pediatrics. *Circulation.* 2007;115(23):3015–3038.
45. Burn J, Brennan P, Little J, et al. Recurrence risks in offspring of adults with major heart defects: results from first cohort of British collaborative study. *Lancet.* 1998;351(9099):311–316.
46. Fesslova V, Brankovic J, Lalatta F, et al. Recurrence of congenital heart disease in cases with familial risk screened prenatally by echocardiography. *J Pregnancy.* 2011;2011:368067.
47. Carvalho JS, Mavrides E, Shinebourne EA, et al. Improving the effectiveness of routine prenatal screening for major congenital heart defects. *Heart.* 2002;88(4):387–391.
48. Simpson LL. Indications for fetal echocardiography from a tertiary-care obstetric sonography practice. *J Clin Ultrasound.* 2004;32(3):123–128.
49. Copel JA, Pilu G, Kleinman CS. Congenital heart disease and extracardiac anomalies: associations and indications for fetal echocardiography. *Am J Obstet Gynecol.* 1986;154(5):1121–1132.
50. Greenwood RD, Rosenthal A, Nadas AS. Cardiovascular malformations associated with omphalocele. *J Pediatr.* 1974;85(6):818–821.
51. Greenwood RD, Rosenthal A, Nadas AS. Cardiovascular malformations associated with imperforate anus. *J Pediatr.* 1975;86(4):576–579.
52. Greenwood RD, Rosenthal A, Nadas AS. Cardiovascular malformations associated with congenital anomalies of the urinary system: observations in a series of 453 infants and children with urinary system malformations. *Clin Pediatr.* 1976;15(12):1101–1104.
53. Greenwood RD, Rosenthal A, Nadas AS. Cardiovascular abnormalities associated with congenital diaphragmatic hernia. *Pediatrics.* 1976;57(1):92–97.
54. Greenwood RD, Rosenthal A, Parisi L, et al. Extracardiac abnormalities in infants with congenital heart disease. *Pediatrics.* 1975;55(4):485–492.
55. Nicolaides KH, Heath V, Cicero S. Increased fetal nuchal translucency at 11–14 weeks. *Prenat Diagn.* 2002;22(4):308–315.
56. Snijders RJ, Noble P, Sebire N, et al. UK multicentre project on assessment of risk of trisomy 21 by maternal age and fetal nuchal-translucency thickness at 10–14 weeks of gestation. Fetal Medicine Foundation First Trimester Screening Group. *Lancet.* 1998;352(9125):343–346.
57. Atzei A, Gajewska K, Huggon IC, et al. Relationship between nuchal translucency thickness and prevalence of major cardiac defects in fetuses with normal karyotype. *Ultrasound Obstet Gynecol.* 2005;26(2):154–157.
58. Bahtiyar MO, Dulay AT, Weeks BP, et al. Prevalence of congenital heart defects in monochorionic/diamniotic twin gestations: a systematic literature review. *J Ultrasound Med.* 2007;26(11):1491–1498.
59. Huhta JC, Paul JJ. Doppler in fetal heart failure. *Clin Obstet Gynecol.* 2010;53(4):915–929.
60. Dhanantwari P, Lee E, Krishnan A, et al. Human cardiac development in the first trimester: a high-resolution magnetic resonance imaging and episcopic fluorescence image capture atlas. *Circulation.* 2009;120(4):343–351.
61. Wloch A, Rozmus-Warcholinska W, Czuba B, et al. Doppler study of the embryonic heart in normal pregnant women. *J Matern Fetal Neonatal Med.* 2007;20(7):533–539.
62. Moon-Grady A, Shahanavaz S, Brook M, et al. Can a complete fetal echocardiogram be performed at 12 to 16 weeks' gestation? *J Am Soc Echocardiogr.* 2012;25(12):1342–1352.
63. Salomon LJ, Baumann C, Delezoide AL, et al. Abnormal abdominal situs: what and how should we look for? *Prenat Diagn.* 2006;26(3):282–285.
64. Chaoui R, Bollmann R, Goldner B, et al. Fetal cardiomegaly: echocardiographic findings and outcome in 19 cases. *Fetal Diagn Ther.* 1994;9(2):92–104.
65. Van Praagh R. Morphologic anatomy. In: Keane JF, Lock JE, Fyler DC, eds. *Nadas Pediatric Cardiology.* Philadelphia, PA: Saunders; 1992:17–26.
66. Rudolph AM, Heymann MA. The circulation of the fetus in utero: methods for studying distribution of blood flow, cardiac output and organ blood flow. *Circ Res.* 1967;21:163–184.
67. Berg C, Bender F, Soukup M, et al. Right aortic arch detected in fetal life. *Ultrasound Obstet Gynecol.* 2006;28(7):882–889.
68. American Institute of Ultrasound in Medicine. AIUM Practice Guideline for the Performance of Fetal Echocardiography. *J Ultrasound Med.* 2013;32:1067–1082.
69. Schneider C, McCrindle BW, Carvalho JS, et al. Development of Z-scores for fetal cardiac dimensions from echocardiography. *Ultrasound Obstet Gynecol.* 2005;26(6):599–605.
70. Sharland GK, Allan LD. Normal fetal cardiac measurements derived by cross-sectional echocardiography. *Ultrasound Obstet Gynecol.* 1992;2(3):175–181.
71. Krishnan A, Pike J, Wilson E, et al. Predictive models for normal fetal cardiac structures. *J Am Soc Echocardiogr.* 2016;29(12):1197–1206.
72. Copel JA, Morotti R, Hobbins JC, et al. The antenatal diagnosis of congenital heart disease using fetal echocardiography: is color flow mapping necessary? *Obstet Gynecol.* 1991;78(1):1–8.
73. Stewart PA, Wladimiroff JW. Fetal echocardiography and color Doppler flow imaging: the Rotterdam experience. *Ultrasound Obstet Gynecol.* 1993;3(3):168–175.
74. Lee W, Allan L, Carvalho JS, et al. ISUOG consensus statement: what constitutes a fetal echocardiogram? *Ultrasound Obstet Gynecol.* 2008;32(2):239–242.
75. Allan LD, Anderson RH, Sullivan ID, et al. Evaluation of fetal arrhythmias by echocardiography. *Br Heart J.* 1983;50(3):240–245.
76. Fouron JC, Fournier A, Proulx F, et al. Management of fetal tachyarrhythmia based on superior vena cava/aorta Doppler flow recordings. *Heart.* 2003;89(10):1211–1216.
77. Strasburger JF, Huhta JC, Carpenter RJ Jr, et al. Doppler echocardiography in the diagnosis and management of persistent fetal arrhythmias. *J Am Coll Cardiol.* 1986;7(6):1386–1391.
78. Pedra SR, Smallhorn JF, Ryan G, et al. Fetal cardiomyopathies: pathogenic mechanisms, hemodynamic findings, and clinical outcome. *Circulation.* 2002;106(5):585–591.
79. Van Mieghem T, DeKoninck P, Steenhaut P, et al. Methods for prenatal assessment of fetal cardiac function. *Prenat Diagn.* 2009;29(13):1193–1203.
80. Friedman D, Buyon J, Kim M, et al. Fetal cardiac function assessed by Doppler myocardial performance index (Tei Index). *Ultrasound Obstet Gynecol.* 2003;21(1):33–36.
81. Gottliebson WM, Border WL, Franklin CM, et al. Accuracy of fetal echocardiography: a cardiac segment-specific analysis. *Ultrasound Obstet Gynecol.* 2006;28(1):15–21.
82. Hornberger LK, Barrea C. Diagnosis, natural history, and outcome of fetal heart disease. *Semin Thorac Cardiovasc Surg Pediatr Card Surg Annu.* 2001;4:229–243.
83. Sivasankaran S, Sharland GK, Simpson JM. Dilated cardiomyopathy presenting during fetal life. *Cardiol Young.* 2005;15(4):409–416.
84. Tworetzky W, McElhinney DB, Margossian R, et al. Association between cardiac tumors and tuberous sclerosis in the fetus and neonate. *Am J Cardiol.* 2003;92(4):487–489.
85. Slodki M, Rychik J, Moszura T, et al. Measurement of the great vessels in the mediastinum could help distinguish true from false-positive coarctation of the aorta in the third trimester. *J Ultrasound Med.* 2009;28(10):1313–1317.

Review of Fetal Cardiac Function Using M-Mode, Pulsed-Doppler, VOCAL, and Speckle-Tracking Software—A Practical Clinical Approach

6

Gregory DeVore • Gary M. Satou • Mark Sklansky

Quantitative evaluation of the fetal cardiovascular system requires analysis of various components affecting cardiac output (CO; the product of multiplying the heart rate/minute by the stroke volume).[1] For example, extremes of fetal heart rate such as congenital heart block (<60/minute) or paroxysmal atrial tachycardia (>200/minute) can result in decreased CO and heart failure.[2–7] Conversely, fetuses with a normal heart rate can have cardiac dysfunction as the result of factors that alter CO resulting from changes in preload, afterload, and ventricular contractility (Fig. 6.1). Although the effect of the factors listed in Figure 6.1 are continuously interactive, the dilemma for the clinician is determining how to approach evaluation of the fetal cardiovascular system for obstetrical care. Currently, there are a number of imaging modalities (M-mode ultrasound [US], 2D US, 4D US, and pulsed-Doppler US) that have been used to examine fetal cardiac function.[1] Depending on the available US equipment, the position of the fetal heart in relation to the transducer beam, and examiner experience, it would be important to understand the various diagnostic tools available, what to measure, and how to interpret the results.

Many investigators have used the term "cardiac function" to refer to evaluation of the heart, whereas others have been more restrictive and defined cardiac function to be equivalent to CO.[1] In this review, we refer to cardiac function as a global term when describing systolic contractility and diastolic relaxation. In addition, we further define specific components of cardiac function as they relate to available diagnostic tests used in fetal echocardiography.[1] This is followed by a discussion of fetal disease states in which these diagnostic US approaches have been used to examine the fetal heart. At the conclusion of this review, the fetal sonologist should be able to identify which US modalities could be incorporated into their clinical practice, how to interpret the significance of the findings, and apply them to the clinical management of the fetus.

HISTORICAL PERSPECTIVE—FETAL HEART RATE MONITORING

For over 40 years, obstetrical care providers have relied on patterns of continuous fetal heart rate tracings (FHRTs) to evaluate the fetus at risk for adverse outcome, both before and during labor.[8,9] Despite the almost universal adaptation of FHRT analysis, there continues to be disagreement about the classification of patterns, as well as the ultimate benefits of this technology.[10–27] In many instances, the correlation of FHRT with pH or adverse outcome has been less than reliable.[28–30] This appears related to the fact that interpretation rests with the subjective impressions of the provider at the bedside. Unfortunately, computer-assisted programs have had inconsistent success in improving the identification of fetuses at risk for adverse outcome.[31,32]

Issues of the relationship of FHRT to adverse outcome and umbilical pH notwithstanding, the object of surveillance is the early detection of impaired organ perfusion in the fetus, especially the vital organs including the brain and the heart. Although there is no direct access to cerebral function other than measuring Doppler blood flow in the middle cerebral artery (MCA), there is access to the fetal heart that avails itself to assessment of cardiac function.[1,33] The importance of understanding cardiac function is demonstrated in Figure 6.2, which illustrates a fetus with normal cardiac function and another with a sinusoidal heart rate pattern secondary to fetal anemia. Although the nadir of the sinusoidal pattern was well within the normal range for both fetuses (120 to 160/minute), the heart of the anemic fetus demonstrated abnormal size, shape, and function of the right ventricle (RV) and left ventricle (LV) 7 days before the development of an increased peak velocity of the MCA, indicating severe anemia and a sinusoidal fetal heart rate pattern (Fig. 6.2B). Therefore, direct evaluation of cardiac function could allow for a more comprehensive understanding of the underlying disease state, in some cases before FHRT deterioration, that could alter management of the high-risk fetus.

SCREENING FOR ABNORMAL CARDIAC FUNCTION

Although quantitative evaluation of cardiac function has focused primarily on fetuses with specific diseases (e.g., growth restriction, risk for fetal anemia, and twin-to-twin transfusion), the question that can be posed is, "How can the clinician identify the fetus at risk for cardiovascular dysfunction that has no underlying clinical risk factors?" Recently, our group described the end-diastolic global sphericity index (GSI) of the four-chamber view, defined as the length divided by the width, as well as the area of the four-chamber view, as screening tools to identify the fetus at risk for fetal abnormalities that have been associated with cardiac dysfunction.[34–36] Figure 6.3A illustrates how the GSI is measured from two end-diastolic linear measurements, easily obtained from current US machines. In addition, the area can be derived from two measurements (Fig. 6.3A) or traced around the epicardial border of the four-chamber view (Fig. 6.3B). Normally, the shape of the four-chamber view is ellipsoid, with a GSI greater than the 5th centile (1.08). Measurement of the end-diastolic area of the four-chamber view correlated with biometric (biparietal diameter [BPD], head circumference [HC], abdominal circumference [AC], femur length [FL], and estimated fetal weight [EFW]) and age measurements. Once an abnormal GSI (<5th centile) or area (>95th centile) is identified, further evaluation of ventricular function should be undertaken.[34–36]

A

Factors Affecting Stroke Volume (SV)		
Preload	**Contractility**	**Afterload**
Raised due to: • fast filling time • increased venous return **Increases end diastolic volume,** Increases stroke volume	• sympathetic stimulation • epinephrine and norepinephrine • high intracellular calcium ions • high blood calcium level • thyroid hormones • glucagon **Decreases end systolic volume,** Increases stroke volume	• increased vascular restistance • semilunar valve damage **Increases end systolic volume** Decreases stroke volume
Lowered due to: • decreased thyroid hormones • decreased calcium ions • high or low potassium ions • high or low sodium • low body temperature • hypoxia • abnormal pH balance • drugs (i.e., calcium channel blockers) **Decreases end diastolic volume,** Decreases stroke volume	• parasympathetic stimulation • acetylcholine • hypoxia • hyperkalemia **Increases end systolic volume** Decreases stroke volume	• decreased vascular resistance **Decreases end systolic volume** Increases stroke volume

B

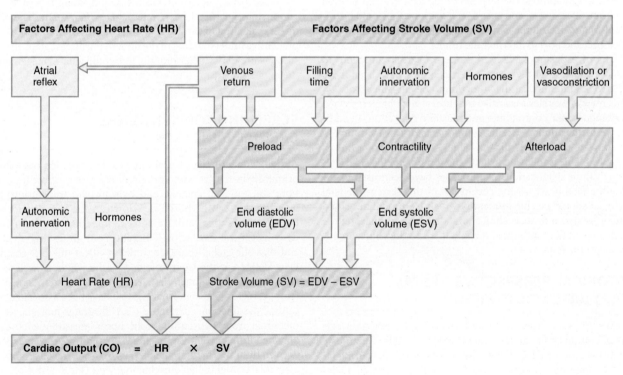

FIGURE 6.1: Factors that alter stroke volume **(A)** and cardiac output **(B)**. (Used Anatomy and physiology. https://openstax.org/details/books/anatomy-and-physiology.)

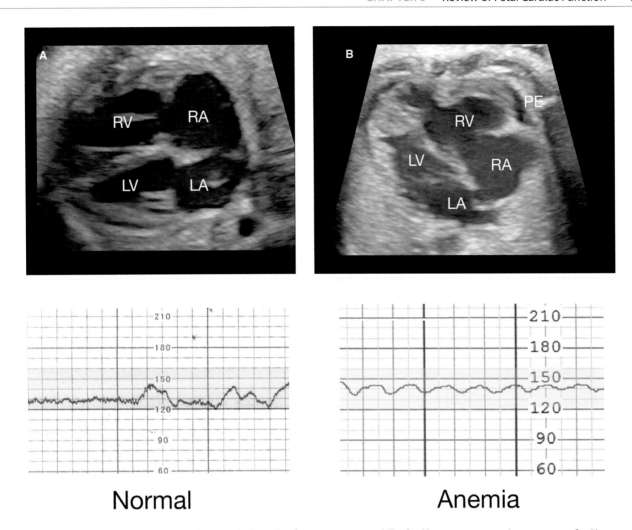

FIGURE 6.2: A: This is from a normal fetus in which cardiac function was normal. The fetal heart rate pattern demonstrates a fetal heart rate varying between 150 and 170 beats/min. **B:** This is from a fetus at 33 weeks with fetal anemia and abnormal changes in size, shape, and contractility of the right and left ventricles. The heart rate varies between 130 and 142, which does not account for the cardiac dysfunction noted in both ventricles and the decreased cardiac output of the left ventricle which was less than the 1st centile, with a heart rate of 133 a week before the appearance of the sinusoidal heart rate pattern. *LA*, left atrium; *LV*, left ventricle; *RA*, right atrium; *RV*, right ventricle. *PE*, pericardial effusion.

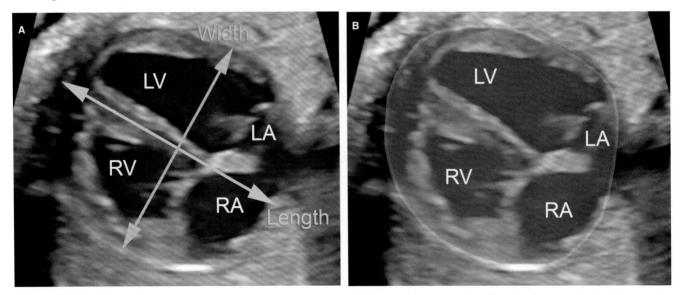

FIGURE 6.3: Computing the Global Sphericity Index (GSI) and area from an end-diastolic image of the four-chamber view. **A:** This illustrates the measurement of two diameters used to compute the GSI. The basal-apical length (*green line*) is divided by the transverse width (*blue line*).[34] A value less than the 5th centile (<1.08) is abnormal, suggesting a globular-shaped four-chamber view. From these two measurements, the area can be computed as follows: Area = (3:14159 * basal-apical length * transverse width)/4.[34,35] **B:** This illustrates the computed area derived using a point-to-point trace around the epicardial border of the four-chamber view.[36] *LA*, left atrium; *LV*, left ventricle; *RA*, right atrium; *RV*, right ventricle.

MYOCARDIAL ANATOMY OF THE RV AND LV

To understand ventricular contractility, it is important to review the orientation of the muscle fibers that comprise the ventricles of the heart. In 2013, Mekkaoui et al. scanned intact cadaver hearts with diffusion magnetic resonance imaging (MRI) tractography to identify the fiber orientation of the myocardium.[37]

They compared the adult heart with the hearts of fetuses at 10 weeks, 14 weeks, 19 weeks, and a newborn at 6 days following birth (Fig. 6.4).[37] They identified three fiber orientations in the adult heart; two opposing helical tracts from the base to the apex of the LV lateral wall, and a nonhelical circumferential tract (Fig. 6.4A and B).[37] The fetal fiber orientation, similar to that of the adult heart, was not present at 10 weeks of

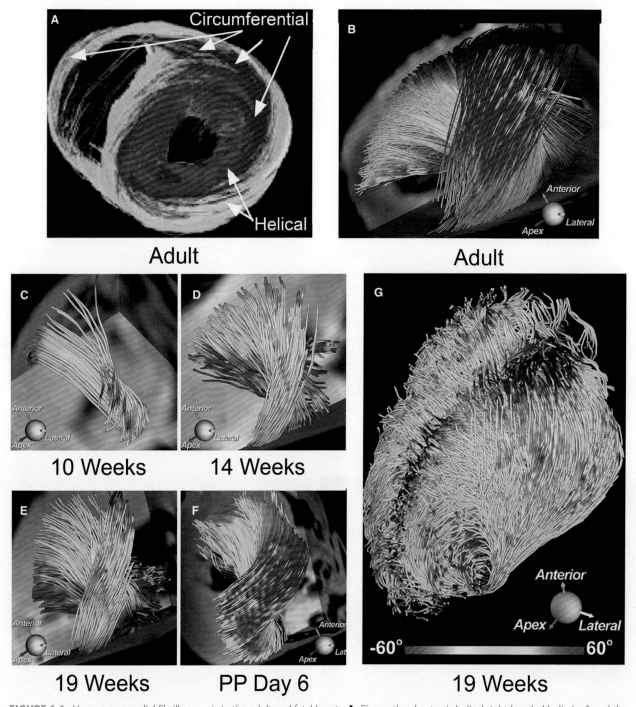

FIGURE 6.4: Human myocardial fibrillogenesis in the adult and fetal hearts. **A:** Shows the short-axis helical right-handed helix (*red*) and the left-handed helix (*green/yellow*). The circumferential fibers (*blue*) have no helix formation. **B:** Shows the left lateral wall in the adult, with similar color interpretation as **(A)**. **C:** Demonstrates the left lateral wall of a 10-week fetus that has the beginning of helical formation. **(D and E)** demonstrate the evolution of helical and circumferential fibers from 14 to 19 weeks of gestation. **F:** Demonstrates a more developed fiber orientation at 6 days postdelivery (PD). **(G)** is the entire heart at 19 weeks. (From Mekkaoui C, Porayette P, Jackowski MP, et al. Diffusion MRI tractography of the developing human fetal heart. *PloS One*. 2013;8(8):e72795. Copyright © 2013 Mekkaoui et al. From Buckberg G, Hoffman JI, Nanda NC, et al. Ventricular torsion and untwisting: further insights into mechanics and timing interdependence: a viewpoint. *Echocardiography*. 2011;28(7):782–804. Copyright © 2011 Wiley Periodicals, Inc. Reprinted by permission of John Wiley & Sons, Inc.)

gestation (Fig. 6.4C), but it evolved to an adult orientation by 19 weeks (Fig. 6.4E).[37] However, the density of fibers did not approach that of the adult heart until after the postnatal period (Fig. 6.4F).[37] The helical structure of the ventricles was recently reviewed by Buckberg et al., who affirmed the findings of Torrent-Guasp and hypothesized that the heart demonstrated two interconnected muscle bands; a basal loop with transverse fibers surrounding the LV and RV, and an apical loop, composed of a right- and left-handed helix that crossed each other at a 60° angle, forming an apical vortex (Fig. 6.5).[38,39] A video, posted online by Buckberg, demonstrates Torrent-Guasp's unraveling of the heart, illustrating the abovementioned anatomy (http://www.mdpi.com/2308-3425/5/2/33/s1).[38] The purpose of the right- and left-handed helix is to provide opposite contraction forces from the base and apex for each ventricle that results in ejecting and filling of blood from each chamber, similar to wringing and unwringing of a cloth towel.

Similar to the apex of the heart, the septum has oblique, opposing helical muscles, resulting in coiling and shortening of the muscles, as is observed in the lateral ventricular walls (Figs. 6.4 to 6.6).[40,41] In addition, the left lateral ventricular wall and LV septum have circumferential fibers that contribute to contraction of the myocardium toward the center of the LV chamber during systole (Fig. 6.6). Therefore, as the result of myocardial fiber and muscle orientation, the interventricular septum (IVS) is committed primarily to the LV. Studies of the RV have suggested that longitudinal shortening from the base to the apex of the chamber develops from coiling and shortening of the apical helix, with little contribution from the lateral wall longitudinal and circumferential fibers.[40,41] In adults and experimental animals, it has been demonstrated that RV heart failure does not occur after elimination of free wall muscle function. However, heart failure occurs when septal ischemia is present.[40–45]

IMAGING TECHNOLOGIES USED TO EVALUATE CARDIAC FUNCTION

Given the abovementioned anatomy of the muscle bands that are responsible for ventricular contractility, the evaluation of the fetal heart can be accomplished from different image acquisition planes. The most common approach is to initially image the four-chamber view, followed by measurements of ventricular contractility using one or more of the following imaging technologies: M-mode US, pulsed-Doppler US, 2D speckle-tracking US, and 4D US (Figs. 6.7–6.9).[46–51] If the LV is imaged in the short-axis plane, perpendicular to the four-chamber view, circumferential and radial contractility can also be computed using speckle-tracking software.[52] For this review, circumferential and radial contractility obtained from the short axis of the LV will not be further addressed because of the paucity of literature describing this technique in the fetus.[52]

ASSESSMENT OF VENTRICULAR FUNCTION

Ejection Fraction

Evaluation of global systolic function of the RV and LV can be measured directly or inferred by sampling specific images of the ventricles obtained from 2D and 4D acquisitions. Irrespective of the imaging technique, the end-diastolic volume (EDV) and end-systolic volume (ESV) are required to compute the ejection fraction (EF) as follows:

$$\text{Ejection Fraction} = ([\text{end-diastolic volume-end-systolic volume}]/\text{end-diastolic volume}).$$

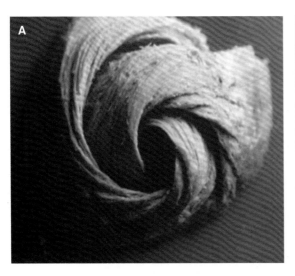

Apex of the Heart

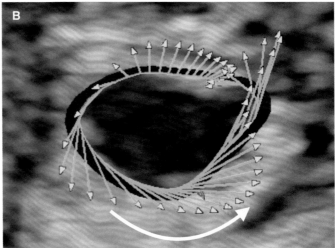

Early Systole of the Apex of the Left Ventricle

FIGURE 6.5: Apical view of the heart muscle. **A:** This illustrates clockwise and counterclockwise spiral formation. (Reprinted from Buckberg GD. Basic science review: The helix and the heart. *J Thorac Cardiovasc Surg.* 2002;124(5):863-883. Copyright © 2002 American Association for Thoracic Surgery. With permission.) **B:** This illustrates the movement of the individual vectors of the apical myocardium in a counterclockwise rotation of the LV during systole.

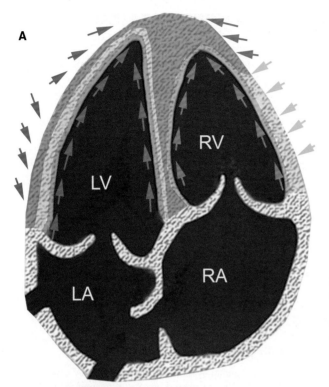

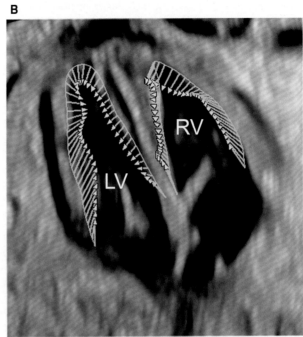

Longitudinal   Helical   Circumferential

FIGURE 6.6: Four-chamber view of myocardial muscle orientation in the fetal heart. **A:** Diagram illustrating the location of the longitudinal, obliquely oriented helical, and circumferential fibers. The circumferential fibers are present along the right and left ventricular free walls as well as the left side of the interventricular septum. **B:** Vector analysis of illustrating the direction and velocity of myocardial segments during systole. The right lateral wall demonstrates longitudinal movement along two-thirds of the wall, with oblique movement of the apical portion of the wall. The left ventricle demonstrates longitudinal movement of the upper one-third of the lateral wall, with circumferential movement of the lateral mid and apical sections of the wall. The septal wall demonstrates movement resulting from circumferential and oblique-helical fibers during systole. *LA*, left atrium; *LV*, left ventricle; *RA*, right atrium; *RV*, right ventricle.

Measurements of RV and LV Volumes Using 4D Ultrasound

Using 4D Spatial Temporal Image Correlation (STIC), and Virtual Organ Computer-aided Analysis (VOCAL), Messing et al., in 2007, obtained 4D volumes of the four-chamber view of the fetal heart and measured EDV and ESV of the RV and LV and computed the EF (Fig. 6.9).[53] They used gestational age (GA) and the EFW as the independent variables and found a low correlation with these independent variables for both the RV and LV EF (R^2 0.050). They reported good intraobserver and interobserver agreement.[53] In 2009, Hamill et al. reaffirmed that measurement of ventricular volumes using VOCAL technology demonstrated an excellent reliability and reproducibility for both intraobserver and interobserver measurements.[54] In 2011, Hamill et al. reported results using 4D VOCAL technology in fetuses between 19 and 40 weeks of gestation and used the HC and AC as well as the FL as their independent variables and found a low correlation coefficient for both the RV and LV.[55] Hamill et al., using VOCAL technology, also found a significant difference between the LV EF (72.2%) and the RV EF (62.4%).[55] Simioni et al. used VOCAL technology and compared LV EF and RV EF between male and female fetuses (LV male = 72.84% vs. LV female = 70.73%; RV male 67.22% vs. RV female 64.76) and demonstrated no significant difference between the sexes.[56]

Measurement of LV Volumes Using 2D Images

The LV is an ellipsoid-shaped structure (Fig. 6.10A). The EDV and ESV have been computed using 2D images from either the four-chamber view or the four-chamber view plus the two-chamber view.[57] A recent study by our group reported measuring the EDV and ESV for the LV using Simpson's rule derived from 24 segments using speckle-tracking analysis of the four-chamber view (Fig. 6.10B).[57] The results identified higher LV values from 20 to 24 weeks of gestation, after which the values were similar from 24 to 40 weeks of gestation (Fig. 6.10C). Data from our group using Simpson's rule demonstrated a narrower distribution band for the 5th and 95th centiles when compared to data from Messing et al. and Hamill et al. using the VOCAL technique (Fig. 6.10D).[57] Schoonderwaldt et al. compared the Simpson's rule method and the VOCAL methodology for evaluating the LV EF and found no significant difference between the two technologies.[58]

Fractional Area Change

Because the shape of the RV chamber is triangular in the coronal plane and crescent shaped in the transverse plane, Simpson's rule cannot be accurately applied to evaluate global contractility of this chamber. Therefore, a surrogate for assessment for global

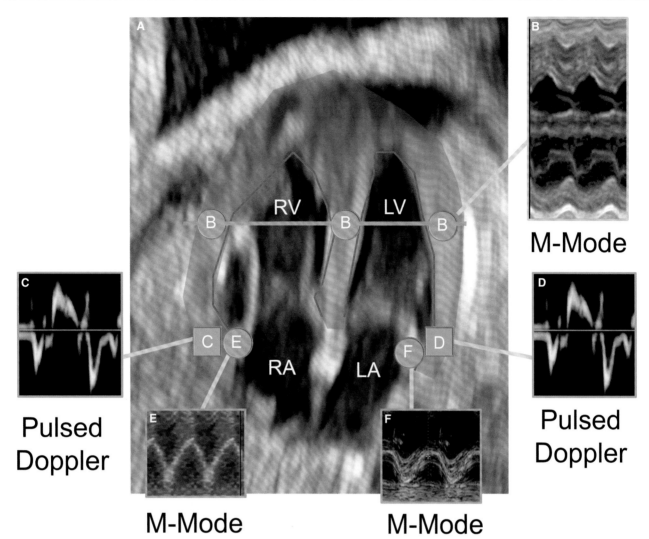

FIGURE 6.7: M-mode and pulsed-Doppler measurements of longitudinal and transverse contractility. **(A)** is the four-chamber view with the apex at 12 o'clock. **B:** Demonstrates the plane of acquisition for the M-mode to measure transverse contractility of the right and left ventricles. **(C and D)** represent placement of the pulsed-Doppler sample volume at the base of the RV and LV walls to record tissue Doppler displacement for computation of longitudinal contractility. **(E and F)** indicate the placement of the M-mode cursor to record annular plane systolic excursion of the tricuspid (TAPSE) and mitral (MAPSE) annulus used to evaluate longitudinal contractility. *LA*, left atrium; *LV*, left ventricle; *RA*, right atrium; *RV*, right ventricle.

contractility, fractional area change (FAC), has been used.[59–65] The equation for computing FAC is as follows:

Fractional area change = ([End-diastolic area − End-systolic area]/End-diastolic area).

The FAC has been used in postnatal evaluation of RV systolic function because it has been shown that it identifies cardiac dysfunction in neonates, pediatric, and adult patients, and is correlated with RV EF computed from MRI.[59,62–65] In a recent study, our group evaluated FAC for the RV and LV and noted that there was a significant correlation with fetal biometric (BPD, HC, AC, FL, EFW) and age variables (Fig. 6.11).[60] The LV FAC was greater than was the RV FAC (Fig. 6.11).[60] The results were validated in fetuses with congenital heart defects.[60] Two prior studies examined FAC, using only the GA as the independent

variable.[61,66] Neither study reported values from 20 to 40 weeks of gestation nor provided additional independent variables for analysis.[61,66] The study reported by Goldinfeld et al. was the only one that provided 5% and 95% intervals for both ventricles between 14 and 29 weeks of gestation, which had lower 5th centile values from 20 to 28 weeks, when compared to the data reported by our group.[61]

Assessment of Transverse Ventricular Contractility

M-Mode Assessment of Transverse Ventricular Contractility

Historically, the first attempts to evaluate transverse contractility involved placing an M-mode cursor perpendicular to the mid IVS and computing the transverse fractional shortening (TFS).[67–72] We have previously demonstrated that the endocardial wall motion of the RV and LV does not move perpendicular to the center of each chamber during systole, but it is

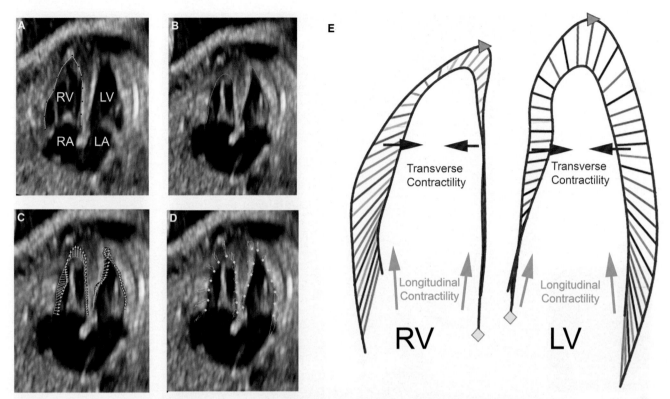

FIGURE 6.8: 2D speckle-tracking analysis used to evaluate global, longitudinal, and transverse contractility. **A:** Demonstrates the automated identification of the endocardial border of the LV. A similar tracing is done for the RV. **B:** The *green lines* indicate the tracking endocardial borders of the RV and LV. **C:** This demonstrates the direction and velocity of the 24 endocardial segments for the RV and LV. **D:** This demonstrates displacement of the 24 endocardial segments during one cardiac cycle, as represented by the *yellow dot* on the *green line*. **E:** Demonstrates the computed displacement of 24 segments along the lateral and septal walls of the RV and LV. The *blue line* represents the position of the endocardium at end diastole and the *red line* the position of the endocardium at end systole. The movement of each of the 24 segments along the lateral and septal walls of the RV and LV is displayed by the colored lines. Global, longitudinal, and transverse contractility can be derived from the 24-segment analysis as well as evaluation of the area of the chamber and the length of the endocardium in diastole and systole.[46–51] *LA*, left atrium; *LV*, left ventricle; *RA*, right atrium; *RV*, right ventricle.

displaced tangentially, having both longitudinal and transverse components (Fig. 6.12A, B).[50,73] Therefore, when the M-mode is used to record TFS, the endocardial segment measured at end diastole is not the same endocardial segment measured at end systole (Fig. 6.12A, B). Previous studies have reported varying results for TFS that range between 26% and 48% for the LV and 21% and 41% for the RV (Fig. 6.12C).[67,68,74–79] The reasons for the variation in fractional shortening between the studies could be explained by the following: (1) tangential displacement of the ventricular walls and septum during systole, (2) not recording the M-mode from the center of the ventricular chambers, (3) placement of the M-mode cursor at different locations distal to the insertion of the atrioventricular valves, and (4) increased fractional shortening of the LV mid and apical portions of the chamber compared to the RV.[50,73] In addition, Simpson and Cook reported the repeatability of M-mode measurements and calculated poor results with limits of agreement between −28% and 32%.[80]

2D 24-Segment Speckle-Tracking Assessment of Transverse Ventricular Contractility

Because M-mode assessment of transverse contractility only focused on the mid chamber, our group examined the TFS of 24

segments distributed from the base to the apex of each ventricle (Fig. 6.13A, B) to obtain a more comprehensive analysis of ventricular contractility.[73] The TFS was computed from the end-diastolic and end-systolic measurements from each of the 24 segments. Because speckle-tracking analysis identifies the end-systolic position for each of the segments, accurate TFS can be computed for each segment (Fig. 6.13C).[73] The measurements were normally distributed for each of the 24 segments for both ventricles. There was not a significant difference in TFS between the RV and LV for segments 1 to 5, representing the base of the ventricles (Fig. 6.13D). However, the LV TFS was significantly increased for segments 6 to 24 when compared to the RV (Fig. 6.13D). This represented the lower base, mid, and apical sections of the chambers (Fig. 6.13C, D). Systolic movement of the lateral and septal wall segments were toward the center of the LV chamber (Fig. 6.13C, D). Systolic movement of the lateral wall of the RV was toward the center of the ventricular chamber (Fig. 6.13C, D). However, the RV septal wall did not move toward the center of the RV chamber (Fig. 6.13C, D). For the examiner who desires to measure TFS but does not have speckle-tracking software to compute the TFS for the 24 segments, end-diastolic and end-systolic measurements obtained from the 2D image at the base (segment 1) and mid portion of the ventricle (segment 12) can be used.[73]

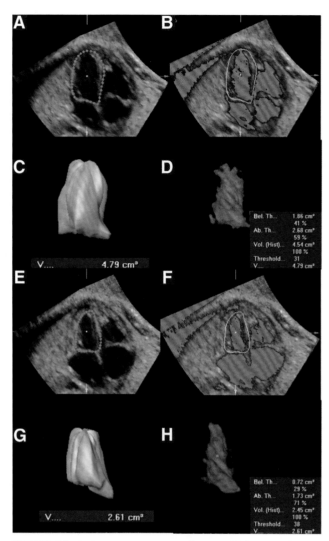

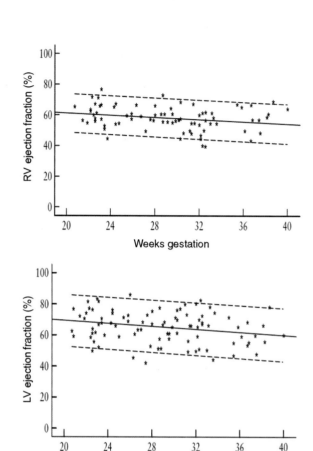

FIGURE 6.9: **A:** Postprocessing quantification of left ventricular volume in end diastole **(A–D)** and end systole **(E–H)**. **(A and E)** The trace in the A-frame at the level of the four-chamber view; **(B and F)** the same frame with the inversion mode activated; **(C and G)** the three-dimensional models created by the Virtual Organ Computer-aided Analysis Tool, which include the entire traced volume; and **(D and H)** the final intraventricular volume models. **B:** Demonstrates the 5th and 95th centiles for the ejection fraction versus weeks of gestation. (From Messing B, Cohen SM, Valsky DV, et al. Fetal cardiac ventricle volumetry in the second half of gestation assessed by 4D ultrasound using STIC combined with inversion mode. *Ultrasound Obstet Gynecol.* 2007;30(2):142–151. Copyright © 2007 ISUOG. Reprinted by permission of John Wiley & Sons, Inc.)

Assessment of Longitudinal Contractility

Assessment of longitudinal movement of the annular base, located at the insertion of the tricuspid and mitral valve leaflets on the lateral walls and septum (Fig. 6.7), toward the apex of each ventricle uses the following imaging modalities: (1) M-mode, (2) tissue Doppler, and (3) speckle-tracking analysis.

M-Mode Ultrasound

Placing the M-mode cursor perpendicular to the atrioventricular valve insertion into the lateral and septal walls identifies movement of the annulus toward the apex of the ventricle during systole (Figs. 6.7 and 6.14). This form of systolic analysis has been termed tricuspid annular plane systolic excursion (TAPSE), and mitral annular plane systolic excursion (MAPSE). Before current technology, the annular movement could only be measured with a conventional M-mode if the apex was at 12 or 6 o'clock (Fig. 6.14A). However, with digital imaging systems, an annular, steerable, M-mode cursor can be placed anywhere on the 2D image to reconstruct the M-mode tracing (Fig. 6.14B).[81,82] In addition, using STIC technology, an M-mode can be computed in a similar manner by placing the M-mode line through the structures of interest (Fig. 6.14C).[79,82] Therefore, with current technology, an M-mode recording of the annuli of the RV and LV lateral walls and septum can be obtained, irrespective of the orientation of the four-chamber view to the US beam. Nomograms for TAPSE and MAPSE have been developed on the basis of the technology used to acquire the M-mode tracing using GA, EFW, and the heart area (Tables 6.1–6.3).[82] Investigators have recently normalized the TAPSE and MAPSE measurements by computing a ratio using the end-diastolic ventricular length, measured from the base to the apex of the chamber (TAPSE/length; MAPSE/length).[83]

2D Speckle Tracking of the RV and LV Lateral and Septal Walls

Our group recently reported measuring the end-diastolic and end-systolic position of the insertion of the atrioventricular valves

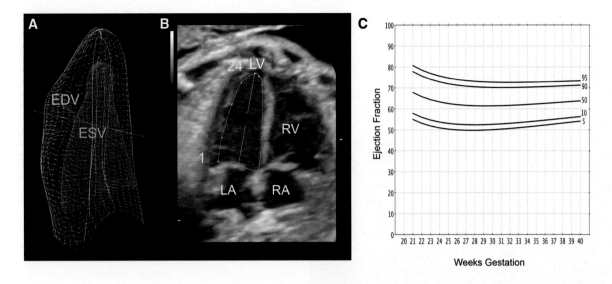

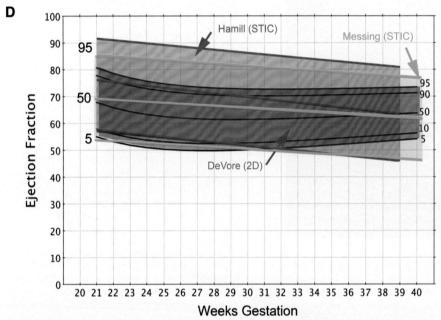

FIGURE 6.10: Computing left ventricular volume using single plane Simpson's rule. **A:** Volume rendering of the end-diastolic volume (EDV) and end-systolic volume (ESV) of the left ventricle. **B:** The EDV and ESV were computed from the speckle-tracking software using Simpson's method of disk analysis. The following illustrates the computation of the left ventricular EDV as follows: (1) end diastole is identified from the 2D image from the four-chamber view. The LV end-diastolic length (EDL) is measured from the base to the apex (*red line*). The EDL is divided into 24 transverse segments that are equidistant from the base to the apex of the ventricle (*yellow lines*). (2) The transverse width (equal to the diameter) of each of the 24 segments (*yellow lines*), perpendicular to the EDL, is measured. (3) The radius is computed by dividing the length by 2. (4) The area for each of the 24 segments is computed using the following equation: ([Length/2] * [Length/2] * 3.14159). (5) The disk volume for each of the 24 segments is computed by multiplying each of the 24 segment lengths by each of the 24 segment areas. (6) The EDV is the sum of each of the 24 transverse disk areas (e.g., 936.53 mm³). (7) The 936.53 mm³ is converted to mL by dividing the value by 1,000 = 0.936.53 mL. (8) At end systole, the same approach. (9) The ejection fraction is computed as follows: (EDV − ESV)/EDV.[57] **C:** Ejection fraction 5% and 95% confidence intervals versus gestational age. (From DeVore GR, Klas B, Satou G, et al. Evaluation of Left Ventricular Size and Function Using Speckle Tracking and Simpson's Rule. *J Ultrasound Med*. 2019;38(5):1209–1221. Copyright © 2018 by the American Institute of Ultrasound in Medicine. Reprinted by permission of John Wiley & Sons, Inc.) **D:** Comparison of the 5th and 95th centiles for the ejection fraction between the study by DeVore et al. and Messing et al. and Hamill et al.[53,55,57] *LA*, left atrium; *LV*, left ventricle; *RA*, right atrium; *RV*, right ventricle.

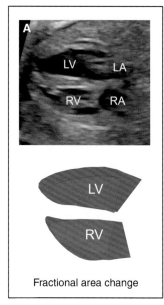

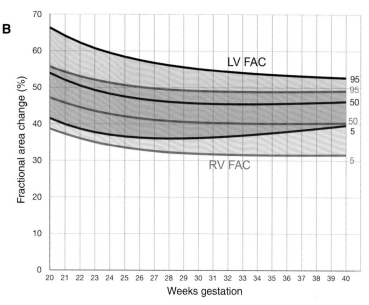

FIGURE 6.11: Right and left ventricular fractional area change (FAC) versus gestational age. **A:** Illustrates the 2D image of the four-chamber view and the corresponding graphic illustrating end-diastolic and end-systolic areas computed from specking tracking analysis.[60] **B:** Centile curves for the LV and RV FAC as a function of gestational age. *LA*, left atrium; *LV*, left ventricle; *RA*, right atrium; *RV*, right ventricle. (From DeVore GR, Klas B, Satou G, et al. Quantitative evaluation of the fetal right and left ventricular fractional area change using speckle tracking technology. *Ultrasound Obstet Gynecol.* 2019;53(2):219–228. Copyright © 2018 ISUOG. Reprinted by permission of John Wiley & Sons, Inc.)

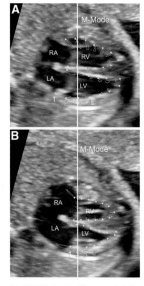

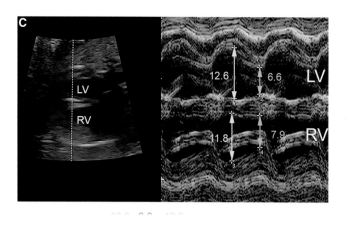

FIGURE 6.12: Tangential displacement of the endocardial wall during ventricular systole. **A:** The end-diastolic frame demonstrates the location of the segments of the left lateral wall and septum (*yellow dots*) and the path that each segment moves throughout the cardiac cycle (*green lines*). The numbers 1 to 4 identify adjacent yellow circles at end diastole. The *white line* represents placement of the M-mode cursor. **B:** The end-systolic frame demonstrates that the *yellow circles* 1 to 4 have moved toward the apex, away from the M-mode cursor line. Number w has replaced number 3, which was previously under the M-mode line. This demonstrates that the portion of the ventricular wall that would be recorded at end diastole during an M-mode examination is not the same portion of the wall that is recorded at end systole. **C:** M-mode evaluation of ventricular function. The M-mode is recorded from the midventricular chambers, perpendicular to the interventricular septum. End-diastolic (*yellow*) and end-systolic (*green*) measurements are made to compute fractional shortening. *LA*, left atrium; *LV*, left ventricle; *RA*, right atrium; *RV*, right ventricle.

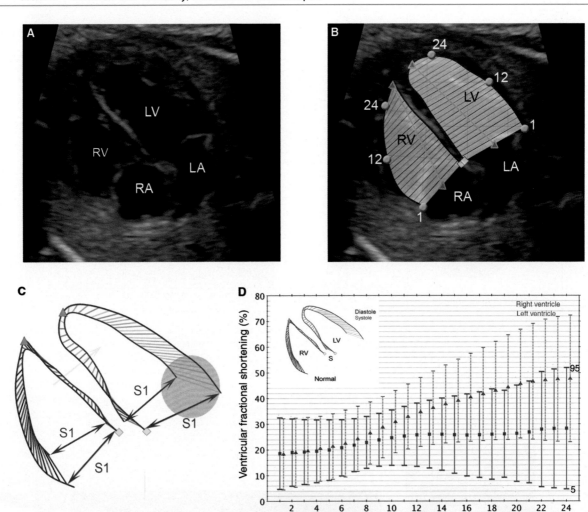

FIGURE 6.13: Measurement of 24 transverse segments to compute the fractional shortening (FS). **A:** Illustrates the four-chamber view from which the images in **B**, **C**, and **D** were derived. **(B)** is an overlay illustrating the location of the 24 segments for each ventricle, with 1 originating at the base and 24 at the apex. **C:** Illustrates the direction for each of the 24 segments that moved from their end-diastolic to the end-systolic position. The value of the end-systolic length (S1, *red line*) was subtracted from the value of the end-diastolic length (S1 *blue line*) to compute the fractional shortening value (ED − ES/ED × 100). **D:** FS for 24 segments of the right and left ventricles. The *blue squares and lines* represent the mean, 5th and 95th centiles for the right ventricle. The *red triangles and lines* represent the mean, 5th and 95th centiles for the left ventricle. The graphic of the four-chamber view demonstrates inward movement toward the center of each chamber for the lateral walls. However, movement of the interventricular septum inward, toward the center of the chamber, occurs only in the left ventricle resulting in a significantly increased FS for segments 6 to 24. *LV*, left ventricle; *RV*, right ventricle; *S*, septum. (From DeVore GR, Klas B, Satou G, et al. Twenty-four Segment Transverse Ventricular Fractional Shortening: a new technique to evaluate fetal cardiac function. *J Ultrasound Med.* 2018;37(5):1129–1141. Copyright © 2017 by the American Institute of Ultrasound in Medicine. Reprinted by permission of John Wiley & Sons, Inc.)

into the lateral and septal walls of the RV and LV to compute the annular plane systolic excursion (APSE) using speckle-tracking analysis (Fig. 6.15A–C).[84] In this study, the APSE was correlated with biometric and age variables, with R^2 values ranging between 0.39 and 0.41 for the RV lateral wall, 0.22 to 0.40 for the RV septal wall, and 0.29 to 0.30 for the LV lateral wall. However, the left septal wall had low R^2 values (0.05 to 0.07). Our study also compared the RV and LV lateral wall APSE with the corresponding septal wall APSE and found the lateral wall was significantly higher ($P < 0.001$) (Fig. 6.15D, E). We also found that the RV lateral and septal wall APSE values were greater than their LV counterparts (Fig. 6.15F, G). In addition, we compared our results with M-mode measurements of the lateral wall tricuspid and mitral APSE from previous studies and found the results were within 1.65 (95th centile) to −1.65 (5th centile) for

the M-mode studies for the RV and LV, except that weeks 34 to 40 for the RV were higher in the study by Messing et al. when compared to our data.[81,82,85]

Tissue Doppler Imaging

Traditionally, pulsed Doppler has been used by the obstetrical community to evaluate blood flow velocity in the umbilical artery (UA) and MCA as well as in the ductus venosus and other fetal vessels.[33,86–92] However, another application of pulsed-Doppler US is insonation of the ventricular walls of the heart to measure wall velocity that occurs during the cardiac cycle.[1] Two approaches have been used in the fetus. The first measures the peak velocity of the ventricular walls from the real-time color Doppler image of the wall movement, with frame rates varying between 20 and 40 frames/s (Fig. 6.16A).[93] The second approach measures wall

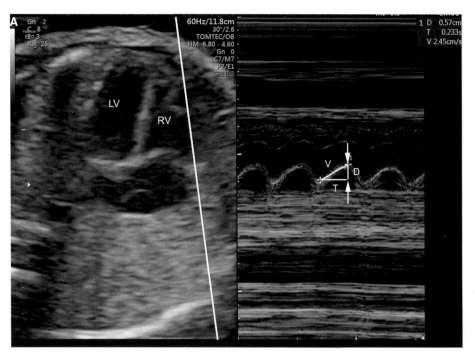

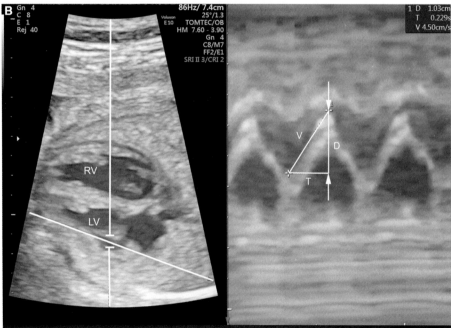

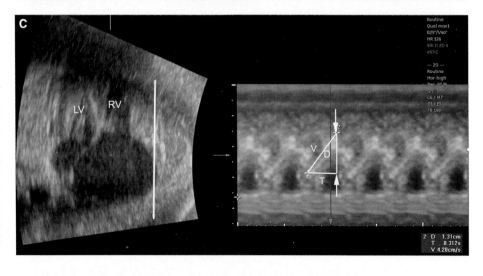

FIGURE 6.14: M-mode recording of annular plane systolic excursion. **A:** M-mode placed through the lateral wall annulus of the RV. **B:** Steered M-mode through the lateral wall annulus of the RV. **C:** STIC M-mode placed through the lateral wall annulus of the RV. The measurement of the annular plane systolic excursion is computed using the "slope" tool that provides the distance (*D*), which is equal to the excursion in centimeters, the slope (cm/s) (*S*) and the time (seconds) (*T*). *LV*, left ventricle; *RV*, right ventricle.

TABLE 6.1   Measurements of TAPSE Using STIC M-Mode

GESTATIONAL WEEK	MESSING ET AL. (n = 241)[82]			TEDESCO ET AL. (n = 300)[79]		
	MEAN (mm)	5TH CENTILE (mm)	95TH CENTILE (mm)	MEAN (mm)	5TH CENTILE (mm)	95TH CENTILE (mm)
20	—	—	5.5	5.3	3.7	6.8
21	3.6	1.4	6.1	5.5	3.9	7.1
22	4.4	2.1	6.3	5.8	4.2	7.5
23	4.4	2.2	6.5	6.1	4.4	7.8
24	4.6	2.5	6.8	6.4	4.6	8.2
25	5.3	2.8	7.1	6.7	4.8	8.5
26	5.4	3.1	7.4	6.9	5	8.9
27	5.6	3.4	7.6	7.2	5.2	9.2
28	5.6	3.6	7.9	7.5	5.4	9.6
29	6.3	3.9	8.2	7.8	5.6	9.9
30	5.8	4.1	8.5	8.1	5.8	10.3
31	6.3	4.5	8.7	8.3	6	10.6
32	6.8	4.7	9.0	8.6	6.3	11
33	6.5	5.0	9.3	8.9	6.5	11.3
34	7.0	5.2	9.5	—	—	—
35	7.7	5.5	9.8	—	—	—
36	7.8	5.8	10.1	—	—	—
37	8.1	6.0	10.4	—	—	—
38	8.7	6.4	10.6	—	—	—
39	8.6	6.6	5.5	—	—	—

Modified from Tedesco GD, de Souza Bezerra M, Barros FSB, et al. Fetal heart function by tricuspid annular plane systolic excursion and ventricular shortening fraction using STIC M-Mode: reference ranges and validation. *Am J Perinatol.* 2017;34(13):1354–1361; Messing B, Gilboa Y, Lipschuetz M, et al. Fetal tricuspid annular plane systolic excursion (f-TAPSE): evaluation of fetal right heart systolic function with conventional M-mode ultrasound and spatiotemporal image correlation (STIC) M-mode. *Ultrasound Obstet Gynecol.* 2013;42(2):182–188.

TABLE 6.2   TAPSE and MAPSE Using Angular M-Mode

GESTATIONAL WEEK	TAPSE			MAPSE		
	MEAN (mm)	5TH CENTILE (mm)	95TH CENTILE (mm)	MEAN (mm)	5TH CENTILE (mm)	95TH CENTILE (mm)
22	4.9	4	5.8	3.9	3.4	4.5
23	5.1	4.2	6	4.1	3.5	4.6
24	5.3	4.4	6.2	4.2	3.7	4.8
25	5.5	4.6	6.5	4.4	3.8	4.9
26	5.7	4.8	6.7	4.5	3.9	5
27	6	5	7	4.6	4.1	5.2
28	6.2	5.1	7.2	4.8	4.2	5.3
29	6.4	5.3	7.4	4.9	4.4	5.5
30	6.6	5.5	7.7	5.1	4.5	5.6

TABLE 6.2 **TAPSE and MAPSE Using Angular M-Mode** (*continued*)

GESTATIONAL WEEK	TAPSE			MAPSE		
	MEAN (mm)	5TH CENTILE (mm)	95TH CENTILE (mm)	MEAN (mm)	5TH CENTILE (mm)	95TH CENTILE (mm)
31	6.8	5.7	7.9	5.2	4.6	5.7
32	7	5.9	8.1	5.3	4.8	5.9
33	7.2	6.1	8.4	5.5	4.9	6
34	7.5	6.3	8.6	5.6	5.1	6.2
35	7.7	6.5	8.9	5.8	5.2	6.3
36	7.9	6.7	9.1	5.9	5.3	6.4
37	8.1	6.9	9.3	6	5.6	6.6
38	8.3	7.1	9.6	6.2	5.6	6.7
39	8.5	7.2	9.8	6.3	5.8	6.9
40	8.7	7.4	10	6.5	5.9	7

From Mao YK, Zhao BW, Wang B. Z-Score reference ranges for angular M-mode displacement at 22-40 weeks' gestation. *Fetal Diagn Ther.* 2017;41(2):115–126.

TABLE 6.3 **TAPSE and MAPSE Using Conventional M-Mode**

GESTATIONAL WEEK	TAPSE			MAPSE		
	MEAN (mm)	5TH CENTILE (mm)	95TH CENTILE (mm)	MEAN (mm)	5TH CENTILE (mm)	95TH CENTILE (mm)
22	4.5	3.5	5.5	3.7	3.1	4.3
23	4.7	3.7	5.8	3.8	3.2	4.5
24	4.9	3.9	6.0	4.0	3.3	4.6
25	5.2	4.1	6.2	4.1	3.5	4.7
26	5.4	4.3	6.4	4.2	3.6	4.9
27	5.6	4.6	6.6	4.4	3.8	5.0
28	5.8	4.8	6.8	4.5	3.9	5.2
29	6.0	5.0	7.1	4.7	4.0	5.3
30	6.2	5.2	7.3	4.8	4.2	5.4
31	6.5	5.4	7.5	4.9	4.3	5.6
32	6.7	5.7	7.7	5.1	4.5	5.7
33	6.9	5.9	7.9	5.2	4.6	5.9
34	7.1	6.1	8.1	5.4	4.7	6.0
35	7.3	6.3	8.4	5.5	4.9	6.1
36	7.6	6.5	8.6	5.6	5.0	6.3
37	7.8	6.7	8.8	5.8	5.2	6.4
38	8.0	7.0	9.0	5.9	5.3	6.6
39	8.2	7.2	9.2	6.1	5.4	6.7
40	8.4	7.4	9.5	6.2	5.6	6.8

From Mao YK, Zhao BW, Wang B. Z-Score reference ranges for angular M-mode displacement at 22-40 weeks' gestation. *Fetal Diagn Ther.* 2017;41(2):115–126.

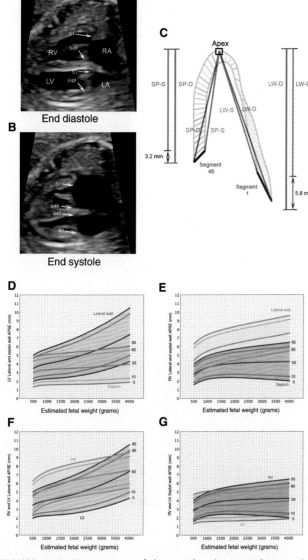

FIGURE 6.15: Measurement of the annular plane systolic excursion for the basal segment of the lateral ventricular wall (segment 1) and the septal segment (48). **A:** Illustrates the end-diastolic four-chamber view. The *arrows* indicate segment 1 (S1) and segment 48 (S48). **B:** Illustrates the end-systolic points for S1 and S48. **C:** Illustrates the computation of the segment lengths. This is done by subtracting SPS-S from SP-D for the septal segment (48) and LW-S from LW-D for the lateral wall segment (1). The *blue lines* represent end-diastolic lengths and the *red lines* the end-systolic lengths. **D:** Compares the left lateral and septal segments. **E:** Compares the right lateral and septal segments. **F:** Illustrates the right and left lateral segments. **G:** Compares the right and left septal segments. The graphs illustrate the 95th, 90th, 50th, 10th, and 5th centiles. *APSE,* annular plane systolic excursion; *LA,* left atrium; *LV,* left ventricle; *RA,* right atrium; *RV,* right ventricle. (From DeVore GR, Klas B, Satou G, et al. Speckle tracking of the basal lateral and septal wall annular plane systolic excursion of the right and left ventricles of the fetal heart. *J Ultrasound Med.* 2019;38(5):1309–1318. Copyright © 2018 by the American Institute of Ultrasound in Medicine. Reprinted by permission of John Wiley & Sons, Inc.)

motion using pulsed-Doppler US, which provides precise measurements of diastolic and systolic velocities of wall movement (Fig. 6.16B–D).[94–96] In 2011, Comas et al. performed a comprehensive study in which they published regression equations, the mean, 5th and 95th centiles, and provided a Z-score calculator for

each of the measurements for the annular basal velocities for the LV, RV, and interventricular septal walls.[96] Figure 6.16E to J illustrates the graphs for the peak systolic velocity (S′) for the LV, RV, and IVS, obtained at the base of the ventricles, using weeks gestation and the EFW as the independent variables.[96] These measurements reflect longitudinal contractility for the base of the heart.

Speckle-Tracking Global and Segmental Strain

The concept of cardiac "strain" can be confusing. However, from a practical perspective, it represents the shortening of the endocardium, myocardium, or epicardium during systole that can be measured with speckle-tracking software. Using the endocardium as an example, the formula for ventricular strain is as follows:

$$\text{Strain} = ([\text{end-systolic length of the endocardium} - \\ \text{end-diastolic length of the endocardium}]/\text{end-} \\ \text{diastolic length of the endocardium}).$$

When computing the FAC or TFS, the systolic measurement is subtracted from the diastolic measurement in the numerator of the equation, resulting in a positive value. However, when measuring strain, many investigators have subtracted the diastolic measurement from the systolic measurement in the numerator of the equation, resulting in a negative number. Therefore, the more negative the strain value (e.g., −40% vs. −25%), the greater the longitudinal contractility. Strain can be measured globally, which includes the entirety of the endocardial length of the chambers, (Fig. 6.17A, B), as well as examining the lateral and septal walls of the chambers (Fig. 6.17C–F). In addition, segmental evaluation, which includes the base, mid, and apical regions of the ventricles can be measured.[50] The strain values for the global, lateral wall, and septal wall measurements from our studies were not correlated with biometric or age variables of the fetus and there were no significant differences between the RV and LV strain values. Tables 6.4 and 6.5 list previous studies in which the global strain has been reported for the LV and RV that include the year of the study, the number of control fetuses examined, the GA range, the software program used to compute global strain, the mean and standard deviation, and the delta Z-score when compared to a recent study from our group.[48,97–108] For the LV, three studies fell within 1 standard deviation, six studies were between 1 and 2 standard deviations, and four studies were 2 or more standard deviations from our mean. Except for the study by Enzenberger, the studies that had values within 1 standard deviation of our data had a higher number of control fetuses (>78). Studies that involved the global strain of the RV demonstrated 5 that had delta Z-score values within 1 standard deviation, 5 with values between 1 and 2 standard deviations, and 1 study greater than 2 standard deviations from our mean. Therefore, our preference is to measure global (LV = −22.93 [3.52]; RV = −22.7 [4.07]) lateral wall (LV = −24.17 [5.2]; RV = −25.82 [4.91]) and septal wall strain (LV = −23.71 [3.5]; RV = −18.89 [6.4]) (Fig. 6.17).

Longitudinal Annular Systolic Displacement Fractional Shortening Using 2D or Speckle-Tracking Software

This technique measures the longitudinal annular systolic displacement fractional shortening (LASD FX) of the mid-length of the ventricular chambers using either measurements obtained by hand or using speckle-tracking software (Fig. 6.18A–C).[48] In a recent study from our group, we reported that the LASD

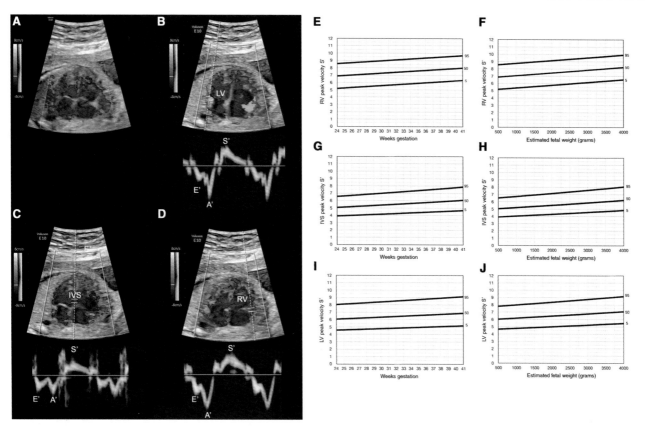

FIGURE 6.16: Tissue Doppler recordings. Recording from the color Doppler image **(A)**, recording from the base of the left lateral wall **(B)**, recording from the base of the interventricular septum **(C)**, and a recording from the base of the right lateral wall **(D)**. **(E–J)** are the mean and 5%, 95% confidence intervals for the S′ for the right ventricle. **(E and F)**, interventricular septum **(G and H)**, and the left ventricle **(I and J)** from Comas et al.[96] for the gestational age and estimated fetal weight.[96]

FX was independent of fetal biometric measurements and GA. The RV LASD FX was 22.94% (±4.73%) and the LV 21.05% (±04.07%). The RV LASD FX was significantly greater than was the LV LASD FX ($P = <0.024$). The LASD FX demonstrated a high correlation with global strain for the RV (0.95) and LV (0.97) (Fig. 6.18E, F). Because the LASD FX is the easiest of the measurements to obtain without any special software or imaging tools, other than a 2D image of the four-chamber view, it is an ideal tool to evaluate longitudinal contractility because it can be used as a surrogate for global longitudinal strain and is not dependent on the orientation of the four-chamber view to the transducer beam. To obtain this measurement, the examiner does the following (Fig. 6.18A, B):

1. Identify the end-diastolic four-chamber view.
2. Draw a line at the base of each ventricular chamber between the annular insertion of the tricuspid and mitral valve leaflets on the septal and lateral walls of each chamber.
3. Draw a line that measures the length from the apex to the middle of the perpendicular line drawn at the base.
4. Repeat steps 1 to 3 for the end-systolic four-chamber view.
5. Compute the LASD FX as follows:

LASD FX = ([end-diastolic longitudinal length/end-systolic longitudinal length]/end-diastolic longitudinal length) × 100

Myocardial Performance Index

In 1995, Tei et al. reported a novel technique for evaluating myocardial function called the myocardial performance index (MPI).[109,110] Because systolic and diastolic dysfunction frequently coexist, it was hypothesized that a combined measure of LV chamber performance could be more reflective of overall cardiac dysfunction than are systolic or diastolic measurements alone. They measured three parameters from the Doppler velocity waveform (Fig. 6.19A, B):

1. Isovolumetric contraction time (ICT). This is the period of time between closure of the atrioventricular valves and the opening of the semilunar valves. During this time, the increased pressure resulting from myocardial contraction opens the aortic and pulmonary valves.
2. Ejection time (ET). This is the time that the aortic valves are open. The ET may be decreased when cardiac dysfunction is present.
3. Isovolumetric relaxation time (IRT). This is the time after all the blood has been ejected from the ventricles following closure of the semilunar valves until the atrioventricular valves open. During this time, the pressure is reduced, and the reuptake of calcium occurs.[111] Reduction in calcium uptake is a manifestation of deterioration of cardiac function. The IRT is the main component that alters the MPI in fetal pathological states. When the IRT is increased, the ET is often decreased.

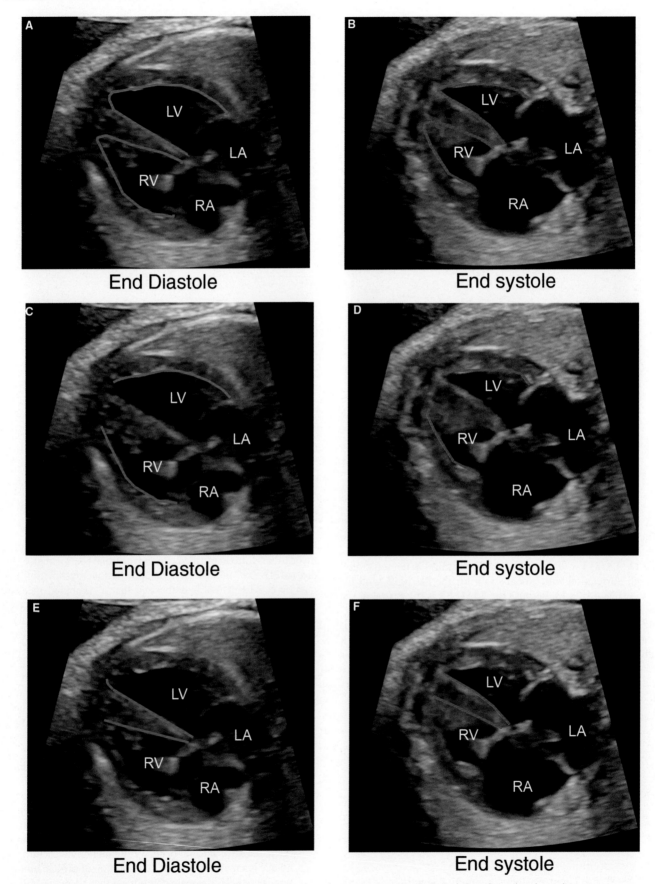

FIGURE 6.17: This illustrates measurements of the endocardium used to compute strain. **A, B:** End-diastolic and end-systolic measurements used to compute global longitudinal strain. **C, D:** End-diastolic and end-systolic measurements used to compute lateral wall strain. **E, F:** End-diastolic and end-systolic measurements used to compute septal wall strain.

TABLE 6.4 **Global Strain of the Left Ventricle from Published Studies**

AUTHOR	YEAR	NO. STUDIED	GESTATIONAL AGE	ANALYSIS PROGRAM[a]	STUDY MEAN	STUDY SD	DELTA Z-SCORE[b]
Di Salvo et al.[100]	2008	100	20–32	GE	−25	4	**−0.59**[b]
Kapusta et al.[104]	2012	78	20–24	GE	−24.89	4.57	**−0.64**[b]
Matsui et al.[105]	2011	93	14–39	Siemens	−21.6	NR	**0.38**[b]
Fan et al.[102]	2014	40	33	Siemens	−18.36	1.11	1.3
Crispi et al.[99]	2014	37	32	GE	−18.2	4.4	1.34
Barker et al.[97]	2009	33	17–38	Siemens	−17.7	6.4	1.49
Enzensberger et al.[101]	2017	101	17–39	Toshiba	−17.54	NR	1.53
Zuo et al.[108]	2012	20	35–40	Siemens	−17.5	1.95	1.54
Brooks et al.[98]	2014	48	18–40	Siemens	−16.7	3.2	1.77
Kapusta	2013	44	30–34	GE	−24.68	4.81	2
Truong et al.[106]	2013	54	15–38	Siemens	−15.6	3.3	2.08
Van Mieghem et al.[107]	2010	59	16–36	GE	−15.1	5.2	2.2
Ishii et al.[103]	2012	81	19–42	Siemens	−15.2	2.7	2.2

NR indicates not reported.
[a] GE Healthcare (Milwaukee, WI); Siemens Medical Solutions (Mountain View, CA); and Toshiba Medical Systems Co. Ltd (Tokyo, Japan).
[b] Delta Z score is computed as (study mean − [−22.93]/3.52). **Delta Z-score values less than 1 and negative values** are not significantly different from the study by DeVore GR, Klas B, Satou G, et al. Longitudinal annular systolic displacement compared to global strain in normal fetal hearts and those with cardiac abnormalities. *J Ultrasound Med.* 2018;37(5):1159–1171.

TABLE 6.5 **Global Strain of the Right Ventricle from Published Studies**

AUTHOR	YEAR	NO. STUDIED	GESTATIONAL AGE	ANALYSIS PROGRAM[a]	STUDY MEAN	STUDY SD	DELTA Z-SCORE[b]
Kapusta et al.[104]	2012	78	20–24	GE	−25.35	NR	**−0.65**[b]
Di Salvo et al.[100]	2008	100	20–32	GE	−24	4	**−0.32**[b]
Kapusta[104]	2013	54	30–34	GE	−23.2	3.9	**−0.12**[b]
Matsui et al.[105]	2011	93	14–39	Siemens	−22.3	NR	**0.07**[b]
Zuo et al.[108]	2012	20	35–40	Siemens	−18.7	2.2	**0.98**[b]
Van Mieghem et al.[107]	2010	59	16–36	GE	−18.5	6.8	1.03
Crispi et al.[99]	2014	37	32	GE	−17.3	4.5	1.33
Truong et al.[106]	2013	54	15–38	Siemens	−16.5	NR	1.52
Enzensberger et al.[101]	2017	101	17–39	Toshiba	−16.47	NR	1.53
Ishii et al.[103]	2012	81	19–42	Siemens	−16	3.3	1.65
Barker et al.[97]	2009	33	17–38	Siemens	−17.4	6.4	4.53

NR indicates not reported.
[a] GE Healthcare (Milwaukee, WI); Siemens Medical Solutions (Mountain View, CA); and Toshiba Medical Systems Co. Ltd (Tokyo, Japan).
[b] Delta Z score is computed as (study mean − [−22.7]/4.07). **Delta Z score values less than 1 and negative values** are not significantly different from the study by DeVore GR, Klas B, Satou G, et al. Longitudinal annular systolic displacement compared to global strain in normal fetal hearts and those with cardiac abnormalities. *J Ultrasound Med.* 2018;37(5):1159–1171.

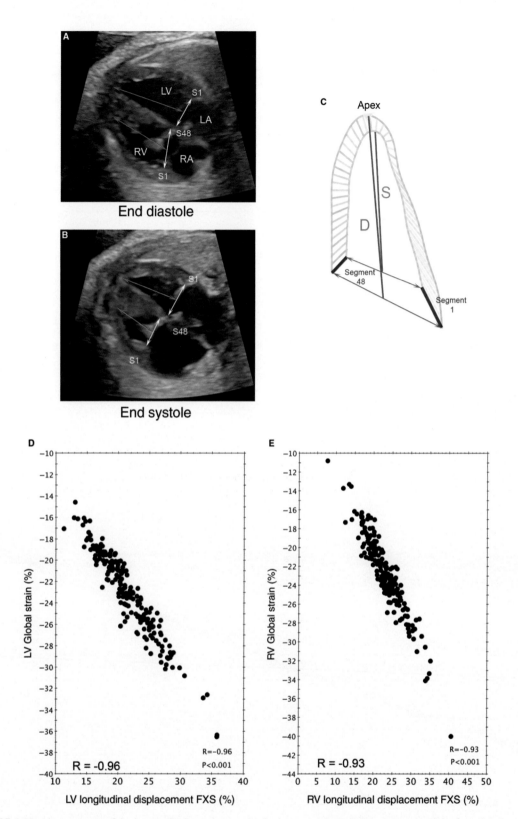

FIGURE 6.18: Measurement of the longitudinal annular systolic displacement. **A:** End-diastolic image of the four-chamber view. The *white lines* are drawn connecting the base of the lateral and septal wall annuli. The *blue lines* are drawn from the apex to the center of the *white lines*, representing the basal-apical measurement. **B:** End-systolic image of the four-chamber view. The *white lines* are drawn connecting the base of the lateral and septal wall annuli. The *red lines* are drawn from the apex to the center of the *white lines*, representing the basal-apical measurement. **C:** Illustrates the graphical representation of the measurements used to compute the longitudinal annular displacement fractional shortening ([End diastole – end systole]/[End diastole] × 100). *S1*, the basal lateral wall segment; *S48*, the basal interventricular basal segment. **D:** Illustrates correlation between LV global strain and LV longitudinal annular displacement fractional shortening. **E:** Illustrates correlation between RV global strain and RV longitudinal annular displacement fractional shortening. *D*, diastole; *LA*, left atrium; *LV*, left ventricle; *RA*, right atrium; *RV*, right ventricle; *S*, systole. (From DeVore GR, Klas B, Satou G, et al. Longitudinal annular systolic displacement compared to global strain in normal fetal hearts and those With cardiac abnormalities. *J Ultrasound Med*. 2018;37(5):1159–1171. Copyright © 2017 by the American Institute of Ultrasound in Medicine. Reprinted by permission of John Wiley & Sons, Inc.)

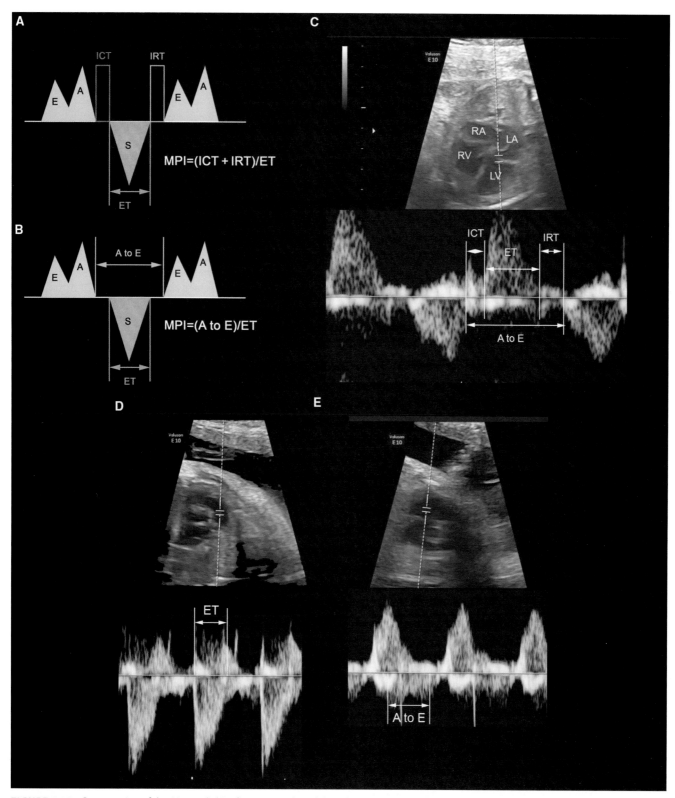

FIGURE 6.19: Computation of the Myocardial Performance Index of the left ventricle. **A:** Illustrates the equation using the isovolumetric contraction time (ICT) and the isovolumetric relaxation time (IRT). **B:** Illustrates using the *A* to *E* measurement. **C:** Illustrates the pulsed-Doppler recording of the LV inflow and outflow tracts to simultaneously record the mitral valve E and A waveforms and the aortic waveform. *A to E*, is the time from the end of the A wave to the beginning of the next E wave; *ET*, ejection time; *ICT*, isovolumetric contraction time; *IRT*, isovolumetric relaxation time. **D, E:** Illustrates the independent recordings of the right ventricular ejection time **(D)** and the right ventricular *A* to *E* time **(E)**. These measurements are used to measure the myocardial performance index. *LA*, left atrium; *LV*, left ventricle; *RA*, right atrium; *RV*, right ventricle.

From these time intervals, the MPI is computed as follows:

$$MPI = (ICT + IRT)/ET$$

Because the ICT + IRT is the difference between the intervals from the closure of the A wave to the beginning of the E wave minus the ET, the MPI equation can be adjusted as follows:

$$MPI = ([\text{Time from closure of the A wave to the beginning of the E wave}] - \text{Ejection time})/\text{Ejection time}$$

In adults, the normal values are 0.39 ± 0.05 (SD), whereas individuals with abnormal cardiac function had increased values of 0.59 (± 0.10 and 1.06 ± 0.24). Tei found that the MPI was not related to heart rate or ventricular size/shape.[109,110,112]

Measuring the MPI for the LV Using Doppler Blood Flow Waveforms

There are several approaches that have been reported for fetal evaluation of the MPI index for the LV.[113,114] At the present time, the best approach is using the "clicks" of the mitral and aortic valve leaflets for measuring the time intervals.[115] In 2005, Hernandez-Andrade et al. reported that using the valve "clicks" improved the reproducibility of the MPI.[115] This approach has been termed the modified MPI.[115] To accomplish this, the pulsed Doppler is placed at a location in which the mitral and aortic valves are simultaneously recorded. The time between the closure of the A wave and the beginning of the E wave is measured from valve "click" to valve "click" (Fig. 6.19C). The pulsed-Doppler waveform of the aorta is recorded, and the ET is measured from "click" to "click" (Fig. 6.19C). The landmarks for the measurements are more accurate than simply evaluating the blood flow waveforms. This technique can be applied to the LV throughout gestation.

Measuring the MPI for the RV Using Doppler Blood Flow Waveforms

Because the tricuspid inflow and the pulmonary outflow tracts are separated, simultaneous recording of the Doppler waveforms is not possible after 20 weeks of gestation because the distance between the tricuspid and pulmonary valves increases such that both valves cannot simultaneously be recorded.[116]

Therefore, the pulsed Doppler can be placed within the RV inflow tract and the waveform recorded (Fig. 6.19D). The time between the closure of the A wave and the beginning of the E wave is measured. The pulsed-Doppler waveform of the pulmonary artery is recorded (Fig. 6.19E) and the ET is measured. From these two measurements the MPI is computed as follows:

$$([\text{Time from closure of the A wave to the beginning of the E wave}] - [\text{Ejection time}]/\text{Ejection time}).^{117-125}$$

MPI in Normal Fetuses Using Blood Flow Waveforms

Table 6.6 lists studies from normal fetuses that have evaluated the MPI for the LV and RV from pulsed-Doppler recordings of blood flow. The 95th percentile has been computed for the MPI.

As the result of refining the technique for obtaining the MPI and measuring "clicks" of the waveforms, as described previously, the studies reported after 2005 may have better reproducibility than those before 2005.[115]

MPI Using TDI

Unlike conventional Doppler imaging of flow through the atrioventricular and semilunar valves, tissue Doppler imaging (TDI) is a measurement of timing of the myocardial wall motion of the RV and LV and the IVS. The recorded waveforms are opposite in direction to the blood flow velocity waveforms (Fig. 6.20A). The recording of TDI is obtained by placing the pulsed-Doppler sample volume at the base of the RV and LV walls or IVS and recording the wall motion (Fig. 6.20). TDI is a sensitive marker of mildly impaired systolic and diastolic function and is useful in the identification of subtle cardiac dysfunction in preclinical stages in postnatal life.[126,127] The TDI measured in adults and children has been shown to predict future cardiovascular disease.[128] Unlike the flow velocity waveform, the TDI demonstrates specific movement of the walls during the ICT and IRT times (Fig. 6.20A–C). The MPI is computed using the same equations for blood flow Doppler recordings (Fig. 6.20C). Normal values for the MPI computed from TDI were reported by Comas et al. in 2011.[96] They examined 213 singleton pregnancies and published the mean, 5th, and 95th percentile ranges for the MPI, using GA and EFW as the independent variables. In addition, they provided regression equations for computing percentiles, as well as a calculator for computing Z-scores for the MPI of the RV, LV, and IVS.[96] Figure 6.20D to F are graphs representing the mean, 5th, and 95th centiles for the MPI of the RV, LV, and IVS versus weeks of gestation.[96]

Cardiac Output

CO is the final common pathway that is determined by the interacting factors listed in Figure 6.1. The LV and RV CO were originally measured using pulsed-Doppler US, followed by 4D VOCAL technology. Simpson's method has also been used to measure CO of the LV.

Pulsed-Doppler Assessment of CO

Measurement of blood volume (Q) requires measurement of the cross-sectional area (A) through which blood is flowing, which is then multiplied by an average velocity.[1]

$$Q = V \times A$$

The average velocity (V) can be computed by multiplying the velocity time integral (VTI) by the heart rate. The VTI is the area under the curve of the Doppler waveform. Multiplying the VTI by the heart rate (beats/min) provides an estimate of the average velocity of blood flow for 1 minute. The second component of the equation to compute blood volume requires measurement of the area of the orifice through which blood is flowing. Because measurements of the aorta and pulmonary artery are circular, measurements of their diameter can be obtained, and the area computed as follows:

$$\text{Area} = ([\text{diameter}/2]^2 \times 3.14)$$

TABLE 6.6 Diastolic Function of the Right and Left Ventricles in Normal Fetuses

Harada et al.[140]	17–24 Wk	25–31 Wk	32–39 Wk
Left Ventricle			
Mitral valve studies	130	91	86
E wave peak velocity (cm/s)	26 ± 4	31 ± 5	38 ± 6
A wave peak velocity (cm/s)	41 ± 6	45 ± 7	47 ± 6
E/A ratio	0.63 ± 0.07[a]	0.70 ± 0.09[a]	0.80 ± 0.10
Right Ventricle			
Tricuspid valve studies	118	71	69
E wave peak velocity (cm/s)	29 ± 5	35 ± 6	39 ± 6
A wave peak velocity (cm/s)	45 ± 6	49 ± 8	51 ± 8
E/A Ratio	0.64 ± 0.07[a]	0.70 ± 0.08[a]	0.77 ± 0.09[a]
Pineda et al.[139]	17–26 Wk	27–32 Wk	33–40 Wk
Left Ventricle			
Mitral valve studies	143	181	161
E wave peak velocity (cm/s)	26.73 ± 6.7	31.01 ± 7.3	34.35 ± 8.7
A wave peak velocity (cm/s)	42.73 ± 8.9	42.81 ± 7.9	42.15 ± 9.2
E/A Ratio	0.62 ± 0.07[a]	0.72 ± 0.09[a]	0.81 ± 0.09[a]
Right Ventricle			
Tricuspid valve studies	143	181	161
E wave peak velocity (cm/s)	30.59 ± 7.2	35.32 ± 7.6	37.88 ± 10.01
A wave peak velocity (cm/s)	49.04 ± 8.4	50.55 ± 8.9	50.04 ± 11.1
E/A Ratio	0.62 ± 0.09[a]	0.69 ± 0.08[a]	0.75 ± 0.09[a]

Values are mean ± 1SD.
[a] $P < 0.05$.
From Tei C, Ling LH, Hodge DO, et al. New index of combined systolic and diastolic myocardial performance: a simple and reproducible measure of cardiac function—a study in normals and dilated cardiomyopathy. *J Cardiol.* 1995;26(6):357–366.

Once these values are measured, then the volume of blood flow can be determined as follows:

$$Q = 3.14 \times (D/2)^2 \times VTI \times HR$$

CO Computed from the Mitral and Tricuspid Inflow Tracts
Investigators have also attempted to measure CO from the mitral and tricuspid Doppler inflow waveforms by measuring the VTI of the combined E and A waveforms using Equation 6.10 (Fig. 6.21A, B).[129–133] Table 6.7 lists the values for CO using the mitral and tricuspid inflow waveforms. The difficulty with this technique, however, is the accurate measurement of the area of the mitral and tricuspid valves that are required in the

abovementioned computation. For this reason, CO determined from the inflow tracts has not been used on a routine basis when evaluating fetal CO.

Aortic and Pulmonary Outflow Tracts
Aortic blood flow velocities can be obtained using the long axis of the five-chamber view of the heart (Fig. 6.22A), whereas pulmonary Doppler flow velocities are best obtained in a plane perpendicular to the long-axis view of the LV, or from the short-axis view of the outflow tracts (Fig. 6.22B). Using these approaches, the blood from the pulmonary artery and the aorta are parallel to the US beam so that accurate Doppler recordings of their respective waveforms can occur (Fig. 6.22C, D). Once the Doppler

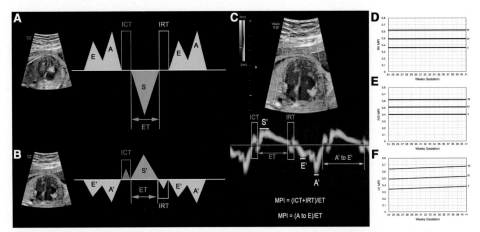

FIGURE 6.20: Blood flow and tissue Doppler waveforms from the left ventricle. **A:** Illustrates the blood flow Doppler waveforms and **(B)** the tissue Doppler waveforms (TDI). The TDI waveforms have lower velocities and are in the opposite direction compared to the blood flow waveforms. In addition, the isovolumetric contraction time (ICT) and isovolumetric relaxation time (IRT) are waveforms in TDI compared to spaces in the blood flow waveform. E and A are the blood flow waveforms for diastole and S for systole for the blood flow waveforms. E' and A' are the blood flow waveforms for diastole and S' for systole for the tissue Doppler waveforms. *E*, ejection time. **C:** Illustrates the tissue Doppler computation of the Myocardial Performance Index (MPI) from the left ventricle. E' and A' are the blood flow waveforms for diastole and S' for systole for the tissue Doppler waveforms. *E*, ejection time. A to E represents the time between the end of the A' waveform to the beginning of the E' waveform. **D to F:** Graphical representation of the mean, 5th, and 95th centiles for the MPI for the right ventricle (RV), interventricular septum (IVS), and the left ventricle (LV) versus weeks of gestation.[96]

waveforms have been obtained, a cross-sectional measurement at the level of the aortic and pulmonary valves is obtained (Fig. 6.22A, B). Investigators have reported that CO increased as a function of GA (Table 6.8).[134–136]

Measurement of LV CO Using 2D Images
The LV is an ellipsoid-shaped structure (Fig. 6.10). The EDV and ESV have been measured using 2D images from either the four-chamber view or the four-chamber view plus the apical two-chamber view.[57] A recent study by our group reported measuring the EDV and ESV for the LV using Simpson's rule computed from the 24 segments derived from speckle-tracking analysis of the four-chamber view (Fig. 6.10), following which the CO for the LV was derived.[57] The results demonstrated an increasing CO when compared to GA, BPD, HC, AC, FL, and EFW. Figure 6.23 illustrates the CO using the HC and FL as the independent variables.[57]

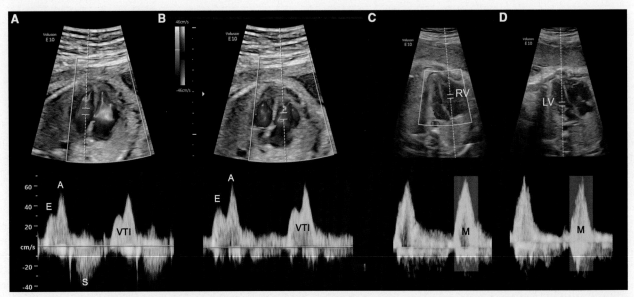

FIGURE 6.21: Mitral and tricuspid pulsed-Doppler waveforms. **A:** Recording from the mitral inflow tract illustrating the E and A waves and the velocity time integral (VTI). **B:** Recording from the tricuspid inflow tract illustrating the E and A waves and the velocity time integral. Monophasic pulsed-Doppler waveform. **(A)** Monophasic Doppler waveform recorded distal to the tricuspid valve. **C:** Monophasic Doppler waveform recorded distal to the tricuspid valve. **D:** Monophasic Doppler waveform recorded distal to the mitral valve. *LV*, left ventricle; *RV*, right ventricle.

TABLE 6.7   Normal Myocardial Performance Index (MPI) Values for the Left and Right Ventricles

REFERENCE	NUMBER OF FETUSES	MPI	GESTATIONAL AGE (wk)	LEFT MPI MEAN (SD)	LEFT MPI 95%	RIGHT MPI MEAN (SD)	RIGHT MPI 95%
Tsutumi et al. (1999)[133]	50	Left ventricle[136]	20 40	0.65 (0.03) 0.43 (0.03)	0.70 0.48		
Eidem et al. (2001)[117]	125	Both ventricles	20–40	0.36 (0.06)	0.46	0.32 (0.03)	0.37
Falkensammer et al. (2001)[118]	23	Both ventricles	24–34	0.41 (0.05)	0.49	0.38 (0.04)	0.45
Friedman et al. (2003)[114]	74	Left ventricle	18–31	0.53 (0.13)	0.74		
Chen et al. (2006)[119]	225	Both ventricles	18–27 +M6 28–36 + 6 37–42	0.37 (0.08) 0.27 (0.05) 0.22 (0.05)	0.50 0.35 0.30	0.39 (0.04) 0.30 (0.05) 0.24 (0.04)	0.46 0.38 0.31
Figueroa-Diesel et al. (2007)[178]	209	Left ventricle	30–40	0.37 (0.06)	0.47		
Wong et al. (2007)[120]	41	Both ventricles	34–37	0.54 (0.16)	0.80	0.58 (0.17)	0.86
Hernandez-Andrade et al. (2005)[115]	557	Left ventricle	19 39	0.35 (0.27) 0.37 (0.29)	0.39 0.42		
Russell et al. (2008)[121]	30	Both ventricles	20 36	0.53 (0.09) 0.57 (0.09)	0.68 0.72	0.54 (0.12) 0.60 (0.11)	0.74 0.78
Acharya et al. (2008)[180]	87	Left ventricle	28 + 3	0.38 (0.1)	0.55		
Van Mieghem et al. (2009)[107]	117	Left ventricle	20–36	0.34 (0.05)	0.42		
Api et al. (2009)[182]	40	Left ventricle	26–40	0.43 (0.045)	0.50		
Wood et al. (2009)[120]	3,200	Left ventricle	11 40	0.4 (0.05) 0.58 (0.05)	0.48 0.66		
Romiti et al. (2010)[122]	49 61 17	Both ventricles	14–26 27–34 35–40	0.42 (0.14) 0.40 (0.17) 0.41 (0.14)	0.65 0.68 0.64	0.49 (0.14) 0.49 (0.16) 0.52 (0.18)	0.72 0.75 0.82
Clur et al. (2011)[123]	120 98 35	Both ventricles	11–15 18–22 28–32	0.36 (0.12) 0.31 (0.12) 0.31 (0.25)	0.56 0.51 0.51	0.35 (0.14) 0.32 (0.16) 0.35 (0.22)	0.58 0.58 0.71
Hamela-Olkowsska and Szymkiewicz-Danger (2011)[124]	117	Both ventricles	18–40	0.47 (0.07)	0.59	0.48 (0.1)	0.65
Ghawi (2013)[125]	250	Both ventricles	2nd and 3rd trimesters (averaged)	0.464 (0.08)	0.60	0.466 (0.09)	0.615

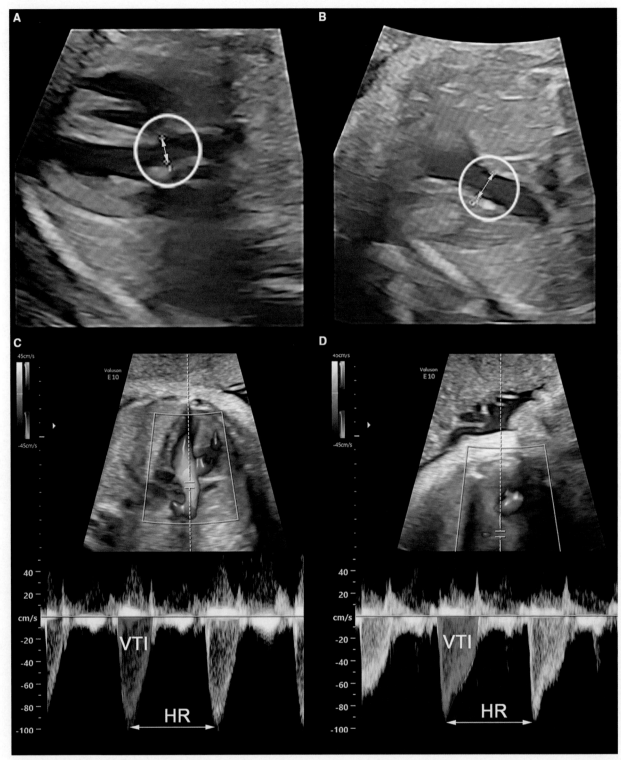

FIGURE 6.22: Cross-sectional measurements of the aorta and pulmonary artery and their corresponding Doppler waveforms. **A:** Demonstrates the level for the cross-sectional measurement of the diameter of the aorta at the level of the aortic valve. **B:** Demonstrates the level for the cross-sectional measurement of the diameter of the main pulmonary artery at the level of the pulmonary valve. **C:** Velocity time interval (VTI) of the aortic outflow tract. **D:** Velocity time interval of the pulmonary outflow tract. *HR*, heart rate.

VOCAL Assessment of CO

Using VOCAL technology, as previously described in this review, Molina et al. in 2008 reported that the CO increased exponentially with GA and the ratio of RV/LV CO increased from 0.97 at 12 weeks to 1.13 at 34 weeks.[137] Hamill et al. in 2011 reported that the CO increased as a function of GA, HC, AC, and FL. However, when the CO was divided by the EFW, there was no increase with GA.[55] Hamill et al. also reported that there was no significant differences observed between the RV and LV CO.[55] Simioni et al., using this technology, reported no significant differences in CO on the basis of the sex of the fetus.[56] In 2012, DeKoninck et al. compared the VOCAL technique with pulsed-Doppler assessment of

		LCO (mL/min)			RCO (mL/min)			
AUTHOR	**SITE OF RECORDING**	**19–21**	**29–31**	**36–40**	**19–21**	**29–31**	**36–40**	**CCO (mL/min/kg)**
De Smedt[132]	AV valves	84	333	820	105	372	915	553
Allan[133]	AV valves	109	333	686	140	428	883	—
Rizzo[184]	AV valves	91	320	693	134	435	890	546

TABLE 6.8 Reported Values of Volume Flow Estimations from the Atrioventricular (AV) Valves for Left Cardiac Output (LCO), Right Cardiac Output (RCO), and Combined Cardiac Output (CCO) Corrected for Fetal Weight

CO (*vide supra*) and found that the results using pulsed Doppler were higher than those using the VOCAL technique.[138] Because of the differences, the VOCAL and pulsed-Doppler normal values cannot be used interchangeably.[138]

ASSESSMENT OF DIASTOLIC FUNCTION OF RV AND LV

Quantitative assessment of diastolic function of the fetal heart initially focused primarily on evaluation of the E and A waveforms, recorded distal to the opening of the tricuspid and mitral valves (Fig. 6.21). Investigators have postulated that ventricular diastolic function reflects ventricular relaxation, compliance, and filling.[139] Several studies have examined the velocities of the E and A wave as a function of GA.[139–145] In one of the largest studies, Fernandez

Pineda et al. examined 485 fetuses from 17 weeks to term and found that the A wave velocity was unchanged throughout pregnancy, suggesting little or no change in compliance.[139] However, the E wave velocity increased, suggesting progressive enhancement of relaxation and elastic recoil, an increase in preload, or both throughout pregnancy.[139] In addition, the E and A wave velocities were higher for the RV than for the LV. From their study, Fernandez Pineda et al. concluded that (1) inflow E wave velocity increased linearly throughout gestation and (2) improvement in active ventricular relaxation or augmented preload was responsible for the change in the E/A ratio as it approached the E/A ratio observed postnatally.[139] It has also been noted that increased ventricular stiffness demonstrates merging of the E and A waveforms into a single waveform, most commonly observed in the RV (Fig. 6.21C, D). Table 6.9 lists normal values for the E wave, A

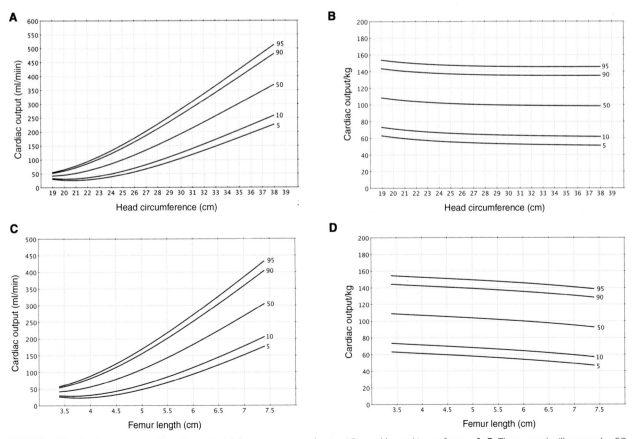

FIGURE 6.23: Cardiac output and cardiac output/kilogram measured using 2D speckle-tracking software. **A, B:** These graphs illustrate the CO **(A)** and (CO/kg) for the head circumference. **C, D:** These graphs illustrate the CO and CO/kg for the femur length.

| TABLE 6.9 | Reported Values of Volume Flow Estimations from the Aorta and Main Pulmonary Artery Outflow Tracts for Left Cardiac Output (LCO), Right Cardiac Output (RCO), and Combined Cardiac Output (CCO) Corrected for Fetal Weight |||||||| |

AUTHOR	SITE OF RECORDING	LCO (mL/min)			RCO (mL/min)			CCO (mL/min/kg)
		19–21	29–31	36–40	19–21	29–31	36–40	
Kenny[135]	Outflow tracts	118	282	676	132	302	692	—
Allan[133]	Outflow tracts	70	269	647	93	361	886	450
Rizzo[130]	Outflow tracts	78	284	670	100	390	866	525

wave, and the E/A ratio from studies by Harada et al. in 1997 and Fernandez Pineda et al. in 2000. The E/A ratios for each of the subgroups between the two studies were almost identical.[138,140]

Another more recent approach used to evaluate diastolic function is to evaluate ventricular and septal wall movement using TDI and examine the peak velocities, which have been labeled E′ and A′, at the base of the lateral walls of the ventricles and the septum (Figure 16).[96] Nomograms for the E′, A′, and E′/A′ have been published from Comas et al. in 2011 using GA and the EFW as the independent variables (Fig. 6.24).[94]

IMPLEMENTATION OF QUANTITATIVE FETAL CARDIAC ASSESSMENT IN CLINICAL CARE

Small-for-Gestational Age (SGA) Fetuses

In the past, SGA fetuses were thought to be constitutionally small versus having intrauterine growth restriction (IUGR) if the Doppler finding of the UA was abnormal. Recent studies, however, have suggested that the SGA fetus may indeed have components of IUGR without abnormal UA Doppler waveforms and have adverse perinatal events and postnatal cardiovascular complications when compared to normal-weight newborns of the same GA.[146–154] Studies have also suggested that echocardiographic and biochemical abnormalities that further deteriorate as the IUGR process becomes more severe are present in subclinical cardiac dysfunction.[66,143,152,155] In 2011, Comas et al. studied 58 SGA fetuses and 58 controls and compared pulsed-Doppler flow velocity variables with pulsed-Doppler tissue Doppler (Table 6.10). They found that the only flow velocity variable that was abnormal was a smaller A wave velocity in both ventricles, whereas tissue Doppler showed significantly lower peak velocities for the right E′, A′, and S′ waves. In addition, the MPI′ for both ventricles was significantly increased in the SGA fetuses. The authors postulated that because the TDI annular peak velocities reflect the motion of the longitudinal myocardial fibers, which are located in the subendocardial layer, TDI measurements are the earliest to be altered in the presence of decreased oxygen.[156] They suggested that TDI measurements are more sensitive than are blood flow velocity measurements.[94] The fetuses with abnormal cardiac function had an increased trend for higher rates of intervention for fetal distress, cesarean section, and preeclampsia, and longer days in the newborn intensive care unit.[94]

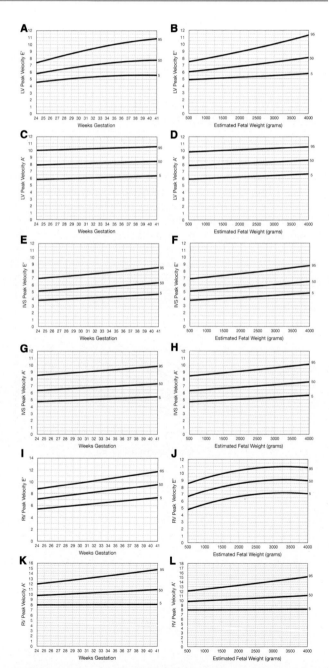

FIGURE 6.24: Graphs of the mean, 5th, and 95th centiles for E′ and A′ for the weeks' gestation and estimated fetal weight for the left ventricle (A–D), interventricular septum (E–H), and the right ventricle (I–L).[96]

TABLE 6.10 Comparison of Doppler Velocity and Ventricular Wall Motion Measurements in the Fetus with Intrauterine Growth Restriction Who Did Not Have Absent Flow in the Umbilical Artery

MEASUREMENTS	CONTROL	IUGR	P VALUE ADJUSTED FOR FETAL WEIGHT
Pulsed-Doppler Flow Velocity			
Variable			
Left E wave velocity (cm/s)	38 (8)	36 (6)	NS
Left A wave velocity (cm/s)	**49 (8)**	**44 (6)**	**<0.001**
Left E/A ratio	0.78 (0.12)	0.83 (0.13)	NS
Right E wave velocity (cm/s)	47 (9)	43 (7)	NS
Right A wave velocity	**59 (10)**	**53 (9)**	**0.007**
Right E/A ratio	0.80 (0.8)	0.82 (0.11)	NS
Left MPI	0.49 (0.08)	0.53 (0.11)	NS
Pulsed Tissue Doppler			
Annular Peak Velocities (cm/s)			
Left PVE' (cm/s)	7.89 (1.56)	7.60 (1.39)	NS
Left PVA' (cm/s)	8.56 (1.37)	8.17 (1.86)	NS
Left PVS' (cm/s)	6.94 (1.19)	6.64 (1.35)	NS
Right PVE' (cm/s)	**9.25 (1.42)**	**8.48 (1.47)**	**0.039**
Right PVA' (cm/s)	**11.23 (2.15)**	**10.13 (1.64)**	**0.033**
Right PVS' (cm/s)	**8.09 (1.29)**	**7.39 (1.29)**	**0.049**
Septal PVE' (cm/s)	6.24 (1.13)	6.11 (1.07)	NS
Septal PVA' (cm/s)	7.41 (1.37)	6.97 (1.34)	NS
Septal PVS' (cm/s)	6.03 (1.02)	5.99 (1.14)	NS
Myocardial Performance Index			
Left MPI'	**0.52 (0.09)**	**0.55 (0.09)**	**0.001**
Right MPI'	**0.49 (0.09)**	**0.56 (0.10)**	**<0.001**
Septal MPI'	0.52 (0.09)	0.59 (0.11)	NS

From Comas M, Crispi F, Cruz-Martinez R, et al. Tissue Doppler echocardiographic markers of cardiac dysfunction in small-for-gestational age fetuses. *Am J Obstet Gynecol.* 2011;205(1):57.e1–57.e6. Bold text represents results that had P values <0.05

Early-Onset IUGR

Fetuses with IUGR have been shown to have cardiac dysfunction, while maintaining appropriate CO for their specific weight.[152,155] Prior studies reported abnormal cardiac dysfunction at more advanced stages of IUGR.[157–160] However, recent studies have suggested that subclinical cardiac dysfunction occurs at earlier stages of fetal deterioration.[95,155,161] In 2010, Comas et al. studied 25 IUGR fetuses whose EFW was below the 10th percentile and UA Pulsatility Index was above the 95th percentile. Fetuses delivered between 26 and 34 weeks of gestation were evaluated. Fetuses with

structural and/or chromosomal anomalies and those with infection were excluded. Fifty fetuses with normal growth, matched for GA, were used as controls. Table 6.11 lists their findings for velocity flow measurements and TDI measurements for diastolic function, systolic function, and combined diastolic and systolic dysfunction. The pulsed-Doppler blood flow measurements demonstrated decreased RV and LV E and A wave velocities, but the E/A ratios were normal. Although the peak velocities for the aorta and pulmonary artery were decreased in the IUGR fetuses, the decrease was not statistically significant. Only the LV demonstrated an increased MPI. The TDI measurements demonstrated similar

TABLE 6.11 Comparison of Doppler Velocity and Ventricular Wall Motion Measurements in Fetuses with Early-Onset Intrauterine Growth Restriction Who Had Abnormal Doppler of the Umbilical Artery

MEASUREMENTS (cm/s)	CONTROL	IUGR	P VALUE ADJUSTED FOR FETAL WEIGHT
Pulsed-Doppler Flow Velocity			
Diastolic Parameters			
Left E wave velocity (cm/s)	**37 (5.4)**	**31 (7.4)**	**<0.002**
Left A wave velocity (cm/s)	**50 (8.5)**	**41 (10.1)**	**<0.001**
Left E/A ratio	0.74 (0.1)	0.78 (0.2)	NS
Right E wave velocity (cm/s)	**43 (7.9)**	**32 (7.5)**	**<0.001**
Right A wave velocity (cm/s)	**57 (9.2)**	**39 (7.2)**	**<0.001**
Right E/A ratio	0.76 (0.1)	0.81 (0.1)	NS
Systolic Parameters			
Aortic peak velocity (cm/s)	94 (20.2)	81 (16.5)	NS
Pulmonary artery peak velocity (cm/s)	91 (20.9)	84 (24.5)	NS
Myocardial Performance Index (Diastolic and Systolic Dysfunction)			
Left MPI	**0.45 (0.06)**	**0.52 (0.09)**	**0.006**
Right MPI	0.47 (0.19)	045 (0.13)	NS
Pulsed Tissue Doppler			
Diastolic Parameters			
Left PVE' (cm/s)	7.3 (1.3)	6.7 (0.8)	NS
Left PVA' (cm/s)	**8.5 (1.4)**	**6.2 (0.7)**	**<0.001**
Left E'/A' (cm/s)	**0.85 (0.13)**	**1.09 (0.17)**	**<0.001**
Right PVE' (cm/s)	**8.5 (1.13)**	**7.2 (1.3)**	**0.007**
Right PVA' (cm/s)	**10.8 (1.5)**	**9.1 (1.2)**	**0.01**
Right E'/A' (cm/s)	0.79 (0.1)	0.82 (0.1)	NS
Septal PVE' (cm/s)	6.3 (1.1)	5.4 (1)	NS
Septal PVA' (cm/s)	**7.4 (1.3)**	**6.2 (0.6)**	**0.049**
Septal E'/A'	0.86 (0.1)	0.88 (0.1)	NS
Systolic Parameters			
Left PVS' (cm/s)	**6.9 (1.2)**	**5.6 (0.6)**	**0.002**
Right PVS' (cm/s)	**7.6 (1.2)**	**6.6 (1.4)**	**0.049**
Septal PVS' (cm/s)	5.8 (0.88)	5.3 (1.1)	NS
Myocardial Performance Index (Diastolic and Systolic Dysfunction)			
Left MPI'	**0.49 (0.08)**	**0.56 (0.09)**	**0.007**
Right MPI'	**0.47 (0.09)**	**0.61 (0.11)**	**0.006**
Septal MPI'	**0.49 (0.06)**	**0.58 (0.05)**	**<0.001**

From Comas M, Crispi F, Cruz-Martinez R, et al. Usefulness of myocardial tissue Doppler vs conventional echocardiography in the evaluation of cardiac dysfunction in early-onset intrauterine growth restriction. *Am J Obstet Gynecol.* 2010;203(1):45.e1–45.e7. Bold text represents results that had P values <0.05

significant decreases for E′ and A′ for both ventricles and an increased MPI′ for both ventricles and septum. This approach also showed a significant decrease in the LV and LV S′. The authors concluded that TDI is a more sensitive tool for evaluating systolic and diastolic dysfunction than was conventional pulsed-Doppler evaluation of the flow velocity waveforms.[95] They also concluded that the aortic and pulmonary artery flow velocities were similar, when corrected for fetal weight.[95]

In 2012, Cruz-Lemini et al. evaluated 157 early-onset (<34 weeks) growth-restricted fetuses to determine Doppler and cardiovascular measurements that predicted perinatal death.[162] An abnormal MPI had an odds ratio of only 1.6.[162] In 2013, Unterscheider et al. examined over 1,100 fetuses with an EFW less than the 10th centile and found an incidence of an abnormal LV MPI in only 12%, compared to 46% that had an abnormal UA and 27% with an abnormal MCA.[163] They did not demonstrate a clinical benefit when the MPI was incorporated into the assessment of these fetuses.[163] A recent study evaluating the MPI in 52 growth-restricted fetuses demonstrated that there was no evidence of the RV or LV MPI correlating with perinatal outcome, and was not useful in triaging fetuses for management when compared to the Doppler of the UA.[164]

Cardiac Function in Fetuses of Mothers with Severe Preeclampsia

In 2017, Bhorat et al. examined fetal cardiac function in 60 fetuses of mothers with severe preeclampsia diagnosed between 27 and 32 weeks of gestation.[161] They found that the LV pulsed-Doppler blood flow MPI values were increased compared to that of controls, irrespective of whether growth restriction was present or absent. In addition, they noted that abnormal MPI values increased as the maternal disease worsened.[161]

Diabetes

In 2008, Hatem et al. examined fetuses of mothers with pregestational diabetes from 25 weeks to term and reported the following[165]:

1. The right and left myocardial velocities of the E′ and A′ were significantly higher in fetuses of diabetic mothers.
2. The E′/A′ ratios were higher than those in normal fetuses.
3. In fetuses of mothers with pregestational diabetes, the ratio of early diastolic peak inflow velocity (E) to peak annular velocity (E′) was lower in fetuses of mothers with diabetes.

They concluded that the changes in diastolic dysfunction were independent of fetal myocardial hypertrophy, and thus an earlier indication of cardiovascular dysfunction.[165]

In 2013, Bui et al. reported a study performed between 17 and 23 weeks of gestation in which they evaluated the MPI for the RV in 69 normal fetuses and 51 fetuses of diabetic mothers.[166] They found that there were no significant differences between the two groups for the E′, A′, E′/A′ ratio, peak E and peak A wave velocities. However, the E/E′ ratio had a P value of <0.05. The RV pulsed-wave blood flow MPI was not statistically significant between the two groups, but the TDI MPI was significantly higher in the diabetic population (0.56 [SD 0.10]) than in controls (0.51 [SD 0.12]), (P < 0.01). They concluded that the MPI of the TDI was more sensitive than was spectral Doppler MPI for detecting cardiac dysfunction in the midtrimester fetus of the diabetic mother.

In 2016, Pilania et al. examined fetuses of mothers who required insulin and found that an abnormal LV MPI and LV CO were more prevalent than that in the control group.[167] In 2017, Aliq et al. examined second-trimester fetuses and found the following abnormalities to be significantly abnormal in fetuses of diabetic mothers: ICT, IRT, MPI, and the mitral E/A ratios (P < 0.03).[168] MAPSE was significantly less in the diabetic group (P = 0.01).[168] Sanhai et al. also reported in 2017 that the LV MPI ratios were higher and the LV E/A ratios were lower in the diabetic group and these were associated with adverse outcome.[169] In 2018, Miranda et al. examined 76 fetuses whose mothers had diabetes and found an increased interventricular septal thickness that had no effect on strain analysis.[170] They examined each fetus using conventional fetal echocardiographic technologies and found no significant differences between the control and study groups. The echocardiographic evaluations included the following: cardiothoracic ratio, left and right atrial atria, GSI, left and right CO, left and right shortening fraction, TAPSE, MAPSE, E/A ratios of the tricuspid and mitral valves, mitral IRT, and RV and LV MPI.[170] When the investigators examined ventricular strain, they identified that RV systolic global strain, and RV and LV early strain rates were significantly different than that in the controls.[170] They concluded the evaluation of ventricular strain was more sensitive than were traditional echocardiographic measurements in identifying fetuses at risk for cardiac dysfunction.[170]

Identification of Pregnancies with Decreased Fetal Movement

Other than high-risk fetuses, recent studies have examined cardiovascular function in fetuses whose mothers complained of decreased fetal movement.[171] In 2018, Ho et al. evaluated the MPI in a case–control study of women complaining of decreased fetal movement.[171] They noted increased RV and LV MPI in fetuses who had an adverse outcome (N = 20) and those who did not (N = 30).[171]

Identification of Non-IUGR Fetuses to Predict Emergency Operative Delivery

In 2017 and 2018, Alsolai et al. examined 284 low-risk fetuses from 36 weeks of gestation until delivery and obtained cardiovascular measurements of RV and LV CO and global strain using speckle-tracking software. The group that required emergency operative delivery demonstrated abnormal LV CO, LV global strain, and LV strain rate when compared to controls.[172–174]

Identification of Adverse Outcome in Fetuses with Idiopathic Polyhydramnios

In 2016, Gezer examined fetuses with concomitant idiopathic polyhydramnios and found that an abnormal IRT, ET, and MPI of the LV were associated with polyhydramnios. An abnormal MPI and polyhydramnios were associated with nonreassuring fetal status, emergency cesarean delivery, and respiratory distress syndrome.[175]

Evaluation of Cardiovascular Function in Twin-to-Twin Transfusion Pregnancies

In 2016, Delabaere et al. examined 77 fetuses before laser ablation and 86 fetuses 4 weeks after the procedure.[176] Overall neonatal survival was 64.9%. The preoperative predictors of neonatal survival for the recipient twin were the UA PI, CPR, absent end-diastolic flow, the ductus venosus A wave, and the RV MPI.[176] For the donor twin, the predictors of neonatal survival were RV MPI, recipient UA EDF, umbilical vein pulsations, and tricuspid regurgitation cardiac hypertrophy.[176]

CONCLUSIONS

For over 40 years, clinicians have focused on interpretation of the FHRT as the primary (or sole) direct cardiovascular parameter to evaluate the well-being of the third-trimester fetus. However, as fetal echocardiography has evolved from simple evaluation of the four-chamber view to detailed assessment of the size and shape of the four-chamber view and evaluation of ventricular size, shape, and contractility, new options are now available to examine both low-risk and high-risk fetuses. Although this review has examined a number of cardiac measurements associated with ventricular contractility and function that have been reported in the literature, the most useful quantitative diagnostic tools that appear to currently be utilized in recent studies are M-mode assessment of TAPSE and MAPSE, Doppler assessment of the LV and RV MPI and MPI', E/A, E'/A', S' of both ventricles, and 2D speckle-tracking strain analysis of both ventricles. One of the difficulties evaluating the fetal heart with pulsed Doppler is the requirement for the four-chamber view to be oriented with the apex at 12 or 6 o'clock. This is problematic because of the prolonged examination time that might be required as the examiner waits for the fetus to be in the proper orientation for examination. In addition, it requires a high level of clinical expertise to accurately acquire the Doppler waveforms for analysis. In contrast, utilization of speckle-tracking software allows for the simultaneous measurements of a number of ventricular measurements (longitudinal contractility, transverse contractility, LV stroke volume

and CO) from a single tracking of the endocardial borders of the RV and LV from the four-chamber view of the heart. In the past, speckle-tracking analysis for ventricular analysis required either dedicated cardiac US machines or offline software. The measurements obtained from speckle tracking reported in our studies allows the examiner, irrespective of their familiarity and skills, to obtain and analyze Doppler waveforms for cardiovascular examination, to use software to obtain RV and LV end-systolic and end-diastolic endocardial measurements (Table 6.12) and measure the size, shape, and function of the ventricles (Table 6.13).

ACKNOWLEDGMENTS

We thank Carrie Grinstead, MLIS, AHIP, Regional Medical Librarian, and Pamela Gay, Library Specialist, Providence Health & Services, and Southern California for assistance procuring references used in this review.

TABLE 6.13 **Fetal Assessment of Ventricular Size and Shape Using Speckle-Tracking Software[46,47,51]**

MEASUREMENTS

RV and LV Shape

End-Diastolic 24-segment Sphericity Index
Base segments 1–8
Mid-segments 9–16
Apical segments 17–24

End-Diastolic Size
End-diastolic longitudinal basal-apical length

End-Diastolic 24-Segment Transverse Width
Base segments 1–8
Mid-segments 9–16
Apical segments 17–24

RV/LV 24 Segment Ratio
Base segments 1–8
Mid-segments 9–16
Apical segments 17–24
RV/LV End-Diastolic Area Ratio
RV/LV Ventricular End-Diastolic Length Ratio

TABLE 6.12 **Evaluation of Ventricular Contractility and Function Using Speckle-Tracking Software[48,49,57]**

MEASUREMENTS

Right and Left Global Ventricular Contractility
Fractional area change

Right and Left Ventricular Longitudinal Contractility
Longitudinal strain
Free wall strain
Septal wall strain
Basal-apical annular systolic displacement
Basal-apical lateral wall annular plane systolic excursion
Basal-apical septal wall annular plane systolic excursion

Right and Left Ventricular Transverse Contractility
24-Segment Transverse Fractional Shortening
Base segments 1–8
Mid-segments 9–16
Apical segments 17–24

Left Ventricular Global Function and Contractility
LV stroke volume
LV cardiac output
LV ejection fraction

REFERENCES

1. Mao YK, Zhao BW, Zhou L, et al. Z-score reference ranges for pulsed-wave Doppler indices of the cardiac outflow tracts in normal fetuses. *Int J Cardiovasc Imaging.* 2019;35(5):811–825.
2. Friedman D, Duncanson L, Glickstein J, et al. A review of congenital heart block. *Images Paediatr Cardiol.* 2003;5(3):36–48.
3. Ho A, Gordon P, Rosenthal E, et al. Isolated complete heart block in the fetus. *Am J Cardiol.* 2015;116(1):142–147.
4. Martin TA. Congenital heart block: current thoughts on management, morphologic spectrum, and role of intervention. *Cardiol Young.* 2014;24 suppl 2:41–46.
5. DeVore GR, Siassi B, Platt LD. Fetal echocardiography. III. The diagnosis of cardiac arrhythmias using real-time-directed M-mode ultrasound. *Am J Obstet Gynecol.* 1983;146(7):792–799.
6. Silber DL, Durnin RE. Intrauterine atrial tachycardia, associated with massive edema in a newborn. *Am J Dis Child.* 1969;117(6):722–726.
7. Silverman NH, Enderlein MA, Stanger P, et al. Recognition of fetal arrhythmias by echocardiography. *J Clin Ultrasound.* 1985;13(4):255–263.

8. Hon EH, Zannini D, Quilligan EJ. The neonatal value of fetal monitoring. *Am J Obstet Gynecol.* 1975;122(4):508–519.

9. Paul RH. Electronic fetal monitoring and later outcome: a thirty-year overview. *J Perinatol.* 1994;14(5):393–395.

10. Ikeda S, Okazaki A, Miyazaki K, et al. Fetal heart rate pattern interpretation in the second stage of labor using the five-tier classification: impact of the degree and duration on severe fetal acidosis. *J Obstet Gynaecol Res.* 2014;40(5):1274–1280.

11. Pinto P, Costa-Santos C, Goncalves H, et al. Improvements in fetal heart rate analysis by the removal of maternal-fetal heart rate ambiguities. *BMC Pregnancy Childbirth.* 2015;15:301.

12. Epstein AJ, Iriye BK, Hancock L, et al. Web-based comparison of historical vs contemporary methods of fetal heart rate interpretation. *Am J Obstet Gynecol.* 2016;215(4):488.e1–488.e5.

13. Rei M, Tavares S, Pinto P, et al. Interobserver agreement in CTG interpretation using the 2015 FIGO guidelines for intrapartum fetal monitoring. *Eur J Obstet Gynecol Reprod Biol.* 2016;205:27–31.

14. Garabedian C, Butruille L, Servan-Schreiber E, et al. Fetal heart-rate variability: validation of a new continuous, noninvasive computerized analysis. *Gynecol Obstet Invest.* 2017;82(5):500–507.

15. Gyllencreutz E, Hulthen Varli I, Lindqvist PG, et al. Reliability in cardiotocography interpretation—impact of extended on-site education in addition to web-based learning: an observational study. *Acta Obstet Gynecol Scand.* 2017;96(4):496–502.

16. Marti Gamboa S, Gimenez OR, Mancho JP, et al. Diagnostic accuracy of the FIGO and the 5-tier fetal heart rate classification systems in the detection of neonatal acidemia. *Am J Perinatol.* 2017;34(5):508–514.

17. Murray H. Antenatal foetal heart monitoring. *Best Pract Res Clin Obstet Gynaecol.* 2017;38:2–11.

18. Pruksanusak N, Thongphanang P, Suntharasaj T, et al. Combined maternal-associated risk factors with intrapartum fetal heart rate classification systems to predict peripartum asphyxia neonates. *Eur J Obstet Gynecol Reprod Biol.* 2017;218:85–91.

19. Ayres-de-Campos D, Arulkumaran S. FIGO consensus guidelines on intrapartum fetal monitoring: physiology of fetal oxygenation and the main goals of intrapartum fetal monitoring. *Int J Gynaecol Obstet.* 2015;131(1):5–8.

20. Ayres-de-Campos D, Spong CY, Chandraharan E. FIGO consensus guidelines on intrapartum fetal monitoring: cardiotocography. *Int J Gynaecol Obstet.* 2015;131(1):13–24.

21. Eden RD, Evans MI, Evans SM, et al. Reengineering electronic fetal monitoring interpretation: using the fetal reserve index to anticipate the need for emergent operative delivery. *Reprod Sci.* 2018;25(4):487–497.

22. Evans MI, Eden RD, Britt DW, et al. Re-engineering the interpretation of electronic fetal monitoring to identify reversible risk for cerebral palsy: a case control series. *J Matern Fetal Neonatal Med.* 2018:1–9.

23. Schifrin BS. The CTG and the timing and mechanism of fetal neurological injuries. *Best Pract Res Clin Obstet Gynaecol.* 2004;18(3):437–456.

24. Schifrin BS, Ater S. Fetal hypoxic and ischemic injuries. *Curr Opin Obstet Gynecol.* 2006;18(2):112–122.

25. Schifrin BS, Cohen WR. The effect of malpractice claims on the use of caesarean section. *Best Pract Res Clin Obstet Gynaecol.* 2013;27(2):269–283.

26. Schifrin BS, Koos B. Defining the limits of electronic fetal heart rate. *Am J Obstet Gynecol.* 2017;216(5):532.

27. Schifrin BS, Soliman M, Koos B. Litigation related to intrapartum fetal surveillance. *Best Pract Res Clin Obstet Gynaecol.* 2016;30:87–97.

28. Di Tommaso M, Seravalli V, Cordisco A, et al. Comparison of five classification systems for interpreting electronic fetal monitoring in predicting neonatal status at birth. *J Matern Fetal Neonatal Med.* 2013;26(5):487–490.

29. Soncini E, Paganelli S, Vezzani C, et al. Intrapartum fetal heart rate monitoring: evaluation of a standardized system of interpretation for prediction of metabolic acidosis at delivery and neonatal neurological morbidity. *J Matern Fetal Neonatal Med.* 2014;27(14):1465–1469.

30. Uccella S, Cromi A, Colombo G, et al. Prediction of fetal base excess values at birth using an algorithm to interpret fetal heart rate tracings: a retrospective validation. *BJOG.* 2012;119(13):1657–1664.

31. Chen CY, Yu C, Chang CC, et al. Comparison of a novel computerized analysis program and visual interpretation of cardiotocography. *PLoS One.* 2014;9(12):e112296.

32. Maeda Mde F, Nomura RM, Niigaki JI, et al. Computerized fetal heart rate analysis in the prediction of myocardial damage in pregnancies with placental insufficiency. *Eur J Obstet Gynecol Reprod Biol.* 2015;190:7–10.

33. DeVore GR. The importance of the cerebroplacental ratio in the evaluation of fetal well-being in SGA and AGA fetuses. *Am J Obstet Gynecol.* 2015;213(1):5–15.

34. DeVore GR, Satou G, Sklansky M. Abnormal fetal findings associated with a global sphericity index of the 4-chamber view below the 5th centile. *J Ultrasound Med.* 2017;36(11):2309–2318.

35. DeVore GR, Satou G, Sklansky M. Area of the fetal heart's four-chamber view: a practical screening tool to improve detection of cardiac abnormalities in a low-risk population. *Prenat Diagn.* 2017;37(2):151–155.

36. DeVore GR, Tabsh K, Polanco B, et al. Fetal heart size: a comparison between the point-to-point trace and automated ellipse methods between 20 and 40 weeks' gestation. *J Ultrasound Med.* 2016;35(12):2543–2562.

37. Mekkaoui C, Porayette P, Jackowski MP, et al. Diffusion MRI tractography of the developing human fetal heart. *PLoS One.* 2013;8(8):e72795.

38. Buckberg GD, Nanda NC, Nguyen C, et al. What is the heart? Anatomy, function, pathophysiology, and misconceptions. *J Cardiovasc Dev Dis.* 2018;5(2).

39. Torrent-Guasp F, Buckberg GD, Clemente C, et al. The structure and function of the helical heart and its buttress wrapping. I. The normal macroscopic structure of the heart. *Semin Thorac Cardiovasc Surg.* 2001;13(4):301–319.

40. Buckberg G, Hoffman JI. Right ventricular architecture responsible for mechanical performance: unifying role of ventricular septum. *J Thorac Cardiovasc Surg.* 2014;148(6):3166.e1-3171.e4.

41. Buckberg GD. The ventricular septum: the lion of right ventricular function, and its impact on right ventricular restoration. *Eur J Cardiothorac Surg.* 2006;29 suppl 1:S272–S278.

42. Kagan A. Dynamic responses of the right ventricle following extensive damage by cauterization. *Circulation.* 1952;5(6):816–823.

43. Cox JL, Bardy GH, Damiano RJ Jr, et al. Right ventricular isolation procedures for nonischemic ventricular tachycardia. *J Thorac Cardiovasc Surg.* 1985;90(2):212–224.

44. Goldstein JA, Tweddell JS, Barzilai B, et al. Importance of left ventricular function and systolic ventricular interaction to right ventricular performance during acute right heart ischemia. *J Am Coll Cardiol.* 1992;19(3):704–711.

45. Hoffman D, Sisto D, Frater RW, et al. Left-to-right ventricular interaction with a noncontracting right ventricle. *J Thorac Cardiovasc Surg.* 1994;107(6):1496–1502.

46. DeVore GR, Klas B, Satou G, et al. Evaluation of the right and left ventricles: an integrated approach measuring the area, length, and width of the chambers in normal fetuses. *Prenat Diagn.* 2017;37(12):1203–1212.

47. DeVore GR, Klas B, Satou G, et al. 24-segment sphericity index: a new technique to evaluate fetal cardiac diastolic shape. *Ultrasound Obstet Gynecol.* 2018;51(5):650–658.

48. DeVore GR, Klas B, Satou G, et al. Longitudinal annular systolic displacement compared to global strain in normal fetal hearts and those with cardiac abnormalities. *J Ultrasound Med.* 2018;37(5):1159–1171.

49. DeVore GR, Klas B, Satou G, et al. Quantitative evaluation of the fetal right and left ventricular fractional area change using speckle tracking technology. *Ultrasound Obstet Gynecol.* 2019;53(2):219–228.

50. DeVore GR, Polanco B, Satou G, et al. Two-dimensional speckle tracking of the fetal heart: a practical step-by-step approach for the fetal sonologist. *J Ultrasound Med.* 2016;35(8):1765–1781.

51. DeVore GR, Zaretsky M, Gumina DL, et al. Right and left ventricular 24-segment sphericity index is abnormal in small-for-gestational-age fetuses. *Ultrasound Obstet Gynecol.* 2018;52(2):243–249.

52. Li L, Craft M, Hsu HH, et al. Left ventricular rotational and twist mechanics in the human fetal heart. *J Am Soc Echocardiogr.* 2017;30(8):773.e1–780.e1.

53. Messing B, Cohen SM, Valsky DV, et al. Fetal cardiac ventricle volumetry in the second half of gestation assessed by 4D ultrasound using STIC combined with inversion mode. *Ultrasound Obstet Gynecol.* 2007;30(2):142–151.

54. Hamill N, Romero R, Hassan SS, et al. Repeatability and reproducibility of fetal cardiac ventricular volume calculations using spatiotemporal image correlation and virtual organ computer-aided analysis. *J Ultrasound Med.* 2009;28(10):1301–1311.

55. Hamill N, Yeo L, Romero R, et al. Fetal cardiac ventricular volume, cardiac output, and ejection fraction determined with 4-dimensional ultrasound using spatiotemporal image correlation and virtual organ computer-aided analysis. *Am J Obstet Gynecol.* 2011;205(1):76.e1–76.e10.

56. Simioni C, Araujo Junior E, Martins WP, et al. Fetal cardiac output and ejection fraction by spatio-temporal image correlation (STIC): comparison between male and female fetuses. *Rev Bras Cir Cardiovasc.* 2012;27(2):275–282.

57. DeVore GR, Klas B, Satou G, et al. Evaluation of left ventricular size and function using speckle tracking and Simpson's rule. *J Ultrasound Med.* 2019;38(5):1209–1221.

58. Schoonderwaldt EM, Groenenberg IA, Hop WC, et al. Reproducibility of echocardiographic measurements of human fetal left ventricular volumes and ejection fractions using four-dimensional ultrasound with the spatio-temporal image correlation modality. *Eur J Obstet Gynecol Reprod Biol.* 2012;160(1):22–29.

59. Anavekar NS, Gerson D, Skali H, et al. Two-dimensional assessment of right ventricular function: an echocardiographic-MRI correlative study. *Echocardiography.* 2007;24(5):452–456.

60. DeVore GR, Klas B, Satou G, et al. Quantitative evaluation of the fetal right and left ventricular fractional area change using speckle tracking technology. *J Ultrasound Obstet Gynecol.* 2019;53(2):219–228.

61. Goldinfeld M, Weiner E, Peleg D, et al. Evaluation of fetal cardiac contractility by two-dimensional ultrasonography. *Prenat Diagn.* 2004;24(10):799–803.

62. Levy PT, Dioneda B, Holland MR, et al. Right ventricular function in preterm and term neonates: reference values for right ventricular areas and fractional area of change. *J Am Soc Echocardiogr.* 2015;28(5):559–569.

63. Rudski LG, Lai WW, Afilalo J, et al. Guidelines for the echocardiographic assessment of the right heart in adults: a report from the American Society of Echocardiography endorsed by the European Association of Echocardiography, a registered branch of the European Society of Cardiology, and the Canadian Society of Echocardiography. *J Am Soc Echocardiogr.* 2010;23(7):685–713; quiz 786-688.

64. Smolarek D, Gruchala M, Sobiczewski W. Echocardiographic evaluation of right ventricular systolic function: the traditional and innovative approach. *Cardiol J.* 2017;24(5):563–572.

65. Kossaify A. Echocardiographic assessment of the right ventricle, from the conventional approach to speckle tracking and three-dimensional imaging, and insights into the "Right Way" to explore the forgotten chamber. *Clin Med Insights Cardiol.* 2015;9:65–75.

66. Tsyvian P, Malkin K, Artemieva O, et al. Cardiac ventricular performance in the appropriate-for-gestational age and small-for-gestational age fetus: relation to

regional cardiac non-uniformity and peripheral resistance. *Ultrasound Obstet Gynecol.* 2002;20(1):35–41.

67. Wladimiroff JW, McGhie JS. M-mode ultrasonic assessment of fetal cardiovascular dynamics. *Br J Obstet Gynaecol.* 1981;88(12):1241–1245.

68. DeVore GR, Siassi B, Platt LD. Fetal echocardiography. IV. M-mode assessment of ventricular size and contractility during the second and third trimesters of pregnancy in the normal fetus. *Am J Obstet Gynecol.* 1984;150(8):981–988.

69. St John Sutton MG, Gewitz MH, Shah B, et al. Quantitative assessment of growth and function of the cardiac chambers in the normal human fetus: a prospective longitudinal echocardiographic study. *Circulation.* 1984;69(4):645–654.

70. Sorensen KE, Borlum KG. Fetal heart function in response to short-term maternal exercise. *Br J Obstet Gynaecol.* 1986;93(4):310–313.

71. Arduini D, Rizzo G, Pennestri F, et al. Modulation of echocardiographic parameters by fetal behaviour. *Prenat Diagn.* 1987;7(3):179–187.

72. Sorensen KE, Borlum KG. Acute effects of maternal smoking on human fetal heart function. *Acta Obstet Gynecol Scand.* 1987;66(3):217–220.

73. DeVore GR, Klas B, Satou G, et al. Twenty-four segment transverse ventricular fractional shortening: a new technique to evaluate fetal cardiac function. *J Ultrasound Med.* 2018;37(5):1129–1141.

74. Luewan S, Yanase Y, Tongprasert F, et al. Fetal cardiac dimensions at 14-40 weeks' gestation obtained using cardio-STIC-M. *Ultrasound Obstet Gynecol.* 2011;37(4):416–422.

75. Hsieh YY, Chang FC, Tsai HD, et al. Longitudinal survey of fetal ventricular ejection and shortening fraction throughout pregnancy. *Ultrasound Obstet Gynecol.* 2000;16(1):46–48.

76. Veille JC, Sivakoff M, Nemeth M. Evaluation of the human fetal cardiac size and function. *Am J Perinatol.* 1990;7(1):54–59.

77. Koyanagi T, Hara K, Satoh S, et al. Relationship between heart rate and rhythm, and cardiac performance assessed in the human fetus in utero. *Int J Cardiol.* 1990;28(2):163–171.

78. Sikkel E, Klumper FJ, Oepkes D, et al. Fetal cardiac contractility before and after intrauterine transfusion. *Ultrasound Obstet Gynecol.* 2005;26(6):611–617.

79. Tedesco GD, de Souza Bezerra M, Barros FSB, et al. Fetal heart function by tricuspid annular plane systolic excursion and ventricular shortening fraction using STIC M-Mode: reference ranges and validation. *Am J Perinatol.* 2017;34(13):1354–1361.

80. Simpson JM, Cook A. Repeatability of echocardiographic measurements in the human fetus. *Ultrasound Obstet Gynecol.* 2002;20(4):332–339.

81. Mao YK, Zhao BW, Wang B. Z-Score reference ranges for angular M-mode displacement at 22-40 weeks' gestation. *Fetal Diagn Ther.* 2017;41(2):115–126.

82. Messing B, Gilboa Y, Lipschuetz M, et al. Fetal tricuspid annular plane systolic excursion (f-TAPSE): evaluation of fetal right heart systolic function with conventional M-mode ultrasound and spatiotemporal image correlation (STIC) M-mode. *Ultrasound Obstet Gynecol.* 2013;42(2):182–188.

83. Cruz-Lemini M, Crispi F, Valenzuela-Alcaraz B, et al. Value of annular M-mode displacement vs tissue Doppler velocities to assess cardiac function in intrauterine growth restriction. *Ultrasound Obstet Gynecol.* 2013;42(2):175–181.

84. DeVore GR, Klas B, Satou G, et al. Speckle tracking of the basal lateral and septal wall annular plane systolic excursion of the right and left ventricles of the fetal heart. *J Ultrasound Med.* 2019;38(5):1309–1318.

85. Gardiner HM, Pasquini L, Wolfenden J, et al. Myocardial tissue Doppler and long axis function in the fetal heart. *Int J Cardiol.* 2006;113(1):39–47.

86. Caradeux J, Martinez-Portilla RJ, Basuki TR, et al. Risk of fetal death in growth-restricted fetuses with umbilical and/or ductus venosus absent or reversed end-diastolic velocities before 34 weeks of gestation: a systematic review and meta-analysis. *Am J Obstet Gynecol.* 2018;218(2s):S774.e21–S782.e21.

87. Figueras F, Caradeux J, Crispi F, et al. Diagnosis and surveillance of late-onset fetal growth restriction. *Am J Obstet Gynecol.* 2018;218(2s):S790.e1–S802.e1.

88. Frusca T, Todros T, Lees C, et al. Outcome in early-onset fetal growth restriction is best combining computerized fetal heart rate analysis with ductus venosus Doppler: insights from the Trial of Umbilical and Fetal Flow in Europe. *Am J Obstet Gynecol.* 2018;218(2s):S783–S789.

89. Hiersch L, Melamed N. Fetal growth velocity and body proportion in the assessment of growth. *Am J Obstet Gynecol.* 2018;218(2s):S700.e1–S711.e1.

90. Khalil A, Morales-Rosello J, Khan N, et al. Is cerebroplacental ratio a marker of impaired fetal growth velocity and adverse pregnancy outcome? *Am J Obstet Gynecol.* 2017;216(6):606.e1–606.e10.

91. McCowan LM, Figueras F, Anderson NH. Evidence-based national guidelines for the management of suspected fetal growth restriction: comparison, consensus, and controversy. *Am J Obstet Gynecol.* 2018;218(2s):S855–S868.

92. Monteith C, Flood K, Mullers S, et al. Evaluation of normalization of cerebro-placental ratio as a potential predictor for adverse outcome in SGA fetuses. *Am J Obstet Gynecol.* 2017;216(3):285.e1–285.e6.

93. Paladini D, Lamberti A, Teodoro A, et al. Tissue Doppler imaging of the fetal heart. *Ultrasound Obstet Gynecol.* 2000;16(6):530–535.

94. Comas M, Crispi F, Cruz-Martinez R, et al. Tissue Doppler echocardiographic markers of cardiac dysfunction in small-for-gestational age fetuses. *Am J Obstet Gynecol.* 2011;205(1):57.e1–57.e6.

95. Comas M, Crispi F, Cruz-Martinez R, et al. Usefulness of myocardial tissue Doppler vs conventional echocardiography in the evaluation of cardiac dysfunction in early-onset intrauterine growth restriction. *Am J Obstet Gynecol.* 2010;203(1):45.e1–45.e7.

96. Comas M, Crispi F, Gomez O, et al. Gestational age- and estimated fetal weight-adjusted reference ranges for myocardial tissue Doppler indices at 24-41 weeks' gestation. *Ultrasound Obstet Gynecol.* 2011;37(1):57–64.

97. Barker PC, Houle H, Li JS, et al. Global longitudinal cardiac strain and strain rate for assessment of fetal cardiac function: novel experience with velocity vector imaging. *Echocardiography.* 2009;26(1):28–36.

98. Brooks PA, Khoo NS, Hornberger LK. Systolic and diastolic function of the fetal single left ventricle. *J Am Soc Echocardiogr.* 2014;27(9):972–977.

99. Crispi F, Bijnens B, Sepulveda-Swatson E, et al. Postsystolic shortening by myocardial deformation imaging as a sign of cardiac adaptation to pressure overload in fetal growth restriction. *Circ Cardiovasc Imaging.* 2014;7(5):781–787.

100. Di Salvo G, Russo MG, Paladini D, et al. Two-dimensional strain to assess regional left and right ventricular longitudinal function in 100 normal foetuses. *Eur J Echocardiogr.* 2008;9(6):754–756.

101. Enzensberger C, Achterberg F, Graupner O, et al. Wall-motion tracking in fetal echocardiography-Influence of frame rate on longitudinal strain analysis assessed by two-dimensional speckle tracking. *Echocardiography.* 2017;34(6):898–905.

102. Fan X, Zhou Q, Zeng S, et al. Impaired fetal myocardial deformation in intrahepatic cholestasis of pregnancy. *J Ultrasound Med.* 2014;33(7):1171–1177.

103. Ishii T, McElhinney DB, Harrild DM, et al. Circumferential and longitudinal ventricular strain in the normal human fetus. *J Am Soc Echocardiogr.* 2012;25(1):105–111.

104. Kapusta L, Mainzer G, Weiner Z, et al. Second trimester ultrasound: reference values for two-dimensional speckle tracking-derived longitudinal strain, strain rate and time to peak deformation of the fetal heart. *J Am Soc Echocardiogr.* 2012;25(12):1333–1341.

105. Matsui H, Germanakis I, Kulinskaya E, et al. Temporal and spatial performance of vector velocity imaging in the human fetal heart. *Ultrasound Obstet Gynecol.* 2011;37(2):150–157.

106. Truong UT, Sun HY, Tacy TA. Myocardial deformation in the fetal single ventricle. *J Am Soc Echocardiogr.* 2013;26(1):57–63.

107. Van Mieghem T, Giusca S, DeKoninck P, et al. Prospective assessment of fetal cardiac function with speckle tracking in healthy fetuses and recipient fetuses of twin-to-twin transfusion syndrome. *J Am Soc Echocardiogr.* 2010;23(3):301–308.

108. Zuo DM, Wang CH, Wang YH. Deformation of the left and right ventricular longitudinal myocardium in fetuses with umbilical cord around neck. *Chin Med J.* 2012;125(9):1608–1613.

109. Tei C, Dujardin KS, Hodge DO, et al. Doppler index combining systolic and diastolic myocardial performance: clinical value in cardiac amyloidosis. *J Am Coll Cardiol.* 1996;28(3):658–664.

110. Tei C, Ling LH, Hodge DO, et al. New index of combined systolic and diastolic myocardial performance: a simple and reproducible measure of cardiac function—a study in normals and dilated cardiomyopathy. *J Cardiol.* 1995;26(6):357–366.

111. Browne VA, Stiffel VM, Pearce WJ, et al. Activator calcium and myocardial contractility in fetal sheep exposed to long-term high-altitude hypoxia. *Am J Physiol.* 1997;272(3 pt 2):H1196–H1204.

112. Tei C, Nishimura RA, Seward JB, et al. Noninvasive Doppler-derived myocardial performance index: correlation with simultaneous measurements of cardiac catheterization measurements. *J Am Soc Echocardiogr.* 1997;10(2):169–178.

113. Tsutsumi T, Ishii M, Eto G, et al. Serial evaluation for myocardial performance in fetuses and neonates using a new Doppler index. *Pediatr Int.* 1999;41(6):722–727.

114. Friedman D, Buyon J, Kim M, et al. Fetal cardiac function assessed by Doppler myocardial performance index (Tei Index). *Ultrasound Obstet Gynecol.* 2003;21(1):33–36.

115. Hernandez-Andrade E, Lopez-Tenorio J, Figueroa-Diesel H, et al. A modified myocardial performance (Tei) index based on the use of valve clicks improves reproducibility of fetal left cardiac function assessment. *Ultrasound Obstet Gynecol.* 2005;26(3):227–232.

116. Hernandez-Andrade E, Benavides-Serralde JA, Cruz-Martinez R, et al. Evaluation of conventional Doppler fetal cardiac function parameters: E/A ratios, outflow tracts, and myocardial performance index. *Fetal Diagn Ther.* 2012;32(1–2):22–29.

117. Eidem BW, Edwards JM, Cetta F. Quantitative assessment of fetal ventricular function: establishing normal values of the myocardial performance index in the fetus. *Echocardiography.* 2001;18(1):9–13.

118. Falkensammer CB, Paul J, Huhta JC. Fetal congestive heart failure: correlation of Tei-index and Cardiovascular-score. *J Perinat Med.* 2001;29(5):390–398.

119. Chen Q, Sun XF, Liu HJ. Assessment of myocardial performance in fetuses by using Tei index. *Zhonghua Fu Chan Ke Za Zhi.* 2006;41(6):387–390 [in Chinese].

120. Wong ML, Wong WH, Cheung YF. Fetal myocardial performance in pregnancies complicated by gestational impaired glucose tolerance. *Ultrasound Obstet Gynecol.* 2007;29(4):395–400.

121. Russell NE, Foley M, Kinsley BT, et al. Effect of pregestational diabetes mellitus on fetal cardiac function and structure. *Am J Obstet Gynecol.* 2008;199(3):312.e1–312.e7.

122. Romiti A, Caforio L, Mappa I, et al. P12.09. Fetal cardiac function assessed by myocardial performance index in normal pregnancy. *Ultrasound Obstet Gynecol.* 2010;36:214.

123. Clur SA, Oude Rengerink K, Mol BW, et al. Fetal cardiac function between 11 and 35 weeks' gestation and nuchal translucency thickness. *Ultrasound Obstet Gynecol.* 2011;37(1):48–56.

124. Hamela-Olkowska A, Szymkiewicz-Dangel J. Quantitative assessment of the right and the left ventricular function using pulsed Doppler myocardial performance index in normal fetuses at 18 to 40 weeks of gestation. *Ginekol Pol.* 2011;82(2):108–113 [in Polish].

125. Ghawi H, Gendi S, Mallula K, et al. Fetal left and right ventricle myocardial performance index: defining normal values for the second and third trimesters-single tertiary center experience. *Pediatr Cardiol.* 2013;34(8):1808–1815.

126. Waggoner AD, Bierig SM. Tissue Doppler imaging: a useful echocardiographic method for the cardiac sonographer to assess systolic and diastolic ventricular function. *J Am Soc Echocardiogr.* 2001;14(12):1143–1152.

127. Price DJ, Wallbridge DR, Stewart MJ. Tissue Doppler imaging: current and potential clinical applications. *Heart.* 2000;84 suppl 2:II11–II18.

128. Ganame J, Claus P, Uyttebroeck A, et al. Myocardial dysfunction late after low-dose anthracycline treatment in asymptomatic pediatric patients. *J Am Soc Echocardiogr.* 2007;20(12):1351–1358.

129. Arduini D, Rizzo G, Romanini C. *Fetal Cardiac Output Measurements in Normal and Pathologic States.* New York, NY: Raven Press; 1995.

130. Rizzo G, Arduini D. Fetal cardiac function in intrauterine growth retardation. *Am J Obstet Gynecol.* 1991;165(4 pt 1):876–882.

131. Copel JA, Grannum PA, Green JJ, et al. Fetal cardiac output in the isoimmunized pregnancy: a pulsed Doppler-echocardiographic study of patients undergoing intravascular intrauterine transfusion. *Am J Obstet Gynecol.* 1989;161(2):361–365.

132. De Smedt MC, Visser GH, Meijboom EJ. Fetal cardiac output estimated by Doppler echocardiography during mid- and late gestation. *Am J cardiol.* 1987;60(4):338–342.

133. Allan LD, Chita SK, Al-Ghazali W, et al. Doppler echocardiographic evaluation of the normal human fetal heart. *Br Heart J.* 1987;57(6):528–533.

134. Mielke G, Benda N. Cardiac output and central distribution of blood flow in the human fetus. *Circulation.* 2001;103(12):1662–1668.

135. Kenny JF, Plappert T, Doubilet P, et al. Changes in intracardiac blood flow velocities and right and left ventricular stroke volumes with gestational age in the normal human fetus: a prospective Doppler echocardiographic study. *Circulation.* 1986;74(6):1208–1216.

136. Kiserud T, Ebbing C, Kessler J, et al. Fetal cardiac output, distribution to the placenta and impact of placental compromise. *Ultrasound Obstet Gynecol.* 2006;28(2):126–136.

137. Molina FS, Faro C, Sotiriadis A, et al. Heart stroke volume and cardiac output by four-dimensional ultrasound in normal fetuses. *Ultrasound Obstet Gynecol.* 2008;32(2):181–187.

138. DeKoninck P, Steenhaut P, Van Mieghem T, et al. Comparison of Doppler-based and three-dimensional methods for fetal cardiac output measurement. *Fetal Diagn Ther.* 2012;32(1–2):72–78.

139. Fernandez Pineda L, Tamariz-Martel Moreno A, Maitre Azcarate MJ, et al. Contribution of Doppler atrioventricular flow waves to ventricular filling in the human fetus. *Pediatr Cardiol.* 2000;21(5):422–428.

140. Harada K, Rice MJ, Shiota T, et al. Gestational age- and growth-related alterations in fetal right and left ventricular diastolic filling patterns. *Am J Cardiol.* 1997;79(2):173–177.

141. Carceller-Blanchard AM, Fouron JC. Determinants of the Doppler flow velocity profile through the mitral valve of the human fetus. *Br Heart J.* 1993;70(5):457–460.

142. Pacileo G, Paladini D, Pisacane C, et al. Role of changing loading conditions on atrioventricular flow velocity patterns in normal human fetuses. *Am J Cardiol.* 1994;73(13):991–993.

143. Reed KL, Sahn DJ, Scagnelli S, et al. Doppler echocardiographic studies of diastolic function in the human fetal heart: changes during gestation. *J Am Coll Cardiol.* 1986;8(2):391–395.

144. Tulzer G, Khowsathit P, Gudmundsson S, et al. Diastolic function of the fetal heart during second and third trimester: a prospective longitudinal Doppler-echocardiographic study. *Eur J Pediatr.* 1994;153(3):151–154.

145. Weiner Z, Efrat Z, Zimmer EZ, et al. Fetal atrioventricular blood flow throughout gestation. *Am J Cardiol.* 1997;80(5):658–662.

146. Barker DJ, Osmond C, Simmonds SJ, et al. The relation of small head circumference and thinness at birth to death from cardiovascular disease in adult life. *BMJ.* 1993;306(6875):422–426.

147. Crispi F, Bijnens B, Figueras F, et al. Fetal growth restriction results in remodeled and less efficient hearts in children. *Circulation.* 2010;121(22):2427–2436.

148. Doctor BA, O'Riordan MA, Kirchner HL, et al. Perinatal correlates and neonatal outcomes of small for gestational age infants born at term gestation. *Am J Obstet Gynecol.* 2001;185(3):652–659.

149. Eixarch E, Meler E, Iraola A, et al. Neurodevelopmental outcome in 2-year-old infants who were small-for-gestational age term fetuses with cerebral blood flow redistribution. *Ultrasound Obstet Gynecol.* 2008;32(7):894–899.

150. Figueras F, Oros D, Cruz-Martinez R, et al. Neurobehavior in term, small-for-gestational age infants with normal placental function. *Pediatrics.* 2009;124(5):e934–e941.

151. Illa M, Coloma JL, Eixarch E, et al. Growth deficit in term small-for-gestational fetuses with normal umbilical artery Doppler is associated with adverse outcome. *J Perinat Med.* 2009;37(1):48–52.

152. Girsen A, Ala-Kopsala M, Makikallio K, et al. Cardiovascular hemodynamics and umbilical artery N-terminal peptide of proB-type natriuretic peptide in human fetuses with growth restriction. *Ultrasound Obstet Gynecol.* 2007;29(3):296–303.

153. Larsen LU, Sloth E, Petersen OB, et al. Systolic myocardial velocity alterations in the growth-restricted fetus with cerebroplacental redistribution. *Ultrasound Obstet Gynecol.* 2009;34(1):62–67.

154. Naujorks AA, Zielinsky P, Beltrame PA, et al. Myocardial tissue Doppler assessment of diastolic function in the growth-restricted fetus. *Ultrasound Obstet Gynecol.* 2009;34(1):68–73.

155. Crispi F, Hernandez-Andrade E, Pelsers MM, et al. Cardiac dysfunction and cell damage across clinical stages of severity in growth-restricted fetuses. *Am J Obstet Gynecol.* 2008;199(3):254.e1–254.e8.

156. Bijnens B, Claus P, Weidemann F, et al. Investigating cardiac function using motion and deformation analysis in the setting of coronary artery disease. *Circulation.* 2007;116(21):2453–2464.

157. Hecher K, Campbell S, Doyle P, et al. Assessment of fetal compromise by Doppler ultrasound investigation of the fetal circulation. Arterial, intracardiac, and venous blood flow velocity studies. *Circulation.* 1995;91(1):129–138.

158. Makikallio K, Vuolteenaho O, Jouppila P, et al. Ultrasonographic and biochemical markers of human fetal cardiac dysfunction in placental insufficiency. *Circulation.* 2002;105(17):2058–2063.

159. Figueras F, Puerto B, Martinez JM, et al. Cardiac function monitoring of fetuses with growth restriction. *Eur J Obstet Gynecol Reprod Biol.* 2003;110(2):159–163.

160. Bhorat IE, Bagratee JS, Pillay M, et al. Determination of the myocardial performance index in deteriorating grades of intrauterine growth restriction and its link to adverse outcomes. *Prenat Diagn.* 2015;35(3):266–273.

161. Bhorat IE, Bagratee JS, Reddy T. Assessment of fetal myocardial performance in severe early onset pre-eclampsia (EO-PET) with and without intrauterine growth restriction across deteriorating stages of placental vascular resistance and links to adverse outcomes. *Eur J Obstet Gynecol Reprod Biol.* 2017;210:325–333.

162. Cruz-Lemini M, Crispi F, Van Mieghem T, et al. Risk of perinatal death in early-onset intrauterine growth restriction according to gestational age and cardiovascular Doppler indices: a multicenter study. *Fetal Diagn Ther.* 2012;32(1–2):116–122.

163. Unterscheider J, Daly S, Geary MP, et al. Predictable progressive Doppler deterioration in IUGR: does it really exist? *Am J Obstet Gynecol.* 2013;209(6):539.e1–539.e7.

164. Henry A, Alphonse J, Tynan D, et al. Fetal myocardial performance index in assessment and management of small-for-gestational-age fetus: a cohort and nested case-control study. *Ultrasound Obstet Gynecol.* 2018;51(2):225–235.

165. Hatem MA, Zielinsky P, Hatem DM, et al. Assessment of diastolic ventricular function in fetuses of diabetic mothers using tissue Doppler. *Cardiol Young.* 2008;18(3):297–302.

166. Bui YK, Kipps AK, Brook MM, et al. Tissue Doppler is more sensitive and reproducible than spectral pulsed-wave Doppler for fetal right ventricle myocardial performance index determination in normal and diabetic pregnancies. *J Am Soc Echocardiogr.* 2013;26(5):507–514.

167. Pilania R, Sikka P, Rohit MK, et al. Fetal cardiodynamics by echocardiography in insulin dependent maternal diabetes and its correlation with pregnancy outcome. *J Clin Diagn Res.* 2016;10(7):QC01–QC04.

168. Atiq M, Ikram A, Hussain BM, et al. Assessment of cardiac function in fetuses of gestational diabetic mothers during the second trimester. *Pediatr Cardiol.* 2017;38(5):941–945.

169. Sanhal CY, Daglar HK, Kara O, et al. Assessment of fetal myocardial performance index in women with pregestational and gestational diabetes mellitus. *J Obstet Gynaecol Res.* 2017;43(1):65–72.

170. Miranda JO, Cerqueira RJ, Ramalho C, et al. Fetal cardiac function in maternal diabetes: a conventional and speckle-tracking echocardiographic study. *J Am Soc Echocardiogr.* 2018;31(3):333–341.

171. Ho D, Wang J, Homann Y, et al. Use of the myocardial performance index in decreased fetal movement assessment: a case-control study. *Fetal Diagn Ther.* 2018;43(3):208–217.

172. Alsolai AA, Bligh LN, Greer RM, et al. Assessment of left ventricular function using the Myocardial Performance Index in term fetuses that develop intrapartum compromise. *J Matern Fetal Neonatal Med.* 2017:1–7.

173. Alsolai AA, Bligh LN, Greer RM, et al. Relationship of prelabor fetal cardiac function with intrapartum fetal compromise and neonatal status at term. *Ultrasound Obstet Gynecol.* 2018;51(6):799–805.

174. Alsolai AA, Bligh LN, Greer RM, et al. Prelabour myocardial deformation and cardiac output in fetuses that develop intrapartum compromise at term: a prospective observational study. *J Matern Fetal Neonatal Med.* 2018:1–9.

175. Gezer C, Ekin A, Ozeren M, et al. Can the myocardial performance index be used as a new predictive factor for a poor prognosis in fetuses with idiopathic polyhydramnios? *J Ultrasound Med.* 2016;35(12):2649–2657.

176. Delabaere A, Leduc F, Reboul Q, et al. Prediction of neonatal outcome of TTTS by fetal heart and Doppler ultrasound parameters before and after laser treatment. *Prenat Diagn.* 2016;36(13):1199–1205.

177. Kapusta L, Mainzer G, Weiner Z, et al. Changes in fetal left and right ventricular strain mechanics during normal pregnancy. *J Am Soc Echocardiogr.* 2013;26(10):1193–1200.

178. Figueroa-Diesel H, Silva MC, Illanes S, et al. OP20.06. Evaluation of the modified myocardial performance index in pregnancies complicated with gestational and pre-gestational diabetes. *Ultrasound Obstet Gynecol.* 2007;30:524.

179. Hernandez-Andrade E, Figueroa-Diesel H, Kottman C, et al. Gestational-age-adjusted reference values for the modified myocardial performance index for evaluation of fetal left cardiac function. *Ultrasound Obstet Gynecol.* 2007;29(3):321–325.

180. Acharya G, Pavlovic M, Ewing L, et al. Comparison between pulsed-wave Doppler- and tissue Doppler-derived Tei indices in fetuses with and without congenital heart disease. *Ultrasound Obstet Gynecol.* 2008;31(4):406–411.

181. Van Mieghem T, Gucciardo L, Lewi P, et al. Validation of the fetal myocardial performance index in the second and third trimesters of gestation. *Ultrasound Obstet Gynecol.* 2009;33(1):58–63.

182. Api O, Emeksiz MB, Api M, et al. Modified myocardial performance index for evaluation of fetal cardiac function in pre-eclampsia. *Ultrasound Obstet Gynecol.* 2009;33(1):51–57.

183. Wood DC, Bisulli M, Ashraf S, et al. OC06.06. Fetal myocardial performance (Tei) index and left ventricular shortening fraction (LVSF). *Ultrasound Obstet Gynecol.* 2009;34:11.

184. Rizzo G, Arduini D, Romanini C. Doppler echocardiographic assessment of fetal cardiac function. *Ultrasound Obstet Gynecol.* 1992;2(6):434–445.

7 Three-Dimensional Ultrasonography

Luis F. Gonçalves

INTRODUCTION

Three-dimensional ultrasonography (3DUS) enhances the examination of anatomical structures and congenital anomalies by providing access to cross-sectional planes that are either difficult or impossible to obtain by two-dimensional ultrasonography (2DUS). The spatial relationships between abnormal findings and adjacent anatomical structures can be more easily appreciated through multiplanar and 3D rendered imaging. Thus, 3DUS may improve the understanding of a complex pathology initially seen by 2DUS. It also frequently facilitates the communication of abnormal findings to patients, family members, and referring providers.[1] Showing patients a realistic 3D image of the fetal face (Fig. 7.1) or other body parts such as the hands and feet when feasible does not substantially increase the examination time and has been shown to increase parental bonding.[2,3] The capability of obtaining multiple 3D images over time and depicting fetal movement is known as four-dimensional ultrasonography (4DUS), whereby the fourth dimension is the temporal dimension or time. 4DUS expands the diagnostic capabilities of 3DUS by making it possible to evaluate complex fetal movements such as facial expressions,[4–6] behavioral patterns in normal and high-risk pregnancies,[7–11] fetal response to stimuli such as music and pain,[12,13] and 4D evaluation of the beating fetal heart.[14–23]

In this chapter, we review the basic principles of 3DUS, provide tips for successful volume acquisition, and describe the most commonly used techniques to explore 3DUS volume datasets, including 4DUS datasets of the fetal heart. Practical examples are provided along with a brief discussion of the complementary roles of 2DUS, 3DUS, fetal magnetic resonance imaging (MRI), and low-dose computed tomography (3D CT) in the prenatal diagnosis of congenital anomalies when applicable.

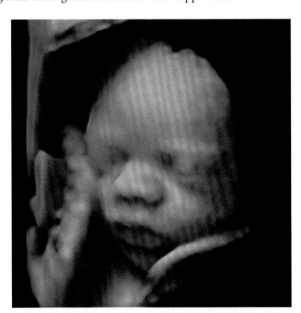

FIGURE 7.1: Three-dimensional rendered image of the fetal face at 29 weeks.

PRINCIPLES OF 3D ULTRASOUND IMAGING

3DUS can be performed in several ways, the most common of which is to generate a 3DUS volume dataset departing from a sequence of 2DUS planar images acquired with mechanical or electronic matrix array probes. A less commonly used technique relies on acquisition of a series of 2DUS images using a regular ultrasound transducer that may or not be attached to a position-sensing device, followed by 3D reconstruction in the ultrasound equipment or external workstations.

Mechanical 3DUS Transducers

Mechanical volumetric probes (Fig. 7.2) are designed to have a 2DUS array mounted on a mechanical wobble contained within a compartment in the transducer head.[24] Once the examiner identifies the structure of interest, the transducer is activated by pressing a button on the ultrasound machine and volume acquisition starts. While the transducer remains stationary in the patient's abdomen,

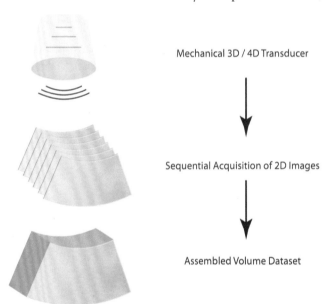

Mechanical 3D / 4D Transducer

Sequential Acquisition of 2D Images

Assembled Volume Dataset

FIGURE 7.2: Scanners equipped with mechanical 3D transducers generate 3D volume datasets by automatically acquiring a sequence of 2D images through a region of interest (ROI) selected by the examiner. The images are reassembled into a final volume dataset that can be explored using postprocessing tools. The examiner can reslice the volume in virtually any plane, either to obtain rendered 3D images or to perform volumetric measurements. Most mechanical 3D transducers are also capable of four-dimensional ultrasonography (4DUS) imaging, whereby multiple volume datasets are continuously acquired and quickly updated on the screen. With this technology, motion (temporal dimension) is added to the three spatial dimensions, allowing real-time visualization of 3D images. The primary limitation of 4DUS is that spatial resolution is often sacrificed at the expense of temporal resolution. (Reproduced by permission from Springer: Gonçalves LF, Joshi A, Mody S, et al. Volume US of the urinary tract in pediatric patients—a pilot study. *Pediatr Radiol.* 2011;41(8):1047–1056. Copyright © 2011 Springer Nature.)

the mechanical wobble drives the array to sweep the region of interest (ROI) at a predetermined interval, sweep angle, and speed. The series of 2DUS images acquired by this process are combined into a volume dataset that can be resliced into any desired plane or segmented using 3D rendering tools.

Matrix Array Transducers

Matrix array transducers contain thousands of transducer elements arranged as a 2D matrix array in the transducer surface (Fig. 7.3). The face of the transducer has either a rectangular or a square shape. Matrix array transducers can scan one line at a time (akin to the mechanical probes described previously), two simultaneous planes (which may be orthogonal to each other or not), or obtain a focused volumetric area of the body by simultaneously activating multiple transducer elements at the same time. Thus, matrix array transducers are capable of real-time volumetric imaging and are well suited for cardiac and obstetric imaging applications.[20,25,26]

Tips for Successful Volume Acquisition

High-Quality 2DUS Is Essential
Regardless of the choice of ultrasound equipment and type of volumetric probe, 3DUS is an extension of 2DUS technology. 3DUS does not compensate for poor image quality caused by common problems such as patient obesity, oligohydramnios, or poor scanning technique. It also does not overcome artifacts that are inherent to the physics of ultrasonography such as, for example, bone shadowing. Thus, attention to detail in gray scale gain, dynamic range, frame rate, focus, magnification, and color Doppler settings, as well as optimization of acoustic windows while scanning are necessary for high-quality 3DUS.

Fetal Movement
Another issue that requires attention during volume acquisition is fetal movement. 3DUS technology has evolved over time to minimize motion-related artifacts. This is accomplished by (1) allowing users to select faster acquisition speeds while still maintaining acceptable image resolution, (2) the development of 4DUS technology for mechanical probes, and (3) real-time volumetric imaging using matrix array probes. Still, excessive fetal movement can be a significant problem, not only because it can degrade image quality but also because it generates artifacts that affect image interpretation.[27,28] Our anecdotal experience is that fetuses tend to move less during the early part of the examination, before the maternal abdomen is manipulated by the act of scanning. Therefore, we recommend beginning the examination with a 3DUS probe in order to take advantage of potentially good acoustic windows and less fetal movement that may be present during the early portion of the examination. Since volume datasets can be manipulated after the scan has ended, the examiner may switch back to a regular 2DUS probe after volume acquisition is accomplished. Another practical tip is to pay careful attention to gentle scanning, avoiding excessive transducer movement and pressure, in an effort to prevent initiation of fetal movements. Once 2DUS imaging has been optimized and a good acoustic window to the structure of interest is present, volume acquisition should start without delay. The examiner should avoid the common misconception that a perfect 2D view (e.g., a perfect facial profile or a perfect four-chamber view) is a prerequisite for high-quality 3DUS imaging. Although ideal, this is not necessary, since once a high-quality volume dataset is acquired, the standard anatomical planes can be obtained offline by image postprocessing. In fact, we propose that all that is needed for a good volume acquisition is a good acoustic window to the structure of interest in the absence of fetal movement. For example, if the target is the fetal face, all that is needed is that the face is oriented toward the transducer, that a fluid interface is present between the fetal face and the transducer, and that the fetus is not moving too much. If the target is the fetal heart, all that is required is that the fetal chest faces the examiner and that no limbs that may cause shadowing are interposed between the fetal chest and the transducer.

Postprocessing

Once the volume dataset is acquired, image postprocessing can take place at the scanner or at a dedicated computer workstation. In the next few sections, we review common approaches to explore 3DUS volume datasets.

Multiplanar Display
The multiplanar display is a simple but practical method to examine 3DUS volume datasets.[24,29] This type of display typically shows three images, one representing the original plane of acquisition and two additional orthogonal planes. A reference "dot" or "cross" marks the intersection of the three orthogonal planes. As the user moves the reference "dot" or "cross" with a mouse or another electronic pointing device, any structure present in the volume dataset can be simultaneously visualized in the other two planes. Figure 7.4 illustrates the basic principles of the multiplanar display method.

Multiple Slice Imaging
An alternative display method presents multiple slices of the volume dataset as a series of images in a single screen.[30,31] This method, variously known as tomographic ultrasound imaging (TUI), Multislice, or iSlice, depending on the manufacturer, permits simultaneous display of several consecutive cross-sectional planes and may facilitate interpretation and/or teaching. Figure 7.5

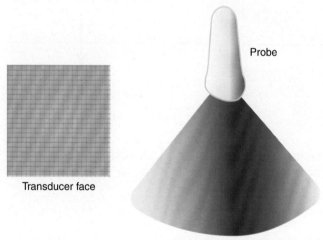

Probe

Transducer face

3D ultrasound "pyramid"

FIGURE 7.3: The "transducer face" diagram illustrates the typical configuration of a matrix array transducer, with thousands of elements arranged as a 2D matrix array, with each tiny square representing a single element. All elements, a portion of them, or two simultaneous lines can be activated simultaneously to produce real-time 3D images. The diagram "3D ultrasound pyramid" illustrates the pyramid of ultrasound that is emitted when all elements are fired simultaneously. The elements can also be fired in sequence, one line at a time, to produce volumetric data in a manner similar to the mechanical probe illustrated in Figure 7.2, just much faster.

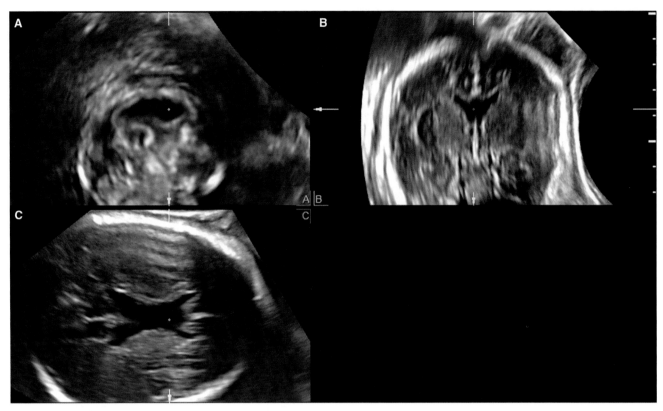

FIGURE 7.4: Multiplanar display of a volume dataset of the fetal brain acquired transabdominally using axial sections through the fetal head. The volume was manipulated so that the sagittal plane is shown in **A**, the coronal plane in **B**, and the original plane of acquisition (the axial plane) in **C**. The original plane of acquisition has the best resolution. The reference *dot* represents the intersection of the three orthogonal planes and, in this example, shows the typical imaging features of absence of the cavum septi pellucidi in the coronal **(A)**, sagittal **(B)**, and axial **(C)** planes.

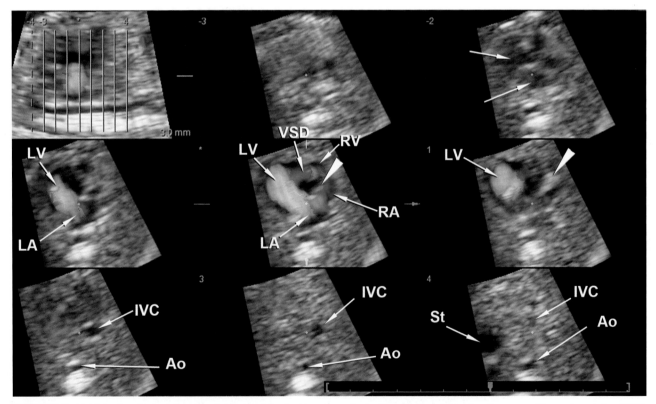

FIGURE 7.5: Multiple slice display of a volume dataset of the fetal heart acquired with color Doppler and spatiotemporal image correlation (STIC). The left upper panel represents the scout sagittal view, with eight consecutive lines representing eight axial planes from the superior mediastinum to the upper abdomen shown in the next eight panels. The *arrowhead* points to the atretic tricuspid valve. *Ao*, abdominal aorta; *IVC*, inferior vena cava; *LA*, left atrium; *LV*, left ventricle; *RA*, right atrium; *RV*, right ventricle; *VSD*, ventricular septal defect: *St*, stomach.

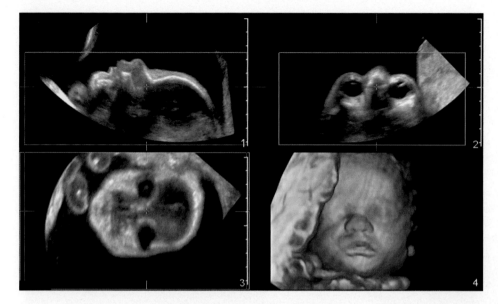

FIGURE 7.6: Multiplanar and volume rendered images of a normal fetal face acquired from a 2DUS facial profile view. **Panels 1–3** show the sagittal, axial, and coronal orthogonal planes, respectively. A generous amount of amniotic fluid is interposed between the transducer and the skin surface of the fetal face. The *boxes* in **panels 1–3**, define the region of interest (ROI). The direction of view (or projection path) is determined by the user and, in this example, is given by the *yellow line*. Therefore, the first echo, brighter than amniotic fluid (the threshold level) along the projection path, is displayed as a pixel in **panel 4** in order to form the rendered view of the fetal face.

shows features of tricuspid atresia with ventricular septal defect (VSD) using the multiple slice display method.

3D Rendering

The term 3D rendering refers to the display method whereby a 3D object is displayed on a 2D screen using 3D photorealistic effects. Images of the fetal face using surface rendering technology have captured the attention of imaging specialists and parents alike, boosting the initial interest in 3DUS for obstetrical imaging.[2,24,29,32]

Surface Rendering: As the name implies, the surface rendering method is used when the intention is to display a 3D image of the surface of an object. This method works by displaying the first hyperechogenic voxel along the projection path of a volume dataset whose brightness is higher than a threshold determined by the user. The typical example is the rendered image of the fetal face (Fig. 7.6).

High-Definition Live Rendering: High-definition live rendering (also known as HDLive, TrueVue, or Realistic Vue depending on US manufacturer) is a technology introduced in 2011 that provides realistic 3D fetal images akin to those seen only by direct visualization with a fetoscope (Fig. 7.7).[33–35] The technology uses a virtual light source whose position can be adjusted by the examiner. The software calculates the speed of sound propagation through structures present along the virtual light path. Selective illumination is produced as the virtual light is reflected, scattered, or attenuated through the different tissues along the propagation path. The images obtained are more natural when compared to traditional surface rendering methods and depth perception is increased. As the virtual light moves toward the front, back, or lateral sides of the volume dataset, different effects are obtained.[36,37]

An additional translucent rendering mode (Silhouette, GlassVue, or CrystalVue depending on the ultrasound manufacturer) that allows inner structures containing fluid to be seen through the outer surface has been developed.[37,38] Figure 7.8A–C shows a volume dataset of an

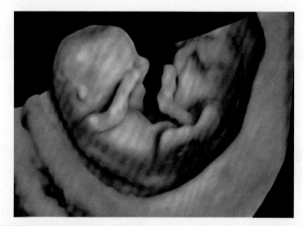

FIGURE 7.7: Three-dimensional rendered view of an 11-week fetus using HDLive.

early monochorionic-monoamniotic twin pregnancy which was postprocessed with realistic rendering and translucent modes. In Figure 7.8A, the light source is positioned in front of the volume dataset (Fig. 7.8A) favoring visualization of the anterior surface of the embryos, yolk sac, vitelline ducts, and umbilical cords. In Figure 7.8B, the light source has been moved to behind the volume dataset, producing a translucent effect. In Figure 7.8C, the silhouette mode was applied, allowing visualization of the second twin through the body of the first twin. Note the exquisite detail that facilitates understanding of the commonly seen feature of monochorionic-monoamniotic twins: a single yolk sac. The images show that the single yolk sac is actually shared and connected to the two embryos by separate vitelline ducts. Figure 7.9 shows rendered images of the stomach and duodenum in a case of duodenal atresia.

Maximum Intensity Projection: In this rendering method, the voxel with the highest brightness signal along the projection path is displayed on the screen.[29,39–41] This is typically used in

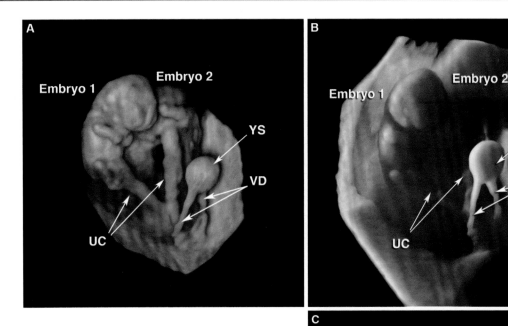

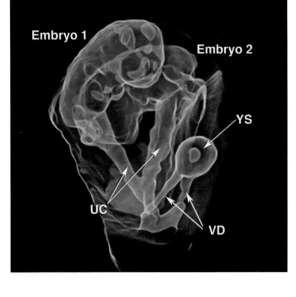

FIGURE 7.8: Monochorionic-monoamniotic twins at 10 weeks. The embryos share a single yolk sac *(YS)* connected to each embryo through a separate vitelline duct *(VD)*. Note the two separate umbilical cords *(UC)* converging to a common origin from the placenta. **A:** HDLive rendering with light positioned in the anterior aspect of the volume dataset favors visualization of the embryonic surfaces. **B:** HDLive rendering with light positioning posterior to the volume dataset produces a translucent effect. **C:** HDLive with silhouette rendering gives a translucent appearance to all visualized structures and allows visualization of embryo 2 projecting behind embryo 1.

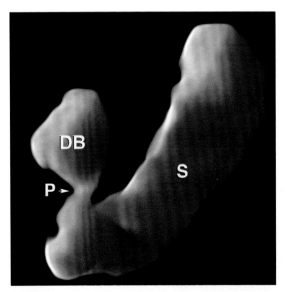

FIGURE 7.9: HDLive three-dimensional rendered view of the stomach *(S)*, pylorus *(P)*, and dilated duodenal bulb *(DB)* in a case of duodenal atresia.

fetal imaging to visualize osseous structures, as illustrated in Figure 7.10.

Minimum Intensity Projection: The minimum intensity projection method, as the name implies, displays the voxel with the lowest brightness signal along the projection path.[29,42] This method is useful to display rendered images of fluid-filled structures. Figure 7.11 shows a rendered view of jejunal atresia in the coronal plane.

Average Intensity Projection: Average intensity projection averages the brightness of voxels along the projection path which are then displayed as a pixel on a 2D screen. This method is useful to obtain rendered views of fetal limbs that simultaneously show the bones and soft tissues. Figure 7.12 shows the same fetal arm, forearm, and hand displayed using just the multiplanar display or volume contrast imaging (VCI, see detailed description later) with a slice thickness of 20 mm using the average intensity projection method.

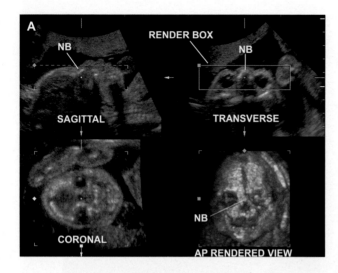

FIGURE 7.10: Normally developed nasal bones in a fetus with no abnormalities at 23 weeks of gestation. Multiplanar and anteroposterior rendered views of the fetal skull using the maximum intensity projection mode. The *render box* delimits the region of interest (ROI), and the *green line* determines the direction of view for reconstruction of the 3D image. The paired nasal bones *(NB)* are visualized as a single structure fused in the midline. (From Gonçalves LF, Espinoza J, Lee W, et al. Phenotypic characteristics of absent and hypoplastic nasal bones in fetuses with Down syndrome: description by 3-dimensional ultrasonography and clinical significance. *J Ultrasound Med.* 2004;23(12):1619–1627. Copyright © 2016 by the American Institute of Ultrasound in Medicine. Reprinted by permission of John Wiley & Sons, Inc.)

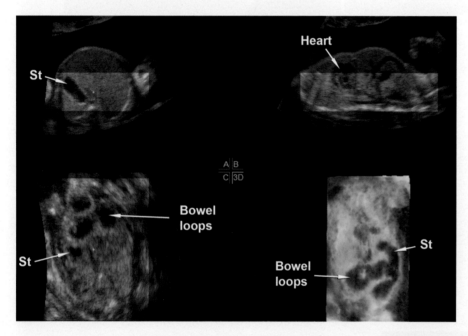

FIGURE 7.11: Multiplanar display of a volume dataset of a fetus with jejunal atresia. **A–C** show axial, sagittal, and coronal views of the fetal abdomen, respectively. The dilated loops of the bowel are seen in the coronal plane. **Panel 3D** shows a rendered view of the abdomen using the minimum intensity projection mode. In this mode, the voxels with the lowest brightness signal along the projection path are preferentially displayed. In this case, a portion of the heart, the stomach *(St)*, and the dilated bowel loops are the structures with the lowest brightness signal. They are simultaneously displayed in a single coronal view, allowing the examiner to compare the relative positions of the bowel loops to the stomach, to determine that there are only a few dilated loops, and to note that the dilated bowel ends as a blind pouch in the left lower quadrant.

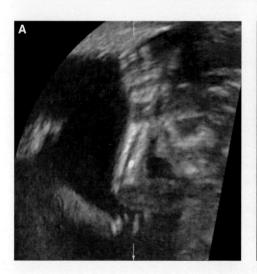

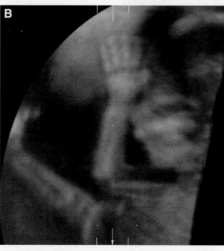

FIGURE 7.12: A: Single view of a fetal arm, forearm, and hand displayed using the multiplanar method. **B:** Volume contrast imaging (VCI) rendered view of the same arm using a 20-mm-thick slab rendered using the average intensity projection method. Note that all fingers and the humerus are better seen on **B** when compared with **A**, with better demonstration of the soft tissues as well.

Inversion Mode: Inversion mode is a rendering method that inverts the grayscale of the voxels with the lowest brightness signal along the projection path. It is used to obtain rendered images of fluid-filled structures.[43–49] Figure 7.13 shows the same case of jejunal atresia previously rendered with minimum intensity projection, now displayed using inversion mode. The fluid-filled structures appear bright, allowing a more realistic depiction of the anatomical relationships between visualized structures.

Volume Contrast Imaging: VCI is a rendering method that combines multiple consecutive frames into a thick slab that can be displayed using any of the rendering methods described previously. Besides the example already provided in Figure 7-12, Figure 7-14 illustrates the improved tissue contrast resolution that can be obtained with this technology.

Postprocessing in the Ultrasound Equipment versus External 3D Workstations: Image postprocessing is an integral part of volumetric imaging and excellent results can only be expected once the examiner becomes comfortable with both volume acquisition and postprocessing. All ultrasound manufacturers provide volume manipulation and rendering capabilities directly in the ultrasound system. However, these tasks can be time consuming and it is not practical to tie the ultrasound equipment for this purpose as it may need to be used to scan other patients. Thus, the availability of computer workstations with 3D rendering software is important to maintain patient throughput. 3DUS education is also facilitated through manipulation of stored volume datasets in external 3D workstations.

FOUR-DIMENSIONAL ULTRASONOGRAPHY

4DUS is a term that describes the addition of a temporal dimension to the three spatial dimensions of a 3DUS volume dataset.[50] Therefore, 4DUS allows sequential display of multiple volumes as they are acquired and hence the capability of capturing motion with volumetric imaging. The technology allows examiners to look not only at gross fetal movements but also at more subtle characteristics such as facial expressions (Fig. 7.15).[4,11,12,51–55] Several investigators have applied this technology to study fetal behavioral states *in utero*, including the effect of adverse maternal and fetal disorders, drug exposure, as well as the effects of external stimuli such as music and touch on the maternal abdomen.[7–9,12,13,56–61]

4DUS of the Fetal Heart

4DUS of the fetal heart is possible with the use of spatiotemporal image correlation (STIC) or real-time volumetric matrix array technology.[14–20,22,23,26,44,62–68] STIC is a rendering algorithm that was developed specifically for fetal echocardiography applications. The algorithm essentially performs retrospective gating of the fetal heart rate to the acquired volume dataset.[15] The end result is that the multiple volumes of the fetal heart obtained in sequence through a single automated sweep of the chest are reshuffled according to the phase of the cardiac cycle in which they were acquired. Provided that there is not excessive fetal motion during acquisition, excellent volume datasets of the fetal heart can be acquired, manipulated, and rendered using any of the methods described in the section "Postprocessing." Figure 7.16 shows multiplanar display and rendered views of the

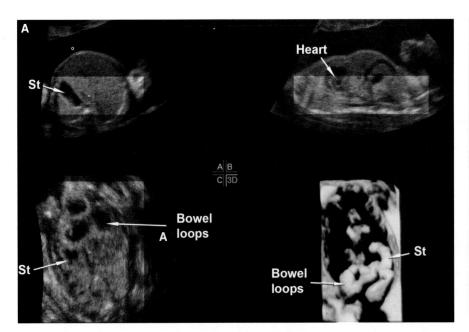
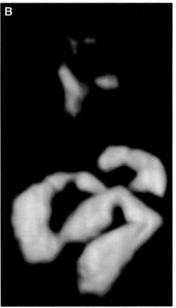

FIGURE 7.13: A: Multiplanar display of a volume dataset of a fetus with jejunal atresia. **A–C** show axial, sagittal, and coronal views, respectively, of the fetal abdomen. The dilated loops of bowel are seen in the coronal plane. **Panel 3D** shows a rendered view of the abdomen using the inversion mode method. The method is analogous to the minimum intensity projection mode, only that the voxels with the lowest brightness along the projection path are displayed with the grayscale inverted. **B:** In this image, further segmentation of the volume dataset was performed to display only the stomach *(St)*, the duodenum, and the proximal jejunum. Part of the fetal heart is included only as a point of reference.

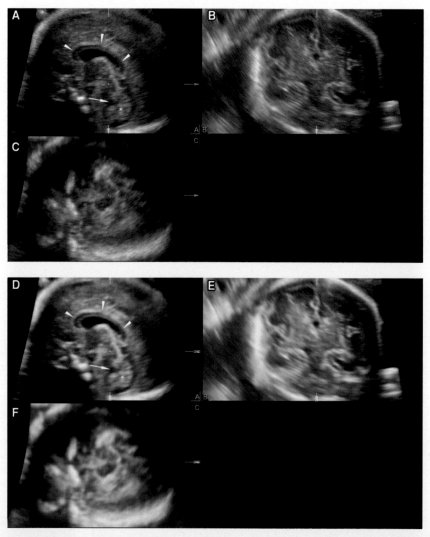

FIGURE 7.14: Multiplanar display of a volume dataset of the fetal brain obtained using a sagittal acquisition through the anterior fontanelle without **(A–C)** and with volume contrast imaging (VCI) **(D–F)**. The corpus callosum (*arrowheads*), cisterna magna, fourth ventricle (*arrow*), and cerebellar vermis (*star*) are well depicted in both images; however, contrast resolution is better with VCI.

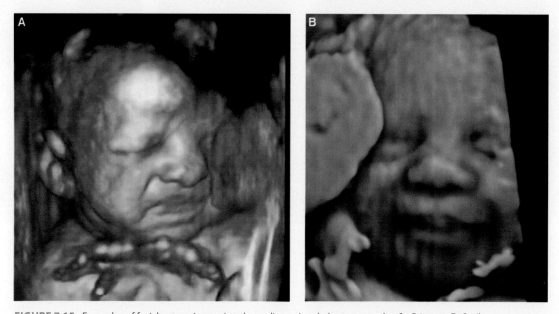

FIGURE 7.15: Examples of facial expressions using three-dimensional ultrasonography. **A:** Grimace. **B:** Smile.

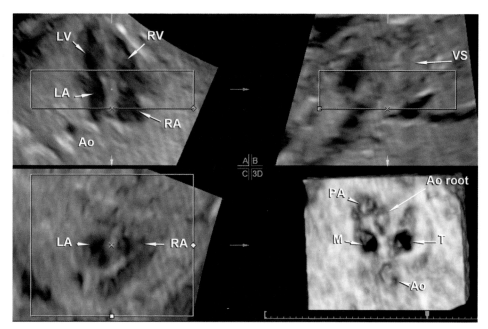

FIGURE 7.16: Volume dataset of the fetal heart acquired with spatiotemporal image correlation (STIC). **A** shows a four-chamber view of the fetal heart, **B** shows an orthogonal sagittal section through the ventricular septum *(VS)* displayed "*en face*," and **C** shows a coronal section at the level of the atrioventricular *(AV)* valves. The rendered view of the *AV* valves is seen in **panel 3D**. Please note that the *green line* that determines the projection path is positioned within the atrial chambers **(panels A and B)** and, therefore, the rendered view is seen as if the examiner is looking at the *AV* valve orifices from the atrial chambers toward the ventricles. *Ao*, descending aorta; *Ao root*, aortic root; *LA*, left atrium; *LV*, left ventricle; *M*, mitral valve orifice; *PA*, pulmonary artery; *RA*, right atrium; *RV*, right ventricle; *T*, tricuspid valve orifice; *VS*, ventricular septum.

atrioventricular valve orifices of a normal fetal heart acquired with a transverse sweep of the fetal chest.

EXAMPLES OF NORMAL AND ABNORMAL FETAL ANATOMY BY VOLUMETRIC IMAGING

In this section, we present a series of images that illustrate examples of normal and abnormal anatomical structures by 3DUS and 4DUS.

Fetal Head

Figure 7.17 shows the sagittal corpus callosum reconstructed from a volume dataset originally acquired using a coronal sweep through the anterior fontanelle. This method is also suited for examination of the neonatal head using volumetric probes.[69–71] Contrast the findings of this normal image with that of a fetus with absent cavum septi pellucidi, shown in Figure 7.4. The same volume dataset is shown in Figure 7.18, now displayed using the multiplanar method with VCI set to a slice thickness of

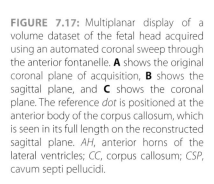

FIGURE 7.17: Multiplanar display of a volume dataset of the fetal head acquired using an automated coronal sweep through the anterior fontanelle. **A** shows the original coronal plane of acquisition, **B** shows the sagittal plane, and **C** shows the coronal plane. The reference *dot* is positioned at the anterior body of the corpus callosum, which is seen in its full length on the reconstructed sagittal plane. *AH*, anterior horns of the lateral ventricles; *CC*, corpus callosum; *CSP*, cavum septi pellucidi.

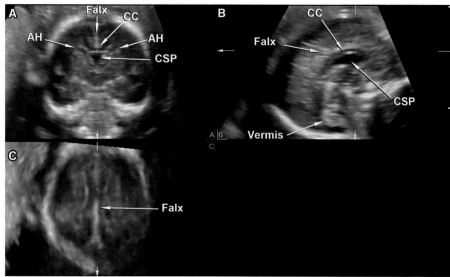

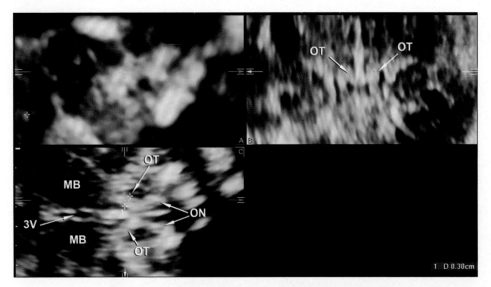

FIGURE 7.18: This image was produced from exactly the same volume dataset of the fetus with absent cavum septi pellucidi shown in Figure 7.17. The view is now magnified and displayed using volume contrast imaging (VCI) with a slice thickness of 3 mm. The sagittal, coronal, and axial orthogonal planes at the level of the suprasellar cistern are shown in **panels A–C.** The optic tracts and optic nerves can be clearly seen. *MB,* mid brain; *ON,* optic nerves; *OT,* optic tracts; *3V,* third ventricle.

3 mm to show the optic nerves and optic tracts at the level of the suprasellar cistern. The optic tracts and nerves can be successfully imaged using 3DUS[72–74] and optic tract measurements in the case of absent cavum septi pellucidi may help identify those fetuses at higher risk for septo-optic dysplasia.[73]

Fetal Face and Calvarium

3DUS is well suited for the evaluation of facial anomalies, with several studies documenting additional diagnostic information or better diagnostic accuracy when compared with 2DUS. 3DUS is useful for the evaluation of cranial sutures,[39,75–77] facial bones,[78–87] as well as cleft lip and palate.[88–99]

Figures 7.1, 7.5, 7.10, and 7.15A and B illustrate the capabilities of 3DUS to depict normal facial structures and demonstrate facial expression. Figure 7.19 shows examples of normal as well as hypoplastic and absent nasal bones in fetuses with trisomy 21.[84,85] Figure 7.20A shows widened cranial sutures in a fetus with cleidocranial dysostosis.[100] The same fetus had pseudoarthrosis of the right clavicle, as shown in Figure 7.20B.

Evaluation of Orofacial Clefts

Orofacial clefts are common birth defects, being second in prevalence only to trisomy 21, according to the Centers of Disease Control of the United States.[101] The most common types of orofacial clefts are isolated cleft lip, cleft lip with cleft palate, and isolated cleft palate. Median clefts are much less common and are usually associated with chromosomal and structural brain anomalies. The adjusted United States prevalence of cleft lip with or without cleft palate between 2004 and 2006 was estimated as 1 in 1,574 live births, and that of

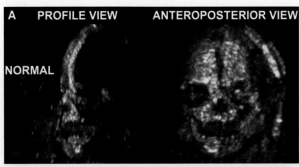

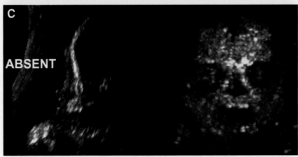

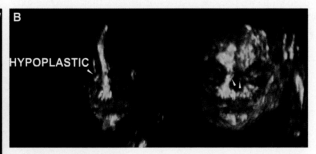

FIGURE 7.19: A: Normally developed nasal bones in a fetus with no abnormalities at 23 weeks of gestation. **B:** Delayed ossification or hypoplastic: Two small ossification centers can be seen away from the midline in the frontal projection and can be seen as a single hyperechogenic linear structure (owing to superimposition) in the sagittal projection. **C:** Absent nasal bones: No ossified nasal bones are present either in the frontal or in the sagittal projection. (From Gonçalves LF, Espinoza J, Lee W, et al. Phenotypic characteristics of absent and hypoplastic nasal bones in fetuses with Down syndrome: description by 3-dimensional ultrasonography and clinical significance. *J Ultrasound Med.* 2004;23(12):1619–1627. Copyright © 2016 by the American Institute of Ultrasound in Medicine. Reprinted by permission of John Wiley & Sons, Inc.)

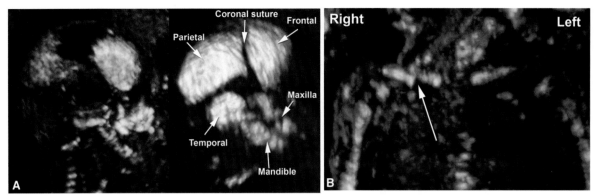

FIGURE 7.20: **A:** Three-dimensional (3D) rendering of the fetal skull at 18 + 3 weeks of gestation using the maximum intensity projection mode demonstrates widening of the coronal suture, absence of the squamous portion of the temporal bone, and absence of the nasal bones. Adjacent 3D image of a normal fetal skull at 18 + 3 weeks for comparison. **B:** 3D rendering of the fetal shoulders using maximum intensity projection. The *arrow* points to the pseudoarthrosis of the right clavicle. (From Soto E, Richani K, Gonçalves LF, et al. Three-dimensional ultrasound in the prenatal diagnosis of cleidocranial dysplasia associated with B-cell immunodeficiency. *Ultrasound Obstet Gynecol.* 2006;27(5):574–579. Copyright © 2006 ISUOG. Reprinted by permission of John Wiley & Sons, Inc.)

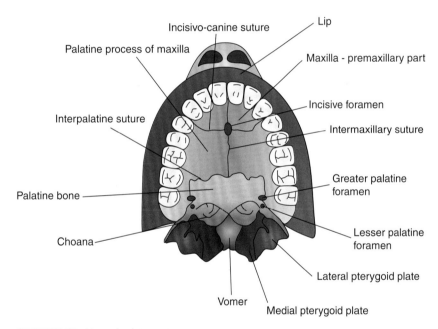

FIGURE 7.21: Normal palate anatomy.

isolated cleft palate as 1 in 940 live births. The prevalence in Asian and Native American populations was higher (as high as 1 in 500), whereas African-derived populations had a lower prevalence, estimated as 1 in 2,500. Approximately 70% of cases of cleft lip and palate and 50% of cases of isolated cleft palate were nonsyndromic. The rest were associated with a wide range of malformation syndromes, chromosomal abnormalities, and teratogen exposure. For a detailed review of the genetics and environmental factors associated with cleft lip and palate, the reader is referred to the excellent review article of Dixon et al.[102]

A diagram illustrating the anatomy of the palate is presented in Figure 7.21. Facial clefts can be unilateral, bilateral, or midline. When clefts involve the lip only, they are called isolated cleft lips or labioalveolar clefts. Clefts can extend to involve the primary palate (alveolus and premaxillary part of the maxilla, anterior to the incisive foramen) and/or the secondary palate (palatine process of the maxillary bones and palatine bone) (Fig. 7.22). In a large prospective ultrasound screening study from the Netherlands that included 35,000 low-risk and 2,800 high-risk patients, 40% of the clefts involved the lip and palate, 29% were isolated cleft lip, and 27% were isolated cleft palate. Median and atypical clefts were observed in only two fetuses. Sixty-one percent of the clefts were unilateral.

Figure 7.23 shows the technique to properly acquire a volume dataset of the hard palate.[90] Figure 7.24 shows how poor volume acquisition leads to shadowing artifact posterior to the tooth buds and, therefore, limited diagnostic value for evaluation of the secondary palate.

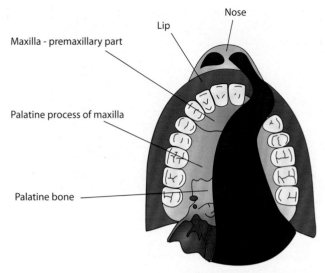

FIGURE 7.22: Diagram illustrating a unilateral cleft lip and palate involving the nose, lip, primary palate (anterior to the incisive foramen), and secondary palate.

Figure 7.25 shows an example of a rendered view of a unilateral cleft lip and Figures 7.26 and 7.27 show extension of the cleft through the primary and secondary palates.

Several investigators have compared the diagnostic performance of 2DUS versus 3DUS for correct classification of the type and extent of orofacial clefts. Collectively, the evidence supports 3DUS as a more accurate method, largely because of better characterization of the extent of hard palate involvement using multiplanar display and/or rendering techniques.[78,88–90,92,93,95–97,99,103–107] In one of the comparative studies, Johnson et al.[93] showed that 2DUS overestimated the severity of the defect in 41.9% (13/31) of the cases. Of interest, a study performed with 3DUS in the first trimester reported sensitivities of 100% and 86% for the diagnosis of clefts of the primary and secondary palate, with a 0.9% false-positive rate.[91]

Pitfalls: 3DUS rendered images of the fetal face provide realistic views of orofacial clefts that may be easier to communicate to parents and surgeons involved in prenatal counseling. However, one must be careful in interpreting 3D rendered images alone and take into consideration the possibility of rendering artifacts

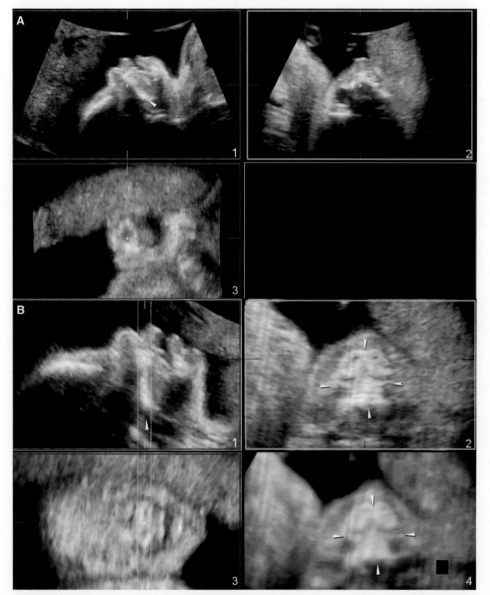

FIGURE 7.23: A: Ideal position of the fetal face for volume acquisition of the secondary palate. Note that the angle between the palate *(arrowhead)* and the transducer is approximately 45° **(panel 1)**. **B:** Manipulation of the volume dataset to show the hard palate in its entirety. In **panel 1**, the volume is rotated around the *z*-axis so that the hard palate *(arrowhead)* is oriented at a 0° angle. In **panel 2**, the full extent of the hard palate can be seen in the axial plane *(four arrowheads)*. **Panel 3** shows the anterior maxillary tooth buds. **Panel 4** shows a rendered view of the hard palate *(four arrowheads)* using the maximum intensity projection method.

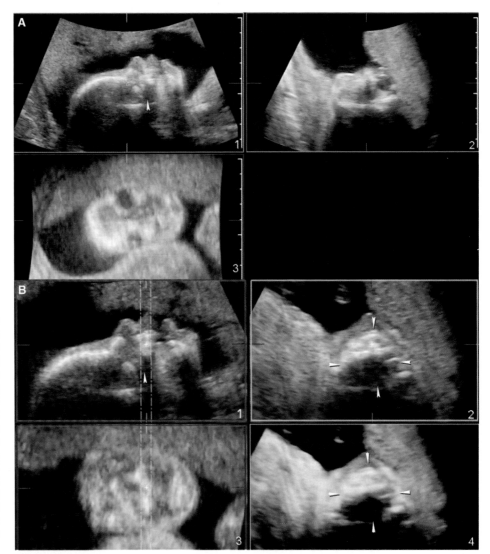

FIGURE 7.24: Contrast the volume acquisition in this figure with that in **Figure 7.23**. **A:** The facial profile is oriented in such a way that the hard palate is oriented parallel (0°) to the transducer and, therefore, a strong acoustic shadow is present posterior to the tooth buds (**panel 1**, *arrowhead*). **B:** As the shadowing artifact is related to poor volume acquisition, it cannot be corrected by postprocessing techniques. The same shadow seen in **panel 1** *(arrowhead)* is seen posterior to the tooth buds in **panel 2** and also in the maximum intensity projection rendered image displayed in **panel 4**. The anterior maxillary tooth buds can be well seen in **panel 3**.

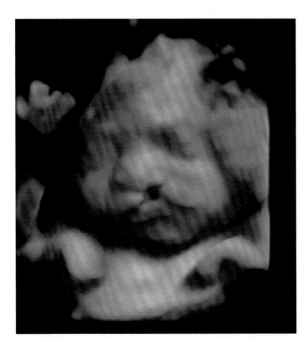

FIGURE 7.25: Three-dimensional rendered view of the fetal face. Unilateral cleft lip is seen on the left side.

related to motion and shadowing that may create artificial clefts.[108–111] In addition, ultrasound has traditionally not performed well for the evaluation of the soft palate, except for a series from Germany that reported on a new sign ("equal sign") for evaluation of the soft palate and uvula. In that study, adequate visualization of the soft palate and uvula was possible in 85.3% and 90.7% of 667 consecutively examined fetuses.[112] Given that assessment of the palate may not be possible in all cases secondary to bone shadowing or persistently unfavorable fetal position, fetal MRI should be considered whenever visualization of the lip and or palate is suboptimal by 2DUS and/or 3DUS. Several studies have demonstrated good consistency of MRI for evaluation of the fetal palate as well as higher diagnostic accuracy and better classification of orofacial clefts when directly compared to ultrasound.[113–120] Figure 7.28 illustrates a case of high-arched palate in a fetus with multiple other abnormalities secondary to arthrogryposis that could not be visualized by either 2DUS or 3DUS.

Fetal Spine

3DUS is a useful adjunct to 2DUS for the examination of the fetal spine. Besides its role in the characterization of segmentation abnormalities and abnormal curvature of the spine, 3DUS has

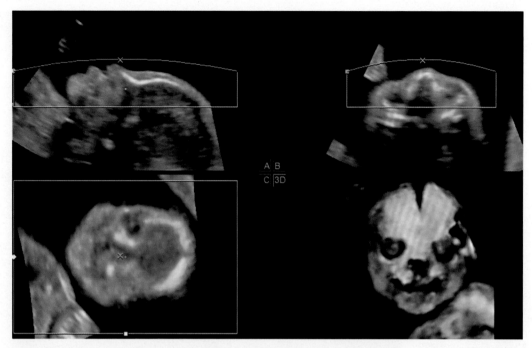

FIGURE 7.26: Multiplanar display and rendered views of the fetal face using the maximum intensity projection method to highlight the skull. A unilateral cleft palate can be seen through the left alveolar ridge.

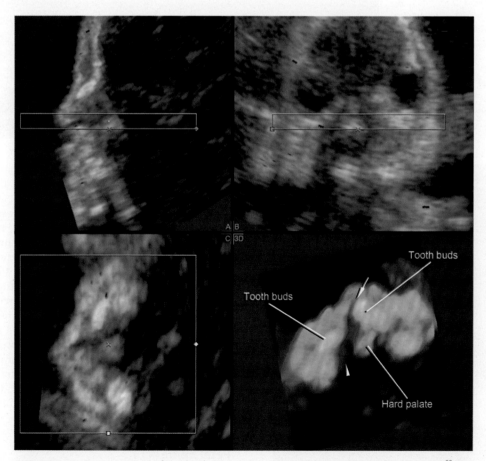

FIGURE 7.27: Reconstruction of the hard palate using the technique proposed by Platt et al.[99] The rendered view using a combination of surface and maximum intensity projection modes shows that the unilateral cleft extends through the primary and secondary palates. *Arrow*, cleft of the primary palate; *arrowhead*, extension to the secondary palate.

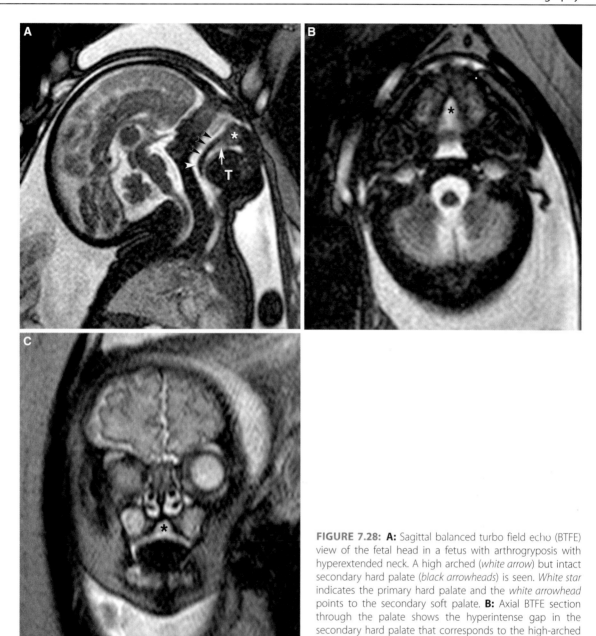

FIGURE 7.28: A: Sagittal balanced turbo field echo (BTFE) view of the fetal head in a fetus with arthrogryposis with hyperextended neck. A high arched (*white arrow*) but intact secondary hard palate (*black arrowheads*) is seen. *White star* indicates the primary hard palate and the *white arrowhead* points to the secondary soft palate. **B:** Axial BTFE section through the palate shows the hyperintense gap in the secondary hard palate that corresponds to the high-arched palate on **A** and **C. C:** Inverted U-shaped gap (*black star*) in the secondary hard palate corresponding to the high-arched palate illustrated on **A** and **B**. T, tongue.

proved accurate with one vertebral segment to determine the level of defect in cases of spinal dysraphism (Fig. 7.29).[41,121–128]

Skeletal Dysplasias

The ability of 3DUS to obtain rendered images of osseous structures makes it a useful adjunctive modality in the diagnostic workup of skeletal dysplasias (see Figs. 7.10, 7.12A, 7.19A–C, 7.20A and B, and 7.29) and isolated musculoskeletal disorders (Figs. 7.30 and 7.31). Several case reports have been published highlighting potential benefits of 3DUS for the visualization of specific features of skeletal abnormalities, for example, enhanced visualization of femoral and tibial bowing in a case of platyspondylic lethal chondrodysplasia, hypoplastic scapulae in campomelic dysplasia, improved characterization of frontal

bossing in thanatophoric dysplasia, demonstration of caudal narrowing of the interpedicular distance of the lumbar spine in achondroplasia, improved visualization of epiphyseal stippling in chondrodysplasia punctata, better characterization of the abnormal spine and ribs in spondylocostal dysostosis, visualization of genu recurvatum in Larsen syndrome, pseudoarthrosis of the clavicle in cleidocranial dysostosis, characteristic hand and feet of Grebe dysplasia (Fig. 7.32), and midface hypoplasia in chondrodysplasia punctata and 3M syndrome.[129–137] Few studies, however, have directly compared 3DUS versus 2DUS for the prenatal diagnosis of skeletal dysplasias, with the exception of the study of Ruano et al.,[138] who showed higher visualization rates for skeletal structures by 3DUS (77.1%) when compared with 2DUS (51.4%), although

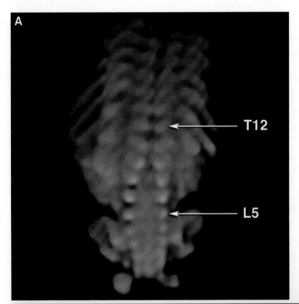

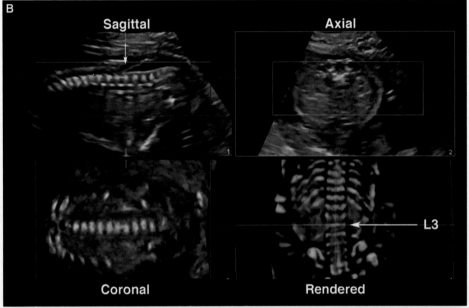

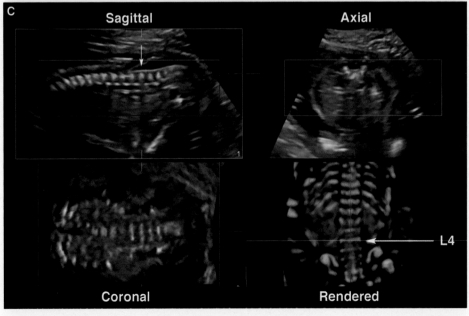

FIGURE 7.29: A: Rendered view of the fetal spine of a fetus with myelomeningocele. T12 is identified by the presence of the 12th rib and L5 is identified counting up from S5. Splaying of the posterior processes of the vertebrae begins at L3. **B:** Multiplanar display and rendered views of the fetal spine in the same fetus shows that the bony defect begins at the level of L3 but, at this level, there is only partial splaying of the posterior laminae and the defect is still covered by soft tissues. **C:** The posterior elements are clearly splayed at the level of L4 and, at this level, there is communication between the contents of the spinal canal and amniotic fluid.

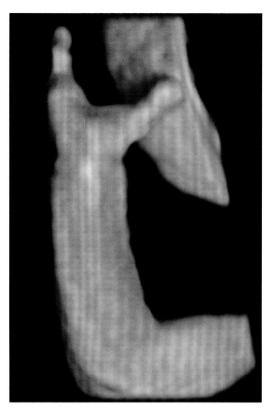

FIGURE 7.30: Three-dimensional rendered view of the fetal hand showing missing central digits in a fetus with ectrodactyly.

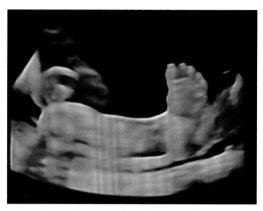

FIGURE 7.31: Three-dimensional rendered view of the fetal leg and feet showing clubfoot.

both showed inferior visualization rates when compared with computed tomography with 3D reconstructions (94.1%).

Congenital Heart Disease

Accurate prenatal diagnosis of congenital heart disease (CHD) is an important goal of prenatal care. Besides affording the parents appropriate and timely counseling, advanced knowledge of ductal-dependent anomalies allows planned delivery at institutions equipped to handle such cases, both from medical as well as surgical standpoints. Indeed, prenatal diagnosis of CHD, including hypoplastic left heart syndrome, D-transposition of the great arteries (D-TGA), and coarctation of the aorta, is associated with improved perinatal morbidity and mortality. Prenatal diagnosis of D-TGA has also been found in one study to be associated with improved long-term neurocognitive outcomes when compared with children diagnosed in the neonatal period.[139–142]

Volumetric Imaging of the Fetal Heart

As briefly described earlier in this chapter, volumetric imaging of the fetal heart can be performed using STIC or real-time matrix array technology.[15,18–20,143,144] Once volume datasets are acquired, the same postprocessing methods that are used to evaluate other fetal organs can be applied to the examination

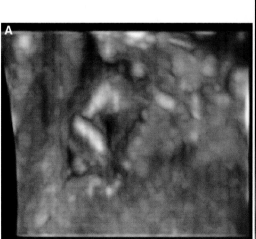

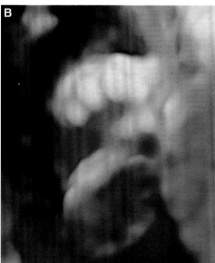

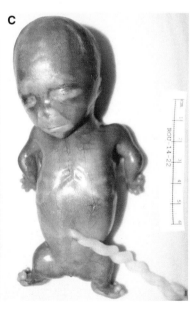

FIGURE 7.32: A: Three-dimensional rendered view of the fetal arm using maximum intensity projection shows shortening and bowing of the humerus and only one shortened and bowed bone in the forearm which turned out to be the radius postnatally. **B:** 3D rendered view of the fetal foot showing globular appearance of the digits which are characteristic of Grebe dysplasia. **C:** Frontal photograph of the fetal body shows the excellent correlation between the 3D rendered view of the fetal toes and the postmortem appearance. (Reproduced by permission from Springer: Goncalves LF, Berger JA, Macknis JK, et al. Grebe dysplasia—prenatal diagnosis based on rendered 3-D ultrasound images of the fetal limbs. *Pediatr Radiol.* 2017;47(1):108–112. Copyright © 2017 Springer Nature.)

of the fetal heart. Because of the complexity of cardiac anatomy and the fact that standardized planes of section are recommended for the examination of the fetal heart, it is natural that several techniques emerged to extract these standardized planes from volume datasets.[18,19,30,31,43,44,145–148] The techniques that we most commonly use in our practice are illustrated in the following sections, along with examples of their application to cases of CHD.

Scrolling through the Volume: Dataset Evaluation of the volume dataset in its original plane of acquisition is an intuitive and easy way to examine the heart. We usually begin our examination with volume datasets acquired through transverse automated sweeps through the fetal chest, since these include an axial section of the upper abdomen, the four-chamber view, the five-chamber view, three-vessel view, and the three-vessel and trachea view, as originally proposed by Yagel et al. using 2DUS (Fig. 7.33).[149]

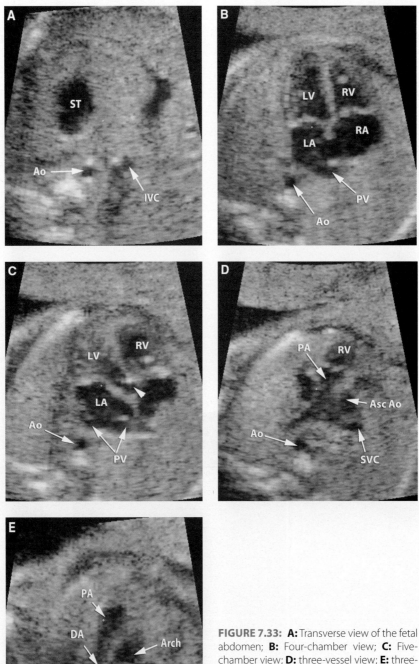

FIGURE 7.33: A: Transverse view of the fetal abdomen; **B:** Four-chamber view; **C:** Five-chamber view; **D:** three-vessel view; **E:** three-vessel and trachea view. *Ao*, descending aorta; *Asc Ao*, ascending aorta; *DA*, ductus arteriosus; *IVC*, inferior vena cava; *LA*, left atrium; *LV*, left ventricle; *PA*, pulmonary artery; *PV*, pulmonary veins; *RA*, right atrium; *RV*, right ventricle; *Short arrow*: aortic root; *ST*, stomach; *SVC*, superior vena cava; *T*, trachea.

Multiple Slice Method: An alternative way to simultaneously display multiple equally spaced planes of section in the same screen is to use the multiple slice method.[30,31] This method automatically slices the volume dataset, and with minimal adjustment, one is usually able to demonstrate the five axial planes of section shown in Figure 7.33 in the majority of cases. Figure 7.34 illustrates the use of this method in a volume dataset of a normal fetal heart and Figure 7.35 shows all planes of section needed to make the diagnosis of hypoplastic right heart due to pulmonary atresia in a single image. A case of tricuspid atresia with VSD is illustrated in Figure 7.5.

Three-Step Technique for Evaluation of the Outflow Tracts: This technique was designed specifically to demonstrate, in the same image, the long-axis view of the left ventricular outflow tract and the short-axis view of the right ventricular outflow tract (Fig. 7.36).[19] This technique has been validated both from the standpoint of reproducibility and clinical applicability.[150,151] It is particularly useful to diagnose conotruncal anomalies, including transposition of the great arteries and conutruncal defects with overriding of the aorta (e.g., tetralogy of Fallot, pulmonary atresia with VSD, truncus arteriosus, and double outlet right ventricle).[151,152] Figure 7.37 shows a case of transposition of the great arteries demonstrated with this technique.

Rendered Images
Cardiac Valves: Rendered images of the cardiac valves can be easily obtained, as illustrated in Figure 7.38, which shows the technique to obtain an *en face* rendered views of the single atrioventricular valve in a case of complete atrioventricular canal. Figure 7.39 shows a comparative example of a rendered *en face* view of a normal atrioventricular valve, a closed single atrioventricular valve, and an open single atrioventricular valve in a case of complete atrioventricular canal. Figure 7.40 show rendered views of the aortic valve in diastole and systole.

Great Vessels: Rendered views of the great vessels, and, for that matter, also of the venous return to the fetal heart can be obtained using several techniques, including inversion mode, color or power Doppler imaging, and B-flow imaging. For volume datasets acquired with color Doppler, the settings should be preadjusted to provide the highest frame rate possible. Failure to do so will result in poor temporal resolution of the volume dataset. Color Doppler optimization includes narrowing the field of view, using a single focal zone adjusted to the depth of the structure of interest, and narrowing the color Doppler ROI. Figures 7.41 to 7.43 illustrate normal outflow tracts displayed using color Doppler, inversion mode, and B-flow imaging.[43,44,64] Figure 7.44 shows the application of 3D rendered reformats to the prenatal diagnosis of transposition of the great arteries.[152]

4D Fetal Echocardiography in Clinical Practice
Among the potential benefits of 4D fetal echocardiography are the ability to obtain anatomical planes not available during 2DUS real-time examination, three-dimensional rendered images that facilitate understanding of complex anatomy, the ability to perform measurements such as mitral and tricuspid annular systolic excursion, as well as volumetric measurements that allow quantification of ventricular size and function.[23] However, questions that are frequently asked before embarking on the clinical use of this technology include how often can volume datasets of sufficient diagnostic quality be obtained and does 3DUS really help compared to conventional 2DUS technology.

A few studies have addressed the feasibility of 4D fetal echocardiography in clinical practice. The first study included 148 high-risk fetuses examined by two experienced sonographers with no more than four acquisition attempts allowed during the examination. Successful volume dataset acquisition was possible in 76% of the cases, with 65% of these volumes deemed to have enough quality for diagnostic purposes.

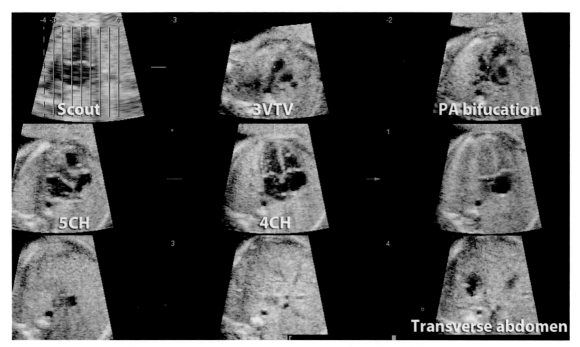

FIGURE 7.34: Multiple slice images of a normal fetal heart applied to the same volume dataset as in Figure 7.33. The "scout view" is sagittal and located in the *left upper corner* of the image. The *vertical lines* represent the planes displayed in the other eight images, from the superior mediastinum to the upper abdomen. Note that most of the planes seen in Figure 2.27 are automatically and simultaneously displayed, except the three-vessel view. *3VTV,* three-vessel and trachea view; *4CH,* four-chamber view; *5CH,* five-chamber view; *PA,* pulmonary artery.

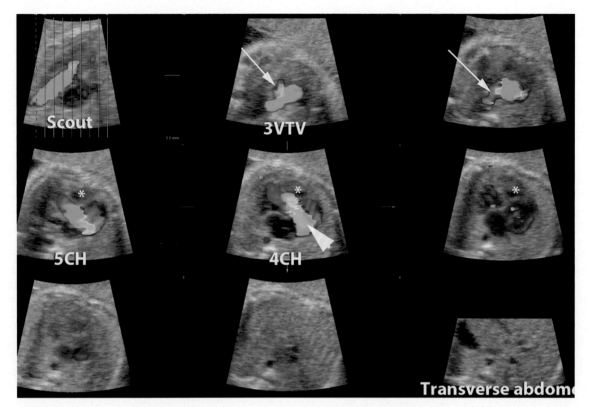

FIGURE 7.35: Volume dataset of an abnormal heart acquired with color Doppler imaging. Tomographic ultrasound imaging sliced from the superior mediastinum to the upper abdomen as in Figure 7.34. Note the hypoplastic right ventricle *(asterisk)*, the severe tricuspid regurgitation *(arrowhead)*, and the retrograde perfusion of the pulmonary artery through the ductus arteriosus *(arrow)* in this case of pulmonary atresia with intact ventricular septum. *3VTV*, three-vessel and trachea view; *4CH*, four-chamber view; *5CH*, five-chamber view.

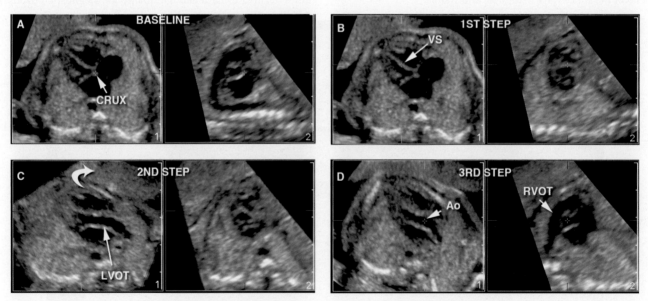

FIGURE 7.36: Simultaneous visualization of the left ventricular outflow tract and right ventricular outflow tract, obtained with the "three-step" technique.[14] Only the original transverse plane of acquisition *(1)* and the reconstructed sagittal plane *(2)* for each step are shown. **Baseline: A** shows the four-chamber view with the fetal spine down and oriented horizontally on *2* (as if the fetus was lying on a flat surface). The reference crosshair is at the crux of the heart. **Step 1:** In **A**, the crosshair has been moved to the middle of the ventricular septum *(VS)*. **Step 2:** Once the crosshair in "anchored" in the middle of the septum, rotating the volume dataset around the *y*-axis *(curved arrow)* will "open up" the septum, showing its normal continuity with the anterior wall of the aorta *(Ao)*. In the same image, the posterior wall of the aorta continues with the anterior leaflet of the mitral valve. Thus, this second step displays the long-axis view of the left ventricular outflow tract *(LVOT)*. **Step 3:** The crosshair is moved to the region of the *Ao*, and the short-axis view of the right ventricular outflow tract *(RVOT)* can be seen on the reconstructed sagittal plane. (Reprinted with permission of Anderson Publishing Ltd. from Gonçalves LF, Espinoza J, Bronsteen R. 3D-4D fetal echocardiography. *Appl Radiol*. 2012;3:31–43. Copyright © 2012 Anderson Publishing Ltd.)

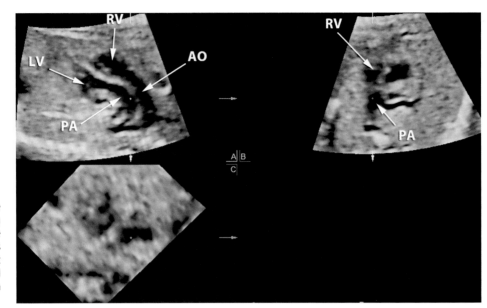

FIGURE 7.37: D-Transposition of the great arteries demonstrated using the three-step technique. Note that the bifurcating pulmonary artery *(PA)* arises from the left ventricle *(LV)*. The vessel that leaves the right ventricle *(RV)* in parallel with the pulmonary artery is the aorta arising transposed. *Ao*, Aorta.

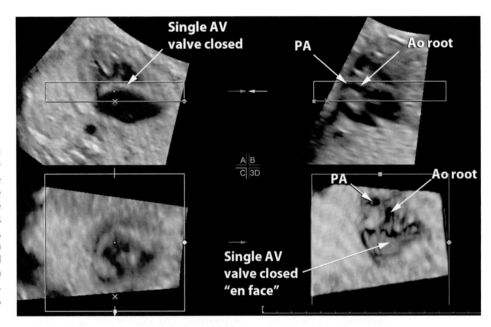

FIGURE 7.38: Multiplanar **(A–C)** and rendered **(3D)** views of the atrioventricular valve seen "*en face*" in a case of complete atrioventricular canal. Note the size of the region of interest (ROI) box as well as the direction of the projection path, which is determined by the *green line*. In this case, the closed single atrioventricular valve in a case of complete atrioventricular canal is seen as if the examiner is looking from the atrial chambers toward the ventricles. *Ao root*, aortic root; *AV*, atrioventricular; *PA*, pulmonary artery.

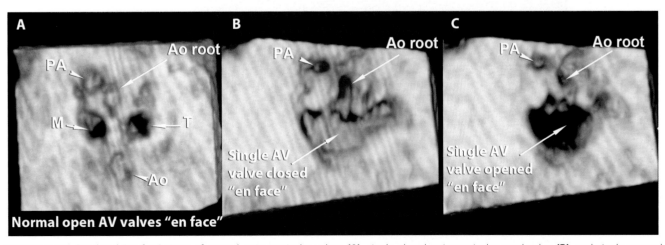

FIGURE 7.39: Rendered "*en face*" views of normal atrioventricular valves **(A)**, single closed atrioventricular canal valve **(B)**, and single opened atrioventricular valve **(C)**. *Ao root*, aortic root; *AV*, atrioventricular; *M*, mitral valve orifice; *PA*, pulmonary artery; *T*, trachea.

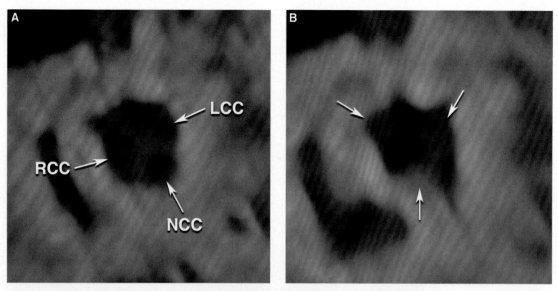

FIGURE 7.40: Rendered views of the aortic valve using TrueVue. The three aortic valve leaflets (LCC, RCC, and NCC) can be appreciated with the valve closed during diastole **(A)**. The hinge points *(arrows)* are appreciated during systole **(B)**. *LCC,* left coronary cusp; *RCC,* right coronary cusp; *NCC,* noncoronary cusp.

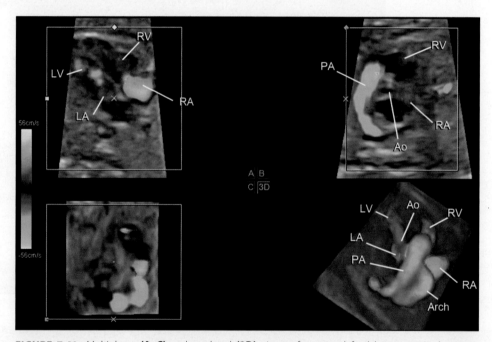

FIGURE 7.41: Multiplanar **(A–C)** and rendered **(3D)** views of a normal fetal heart acquired using a transverse sweep through the fetal chest and color Doppler imaging. Note the region of interest (ROI) box adjusted in **panels A–C** to include the entire heart. Also note the projection direction given in **panels B** and **C** by the position of the *green line*. In this case, the projection direction is from the superior mediastinum down toward the abdomen. Therefore, the resulting rendered image **(3D)** displays, in sequence, the pulmonary artery crossing over the aortic root, the ascending aorta and part of the arch, and then the atrial and ventricular chambers seen in the background in *red*. *Ao,* aorta; *LA,* left atrium; *LV,* left ventricle; *PA,* pulmonary artery; *RA,* right atrium; *RV,* right ventricle.

However, only 25% of the volume datasets were considered high quality.[153] The second study allowed 40 minutes for volume dataset acquisition per examination, and showed that the four-chamber view and outflow tracts could be adequately visualized in 70% and 83% of the cases, respectively.[154] The main factors associated with poor volume dataset quality were maternal obesity, anterior placenta, and unfavorable fetal position (spine up).[153,154] A more recent study including 1,124 fetuses reported unsuccessful volume acquisition in 18.6% of the cases,

with the most important contributing factors being shadowing artifacts from unexpected fetal limb movements during volume acquisition, maternal BMI greater than 28 kg/m^2, anterior placenta, estimated fetal weight (EFW) greater than 1,300 g, and not imaging the fetal body with 4D rendered images prior to volume acquisition to exclude sources of obstruction to insonation of the fetal heart such as fetal limbs.[155]

Regarding the applicability of 4D fetal echocardiography to clinical practice, the evidence available to date indicates that

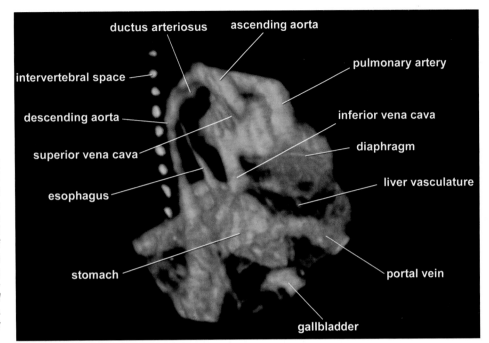

FIGURE 7.42: Three-dimensional rendered image of the aortic and ductal arches in a normal fetus at 22 + 2 weeks using the inversion mode technique. (From Gonçalves LF, Espinoza J, Lee W, et al. Three- and four-dimensional reconstruction of the aortic and ductal arches using inversion mode: a new rendering algorithm for visualization of fluid-filled anatomical structures. *Ultrasound Obstet Gynecol.* 2004;24(6):696–698. Copyright © 2004 ISUOG. Reprinted by permission of John Wiley & Sons, Inc.)

examiners can rely on volume datasets of the fetal heart for diagnostic purposes. Viñals et al.[17,22] conducted studies in Chile with volume datasets of the fetal heart obtained by examiners with little experience in fetal echocardiography and then transmitted to a remote server via an Internet link. Volumes were evaluated by an expert in fetal echocardiography, with a complete examination possible in 96.2% of the cases obtained in the second trimester[17] and a high degree of interobserver concordance

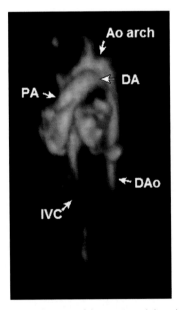

FIGURE 7.43: Rendered image of the aortic and ductal arches obtained from a volume dataset acquired with B-flow imaging. *Ao arch,* aortic arch; *DA,* ductus arteriosus; *Dao,* descending aorta; *IVC,* inferior vena cava; *PA,* pulmonary artery. (From Gonçalves LF, Lee W, Espinoza J, et al. Examination of the fetal heart by four-dimensional [4D] ultrasound with spatiotemporal image correlation [STIC]. *Ultrasound Obstet Gynecol.* 2006;27(3):336–348. Copyright © 2006 ISUOG. Reprinted by permission of John Wiley & Sons, Inc.)

for fetal echocardiography views extracted from volume datasets obtained between 11 and 14 weeks of gestation.[22] Bennasar et al.[156] compared 4DUS against 2DUS for diagnostic accuracy in detecting CHD. Volume datasets were analyzed blindly 1 year after acquisition. The study included 342 fetuses with suspected CHD and showed similar diagnostic accuracy for both methods (91% for 4DUS vs. 94.2% for 2DUS, $P > 0.05$), with 10 false-negative diagnoses by 4DUS (VSD [$n = 9$], interrupted aortic arch [$n = 1$]) and 3 by 2DUS (VSD [$n = 2$], persistent left superior vena cava [$n = 1$]). 4DUS had 19 false-positive diagnoses (VSD [$n = 10$], coarctation of the aorta [$n = 4$], persistent left superior vena cava [$n = 2$], pulmonary stenosis [$n = 1$], tricuspid dysplasia [$n = 1$], rhabdomyoma [$n = 1$]), while 2DUS have 17 false-positive diagnoses (VSD [$n = 11$], coarctation of the aorta [$n = 4$], tricuspid dysplasia [$n = 1$], ostium primum atrial septal defect [$n = 1$]). Espinoza et al.[157] conducted a multicenter study that included experts at seven international institutions. Ninety volume datasets of fetuses with and without CHD were uploaded to a server and examined blindly by the experts. The study showed very good sensitivity and specificity for the diagnosis of CHD (93% and 96%, respectively) with excellent inter-center agreement (kappa = 0.97). The study conducted by Shen and Yagel[158] demonstrated the additional value of 4DUS when compared with 2DUS in 193 cases of CHD analyzed blindly. The study showed that 12 cardiac anomalies were correctly diagnosed only by 4DUS, including a right aortic arch with anomalous branching, transposition of the great arteries with pulmonary atresia, interrupted aortic arch, right ventricular aneurysm, and total anomalous pulmonary venous return. In that study, the sensitivity of 2DUS was 87.6% (95% confidence interval [CI], 81.8% to 91.7%), and the sensitivity of 4DUS was 93.8% (95% CI, 89.1% to 96.6%). Both imaging modalities had a specificity of 100% (95% CI, 99.9% to 100%).

Automation: Software-based automatic segmentation of the fetal heart is possible. Abuhamad et al.[159,160] were the first to develop such a system with successful display of the ventricular outflow

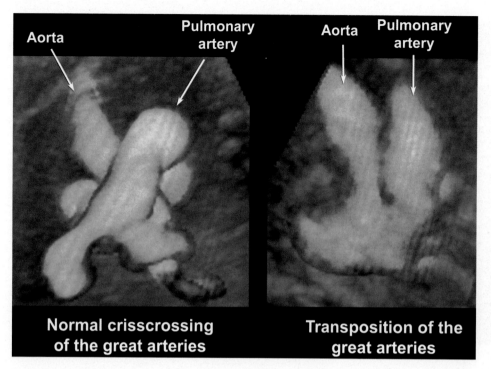

FIGURE 7.44: Rendered images from volume datasets of the fetal heart in a normal case **(A)** and transposition of the great arteries (TGA) (Reproduced from Gonçalves LF, Romero R, Espinoza J, et al. Four-dimensional ultrasonography of the fetal heart using color Doppler spatio-temporal image correlation. *J Ultrasound Med* 2004;23(4):473–481. Copyright © 2016 by the American Institute of Ultrasound in Medicine. Reprinted by permission of John Wiley & Sons, Inc.) **(B)**. The volumes were acquired through a transverse sweep of the fetal chest using power Doppler four-dimensional ultrasonography with spatiotemporal image correlation. In the normal case, normal crisscrossing of the great arteries is observed, whereas in TGA, the vessels leave the ventricles in parallel. The technique used to render the volume datasets is explained in Figure 7.41. (Reproduced from Gonçalves LF, Espinoza J, Romero R, et al. A systematic approach to prenatal diagnosis of transposition of the great arteries using 4-dimensional ultrasonography with spatiotemporal image correlation. *J Ultrasound Med.* 2004;23(9):1225–1231. Copyright © 2016 by the American Institute of Ultrasound in Medicine. Reprinted by permission of John Wiley & Sons, Inc.)

tract, right ventricular outflow tract, and abdominal circumference in 94.4%, 91.7%, and 97.2% of 72 volume datasets that included the four-chamber view acquired between 18 and 23 weeks. A more recently developed method, named fetal intelligent navigation (FINE), automatically generates and displays nine standard fetal echocardiography views from volume datasets acquired with the use of STIC technology. The reported successful visualization rates of the nine views is 96% to 100% for second-trimester[161] and 98% to 100% for third-trimester fetuses.[148,162] High-quality volume datasets are required, with the following criteria recommended by the authors: (1) fetal spine between 4- and 8-o'clock, (2) enough sweep angle to include images from the stomach to the superior mediastinum, (3) optimized 2DUS imaging such that the anatomy can be visualized, and (4) absence of excessive motion artifacts.[163] In a recent case-control study of 100 normal fetuses and 50 fetuses with CHD, including fetuses with conutruncal anomalies ($n = 21$), left heart anomalies ($n = 10$), right heart anomalies ($n = 8$), complex cardiac defects ($n = 6$), and septal defects ($n = 5$), FINE achieved an overall sensitivity of 98% and specificity of 93% for detection of CHDs. False-positive diagnoses included VSDs ($n = 6$) and a suspected cardiac tumor in the right ventricle ($n = 1$). The only false-negative diagnoses occurred in a fetus with branch pulmonary artery stenosis and a small secundum atrial septal defect. Complete concordance was achieved in 74% of the cases with minor or major discrepancies seen in 12% and 14% of the cases, respectively. Importantly, the high diagnostic accuracy in this study was achieved despite suboptimal volume datasets that were partially compromised by shadowing and/or motion artifacts in 21% and 23% of the cases, respectively.[163]

VOLUMETRIC MEASUREMENTS

Before widespread availability of 3DUS equipment, fetal volumetric measurements of an anatomical structure could only be estimated from 2DUS images. These estimations are still accomplished today with the use of the ellipsoid formula

(transverse $\times$ anteroposterior $\times$ longitudinal dimensions $\times \pi/6$), which assumes an approximate ellipsoid shape and regular contour of the structure of interest. While this may work for volumetric measurements of the ovary, for example, it does not fit perfectly the contour of more complex anatomical structures such as the left and right ventricles of the heart, where measurement errors as high as 25% have been reported.[164] Direct volumetric measurements can be performed from 3DUS and 4DUS volume datasets acquired with most commercially available equipment. Two methods are generally used: (1) multiplanar or multiple parallel plane measurements or (2) rotational virtual organ computer-aided analysis (VOCAL, GE Healthcare, Milwaukee, WI).[45,165–176]

Even though *in vitro* studies evaluating the accuracy of 3DUS volumetric measurement accuracy have shown excellent accuracy and reliability,[177–179] a review of published nomograms for volumetric measurements of various fetal organs revealed remarkable variability.[167] To illustrate the point, suppose an examiner wants to know what is the expected mean fetal lung volume for a 28-week fetus. After a literature search is conducted, the examiner will find out that reported mean fetal lung volumes for a 28-week fetus varies between 17.2 and 43.3 mL (based on 15 peer-reviewed articles).[167,169,180–191] The implications of this observation are clinically important: a fetal lung volume of 36.12 mL at 28 weeks may lie anywhere between −2.94 standard deviations and +1.11 standard deviations of the mean for gestational age, depending on the chosen nomogram. Such a wide discrepancy makes it difficult to diagnose true pathology with confidence. Consequently, volumetric measurements by 3DUS must be approached with caution. Methodological sources of error, rather than true biological differences, are likely the explanation for the wide variation in reported normal values. One such source of variation is inherent to the physical principles underlying ultrasonography, a reflective technique that suffers from artifacts related to bone shadowing that limit the ability to precisely define the borders of soft-tissue structures (e.g., rib shadows impairing precise tracing of lung contours or shadowing from skull bones that prevent perfect visualization and tracing of the brain parenchyma). Other potential sources of variability include the heterogeneity of 3DUS system platforms, inconsistency in the interpretation of ultrasonographic images, problems with data analysis and reporting of measurement errors, as well as issues related to method validation.[167] To complicate matters further, there are a multitude of mutually incompatible 3DUS imaging formats and software measuring tools, an issue that is unlikely to improve until US volume datasets stored using the DICOM standard can be opened by any commercially or freely available software with 3D volumetric measurement and rendering capabilities.

In the following sections, we review the clinical applications of 3DUS volumetry to two clinically relevant scenarios: fetal weight estimation using limb volumes and volumetric measurements of the fetal heart to evaluate cardiac function.

Fetal Weight Estimation Using Volumetric Imaging

EFW is routinely obtained in the second and third trimesters to assess fetal size and nutritional status. Most methods used to estimate fetal weight are based on 2D measurements of the fetal biparietal diameter (BPD), head circumference (HC), abdominal circumference (AC), and femur length (FL). When compared with actual fetal weight, ultrasonographic EFW is associated with random errors in the order of 8.1% to 11.8%.[192]

3DUS has been proposed as an alternative method for fetal weight estimation and to evaluate fetal body composition.[170,193–202] Initial studies used total limb volumetry to predict fetal weight.[178,203] However, total limb volumetry is technically cumbersome, largely due to poor visualization of soft-tissue borders at the distal ends of the limbs, and the large number of manual tracings to obtain a volume measurement. To overcome these obstacles, fractional limb volumetry (FLV) was introduced in 2001.[170] In FLV, only the midportion of the limb is measured as a fixed percentage (50%) of the diaphysis length. Either fractional thigh (T_{vol}) or fractional arm volume (A_{vol}) can be measured, as illustrated in Figures 7.45 and 7.46. Initial investigations found

that a combination of either T_{vol} or A_{vol} and AC could predict actual birth weight much more reliably than do conventional 2DUS measurements.[170] Furthermore, T_{vol} correlates strongly with the percentage of neonatal body fat measured within 48 hours of delivery by air displacement plethysmography.[201]

Subsequent studies found that A_{vol} and T_{vol} measurements could be performed with good intraobserver and interobserver bias and agreement [intraobserver bias and agreement: A_{vol} 2.2% ± 4.2% (95% limits of agreement, −6.0% to 10.5%), T_{vol} 2.0% ± 4.2% (95% limits of agreement, −6.3% to 10.3%);

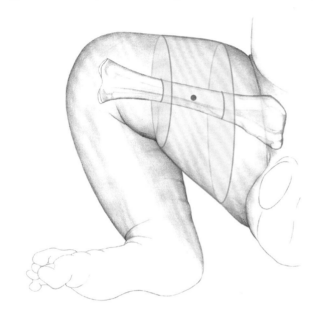

FIGURE 7.45: Illustration of fractional thigh volume (T_{vol}). T_{vol} is a subvolume that includes 50% of the femoral diaphysis length. The volume is centered on the midfemoral shaft *(small circle)*. The principle is the same for fractional arm volume (A_{vol}). (From Lee W, Deter RL, McNie B, et al. Individualized growth assessment of fetal soft tissue using fractional thigh volume. *Ultrasound Obstet Gynecol.* 2004;24(7):767–774. Copyright © 2004 ISUOG. Reprinted by permission of John Wiley & Sons, Inc.)

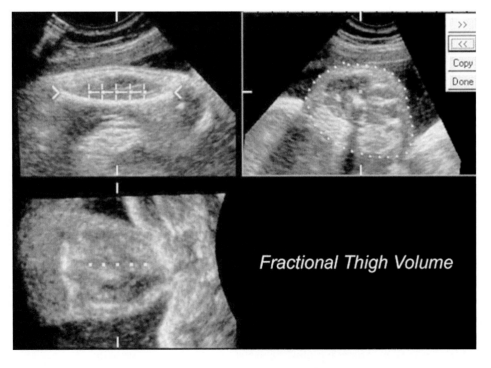

FIGURE 7.46: Fractional thigh volume by three-dimensional ultrasonography. Orthogonal viewing planes (sagittal, upper left window; axial, upper right window; coronal, lower left window) are used to examine the fetal thigh by multiplanar imaging. The *arrowheads* are electronically positioned at both ends of the femoral diaphysis in the sagittal plane. A midthigh subvolume is based on 50% of the diaphysis length and is split into five sections that are manually traced from axial views. The principle is the same for fractional arm volume (A_{vol}). (From Lee W, Deter RL, McNie B, et al. Individualized growth assessment of fetal soft tissue using fractional thigh volume. *Ultrasound Obstet Gynecol.* 2004;24(7):767–774. Copyright © 2004 ISUOG. Reprinted by permission of John Wiley & Sons, Inc.)

interobserver bias and agreement: A_{vol} $-1.9\% \pm 4.9\%$ (95% limits of agreement, -11.6% to 7.8%), T_{vol} $-2.0\% \pm 5.4\%$ (95% limits of agreement, -12.5% to 8.6%)]. Normal reference ranges for A_{vol} and T_{vol} during pregnancy have been established in 2009 and are reproduced in Appendices 15 and 16.[193]

More recently, new fetal weight estimation models based on FLV and conventional 2DUS were developed[204] and subsequently validated[195] in a different population. The validation study included 164 pregnant women who delivered between 21 and 42 weeks of menstrual age and who had T_{vol}, A_{vol}, BPD, AC, and FL measured within 4 days of delivery. The best model to predict actual birth weight was a combination of the BPD, AC, and T_{vol}.[195] The model correctly classified a greater proportion of EFW within 5% (55.1% vs. 43.7%, $P = 0.03$) and 10% (86.5% vs. 75.9%, $P < 0.05$) of actual birth weight when compared with EFW calculated using formulas derived from 2DUS measurements (modified Hadlock formula using BPD, AC, and FL with coefficients derived from the same population).[204]

The formulas to estimate birth weight based on a combination of 2DUS parameters and T_{vol} and A_{vol} are provided here:[195]

$$T_{vol} : \ln BW = -0.8297 + 04.0344\,(\ln BPD) - 0.7820\,(\ln BPD)^2$$
$$+ 0.7853\,(\ln AC) + 0.0528\,(\ln T_{vol})^2$$

$$A_{vol} :$$
$$\ln BW = 0.5046 + 1.9665\,(\ln BPD) - 0.3040\,(\ln BPD)^2$$
$$+ 0.9675\,(\ln AC) + 0.3557\,(\ln A_{vol})$$

Functional Evaluation of the Fetal Heart by 4DUS

Stroke volume (SV), cardiac output (CO), and ejection fraction (EF) are important parameters to evaluate fetal cardiac function. Until recently, these could only be estimated from 2DUS measurements that rely on imperfect geometric assumptions about ventricular shape (orthogonal measurements, multiple disk method—Simpson's rule),[205,206] or by using a combination of 2DUS and Doppler.[207] Simpson and Cook[208] showed that the repeatability of volumetric measurements using the multiple disk method is poor (the coefficient of variation exceeded 10% for the estimation for both the left ventricular end-diastolic volume [13%] and the SV [14%]), with intraobserver errors consistently higher than intraobserver errors. Furthermore, formulas that rely on geometric assumptions about ventricular morphology apply only to the left ventricle, since the right ventricle has a complex morphology.

Doppler calculations of SV and CO are accomplished by multiplying the Doppler velocity time integral (VTI) by the 2D cross-sectional valve area of either the atrioventricular or the semilunar valves. The formulas are as given:

$$SV = VTI \times \frac{\pi d^2}{4}, \text{where } d \text{ is the diameter of the valve}$$

$$CO = SV \times \text{heart rate}$$

Several sources of error are possible with the combination of 2DUS and Doppler measurements. These include (1) poor angle of insonation ($<20°$), which may result in underestimation of the Doppler VTI, and (2) the derivation of valve area from its radius squared, which tends to amplify measurement errors, even if minimal. Poor reproducibility of Doppler measurements

to evaluate SV and CO has been previously reported, with interobserver errors consistently higher than intraobserver errors.[208]

With the advent of 4DUS fetal echocardiography, left and right ventricular volumes can now be directly measured during systole and diastole, allowing direct calculation of SV, CO, and EF. The first attempt to measure ventricular volumes using 4DUS was reported by Meyer-Wittkopf et al.[209] in 2001. In that study, the investigators used a free-hand volume acquisition system composed of standard 2DUS equipment interfaced with a magnetic tracking system. Volumetric measurements were obtained in 57 normal fetuses and in 22 fetuses with CHD. The authors found that end-systolic and end-diastolic volumes increased exponentially with gestational age for both groups. Fetuses with CHD and inequality of ventricular sizes tended to have smaller combined end-diastolic volume and SV than normal fetuses. Free-hand volumetric measurements of the fetal hearts was also attempted by Esh-Broder et al.,[210] who found mean right and left ventricular EF of 54% $\pm$ 11.2% and 57.5% $\pm$ 14.6% between 20 and 24 weeks of gestation.

After the introduction of STIC technology in 2003,[17,18] several groups have reported on the ability to obtain volumetric measurements of the fetal heart using this technology. Experiments *in vitro* using pulsatile balloon models have validated the accuracy of STIC for measurements of small volumes such as those found in second- and third-trimester fetal hearts.[211,212] Several subsequent studies performed in human fetuses collectively showed that (1) the intraobserver and interobserver repeatability and reproducibility for volumetric measurements of the fetal heart using STIC are high;[176,213–217] (2) that EF tends to remain stable through gestation;[213–215] (3) that SV and CO for both the right and the left ventricles increase exponentially with gestation, except when corrected for EFW;[168,176,214–216] and that increased placental resistance to blood flow assessed by abnormal umbilical artery Doppler velocimetry is associated with changes in fetal cardiac function (Table 7.1).[218]

Of interest is the large study of Hamill et al.,[168] who applied one of the 4D segmentation methods with best repeatability and reproducibility, namely VOCAL with contour finder, to measure end-diastolic and end-systolic volumes of the right and left ventricles in 184 fetuses examined between 19 and 42 weeks (Fig. 7.47). SV, CO, and EF were calculated. The study confirmed prior observations that ventricular volumes, SV and CO increase with advancing gestational age. However, it also showed no difference between left and right ventricles for SV and CO, as well as a drop in EF with advancing gestation, with the left EF significantly greater than the right, findings that have not been previously reported.

Regarding the feasibility of 4DUS with STIC to measure cardiac volumes in clinical practice, a few reports comment on pitfalls related to volume acquisition. Hamill et al.,[168] for example, rejected 33/217 (15%) volumes based on poor image quality, whereas Schoonderwaldt et al.[219] reported poor success rate for STIC acquisitions in a study of 84 pregnancies scanned between 20 and 34 weeks of gestation. In that study, only 30/84 volumes (36%) had sufficient quality to allow volumetric measurements. The other volumes had to be excluded due to unfavorable fetal position with the spine projecting anterior or lateral, and/or fetal movements that resulted in acoustic shadows and movement artifacts. Uittenbogaard et al.[213] also noted low-image resolution at early gestational age, and a high failure rate after 30 weeks' gestation.

TABLE 7.1			Volumetric Measurements of the Fetal Heart Using Spatiotemporal Image Correlation (STIC)		
AUTHOR	**YEAR**	**N**	**GA RANGE (WEEKS)**	**METHOD**	**MAIN FINDINGS**
Messing[215]	2007	100	20–40	Inversion mode	• ESV, EDV, and SV for both ventricles correlated strongly with GA • No significant change in EF change with GA, with left EF slightly larger than the right • Good intraobserver and interobserver reproducibility
Rizzo[217]	2007	56	20–32	VOCAL manual trace	• Good intra- and interobserver agreement for SV measured with either Doppler or STIC • STIC significantly faster than Doppler (3.1 ± 0.84 min vs. 7.9 ± 2.3 min, $P < 0.0001$)
Molina[216]	2008	140	12–34	VOCAL manual trace	• SV and CO increased with GA • Ratio of right to left SV increased with GA from 0.97 at 12 wk to 1.13 at 34 wk
Uittenbogaard[213]	2009	63	12–30	3D slice method	• Longitudinal study involving 202 STIC volumes • Ratio of right to left SV of about 1.2
Hamill[176]	2009	25		VOCAL contour trace VOCAL manual trace Inversion	• Better intra- and interobserver agreement for the contour trace method • Better agreement between measurements with 15° rotation increments • Ventricular volume measurements were repeatable and reproducible
Rizzo[217]	2010	45	19–32	VOCAL manual trace VOCAL SonoAVC	• Good reliability between manual trace and SonoAVC • SonoAVC significantly faster (2.8 ± 1.9 min vs. 11.7 ± 4.8 min $P < 0.0001$)
Hamill[168]	2011	184	19–42	VOCAL contour trace	• In this study, normal fetal cardiovascular physiology was characterized by a larger right ventricular volume and a greater left ventricular ejection fraction, resulting in similar left ventricular and right ventricular stroke volume and cardiac output
Hamill[218]	2013	34	20–36	VOCAL contour trace	• End-systolic and end-diastolic volumes, cardiac output, and adjusted cardiac output were compared between 34 fetuses with umbilical artery Doppler pulsatility index > 95th percentile and 184 control fetuses. Mean left and right stroke volume and cardiac output were lower for fetuses with abnormal umbilical artery Doppler. Right ventricular volume, stroke volume, and cardiac output were higher for the right ventricle where ejection fraction was higher for the left ventricle

CO, cardiac output; EDV, end-diastolic volume; EF, ejection fraction; ESV, end-systolic volume; GA, gestational age; SV, stroke volume; VOCAL, Virtual Organ Computer-Aided Analysis.

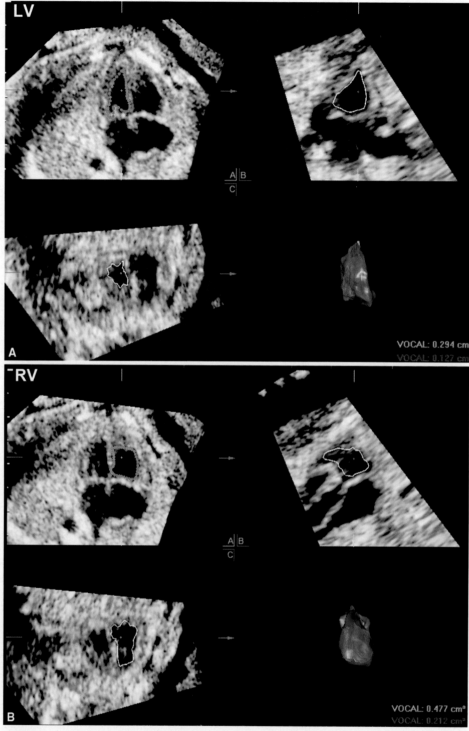

FIGURE 7.47: A: Left *(LV)* and **B:** right *(RV)* ventricular volume measurements obtained VOCAL (Virtual Organ Computed Aided Analysis, 4DView, GE Healthcare, Milwaukee, Wisconsin, USA) during systole and diastole. Once the measurements are obtained, several hemodynamic parameters can be calculated. For example, (1) ejection fraction *(EF)* for the right ventricle *(RV)* is calculated as follows: RV end-diastolic volume (0.477 mL)—RV end-systolic volume (0.212 mL)/RV end-diastolic volume (0.477 mL) = 55.5%; (2) EF for the left ventricle *(LV)* is LV end-diastolic volume (0.294 mL)—LV end-systolic volume (0.127 mL)/LV end-diastolic volume (0.294 mL) = 56.8%; (3) stroke volume for the RV is RV end-diastolic volume (0.477 mL)—RV end-systolic volume (0.212 mL) = 0.265 mL and RV cardiac output for a fetal heart rate of 140 bpm is 37.1 mL; (4) stroke volume for the LV is LV end-diastolic volume (0.294 mL)—LV end-systolic volume (0.127 mL) = 0.167 mL and LV cardiac output for a fetal heart rate of 140 bpm is 23.4 mL.

CONCLUSION

3DUS provides the obstetrical imager with a tool that can improve diagnosis by enhancing the display of anatomical structures imaged by 2DUS. The multiplanar format allows visualization of a structure or lesion simultaneously in three planes. Realistic renditions of the structures of interest enhance the capabilities of the examiner in several conditions, including facial clefts and skeletal abnormalities. Clinical applicability of 3DUS and 4DUS has been demonstrated in several areas, including facial defects, skeletal abnormalities and CHD. The ability to obtain volumetric measurements also aids with more precise estimation of fetal weight using fractional thigh or arm volumes. The reader is reminded, however, that 3D imaging only enhances 2DUS, and, therefore, artifacts and limitations inherent to ultrasonography are unlikely to be overcome by 3D/4D technology.

REFERENCES

1. Gonçalves LF, Lee W, Espinoza J, et al. Three- and 4-dimensional ultrasound in obstetric practice: does it help? *J Ultrasound Med.* 2005;24(12):1599–1624. doi:10.7863/jum.2005.24.12.1599.
2. Pretorius DH, Gattu S, Ji E-K, et al. Preexamination and postexamination assessment of parental-fetal bonding in patients undergoing 3-/4-dimensional obstetric ultrasonography. *J Ultrasound Med.* 2006;25(11):1411–1421.
3. de Jong-Pleij EAP, Ribbert LSM, Pistorius LR, et al. Three-dimensional ultrasound and maternal bonding, a third trimester study and a review. *Prenat Diagn.* 2013;33(1):81–88. doi:10.1002/pd.4013.
4. Kurjak A, Azumendi G, Vecek N, et al. Fetal hand movements and facial expression in normal pregnancy studied by four-dimensional sonography. *J Perinat Med.* 2003;31(6):496–508. doi:10.1515/JPM.2003.076.
5. Kurjak A, Azumendi G, Andonotopo W, et al. Three- and four-dimensional ultrasonography for the structural and functional evaluation of the fetal face. *Am J Obstet Gynecol.* 2007;196(1):16–28. doi:10.1016/j.ajog.2006.06.090.
6. Hata T, Hanaoka U, Mashima M, et al. Four-dimensional HDlive rendering image of fetal facial expression: a pictorial essay. *J Med Ultrason (2001).* 2013;40(4):437–441. doi:10.1007/s10396-013-0441-8.
7. Kurjak A, Stanojevic M, Andonotopo W, et al. Behavioral pattern continuity from prenatal to postnatal life—a study by four-dimensional (4D) ultrasonography. *J Perinat Med.* 2004;32(4):346–353. doi:10.1515/JPM.2004.065.
8. Kurjak A, Andonotopo W, Hafner T, et al. Normal standards for fetal neurobehavioral developments—longitudinal quantification by four-dimensional sonography. *J Perinat Med.* 2006;34(1):56–65. doi:10.1515/JPM.2006.007.
9. Miskovic B, Vasilj O, Stanojevic M, et al. The comparison of fetal behavior in high risk and normal pregnancies assessed by four dimensional ultrasound. *J Matern Fetal Neonatal Med.* 2010;23(12):1461–1467. doi:10.3109/14767051003678200.
10. Mori N, Kanenishi K, AboEllail MAM, et al. Neurological development may be accelerated in growth-restricted fetuses: a 4D ultrasound study. *J Perinat Med.* 2019;47(4):429–433. doi:10.1515/jpm-2018-0379.
11. Mori N, AboEllail MAM, Tenkumo C, et al. Fetal facial expressions in small-for-gestational-age and growth-restricted fetuses. *J Matern Fetal Neonatal Med.* 2019;32(9):1426–1432. doi:10.1080/14767058.2017.1410788.
12. Lopez-Teijon M, Garcia-Faura A, Prats-Galino A. Fetal facial expression in response to intravaginal music emission. *Ultrasound.* 2015;23(4):216–223. doi:10.1177/1742271X15609367.
13. Bernardes LS, Ottolia JF, Cecchini M, et al. On the feasibility of accessing acute pain-related facial expressions in the human fetus and its potential implications: a case report. *Pain Reports.* 2018;3(5):e673. doi:10.1097/PR9.0000000000000673.
14. Deng J, Gardener JE, Rodeck CH, et al. Fetal echocardiography in three and four dimensions. *Ultrasound Med Biol.* 1996;22(8):979–986.
15. Nelson TR, Pretorius DH, Sklansky M, et al. Three-dimensional echocardiographic evaluation of fetal heart anatomy and function: acquisition, analysis, and display. *J Ultrasound Med.* 1996;15(1):1–2.
16. Sklansky MS, Nelson T, Strachan M, et al. Real-time three-dimensional fetal echocardiography: initial feasibility study. *J Ultrasound Med.* 1999;18(11):745–752.
17. Vinals F, Poblete P, Giuliano A, et al. Spatio-temporal image correlation (STIC): a new tool for the prenatal screening of congenital heart defects. *Ultrasound Obstet Gynecol.* 2003;22(4):388–394. doi:10.1002/uog.883.
18. DeVore GR, Falkensammer P, Sklansky MS, et al. Spatio-temporal image correlation (STIC): new technology for evaluation of the fetal heart. *Ultrasound Obstet Gynecol.* 2003;22(4):380–387. doi:10.1002/uog.217.
19. Goncalves LF, Lee W, Chaiworapongsa T, et al. Four-dimensional ultrasonography of the fetal heart with spatiotemporal image correlation. *Am J Obstet Gynecol.* 2003;189(6):1792–1802.
20. Maulik D, Nanda NC, Singh V, et al. Live three-dimensional echocardiography of the human fetus. *Echocardiography.* 2003;20(8):715–721.
21. Chaoui R, Hoffmann J, Heling KS. Three-dimensional (3D) and 4D color Doppler fetal echocardiography using spatio-temporal image correlation (STIC). *Ultrasound Obstet Gynecol.* 2004;23(6):535–545. doi:10.1002/uog.1075.
22. Vinals F, Ascenzo R, Naveas R, et al. Fetal echocardiography at 11 + 0 to 13 + 6 weeks using four-dimensional spatiotemporal image correlation telemedicine via an Internet link: a pilot study. *Ultrasound Obstet Gynecol.* 2008;31(6):633–638. doi:10.1002/uog.5350.
23. DeVore GR, Satou G, Sklansky M. 4D fetal echocardiography: an update. *Echocardiography.* 2017;34(12):1788–1798. doi:10.1111/echo.13708.
24. Merz E, Bahlmann F, Weber G, et al. Three-dimensional ultrasonography in prenatal diagnosis. *J Perinat Med.* 1995;23(3):213–222.
25. von Ramm OT, Smith SW. Real time volumetric ultrasound imaging system. *J Digit Imaging.* 1990;3(4):261–266. doi:10.1007/BF03168124.
26. Goncalves LF, Espinoza J, Kusanovic JP, et al. Applications of 2-dimensional matrix array for 3- and 4-dimensional examination of the fetus: a pictorial essay. *J Ultrasound Med.* 2006;25(6):745–755.
27. Hull AD, Pretorius DH, Lev-Toaff A, et al. Artifacts and the visualization of fetal distal extremities using three-dimensional ultrasound. *Ultrasound Obstet Gynecol.* 2000;16(4):341–344. doi:10.1046/j.1469-0705.2000.00187.x.
28. Miric Tesanic D, Merz E. Artifacts in 3D prenatal sonography. *Ultraschall Med.* December 2018. doi:10.1055/a-0790-8163.
29. Riccabona M, Pretorius DH, Nelson TR, et al. Three-dimensional ultrasound: display modalities in obstetrics. *J Clin Ultrasound.* 1997;25(4):157–167.
30. Devore GR, Polanko B. Tomographic ultrasound imaging of the fetal heart: a new technique for identifying normal and abnormal cardiac anatomy. *J Ultrasound Med.* 2005;24(12):1685–1696.
31. Goncalves LF, Espinoza J, Romero R, et al. Four-dimensional ultrasonography of the fetal heart using a novel Tomographic Ultrasound Imaging display. *J Perinat Med.* 2006;34(1):39–55. doi:10.1515/JPM.2006.006.
32. Kratochwil A. Attempt at three-dimensional imaging in obstetrics. *Ultraschall Med.* 1992;13(4):183–186. doi:10.1055/s-2007-1005306.
33. Kagan KO, Pintoffl K, Hoopmann M. First-trimester ultrasound images using HDlive. *Ultrasound Obstet Gynecol.* 2011;38(5):607. doi:10.1002/uog.10112.
34. Merz E. Surface reconstruction of a fetus (28 + 2 GW) using HDlive technology. *Ultraschall Med.* 2012;33(3):211.
35. Hata T, Hanaoka U, Tenkumo C, et al. Three- and four-dimensional HDlive rendering images of normal and abnormal fetuses: pictorial essay. *Arch Gynecol Obstet.* 2012;286(6):1431–1435. doi:10.1007/s00404-012-2505-1.
36. Grigore M, Mares A. The role of HDlive technology in improving the quality of obstetrical images. *Med Ultrason.* 2013;15(3):209–214.
37. Pooh RK. First trimester scan by 3D, 3D HDlive and HDlive silhouette/flow ultrasound imaging. *Donald Sch J Ultrasound Obstet Gynecol.* 2015;9(4):361–371. doi:10.5005/jp-journals-10009-1423.
38. Hata T, AboEllail MAM, Sajapala S, et al. HDlive Silhouette mode with spatiotemporal image correlation for assessment of the fetal heart. *J Ultrasound Med.* 2016;35(7):1489–1495. doi:10.7863/ultra.15.08061.
39. Pretorius DH, Nelson TR. Prenatal visualization of cranial sutures and fontanelles with three-dimensional ultrasonography. *J Ultrasound Med.* 1994;13(11):871–876.
40. Lee A, Kratochwil A, Deutinger J, et al. Three-dimensional ultrasound in diagnosing phocomelia. *Ultrasound Obstet Gynecol.* 1995;5(4):238–240. doi:10.1046/j.1469-0705.1995.05040238.x.
41. Johnson DD, Pretorius DH, Riccabona M, et al. Three-dimensional ultrasound of the fetal spine. *Obstet Gynecol.* 1997;89(3):434–438. doi:10.1016/S0029-7844(96)00498-x.
42. Espinoza J, Gonçalves LF, Lee W, et al. The use of the minimum projection mode in 4-dimensional examination of the fetal heart with spatiotemporal image correlation. *J Ultrasound Med.* 2004;23(10):1337–1348.
43. Goncalves LF, Espinoza J, Lee W, et al. Three- and four-dimensional reconstruction of the aortic and ductal arches using inversion mode: a new rendering algorithm for visualization of fluid-filled anatomical structures. *Ultrasound Obstet Gynecol.* 2004;24(6):696–698. doi:10.1002/uog.1754.
44. Goncalves LF, Espinoza J, Lee W, et al. A new approach to fetal echocardiography: digital casts of the fetal cardiac chambers and great vessels for detection of congenital heart disease. *J Ultrasound Med.* 2005;24(4):415–424.
45. Lee W, Goncalves LF, Espinoza J, et al. Inversion mode: a new volume analysis tool for 3-dimensional ultrasonography. *J Ultrasound Med.* 2005;24(2):201–207.
46. Chaoui R, Heling KS. New developments in fetal heart scanning: three- and four-dimensional fetal echocardiography. *Semin Fetal Neonatal Med.* 2005;10(6):567–577. doi:10.1016/j.siny.2005.08.008.
47. Espinoza J, Goncalves LF, Lee W, et al. A novel method to improve prenatal diagnosis of abnormal systemic venous connections using three- and four-dimensional ultrasonography and "inversion mode." *Ultrasound Obstet Gynecol.* 2005;25(5):428–434. doi:10.1002/uog.1877.
48. Ghi T, Cera E, Segata M, et al. Inversion mode spatio-temporal image correlation (STIC) echocardiography in three-dimensional rendering of fetal ventricular septal defects. *Ultrasound Obstet Gynecol.* 2005;26(6):679–680. doi:10.1002/uog.2613.
49. Benacerraf BR. Inversion mode display of 3D sonography: applications in obstetric and gynecologic imaging. *AJR Am J Roentgenol.* 2006;187(4):965–971. doi:10.2214/AJR.05.1462.
50. Deng J. Terminology of three-dimensional and four-dimensional ultrasound imaging of the fetal heart and other moving body parts. *Ultrasound Obstet Gynecol.* 2003;22(4):336–344. doi:10.1002/uog.890.

51. Kanenishi K, Hanaoka U, Noguchi J, et al. 4D ultrasound evaluation of fetal facial expressions during the latter stages of the second trimester. *Int J Gynaecol Obstet.* 2013;121(3):257–260. doi:10.1016/j.ijgo.2013.01.018.

52. Sato M, Kanenishi K, Hanaoka U, et al. 4D ultrasound study of fetal facial expressions at 20–24 weeks of gestation. *Int J Gynaecol Obstet.* 2014;126(3):275–279. doi:10.1016/j.ijgo.2014.03.036.

53. AboEllail MAM, Hata T. Fetal face as important indicator of fetal brain function. *J Perinat Med.* 2017;45(6):729–736. doi:10.1515/jpm-2016-0377.

54. Grigore M, Gafitanu D, Socolov D, et al. The role of 4D US in evaluation of fetal movements and facial expressions and their relationship with fetal neurobehaviour. *Med Ultrason.* 2018;1(1):88–94. doi:10.11152/mu-1350.

55. AboEllail MAM, Kanenishi K, Mori N, et al. 4D ultrasound study of fetal facial expressions in the third trimester of pregnancy. *J Matern Fetal Neonatal Med.* 2018;31(14):1856–1864. doi:10.1080/14767058.2017.1330880.

56. Hata T, Kanenishi K, AboEllail MAM, et al. Effect of psychotropic drugs on fetal behavior in the third trimester of pregnancy. *J Perinat Med.* 2019;47(2):207–211. doi:10.1515/jpm-2018-0114.

57. Kurjak A, Stanojevic M, Andonotopo W, et al. Fetal behavior assessed in all three trimesters of normal pregnancy by four-dimensional ultrasonography. *Croat Med J.* 2005;46(5):772–780.

58. Salihagic-Kadic A, Kurjak A, Medic M, et al. New data about embryonic and fetal neurodevelopment and behavior obtained by 3D and 4D sonography. *J Perinat Med.* 2005;33(6):478–490. doi:10.1515/JPM.2005.086.

59. Kurjak A, Miskovic B, Stanojevic M, et al. New scoring system for fetal neurobehavior assessed by three- and four-dimensional sonography. *J Perinat Med.* 2008;36(1):73–81. doi:10.1515/JPM.2008.007.

60. Kurjak A, Talic A, Stanojevic M, et al. The study of fetal neurobehavior in twins in all three trimesters of pregnancy. *J Matern Fetal Neonatal Med.* 2013;26(12):1186–1195. doi:10.3109/14767058.2013.773306.

61. Marx V, Nagy E. Fetal behavioral responses to the touch of the mother's abdomen: a frame-by-frame analysis. *Infant Behav Dev.* 2017;47:83–91. doi:10.1016/j.infbeh.2017.03.005.

62. Sklansky MS, Nelson TR, Pretorius DH. Usefulness of gated three-dimensional fetal echocardiography to reconstruct and display structures not visualized with two-dimensional imaging. *Am J Cardiol.* 1997;80(5):665–668.

63. Scharf A, Geka F, Steinborn A, et al. 3D real-time imaging of the fetal heart. *Fetal Diagn Ther.* 2000;15(5):267–274. doi:10.1159/000021020.

64. Goncalves LF, Romero R, Espinoza J, et al. Four-dimensional ultrasonography of the fetal heart using color Doppler spatiotemporal image correlation. *J Ultrasound Med.* 2004;23(4):473–481.

65. Sklansky MS, DeVore GR, Wong PC. Real-time 3-dimensional fetal echocardiography with an instantaneous volume-rendered display: early description and pictorial essay. *J Ultrasound Med.* 2004;23(2):283–289.

66. Hata T, Kanenishi K, Tanaka H, et al. Real-time 3-D echocardiographic evaluation of the fetal heart using instantaneous volume-rendered display. *J Obstet Gynaecol Res.* 2006;32(1):42–46. doi:10.1111/j.1447-0756.2006.00349.x.

67. Volpe P, Campobasso G, Stanziano A, et al. Novel application of 4D sonography with B-flow imaging and spatio-temporal image correlation (STIC) in the assessment of the anatomy of pulmonary arteries in fetuses with pulmonary atresia and ventricular septal defect. *Ultrasound Obstet Gynecol.* 2006;28(1):40–46. doi:10.1002/uog.2818.

68. Yeo L, Romero R. Intelligent navigation to improve obstetrical sonography. *Ultrasound Obstet Gynecol.* 2016;47(4):403–409. doi:10.1002/uog.12562.

69. Salerno CC, Pretorius DH, Hilton SW, et al. Three-dimensional ultrasonographic imaging of the neonatal brain in high-risk neonates: preliminary study. *J Ultrasound Med.* 2000;19(8):549–555. doi:10.7863/jum.2000.19.8.549.

70. Riccabona M, Nelson TR, Weitzer C, et al. Potential of three-dimensional ultrasound in neonatal and paediatric neurosonography. *Eur Radiol.* 2003;13(9):2082–2093. doi:10.1007/s00330-003-1845-4.

71. Riccabona M, Fritz G, Ring E. Potential applications of three-dimensional ultrasound in the pediatric urinary tract: pictorial demonstration based on preliminary results. *Eur Radiol.* 2003;13(12):2680–2687. doi:10.1007/s00330-003-2075-5.

72. Bault J-P. Visualization of the fetal optic chiasma using three-dimensional ultrasound imaging. *Ultrasound Obstet Gynecol.* 2006;28(6):862–864. doi:10.1002/uog.3868.

73. Bault JP, Salomon LJ, Guibaud L, et al. Role of three-dimensional ultrasound measurement of the optic tract in fetuses with agenesis of the septum pellucidum. *Ultrasound Obstet Gynecol.* 2011;37(5):570–575. doi:10.1002/uog.8847.

74. Paladini D, Birnbaum R, Donarini G, et al. Assessment of fetal optic chiasm: an echoanatomic and reproducibility study. *Ultrasound Obstet Gynecol.* 2016;48(6):727–732. doi:10.1002/uog.17227.

75. Faro C, Benoit B, Wegrzyn P, et al. Three-dimensional sonographic description of the fetal frontal bones and metopic suture. *Ultrasound Obstet Gynecol.* 2005;26(6):618–621. doi:10.1002/uog.1997.

76. Devonald KJ, Ellwood DA, Griffiths KA, et al. Volume imaging: three-dimensional appreciation of the fetal head and face. *J Ultrasound Med.* 1995;14(12):919–925.

77. Tutschek B, Blaas H-GK, Abramowicz J, et al. Three-dimensional ultrasound imaging of the fetal skull and face. *Ultrasound Obstet Gynecol.* 2017;50(1):7–16. doi:10.1002/uog.17436.

78. Mangione R, Lacombe D, Carles D, et al. Craniofacial dysmorphology and three-dimensional ultrasound: a prospective study on practicability for prenatal diagnosis. *Prenat Diagn.* 2003;23(10):810–818. doi:10.1002/pd.681.

79. Nicot R, Druelle C, Hurteloup E, et al. Prenatal craniofacial abnormalities: from ultrasonography to 3D-printed model. *Ultrasound Obstet Gynecol.* February 2019. doi:10.1002/uog.20242.

80. Mak ASL, Leung KY. Prenatal ultrasonography of craniofacial abnormalities. *Ultrason (Seoul, Korea).* 2019;38(1):13–24. doi:10.14366/usg.18031.

81. Rotten D, Levaillant JM. Two- and three-dimensional sonographic assessment of the fetal face. 2. Analysis of cleft lip, alveolus and palate. *Ultrasound Obstet Gynecol.* 2004;24(4):402–411. doi:10.1002/uog.1718.

82. Lee W, DeVore GR, Comstock CH, et al. Nasal bone evaluation in fetuses with Down syndrome during the second and third trimesters of pregnancy. *J Ultrasound Med.* 2003;22(1):55–60.

83. Sleurs E, Goncalves LF, Johnson A, et al. First-trimester three-dimensional ultrasonographic findings in a fetus with frontonasal malformation. *J Matern Fetal Neonatal Med.* 2004;16(3):187–197. doi:10.1080/14767050400009139.

84. Goncalves LF, Espinoza J, Lee W, et al. Phenotypic characteristics of absent and hypoplastic nasal bones in fetuses with Down syndrome: description by 3-dimensional ultrasonography and clinical significance. *J Ultrasound Med.* 2004;23(12):1619–1627.

85. Benoit B, Chaoui R. Three-dimensional ultrasound with maximal mode rendering: a novel technique for the diagnosis of bilateral or unilateral absence or hypoplasia of nasal bones in second-trimester screening for Down syndrome. *Ultrasound Obstet Gynecol.* 2005;25(1):19–24. doi:10.1002/uog.1805.

86. Pilu G, Visentin A, Ambrosini G, et al. Three-dimensional sonography of unilateral Tessier number 7 cleft in a mid-trimester fetus. *Ultrasound Obstet Gynecol.* 2005;26(1):98–99. doi:10.1002/uog.1903.

87. McGahan MC, Ramos GA, Landry C, et al. Multislice display of the fetal face using 3-dimensional ultrasonography. *J Ultrasound Med.* 2008;27(11):1573–1581.

88. Pretorius DH, House M, Nelson TR, et al. Evaluation of normal and abnormal lips in fetuses: comparison between three- and two-dimensional sonography. *AJR Am J Roentgenol.* 1995;165(5):1233–1237. doi:10.2214/ajr.165.5.7572510.

89. Merz E, Weber G, Bahlmann F, et al. Application of transvaginal and abdominal three-dimensional ultrasound for the detection or exclusion of malformations of the fetal face. *Ultrasound Obstet Gynecol.* 1997;9(4):237–243. doi:10.1046/j.1469-0705.1997.09040237.x.

90. Pilu G, Segata M. A novel technique for visualization of the normal and cleft fetal secondary palate: angled insonation and three-dimensional ultrasound. *Ultrasound Obstet Gynecol.* 2007;29(2):166–169. doi:10.1002/uog.3877.

91. Martinez-Ten P, Adiego B, Illescas T, et al. First-trimester diagnosis of cleft lip and palate using three-dimensional ultrasound. *Ultrasound Obstet Gynecol.* 2012;40(1):40–46. doi:10.1002/uog.10139.

92. Ulm MR, Kratochwil A, Ulm B, et al. Three-dimensional ultrasonographic imaging of fetal tooth buds for characterization of facial clefts. *Early Hum Dev.* 1999;55(1):67–75.

93. Johnson DD, Pretorius DH, Budorick NE, et al. Fetal lip and primary palate: three-dimensional versus two-dimensional US. *Radiology.* 2000;217(1):236–239. doi:10.1148/radiology.217.1.r00oc18236.

94. Lee W, Kirk JS, Shaheen KW, et al. Fetal cleft lip and palate detection by three-dimensional ultrasonography. *Ultrasound Obstet Gynecol.* 2000;16(4):314–320. doi:10.1046/j.1469-0705.2000.00181.x.

95. Chmait R, Pretorius D, Jones M, et al. Prenatal evaluation of facial clefts with two-dimensional and adjunctive three-dimensional ultrasonography: a prospective trial. *Am J Obstet Gynecol.* 2002;187(4):946–949.

96. Campbell S, Lees C, Moscoso G, et al. Ultrasound antenatal diagnosis of cleft palate by a new technique: the 3D "reverse face" view. *Ultrasound Obstet Gynecol.* 2005;25(1):12–18. doi:10.1002/uog.1819.

97. Benacerraf BR, Sadow PM, Barnewolt CE, et al. Cleft of the secondary palate without cleft lip diagnosed with three-dimensional ultrasound and magnetic resonance imaging in a fetus with Fryns' syndrome. *Ultrasound Obstet Gynecol.* 2006;27(5):566–570. doi:10.1002/uog.2778.

98. Chmait R, Pretorius D, Moore T, et al. Prenatal detection of associated anomalies in fetuses diagnosed with cleft lip with or without cleft palate in utero. *Ultrasound Obstet Gynecol.* 2006;27(2):173–176. doi:10.1002/uog.2593.

99. Platt LD, Devore GR, Pretorius DH. Improving cleft palate/cleft lip antenatal diagnosis by 3-dimensional sonography: the "flipped face" view. *J Ultrasound Med.* 2006;25(11):1423–1430.

100. Soto E, Richani K, Gonçalves LF, et al. Three-dimensional ultrasound in the prenatal diagnosis of cleidocranial dysplasia associated with B-cell immunodeficiency. *Ultrasound Obstet Gynecol.* 2006;27(5):574–579. doi:10.1002/uog.2770.

101. Parker SE, Mai CT, Canfield MA, et al. Updated national birth prevalence estimates for selected birth defects in the United States, 2004–2006. *Birth Defects Res Part A Clin Mol Teratol.* 2010;88(12):1008–1016. doi:10.1002/bdra.20735.

102. Dixon MJ, Marazita ML, Beaty TH, et al. Cleft lip and palate: understanding genetic and environmental influences. *Nat Publ Gr.* 2011;12(3):167–178. doi:10.1038/nrg2933.

103. Mueller GM, Weiner CP, Yankowitz J. Three-dimensional ultrasound in the evaluation of fetal head and spine anomalies. *Obstet Gynecol.* 1996;88(3):372–378. doi:10.1016/0029-7844(96)00207-4.

104. Ghi T, Perolo A, Banzi C, et al. Two-dimensional ultrasound is accurate in the diagnosis of fetal craniofacial malformation. *Ultrasound Obstet Gynecol.* 2002;19(6):543–551. doi:10.1046/j.1469-0705.2002.00721.x.

105. Sommerlad M, Patel N, Vijayalakshmi B, et al. Detection of lip, alveolar ridge and hard palate abnormalities using two-dimensional ultrasound enhanced with the three-dimensional reverse-face view. *Ultrasound Obstet Gynecol.* 2010;36(5):596–600. doi:10.1002/uog.7739.

106. Faure JM, Captier G, Baumler M, et al. Sonographic assessment of normal fetal palate using three-dimensional imaging: a new technique. *Ultrasound Obstet Gynecol.* 2007;29(2):159–165. doi:10.1002/uog.3870.

107. Faure J-M, Baumler M, Boulot P, et al. Prenatal assessment of the normal fetal soft palate by three-dimensional ultrasound examination: is there an objective technique? *Ultrasound Obstet Gynecol.* 2008;31(6):652–656. doi:10.1002/uog.5371.

108. Timor-Tritsch IE, Platt LD. Three-dimensional ultrasound experience in obstetrics. *Curr Opin Obstet Gynecol.* 2002;14:569–575. doi:10.1097/00001703-200212000-00001.

109. Ramos GA, Romine LE, Gindes L, et al. Evaluation of the fetal secondary palate by 3-dimensional ultrasonography. *J Ultrasound Med.* 2010;29(3):357–364.

110. Leung KY, Ngai CSW, Tang MHY. Facial cleft or shadowing artifact? *Ultrasound Obstet Gynecol.* 2006;27(2):231–232. doi:10.1002/uog.2696.

111. Gindes L, Weissmann-brenner A, Zajicek M, et al. Three-dimensional ultrasound demonstration of the fetal palate in high-risk patients: the accuracy of prenatal visualization. 2013:436–441. doi:10.1002/pd.4083.

112. Wilhelm L, Borgers H. The "equals sign": a novel marker in the diagnosis of fetal isolated cleft palate. *Ultrasound Obstet Gynecol.* 2010;36(4):439–444. doi:10.1002/uog.7704.

113. Ghi T, Tani G, Savelli L, et al. Prenatal imaging of facial clefts by magnetic resonance imaging with emphasis on the posterior palate. *Prenat Diagn.* 2003;23(12):970–975. doi:10.1002/pd.737.

114. Kazan-Tannus JFF, Levine D, McKenzie C, et al. Real-time magnetic resonance imaging aids prenatal diagnosis of isolated cleft palate. *J Ultrasound Med.* 2005;24(11):1533–1540. doi:10.1002/pd.737.

115. Mailáth-Pokorny M, Worda C, Krampl-Bettelheim E, et al. What does magnetic resonance imaging add to the prenatal ultrasound diagnosis of facial clefts? *Ultrasound Obstet Gynecol.* 2010;36(4):445–451. doi:10.1002/uog.7743.

116. Wang G, Shan R, Zhao L, et al. Fetal cleft lip with and without cleft palate: comparison between MR imaging and US for prenatal diagnosis. *Eur J Radiol.* 2011;79(3):437–442. doi:10.1016/j.ejrad.2010.03.026.

117. Manganaro L, Tomei A, Fierro F, et al. Fetal MRI as a complement to US in the evaluation of cleft lip and palate. *Radiol Med.* 2011;116:1134–1148. doi:10.1007/s11547-011-0683-8.

118. Arangio P, Manganaro L, Pacifici A, et al. Importance of fetal MRI in evaluation of craniofacial deformities. *J Craniofac Surg.* 2013;24(3):773–776. doi:10.1097/SCS.0b013e318286988c.

119. Dabadie A, Quarello E, Degardin N, et al. Added value of MRI for the prenatal diagnosis of isolated orofacial clefts and comparison with ultrasound. *Diagn Interv Imaging.* 2016;97(9):915–921. doi:10.1016/j.diii.2015.11.015.

120. Zheng W, Li B, Zou Y, et al. The prenatal diagnosis and classification of cleft palate: the role and value of magnetic resonance imaging. *Eur Radiol.* 2019;29(10):5600–5606. doi:10.1007/s00330-019-06089-9.

121. Nelson TR, Pretorius DH. Visualization of the fetal thoracic skeleton with three-dimensional sonography: a preliminary report. *AJR Am J Roentgenol.* 1995;164(6):1485–1488. doi:10.2214/ajr.164.6.7754898.

122. Riccabona M, Johnson D, Pretorius DH, et al. Three dimensional ultrasound: display modalities in the fetal spine and thorax. *Eur J Radiol.* 1996;22(2):141–145.

123. Schild RL, Wallny T, Fimmers R, et al. Fetal lumbar spine volumetry by three-dimensional ultrasound. *Ultrasound Obstet Gynecol.* 1999;13(5):335–339. doi:10.1046/j.1469-0705.1999.13050335.x.

124. Lee W, Chaiworapongsa T, Romero R, et al. A diagnostic approach for the evaluation of spina bifida by three-dimensional ultrasonography. *J Ultrasound Med.* 2002. doi:10.7863/jum.2002.21.6.619.

125. Yang XH, Chen M, Leung TY, et al. Use of three-dimensional (3D) sonography to assess the true midsagittal plane of the fetal spine. *J Matern Fetal Neonatal Med.* 2011;24(2):297–300. doi:10.3109/14767058.2010.487139.

126. Huissoud C, Bisch C, Charrin K, et al. Prenatal diagnosis of partial lumbar asoma by two- and three-dimensional ultrasound and computed tomography: embryological aspects and perinatal management. *Ultrasound Obstet Gynecol.* 2008;32(4):579–581. doi:10.1002/uog.6136.

127. Alvarez de la Rosa M, Padilla Perez AI, de la Torre Fernandez de Vega FJ, et al. Genetic counseling in a case of congenital hemivertebrae. *Arch Gynecol Obstet.* 2009;280(4):653–658. doi:10.1007/s00404-009-0969-4.

128. Haratz K, Vinkler C, Lev D, et al. Hemifacial microsomia with spinal and rib anomalies: prenatal diagnosis and postmortem confirmation using 3-D computed tomography reconstruction. *Fetal Diagn Ther.* 2011;30(4):309–313. doi:10.1159/000330121.

129. Steiner H, Spitzer D, Weiss-Wichert PH, et al. Three-dimensional ultrasound in prenatal diagnosis of skeletal dysplasia. *Prenat Diagn.* 1995;15(4):373–377.

130. Garjian KV, Pretorius DH, Budorick NE, et al. Fetal skeletal dysplasia: three-dimensional US—initial experience. *Radiology.* 2000;214(3):717–723. doi:10.1148/radiology.214.3.r00mr23717.

131. Chen CP, Chern SR, Shih JC, et al. Prenatal diagnosis and genetic analysis of type I and type II thanatophoric dysplasia. *Prenat Diagn.* 2001;21(2):89–95.

132. Moeglin D, Benoit B. Three-dimensional sonographic aspects in the antenatal diagnosis of achondroplasia. *Ultrasound Obstet Gynecol.* 2001;18(1):81–83. doi:10.1046/j.1469-0705.2001.00482.x.

133. Viora E, Sciarrone A, Bastonero S, et al. Three-dimensional ultrasound evaluation of short-rib polydactyly syndrome type II in the second trimester: a case report. *Ultrasound Obs Gynecol.* 2002;19(1):88–91.

134. Krakow D, Williams J, Poehl M, et al. Use of three-dimensional ultrasound imaging in the diagnosis of prenatal-onset skeletal dysplasias. *Ultrasound Obstet Gynecol.* 2003;21(5):467–472. doi:10.1002/uog.111.

135. Shih JC, Peng SS, Hsiao SM, et al. Three-dimensional ultrasound diagnosis of Larsen syndrome with further characterization of neurological sequelae. *Ultrasound Obstet Gynecol.* 2004;24(1):89–93. doi:10.1002/uog.1080.

136. Goncalves LF, Berger JA, Macknis JK, et al. Grebe dysplasia—prenatal diagnosis based on rendered 3-D ultrasound images of fetal limbs. *Pediatr Radiol.* 2017;47(1):108–112. doi:10.1007/s00247-016-3705-9.

137. Vimercati A, Chincoli A, de Gennaro AC, et al. 2D and 3D ultrasonographic evaluation of fetal midface hypoplasia in two cases with 3-M syndrome. *Geburtshilfe Frauenheilkd.* 2016;76(7):814–818. doi:10.1055/s-0042-105285.

138. Ruano R, Molho M, Roume J, et al. Prenatal diagnosis of fetal skeletal dysplasias by combining two-dimensional and three-dimensional ultrasound and intrauterine three-dimensional helical computer tomography. *Ultrasound Obstet Gynecol.* 2004;24(2):134–140. doi:10.1002/uog.1113.

139. Bonnet D, Coltri A, Butera G, et al. Detection of transposition of the great arteries in fetuses reduces neonatal morbidity and mortality. *Circulation.* 1999;99(7):916–918. doi:10.1161/01.CIR.99.7.916.

140. Calderon J, Angeard N, Moutier S, et al. Impact of prenatal diagnosis on neurocognitive outcomes in children with transposition of the great arteries. *J Pediatr.* 2012;161(1):94–99. doi:10.1016/j.jpeds.2011.12.036.

141. Franklin O, Burch M, Manning N, et al. Prenatal diagnosis of coarctation of the aorta improves survival and reduces morbidity. *Heart.* 2002;87(1):67–69. doi:10.1136/heart.87.1.67.

142. Tworetzky W, McElhinney DB, Reddy VM, et al. Improved surgical outcome after fetal diagnosis of hypoplastic left heart syndrome. *Circulation.* 2001;103(9):1269–1273. doi:10.1186/1750-1172-2-23.

143. Sklansky MS, Nelson TR, Pretorius DH. Three-dimensional fetal echocardiography: gated versus nongated techniques. *J Ultrasound Med.* 1998;17(7):451–457.

144. Sklansky M, Miller D, Devore G, et al. Prenatal screening for congenital heart disease using real-time three-dimensional echocardiography and a novel "sweep volume" acquisition technique. *Ultrasound Obstet Gynecol.* 2005;25(5):435–443. doi:10.1002/uog.1858.

145. Espinoza J, Kusanovic JP, Goncalves LF, et al. A novel algorithm for comprehensive fetal echocardiography using 4-dimensional ultrasonography and tomographic imaging. *J Ultrasound Med.* 2006;25(8):947–956.

146. Yeo L, Romero R, Jodicke C, et al. Simple targeted arterial rendering (STAR) technique: a novel and simple method to visualize the fetal cardiac outflow tracts. *Ultrasound Obstet Gynecol.* 2011;37(5):549–556. doi:10.1002/uog.8841.

147. Yeo L, Romero R, Jodicke C, et al. Four-chamber view and "swing technique" (FAST) echo: a novel and simple algorithm to visualize standard fetal echocardiographic planes. *Ultrasound Obstet Gynecol.* 2011;37(4):423–431. doi:10.1002/uog.8840.

148. Yeo L, Romero R. Fetal Intelligent Navigation Echocardiography (FINE): a novel method for rapid, simple, and automatic examination of the fetal heart. *Ultrasound Obstet Gynecol.* 2013;42(3):268–284. doi:10.1002/uog.12563.

149. Yagel S, Cohen SM, Achiron R. Examination of the fetal heart by five short-axis views: a proposed screening method for comprehensive cardiac evaluation. *Ultrasound Obstet Gynecol.* 2001;17(5):367–369.

150. Goncalves LF, Espinoza J, Romero R, et al. Four-dimensional fetal echocardiography with spatiotemporal image correlation (STIC): a systematic study of standard cardiac views assessed by different observers. *J Matern Fetal Neonatal Med.* 2005;17(5):323–331. doi:10.1080/1476705500127765.

151. Rizzo G, Capponi A, Muscatello A, et al. Examination of the fetal heart by four-dimensional ultrasound with spatiotemporal image correlation during routine second-trimester examination: the "three-steps technique." *Fetal Diagn Ther.* 2008;24(2):126–131. doi:10.1159/000142142.

152. Gonçalves LF, Espinoza J, Romero R, et al. A systematic approach to prenatal diagnosis of transposition of the great arteries using 4-dimensional ultrasonography with spatiotemporal image correlation. *J Ultrasound Med.* 2004;23(9):1225–1231.

153. Uittenbogaard LB, Haak MC, Spreeuwenberg MD, et al. A systematic analysis of the feasibility of four-dimensional ultrasound imaging using spatiotemporal image correlation in routine fetal echocardiography. *Ultrasound Obstet Gynecol.* 2008;31(6):625–632. doi:10.1002/uog.5351.

154. Cohen L, Mangers K, Grobman WA, et al. Satisfactory visualization rates of standard cardiac views at 18 to 22 weeks' gestation using spatiotemporal image correlation. *J Ultrasound Med.* 2009;28(12):1645–1650.

155. Inubashiri E, Tatedo S, Nishiyama N, et al. Feasibility assessment for successfully visualizing the fetal heart utilizing spatiotemporal image correlation. *J Med Ultrason.* 2018;45(2):269–279. doi:10.1007/s10396-017-0818-1.

156. Bennasar M, Martínez JM, Gómez O, et al. Accuracy of four-dimensional spatiotemporal image correlation echocardiography in the prenatal diagnosis of congenital heart defects. *Ultrasound Obstet Gynecol.* 2010;36(4):458–464. doi:10.1002/uog.7720.

157. Espinoza J, Lee W, Comstock C, et al. Collaborative study on 4-dimensional echocardiography for the diagnosis of fetal heart defects: the COFEHD study. *J Ultrasound Med.* 2010;29(11):1573–1580.

158. Shen O, Yagel S. The added value of 3D/4D ultrasound imaging in fetal cardiology: has the promise been fulfilled? *Ultrasound Obstet Gynecol.* 2010;35(3):260–262. doi:10.1002/uog.7569.

159. Abuhamad A, Falkensammer P, Reichartseder F, et al. Automated retrieval of standard diagnostic fetal cardiac ultrasound planes in the second trimester of pregnancy: a prospective evaluation of software. *Ultrasound Obstet Gynecol.* 2008;31(1):30–36. doi:10.1002/uog.5228.

160. Abuhamad A, Falkensammer P, Zhao Y. Automated sonography: defining the spatial relationship of standard diagnostic fetal cardiac planes in the second trimester of pregnancy. *J Ultrasound Med.* 2007;26(4):501–507.

161. Veronese P, Bogana G, Cerutti A, et al. A prospective study of the use of Fetal Intelligent Navigation Echocardiography (FINE) to obtain standard fetal echocardiography views. *Fetal Diagn Ther.* 2017;41(2):89–99. doi:10.1159/000446982.

162. Garcia M, Yeo L, Romero R, et al. Prospective evaluation of the fetal heart using Fetal Intelligent Navigation Echocardiography (FINE). *Ultrasound Obstet Gynecol.* 2016;47(4):450–459. doi:10.1002/uog.15676.

163. Yeo L, Luewan S, Romero R. Fetal Intelligent Navigation Echocardiography (FINE) detects 98% of congenital heart disease. *J Ultrasound Med.* 2018;37(11):2577–2593. doi:10.1002/jum.14616.

164. Riccabona M, Nelson TR, Pretorius DH, et al. Distance and volume measurement using three-dimensional ultrasonography. *J Ultrasound Med.* 1995;14(12):881–886. doi:10.7863/jum.1995.14.12.881.

165. Riccabona M, Nelson TR, Pretorius DH, et al. In vivo three-dimensional sonographic measurement of organ volume: validation in the urinary bladder. *J Ultrasound Med.* 1996;15(9):627–632. doi:10.7863/jum.1996.15.9.627.

166. Barreto EQ, Milani HF, Araujo Júnior E, et al. Reproducibility of fetal heart volume by 3D-sonography using the XI VOCAL method. *Cardiovasc Ultrasound.* 2010;8:17. doi:10.1186/1476-7120-8-17.

167. Ioannou C, Sarris I, Salomon LJ, et al. A review of fetal volumetry: the need for standardization and definitions in measurement methodology. *Ultrasound Obstet Gynecol.* 2011;38(6):613–619. doi:10.1002/uog.9074.

168. Hamill N, Yeo L, Romero R, et al. Fetal cardiac ventricular volume, cardiac output, and ejection fraction determined with 4-dimensional ultrasound using spatiotemporal image correlation and virtual organ computer-aided analysis. *Am J Obstet Gynecol.* 2011;205(1):76.e1–76.e10. doi:10.1016/j.ajog.2011.02.028.

169. Laudy JA, Janssen MM, Struyk PC, et al. Three-dimensional ultrasonography of normal fetal lung volume: a preliminary study. *Ultrasound Obstet Gynecol.* 1998;11(1):13–16. doi:10.1046/j.1469-0705.1998.11010013.x.

170. Lee W, Deter RL, Ebersole JD, et al. Birth weight prediction by three-dimensional ultrasonography: fractional limb volume. *J Ultrasound Med.* 2001;20(12):1283–1292.

171. Kalache KD, Espinoza J, Chaiworapongsa T, et al. Three-dimensional ultrasound fetal lung volume measurement: a systematic study comparing the multiplanar method with the rotational (VOCAL) technique. *Ultrasound Obstet Gynecol.* 2003;21(2):111–118. doi:10.1002/uog.39.

172. Ruano R, Joubin L, Sonigo P, et al. Fetal lung volume estimated by 3-dimensional ultrasonography and magnetic resonance imaging in cases with isolated congenital diaphragmatic hernia. *J Ultrasound Med.* 2004;23(3):353–358.

173. Lee W, Deter RL, McNie B, et al. Individualized growth assessment of fetal soft tissue using fractional thigh volume. *Ultrasound Obstet Gynecol.* 2004;24(7):766–774. doi:10.1002/uog.1779.

174. Lee W, Deter RL, McNie B, et al. The fetal arm: individualized growth assessment in normal pregnancies. *J Ultrasound Med.* 2005;24(6):817–828.

175. Peralta CFA, Cavoretto P, Csapo B, et al. Lung and heart volumes by three-dimensional ultrasound in normal fetuses at 12-32 weeks' gestation. *Ultrasound Obstet Gynecol.* 2006;27(2):128–133. doi:10.1002/uog.2670.

176. Hamill N, Romero R, Hassan SS, et al. Repeatability and reproducibility of fetal cardiac ventricular volume calculations using spatiotemporal image correlation and virtual organ computer-aided analysis. *J Ultrasound Med.* 2009;28(10):1301–1311.

177. Liang RI, Chang FM, Yao BL, et al. Predicting birth weight by fetal upper-arm volume with use of three-dimensional ultrasonography. *Am J Obstet Gynecol.* 1997;177(3):632–638.

178. Ioannou C, Sarris I, Yaqub MK, et al. Surface area measurement using rendered three-dimensional ultrasound imaging: an in-vitro phantom study. *Ultrasound Obstet Gynecol.* 2011;38(4):445–449. doi:10.1002/uog.8984.

179. Raine-Fenning NJ, Clewes JS, Kendall NR, et al. The interobserver reliability and validity of volume calculation from three-dimensional ultrasound datasets in the in vitro setting. *Ultrasound Obstet Gynecol.* 2003;21(3):283–291. doi:10.1002/uog.61.

180. Ruano R, Benachi A, Joubin L, et al. Three-dimensional ultrasonographic assessment of fetal lung volume as prognostic factor in isolated congenital diaphragmatic hernia. *BJOG.* 2004;111(5):423–429. doi:10.1111/j.1471-0528.2004.00100.x.

181. Sabogal JC, Becker E, Bega G, et al. Reproducibility of fetal lung volume measurements with 3-dimensional ultrasonography. *J Ultrasound Med.* 2004;23(3):347–352.

182. Araujo Junior E, Nardozza LMM, Pires CR, et al. Comparison of the two-dimensional and multiplanar methods and establishment of a new constant for the measurement of fetal lung volume. *J Matern Fetal Neonatal Med.* 2008;21(1):81–88. doi:10.1080/14767050701831280.

183. Britto ISW, de Silva Bussamra LCC, Araujo Júnior E, et al. Fetal lung volume: comparison by 2D- and 3D-sonography in normal fetuses. *Arch Gynecol Obstet.* 2009;280(3):363–368. doi:10.1007/s00404-008-0908-9.

184. Gerards FA, Engels MAJ, Twisk JWR, et al. Normal fetal lung volume measured with three-dimensional ultrasound. *Ultrasound Obstet Gynecol.* 2006;27(2):134–144. doi:10.1002/uog.2672.

185. Bahmaie A, Hughes SW, Clark T, et al. Serial fetal lung volume measurement using three-dimensional ultrasound. *Ultrasound Obstet Gynecol.* 2000;16(2):154–158. doi:10.1046/j.1469-0705.2000.00193.x.

186. Chang C-H, Yu C-H, Chang F-M, et al. Volumetric assessment of normal fetal lungs using three-dimensional ultrasound. *Ultrasound Med Biol.* 2003;29(7):935–942.

187. Hughes SW, D'Arcy TJ, Maxwell DJ, et al. Volume estimation from multiplanar 2D ultrasound images using a remote electromagnetic position and orientation sensor. *Ultrasound Med Biol.* 1996;22(5):561–572.

188. Hata T, Kuno A, Dai S-Y, et al. Three-dimensional sonographic volume measurement of the fetal spleen. *J Obstet Gynaecol Res.* 2007;33(6):793–798. doi:10.1111/j.1447-0756.2007.00658.x.

189. Moeglin D, Talmant C, Duyme M, et al. Fetal lung volumetry using two- and three-dimensional ultrasound. *Ultrasound Obstet Gynecol.* 2005;25(2):119–127. doi:10.1002/uog.1799.

190. Osada H, Iitsuka Y, Masuda K, et al. Application of lung volume measurement by three-dimensional ultrasonography for clinical assessment of fetal lung development. *J Ultrasound Med.* 2002;21(8):841–847.

191. Pohls UG, Rempen A. Fetal lung volumetry by three-dimensional ultrasound. *Ultrasound Obstet Gynecol.* 1998;11(1):6–12. doi:10.1046/j.1469-0705.1998.11010006.x.

192. Melamed N, Yogev Y, Meizner I, et al. Sonographic fetal weight estimation. *J Ultrasound Med.* 2009;28(5):617–629. doi:10.7863/jum.2009.28.5.617.

193. Lee W, Balasubramaniam M, Deter RL, et al. Fractional limb volume—a soft tissue parameter of fetal body composition: validation, technical considerations and normal ranges during pregnancy. *Ultrasound Obstet Gynecol.* 2009;33(4):427–440. doi:10.1002/uog.6319.

194. Song TB, Moore TR, Lee JI, et al. Fetal weight prediction by thigh volume measurement with three-dimensional ultrasonography. *Obstet Gynecol.* 2000;96(2):157–161.

195. Lee W, Deter R, Sangi-Haghpeykar H, et al. Prospective validation of fetal weight estimation using fractional limb volume. *Ultrasound Obstet Gynecol.* 2013;41(2):198–203. doi:10.1002/uog.11185.

196. Matsumoto M, Yanagihara T, Hata T. Three-dimensional qualitative sonographic evaluation of fetal soft tissue. *Hum Reprod.* 2000;15(11):2438–2442.

197. Chang C-H, Yu C-H, Chang F-M, et al. Three-dimensional ultrasound in the assessment of normal fetal thigh volume. *Ultrasound Med Biol.* 2003;29(3):361–366.

198. Patipanawat S, Komwilaisak R, Ratanasiri T. Correlation of weight estimation in large and small fetuses with three-dimensional ultrasonographic volume measurements of the fetal upper-arm and thigh: a preliminary report. *J Med Assoc Thai.* 2006;89(1):13–19.

199. Schild RL, Maringa M, Siemer J, et al. Weight estimation by three-dimensional ultrasound imaging in the small fetus. *Ultrasound Obstet Gynecol.* 2008;32(2):168–175. doi:10.1002/uog.6111.

200. Siemer J, Peter W, Zollver H, et al. How good is fetal weight estimation using volumetric methods? *Ultraschall Med.* 2008;29(4):377–382. doi:10.1055/s-2008-1027191.

201. Lee W, Balasubramaniam M, Deter RL, et al. Fetal growth parameters and birth weight: their relationship to neonatal body composition. *Ultrasound Obstet Gynecol.* 2009;33(4):441–446. doi:10.1002/uog.6317.

202. Nardozza LMM, Vieira MF, Araujo Junior E, et al. Prediction of birth weight using fetal thigh and upper-arm volumes by three-dimensional ultrasonography in a Brazilian population. *J Matern Fetal Neonatal Med.* 2010;23(5):393–398. doi:10.1080/14767050903184215.

203. Chang FM, Liang RI, Ko HC, et al. Three-dimensional ultrasound-assessed fetal thigh volumetry in predicting birth weight. *Obstet Gynecol.* 1997;90(3):331–339.

204. Lee W, Balasubramaniam M, Deter RL, et al. New fetal weight estimation models using fractional limb volume. *Ultrasound Obstet Gynecol.* 2009;34(5):556–565. doi:10.1002/uog.7327.

205. Schmidt KG, Silverman NH, Hoffman JIE. Determination of ventricular volumes in human fetal hearts by two-dimensional echocardiography. *Am J Cardiol.* 1995;76(17):1313–1316. doi:10.1016/S0002-9149(99)80365-8.

206. Wadimiroff JW, McGnie J. Ultrasonic assessment of cardiovascular geometry and function in the human fetus. *BJOG.* 1981;88(9):870–875. doi:10.1111/j.1471-0528.1981.tb02221.x.

207. De Smedt MCH, Visser GHA, Meijboom EJ. Fetal cardiac output estimated by Doppler echocardiography during mid- and late gestation. *Am J Cardiol.* 1987;60(4):338–342. doi:10.1016/0002-9149(87)90238-4.

208. Simpson JM, Cook A. Repeatability of echocardiographic measurements in the human fetus. *Ultrasound Obstet Gynecol.* 2002:332–339.

209. Meyer-Wittkopf M, Cole A, Cooper SG, et al. Three-dimensional quantitative echocardiographic assessment of ventricular volume in healthy human fetuses and in fetuses with congenital heart disease. *J Ultrasound Med.* 2001;20(4):317–327.

210. Esh-Broder E, Ushakov FB, Imbar T, et al. Application of free-hand three-dimensional echocardiography in the evaluation of fetal cardiac ejection fraction: a preliminary study. *Ultrasound Obstet Gynecol.* 2004;23(6):546–551. doi:10.1002/uog.1059.

211. Bhat AH, Corbett VN, Liu R, et al. Validation of volume and mass assessments for human fetal heart imaging by 4-dimensional spatiotemporal image correlation echocardiography: in vitro balloon model experiments. *J Ultrasound Med.* 2004;23(9):1151–1159.

212. Uittenbogaard LB, Haak MC, Peters RJH, et al. Validation of volume measurements for fetal echocardiography using four-dimensional ultrasound imaging and spatiotemporal image correlation. *Ultrasound Obstet Gynecol.* 2010;35(3):324–331. doi:10.1002/uog.7561.

213. Uittenbogaard LB, Haak MC, Spreeuwenberg MD, et al. Fetal cardiac function assessed with four-dimensional ultrasound imaging using spatiotemporal image correlation. *Ultrasound Obstet Gynecol.* 2009;33(3):272–281. doi:10.1002/uog.6287.

214. Simioni C, Nardozza LMM, Araujo Júnior E, et al. Heart stroke volume, cardiac output, and ejection fraction in 265 normal fetus in the second half of gestation assessed by 4D ultrasound using spatio-temporal image correlation. *J Matern Fetal Neonatal Med.* 2011;24(9):1159–1167. doi:10.3109/14767058.2010.545921.

215. Messing B, Cohen SM, Valsky DV, et al. Fetal cardiac ventricle volumetry in the second half of gestation assessed by 4D ultrasound using STIC combined with inversion mode. *Ultrasound Obstet Gynecol.* 2007;30(2):142–151. doi:10.1002/uog.4036.

216. Molina FS, Faro C, Sotiriadis A, et al. Heart stroke volume and cardiac output by four-dimensional ultrasound in normal fetuses. *Ultrasound Obstet Gynecol.* 2008;32(2):181–187. doi:10.1002/uog.5374.

217. Rizzo G, Capponi A, Pietrolucci ME, et al. Role of sonographic automatic volume calculation in measuring fetal cardiac ventricular volumes using 4-dimensional sonography: comparison with virtual organ computer-aided analysis. *J Ultrasound Med.* 2010;29(2):261–270.

218. Hamill N, Romero R, Hassan S, et al. The fetal cardiovascular response to increased placental vascular impedance to flow determined with 4-dimensional ultrasound using spatiotemporal image correlation and virtual organ computer-aided analysis. *Am J Obstet Gynecol.* 2013;208(2):153.e1–153.e13. doi:10.1016/j.ajog.2012.11.043.

219. Schoonderwaldt EM, Groenenberg IAL, Hop WCJ, et al. Reproducibility of echocardiographic measurements of human fetal left ventricular volumes and ejection fractions using four-dimensional ultrasound with the spatio-temporal image correlation modality. *Eur J Obstet Gynecol Reprod Biol.* 2012;160(1):22–29. doi:10.1016/j.ejogrb.2011.09.036.

8

Fetal Magnetic Resonance Imaging Techniques and Safety

Dorothy I. Bulas • Teresa Victoria • Timothy P. L. Roberts

BACKGROUND

Magnetic resonance imaging (MRI) is an alternative modality to evaluate the fetus. It uses no ionizing radiation, has excellent tissue contrast, provides a large field of view (FOV), is not limited by maternal body habitus or overlying bone, and can image the fetus in multiple planes no matter where the fetal lie. Fetal MRI was initially attempted in the 1980s but was limited because of slow sequences requiring fetal and/or maternal sedation. Since then, the development of faster sequences has been fundamental in the success of imaging the moving fetus without the use of sedation.[1-3] Faster scanning techniques now allow studies to be performed without sedation in the second and third trimesters, with excellent tissue contrast, good signal-to-noise ratio (SNR), and minimal motion artifact.

Utility

With advances in fetal management, there is an increasing need for precise depiction of abnormalities. Ultrasound (US) remains the screening modality of choice in the assessment of the fetus.[4]

When additional information is needed, MRI has become a useful adjunct in the assessment of complex fetal anomalies. The use of fetal MRI can help confirm or exclude the presence of lesions noted by US. MRI can demonstrate additional subtle anomalies not visualized by US that may alter outcome. These additional findings can aid in the planning of fetal intervention, delivery, and postnatal therapeutic planning as well as in counseling parents regarding long-term prognosis.

MRI has numerous advantages that make it a complementary study in the evaluation of the fetus. MRI, in comparison with US, is not limited by fetal lie, overlying maternal or fetal bone, obesity, or oligohydramnios. MRI offers excellent soft-tissue contrast and multiplanar visualization of all organs. Evidence-based data for the performance of fetal MRI are strongest for central nervous system (CNS) anomalies and for cases being considered for fetal intervention, such as neural tube defects.[5,6] Advanced techniques are being developed that may provide physiological information, including fetal spectroscopy and functional MRI (fMRI)[7,8] (see Chapter 10). Much research is currently being performed on the use of MRI to estimate lung volumes, particularly in cases of congenital diaphragmatic hernia as well as lung masses and lung hypoplasia.[9,10] With the airway filled with fluid in fetal life, MRI can directly visualize the larynx, pharynx, and trachea, assessing the need for ex utero intrapartum treatment (EXIT) procedure when an oral or neck mass is present compressing the airway.[2,3] Various T1, T2, and echo planar sequences can distinguish blood, fat, meconium, and cartilage, thus increasing the accuracy of diagnosis.[11] Large FOV with multiplanar capability enables other specialists as well as family members to better visualize and understand the abnormalities. The ability to view images as a team is a powerful tool in counseling families and planning potential interventions.[5,6,12] Indeed, the ability to view images has pulled many specialists into fetology, including neonatologists, pediatric surgeons, neurosurgeons, neurologists, and urologists who may feel more comfortable reviewing MRI images.[13-15] This team approach is particularly useful in planning fetal surgery or complex deliveries in cases of neck masses, sacrococcygeal teratomas, and conjoined twins.[16-18] In addition, fetal studies can be used for postnatal surgical planning, decreasing the need for emergent studies in the unstable newborn.

Timing

MRI can be a useful adjunct when a targeted sonogram performed by an experienced sonographer raises questions that could benefit from further assessment. MRI may provide additional information when an abnormality is identified by US or when findings are equivocal and require clarification.[5,14] The optimal timing of a fetal MRI depends on what questions need to be answered.

As the theoretical risk of MRI is potentially highest during organogenesis, and the size of the developing fetus is so small early gestation, fetal MRI in the first trimester is not recommended.[19-21] At times, owing to maternal indications, MRI has been performed early in the first trimester, with limited visualization of the embryo. Anomalies are better visualized by US during this gestation.

From 12 to 16 weeks, fetal MRI remains limited because of the small size of the fetus, increased fetal motion, and the fact that some anomalies may have not yet evolved (such as cortical dysplasias).

MRI between 17 and 24 weeks' gestation is useful to further evaluate or confirm findings noted on target sonograms that can impact pregnancy planning and intervention.

MRI in the third trimester is optimal for the assessment of many anomalies, particularly of the cerebral cortex, owing to improved spatial resolution. Decreased motion, head engagement in the lower pelvis, and larger targets allow for advanced imaging such as spectroscopy, diffusion tension imaging (DTI), and fMRI. Later studies, however, risk identifying anomalies too late for optimal intervention. MRI studies performed in the second trimester may, at times, benefit from a follow-up examination in the third trimester, particularly those requiring complex delivery planning such as neck masses.

Limitations

Technical challenges include motion artifact, limited fast sequences, optimizing SNR, and lack of technical expertise. Motion comes mainly from the fetus but also from the mother, who can be uncomfortable and anxious, making it difficult to obtain adequate images. The moving fetus makes obtaining appropriate planes challenging for the technologist, and repeat sequences are often required to obtain a quality image. If the MRI technologist is inexperienced, the physician will need to help, as anatomy can be confusing in a moving fetus, particularly when complex anomalies are distorting normal landmarks.

Fast scanning sequences are limited. T1 and T2 sequences must be optimized to decrease the scanning time and motion artifact. Some sequences require the breath to be held to improve image quality (T1). This can be difficult for a mother lying uncomfortably with diaphragms elevated by the gravid uterus. Fetal gating is currently not commercially available, limiting evaluation of the fetal heart. Various centers, however, have been working on methods to fetal gating examinations using US.[22–25] When fetal motion is problematic, particularly when polyhydramnios is present, dynamic steady-state free precession (SSFP) can be useful.

Interpreting fetal MRIs can be challenging as structures are small and change with fetal maturation. Great care must be taken when interpreting as well as performing these studies. Prognosis of abnormalities can be highly varied with limited long-term data available. This can make counseling difficult at times, even when anomalies are well delineated. Additional long-term follow-up studies are necessary to provide more accurate data for improved counseling.[5,26]

SAFETY

While there is currently no evidence that fetal MRI produces harmful effects to the fetus, long-term safety has not been firmly established. There is a lack of consensus as to whether there are true risks to the fetus.[19–21,27,28]

While no adverse effects have been consistently demonstrated, the evidence is inconclusive, numbers are small, and data variable with potential confounders.[28]

Several potential safety issues have been raised. These include acoustic damage and teratogenic effects due to torque, acceleration by the static field, nerve stimulation by the gradient fields, and/or tissue heating by radio frequency (RF) fields.[19–22,27–31]

In terms of acoustic damage, MRI produces a loud tapping noise when coils are exposed to rapidly oscillating electromagnetic currents. Initially, concern was raised regarding potential acoustic damage to the developing ear. More recent studies, including those assessing 3T which is associated with increased noise, have been reassuring with no evidence that there is an increased risk of clinically detected hearing abnormalities.[32,33]

Some studies have raised the concern for teratogenic effects of MRI when performed early in pregnancy, secondary to the heating effect of MRI gradient changes and a direct nonthermal interaction of the electromagnetic field.[34,35,28] Static magnetic fields produce short-term high-field exposure to the patient from 0.2 to 3 T and long-term low-field exposure to MRI staff (0.5 to 200 mT). Animal studies have demonstrated effects such as a decrease in crown-rump length when mice were exposed to MRI in midgestation,[34] eye malformations in genetically predisposed mice,[35] and demise of chick embryos when exposed to strong magnetic fields.[19] These studies are not applicable to humans and cannot be extrapolated, but they do raise concerns.

RF fields generate heat and are measured by specific absorption rate (SAR). Mathematical models on simulations have identified RF levels that are tolerable to humans; however, fetal dosimetry is only now being developed.[36–38] Fast sequences use high-specification magnetic field gradients. dB/dt exposure needs to be further researched not only in adults but in the fetus as well. Murbach et al.[30] investigated whether children and fetuses were at higher risk than adults when current RF regulations were applied. In their limited series, they noted local exposure was smaller for children and fetuses than adults. Local thermal load, however, could be increased to the fetus because of high exposure average of the nonperfused amniotic fluid.[30]

Effective exposure time during a fetal MRI has not been well studied, making estimation of RF deposition and noise exposure difficult. Brugger and Prayer noted that actual imaging time accounts for only about 33% of total study time. Exposure time is not continuous, with the remaining time taken up by repositioning of the coil/mother and planning sequences.[39]

Kanal et al.[40] produced a worker survey on female MRI technologists concerning low-field exposure. There were over 1,900 responses, with no statistically significant associations revealed.

3 Tesla Safety

A survey of the pediatric radiologists of North America shows that approximately 25% of the responders use 1.5 and 3T magnet strength platforms interchangeably for fetal MR, while about 7% use 3T magnets exclusively.[1] Better SNR is gently pushing some centers to do more fetal scanning at the higher magnet strength. As the older generation scanners are being replaced by the newer and more versatile versions, institutions tend to acquire the higher magnet strength to scan all of their patients, including the gravid patient.[41] To date, the Food and Drug Administration (FDA) has not issued a document specifically addressing the safety of fetal MR at 3 T; it has, however, suggested that when evaluating the safety of any MR device, the following four areas of concern should be explored and evaluated:

1. RF power deposition
2. Static field exposure
3. Gradient field switching
4. Noise and fetal acoustic effect

Radio Frequency Power Deposition

Excitation and refocusing MR RF pulses generate signals that form an image. These pulses consist of oscillating electromagnetic fields, which, in turn, generate electrical currents. These electrical currents produce energy that translates into heat transferred through the soft tissues of the imaged subject; in this case, the mother and her fetus. Hyperthermia during pregnancy has been associated with untoward effects to the fetus, with the threshold of effect at about $1.5°C$ above normal core body temperature. These untoward effects have been reviewed[42] with the most profound and devastating effects manifested in the embryonic rather than the fetal stage. Generally speaking, in humans, an elevation of the maternal body temperature by $2°C$ for at least 24 hours may cause a range of developmental effects, with not much additional information available for shorter exposure times. With regard to direct RF exposure to the fetus, significant heat absorption by the mother as well as heat dissipation due to conductive and convective exchanges offer significant protection to the fetus.[43] Yet, it is difficult to measure patient's temperature changes in vivo, both in the mother and particularly in the fetus; thus, a surrogate, the SAR, is utilized to reflect the amount of energy (and by default, heat) that is produced and deposited in the tissues while scanning.

The main safety concern in fetal MR is the absorption of so much RF energy or SAR that it causes harm to the fetus. For this reason, fetal MRI is always performed in the lowest SAR level or "normal mode." The SAR, which is defined as RF energy per unit time per kg and is measured in Watts/kg, is defined by the following relationship:

$$\text{SAR} \propto B_0^2\ \alpha^2 \Delta f$$

The SAR is proportional to the main magnetic field strength (B_0), the flip angle (α), and the RF bandwidth (Δf).[44] Thus, doubling the field strength from 1.5 to 3 T leads to quadrupling the SAR. However, there are ways to decrease the SAR while scanning, which include decreasing the flip angle or increasing the repetition time (TR), although, by doing so, the SNR or scan speed advantages gained at higher magnet strength may be compromised. The use of multielement RF hardware/reconstruction techniques, such as parallel imaging, can also decrease the SAR level. Despite this, the SAR levels on a clinical basis stay within the safety limit of 4 W/kg allowed by the FDA mainly because clinical MR systems have a fail-safe mechanism that does not allow scanning if the limit is to be exceeded.[45]

The overall body SAR is thus not the real impediment to fetal scanning at 3 T, as the subject is protected by the fail-safe mechanism present in all MR scanners. There is, however, a concern in the inhomogeneous distribution of energy or heat within the fetal tissue, the so-called hotspots or local SAR. This occurs as the absorbed energy is applied to one body region more than others. Practically speaking, it is difficult to calculate hotspots, just as it is difficult to calculate temperature of different tissues in vivo; thus, modeling has been used as best surrogate. Using modeling, Hand et al. utilized a 28-week pregnant model and subjected it to birdcage coils operating at 64 and 127 MHz (the equivalent of 1.5 and 3 T, respectively).[46] They showed that, as long as using normal mode, the highest local SAR was on the mother, with the fetus being exposed to approximately 40% to 60% at 64 MHz and 50% to 70% at 127 MHz. In a subsequent paper, the group also predicted that procedures compliant with International Electrotechnical Commission (IEC) and as long as scanning is done in *normal mode* (maternal whole-body averaged $\text{SAR}_{\text{MWB}} \leq 2$ W/kg [continuous or time averaged over 6 minutes]), whole fetal SAR, local fetal SAR_{10g}, and average fetal temperature are within international safety limits.[38]

The above experiments by Hand et al. were conducted using a circularly polarized (CP) mode of scanning. Murbach et al. evaluated the RF deposition and temperature changes in pregnant models using a two-port body coils at 3 T.[47] They postulated that, in contrast to CP B_1 fields, the polarization in RF shimmed (two-port excitation) body coils would become linear, thereby significantly increasing local RF absorption. What they found is that in this two-port scenario, the conclusion that the mother receives the highest local SAR exposure would no longer hold and that, in fact, both mother and fetus would get similar SAR exposure. They also report that in this static model, the basic restrictions of the International Commission of Non-Ionizing Radiation Protection (IC-NIRP) of wbSAR = 0.08 W/kg and psSAR10g = 2 to 4 W/kg (whereas wbSAR stands for whole-body SAR, and psSAR10g is peak special SAR averaged over any 10 g) is exceeded by a factor of 2 for the fetus while in normal operating mode. The authors did not explain how these findings would change if parallel transmit is utilized, in which the two-port excitation system is split into a number of excitation ports. Further, when evaluating temperature change, these authors showed that in worst-case scenarios, at the constant maximum temperature, the proposed thermal dose may be reached. There are a number of limitations to this study, namely, the study is done in static models in which the amniotic fluid is stationary (thus not able to take advantage of the dispersive capabilities of convection and dispersion of heat with movement), does not take into account the different properties and dynamics of the different soft tissues of the real patient (both mother and fetus), and finally does not take into account fetal movement, by which hotspots are unlikely to remain in the same location for prolonged periods of time. Still, the findings by Murbach et al. are concerning despite the dissimilarities between the static model and the in vivo patient, making its practical translation to a real patient difficult to discern.

In 2016, a study by Cannie et al. attempted to evaluate in vivo temperature changes in a group of miniature pigs during MRI at 3T magnet strength,[48] similar to how Levin et al. had done at 1.5 T.[36] Their conclusions state that when using normal mode, 3T fetal imaging does not result in temperature increases above 1°C when normal SAR regimens (that is, clinical imaging parameters) are used, with imaging times less than 30 minutes. High SAR regimens, however, the authors postulate, may lead to a cumulative temperature increase over 1 hour of imaging time of up to 2.5°C. These findings immediately raised concern in the obstetric imaging population. However, when analyzing the paper, one must realize that (1) the 2.5°C was a cumulative temperature of various pigs (and not a single organ of a single subject), (2) the study was done under scanning parameters that would not happen practically speaking (nonstop scanning, no breaks, for an hour), and (3) there were no 1.5T control subjects included in the study.

RF deposition, energy transfer, and heat rise are a real concern when scanning the fetus at 3 T. There are still many questions about what is safe, and the question whether the temperature rises to unacceptable levels when scanning the fetus at 3 T remains. For now, certain safety parameters should be considered:

1. To always scan the fetus in normal mode,
2. To minimize the time of scanning,
3. To intercalate high SAR sequences (single-shot turbo spin-echo mainly) with lower SAR sequences such as echo planar imaging (EPI), as clinically indicated.

Static Field Exposure

The risks associated with high static magnetic fields are mainly biological. In a review from 2004, de Wilde does a comprehensive review on this subject, concluding that fields up to 8 T do not affect rapid embryonic cleavage, cell multiplication, and differentiation, nor any effect on the dielectric properties of chick-embryo myoblast membranes and that up to 8 T, there is no adverse effect from exposure to static magnetic fields on neurocognitive testing or vital sign changes of volunteers.[49] The fourth edition of the Safety Guidelines for Magnetic Resonance Imaging Equipment in Clinical Use (http://www.ismrm.org/smrt/files/con2033065.pdf) published in 2014 also reviews this topic and concludes that the biological effects most likely to occur in patients and volunteers undergoing MRI procedures are the production of vertigo-like sensations and that the probability of clinically relevant physiological effects or of significant changes in cognitive functions occurring in fields of up to 4 T appear to be low. Furthermore, the guidelines state that the accumulated experience of MRI procedures in clinical situations, where exposures using fields of 3 T are becoming increasingly common, does not suggest that any obvious detrimental field–related effects occur, especially in the short term (of note, and following this line of thinking, to date, there has been no report of untoward clinical effects in the gravid patient or the fetus in the past decade, when 3T scanning became more mainstream). Lastly, the 2009 ICNIRP guidelines conclude that, regarding the static field, "current information does not indicate any serious health effects resulting from acute exposure to static magnetic fields up to 8 T" (http://www.icnirp.org/en/publications/index.html).

It is important to note that these studies have not been done in vivo or in a human fetus. Thus, the actual translation of the research to the human conceptus is not truly known, and care must always be taken when scanning the fetus at 3 T.

Gradient Field Switching
The hazards of pulsed electromagnetic fields are biological effects, namely, the risk of peripheral nerve stimulation (PNS) and acoustic damage.

The risk of PNS arises from the interaction of the magnetic fields of the gradient coil with the nerve fibers in the human body inducing electric currents.[50] Magnetic field gradients can be in the order of 10s of mT/m and can switch at a rate up to 200 mT/m/ms. If an electric potential is applied to a nerve, its membrane will be charged, which may, in turn, generate an action potential and a subsequent unwanted action, such as muscle contractions and sensory perceptions that may lead to seizures, cardiac arrhythmias, and pain. This may manifest as a tingling sensation. The effects of MR scanning at 3 T on the fetal PNS are not thought to be deleterious as the gradient design of a 1.5 and 3T scanner is equivalent (Ellen Grant, MD, "Potential Risk of Fetal Magnetic Resonance Imaging: 3 Tesla compared to 1.5 Tesla," unpublished manuscript). In addition, PNS has the greatest effect in the periphery of the gradient coil rather than isocenter, where the fetus is always placed (if the magnetic field gradient applied is 10 mT/m, then the actual field experienced even 10 cm from isocenter is only 1 mT).

Noise and Fetal Acoustic Effect
The fetus appears to be physically protected from noise by a double insulating barrier: the maternal abdomen and the amniotic fluid, which surrounds the fetus and bathes the fetal auditory canal. These physical barriers attenuate sound, similar to when someone outside a pool talks to a person who is completely submerged in the water.

One study contrasted the prevalence of congenital hearing loss in neonates who had a 3T prenatal MR with those who had a 1.5T prenatal MR.[51] The study was done by comparing the fail rates of their neonatal hearing screening programs. These studies, which are mandated by the state's government legislation for all newborns, consist of the transient otoacoustic emission test and the auditory brainstem response test. The study showed that when comparing 128 patients, there was no significant difference in the fail rate of those who had had a prenatal scan at 3T magnet strength with those that had had a 1.5T scan, supporting the argument that the increase noise associated with 3 T does not increase the rate of clinically detectable hearing abnormalities. Notably, several manufacturers are exploring a variety of techniques,

both through hardware and optimized pulse sequence design, to reduce the acoustic noise of clinical MRI.

Precautions must be taken including insuring that normal MR mode is always used, that the shortest amount of scanning time is achieved to reach a diagnosis, and that high SAR sequences are intercalated with low SAR sequences. It is important to remember that while several series have described no adverse long-term effects of fetal MRI in children imaged as fetus, the samples have been small, and no long-term studies are currently available regarding higher strength magnets greater than 3 T.[32,33,49,52–55]

With no conclusive documentation of deleterious effects of MRI at 1.5 T, no specific recommendations may be required for any trimester in pregnancy.[56] Pregnant patients should undergo an MRI, if the attending radiologist determines a need and benefits outweigh any potential risks. However, with the advent of higher Tesla magnets, radiologists should be aware of increased power deposition with high-field studies and ensure that established guidelines are not exceeded.[56–59]

Gadolinium
MRI contrast agents should not be routinely administered to the pregnant patient. While there are no specific fetal indications for the use of MRI contrast, rarely, contrast may be needed for assessing maternal pathology.

The use of intravenous gadolinium and its toxic effects to the fetus has been tested in animals with limited studies in humans. Gadolinium crosses the placenta and is excreted in urine by the fetus and later reabsorbed/swallowed, prolonging the elimination time.[60–66] When excreted into the amniotic fluid, the gadolinium chelate molecules may remain for an indeterminate amount of time before being eliminated. The longer the chelate molecule remains in the amniotic fluid, the greater the potential of dissociation of the gadolinium ion from its chelate molecule.

In a study with rabbits, a high concentration of gadolinium was noted 5 minutes after its administration, with a subsequent decrease of 50% after 60 minutes.[63,65] At high (two to seven times the dose used in humans) and repeated doses, teratogenic effects (including growth retardation, visual problems, and bone and visceral anomalies) have been described in animals.[60,63–65] No carcinogenic or mutagenic effects have been noted.[60] Other preclinical studies using contrast have not shown negative effects on the fetus, including detectable chromosomal damage, abortions, stillbirth, and grossly detectable anomalies, even at 11 to 16 times the clinical dose.[60]

In the human fetus, the concentration of gadolinium in different organs is low, except for the kidneys, which show an increase in concentration over the first 60 minutes.[60,66] A few human clinical studies using contrast have been performed with no adverse effects to the fetus or neonate reported, even when given during the first trimester.[60,67,68] However, in a more recent large Canadian review, gadolinium MRI at any time during pregnancy was shown to be associated with an increased risk of a broad set of rheumatological, inflammatory, or infiltrative skin conditions and for stillbirth or neonatal death.[69]

In the past few years, reports have emerged of gadolinium deposits in the brain on T1 images long after contrast had been given. There is now evidence that gadolinium will deposit throughout the body, including the brain, in people with normal renal function. The highest concentrations have been found in bones, followed by that in the brain, skin, kidney, liver, and spleen. The clinical effects of this deposition remain unknown, with no current evidence of neurotoxicity. However, as of May 2018, the FDA has asked health care providers to inform patients about potential risks that could be associated with gadolinium-based contrast agents (GBCAs). As the length of time gadolinium can stay in the body appears to be prolonged, administration of gadolinium particularly with pregnant women and children should be carefully assessed.[70,71]

The use of gadolinium late in gestation may be appropriate for specific maternal or obstetric indications. The decision to administer MRI contrast to the pregnant patient, however, should be well documented with thoughtful risk-to-benefit analysis. Benefits should outweigh theoretical risks of fetal exposure to free gadolinium ions.[60,69,70]

TECHNIQUE

Patient Positioning (Table 8.1)

The patient should go through appropriate metal screening. Heavy clothing should be removed and light gowns offered to increase comfort during the study. The bladder should be emptied just prior to getting on the scanner.

The patient can lie either supine with a pillow under her knees or in a decubitus position. The left lateral position has been thought to reduce the risk of vena cava compression syndrome. However, a study by Kienzl et al. has suggested that vena cava compression syndrome is actually rare during MRI scanning in the supine position. Despite narrowing of the inferior vena cava (IVC), there appear to be physiological compensatory mechanisms.[72] Nonetheless, the lateral decubitus position can have additional advantages. It can help in patients with back pain or sciatica, or in the third trimester when the mother may have shortness of breath lying supine due to elevation of the diaphragms.

Because of claustrophobia, most patients prefer to go into the bore of the magnet feet first. This allows the uterus to be in

---

TABLE 8.1   Fetal MR Technique Tips

- USE the largest bore magnet available.
- POSITION the patient so that he or she is comfortable, feet first.
- USE distracting techniques. Have a family member accompany the patient in the scanner.
- PLACE a surface coil when possible. Multichannel better, more elements better. Two surface coils work well in series, especially with larger patients.
- LOCALIZE to the uterus with a large field of view. Check cervical length and placental location.
- REDUCE field of view.
- 3-Point PLAN a standard plane in the fetus.
- HAVE a protocol planned, but remain flexible with the order of sequences. Acquire the sequences most likely to answer the question first. Consider leaving the loudest sequences and breath-hold sequences until last. If there is significant fetal motion, consider repeating a key sequence until the fetus rests, or use dynamic SSFP.
- OBTAIN images of the entire fetus.
- REVIEW images with the technologist before ending the examination.

SSFP, steady-state free precession.

---

the center of the bore with the mother's head at the level of the flanged opening so they can see out into the room. Having a family member accompany the mother into the scanning room can be extremely helpful. If the mother is anxious, holding her hand may be calming. An alarm ball or other method of direct communication to the technologist should be offered. Listening to music or watching a movie can be a useful distraction technique. If a patient is extremely claustrophobic or anxious, oral sedation and/or oxygen supplementation may be required.

Coils

Depending on the size of the mother and fetal gestation, either a torso or cardiac-phased array surface coil is placed over the gravid uterus. One or two flexible phased array surface coils can be wrapped over the patient, sandwiching the uterus between the tabletop coils and surface coils.[73] Elements closest to the uterus can then be selected, which can increase the SNR. If the patient is too large to fit into the magnet with a surface coil, the coil intrinsic to the magnet may be used. Large-bore magnets are particularly advantageous when the body mass index (BMI) is high or there are multiple gestations.

Imaging Protocol (Table 8.2)

The development of single-shot rapid acquisition with relaxation enhancement sequences has been key to decreasing fetal and maternal movement artifact. A series of images can be performed in as little as 15 to 20 seconds. Slices are acquired one at a time, each slice produced in less than 400 milliseconds by a single-excitation pulse. Examination times overall average 20 to 40 minutes, depending on how many sequences have to be repeated owing to fetal movement and protocol.

An initial three-plane localizer sequence should be performed. This will demonstrate the cranial and caudal extent of the uterus and can be followed with T2 half Fourier single-shot echo (SSFSE/Haste/ssTSE/Fast FE) (Table 8.2), large FOV,[45,59] thick (5 to 10 mm) sections through the entire uterus, coronal to the mother. This can be followed by T2 SSFSE or steady state free precession (SSFP) sagittal and/or axial planes of the maternal pelvis. These sequences will allow assessment of fetal lie, placental position and signal, cervix, and fetal situs. These sequences also help determine whether the surface coils need to be repositioned to get the best signal from the fetal anatomy in question.

At this point, there are several ways to get into a fetal orthogonal plane. Advanced technology allows user selection of three points within the images that will appear on the same plane in the next sequence. For example, two points can be selected in the lumbar spinal canal, and one at the umbilicus, which would result in a perfect sagittal stack. If this technology is not available, it is possible to pick two points that are symmetric on either side of the body; for example, the orbits place the center "eye" of the stack on the one point, then page through the images until the second point is visible and rotate the stack so that the center line passes through the second point. This will result in images between axial and coronal, from which a perfect sagittal can then be obtained.[74] If this technology is not available, then landmarks of the spine and interhemispheric fissure in the brain may be helpful to obtain anatomic imaging.

Because the fetus continues to move throughout the study, each sequence is typically planned using a plane perpendicular to the prior sequence. Images of the head, then body or vice versa, should be protocoled depending on which anomaly needs to be

TABLE 8.2	**Vendor Sequences Used in Fetal MRI**				
SEQUENCE TYPE	**GE**	**SIEMENS**	**PHILIPS**	**HITACHI**	**CANON**
Half Fourier single-shot echo (T2)	SSFSE	HASTE	SSTSE	SSFSE	FASE
Steady-state free precession (SSFP) (T2)	FIESTA	TruFISP	Balanced FFE	Balanced SARGE	True SSFP
Spoiled gradient echo (T1)	SPGR	FLASH	T1-FFE	RF spoiled SARGE, RSSG	FastFE
3D ultrafast (T1)	3D FGRE, 3D Fast SPGR	MPRAGE	3D TFE	MPRAGE	3D Fast FE
Ultrafast gradient echo (GRE)	Fast GRE, Fast SPGR	Turbo FLASH		RGE	FastFE
Rapid acquisition relaxation enhancement	FSE	TSE	TSE	FSE	FSE
Diffusion-weighted imaging (DWI)	DWI	DWI	DWI	DWI	DWI
Diffusion tension imaging (DTI)	DTI	DTI	DTI		DTI
Echo planar imaging (EPI)	EPI	EPI	EPI	EPI	EPI
Susceptibility-weighted imaging (SWI)	SWAN	SWI			
Parallel imaging	ASSET	iPAT, mSENSE	SENSE	RAPID	SPEEDER

MRI, magnetic resonance imaging; *3D*, three-dimensional; *RF*, radio frequency.

evaluated first. In the sagittal and coronal planes, the entire head, chest, and abdomen can often be included, particularly in earlier gestation. Dedicated axial sequences of the fetal brain and abdomen, however, are typically needed for optimal image interpretation. At times, the fetus will move, but then quickly return to its initial position. Therefore, it can be helpful to simply repeat the sequence without changing parameters. If the fetus truly has moved into another position, the above techniques can be used to rapidly get another appropriate orthogonal plane.

Quiet maternal breathing is typically adequate; however, breath-hold techniques are needed for certain series, particularly T1 gradient echo (GRE) sequences. Breath-holding can be useful if the fetus is breech, when the maternal diaphragmatic motion is more readily transmitted to the fetus. Breath-holding is successful only if the length of the sequence is relatively short, less than 20 seconds. Allowing the mother to gently release the breath-hold toward the end of the series can help if the sequence is longer than this.

Phase oversampling is often used in fetal MRI. It has the advantages of reducing the FOV to include just the fetus and exclude maternal anatomy by eliminating phase wrap, and it also increases the SNR, which can be particularly important early in gestation when the fetus is small. The disadvantage is that it increases the scan time according to the number of phase-encoding steps. If this is problematic, the phase oversampling ratio can be reduced or turned off completely. This will result in phase wrap, but with careful positioning and sizing of the FOV, often the maternal structures will only phase wrap into the maternal

structures on the opposite side of the body and not overlie onto the fetal anatomy.

When scanning the fetus, a smaller 24- to 30-cm FOV should be used. Slices as thin as 2 to 3 mm can be obtained; however, the smaller the slice thickness, the lower the SNR. In larger fetuses, slice thicknesses of 4 to 6 mm work well, decreasing time per series and improving signal.

A typical matrix size is 256 pixels. Counterintuitively, increasing the matrix size in the attempt to increase in-plane resolution will typically have the opposite effect because of loss of signal from smaller voxels. This can be partly countered by increasing the slice thickness but results in more volume averaging.

T2 SSFSE/HASTE/ssTSE/SsFSE/FASE sequences (Table 8.2) provide the highest SNR and resolution and are fast.[74] Slices as thin as 2 to 3 mm with no skip can be obtained. These T2 images are most useful for anatomic detail, particularly of the fetal surface structures at the interface with amniotic fluid and the various body cavities that are fluid filled, such as the brain, ventricles, eyes, nasal cavities, oral cavity, airway, gastrointestinal (GI) tract, and genitourinary (GU) tract. Typically, axial, sagittal, and coronal images angled to the brain and then the body should be obtained.

Heavy T2 hydrography takes longer to acquire, but produces excellent SNR contrast. Slice thickness choices are dependent on gestational age (GA); 3 mm works well at <24 weeks, and 4 mm at >24 weeks decreases the length of this longer sequence.[75–77]

SSFP/FIESTA/TruFISP/Balanced FFE/Balanced SARGE/ True SSFP images demonstrate bright blood imaging. The cardiac chambers and great vessels may be discretely identified.

Images can be obtained in all three planes at 3- to 4-mm increments. This sequence is also quite useful for the assessment of fluid-filled structures, such as dilated renal collecting systems or cystic masses. Because of its high contrast, inner ear anatomy, clefts of the palate, and fluid surrounding the spinal cord are particularly well demonstrated. Extremities are outlined by the amniotic fluid, with fingers and toes often visualized. There is less contrast between gray and white matter in the brain and meconium in the abdomen due to lower flip angles and banding artifacts.

Thick-slab T2 sequences are useful for assessing fetal surface contours. Thick-slab acquisitions of 40 to 60 mm give an overall three-dimensional (3D) effect. Transparency is increased using shorter echo times or using SSFP sequences that can similarly be acquired with thick slices. To maximize SNR, overlapping slices of 5- to 6-mm thickness can be used; however, this approach typically makes this sequence less useful for volumetry. These images can be useful for parents and health care workers not used to evaluation of two-dimensional (2D) anatomy.[78]

T1 sequences are fast multiplanar spoiled gradient recall acquisitions in the steady-state (SPGR/FLASH/T1-FFE/Fast FE) sequences (Table 8.2) that require breath-hold with thicker slices (5 to 7 skip 0) for sufficient SNR. It can be useful to perform a T1 sequence immediately after a T2 sequence with the same slice parameters so they can be directly compared. T1 images are particularly useful for detecting hemorrhage, calcification, meconium, thyroid tissue, and fat.

Dynamic SSFP sequences (Cine, real time) can be used to assess fetal movements. Multiple frames per second can be obtained at each slice, with slice thicknesses ranging from 7 to 50 mm. Assessment of fetal breathing, swallowing, cardiac motion, and GI activity is possible. When there is a burst of fetal activity that precludes the use of other imaging sequences, it can be a useful backup sequence. When the fetus settles down, other sequences can then be acquired.

EPI is useful in the assessment of the musculoskeletal system with high-signal cartilage and low-signal bone. The fetal liver has significant hypointense signal, while other organs are intermediate in signal. Flow voids make vessels and heart hypointense. Susceptibility-weighted imaging can be used to detect hemorrhage and calcification.[11]

Long-Tau inversion recovery sequences can be useful to further characterize fluid that appears high intensity on T2 imaging, but that may contain proteinaceous fluid such as hemorrhage.

Diffusion-weighted imaging (DWI) sequences can be acquired with three phase-encoding directions. The area of interest should be as centered as possible. DWI can demonstrate ischemic lesions in white matter. It can be used in the identification of renal tissue, particularly if kidneys are not visible sonographically or by routine MRI.

Advanced imaging with **spectroscopy and DTI** is becoming available and is discussed in Chapter 10.

Whatever the indication for the fetal MRI is, the entire fetus from head to toe should be examined. Fetal pathologies and malformations frequently involve multiple organs. Thus, identification of other anomalies can further elucidate an underlying genetic or chromosomal syndrome.

Because of the risk of maternal fatigue, anxiety, or discomfort, it is important to complete the study as quickly and efficiently as possible. Protocols should be well thought out prior to placing the mother on the scanner. If a brain anomaly is present, planes angled to the brain should first be obtained, then sequences angled

to the chest and abdomen. Most protocols benefit from a combination of T2 sequences (SSFSE and/or SSFP) in all three planes and T1 imaging in at least one plane.

Postprocessing

Volumetry of fetal organs by MRI has become a useful tool, particularly in the determination of fetal lung volumes (see Chapter 25). A region of interest can be manually segmented and its total area multiplied by the slice thickness to calculate volumes. Continuous motion–free images are needed for accurate volumetry. Sequences may need to be repeated to ensure continuity of images if volumes are to be obtained. Spatial resolution of reformatted images can be limited owing to large-slice thickness. Advanced methods to develop 3D volume images are being developed so that even when motion occurs, accurate data can be generated (see Chapter 10).[8]

3D virtual model reconstruction using techniques such as stereolithography or fused deposition modeling can create life-size physical models using T2 MRI data (see Chapter 12).[79,80]

3 Tesla MRI

As the push for improved resolution and increased signal continues, and more 3T scanners become available for use, centers have begun to address the use of 3T scanners for fetal imaging. The use of 3T magnets, however, represents another technical challenge, with its increased susceptibility to motion artifact and the need to closely follow SAR limits.[58,59]

The US FDA approved the use of 3 T for human use in 2002. Advantages include improved SNR at higher strengths as more protons are available to increase magnetization. The gain of SNR may be up to 1.7 to 1.8 times that of 1.5 T.[45,81] Image quality and temporal and/or special resolution can thus be improved. With greater SNR, parallel imaging can be implemented to speed SSFSE protocols, reduce echo time, and potentially decrease RF heating by decreasing the number of pulses required.[45]

With 3 T, unfortunately, more artifacts are encountered. RF field inhomogeneity is a major challenge, with the larger the FOV, the worse the artifact. RF shielding artifact "conductivity effect" from amniotic fluid results in blackout areas often where the fetus is lying. Dielectric pads, RF cushions, or saline pads can help decrease these dielectric resonance artifacts.[45,82] Multichannel transmission coils, RF shimming with parallel imaging, may also help decrease RF field inhomogeneity.

Magnetic susceptibility artifacts and chemical shift artifacts are also accentuated with 3 T, requiring additional modifications. Changing the FOV, scan orientation, frequency, or bandwidth may move the artifact away from the fetal area of interest.

The US FDA limits of exposure to changing magnetic fields are independent of magnetic field strength. FDA safety limits prevent exposure to changing magnetic fields (dB/dt) of more than 60 T per second with fail-safe software limiting scanners from exposures above these limits. With the fetus near the center of the FOV exposure, dB/dt changes are usually low, with slew rates similar at both 1.5 and 3 T (see section "3 Tesla Safety" above)[45]

RF pulses deposit energy into the imaged subject. The energy deposition is measured by the SAR reported in Watts per kilogram. The amplitude of applied RF fields increases with increasing magnetic field strength and quadruples from 1.5 to 3 T. Decreasing number of slices, lowering flip angles, increasing TR, and shorter echo train length can decrease SAR. The FDA safety limits are set at 4 W/kg, independent of magnetic field strength with fail-safe controls prohibiting additional exposure. Studies by Victoria et al.[45] have demonstrated SAR well below whole-body exposure limits for both 1.5 and 3 T.

Focal SAR hotspots are of concern because of RF field inhomogeneity, dielectric, and standing wave effects. Modeling of fetal environment by Hand et al.[38,46] suggests that maximum energy deposited to the fetus is a fraction of that received by the mother. The fetus may be exposed to a peak of 50% to 70% of maternal SAR at 3 T. In their study, average temperature of the fetus remained below 38°C. However, they noted that continuous exposures over 7.5 minutes can exceed the 38°C limit, so long continuous exposures should be avoided.[46]

While 3 T has inherent artifact issues and potential increased safety risks, limiting SAR levels to those associated with 1.5 T and developing methods to decrease inhomogeneity have progressed.

Indications (Table 8.3)

Fetal MRI is a valuable complement to prenatal US. Because of higher contrast resolution, large FOV, and ability to image both sides of the fetus at once, fetal MRI can be more precise than US for anatomic evaluation. There are multiple indications for performing a fetal MRI, some of which are listed in Table 8.3. As MRI technology advances, additional indications will continue to develop, many of which are described in the chapters of this book.

TABLE 8.3	Fetal MRI Indications
Brain	Congenital anomalies such as ventriculomegaly, agenesis of the corpus callosum, holoprosencephaly, posterior fossa anomalies, cortical dysplasias, tuberous sclerosis, lissencephaly, microcephaly, family history
	Vascular abnormalities such as malformations, infarctions, hydranencephaly, twin-to-twin complications
	Craniosynostosis
	Tumors
	Infection
Spine	Neural tube defects/vertebral anomalies
	Sacrococcygeal teratoma
	Caudal regression/sirenomelia
Face and neck	Facial and palate clefts, micrognathia, dacryocystocele, anophthalmia
	Masses—lymphatic malformations, hemangioma, teratoma, goiter
	Airway obstruction
Thorax	Masses—congenital pulmonary airway malformations, congenital diaphragmatic hernia, effusions
	Lung hypoplasia—oligohydramnios, skeletal dysplasia
	Cardiac—heterotaxy
Abdomen	Masses/cysts
	Complex ventral wall defects
	Genitourinary anomalies/cloaca
	Bowel anomalies
Musculoskeletal	Limb anomalies
	Muscle abnormalities
	Soft-tissue masses—lymphangiomas, hemangiomas
	Skeletal dysplasia
Twins	Monochorionic, twin-to-twin complications
	Conjoined
Fetal intervention/surgery Delivery planning Postnatal surgical planning	EXIT procedures for airway obstruction Congenital diaphragmatic hernia repair Myelomeningocele repair Complex lesions requiring immediate neonatal surgery
Maternal	Placenta implantation abnormalities Poor evaluation due to obesity/oligohydramnios

MRI, magnetic resonance imaging; *EXIT,* ex utero intrapartum treatment *T2.*

Maternal

Initial large FOV images are an opportunity to identify maternal abnormalities, such as fibroids and ovarian pathology (Figs. 8.1 and 8.2). At times, maternal renal or skeletal anomalies are identified that should be described if noted. Pelvic inlet measures can be obtained as needed but require large FOV pelvic images in all three planes for complete assessment of sagittal inlet and outlet, transverse inlet diameter, and interspinous distance.[83–86]

Placenta/Umbilical Cord

Placental location and thickness are well delineated by MRI (Fig. 8.3). When a placental anomaly is present, all three planes of the uterus should be obtained for adequate assessment.[87,88] The placenta appears as an intermediate-signal soft-tissue structure along the margin of the uterus. The myometrial decidual interface is visible as a low-signal intensity line deep to the placenta.

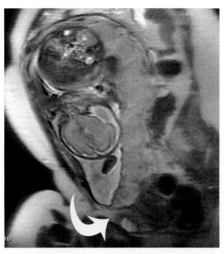

FIGURE 8.3: Placenta previa. Sagittal SSFSE image of a gravid uterus demonstrates the placenta completely covering the cervix (*curved arrow*).

MRI has been used to evaluate placenta accreta, with an overall sensitivity of 80% to 88% and a specificity of 65% to 100%.[89–91] MRI features include uterine bulging, heterogeneous placental signal, and dark intraplacental bands.[90–92] Some studies have used intravenous gadolinium contrast to assess for accreta, though the use remains controversial due to safety concerns. If contrast is being considered, the study should be timed as close to delivery as possible[87] (see Chapter 13.2).

Cervical length can be measured in the sagittal plane with location of placenta in relation to the cervix best noted on this view.

While MRI volumetry of amniotic fluid can be calculated, simple estimation of amniotic fluid is usually adequate.[93] Uterine synechia and amniotic sheets may be well visualized in all three planes[94] (Figs. 8.4 and 8.5).

The number of umbilical vessels is best determined in a transverse plane either by SSFSP or SSFP. The two umbilical arteries can be followed as they course along the fetal bladder. Placental cord insertion and fetal cord insertion should be identified, noting the length and configuration of the umbilical cord (Fig. 8.6).

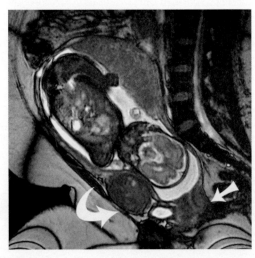

FIGURE 8.1: Fibroid. Sagittal SSFP image of a gravid uterus demonstrates an anterior fibroid compressing the fetal head (*curved arrow*). *Straight arrow* points to the closed cervix.

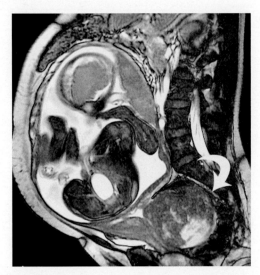

FIGURE 8.2: Fibroid. Sagittal SSFP image of a gravid uterus demonstrates a large cervical fibroid (*curved arrow*) deep in the pelvis.

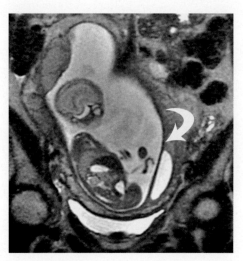

FIGURE 8.4: Uterine synechia. Coronal SSFSE image of a gravid uterus at 21 weeks' gestation demonstrates a thick band (*curved arrow*) along the lateral inferior uterus. No fetal entrapment was noted.

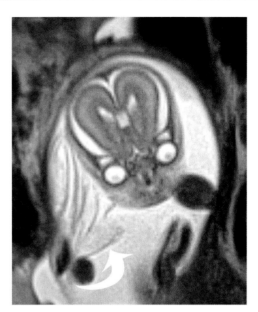

FIGURE 8.5: Amniotic bands. Numerous thin sheets (*curved arrow*) are adjacent to the fetal face. There were limb deformities, but no facial cleft was noted.

Situs

Fetal orientation should be evaluated on the basis of fetal and maternal anatomy using the initial large FOV sequences. Identifying the location of the fetal heart and stomach may not automatically identify the left side of the fetus in cases of heterotaxy.

Brain (see Chapters 9 and 10)

Coronal, axial, and sagittal orthogonal planes should be acquired with T2 sequences. T1 and diffusion-weighted sequences may provide additional information. Long-Tau inversion recovery, spectroscopy, volumetric data, and DTI are advanced techniques that may be useful in cranial assessment and are described further in Chapter 10.

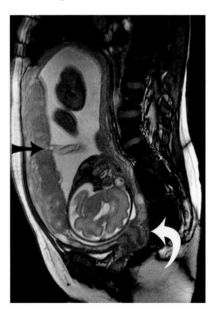

FIGURE 8.6: Placental cord insertion. Sagittal SSFP image of a gravid uterus demonstrates an anterior placenta with central cord insertion (*black arrow*). Note the closed cervix (*curved white arrow*).

Face (Table 8.4)

The sagittal midline plane is important for assessing the facial profile, including the nose, chin, and soft palate (Fig. 8.7). Fluid motion may be seen because of fetal exhalation. Coronal planes of the face are useful in assessing symmetry of the face, lips (for clefts), orbits, and nose (Fig. 8.8). External ears should be evaluated for their presence, location, and shape. Axial plane of the maxilla demonstrates tooth buds as a continuous arc (Fig. 8.9). The primary palate is triangular and includes the alveolar ridge. The secondary palate includes the remaining hard and soft palates.

TABLE 8.4	Fetal Face
ANATOMY	**SEQUENCES**
Craniofacial ratio, profile	Sagittal T2 SSFSE, SSFP
Nose	Sagittal, coronal T2 SSFSE, SSFP
Lips, palate, teeth	Coronal, axial T2 SSFSE, SSFP
Pharynx	Sagittal T2 SSFSE, SSFP
Swallow, breathing	Sagittal dynamic SSFP

SSFSE, single-shot fast spin-echo; *SSFP*, steady-state free precession.
Reproduced by permission from Springer: Prayer D, Brugger P. Investigation of normal organ development with fetal MRI. *Eur Radiol.* 2007;17(10):2458–2471. Copyright © 2007 Springer-Verlag.

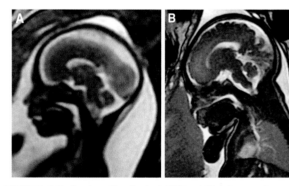

FIGURE 8.7: Fetal profile. Sagittal SSFP midline image demonstrates fetal lips, chin, soft palate, and pharynx at 21 **(A)** and 32 weeks' gestational age (GA) **(B)**.

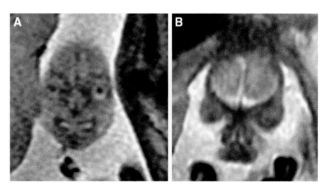

FIGURE 8.8: Fetal face coronal SSFSE. **A:** 21-week' gestation demonstrates the orbits, nose, and mouth. **B:** Slightly more superficial coronal section at 29 weeks' gestation demonstrates intact lip and nares.

Neck (Table 8.5)

Axial and sagittal T2 imaging best detect the fluid-filled larynx and trachea. Epiglottis and laryngeal folds are typically noted only in the late second and third trimesters (Fig. 8.10). The cervical esophagus is usually not seen unless caught during a swallow. The

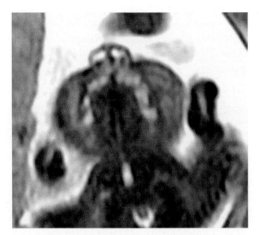

FIGURE 8.9: Fetal face axial SSFSE at 29 weeks' gestation demonstrates the maxilla with tooth buds in a continuous arc.

TABLE 8.5	Fetal Neck
ANATOMY	**SEQUENCES**
Larynx, trachea	Sagittal, coronal, axial T2 SSFSE, SSFP
Thyroid	Axial, coronal T1 GRE
Vessels	Axial, coronal, sagittal SSFP, GRE

SSFSE, single-shot fast spin-echo; SSFP, steady-state free precession; GRE, gradient echo.
Reproduced by permission from Springer: Prayer D, Brugger P. Investigation of normal organ development with fetal MRI. *Eur Radiol.* 2007;17(10):2458–2471. Copyright © 2007 Springer-Verlag.

thyroid gland is poorly seen on T2 sequences but is high signal on T1 imaging from 18 weeks' GA onward (Fig. 8.11). Cervical vessels can be identified on all three planes using SSFP sequences (Fig. 8.12).

Thorax (Table 8.6)

Fetal lungs increase in volume throughout gestation and can be measured with MRI volumetry. Normal lung volumes have been documented by MRI as demonstrating growth proportionate to fetal body size.

The trachea, carina, and bronchi are often seen filled with fluid on T2 imaging. Repeating sequences with thinner slices may be required for adequate evaluation as needed (Fig. 8.13).

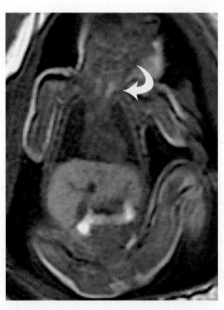

FIGURE 8.11: Coronal T1 at 29 weeks' gestation demonstrates high-signal thyroid glands (*curved arrow*), high-signal meconium in the transverse colon, and intermediate-signal liver.

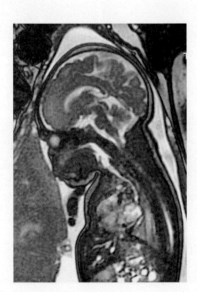

FIGURE 8.10: Sagittal SSFP at 32 weeks' gestation demonstrates the larynx, epiglottis, and trachea.

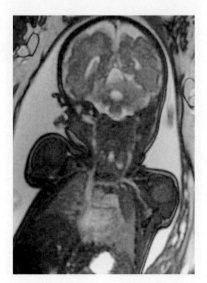

FIGURE 8.12: Coronal SSFP at 32 weeks' gestation demonstrates bilateral subclavian and jugular veins as well as superior vena cava.

TABLE 8.6	Fetal Thorax
ANATOMY	SEQUENCES
Lung parenchyma	Coronal, axial, sagittal SSFSE; volumetry
Diaphragmatic hernia	Coronal, axial, sagittal SSFSE; volumetry; coronal, sagittal T1 GRE
Heart	Axial, long- and short-axis SSFP, dynamic SSFP
Thymus	Axial, coronal T2 SSFSE
Diaphragm	Coronal, sagittal SSFSE, dynamic SSFP
Esophagus	Thick-slab sagittal SSFSE, SSFP; axial SSFSE, SSFP; dynamic SSFP

SSFSE, single-shot fast spin-echo; *SSFP*, steady-state free precession; *GRE*, gradient echo.
Reproduced by permission from Springer: Prayer D, Brugger P. Investigation of normal organ development with fetal MRI. *Eur Radiol.* 2007;17(10):2458–2471. Copyright © 2007 Springer-Verlag.

Lung parenchyma is homogeneously brighter than muscle on T2 imaging and increases in signal after 24 weeks' gestation, while T1 signal decreases with GA (Fig. 8.14). Apparent diffusion coefficient has been used in addition to T2 signal to assess lung maturation.[95]

The diaphragms are dome-shaped bands between the lungs and the abdomen. They have low signal on T2, slightly lower than adjacent liver. Breathing may be noted on dynamic SSFP sequences. The esophagus is rarely seen unless caught during a swallow (Fig. 8.15). If an atresia is present, fluid may be identified proximal to the obstruction but is not a constant finding. Thick dynamic SSFP sequences in the sagittal midline plane may best demonstrate transient dilatation of a proximal esophageal pouch.

The thymus is homogeneous, intermediate signal in the anterior mediastinum. It is best seen in the third trimester and

should not have any mass effect on adjacent vessels or the trachea (Fig. 8.16).

The heart is low signal on T2 SSFSE due to flowing blood. This sequence is limited to identification of the position and size of the heart. SSFP sequences are more useful in delineating the myocardium, septum, and valves (Fig. 8.17). Dynamic SSFP sequences can demonstrate cardiac motion. These sequences may be particularly useful in cases of oligohydramnios and maternal obesity when fetal echocardiography may be limited. While US remains the primary method of assessing fetal heart dynamics, Chapter 11 describes advances in cardiac MRI that may provide additional information.

Abdomen (Tables 8.7 and 8.8)

The fetal abdomen is well visualized by MRI, with progressive changes as gestation advances. The dominant fluid-filled abdominal structures throughout the second and third trimesters include the stomach, gallbladder, and bladder (Fig. 8.18). The stomach is a fluid-filled structure in the left upper quadrant, high signal on T2, and low signal on T1. While the stomach may be transiently small, it should always be seen during a 30-minute scan.

Before 25 weeks' gestation, small bowel is typically collapsed containing minimal fluid. In the third trimester, small bowel becomes fluid filled, high signal on T2, and low signal on T1 (Fig. 8.19). Meconium, which is typically low signal on T2 and high signal on T1 likely because of protein and/or paramagnetic minerals, initially fills the rectum at 19 to 20 weeks' gestation. There is progression from the rectum to the descending colon by 22 to 23 weeks.[96] Meconium will variably extend to the transverse and ascending colon during the third trimester, usually around 25 weeks, with continuous colonic filling closer to term (Fig. 8.20) (see Chapter 26.1). MRI can provide information regarding the level of bowel obstruction if present and assess size of colon and rectum in later gestation.

The liver is homogeneous, low-to-intermediate signal on T2, slightly high signal on T1 (Fig. 8.21) (Table 8.8). Iron causes low signal on T2. Thus, early in gestation when there

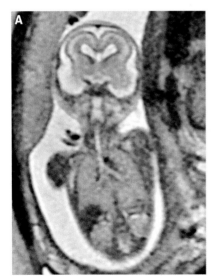
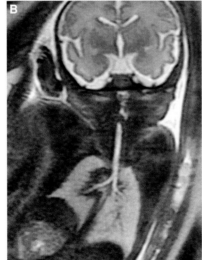
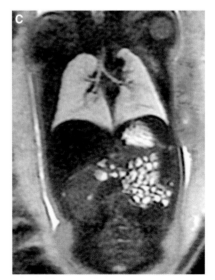

FIGURE 8.13: Trachea and bronchi. Coronal SSFSE images at at 21 weeks **(A)**, 31 weeks **(B)**, 37 weeks **(C)** gestation.

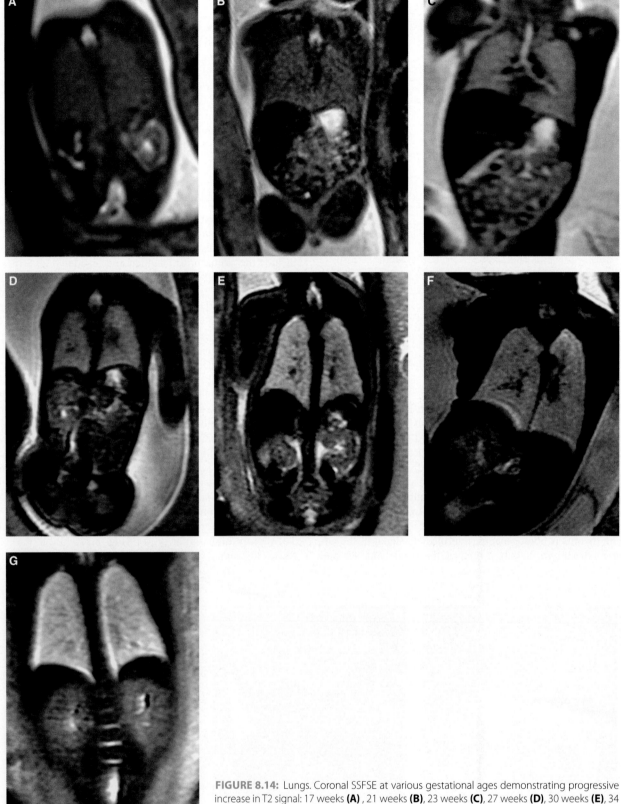

FIGURE 8.14: Lungs. Coronal SSFSE at various gestational ages demonstrating progressive increase in T2 signal: 17 weeks **(A)** , 21 weeks **(B)**, 23 weeks **(C)**, 27 weeks **(D)**, 30 weeks **(E)**, 34 weeks **(F)**, 37 weeks **(G)** gestation.

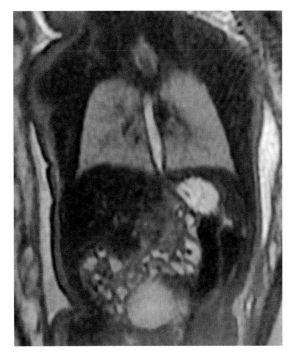

FIGURE 8.15: Fluid-filled esophagus. Coronal SSFSE image at 33 weeks' gestation.

TABLE 8.7 Fetal Abdomen

ANATOMY	SEQUENCES
Liver, spleen	Coronal, axial, sagittal T2 SSFSE; coronal T1 GRE, EPI
Gallbladder	Axial, sagittal T2 SSFSE, SSFP
Bowel/meconium	Axial, coronal, sagittal T2 SSFSE; coronal, sagittal T1 GRE
Kidneys, adrenals	Coronal, sagittal, axial T2 SSFSE; coronal thick-slab SSFP; axial DWI
Bladder	Axial, sagittal, coronal T2 SSFSPR, SSFP
Vessels—aorta, IVC, umbilical, azygous	Coronal, sagittal, axial SSFP
Internal genitalia	Not well visualized; axial, sagittal T2 SSFSE
External genitalia	Sagittal, axial T2 SSFSE, SSFP

SSFSE, single-shot fast spin-echo; *SSFP*, steady-state free precession; *GRE*, gradient echo; *DWI*, diffusion-weighted imaging; *EPI*, echo planar imaging; *IVC*, inferior vena cava.

Reproduced by permission from Springer: Prayer D, Brugger P. Investigation of normal organ development with fetal MRI. *Eur Radiol.* 2007;17(10):2458–2471. Copyright © 2007 Springer-Verlag.

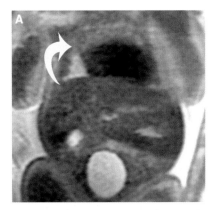
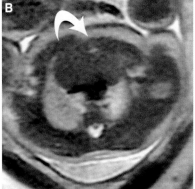

FIGURE 8.16: Thymus. Coronal **(A)** and axial **(B)** SSFSE images at 32 weeks' gestation demonstrate an intermediate-signal soft-tissue mass (*curved arrow*) in the anterior mediastinum consistent with thymus.

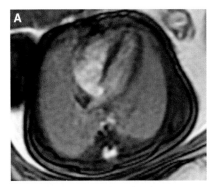
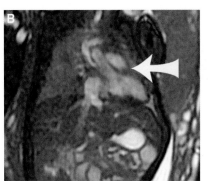
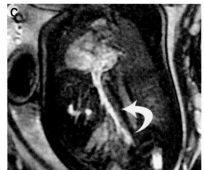

FIGURE 8.17: Fetal heart. **A:** Axial SSFP image of the four chambers. **B:** Oblique SSFP demonstrates the left ventricular outflow track (*straight arrow*). **C:** Oblique coronal SSFP demonstrates the inferior vena cava (*curved arrow*) draining into the right atrium.

TABLE 8.8   **T1 and T2 weighted Appearance of Organs**

	T2	T1
Orbits (vitreous)	High signal	Low signal
Nasopharynx, oropharynx, trachea	High-signal lumen, low-signal wall	Low signal
Thyroid gland	Intermediate signal	High signal
Thymus	Intermediate signal	Intermediate signal
Lungs	Intermediate signal, increasing with GA	Low signal, decreasing with GA
Aorta, heart, vessels	Low signal (flow void)	
Stomach	High signal	Low signal
Fluid-filled bowel	High signal	Low signal
Meconium	Low signal	High signal
Liver, spleen, gallbladder	Low or high signal in the second trimester, intermediate or high signal in the third trimester	Slightly high signal or low signal
Kidneys	Cortex = intermediate signal Medulla = slightly high signal	
Bladder	High signal	Low signal
Bone, cartilage	Low signal/high signal—EPI	Low signal

EPI, echo planar imaging; *GA*, gestational age.

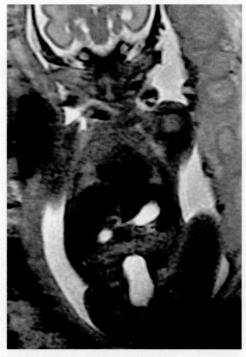

FIGURE 8.18: Fluid-filled stomach, gallbladder, and bladder. Coronal SSFSE image at 30 weeks' gestation.

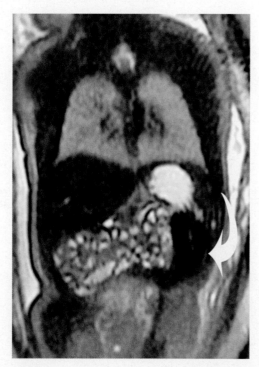

FIGURE 8.19: Fluid filled small bowel. Coronal SSFSE at 32 weeks' gestation demonstrates fluid-filled high-signal small bowel and low-signal meconium-filled descending colon (*curved arrow*).

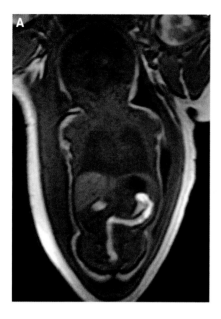
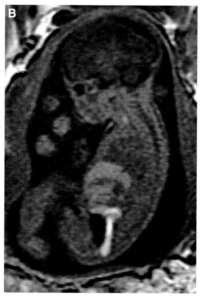

FIGURE 8.20: T1 bowel. Coronal **(A)** and sagittal **(B)** images at 30 weeks' gestation demonstrate high-signal meconium in the rectum, sigmoid, and descending colon.

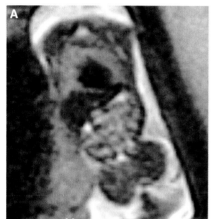
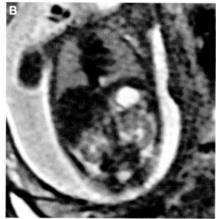
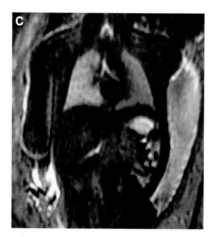

FIGURE 8.21: Liver. Coronal SSFSE images of the liver and spleen at 17 weeks **(A)**, 21 weeks **(B)** 29 weeks **(C)** gestation.

is a large amount of iron bound to fetal hemoglobin in the liver, parenchyma is relatively low in signal best assessed by echo planar sequences. By the third trimester, there is less iron, a change that can help assess fetal physiology.[96,97] Splenic signal changes may also be noted on echo planar sequences, possibly due to red pulp volume in the third trimester.[96] The spleen is noted posterior to the stomach, best seen on sagittal and axial images. The two hepatic lobes are equal in size, with the ductus venosus and portal vein noted best on SSFP sequences.

MRI appearance of the fetal gallbladder is variable. Signal intensity changes over time, likely due to accumulation of paramagnetic substances/sludge in bile. Brugger et al.[98] described T2 high signal exclusively in fetuses younger than 27 weeks' gestation. Lower signal gallbladders were noted only after 30 weeks' gestation and may cause nonvisualization of an otherwise normal gallbladder. When the gallbladder is not visualized in the second trimester, diagnosis of biliary atresia, particularly in

cases of heterotaxy, should be considered. Cystic fibrosis should also be included in the differential.

The cord insertion is best visualized by axial or sagittal SSFSE or SSFP sequences (Fig. 8.22). In the third trimester, the cord insertion may be difficult to identify owing to overlying limbs.

The GU track requires assessment of the kidneys, adrenal glands, ureters, bladder, and genitalia. The fetal kidneys are relatively well seen early in the second trimester, intermediate in signal on T2. Perinephric fat is high signal on T2 and can be mistaken for perirenal fluid. Fluid in the renal pelvis is well depicted separate from the renal tissue. With maturation, the renal cortex and the medulla become more differentiated (Fig. 8.23). DWI is useful in identifying renal parenchyma, particularly if not in the expected location (Fig. 8.24). Apparent diffusion coefficient of the kidneys increases with advancing gestation.[99] The adrenal glands are noted above the kidneys. In the early second trimester, the adrenal are hypointense on T2 and relatively well seen because of surrounding hyperintense perirenal fat

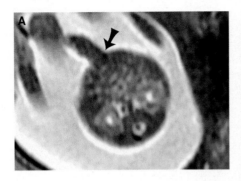

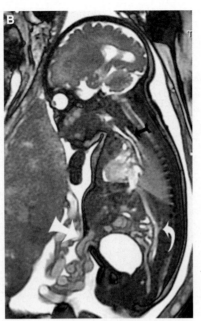

FIGURE 8.22: Cord insertion. **A:** Axial SSFSE at 20 weeks' gestation demonstrates cord insertion (*black arrow*) at the ventral abdomen. **B:** Sagittal (SSFP) image at 32 weeks' gestation demonstrates cord insertion (*straight arrow*), inferior vena cava draining into the right atrium (*white curved arrow*) as well as the fluid-filled trachea and partially filled proximal esophagus (*black arrow*).

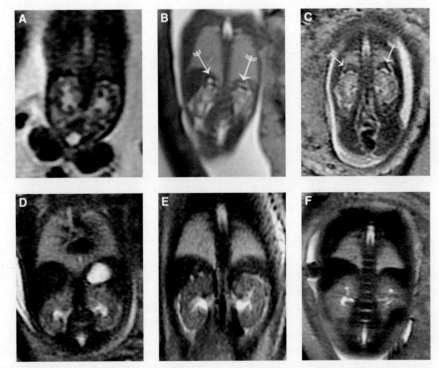

FIGURE 8.23: Kidneys. Coronal SSFSE at various gestational ages: 17 **(A)**, 20 **(B)**, 23 **(C)**, 28 **(D)**, 32 **(E)**, and 37 weeks **(F)**. Note low-signal adrenals surrounding by high-signal fat at 20 and 23 weeks' gestation (*arrows*).

(Fig. 6.1-23). They can be triradiate or lambda-shaped. As they grow becoming pyramidal in shape, they become higher in signal, becoming more difficult to visualize in the third trimester.

The ureters are typically not visualized. When dilated, sagittal and coronal T2 SSFSE and SSFP sequences help document the level of ureteral insertion. Thick-slab coronal imaging can simulate MRI urography[78] (Fig. 8.25).

The bladder should always contain high-signal fluid on T2 sequences and should be identified some time during a 30-minute examination.

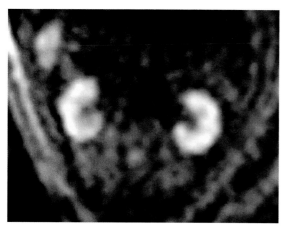

FIGURE 8.24: Oblique diffusion-weighted image of both kidneys at 32 weeks' gestation.

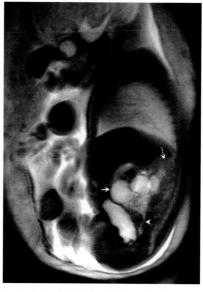

FIGURE 8.25: Sagittal thick-slab SSFSE of a kidney with hydro-ureteronephrosis (*dotted arrow*) and a contralateral multicystic dysplastic kidney (*solid arrow*). *Arrowhead* points to the distal hydroureter.

The uterus, vagina, ovaries, and prostate are not well separated from surrounding tissues. If ascites or an anomaly such as an ovarian cyst or hydrometrocolpos is present, they can be depicted. Identifying labia or penis and scrotum is best noted on axial or sagittal T2 sequences, with amniotic fluid outlining the surface (Fig. 8.26) (see Chapter 27.3). Testicles within the scrotum may be seen after 28 weeks' gestation.[100,101]

Musculoskeletal (Table 8.9)

While US remains the cornerstone of fetal skeletal assessment, MRI has become an important adjunct. Large FOV can help assess configuration of limbs, with thick-slab delineating fetal surface contours[78,102–104] (Figs. 8.27 and 8.28). Dynamic SSFP images may characterize extremity movement.

T2 sequences demonstrate skin and muscle. Muscle is relatively homogeneous, hypointense on T2, so discreet muscles cannot be delineated. High signal or thin musculature may suggest an abnormality[69,104] (Fig. 8.29). The subcutaneous tissue layer becomes more prominent as subcutaneous fat

TABLE 8.9	Fetal Musculoskeletal
ANATOMY	SEQUENCES
Hands, feet	Coronal, sagittal SSFP; dynamic SSFP; thick-slab SSFP; EPI
Arms, legs	Sagittal, coronal EPI, SSFP; dynamic SSFP
Spine	Axial, sagittal T2 SSFSE; EPI; T1 GRE to look for fat

SSFSE, Single-shot fast spin-echo; *SSFP*, steady-state free precession; *GRE*, gradient echo; *EPI*, echo planar imaging.
Reproduced by permission from Springer: Prayer D, Brugger P. Investigation of normal organ development with fetal MRI. *Eur Radiol.* 2007;17(10):2458–2471. Copyright © 2007 Springer-Verlag.

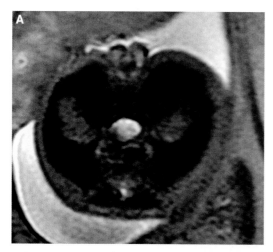
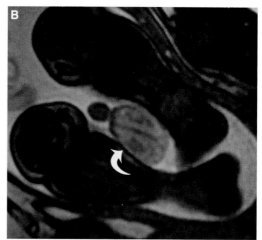

FIGURE 8.26: Genitalia. **A:** Axial SSFSE demonstrates labia at 33 weeks' gestation. **B:** Oblique (SSFP) image of testes within the scrotal sacs (*curved arrow*) in a 32-week male fetus.

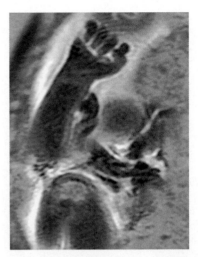

FIGURE 8.27: Coronal SSFSE image of the arm at 26 weeks' gestation demonstrates amniotic fluid outlining the fingers of the hand.

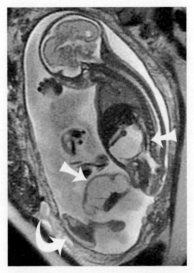

FIGURE 8.28: Lymphangioma. Large field of view SSFSE sagittal image at 24 weeks' gestation demonstrates large subcutaneous cysts along the femur, loculated septated cysts within the abdomen (*straight arrows*) as well as swelling of the foot (*curved arrow*) in a fetus with extensive lymphangioma.

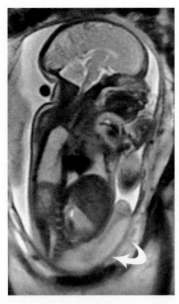

FIGURE 8.29: Amyoplasia. Sagittal SSFSE image at 34 weeks' gestation demonstrates abnormal high signal of the muscles of the thigh (*curved arrow*). Amyoplasia is characterized by the absence of limb muscles that are replaced by fibrous and fatty tissue. Fetal activity was decreased.

develops in the third trimester, with high signal on T1 imaging (Fig. 8.30).[105]

EPI sequences provide a way of evaluating bone (low-signal) and cartilage (high-signal) maturation[80] (Fig. 8.31). With US only moderately accurate in the diagnosis of specific skeletal dysplasias, fetal MRI may become a useful adjunct in arriving at a more definitive diagnosis (see Chapter 29 skeletal chapter).[106]

Normal Measurements

Reference values of fetal organs are available from numerous US studies. Various studies evaluating measurements either by fetal MRI alone or by comparison with US have been performed. MRI measurements have shown good correlation with US.[107–111] Volumetric data for lung and fetal weight may be more accurate by MRI than US.[112–114] MRI measures continue to be established, including the brain, lungs, liver, and kidney.

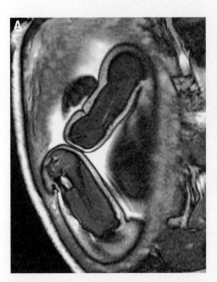
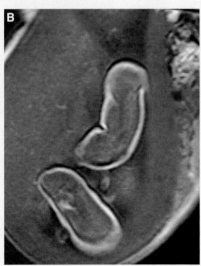

FIGURE 8.30: Subcutaneous fat at 37- weeks' gestation. **A:** Sagittal SSFP image demonstrates low-signal muscle bone and cartilage. **B:** T1 image in the same plane delineates high-signal subcutaneous fat that develops in the third trimester.

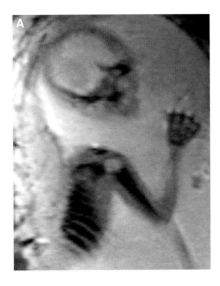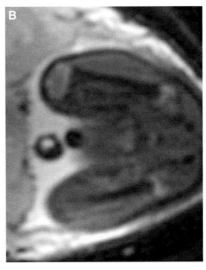

FIGURE 8.31: Skeleton. **A:** Sagittal echo planar imaging (EPI) of a 21-week fetus demonstrates hyperintense cartilage and hypointense bone that is well delineated against the adjacent high-signal muscle. **B:** Axial EPI of both femurs at 33 weeks' gestation demonstrates less contrast between the muscle and the bone.

CONCLUSION

MRI has been increasingly used as a problem-solving tool in the assessment of the fetus. When using this modality, it is important to be aware of potential safety risks, know how to optimize protocols, and understand how fetal anatomy develops over gestation. With appropriate use, this exciting modality will continue to evolve, further advancing the care of the fetus.

REFERENCES

1. Coakley FV, Glenn OA, Qayyum A, et al. Fetal MRI: a developing technique for the developing patient. *AJR Am J Roentgenol.* 2004;182(1):243–252.
2. Reddy UM, Filly RA, Copel JA. Prenatal imaging: ultrasonography and magnetic resonance imaging. *Clin Obstet Gynecol.* 2008;112(1):145–157.
3. Levine D. Obstetric MRI. *J Magn Reson Imaging.* 2006;24:1–15.
4. Griffiths PD, Bradburn M, Mandefield L, et al. The rate of brain abnormalities on in utero MRI studies in fetuses with normal US examinations of the brain and calculation of indicators of diagnostic performance. *Clin Radiol.* 2019;74(7):527–533.
5. Bulas D. Imaging of fetal anomalies. In: Medina LS, Applegate KE, Blackmore CC, eds. *Evidence Based Imaging.* New York, NY: Springer; 2009:615–632.
6. Griffiths PD, Bradburn M, Campbell MJ, et al. Use of MRI in the diagnosis of fetal brain abnormalities in utero (MERIDIAN): a multicenter, prospective cohort study. *Lancet.* 2017;389:538–546.
7. Garel C. Fetal MRI: what is the future? *Ultrasound Obstet Gynecol.* 2008; 31(2):123–128.
8. Clouchoux C, Limperopoulos C. Novel applications of quantitative MRI for the fetal brain. *Pediatr Radiol.* 2012;42(suppl 1):S24–S32.
9. Kline-Fath BM. Current advances in prenatal imaging of congenital diaphragmatic hernia. *Pediatr Radiol.* 2012;42(suppl 1):S74–S90.
10. Meyers ML, Garcia JR, Blough KL, et al. Fetal lung volumes by MRI: normal weekly values from 18 through 38 weeks' Gestation. *AJR Am J Roentgenol.* 2018;211(2):432–438.
11. Diogo MC, Prayer D, Gruber GM, et al. Echo-planar FLAIR sequence improves subplate visualization in fetal MRI of the brain. *Radiology.* 2019;292(1).
12. Griffiths PD, Bradburn M, Campbell MJ, et al; MERIDIAN Collaborative Group. Change in diagnostic confidence brought about by using in utero MRI for fetal structural brain pathology: analysis of the MERIDIAN cohort. *Clin Radiol.* 2017;72(6):451–457.
13. Benacerraf BR, Shipp TD, Bromley B, et al. What does magnetic resonance imaging add to the prenatal sonographic diagnosis of ventriculomegaly? *J Ultrasound Med.* 2007;26(11):1513–1522.
14. Garel C, Brisse H, Sebag G, et al. Magnetic resonance imaging of the fetus. *Pediatr Radiol.* 1998;28:201–211.
15. Chapman T, Alazraki AL, Eklund MJ. A survey of pediatric diagnostic radiologists in North America: current practices in fetal magnetic resonance imaging. *Pediatr Radiol.* 2018;48(13):1924–1935.
16. Werner H, Gasparetto TD, Daltro P, et al. Typical lesions in the fetal nervous system: correlations between fetal magnetic resonance imaging and obstetric ultrasonography findings. *Ultrasonography.* 2018;37(3):261–274.
17. Peiró JL, Sbragia L, Scorletti F, et al. Management of fetal teratomas. *Pediatr Surg Int.* 2016;32(7):635–647.
18. Mehollin-Ray AR. Prenatal and postnatal radiologic evaluation of conjoined twins. *Semin Perinatol.* 2018;42(6):369–380.
19. Yip YP, Capriotti C, Talagala SL, et al. Effects of MR exposure at 1.5 T on early embryonic development of the chick. *J Magn Reson Imaging.* 1994;4:742–748.
20. Yip YP, Capriotti C, Yip JW. Effects of MR exposure on axonal outgrowth in the sympathetic nervous system of the chick. *J Magn Reson Imaging.* 1995;5:457–462.
21. Mevissen M, Buntenkotter S, Loscher W. Effects of static and time varying (50-Hz) magnetic fields on reproduction and fetal development in rats. *Teratology.* 1994;50:229–237.
22. Schoennagel BP, Yamamura J, Kording F, et al. Fetal dynamic phase-contrast MR angiography using ultrasound gating and comparison with Doppler ultrasound measurements. *Eur Radiol.* 2019;29(8):4169–4176.
23. Tavares de Sousa M, Hecher K, Yamamura J, et al. Dynamic fetal cardiac magnetic resonance imaging in four-chamber view using Doppler ultrasound gating in normal fetal heart and in congenital heart disease: comparison with fetal echocardiography. *Ultrasound Obstet Gynecol.* 2019;53(5):669–675.
24. Kording F, Yamamura J, de Sousa MT, et al. Dynamic fetal cardiovascular magnetic resonance imaging using Doppler ultrasound gating. *J Cardiovasc Magn Reson.* 2018;20(1):17.
25. Kording F, Schoennagel BP, de Sousa MT, et al. Evaluation of a portable Doppler ultrasound gating device for fetal cardiac MR imaging: initial results at 1.5T and 3T. *Magn Reson Med Sci.* 2018;17(4):308–317.
26. Batty R, Gawne-Cain ML, Mooney C, et al. Analysis of errors made on in utero MR studies of the fetal brain in the MERIDIAN study. *Eur Radiol.* 2019;29(1):195–201.
27. Magin RL, Lee JK, Klintsova A, et al. Biological effects of long-duration, high-field (4 T) MRI on growth and development of the mouse. *J Magn Reson Imaging.* 2000;12:140–149.
28. Saunders R. Static magnetic fields: animal studies. *Prog Biophys Mol Biol.* 2005;87(2–3):225–239.
29. Mervak BM, Altun E, McGinty KA, et al. MRI in pregnancy: indications and practical considerations. *J Magn Reson Imaging.* 2019;49:621–630.
30. Murbach M, Cabot E, Neufeld E, et al. Local SAR enhancements in anatomically correct children and adult models as a function of position within 1.5 T MR body coil. *Prog Biophys Mol Biol.* 2011;107(3):428–433.
31. Neufeld E, Gosselin MC, Murbach M, et al. Analysis of the local worst case SAR exposure caused by an MRI multi transmit body coil in anatomical models of the human body. *Phys Med Biol.* 2011;56(15):4649–4659.
32. Jaimes C, Delgado J, Cunnane MB. Does 3-T fetal MRI induce adverse acoustic effects in the neonate? A preliminary study comparing postnatal auditory test performance of fetuses scanned at 1.5 and 3 T. *Pediatr Radiol.* 2019 Jan;49(1):37–45.
33. Chartier AL, Bouvier MJ, McPherson DR et al .The Safety of Maternal and Fetal MRI at 3 T. *AJR Am J Roentgenol.* 2019 Nov;213(5):1170–1173.
34. Heinrichs WL, Fong P, Flannery M, et al. Midgestational exposure of pregnant BALB/c mice to magnetic resonance imaging conditions. *Magn Reson Imaging.* 1988;6(3):305–313.
35. Tyndall DA, Sulik KK. Effects of magnetic resonance imaging on eye development in the C57BL/6J mouse. *Teratology.* 1991;43:263–275.
36. Levine D, Zuo C, Faro CB, et al. Potential heating effect in the gravid uterus during MR HASTE imaging. *J Magn Reson Imaging.* 2001;13(6):856–861.
37. Dimbylow P. Development of pregnant female, hybrid voxel-mathematical models and their application to the dosimetry of applied magnetic and electric fields at 50 Hz. *Phys Med Biol.* 2006;51(10):2383–2394.
38. Hand JW, Li Y, Hajnal JV. Numerical study of RF exposure and the resulting temperature rise in the foetus during a magnetic resonance procedure. *Phys Med Biol.* 2010;55(4):913–930.
39. Brugger PC, Prayer D. Actual imaging time in fetal MRI. *Eur J Radiol.* 2012; 81(3):e194–e196.
40. Kanal E, Gillen J, Evans JA, et al. Survey of reproductive health among female MR workers. *Radiology.* 1993;187(2):395–399.

41. Weisstanner C, Gruber GM, Brugger PC, et al. Fetal MRI at 3T-ready for routine use? *Br J Radiol.* 2017;90(1069):20160362.

42. Edwards MJ, Saunders RD, Shiota K. Effects of heat on embryos and foetuses. *Int J Hyperthermia.* 2003;19:295–324.

43. Ziskin MC, Morrissey J. Thermal thresholds for teratogenicity, reproduction, and development. *Int J Hyperthermia.* 2011;27:374–387.

44. Gholipour A, Estroff JA, Barnewolt CE, et al. Fetal MRI: a technical update with educational aspirations. *Concepts Magn Reson Part A Bridg Educ Res.* 2014;43:237–266.

45. Victoria T, Jaramillo D, Roberts TP, et al. Fetal magnetic resonance imaging: jumping from 1.5 to 3 tesla (preliminary experience). *Pediatr Radiol.* 2014;44:376–386.

46. Hand JW, Li Y, Thomas EL, et al. Prediction of specific absorption rate in mother and fetus associated with MRI examinations during pregnancy. *Magn Reson Med.* 2006;55:883–893.

47. Murbach M, Neufeld E, Samaras T, et al. Pregnant women models analyzed for RF exposure and temperature increase in 3T RF shimmed birdcages. *Magn Reson Med.* 2017;77:2048–2056.

48. Cannie MM, De Keyzer F, Van Laere S, et al. Potential heating effect in the gravid uterus by using 3-T MR imaging protocols: experimental study in miniature pigs. *Radiology.* 2016;279:754–761.

49. De Wilde JP, Rivers AW, Price DL. A review of the current use of magnetic resonance imaging in pregnancy and safety implications for the fetus. *Prog Biophys Mol Biol.* 2005;87:335–353.

50. Davids M, Guerin B, Malzacher M, et al. Predicting magnetostimulation thresholds in the peripheral nervous system using realistic body models. *Sci Rep.* 2017;7:5316.

51. Jaimes C, Delgado J, Cunnane MB, et al. Does 3-T fetal MRI induce adverse acoustic effects in the neonate? A preliminary study comparing postnatal auditory test performance of fetuses scanned at 1.5 and 3 T. *Pediatr Radiol.* 2019;49:37–45.

52. Myers C, Duncan KR, Gowland PA, et al. Failure to detect intrauterine growth restriction following in utero exposure to MRI. *Br J Radiol.* 1998;71:549–551.

53. Clements H, Duncan KR, Fielding K, et al. Infants exposed to MRI in utero have a normal paediatric assessment at 9 months of age. *Br J Radiol.* 2000;73:190–194.

54. Kok RD, de Vries MM, Heerschap A, et al. Absence of harmful effects of magnetic resonance exposure at 1.5 T in utero during the third trimester of pregnancy: a follow-up study. *Magn Reson Imaging.* 2004;22:851–854.

55. International Commission on Non-Ionizing Radiation Protection. Medical magnetic resonance (MR) procedures: protection of patients. *Health Phys.* 2004;87(2):197–216.

56. Kanal E, Borgstede JP, Barkovich AJ, et al. American College of Radiology white paper on MR safety. *AJR Am J Roentgenol.* 2002;178(6):1335–1347.

57. Bulas D, Egloff A. Benefits and risks of MRI in pregnancy. *Semin Perinatol.* 2013;37(5):301–304.

58. Welsh R, Nemec U, Thomason M. Fetal magnetic resonance imaging at 3.0 T. *Top Magn Reson Imaging.* 2011;1:1–13.

59. Merkle EM, Dale BM, Paulson EK. Abdominal MR imaging at 3 T. *Magn Reson Imaging Clin N Am.* 2006;14(1):17–26.

60. Sundgren PC, Leander P. Is administration of gadolinium-based contrast media to pregnant women and small children justified? *J Magn Reson Imaging.* 2011;34(4):750–757.

61. Runge VM. Safety of approved MR contrast media for intravenous injection. *J Magn Reson Imaging.* 2000;12:205–213.

62. Webb JAW, Thomsen HS, Morcos SK. The use of iodinated and gadolinium contrast media during pregnancy and lactation. *Eur Radiol.* 2005;15(6):1234–1240.

63. Okuda Y, Sagami F, Tirone P, et al. Reproductive and developmental toxicity study of gadobenate dimeglumine formulation (E7155) (3): study of embryo-fetal toxicity in rabbits by intravenous administration [in Japanese]. *J Toxicol Sci.* 1999;24(suppl 1):79–87.

64. Rofsky NM, Pizzarello DJ, Weinreb JC, et al. Effect on fetal mouse development of exposure to MR imaging and gadopentate dimeglumine. *J Magn Reson Imaging.* 1994;4:805–807.

65. Novak Z, Thurmond AS, Ross PL, et al. Gadolinium DTPA transplacental transfer and distribution in fetal tissue in rabbits. *Invest Radiol.* 1993;28:828–830.

66. Vanhaesebrouck P, Verstraete AG, De Praeter C, et al. Transplacental passage of a nonionic contrast agent. *Eur J Pediatr.* 2005;164:408–410.

67. Marcos HB, Semelka RC, Worawattanakul S. Normal placenta: gadolinium enhanced dynamic MR imaging. *Radiology.* 1997;205:493–496.

68. Prayer C, Brugger P. Investigation of normal organ development with fetal MRI. *Eur Radiol.* 2007;17:2458–2471.

69. Ray JG, Vermeulen MJ, Bharatha, A et al. Association Between MRI Exposure During Pregnancy and Fetal and Childhood Outcomes. *JAMA.* 2016; 316(9):952–961.

70. Fraum TJ, Ludwig DR, Bashir MR, et al. Gadolinium-based contrast agents: a comprehensive risk assessment. *J Magn Reson Imaging.* 2017;46:338–353.

71. Rozenfeld MN, Podberesky DJ. Godolinium-based contrast agents in children. *Pediatr Radiol.* 2018;48:1188–1196.

72. Kienzl D, Berger-Kulemann V, Kasprian G, et al. Risk of inferior vena cava compression syndrome during fetal MRI in the supine position: a retrospective analysis. *J Perinat Med.* 2013;16:1–6.

73. Serai SD, Merrow AC, Kline-Fath BM. Fetal MRI on a multi-element digital coil platform. *Pediatr Radiol.* 2013;43(9):1213–1217.

74. Hosseinzadeh K, Owens E. Optimization of acquisition time for MRI of fetal head: the eyes have it. *AJR Am J Roentgenol.* 2005;185(4):1060–1062.

75. Chaumoitre K, Wikberg E, Shojai R, et al. Fetal magnetic resonance hydrography: evaluation of a single-shot thick-slab RARE (rapid acquisition with relaxation enhancement) sequence in fetal thoracoabdominal pathology. *Ultrasound Obstet Gynecol.* 2006;27(5):537–544.

76. Huisman TA, Solopova A. MR fetography using heavily T2-weighted sequences: comparison of thin- and thick-slab acquisitions. *Eur J Radiol.* 2009;71(3):557–563.

77. Kline-Fath BM, Calvo-Garcia MA, O'Hara SM, et al. Water imaging (hydrography) in the fetus: the value of a heavily T2-weighted sequence. *Pediatr Radiol.* 2007;37(2):133–140.

78. Brugger PC, Mittermayer C, Prayer D. A new look at the fetus thick slab T2w sequence in fetal MRI. *Eur J Radiol.* 2006;57:182–186.

79. Werner H, Lopes dos Santos JR, Fontes R, et al. Virtual bronchoscopy for evaluating cervical tumors of the fetus. *Ultrasound Obstet Gynecol.* 2013;41(1):90–94.

80. Werner H, dos Santos JR, Fontes R, et al. Additive manufacturing models of fetuses built from three-dimensional ultrasound, MRI and CT scan data. *Ultrasound Obstet Gynecol.* 2010;36(3):355.

81. Barth MM, Smith MP, Pedrosa I, et al. Body MR imaging at 3.0 T: understanding the opportunities and challenges. *Radiographics.* 2007;27:1445–1462.

82. Kataoka M, Isoda H, Maetani Y, et al. MR imaging of the female pelvis at 3 Tesla: evaluation of image homogeneity using different dielectric pads. *J Magn Reson Imaging.* 2007;26:1572–1577.

83. Zaretsky MV, Alexander JM, McIntire DD, et al. MRI pelvimetry and the prediction of labor dystocia. *Obstet Gynecol.* 2005;106:919–926.

84. Korhonen U, Solja R, Laitinen J, et al. MR pelvimetry measurements, analysis of inter and intraobserver variation. *Eur J Radiol.* 2010;75:56–61.

85. Keller T, Rake A, Michel S, et al. Obstetric MR pelvimetry: reference values and evaluation of inter- and intraobserver error and intraindividual variability. *Radiology.* 2003;227:37–43.

86. Tukeva TA, Aronen HJ, Karjalainen PT, et al. Low field MRI pelvimetry. *Eur Radiol.* 1997;7:230–234.

87. Gowlan P. Placental MRI. *Semin Fetal Neonatal Med.* 2005;10:485–490.

88. Nguyen D, Nguyen C, Yavobozzi M, et al. Imaging of the placenta with pathologic correlation. *Semin Ultrasound CT MR.* 2012;33:65–77.

89. Elsayes KM, Trout A, Friedkin A, et al. Imaging of the placenta: a multimodality pictorial review. *Radiographics.* 2009;29:1371–1391.

90. Baughman WC, Corteville JE, Shah RR. Placenta accrete: spectrum of US and MR findings. *Radiographics.* 2008;28:1905–1916.

91. Warshak CR, Eskander R, Hull AD, et al. Accuracy of US and MRI in the diagnosis of placenta accrete. *Obstet Gynecol.* 2006;108:573–581.

92. Jha P, Rabban J, Chen LM, et al. Placenta accreta spectrum: value of placental bulge as a sign of myometrial invasion on MR imaging. *Abdom Radiol.* 2019;44:2572–2581.

93. Zaretsky MV, McIntire DD, Reichel TF, et al. Correlation of measured amniotic fluid volume to sonographic and MR predictions. *Am J Obstet Gynecol.* 2004;191:2148–2153.

94. Kato K, Shiozawa T, Ashida T, et al. Prenatal diagnosis of amniotic sheets by MRI. *Am J Obstet Gynecol.* 2005;193:881–884.

95. Moore RJ, Stradchan B, Tyler DJ, et al. In vivo diffusion measurements as an indication of fetal lung maturation using echo planar imaging at 0.5 T. *Magn Reson Med.* 2001;45:247–253.

96. Brugger P, Prayer D. Fetal abdominal MRI. *Eur J Radiol.* 2006;57:278–293.

97. Goitein O, Eshet Y, Hoffmann C, et al. Fetal liver T2* values: defining a standardized scale. *J Magn Reson Imaging.* 2013;38(6):1342–1345.

98. Brugger PC, Weber M, Prayer D. MRI of the fetal gallbladder and bile. *Eur Radiol.* 2010;20:2862–2869.

99. Witzani L, Brugger P, Horman M, et al. Normal renal development investigated with fetal MRI. *Eur J Radiol.* 2006;57:294–302.

100. Nemec SF, Nemec U, Weber M, et al. Female external genitalia on fetal MRI. *Ultrasound Obstet Gynecol.* 2011;38:695–700.

101. Nemec SF, Nemec U, Weber M, et al. Penile biometry on prenatal MRI. *Ultrasound Obstet Gynecol.* 2012;39:330–335.

102. Nemec SF, Nemec U, Grugger PC, et al. Skeletal development on fetal MRI. *Top Magn Reson Imaging.* 2011;22:101–106.

103. Nemec SF, Nemec U, Brugger PC, et al. MR imaging of the fetal musculoskeletal system. *Prenat Diagn.* 2012;32:205–213.

104. Witters I, Moerman P, Fryns FP. Fetal akinesia deformation sequence: a study of 30 consecutive in utero diagnoses. *Am J Med Genet.* 2002;113:23–28.

105. Anblagan D, Deshpande R, Jones NW, et al. Measurement of fetal fat in utero in normal and diabetic pregnancies using magnetic resonance imaging. *Ultrasound Obstet Gynecol.* 2013;42(3):335–340.

106. Applegate KE. Can MR imaging be used to characterize fetal musculoskeletal development? *Radiology.* 2004;233:305–306.

107. Garel C. Fetal cerebral biometry: normal parenchymal findings and ventricular size. *Eur Radiol.* 2005;15:809–813.

108. Parazzini C, Righini A, Rustico M, et al. Prenatal MRI: brain normal linear biometric values below 24 gestation weeks. *Neuroradiology.* 2008;50:877–883.

109. Duncan KR, Issa B, Moore R, et al. A comparison of fetal organ measurement by echo-planar magnetic resonance imaging and ultrasound. *BJOG.* 2005;112:43–49.

110. Michielsen K , Meersschaert J, De Keyzer F et al , MR Volumetry of the Normal Fetal Kidney: Reference Values *Prenat Diagn* 2010,30(11), 1044–8.

111. Kacem Y, Cannie MM, Kadji C, et al. Fetal weight estimation: comparison of 2 dimensional US and MRI assessment. *Radiology.* 2013;267:902–910.

112. Lo Zito L, Kadfi C, Cannie M, et al. Determination of fetal body volume measurement at term with MRI effect of various factors. *J Matern Fetal Neonatal Med.* 2013;26:1254–1258.

113. Meyers M, Garcia JR, Blough K et al. Fetal Lung Volumes by MRI: Normal Weekly Values From 18 Through 38 Weeks' Gestation. *AJR.* 2018 ; 211(2), 432–438.

114. Rubesova E. Why Do We Need More Data on MR Volumetric Measurements of the Fetal Lung? *Pediatr Radiol.* 2016; 46(2), 167–71.

9 Magnetic Resonance Imaging of the Normal Fetal Brain

Beth M. Kline-Fath

BACKGROUND

Magnetic resonance imaging (MRI) of the fetal brain is essentially imaging neuroembryology. Given the complexities of development, the fetal brain changes dramatically from the first trimester to birth. Knowing the appearance of the normal fetal brain at each gestational age is essential before abnormalities in central nervous system (CNS) development can be diagnosed. An understanding of CNS embryology is imperative to accurate interpretation of fetal neuroimaging. In this chapter, embryology of the brain is covered prior to MRI. At the end of the chapter, an atlas of normal fetal brain MRI in 2-week increments is provided to reinforce the changes over each gestation.

Imaging

Fetal brain imaging can be performed on both 1.5 and 3 Tesla (T) magnets. Imaging at 1.5 T in general is easier as it is not as susceptible to artifacts from field inhomogeneity, standing wave, or radiofrequency shield artifacts, which may result in areas of black signal in the area imaged.[1] 3T fetal MRI may be especially difficult in multiple gestations or a pregnancy complicated by polyhydramnios. Higher field strength, however, provides improved resolution, and new data suggests that 3T fetal MRI may provide better CNS detail than 1.5T fetal MRI.[2]

The fetal brain has higher water and lower protein content than the normal adult brain, with total water dropping precipitously intrauterine over time in converse to the reciprocal rise in lipid concentration.[3] Therefore, subtle differences in the brain parenchyma are best depicted by utilizing T2 imaging. The greatest depiction of fetal brain morphology and signal intensity is achieved with a T2 Single-shot Rapid Acquisition with Refocused Echos/Fast Spin Echo (SS-RARE or SS-FSE) or Half-Fourier Acquisition Single-shot Turbo spin Echo (HASTE), which provides the highest signal-to-noise ratio and resolution. Imaging of the fetal brain should include all three planes ideally at slice thickness of 3 mm with no gap and field of view (FOV) of 24 to 30. At least two sets, particularly of the sagittal plane, are useful due to fetal motion. Optimizing anatomical imaging is important, as symmetry of the fetal brain can be utilized to verify normal. The interhemispheric fissure is an excellent midline landmark to set up the anatomical sequences. If the fetal gestational age is greater than 25 weeks and more signal-to-noise ratio is desired, then a 4-mm slice thickness with no gap may be used. A 2-mm slice thickness can also be helpful, especially in evaluation of the fetal posterior fossa.

Fluid-attenuated inversion recovery (FLAIR) sequences may provide additional information with regard to the fetal brain, but most imagers utilize true fast imaging with Steady-State Free Precession (SSFP) or two-dimensional (2D) Fiesta imaging as it offers good resolution, bright-blood imaging, and high definition between fluid and soft-tissue interfaces. It is excellent in evaluating the midline anatomy, the fetal palate, and the skull base, including temporal bones. The disadvantages include less

signal and contrast between gray matter and white matter (WM), compared to single-shot fast spin-echo (SSFSE), due to lower flip angle and banding artifacts.[4] SSFP imaging is typically obtained at slice thickness of 3 to 4 mm in axial, coronal, and/or sagittal plane. 3D SSFP imaging with thin slices may provide detailed midline anatomy and cortical sulcation.[5] Cine SSFP can evaluate swallowing and fetal movement, which has been found useful in evaluation of neurological integrity.[6]

Axial or coronal gradient echo planar T2 images (3 to 4 mm skip 0) are utilized to help detect hemorrhage. Echo planar imaging (EPI) can be helpful in the evaluation of calvarium. Fast spoiled gradient recalled acquisition in the steady-state (FSPGR) T1 images (5 mm skip 0) are important for identification of hemorrhage, fat, or calcification and the normal pituitary gland.

Diffusion-weighted imaging (DWI) is extremely useful when evaluating the fetal brain. Diffusion exploits the properties of randomly moving water molecules in a magnetic field. Within tissue, diffusion of water can be restricted by many sources, including cell membranes, axons, and small vessels. The components that do not allow water to move in all directions move anisotropically. A high fractional anisotropy (FA) value reflects water motion limited in direction. The apparent diffusion coefficient (ADC) serves as a measure of freedom of diffusion of protons. Low ADC values reflect a restriction in diffusion of water, while high ADC values reflect little restriction in water diffusion. The T2 trace or DWI image reflects similar changes but with opposite high signal. Diffusion allows for depiction of fetal brain development, including areas of early myelination and cytotoxic and/or vasogenic edema related to injury or ischemia. The T2* image can be utilized to detect hemorrhagic products. Imaging is typically obtained at slice thickness of 5 mm with no gap and FOV of 32 to 40. Table 9.1 provides typical imaging sequences and anatomy depicted.

Diffusion tensor imaging is increasingly being utilized to understand WM development as it provides magnitude, anisotropy, and orientation of the diffusion by a 3D ellipsoid. This modality takes into account the length of the longest, middle, and shortest axis (eigenvalues) and their orientations (eigenvectors). FA value is utilized to characterize the shape of ellipsoid, particularly WM microstructure. Mean diffusivity (MD), an average of all eigenvalues, represents the magnitude of water diffusion along all directions.

Fetal brain measurements (Table 21 in Appendix A1) are imperative to ensure normal growth. The entire fetus should be examined, as malformations frequently involve multiple organs that may provide a clue to underlying genetic or chromosomal syndromes.

Higher level MRI techniques, including spectroscopy, diffusion tractography, and functional imaging, will be covered in Chapter 10. Multiple postprocessing techniques, such as motion correction, automated tissue delineation, 3D printing (Chapter 12), and artificial intelligence, are new innovations that will not be stressed in this chapter.

TABLE 9.1	Fetal Brain Imaging
ANATOMY	**SEQUENCES**
Cerebrum	T2 SSFSE (primary), SSFP, FLAIR
Midline and sulcation	T2 SSFSE, SSFP
Blood, fat, or calcification	T1, GRE, T2* from diffusion
Ischemia	Diffusion
Myelination	T1, T2 SSFSE, diffusion
Pituitary	T1
Temporal bone	SSFP
Calvarium	EPI
Fetal swallowing/motion	Cine SSFP

SSFSE, single-shot fast spin-echo; *SSFP*, Steady-state free precession; *GRE*, gradient echo; *EPI*, echo planar imaging, * means star.

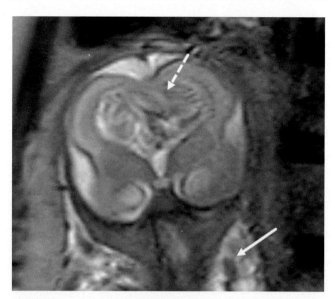

FIGURE 9.1: Coronal T2 image of a fetus at 25 weeks with severe ventriculomegaly. Dark signal within the ventricles (*dotted arrow*) is related to cerebrospinal fluid pulsation artifact in large spaces, similar to heterogeneous signal in amniotic fluid (*solid arrow*).

Indications

MRI is a valuable complement to prenatal ultrasound (US) in the evaluation of the fetal brain. Because of higher contrast resolution, large FOV, and ability to image both sides of the fetus at once, fetal MRI is excellent at evaluating parenchymal architecture, cortical development, sulcation, brainstem, and cerebellar anatomy. Most fetal brain MR examinations are performed after identification of an abnormality on prenatal sonography. Common indications are to investigate cause for ventriculomegaly or to verify a suspected CNS malformation, while excluding associated anomalies. Fetal MRI may be performed in the presence of a known disorder that predisposes the fetus to brain injury. Examples would include twin gestations with twin–twin transfusion syndrome or pregnancies exposed to maternal infection, trauma, or coagulation disorder. Sometimes, fetal MRI is requested if there is a family history of a chromosomal or genetic disorder or if there are extracerebral malformations that are linked to known intracranial anomalies, especially in the workup of a genetic syndrome.

Limitations

Fetal MRI can be operator dependent and can be limited if appropriate anatomical imaging is not obtained. Fetal MRI can be hampered by fetal, maternal, and/or amniotic fluid movement, especially in the presence of polyhydramnios. The study can be restricted by small fetal size, especially less than 20 weeks' gestation, and partial volume averaging. The smallest FOV without wraparound, standard anatomical planes, and the thinnest slices are necessary for optimal diagnostic fetal imaging.

Pitfalls in interpretation are possible if one is not familiar with the MRI appearance of the normal brain at each gestational age. Two possible misdiagnoses include lissencephaly prior to 24 weeks and misinterpreting the germinal matrix as hemorrhage early in gestation.[7] Correct interpretation may be limited if the gestational age of the fetus is not correct or known. Imaging early when the architecture of the fetal brain is primitive also may prevent detection of developing malformations. Artifacts related to maternal and fetal motion can make interpretation difficult. Flow artifact related to amniotic fluid and cerebrospinal fluid (CSF) in the ventricles should not be interpreted as hemorrhage (Fig. 9.1).

Typically, imaging should be performed at least twice in each plane and pathology confirmed on two different imaging planes and/or sequences.

BASIC EMBRYOLOGY

The first 8 weeks of development is represented by the embryonic period, which is the time when there is formation of the body and somites, closure of the neural tube, and establishment of primitive organs systems, including the cerebral cortex. The fetal period is often considered the time from the embryonic period to birth. Embryology timelines tend to reflect postconception or postovulatory dating, whereas in fetal imaging, we refer to age via last menstrual period, which can allow for a 2-week difference. Please note that embryology in this chapter is dated by postconception age and fetal MRI reflects fetal age by last menstrual period.

The stages of embryonic development are primary neurulation (also known as dorsal induction), ventral induction, neuronal cell lineage, proliferation, differentiation, neuronal migration, organization, and, finally, brain myelination (Table 9.2). Primary neurulation (dorsal induction) and ventral induction are described in this chapter as it relates to fetal imaging.

Initially, ectodermal cells at day 23, through dorsal induction, differentiate into a neural plate. The plate will thicken and fold to the midline, giving rise to a neural tube with a central embryonic vesicle (Fig. 9.2). The neural tube closes at the anterior neuropore (lamina terminalis) at day 24 and posterior neuropore (lumbosacral) on day 26. During this time, development of the ear and eye is noted by visualization of the otic disc and optic sulcus, respectively. The final phase of primary neurulation is separation of the neural tissue and surface ectoderm.[8]

At the end of the fourth week, the cranial aspect of the neural tube forms three primary vesicles: prosencephalon (forebrain), mesencephalon (midbrain), and rhombencephalon (hindbrain). At the same time, two flexures develop: the cervical flexure at the junction of the hindbrain and spinal cord and cephalic flexure at the level of the midbrain. During the fifth week, the

TABLE 9.2	Stages of Embryonic Development
MAJOR DEVELOPMENTAL EVENT	**TIME OF OCCURRENCE**
Primary Neurulation	3–5 wk
Anterior neuropore closure	24 d
Posterior neuropore closure	26 d
Development of prosencephalon/ rhombencephalon	4–5 wk
Ventral induction[a]	5–6 wk
Midline/commissure	8–20 wk
Anterior commissure	8–9 wk
Hippocampal	9–11 wk
Septum pellucidum	10–17 wk
Corpus callosum	10–17 wk
Neuronal lineage, proliferation, and migration	
Cerebral	5–24 wk
Ventricular zone	5–14 wk
Subventricular zone	14–24 wk
Cerebellum Ventricular/rhombic lips	8 wk-postnatal
Neuronal organization	24 wk to postnatal
Myelination	20 wk to postnatal

[a]Formation of cerebral hemispheres, cerebellum, brainstem, optic vesicles, olfactory bulbs and tracts, pituitary gland and stalk, and face.

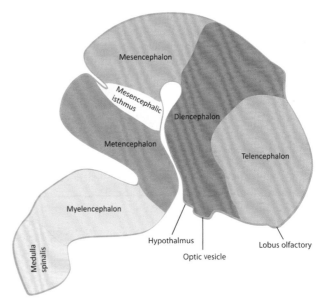

FIGURE 9.3: The primitive brain denoting embryological origins and flexures.

prosencephalon divides into telencephalon and diencephalon, distinguished by further visualization of the optic vesicles. The mesencephalon remains unchanged, but an area is defined between the hindbrain and midbrain, known as the mesencephalic isthmus. The rhombencephalon will further differentiate into the metencephalon and myelencephalon. Flexure in the hindbrain (pontine) will occur with this division (Fig. 9.3). Persistence of the central embryonic canal in each of these areas will give rise to the ventricular system: telencephalon—lateral ventricles, diencephalon—third ventricle, mesencephalon—cerebral aqueduct, and rhombencephalon—fourth ventricle (Fig. 9.4). As the vesicles form, the choroid plexus will develop from blood vessels that invade the ventricular walls.

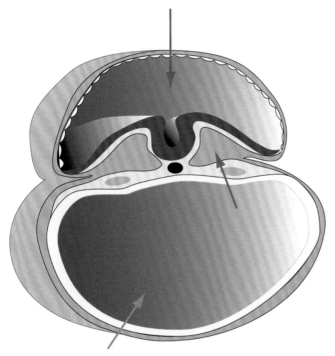

FIGURE 9.2: Section through the trilaminar germ disc. The neural tissue, blue layer marked by green arrow, arises from ectoderm along the dorsal aspect of the embryo and contains amniotic fluid due to continuity with the amniotic sac. The mesodermal layer is delineated by blue arrow and yolk sac by brown arrow.

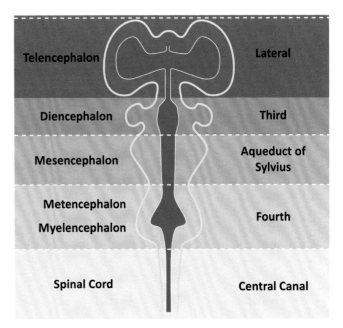

FIGURE 9.4: The primitive cerebral vesicles and associated ventricular origins.

A sulcus hemispheric divides the developing telencephalon and diencephalon. The dorsal medial corresponds to the velum interpositum, and the basal medial corresponds to the lamina terminalis. A loose mesenchyme will form primary meninges at 5 weeks. As a result of growth in the sagittal midline, the falx cerebri, sagittal sinus, and leptomeninges will deepen in the interhemispheric fissure. The dural layer is present at 6 weeks, and as the dura develops, the attachment between the tentorium cerebelli and falx moves more caudal, causing reduction in the size of the posterior fossa relative to supratentorial brain.[8] The internal carotid vessels will give rise to five terminal branches: anterior, middle, and posterior cerebral arteries; choroidal artery, and ophthalmic artery. The posterior cerebral artery will detach and fuse to the rostral basilar artery, embryonic origination from paired longitudinal neural arteries.

The walls of the telencephalic cerebral vesicle are extremely thin but are connected in the midline by the lamina terminalis, the site of anterior neuropore closure. Ventral induction is the formation of the brain into two cerebral hemispheres. The telencephalon does not cleave, but instead at the beginning of the fifth week, bilateral evaginations around the foramina of Monro develop as outgrowths of the dorsolateral walls of the prosencephalon, forming caudal wards and bending in ventral and rostral directions, eventually completely covering the diencephalon and encircling the thalamus. With this C-shaped growth, the temporal lobes that initially were the posterior pole of the telencephalon are now ventral, the occipital lobe lies dorsal posterior telencephalon, and the hippocampus rotates dorsomedial to ventromedial. The interhemispheric fissure will be present at approximately 10 weeks, forming anterior to posterior.[9] Concurrently during ventral induction, the cerebellum, brainstem, olfactory bulbs (OBs) and tract, pituitary gland and stalk, and face are forming.

The development of the brain is influenced and directed by innumerable genes and signaling molecules that are essential for normal cell proliferation, differentiation, migration, organization, and myelination. However, the discussion of genetic embryology and molecular dynamics is beyond the space allotment and will not be discussed further here.

VENTRICLES AND CAVUM SEPTUM PELLUCIDUM

The ventricles arise from the cavities of the primitive cerebral vesicles. Life begins in water, so it is not surprising that neuronal and

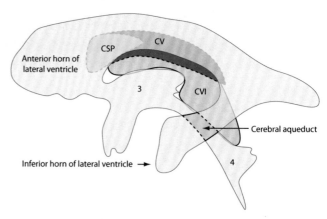

FIGURE 9.5: Lateral figure of the ventricles (lateral, third, aqueduct, and fourth). *CSP*, cavum septum pellucidum; *CV*, cavum vergae; *CVI*, cavum velum interpositum.

glial cells for the developing brain originate in or near the walls of the ventricles in a structure known as the germinal matrix.

Lateral Ventricles

Embryology

The lateral ventricles begin as a primitive cerebral cavity, which becomes paired with cleavage of the telencephalon. The cavities communicate with each other and the third ventricle through the intraventricular foramina (Fig. 9.5). Along the medial wall of the primitive ventricles, the choroid plexus develops as a fold covered by pseudostratified epithelium with proliferation of underlying blood vessels. The choroid is anchored at the foramen of Monro and present in the body, atrium, and temporal horns of the lateral ventricles. Early in the pregnancy, the choroid has a high glycogen content, which is believed to be a major energy supply for the growing cerebrum, but after 19 weeks, the choroid will also be responsible for CSF production.

Magnetic Resonance Imaging

The lateral ventricles are visible at 13 to 14 weeks and change dramatically with the development of the cerebrum. Before 16 weeks, the primitive lateral ventricles appear large and are composed of globular frontal horns, body, and atrium (Fig. 9.6A). With growth of the occipital and temporal lobes, periventricular structures, and corpus callosum, the ventricles narrow gradually, achieving

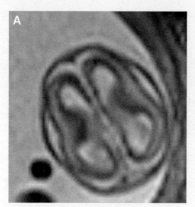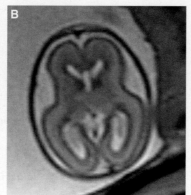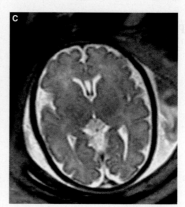

FIGURE 9.6: Axial T2 MRI of fetuses showing change in ventricular configuration. **A:** 17 weeks with large rudimentary ventricles **B:** 23 weeks with prominent occipital horns **C:** 34 weeks with small mature ventricular system.

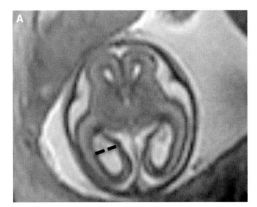
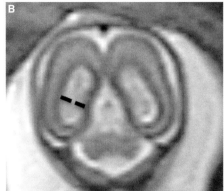

FIGURE 9.7: A: Axial T2 of a fetus at 18 weeks demonstrating lateral ventricle atrial measurement inside the wall at the level of the choroid. **B:** Coronal SSFSE T2 in the same fetus demonstrating atrial measurement.

an adult configuration. The growth of the thalamus and corpus striatum results in the development of the foramen of Monro. The caudate nuclei reshape the frontal horn so that they appear biconcave rather than lobular. The occipital horns may appear prominent until 24 weeks (Fig. 9.6B) but demonstrate typical internal and medial deviation in the early third trimester due to evolution of the calcar avis.[10] Between 24 and 28 weeks, the lateral ventricles appear less prominent, and by 34 to 36 weeks, the ventricles appear small (Fig. 9.6C). Despite the apparent change in the lateral ventricles and a twofold increase in CSF volume, the atrial diameter is relatively constant, ranging from 14 to 40 weeks' gestation, with normal values being <10 mm on prenatal US.[11,12] Measurements performed with fetal MRI have confirmed that atrial width is not dependent on gestational age, with average normal values of 6 to 7 mm, with threshold for ventriculomegaly being greater than 10 mm.[10,13,14] Axial measurements on fetal MRI at the level of the thalamic nuclei can be obtained but may be 1 to 2 mm inconsistent with US measurements (Fig. 9.7A).[13] Coronal measurements inside the lateral ventricular wall at the level of the choroid plexus are highly concordant between both US and MRI (Fig. 9.7B).[14] Atrio-cerebral ratio (ratio of the atrium diameter and brain biparietal diameter [BPD]) progressively decrease during gestation, reflecting fetal brain growth in the presence of constant ventricular size.

Cavum Septum Pellucidum

Embryology
The cavum septum pellucidum (CSP) is an important space defined by two thin translucent membranes that extend from the anterior part of the body, genu, and rostrum of the corpus callosum, inferior to the superior surface of the fornix and lateral along the inner walls of the lateral ventricles. The cavum vergae is a cavity within the septum pellucidum, located posterior to the foramina of Monro or, anatomically, the vertical plane, formed by the anterior columns of the fornix (Fig. 9.5). The embryological development of the CSP is closely associated with the formation of the corpus callosum, thought to represent a space caused by thinning of the commissural plate and disappearance of the glial sling and may be understood as the bridge scaffolding that remains after the corpus callosum has formed.[15,16] The structure begins to develop at 10 to 12 weeks and is present by 17 weeks.[15] Although, visually the cavum is a CSF space, the septal leaflets, which contain neurons, are important, serving as a relay station for the hippocampus and hypothalamus.

Magnetic Resonance Imaging
The CSP can be visualized as early as 15 weeks but should be apparent by 18 weeks, with the space increasing in size from 19 to 27 weeks, plateauing at 28 weeks (Fig. 9.8).[17] The CSP is best depicted on coronal or axial plane as a cystic space lined by two parallel intermediate T2 signal leaflets, measuring transversely between 2 and 10 mm in size. Closure of cavum begins at approximately 24 weeks from posterior to anterior. The cavum vergae fuses by 40 weeks and, the CSP as early as 37 weeks but sometimes as late as 3 to 6 months postnatal.[15,17] On imaging, the cavum can become prominent late fetal period and resemble an interhemispheric cyst.

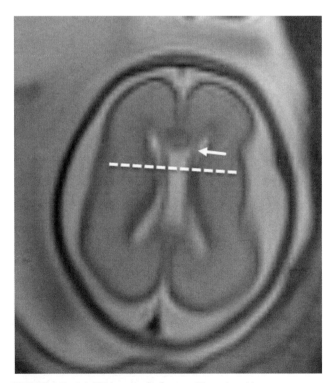

FIGURE 9.8: Axial T2 image of a fetus at 25 weeks with cavum septum pellucidum and vergae. The septal leaflets of the septum pellucidum are defined by arrows. The cavum pellucidum is anterior to the foramen of Monro (*anterior to dotted line*), and cavum vergae is posterior (*posterior to dotted line*).

Third Ventricle and Aqueduct

The third ventricle becomes visible in the late first trimester. Although the volume of the third ventricle increases 23-fold over gestation, the size is relatively stable, appearing as a slit-like CSF structure located between the thalamic nuclei.[11] A normal third ventricle should measure less than 4 mm in transverse dimension, being easiest to visualize on the coronal plane (Fig. 9.9).[18,19] The aqueduct of Sylvius is closely related to development of the mesencephalon, representing a thin linear CSF space between the tectum and midbrain, best depicted on anatomical midline sagittal image (Fig. 9.10).

Fourth Ventricle

Embryology

The fourth ventricle undergoes unusual development. Between 5 and 7 weeks, a large ellipsoid CSF cavity develops due to focal dilatation of the central canal of the hindbrain neural tube.[20,21] Choroid plexus will develop within the primitive vesicle. The inferior roof of this rhombencephalic vesicle will evaginate caudal and dorsal to the developing cerebellar vermis as a diverticulum known as Blake pouch (Fig. 9.11).[20,21] The pouch contains an inner layer of ependymal, middle layer of attenuated neuroglial tissue, and outer layer of pia-arachnoid. Blake pouch will fenestrate down to the obex, leaving a hole which is termed Blake metaphor or the primitive foramen of Magendie. By 4 months, the foramen of Luschka will open, resulting in equilibration of the CSF between ventricles and the subarachnoid spaces. Before fenestration, there is likely transient increase in intra-axial CSF pressure, resulting in enlargement of the fourth ventricle from 14 to 16 weeks, which then decreases to normal size around 22 to 23 weeks.[21] There is an eightfold increase in volume by term.[11] The septae in the cisterna magna are remnants of Blake pouch walls.[21]

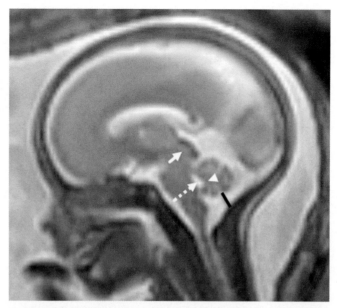

FIGURE 9.10: Sagittal T2 image at 24 weeks with fluid in the aqueduct of Sylvius (*white arrow*). The fourth ventricle (*dotted white arrow*) is normal in size and configuration. Fastigial point denoted with *a white arrowhead*. Cisterna magna is labeled with *a black line*.

Magnetic Resonance Imaging

The fourth ventricle is a triangular CSF space between the brainstem and the vermis, best evaluated on a sagittal midline image of the fetal brain. The pointed posterior recess of the fourth ventricle is known as the fastigial point. Normal dimensions (Table 21 in Appendix A1) on sagittal plane anterior to posterior from the dorsal pons to fastigial point average 4.5 ± 2.5 mm with a maximum dimension <7 mm (Fig. 9.10).[19]

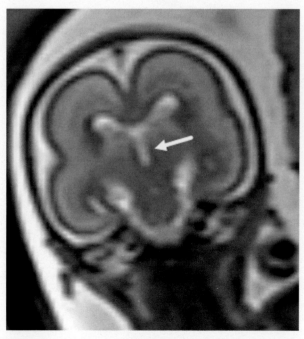

FIGURE 9.9: Coronal T2 image at 25 weeks with slit-like normal third ventricle (*arrow*).

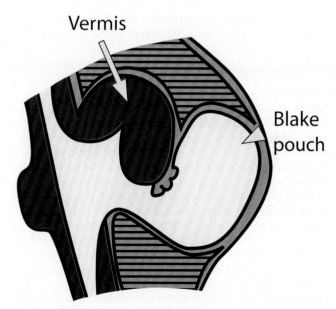

FIGURE 9.11: Blake pouch. Rhombencephalic vesicle known as Blake pouch is present early in the development of the fourth ventricle. The subarachnoid space (*striped purple*) does not communicate with Blake pouch.

SUBARACHNOID SPACES

Supratentorial

Embryology

Early in gestation, the subarachnoid spaces appear enlarged because of immaturity and small size of the fetal brain (Fig. 9.12). As the brain develops and increases in weight, the spaces appear less prominent, even though there is an 11-fold increase in volume to term.[11] The extra-axial spaces remain constant until 30 weeks from which they decrease in size, although prominent spaces can persist in some fetuses in the parieto-occipital area.[22]

Magnetic Resonance Imaging

Subarachnoid spaces can be measured from the cortex of the brain to the inner table of the cranium anterior frontal or parietal. The frontal subarachnoid space measured on axial plane at the level of the frontal lobes and superior anterior gyrus should measure maximum width of 6 mm, with the space decreasing in size after 32 weeks, with mean values at 18 to 30 weeks of 3 to 4 mm and after 32 weeks 1.7 to 2.1 mm.[23] The parieto-occipital space measured on a sagittal image at the level of the parieto-occipital sulcus reaches a maximum of 11 mm between 26 and 28 weeks and decreases in size after 34 weeks to 5 to 7 mm.[23] Interhemispheric dimensions by gestational age are present in Table 21 Appendix A1. Comparing brain BPD-to-bone BPD ratio may also provide clues to enlarged spaces.

Infratentorial

Embryology

The tentorium demonstrates definitive orientation perpendicular to the occipital bone, inserting adjacent to the torcula by 20 to 21 weeks.[24] The cisterna magna has two compartments. The mesial compartment between the cisterna magna septa is derived from Blake pouch. The lateral compartment is derived from cavitation of the meninx primitiva to form subarachnoid space. The remnant walls of Blake pouch can be identified on fetal MRI as bridging septae within the cisterna magna on a heavily T2 sequence (Fig. 9.13).

Magnetic Resonance Imaging

The cisterna magna is measured on an axial or sagittal image from midline posterior cerebellar vermis to inner margin of the occiput (Fig. 9.10). The cisterna magna increases with gestational age but normal size should be greater than 2 and less 10 mm.[13,23]

SUPRATENTORIAL BRAIN

Cerebral Parenchyma

Embryology

Neuronal Migration: The supratentorial brain (forebrain) is derived from the telencephalon and diencephalon, subdivided into distinct dorsoventral and rostral caudal (frontal to occipital) domains. The dorsal telencephalon (pallium) gives rise to the cerebral cortex and hippocampus, and the ventral telencephalon (subpallium) to the striatum, pallidum, and telencephalic stalk. The diencephalon develops into the thalamus and hypothalamus (Fig. 9.14). Neurons and glial cells arise in two germinal matrices, the ventricular zone (VZ) and the subventricular zone (SVZ). Important cortical neurons include motor or pyramidal neurons of excitatory type, which are glutamate mediated. Interneurons or sensory granule cells are inhibitory

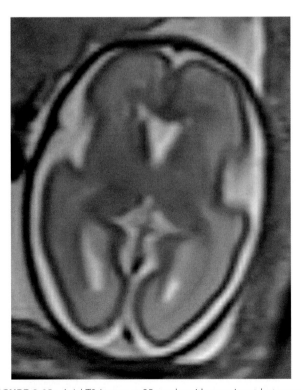

FIGURE 9.12: Axial T2 image at 25 weeks with prominent but normal extra-axial fluid spaces.

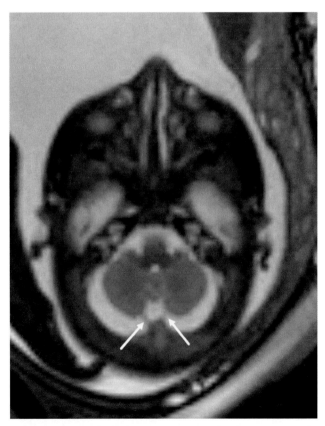

FIGURE 9.13: Axial SSFP image at 24 weeks demonstrating thin septations paramidline (*arrows*) that are septal leaflets remnant of Blake pouch.

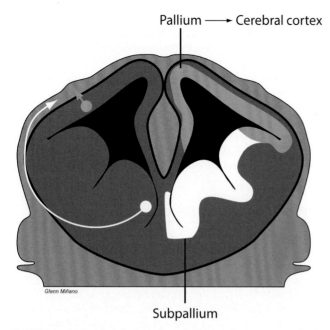

Pallium ——→ Cerebral cortex

Subpallium

Glenn Miñano

FIGURE 9.14: On the left, the pallium and subpallium. On the right, the primary mode of neural migration for each region.

or gamma-aminobutyric acid (GABA) mediated. Glutamatergic contributes 70% to 80% and GABAeric 20% to 30% of neurons.[25] Astrocytes are present for neuronal support, and oligodendrocytes are important for myelination.

Two types of neuronal migration are described by pathology: radial and tangential. Radial migration is perpendicular to the neuroepithelial surface, and tangential is parallel to the pial surface. However, these types of migration are dynamic, with radial migration possible in two opposing directions, tangential being either directed or nondirected and cells switching between these two types of migration, sometimes known as random walk. Beginning in the embryonic and continuing in the fetal period to 24 weeks, the time is dominated by neuronal proliferation and migration.[26] From 24 weeks to term, structural

neuronal organization and maturation ensues.[26] Beginning in the fetal period and continuing postnatal is a time of myelination (Table 9.2).

In the embryonic period, prior to closure of the neural tube, predecessor neurons migrate tangential from the subpallium to lie beneath the pial surface.[27] These cells give rise to the preplate, which acts as a scaffold for future cellular and axonal navigation.[28] At embryonic day 30 with closure of the neural tube, the forebrain is composed of two layers: the cerebral vesicle lined by a single layer of cells, the primitive germinal matrix or VZ, and the more superficial preplate layer. The VZ contains homogeneous pseudostratified epithelium with radial processes that will undergo extensive proliferation with cells dividing symmetrically. At approximately 6.5 weeks, the cells in the VZ will have the ability to transform into neural stem cells known as apical radial glia (aRG), switching to asymmetrical mode of division where one cell remains a progenitor and the other a destined neuron or glial cell (Fig. 9.15).[25] One week before the presence of the cortical plate (CP), the VZ will also give rise to dividing cells that are not attached to the ventricular surface in a germinal matrix known as the subventricular zone (SVZ). Both the VZ and the SVZ will provide excitatory neurons that migrate radial to the CP.

The aRG in the VZ is bipolar in shape with nucleus near the ventricle, a short process connecting to the lateral ventricle and a long process to the outer surface of the brain.[27,28] These neurons extend along RG filaments to the preplate, separating it into a thin superficial layer, known as the marginal zone (MZ) or CP layer I and a deep layer termed presubplate (PSP). This migration of cells at 7 to 8 weeks marks the onset of neurogenesis and transition from embryonic to fetal period.[26] With migration of these cells, the primitive WM, known as the intermediate zone (IZ), will develop as a compartment between proliferative layers and postmigratory cells containing afferent axons originating from the forebrain and thalamus and efferent from the CP and PSP. As neurogenesis progresses, aRG will give rise to apical intermediate cells that divide symmetrically to form a pair of neurons.

The surface and volume expansion of the human cortex in the second half of gestation is primarily related to cell proliferation

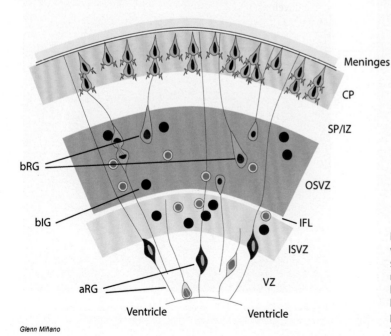

Glenn Miñano

FIGURE 9.15: There is radial migration of cells from the ventricular zone (VZ) and subventricular zone (SVZ). The neural stem cell in the VZ is the apical radial glia (aRG), which will give rise to intermediate progenitors (bIG) and stem cells in the SVZ known as basal radial glia (bRG). The SVZ is classified into three layers: the inner layer (iSVZ), inner fiber layer (iFL) also known as periventricular-rich zone, and outer layer (oSVZ). *IZ,* intermediate zone; *SP,* subplate; *CP,* cortical plate.

in the SVZ.[25] The SVZ is divided into an inner and outer zone, split by a thin inner fibrous layer, also known as the periventricular-rich zone (PVRZ), which contains growing fibers, many callosal in origin.[29] Two types of radial migrating cells are noted in the SVZ. Arising from the aRG cells, basal intermediate progenitor (bIP) will move into the inner SVZ (iSVZ) and undergo symmetric proliferative divisions before a terminal symmetric neurogenic division. Superficial to the PVRZ, in a cellular layer known as the outer SVZ (oSVZ), the aRG will give rise to a cell type termed basal radial glial (bRG) cell, a mammalian-specific cell, especially pronounced in humans.[30] These cells are monopolar and lack connection with the ventricle but contact the basal lamina. bRG cells represent neural stem cells that can self-renew, give rise to bIP, and also provide a broad lineage of neuronal and glial cells (Fig. 9.15).[25,28] The iSVZ is fairly constant in size; however, the oSVZ grows progressively larger during neurogenesis.[25]

Neurons are primarily formed from 5 to 25 weeks, with majority reaching the CP by 20 weeks.[28] The VZ cells are direct descendent neurons for the neural plate, differentiating into radial glia, neurons, astrocytes, and stem cells in the oSVZ. Continuing to 14 weeks, waves of glutaminergic projection (pyramidal) neurons migrate along specialized RG fibers to the interface between the MZ and the CP where they interact with waiting afferent fibers from nucleus basalis, monoamine nucleus, thalamus, and corpus callosum and then detach to form layers of the CP in an inside-out manner, with the first neurons residing in future layer VI and later migrating neurons in the superficial layer II of the cortex (Fig. 9.16).[30,31] The MZ

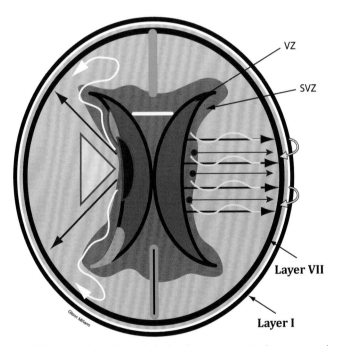

FIGURE 9.16: Cerebral cortical development ventricular zone and subventricular zone in pallium and subpallium. *Pallium (right side):* Migration from the ventricular (VZ) and subventricular zone (SVZ) demonstrate neurons traveling radial from the ependymal and subependymal areas with guidance by radial glial cells (yellow curvy lines) to the cortex. The neurons then migrate in an inside out configuration (yellow curved arrows) after splitting the preplate into layers 1 and VII. *Subpallium (left side):* Neurons arising from the ganglionic eminences avoid the striatum (light tan) to migrate tangentially (red and white lines). Gangionic eminences are medial (red), lateral (light blue) and caudal (orange).

present below the pial surface is composed largely of fibers, dendrites of immature pyramidal neurons, and Cajal–Retzius cells, which secrete a protein Reelin that is required for normal inside-to-outside positioning of the cells.[32] Over time, aRG cells will switch from proliferative to differentiative divisions. The SVZ, after approximately 15 to 16 weeks, in the mid- to later fetal period becomes the remaining source of neurons for the CP. However, the SVZ also supports the formation of a transient layer important for CP development (Fig. 9.16).[33] As afferent fibers penetrate the CP, particularly thalamocortical, at weeks 13 to 15, there is dispersion of cells with development of a deep zone that is loosely packed with cells, known as the subplate (SP), also cortical layer VII.[30]

Interneurons comprise 20% to 30% of the cortex and are important for modulating cortical output, leading to higher executive movement, thinking, and emotion.[34] These inhibitory cells are diverse cells of VZ and SVZ etiology that predominately migrate tangentially and arise in the ventral portion of the brain in the ganglionic eminence (GE), preoptic area (POa) (region of the hypothalamus), and septal anlage of the developing septum. The VZ in each of these areas promote RG cells to differentiate into GABAergic fate progenitor intermediate cells, which encode enzymes that convert glutamate to GABA.[35] Interneurons can exit through many pathways, dorsally to the cortex, ventrolaterally to the striatum, caudal to the hippocampus, and ventral to the OB.

The cells in thickened GE are small and compact and lie along the lateral walls of the frontal and lesser extent temporal/occipital horns of the lateral ventricles. Two eminences lie along the subpallium. The medial GE (MGE) lies closer to midline at the level of the globus pallidus near the developing third ventricle, and the lateral GE (LGE) is adjacent but continues along the frontal horn more superior. The caudal GE (CGE) lies along the temporal/occipital horns. Interneurons derived from these areas may have short axons connecting one neuron to another or long axons as in projection interneurons, linking distant brain regions.[32,36]

The MGE (50% to 60%) and CGE (30% to 40%) and, to lesser extent, POa (10%) and questionable LGE contribute cells for the developing neocortex through a long tangential migratory path up to 20 weeks' gestation (Fig. 9.16).[31,32,36] Cells from primarily the MGE migrate through two migratory streams, the SVZ/IZ and MZ ventral to dorsal, some with the guidance of axons, avoiding the striatum to provide interneurons in the middle and deep layers of the CP. Caudal cells migrate later through multiple migratory streams to provide cells to superficial layers of the CP.[37] Interneurons will switch the mode of migration from tangential to radial to contact RG fibers and reach final CP position. MGE and POa interneurons migrate inside to out, whereas CGE interneurons outside-in, but both will delay until corresponding excitatory pyramidal cells are in appropriate laminar distribution and have provided signaling to the interneuron.[31,37] In the absence of appropriate interaction, interneuron cell death ensues, which is likely an important regulator of CP specialization.[37] The complex migration of these cells to the cerebral cortex is complete by 24 weeks.[27] Given the diversity of function of interneurons, there are many different subtypes, separated by marker, origin, cell morphology, and axonal targeting.

Because each GE is not clearly demarcated from each other, the origin of interneuron populations can be difficult to define, but new molecular markers are proving helpful (Table 9.3).

TABLE 9.3   Sites of Developing Cells and Originating Structures

Lateral GE:	GABA projection striatum (caudate, putamen, globus pallidus)
	GABAergic olfactory bulb
	Late GABAergic neocortex
	Glial
Medial GE:	GABA projection globus pallidus and amygdala
	GABAergic cortex, hippocampus, amygdala, striatum
	Cholinergic striatum
	Glial
Caudal GE:	GABAergic hippocampus, amygdala, cortex, striatum
	GABA projection striatum
Preoptic:	GABAergic cortex
	Cholinergic caudate and putamen

GE, ganglionic eminence.

The MGE primarily provides interneurons to the globus pallidus.[38] The LGE is responsible for the striatum, especially caudate, putamen and OB.[38] CGE and, to a lesser amount, MGE cells are also a source of interneurons for the hippocampus and amygdala. The POa also provides interneurons to the caudate and putamen.[39]

In the diencephalon, the ventral tissue early on differentiates into nuclear territories for the hypothalamus. The dorsal diencephalon gives rise to the thalamus, initially a compact undivided mass and the lateral geniculate body.[30] With enlargement of the cortex, there is corresponding increase in thalamic nuclei during embryonic and early fetal time due to cell proliferation and migration in VZ, SVZ, and MZ of the diencephalon.[34,40] At 13 weeks, with tangential migration of neurons in the MGE and LGE, a corridor is created, which allows the thalamocortical fibers, conveying motor and sensory input to the CP, to navigate the GE deep to the developing globus pallidus and advance through the striatum to reach the developing cortex.[41] From 15 to 34 weeks, cells will also migrate tangential from the GE to contribute GABAergic neurons to the thalamus via a transient fetal structure beneath the thalamic surface called the gangliothalamic body.[40] These cells give rise to associated nuclei, such as the pulvinar and mediodorsal, as well as anterior (limbic) and other relay nuclei.

Neuronal Organization: Following proliferation and migration, cortical organization, axonal growth, and early fetal circuitry in the CP are orchestrated by a transient layer termed the subplate (SP).[30] The SP, representing layer VII of the developing CP, is composed of one of the oldest population of neurons in the developing forebrain as well as neurotransmitters, transient synapsis, and abundant hydrophilic extracellular matrix for axonal guidance.[30,42] At 10 to 12 weeks, in the PSP stage, the earliest generated neurons develop synaptic activity, and there are afferent fibers from brainstem nuclei and basal forebrain and efferent fibers connecting to the thalamus and subcortical

areas.[43,44] At 13 to 15 weeks, the SP proper is defined due to the addition of neurons, which have migrated radial from the VZ with those for CP layer VI, and ingrowth of thalamocortical fibers, which are responsible for dispersion of SP neurons.[43] There are also corticocortical and monoamine followed by later callosal fiber ingrowth, which further increase the size of the SP to 22 weeks. When fibers arrive to the SP, there is a long waiting period where axons interact with SP neurons and interdigitate with afferent callosal fibers from the PVRZ.[30] After 23 to 24 weeks, the thalamocortical fibers demonstrate growth into the CP at the same time as neuronal lamination, being earlier in the somatosensory than frontal and occipital lobes.[30,43] In this late phase, neuronal differentiation and circuitry is initiated directly though thalamocortical and basal forebrain axon fiber synapsis with CP neurons and indirectly via interactions with SP neurons which then innervate and potentially regulate radial migration of neocortical neurons.[43,45]

The SP layer peak development is between 13 and 31 weeks, being thickest at 30 weeks, occupying 45% of the telencephalon.[46] With relocation of fibers to the CP, death of SP neurons, and later neocortical neurons migration to the CP, the SP decreases in size.[44] The large extracellular matrix disappears around 32 to 34 weeks, occurring first in primary sensory and motor areas and last in associative areas. SP persists longest in the crowns of developing gyri and prefrontal and opercular cortical regions.[43] SP neurons that persist and grow postnatal will gradually be transformed to interstitial neurons in the destined subcortical WM.[42,43]

After production of neurons, a gliotic switch occurs, and from 29 to 34 weeks, glial progenitors arise from primarily the SVZ, which differentiate into astrocytes and oligodendrocytes for the neocortex, striatum, and WM.[30,36,47] Astrocytes are the most abundant diverse cell in the CNS, present in both gray and WM, and support neuronal migration, survival, and synapsis turnover.[48] Oligodendrocyte progenitor can be seen arising early in the MGE and LGE and other areas of the dorsal VZ/SVZ. These glial precursors differentiate into preoligodendrocytes, which make up 90% of the population until 28 weeks.[49] The astrocyte and likely neurons in contact with the preoligodendrocyte cell play a major role in initiation of the myelination process (also known as myelination gliosis). Microglia, unlike astrocytes and oligodendrocytes, are born during embryogenesis from the yolk sac as primitive macrophages, which migrate into the developing brain to differentiate into microglia.[48] Microglia and astrocytes are essential for eliminating unnecessary synapsis so that precise wiring is obtained.[48]

The prospective central WM, or IZ, is generated by the VZ at 8 weeks but increases dramatically in size from 13 to 20 weeks.[50] Multiple migrating neurons and glia pass through the IZ, but the IZ is especially important for growing axonal pathways, which are crucial to the development of the expanded cerebral cortex. With axonal growth, fibers must pass through the diencephalic–telencephalic border and corticostriatal junction to pass through periventricular crossroads prior to waiting in the SP before penetrating CP. Peak growth of axons is between 22 and 34 weeks.[51]

WM tracts can be divided in five function categories, including brainstem, limbic, projection, commissural, and association, and have been studied by histology and diffusion tensor imaging.[52] In the late embryonic period, a prominent projection fiber known as the hemispheric stalk will emanate from the ventrolateral thalamus and be joined by fibers from the basal telencephalon to give rise to the internal capsule and external capsule.[30,51] Before 10 weeks, brainstem tracts and limbic fibers arise likely since they support basic life functions.[52] Growth of the internal capsule and projection thalamic radiations are noted at 11 to 13 weeks, and corticospinal tract by 17 weeks.[52] The commissural fiber system is present in the PVRZ in conjunction with fronto-occipital, frontal pontine, and subcallosal fibers.[52,53] From 15 to 18 weeks, six periventricular crossroads containing hydrophilic extracellular matrix for axon guidance become evident, representing areas of efferent fibers and afferent crossing projection or thalamocortical (radial), associative (sagittal), and callosal (transverse) pathways.[51,54] The most numerous are projection fibers of the corona radiata that develops anterior, superior, and last posterior from 13 to 34 weeks due to enlargement of the thalamocortical, commissural, and associative fibers. As the afferent fibers relocate from the SP to cortex, the WM architecture changes from predominately tangential to radial, and sulcation becomes active.[51,54] The superior longitudinal fasciculus arises during the third trimester and long-range corticocortical fibers around 33 to 35 weeks, given that they contribute to higher level functioning.[52]

Neuronal Differentiation: Prior to 24 weeks, the CP is devoid of synapsis.[51] After 24 weeks, the neurons have settled into the CP with laminar position. Differentiation of cells is complex requiring production of axons, dendrites, and synapsis with neurotransmitters from deep to superficial layers of the CP.[55] The acceleration of dendritic differentiation in the CP accompanies ingrowth of many other afferent fibers, especially commissural and associative corticocortical fibers. With differentiation, the CP will organize in six final vertical layers of differentiated neurons and axonal networks. Layers II and III will connect with ipsilateral or contralateral cortex, layer IV is afferent from thalamus and layer VI efferent to thalamus, and layer V provides connection with structures other than the thalamus. These changes result in further development of the cortex with appearance of sulci, accelerated at weeks 25 to 26, and increase in brain weight and volume.[30] Final cortical circuitry is present 3 months postnatal in the primary motor, sensory, and visual cortices but will be delayed till more than 1 year in associative prefrontal cortex.[44]

The germinal matrix compartments decrease dramatically after 25 weeks.[46] The VZ, after exhaustion at about 16 weeks, transforms into ependymal cells, while the involution of the SVZ and GE at approximately 34 to 36 weeks results in a subependymal layer and mature basal ganglia.[34] Migration is for most part complete by birth, with exception of small quantities of pluripotent SVZ cells that persist along the ventricular walls postnatal, including a population along the rostral lateral ventricle that generates olfactory neurons and glia after birth and migrate to the OB within the rostral migratory stream (RMS).[34,56]

Magnetic Resonance Imaging

Reflecting embryology, the fetal brain grows, demonstrating changing lamination and architecture over gestation. Timelines for lamination in this chapter reflects those expected when performing imaging at 1.5 and 3 T, although higher field strength and postmortem MRI can provide different lamination dating that will not be covered herein. Fetal brain biometry is essential to confirm normal growth and should be a standard part of interpretation and reporting (Table 21 in Appendix A1).

Areas such as the germinal matrix (VZ and SVZ) and cortex will be represented by T1 hyperintense and T2 hypointense

signal and demonstrate high signal on diffusion and low signal on ADC map due to high cell density, radial organization, and microvascularity.[57,58] The IZ demonstrates T1 hypointense and T2 hyperintense signal due to lack of myelination and high water content. The PVRZ and SP due to high hydrophilic extracellular matrix also demonstrate T1 hypointense and T2 hyperintense signal. Both the IZ and the SP with low cellularity will appear hypointense on diffusion and hyperintense on ADC map.[58,59]

16 to 20 Weeks: Imaging at this time demonstrates a **three-layer pattern** likely due to the limited spatial resolution in the presence of a small fetal brain (Figs. 9.17, 9.18, and 9.19).[60,61] The three-layer pattern on T2 imaging is comparable to an oreo cookie, dark on the ends and white in the middle. The three layers from deep to superficial are listed herein below. The MZ is too thin to be separated from the CP on MRI.

Three-Layer Pattern (Central to Peripheral)
VZ/SVZ: Dark T2, *bright T1, high diffusion, low ADC*
IZ: Bright T2, *dark T1, low diffusion, high ADC*
CP: Dark T2, *bright T1, high diffusion, low ADC*

At this early gestation, the germinal matrix is thick due to high neuronal proliferation and incomplete migration. Both the VZ and the SVZ cannot be separated; however, there may be subtle gradation of T2 dark signal, being greatest at the ventricular wall and decreasing more peripheral.[62] The GE is extremely dark and thick at the caudothalamic groove and along the

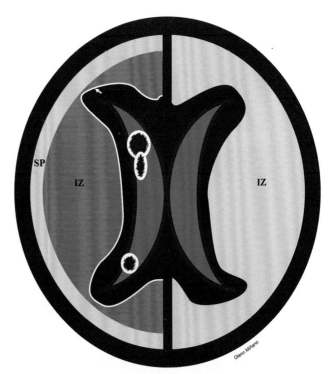

5 layer (20-28 wks)   3 layer (<20 wks)

FIGURE 9.17: The layers of the fetal brain less than 20 weeks and between 20 and 28 weeks. *Less than 20 weeks or three-layer pattern:* germinal matrix (GM), intermediate zone (IZ), and cortical plate (CP). *20 to 28 weeks or five-layer pattern:* GM, ganglionic eminences (starry structures), periventricular-rich zone or cell sparse layer of the SVZ (PVRZ), IZ containing cell dense SVZ, subplate (SP), and CP.

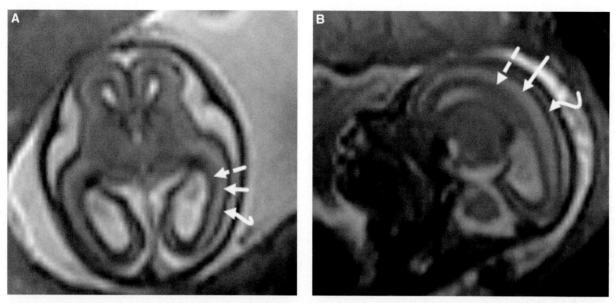

FIGURE 9.18: **A:** Axial T2 image of a 19-week fetus with three-layer pattern. *Dotted arrow* is germinal matrix, *solid* intermediate zone or white matter, and *curved arrow* cortex. **B:** Sagittal T2 image of the same fetus showing germinal matrix (*dotted arrow*), intermediate zone (*solid arrow*), and cortex (*curved arrow*).

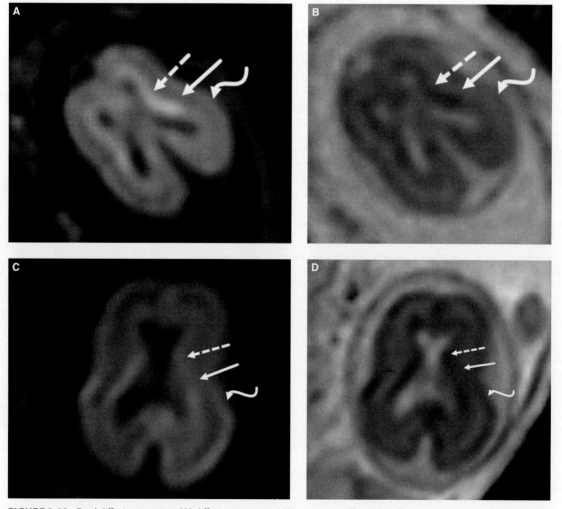

FIGURE 9.19: Fetal diffusion imaging: **(A)** diffusion image and **(B)** apparent diffusion coefficient (ADC) of a fetus at 19 weeks' gestation and **(C)** diffusion image and **(D)** ADC of a fetus at 24 weeks' gestation. The germinal matrix (*dotted arrow*) and cortex (*curved arrow*) demonstrate high diffusion and low ADC and intermediate zone (*solid arrow*) is low diffusion and high ADC. Notice the thicker germinal matrix in a 19-week fetus but thicker cortex in a 24-week fetus.

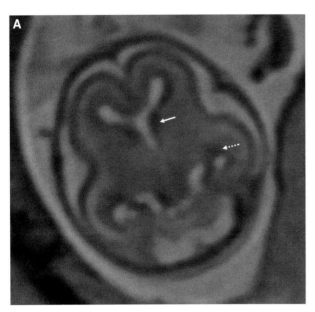 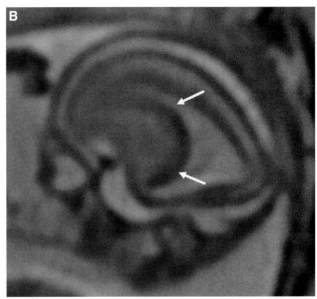

FIGURE 9.20: Fetus at 18 weeks' gestation. **A:** Coronal image demonstrating thick germinal matrix with prominent ganglionic eminences medial/lateral (*solid short arrow*) and caudal (*dotted arrow*) **B:** On sagittal oblique T2 imaging, the germinal matrix has a "C" configuration (*arrows*).

temporal/occipital horn, appearing fused on sagittal imaging, as a "C" configuration (Fig. 9.20). The GE is extremely prominent and should not be confused with hemorrhage (which also appears dark on T2 in the germinal matrix). The germinal matrix should be smooth without nodularity. The cortex of the brain is thin due to incomplete neuronal substrate.

20 to 30 Weeks: From 20 to 28 weeks, a **five-layer pattern** is observed (Fig. 9.17).[60,61,63–67] The pattern on T2 imaging appears similar to a tiramisu, being dark, white, hazy dark, white and dark from deep to superficial (Fig. 9.21). With the growth of the brain, the SVZ compartments are evident with the inner (iSVZ) containing the GEs inseparable from the VZ, a middle PVRZ where fibers of the corpus callosum are growing and the cellular outer (oSVZ) merging and inseparable from the IZ.[54] The oSVZ is marginated by the external capsule, and the IZ contains tangentially oriented thalamo-cortical fibers. The hazy dark T2 signal of the oSVZ and IZ during this time is likely due to proliferation and migration of bRG cells in the oSVZ as well as migrating neurons and glial cells into the IZ.[67] The SP is extremely prominent due to large extracellular hydophilic matrix and migration of neurons, awaiting organization.

Five-Layer Pattern (Central to Peripheral)
VZ/iSVZ/GE: Dark T2, *bright T1, high diffusion, low ADC*
PVRZ: Bright T2, *dark T1, low diffusion, high ADC* (diffusion can be difficult to separate due to small size)[59]
oSVZ/IZ: Hazy dark T2, *mildly bright T1, slightly high diffusion, low ADC*
SP: Bright T2, *dark T1, low diffusion, high ADC*
CP: Dark T2, *bright T1, high diffusion, low ADC*

Although the five-layer pattern is present throughout this time, changes in the individual layers can be noted which reflect migration and organization of neurons. The germinal matrix, especially the GE, will early appear very prominent, with the volume increasing exponentially up to 23 weeks, but then

one-half of the volume is lost from 26 to 28 weeks, thus causing diminution in signal and size.[68] The VZ and iSVZ have abundant radial fibers with high FA, but show inverse correlation with gestational age due to loss of proliferating radially oriented cells migrating to the cortex.[69,70] The oSVZ and IZ contains both radial and tangential fibers; therefore, the FA is lower than the germinal matrix near the ventricular wall (VZ and iSVZ). After 22 weeks, the neuronal and glial cells population diminishes in the oSVZ and IZ, and there is an increase in projecting fibers and acid mucopolysaccharide, resulting in higher T2 and lower T1 signal. The ADC values show a slow decline in the WM with increase in FA with gestation, which may reflect organization of the WM and axons.[71,72]

The SP thickness can be seen to vary in time, and when maximum in size, the SP takes over outer half of the cerebrum. The SP is also heterogeneous in distribution being thicker lateral frontal, temporal, and dorsal parietal (somatosensory areas) and thinner medial frontal and occipital lobes.[73,74] However, the posterior regions, including occipital pole, ventral occipitotemporal region, and planum temporale (heart of Wernicke area), have the greatest increases in SP thickness.[74] After 25 weeks' gestation, the hydrophilic extracellular matrix in the SP diminishes in conjunction with the thalamocortical fibers relocating to the cortex. As a result, the FA values in the SP are low but increase from 18 to 25 weeks.[57] At 25 weeks, there is blurring of layers with decreased discrimination of the IZ and SP, although diffusion imaging can discriminate by demonstrating tangentially oriented IZ fibers compared to the adjacent SVZ and SP.[72,75]

The cortex thickens with increasing gestational age due to increase in cell number and organization of the six cellular layers. The FA values are initially high, corresponding with radial organization of the cells, most dominant at 26 weeks.[69,75] However, the FA in the cortex is noted to decline to approximately 35 weeks, reflecting the less evident radial organization due elaboration of dendrites, formation of synapses, and proliferation and transition of glia to astrocytes.[70] The FA value declines later in areas of high association, such as the frontal cortex, and earlier in central somatosensory areas.[70]

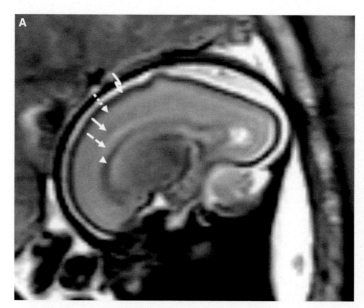
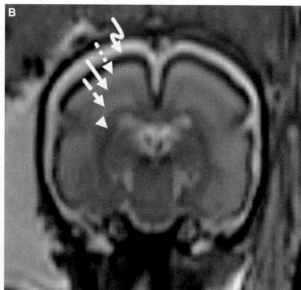

FIGURE 9.21: Fetus at 25 weeks' gestation on **(A)** sagittal and **(B)** coronal T2 imaging. The brain demonstrates a five-layer lamination with dark germinal matrix (*arrowhead*), thin high-signal periventricular-rich zone (*dashed arrows*), dark intermediate zone (*solid arrow*), thick high T2 signal subplate (*dotted arrow*), and cortex (*curved arrow*).

In the developing fetal WM, encompassing the PVRZ, IZ, and SP, there are six periventricular crossroads that represent areas of major intersecting developing fibers. These crossroads can be identified by 22 weeks and contain abundant hydrophilic extracellular matrix similar to the SP and are thus with decreased signal on T1 and hyperintense on T2 imaging. The six crossroads are located: *frontal* along lateral margin of the frontal horn and body of lateral ventricle, *frontal* along the dorsal aspect of the lateral ventricle, *frontal* inferolateral to the frontal horn and ventral to the putamen, *occipital* lateral to the atrium/occipital horn, *parietal* anterolateral to the atrium and centered over the retrolenticular internal capsule, and *temporal* anterolateral to the temporal horn.[54] The two main crossroads that are most evident on fetal imaging are the frontal, lateral to frontal horn, and parietal, posterior at the fountainhead of the anterior and posterior limbs of internal capsule, also known as Wetterwinkel (Fig. 9.22).[61]

At 28 weeks, the SVZ/VZs have decreased significantly in size, and the hydrophilic extracellular matrix in the SP and periventricular crossroads has diminished. With decline in migrating neurons in the IZ, there is blurring and loss of the multilayer pattern.[57,67] However, the multilayer pattern often persists longer in the frontal and anterior temporal lobes due to persistence of the SP.[43] As a result, the SP in the anterior temporal lobes can be noted at 30 to 32 weeks.[7]

30 to 40 Weeks: After 30 weeks, there is continued blurring and loss of the multilayer pattern. The germinal matrix completely surrounds the ventricular walls until 30 weeks' gestation.[59] At approximately 33 weeks, small rests of the GE persist caudothalamic and in the roof of the temporal horn and lateral wall of the occipital horn (Fig. 9.23). At 36 weeks, germinal matrix is increasing less evident with only small rests of cells at the caudate heads in the GE. However, small quantities of cells from the SVZ will persist late gestation and postnatal within the WM along the frontal horns, representing progenitors that will travel to the OB (Fig. 9.23A). Thus, the layered pattern is three in areas of residual germinal matrix and appears as two layered, white and cortical gray, in most areas of the fetal brain.[60] From 28 to 40 weeks, the WM, including corona radiata, increases in size. The development of the WM is associated with high ADC values that decline with increasing gestational age, except, to lesser extent, frontal WM.[76,77] These changes reflect WM maturation related to reduced water content and increase in lipid important

FIGURE 9.22: Periventricular crossroads. Axial T2 image of a fetus at 25 weeks showing periventricular crossroad lateral to the atrium (*long arrow*) and adjacent to the frontal horns (*short arrow*).

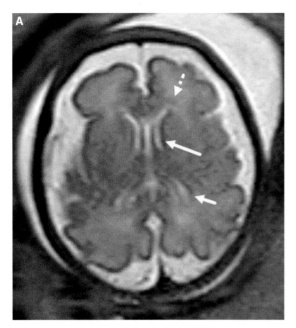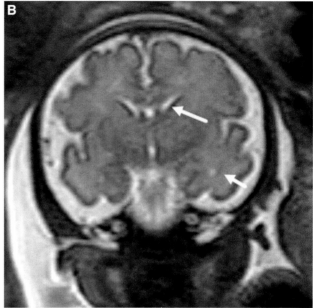

FIGURE 9.23: Fetus at 32 weeks. **A:** Axial T2 image demonstrating small germinal matrix at the caudothalamic groove (*long arrow*) and by the temporal horns (*short arrow*). Note small germinal matrix by frontal horns, which is olfactory in origin and will persist postnatal (*dotted arrow*). **B:** Coronal T2 denoting germinal matrix at the caudothalamic groove (*long arrow*) and by the temporal horns (*short arrow*).

for myelination. The cortex of the brain reaches maximum thickness, and gyration/sulcation is increasingly evident.

Deep Gray Nuclei

Embryology

As described earlier, the caudate, putamen, and globus pallidus arise from ventral telencephalon. The thalamus originates from the diencephalon, with contribution from the ventral telencephalon via cells arising from the GE and migrating to the thalamus through a transient structure known as the gangliothalamic body.

Magnetic Resonance Imaging

The deep gray nuclei are variable in signal depending on gestational age. Before 27 weeks, the pallidum demonstrates isointense signal on T1 and T2 imaging similar to the internal capsule and WM (Fig. 9.24A).[60] The thalamus is heterogeneous in MRI signal. Early in gestation, the dorsal aspect demonstrates signal similar to the WM, but the ventral portion is T2 hyperintense.[62] In my experience, thalamic T2 hyperintensity is noted typically before 22 to 24 weeks and may to be related to fiber interactions with the SP (Fig. 9.24B). After that time, the signal of the thalamus is homogeneously isointense with WM.

With further development, the pallidum and thalamus appear hyperintense on T1 and hypointense on T2 imaging from 26 to 28 weeks onward (Fig. 9.24C). The putamen and caudate are T1 hypointense and T2 hyperintense with regard to the internal capsule until 34 weeks. After that time, similar to the thalamus and pallidum, the two structures appear high on T1 and dark on T2 imaging (Fig. 9.24D).[60] With change in signal of the basal ganglia and thalamus, the internal capsule becomes an unmyelinated T1 hypointense and T2 hyperintense structure. Diffusion ADC values decrease and FA increases in the basal ganglia and thalamus, with advancing gestational age related to the increase in neuronal cell density, membrane proliferation, and fiber myelination.[52,57,71]

COMMISSURES/CORPUS CALLOSUM

Embryology

Commissures are bundles of WM connecting structures on both sides of the CNS (Fig. 9.25). The commissures develop in the area of the supratentorial brain in closest apposition to the anterior wall of the third ventricle or lamina terminalis. During the eighth week, in the upper/dorsal area of the lamina terminalis, active cellular proliferation results in a joining plate, also known as the lamina reuniens of His. There are three main commissures: the anterior (olfactory and inferior temporo-occipital cortex), hippocampal (hippocampal and posterior neocortex), and corpus callosum (hemispheric neocortex). The anterior commissure forms from the ventral lamina reuniens during weeks 8 to 10. The fornix and the hippocampal commissures arise in the dorsal lamina reuniens at 9 to 11 weeks.[15,16]

The development of the largest commissure, the corpus callosum, is initiated at 10 weeks in the interhemispheric midline, which is filled with primitive meninges. Deeping in the interhemispheric fissure results in a cleft, known as the sulcus medianus telencephali medii, which is in continuity with the upper lamina reuniens of His. The banks of this groove approximate and form the massa commissuralis. Glial and neuronal cells migrate medially from the SVZ to midline to form a glial sling/zipper at the corticoseptal boundary.[16] Axons of callosal neurons will extend through IZ and navigate a path along the medial ventricle to the glial sling cells, which express surface molecules and secrete chemicals that guide axons across midline. Two additional specialized glial structures also direct axons to the midline and glial sling. These include the indusium griseum glia (vestigial hippocampal cells left behind due to telencephalic flexure) anterior at corticoseptal boundary and the glial wedge along the dorsomedial aspect of the lateral ventricle. From 13 to 20 weeks, these glial cells will, with chemorepulsion and chemoatttractive factors, channel the axons toward the glial sling.

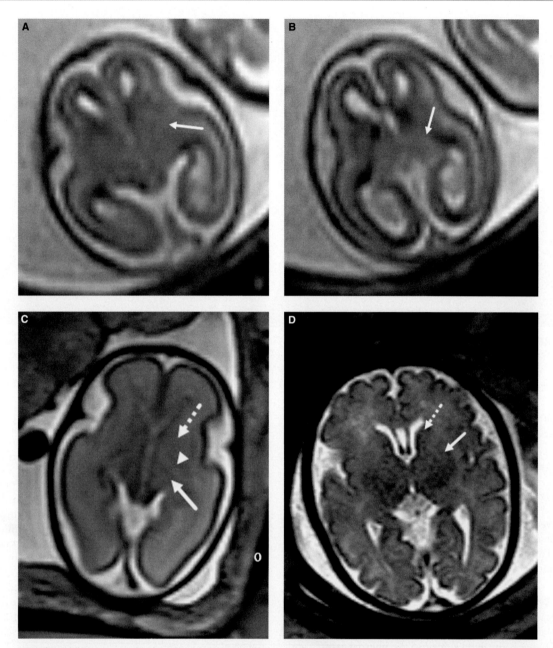

FIGURE 9.24: Deep gray nuclei. **A:** Axial T2 image of a fetus at 18 weeks demonstrating homogeneous signal in the basal ganglia and internal capsule (*arrow*). **B:** Axial T2 in the same fetus, with accentuated high T2 signal in the area of the superior thalami (*arrow*). **C:** Axial T2 image of a fetus at 26 weeks showing the thalamus (*solid arrow*) and pallidum (*dotted arrow*) being hypointense with regard to the internal capsule (*arrowheads*). **D:** Axial T2 image of a fetus at 35 weeks showing caudate (*dotted arrow*) and putamen (*solid arrow*) hypointense on T2 imaging, and there is definition of the T2 hyperintense internal capsule.

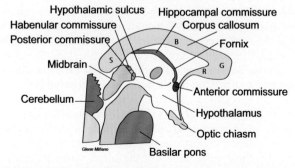

FIGURE 9.25: Diagram of the midline brain and commissures. The parts of the corpus callosum. *R*, rostrum; *G*, genu, *B*, body; *S*, splenium.

Beginning at 12 to 13 weeks, the axons will follow the sling to cross the midline. The first axons to cross arise from the area of the cingulate cortex, followed by neocortical areas.[16,78] At week 14, the corpus callosum is short and stretches from the anterior to hippocampal commissure, anatomically representing the anterior body of the corpus callosum.[79]

Thereafter, growth of the structure occurs by addition of fibers. Rather than growing from front to back, as previously described, the corpus callosum grows as two independent portions, with the anterior crossing by the glial sling and the posterior via the hippocampal commissure. The two then meet in the midline posterior body area. However, due to disproportionate growth of the frontal lobes, the hippocampus and splenium are shifted posterior above the dorsal third ventricle and the anterior aspect of the corpus callosum appears prominent.[79] As a result, the anterior sections of the corpus callosum are identified by 14 to 15 weeks and posterior at 18 to 19 weeks. At 20 weeks, the shape of the corpus callosum is complete but only 5% of its mature sagittal section.[16] Continued growth is noted throughout fetal and into postnatal life.

Magnetic Resonance Imaging

The corpus callosum is visualized as a hypointense structure of uniform thickness superior to the fornix on a sagittal T2 image.[61,63] Prior to 20 weeks, the corpus callosum is short in the midline and rather horizontal in shape (Fig. 9.26A). After 20 weeks, the structure shows a crescent shape and can be identified above the septum pellucidum (Fig. 9.26B). Its length grows through gestation,

and normal values are present in Table 21 of Appendix A1. The genu, body, and splenium should be apparent; however, the rostrum is difficult to define in greater than 50% of cases, and the flexion of the genu is frequently poorly identified in early gestation (Fig. 9.26B,C).[80] The structure is verified on coronal imaging as a crescent of tissue crossing above the walls of the lateral ventricles and the lower margin of the interhemispheric fissure (Fig. 9.26D). It is important to separate the corpus callosum from the fornix. The anterior commissure may not be well delineated until the third trimester. Crossing fibers of the corpus callosum demonstrate low ADC and high FA values, greater in the splenium than genu.[59,81] Diffusion tractography may also demonstrate the normal development of the corpus callosum, with accuracy values of 67% to 75% and a positive predictive value in identification of all four segments between 50% and 100%.[82]

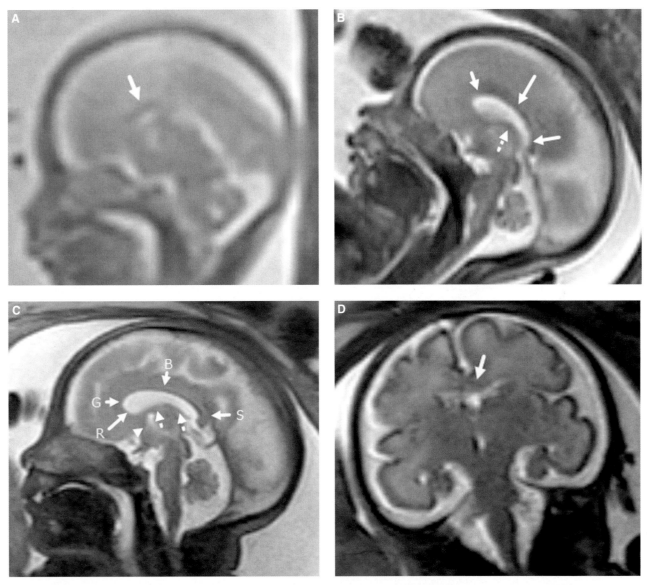

FIGURE 9.26: A: Sagittal T2 of a 16-week fetus. The corpus callosum is seen but short, horizontal, and incompletely formed (*arrow*). **B:** Sagittal T2 of a 24-week fetus. The corpus callosum is crescentic and fully formed (*arrows*). Note the rostrum is not well delineated. The fornix is identified inferior (*dotted arrow*). **C:** Sagittal T2 of a 30-week fetus. The corpus callosum is elongated and C shaped. All parts are clearly delineated with portions labeled: *R*, rostrum; *G*, genu; *B*, body; *S*, splenium. The dotted arrows represent fornix and arrowhead anterior commissure. **D:** Coronal T2 image of a 30-week fetus showing the crossing fibers of the corpus callosum (*arrows*).

TEMPORAL LOBE

Embryology

The hippocampus can be identified at 9 weeks, with a prominent VZ but relative lack of SVZ.[83] The parahippocampus gyrus, like the neocortex, contains both the VZ and the SVZ. Neurons in the hippocampus arise from the VZ and migrate along RG cells to form the cortex of the cornu ammonis in an inside-out manner, similar to the neocortex.[84] The dentate CP does not follow the inside-out pattern and develops in a protracted pattern into adulthood.[84] The marginal layer is increased in size in the hippocampus compared to other areas of the neocortex, with prominent hydrophilic extracellular matrix and large number of Cajal–Retzius cells, as it is the primary site of afferent synapse formation rather than the SP, which is significantly thinner.[67,84] Interneurons arise from the CGE and MGE. In the hippocampus, the pioneering fibers essential for neuron migration are the septo-hippocampal fibers.[84] WM tracts of the hippocampus merge and extend via fimbria to the hippocampal commissure/fornix. Limbic pathways, especially those to the cingulate cortex, develop early, being present at mid-fetal period.[51]

The hippocampal sulcus is one of the oldest sulci forming as a shallow structure around 10 weeks between the cornu ammonis containing pyramidal cells and the dentate gyrus, a granular cell layer.[85] The sulcus is initially wide and vertical, but at 12 to 16 weeks, the hippocampus sulcus is deep due to rotation toward the cornu ammonis caused by increasing thickness of the dentate gyrus.[85] The sulcus becomes progressively smaller and more horizontal with infolding of the dentate gyrus. By 18 to 21 weeks, the hippocampus demonstrates the typical C-shaped configuration with near-complete obliteration of the hippocampal sulcus.[85]

The amygdala is a nuclei, anterior to the hippocampus, which develops primarily from the GE of the SVZ. The ventrolateral portion of the amygdala is covered by VZ and SVZ and the dorsolateral by complex crossroad fibers. The amygdala complex fiber systems connect to the orbital and temporal cortex.[51]

Magnetic Resonance Imaging

The cortex of the hippocampus demonstrates T2 hypointensity. The marginal layer due to high hydrophilic extracellular matrix can be visualized as a band of T2 hyperintensity.[50] The SP is small and thus not well delineated.

The hippocampus is best depicted on coronal T2 imaging. As early as 18 weeks, the hippocampus appears as a slim "C"-shaped T2 hypointense structure along the medial temporal lobe (Fig. 9.27A).[63] Due to growth of the cortex, there is progressive infolding, which results in a horizontal oval hippocampal configuration and deepening of the hippocampal sulcus.[64] Closure of the hippocampal sulcus is variable in the fetus, being open in some up to 32 weeks.[86] The oval hippocampal configuration can be seen as early as 21 weeks but not typically until after 27 weeks (Fig. 9.27B).

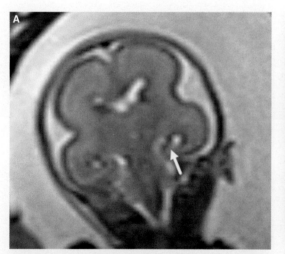

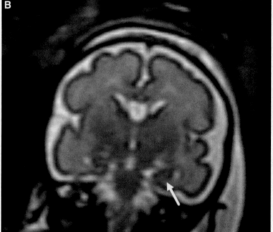

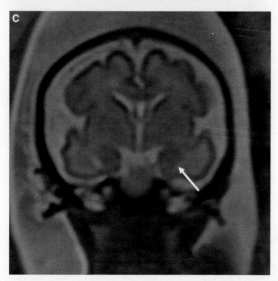

FIGURE 9.27: A: Coronal T2 of a 22-week fetus with open hippocampal fissures and dark C-shaped hippocampi, denoted on the left with *arrow*. **B:** Coronal T2 of a 30-week fetus with horizontal oval hippocampi, denoted on the left with *arrow*. Hippocampal fissure is closed. **C:** Coronal T2 of a 30-week fetus demonstrating dark T2 amygdala (*left denoted with arrow*).

A nonoval or incompletely inverted/rotated hippocampus, particularly on the left, can be observed in 33% of fetal cases as described postnatal.[86] Hippocampal development, including the sulcus and inverted formation, develops faster on the right than on the left. The collateral sulcus also develops earlier on the right and may be horizontal or vertical, especially when the hippocampus is nonoval.[86]

The amygdala is a cellular but inhomogeneous nucleus showing primarily T2 hyperintensity, located anterior to the temporal horn on coronal imaging and anterior to the hippocampus on axial plane (Fig. 9.27C).[61] The amygdala signal is stable throughout gestation.

SULCATION

Embryology

The folding process of the CP is extremely important as it provides a vast expansion of surface area for the cortex. The exact mechanism by which sulcation occurs is still poorly understood with hypothesis including differential CP growth, axon–axon connections creating tension, and genetic guidance. Current investigation suggests that the SP may facilitate sulci and gyri formation by axonal guidance.[87] This theory may be further supported in that the SP development occurs at the time when the CP begins to acquire sulci and gyri and that dissolution of the SP is first noted in regions underlying sulci but persisting longer below tips of the gyri.[87]

The fountain head for expansion of the cerebral cortex is the primordium of the insula.[30] Early in gestation, the Sylvian fissure is wide with obtuse angle and appears as a shallow fossa. Over time, the fissure becomes deeper and longer. Around 19 weeks, the circular sulcus, which grows into circular shape, appears on the superior aspect of the Sylvian fissure. As the frontal lobe grows, the circular sulcus will lose its shape and join the Sylvian as a single deep fissure.[9] With accelerated growth of the frontal and parietal lobes in an anterior-to-posterior direction, the Sylvian fissure will change from an open and shallow to deep, narrow, and horizontal configuration. The operculum is the stage in which the two lips have yet to come together. As the Sylvian fossa expands, from 15 to 23 weeks, the frontal, parietal, and temporal lobes develop opercular (perisylvian) cortex adjacent. The frontal and temporal lips come together at 37 to 38 weeks to create the Sylvian fissure.[88]

In general, fissures and sulci are not alternative terms. Fissures generally form earlier due to external forces on the brain, whereas sulci result predominately from internal forces such as increased neurons and glial cells. Primary supratentorial fissures include interhemispheric, choroidal, hippocampal, Sylvian, and calcarine.[88] The primary sulci are the superior and inferior frontal and temporal sulci that divide the region into superior, middle, and inferior gyri. Somatosensory area includes central, precentral, and postcentral sulcus. The intraparietal sulcus separates superior from inferior parietal lobules. Medially, the callosal and cingulate including marginal, subparietal, and parieto-occipital sulci are present, and inferiorly, the brain is separated laterally by occipitotemporal and medially by collateral sulcus.

The appearance of the primary sulci is from 16 to 29 weeks, but the majority coincides with ingrowth of the thalamocortical axons to the CP at 25 weeks.[51,87] The secondary gyri are noted at the time of development of corticocortical connections around 32 weeks.[65] The tertiary sulci begin to appear around 36 weeks.[87] The primary sulci are constant between individuals, whereas the secondary sulci show some differences and the tertiary higher variability in shape and position.[9] Cortical sulcation is asymmetric with differences between the right and left hemisphere noted, particularly with earlier development of sulci along the right perisylvian region.[9]

Magnetic Resonance Imaging

Cortical sulcation is one of the most accurate ways to date a pregnancy on fetal MRI as it follows a predictable pattern, delayed by an average of 1 to 2 weeks behind the neuropathological correlative.[9,89,90] A larger lag of 2 to 3 weeks has been described in twin gestations though in my experience not common unless there is growth restriction.[89] Cortical gyration, however, can be dated close to the neuropathological model when utilizing motion corrected 3D reconstruction with quantitative analysis.[91]

When imaging a fetus, it is important to remember that there can be a delay of 2 weeks from the time the sulcus is identified on MRI to when it is present in 75% of fetuses.[9] Cortical sulcation on MRI has also been noted to be asymmetric, with the right sulci including the frontoparietal operculum and superior temporal gyrus appearing prior to that on the left.[9,91,93]

On imaging, primary sulci develop first as a shallow depression. With time, the sulcus becomes deeper and the adjacent surface more angular, resulting in a V-shaped configuration. As the sulcus deepens and narrows, the gyrus transforms from a round to square configuration.[94] The primary sulcus with maturation develops branches, which become secondary sulci. The secondary sulci will also branch creating tertiary sulci.[94]

Cortical gyration occurs late in fetal life. In the first half, less than 20 weeks, the brain is smooth and lissencephalic in appearance. In the second half of pregnancy, the brain develops sulci and becomes complex in appearance. The appearance of the fetal brain, therefore, provides important information with regard to gestational age and can be utilized as a timeline for normal fetal development, with sulci identified in 75% of fetuses at ages described below and listed in Table 9.4.[89,92] The SSFSE T2 images are very sensitive to detection of the fissures. SSFP is excellent, given separation of the CSF from the

TABLE 9.4	Fetal Sulcation in Weeks
GESTATIONAL AGE	**NEW SULCI (DETECTED IN 75% OF FETUSES)**
14–15	Interhemispheric
16	Sylvian
22–23	Callosal Parieto-occipital Hippocampal
24–25	Calcarine Cingular
26	Central Collateral
27	Precentral Superior temporal Marginal
28	Postcentral Intraparietal
29	Superior frontal Inferior frontal
33–34	Inferior temporal Occipitotemporal

adjacent cortical indentation. Motion correction, 3D reformation, tissue segmentation, and quantitation folding measures are additional techniques that may improve cortical folding assessment.[91,95]

14 to 15 Weeks: Pathologically, the first fissure to develop is the **interhemispheric fissure**, which appears at 8 weeks, forming anteriorly and extending posterior by 10 weeks and can be identified as early as 14 to 15 weeks' gestation. The fetal brain is absent of other sulci, smooth in configuration (Fig. 9.28A).

16 Weeks: The first sulcus to become evident is the **Sylvian fissure**, visualized as a shallow infolding along the surface of the brain (Fig. 9.28B).

17 to 21 Weeks: Only the interhemispheric and Sylvian fissures are identified, although the Sylvian fissures increase in depth with increase in gestational age (Fig. 9.28C).

22 to 23 Weeks: The **callosal, parieto-occipital,** and **hippocampal fissures** can be identified. The callosal and hippocampal

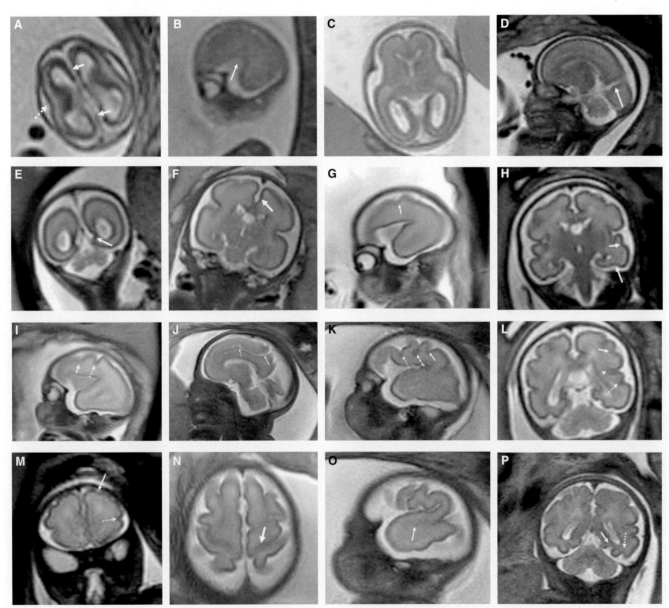

FIGURE 9.28: Multiple SSFSE T2 images of fetal sulcation. **A:** Axial: A 17-week fetus with interhemispheric (*solid arrows*) and shallow Sylvian fissure (*dotted arrow*). **B:** Sagittal image of a fetus at 18 weeks with shallow Sylvian fissure (*arrow*). **C:** Axial image of a fetus at 21 weeks with deeper Sylvian fissure, but the brain is otherwise smooth. **D:** Sagittal: Parieto-occipital fissure (*arrow*) in a 24-week fetus. **E:** Coronal: Calcarine (*arrow*) in a 24-week fetus. **F:** Coronal: Cingulate fissure (*arrow*) in a 25-week fetus. Notice continued narrowing of the Sylvian fissures. **G:** Sagittal: Central sulcus (*arrow*) in a 26-week fetus. **H:** Coronal: Collateral sulcus (*long arrow*) and superior temporal sulcus (*short arrow*) in a 27-week fetus. Notice asymmetry in development with collateral and superior temporal sulcus deeper on the right than on the left. **I:** Sagittal: Precentral (*solid arrow*) sulcus at 27 weeks. Note deeper central sulcus (*dotted arrow*). **J:** Sagittal image of the marginal (*solid arrows*) extending from the cingulate sulcus (*dotted arrow*). **K:** Sagittal: postcentral (*solid arrow*) is shallow in a 28-week fetus. Note deep central (*dashed arrow*) and moderately undulated precentral sulcus (*dotted arrow*). **L:** Coronal: Intraparietal sulcus (*solid arrow*) is present at 28 weeks. Also note deep posterior Sylvian (*arrowhead*) and superior temporal (*dotted arrow*). **M:** Coronal: Superior (*solid arrows*) and inferior frontal sulcus (*dotted arrow*) at 29 weeks. **N:** Axial image demonstrating medial extension of the central sulcus (*solid arrow*). **O:** Sagittal: Deep cortical indentation of the superior temporal sulcus (*arrow*) in a 30-week fetus. **P:** Coronal: Occipitotemporal sulcus (*dotted arrows*) and posterior collateral sulcus (*solid arrow*).

fissures are best depicted on coronal imaging (Fig. 9.27A). In general, the callosal fissure is more difficult to visualize. The parieto-occipital is defined on sagittal plane (Fig. 9.28D). The Sylvian fissure has become angular in configuration with increased formation of the posterior operculum (Fig. 9.27A).

24 to 25 Weeks: The **calcarine fissure** (Fig. 9.28E) and **cingulate sulcus** (Fig. 9.28F) are evident, both best depicted on coronal plane.

26 Weeks: The **central sulcus** (Fig. 9.28G) is identified as a shallow indentation along the lateral aspect of the brain. This sulcus is best depicted on sagittal and axial imaging. The **collateral sulcus** (Fig. 9.28H) is noted, on a coronal sequence, along the inferior temporal lobe.

27 Weeks: The posterior portion of the **superior temporal sulcus** (Fig. 9.28H) is noted, best depicted on a sagittal or coronal imaging. The **precentral sulcus** (Fig. 9.28I) is seen as a shallow indentation on the lateral aspect of the cerebral hemisphere ventral to the central sulcus. The **marginal sulcus** (Fig. 9.28J) is also best identified on a sagittal imaging, representing posterior extension of the cingulate sulcus.

28 Weeks: The **postcentral sulcus** (Fig. 9.28K) is now identified dorsal to the central sulcus as a lateral indentation along the lateral cerebral hemisphere, best appreciated on axial and sagittal imaging. The **intraparietal sulcus**, located on the lateral surface of the brain, runs perpendicular and dorsal to the postcentral sulcus and is best depicted on a coronal or sagittal imaging (Fig. 9.28L).

29 Weeks: The **superior** and **inferior frontal sulci** (Fig. 9.28M) are identified, best depicted on a coronal imaging.

30 to 32 Weeks: The central sulcus has extended medially such that it abuts the interhemispheric fissure (Fig. 9.28N). The anterior portion of the superior temporal sulcus is now present (Fig. 9.28O). There is continued evolution of primary sulcation with development of multiple secondary gyri.

33 to 34 Weeks: The **inferior temporal sulcus** and the **occipitotemporal sulcus,** medial to the inferior temporal and lateral to the collateral sulcus, are now identified (Fig. 9.28P). At 34 weeks, all primary and most of the secondary gyri are present.

35 to 40 Weeks: Fetal brain demonstrates appearance similar to term infant. The sulci continue to deepen, and gyri become square in configuration. Tertiary sulci are evident.

If sulcation is abnormal, follow-up imaging in 4 to 6 weeks should be considered to reassess development. As gyration progresses later in gestation, performing MRI in the fetus beyond 25 to 28 weeks typically provides further information with regard to cortical development.

PITUITARY AND OLFACTORY BULBS

Embryology

During ventral induction from 5 to 6 weeks postconception, there is development of the optic vesicles, pituitary gland and stalk, and olfactory bulbs (OBs).

The optic chiasm develops from the rostral wall of the diencephalon, and optic sulci arise as invaginations on inner surface of the diencephalon.[8] The optic sulci will transform into optic vesicles, and with constriction at attachment to forebrain, the optic stalk or optic nerve arises.

The pituitary is derived from two areas. The adenohypophysis is formed from an ectodermal outpouching of the oral cavity, known as Rathke pouch. At 3 weeks, Rathke pouch appears as an evagination of the stomodeum and grows through a patent canal connecting the sella turcica and pharynx, known as the craniopharyngeal canal. By the end of the second month, the tissue loses connection with the oral cavity, the canal obliterates, and cells proliferate to form the adenohypophysis. The neurohypophysis is derived from neural ectoderm as a downward extension of the diencephalon, resulting in the infundibular process. The infundibulum gives rise to the stalk and later the posterior lobe of the pituitary.[8]

OB development is primarily through stimulation of olfactory sensory afferents that arise in the epithelium of the nasal cavity. These axons pass through the cribriform plate to the rostral forebrain and form a superficial layer that induces neurogenesis. The primordial bulbs are present at 4.5 weeks as a ventro-rostrol overgrowth of neuroepithelium of the primitive telencephalon. As the bulbs form, neurons from the LGE SVZ migrate into each bulb along the RMS.[96] The olfactory lamination is six layered, similar to other cortex; however, it is the only sensory system that does not project to the thalamus.[96] The olfactory sulcus is a horizontal structure separating the medial rectus gyrus and lateral orbital gyrus, being present at 16 weeks initially as shallow open indentations.[9] The sulci will increases in depth from a posterior to anterior direction.[9]

The areas of residual GE tissue from the SVZ adjacent to the frontal horns represent RMS. This specialized migratory route, along which neuronal precursors, continue to travel to reach the olfactory cortex, tract, and bulb, and will be present postnatal, representing a source of postnatal neurogenesis.[96]

Magnetic Resonance Imaging

The normal expansion of the subarachnoid space in the frontal and suprasellar area allows for reliable visualization of the optic chiasm, pituitary, and OBs.

Optic Chiasm/Nerves

The optic chiasm can be seen in 89% of fetal cases, increasing in detection with increase in gestational age.[97] Early in gestation, it is often difficult to separate the chiasm from the floor of the third ventricle/hypothalamic tissue (Fig. 9.29A). All three planes of T2 imaging can be utilized for optic chiasm anatomy (Fig. 9.29B–D). Optic nerve diameters increase with gestational age.[98]

Pituitary Gland and Stalk

The pituitary stalk, a thin T2 and T1 isointense structure, is well delineated on fetal MRI, best detected on sagittal and coronal planes (Fig. 9.29A–D).[97] An increase in detection is noted with gestational age, with sensitivity at 72% below 25 weeks and 100% beyond 26 weeks.[99] The pituitary gland on T2 imaging demonstrates homogeneous dark signal (Fig. 9.29B). On T1 images, the gland can be detected in 60% of fetuses and is noted to increase in diameter (2 to 6 mm) with increasing gestational age.[97] The gland demonstrates increased T1 signal such that the anterior and posterior lobes cannot be separated, similar in appearance to the neonate pituitary (Fig. 9.29E).[100] The posterior lobe is normal high T1 signal due to neurosecretory granules and phospholipids; however, the anterior lobe is believed to demonstrate high T1 signal due to higher hormonal synthetic activity and less free water molecules.[100] Postsphenoid ossification, noted as T1 hyperintensity inferior to the sella, can be demonstrated, increasing in size with gestational age.[101]

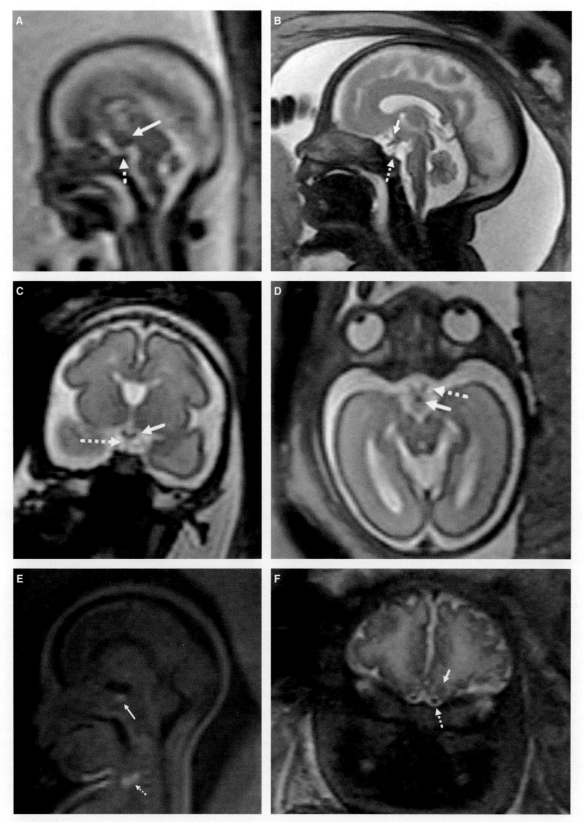

FIGURE 9.29: Optic chiasm, nerve, pituitary, and olfactory. **A:** Sagittal SSFSE T2 of a 17-week fetus. It is difficult to separate the optic chiasm (*solid arrow*) from hypothalamic tissue. The infundibulum is well delineated (*dotted arrow*). **B:** Sagittal T2 in a fetus at 30 weeks showing optic chiasm (*solid arrow*), infundibulum and dark pituitary (*dotted arrow*). **C:** Coronal T2 in a fetus at 29 weeks demonstrating optic chiasm (*solid arrow*) and infundibulum (*dotted arrow*). **D:** Axial T2 image demonstrating the left prechiasmatic optic nerve (*dotted arrow*) and infundibulum at the median eminence (*solid arrow*). **E:** Sagittal T1 image in a fetus at 24 weeks showing homogeneous hyperintense pituitary gland (*solid arrow*). Note hyperintense T1 signal in the thyroid gland (*dotted arrow*). **F:** Coronal SSFSE in a fetus at 34 weeks showing left olfactory sulci (*solid arrow*) and olfactory bulb (*dotted arrow*).

Olfactory System

Coronal T2 imaging provides best visualization of the OBs as punctate structures with lower T2 signal intensity ventral to the frontal lobes (Fig. 9.29F).[97,102] The sensitivity in detection of the OBs increases with gestational age to approximately 35 weeks, being approximately 85% to 90% between 30 and 34 weeks. After 35 weeks, the detection falls to 66%, likely due to decrease in frontal subarachnoid space.[102]

The olfactory sulci are also best delineated on coronal T2 imaging and can be detected in 47% of fetuses prior to 30 weeks and 90% to 100% of fetuses thereafter (Fig. 9.29F).[102] Prior to 31 weeks, the sulci appear open and shallow. From 32 weeks, the sulci become progressively deeper, visualized on more anterior slices with increasing gestational age.[102]

The cells that travel the RMS can be defined from 24 weeks to postnatal as medial caps of low T2 and high T1 signal and lateral high T2 and low T1 signal adjacent to the frontal horns of the lateral ventricles (Fig. 9.23A).[103]

INFRATENTORIAL

The infratentorial brain is derived from the mesencephalon and the rhombencephalon. The rhombencephalon is further divided into the metencephalon, future pons and cerebellum, and myelencephalon, which will become the medulla oblongata. The mesencephalon gives rise to the midbrain, and at the midbrain–hindbrain boundary, there is an area known as the isthmic organizer that influences the development of the cerebellar hemispheres, vermis, and pons.[104] The cerebellar hemispheres are derived primarily from the metencephalon, while the vermis is derived at least partly from the mesencephalon.[105]

Cerebellum Parenchyma

Embryology

Neuronal Migration: The cerebellum plays a central role in coordination of motion and control of balance and is also important in learning and higher cognitive functions. The flocculonodular or vestibulocerebellum participates primarily in balance and spatial orientation via vestibular nuclei. The vermis or spinocerebellum (paleocerebellum) mainly functions to fine-tune body and limb movements via input from the dorsal column of the spinal cord and trigeminal nerve. The cerebellar hemispheres or cerebrocerebellum (neocerebellum) receive input from cerebral cortex via pontine nuclei and send output to the red nucleus and premotor and primary motor area via the ventral lateral thalamus.

The cerebellar system includes the precerebellar nuclei afferent pathway, centrally placed deep cerebellar nuclei (DCN), efferent cerebellar pathway, and the cerebellar cortex. The cerebellar cortex has five different cellular populations in a three-layered laminar pattern encompassing from deep to superficial, the granule cell layer (GCL), Purkinje cell layer (PCL), and molecular layer (ML). The dominant neurons are the Purkinje cells (PCs) and granule cells (GCs). The PC is the heart of the cerebellar circuit and represents the efferent neurons with projections to the DCN. Although the cell body is primarily present in the PCL, the dendrite arborization spreads out into the ML. The stellate and basket interneurons in the ML modulate the activity of the PC. The GCs are small, numerous, and spherical but have axons that extend to the ML and bifurcate in a T shape to communicate via parallel fibers with Purkinje dendrites. The precerebellar nuclei, present within brainstem, interact with two afferent axons known as the mossy and climbing fibers. The mossy fibers rise from multiple precerebellar nuclei and innervate dendrites of GC, which then connect via parallel fibers to the PC and finally DCN. For example, in the cerebellar hemispheres, the mossy fibers extending from pontine nuclei, which have received afferent input from the cerebrum, relay to the GC and then PC, which communicate with the dentate nuclei that connect to the thalamus and cerebral cortex, important for higher cognitive and emotional functions. The climbing fibers arise from the inferior olivary nucleus and project directly to PC dendrites. PCs gather the information and send information via axons to the DCN and vestibular nuclei, necessary for control of balance.

The cerebellum is one of the first structures in the brain to develop but one of the last to mature, with cellular organization continuing for many months after birth in a transient layer known as the external granular layer (EGL). The cerebellum develops from two germinal matrix locations: a VZ and the rhombic lips (RLs) (Fig. 9.30). The VZ is in the roof of the fourth ventricle and provides inhibitory neurons or GABAergic neurons that migrate radial with the help of glial cells, giving rise to DCN, PCs, Golgi cells,

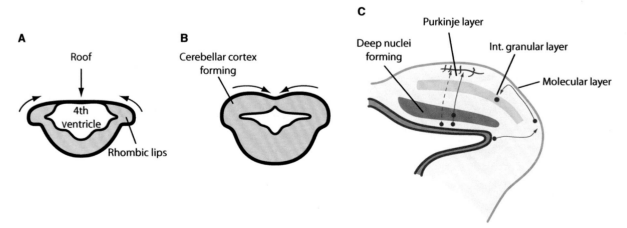

FIGURE 9.30: A: The germinal matrix of the cerebellum includes the roof of the fourth ventricle and rhombic lips. **B:** With continued growth, the hemispheres form first. **C:** Image demonstrating the migration of cells with development of final cell layers, including deep nuclei, internal granular, Purkinje cells, and molecular cells.

stellate cells, and basket cells. In addition, oligodendrocytes and glial cells, including specialized Bergmann glia, arise from the VZ. The RLs are dorsolaterally located in the metencephalon between the roof plate and neuroepithelium at the caudal aspect of the fourth ventricle and give rise to glutamatergic or excitatory neurons that migrate tangential and provide precursor for large neurons of DCN, unipolar brush cells, GC, and precerebellar nuclei.[106]

The DCN relay all output from the cerebellar cortex to cortical and subcortical targets. There are three DCNs, the fastigial that receive from the vermis, the interposed (emboliform and globose) from paravermis, and large dentate from lateral cerebellar hemispheres. The first neurons born are the DCNs at approximately 5 weeks. Precursor neurons migrate tangential from the upper RL, and interneurons migrate radial from the VZ to form the DCN with the dentate nuclei present at approximately 7 to 8 weeks. Mesencephalic neural crest cells are also a source of neurons for the DCN.[106]

The VZ will give rise to the PC beginning at 7 weeks postconception.[106,107] The PCs predominately migrate along RG cells to form a multicellular thick cluster.[106] The full number of PCs is present early, but cells will arrange into a single monolayer with expansion of the vermis and hemispheres in conjunction with extensive dendritic arborization and synaptogenesis from 16 to 28 weeks.[106] Bergman glia cells are essential for forming the PC monolayer and assisting dendrite growth to the EGL and synapse formation. Till after birth, the Purkinje neurons will mature, projecting their axons to the DCN.

From late embryonic to postnatal, interneurons will migrate from the VZ to the cerebellar parenchyma in an inside-out sequence to give rise to neurons in the DCN, GCL (Golgi and Lugaro cells), and, finally, ML (stellate and basket cells). These progenitors continue to divide while migrating through the WM to their final destination in the nuclei or cortex. Stellate and basket cells will reside first in the EGL and then migrate tangentially to their final position in the ML where they become postmitotic postnatal.[106,108] At the end of the embryonic period, the upper RL will give rise to unipolar brush cells, which interact with GC to amplify vestibular

inputs to the cerebellum. The unipolar brush cells migrate tangential but, similar to VZ neurons, will colonize the cerebellar WM before transitioning to their final location in the GL.[106] The lower RL gives rise to the precerebellar nuclei, including the pontine and inferior olivary nuclei, which will migrate primarily tangential but over complex pathways.[108] The pontine nuclei migrate later than other precerebellar nuclei, at 12.5 weeks with earlier born neurons situated in the dorsal and later ventral pons.[108]

Neuronal Organization/Differentiation: At approximately 11 to 13 weeks, the upper portion of the RL will give rise to GC precursors, which will migrate tangentially through a subpial stream pathway to the superficial aspect of the cerebellum forming the EGL, a distinct layer present between 10 weeks and 2 months postnatal.[106] The outer EGL will become a germinative zone along the pial surface, with proliferative activity generating large number of GC. Granule neuron precursors migrate from the outer EGL to the inner area where they become postmitotic. The EGL cells will then migrate radial along Bergmann glia cells to the definitive internal GL beginning at 16 weeks. A transient layer known as the lamina dissecans is visible superficial to the GCL and deep to the PCL from 20 to 32 weeks.[109] This layer acts as a transient zone for proliferating and migrating cells and disappears first from the vermis and last cerebellar hemispheres. The EGL will disappear 1.5 years after birth, leaving a three-layered cerebellar cortex.[106] While the rate of differentiation of neuronal groups in the vermis precedes the hemispheres, the overall bulk growth of the vermis lags behind that of the hemispheres by approximately 12 weeks.[109] Cortical organization occurs in all areas, resulting in development of dendrites and synapsis to form a functioning neuron.[108]

With the appearance of the pontine flexure at approximately the fifth gestational weeks, the cerebellum arises due to bending of the fourth ventricle (Fig. 9.4). As this occurs between 28th and 32nd postconception days, tissue develops in the form of an inverted V, resulting in a thin roof and dorsal alar plate that represents the cerebellar primordium (tuberculum cerebelli [TC]) (Fig. 9.31).[105,109] At 6 weeks postconception, the TC first grows

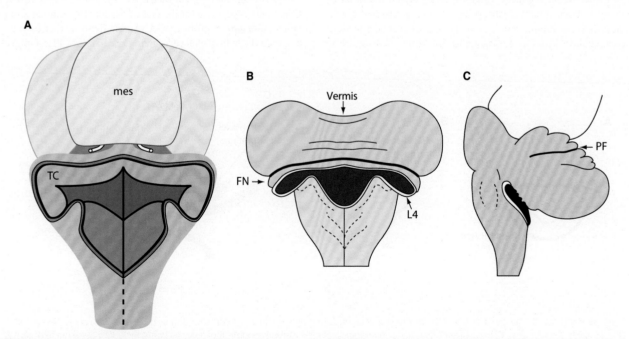

FIGURE 9.31: A: Below the mesencephalon (mes) is the tuberculum cerebelli (TC), which is an inverted V-shaped tissue that develops into the cerebellum. **B:** The hemispheres and flocculonodular lobe (FN) develop first, followed by the vermis. L4 is lateral recess of fourth ventricle. **C:** First fissure on the vermis is the primary fissure (PF).

laterally and caudally, giving rise to an inner cerebellar bulge that will represent the hemispheres. An external bulge will develop in the seventh week, which will represent the flocculi delineated by the posterolateral fissures. This fissure is the first fissure to appear and separates the cerebellum from the flocculonodular lobe.[110] The midline component then accelerates, resulting in formation of the vermis at 9 weeks (Fig. 9.31).[111] Fissures then begin to form transversely across the cerebellum, first on the vermis and then laterally into the hemispheres. The second fissure to develop, the primary fissure, divides the cerebellar vermis and hemispheres into anterior and posterior lobes and is present by 11 to 12 weeks.[107,110,111] The primary fissure is first identified midline, penetrating deeply into the vermis and extending laterally onto the medial cerebellar hemispheres where it will remain as a shallow fissure. The vermis and cerebellar hemispheres share the same fissures; however, the horizontal fissure is the deepest fissure within the hemispheres. Main fissures and nine vermian subdivisions are present at approximately 14 weeks (Fig. 9.32).[107] The foliated appearance of the hemispheres is detected by 30 weeks' gestation.[112] Inferior and middle cerebellar peduncles are noted at 13 weeks.[113]

Magnetic Resonance Imaging
The cerebellum changes signal, architecture, and sulcation depending on gestational age.

16 to 20 Weeks: The cerebellum and vermis are small and demonstrates **homogeneous intermediate T2 signal** (Fig. 9.33A).[114] The germinal matrix, likely due to size and technique limitation, is not delineated.

Initially, the cerebellar hemispheres and vermis are thin but will enlarge, with growth first noted in the hemispheres dorsolaterally and then later caudolaterally. The fourth ventricle is large and in continuity with the cisterna magna (Fig. 9.33B). As the vermis grows exophytically from the roof of the rhombencephalic vesicle, the ventricle will decrease in size. The vermis should cover the developing fourth ventricle accentuating the posterior recess known as the fastigial point as early as 18 to 20 weeks.[21,107] At this time, the craniocaudal length of the vermis should be nearly equal to the cerebellar hemispheres.[115] The primary fissure can be recognized by 17.5 weeks (Fig. 9.33C).[21]

20 to 30 Weeks: A **three-layer pattern** in the cerebellum is identified with the development of the DCN, WM, and cerebellar cortex (Fig. 9.33D).[107,111] Cellular areas including the DCN and cerebellar cortex will demonstrate hyperintense T1 and hypointense T2 signal. The cerebellar WM is predominantly water and demonstrates T1 hypointense and T2 hyperintense. However, the middle cerebellar peduncles appear as low T2 signal between 23 to 26 weeks due to high cellularity.[61,112] In the cerebellar cortex, there is a lack of anisotropy due to different directions of migrating neurons.[61] Progressive decline in mean diffusivity is noted with increasing gestational age, reflecting neuron proliferation and organization.[76,77]

From deep to superficial, the layers include the following:

DCN: Dark T2, *bright T1*
Cerebellar WM: Bright T2, *dark T1*
Cerebellar cortex: Dark T2, *bright T1*

By 21 weeks, the tentorium has a definitive orientation perpendicular to the occipital bone with insertion at the level of the torcula.[112] The fissures of the cerebellum become increasingly evident (Table 9.5). By 27 weeks, all vermian foliation will be detected (Fig. 9.33E,F). The hemisphere foliation will follow a few weeks later appearing between 24 and 29 weeks (Fig. 9.33G).[107,115]

30 to 40 Weeks: Three-layer pattern persists, but gyration of the DCN results in signal changes such that the central core is T2 hyperintense and peripheral gyri hypointense (Fig. 9.33H).[61,112] By 30 to 33 weeks, prominent folia can be identified throughout the vermis, though the hemispheres surface remains relatively smooth.[22,112] The flocculonodular lobule is T2 hypointense at 30 to 31 weeks (Fig. 9.33I).[112] After 34 weeks, the lateral cerebellum becomes convoluted.

Growth and development of the cerebellum should be assessed by measurements as, between 19 and 37 weeks, the cerebellum grossly doubles in diameter.[111] The transverse cerebellar diameter should be obtained on either axial or coronal plane with greatest cerebellar diameter. The vermis should be measured craniocaudal and anterior posterior on midsagittal section as greatest

CEREBELLAR VERMIS FISSURES AND LOBULES

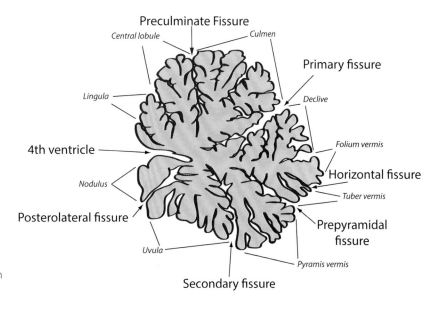

FIGURE 9.32: Fissures and lobules of the cerebellum with attention to vermis.

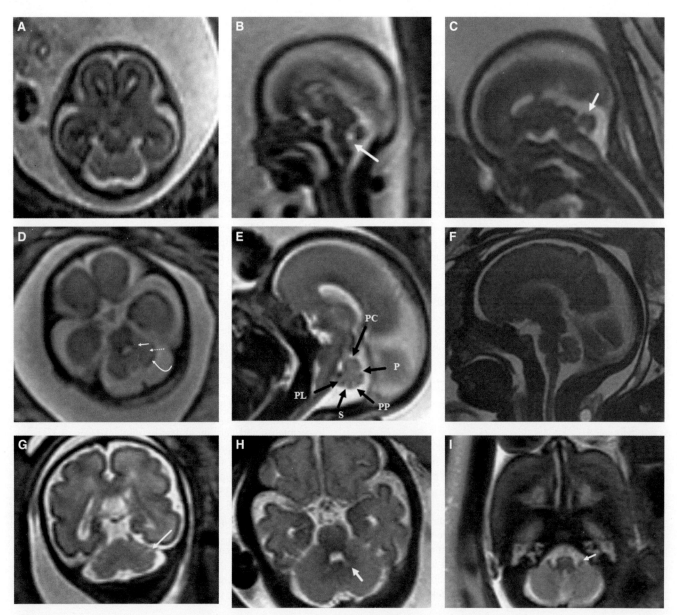

FIGURE 9.33: T2 images of cerebellum. **A:** Axial SSFSE of a fetus at 19 weeks with homogeneous cerebellum. **B:** Sagittal SSFSE of a fetus at 17 weeks with fastigial point and incomplete coverage of the fourth ventricle by vermis (*arrow*). **C:** Sagittal SSFP image showing vermis covers the fourth ventricle and primary fissure is seen (*arrow*) in a fetus at 19 weeks. **D:** Axial SSFSE showing cerebellum three-layer pattern in a fetus at 24 weeks. Cerebellar nuclei (DCN) (*solid arrow*), white matter (*dotted arrow*), and cortex (*curved arrow*). **E:** Sagittal SSFSE showing vermian fissures in a fetus at 25 weeks. *P*, primary; *PP*, prepyramidal; *S*, secondary, *PL*, posterolateral, *PC*, preculminate. **F:** Sagittal SSFP with all vermian foliation present in a fetus at 28 weeks. **G:** Coronal SSFSE showing prominent foliation of the cerebellar hemispheres in a fetus at 30 weeks. *Arrow* denotes deepest horizontal fissure. **H:** Axial SSFSE demonstrating central high T2 (*arrow*) and peripheral dark signal in the DCN in a fetus at 33 weeks. **I:** Axial SSFSE showing the flocculus lobes (*arrow*) in a fetus at 33 weeks.

height and distance from the fastigial point to posterior surface of the vermis (Table 21 in Appendix A1).[112]

The tegmento-vermian angle is an excellent way to follow normal vermian development. The angle is obtained by drawing a line along the dorsal surface of the brainstem parallel to the tegmentum and should transect at the obex. Second line is drawn along the ventral surface of the vermis. The normal fetal tegmento-vermian angle is close to 0 degrees, with average values of 2.5° ± 2.3° (Fig. 9.34).[115,116] A significantly elevated angle (>40 degrees) is associated with pathology. The superior fossa angle is also independent of gestational age and is measured

via angle created by lines from dorsum sella to great cerebral vein and great cerebral vein to torcula. Normal values averaged 100.9° ± 8°.[116]

Another helpful line is one drawn through the fastigial point and declive (lobule below primary fissure) (Fig. 9.35). The anterior and posterior lobes are defined, and normal ratios should be 47% above and 53% below or subjectively 1:2, respectively.[107,115] After 20 weeks, the vermis lags in growth compared to the hemispheres, so a normal height ratio of the vermis to hemisphere is on average 0.8 but should definitely be greater than 0.7.[117]

TABLE 9.5   Visualization of Fissures for the Cerebellar Vermis in Weeks

TIMING	FISSURE	LANDMARKS/ADJACENT LOBULES
17.5	Primary	Culmen and Declive
≤20	Posterolateral	Uvula and Nodulus
21	Prepyramidal	Tuber and Pyramis
21–22	Preculminate	Central and Culmen
24	Secondary/ Postpyramidal	Pyramis and Uvula
27	Horizontal	Folium and Tuber

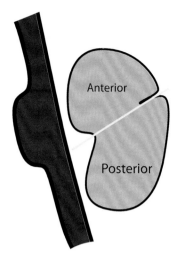

FIGURE 9.35: Fastigial and declive line (*yellow line*) to separate anterior and posterior lobes.

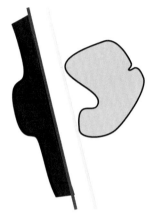

FIGURE 9.34: Tegmento-vermian angle should be close to 0 degrees. The tegmentum (*red line*) should be parallel to the line drawn along the ventral vermis (*yellow line*).

BRAINSTEM

Embryology

During the fourth week, a longitudinal groove called the sulcus limitans appears in the lateral wall of the neural tube dividing the structure into ventral and dorsal halves, which, with thickening, will give rise to basal (motor) and alar (sensory) plates. The myelencephalon, metencephalon, and mesencephalon are responsible for development of the brainstem, which arises from 6 to 7 postconception weeks and matures caudal to rostral, thus forming first the medulla, then pons, and finally midbrain.[61] Formation results from direct and indirect migration of cells from the periventricular germinal zones. The alar plate that fuses by 4 weeks extraventricular will give rise to the cerebellum and the basal to the tegmentum of the pons.

There is significant interval growth of the pons after 13 weeks' gestation with development of pontine nuclei.[118] The corticospinal tracts and crossing pontine tracts are also present at 13 weeks.[113] For the most part, direct migration results in cells destined to become motor and sensory brainstem nuclei.[119] The midbrain develops directly from the primary brain vesicle, with thickening of cells in the alar plate giving rise to tectum (inferior and superior colliculi). The cerebral peduncles form as a result of neuronal descent from the cerebral cortex.[118] Although the

cranial nerves originate early in the fourth week, their eventual positions change as a result of ingrowth of fiber tracts and migration of neurons from the RLs.[119] The olfactory arises from the telencephalon and optic from the diencephalon. The oculomotor nerve arises from the mesencephalon. The remaining cranial nerves are derived from rhombencephalon.[120] The pontine, cervical, and mesencephalic flexures disappear at 14 to 15 weeks, resulting in the straight configuration of the brainstem.[118] The brainstem does not mature before the seventh postnatal month.

Magnetic Resonance Imaging

The brainstem prior to myelination is **homogeneous T2 isointense,** except the tectum and solitary nucleus that are T2 hypointense due to high cellularity (Fig. 9.36).[107,114] The inferior colliculus is the relay station for auditory input and is T2 hypointense as early as 16 weeks but reliably by 20 weeks. The solitary nucleus/tract is located in the dorsal medulla and receives cardiovascular, visceral, respiratory, gustatory, and orotactile information and demonstrates decreased T2 signal as early as 18 weeks.[107] The brainstem appears high on diffusion and low signal on ADC maps.[59] Progressive

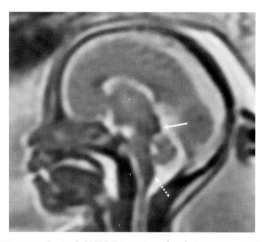

FIGURE 9.36: Sagittal SSFSE T2 image of a fetus at 21 weeks with homogeneous isointense brainstem, except dark signal in tectum/inferior colliculus (*solid arrow*) and medulla/solitary nucleus (*dotted arrow*). Note that the brainstem is straight, and the pons is rounded in contour.

decline in mean diffusivity is noted in the pons with increasing gestational age, reflecting neuron proliferation and organization.[76,77]

It is important to evaluate the configuration of the brainstem, which should be straight, and the contour of the pons, which should be rounded at every gestational age (Fig. 9.36). The brainstem grows significantly; therefore, pontine measurements in anterior to posterior and craniocaudal dimension (Table 21 in Appendix A1) are helpful to ensure normalcy.

MYELINATION

Embryology

Myelin is an organized multilamellar structure formed by the plasma membrane of the oligodendrocyte. The membrane surrounds neuronal axons and facilitates electric impulse conduction. The process of myelination includes proliferation and differentiation of oligodendrocytes, proliferation of astrocytes for neuronal support and connection, and increased lipid synthesis of oligodendrocytes. Myelin is rich in lipids and, to a lesser extent, proteins, and with its development, water content decreases. Myelination follows an organized pattern, progressing from caudal to cranial, central to peripheral, and occipital to frontal and then temporal. Areas important to sensory function show myelination prior to motor and projection fibers demonstrate myelination prior to associative fibers.

Magnetic Resonance Imaging

Myelination in axons results in high signal on T1 and low signal on T2, likely related to increase in cholesterol and glycolipid content but also due to increase in cellular density. Myelination begins at 12 to 13 weeks in the spinal cord, followed by the brainstem, and progresses cranially (Fig. 9.37).[97] Prior to 18 weeks, the brainstem is homogeneous in signal, with exception of low signal in the tectum.[107,114]

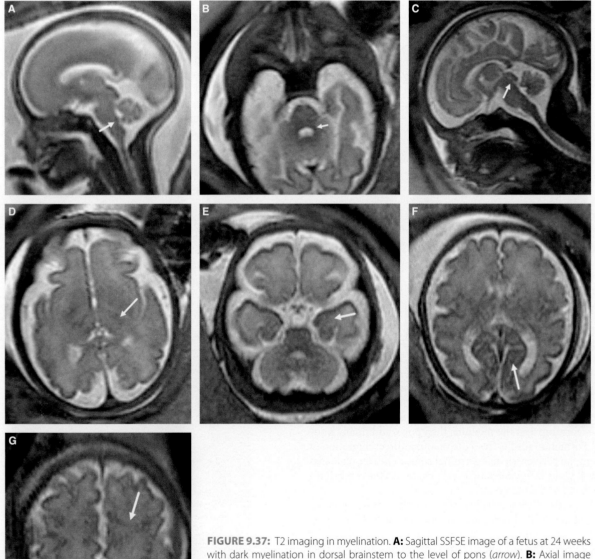

FIGURE 9.37: T2 imaging in myelination. **A:** Sagittal SSFSE image of a fetus at 24 weeks with dark myelination in dorsal brainstem to the level of pons (*arrow*). **B:** Axial image of a fetus at 29 weeks with dark myelinated superior cerebellar peduncles (*arrows*). **C:** Sagittal image of a fetus at 32 weeks with myelination now dorsal midbrain (*arrow*). Note myelination along the entire brainstem. **D:** Axial image of a fetus at 32 weeks with dark signal in posterior lateral thalami (*arrow*). **E:** Axial MRI showing early myelination medial temporal (*arrow*). **F:** Axial MRI showing early myelination medial occipital (*arrow*). **G:** Early myelination perirolandic (*arrow*).

Myelination progresses as noted below:

18 Weeks: Dorsal medulla in the ventral ascending sensory tracts and dorsal solitary nucleus tract[107]

20 Weeks: Posterior medial medulla and dorsal pons, in the area of the medial longitudinal fasciculus (MLF), medial and lateral lemniscus[59,114] (Fig. 9.37A)

28 to 29 Weeks: Inferior and superior cerebellar peduncles (Fig. 9.37B)[112]

32 Weeks: Dorsal midbrain (Fig. 9.37C)[96]

32 to 33 Weeks: Inferior colliculus, lateral putamen, and ventrolateral thalami (Fig. 9.37D).[114] Hyperintense T1 signal dot possible in the posterior limb of the internal capsule[5,59]

35 Weeks: T1 bright dot in the posterior limb of the internal capsule.[5,59] Optic tracts and areas of high metabolic activity in the perirolandic, calcarine, and medial temporal subcortical WM (Fig. 9.37E–G)[5,22]

38 to 40 Weeks: T2 dark dot posterior limb of the internal capsule and superior vermis[112]

REFERENCES

1. Tocchio S, Kline-Fath B, Danal E, et al. MRI evaluation and safety in the developing brain. *Semin Perinatol.* 2015;29(2):73–104.
2. Priago G, Barrowman NJ, Hurteau-Miller J, et al. Does 3T Fetal MRI improve image resolution of the normal brain structures between 20 and 24 weeks' gestational age? *AJNR Am J Neuroradiol.* 2017;38:1636–1642.
3. Dobbing, J, Sands J. Quantitative growth and development of human brain. *Arch Dis Child.* 1973;48:757–767.
4. Chung HW, Chen CY, Zimmerman RA, et al. T2-weighted fast MR imaging with true FISP versus HASTE: Comparative efficacy in the evaluation of normal fetal brain maturation. *AJR Am J Roentgenol.* 2000;175:1375–1380.
5. Fogliarini C, Chaumoitre K, Chapon F, et al. Assessment of cortical maturation with prenatal MRI. Part I: normal and cortical maturation. *Eur Radiol.* 2005;15:1671–1685.
6. Hayat TTA, Martinz-Biarge M, Kyriakopoulou V, et al. Neurodevelopmental correlates of fetal motor behavior assessed using cine MR imaging. *AJNR Am J Neuroradiol.* 2018;39:1519–1522.
7. Al-Mukhtar A, Kasprian G, Schmook MT, et al. Diagnostic pitfalls in fetal brain MRI. *Semin Perinatol.* 2009;33:251–258.
8. Ten Donkelaar H, Lammens M, Hori A. *Clinical Neuroembryology.* Berlin Heidelberg: Springer-Verlag; 2006.
9. Chi JG, Dooling EC, Gilles FH. Gyral development of the human brain. *Ann Neurol.* 1977;1:86–93.
10. Levine D, Trop I, Mehta TS, et al. MR imaging appearance of fetal cerebral ventricular morphology. *Radiology.* 2002;223:652–660.
11. Andescavage NN, DuPlessis A, McCarter R, et al. Cerebrospinal fluid and parenchymal brain development and growth in the healthy fetus. *Dev Neurosci.* 2016;38:420–429.
12. Farrell TA, Hertzberg BS, Kliewer MA, et al. Fetal lateral ventricles: reassessment of normal values for atrial diameter at US. *Radiology.* 1994;193:409–411.
13. Twickler DM, Riechel T, Mcintire DD, et al. Fetal central nervous system ventricle and cisterna magna measurements by magnetic resonance imaging. *Am J Obstet Gynecol.* 2002;187:927–931.
14. Garel C, Alberti C. Coronal measurement of the fetal lateral ventricles: comparison between ultrasonography and magnetic resonance imaging. *Ultrasound Obstet Gynecol.* 2006;27:23–27.
15. Sarwar M. The septum pellucidum: normal and abnormal. *AJNR Am J Neuroradiol.* 1989;10:989–1005.
16. Raybaud C. The corpus callosum, the other great forebrain commissures, and the septum pellucidum: anatomy, development, and malformation. *Neuroradiology.* 2010;52:447–477.
17. Jou HJ, Shyu MK, Wu SC, et al. Ultrasound measurement of the fetal cavum septi pellucidi. *Ultrasound Obstet Gynecol.* 1998;12:419–421.
18. Sari A, Ahmetoglu A, Dinc H, et al. Fetal biometry: size and configuration of the third ventricle. *Acta Radiol.* 2005;46(6):631–635.
19. Garel C. Fetal cerebral biometry: normal parenchymal findings and ventricular size. *Eur Radiol.* 2005;15:809–813.
20. Blake JA. The roof and lateral recesses of the fourth ventricle, considered morphologically and embryologically. *J Comparative Neurol.* 1900;10(1):78–108.
21. Robinson AJ, Goldstein R. The cisterna magna septa: vestigial remnants of Blake's pouch and a potential new marker for normal development of the rhombencephalon. *J Ultrasound Med.* 2007;26:83–95.
22. Girard NJ, Chaumoitre K. The brain in the belly: what and how of fetal neuroimaging. *J Magn Reson Imaging.* 2012;36:788–804.
23. Watanabe Y, Abe S, Takagi K, et al. Evolution of subarachnoid space in normal fetuses using magnetic resonance imaging. *Prenat Diagn.* 2005;25:1217–1222.
24. Triulzi F, Parazzini C, Righini A. MRI of fetal and neonatal cerebellar development. *Sem Fetal Neonatal Med.* 2005;10:411–420.
25. Florio M, Huttner WB. Neural progenitors, neurogenesis and the evolution of the neocortex. *Development.* 2014;141:2182–2194.
26. Marin-Padilla M. Origin, formation, and prenatal maturation of the human cerebral cortex: an overview. *J Craniofacial Genet Dev Biol.* 1990;10;137–146.
27. Bystron I, Rakic P, Molnar Z, et al. The first neurons of the human cerebral cortex. *Nat Neurosci.* 2006;9:880–886.
28. Bystron I, Blakemore C, Rakic P. Development of the human cerebral cortex: boulder Committee revisited. *Nat Rev Neurosci.* 2008;9:110–122.
29. Smart I, Dehay C, Giroud P, et al. Unique morphological features of the proliferative zones and postmitotic compartments of the neural epithelium giving rise to the striate and extrastriate cortex in the monkey. *Cereb Cortex.* 2202;12(1);37–53.
30. Kostovic I, Sedmak G, Juas M. Neural histology and neurogenesis of the human fetal and infant brain. *Neuroimage.* 2019;188:743–773.
31. Azzarelli R, Oleari R, Lettieri A, et al. In vitro, ex vivo and in vivo techniques to study normal neuronal migration in the developing cerebral cortex. *Brain Sci.* 2017;7(48):1–20.
32. Marin O, Rubenstein JL. Cell migration in the forebrain. *Annu Rev Neurosci.* 2003;26:441–483.
33. Zecevic N, Chen Y, Filipovic R. Contributions of cortical subventricular zone to the development of the human cerebral cortex. *J Comp Neurol.* 2005;491:109–122.
34. Petanjek Z, Dujmovic A, Kostovic I, et al. Distinct origin of GABA-ergic neurons in forebrain of man, nonhuman primates and lower mammals. *Coll Antropol.* 2008;32(suppl 1):9–17.
35. Lim L, Mi D, Llorca A, et al. Development and functional diversification of cortical interneurons. *Neuron.* 2018;100(2):294–313.
36. Del Bigio MR. Cell proliferation in human ganglionic eminence and suppression after prematurity-associated haemorrhage. *Brain.* 2011;134:1344–1361.
37. Guo J, Anton ES. Decision making during interneuron migration in the developing cerebral cortex. *Trends Cell Biol.* 2014;24(6):342–351.
38. Bandler RC, Mayer C, Fishell G. Cortical interneuron specification: the juncture of genes, time and geometry. *Curr Opin Neurobiol.* 2017;42:17–24.
39. Medina L, Abellán A, Vicario A, et al. Evolutionary and developmental contributions for understanding the organization of the basal ganglia. *Brain Behav Evol.* 2014;83:112–125.
40. Letinić K, Kostović I. Transient fetal structure, the gangliothalamic body, connects telencephalic germinal zone with all thalamic regions in the developing human brain. *J Comp Neurol.* 1997;384:373–395.
41. Lopez-Bendito G, Cautinat A, Sanchez JA, et al. Tangential neuronal migration controls axon guidance: a role for neuregulin-1 in thalamocortical axon navigation. *Cell.* 2006;125:127–142.
42. Kostović I, Jovanov-Milosević N. Subplate zone of the human brain: historical perspective and new concepts. *Coll Antropol.* 2008;32(suppl 1):3–8.
43. Kostović I, Judaš M, Sedmak G. Developmental history of the suplate zone, subplate neurons and interstitial white matter neurons: relevance for schizophrenia. *Int J Dev Neurosci.* 2011;29:193–205.
44. Hadders-Algra M. Early human brain development: starring the subplate. *Neurosci Biobehav Rev.* 2018;92:276–290.
45. Ohtaka-Maruyama C, Okamoto M, Endo K, et al. Synaptic transmission from subplate neurons controls radial migration of neocortical neurons. *Science.* 2018;360:313–317.
46. Vasung L, Lepage C, Rados M, et al. Quantitative and qualitative analysis of transient fetal compartments during prenatal human brain development. *Front Neuroanat.* 2016;10(11):1–17.
47. Brazel CY, Romanko MJ, Rothstein RP, et al. Roles of mammalian subventricular zone in brain development. *Prog Neurobiol.* 2003;69:49–69.
48. Zuchero JB, Barres BA. Glia in mammalian development and disease. *Development.* 2015;142:3805–3809.
49. Back SA, Han BH, Luo NL, et al. Selective vulnerability of late oligodendrocyte progenitors to hypoxia-ischemia. *J Neurosci.* 2002;22:455–463.
50. Samuelsen GB, Larsen BK, Bogdanovic N, et al. The changing number of cells in the human fetal forebrain and its subdivisions: a stereological analysis. *Cereb Cortex.* 2003;13:115–122.
51. Vasung L, Juang H, Jovanov-Milosevic N, et al. Development of axonal pathways in the human fetal fronto-limbic brain: histochemical characterization and diffusion tensor imaging. *J Anat.* 2010;217: 400–417.
52. Ouyang M, Dubois J, Yu Q, et al. Delineation of early brain development from fetuses to infant with diffusion MRI and beyond. *Neuroimage.* 2019;185:836–850.
53. Vasung L, Jovanov-Milošević N, Pletikos M, et al. Prominent periventricular fiber system related to ganglionic eminence and striatum in the human fetal cerebrum. *Brain Struct Funct.* 2011;215:237–253.
54. Judas M, Rados M, Jovanov-Milosevic N, et al. Structural, immunocytochemical and MR imaging properties of periventricular crossroads of growing cortical pathways in preterm infants. *AJNR Am J Neuroradiol.* 2005;26:2671–2784.

55. Kostović I, Judaš M. Correlation between the sequential ingrowth of afferents and transient patterns of cortical lamination in preterm infants. *Anat Rec.* 2002;267:1–6.

56. Kam M, Curtis MA, McGlashan SR, et al. The cellular composition and morphological organization of the rostral migratory stream in the adult human brain. *J Chem Neuroanat.* 2009;37:196–205.

57. Widjaja E, Geibprasert S, Mahmoodabadi SZ, et al. Alteration of human fetal subplate layer and intermediate zone during normal development on MR and diffusion tensor imaging. *AJNR Am J Neuroradiol.* 2010;31:1091–1099.

58. Maas LC, Mukherjee P, Carballido-Gamio J, et al. Early laminar organization of the human cerebrum demonstrated with diffusion tensor imaging in extremely premature infants. *Neuroimage.* 2004;22:1134–1140.

59. Girard N, Confort-Gouny S, Schneider J, et al. MR imaging of brain maturation. *J Neuroradiol.* 2007;34:290–310.

60. Brisse H, Fallet C, Sebag G, et al. Supratentorial parenchyma in the developing fetal brain: in vitro MR study with histologic comparison. *AJNR Am J Neuroradiol.* 1997;18:1491–1497.

61. Prayer D, Kasprian G, Krampl E, et al. MRI of normal fetal brain development. *Eur J Radiol.* 2006;57:199–216.

62. Wang R, Dai G, Takahashi E. High resolution MRI reveals detailed layer structures in early human fetal stages: in vitro studies with histologic correlation. *Front Neuroanat.* 2015;9:150.

63. Glenn OA. Normal development of the fetal brain by MRI. *Semin Perinatol.* 2009;33:208–219.

64. Girard N, Raybaud C, Poncet M. In vivo MR study of brain maturation in normal fetuses. *AJNR Am J Neuroradiol.* 1995;16:407–413.

65. Kostović I, Judaš M, Radoš M, et al. Laminar organization of the human fetal cerebrum revealed by histochemical markers and magnetic resonance imaging. *Cereb Cortex.* 2002;12:536–544.

66. Kostovic I, Vasung L. Insights from in vitro fetal magnetic resonance imaging of the cerebral development. *Semin Perinatol.* 2009;33:220–233.

67. Rados M, Judas M, Kostović I. In vitro MRI of brain development. *Eur J Radiol.* 2006;57:187–198.

68. Kinoshita Y, Okudera T, Tsuru E, et al. Volumetric analysis of the germinal matrix and lateral ventricles performed using MR images of postmortem fetuses. *AJNR Am J Neuroradiol.* 2001;22:382–388.

69. Gupta RK, Hasan KM, Trivedi R, et al. Diffusion tensor imaging of the developing human cerebrum. *J Neurosci Res.* 2005;81:172–178.

70. Huang H, Vasung L. Gaining insight of fetal brain development with diffusion MRI and histology. *Int J Dev Neurosci.* 2014;32:11–22.

71. Righini A, Bianchini E, Parazzini C, et al. Apparent diffusion coefficient determination in normal fetal brain: a prenatal MR imaging study. *AJNR Am J Neuroradiol.* 2003;24:799–804.

72. Glenn O. Contributions of diffusion-weighted imaging to fetal and neonatal imaging. *Top Magn Reson Imaging.* 2011;22:3–9.

73. Zhan J, Dinov ID, Li J, et al. Spatial-temporal atlas of human fetal brain development during the early second trimester. *Neuroimage.* 2013;82:115–126.

74. Corbett-Detig J, Habas PA, Scott JA, et al. 3D global and regional patterns of human fetal subplate growth determined in utero. *Brain Struct Funct.* 2011;215:255–263.

75. Wang X, Pattersson DR, Studholme C, et al. Characterization of laminar zones in the mid-gestation primate brain with magnetic resonance imaging and histological methods. *Front Neuroanat.* 2015;9:147.

76. Schneider JF, Confort-Gouny S, Le Fur Y, et al. Diffusion-weighted imaging in normal fetal brain maturation. *Eur Radiol.* 2007;17:2422–2429.

77. Schneider MM, Berman JI, Baumer FM, et al. Normative apparent diffusion coefficient values in the developing fetal brain. *AJNR Am J Neuroradiol.* 2009;30:1799–1803.

78. Koester SE, O'Leary DDM. Axons of early generated neurons in cingulate cortex pioneer the corpus callosum. *J Neurosci.* 1994;14:6608–6620.

79. Kier EL, Truwit CL. The normal and abnormal genu of the corpus callosum: an evolutionary, embryologic, anatomic and MR analysis. *AJNR Am J Neuroradiol.* 1996;17:1631–1641.

80. Harreld JH, Bhore R, Chason DP, et al. Corpus callosum length by gestational age as evaluated by fetal MR imaging. *AJNR Am J Neuroradiol.* 2011;32:490–494.

81. Kasprian G, Brugger PC, Weber M, et al. In utero tractography of fetal white matter development. *Neuroimage.* 2008;43:213–234.

82. Song JW, Gruber GM, Patsch JM, et al. How accurate are prenatal tractography results? A postnatal in vivo follow-up study using diffusion tensor imaging. *Pediatr Radiol.* 2018;48:486–498.

83. Arnold SE, Trojanowski JQ. Human fetal hippocampal development: I. Cytoarchitecture, myeloarchitecture, and neuronal morphologic features. *J Comp Neurol.* 1996;367:274–292.

84. Supèr H, Soriano E, Uylings HBM. The functions of the preplate in development and evolution of the neocortex and hippocampus. *Brain Res Brain Res Rev.* 1998;27:40–64.

85. Kier EL, King JH, Fulbright RK, et al. Embryology of the human fetal hippocampus: MR imaging, anatomy and histology. *AJNR Am J Neuroradiol.* 1997;18:525–532.

86. Bajic D, Canto Moreira NC, Wikström J, et al. Asymmetric development of the hippocampal region is common: a fetal MR imaging study. *AJNR Am J Neuroradiol.* 2012;33:513–518.

87. Rana S, Shishegar R, Quezada S, et al. The subplate: a potential driver of cortical folding? *Cereb Cortex.* 2019;29(11):4697–4708.

88. Sarnat HB, Flores-Sarnat L. Telencephalic flexure and malformations of the lateral cerebral (sylvian) fissure. *Pediatr Neurol.* 2016;63:23–38.

89. Levine D, Barnes PD. Cortical maturation in normal and abnormal fetuses as assessed with prenatal MR imaging. *Radiology.* 1999;210:751–758.

90. Garel C, Chantrel E, Brisse H, et al. Fetal cerebral cortex: normal gestational landmarks identified using prenatal MR imaging. *AJNR Am J Neuroradiol.* 2001;22:184–189.

91. Habas PA, Scott JA, Roosta A, et al. Early folding patterns and asymmetries of the normal human brain detected from in utero MRI. *Cereb Cortex.* 2012;22:13–25.

92. Garel C, Chantrel E, Elmaleh M, et al. Fetal MRI: normal gestational landmarks for cerebral biometry, gyration and myelination. *Childs Nerv Syst.* 2003;19:422–425.

93. Kasprian G, Langs G, Brugger PC, et al. The prenatal origin of hemispheric asymmetry: an in utero neuroimaging study. *Cereb Cortex.* 2011;21:1076–1083.

94. Van der Knaap MS, van Wezel-Meijler G, Barth PC, et al. Normal gyration and sulcation in preterm and term neonates: appearance on MR images. *Radiology.* 1996;200:389–396.

95. Wu, J, Awate SP, Licht DF, et al. Assessment of MRI-based automated fetal cerebral cortical folding measures in prediction of gestation age in the third trimester. *AJNR Am J Neuroradiol.* 2015;36:1369–1374.

96. Sarnat HB, Flores-Sarnat L. Olfactory development, part 2: neuroanatomic maturation and dysgeneses. *J Child Neurol.* 2017;32(6):579–591.

97. Schmook MT, Brugger PC, Weber M, et al. Forebrain development in fetal MRI: evaluation of anatomical landmarks before gestational week 27. *Neuroradiology.* 2010;52:495–504.

98. Soo A, Taha S, Lally P, et al. Assessment of optic nerve development using post-mortem MRI in fetuses and newborns. *Prenat Diagn.* 2015;35:1262–1264.

99. Righini A, Parazzini C, Doneda C, et al. Prenatal MR imaging of the normal pituitary stalk. *AJNR Am J Neuroradiol.* 2009;30:1014–1016.

100. Dietrich RB, Lis LE, Greensite FS, et al. Normal MR appearance of the pituitary gland in the first 2 years of life. *AJNR Am J Neuroradiol.* 1995;16:1413–1419.

101. Mehemed TM, Fushimi Y, Okada T, et al. MR imaging of the pituitary gland and postsphenoid ossification in fetal specimens. *AJNR Am J Neuroradiol.* 2016;37:1523–1527.

102. Azoulay R, Fallet-Bianco C, Garel C, et al. MRI of the olfactory bulbs and sulci in human fetuses. *Pediatr Radiol.* 2006;36:97–107.

103. Battin M, Rutherford MA. Magnetic resonance imaging of the brain in preterm infants: 24 weeks' gestation to term. In: Rutherford MA, ed. *MRI of the Neonatal Brain.* Philadelphia, PA: W.B. Saunders; 2000:1–28.

104. Nakamura H, Katahira T, Matsunaga E, et al. Isthmus organizer for midbrain and hindbrain development. *Brain Res Rev.* 2005;49:120–126.

105. Hashimoto M, Hibi M. Development and evolution of cerebellar neural circuits. *Develop Growth Differ.* 2012;54:373–389.

106. Rahimi-Balaei M, Bergen H, Kong J, et al. Neuronal migration during development of the cerebellum. *Front Cell Neurosci.* 2018;121:484.

107. Adamsbaum C, Moutard ML, André C, et al. MRI of the fetal posterior fossa. *Pediatr Radiol.* 2005;35:124–140.

108. Hatanaka Y, Zhu Y, Torigoe M, et al. From migration to settlement: the pathways, migration modes and dynamics of neurons in the developing brain. *Proc Jpn Acad Ser B Phys Biol Sci.* 2016;92:1–19.

109. Ten Donkelaar HJ, Lammens M, Wesseling P, et al. Development and developmental disorders of the human cerebellum. *J Neurol.* 2003;250:1025–1036.

110. Ten Donkelaar HJ, Lammens M. Development of the human cerebellum and its disorders. *Clin Perinatol.* 2009;36:513–530.

111. Triulzi F, Parazzini C, Righini A. Magnetic resonance imaging of fetal cerebellar development. *Cerebellum.* 2006;5:199–205.

112. Triulzi F, Parazzini C, Righini A. MRI of fetal and neonatal cerebellar development. *Sem Fetal Neonatal Med.* 2005;10:411–420; Fink AJ, Englund C, Daza RAM, et al. Development of the deep cerebellar nuclei: transcription factors and cell migration from the rhombic lip. *J Neurosci.* 2006;26:3066–3076.

113. Huang H. Structure of the fetal brain: what we are learning from diffusion tensor imaging. *Neuroscientist.* 2010;16(6):634–649.

114. Stazzone MM, Hubbard AM, Bilaniuk LT, et al. Ultrafast MR imaging of the normal posterior fossa in fetuses. *AJR Am J Roentgenol.* 2000;175:835–839.

115. Robinson AJ, Blaser S, Toi A, et al. The fetal cerebellar vermis: assessment for abnormal development by ultrasonography and magnetic resonance imaging. *Ultrasound Q.* 2007;23:211–223.

116. Chapman T, Menashe SJ, Zare M, et al. Establishment of normative values for the posterior fossa by magnetic resonance imaging. *Prenat Diagn.* 2018;38:1035–1041.

117. Kapur RP, Mahony BS, Finch L, et al. Normal and abnormal anatomy of the cerebellar vermis in midgestational human fetuses. *Birth Defects Res A Clin Mol Teratol.* 2009;85:700–709.

118. Haratz KK, Lerman-Sagie T. Prenatal diagnosis of brainstem anomalies. *Eur J Paediatr Neurol.* 2018;22:1016–1026.

119. Yachnis AT, Rorke LB. Cerebellar and brainstem development: an overview in relation to Joubert syndrome. *J Child Neurol.* 1999;14:570–573.

120. Barkovich AJ, Millen KJ, Dobyns WB. A developmental and genetic classification for midbrain-hindbrain malformations. *Brain.* 2009;132:3199–3230.

16 TO 17 WEEKS

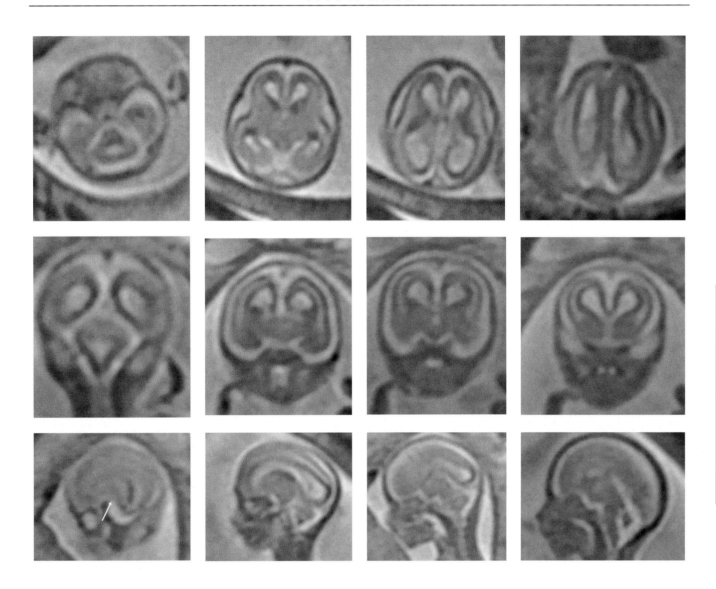

SUPRATENTORIAL

Sulcation: Interhemispheric, Sylvian (arrow)

Parenchyma: Three layer

Basal ganglia: Difficult to separate from germinal matrix

Germinal matrix: Thick, prominent GE

Corpus callosum: Short and horizontal

Lateral ventricles: Primitive lateral

INFRATENTORIAL

Parenchyma: Homogeneous

Vermis: Incomplete coverage of fourth

  Sulcation: Smooth

Cerebellar hemispheres:

  Sulcation: Smooth

Myelination: Possible medulla

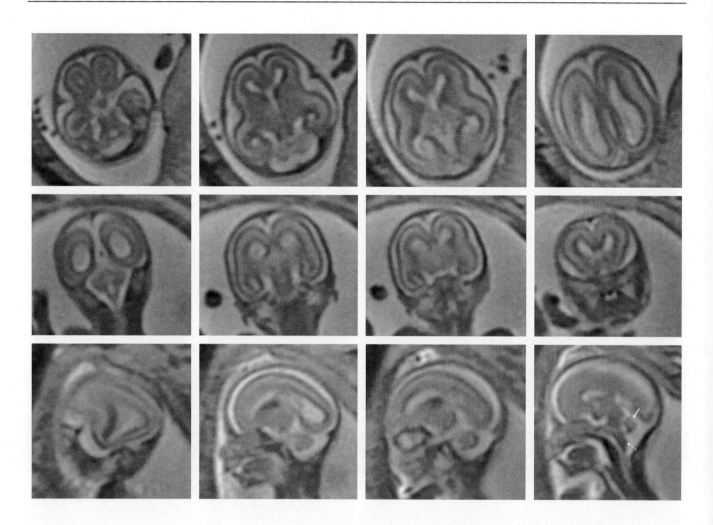

SUPRATENTORIAL

Sulcation: Interhemispheric, Sylvian

Parenchyma: Three layer

Basal ganglia: Homogeneous to white matter

Germinal matrix: Thick, prominent GE

Corpus callosum: Short

Lateral ventricles: Biconcave frontal, but occipital horns prominent

INFRATENTORIAL

Parenchyma: Homogeneous

Vermis: Near coverage of fourth

   Sulcation: Primary (arrow)

Cerebellar hemispheres:

   Sulcation: Smooth

Myelination: Medulla (dotted arrow)

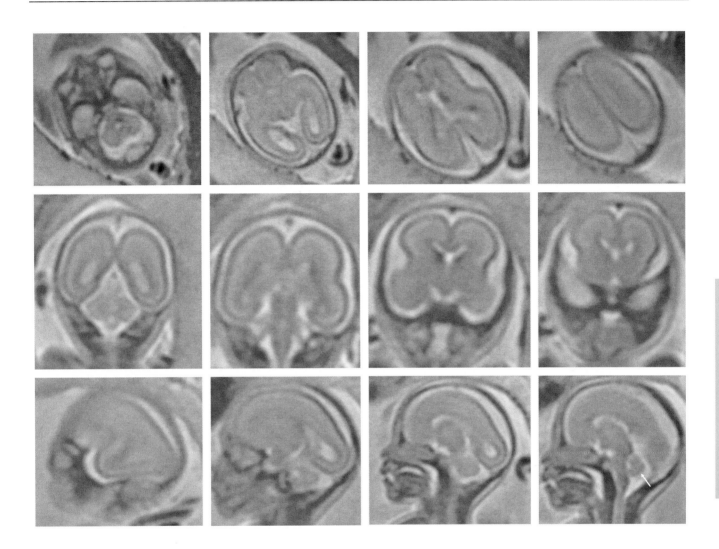

SUPRATENTORIAL

SULCATION: Interhemispheric, **Sylvian deepens**

PARENCHYMA: Five layer

BASAL GANGLIA: Homogeneous to white matter with thalamus mildly T2 hyperintense

GERMINAL MATRIX: Thick, prominent GE

CORPUS CALLOSUM: Crescentic, short but fully formed

LATERAL VENTRICLES: Mature configuration but prominent occipital horns

INFRATENTORIAL

PARENCHYMA: Three layer

VERMIS: Coverage of fourth

SULCATION: Primary, **prepyramidal (arrow)**

CEREBELLAR HEMISPHERES:

SULCATION: Flocculonodular, hemispheres smooth

MYELINATION: Medulla, **pons**

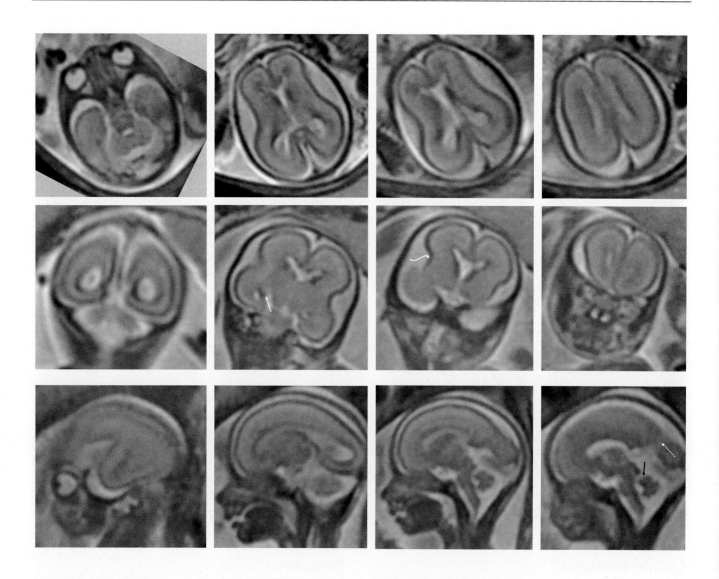

SUPRATENTORIAL

SULCATION: Interhemispheric, **Sylvian angular (curved white arrow)**, **callosal**, **parieto-occipital (dotted white arrow)**, hippocampal (white solid arrow)

PARENCHYMA: Five layer

BASAL GANGLIA: Homogeneous to white matter with thalamus mildly hyperintense

GERMINAL MATRIX: Thinning, less prominent GE

CORPUS CALLOSUM: Crescentic

LATERAL VENTRICLES: Mature configuration but prominent occipital horns

INFRATENTORIAL

PARENCHYMA: Three layer

VERMIS: Coverage of fourth

    SULCATION: Primary, prepyramidal, **preculminate (black arrow)**

CEREBELLAR HEMISPHERES:

    SULCATION: Flocculonodular, hemispheres smooth

MYELINATION: Medulla, pons

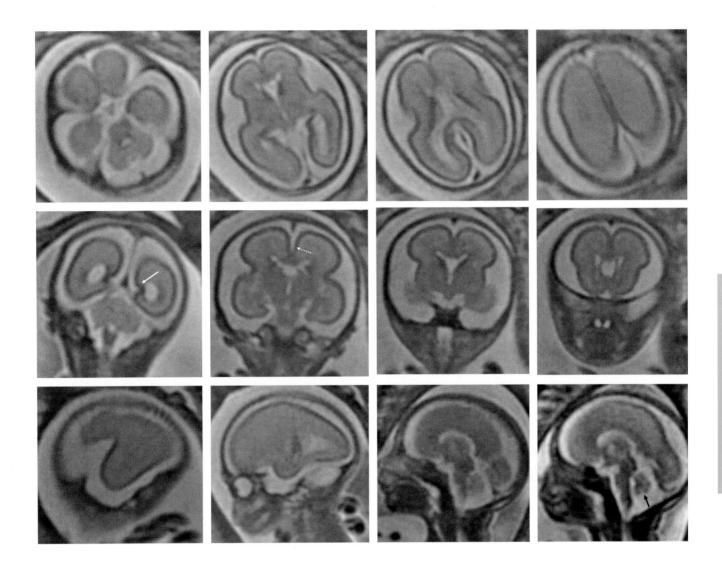

SUPRATENTORIAL

SULCATION: Interhemispheric, Sylvian, callosal, parieto-occipital, hippocampal, **calcarine (solid arrow), cingular (dotted arrow)**

PARENCHYMA: Five layer

BASAL GANGLIA: Homogeneous to white matter with thalamus mildly hyperintense

GERMINAL MATRIX: Moderate prominent

CORPUS CALLOSUM: Crescentic

LATERAL VENTRICLES: Normal configuration and less prominent

INFRATENTORIAL

PARENCHYMA: Three layer

VERMIS: Coverage of fourth

SULCATION: Primary, prepyramidal, preculminate, **postpyramidal or secondary (black arrow)**

CEREBELLAR HEMISPHERES:

SULCATION: Early foliation

MYELINATION: Medulla, pons

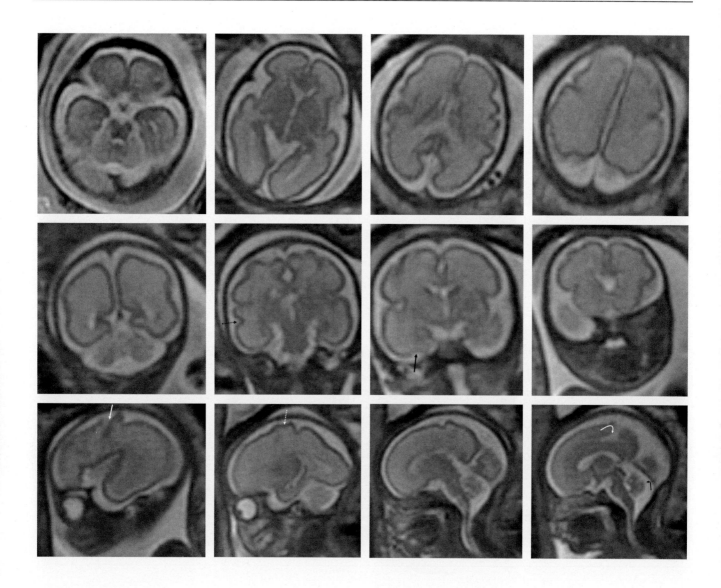

SUPRATENTORIAL

SULCATION: Interhemispheric, Sylvian, callosal, parieto-occipital, hippocampal, calcarine, cingular, **central (solid white arrow), collateral (black solid arrow), precentral (dotted white arrow), superior temporal (dotted black arrow), marginal (curved white arrow)**

PARENCHYMA: Five layer

BASAL GANGLIA: Homogeneous to white matter

GERMINAL MATRIX: Less prominent

CORPUS CALLOSUM: Crescentic

LATERAL VENTRICLES: Normal configuration and less prominent

INFRATENTORIAL

PARENCHYMA: Three layer

VERMIS: Coverage of fourth

SULCATION: Primary, prepyramidal, preculminate, postpyramidal (secondary), **horizontal (curved black arrow)**

CEREBELLAR HEMISPHERES:

SULCATION: Partial foliation

MYELINATION: Medulla, pons

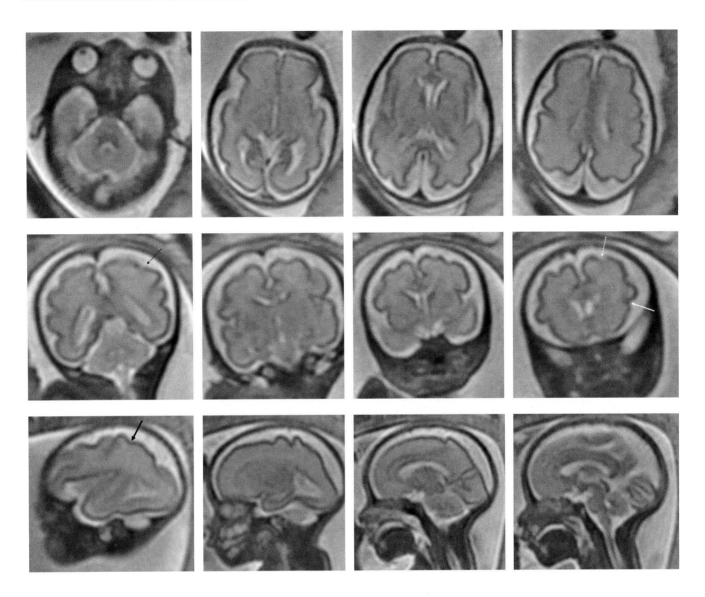

SUPRATENTORIAL

SULCATION: Interhemispheric, Sylvian, callosal, parieto-occipital, hippocampal, calcarine, cingular, central, collateral, precentral, superior temporal, marginal, **postcentral (black solid arrow), intraparietal (dotted black arrow), superior frontal (dotted white arrow), and inferior frontal (solid white arrow)**

PARENCHYMA: Blurring of multilayer with residual five-layer frontal and temporal

BASAL GANGLIA: Thalamus and pallidum T2 hypointense

GERMINAL MATRIX: Less prominent but still along lateral ventricles

CORPUS CALLOSUM: Crescentic

LATERAL VENTRICLES: Normal

INFRATENTORIAL

PARENCHYMA: Three layer

VERMIS: Coverage of fourth

SULCATION: All fissures

CEREBELLAR HEMISPHERES:

SULCATION: Completely foliated

MYELINATION: Medulla, pons, **inferior and superior cerebellar peduncles**

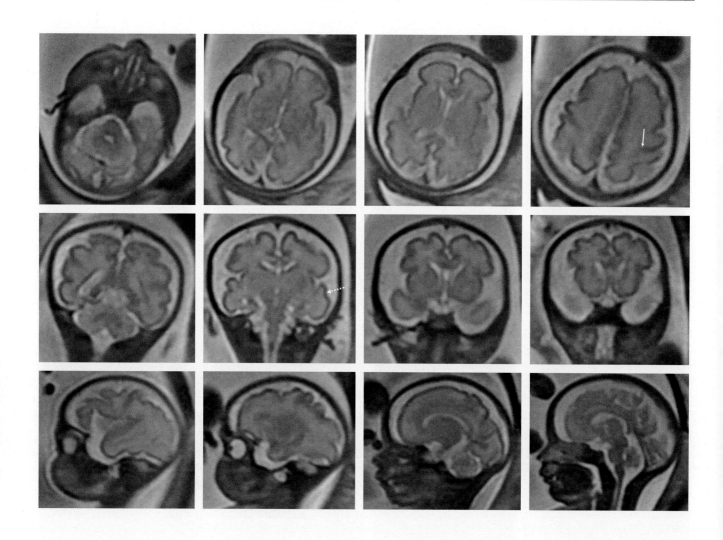

SUPRATENTORIAL

SULCATION: Interhemispheric, Sylvian, callosal, parieto-occipital, hippocampal, calcarine, cingular, central, collateral, precentral, superior temporal, marginal, postcentral, intraparietal, superior frontal, and inferior frontal. **Central sulcus now extends medially (solid white arrow) and superior temporal anteriorly (dotted white arrow)**

PARENCHYMA: Blurring of layers with residual five-layer anterior temporal lobes

BASAL GANGLIA: Thalamus and pallidum T2 hypointense

GERMINAL MATRIX: Inconsistent along lateral ventricles

CORPUS CALLOSUM: Crescentic

LATERAL VENTRICLES: Normal

INFRATENTORIAL

PARENCHYMA: Three layer with T2 hyperintense central and peripheral hypointense DCN

VERMIS: Coverage of fourth

   SULCATION: All fissures

CEREBELLAR HEMISPHERES:

   SULCATION: Folia diffusely

MYELINATION: Medulla, pons, inferior and superior cerebellar peduncles

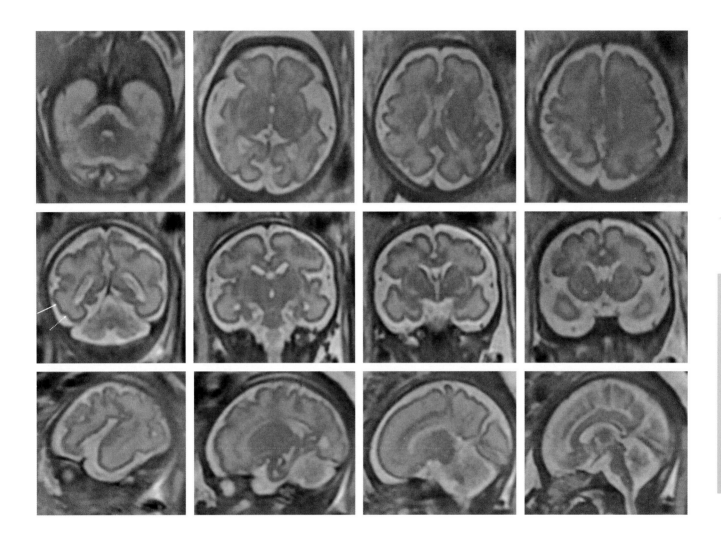

SUPRATENTORIAL

SULCATION: Interhemispheric, Sylvian, callosal, parieto-occipital, hippocampal, calcarine, cingular, central, collateral, precentral, superior temporal, marginal, postcentral, intraparietal, superior frontal, and inferior frontal. Central sulcus now extends medially and superior temporal anteriorly. **Inferior temporal (solid arrow) and occipitotemporal (dotted arrow)**

PARENCHYMA: Two layer in absence of germinal matrix

BASAL GANGLIA: Thalamus and pallidum T2 hypointense

GERMINAL MATRIX: Small rests at caudate head and temporal/occipital horn in the ganglionic eminences

CORPUS CALLOSUM: Crescentic

LATERAL VENTRICLES: Normal

INFRATENTORIAL

PARENCHYMA: Three layer with T2 hyperintense central and peripheral hypointense DCN

VERMIS: Coverage of fourth

SULCATION: All fissures

CEREBELLAR HEMISPHERES:

SULCATION: Folia diffusely

MYELINATION: Medulla, pons, inferior and superior cerebellar peduncles, **dorsal midbrain, inferior colliculus, ventrolateral thalami, possible T1 high-signal dot posterior limb of internal capsule**

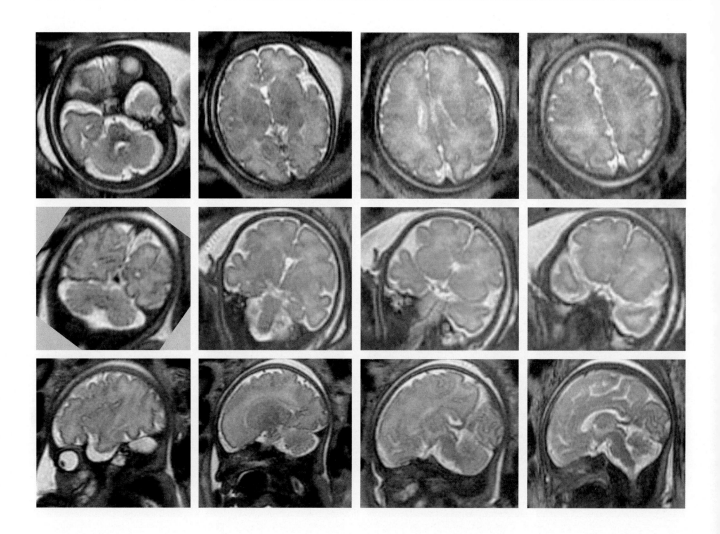

SUPRATENTORIAL

SULCATION: **All primary with most secondary**

PARENCHYMA: Two layer in absence of germinal matrix

BASAL GANGLIA: Thalamus, pallidum, caudate, and putamen T2 hypointense

GERMINAL MATRIX: Small rest at caudate heads

CORPUS CALLOSUM: Crescentic

LATERAL VENTRICLES: Normal

INFRATENTORIAL

PARENCHYMA: Three layer with T2 hyperintense central and peripheral hypointense DCN

VERMIS: Coverage of fourth

SULCATION: All fissures

CEREBELLAR HEMISPHERES:

SULCATION: Folia diffusely

MYELINATION: Medulla, pons, inferior and superior cerebellar peduncles, dorsal midbrain, inferior colliculus, lateral putamen, ventrolateral thalami, T1 high-signal posterior limb of internal capsule, **optic tracts and subcortical white matter perirolandic, calcarine, medial temporal lobe**

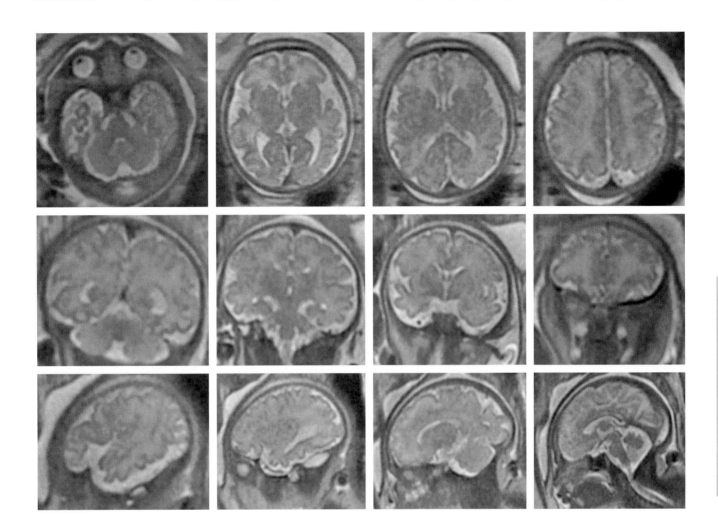

SUPRATENTORIAL

SULCATION: All primary, secondary, and tertiary sulci

PARENCHYMA: Two layer

BASAL GANGLIA: Thalamus, pallidum, caudate, and putamen T2 hypointense

GERMINAL MATRIX: Nearly absent

CORPUS CALLOSUM: Crescentic

LATERAL VENTRICLES: Normal

INFRATENTORIAL

PARENCHYMA: Three layer with T2 hyperintense central and peripheral hypointense DCN

VERMIS: Coverage of fourth

   SULCATION: All fissures

CEREBELLAR HEMISPHERES:

   SULCATION: Folia diffusely

MYELINATION: Medulla, pons, inferior and superior cerebellar peduncles, dorsal midbrain, inferior colliculus, lateral putamen, ventrolateral thalami, T1 high-signal posterior limb of internal capsule, optic tracts and subcortical white matter perirolandic, calcarine, medial temporal lobes

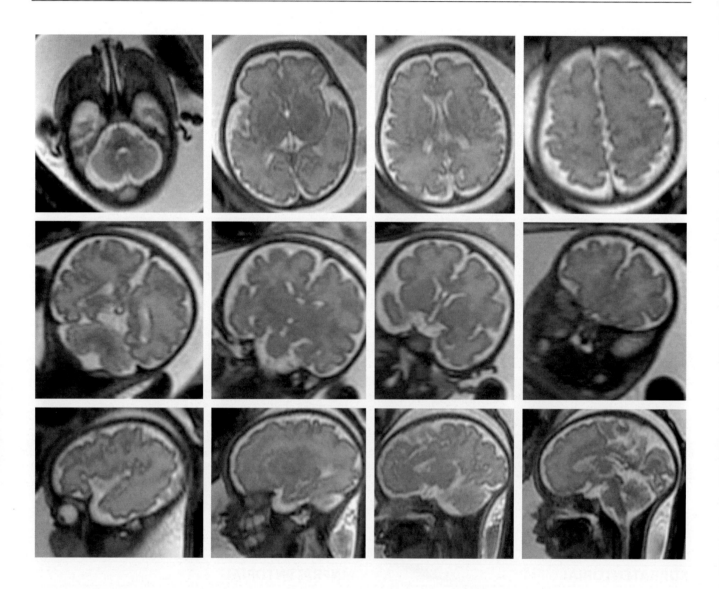

SUPRATENTORIAL

SULCATION: All primary, secondary, and tertiary sulci

PARENCHYMA: Two layer

BASAL GANGLIA: Thalamus, pallidum, caudate, and putamen T2 hypointense

GERMINAL MATRIX: Absent

CORPUS CALLOSUM: Crescentic

LATERAL VENTRICLES: Normal

INFRATENTORIAL

PARENCHYMA: Three layer with T2 hyperintense central and peripheral hypointense DCN

VERMIS: Coverage of fourth

  SULCATION: All fissures

CEREBELLAR HEMISPHERES:

  SULCATION: Folia diffusely

MYELINATION: Medulla, pons, inferior and superior cerebellar peduncles, dorsal midbrain, inferior colliculus, lateral putamen, ventrolateral thalami, T1 high-signal posterior limb of internal capsule, optic tracts and subcortical white matter perirolandic, calcarine, medial temporal lobes. **T2 focal dark signal in the posterior limb of the internal capsule and superior vermis**

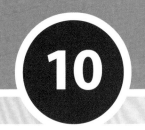

10 Advanced Brain and Placenta Imaging

Nickie Andescavage • Catherine Limperopoulos

The successful application of *in vivo* magnetic resonance imaging (MRI) in the living fetus has led to unprecedented advances in our understanding of the elaborate maturational processes that take place in the healthy fetal brain, and in how these critical maturational events can be derailed by developmental aberrations and acquired injury. The availability of a growing set of MRI sequences, together with the advent of dedicated image-processing pipelines, is providing us with unparalleled access to fetal brain micro- and macrostructure, metabolism, function, and behavior. These quantitative methods are affording us with increasingly reliable and reproducible quantitative neuroimaging biomarkers of the healthy and high-risk fetus. This section presents advances in *in vivo* fetal quantitative neuroimaging techniques and demonstrates their clinical application in the high-risk fetus.

TECHNIQUE

Image degradation frequently accompanies nonsedated fetal MRI studies.[1,2] Although the most common culprit for image degradation is fetal and maternal motion occurring during the acquisition, the inherent high water content of the fetal brain and surrounding intrauterine tissue also negatively impacts the signal. Consequently, fetal MR images are often corrupted by motion artifact and resulting low tissue contrast (Fig. 10.1).[3–5]

A common strategy to counteract the effects of motion is to reduce the acquisition time.[4] However, MRI in nonsedated patients often involves a trade-off between high-image quality and resolution, and fast scanning. A reduced acquisition time leads to the use of increased slice thickness and lower resolution images. Current research efforts are focused on implementing new acquisition protocols in order to decrease scanning time, increase tissue contrast, and to develop specific image postprocessing algorithms that are dedicated to collectively enhance image quality, signal-to-noise (SNR) ratio, contrast, and spatial resolution.

Fetal MRI Acquisitions

A number of fetal-specific MRI acquisition protocols have been developed, providing a large set of modalities with which to study fetal brain *in vivo*,[4,6–8] particularly half Fourier

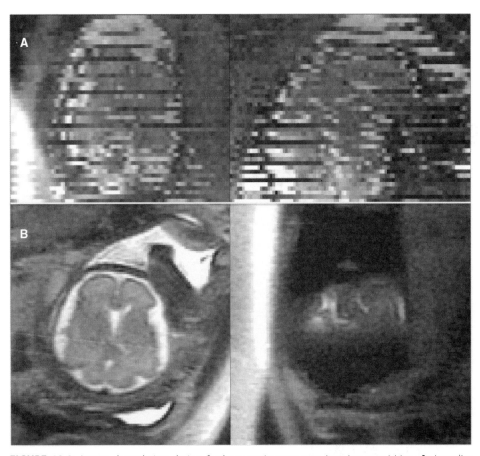

FIGURE 10.1: Image degradation during fetal magnetic resonance imaging acquisition. **A:** Interslice motion, observed from out-of-plane directions. **B:** Intraslice motion, resulting in a loss of image contrast and intensity.

single-shot fast spin echo (SSFSE) T2 sequences. Standard T1 imaging in the *in utero* fetus is not always feasible as T1 sequences require a longer acquisition time, are prone to image degradation, and offer a low gray and white matter contrast.[8] As an alternative, snapshot inversion recovery (SNAPIR) imaging has been shown to effectively overcome motion artifact, and offers improved anatomical detail in comparison with standard T1 acquisitions. Other imaging modalities, including diffusion-weighted imaging (DWI) and diffusion tensor imaging (DTI), functional MRI, and spectroscopy, are actively being developed and refined, and are described further in this section.

Similarly, there are emerging reports of using 3.0 Tesla (T) magnets in studying the human pregnancy, compared to typical 1.5 T.[9–11] While the 3 T magnet has been in regular use for neonates and pediatrics due to better SNR, its use has been limited in pregnancy due to potential increase in energy deposition compared to 1.5 T. While early reports suggest that whole-body energy deposition (specific absorption rate, or SAR) may be lower at 3.0 T with concurrent improvement in SNR,[11] ongoing evaluations for safety and utility are warranted. In particular, susceptibility-related artifacts may increase at higher field strengths, so that ongoing sequence optimization at 3.0 T is needed.

Fetal MR Image Processing

Once the raw MR images have been acquired, the quality is often suboptimal for subsequent quantitative analysis, particularly as it relates to decreased spatial resolution and tissue contrast. A recent body of work that focuses on developing fetal-specific imaging processing pipelines has emerged and it addresses the unique complexities encountered with fetal imaging, including specific image artifacts, noise, poor SNR, low voxel resolution, low tissue contrast, and intensity field nonuniformity.[3,5,12,13]

A common artifact encountered in fetal MRI is the inhomogeneity of the voxel intensities. This degradation is due to several factors, including coil design, poor radio frequency field uniformity, loss of signal (due to the position of the coil and the distance between the fetus and the coil), and/or patient anatomy. Consequently, this leads to variation in the signal intensity across the image. Intensity nonuniformity can be particularly strong in fetal imaging, in situations where the coil is not often properly positioned, or if the fetus is too far from the coil. Another common artifact encountered in fetal MRI is "noise," which gives the images a grainy appearance, frequently making brain tissue boundary (e.g., white matter/gray matter) delineation difficult to achieve. Several algorithms have been proposed to compensate for these artifacts,[12–16] and are summarized later.

Novel methods that increase fetal MR image contrast and resolution have been developed.[3,17,18] These methods typically rely on multiple low-resolution acquisitions of the same fetal brain (typically 2- to 4-mm slice thickness), in all three directions (coronal, axial, and sagittal). The in-plane resolution of these images usually ranges from 0.8 to 1.6 mm. Several approaches have been proposed to overcome this issue, either by compensating interslice motion or by reconstructing a single high-resolution isotropic volume, using the available multiple low-resolution MR images of a single fetal brain.[3,18] These super-resolution methods result in the creation of a single high-resolution volume as well as an increase in tissue contrast (Fig. 10.2), and are now readily incorporated in advanced fetal brain imaging pipelines,[18,19] to allow for an accurate representation of the fetal brain anatomy, which is mandatory in order to delineate brain tissues and extract quantitative features such as brain volumes.

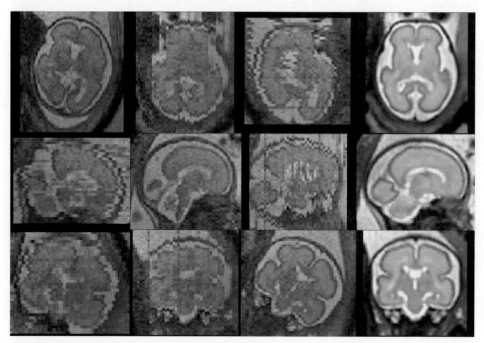

FIGURE 10.2: High-resolution reconstruction of a fetal brain magnetic resonance image (*right column*), using initial low-resolution images, acquired in three different (axial, sagittal, and coronal) directions (*three left columns, left to right*).

QUANTIFYING FETAL BRAIN STRUCTURE

Brain Volumetry

The availability of high-resolution image reconstruction is enabling us to accurately quantify *in utero* brain development, by extracting anatomical features such as brain tissue (e.g., cortical gray matter, white matter) volumes, and regional brain structures (e.g., cerebellum, brainstem). Although previous studies have reported three-dimensional (3D) fetal brain growth measurements using manual delineation of brain volumes,[20–22] manual segmentations remain problematic, mainly for two reasons: the resulting labeling can be operator biased; and manual editing of a high-resolution segmentation is a very tedious and time-consuming process. For example, segmenting a single fetal brain can take several hours, even for a well-trained operator.[23] Consequently, this cannot be applied to large-scale databases.

A growing number of methods are becoming available to automatically localize and extract the fetal brain from surrounding tissue for reconstruction, along with methods to delineate and quantify global and regional brain volumes in the fetus, including intracranial cavity volume, total brain volume, cerebellar volume, cerebral volume, lateral ventricular volume, and brainstem volume (Fig. 10.3).[3,24–26] The quantification of brain tissue volumes, including cortical gray matter, unmyelinated white matter, and basal ganglia, has also been investigated.[27,28] These methods may be single-[19,24,25,28] or multiatlas based.[29] However, caution must be used when applying these methods to the fetus, where there are rapid changes in size and shape across gestation, along with increasing complexity of fetal brain development, lamination, and gyrification. Recent advances in preprocessing methods and the development of robust atlases specific to the fetal brain now allow for automated segmentations for fetuses between 19 and 39 weeks' gestation.[19,30–32] However, manual inspection and editing may still be required, particularly for the fetus with significant malformations, and for the fetus evaluated at very early or very late gestations.

Quantification of fetal brain growth is relevant in the clinical setting in order to reliably ascertain the timing and progression of aberrant brain trajectories. Recent studies have employed sophisticated segmentation tools to characterize normal *in utero* brain maturation, and to compare cerebral tissue development in healthy and high-risk fetal populations. In fact, normative fetal brain growth trajectories are now readily available (Fig. 10.4).[24,25,33–35] These normative curves demonstrate exponential brain growth between 18 and 39 weeks' gestation (Fig. 10.4). These segmentation methods have also been shown to be very informative when studying high-risk fetuses.[25,27,29,36,37] For example, Limperopoulos and colleagues[22] showed a progressive third-trimester impairment in brain growth in fetuses with complex congenital heart disease (CHD) compared with healthy control fetuses. Noteworthy is the fact that the conventional brain MRI studies of these fetuses were considered normal. These findings were extended in a subgroup of fetuses with hypoplastic left heart syndrome (HLHS),[27] and delayed development of the cortical gray matter, subcortical gray matter, and white matter volumes was also reported in the third trimester. Automated fetal brain segmentation methods have also been applied to characterize lateral ventricular volume, shape, and surface features in fetuses with ventriculomegaly.[29,37] Normative fetal datasets have also served as important references for the development of the *ex utero* fetus, comparing brain growth in premature infants to gestational age-matched fetal controls.[38]

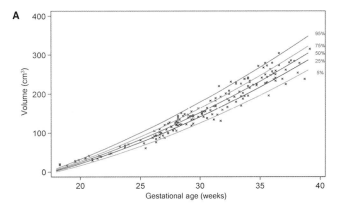
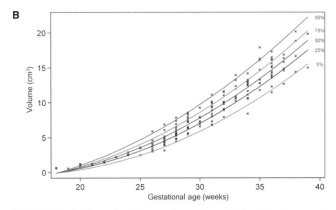

FIGURE 10.4: Example of normative volumetric fetal brain growth curves for the cerebral cortex and cerebellum between 18 and 40 weeks' gestation. **A:** Cerebral cortex. **B:** Cerebellum. (From Andescavage N, duPlessis A, McCarter R, et al. Complex trajectories of brain development in the healthy human fetus. *Cereb Cortex.* 2017;27(11):5274–5283. Copyright © 2016 The Author. Reproduced by permission of Oxford University Press.)

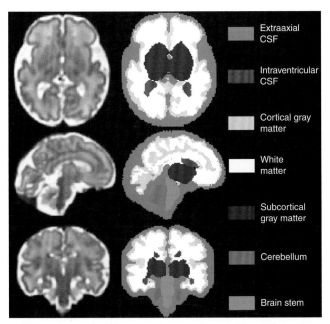

FIGURE 10.3: Segmentation of a high-resolution reconstructed fetal brain (*left*) in seven tissue classes (*right*). *CSF,* cerebrospinal fluid.

Taken together, MRI volumetric methods are increasingly demonstrating valuable clinical utility. Ongoing clinical implementation will largely depend on the ability to decrease computational burden associated with quantitative MRI in order to provide expedited diagnostic information to the clinical team.

Cortical Development

Cerebral cortical anatomy has been directly related to cytoarchitecture and brain function.[39–41] From a developmental perspective, cortical gyrification is closely linked to the maturation of underlying brain structures.[42] The formation of gyri and sulci follows a highly orchestrated developmental process, which was first described in *postmortem* fetuses.[43] Initial studies relied on conventional MRI to describe the timetable of cortical folding using visual/clinical descriptions[44] or geometric measurements in *ex vivo*[45] and *in vivo* fetuses.[46] More recently, advances in brain imaging have permitted the development of quantitative methods to delineate the emergence of the sulcal pattern *in vivo*.

Several studies have characterized cortical folding processes using 3D reconstruction of the fetal cortical surface.[19,28] These techniques offer not only global measurements of the cortical surface, including surface area and gyrification index, but also very specific measurements of the sulci and gyri, including shape, location, curvature, depth, or length, and offer probabilistic maps of the sulcal patterns.[19] It has been demonstrated that during the second and third trimesters of pregnancy, the complexity of the cortical surface is dramatically increasing in several regions, including the frontal, temporal, and occipital lobes.[19,28] As with volumetry, there are emerging methods for the automated quantification of cortical folding that can be used to assess cerebral maturation and development.[47,48]

Clinically, surface-based methods have demonstrated their potential to provide unique insights into developmental brain disturbances. Clouchoux et al.[27] investigated differences in cortical maturation between healthy fetuses and fetuses with HLHS. The study demonstrated delayed cortical folding in fetuses with HLHS compared with the controls in several cortical areas, including the frontal, parietal, calcarine, temporal, and collateral regions (Fig. 10.5). Interestingly, this cortical folding delay appears to precede volumetric growth impairments, and it may represent an important, early marker for subsequent disturbances in growth. Similar studies in fetuses with ventriculomegaly have shown reduced cortical folding in the parieto-occipital region compared with healthy controls, including reductions in cortical folding of the insula, posterior temporal lobe, and occipital lobe for fetuses with mild, isolated ventriculomegaly.[37,49] Furthermore, reductions in sulcal patterns detected through automated methods in fetal life were associated with abnormalities confirmed on qualitative postnatal neuroimaging.[50]

In summary, available studies suggest that cortical folding quantification provides a promising and powerful tool for investigating the timing and extent of cerebral cortical aberrations in high-risk fetuses.

Fetal Brain Microstructure

During fetal brain maturation, the cerebral white matter undergoes a rapid set of changes in its microstructural organization.[51–56] These changes can be observed and quantified using DWI and DTI. DWI allows us to characterize the diffusion of water molecules in the brain, reflecting the degree of organization of the white matter fibers, and can be measured by calculating the apparent diffusion coefficient (ADC). Several studies

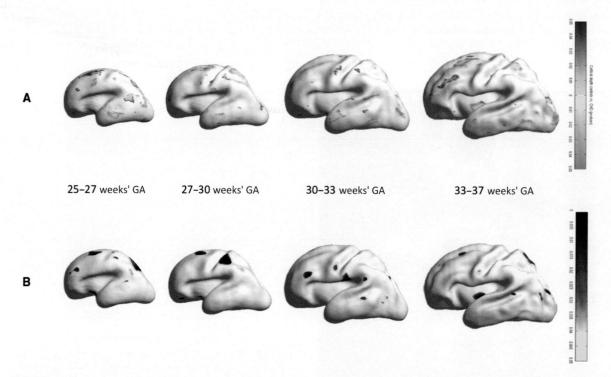

FIGURE 10.5: Local cortical development delays in fetuses with hypoplastic left heart syndrome, compared with healthy controls. **A:** Delays in cortical depth. **B:** Delays in sulcation. *GA*, gestational age. (From Clouchoux C, du Plessis AJ, Bouyssi-Kobar M, et al. Delayed cortical development in fetuses with complex congenital heart disease. *Cereb Cortex.* 2013;23(12):2932–2943. Copyright © 2012 The Author. Reproduced by permission of Oxford University Press.)

have described normal and abnormal microstructure using DWI. These studies have reported a decrease in ADC from 30 weeks of gestation onward.[56–59] DWI has been shown to provide valuable information in cases of fetal brain hemorrhage and acute ischemia.[52,53,56] In CHD fetuses, ADC values have been shown to be higher when compared with the controls.[60] DWI has also been used to investigate brain maturation between fetuses and infants born prematurely.[61] Differences in ADC were reported between the two groups in the pons and the parietal white matter, where higher ADC values were reported in fetuses, suggesting increased regional brain maturation in *in utero* fetuses compared with *ex utero* preterm infants.

DTI allows us to quantify the direction and magnitude of water molecule diffusion, and is measured using fractional anisotropy (FA).[61] Complementary to DWI, DTI provides an indirect assessment of axonal/fiber connectivity in the developing brain.[54,60,62–66] Although DTI can provide important insights into fetal brain microstructural development, its successful application to the living fetus remains technically challenging secondary to fetal and maternal motion, and low voxel resolution. Consequently, very few studies have investigated this modality *in vivo*.[67–74] Hierarchical regional distribution of FA values has been described in the *in utero* fetal brain, with gradually decreasing FA in the splenium, the genu of the corpus callosum, and, lastly, the internal capsule with increasing gestational age.[67] Zanin and colleagues[75] also reported a gradual maturation of the cerebral white matter, which they divided into three different phases, potentially reflecting axonal organization, myelination gliosis, and myelination. Similarly, there are descriptions of abnormalities in the cortico-cortical and cortico-subcortical tracts for fetuses with agenesis of the corpus callosum.[68] Validation of fetal DTI studies remains challenging. Mitter et al. report good correspondence of *in utero* tractography of the internal capsule and corona radiata with postmortem histology-based tractography in a small series of subjects; however, the authors also report multiple limitations of *in utero* DTI for the other brain regions, particularly for tracts with crossing fibers.[72] Song et al. present another series of 12 subjects with fetal and postnatal DTI examinations of the corpus callosum and corticospinal tracts; here, the authors report a wide range of both negative and positive predictive values from fetal to postnatal studies, highlighting the significant challenges that remain in characterizing emerging white matter tracts of the fetal brain.[74]

QUANTIFYING FETAL BRAIN METABOLISM AND FUNCTION

Spectroscopy

Metabolite mapping of the fetal brain can provide crucial insights into brain maturation, in both healthy and high-risk pregnancies. The recent successful application of proton magnetic resonance spectroscopy (^{1}HMRS) has enabled the quantification of metabolic profiles in the living fetus.[22,76–79] Despite the length of the acquisition (~3 to 4 minutes), recent studies showed that unsedated single-voxel spectroscopy can be successfully performed in about two-thirds of fetuses.[22,78]

The most commonly reported metabolites in the fetal brain include creatine (Cr), reflecting cellular mitochondrial metabolism, choline (Cho), a marker of myelination, and *N*-acetylaspartate (NAA), a neuroaxonal marker reflecting dendrites and synapse development (Fig. 10.6).[77,80–85] Cr and NAA increase between 18 and 40 weeks' gestation, while Cho remains relatively stable. This evolution in metabolic concentrations is associated with myelination and the development of synapses and dendrites. Lactate, the product of anaerobic metabolism, has been reported in compromised fetuses, including those with intrauterine growth restriction (IUGR) and complex CHD.[22,76,77,79,80] Moreover, decreased NAA:Cr and NAA:Cho ratios have also been found to be lower in these high-risk fetuses.[22,79,86] These emerging studies suggest that fetal brain ^{1}HMRS may serve as an important early marker of fetal compromise.

Fetal Resting-State Functional MRI

Functional magnetic resonance imaging (fMRI) is a noninvasive MRI modality that enables the quantification of local blood oxygenation, using the blood oxygen level–dependent (BOLD) response. Functional MRI provides an indirect measure of regional activation of the brain. To date, functional assessment of the living fetus has been largely limited to Doppler ultrasound, changes in fetal activity or heart rate, or magnetoencephalography (MEG).[87–90] Understandably, task-related fMRI is not possible in the fetus. A very small number of stimulus-driven fetal fMRI experiments have been performed to date, where fetal brain oxygenation level was measured during auditory,[91–93] vibroacoustic,[94] or visual stimuli.[95] For example, Jardri and colleagues[92] reported fetal

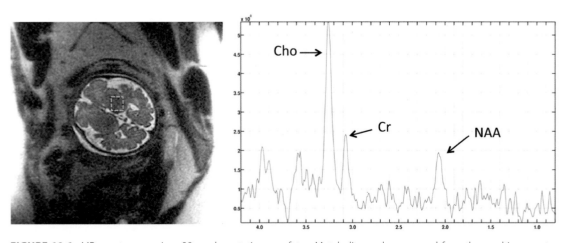

FIGURE 10.6: MR spectroscopy in a 32-week gestation age fetus. Metabolite peaks measured from the resulting spectra (*right*), including Choline (*Cho*), Creatine (*Cr*), and *N*-acetylaspartate (*NAA*).

activation in the left temporal cortex in six fetuses (33 weeks of gestation), when an auditory stimulus was applied. Noteworthy is the fact that mothers were sedated during the study, and the authors reported that signal variance was not corrupted by fetal motion during the acquisition.

More recently, resting-state fMRI has been explored in the living fetus.[96–98] Resting-state fMRI is designed to quantify regional brain activity and interactions when the subject is not performing any given task.[99] The goal is then to extract the "default mode" functional network, representing regions with a functional activity, even when the subject is not performing an explicit task.[100] Schopf and colleagues[96] used resting-state fMRI in a cohort of 16 healthy fetuses from 16 to 36 weeks of gestation, to analyze fetal brain networks. This study reported a bilateral occipital network, as well as medial and lateral prefrontal networks. Thomason and colleagues reported bilateral connectivity in 20 cortical regions, including visual, somatosensory, ventral, dorsal, and cingulate cortex using resting-state fMRI in healthy fetuses.[97] Functional connectivity was shown to increase with gestational age.[101] Interestingly, a more recent study found decreased systems-level functional connectivity in fetuses that would later be born prematurely.[102] Although fMRI remains technically challenging, available studies are demonstrating the feasibility of measuring functional brain connectivity *in utero*, and will likely provide a critical foundation for understanding the role of early life insults on later disturbances in neural functional connectivity.

Fetal Behavior

Fetal movements, reflexive and voluntary, are closely related to fetal brain function.[2] With advancing gestational age, these movements become increasingly complex, and specific patterns of movements have been described at each developmental stage.[2,103] Given that fetal movements rely on an intact central nervous system,[103,104] their quantification can potentially provide important biomarkers of fetal health and well-being (Fig. 10.7).

Dynamic MRI cine sequences have been used to investigate fetal movements.[105,106] Hayat and colleagues[106] reported a multislice balanced steady-state free precision cine sequence, originally developed for adult cardiac dynamic MRI, to image fetal movements in 37 healthy fetuses (10 to 37 weeks of gestation). The study demonstrated three levels of fetal activity at 22, 28, and 36 weeks of gestation. These stages were described as (a) whole-body movements, (b) low-intensity movements (single limb), and (c) complete inactivity. Moreover, a gradual decrease in activity was associated with decreasing free space available in the uterus. Guo and colleagues[105] also investigated fetal movements using cine MRI in 25 fetuses, from 18 to 33 weeks of gestation, with and without central nervous system abnormalities. The study

demonstrated significantly diminished and/or abnormal fetal movements among fetuses with major central nervous system abnormalities. More recently, a long-term follow-up study revealed that abnormal fetal movements were associated with abnormal neurodevelopmental outcomes up to 4 years postnatally.[107] Although ongoing development of MRI sequences is needed, alongside the quantification of fetal movements, cine MRI may provide clinically important, adjunct four-dimensional information for high-risk fetuses.

QUANTIFYING PLACENTAL STRUCTURE AND FUNCTION

The placenta is an essential organ that provides nutrients to the fetus and plays important immune and endocrine functions.[108] Abnormal placental anatomy has been associated with neonatal death and small-for-gestational age (SGA) neonates.[109,110] Moreover, vascular placental pathologies detected through T1 MRI have also been shown to be strongly predictive of adverse neonatal outcome, including fetal demise.[110] *In vivo* placental anatomy and perfusion is conventionally assessed using Doppler ultrasound. Recently, different MRI modalities that are beginning to quantify placental anatomy, microstructure, perfusion, and metabolism have emerged. These are summarized later.

Placental Volume/Microstructure

The relationship between placental volume and outcome has been recently investigated in a small number of high-risk pregnancies.[109,111,112] Decreased placental volume has been reported in association with maternal smoking during pregnancy,[111] IUGR,[36,110] and SGA neonates.[109] Interestingly, Andescavage and colleagues[36] also demonstrated a concomitant reduction in volumetric growth of the fetal brain overall, along with specific regional decreases in cerebral and cerebellar volumes. Placental volume has also been associated with birth outcomes for the fetus with CHD, where pregnancies with smaller placentas were associated with lower birth weights and premature delivery.[113]

Placental microstructure has also been explored using both structural and diffusion MRI. Texture analysis allows for the quantitative analysis of digital images and may act as a surrogate for detecting structural aberrations beyond typical qualitative assessments.[114] Textural analyses of placenta development in IUGR reveal significant differences in image texture, suggestive of accelerated tissue heterogeneity and placental maturation.[115] In a study by Dahdouh et al.,[116] machine learning–based algorithms using shape and textural features of the placenta were able to accurately identify pregnancies complicated by fetal growth restriction (FGR) and better estimate subsequent birth weight compared to traditional clinical and sonographic metrics.

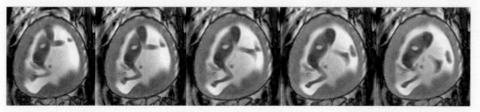

FIGURE 10.7: Sample frames of a cine-magnetic resonance imaging acquisition in a 32-week gestational age fetus.

DWI of the placenta has been used to investigate placental invasion, and to determine the microarchitecture of the myometrium.[117] Placental DWI has also been studied in fetuses with placental insufficiency.[118] Restricted diffusion and reduced ADC were found in IUGR pregnancies when compared with healthy fetus controls, as well as in the growth restricted fetus of monochorionic twins.[118,119] Regional diffusion and perfusion metrics extracted from DWI have also been reported in healthy gestations, as well as in pregnancies complicated by IUGR or preeclampsia.[120–122] These findings suggest that diffusion MRI may have an important role for early detection of placental-based disorders.

Placental Function

The placenta represents the primary source of nutrients for the developing fetus, and therefore the ability to noninvasively quantify placental function, including blood flow, oxygenation, and metabolism, is critical. *In vivo* placental perfusion has been explored using the intravoxel incoherent motion (IVIM) technique.[121,123,124] Indirectly, the volume of blood moving in the placental capillary networks can be measured using IVIM.[123] Using the same technique, decreased placental perfusion fraction, reflecting the percent of moving blood, has been described in pregnancies complicated by IUGR and preeclampsia.[121,122,124] Placental perfusion has also been measured through several arterial spin labeling (ASL) techniques. In a study using a flow-sensitive alternating inversion recovery (FAIR), the sequence of ASL reported reduced placental perfusion in SGA newborns when compared with healthy control pregnancies using both ASL and IVIM techniques, and were further correlated with uterine artery pulsatility index measured by Doppler sonography.[125] Another study of velocity-selective ASL revealed decreased global placental perfusion and increased regional variation in pregnancies with fetal CHD compared to healthy controls.[126] These studies suggest that placental perfusion MRI measurements in high-risk pregnancies may reliably predict pregnancy outcomes.

Oxygenation measurements of placental tissue have also been the focus of recent studies.[127,128] Intact placental oxygenation is critical for normal fetal growth and development; however, the relationship between placental oxygenation and supply of oxygen to the fetal organs is not yet fully understood. Huen and colleagues[127] investigated the feasibility of placental oxygenation quantification using oxygen-enhanced MRI (R1 contrast) and BOLD MRI (R2* contrast) *in vivo*. The study showed an increase in R1 and a concomitant decrease in R2* signals in the placenta when oxygen was administered to pregnant women compared with breathing in room air.[127] Placental oxygenation using BOLD MRI in a second study was found to increase by 6.5% when oxygen was delivered to the mother over 10 minutes (12 L O_2/min).[128] Interestingly, other fetal organs showed an increase in oxygen levels, including liver, spleen, and kidney; however, no change in oxygenation was detected in the fetal brain. The authors speculate that reduced fetal brain perfusion may reflect a "reverse" brain-sparing mechanism.[128] Time-to-plateau studies of placental-fetal oxygenation studies have also shown a positive correlation with placental pathology and a negative correlation with fetal liver and brain volumes as well as infant birth weights.[129] Additional studies of oxygen transfer from the maternal-placental-fetal units are needed to better understand physiological changes of the placenta and fetus in healthy and high-risk pregnancies.

Placental Metabolism

Few studies have reported ^{1}HMRS as a potential noninvasive method to assess placental metabolism.[130,131] In a preliminary study by Denison,[130] ^{1}HMRS was used to quantify metabolic profiles of the placenta in three women with IUGR and three matched controls. When compared with the controls, the IUGR placenta showed a lower Cho/lipid ratio compared with healthy control pregnancies, suggesting that ^{1}HMRS could be used to detect early signs of critical placental insufficiency. A second study showed a decrease in NAA/lipid and Cho/lipid ratios in IUGR compared to healthy controls. Ongoing development of MRI sequences and postprocessing techniques to mitigate maternal-placental motion is needed for the better evaluation of placental metabolism in high-risk pregnancies.[131]

Collectively, these preliminary studies suggest that the application of advanced placental MRI techniques has the potential to provide important, currently unavailable diagnostic information of placental functional integrity. However, these exciting placental-based MR techniques need ongoing validation before they can be translated into the clinical milieu.

CONCLUSION

Advanced fetal MRI is becoming a powerful obstetrical tool that is transforming our ability to noninvasively assess health and wellness in the living fetus. Faster, more robust MRI pulse sequences are now adept at freezing fetal motion, while advanced postprocessing pipelines are capable of reconstructing 3D representations of the fetal brain, allowing for the precise delineation of critical maturational processes that occur throughout pregnancy. The increasing availability of normative values for fetal brain structure, microstructure, and metabolic function is revolutionizing our ability to accurately identify and monitor the compromised fetus. The successful streamlining and adoption of these emerging fetal imaging biomarkers in the clinical setting will require ongoing validation and necessitate a significant reduction in the current computational encumbrance that is inherent to these techniques. This, in turn, will offer advanced fetal diagnostic capabilities to guide clinical management of the high-risk fetus and the development of prenatal interventions.

REFERENCES

1. Garel C. Fetal MRI: what is the future? *Ultrasound Obstet Gynecol.* 2008;31(2):123–128.
2. Prayer D, Brugger PC. Investigation of normal organ development with fetal MRI. *Eur Radiol.* 2007;17(10):2458–2471.
3. Gholipour A, Estroff JA, Warfield SK. Robust super-resolution volume reconstruction from slice acquisitions: application to fetal brain MRI. *IEEE Trans Med Imaging.* 2010;29(10):1739–1758.
4. Jiang S, Xue H, Counsell S, et al. In-utero three dimension high resolution fetal brain diffusion tensor imaging. *Med Image Comput Comput Assist Interv.* 2007;10(pt 1):18–26.
5. Rousseau F, Glenn OA, Iordanova B, et al. Registration-based approach for reconstruction of high-resolution in utero fetal MR brain images. *Acad Radiol.* 2006;13(9):1072–1081.
6. Li Y, Pang Y, Vigneron D, Glenn O, Xu D, Zhang X. Investigation of multichannel phased array performance for fetal MR imaging on 1.5T clinical MR system. *Quant Imaging Med Surg.* 2011;1(1):24–30.

7. Malamateniou C, McGuinness AK, Allsop JM, O'Regan DP, Rutherford MA, Hajnal JV. Snapshot inversion recovery: an optimized single-shot T1-weighted inversion-recovery sequence for improved fetal brain anatomic delineation. *Radiology*. 2011;258(1):229–235.

8. Sandrasegaran K, Lall C, Aisen AA, Rajesh A, Cohen MD. Fast fetal magnetic resonance imaging. *J Comput Assist Tomogr*. 2005;29(4):487–498.

9. Victoria T, Jaramillo D, Roberts TP, et al. Fetal magnetic resonance imaging: jumping from 1.5 to 3 tesla (preliminary experience). *Pediatr Radiol*. 2014; 44(4):376–386; quiz 3-5.

10. da Silva NA Jr, Vassallo J, Sarian LO, Cognard C, Sevely A. Magnetic resonance imaging of the fetal brain at 3 Tesla: preliminary experience from a single series. *Medicine (Baltimore)*. 2018;97(40):e12602.

11. Krishnamurthy U, Neelavalli J, Mody S, et al. MR imaging of the fetal brain at 1.5T and 3.0T field strengths: comparing specific absorption rate (SAR) and image quality. *J Perinat Med*. 2015;43(2):209–220.

12. Coupe P, Yger P, Prima S, Hellier P, Kervrann C, Barillot C. An optimized block-wise nonlocal means denoising filter for 3-D magnetic resonance images. *IEEE Trans Med Imaging*. 2008;27(4):425–441.

13. Tustison NJ, Avants BB, Cook PA, et al. N4ITK: improved N3 bias correction. *IEEE Trans Med Imaging*. 2010;29(6):1310–1320.

14. Erturk MA, Bottomley PA, El-Sharkawy AM. Denoising MRI using spectral subtraction. *IEEE Trans Biomed Eng*. 2013;60(6):1556–1562.

15. Kim K, Habas P, Rajagopalan V, et al. Non-iterative relative bias correction for 3D reconstruction of in utero fetal brain MR imaging. *Conf Proc IEEE Eng Med Biol Soc*. 2010;2010:879–882.

16. Sled JG, Zijdenbos AP, Evans AC. A nonparametric method for automatic correction of intensity nonuniformity in MRI data. *IEEE Trans Med Imaging*. 1998;17(1):87–97.

17. Kim K, Habas PA, Rousseau F, Glenn OA, Barkovich AJ, Studholme C. Intersection based motion correction of multislice MRI for 3-D in utero fetal brain image formation. *IEEE Trans Med Imaging*. 2010;29(1):146–158.

18. Rousseau F, Oubel E, Pontabry J, et al. BTK: an open-source toolkit for fetal brain MR image processing. *Comput Methods Programs Biomed*. 2013;109(1):65–73.

19. Clouchoux C, Kudelski D, Gholipour A, et al. Quantitative in vivo MRI measurement of cortical development in the fetus. *Brain Struct Funct*. 2012;217(1):127–139.

20. Grossman R, Hoffman C, Mardor Y, Biegon A. Quantitative MRI measurements of human fetal brain development in utero. *Neuroimage*. 2006;33(2):463–470.

21. Kazan-Tannus JF, Dialani V, Kataoka ML, et al. MR volumetry of brain and CSF in fetuses referred for ventriculomegaly. *AJR Am J Roentgenol*. 2007;189(1):145–151.

22. Limperopoulos C, Tworetzky W, McElhinney DB, et al. Brain volume and metabolism in fetuses with congenital heart disease: evaluation with quantitative magnetic resonance imaging and spectroscopy. *Circulation*. 2010;121(1):26–33.

23. Fischl B, Dale AM. Measuring the thickness of the human cerebral cortex from magnetic resonance images. *Proc Natl Acad Sci U S A*. 2000;97(20):11050–11055.

24. Clouchoux C, Guizard N, Evans AC, du Plessis AJ, Limperopoulos C. Normative fetal brain growth by quantitative in vivo magnetic resonance imaging. *Am J Obstet Gynecol*. 2012;206(2):173.e1–e8.

25. Jacob FD, Habas PA, Kim K, et al. Fetal hippocampal development: analysis by magnetic resonance imaging volumetry. *Pediatr Res*. 2011;69(5 pt 1):425–429.

26. Tourbier S, Velasco-Annis C, Taimouri V, et al. Automated template-based brain localization and extraction for fetal brain MRI reconstruction. *Neuroimage*. 2017;155:460–472.

27. Clouchoux C, du Plessis AJ, Bouyssi-Kobar M, et al. Delayed cortical development in fetuses with complex congenital heart disease. *Cereb Cortex*. 2013;23(12):2932–2943.

28. Habas PA, Scott JA, Roosta A, et al. Early folding patterns and asymmetries of the normal human brain detected from in utero MRI. *Cereb Cortex*. 2012;22(1):13–25.

29. Gholipour A, Akhondi-Asl A, Estroff JA, Warfield SK. Multi-atlas multi-shape segmentation of fetal brain MRI for volumetric and morphometric analysis of ventriculomegaly. *Neuroimage*. 2012;60(3):1819–1831.

30. Corbett-Detig J, Habas PA, Scott JA, et al. 3D global and regional patterns of human fetal subplate growth determined in utero. *Brain Struct Funct*. 2011;215(3–4):255–263.

31. Gholipour A, Rollins CK, Velasco-Annis C, et al. A normative spatiotemporal MRI atlas of the fetal brain for automatic segmentation and analysis of early brain growth. *Sci Rep*. 2017;7(1):476.

32. Rajagopalan V, Scott J, Habas PA, et al. Local tissue growth patterns underlying normal fetal human brain gyrification quantified in utero. *J Neurosci*. 2011;31(8):2878–2887.

33. Andescavage NN, du Plessis A, McCarter R, et al. Complex trajectories of brain development in the healthy human fetus. *Cereb Cortex*. 2017;27(11):5274–5283.

34. Andescavage NN, du Plessis A, McCarter R, Vezina G, Robertson R, Limperopoulos C. Cerebrospinal fluid and parenchymal brain development and growth in the healthy fetus. *Dev Neurosci*. 2016;38(6):420–429.

35. Scott JA, Habas PA, Kim K, et al. Growth trajectories of the human fetal brain tissues estimated from 3D reconstructed in utero MRI. *Int J Dev Neurosci*. 2011;29(5):529–536.

36. Andescavage N, du Plessis A, Metzler M, et al. In vivo assessment of placental and brain volumes in growth-restricted fetuses with and without fetal Doppler changes using quantitative 3D MRI. *J Perinatol*. 2017;37(12):1278–1284.

37. Scott JA, Habas PA, Rajagopalan V, et al. Volumetric and surface-based 3D MRI analyses of fetal isolated mild ventriculomegaly: brain morphometry in ventriculomegaly. *Brain Struct Funct*. 2013;218(3):645–655.

38. Bouyssi-Kobar M, du Plessis AJ, McCarter R, et al. Third trimester brain growth in preterm infants compared with in utero healthy fetuses. *Pediatrics*. 2016;138(5).

39. Dubois J, Benders M, Borradori-Tolsa C, et al. Primary cortical folding in the human newborn: an early marker of later functional development. *Brain*. 2008;131(pt 8):2028–2041.

40. Fischl B, Rajendran N, Busa E, et al. Cortical folding patterns and predicting cytoarchitecture. *Cereb Cortex*. 2008;18(8):1973–1980.

41. Kostovic I, Judas M. Correlation between the sequential ingrowth of afferents and transient patterns of cortical lamination in preterm infants. *Anat Rec*. 2002;267(1):1–6.

42. Van Essen DC. A tension-based theory of morphogenesis and compact wiring in the central nervous system. *Nature*. 1997;385(6614):313–318.

43. Chi JG, Dooling EC, Gilles FH. Gyral development of the human brain. *Ann Neurol*. 1977;1(1):86–93.

44. Garel C, Chantrel E, Brisse H, et al. Fetal cerebral cortex: normal gestational landmarks identified using prenatal MR imaging. *AJNR Am J Neuroradiol*. 2001;22(1):184–189.

45. Batchelor PG, Castellano Smith AD, Hill DL, Hawkes DJ, Cox TC, Dean AF. Measures of folding applied to the development of the human fetal brain. *IEEE Trans Med Imaging*. 2002;21(8):953–965.

46. Hu HH, Guo WY, Chen HY, et al. Morphological regionalization using fetal magnetic resonance images of normal developing brains. *Eur J Neurosci*. 2009;29(6):1560–1567.

47. Wright R, Kyriakopoulou V, Ledig C, et al. Automatic quantification of normal cortical folding patterns from fetal brain MRI. *Neuroimage*. 2014;91:21–32.

48. Wu J, Awate SP, Licht DJ, et al. Assessment of MRI-based automated fetal cerebral cortical folding measures in prediction of gestational age in the third trimester. *AJNR Am J Neuroradiol*. 2015;36(7):1369–1374.

49. Benkarim OM, Hahner N, Piella G, et al. Cortical folding alterations in fetuses with isolated non-severe ventriculomegaly. *Neuroimage Clin*. 2018;18:103–114.

50. Im K, Guimaraes A, Kim Y, et al. Quantitative folding pattern analysis of early primary sulci in human fetuses with brain abnormalities. *AJNR Am J Neuroradiol*. 2017;38(7):1449–1455.

51. Agid R, Lieberman S, Nadjari M, Gomori JM. Prenatal MR diffusion-weighted imaging in a fetus with hemimegalencephaly. *Pediatr Radiol*. 2006;36(2):138–140.

52. Baldoli C, Righini A, Parazzini C, Scotti G, Triulzi F. Demonstration of acute ischemic lesions in the fetal brain by diffusion magnetic resonance imaging. *Ann Neurol*. 2002;52(2):243–246.

53. Brunel H, Girard N, Confort-Gouny S, et al. Fetal brain injury. *J Neuroradiol*. 2004;31(2):123–137.

54. Bui T, Daire JL, Chalard F, et al. Microstructural development of human brain assessed in utero by diffusion tensor imaging. *Pediatr Radiol*. 2006;36(11):1133–1140.

55. Kim DH, Chung S, Vigneron DB, Barkovich AJ, Glenn OA. Diffusion-weighted imaging of the fetal brain in vivo. *Magn Reson Med*. 2008;59(1):216–220.

56. Righini A, Bianchini E, Parazzini C, et al. Apparent diffusion coefficient determination in normal fetal brain: a prenatal MR imaging study. *AJNR Am J Neuroradiol*. 2003;24(5):799–804.

57. Manganaro L, Perrone A, Savelli S, et al. Evaluation of normal brain development by prenatal MR imaging. *Radiol Med*. 2007;112(3):444–455.

58. Schneider JF, Confort-Gouny S, Le Fur Y, et al. Diffusion-weighted imaging in normal fetal brain maturation. *Eur Radiol*. 2007;17(9):2422–2429.

59. Schneider MM, Berman JI, Baumer FM, et al. Normative apparent diffusion coefficient values in the developing fetal brain. *AJNR Am J Neuroradiol*. 2009;30(9):1799–1803.

60. Berman JI, Hamrick SE, McQuillen PS, et al. Diffusion-weighted imaging in fetuses with severe congenital heart defects. *AJNR Am J Neuroradiol*. 2011;32(2):E21–E22.

61. Ozcan UA, Isik U, Dincer A, Erzen C. Identification of fetal precentral gyrus on diffusion weighted MRI. *Brain Dev*. 2013;35(1):4–9.

62. Anjari M, Srinivasan L, Allsop JM, et al. Diffusion tensor imaging with tract-based spatial statistics reveals local white matter abnormalities in preterm infants. *Neuroimage*. 2007;35(3):1021–1027.

63. Basser PJ, Mattiello J, LeBihan D. MR diffusion tensor spectroscopy and imaging. *Biophys J*. 1994;66(1):259–267.

64. Huang H, Xue R, Zhang J, et al. Anatomical characterization of human fetal brain development with diffusion tensor magnetic resonance imaging. *J Neurosci*. 2009;29(13):4263–4273.

65. Huppi PS, Warfield S, Kikinis R, et al. Quantitative magnetic resonance imaging of brain development in premature and mature newborns. *Ann Neurol*. 1998;43(2):224–235.

66. Partridge SC, Mukherjee P, Henry RG, et al. Diffusion tensor imaging: serial quantitation of white matter tract maturity in premature newborns. *Neuroimage*. 2004;22(3):1302–1314.

67. Dubois J, Dehaene-Lambertz G, Soares C, Cointepas Y, Le Bihan D, Hertz-Pannier L. Microstructural correlates of infant functional development: example of the visual pathways. *J Neurosci*. 2008;28(8):1943–1948.

68. Jakab A, Kasprian G, Schwartz E, et al. Disrupted developmental organization of the structural connectome in fetuses with corpus callosum agenesis. *Neuroimage.* 2015;111:277–288.

69. Kasprian G, Brugger PC, Weber M, et al. In utero tractography of fetal white matter development. *Neuroimage.* 2008;43(2):213–224.

70. Khan S, Vasung L, Marami B, et al. Fetal brain growth portrayed by a spatiotemporal diffusion tensor MRI atlas computed from in utero images. *Neuroimage.* 2019;185:593–608.

71. Marami B, Mohseni Salehi SS, Afacan O, et al. Temporal slice registration and robust diffusion-tensor reconstruction for improved fetal brain structural connectivity analysis. *Neuroimage.* 2017;156:475–488.

72. Mitter C, Jakab A, Brugger PC, et al. Validation of in utero tractography of human fetal commissural and internal capsule fibers with histological structure tensor analysis. *Front Neuroanat.* 2015;9:164.

73. Mitter C, Kasprian G, Brugger PC, Prayer D. Three-dimensional visualization of fetal white-matter pathways in utero. *Ultrasound Obstet Gynecol.* 2011;37(2):252–253.

74. Song JW, Gruber GM, Patsch JM, Seidl R, Prayer D, Kasprian G. How accurate are prenatal tractography results? A postnatal in vivo follow-up study using diffusion tensor imaging. *Pediatr Radiol.* 2018;48(4):486–498.

75. Zanin E, Ranjeva JP, Confort-Gouny S, et al. White matter maturation of normal human fetal brain. An in vivo diffusion tensor tractography study. *Brain Behav.* 2011;1(2):95–108.

76. Andescavage N, Limperopoulos C, Evangelou I, Murnick J, du Plessis A. Pregnancy outcomes in two growth restricted fetuses with in utero cerebral lactate. *J Neonatal Perinatal Med.* 2015;8(3):269–273.

77. Borowska-Matwiejczuk K, Lemancewicz A, Tarasow E, et al. Assessment of fetal distress based on magnetic resonance examinations: preliminary report. *Acad Radiol.* 2003;10(11):1274–1282.

78. Story L, Damodaram MS, Allsop JM, et al. Brain metabolism in fetal intrauterine growth restriction: a proton magnetic resonance spectroscopy study. *Am J Obstet Gynecol.* 2011;205(5):483.e1–e8.

79. Wolfberg AJ, Robinson JN, Mulkern R, Rybicki F, du Plessis AJ. Identification of fetal cerebral lactate using magnetic resonance spectroscopy. *Am J Obstet Gynecol.* 2007;196(1):e9–e11.

80. Azpurua H, Alvarado A, Mayobre F, Salom T, Copel JA, Guevara-Zuloaga F. Metabolic assessment of the brain using proton magnetic resonance spectroscopy in a growth-restricted human fetus: case report. *Am J Perinatol.* 2008;25(5):305–309.

81. Berger-Kulemann V, Brugger PC, Pugash D, et al. MR spectroscopy of the fetal brain: is it possible without sedation? *AJNR Am J Neuroradiol.* 2013;34(2):424–431.

82. Fenton BW, Lin CS, Macedonia C, Schellinger D, Ascher S. The fetus at term: in utero volume-selected proton MR spectroscopy with a breath-hold technique—a feasibility study. *Radiology.* 2001;219(2):563–566.

83. Kok RD, van den Berg PP, van den Bergh AJ, Nijland R, Heerschap A. Maturation of the human fetal brain as observed by 1H MR spectroscopy. *Magn Reson Med.* 2002;48(4):611–616.

84. Kok RD, van den Bergh AJ, Heerschap A, Nijland R, van den Berg PP. Metabolic information from the human fetal brain obtained with proton magnetic resonance spectroscopy. *Am J Obstet Gynecol.* 2001;185(5):1011–1015.

85. Evangelou IE, du Plessis AJ, Vezina G, Noeske R, Limperopoulos C. Elucidating metabolic maturation in the healthy fetal brain using 1H-MR spectroscopy. *AJNR Am J Neuroradiol.* 2016;37(2):360–366.

86. Sanz-Cortes M, Egana-Ugrinovic G, Simoes RV, Vazquez L, Bargallo N, Gratacos E. Association of brain metabolism with sulcation and corpus callosum development assessed by MRI in late-onset small fetuses. *Am J Obstet Gynecol.* 2015;212(6):804.e1–e8.

87. Blum T, Saling E, Bauer R. First magnetoencephalographic recordings of the brain activity of a human fetus. *Br J Obstet Gynaecol.* 1985;92(12):1224–1229.

88. Eswaran H, Wilson J, Preissl H, et al. Magnetoencephalographic recordings of visual evoked brain activity in the human fetus. *Lancet.* 2002;360(9335):779–780.

89. Lengle JM, Chen M, Wakai RT. Improved neuromagnetic detection of fetal and neonatal auditory evoked responses. *Clin Neurophysiol.* 2001;112(5):785–792.

90. Preissl H, Lowery CL, Eswaran H. Fetal magnetoencephalography: current progress and trends. *Exp Neurol.* 2004;190 suppl 1:S28–S36.

91. Hykin J, Moore R, Duncan K, et al. Fetal brain activity demonstrated by functional magnetic resonance imaging. *Lancet.* 1999;354(9179):645–646.

92. Jardri R, Pins D, Houfflin-Debarge V, et al. Fetal cortical activation to sound at 33 weeks of gestation: a functional MRI study. *Neuroimage.* 2008;42(1):10–18.

93. Moore RJ, Vadeyar S, Fulford J, et al. Antenatal determination of fetal brain activity in response to an acoustic stimulus using functional magnetic resonance imaging. *Hum Brain Mapp.* 2001;12(2):94–99.

94. Fulford J, Vadeyar SH, Dodampahala SH, et al. Fetal brain activity and hemodynamic response to a vibroacoustic stimulus. *Hum Brain Mapp.* 2004;22(2):116–121.

95. Fulford J, Vadeyar SH, Dodampahala SH, et al. Fetal brain activity in response to a visual stimulus. *Hum Brain Mapp.* 2003;20(4):239–245.

96. Schopf V, Kasprian G, Brugger PC, Prayer D. Watching the fetal brain at 'rest'. *Int J Dev Neurosci.* 2012;30(1):11–17.

97. Thomason ME, Dassanayake MT, Shen S, et al. Cross-hemispheric functional connectivity in the human fetal brain. *Sci Transl Med.* 2013;5(173):173ra24.

98. van den Heuvel MI, Thomason ME. Functional connectivity of the human brain in utero. *Trends Cogn Sci.* 2016;20(12):931–939.

99. Biswal BB, Van Kylen J, Hyde JS. Simultaneous assessment of flow and BOLD signals in resting-state functional connectivity maps. *NMR Biomed.* 1997;10(4–5):165–170.

100. Mak LE, Minuzzi L, MacQueen G, Hall G, Kennedy SH, Milev R. The default mode network in healthy individuals: a systematic review and meta-analysis. *Brain Connect.* 2017;7(1):25–33.

101. Thomason ME, Grove LE, Lozon TA Jr, et al. Age-related increases in long-range connectivity in fetal functional neural connectivity networks in utero. *Dev Cogn Neurosci.* 2015;11:96–104.

102. Thomason ME, Scheinost D, Manning JH, et al. Weak functional connectivity in the human fetal brain prior to preterm birth. *Sci Rep.* 2017;7:39286.

103. Prechtl HF, Einspieler C. Is neurological assessment of the fetus possible? *Eur J Obstet Gynecol Reprod Biol.* 1997;75(1):81–84.

104. Olesen AG, Svare JA. Decreased fetal movements: background, assessment, and clinical management. *Acta Obstet Gynecol Scand.* 2004;83(9):818–826.

105. Guo WY, Ono S, Oi S, et al. Dynamic motion analysis of fetuses with central nervous system disorders by cine magnetic resonance imaging using fast imaging employing steady-state acquisition and parallel imaging: a preliminary result. *J Neurosurg.* 2006;105(2 suppl):94–100.

106. Hayat TT, Nihat A, Martinez-Biarge M, et al. Optimization and initial experience of a multisection balanced steady-state free precession cine sequence for the assessment of fetal behavior in utero. *AJNR Am J Neuroradiol.* 2011;32(2):331–338.

107. Hayat TTA, Martinez-Biarge M, Kyriakopoulou V, Hajnal JV, Rutherford MA. Neurodevelopmental correlates of fetal motor behavior assessed using cine MR imaging. *AJNR Am J Neuroradiol.* 2018;39(8):1519–1522.

108. De Bonis M, Torricelli M, Severi FM, Luisi S, De Leo V, Petraglia F. Neuroendocrine aspects of placenta and pregnancy. *Gynecol Endocrinol.* 2012;28 suppl 1:22–26.

109. Derwig IE, Akolekar R, Zelaya FO, Gowland PA, Barker GJ, Nicolaides KH. Association of placental volume measured by MRI and birth weight percentile. *J Magn Reson Imaging.* 2011;34(5):1125–1130.

110. Messerschmidt A, Baschat A, Linduska N, et al. Magnetic resonance imaging of the placenta identifies placental vascular abnormalities independently of Doppler ultrasound. *Ultrasound Obstet Gynecol.* 2011;37(6):717–722.

111. Anblagan D, Jones NW, Costigan C, et al. Maternal smoking during pregnancy and fetal organ growth: a magnetic resonance imaging study. *PLoS One.* 2013;8(7):e67223.

112. Javor D, Nasel C, Schweim T, Dekan S, Chalubinski K, Prayer D. In vivo assessment of putative functional placental tissue volume in placental intrauterine growth restriction (IUGR) in human fetuses using diffusion tensor magnetic resonance imaging. *Placenta.* 2013;34(8):676–680.

113. Andescavage N, Yarish A, Donofrio M, et al. 3-D volumetric MRI evaluation of the placenta in fetuses with complex congenital heart disease. *Placenta.* 2015;36(9):1024–1030.

114. Di Cataldo S, Ficarra E. Mining textural knowledge in biological images: applications, methods and trends. *Comput Struct Biotechnol J.* 2017;15:56–67.

115. Andescavage N, Dahdouh S, Jacobs M, et al. In vivo textural and morphometric analysis of placental development in healthy & growth-restricted pregnancies using magnetic resonance imaging. *Pediatr Res.* 2019;85:974–981.

116. Dahdouh S, Andescavage N, Yewale S, et al. In vivo placental MRI shape and textural features predict fetal growth restriction and postnatal outcome. *J Magn Reson Imaging.* 2018;47(2):449–458.

117. Morita S, Ueno E, Fujimura M, Muraoka M, Takagi K, Fujibayashi M. Feasibility of diffusion-weighted MRI for defining placental invasion. *J Magn Reson Imaging.* 2009;30(3):666–671.

118. Bonel HM, Stolz B, Diedrichsen L, et al. Diffusion-weighted MR imaging of the placenta in fetuses with placental insufficiency. *Radiology.* 2010;257(3):810–819.

119. Fu L, Zhang J, Xiong S, Sun M. Decreased apparent diffusion coefficient in the placentas of monochorionic twins with selective intrauterine growth restriction. *Placenta.* 2018;69:26–31.

120. Capuani S, Guerreri M, Antonelli A, et al. Diffusion and perfusion quantified by Magnetic Resonance Imaging are markers of human placenta development in normal pregnancy. *Placenta.* 2017;58:33–39.

121. Siauve N, Hayot PH, Deloison B, et al. Assessment of human placental perfusion by intravoxel incoherent motion MR imaging. *J Matern Fetal Neonatal Med.* 2019;32(2):293–300.

122. Sohlberg S, Mulic-Lutvica A, Lindgren P, Ortiz-Nieto F, Wikstrom AK, Wikstrom J. Placental perfusion in normal pregnancy and early and late preeclampsia: a magnetic resonance imaging study. *Placenta.* 2014;35(3):202–206.

123. Moore RJ, Issa B, Tokarczuk P, et al. In vivo intravoxel incoherent motion measurements in the human placenta using echo-planar imaging at 0.5 T. *Magn Reson Med.* 2000;43(2):295–302.

124. Moore RJ, Strachan BK, Tyler DJ, et al. In utero perfusing fraction maps in normal and growth restricted pregnancy measured using IVIM echo-planar MRI. *Placenta.* 2000;21(7):726–732.

125. Derwig I, Barker GJ, Poon L, et al. Association of placental T2 relaxation times and uterine artery Doppler ultrasound measures of placental blood flow. *Placenta*. 2013;34(6):474–479.

126. Zun Z, Zaharchuk G, Andescavage NN, Donofrio MT, Limperopoulos C. Non-invasive placental perfusion imaging in pregnancies complicated by fetal heart disease using velocity-selective arterial spin labeled MRI. *Sci Rep*. 2017;7(1):16126.

127. Huen I, Morris DM, Wright C, et al. R1 and R2 * changes in the human placenta in response to maternal oxygen challenge. *Magn Reson Med*. 2013;70(5): 1427–1433.

128. Sorensen A, Peters D, Simonsen C, et al. Changes in human fetal oxygenation during maternal hyperoxia as estimated by BOLD MRI. *Prenat Diagn*. 2013;33(2):141–145.

129. Luo J, Abaci Turk E, Bibbo C, et al. In vivo quantification of placental insufficiency by BOLD MRI: a human study. *Sci Rep*. 2017;7(1):3713.

130. Denison FC, Semple SI, Stock SJ, Walker J, Marshall I, Norman JE. Novel use of proton magnetic resonance spectroscopy (1HMRS) to non-invasively assess placental metabolism. *PLoS One*. 2012;7(8):e42926.

131. Song F, Wu W, Qian Z, Zhang G, Cheng Y. Assessment of the placenta in intrauterine growth restriction by diffusion-weighted imaging and proton magnetic resonance spectroscopy. *Reprod Sci*. 2017;24(4):575–581.

11 Fetal Cardiovascular Magnetic Resonance

Mike T. M. Seed • Davide Marini

In recent years, technological advances have resulted in acquisition of high spatial and temporal resolution cardiac magnetic resonance (CMR) imaging in the fetus. Fetal CMR has emerged as an alternative to ultrasound, which may be helpful to confirm a diagnosis of congenital heart disease (CHD) when the ultrasound assessment is limited by poor acoustic windows, for example, in late gestation or in the setting of oligohydramnios. Magnetic resonance imaging (MRI) also provides unique physiologic information, including vessel blood flow, oxygen saturation, and hematocrit, which may be helpful to investigate fetal cardiovascular, hematological, and placental conditions. In this chapter, we summarize some of the main techniques employed in fetal CMR, describe some of settings in which it has been used, and consider what other clinical applications may emerge in the future.

BACKGROUND

Over the past four decades, CMR has gained increasing importance as a useful noninvasive adjunct for the assessment of the cardiovascular system in adults and children.[1,2] Popular CMR techniques include the quantification of cardiac chamber volumes, vascular flow measurements, three-dimensional angiography, and myocardial tissue characterization. In prenatal patients, ultrasound has remained the mainstay of cardiovascular imaging, with initial attempts to explore the feasibility of fetal CMR hampered by technical limitations.[3–5] However, in concert with other rapidly evolving imaging and laboratory techniques for prenatal diagnosis, innovative new fetal CMR techniques have overcome many of the technical challenges involved in imaging the fetal cardiovascular system, prompting an increasing number of groups to investigate the potential clinical utility of this imaging modality as an adjunct to ultrasound. Fetal CMR can now precisely define cardiac anatomy and is currently being used in some centers to define fetal cardiac malformations when a comprehensive diagnosis cannot be achieved using ultrasound.[6–8] Cardiac MRI also provides a unique opportunity to collect information about the impact of cardiac malformations and placental dysfunction on fetal cardiovascular physiology. Cine phase-contrast analysis is the noninvasive gold standard technique for the measurement of vessel blood flow in postnatal subjects. Similarly, MRI is better suited to quantifying blood flow in the major fetal arteries and veins than is ultrasound due to the intrinsic nature of the technique, which accounts for the different flow velocities across the vessel lumen.[9,10] Moreover, by exploiting the paramagnetic effect of deoxyhemoglobin on T2 relaxation, MRI can provide direct information about fetal oxygenation, while diffusion-weighted imaging and magnetic resonance (MR) spectroscopy offer the potential to evaluate cerebral tissue microstructure and metabolism.[11–13] Pre- and postnatal brain imaging incorporating these quantitative techniques has been used to explore the impact of fetal CHD and intrauterine growth restriction (IUGR) on brain development *in utero*.[12,13] Many of these MRI applications are currently mainly being undertaken in the setting of perinatal research. However, with the current rapid growth of fetal therapy, it seems likely that in the future more sophisticated fetal imaging methods will play an increasingly important role in the diagnosis and management of fetal conditions.

FETAL CARDIAC MRI METHODS

To image the fetal heart using MRI, a number of problems must be addressed. With average fetal heart rates of 140 to 150 beats/minute and a total length of between 2 and 4 cm depending on gestational age, there are increased requirements for spatial and temporal resolution. Meanwhile, the usual approach to overcoming cardiac motion, which is to use the electrocardiographic signal to "trigger" or "gate" the acquisition, is not readily available in the case of the fetus, due to interference from maternal cardiac electrical activity. Even when an alternative system for cardiac triggering can be applied, fetal body movements and maternal respiration can significantly degrade image quality.

Static Imaging of the Fetal Thorax and Heart

Two of the most popular pulse sequences used in fetal MRI studies of the brain and body are single-shot T2 fast spin-echo (SS-T2-FSE) and steady-state free precession (SSFP). Using single-shot T2 fast spin echo with half Fourier reconstruction, a high-resolution image of the fetus can be acquired within 2 seconds, and this approach provides excellent contrast between the vessels, which appear black due to the loss of any signal from flowing blood and surrounding structures such as the lungs, which are bright.[14] However, to achieve images that depict the intracardiac anatomy, a "bright blood" sequence such as SSFP is the best option since this provides good contrast between the myocardium and blood and has the shortest repetition time, allowing for a single slice to be acquired in approximately 1 second. Examples of these sequences with some proposed imaging parameters are listed in Table 11.1.[15] Although some detail regarding cardiac anatomy can be achieved with static nongated static SSFP images, artifacts do arise from cardiac motion. Thus, for high-quality anatomical imaging that also provides information about cardiac function, a system for cardiac triggering is required.

High-Resolution Cine Imaging of the Fetal Heart

Over the past decade, a series of technical innovations have resulted in steady progress toward the routine acquisition of high-quality cine CMR in the fetus. In 2010, an artificial cardiac triggering, or "gating" system, called metric optimized gating (MOG), was developed for use in the fetus.[16] MOG involves the acquisition of k-space data for cine imaging using a synthetic trigger that is deliberately arranged to have a longer R–R interval than that expected in the fetal subject. Hypothetic trigger locations are then retrospectively applied to the data, until an image metric identifies the correct average fetal heart rate present during the acquisition by selecting the reconstruction with least artifacts in the resulting images (Fig. 11.1). MOG algorithms have

Oversampled Data Acquisition

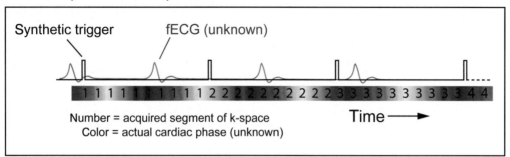

Iterative Reconstruction

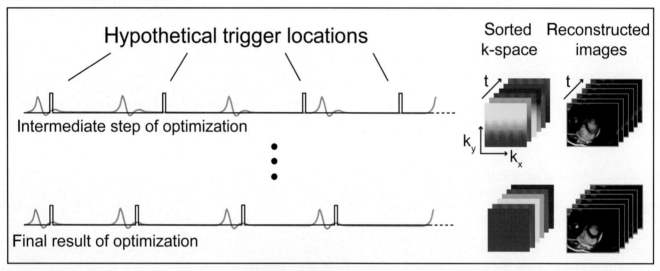

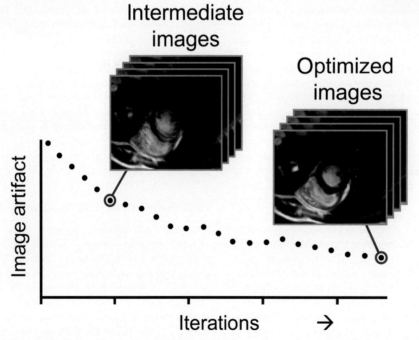

FIGURE 11.1: Metric optimized gating. A synthetic trigger with longer R–R interval is used to acquire the k-space data. Hypothetic trigger locations are then retrospectively applied to the data and iteratively reconstructed with the correct average R–R interval identified as the reconstruction with the least image artifact.

been developed for cine phase-contrast flow measurements and for anatomical imaging of the beating heart.[8,9,11,17] The MOG reconstruction algorithm is available as an open-source software for use with one of the commercial vendor MRI systems (http://metricoptimizedgating.github.io/MOG-Public), and its accuracy and reproducibility have recently been validated by an independent group.[18] However, although MOG overcomes cardiac motion, it does not address fetal or maternal body motion. In order to minimize artifacts resulting from fetal and maternal movements, additional approaches have been deployed. These can be summarized as methods designed to accelerate the acquisition and approaches to correcting for fetal motion. The use of an undersampling approach known as compressed sensing can result in a dramatic reduction in scan time, providing excellent agreement between the fully sampled and retrospectively undersampled reconstructions of Cartesian data with acceleration factors of up to 4.[19] In addition, the use of a golden-angle radial acquisition combined with compressed sensing yields acceleration factors of up to 16.[19–23] Fetal data are acquired using a continuous golden-angle radial trajectory, while preliminary time-averaged reconstructions for each slice are used to confirm slice prescription and provide an initial assessment of gross fetal movement. Following the MRI examination, offline real-time reconstruction of the data enables assessment and correction of translational in-plane motion and rejection of through-plane motion and calculation of the fetal heart rate using MOG.[24–26] The motion and gating information are then used to reconstruct high-resolution cine imaging.[26] Both real-time and cine reconstructions of the data rely on compressed sensing to suppress streaking artifacts from radial undersampling and provide acceleration factors of up to 27.[10,26] This technique has also recently been used to implement phase-contrast fetal blood flow analysis, reducing scan time and the need to repeat phase-contrast flow acquisitions because of excessive artifacts.[27] Using a novel phase-contrast MR acquisition scheme with golden-angle radial sampling while continuously updating the velocity encode, a pipeline similar to the one described previously has achieved the first motion-corrected multidimensional flow measurement in the fetus, allowing for a more comprehensive assessment of intracardiac flow patterns.[27]

Doppler Ultrasound Gated Fetal Cardiovascular MR

An alternative technology for obtaining triggered acquisitions involves measurement of the fetal cardiac cycle using a Doppler ultrasound transducer placed over the maternal abdomen.[28] This portable Doppler ultrasound cardiotocographic gating device has proved to be safe, MRI compatible, and reliable at different field strengths when applied in human fetuses.[29,30] Dynamic fetal cardiac four-chamber cardiac imaging acquired using cardiotocographic gating has been used to evaluate the cardiac anatomy in fetuses with CHD, yielding good agreement with fetal echocardiography in terms of the dimensions of structures and cardiac diagnosis.[31]

FETAL CMR AS AN ADJUNCT TO FETAL ECHOCARDIOGRAPHY

Transabdominal echocardiography is the cornerstone of fetal cardiovascular assessment throughout pregnancy. However, it may be limited by fetal position, oligohydramnios, overlying bone,

and obesity. The diagnostic role of fetal MRI, as a complementary tool when the ultrasound is hampered by inadequate acoustic window, has recently been proposed by several groups.[7,32–36] In a prospective single-center study, a combination of SSFP and (SS-T2-FSE) sequences identified the same diagnosis as postnatal findings in 79% of fetuses with CHD at a mean gestational age of 25.5 weeks.[32] The diagnosis established with both ultrasound and fetal CMR were incorrect when compared with postnatal diagnosis in just 2/68 (3%) of cases. In 10 (15%) cases, the diagnosis at echocardiography was incorrect but correct by MRI. In 12 (18%) cases, the diagnosis by echocardiography was correct and by MRI was incorrect.[32]

Other researchers have investigated the clinical utility of fetal cardiac MRI at a mean gestational age of 32 weeks (range 26 to 38 weeks) to clarify the diagnosis when the echocardiography assessment was not exhaustive.[7] The majority of referrals were for suspected vascular abnormalities (17/22), particularly those involving the aortic arch ($n = 10$) and pulmonary vessels ($n = 4$). SS-T2-FSE sequences produced "black-blood" images, useful for examining the extracardiac vasculature in these cases. SSFP sequences were more useful for intracardiac structures. Real-time SSFP allowed for dynamic assessment of structures such as cardiac masses, with MRI signal relaxation patterns also allowing for tissue characterization in these cases.[7]

In a retrospective review of a large series of 7,282 fetal CMR examinations performed from June 2006 to March 2017, nine cases of anomalous courses of the left brachiocephalic vein (LBCV), including two retroesophageal LBCV, were correctly diagnosed by fetal CMR.[33] One case of an abnormal retroaortic LBCV was missed by fetal CMR and identified postnatally during further imaging for the associated tetralogy of Fallot. Prenatal cardiac ultrasound correctly diagnosed five cases of retroaortic and one retroesophageal LBCV as well as the associated intracardiac anomalies.[33] In a single-center series of 23 aortic arch anomalies, the accuracy of fetal cardiac MRI was 95.6%, which was significantly higher than that of standard ultrasound (60.8%).[35]

Three-dimensional volume-rendering reconstructions derived from postnatal computed tomography (CT) and MRI have been used in clinical practice for at least 40 years. Recently, MRI data were acquired in 85 fetuses, as overlapping stacks of standard 2D SS-T2-FSE images. These images were then processed with an open-source reconstruction algorithm including motion correction to produce a high-resolution three-dimensional volume of the fetal thorax. The imaging produced showed good spatial agreement with ultrasound, and significantly improved visualization and diagnostic quality compared with source 2D MRI data, providing an additional diagnostic tool.[37]

Although fetal CMR has not been shown to provide useful diagnostic information early in the second trimester, when decision-making about the continuation of a pregnancy affected by CHD in the fetus typically takes place, these clinical studies perhaps provide an indication of how MRI might find a role as an adjunct to the routine ultrasound examination in the diagnosis of CHD in the future. This has been particularly valuable in the last weeks of pregnancy, when the acoustic window usually worsens, for example, in an unusual case of a right ventricular diverticulum with pulmonary stenosis and an inlet ventricular septal defect (Fig. 11.2).

In a recent case of a giant rhabdomyoma, fetal CMR allowed for a superior assessment of the patency of the left ventricular outflow tract and provided an accurate measurement of the

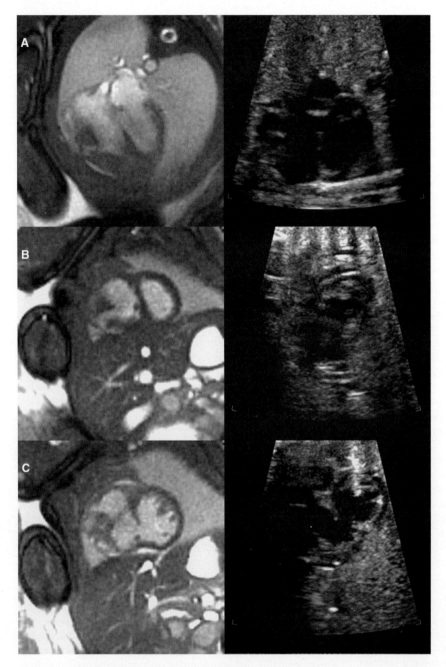

FIGURE 11.2: Anatomical imaging with fetal cine CMR compared with echocardiography in late gestation. **A.** Four chamber view showing a right ventricular diverticulum. **B.** Short-axis view at the level of the diverticulum. **C.** Basal short axis showing the inlet ventricular septal defect.

volume of the mass.[38] In complex cases such as these, MRI may also provide additional relevant information regarding extra-cardiac malformations. For example, in the rhabdomyoma case described, dedicated fetal brain sequences revealed multiple cerebral masses, as are typically seen in tuberous sclerosis. Additional information regarding lung pathology, including the pulmonary lymphangiectasia seen in the setting of pulmonary venous obstruction (Fig. 11.3) or the airway compression and lung hyperinflation seen in tetralogy of Fallot with absent pulmonary valve (Fig. 11.4), may be very relevant in perinatal clinical decision-making.[39-44]

MR OXIMETRY

The dependence of the transverse relaxation time (T2 and T2*) of blood on the oxygenation state of hemoglobin in erythrocytes

was discovered in the 1980s by MRI spectroscopy at high field strength.[45,46] A decade later, the extravascular T2* imaging characteristics of the blood oxygenation effect was identified, and associated with modifications of regional cerebral function.[47,48] This observation is referred to as the blood oxygenation level–dependent (BOLD) contrast, and was successively recognized to be the pivotal mechanism of localized MR signal changes associated with local brain function.[49] This connection opened the door to functional brain MRI, which has revolutionized human neuroscience, and aided in neurosurgical planning. Similarly, the BOLD signal has been measured in human and animal fetuses to compare tissue oxygenation in various fetal organs at baseline and during episodes of hypoxia and hyperoxia.[50,51]

While the BOLD signal is robust and provides information about tissue oxygenation, particularly in terms of showing a response to a provocative challenge, it does not provide truly

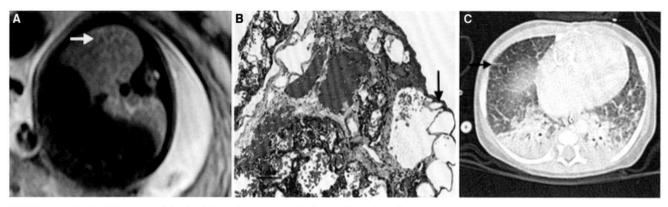

FIGURE 11.3: **A:** Axial T2 image of the fetal chest demonstrates high-signal branching linear structures extending to the surface of the lung (*arrow*) suggestive of pulmonary lymphangiectasia. **B:** The diagnosis was confirmed by lung biopsy showing dilated lymphatics (*arrow*). **C:** Postnatal high-resolution computed tomography in this patient, showing thickening of the interlobular septae (*arrow*).

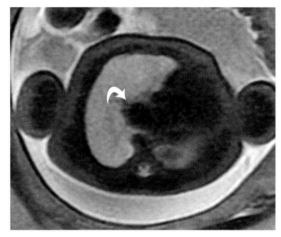

FIGURE 11.4: Tetralogy of Fallot with absent pulmonary valve. Axial T2 image through the thorax demonstrates hyperinflation of the right lung, which is high in signal with deviation of the heart to the left. The left lung is small and darker in signal. The pulmonary artery is prominent (*arrow*).

quantitative data regarding blood oxygen content and saturation. However, by measuring the T2 of blood within vessels, it is possible to estimate oxygen saturation. The accuracy of this approach is dependent on a reliable value for hemoglobin concentration or hematocrit (Hct), although it is possible to estimate both oxygen saturation and hemoglobin concentration by acquiring a combination of T1 and T2 measurements of blood. The T2 of blood is primarily determined by its oxygen saturation, although this relationship is dependent on the magnetic field strength, the refocusing interval of the T2 preparation pulse used to quantify T2, and hemoglobin concentration, with increases in hematocrit resulting in a T2 shortening effect.[52,53] By contrast, the T1 of blood is more strongly related to hematocrit, with higher Hct associated with a shortening of T1, although this relationship is also influenced by oxygen saturation. Using cubic polynomial equations, it is possible to calculate both the oxygen saturation and Hct of the blood in a vessel by measuring the T1 and T2 of the blood. Blood oxygen content then is the product of oxygen saturation and hemoglobin concentration:

$$Oxygen\ content = Oxygen\ saturation \times Hemoglobin$$
$$concentration \times 1.36$$

where 1.36 is the number of milliliters of oxygen bound to 1 g of hemoglobin at 1 atm.[54,55] This calculation ignores the amount of oxygen dissolved in plasma, which is negligible in the fetus. The combination of this method for measuring blood oxygen content with cine phase-contrast flow quantification provides a unique approach to measuring oxygen transport in fetal vessels.[55]

Early applications of MR oximetry included the quantification of postnatal cerebral oxygen consumption using the Fick principle, which measures cerebral oxygen consumption by combining a measurement of cerebral blood flow with arterial and venous oxygen saturation.[56] Cerebral venous oxygen saturation (SaO_2) has usually been quantified by interrogating the superior sagittal sinus.[57] Oxygen content in the umbilical vein and descending aorta can be used to calculate fetal oxygen delivery (DO_2) and consumption (VO_2) as follows:

$$Fetal\ DO_2 = UV\ flow \times UV\ SaO_2 \times 1.36 \times Hb/100$$

$$Fetal\ VO_2 = UV\ flow \times (UV\ SaO_2 - DAO$$
$$SaO_2) \times 1.36 \times Hb/100$$

Similarly, oxygen content in the ascending aorta and superior vena cava and superior vena cava flow can be used to approximate cerebral oxygen delivery:

$$Cerebral\ DO_2 = SVC\ flow \times AAO\ SaO_2 \times 1.36 \times Hb/100$$
$$Cerebral\ VO_2 = SVC\ flow \times (AAO\ SaO_2 - SVC$$
$$SaO_2) \times 1.36 \times Hb/100$$

Initial attempts to perform fetal MR oximetry employed prior calibration data derived from *in vitro* experiments using adult blood to derive the relationship between T2 and oxygen saturation. However, these relationships are not necessarily applicable to fetal blood, which differs from its adult counterpart in several respects. Specifically, fetal blood is rich in the fetal form of hemoglobin (HbF), which has a greater affinity for oxygen, and this facilitates the transfer of oxygen from maternal to fetal blood within the placenta.[55] In addition, fetal erythrocytes are 20% larger and 50% less permeable to water, while fetal plasma is less viscous (by 20% at late gestation), due to a lower protein concentration.[55,57] In recognition that these differences are likely to affect MRI relaxation properties, the relationships between fetal blood relaxation times and SaO_2 and Hct at 1.5 and 3T have been characterized using umbilical cord blood samples harvested from elective human caesarean deliveries. This approach has confirmed the reliability of a method for calculating Hct and SaO$_2$ that is based on measurements of the T1 and T2 relaxation times of fetal blood.[53,58,59]

HEMODYNAMICS OF THE HUMAN FETAL CIRCULATION BY CMR

The first phase-contrast MRI measurements of the distribution of blood flow in the late-gestation human fetus have been obtained using MOG. The results are in keeping with prior animal and human ultrasound studies showing that the fetal circulation operates in parallel with shunts at the foramen ovale and ductus arteriosus.[9] Reference ranges for phase-contrast measured flows in the major fetal vessels of the late-gestation human fetus have since been established.[10] Other studies have investigated fetal blood flow distribution in fetuses with different forms of CHD and in those with late-onset IUGR, demonstrating a link between fetal blood flow distribution and postnatal course, and exploring the relationship between fetal hemodynamics with lung and brain development.[12,41,60] With the development of fetal MR oximetry using T2 mapping, it has become possible to estimate the oxygen saturations in the different extracardiac vessels and define the entire circulatory system of normal fetuses and those with various forms of CHD and IUGR.[11] Using this approach, it has been possible to confirm the presence of streaming in the human fetal circulation, whereby oxygenated blood returning to the heart from the placenta via the umbilical vein and ductus venosus is preferentially directed toward the foramen ovale and left heart, while more desaturated blood returning from the upper and lower body venous system passes from the right atrium into the right ventricle (Fig. 11.5). Thus, the most metabolically active fetal organs, the brain and heart, are supplied with a reliable source of oxygen, while the desaturated blood returning

from fetal organs is directed back to the placenta. Virtually all important CHD subtypes interrupt this streaming mechanism leading to desaturation of the blood supplied to the developing brain. In fetuses with more severe forms of CHD collectively referred to as single-ventricle physiology, further reductions in fetal oxygenation result from diminished combined ventricular output and umbilical blood flow. A modest reduction in umbilical venous oxygen saturation also points to subtle placental dysfunction in pregnancies affected by fetal CHD. In pregnancies affected by CHD and IUGR, reductions in fetal oxygen delivery and ascending aortic saturation are usually offset by some degree of cerebral vasodilation and increased cerebral blood flow. This mechanism, often referred to as "brain-sparing physiology," may protect the brain against hypoxic ischemic injury but is associated with reductions in brain growth and maturation, although the long-term neurodevelopmental consequences of this remain uncertain.[11,12]

The recognition that neurodevelopmental disorders in children with CHD may have their origins in the prenatal period has led to interest in the potential of fetal interventions to improve *in utero* brain development. Acute maternal hyperoxygenation in human fetuses with and without CHD results in increased oxygen saturations in the umbilical vein and increased pulmonary blood flow, and studies are currently under way to investigate the potential neuroprotective efficacy of chronic transplacental oxygen therapy in fetuses with single-ventricle CHD.[61] Fetal CMR has recently confirmed a positive hemodynamic influence of ductal constriction induced with nonsteroidal anti-inflammatory drugs for the treatment of fetal circular shunting in severe forms of Ebstein anomaly and tricuspid valve dysplasia.[62] Left atrial decompression by radiofrequency perforation septostomy with/without stenting of the atrial septum is

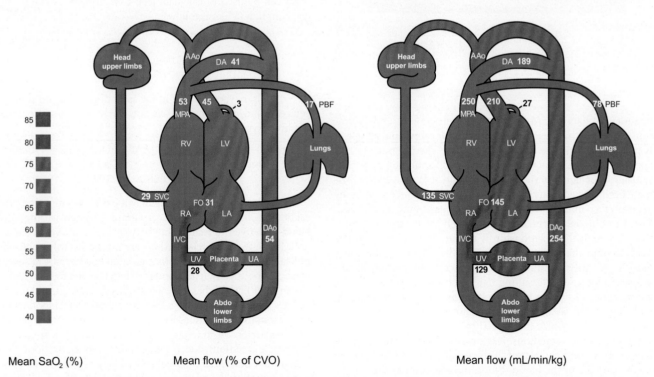

FIGURE 11.5: Mean flows and oxygen saturations in the late-gestation human fetus by magnetic resonance imaging. Mean flows as percentage of the combined ventricular output (CVO) (*left*) and in mL/min/kg (*right*). AAo, ascending aorta; DA, ductus arteriosus; MPA, main pulmonary artery; RV, right ventricle; LV, left ventricle; SVC, superior vena cava; FO, foramen ovale; LA, left atrium; PBF, pulmonary blood flow; RA, right atrium; IVC, inferior vena cava; UV, umbilical vein; UA, umbilical vein; DAo, descending aorta.

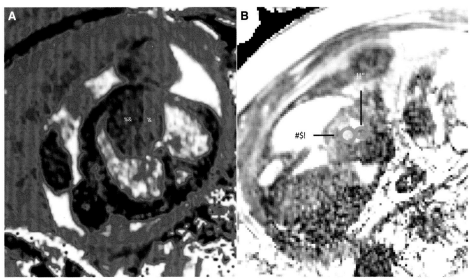

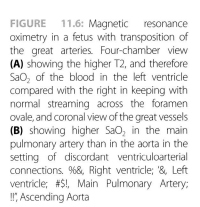

FIGURE 11.6: Magnetic resonance oximetry in a fetus with transposition of the great arteries. Four-chamber view **(A)** showing the higher T2, and therefore SaO$_2$ of the blood in the left ventricle compared with the right in keeping with normal streaming across the foramen ovale, and coronal view of the great vessels **(B)** showing higher SaO$_2$ in the main pulmonary artery than in the aorta in the setting of discordant ventriculoarterial connections. %&, Right ventricle; '&, Left ventricle; #$!, Main Pulmonary Artery; !!', Ascending Aorta

now an option for fetuses with hypoplastic left heart syndrome with pulmonary vein Doppler evidence of left atrial hypertension secondary to an intact or highly restrictive atrial septum.[63] Fetal MRI has become part of pre- and postintervention assessment in this setting, particularly when there is uncertainty about the severity of pulmonary venous obstruction, as it identifies secondary pulmonary lymphangiectasia[41,42,63] (Fig. 11.3).

Newborns with transposition of the great arteries may also be at high risk for hypoxic ischemic injury or demise in the delivery room because of an intact or highly restrictive atrial septum, and this has led to exploration of the utility of fetal atrial septostomy prior to birth in selected cases.[64,65] Fetal CMR may be helpful to exclude significant atrial septal restriction using

MR oximetry. The finding of higher oxygen saturations in the left ventricle compared to that in the right is in keeping with the expected preferential streaming of oxygenated blood across a patent foramen ovale, which may predict stable oxygenation following birth (Fig. 11.6).

APPROACH TO PERFORMING A FETAL CMR EXAMINATION

As previously described, there are now many MRI sequences available for imaging the fetal heart (Table 11.1). The examination should be tailored to the main goal of the study, prioritizing those acquisitions most essential to the specific objective.

TABLE 11.1   Imaging Parameters for Fetal Cardiovascular MRI

SEQUENCE	TYPE	ECG TRIGGER	RESP.	PARALLEL IMAGING FACTOR	NSA	TE (ms)	TR (ms)	SLICE THICK (mm)	MATRIX SIZE	FOV (mm)	TEMP. RESOL. (ms)	SCAN TIME (S)
3D-SSFP	3D	—	Breath-hold	2	1	1.74	3.99	2	256 × 205 × 80	400	—	13
Static SSFP	2D	—	Free breathing	—	1	1.3	6.33	4	320 × 211	350	1,336	24 (15 slices)
Cine SSFP	2D	MOG[a]	Free breathing	2	1	1.26	3.04	5	340 × 310	340	46	55 (10 slices)
Phase contrast[b]	2D	MOG[a]	Free breathing	—	1	3.15	6.78	3	240 × 240	240	54	36
T2 mapping[c]	2D	PG	Free breathing	2	1	1.15	3.97	6	224 × 136	350	4,000	16
T1 mapping[d]	2D	PG	Free breathing	2	1	1.15	3.97	6	224 × 136	350	4,000	16

[a]R–R interval 545 ms.
[b]Velocity encoding sensitivity: arteries 150 cm/s, veins 100 cm/s, umbilical vein 50 cm/s. Segments per cardiac cycle: 4.
[c]T2 mapping: five preparation times (0 ms, 0.33 × T2, 0.66*T2, 1.00*T2, 1.33*T2) with 4,000 ms of magnetization recovery between the T2 preparations.
[d]The start time and inversion time increment for the T1 sequence were 100 and 400 ms, respectively.
FOV, field of view; MOG, metric optimized gating; NSA, number of signal average; PG, pseudogating; SSFP, steady-state free precession; TE, echo time; TR, repetition time.

Despite technological advances, gross fetal movements are still a major problem and these are unpredictable and may appear suddenly. One approach is to start with a stack of parallel static SSFP images of the fetal thorax in the three standard planes shown in Figure 11.7. These are useful to prescribe the phase-contrast and oximetry sequences shown in the figure when a hemodynamic assessment is required. An open-source software to measure T1 and T2 is available from https://github.com/shportnoy/blood_roi_tool. The conversion from T1 and T2 into Hct and Hb values can be obtained from https://github.com/shportnoy/oximetry_calculator. Since flow and oxygen delivery and consumption calculations need to be indexed to fetal body weight, standard

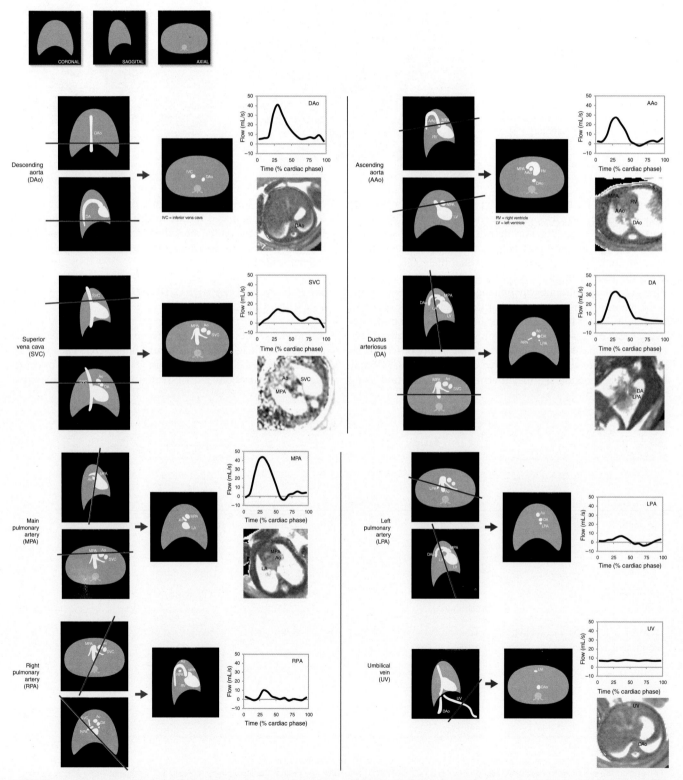

FIGURE 11.7: Slice prescriptions for fetal cardiovascular magnetic resonance. Orientation of slices for phase-contrast and T2 mapping of the major fetal vessels is based on three-plane static steady-state free precession (SSFP) survey of the fetal thorax showing representative flow curves and T2 maps. *LA*, left atrium; *LV*, left ventricle; *MPA*, main pulmonary artery; *RV*, right ventricle.

segmentation of a 3D-SSFP acquisition covering the entire fetal body can provide both fetal and fetal brain volumes. These are necessary to obtain fetal and fetal brain weights through standardized conversion factors derived from autopsy studies.[66,67]

If the fetal MRI study has been requested to confirm the cardiac anatomy, cine SSFP is likely to be helpful. Motion compensated cine CMR of the fetal heart using undersampled radial acquisition with compressed sensing has the advantage of providing excellent images of both intra- and extracardiac vascular anatomy and also provides an assessment of systolic ventricular function. One current drawback of this approach is that the cine SSFP images require extensive postprocessing for reconstruction, and are therefore not available during the examination. However, in the absence of fetal motion, the quality of the static sequences is often sufficient for the planning of other sequences and provides an overview of the cardiac anatomy before the postprocessing reconstructions are available.

FUTURE DIRECTIONS

With ongoing improvements in the quality of anatomical cine imaging, volumetric ventricular segmentation may become feasible with fetal CMR. The ability to accurately measure ventricular mass, end-diastolic and systolic volumes, and right and left ventricular ejection fractions could be of considerable interest in a number of situations. The utility of this approach has been explored in the setting of a fetal sheep model of myocardial infarction.[68] In this study, myocardial infarcts induced by ligation of a branch of the left anterior coronary artery resulted in regional wall motion abnormalities evident on cine imaging.[69] The extent of infarction was also revealed by late gadolinium enhancement. The application of this kind of imaging technology in animal models represents an exciting advance in the development of fetal CMR. For example, the combination of fetal surgical preparation and four-dimensional cine phase-contrast measurement has made it possible to characterize and quantify complex *in utero* blood flow patterns including the preferential streaming of oxygenated blood across the foramen ovale.[70] Ultimately, fetal CMR acquisitions will likely move toward a single, motion-robust, four-dimensional flow-encoded acquisition that allows for simultaneous assessment of the anatomy, ventricular volumes, and vessel flows in a single sequence, using motion-corrected 3D volumetric reconstructions of 2D multiplanar MRI.[71]

Fetal anemia secondary to alloimmunization, parvovirus, and hemoglobinopathies results in tissue hypoxia, hydrops, and fetal demise. However, *in utero* transfusion is an effective treatment and prevents adverse outcomes. Screening for maternal autoantibodies and Doppler ultrasound for measurement of the peak systolic velocity in the middle cerebral artery (MCA-PSV), which reveals elevated velocities in the anemic fetus resulting from a hyperdynamic circulation and reduced blood viscosity, are highly effective in detecting fetal anemia. However, multiple transfusions are often required for the effective treatment of fetal anemia, and the MCA-PSV becomes less specific for anemia following multiple prior transfusions and in late gestation. The gold standard test for fetal anemia is fetal blood sampling, although this carries a 1% to 2% risk of fetal loss. The combination of T1 and T2 mapping of blood in the umbilical vein by MRI, as described previously, has therefore been investigated as a potential approach to improving the specificity of noninvasive testing for fetal anemia. Preliminary findings in a group of 22 anemic fetuses suggest that MRI provides improved specificity over MCA-PSV in fetuses with anemia and could therefore be considered as an adjunct to

ultrasound, particularly in the setting of a high MCA-PSV result in late gestation and following prior transfusions.[72]

LIMITATIONS OF FETAL CMR

Despite technologic improvements, the intrinsic trade-off between spatial resolution, signal-to-noise ratio, and scan time inherent to MRI continues to be a challenge for fetal applications. This is particularly true for early second-trimester imaging, at which stage the fetus is much smaller and more vigorous in its body movements. However, this is the period of the pregnancy when much of the important decision-making about a pregnancy occurs, and so future fetal cardiac MRI technical development should include a focus on enhancing our capability to image the heart at earlier gestations.

SUMMARY

Thanks to recent advances in MRI technology, fetal cardiac MRI is now a rapidly evolving modality that promises to improve visualization of fetal cardiac anatomy and define cardiovascular physiology through a combination of cine imaging, vessel blood flow, and oximetry and hematocrit measurements. Although there are currently no established clinical indications for fetal CMR, the technique holds the potential to supplement ultrasound in the assessment of prenatal cardiovascular disease. As researchers seek to evaluate new forms of fetal treatment for CHD such as *in utero* cardiac interventions, maternal hyperoxygenation, and nonsteroidal anti-inflammatory drugs, there would appear to be potential utility for a modality that allows for the direct quantification of fetal cardiac function, oxygenation, and vascular distribution. Similarly, some approach that exploits the magnetic properties of deoxyhemoglobin as a biomarker of fetal and/or placental hypoxemia is likely to play an increasing role in the diagnosis and assessment of fetal growth restriction.[12,73]

REFERENCES

1. Goldman MR, Pohost GM, Ingwall JS, et al. Nuclear magnetic resonance imaging: potential cardiac applications. *Am J Cardiol.* 1980;46:1278–1283.
2. Forder JR, Pohost GM. Cardiovascular nuclear magnetic resonance: basic and clinical applications. *J Clin Invest.* 2003;111:1630–1639.
3. Gorincour G, Bourlière-Najean B, Bonello B, et al. Feasibility of fetal cardiac magnetic resonance imaging: preliminary experience. *Ultrasound Obstet Gynecol.* 2007;29:105–108.
4. Manganaro L, Savelli S, Di Maurizio M, et al. Assessment of congenital heart disease (CHD): is there a role for fetal magnetic resonance imaging (MRI)? 2009;72:172–180.
5. Manganaro L, Savelli S, Di Maurizio M, et al. Potential role of fetal cardiac evaluation with magnetic resonance imaging: preliminary experience. *Prenat Diagn.* 2008;28:148–156.
6. Manganaro L, Vinci V, Bernardo S, et al. Magnetic resonance imaging of fetal heart: anatomical and pathological findings. *J Matern Fetal Neonatal Med.* 2014;27:1213–1219.
7. Lloyd DFA, van Amerom JFP, Pushparajah K, et al. An exploration of the potential utility of fetal cardiovascular MRI as an adjunct to fetal echocardiography. *Prenat Diagn.* 2016;36:916–925.
8. Roy C, Marini D, Lloyd D, et al. Preliminary experience using motion compensated CINE magnetic resonance imaging to visualise fetal congenital heart disease. *Circ Cardiovasc Imaging.* 2018;11:e007745. doi:10.1161/CIRCIMAGING.118.007745.
9. Seed M, van Amerom J, Yoo SJ, et al. Feasibility of quantification of the distribution of blood flow in the normal human fetal circulation using CMR: a cross-sectional study. *J Cardiovasc Magn Reson.* 2012;14:79.
10. Prsa M, Sun L, Van Amerom J, et al. Reference ranges of blood flow in the major vessels of the normal human fetal circulation at term by phase-contrast magnetic resonance imaging. *Circ Cardiovasc Imaging.* 2014;7:663–670.
11. Sun L, Macgowan CK, Sled JG, et al. Reduced fetal cerebral oxygen consumption is associated with smaller brain size in fetuses with congenital heart disease. *Circulation.* 2015;131:1313–1323.
12. Zhu MY, Milligan N, Keating S, et al. The hemodynamics of late-onset intrauterine growth restriction by MRI. *Am J Obstet Gynecol.* 2016;214:367.e1–367.e17.

13. Limperopoulos C, Tworetzky W, McElhinney DB, et al. Brain volume and metabolism in fetuses with congenital heart disease: evaluation with quantitative magnetic resonance imaging and spectroscopy. *Circulation.* 2010;121:26–33.

14. Prayer D. *Fetal MRI.* Heidelberg, Germany: Springer; 2011.

15. Yagel S, Silverman N, Gembruch U. *Fetal Cardiology: Embryology, Genetics, Physiology, Echocardiographic Evaluation, Diagnosis and Perinatal Management of Cardiac Disease.* 3rd ed. Boca Raton, FL: CRC Press, Taylor & Francis Group; 2018.

16. Jansz MS, Seed M, Van Amerom JFP, et al. Metric optimized gating for fetal cardiac MRI. *Magn Reson Med.* 2010;64:1304–1314.

17. Tsai-Goodman B, Zhu MY, Al-Rujaib M, et al. Foetal blood flow measured using phase contrast cardiovascular magnetic resonance—preliminary data comparing 1.5 T with 3.0 T. *J Cardiovasc Magn Reson.* 2015;17:30.

18. Bidhult S, Töger J, Heiberg E, et al. Independent validation of metric optimized gating for fetal cardiovascular phase-contrast flow imaging. *Magn Reson Med.* 2019;81:495–503.

19. Roy CW, Seed M, Macgowan CK. Accelerated MRI of the fetal heart using compressed sensing and metric optimized gating. *Magn Reson Med.* 2017;77:2125–2135.

20. Roy CW, Seed M, Kingdom JC, et al. Motion compensated cine CMR of the fetal heart using radial undersampling and compressed sensing. *J Cardiovasc Magn Reson.* 2017;19:1–14.

21. van Amerom JFP, Lloyd DFA, Price AN, et al. Fetal cardiac cine imaging using highly accelerated dynamic MRI with retrospective motion correction and outlier rejection. *Magn Reson Med.* 2018;79:327–338.

22. Chaptinel J, Yerly J, Mivelaz Y, et al. Fetal cardiac cine magnetic resonance imaging in utero. *Sci Rep.* 2017;7:1–10.

23. Haris K, Hedström E, Bidhult S, et al. Self-gated fetal cardiac MRI with tiny golden angle iGRASP: a feasibility study. *J Magn Reson Imaging.* 2017;46:207–217.

24. Kellman P, Chefd'hotel C, Lorenz CH, et al. High spatial and temporal resolution cardiac cine MRI from retrospective reconstruction of data acquired in real time using motion correction and resorting. *Magn Reson Med.* 2009;62:1557–1564.

25. Hansen MS, Sørensen TS, Arai AE, et al. Retrospective reconstruction of high temporal resolution cine images from real-time MRI using iterative motion correction. *Magn Reson Med.* 2012;68:741–750.

26. Roy CW, Seed M, Van Amerom JFP, et al. Dynamic imaging of the fetal heart using metric optimized gating. *Magn Reson Med.* 2013;70:1598–1607.

27. Goolaub DS, Roy CW, Schrauben E, et al. Multidimensional fetal flow imaging with cardiovascular magnetic resonance: a feasibility study. *J Cardiovasc Magn Reson.* 2018;20:77.

28. Yamamura J, Kopp I, Frisch M, et al. Cardiac MRI of the fetal heart using a novel triggering method: Initial results in an animal model. *J Magn Reson Imaging.* 2012;35:1071–1076.

29. Kording F, Schoennagel BP, de Sousa MT, et al. Evaluation of a portable Doppler ultrasound gating device for fetal cardiac MR imaging: initial results at 1.5T and 3T. *Magn Reson Med Sci.* 2018;17:308–317.

30. Kording F, Yamamura J, De Sousa MT, et al. Dynamic fetal cardiovascular magnetic resonance imaging using Doppler ultrasound gating. *J Cardiovasc Magn Reson.* 2018;20:1–10.

31. Tavares de Sousa M, Hecher K, Yamamura J, et al. Dynamic fetal cardiac magnetic resonance four chamber view imaging using Doppler ultrasound gating in the normal fetal heart and in congenital heart disease: comparison to fetal echocardiography. *Ultrasound Obstet Gynecol.* 2019;53:669–675. doi:10.1002/uog.20167.

32. Dong SZ, Zhu M, Li F. Preliminary experience with cardiovascular magnetic resonance in evaluation of fetal cardiovascular anomalies. *J Cardiovasc Magn Reson.* 2013;15:40.

33. Dong SZ, Zhu M. MR imaging of subaortic and retroesophageal anomalous courses of the left brachiocephalic vein in the fetus. *Sci Rep.* 2018;8:6–11.

34. Dong SZ, Zhu M. Magnetic resonance imaging of fetal persistent left superior vena cava. *Sci Rep.* 2017;7:1–9.

35. Li X, Li X, Hu K, et al. The value of cardiovascular magnetic resonance in the diagnosis of fetal aortic arch anomalies. *J Matern Fetal Neonatal Med.* 2017;30:1366–1371.

36. Li X, Li X, Saul D, et al. Fetal MRI diagnosis of 2 types of left pulmonary artery sling. *Radiol Case Rep.* 2017;12:653–657.

37. Lloyd DFA, Pushparajah K, Simpson JM, et al. Three-dimensional visualisation of the fetal heart using prenatal MRI with motion-corrected slice-volume registration: a prospective, single-centre cohort study. *Lancet.* 2019;393:1619–1627.

38. Roy C, Macgowan C. Dynamic MRI of a large fetal cardiac mass. *Radiology.* 2019;290:288.

39. Lam CZ, Bhamare TA, Gazzaz T, et al. Diagnosis of secondary pulmonary lymphangiectasia in congenital heart disease: a novel role for chest ultrasound and prognostic implications. *Pediatr Radiol.* 2017;47:1441–1451.

40. Seed M, Bradley T, Bourgeois J, et al. Antenatal MR imaging of pulmonary lymphangiectasia secondary to hypoplastic left heart syndrome. *Pediatr Radiol.* 2009;39:747–749.

41. Al Nafisi B, Van Amerom JF, Forsey J, et al. Fetal circulation in left-sided congenital heart disease measured by cardiovascular magnetic resonance: a case-control study. *J Cardiovasc Magn Reson.* 2013;15:65.

42. Victoria T, Andronikou S. The fetal MR appearance of 'nutmeg lung': findings in 8 cases linked to pulmonary lymphangiectasia. *Pediatr Radiol.* 2014;44:1237–1242.

43. Saul D, Degenhardt K, Iyoob SD, et al. Hypoplastic left heart syndrome and the nutmeg lung pattern in utero: a cause and effect relationship or prognostic indicator? *Pediatr Radiol.* 2016;46:483–489.

44. Chelliah A, Berger JT, Blask A, et al. Clinical utility of fetal magnetic resonance imaging in tetralogy of Fallot with absent pulmonary valve. *Circulation.* 2013;127:757–759.

45. Thulborn KR, Waterton JC, Matthews PM, et al. Oxygenation dependence of the transverse relaxation time of water protons in whole blood at high field. *Biochim Biophys Acta.* 1982;714:265–270.

46. Thulborn KR. My starting point: the discovery of an NMR method for measuring blood oxygenation using the transverse relaxation time of blood water. *Neuroimage.* 2012;62:589–593.

47. Ogawa S, Lee T, Kay A, et al. Brain magnetic resonance imaging with contrast dependent on blood oxygenation. *Proc Natl Acad Sci USA.* 1990;87:9868–9872.

48. Ogawa S, Menon R, Tank D, et al. Functional brain mapping by blood oxygenation level-dependent contrast magnetic resonance imaging. A comparison of signal characteristics with a biophysical model. *Biophys J.* 1993;64:803–812.

49. He X, Yablonsky A. Quantitative BOLD: Mapping of human cerebral deoxygenated blood volume and oxygen extraction fraction: default state. *Magn Reson Med.* 2007;57:115–126.

50. Sørensen A, Peters D, Fründ E, et al. Changes in human fetal oxygenation during maternal hyperoxia as estimated by BOLD MRI. *Prenat Diagn.* 2013;33:141–145.

51. Wedegärtner U, Tchirikov M, Schäfer S, et al. Functional MR imaging: comparison of BOLD signal intensity changes in fetal organs with fetal and maternal oxyhemoglobin saturation during hypoxia in sheep. *Radiology.* 2006;238:872–880.

52. Wright GA, Hu BS, Macovski A. 1991 I.I. Rabi Award. Estimating oxygen saturation of blood in vivo with MR imaging at 1.5 T. *J Magn Reson Imaging.* 1991;1:275–283.

53. Portnoy S, Seed M, Sled J, et al. Non-invasive evaluation of blood oxygen saturation and hematocrit from T1 and T2 relaxation times: In-vitro validation in fetal blood. *Magn Reson Med.* 2017;78:2352–2359.

54. Wilkinson J. Haemodynamic calculations in the catheter laboratory. *Heart.* 2001;85:113–120.

55. Rudolph A. *Congenital Diseases of the Heart—Clinical-Physiological Considerations.* 3rd ed. Chichester, England: Wiley-Blackwell; 2009:1–24.

56. Ge Y, Zhang Z, Lu H, et al. Characterizing brain oxygen metabolism in patients with multiple sclerosis with T2-relaxation-under-spin-tagging MRI. *J Cereb Blood Flow Metab.* 2012;32:403–412.

57. Giombi A, Burnard E. Rheology of human foetal blood with reference to haematocrit, plasma viscosity, osmolality and pH. *Biorheology.* 1970;6:315–328.

58. Portnoy S, Osmond M, Zhu MY, et al. Relaxation properties of human umbilical cord blood at 1.5 Tesla. *Magn Reson Med.* 2017;77:1678–1690.

59. Portnoy S, Milligan N, Seed M, et al. Human umbilical cord blood relaxation times and susceptibility at 3 T. *Magn Reson Med.* 2018;79:3194–3206.

60. Porayette P, Van Amerom JFP, Yoo SJ, et al. MRI shows limited mixing between systemic and pulmonary circulations in foetal transposition of the great arteries: a potential cause of in utero pulmonary vascular disease. *Cardiol Young.* 2015;25:737–744.

61. Porayette P, Madathil S, Sun L, et al. MRI reveals hemodynamic changes with acute maternal hyperoxygenation in human fetuses with and without congenital heart disease. *Prenat Diagn.* 2016;36:274–281.

62. Torigoe T, Mawad W, Seed M, et al. Treatment of fetal circular shunt with non-steroidal anti-inflammatory drugs. *Ultrasound Obstet Gynecol.* 2019;53:841–846. doi:10.1002/uog.20169.

63. Chaturvedi R, Ryan G, Seed M, et al. Fetal stenting of the atrial septum: technique and initial results in cardiac lesions with left atrial hypertension. *Int J Cardiol.* 2013;168:2029–2036.

64. Jouannic JM, Gavard L, Fermont L, et al. Sensitivity and specificity of prenatal features of physiological shunts to predict neonatal clinical status in transposition of the great arteries. *Circulation.* 2004;110:1743–1746.

65. Mawad W, Chaturvedi RR, Ryan G, et al. Percutaneous fetal atrial balloon septoplasty for simple transposition of the great arteries with an intact atrial septum. *Can J Cardiol.* 2018;34:342.e9–342.e11.

66. Roelfsema NM, Hop WCJ, Boito SME, et al. Three-dimensional sonographic measurement of normal fetal brain volume during the second half of pregnancy. *Am J Obstet Gynecol.* 2004;190:275–280.

67. Baker PN, Johnson IR, Gowland PA, et al. Fetal weight estimation by echo-planar magnetic resonance imaging. *Lancet.* 1994;343:644–645.

68. Duan A, Darby J, Soo J, et al. Feasibility of phase-contrast cine magnetic resonance imaging for measuring blood flow in the sheep fetus. *Am J Physiol Regul Integr Comp Physiol.* 2019;371:R780–R792.

69. Duan AQ, Lock MC, Perumal SR, et al. Feasibility of detecting myocardial infarction in the sheep fetus using late gadolinium enhancement CMR imaging. *J Cardiovasc Magn Reson.* 2017;19:1–11.

70. Schrauben EM, Saini BS, Darby JRT, et al. Fetal hemodynamics and cardiac streaming assessed by 4D flow cardiovascular magnetic resonance in fetal sheep. *J Cardiovasc Magn Reson.* 2019;21:8.

71. van Amerom JF, Lloyd DF, Deprez M, et al. Fetal whole-heart 4D imaging using motion-corrected multi-planar real-time MRI. *Magn Reson Med.* 2019;82:1055–1072.

72. Duan A, Keunen J, Portnoy S, et al. P22.01: Preliminary investigation of the utility of MRI for measuring the hematocrit in fetal anemia. *Ultrasound Obstet Gynecol.* 2016;48:237.

73. Sinding M, Peters DA, Frøkjær JB, et al. Prediction of low birth weight: comparison of placental T2* estimated by MRI and uterine artery pulsatility index. *Placenta.* 2017;49:48–54.

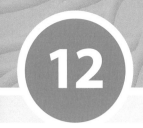

12

Three-Dimensional Printing/Additive Manufacturing in Advanced Fetal Imaging

Heron Werner Jr • Jorge Lopes • Gerson Ribeiro

The earliest records of graphical representation of the fetus date back to the year 1500. As examples, artistic drawings are scattered in museums and private collections around the world. Among the artists who achieved a refined quality in terms of visual representation of the fetus is Leonardo da Vinci, who through various anatomical studies displayed the process of fetal development.

The use of physical models in medicine for didactic purposes began in Italy at the time of the Renaissance period. Wax models representing different parts of the human body emerged with great visual realism and included the changes of a woman's body during pregnancy.[1]

With the advent of three-dimensional (3D) printing, also known as additive manufacturing (AM) technologies, noninvasive fetal imaging techniques can be enhanced. Uterine morphology and fetal anatomy can be better visualized, improving the understanding of various malformations and pathologies. These models can aid in interdisciplinary discussions and help guide medical and surgical interventions.[2–20]

ADDITIVE MANUFACTURING TECHNOLOGIES

Data that can be converted to 3D files needs to be obtained via ultrasound or magnetic resonance imaging. The actual AM method is based on the successive overlapping of thin layers of specific material substances, according to the appropriate technical method, and is carried out by transforming the 3D files into a Standard Triangulation Language (STL) extension, which consists basically of X, Y, and Z coordinates.[8,11] Once the STL file is generated, the next step is the horizontal slicing of the whole 3D volumetric file using an appropriate software for the designated hardware and calculating the supporting structures when necessary. The building process starts with the sequential deposition of layers of material, the layer width ranging from microns to fractions of millimeters, depending on the technology chosen. Then a postprocessing step starts, an essential procedure in all current rapid prototyping (RP) technologies, where the model has to be cleaned to remove the support material and/or residues used during the building process.[2,6]

There are currently several different systems of AM technologies on the market which, although using dissimilar material procedures, are based on the same principle of manufacturing by layer deposition. One of the most important features of AM is the possibility of manufacturing parts with significant geometrical complexity, a process in which conventional technologies are more expensive and lengthy, affecting both the time taken to launch the product commercially and the total costs of production.[5]

An interesting current trend (the makers' movement[1]) related to additive equipment is the creation, modification, and customization of AM, now a rapidly growing market. Being smaller in terms of overall size than regular equipment, and, consequently, having a reduced area for construction, this AM equipment is more office friendly and also less expensive, similar to the laser and inkjet paper printers in common use in offices.

The main AM technologies currently marketed are classified into three categories, designated by physical state of the materials to be transformed: liquid-based systems (associated with photosensitive resins), powder-based systems (associated with sintering or agglutination of grain particles), and solid-based systems (associated with nonpowder formats, such as sheets or thermoplastic extruded filaments) (Fig. 12.1).[5]

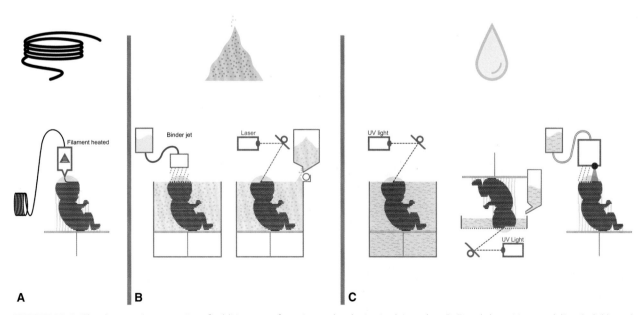

FIGURE 12.1: The three main categories of additive manufacturing technologies in the market. **A:** Fused deposition modeling (solid-based system). **B:** Selective laser sintering (powder-based system). **C.** Stereolithography (liquid-based system). *UV*, ultraviolet.

In order to exemplify the categories, three different AM technologies are described:

1. Stereolithography (liquid-based system), or SLA, was the very first additive technology commercially available, introduced in 1988 in California in the United States. The technique is based on the polymerization of photosensitive resins by means of ultraviolet (UV) light emitted from a laser source and focused on a polymer bath surface.[10]

   When exposed to the laser beam, the photocurable resin changes from a liquid to a solid state, generating a physical slice. This procedure is then repeated sequentially until it reaches the final dimension of the physical model to be built. Currently, this technology is one of the most accurate, presenting in general a very high surface quality (Fig. 12.2).

   This process also requires the addition of physical supports during the construction of the prototype (which are manually removed after it has been built) as well as exposure to UV lamps after production to completely harden the model. There is a wide range of available materials utilized with this technology, with the most common being high-performance polymers and acrylic and epoxy resins.

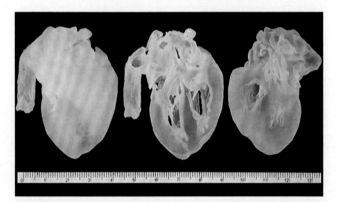

FIGURE 12.2: Fetal heart: additive manufacturing physical model built on stereolithography technology.

2. Selective laser sintering (powder-based system) or SLS, uses a range of materials (nylon, metallic materials, and other) in powder form that generate prototypes by heating material to below its melting point until its particles adhere to each other.[20]

   In the SLS process, a laser beam is focused on the surface of the material which fuses the powder, creating one slice on the surface of a powder bed. After each layer is built, the powder bed is lowered by the thickness of one layer, and a new layer of material is applied on top, the process being repeated until the model is completed (Fig. 12.3).

   One of the advantages of SLS is the strength of the prototypes, which can function in some cases as a final product, to be tested in real conditions. In addition, the postprocessing phase is very simple. Since the parts are strong enough to be manipulated, the model only requires removal from the powder bed and then vacuuming to remove excess powder. The nonfused material can be reused for other kinds of prototype, although the material loses some of its physical properties when it is exposed to heat.

3. Fused deposition modelling (solid-based system) or FDM, works through the microextrusion of thermoplastic materials, which is sequentially deposited in layers. The thermoplastic filament (the most common being acrylonitrile butadiene styrene or ABS) is melted and extruded through a heated nozzle, which moves according to the X and Y coordinates to produce one slice of the model (a profile). Continuing the process, the elevator moves down and the next layer is built on the top of the previous one until the prototype model is fully built.[10]

   This technology requires the construction of supports that are matched to the shape of the prototype and then removed in the postprocessing phase (Fig. 12.4).

   In terms of didactic purposes, this is one of few processes that allow observation of the deposition process through a window, which can be stopped if something becomes visibly wrong with the model. Depending on their built shape, FDM prototypes are strong enough to be used as a final product, or

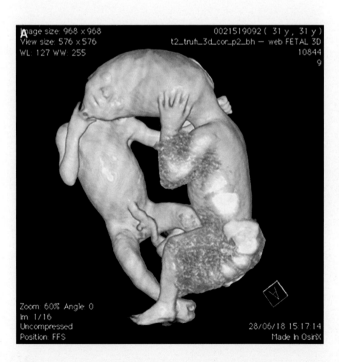

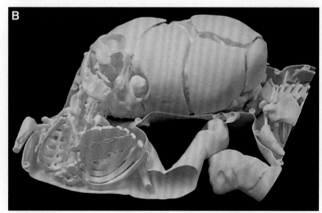

FIGURE 12.3: Conjoined twins (craniopagus): 3D magnetic resonance imaging **(A)** and additive manufacturing model demonstrating bone anatomy built on selective laser sintering technology **(B)**.

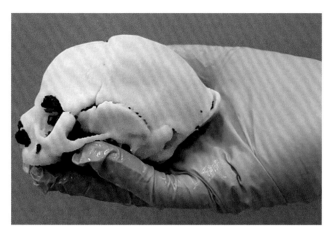

FIGURE 12.4: Fetus at 37 weeks with microcephaly due to Zika infection: additive manufacturing model of the skull built on fused deposition modeling technology.

even tested in real conditions, taking into consideration the characteristics of the thermoplastics to be simulated.

ADDITIVE MANUFACTURING AND NONINVASIVE IMAGE TECHNOLOGIES COMBINED IN FETAL MEDICINE

The importance of AM in the biomedical sector has increased steadily in the past few years. Utilization of AM models has been reported widely in the medical scientific literature, especially with regard to surgical planning, biomedical research, and medical education.[3,11]

Ultrasound (US) is currently the primary method for fetal assessment during pregnancy because it is user friendly, accurate, cost-effective, and safe.[9] During the past two decades, three-dimensional ultrasound (3DUS) has been used as an important complementary tool for confirming the diagnosis, assessing the prognosis, and counseling the parents.[18]

Magnetic resonance imaging (MRI) is a diagnostic modality that complements US, particularly for inconclusive cases that require further diagnostic investigation. In contrast to US, MRI is not affected by fetal position, oligohydramnios, bone overlay, or maternal obesity.[4,7,18] With the advent of fast sequences, software dedicated to 3D reconstruction has enabled the study of more complex fetal abnormalities. The aim of this chapter is to demonstrate physical fetal models using images obtained by 3DUS and MRI to guide 3D printing technology (Figs. 12.5 to 12.10). In order to construct physical models from the medical examinations (3DUS and MRI), the first step is the production of 3D virtual models. All 3DUS and MRI files are exported to a workstation in Digital Imaging and Communications in Medicine (DICOM) format for segmentation to be done by a 3D modeling technician and supervised by the physician in charge. The 3D structure of the fetus is reconstructed by generating software manipulation known as skinning surfaces that join the resulting profiles. Segmentation software that converts medical images into numerical models can be used for 3D virtual model reconstruction, and the models are exported into an STL format and converted into an "OBJ" extension for postprocessing surface adjustment. The volumetric surface can be smoothed, to be later compared and analyzed as a topographic construction. It is important to highlight that the imaging fusion of real-time 3DUS and MRI is feasible and may improve the fetal diagnosis.[11] Recently, new US systems and their external volume manipulation programs have become available, permitting automatic conversion by direct export in STL format (Fig. 12.11).[8]

AM has become a very useful and potentially transformative tool in a number of different fields, including medicine. The use of AM is becoming important for educational purposes. The technique can provide better interaction between parents and their unborn child during pregnancy, by physically recreating the interior of the womb during gestation, including physical appearance, actual size, and malformations in some cases (Fig. 12.12).

The study of fetal malformations through 3D reconstruction using US and MRI can assist in guiding counseling, medical, and/or surgical interventions. We believe that physical models will shortly help in the tactile and interactive study of many medical disciplines. These techniques may be useful for prospective parents—especially visually disabled parents—as they recreate a 3D model with the physical characteristics of the fetus, allowing a more direct emotional connection with the unborn baby.

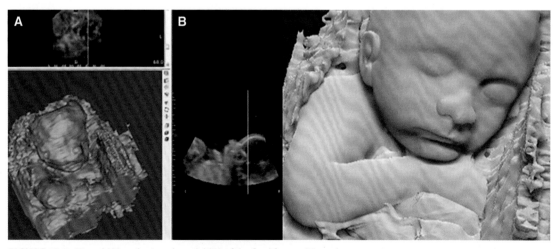

FIGURE 12.5: Virtual **(A)** and printed model **(B)** of the fetal face at 27 weeks.

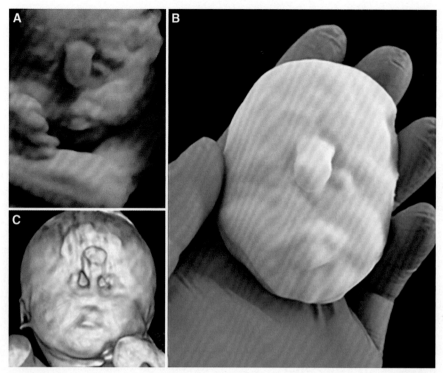

FIGURE 12.6: Alobar holoprosencephaly at 25 weeks: 3D fetal reconstruction obtained by ultrasound (HDlive) **(A)**, magnetic resonance imaging **(B)** and the printed model **(C)**.

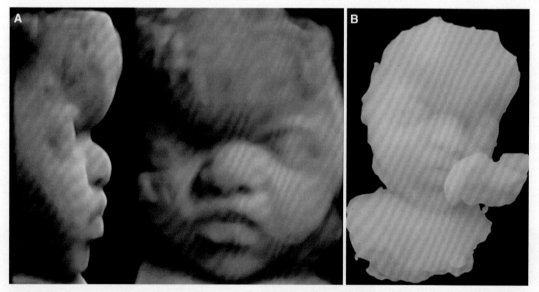

FIGURE 12.7: Apert syndrome at 26 weeks: 3D view of the fetal face and profile obtained from 3D ultrasound (HDlive) **(A)** and the printed model **(B)**.

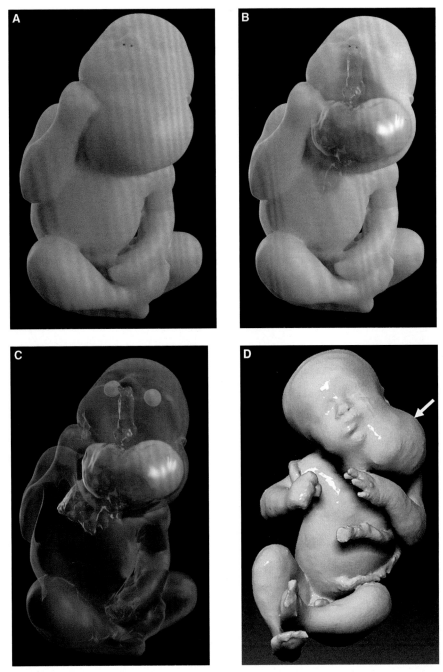

FIGURE 12.8: Cervical teratoma at 37 weeks: 3D virtual model showing the airway path **(A–C)** and 3D fetal model obtained by magnetic resonance imaging **(D)**.

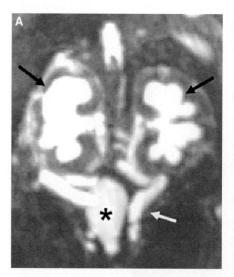
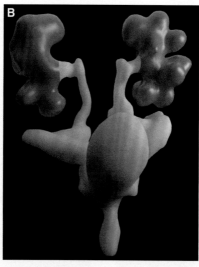
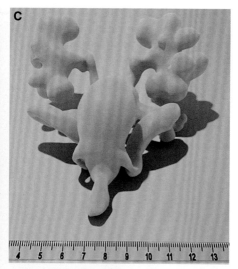

FIGURE 12.9: Lower urinary tract obstruction at 31 weeks of gestation: Coronal T2 magnetic resonance imaging showing the increased volume bladder (*asterisk*), hydronephrosis (*black arrows*), and dilated ureters (*white arrow*) **(A)**. 3D virtual reconstruction **(B)** and 3D printed model **(C)**.

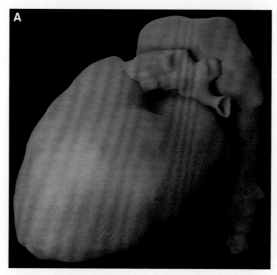
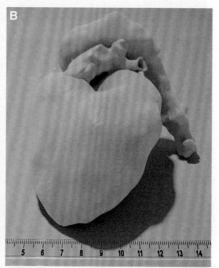

FIGURE 12.10: Fetal heart at 28 weeks: 3D reconstruction obtained by ultrasound spatiotemporal image correlation **(A)** and 3D printed model **(B)**.

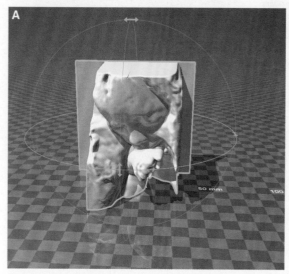
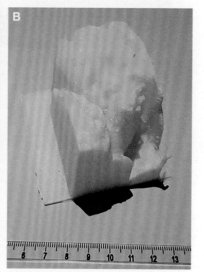

FIGURE 12.11: Fetal face: Automatic conversion by direct export in Standard Triangulation Language format obtained by Voluson E10, GE Medical. Virtual **(A)** and printed model **(B)**.

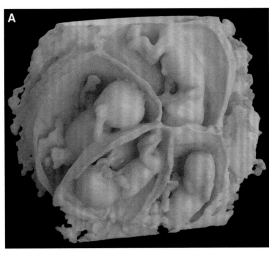 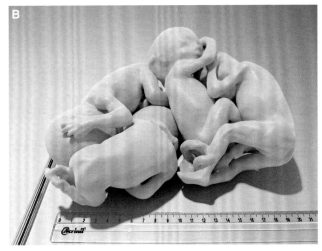

FIGURE 12.12: Monochorionic diamniotic quadruplet pregnancy at 26 weeks: 3D printed model obtained by ultrasound at 12 weeks **(A)** and 3D printed model obtained by magnetic resonance imaging **(B)**.

REFERENCES

1. Santos JRL. *3D Modelling Tools: The Experimental Application of Digital Model Making Technologies in Fetal Medicine.* London, England: The Royal College of Art; 2009.
2. Farzadi A, Solati-Hashjin M, Asadi-Eydivand M, Abu Osman NA. Effect of layer thickness and printing orientation on mechanical properties and dimensional accuracy of 3D printed porous samples for bone tissue engineering. *PLoS One.* 2014;9(9):e108252.
3. George E, Liacouras P, Rybicki FJ, Mitsouras D. Measuring and establishing the accuracy and reproducibility of 3D printed medical models. *Radiographics.* 2017:160165. doi:10.1148/rg.2017160165.
4. Hellinger JC, Epelman M. Fetal MRI in the third dimension. *Appl Radiol.* 2010;39:8–22.
5. Hopkinson R, Hague RJM, Dickens PM. *Rapid Manufacturing—An Industrial Revolution for the Digital Age, Loughborough University.* London, England: John Wiley and Sons; 2006:57.
6. Leng S, McGee K, Morris J, et al. Anatomic modeling using 3D printing: quality assurance and optimization. *3D Print Med.* 2017;3:1–14.
7. Prayer D, Malinger G, Brugger PC, et al. ISUOG Practice Guidelines: performance of fetal magnetic resonance imaging. *Ultrasound Obstet Gynecol.* 2017;49:671–680. doi:10.1002/uog.17412.
8. Tutschek B. 3D prints from ultrasound volumes. *Ultrasound Obstet Gynecol.* 2018;52(6):691–698.
9. Tutschek B. Three-dimensional ultrasound: techniques and clinical applications. In: Copel J, D'Alton ME, Feltovich H, et al., eds. *Obstetric Imaging.* Philadelphia, PA: Elsevier; 2017:712–721.
10. Watmough M, Aldersey-Williams H. *Rapid Manufacturing—New Possibilities for Materials and Design—Essays to Accompany the MADE Workshop.* London, England: Royal College of Art; 2007:14.
11. Werner H, Lopes dos Santos JR, Fontes R, et al. Additive manufacturing models of fetuses built from three-dimensional ultrasound, magnetic resonance imaging and computed tomography scan data. *Ultrasound Obstet Gynecol.* 2010;36:355–361.
12. Werner H, Lopes dos Santos JR, Fontes R, et al. Virtual bronchoscopy for evaluating cervical tumors of the fetus. *Ultrasound Obstet Gynecol.* 2013;41(1):90–94.
13. Werner H, Lopes J, Tonni G, Araujo Junior E. Physical model from 3D ultrasound and magnetic resonance imaging scan data reconstruction of lumbosacral myelomeningocele in a fetus with Chiari II malformation. *Childs Nerv Syst.* 2015;31:511–513.
14. Werner H, Castro P, Daltro P, et al. Monochorionic diamniotic quadruplet pregnancy: physical models from prenatal three-dimensional ultrasound and magnetic resonance imaging data. *Ultrasound Obstet Gynecol.* 2017;49(6):812–814.
15. Werner H, Lopes J, Tonni G, Araujo Junior E. Maternal-fetal attachment in blind women using physical model from three-dimensional ultrasound and magnetic resonance scan data: six serious cases. *J Matern Fetal Neonatal Med.* 2016;29:2229–2232.
16. Werner H, Lopes J, Ribeiro G, et al. Three-dimensional virtual cystoscopy: noninvasive approach for the assessment of urinary tract in fetuses with lower urinary tract obstruction. *Prenat Diagn.* 2017;37:1350–1352.
17. Werner H, Lopes dos Santos JR, Ribeiro G, Belmonte SL, Daltro P, Araujo Júnior E. Combination of ultrasound, magnetic resonance imaging and virtual reality technologies to generate immersive three-dimensional fetal images. *Ultrasound Obstet Gynecol.* 2017;50:271–273.
18. Werner H, Marcondes M, Daltro P, et al. Three-dimensional reconstruction of fetal abnormalities using ultrasonography and magnetic resonance imaging. *J Matern Fetal Neonatal Med.* 2019;32:3502–3508. doi:10.1080/14767058.2018.1465558.
19. Werner H, Arcoverde V, Ribeiro G, et al. An interactive experiment combining ultrasound, magnetic resonance imaging, and force feedback technology to physically feel the fetus during pregnancy. *Eur J Radiol.* 2019;110:128–129.
20. Werner H, Lopes J, Ribeiro G, Raposo AB, Trajano E, Araujo Júnior E. Three-dimensional virtual traveling navigation and three dimensional printing models of a normal fetal heart using ultrasonography data. *Prenat Diagn.* 2019;1–3.

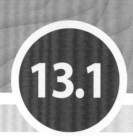

Ultrasound Evaluation of the Placenta, Amniotic Fluid, Umbilical Cord, and Amniotic Membranes

13.1

Edgar Hernandez-Andrade • Eleazar E. Soto Torres • Dan Tirosh

A complete ultrasound (US) evaluation during pregnancy requires a detailed examination of the placenta, umbilical cord, and amniotic fluid (AF).[1,2] Placental and umbilical cord anomalies are highly related to obstetric complications such as placenta and vasa previa, placenta accreta, placental abruption, preeclampsia, fetal growth restriction, and perinatal death.[3] In twin pregnancies, an accurate diagnosis of chorionicity is required to identify cases at a higher risk of serious complications such as twin-to-twin transfusion syndrome (TTTS) and selective growth restriction. Placental anomalies might also affect the fetal programming and increase the risk of metabolic and cardiovascular diseases in children and adult life.[4] Nevertheless, and despite different proposals for a systematic evaluation of the placenta,[5] in most cases, this evaluation is commonly limited to its location in the uterus.

PLACENTA

Basic Development

The placenta is a multifunctional organ responsible for the interchange of oxygen and nutrients between the fetus and the mother. This interchange takes place in the terminal villi through the syncytiotrophoblast. The fetal vessels are contained in the terminal villi, which is surrounded by maternal blood. Other metabolic processes such as the production of peptide and steroid hormones also occur in the syncytiotrophbloblast.[6] Due to its high metabolic rate, the syncytiotrophoblast consumes approximately 40% of oxygen of the fetoplacental unit.[7]

Two important processes should occur for having a functional placental unit: (1) transformation of the spiral arteries and (2) an adequate development of the villi and of the intervillous space. After implantation, the trophectoderm generates a layer of cells around the blastocyst called trophoblast cells. These cells differentiate into villus and extravillous trophoblasts. Villus trophoblasts form the chorionic villi that will perform the metabolite exchange between the fetus and the mother. The extravillous trophoblast migrates into the decidua and myometrium, invading the maternal spiral arteries transforming them into low-vascular resistance vessels through a sequence of anatomical changes: (1) lumen dilatation, (2) transformation of the media and the endothelial layers of the artery, and (3) replacement of the muscular and elastic walls by fibrinoid material.[8] Two periods of trophoblast invasion have been described: (1) transformation of the decidual segment of the spiral arteries occurring during the first trimester of pregnancy, and (2) transformation of the myometrial segments of the spiral arteries in the second trimester of pregnancy. Abnormal transformation of the spiral arteries is related to the development of perinatal complications

such as preeclampsia,[9,10] preterm delivery,[11] spontaneous abortion, fetal death, preterm labor with intact membranes, preterm premature rupture of the membranes (PPROM), and placental abruption.[3,12]

Placental Size, Shape, and Appearance

Biometric measurements of the placenta such as length, thickness, area, and volume have been proposed as potentially useful methods to estimate the risk of perinatal complications.[13,14] These measurements, while seeming to be simple, might have a significant variation due to the location of the placenta. Placenta thickness is measured in the center of the placenta, which is usually defined as the site of umbilical cord insertion (Fig. 13.1-1); however, in approximately 20% of all pregnancies, the umbilical cord is not inserted in the center of the placenta. The shape of the placenta is mainly circular (90%), the remaining 10% have either a multilobulated or a star-shaped placenta. These anatomic differences, together with variations in placenta location and an irregular fetal surface, might affect the biometric measurements of the placenta.[15] Lee et al. reported a mean placental thickness of 24.6 mm at 18 to 22 weeks of gestation, and that posterior placentas are, in average, 6 mm thicker than anterior placentas.[15] Hoddick et al. reported that an anterior placenta thickness greater than 33 mm, or a posterior placenta thickness greater than 40 mm in the midtrimester of pregnancy, should be considered abnormal.[16] Increased placental thickness has been associated with uncontrolled diabetes, fetal anemia, fetal hydrops, alpha-thalassemia, and placental floor infarction.[17] In contrast, reduced placental thickness has been associated with intrauterine growth restriction and preeclampsia.[18] Milligan et al. evaluated the reproducibility of measuring

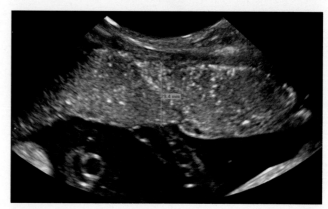

FIGURE 13.1-1: Placental thickness measured at the site of the umbilical cord insertion at 35 weeks of gestation.

placenta thickness and placenta length in the second trimester of pregnancy. They reported an intraoperator correlation coefficient (ICC) of 0.97 for placental length using a curvilinear approach, and an ICC of 0.95 for placenta thickness. The authors also proposed reference values for placenta length and thickness at 20 to 23 weeks of gestation.[19]

Placental Volume

Calculation of the complete placental volume can be done before 24 weeks of gestation as the entire placenta can be obtained using 3D US (Fig. 13.1-2).[20,21] Placenta volume can be calculated using 3D or 2D US techniques.[20,22–32] The most used 3D technique for volume calculation is VOCAL (virtual organ computer-aided analysis), but a multiplanar technique has also been proposed, where parallel 2D images combine biometric measurements obtained at different placental planes to estimate the placental volume. However, and despite some reports showing a significant association with perinatal complications[24,28,31] and chromosomal anomalies,[22,23] the placental volume has not yet shown a consistent performance for identification of fetuses at risk for perinatal complications.[26,27,30]

Placental Echogenicity

Grannum et al.[33] proposed the first grading system of placental echogenicity: grade 0, smooth chorionic plate; grade I, subtle indentation of echogenic lines in the chorionic plate; grade II, marked incomplete indentation from the chorionic plate to the basal layer and basal echogenic densities; and grade III, continuous and marked echogenic densities from the chorionic plate to the basal layer (Fig. 13.1-3). In earlier studies, grade III placentas were found to be significantly correlated with lung maturity, postterm pregnancies, and intrauterine growth restriction.[33,34] Despite that evaluation of placental echogenicity has lost popularity due to its weak correlation with adverse perinatal outcomes and

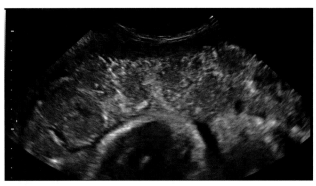

FIGURE 13.1-3: Placenta Grannum grade III showing continuous echogenic densities from the chorionic plate to the basal layer.

poor agreement between operators,[35–37] recent studies showed that increased echogenicity can be related to fetal–placental hemorrhage,[38,39] TTTS,[40] and anemia polycythemia sequence in monochorionic twins.[41] Furthermore, Chen et al. evaluated 15,122 pregnancies and reported an adjusted odds ratio (OR) of 7.62 (95% CI 5.0 to 11.62) for stillbirth when a grade III placenta was observed.[42]

A jellylike consistency of the placenta, defined as a thick placenta with a patchy decrease in echogenicity (Fig. 13.1-4), has been associated with preeclampsia, subchorial thrombosis with massive fibrin deposition, and fetal demise.[13,43] Janiaux et al.[18] reported that US identification of a jellylike placenta at 18 to 26 weeks of gestation was more prevalent in women who later developed preeclampsia, and that these placentas showed subchorial thrombosis and massive fibrin deposition.[18]

Placental Anatomical Anomalies

Succenturiate Placenta is characterized by the presence of one or several accessory placental lobes separated from the main

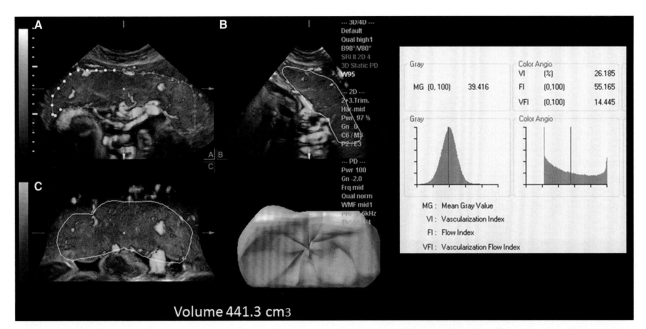

FIGURE 13.1-2: Placental volume obtained using virtual organ computer-aided analysis (VOCAL). The **A**, **B**, and **C** images show the multiplanar visualization of the placenta with the selected region of interest where VOCAL was calculated. The rendered image is created by delineating the placenta in 12 planes separated by 30° in a rotational process. Placental blood perfusion is calculated from the voxels containing power Doppler information. Three indices estimating blood perfusion are provided from the power Doppler signal analysis: vascular index (VI: percentage of voxels with power Doppler ultrasound [PDU] information over the total number of voxels), flow index (FI: averaged value of all voxels with PDU information) and vascular flow index (*VFI*).

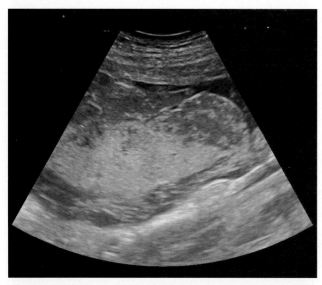

FIGURE 13.1-4: Thick jellylike placenta with patchy decrease reduced echogenicity and quivering to abdominal pressure.

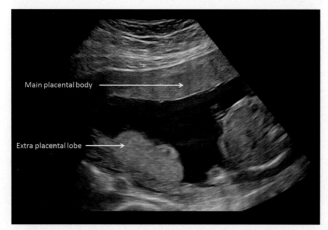

Main placental body

Extra placental lobe

FIGURE 13.1-5: Bilobed placenta (subcenturiata); the main placental body is in the anterior wall of the uterus, and the extra lobe is located in the posterior wall of the uterus.

placental area (Fig. 13.1-5). The vascular connection between the accessory lobes and the main placenta may be a risk factor for vasa previa when these vessels are near the internal cervical os.[44-46] Succenturiate placentas are more frequently found in pregnancies from assisted reproduction techniques and are significantly correlated with retained placenta, postpartum hemorrhage, and cesarean section for nonreassuring fetal status.[45,47,48]

Circumvallate Placenta is characterized by a small chorionic plate with an extension of placental tissue beyond the margins of the membrane insertion where a double layer of amnion and chorion form a raised, rolled edge.[14,49] The placental membranes are attached to the fetal surface of the placenta instead of the underlying villous placental margin. The US appearance is irregular with an uplifted edge of the placenta (where the placental margin is rounded); a marginal shelf, rim, or band (where the placental edge is thin or sheetlike); and a bright border at the periphery of the placenta due to a thickened membranous rim[32,50] (Fig. 13.1-6). This type of placenta is associated with premature delivery, oligohydramnios, placental abruption, and fetal death.[51] The presence of a placental shelf suggesting a circumvallate placenta is frequent in the first trimester of pregnancy. Shen et al. reported 11.2% (17/152) placentas between 13 and 16 weeks of gestation with a placental shelf; two of them remained at 20 to 22 weeks, and all disappear in the third trimester of pregnancy.[52]

Placenta Membranacea or Placenta Diffusa is suspected when placental tissue extends over most of the uterine cavity on US examination.[53] The reported incidence is about 1 in 21,500 deliveries increasing to 1 in 184 in cases of placenta previa.[54] Placenta membranacea can be related to antepartum bleeding, spontaneous abortion, preterm delivery, fetal death, fetal growth restriction, postpartum hemorrhage, and placental retention.

Placental Circulation/Perfusion

Evaluation of blood movement within the intraplacental vessels or within placental lakes can be done using spectral and color Doppler techniques[55] (Fig. 13.1-7). Semiquantitative analysis of blood flow perfusion using 3D power Doppler ultrasound (PDU) has been proposed as a useful clinical tool for identifying cases at risk for perinatal complications[56,57] (Fig. 13.1-2). Three indices are calculated: (1) vascular index, representing the number of voxels containing power Doppler information, (2) flow index, indicating the averaged intensity of the voxels containing PDU information, and (3) the vascular/flow index, which is the ratio between the two indices.[26] The vascular index has been reported significantly reduced in women who later developed preeclampsia and uncontrolled diabetes.[26,27,30] Farina et al. showed a moderate prediction for fetal growth restriction when the perfusion indices were evaluated in the first trimester of pregnancy with a detection rate of 51% to 53% and a false-positive rate of 10% for small for gestational age fetuses in the third trimester of pregnancy.[58] One of the main concerns of 3D PDU volume reconstruction is the low reproducibility between operators. Cheong et al.[25] reported a correlation coefficient of 0.33 among operators in the calculation of the blood flow indices, whereas Bujold et al.[59] reported a good interobserver correlation ($R^2 > 0.8$) for all vascular indices during the first trimester of pregnancy. Several authors have proposed intraplacental Doppler velocimetry for identification of women

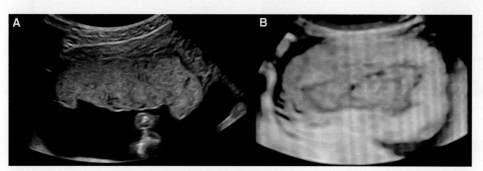

A   B

FIGURE 13.1-6: Placenta circumvallate; the edges of the placenta create a ring formed by a double fold of the amniotic and chorionic membranes: **(A)** Two-dimensional image with the edges of the placenta located above the principal body of the placenta; **(B)** 3D rendering showing the complete ring around the placenta.

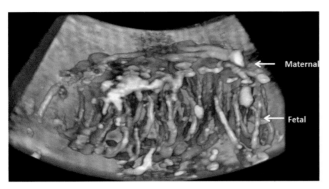

FIGURE 13.1-7: Placenta vascularity shown using 3D high-definition flow ultrasound. The maternal vessels are located in the basal plate, whereas the fetal vessels create an extensive network inside the placenta.

at risk for preeclampsia and/or fetal growth restriction.[60–66] Nevertheless, no consensus still exists on where in the placenta the Doppler gate should be located, and on how reproducible is this evaluation. Babic et al. suggested the acquisition of three intra-placental arterial Doppler waveforms: (1) in the fetal part of the placenta at the insertion of the umbilical cord, (2) at 1 cm from the insertion of the cord and; and (3) at 4 cm from the umbilical cord insertion.[66]

Key points

- Nine out of ten placentas have a circular shape and a central cord insertion.
- Placenta thickness can be measured at the site of umbilical cord insertion. The normal thickness ranges from 2 to 4 cm.
- Increased placental thickness is associated with fetal hydrops, uncontrolled diabetes, and placental floor infarction.
- Reduced placenta thickness can be related to preeclampsia and intrauterine growth restriction.

Placental Location and Placenta Previa

Placental location is the most frequent placental characteristic evaluated during US scanning. Maternal bleeding represents a major cause of death worldwide and is strongly associated with a low-lying placenta and placenta previa.[67,68] A low-lying placenta is also related to breech presentation.[69] Several factors increase the risk of placenta previa, i.e., multiparity, previous abortion, smoking, advanced maternal age, and previous uterine surgical procedures. It has been estimated that from 359 women with a prior cesarean section, one will have placenta previa in further pregnancies (OR 1.60, 95% CI 1.44 to 1.76).[70] This rate increases with the number of previous cesarean sections. Patients with a history of placenta previa also have an increased risk for placenta previa in further pregnancies.[70] Gurol-Urganci et al.[70] reported an OR of 4.77 (95% CI 3.55 to 6.42) for repeated placenta previa. In women with placenta previa, a cervical length less than 30 mm increases the risk of vaginal bleeding <34 weeks of gestation as compared to women with placental previa but with a longer cervix.[71] In some cases, the diagnosis of complete placenta previa can be made early in pregnancy[72]; however, confirmation by US in the third trimester of pregnancy is always required.[73]

The risk of maternal bleeding is related to the distance from the placental edge to the internal cervical os (ICO), which can be can be better visualized using transvaginal US.[74,75] In cases in which the edge of the placenta is located close to the ICO, the following classic classification was proposed[67]: (1) low-lying, the placenta is located at less than or equal to 2 cm from the ICO

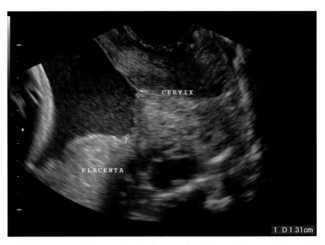

FIGURE 13.1-8: Transvaginal US of a low-lying placenta. Note the distance from the placental edge to the internal cervical os is less than 2 cm.

(Fig. 13.1-8); (2) marginal previa, the placenta is close to the ICO but does not cover it (Fig. 13.1-9); (3) partial previa, only part of the ICO is covered by the placenta (Fig. 13.1-10); and (4) complete previa, the entire ICO is covered by placental tissue (Fig. 13.1-11). However, on a recent expert committee, this terminology was updated as follows: (1) *Normal placental* location when the edge of the placenta is more than 2 cm away from the ICO (>16 weeks); (2) *low-lying placenta* was defined when the edge of the placenta is less than 2 cm away from the ICO without covering it; and (3) placenta previa was defined when the edge of the placenta covers the ICO. For low-lying placenta and placenta previa, a follow-up US at 30 to 32 weeks is recommended with transvaginal US.

Bronsteen et al.[76] found that when the placenta is within 1 cm of the ICO, 73% of women required cesarean section due to vaginal bleeding, whereas among pregnant women with a placenta lying between 1 and 2 cm, only 23% required cesarean section due to maternal bleeding. Therefore, a vaginal delivery may be considered if the edge of a low-lying placenta is located >1 cm away from the ICO. If the distance between the edge of the placenta and the ICO is >2 cm, the risk of vaginal bleeding before and during labor is not increased, and a vaginal delivery is not contraindicated.[77]

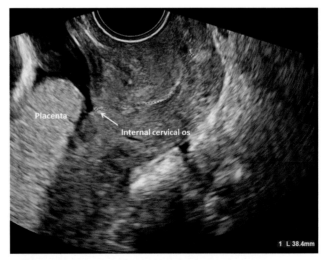

FIGURE 13.1-9: Placenta previa, the edge of the placenta is at the border of the internal cervical os.

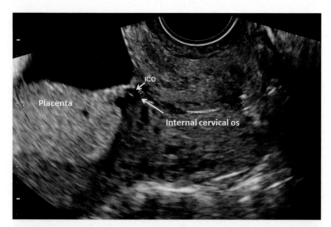

FIGURE 13.1-10: Placenta previa, the edge of the placenta is over the internal cervical os.

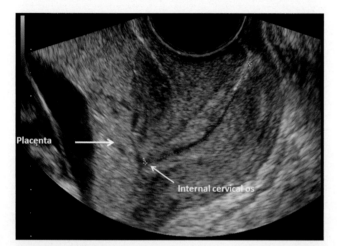

FIGURE 13.1-11: Placenta previa totalis; placental tissue covering the entire internal cervical os.

Measuring the distance between the edge of the placenta and the ICO should be done with transvaginal US. Farine et al.[74] reported that transvaginal US allowed a better visualization of the ICO and of the lower margin of the placenta as compared to transabdominal US. Transvaginal US increased by twofold the positive predictive value for placenta previa as compared with transabdominal US. Transvaginal US does not increase the risk of bleeding in women with a low-lying placenta.[68,78,79]

Placental Migration: Changes in placenta location in relation to the ICO are referred to as "placental migration."[80,81] This slight displacement can be related to (1) a progressive increase in uterine volume resulting in the movement of the placental edge away from the ICO; (2) development of the lower uterine segment during the third trimester of pregnancy; (3) continuous renovation and reformation of placental tissue; and (4) necrosis of marginal placental tissue.[80] Cho et al.[82] reported that posterior placentas migrate at an average rate of 1.6 mm (SD, 0.9 mm) per week, whereas anterior placentas migrate approximately at a rate of 2.6 mm (SD 1.5 mm) per week. A weekly rate of placental migration lower than 2 mm per week is significantly associated with an increased risk of cesarean section due to maternal bleeding.[77,83]

Confirmation of placental location in the third trimester of pregnancy has shown that 95% of women with a placental edge located within 2 cm from the ICO during the second trimester scan were no longer considered as low-lying placentas.[84] Among women identified as complete placenta previa in the second trimester, 67% of them will have a vaginal delivery, and among those considered as marginal previa, 73% of them will have a vaginal delivery. Only a few women with a low-lying placenta identified in the second trimester of pregnancy will have a cesarean section due to antepartum hemorrhage. Women with complete placenta previa showed no placental migration after 28 to 32 weeks of gestation,[85] whereas patients with partial placenta previa showed a reduced placenta migration even after 36 weeks of gestation.[83,86]

Recommendation for US Evaluation: The bladder should be empty, avoid pressing the cervix with the US transducer, visualize the entire endocervical canal (the anterior and posterior cervical lips should be of similar size), make a detailed sweep from side to side to document the location of the placental edge, measure the shortest distance between placental edge and the ICO, do not measure during contractions or during dynamic cervical changes, repeat the measurement, and select the shortest. Sonographers should report the distance in millimeters between the cervix and the placental edge. The risk of bleeding increases according to the distance.[68] A placental edge reaching the border of the ICO should be considered to be at 0 mm. If the placenta edge is within 20 mm from the cervix, a follow-up US is recommended; in these patients, the risk of cesarean section for vaginal bleeding is increased. When the placenta reaches or is located over the internal os at 18 to 24 weeks of pregnancy, a follow-up examination in the third trimester should be performed.[87]

Key points
- Low-lying placenta is diagnosed when the placental edge is within 2 cm of the ICO.
- The distance between the ICO and the lower placental edge should be confirmed by transvaginal US.
- Most cases of placenta previa diagnosed during the second trimester will resolve in the third trimester.
- The diagnosis of placenta previa should be confirmed during the third trimester of pregnancy.
- The risk of placenta previa increases in accordance with the number of previous cesarean sections and/or a history of previous placenta previa.
- The risk of bleeding during labor increases in relation to the distance between the ICO and the placenta edge when the measurement is less than or equal to 2 cm.
- A distance greater than 2 cm between the ICO and the placenta border should be considered normal and safe for vaginal delivery.

Vasa Previa

Vasa previa is diagnosed when fetal chorionic blood vessels are exposed coursing through the membranes and are interposed between the fetal presenting part and the internal os (Fig. 13.1-12).[88–90] Vasa previa is a life-threatening fetal condition, as rupture of the membranes might lead to rupture of the fetal vessel and exsanguination. The prevalence of vasa previa is approximately 1.5 to 4 in 10,000 pregnancies[91] and is more frequently observed in pregnancies from assisted reproductive techniques.[92] Most cases are found in association with low-lying placenta, velamentous insertion of the cord, bilobed placenta,

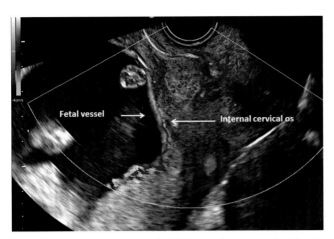

FIGURE 13.1-12: Vasa previa; the fetal vessels are attached by the amniotic membranes close to the internal cervical os.

and multiple gestations.[93–96] Current classification defines two types of vasa previa.[97] Type I occurs when there is a velamentous cord insertion and fetal vessels run within the amniotic membranes over the cervix or are in close proximity to it. Pregnancies with resolved placenta previa or low-lying placenta are also at risk for type I vasa previa due to the higher prevalence of velamentous insertion of the cord. Type II occurs when there is a bilobed placenta and fetal vessels connecting the two placental lobes course over or near the cervix. The classic criteria to define a vasa previa is similar to that for placenta previa, the fetal vessels must be within 2 cm of the ICO; however, pregnancies with a fetal vessel 3 to 4 cm from the ICO should be closely followed up to exclude/confirm vasa previa.

The US finding associated with vasa previa is presence of an echolucent area at the placental edge suggestive of blood vessels outside of the umbilical cord in proximity to the ICO (up to 3 to 4 cm) confirmed using color and spectral Doppler.[98] Spectral Doppler demonstrates a venous or arterial waveform from fetal origin, and no association between movement of the vascular structure and fetal movements.[99] The prenatal diagnosis of vasa previa is of extreme importance as it is associated with a 97% neonatal survival as compared to 43% of those who are diagnosed intrapartum or the diagnosis is done after a catastrophic bleeding.[94] Serial US evaluation can be helpful to determine a fixed location of the vascular structure. When the placenta is not in the lower part of the uterus, or in the absence of extra placenta lobes, the fetal vessels seen between the presenting part and the cervix are most probably a normal umbilical cord in a funic presentation. Other differential diagnoses include chorioamniotic separation, folding of the amniotic membranes, amniotic bands, or

varicosities of the uterine veins.[100,101] Due to the high risk of fetal/neonatal mortality, women diagnosed with vasa previa should stay in the hospital after 30 weeks of gestation with frequent monitoring of the fetal heart rate and uterine contractions, steroid therapy for lung maturation, and delivery by cesarean section at 34 to 35 weeks of gestation.[94,102]

Key points
- Vasa previa is suspected when a vascular structure between the fetal presenting part and the ICO is observed.
- Vasa previa should be confirmed by transvaginal US and may be associated with low-lying placenta, velamentous insertion of the cord, multiple pregnancies, and bilobed placenta.
- Absence of movement of the vessels with fetal movements is highly suspicious of vasa previa.
- Vasa previa increases the risk of fetal bleeding and death.

Placental Hematomas

There is no standard ultrasonographic definition of placental hematomas.[103–105] They are usually referred to as hypoechoic or anechoic areas behind the placenta or the membranes. Hematomas are classified by their location as retroplacental, subchorionic, and subamniotic[106,107] (Fig. 13.1-13) and are seen in 1% to 3% of all pregnancies, being more frequent in the first trimester of pregnancy.[106] The presence of a placental hematoma has been associated with an increased risk of spontaneous abortion, stillbirth, placental abruption, premature rupture of membranes, and preterm delivery.[108,109] Nagy et al.[110] reported a significant risk for placental abruption (relative risk [RR] 5.0; 95% CI, 2.8 to 11.1), preeclampsia (RR 4.0; 95% CI, 2.4 to 6.7), cotyledon retention or fragmented placenta (RR 3.2; 95% CI, 2.2 to 4.7), manual placental extraction (RR 3.4; 95% CI, 2.1 to 5.8), and neonatal intensive care unit (NICU) admission (RR 5.6; 95% CI 4.1 to 7.6) when a large placental hematoma (>50% of the gestational sac size) was observed. A massive subchorionic hematoma has been associated with a 40% risk of perinatal death.[111] Placental hematomas are highly related to placental abruption.

Placental Abruption

Placental abruption is defined as a premature separation of a normally implanted placenta (Fig. 13.1-14). The overall prevalence of placental abruption is about 1%, but it increases by 10-fold in preterm deliveries.[112,113] Placental abruption greatly increases the risk of fetal and antenatal death and morbidity.[114] Ananth et al.[115] reported an overall incidence of placental abruption of 9.6/1,000 deliveries. They proposed a classification based on the presence/absence of associated perinatal complications

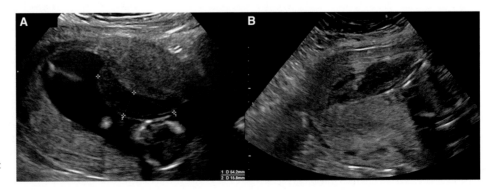

FIGURE 13.1-13: Placental hematomas: **(A)** Subamniotic; **(B)** Retroplacental.

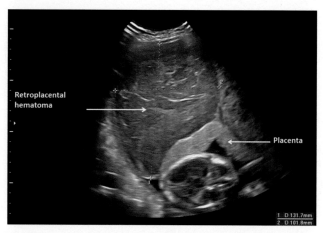

FIGURE 13.1-14: Placental abruption; note the large retroplacental hematoma (13 × 10 cm) and the relatively small placenta.

as severe placental abruption defined by the presence of at least one of the following: disseminated intravascular coagulation, hypovolemic shock, blood transfusion, hysterectomy, renal failure, or maternal death, intrauterine growth restriction, and fetal or neonatal death. Mild abruptions were those with none of the previously mentioned complications.

Risk factors for placental abruption include chronic hypertension, preeclampsia, superimposed preeclampsia, multiple gestation, oligohydramnios, polyhydramnios, myometrial tumors, thrombophilia disorders, premature rupture of membranes, cocaine and drug abuse, and chorioamnionitis.[112,116] History of abruption in a previous pregnancy is an important risk factor for recurrence in future pregnancies.[116] Ruiter reported an adjusted odds ratio of 93 (95% CI 62 to 139) for repeated placenta abruption.[117] There is no direct association between transvaginal bleeding and the degree of abruption, as a large amount of blood can be collected in the uterus; therefore, pain and contractions are the most reliable clinical signs for clinical diagnosis. The abruption can be revealed (transvaginal bleed) or concealed (accumulation of blood within the placenta or in the retroplacental space with abdominal pain). The risk of fetal demise increases when the abruption involves more than 50% of the placental surface.[112] The fetal heart rate shows different pathological patterns, i.e., variable decelerations, bradycardia, and a sinusoidal pattern. US has a sensitivity of 24%, and a positive predictive value of 88% for placental abruption.[118] Oyelese et al.[112] evaluated more than 7,000 placentas after delivery and reported a prevalence of 3.8% of abruption with a majority of patients presenting without clinical symptoms; therefore, they recommended that placental abruption should be diagnosed only when clinical symptoms are present. The same authors reported that the risk of placental abruption increases from 20 weeks onward, reaching its highest prevalence between 24 and 26 weeks followed by a reduction until the end of the pregnancy. They also reported that after 24 weeks of gestation, fetal death is significantly correlated with placental abruption. In the majority of patients, the location of the abruption is subchorionic (80%), followed by retroplacental (16%) and preplacental (4%). The echogenicity of the placenta can change in relation to the severity of the hemorrhage: acute hemorrhage shows a hyperechoic area, and resolving hematomas a hypoechoic appearance.[119] Changes from echodense to echolucid seemed to occur within 2 weeks of the hemorrhage.[48,119]

Key points
- The contribution of sonographic findings in the diagnosis of placental abruption is limited; therefore the diagnosis should rely on clinical findings.

Placental Lakes and Placental Lesions

Placental Venous Lakes are hypoechoic areas without villus structures that are usually larger than 2 cm containing turbulent low velocity flow (swirling) (Fig. 13.1-15). They are mainly seen during the third trimester of pregnancy and seem not to increase the risk of perinatal complications[120,121]; however, some authors have reported a mild association with fetal growth restriction, mainly with lakes larger than 5 cm.[122–124] The shape of the lake changes dynamically and can be seen surrounded by a rich network of vessels.

Placental Infarcts: Placental infarcts can be seen in approximately 20% of uncomplicated pregnancies and in 40% and 70% of patients with mild and severe preeclampsia, respectively.[125–127] Placental infarcts are mainly due to (a) occlusion of the spiral arteries by thrombus; (b) strangulation of the placental villi due to increased perivillous or intervillous fibrin/fibrinoid deposition; and (c) impairment of the fetal circulation due to fetal thrombotic vasculopathy.[128–131] Placental infarcts can be observed as echodense or echolucent avascular areas (Fig. 13.1-16). Fitzgerald et al.[132] reported that 50% of well-defined rounded cystic areas were associated with placental infarcts reflecting maternal vascular underperfusion, and that these patients had a higher risk of preeclampsia and fetal growth restriction. Cystic images highly suspicious of placental infarcts can be observed in 72% of fetuses with absent end diastolic flow in the umbilical artery (UA).[133] Echogenic cystic lesions had a 37% sensitivity for confirmed villous infarcts, and when combined with abnormal uterine artery Doppler velocimetry, a 53% positive predictive value for fetal death.

Placental Floor Infarction and Massive Perivillous Fibrin Deposition are linked to the accumulation of serum-derived fibrin and trophoblast-derived extracellular matrix around the distal villi.[134] The reported incidence is 0.09% in all pregnant women and has been associated with adverse pregnancy outcomes such as fetal death, fetal growth restriction, preterm delivery, preeclampsia, and recurrent spontaneous abortion.[135–137] US findings suggestive of massive perivillous deposition include

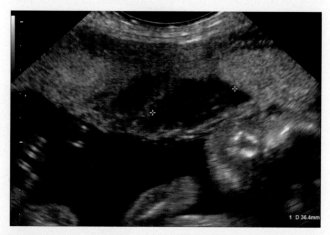

FIGURE 13.1-15: Placenta lakes: hypoechoic areas of irregular shape with no echogenic rim, and turbulent swirling blood flow inside.

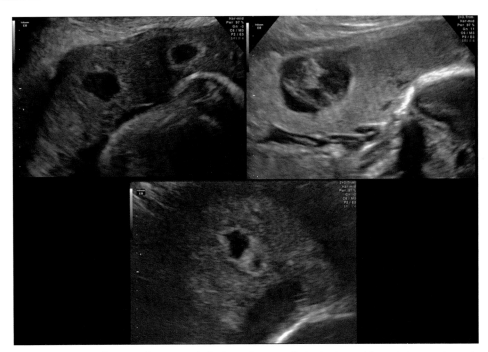

FIGURE 13.1-16: Placenta infarcts: rounded or irregular areas of mixed echogenicity and a hyperechogenic rim with no blood movement inside.

cystic hypoechoic areas larger than 1 cm, surrounded by an echogenic rim without blood flow inside the cyst (Fig. 13.1-17). The hyperechogenic rim represents villi compressed by laminated fibrin and erythrocytes. The majority of echogenic cystic lesions (72%) are 1 to 2 cm in length with a mean thickness of the echogenic rim measuring about 0.25 mm. In complicated pregnancies with echogenic lesions, Proctor et al.[138] reported a 79% prevalence of abnormal perinatal outcome, 61% of preterm delivery, 18% of severe fetal growth restriction, and 4% of perinatal death. Histopathology studies showed that 60 to 75% of placental cystic lesions are associated with intervillous thrombosis.[138]

Placental Mesenchymal Dysplasia is an anomaly characterized by a mesenchymal villus hyperplasia and dilatation of the chorionic vessels. The histological findings consist of enlarged stem villi with loose connective tissue and cistern-like formations.[139,140]

Mesenchymal dysplasia has a prevalence of 0.2% and is associated with overgrowth syndromes such as Beckwith–Wiedemann, to fetal growth restriction, fetal demise, and elevated serum alpha fetoprotein.[141] The diagnosis is mainly done in the third trimester of pregnancy based on US findings such as placentomegaly, thick placenta with hypoechoic areas, increased vascularity, and elevated alpha fetoprotein in maternal serum[142] (Fig. 13.1-18). Differential diagnoses include molar pregnancy, chorioangioma, and placental hematomas

Trophoblastic Disease

Trophoblastic disease refers to a group of clinical entities related to an abnormal development of the trophoblast classified as complete hydatidiform mole, partial hydatidiform mole, and choriocarcinoma.[143]

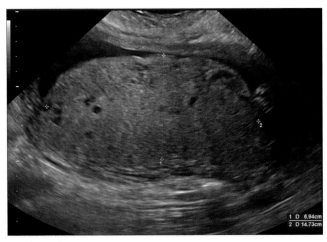

FIGURE 13.1-17: Perivillous fibrin deposition (placenta floor infarction); thickened placenta with areas of increased echogenicity, the fetus is small and the amniotic fluid is reduced.

FIGURE 13.1-18: Placental mesenchymal dysplasia; thick and enlarged placenta with cystic images; the fetus has an increased size.

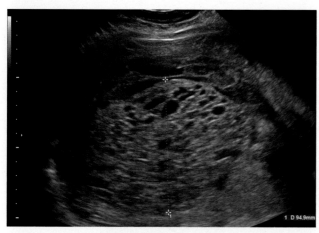

FIGURE 13.1-19: Complete mole: mixed echogenic multicystic avascular areas; there is no fetus.

A complete hydatidiform mole is characterized by swelling of the villus tissue and trophoblastic hyperplasia with no embryonic or fetal tissue (Fig. 13.1-19).[144,145] The hydropic trophoblast tissue fills the uterus with the US appearance of multiple sonolucencies that gives the classical "cluster of grapes" appearance.[144] The coexistence of a complete mole and a normal fetus can be seen in dichorionic twin pregnancies with a molar degeneration of one of the twins.[146] A complete molar pregnancy is associated with severe vaginal bleeding and persistent gestational trophoblastic disease.[147]

A partial mole is the degeneration of one or several regions of the placenta coexisting with normal placental tissue and a live fetus[144] (Fig. 13.1-20). The degenerated trophoblastic tissue gives an image of multiple vesicles surrounded by normal placental tissue. These pregnancies are related to fetal triploidy, pregnancy-induced hypertension, and persistent gestational trophoblastic disease.

Choriocarcinoma is a highly malignant tumor originating from trophoblastic epithelial cells. Approximately 50% of choriocarcinomas occur in the setting of a molar pregnancy, 30% after a miscarriage, and 20% after an apparent normal pregnancy.[148,149] Clinical presentation includes vaginal bleeding, respiratory symptoms/dyspnea, and abdominal pain. The tumor is frequently metastatic to the lung and brain.[123,150–152] Detailed placental evaluation with US might identify the primary tumor in the placenta that usually measures 2.5 to 8 mm.[153] The sonographic appearance of this tumor is heterogeneous, echogenic, with myometrium invasion and low-impedance circulation, and areas of marked vascularization within the mass documented with color and power Doppler imaging.[154]

Placental Tumors

Chorioangiomas are the most common and benign vascular placental tumors; small chorioangiomas are identified in about 1% of placentas[155] (Fig. 13.1-21). They are usually asymptomatic, but if the tumor is "large" (>4 cm), it can be associated with increased fetal and neonatal morbidity including anemia, polyhydramnios, hydrops, growth restriction, and perinatal death.[156,157] Chorioangiomas are generally diagnosed incidentally by US and have been associated with increased alpha-fetoprotein (AFP) concentrations in maternal serum and amniotic fluid (AF). The tumors appear solid and well circumscribed and can be either hyperechoic or hypoechoic, protruding from the fetal surface of the placenta or near the umbilical cord insertion site. Areas of hemorrhage, infarction, or calcification can be visualized within the mass. In addition, abundant blood flow determined by color and power Doppler is a common characteristic.[158–160] Some of the differential diagnosis when evaluating a solid mass of the placenta include placental teratoma, placental hematoma, partial hydatidiform mole, and metastasis.[161] Prenatal surgery attempting to obliterate the feeding vessel of the tumor has been reported with mixed results.[162,163] Due to the potential for adverse outcome associated with chorioangiomas, serial evaluation of fetal growth and fetal cardiac function are recommended.

Teratoma: It is a very rare tumor originated from the primitive germinal cells that derivate in multiple tissues within the tumor. Sonographic findings are a heterogeneous cyst of variable size with the presence of tissues of variable echogenicity, or echogenic areas suggestive of calcification or fat, alternating with hypoechoic areas filled with fluid.[164–166] Color Doppler sonography showed lower vascularization within the lesion than in the rest of the placenta. The distinction between a teratoma and an acardiac fetus can be challenging.

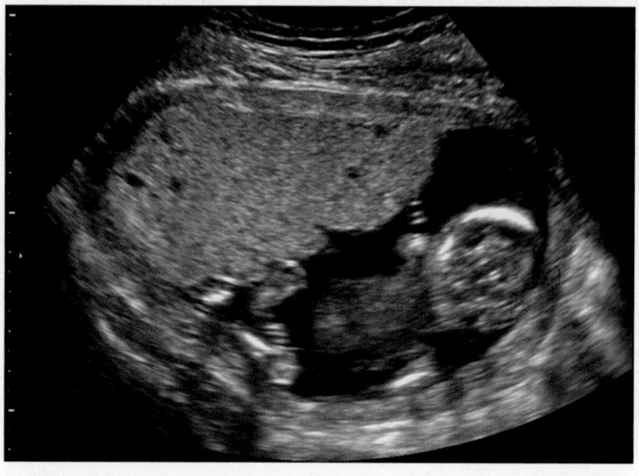

FIGURE 13.1-20: Partial mole, enlarged placenta with cystic avascular areas, the fetus is very small for gestational age due to the association with fetal triploidy.

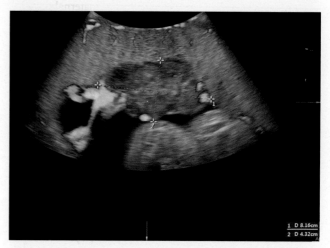

FIGURE 13.1-21: Chorioangioma; placental tumor located near the insertion of the umbilical cord with irregular echogenicity; the tumor can show increased or reduced vascularization.

Placenta in Multiple Pregnancies

Clinical management of twin pregnancies is based on an accurate determination of chorionicity (number of placentas). This is better performed during the first trimester of gestation by the identification of the lambda or T signs.[167,168] The lambda sign is created by proliferating chorionic villi growing into the space between the two layers of chorion at the site of placental insertion.[169] A lambda sign is characteristic of dichorionic twins with a sensitivity and specificity close to 100%. A clear T sign, which is due to the apposed amnion of the gestational sacs without chorionic tissue between the amnion layers, is highly suggestive of monochorionic twins (Fig. 13.1-22). When either the T or lambda signs cannot be clearly defined, that pregnancy should be considered as monochorionic and followed up closely.

Dichorionic twins have two separate placentas with no vascular communications between them. Theoretically, there is no risk of TTTS in these twins[170]; however, placental vascular communications have been reported in one case of dichorionic monozygotic twins.[171] In dichorionic twins, a disproportion in placental size may lead to selective fetal growth restriction.[172] All monochorionic twins have placental vascular anastomosis[173]; it is the imbalance in the number and type of anastomosis and differences in the insertion of the umbilical cords that increases the risk of complications (Fig. 13.1-23). There are two types of placental vascular anastomoses: unidirectional (arterial/venous), also called deep communications, and bidirectional (arterial–arterial, venous–venous), also called superficial communications. Unidirectional communications are mainly related to TTTS, while bidirectional communications are associated with selective intrauterine growth restriction.[173] In monochorionic twins, differences in the placental territory for each twin have been also associated with discordant fetal growth. In selective fetal growth restriction, there is usually a large disproportion in placental area for each twin.[173]

Placenta Conclusions

Three main components of the placental US evaluation should be routinely conducted: (1) location (in relation to the uterus and ICO); (2) appearance; and (3) consistency. If any of these parameters appear abnormal, additional placental evaluation is needed including placental biometry, transvaginal US to define the precise location of the placenta and umbilical vessels, and application of accessory techniques such as color Doppler US, to identify placental lesions that might increase the risk of maternal and fetal morbidity and mortality.

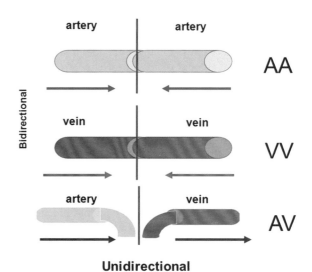

FIGURE 13.1-23: Placenta vascular anastomoses in monochorionic twins; arterial–arterial (AA), and venous–venous (VV) are bidirectional communications occurring in the surface of the placenta. Arterial–venous (AV) are unidirectional communications, the vessels run in the surface of the placenta, but the interchange of blood occurs deep in the placental tissue (deep anastomoses)

AMNIOTIC FLUID (AF)

The AF provides a supportive environment for the fetus. AF is fundamental for the development of the fetal respiratory, gastrointestinal, and musculoskeletal systems. AF protects the fetus from trauma and infection through its bacteriostatic properties and prevents compression of the umbilical cord. It is also believed that AF formation and maintenance reflects the integrity of the fetal cardiopulmonary and urogenital systems.

The Origin of Amniotic Fluid

The dynamics of the AF are complex and not entirely understood. At the beginning of pregnancy, there is free transport of water, electrolytes, and other components through the chorioamniotic membranes. In addition, there is passage of water across the embryonic skin until fetal keratinization is established at around 24 to 26 weeks.[174,175]

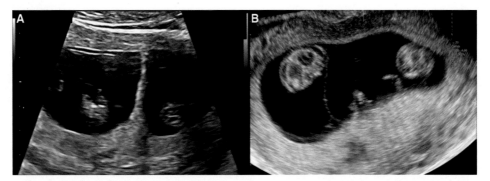

FIGURE 13.1-22: Diamnioitc twins: **(A)** Lambda sign from dichorionic pregnancies, the increase in thickness at the site of the placental insertion of the membranes is due to the chorionic tissue between the two amniotic membranes; **(B)** "T" sign from monochorionic pregnancies representing the two amnion layers without chorion in the middle.

The kidneys and the lungs are two primary sources of AF later in pregnancy. By the ninth week of gestation hypo-osmolar urine is first produced by the kidneys but does not greatly contribute to the total amount of AF. However, after 14 weeks of gestation, approximately two-thirds of the AF is produced by fetal urination and one-third from pulmonary fluid. At term, urine output ranges from 400 to 1,200 mL/day[176,177] and the fetal lungs secrete fluid at a rate of 300 to 400 mL/day.[178] The AF volume increases steadily during the first half of pregnancy, and in the second half, the AF becomes hypotonic in comparison to maternal plasma.[179]

AF volume measured during the first half of pregnancy increases logarithmically with advancing gestation.[180] It is estimated that at 8 weeks, there is about 23 mL of fluid, and at 14 weeks this has increased to approximately 100 mL.[180] A 38 to 41 weeks of gestation, the amount of AF has been estimated in 532 mL[181]; whereas after 42 weeks of gestation AF decreases approximately 150 to 170 mL per week.[182] Using an US approach (maximal vertical pocket [MVP] or 2-diameter pocket), the AF increases from 14 to 20 weeks' gestation, plateaus between 20 and 37 weeks, and then gradually declines through the 41st week of gestation.[183]

AF volume is maintained through a balance between fetal fluid production (lung liquid and urine) and fluid resorption (fetal swallowing and outflow across the amniotic and/or chorionic membranes). It is estimated that, near term, the fetus remove 200 to 500 mL of AF per day by swallowing.[184,185] Several fetal endocrine factors such as fetal vasopressin and catecholamines affect fetal renal blood flow, glomerular filtration rate, and urine flow rate.[186,187] In addition, reduction of blood flow to the fetus may elicit an endocrine response that leads to flow redistribution with reduction in fetal urine output and AF volume.[188]

US Methods to Assess Amniotic Fluid

Several semiquantitative US techniques have been described to determine the amount of AF fluid during pregnancy. These techniques are not intended to define the exact amount of AF, but rather to provide a numerical reference that can be used for diagnosis and prognosis.

The Largest Vertical Pocket was described by Manning et al.[189] as part of the biophysical profile (BPP). A normal vertical pocket was defined as that greater than 1 cm in vertical diameter visualized in any region of the uterine cavity. Subsequently, in 1984, Chamberlain et al.[190] described it as the MVP. The authors described that the depth of the pocket should be measured at a right angle to the uterine contour (to exclude errors related to the umbilical cord). The depth of the pocket ($<$1.0 cm, 1.0 to 2.0 cm, and $>$2 cm to $<$8.0 cm) was used for the classification of cases into "decreased," "marginal," or "normal" AF groups, respectively. The authors acknowledged that the choice of less than 8 cm as the upper margin for normal AF estimate was arbitrary.[190] Based on this study, the original measurement described by Manning et al.[189] used in the BPP to define oligohydramnios was changed to a pocket of less than 2 cm.

The Amniotic Fluid Index (AFI) (Fig. 13.1-24) was then described by Phelan et al.[191] For this technique, the measurements are performed with the patient in supine position and the transducer perpendicular to the floor.[191] Real time B-scanning is used to divide the uterus into four quadrants (defined by the linea nigra into right and left halves, and by the umbilicus into upper and lower halves). The largest vertical pocket free of umbilical cord or fetal parts is measured in each quadrant, and the sum of the four measurements expressed in centimeters equals the AFI. Phelan et al.[192] suggested that for pregnancies before 20 weeks of gestation, the abdomen can be divided into two halves using the *linea*

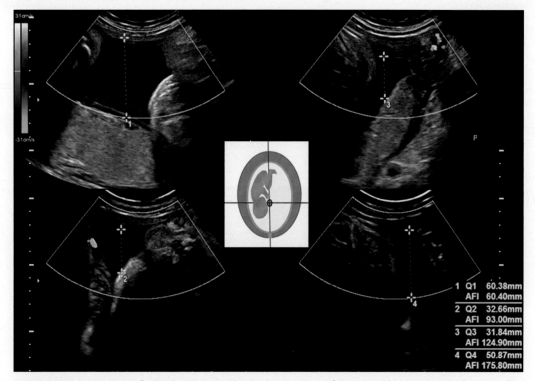

FIGURE 13.1-24: Amniotic fluid index, estimated by the measurement of the maximal accumulation of amniotic fluid in each of the four quadrants of the uterus (as shown in the figure in the *center*).

nigra and adding each half to determine the AFI.[192] In clinical practice, both AFI and MVP are widely used. The AFI and MVP values are not normally distributed during pregnancy across gestational age[183,192,193] (Tables 4A and 4B in Appendix A1).

The original studies to assess AFI and MVP were performed without color Doppler. The idea of using color Doppler to exclude the presence of the umbilical cord was felt to improve the accuracy in the diagnosis. However, the use of color Doppler has led to an overdiagnosis of oligohydramnios without improving neonatal outcomes in patients who would have been labeled as normal without the use of color Doppler.[194,195]

The American College of Obstetricians and Gynecologists recommended that either the MVP or the AFI can be used for assessment of the amount of AF.[196] However, The Society of Obstetricians and Gynecologists of Canada, in a recent publication, recommends the use of single deepest pocket (SDP) or the MVP for the diagnosis of oligohydramnios or polyhydramnios instead of AFI.[197] The Cochrane collaboration reported no difference in the performance of the MVP and the AFI for identification of women at risk of: newborn admission to the NICU, UA pH <7.1 at birth, presence of meconium, and Apgar score less than 7 at 5 minutes based on five trials including 3,226 patients. However, using AFI more pregnancies were diagnosed with oligohydramnios, and an increased rate of inductions of labor and cesarean sections were noted without improving neonatal outcomes as compared to those in which MVP was used to diagnose oligohydramnios.[198]

Recommendations for Semiquantitatively Assessing the AF Volume during Pregnancy

Technical considerations:

1. The transducer should be located in a parasagittal plane in each of the four quadrants of the maternal abdomen.
2. The sonographer should look for the largest unobstructed AF pocket and measure the vertical diameter.
3. The sonographer should avoid measuring gray areas on the screen, because AF is usually black on the gray scale.
4. The sonographer should not measure between fetal anatomical structures (i.e., arm, legs, umbilical cord) and between narrow spaces between fetal structures and the uterus.
5. Color Doppler may be used in areas where the umbilical cord is not clearly visualized; however, this may lead to overdiagnosis of oligohydramnios.

OLIGOHYDRAMNIOS

The importance of the diagnosis of oligohydramnios in obstetrics is due to its association with adverse perinatal outcomes as compared to women with normal AF[190,199–201] including stillbirth (1.4% vs. 0.3% $p<0.03$), nonreassuring fetal heart rate (48% vs. 39%; $p<0.03$), admission to the NICU (7% vs. 2%; $p<0.001$), meconium aspiration syndrome (1% vs. 0.1%; $p<0.001$), increased rate of induction of labor, birthweight less than 10th centile, higher prevalence of cesarean section, NICU admission and neonatal death (5% vs. 0.3%; $p<0.001$).[201] In a recent systematic review and metanalaysis[202] including 15 studies; oligohydramnios (defined as AFI <5 cm) was associated with meconium aspiration syndrome (RR, 2.8; 95% CI, 1.4 to 5.8), cesarean delivery for fetal distress (RR, 2.2; 95% CI, 1.6 to 2.8), and admission to the

NICU (RR, 1.7; 95% CI, 1.2 to 2.4). Patients with oligohydramnios and comorbidities were more likely to have a newborn with low birth weight (RR, 2.4; 95% CI, 1.3 to 4.3).

In cases of preterm labor, intact membranes and oligohydramnios (AFI <5 cm) the rate of intra-amniotic infection/inflammation was higher [85.7% (6/7) vs. 32.8% (87/265); $p<0.01$] and the interval-to-delivery was shorter (median 18 hours vs. median 311 hours; $p<0.01$) compared to those with an AFI greater than 5 cm.[203]

US Assessment of Oligohydramnios

The most common criteria used to define oligohydramnios based on the AFI are either a fixed value of <5 cm[192], or a value <5th percentile according to gestational age charts[193,204] (Table 4A in Appendix A1). When using the MVP, a fixed value <2 cm or a value <5th percentile for gestational age can be used to define oligohydramnios[204] (Table 4B in Appendix A1). The accuracy of the AFI, MVP, and the 2-diameter pocket by US was reported by Magann et al.[183] The authors concluded that the MVP technique was less likely to classify patients as having oligohydramnios (1%) than either AFI (8%) or the 2-diameter pocket (30%).[183] Similar findings, noted by Alfirevic et al.,[205] who reported more women diagnosed with oligohydramnios when the AFI was used (25/250, 10%) than with the MVP (6/250, 2%).[205] In a randomized clinical trial, Moses et al.[206] concluded that oligohydramnios was diagnosed more frequently in patients in which the AFI was used (25%), versus those in whom the MVP was used (8%).

A systematic review and meta-analysis[207] including four randomized trials[205,206,208,209] and 3,125 pregnant women (low risk and high risk) showed that when the AFI was used, more cases of oligohydramnios were diagnosed (risk ratio [RR] 2.33, 95% CI 1.67 to 3.24), more women had induction of labor (RR 2.10; 95% CI 1.60 to 2.76), and there were more cesarean deliveries for fetal distress (RR 1.45; 95% CI 1.07 to 1.97) in comparison to the MVP; and (2) there was no evidence that any method was superior in preventing poor perinatal outcomes, such as admission to NICU; UA pH less than 7.1; presence of meconium fluid; or Apgar score less than 7 at 5 minutes. Similarly, in a recent multicenter, open-label, randomized controlled trial (SAFE trial)[210] comparing an MVP versus AFI to predict pregnancy outcomes in 1,052 pregnant women demonstrated that more cases of oligohydramnios were diagnosed using the AFI vs. the MVP (9.8% vs. 2.2%; RR, 4.51 (95% CI, 2.2 to 8.57)) and more cases of labor induction for oligohydramnios were performed when using the AFI vs. the MVP (12.7% vs. 3.6%; RR, 3.50 (95% CI, 1.76 to 6.96)). Interestingly, abnormal cardiotocography was seen more often in the AFI group than in the MVP group [32.3% vs. 26.2%; RR, 1.23 (95% CI, 1.02 to 1.50)]. There was no difference in the primary outcome, which was newborn admission to the NICU [4.2% vs. 5.0%; RR, 0.85 (95% CI, 0.48 to 1.50)].

Several authors have reported that the outcome of pregnancies complicated with "isolated oligohydramnios" is comparable to that of low-risk pregnancies with normal AF levels.[211–215] Based on the current available information derived from randomized studies and meta-analysis; the authors recommend the use of MVP less than or equal to 2 cm for diagnosing oligohydramnios as it reduces the rate of false-positive diagnosis, leading to less induction without increasing neonatal morbidity. The use of AFI for diagnosis of oligohydramnios or reduced AF may have a role when significant changes are noted; however, clinical correlation is strongly recommended.

Clinical Assessment of Oligohydramnios

The reported incidence of oligohydramnios varies widely (3% to 40%) depending on the study population, whether it was determined intrapartum or antepartum, and on the US technique used.[200] When the AF is found to be decreased or absent on US examination, several considerations should be taken into account (Table 13.1-1).

Most importantly, a thorough maternal history to determine rupture of amniotic membranes should be obtained. A history consistent or suspicious of rupture of membranes requires a complete examination that includes a sterile speculum examination to determine the presence of vaginal pooling, along with nitrazine ferning testing, and/or immunoassay fluid testing (Amnisure or Rom Plus).[216] If rupture of membranes is ruled out, maternal medication intake should be investigated as several drugs have been associated with decrease AF such as angiotensin-converting

enzyme (ACE) inhibitor,[217] and chronic use of indomethacin.[218] A significant group of patients may also have oligohydramnios associated with preeclampsia,[219] diabetes,[220] and growth restriction.[183] US growth assessment to determine fetal growth restriction is essential. If the workup shows a negative result, the fetal renal anatomy and bladder should be assessed by US, as decreased or absent AF may be a consequence of bilateral renal agenesis,[221] bilateral multi-/polycystic kidneys,[222] or urinary tract obstruction.[223] It is important not to mistake the adrenal glands for the kidneys as the adrenal glands can be enlarged and displaced downward ("lying down") in cases of renal agenesis, giving the false impression of a kidney when the kidneys are not present.[224,225] In addition, an ectopic location of a nonfunctional kidney should be suspected. Of note, the outcomes of pregnancies complicated by chronic oligohydramnios or anhydramnios of renal origin are extremely poor, with a few number of survivors due to the association with pulmonary hypoplasia.[222] Another reported cause of decreased AF is maternal dehydration[226]; in these cases, the maternal hydration status should be assessed (physical examination and urinalysis), and a fluid challenge may be considered. If any of these findings are not present, oligohydramnios can be referred to as unexplained or idiopathic oligohydramnios.

Clinical Management of Oligohydramnios in the Third Trimester

Several randomized studies have reported that the use of oral or intravenous (IV) hydration can improve or increase the AFI in pregnancies that appear to be complicated by oligohydramnios or decreased AF in the third trimester and intact membranes.[227–230] Others have reported that IV hydration improves the uteroplacental perfusion.[188]

Doppler velocimetry has been used in the management of pregnancies complicated by oligohydramnios. A retrospective study including 76 pregnancies[231] reported that 80% of those complicated by oligohydramnios (AFI <5th percentile) and abnormal Doppler velocimetry of the UA had associated perinatal morbidity, whereas in those with oligohydramnios but normal UA Doppler, only 37% had associated perinatal morbidity 25 ($p = 0.001$). Patients with abnormal umbilical Doppler velocimetry were delivered earlier (31.4 weeks) than were patients with normal UA Doppler (33.8 weeks); ($p < 0.005$). Of note, no fetal deaths were reported in either group, but 73% of patients had fetal growth restriction in the abnormal Doppler group versus 13% in the normal Doppler group. The authors concluded that pregnancies with oligohydramnios and normal UA Doppler can be managed more conservatively, with intervention only for indications other than oligohydramnios.[231] Furthermore, this study suggests that avoiding intervention in pregnancies with oligohydramnios and normal UA Doppler velocimetry may decrease iatrogenic morbidity related to prematurity, especially in cases where no fetal growth restriction is evident.[231] Once idiopathic oligohydramnios is diagnosed, serial AF measurements, fetal growth evaluation, fetal Doppler evaluation, and antenatal testing (including nonstress test and BPP) should be initiated.

Borderline Oligohydramnios

Borderline AF has different definitions; some authors use an AFI between 5.1 and 8 cm, and others have used a definition of an AFI between 5.1 and 10 cm.[232] In uncomplicated pregnancies, borderline oligohydramnios has been associated with fetal growth

---

TABLE 13.1-1   Factors Associated with Oligohydramnios

MATERNAL

Maternal dehydration

Hypertensive disorders

Antiphospholipid syndrome

Dialysis

Myotonic dystrophy

Medications

- Angiotensin-converting enzyme (ACE) inhibitors
- Long-term use of nonsteroidal anti-inflammatory drugs (i.e., indomethacin, sulindac)
- Thiazide diuretics

FETAL

Premature rupture of membranes

Growth restriction

Post-term pregnancy

Twin-to-twin transfusion syndrome (donor)

Meckel–Gruber syndrome

Triploidy

Inborn errors of metabolism

Chorioamniotic separation

Abdominal pregnancy

Chronic abruption–oligohydramnios sequence (CHAOS)

Fetal infections

- Rubeola infection

Renal malformations

- Polycystic horseshoe-shaped kidney
- Urethral obstruction
- Polycystic kidneys
- Multicystic dysplastic kidneys
- Bilateral renal agenesis

restriction, small for gestational age newborns, induction of labor, and admission to the NICU.[232] Others, however, suggest that there is no association with an increased risk of adverse perinatal outcomes in uncomplicated pregnancies with borderline oligohydramnios in late preterm[233] or at term gestation.[234] However, it is associated with a higher rate of induction of labor and small for gestational age fetuses at term in uncomplicated pregnancies.[234] There are no clear guidelines for the clinical management of borderline oligohydramnios.

Key points
- Oligohydramnios is defined as an MVP less than 2 cm.
- MVP (<2 cm) reduces the rate of false-positive diagnosis of oligohydramnios compared to AFI (<5 cm).
- In the presence of oligohydramnios, evaluate for rupture of membranes, maternal medication intake, evidence of growth restriction or preeclampsia, and the fetal genitourinary system.
- Use of AFI instead of MVP to define oligohydramnios at term may lead to higher rate of induction of labor and cesarean section without improving neonatal outcomes.
- UA Doppler examination appears to be of value in the antenatal care of women with idiopathic oligohydramnios.

POLYHYDRAMNIOS

The reported incidence of polyhydramnios is approximately 1 to 2%.[235,236] Several measurements have been suggested to define polyhydramnios using US; by a fixed MVP value of greater than 8 cm[237] (Fig. 13.1-25); an AFI greater than 20 cm (between 36 and 40 weeks of gestation); or AFI greater than 24 cm that represents the 97.5th percentile between 20 and 42 weeks.[193,238] Magann et al. concluded that both, the MVP and the AFI, performed similarly to identify polyhydramnios (both <1%).[183] Odibo et al. noted that an MVP greater than 8 cm classified more cases as polyhydramnios despite that the AFI was still within normal range (<24 cm).[195] Other authors have arbitrarily categorized pregnancies with polyhydramnios into three groups based on the AFI: mild (AFI 25.1 to 30.0 cm); moderate (AFI 30.1 to 35.0 cm); or severe (AFI >35.1 cm).[239] This classification showed a significant association with the RR of congenital anomalies: polyhydramnios mild: 3.2 (95% CI 1.5 to 6.8); moderate 5.7 (95% CI 2.4 to 13.3), and severe 13.1 (95% CI 5.8 to 29.5).[239] However, the rate of preterm delivery did not differ significantly according to the severity of polyhydramnios

unless the pregnancy was complicated with congenital anomalies and/or diabetes.[239] On the contrary, the association of fetal anomalies seem not to be related to a classification of polyhydramnios based on the MVP as mild (8 to 11 cm), moderate (12 to 14 cm), and severe (>15 cm).[235] Based on this classification, more than 60% of patients with mild polyhydramnios will not have an identifiable cause (idiopathic), and more than 70% will end with a normal healthy infant at term.[235]

Polyhydramnios is associated with an increased risk of macrosomia (birth weight >4,000 gm),[240–242] preterm delivery,[243] NICU admission,[243] meconium-stained AF,[243] small for gestational age,[244] and low birth weight[243] accounting for two- to fivefold increase in perinatal and neonatal mortality.[235–237,243–245] Moreover, the rate of cesarean section has been reported to be increased in pregnancies complicated with polyhydramnios,[236,242,245] primarily due to abnormal fetal heart rate,[236] suspected macrosomia,[236] and failure to labor progress.[242] Of note, the combination of small for gestational age and polyhydramnios has been considered to be ominous for the fetus as it represents an independent risk factor for neonatal mortality (59%) and chromosomal abnormalities (38%).[244,246] A systematic review and meta-analysis by Morris et al. reported a strong association between polyhydramnios (MVP >8 cm or AFI >24 cm) and birthweight greater than 90th centile (OR 11.41, 95% CI 7.09 to 18.36).[247]

Chen et al. showed that the rate of placental abruption and placenta accreta was higher in pregnancies complicated with polyhydramnios.[243] It has been reported that the rate of fetal aneuploidy in cases of isolated polyhydramnios is around 1%[236,248] and 10% in the presence of associated anomalies.[248] In retrospective studies, 9.3% to 28.4% of isolated polyhydramnios had an anomaly or a syndrome detected after birth (Table 13.1-2).[249,250] Therefore, caution should be considered when establishing "idiopathic" polyhydramnios with a very good prognosis. In a series of 113 cases with polyhydramnios, 42.8% of cases showed a reduction to mild polyhydramnios or normal AF volume with advancing gestation. In those cases, the morbidity (i.e., preterm

TABLE 13.1-2 Fetal Anomalies and Syndromes Diagnosed after Birth in Idiopathic Polyhydramnios

Beckwith–Wiedemann syndrome	Trisomy 21
Pulmonary valve stenosis	Cheiloschisis
Bartter syndrome	Pierre Robin sequence
Hypospadias	Palatoschisis
X-linked myotubular myopathy	Gastrointestinal atresia (esophageal atresia)
Developmental and motor disorder	Intrahepatic atrioventricular shunt
Hemiplegia (cerebral bleeding *in utero*)	Pierre Robin sequence with cleft palate
Noonan syndrome	Hydrocephalus

Data obtained from Dorleijn DM, Cohen-Overbeek TE, Groenendaal F, et al. Idiopathic polyhydramnios and postnatal findings. *J Matern Fetal Neonatal Med.* 2009;22:315–320; Abele H, Starz S, Hoopmann M, et al. Idiopathic polyhydramnios and postnatal abnormalities. *Fetal Diagn Ther.* 2012;32:251–255.

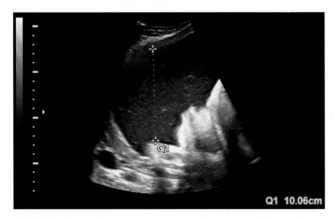

FIGURE 13.1-25: Increased amniotic fluid measured by the maximal vertical amniotic fluid pocket.

delivery, preeclampsia, cesarean delivery) and neonatal mortality was lower in comparison to women who had persistent polyhydramnios.[251]

The increased AF pressure due to polyhydramnios may lead to fetal acidemia and hypoxia (determined by cordocentesis)[252] due to abnormal uteroplacental perfusion, umbilical venous compression, or distortion of the vascular structure in the placenta villi, to uterine contractions and preterm labor, and to placental abruption.[252]

In conclusion, based on the current literature, an acceptable definition of polyhydramnios in the late second and the third trimester in both singleton and multiple gestations is an MVP greater than 8 cm[253] or a AFI greater than 24 cm.

Clinical Evaluation of Polyhydramnios

Polyhydramnios may be caused either by excess fetal urine or lung fluid production, or by a defect in AF resorption. One of the typical clinical findings associated with polyhydramnios is a fundal height greater than the current gestational age. This should prompt the clinician to perform a US examination to evaluate for polyhydramnios, a large for gestational age fetus, unrecognized multiple pregnancies, or any potential anomaly. The prevalence of either pregestational[236,254] or gestational diabetes[255–257] and polyhydramnios has been reported to be 5 to 64%[236,248,254] and 2 to 12%,[248,257] respectively. There is a strong association between polyhydramnios and central nervous system (CNS) abnormalities (i.e., anencephaly, encephalocele, hydranencephaly).[258] Gastrointestinal anomalies such as atresia or obstructions (i.e., esophagus, duodenal, tracheoesophageal fistulas) should be suspected.[258] A characteristic sign of fetuses with gastrointestinal obstructions or atresia is that polyhydramnios usually develops after the second trimester. The absence of the stomach bubble with polyhydramnios is associated with esophageal atresia and tracheoesophageal fistula.[259] Of note, if the stomach is not seen, the US scan should be repeated after 30 to 60 minutes, giving time for the stomach to fill. An enlarged thyroid (fetal goiter) may cause esophageal obstruction and polyhydramnios.[260,261] Space-occupying thoracic lesions, such as bronchopulmonary sequestration (BPS) or congenital cystic adenomatoid malformation (CCAM), can cause compression of the gastrointestinal tract and lead to polyhydramnios.[262,263] These lesions can also cause compression and/or obstruction of the fetal circulation or lymphatics resulting in hydrops and polyhydramnios.[262]

Conditions that can affect the musculoskeletal system (particularly those affecting fetal tone or fetal movements, i.e., akinesia, hypokinesia, hypotonia) can be associated with polyhydramnios. Polyhydramnios and abnormal fetal posture is also associated with Pena–Shokeir, Freeman–Sheldon syndrome, arthrogryposis, or to an inherited neuromuscular disorder.[264–267] In cases of Prader–Willi syndrome, polyhydramnios, decreased fetal movements, resulting in an abnormal fetal posture[268,269] (Table 13.1-3).

If the fetus is affected with Bartter syndrome (fetal polyuria due to an abnormal loop of Henle), the nephrons' ability to control urinary sodium, potassium, and chloride will be affected and lead to fetal polyuria and subsequent polyhydramnios.[270]

In the case of fetal growth restriction and polyhydramnios, chromosomal aneuploidy should be suspected, especially trisomy 18.[246] Overgrowth syndromes such as Perlman syndrome and Beckwith–Wiedemann syndrome (BWS) are inherited disorders that can present with polyhydramnios.[271,272] Additional US findings of Perlman syndrome are macrosomia and nephromegaly; in BWS, there is also macrosomia, renal anomalies,

abdominal wall defects, and macroglosia. For these rare cases of polyhydramnios, prenatal diagnosis through AF chromosomal microarray is available. Persistent abnormal heart rate (tachyarrhythmia) that leads to increased cardiac output and subsequent hydrops can also be associated with polyhydramnios.[273] Large placental chorioangiomas can increase the fetal cardiac output, which may lead to hydrops and polyhydramnios.[274] In some cases of cytomegalovirus (CMV), parvovirus B19, and varicella zoster infections, polyhydramnios can be observed.[275] Maternal ingestion of lithium has been reported to cause polyhydramnios probably due to a form of fetal nephrogenic diabetes.[276]

Management of Polyhydramnios

The management should be focused on the specific clinical condition (diabetic control, obstructive lesion), with the primary goal to improve maternal symptoms (such as reducing preterm contractions, improving respiratory symptoms), or to reverse/treat the fetal condition associated with polyhydramnios. Usually, mild and moderate polyhydramnios do not require intervention as the symptoms are usually not severe. In contrast, severe polyhydramnios (leading to significant symptomology such as preterm labor, maternal respiratory compromise, and maternal discomfort) may require some form of therapy.

Polyhydramnios can be treated by removing the AF via amniocentesis (amnioreduction); two protocols have been described, the standard and the aggressive.[277] The standard protocol consists of removing the AF at a rate of 45 to 90 mL/min for 60 to 120 minutes using a 20-gauge needle until an MVP below 7 to 8 cm is measured. The aggressive protocol consists of using an 18-gauge needle, removing the AF at a rate of 140 mL/min until oligohydramnios is obtained.[277] Potential complications such as contractions, rupture of membranes, chorioamnionitis, and placental abruption are present in approximately 1.5% of procedures.[278] Due to the risk of polyhydramnios recurrence after an amnioreduction, this treatment is usually performed only in severe cases.

Once no fetal anomalies have been detected and other potential etiologies have been excluded, the AF can be monitored every 10 to 14 days, in combination with nonstress test, and/or fetal BPP.[279] However, according to a recent publication of the Society of Maternal-Fetal Medicine, antenatal testing is not recommended in cases of mild isolated polyhydramnios.[280] Unfortunately, a percentage (between 5 and 28%) of fetuses with idiopathic polyhydramnios may have a significant anomaly, syndrome, or morbidity that may not be detected prenatally[249,250,281] but the pregnancy course is likely to be uneventful.

Key points
- Definition of polyhydramnios: MVP greater than 8 cm, AFI greater than 24 cm.
- Isolated polyhydramnios is associated with increased risk of macrosomia. In most cases of mild polyhydramnios, the outcome is favorable.
- In the presence of polyhydramnios, evaluate for maternal diabetes and fetal anomalies (i.e., gastrointestinal, pulmonary, renal, or CNS).
- The rate of aneuploidy in idiopathic polyhydramnios is 1%, and 10% when structural anomalies are detected.
- Idiopathic polyhydramnios may be associated with increased postnatal morbidity due to anomalies or syndromes not detected prenatally.
- Amnioreduction is reserved for severe cases of polyhydramnios when patients are symptomatic.

TABLE 13.1-3	Factors Associated with Polyhydramnios

Maternal	Encephalocele
Diabetes mellitus (preexisting and gestational)	Microcephaly
Lithium intake	Sacrococcygeal teratoma
Fetal Causes	*Gastrointestinal (GI) tract*
Erythroblastosis fetalis	Astomia
Fetal arrhythmias	Congenital diaphragmatic hernia
Macrosomia	Annular pancreas
Placental abnormalities—chorioangioma	Omphalocele
Cystic hygromas	Small bowel atresia
Beckwith–Wiedemann syndrome, Perlman syndrome	Tracheoesophageal fistula
Achondrogenesis type 1-B	Esophageal atresia
Fetal infections	Duodenal stenosis
Cytomegaloviruses infection	Gastroschisis
Varicella zoster	Cleft palate
Parvovirus B19	Fetal goiter occluding the GI tract
Toxoplasmosis	*Respiratory tract*
Noonan syndrome	Cystic adenomatoid malformation of the lung
Bartter syndrome	Chylothorax
Multiple pregnancies	Bronchopulmonary sequestration
Twin-to-twin transfusion syndrome (recipient)	*Cardiovascular system*
Twin reversed arterial perfusion sequence	Valvular incompetence
Idiopathic	Valvular stenosis
Fetal malformations	Ebstein anomaly
Central nervous system	*Musculoskeletal System*
Anencephaly	Skeletal dysplasia
Hydrocephaly	Pena–Shokeir syndrome
Iniencephaly	Myotonic dystrophy
Intracerebral arteriovenous malformations	Fetal akinesia/hypokinesia syndrome
Hydranencephaly	

Other US Findings in the Amniotic Fluid

Occasionally, the AF may appear to contain homogeneous echogenic material, particulate matter, or free-floating particles. Particulate matter in the first two trimesters of pregnancy has been associated with intra-amniotic bleeding.[282,283] Moreover, free-floating particulate matter has also been described in uncommon cases such as excessive desquamation of the skin in congenital ichthyosis,[284] epidermolysis bullosa letalis,[285] or the acrania–anencephaly sequence.[286]

Some authors have described that this echogenic material is suggestive of the presence of meconium in the AF (especially in the third trimester).[286] However, other authors do not support this statement,[287] and suggested that this echogenic material is vernix.[288] The reason for these differences is that meconium and vernix can have a similar appearance on US.[289]

The presence of free-floating hyperechogenic material within the AF in close proximity to the uterine cervix has been described in women with an episode of preterm labor,[290] in women with a history of preterm delivery or threatened preterm labor,[291] and in asymptomatic women at risk for spontaneous preterm delivery in the midtrimester of pregnancy.[292] This particulate matter is known as AF "sludge" (Fig. 13.1-26) and is an independent risk factor for preterm delivery, histological chorioamnionitis, and microbial invasion of the amniotic cavity in patients with spontaneous preterm labor or with a short cervix and intact membranes.[290,292–294]

Amniotic Fluid Assessment of Preterm Prelabor Rupture of Membranes (PPROM)

The sonographic examination of fetuses with PPROM may be challenging due to the reduced AF volume. However, contrary to what is generally believed, rupture of membranes is not always associated with severe immediate oligohydramnios. Harding et

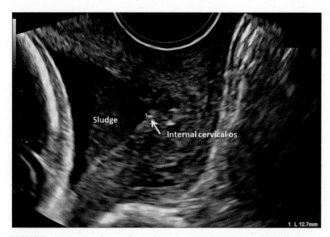

FIGURE 13.1-26: Cervical sludge; hyperechogenic material in the amniotic fluid located over the internal cervical os. The sludge moves with the maternal or fetal movements but tends to return to the same location.

al.[295] noted that the AFI in patients with preterm PPROM remained stable with a mean AFI on admission of 5.9 ± 2.5 cm, and of 5.4 ± 2.0 cm on the day of delivery. Moreover, Vintzileos et al.[296] reported that 65.5% of patients with PPROM had an MVP greater than 2 cm, while 15.5% had a MVP between 1 and 2 cm. Only 19% of women with PPROM had an MVP less than 1 cm. Patients with an AF pocket less than 1 cm had a shorter latency to delivery period, and higher incidence of chorioamnionitis and neonatal sepsis than did patients with PPROM and a MVP greater than 2 cm.[296] Similar findings were reported in another study, which found that women with an MVP of less than 1 × 1 cm had a higher incidence of chorioamnionitis and endometritis than did those with an AF pocket greater than 1 × 1 cm.[297] Notably, no difference in the duration of the latency period between the two groups was found, but a higher proportion of patients with reduced fluid were in labor at the time of admission.[297] Storness–Bliss et al.[298] evaluated women with periviable PPROM (<24 weeks), those who had an MVP >1 cm had a longer latency to delivery period than did those with an MVP less than 1 cm (57 days vs. 13 days; $p = 0.014$), and there were more surviving fetuses in the group with an MVP > 1 cm than in the group with MVP < 1 cm [6/10 (60%) vs. 1/12 (8.3%); $p = 0.02$]. The gestational age at rupture of membranes was similar in both groups (19 weeks); however, the gestational age at delivery was different (27.5 weeks vs. 22.9 weeks) but did not reach statistical significance ($p = 0.07$).[298] Hadi et al.[299] also reported that patients with PPROM between 20 and 25 weeks of gestation with higher AFI had a longer latency to delivery and higher neonatal survival. However, others have reported that US assessment of AF is a poor predictor of survival in cases of previable PPROM.[300]

Patients with PPROM and fetal heart decelerations have a lower AFI than do those without decelerations (4.32 cm ± 1.67 vs. 6.47 cm ± 3.59, $p<0.01$).[301] This observation suggests that cord compression due to oligohydramnios may be the mechanism behind variable decelerations observed in patients with PPROM.

AMNIOTIC MEMBRANES

The fetal membranes are formed primarily by the chorion and amnion, and are physiologically separated during the first 12 to 13 weeks of fetal life by the extra-embryonic celomic cavity. After

13 weeks of gestation, the amnion and chorion start attaching to each other to form the amniotic membrane that surrounds the amniotic cavity, and by 16 weeks, they are usually fused. When the chorioamniotic membranes remain unfused after 16 weeks of gestation, there is an association with chromosomal abnormalities including trisomy 21, trisomy 18, and Turner syndrome, and to fetal structural abnormalities such as cystic hygroma, and exomphalos[302,303] (Fig. 13.1-27).

Amniotic sheets (synechia) are fibrous scar bands covered with two layers of chorion and amnion. These are different from amniotic bands, as they cause no restriction of fetal motion or subsequent fetal deformity. The length of the sheets is between 3 and 10 cm (average 7 cm), and the thickness ranges from 3 to 8 mm (average 6 mm).[304] The reported incidence on US is approximately 0.14 to 0.6%.[304–306] Many patients who have synachia have a clinical history of uterine instrumentation (voluntary termination, and dilatation and curettage) or uterine infections to explain scar formation.[305] Amniotic sheets have the appearance of a thick amniotic band with a broad base (Fig. 13.1-28). They can be seen with either a free edge or appear to traverse the entire length of the sac.[306] Although the amniotic sheet appears to be within the AF, it is anatomically external to the amniotic sac.[307] Color Doppler in the thick portions of the amniotic sheets will show maternal vessels within the thickest portion of the synachiae.[308] The overall consensus is that the presence of amniotic sheets is a benign finding; however, a higher rate of malpresentation (especially when the amniotic sheet is perpendicular to the placenta) has been reported.[305]

Amniotic band syndrome occurs when the amnion ruptures, leading to formation of fibrous bands that can cross fetal parts and cause or are associated with significant anomalies in the fetus. It has a prevalence of 1/10,000 pregnancies and the anomalies can range from very mild defects to severe limb amputation, body wall defects, or craniofacial anomalies[309] (Fig. 13.1-29). The possible etiologies include early disruption of the amnios, a primary mesodermal defect, or a vascular endothelial injury.

A characteristic US feature is the presence of an amniotic band attached to the fetus with restriction of movement or deformity. However, sometimes the band is not visible, and the most common findings suggestive of this condition are constriction rings in body parts, distal lymphedema, syndactyly, clubbed feet, and

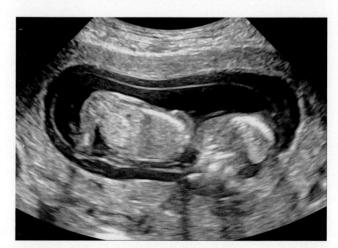

FIGURE 13.1-27: Lack of fusion of the chorioamniotic membranes (amniotic membrane separation). This is an abnormal finding after 16 weeks of gestation or after fetal invasive procedures. Fetal movement may cause the membrane to undulate.

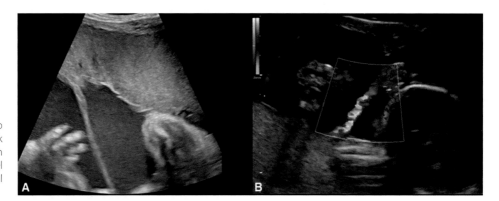

FIGURE 13.1-28: Amniotic sheets, also referred to as amniotic synechia; **(A)** thick amniotic sheet crosses the entire length of the gestational sac; **(B)** maternal vessel within the synechia. There is no fetal restriction or fetal deformity

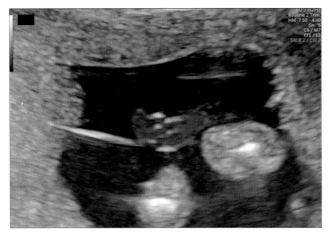

FIGURE 13.1-29: Amniotic band, thin membrane inserting in the placenta and in the umbilical cord. The amniotic band keeps attached to the umbilical cord even after intense fetal movements. Amniotic bands can create disruptions, amputations, and deformities.

asymmetric cranial defects.[310] Amniotic band syndrome is considered as part of the ADAM complex (amniotic deformity, adhesions, mutilations) integrated by amniotic band syndrome, congenital constriction bands, pseudoainhum, and Streeter dysplasia.[311] Some authors have suggested fetoscopic treatment for amniotic band release.[312]

UMBILICAL CORD

The umbilical cord consists of an outer layer of epithelium from the amnion containing a gelatinous substance known as Wharton jelly mainly formed by mucopolysaccharides.[313] Within this

jelly structure, there are the allantois, the vitelline duct, and the umbilical vessels. The umbilical cord is formed at 4 to 6 weeks' postconception by the connection between the body stalk and the yolk stalk (ductus omphaloentericus).[313] The helical course of the umbilical vessels can be observed as early as 28 days postconception, and is clearly visible from 7 weeks in 95% of fetuses (Fig. 13.1-30). The umbilical cord is inserted in the center of the placenta in about 90% of cases, and marginal insertion occurs within 1 cm of the placental edge. A velamentous insertion of the placenta is when the vessels start branching still in the amniotic membranes before the placental insertion (Fig. 13.1-31). The origin of the coiling is unknown, but it has been related to active or passive torsion of the embryo, differential umbilical vascular growth rates, fetal movements, and to fetal hemodynamic forces and the muscular fibers in the arterial wall. There are two umbilical arteries and one vein; generally the right vena umbilicalis becomes obliterated and the left persists. The intra-abdominal portions of the umbilical vessels degenerate after birth; the umbilical arteries become the lateral ligaments of the bladder, and the umbilical vein becomes the round ligament of the liver. In the majority of umbilical cords, there is an anastomosis within 1.5 cm of the placental insertion site called Hyrtl anastomosis.[313,314]

Single Umbilical Artery (SUA)

It is reported to have an incidence between 0.1 and 0.6% in singleton pregnancies,[315-317] 9.2% in twin pregnancies,[318] and 5.9% in women older than 37 years old and increased nuchal translucency.[319] A single umbilical artery (SUA) is the result of obliteration or atrophy of one of the arteries. The diagnosis is done by direct visualization of the umbilical cord where two round structures are identified (one vein and one artery) (Fig. 13.1-32). The use of color Doppler facilitates the visualization of the vessels.

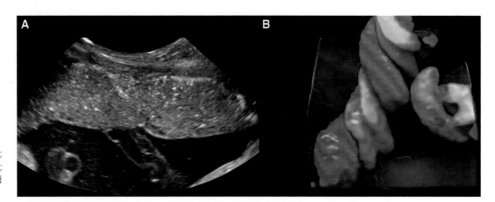

FIGURE 13.1-30: Normal umbilical cord; **(A)** insertion in the middle of the placenta; **(B)** normal anatomy of the umbilical cord with two arteries and one vein.

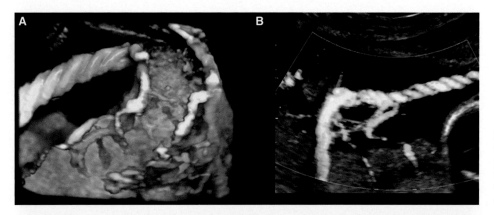

FIGURE 13.1-31: (A) Marginal insertion of the umbilical cord within 1 cm of the placental edge; **(B)** velamentous insertion, the cord inserts in the membranes and the vessels start branching before entering the placenta.

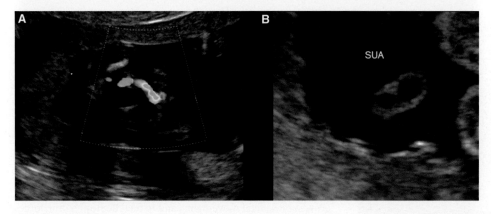

FIGURE 13.1-32: Single umbilical artery *(SUA)* visualized in **(A)** a cross-sectional plane of the fetal pelvis and the bladder; and **(B)** cross section of a free loop of the umbilical cord.

Another approach is to obtain a transverse view of the fetal bladder and use color. Normally, the umbilical arteries will be seen each at each side of the fetal bladder. This approach may have certain benefits because it can identify the side where the UA is absent. The left UA was detected more frequently absent than was the right side (61.7% vs. 38.3%).[320]

SUA is associated with many other congenital anomalies including cardiac, genitourinary, gastrointestinal, skeletal, and CNS.[316,320,321] SUA was associated with an increased risk of intrauterine growth restriction (adjusted OR 2.1, 95% CI 1.6 to 2.7, $P < 0.01$) and preterm delivery before 34 weeks (adjusted OR 3.1, 95% CI 2.1 to 4.8, $P<0.01$).[315-317]

Once an SUA is detected, a detailed fetal US evaluation of the fetus should be performed. Some authors recommend a screening echocardiogram, while other suggest that evaluation of the fetal heart with the standard views (four-chamber view, outflow tracts, and transverse arches) is enough to detect the cardiac defects present in fetuses with SUA.[321] Evaluation of the fetal growth in the third trimester around 32 weeks is also recommended.

Key points

- The incidence of SUA is between 0.1 and 0.6%.
- Color Doppler is useful for diagnosis of SUA. Use transverse view of the umbilical cord or evaluate at the cord insertion at the level of the fetal bladder.
- SUA is associated with a mild increase in the risk of fetal anomalies (cardiac and genitourinary primarily) and growth restriction.

Umbilical Cord Coiling Index

The coiling index (CI) is the number of complete coils per centimeter of umbilical cord measured after delivery. Coiling is a characteristic of the umbilical cord that is established by 9

menstrual weeks. Strong et al.[322] were the first to describe the CI after birth and reported an estimated mean of 0.21 (SD 0.07) (Fig. 13.1-33). The authors reported that a CI less than 10th or greater than 90th centiles was associated with a high prevalence of perinatal complications such as chromosomal abnormalities, operative delivery for fetal stress, and severe heart rate decelerations during labor. The physiological explanation for the coiling and the direction of coiling in the umbilical cord is still not known. Some authors considered that the fetal movements can influence the coiling, as fetuses with polyhydramnios have an increased CI.[323] Others suggested that the amount of Wharton jelly, the presence of the Roach muscle (a small muscle bundle lying just beside the UA)[324] and the thickness of the umbilical cord[86] might influence the coiling of the umbilical cord.[325] Increased CI (hypercoiling) or reduced CI (hypocoiling) is considered when the CI is greater than 90th or less than 10th

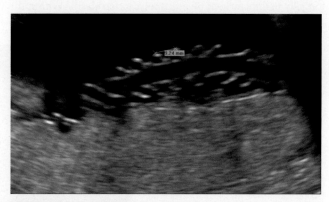

FIGURE 13.1-33: Umbilical cord coiling index calculated as 1/distance in cm, [1/0.924 = 1.08], hypercoiled, (normal 0.44).

centiles, respectively.[326] There is no a clear difference in the association between increased or reduced CI and specific perinatal complications; however, both have been correlated with an increased risk of perinatal death, intrauterine growth restriction, and polyhydramnios.

Degani et al.[327] estimated the CI just before delivery using US. As it is not possible to measure the total length of the umbilical cord, the authors proposed the estimation of the CI in a clearly visualized segment of the umbilical cord. The calculation is by estimating the ratio 1/length of one complete coil (i.e., distance 2.26 cm; CI = 1/2.26 mm = 0.44) with an estimated CI mean of 0.44 (SD 0.11). The authors reported a significant correlation between the prenatal and postnatal CI.[327] There is no consistent data on the clinical significance of an abnormal CI evaluated prenatally.[328] Moreover, the CI can vary in the same fetus according to the anatomical location and gestational age. Still more data on the reliability of the CI and on the clinical implications are necessary for establishing its clinical value.

Umbilical Cord Cysts and Tumors

Visualization of an umbilical cord cyst in early pregnancy is relatively frequent, with an estimated prevalence of 3 to 5% before 12 weeks of gestation. Most of the cysts disappear after the first trimester of pregnancy. The histological examination of the cysts shows two types: pseudocysts formed either by a localized increased in Wharton jelly or by fluid collection related to urachal malformations, and true cysts derived from epithelial cells such as omphalomesenteric and vesicoallantoic cysts. There are no clear US differences between pseudocysts and true cysts as both have similar size and characteristics; however, true cysts are mainly seen in the fetal insertion of the umbilical cord and at early gestational ages. The common US findings are a regular echolucid structure with a mean diameter of 2 cm, with no blood flow inside (Fig. 13.1-34).[329,330]

Ghezzi et al.[331] reported a prevalence of umbilical cord cysts of 2.1% (21/1,159) between 6 and 14 weeks of gestation. All women presenting a single cyst ended having a healthy newborn with no structural anomalies. However, among those presenting more than one cord cyst (n = 6), four had a miscarriage before 14 weeks of gestation, one presented an obstructive uropathy, and one had a normal uncomplicated newborn. Ross et al.[332] reported a prevalence of umbilical cord cysts of 29/859 (3.4%) in pregnancies evaluated between 7 and 13 weeks of gestation. In most of the cases, the cyst resolved

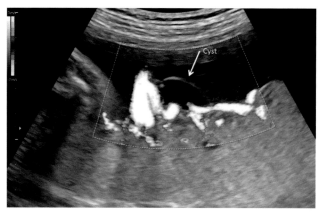

FIGURE 13.1-34: Umbilical cord cyst; a regular rounded, echolucid structure within the cord without blood flow, located near the cord insertion.

after 12 weeks. Among cases with a persistent cyst until the end of the pregnancy (n = 27), seven (26%) had structural or chromosomal anomalies, including obstructive urinary malformations, exomphalos, trisomy 18, and arthrogryposis. The authors also mentioned that in cases of cysts with no structural defects, the risk of complications at birth was very low. The risk of perinatal complications seemed to be increased when the cyst was located close to the placental or fetal umbilical cord insertions.

Although rare, hemangiomas are one of the most common tumors of the umbilical cord.[333] They are benign tumors which may be associated with increased AFP, polyhydramnios, congenital anomalies, and increased perinatal mortality.[333] Noniatrogenic umbilical cord hematoma is usually secondary to invasive procedures, such as cordocentesis with a poor prognosis for the fetus.[334]

UA aneurysm is an extremely rare vascular anomaly.[335,336] It is a cystic structure with nonpulsatile turbulent blood flow. There is a high prevalence of aneuploidy, fetal structural anomalies, and there is a risk of fetal death due to acute umbilical venous compression.[337,338] Other tumors can include umbilical vein varix,[339] teratoma,[340] and angiomyxomas.[341]

Nuchal Cord

Nuchal cord is a common finding at the time of US assessment or at the time of delivery and it is considered a benign finding. Single and double nuchal cords are reported to be present

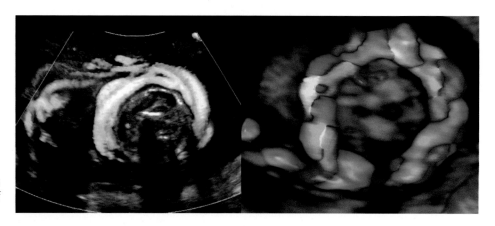

FIGURE 13.1-35: Nuchal cord; transverse view of the fetal neck, and visualization of the nuchal cord with color Doppler.

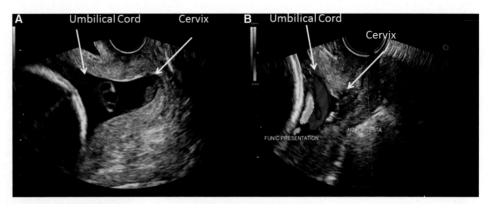

FIGURE 13.1-36: Funic presentation **(A)** transvaginal ultrasound of a patient with a short cervix, the umbilical cord can be seen floating between the fetal head and the cervix; **(B)** visualization of the umbilical cord with color Doppler ultrasound in patient with a normal cervix.

in 33.7 and 5.8% of deliveries, respectively.[342] A nuchal cord should be identified by presence of the cord in the transverse and sagittal planes of the neck and lying around at least three of the four sides of the neck. For accurate diagnosis, both sagittal and transverse sections (linear and circular sections, respectively, of the cord) are required to avoid overdiagnosis of this condition[343] (Fig. 13.1-35). The diagnosis should rely on color Doppler.[344] The presence of a nuchal cord in the first trimester is not associated with fetal hemodynamic changes.[345] Nuchal cord diagnosed by US remote from delivery will spontaneously reduce later in gestation[346] and is not usually associated with adverse neonatal outcomes.[347] The differential diagnoses of a nuchal cord include a posterior cystic neck mass, nuchal folds of the fetal skin, or AF pockets.[343] The management and recommendations are controversial, with some suggesting increased antenatal testing and others not recommending additional surveillance.[348]

Funic (Cord) Presentation

A funic or cord presentation is when the umbilical cord floats or is visualized in front of the presenting part in the lower uterine segment close to the ICO (Fig. 13.1-36). It is usually associated with fetal malpresentation (breech or transverse), with a low-lying placenta or with a marginal cord insertion. If the amniotic sac ruptures, a cord prolapse can occur with subsequent cord compression and hypoxia to the fetus. In a retrospective study, the reported incidence of funic presentation in the third trimester was 0.16% (13/8,122).[349,350]

CONCLUSION

The obstetric US scan is traditionally dedicated to anatomical and hemodynamic fetal evaluation, with less time spent on the evaluation of the placenta, umbilical cord, and membranes. While obvious abnormalities such as large placental abruption, umbilical cord cysts, or detachment of the amniotic membranes tend to be recognized immediately, other abnormalities tend to be overlooked. Given the association with adverse perinatal outcomes, a detailed evaluation including location of the placenta and its relation with ICO, placental thickness, placental shape, placental umbilical cord insertion, and presence of sonographic findings suggestive of morbidly adherent placenta, together with the amount and characteristics of the AF, umbilical cord, and amniotic membranes, is of paramount importance to identify potential complications that can increase the risk of adverse perinatal outcomes and maternal morbidity and mortality.

REFERENCES

1. Bowman ZS, Kennedy AM. Sonographic appearance of the placenta. *Curr Probl Diagn Radiol.* 2014;43:356–373.
2. Rheinboldt M, Delproposto Z. Sonography of placental abnormalities: a pictorial review. *Emerg Radiol.* 2015;22:401–408.
3. Bukowski R, Hansen NI, Pinar H, et al. Altered fetal growth, placental abnormalities, and stillbirth. *PLoS One.* 2017;12:e0182874.
4. Thornburg KL, Kolahi K, Pierce M, et al. Biological features of placental programming. *Placenta.* 2016;48(suppl 1):S47–S53.
5. Kingdom JC, Audette MC, Hobson SR, et al. A placenta clinic approach to the diagnosis and management of fetal growth restriction. *Am J Obstet Gynecol.* 2018;218:S803–S817.
6. Burton GJ, Fowden AL. The placenta: a multifaceted, transient organ. *Philos Trans R Soc Lond B Biol Sci.* 2015;370:20140066.
7. Carter AM. Placental oxygen consumption. Part I: in vivo studies—a review. *Placenta.* 2000;21(suppl 1):S31–S37.
8. Espinoza J, Romero R, Mee Kim Y, et al. Normal and abnormal transformation of the spiral arteries during pregnancy. *J Perinat Med.* 2006;34:447–458.
9. Robertson WB, Brosens I, Dixon G. Uteroplacental vascular pathology. *Eur J Obstet Gynecol Reprod Biol.* 1975;5:47–65.
10. Pijnenborg R, Bland JM, Robertson WB, et al. Uteroplacental arterial changes related to interstitial trophoblast migration in early human pregnancy. *Placenta.* 1983;4:397–413.
11. Kim YM, Bujold E, Chaiworapongsa T, et al. Failure of physiologic transformation of the spiral arteries in patients with preterm labor and intact membranes. *Am J Obstet Gynecol.* 2003;189:1063–1069.
12. Romero R, Kusanovic JP, Chaiworapongsa T, et al. Placental bed disorders in preterm labor, preterm PROM, spontaneous abortion and abruptio placentae. *Best Pract Res Clin Obstet Gynaecol.* 2011;25:313–327.
13. Jauniaux E, Moscoso G, Campbell S, et al. Correlation of ultrasound and pathologic findings of placental anomalies in pregnancies with elevated maternal serum alpha-fetoprotein. *Eur J Obstet Gynecol Reprod Biol.* 1990;37:219–230.
14. Elsayes KM, Trout AT, Friedkin AM, et al. Imaging of the placenta: a multimodality pictorial review. *Radiographics.* 2009;29:1371–1391.
15. Lee AJ, Bethune M, Hiscock RJ. Placental thickness in the second trimester: a pilot study to determine the normal range. *J Ultrasound Med.* 2012;31:213–218.
16. Hoddick WK, Mahony BS, Callen PW, et al. Placental thickness. *J Ultrasound Med.* 1985;4:479–482.
17. Leung KY, Cheong KB, Lee CP, et al. Ultrasonographic prediction of homozygous alpha0-thalassemia using placental thickness, fetal cardiothoracic ratio and middle cerebral artery Doppler: alone or in combination? *Ultrasound Obstet Gynecol.* 2010;35:149–154.
18. Jauniaux E, Ramsay B, Campbell S. Ultrasonographic investigation of placental morphologic characteristics and size during the second trimester of pregnancy. *Am J Obstet Gynecol.* 1994;170:130–137.
19. Milligan N, Rowden M, Wright E, et al. Two-dimensional sonographic assessment of maximum placental length and thickness in the second trimester: a reproducibility study. *J Matern Fetal Neonatal Med.* 2015;28:1653–1659.
20. Hafner E, Metzenbauer M, Dillinger-Paller B, et al. Correlation of first trimester placental volume and second trimester uterine artery Doppler flow. *Placenta.* 2001;22:729–734.
21. Hata T, Tanaka H, Noguchi J, et al. Three-dimensional ultrasound evaluation of the placenta. *Placenta.* 2011;32:105–115.
22. Metzenbauer M, Hafner E, Schuchter K, et al. First-trimester placental volume as a marker for chromosomal anomalies: preliminary results from an unselected population. *Ultrasound Obstet Gynecol.* 2002;19:240–242.
23. Wegrzyn P, Faro C, Falcon O, et al. Placental volume measured by three-dimensional ultrasound at 11 to 13 + 6 weeks of gestation: relation to chromosomal defects. *Ultrasound Obstet Gynecol.* 2005;26:28–32.
24. Hafner E, Metzenbauer M, Hofinger D, et al. Comparison between three-dimensional placental volume at 12 weeks and uterine artery impedance/notching at 22 weeks in screening for pregnancy-induced hypertension, pre-eclampsia and fetal growth restriction in a low-risk population. *Ultrasound Obstet Gynecol.* 2006;27:652–657.

25. Cheong KB, Leung KY, Li TK, et al. Comparison of inter- and intraobserver agreement and reliability between three different types of placental volume measurement technique (XI VOCAL, VOCAL and multiplanar) and validity in the in-vitro setting. *Ultrasound Obstet Gynecol.* 2010;36:210–217.
26. Odeh M, Ophir E, Maximovsky O, et al. Placental volume and three-dimensional power Doppler analysis in prediction of pre-eclampsia and small for gestational age between Week 11 and 13 weeks and 6 days of gestation. *Prenat Diagn.* 2011;31:367–371.
27. Odibo AO, Goetzinger KR, Huster KM, et al. Placental volume and vascular flow assessed by 3D power Doppler and adverse pregnancy outcomes. *Placenta.* 2011;32:230–234.
28. Pomorski M, Zimmer M, Florjanski J, et al. Comparative analysis of placental vasculature and placental volume in normal and IUGR pregnancies with the use of three-dimensional Power Doppler. *Arch Gynecol Obstet.* 2012;285:331–337.
29. Rijken MJ, Moroski WE, Kiricharoen S, et al. Effect of malaria on placental volume measured using three-dimensional ultrasound: a pilot study. *Malar J.* 2012;11:5.
30. Rizzo G, Capponi A, Pietrolucci ME, et al. First trimester placental volume and three dimensional power doppler ultrasonography in type I diabetic pregnancies. *Prenat Diagn.* 2012;32:480–484.
31. Effendi M, Demers S, Giguere Y, et al. Association between first-trimester placental volume and birth weight. *Placenta.* 2014;35:99–102.
32. Titapant V, Cherdchoogieat P. Nomogram of placental thickness, placental volume and placental vascular indices in healthy pregnant women between 12 and 20 weeks of gestation. *J Med Assoc Thai.* 2014;97:267–273.
33. Grannum PA, Berkowitz RL, Hobbins JC. The ultrasonic changes in the maturing placenta and their relation to fetal pulmonic maturity. *Am J Obstet Gynecol.* 1979;133:915–922.
34. Grannum PA. The placenta. *Clin Diagn Ultrasound.* 1989;25:203–219.
35. Sau A, Seed P, Langford K. Intraobserver and interobserver variation in the sonographic grading of placental maturity. *Ultrasound Obstet Gynecol.* 2004;23:374–377.
36. Moran M, Ryan J, Higgins M, et al. Poor agreement between operators on grading of the placenta. *J Obstet Gynaecol.* 2011;31:24–28.
37. Mirza FG, Ghulmiyyah LM, Tamim H, et al. To ignore or not to ignore placental calcifications on prenatal ultrasound: a systematic review and meta-analysis. *J Matern Fetal Neonatal Med.* 2018;31:797–804.
38. Maeda K, Utsu M, Kihaile PE. Quantification of sonographic echogenicity with grey-level histogram width: a clinical tissue characterization. *Ultrasound Med Biol.* 1998;24:225–234.
39. Kuo PL, Lin CC, Lin YH, et al. Placental sonolucency and pregnancy outcome in women with elevated second trimester serum alpha-fetoprotein levels. *J Formos Med Assoc.* 2003;102:319–325.
40. Kusanovic JP, Romero R, Gotsch F, et al. Discordant placental echogenicity: a novel sign of impaired placental perfusion in twin-twin transfusion syndrome? *J Matern Fetal Neonatal Med.* 2010;23:103–106.
41. Movva VC, Rijhsinghani A. Discrepancy in placental echogenicity: a sign of twin anemia polycythemia sequence. *Prenat Diagn.* 2014;34:809–811.
42. Chen KH, Seow KM, Chen LR. The role of preterm placental calcification on assessing risks of stillbirth. *Placenta.* 2015;36:1039–1044.
43. Raio L, Ghezzi F, Cromi A, et al. The thick heterogeneous (jellylike) placenta: a strong predictor of adverse pregnancy outcome. *Prenat Diagn.* 2004;24:182–188.
44. Meizner I, Mashiach R, Shalev Y, et al. Blood flow velocimetry in the diagnosis of succenturiate placenta. *J Clin Ultrasound.* 1998;26:55.
45. Suzuki S, Igarashi M. Clinical significance of pregnancies with succenturiate lobes of placenta. *Arch Gynecol Obstet.* 2008;277:299–301.
46. Cavaliere AF, Rosati P, Ciliberti P, et al. Succenturiate lobe of placenta with vessel anomaly: a case report of prenatal diagnosis and literature review. *Clin Imaging.* 2014;38:747–750.
47. Hata K, Hata T, Aoki S, et al. Succenturiate placenta diagnosed by ultrasound. *Gynecol Obstet Invest.* 1988;25:273–276.
48. Shukunami K, Tsunezawa W, Hosokawa K, et al. Placenta previa of a succenturiate lobe: a report of two cases. *Eur J Obstet Gynecol Reprod Biol.* 2001;99:276–277.
49. Harris RD, Wells WA, Black WC, et al. Accuracy of prenatal sonography for detecting circumvallate placenta. *AJR Am J Roentgenol.* 1997;168:1603–1608.
50. AboEllail MA, Kanenishi K, Mori N, et al. HDlive imaging of circumvallate placenta. *Ultrasound Obstet Gynecol.* 2015;46:513–514.
51. Suzuki S. Clinical significance of pregnancies with circumvallate placenta. *J Obstet Gynaecol Res.* 2008;34:51–54.
52. Shen O, Golomb E, Lavie O, et al. Placental shelf—a common, typically transient and benign finding on early second-trimester sonography. *Ultrasound Obstet Gynecol.* 2007;29:192–194.
53. Molloy CE, McDowell W, Armour T, et al. Ultrasonic diagnosis of placenta membranacea in utero. *J Ultrasound Med.* 1983;2:377–379.
54. Hurley VA, Beischer NA. Placenta membranacea. Case reports. *Br J Obstet Gynaecol.* 1987;94:798–802.
55. Collins SL, Stevenson GN, Noble JA, et al. Developmental changes in spiral artery blood flow in the human placenta observed with colour Doppler ultrasonography. *Placenta.* 2012;33:782–787.
56. Yu CH, Chang CH, Ko HC, et al. Assessment of placental fractional moving blood volume using quantitative three-dimensional power doppler ultrasound. *Ultrasound Med Biol.* 2003;29:19–23.
57. Hafner E, Metzenbauer M, Stumpflen I, et al. Measurement of placental bed vascularization in the first trimester, using 3D-power-Doppler, for the detection of pregnancies at-risk for fetal and maternal complications. *Placenta.* 2013;34:892–898.
58. Farina A. Placental vascular indices (VI, FI and VFI) in intrauterine growth retardation (IUGR). A pooled analysis of the literature. *Prenat Diagn.* 2015;35:1065–1072.
59. Bujold E, Effendi M, Girard M, et al. Reproducibility of first trimester three-dimensional placental measurements in the evaluation of early placental insufficiency. *J Obstet Gynaecol Can.* 2009;31:1144–1148.
60. Hsieh FJ, Kuo PL, Ko TM, et al. Doppler velocimetry of intraplacental fetal arteries. *Obstet Gynecol.* 1991;77:478–482.
61. Kirkinen P, Kurmanavichius J, Huch A, et al. Blood flow velocities in human intraplacental arteries. *Acta Obstet Gynecol Scand.* 1994;73:220–224.
62. Lacin S, Demir N, Koyuncu F, et al. Value of intraplacental villous artery Doppler measurements in severe preeclampsia. *J Postgrad Med.* 1996;42:101–104.
63. Jaffe R, Woods JR. Doppler velocimetry of intraplacental fetal vessels in the second trimester: improving the prediction of pregnancy complications in high-risk patients. *Ultrasound Obstet Gynecol.* 1996;8:262–266.
64. Haberman S, Friedman ZM. Intraplacental spectral Doppler scanning: fetal growth classification based on Doppler velocimetry. *Gynecol Obstet Invest.* 1997;43:11–19.
65. Mu J, Kanzaki T, Tomimatsu T, et al. Investigation of intraplacental villous arteries by Doppler flow imaging in growth-restricted fetuses. *Am J Obstet Gynecol.* 2002;186:297–302.
66. Babic I, Ferraro ZM, Garbedian K, et al. Intraplacental villous artery resistance indices and identification of placenta-mediated diseases. *J Perinatol.* 2015;35:793–798.
67. Oppenheimer LW, Farine D, Ritchie JW, et al. What is a low-lying placenta? *Am J Obstet Gynecol.* 1991;165:1036–1038.
68. Dashe JS. Toward consistent terminology of placental location. *Semin Perinatol.* 2013;37:375–379.
69. Filipov E, Borisov I, Kolarov G. Placental location and its influence on the position of the fetus in the uterus [in Bulgarian]. *Akush Ginekol (Sofiia).* 2000;40:11–12.
70. Gurol-Urganci I, Cromwell DA, Edozien LC, et al. Risk of placenta previa in second birth after first birth cesarean section: a population-based study and meta-analysis. *BMC Pregnancy Childbirth.* 2011;11:95.
71. Ghi T, Contro E, Martina T, et al. Cervical length and risk of antepartum bleeding in women with complete placenta previa. *Ultrasound Obstet Gynecol.* 2009;33:209–212.
72. Ben Nagi J, Ofili-Yebovi D, Marsh M, et al. First-trimester cesarean scar pregnancy evolving into placenta previa/accreta at term. *J Ultrasound Med.* 2005;24:1569–1573.
73. Kapoor S, Thomas JT, Petersen SG, et al. Is the third trimester repeat ultrasound scan for placental localisation needed if the placenta is low lying but clear of the os at the mid-trimester morphology scan? *Aust N Z J Obstet Gynaecol.* 2014;54:428–432.
74. Farine D, Peisner DB, Timor-Tritsch IE. Placenta previa is the traditional diagnostic approach satisfactory? *J Clin Ultrasound.* 1990;18:328–330.
75. Olive EC, Roberts CL, Algert CS, et al. Placenta praevia: maternal morbidity and place of birth. *Aust N Z J Obstet Gynaecol.* 2005;45:499–504.
76. Bronsteen R, Valice R, Lee W, et al. Effect of a low-lying placenta on delivery outcome. *Ultrasound Obstet Gynecol.* 2009;33:204–208.
77. Oppenheimer L, Holmes P, Simpson N, et al. Diagnosis of low-lying placenta: can migration in the third trimester predict outcome? *Ultrasound Obstet Gynecol.* 2001;18:100–102.
78. Tan NH, Abu M, Woo JL, et al. The role of transvaginal sonography in the diagnosis of placenta praevia. *Aust N Z J Obstet Gynaecol.* 1995;35:42–45.
79. Oyelese Y, Smulian JC. Placenta previa, placenta accreta, and vasa previa. *Obstet Gynecol.* 2006;107:927–941.
80. Grappell PM. Placenta praevia and placental migration. *Radiology.* 1980;134:263–264.
81. Bhide A, Thilaganathan B. Recent advances in the management of placenta previa. *Curr Opin Obstet Gynecol.* 2004;16:447–451.
82. Cho JY, Lee YH, Moon MH, et al. Difference in migration of placenta according to the location and type of placenta previa. *J Clin Ultrasound.* 2008;36:79–84.
83. Ohira S, Kikuchi N, Kobara H, et al. Predicting the route of delivery in women with low-lying placenta using transvaginal ultrasonography: significance of placental migration and marginal sinus. *Gynecol Obstet Invest.* 2012;73:217–222.
84. Blouin D, Rioux C. Routine third trimester control ultrasound examination for low-lying or marginal placentas diagnosed at mid-pregnancy: is this indicated? *J Obstet Gynaecol Can.* 2012;34:425–428.
85. Lodhi SK, Khanum Z, Watoo TH. Placenta previa: the role of ultrasound in assessment during third trimester. *J Pak Med Assoc.* 2004;54:81–83.
86. Predanic M, Perni SC. Absence of a relationship between umbilical cord thickness and coiling patterns. *J Ultrasound Med.* 2005;24:1491–1496.
87. Oppenheimer L. Diagnosis and management of placenta previa. *J Obstet Gynaecol Can.* 2007;29:261–266.
88. Lijoi AF, Brady J. Vasa previa diagnosis and management. *J Am Board Fam Pract.* 2003;16:543–548.
89. Derbala Y, Grochal F, Jeanty P. Vasa previa. *J Prenat Med.* 2007;1:2–13.
90. Breborowicz GH, Markwitz W, Szpera-Gozdziewicz A, et al. Prenatal diagnosis of vasa previa. *J Matern Fetal Neonatal Med.* 2015;28:1806–1808.

91. Lee W, Lee VL, Kirk JS, et al. Vasa previa: prenatal diagnosis, natural evolution, and clinical outcome. *Obstet Gynecol.* 2000;95:572–576.
92. Al-Khaduri M, Kadoch IJ, Couturier B, et al. Vasa praevia after IVF: should there be guidelines? Report of two cases and literature review. *Reprod Biomed Online.* 2007;14:372–374.
93. Catanzarite V, Maida C, Thomas W, et al. Prenatal sonographic diagnosis of vasa previa: ultrasound findings and obstetric outcome in ten cases. *Ultrasound Obstet Gynecol.* 2001;18:109–115.
94. Oyelese Y, Catanzarite V, Prefumo F, et al. Vasa previa: the impact of prenatal diagnosis on outcomes. *Obstet Gynecol.* 2004;103:937–942.
95. Baulies S, Maiz N, Munoz A, et al. Prenatal ultrasound diagnosis of vasa praevia and analysis of risk factors. *Prenat Diagn.* 2007;27:595–599.
96. Ruiter L, Kok N, Limpens J, et al. Systematic review of accuracy of ultrasound in the diagnosis of vasa previa. *Ultrasound Obstet Gynecol.* 2015;45:516–522.
97. Sinkey RG, Odibo AO, Dashe JS. #37: diagnosis and management of vasa previa. *Am J Obstet Gynecol.* 2015;213:615–619.
98. Gagnon R, Morin L, Bly S, et al. SOGC clinical practice guideline: guidelines for the management of vasa previa. *Int J Gynaecol Obstet.* 2010;108:85–89.
99. Baschat AA, Gembruch U. Ante- and intrapartum diagnosis of vasa praevia in singleton pregnancies by colour coded Doppler sonography. *Eur J Obstet Gynecol Reprod Biol.* 1998;79:19–25.
100. Clerici G, Burnelli L, Lauro V, et al. Prenatal diagnosis of vasa previa presenting as amniotic band. 'A not so innocent amniotic band'. *Ultrasound Obstet Gynecol.* 1996;7:61–63.
101. Daly-Jones E, Hollingsworth J, Sepulveda W. Vasa praevia: second trimester diagnosis using colour flow imaging. *Br J Obstet Gynaecol.* 1996;103:284–286.
102. RCOG. Placenta Praevia, placenta praevia accreta and vasa previa. Royal College of Obstetrics and Gynecology Green-Top Guidelines. 2011:2–26.
103. Windrim C, Athaide G, Gerster T, et al. Sonographic findings and clinical outcomes in women with massive subchorionic hematoma detected in the second trimester. *J Obstet Gynaecol Can.* 2011;33:475–479.
104. Satomi M, Hiraizumi Y, Suzuki S. Subchorionic haematoma distinct from the placental tissue at 39 weeks' gestation. *J Obstet Gynaecol.* 2012;32:304–305.
105. Alanjari A, Wright E, Keating S, et al. Prenatal diagnosis, clinical outcomes, and associated pathology in pregnancies complicated by massive subchorionic thrombohematoma (Breus' mole). *Prenat Diagn.* 2013;33:973–978.
106. Deans A, Jauniaux E. Prenatal diagnosis and outcome of subamniotic hematomas. *Ultrasound Obstet Gynecol.* 1998;11:319–323.
107. Shukunami K, Orisaka M, Orisaka S, et al. A subamniotic hematoma resembling a deflated balloon. *J Matern Fetal Neonatal Med.* 2004;16:373–375.
108. Xiang L, Wei Z, Cao Y. Symptoms of an intrauterine hematoma associated with pregnancy complications: a systematic review. *PLoS One.* 2014;9:e111676.
109. Ott J, Pecnik P, Promberger R, et al. Intra- versus retroplacental hematomas: a retrospective case-control study on pregnancy outcomes. *BMC Pregnancy Childbirth.* 2017;17:366.
110. Nagy S, Bush M, Stone J, et al. Clinical significance of subchorionic and retroplacental hematomas detected in the first trimester of pregnancy. *Obstet Gynecol.* 2003;102:94–100.
111. Fung TY, To KF, Sahota DS, et al. Massive subchorionic thrombohematoma: a series of 10 cases. *Acta Obstet Gynecol Scand.* 2010;89:1357–1361.
112. Oyelese Y, Ananth CV. Placental abruption. *Obstet Gynecol.* 2006;108:1005–1016.
113. Melchiorre K, Thilaganathan B. Maternal cardiac function in preeclampsia. *Curr Opin Obstet Gynecol.* 2011;23:440–447.
114. Hall DR. Abruptio placentae and disseminated intravascular coagulopathy. *Semin Perinatol.* 2009;33:189–195.
115. Ananth CV, Lavery JA, Vintzileos AM, et al. Severe placental abruption: clinical definition and associations with maternal complications. *Am J Obstet Gynecol.* 2016;214:272.e271–272.e279.
116. Boisrame T, Sananes N, Fritz G, et al. Placental abruption: risk factors, management and maternal-fetal prognosis. Cohort study over 10 years. *Eur J Obstet Gynecol Reprod Biol.* 2014;179:100–104.
117. Ruiter L, Ravelli AC, de Graaf IM, et al. Incidence and recurrence rate of placental abruption: a longitudinal linked national cohort study in the Netherlands. *Am J Obstet Gynecol.* 2015;213:573.e571–e578.
118. Glantz C, Purnell L. Clinical utility of sonography in the diagnosis and treatment of placental abruption. *J Ultrasound Med.* 2002;21:837–840.
119. Nyberg DA, Cyr DR, Mack LA, et al. Sonographic spectrum of placental abruption. *AJR Am J Roentgenol.* 1987;148:161–164.
120. Thompson MO, Vines SK, Aquilina J, et al. Are placental lakes of any clinical significance? *Placenta.* 2002;23:685–690.
121. Reis NS, Brizot ML, Schultz R, et al. Placental lakes on sonographic examination: correlation with obstetric outcome and pathologic findings. *J Clin Ultrasound.* 2005;33:67–71.
122. Jauniaux E, Nicolaides KH. Placental lakes, absent umbilical artery diastolic flow and poor fetal growth in early pregnancy. *Ultrasound Obstet Gynecol.* 1996;7:141–144.
123. Huang CY, Chen CA, Hsieh CY, et al. Intracerebral hemorrhage as initial presentation of gestational choriocarcinoma: a case report and literature review. *Int J Gynecol Cancer.* 2007;17:1166–1171.
124. Muramatsu K, Itoh H, Yamasaki T, et al. A case of a huge placental lake; prenatal differential diagnosis and clinical management. *J Obstet Gynaecol Res.* 2010;36:165–169.
125. Moldenhauer JS, Stanek J, Warshak C, et al. The frequency and severity of placental findings in women with preeclampsia are gestational age dependent. *Am J Obstet Gynecol.* 2003;189:1173–1177.
126. Vinnars MT, Nasiell J, Ghazi S, et al. The severity of clinical manifestations in preeclampsia correlates with the amount of placental infarction. *Acta Obstet Gynecol Scand.* 2011;90:19–25.
127. Krielessi V, Papantoniou N, Papageorgiou I, et al. Placental pathology and blood pressure's level in women with hypertensive disorders in pregnancy. *Obstet Gynecol Int.* 2012;2012:684083.
128. Brosens I, Renaer M. On the pathogenesis of placental infarcts in pre-eclampsia. *J Obstet Gynaecol Br Commonw.* 1972;79:794–799.
129. Fox H, Sebire N. Macroscopic abnormalities of the placenta. In: Fox H, Sebire N, eds. *Pathology of the Placenta.* 3rd ed. Philadelphia: Saunders Elseviere; 2007:95–146.
130. Ogge G, Chaiworapongsa T, Romero R, et al. Placental lesions associated with maternal underperfusion are more frequent in early-onset than in late-onset preeclampsia. *J Perinat Med.* 2011;39:641–652.
131. Aurioles-Garibay A, Hernandez-Andrade E, Romero R, et al. Prenatal diagnosis of a placental infarction hematoma associated with fetal growth restriction, preeclampsia and fetal death: clinicopathological correlation. *Fetal Diagn Ther.* 2014;36:154–161.
132. Fitzgerald B, Shannon P, Kingdom J, et al. Rounded intraplacental haematomas due to decidual vasculopathy have a distinctive morphology. *J Clin Pathol.* 2011;64:729–732.
133. Viero S, Chaddha V, Alkazaleh F, et al. Prognostic value of placental ultrasound in pregnancies complicated by absent end-diastolic flow velocity in the umbilical arteries. *Placenta.* 2004;25:735–741.
134. Hung NA, Jackson C, Nicholson M, et al. Pregnancy-related polymyositis and massive perivillous fibrin deposition in the placenta: are they pathogenetically related? *Arthritis Rheum.* 2006;55:154–156.
135. Andres RL, Kuyper W, Resnik R, et al. The association of maternal floor infarction of the placenta with adverse perinatal outcome. *Am J Obstet Gynecol.* 1990;163:935–938.
136. Sebire NJ, Backos M, Goldin RD, et al. Placental massive perivillous fibrin deposition associated with antiphospholipid antibody syndrome. *BJOG.* 2002;109:570–573.
137. Jindal P, Regan L, Fourkala EO, et al. Placental pathology of recurrent spontaneous abortion: the role of histopathological examination of products of conception in routine clinical practice: a mini review. *Hum Reprod.* 2007;22:313–316.
138. Proctor LK, Whittle WL, Keating S, et al. Pathologic basis of echogenic cystic lesions in the human placenta: role of ultrasound-guided wire localization. *Placenta.* 2010;31:1111–1115.
139. Moscoso G, Jauniaux E, Hustin J. Placental vascular anomaly with diffuse mesenchymal stem villous hyperplasia. A new clinico-pathological entity? *Pathol Res Pract.* 1991;187:324–328.
140. Jauniaux E, Nicolaides KH, Hustin J. Perinatal features associated with placental mesenchymal dysplasia. *Placenta.* 1997;18:701–706.
141. Robinson WP, Slee J, Smith N, et al. Placental mesenchymal dysplasia associated with fetal overgrowth and mosaic deletion of the maternal copy of 11p15.5. *Am J Med Genet A.* 2007;143A:1752–1759.
142. Vaisbuch E, Romero R, Kusanovic JP, et al. Three-dimensional sonography of placental mesenchymal dysplasia and its differential diagnosis. *J Ultrasound Med.* 2009;28:359–368.
143. Loh KY, Sivalingam N, Suryani MY. Gestational trophoblastic disease. *Med J Malaysia.* 2004;59:697–702; quiz 703.
144. Jauniaux E. Ultrasound diagnosis and follow-up of gestational trophoblastic disease. *Ultrasound Obstet Gynecol.* 1998;11:367–377.
145. Candelier JJ. The hydatidiform mole. *Cell Adh Migr.* 2016;10:226–235.
146. Wang PS, Horrow MM. Twin pregnancy with complete hydatidiform mole and normal coexisting fetus. *Ultrasound Q.* 2013;29:219–220.
147. van Cromvoirt SM, Thomas CM, Quinn MA, et al. Identification of patients with persistent trophoblastic disease after complete hydatidiform mole by using a normal 24-hour urine hCG regression curve. *Gynecol Oncol.* 2014;133:542–545.
148. Seckl MJ, Sebire NJ, Berkowitz RS. Gestational trophoblastic disease. *Lancet.* 2010;376:717–729.
149. Shanbhogue AK, Lalwani N, Menias CO. Gestational trophoblastic disease. *Radiol Clin North Am.* 2013;51:1023–1034.
150. Guvendag Guven ES, Guven S, Esinler I, et al. Placental site trophoblastic tumor in a patient with brain and lung metastases. *Int J Gynecol Cancer.* 2004;14:558–563.
151. Ibi T, Hirai K, Bessho R, et al. Choriocarcinoma of the lung: report of a case. *Gen Thorac Cardiovasc Surg.* 2012;60:377–380.
152. Mittal S, Aird I, Haugk B. Gestational choriocarcinoma in liver mimicking ruptured ectopic pregnancy. *J Obstet Gynaecol.* 2012;32:499.
153. Sebire NJ, Jauniaux E. Fetal and placental malignancies: prenatal diagnosis and management. *Ultrasound Obstet Gynecol.* 2009;33:235–244.
154. Savelli L, Pollastri P, Mabrouk M, et al. Placental site trophoblastic tumor diagnosed on transvaginal sonography. *Ultrasound Obstet Gynecol.* 2009;34:235–236.
155. Wallenburg HC. Chorioangioma of the placenta. Thirteen new cases and a review of the literature from 1939 to 1970 with special reference to the clinical complications. *Obstet Gynecol Surv.* 1971;26:411–425.
156. Sepulveda W, Alcalde JL, Schnapp C, et al. Perinatal outcome after prenatal diagnosis of placental chorioangioma. *Obstet Gynecol.* 2003;102:1028–1033.

157. Zanardini C, Papageorghiou A, Bhide A, et al. Giant placental chorioangioma: natural history and pregnancy outcome. *Ultrasound Obstet Gynecol.* 2010;35:332–336.

158. Jauniaux E, Ogle R. Color Doppler imaging in the diagnosis and management of chorioangiomas. *Ultrasound Obstet Gynecol.* 2000;15:463–467.

159. Zalel Y, Weisz B, Gamzu R, et al. Chorioangiomas of the placenta: sonographic and Doppler flow characteristics. *J Ultrasound Med.* 2002;21:909–913.

160. Saksiriwutho P, Ratanasiri T, Doankum C, et al. Prenatal three dimensional ultrasonography and expectant management of placental chorioangioma: a case report. *J Med Assoc Thai.* 2013;96:496–500.

161. Wolfe BK, Wallace JH. Pitfall to avoid: chorioangioma of the placenta simulating fetal tumor. *J Clin Ultrasound.* 1987;15:405–408.

162. Quintero RA, Reich H, Romero R, et al. In utero endoscopic devascularization of a large chorioangioma. *Ultrasound Obstet Gynecol.* 1996;8:48–52.

163. Sepulveda W, Wong AE, Herrera L, et al. Endoscopic laser coagulation of feeding vessels in large placental chorioangiomas: report of three cases and review of invasive treatment options. *Prenat Diagn.* 2009;29:201–206.

164. Williams VL, Williams RA. Placental teratoma: prenatal ultrasonographic diagnosis. *J Ultrasound Med.* 1994;13:587–589.

165. Ahmed N, Kale V, Thakkar H, et al. Sonographic diagnosis of placental teratoma. *J Clin Ultrasound.* 2004;32:98–101.

166. Buyukkurt S, Evruke C, Zeren H, et al. Prenatal diagnosis of placental teratoma: a case report. *Eur J Obstet Gynecol Reprod Biol.* 2009;146:233–234.

167. Sepulveda W, Sebire NJ, Hughes K, et al. The lambda sign at 10-14 weeks of gestation as a predictor of chorionicity in twin pregnancies. *Ultrasound Obstet Gynecol.* 1996;7:421–423.

168. Carroll SG, Soothill PW, Abdel-Fattah SA, et al. Prediction of chorionicity in twin pregnancies at 10-14 weeks of gestation. *BJOG.* 2002;109:182–186.

169. Finberg HJ. The "twin peak" sign: reliable evidence of dichorionic twinning. *J Ultrasound Med.* 1992;11:571–577.

170. Gratacos E, Deprest J. Current experience with fetoscopy and the Eurofoetus registry for fetoscopic procedures. *Eur J Obstet Gynecol Reprod Biol.* 2000;92:151–159.

171. Quintero R, Kontopoulos EV, Barness E, et al. Twin-twin transfusion syndrome in a dichorionic-monozygotic twin pregnancy: the end of a paradigm? *Fetal Pediatr Pathol.* 2010;29:81–88.

172. Acosta-Rojas R, Becker J, Munoz-Abellana B, et al. Twin chorionicity and the risk of adverse perinatal outcome. *Int J Gynaecol Obstet.* 2007;96:98–102.

173. Lewi L, Deprest J, Hecher K. The vascular anastomoses in monochorionic twin pregnancies and their clinical consequences. *Am J Obstet Gynecol.* 2013;208:19–30.

174. Parmley TH, Seeds AE. Fetal skin permeability to isotopic water (THO) in early pregnancy. *Am J Obstet Gynecol.* 1970;108:128–131.

175. Lind T, Kendall A, Hytten FE. The role of the fetus in the formation of amniotic fluid. *J Obstet Gynaecol Br Commonw.* 1972;79:289–298.

176. Gresham EL, Rankin JH, Makowski EL, et al. An evaluation of fetal renal function in a chronic sheep preparation. *J Clin Invest.* 1972;51:149–156.

177. Rabinowitz R, Peters MT, Vyas S, et al. Measurement of fetal urine production in normal pregnancy by real-time ultrasonography. *Am J Obstet Gynecol.* 1989;161:1264–1266.

178. Mescher EJ, Platzker AC, Ballard PL, et al. Ontogeny of tracheal fluid, pulmonary surfactant, and plasma corticoids in the fetal lamb. *J Appl Physiol.* 1975;39:1017–1021.

179. Brace RA, Wolf EJ. Normal amniotic fluid volume changes throughout pregnancy. *Am J Obstet Gynecol.* 1989;161:382–388.

180. Smith DL. Amniotic fluid volume. A measurement of the amniotic fluid present in 72 pregnancies during the first half of pregnancy. *Am J Obstet Gynecol.* 1971;110:166–172.

181. Horsager R, Nathan L, Leveno KJ. Correlation of measured amniotic fluid volume and sonographic predictions of oligohydramnios. *Obstet Gynecol.* 1994;83:955–958.

182. Beischer NA, Brown JB, Townsend L. Studies in prolonged pregnancy. 3. Amniocentesis in prolonged pregnancy. *Am J Obstet Gynecol.* 1969;103:496–503.

183. Magann EF, Sanderson M, Martin JN, et al. The amniotic fluid index, single deepest pocket, and two-diameter pocket in normal human pregnancy. *Am J Obstet Gynecol.* 2000;182:1581–1588.

184. Pritchard JA. Deglutition by normal and anencephalic fetuses. *Obstet Gynecol.* 1965;25:289–297.

185. Abramovich DR, Garden A, Jandial L, et al. Fetal swallowing and voiding in relation to hydramnios. *Obstet Gynecol.* 1979;54:15–20.

186. Lingwood B, Hardy KJ, Coghlan JP, et al. Effect of aldosterone on urine composition in the chronically cannulated ovine foetus. *J Endocrinol.* 1978;76:553–554.

187. Robillard JE, Weitzman RE. Developmental aspects of the fetal renal response to exogenous arginine vasopressin. *Am J Physiol.* 1980;238:F407–F414.

188. Flack NJ, Sepulveda W, Bower S, et al. Acute maternal hydration in third-trimester oligohydramnios: effects on amniotic fluid volume, uteroplacental perfusion, and fetal blood flow and urine output. *Am J Obstet Gynecol.* 1995;173:1186–1191.

189. Manning FA, Platt LD, Sipos L. Antepartum fetal evaluation: development of a fetal biophysical profile. *Am J Obstet Gynecol.* 1980;136:787–795.

190. Chamberlain PF, Manning FA, Morrison I, et al. Ultrasound evaluation of amniotic fluid volume. I. The relationship of marginal and decreased amniotic fluid volumes to perinatal outcome. *Am J Obstet Gynecol.* 1984;150:245–249.

191. Phelan JP, Smith CV, Broussard P, et al. Amniotic fluid volume assessment with the four-quadrant technique at 36-42 weeks' gestation. *J Reprod Med.* 1987;32:540–542.

192. Phelan JP, Ahn MO, Smith CV, et al. Amniotic fluid index measurements during pregnancy. *J Reprod Med.* 1987;32:601–604.

193. Moore TR, Cayle JE. The amniotic fluid index in normal human pregnancy. *Am J Obstet Gynecol.* 1990;162:1168–1173.

194. Magann EF, Chauhan SP, Whitworth NS, et al. Subjective versus objective evaluation of amniotic fluid volume of pregnancies of less than 24 weeks' gestation: how can we be accurate? *J Ultrasound Med.* 2001;20:191–195.

195. Odibo IN, Whittemore BS, Hughes DS, et al. Addition of color Doppler sonography for detection of amniotic fluid disturbances and its implications on perinatal outcomes. *J Ultrasound Med.* 2017;36:1875–1881.

196. ACOG. ACOG Practice Bulletin No. 101: ultrasonography in pregnancy. *Obstet Gynecol.* 2009;113:451–461.

197. Lim KI, Butt K, Naud K, et al. Amniotic fluid: technical update on physiology and measurement. *J Obstet Gynaecol Can.* 2017;39:52–58.

198. Nabhan AF, Abdelmoula YA. Amniotic fluid index versus single deepest vertical pocket as a screening test for preventing adverse pregnancy outcome. *Cochrane Database Syst Rev.* 2008:Cd006593.

199. Manning FA, Hill LM, Platt LD. Qualitative amniotic fluid volume determination by ultrasound: antepartum detection of intrauterine growth retardation. *Am J Obstet Gynecol.* 1981;139:254–258.

200. Chauhan SP, Sanderson M, Hendrix NW, et al. Perinatal outcome and amniotic fluid index in the antepartum and intrapartum periods: a meta-analysis. *Am J Obstet Gynecol.* 1999;181:1473–1478.

201. Casey BM, McIntire DD, Bloom SL, et al. Pregnancy outcomes after antepartum diagnosis of oligohydramnios at or beyond 34 weeks' gestation. *Am J Obstet Gynecol.* 2000;182:909–912.

202. Rabie N, Magann E, Steelman S, et al. Oligohydramnios in complicated and uncomplicated pregnancy: a systematic review and meta-analysis. *Ultrasound Obstet Gynecol.* 2017;49:442–449.

203. Kim BJ, Romero R, Mi Lee S, et al. Clinical significance of oligohydramnios in patients with preterm labor and intact membranes. *J Perinat Med.* 2011;39:131–136.

204. Magann EF, Doherty DA, Chauhan SP, et al. How well do the amniotic fluid index and single deepest pocket indices (below the 3rd and 5th and above the 95th and 97th percentiles) predict oligohydramnios and hydramnios? *Am J Obstet Gynecol.* 2004;190:164–169.

205. Alfirevic Z, Luckas M, Walkinshaw SA, et al. A randomised comparison between amniotic fluid index and maximum pool depth in the monitoring of post-term pregnancy. *Br J Obstet Gynaecol.* 1997;104:207–211.

206. Moses J, Doherty DA, Magann EF, et al. A randomized clinical trial of the intrapartum assessment of amniotic fluid volume: amniotic fluid index versus the single deepest pocket technique. *Am J Obstet Gynecol.* 2004;190:1564–1569; discussion 1569–1570.

207. Nabhan AF, Abdelmoula YA. Amniotic fluid index versus single deepest vertical pocket: a meta-analysis of randomized controlled trials. *Int J Gynaecol Obstet.* 2009;104:184–188.

208. Chauhan SP, Doherty DD, Magann EF, et al. Amniotic fluid index vs single deepest pocket technique during modified biophysical profile: a randomized clinical trial. *Am J Obstet Gynecol.* 2004;191:661–667; discussion 667–668.

209. Magann EF, Doherty DA, Field K, et al. Biophysical profile with amniotic fluid volume assessments. *Obstet Gynecol.* 2004;104:5–10.

210. Kehl S, Schelkle A, Thomas A, et al. Single deepest vertical pocket or amniotic fluid index as evaluation test for predicting adverse pregnancy outcome (SAFE trial): a multicenter, open-label, randomized controlled trial. *Ultrasound Obstet Gynecol.* 2016;47:674–679.

211. Conway DL, Adkins WB, Schroeder B, et al. Isolated oligohydramnios in the term pregnancy: is it a clinical entity? *J Matern Fetal Med.* 1998;7:197–200.

212. Rainford M, Adair R, Scialli AR, et al. Amniotic fluid index in the uncomplicated term pregnancy. Prediction of outcome. *J Reprod Med.* 2001;46:589–592.

213. Locatelli A, Vergani P, Toso L, et al. Perinatal outcome associated with oligohydramnios in uncomplicated term pregnancies. *Arch Gynecol Obstet.* 2004;269:130–133.

214. Zhang J, Troendle J, Meikle S, et al. Isolated oligohydramnios is not associated with adverse perinatal outcomes. *BJOG.* 2004;111:220–225.

215. Ek S, Andersson A, Johansson A, et al. Oligohydramnios in uncomplicated pregnancies beyond 40 completed weeks. A prospective, randomised, pilot study on maternal and neonatal outcomes. *Fetal Diagn Ther.* 2005;20:182–185.

216. Sean Esplin M, Hoffman MK, Theilen L, et al. Prospective evaluation of the efficacy of immunoassays in the diagnosis of rupture of the membranes. *J Matern Fetal Neonatal Med.* 2019:1–7.

217. Bullo M, Tschumi S, Bucher BS, et al. Pregnancy outcome following exposure to angiotensin-converting enzyme inhibitors or angiotensin receptor antagonists: a systematic review. *Hypertension.* 2012;60:444–450.

218. Kirshon B, Moise KJ Jr, Mari G, et al. Long-term indomethacin therapy decreases fetal urine output and results in oligohydramnios. *Am J Perinatol.* 1991;8:86–88.

219. Schucker JL, Mercer BM, Audibert F, et al. Serial amniotic fluid index in severe preeclampsia: a poor predictor of adverse outcome. *Am J Obstet Gynecol.* 1996;175:1018–1023.

220. Kjos SL, Leung A, Henry OA, et al. Antepartum surveillance in diabetic pregnancies: predictors of fetal distress in labor. *Am J Obstet Gynecol.* 1995;173:1532–1539.

221. Sepulveda W, Stagiannis KD, Flack NJ, et al. Accuracy of prenatal diagnosis of renal agenesis with color flow imaging in severe second-trimester oligohydramnios. *Am J Obstet Gynecol.* 1995;173:1788–1792.

222. Grijseels EW, van-Hornstra PT, Govaerts LC, et al. Outcome of pregnancies complicated by oligohydramnios or anhydramnios of renal origin. *Prenat Diagn.* 2011;31:1039–1045.

223. Oliveira EA, Diniz JS, Cabral AC, et al. Predictive factors of fetal urethral obstruction: a multivariate analysis. *Fetal Diagn Ther.* 2000;15:180–186.

224. Hoffman CK, Filly RA, Callen PW. The "lying down" adrenal sign: a sonographic indicator of renal agenesis or ectopia in fetuses and neonates. *J Ultrasound Med.* 1992;11:533–536.

225. Bronshtein M, Amit A, Achiron R, et al. The early prenatal sonographic diagnosis of renal agenesis: techniques and possible pitfalls. *Prenat Diagn.* 1994;14:291–297.

226. Goodlin RC, Anderson JC, Gallagher TF. Relationship between amniotic fluid volume and maternal plasma volume expansion. *Am J Obstet Gynecol.* 1983;146:505–511.

227. Kilpatrick SJ, Safford KL, Pomeroy T, et al. Maternal hydration increases amniotic fluid index. *Obstet Gynecol.* 1991;78:1098–1102.

228. Doi S, Osada H, Seki K, et al. Effect of maternal hydration on oligohydramnios: a comparison of three volume expansion methods. *Obstet Gynecol.* 1998;92:525–529.

229. Yan-Rosenberg L, Burt B, Bombard AT, et al. A randomized clinical trial comparing the effect of maternal intravenous hydration and placebo on the amniotic fluid index in oligohydramnios. *J Matern Fetal Neonatal Med.* 2007;20:715–718.

230. Patrelli TS, Gizzo S, Cosmi E, et al. Maternal hydration therapy improves the quantity of amniotic fluid and the pregnancy outcome in third-trimester isolated oligohydramnios: a controlled randomized institutional trial. *J Ultrasound Med.* 2012;31:239–244.

231. Carroll BC, Bruner JP. Umbilical artery Doppler velocimetry in pregnancies complicated by oligohydramnios. *J Reprod Med.* 2000;45:562–566.

232. Magann EF, Chauhan SP, Hitt WC, et al. Borderline or marginal amniotic fluid index and peripartum outcomes: a review of the literature. *J Ultrasound Med.* 2011;30:523–528.

233. Sahin E, Madendag Y, Tayyar AT, et al. Perinatal outcomes in uncomplicated late preterm pregnancies with borderline oligohydramnios. *J Matern Fetal Neonatal Med.* 2018;31:3085–3088.

234. Choi SR. Borderline amniotic fluid index and perinatal outcomes in the uncomplicated term pregnancy. *J Matern Fetal Neonatal Med.* 2016;29:457–460.

235. Hill LM, Breckle R, Thomas ML, et al. Polyhydramnios: ultrasonically detected prevalence and neonatal outcome. *Obstet Gynecol.* 1987;69:21–25.

236. Biggio JR Jr, Wenstrom KD, Dubard MB, et al. Hydramnios prediction of adverse perinatal outcome. *Obstet Gynecol.* 1999;94:773–777.

237. Chamberlain PF, Manning FA, Morrison I, et al. Ultrasound evaluation of amniotic fluid volume. II. The relationship of increased amniotic fluid volume to perinatal outcome. *Am J Obstet Gynecol.* 1984;150:250–254.

238. Machado MR, Cecatti JG, Krupa F, et al. Curve of amniotic fluid index measurements in low-risk pregnancy. *Acta Obstet Gynecol Scand.* 2007;86:37–41.

239. Lazebnik N, Many A. The severity of polyhydramnios, estimated fetal weight and preterm delivery are independent risk factors for the presence of congenital malformations. *Gynecol Obstet Invest.* 1999;48:28–32.

240. Smith CV, Plambeck RD, Rayburn WF, et al. Relation of mild idiopathic polyhydramnios to perinatal outcome. *Obstet Gynecol.* 1992;79:387–389.

241. Sohaey R, Nyberg DA, Sickler GK, et al. Idiopathic polyhydramnios: association with fetal macrosomia. *Radiology.* 1994;190:393–396.

242. Panting-Kemp A, Nguyen T, Chang E, et al. Idiopathic polyhydramnios and perinatal outcome. *Am J Obstet Gynecol.* 1999;181:1079–1082.

243. Chen KC, Liou JD, Hung TH, et al. Perinatal outcomes of polyhydramnios without associated congenital fetal anomalies after the gestational age of 20 weeks. *Chang Gung Med J.* 2005;28:222–228.

244. Erez O, Shoham-Vardi I, Sheiner E, et al. Hydramnios and small for gestational age are independent risk factors for neonatal mortality and maternal morbidity. *Arch Gynecol Obstet.* 2005;271:296–301.

245. Maymon E, Ghezzi F, Shoham-Vardi I, et al. Isolated hydramnios at term gestation and the occurrence of peripartum complications. *Eur J Obstet Gynecol Reprod Biol.* 1998;77:157–161.

246. Sickler GK, Nyberg DA, Sohaey R, et al. Polyhydramnios and fetal intrauterine growth restriction: ominous combination. *J Ultrasound Med.* 1997;16:609–614.

247. Morris RK, Meller CH, Tamblyn J, et al. Association and prediction of amniotic fluid measurements for adverse pregnancy outcome: systematic review and meta-analysis. *BJOG.* 2014;121:686–699.

248. Dashe JS, McIntire DD, Ramus RM, et al. Hydramnios: anomaly prevalence and sonographic detection. *Obstet Gynecol.* 2002;100:134–139.

249. Dorleijn DM, Cohen-Overbeek TE, Groenendaal F, et al. Idiopathic polyhydramnios and postnatal findings. *J Matern Fetal Neonatal Med.* 2009;22:315–320.

250. Abele H, Starz S, Hoopmann M, et al. Idiopathic polyhydramnios and postnatal abnormalities. *Fetal Diagn Ther.* 2012;32:251–255.

251. Golan A, Wolman I, Sagi J, et al. Persistence of polyhydramnios during pregnancy – its significance and correlation with maternal and fetal complications. *Gynecol Obstet Invest.* 1994;37:18–20.

252. Fisk NM, Vaughan J, Talbert D. Impaired fetal blood gas status in polyhydramnios and its relation to raised amniotic pressure. *Fetal Diagn Ther.* 1994;9:7–13.

253. Moise KJ Jr. Toward consistent terminology: assessment and reporting of amniotic fluid volume. *Semin Perinatol.* 2013;37:370–374.

254. Idris N, Wong SF, Thomae M, et al. Influence of polyhydramnios on perinatal outcome in pregestational diabetic pregnancies. *Ultrasound Obstet Gynecol.* 2010;36:338–343.

255. Jacobson JD, Cousins L. A population-based study of maternal and perinatal outcome in patients with gestational diabetes. *Am J Obstet Gynecol.* 1989;161:981–986.

256. Bar-Hava I, Scarpelli SA, Barnhard Y, et al. Amniotic fluid volume reflects recent glycemic status in gestational diabetes mellitus. *Am J Obstet Gynecol.* 1994;171:952–955.

257. Bartha JL, Martinez-Del-Fresno P, Comino-Delgado R. Early diagnosis of gestational diabetes mellitus and prevention of diabetes-related complications. *Eur J Obstet Gynecol Reprod Biol.* 2003;109:41–44.

258. Barkin SZ, Pretorius DH, Beckett MK, et al. Severe polyhydramnios: incidence of anomalies. *AJR Am J Roentgenol.* 1987;148:155–159.

259. McKelvey A, Stanwell J, Smeulders N, et al. Persistent non-visualisation of the fetal stomach: diagnostic and prognostic implications. *Arch Dis Child Fetal Neonatal Ed.* 2010;95:F439–F442.

260. Agrawal P, Ogilvy-Stuart A, Lees C. Intrauterine diagnosis and management of congenital goitrous hypothyroidism. *Ultrasound Obstet Gynecol.* 2002;19:501–505.

261. Koyuncu FM, Tamay AG, Bugday S. Intrauterine diagnosis and management of fetal goiter: a case report. *J Clin Ultrasound.* 2010;38:503–505.

262. Pumberger W, Hormann M, Deutinger J, et al. Longitudinal observation of antenatally detected congenital lung malformations (CLM): natural history, clinical outcome and long-term follow-up. *Eur J Cardiothorac Surg.* 2003;24:703–711.

263. Chen WS, Yeh GP, Tsai HD, et al. Prenatal diagnosis of congenital cystic adenomatoid malformations: evolution and outcome. *Taiwan J Obstet Gynecol.* 2009;48:278–281.

264. MacMillan RH, Harbert GM, Davis WD, et al. Prenatal diagnosis of Pena-Shokeir syndrome type 1. *Am J Med Genet.* 1985;21:279–284.

265. Zelop C, Benacerraf B. Sonographic diagnosis of fetal upper extremity dysmorphology: significance and outcome. *Ultrasound Obstet Gynecol.* 1996;8:391–396.

266. Rudnik-Schoneborn S, Nicholson GA, Morgan G, et al. Different patterns of obstetric complications in myotonic dystrophy in relation to the disease status of the fetus. *Am J Med Genet.* 1998;80:314–321.

267. Jungbluth H, Wallgren-Pettersson C, Laporte J. Centronuclear (myotubular) myopathy. *Orphanet J Rare Dis.* 2008;3:26.

268. Dudley O, Muscatelli F. Clinical evidence of intrauterine disturbance in Prader-Willi syndrome, a genetically imprinted neurodevelopmental disorder. *Early Hum Dev.* 2007;83:471–478.

269. Geysenbergh B, De Catte L, Vogels A. Can fetal ultrasound result in prenatal diagnosis of Prader-Willi syndrome? *Genet Couns.* 2011;22:207–216.

270. Bhat YR, Vinayaka G, Sreelakshmi K. Antenatal bartter syndrome: a review. *Int J Pediatr.* 2012;2012:857136.

271. Williams DH, Gauthier DW, Maizels M. Prenatal diagnosis of Beckwith-Wiedemann syndrome. *Prenat Diagn.* 2005;25:879–884.

272. Alessandri JL, Cuillier F, Ramful D, et al. Perlman syndrome: report, prenatal findings and review. *Am J Med Genet A.* 2008;146a:2532–2537.

273. Maxwell DJ, Crawford DC, Curry PV, et al. Obstetric importance, diagnosis, and management of fetal tachycardias. *BMJ.* 1988;297:107–110.

274. Zalel Y, Gamzu R, Weiss Y, et al. Role of color Doppler imaging in diagnosing and managing pregnancies complicated by placental chorioangioma. *J Clin Ultrasound.* 2002;30:264–269.

275. Degani S. Sonographic findings in fetal viral infections: a systematic review. *Obstet Gynecol Surv.* 2006;61:329–336.

276. Ang MS, Thorp JA, Parisi VM. Maternal lithium therapy and polyhydramnios. *Obstet Gynecol.* 1990;76:517–519.

277. Coviello D, Bonati F, Montefusco SM, et al. Amnioreduction. *Acta Biomed.* 2004;75(suppl 1):31–33.

278. Elliott JP, Sawyer AT, Radin TG, et al. Large-volume therapeutic amniocentesis in the treatment of hydramnios. *Obstet Gynecol.* 1994;84:1025–1027.

279. ACOG. ACOG practice bulletin. Antepartum fetal surveillance. Number 9, October 1999 (replaces Technical Bulletin Number 188, January 1994). Clinical management guidelines for obstetrician-gynecologists. *Int J Gynaecol Obstet.* 2000;68:175–185.

280. Dashe JS, Pressman EK, Hibbard JU. SMFM Consult Series #46: evaluation and management of polyhydramnios. *Am J Obstet Gynecol.* 2018;219:B2–B8.

281. Touboul C, Boileau P, Picone O, et al. Outcome of children born out of pregnancies complicated by unexplained polyhydramnios. *BJOG.* 2007;114:489–492.

282. Sepulveda W, Reid R, Nicolaidis P, et al. Second-trimester echogenic bowel and intraamniotic bleeding: association between fetal bowel echogenicity and amniotic fluid spectrophotometry at 410 nm. *Am J Obstet Gynecol.* 1996;174:839–842.

283. Vengalil S, Santolaya-Forgas J, Meyer W, et al. Ultrasonically dense amniotic fluid in early pregnancy in asymptomatic women without vaginal bleeding. A report of two cases. *J Reprod Med.* 1998;43:462–464.

284. Vohra N, Rochelson B, Smith-Levitin M. Three-dimensional sonographic findings in congenital (harlequin) ichthyosis. *J Ultrasound Med.* 2003;22:737–739.

285. Dolan CR, Smith LT, Sybert VP. Prenatal detection of epidermolysis bullosa letalis with pyloric atresia in a fetus by abnormal ultrasound and elevated alpha-fetoprotein. *Am J Med Genet.* 1993;47:395–400.
286. Timor-Tritsch IE, Greenebaum E, Monteagudo A, et al. Exencephaly-anencephaly sequence: proof by ultrasound imaging and amniotic fluid cytology. *J Matern Fetal Med.* 1996;5:182–185.
287. Sherer DM, Abramowicz JS, Smith SA, et al. Sonographically homogeneous echogenic amniotic fluid in detecting meconium-stained amniotic fluid. *Obstet Gynecol.* 1991;78:819–822.
288. Brown DL, Polger M, Clark PK, et al. Very echogenic amniotic fluid: ultrasonography-amniocentesis correlation. *J Ultrasound Med.* 1994;13:95–97.
289. DeVore GR, Platt LD. Ultrasound appearance of particulate matter in amniotic cavity: vernix or meconium? *J Clin Ultrasound.* 1986;14:229–230.
290. Espinoza J, Goncalves LF, Romero R, et al. The prevalence and clinical significance of amniotic fluid 'sludge' in patients with preterm labor and intact membranes. *Ultrasound Obstet Gynecol.* 2005;25:346–352.
291. Bujold E, Pasquier JC, Simoneau J, et al. Intra-amniotic sludge, short cervix, and risk of preterm delivery. *J Obstet Gynaecol Can.* 2006;28:198–202.
292. Kusanovic JP, Espinoza J, Romero R, et al. Clinical significance of the presence of amniotic fluid 'sludge' in asymptomatic patients at high risk for spontaneous preterm delivery. *Ultrasound Obstet Gynecol.* 2007;30:706–714.
293. Romero R, Kusanovic JP, Espinoza J, et al. What is amniotic fluid 'sludge'? *Ultrasound Obstet Gynecol.* 2007;30:793–798.
294. Romero R, Schaudinn C, Kusanovic JP, et al. Detection of a microbial biofilm in intraamniotic infection. *Am J Obstet Gynecol.* 2008;198:135.e131–e135.
295. Harding JA, Jackson DM, Lewis DF, et al. Correlation of amniotic fluid index and nonstress test in patients with preterm premature rupture of membranes. *Am J Obstet Gynecol.* 1991;165:1088–1094.
296. Vintzileos AM, Campbell WA, Nochimson DJ, et al. Degree of oligohydramnios and pregnancy outcome in patients with premature rupture of the membranes. *Obstet Gynecol.* 1985;66:162–167.
297. Gonik B, Bottoms SF, Cotton DB. Amniotic fluid volume as a risk factor in preterm premature rupture of the membranes. *Obstet Gynecol.* 1985;65:456–459.
298. Storness-Bliss C, Metcalfe A, Simrose R, et al. Correlation of residual amniotic fluid and perinatal outcomes in periviable preterm premature rupture of membranes. *J Obstet Gynaecol Can.* 2012;34:154–158.
299. Hadi HA, Hodson CA, Strickland D. Premature rupture of the membranes between 20 and 25 weeks' gestation: role of amniotic fluid volume in perinatal outcome. *Am J Obstet Gynecol.* 1994;170:1139–1144.
300. Hunter TJ, Byrnes MJ, Nathan E, et al. Factors influencing survival in pre-viable preterm premature rupture of membranes. *J Matern Fetal Neonatal Med.* 2012;25:1755–1761.
301. Smith CV, Greenspoon J, Phelan JP, et al. Clinical utility of the nonstress test in the conservative management of women with preterm spontaneous premature rupture of the membranes. *J Reprod Med.* 1987;32:1–4.
302. Ulm B, Ulm MR, Bernaschek G. Unfused amnion and chorion after 14 weeks of gestation: associated fetal structural and chromosomal abnormalities. *Ultrasound Obstet Gynecol.* 1999;13:392–395.
303. Lewi L, Hanssens M, Spitz B, et al. Complete chorioamniotic membrane separation. Case report and review of the literature. *Fetal Diagn Ther.* 2004;19:78–82.
304. Sistrom CL, Ferguson JE. Abnormal membranes in obstetrical ultrasound: incidence and significance of amniotic sheets and circumvallate placenta. *Ultrasound Obstet Gynecol.* 1993;3:249–255.
305. Lazebnik N, Hill LM, Many A, et al. The effect of amniotic sheet orientation on subsequent maternal and fetal complications. *Ultrasound Obstet Gynecol.* 1996;8:267–271.
306. Tan KB, Tan TY, Tan JV, et al. The amniotic sheet: a truly benign condition? *Ultrasound Obstet Gynecol.* 2005;26:639–643.
307. Mahony BS, Filly RA, Callen PW, et al. The amniotic band syndrome: antenatal sonographic diagnosis and potential pitfalls. *Am J Obstet Gynecol.* 1985;152:63–68.
308. Ozkavukcu E, Haliloglu N. Gray-scale and color Doppler US findings of amniotic sheets. *Diagn Interv Radiol.* 2012;18:298–302.
309. Orioli IM, Ribeiro MG, Castilla EE. Clinical and epidemiological studies of amniotic deformity, adhesion, and mutilation (ADAM) sequence in a South American (ECLAMC) population. *Am J Med Genet A.* 2003;118A:135–145.
310. Rushton DI. Amniotic band syndrome. *Br Med J (Clin Res Ed).* 1983;286:919–920.
311. Shetty P, Menezes LT, Tauro LF, et al. Amniotic band syndrome. *Indian J Surg.* 2013;75:401–402.
312. Belfort MA, Whitehead WE, Ball R, et al. Fetoscopic amniotic band release in a case of chorioamniotic separation: an innovative new technique. *AJP Rep.* 2016;6:e222–e225.
313. de Laat MW, Franx A, van Alderen ED, et al. The umbilical coiling index, a review of the literature. *J Matern Fetal Neonatal Med.* 2005;17:93–100.
314. Fujikura T. Fused umbilical arteries near placental cord insertion. *Am J Obstet Gynecol.* 2003;188:765–767.
315. Gornall AS, Kurinczuk JJ, Konje JC. Antenatal detection of a single umbilical artery: does it matter? *Prenat Diagn.* 2003;23:117–123.
316. Hua M, Odibo AO, Macones GA, et al. Single umbilical artery and its associated findings. *Obstet Gynecol.* 2010;115:930–934.
317. Burshtein S, Levy A, Holcberg G, et al. Is single umbilical artery an independent risk factor for perinatal mortality? *Arch Gynecol Obstet.* 2011;283:191–194.
318. Klatt J, Kuhn A, Baumann M, et al. Single umbilical artery in twin pregnancies. *Ultrasound Obstet Gynecol.* 2012;39:505–509.
319. Rembouskos G, Cicero S, Longo D, et al. Single umbilical artery at 11-14 weeks' gestation: relation to chromosomal defects. *Ultrasound Obstet Gynecol.* 2003;22:567–570.
320. Santillan M, Santillan D, Fleener D, et al. Single umbilical artery: does side matter? *Fetal Diagn Ther.* 2012;32:201–208.
321. DeFigueiredo D, Dagklis T, Zidere V, et al. Isolated single umbilical artery: need for specialist fetal echocardiography? *Ultrasound Obstet Gynecol.* 2010;36:553–555.
322. Strong TH Jr, Elliott JP, Radin TG. Non-coiled umbilical blood vessels: a new marker for the fetus at risk. *Obstet Gynecol.* 1993;81:409–411.
323. Cromi A, Ghezzi F, Durig P, et al. Sonographic umbilical cord morphometry and coiling patterns in twin-twin transfusion syndrome. *Prenat Diagn.* 2005;25:851–855.
324. de Laat MW, Nikkels PG, Franx A, et al. The Roach muscle bundle and umbilical cord coiling. *Early Hum Dev.* 2007;83:571–574.
325. Di Naro E, Ghezzi F, Raio L, et al. Umbilical vein blood flow in fetuses with normal and lean umbilical cord. *Ultrasound Oste Gynecol.* 2001;17:224–228.
326. Strong TH Jr, Jarles DL, Vega JS, et al. The umbilical coiling index. *Am J Obstet Gynecol.* 1994;170:29–32.
327. Degani S, Lewinsky RM, Berger H, et al. Sonographic estimation of umbilical coiling index and correlation with Doppler flow characteristics. *Obstet Gynecol.* 1995;86:990–993.
328. Sebire NJ. Pathophysiological significance of abnormal umbilical cord coiling index. *Ultrasound Obstet Gynecol.* 2007;30:804–806.
329. Heifetz SA, Rueda-Pedraza ME. Omphalomesenteric duct cysts of the umbilical cord. *Pediatr Pathol.* 1983;1:325–335.
330. Shukunami K, Tsuji T, Kotsuji F. Prenatal sonographic features of vesicoallantoic cyst. *Ultrasound Obstet Gynecol.* 2000;15:545–546.
331. Ghezzi F, Raio L, Di Naro E, et al. Single and multiple umbilical cord cysts in early gestation: two different entities. *Ultrasound Obstet Gynecol.* 2003;21:215–219.
332. Ross JA, Jurkovic D, Zosmer N, et al. Umbilical cord cysts in early pregnancy. *Obstet Gynecol.* 1997;89:442–445.
333. Papadopoulos VG, Kourea HP, Adonakis GL, et al. A case of umbilical cord hemangioma: Doppler studies and review of the literature. *Eur J Obstet Gynecol Reprod Biol.* 2009;144:8–14.
334. Jauniaux E, Nicolaides KH, Campbell S, et al. Hematoma of the umbilical cord secondary to cordocentesis for intrauterine fetal transfusion. *Prenat Diagn.* 1990;10:477–478.
335. Sepulveda W, Leible S, Ulloa A, et al. Clinical significance of first trimester umbilical cord cysts. *J Ultrasound Med.* 1999;18:95–99.
336. Sepulveda W, Corral E, Kottmann C, et al. Umbilical artery aneurysm: prenatal identification in three fetuses with trisomy 18. *Ultrasound Obstet Gynecol.* 2003;21:292–296.
337. Berg C, Geipel A, Germer U, et al. Prenatal diagnosis of umbilical cord aneurysm in a fetus with trisomy 18. *Ultrasound Obstet Gynecol.* 2001;17:79–81.
338. Doehrman P, Derksen BJ, Perlow JH, et al. Umbilical artery aneurysm: a case report, literature review, and management recommendations. *Obstet Gynecol Surv.* 2014;69:159–163.
339. Mankuta D, Nadjari M, Pomp G. Isolated fetal intra-abdominal umbilical vein varix: clinical importance and recommendations. *J Ultrasound Med.* 2011;30:273–276.
340. Keene DJ, Shawkat E, Gillham J, et al. Rare combination of exomphalos with umbilical cord teratoma. *Ultrasound Obstet Gynecol.* 2012;40:481.
341. Cheng HP, Hsu CY, Chen CP, et al. Angiomyxoma of the umbilical cord. *Taiwan J Obstet Gynecol.* 2006;45:360–362.
342. Schaffer L, Burkhardt T, Zimmermann R, et al. Nuchal cords in term and postterm deliveries—do we need to know? *Obstet Gynecol.* 2005;106:23–28.
343. Sherer DM, Manning FA. Prenatal ultrasonographic diagnosis of nuchal cord(s): disregard, inform, monitor or intervene? *Ultrasound Obstet Gynecol.* 1999;14:1–8.
344. Jauniaux E, Mawissa C, Peellaerts C, et al. Nuchal cord in normal third-trimester pregnancy: a color Doppler imaging study. *Ultrasound Obstet Gynecol.* 1992;2:417–419.
345. Petousis S, Margioula-Siarkou C, Mamopoulos A, et al. Does first-trimester nuchal cord affect the blood flow in the ductus venosus? A prospective observational study. *J Matern Fetal Neonatal Med.* 2018;31:3115–3118.
346. Schaefer M, Laurichesse-Delmas H, Ville Y. The effect of nuchal cord on nuchal translucency measurement at 10-14 weeks. *Ultrasound Obstet Gynecol.* 1998;11:271–273.
347. Gonzalez-Quintero VH, Tolaymat L, Muller AC, et al. Outcomes of pregnancies with sonographically detected nuchal cords remote from delivery. *J Ultrasound Med.* 2004;23:43–47.
348. Moshiri M, Zaidi SF, Robinson TJ, et al. Comprehensive imaging review of abnormalities of the umbilical cord. *Radiographics.* 2014;34:179–196.
349. Raga F, Osborne N, Ballester MJ, et al. Color flow Doppler: a useful instrument in the diagnosis of funic presentation. *J Natl Med Assoc.* 1996;88:94–96.
350. Ezra Y, Strasberg SR, Farine D. Does cord presentation on ultrasound predict cord prolapse? *Gynecol Obstet Invest.* 2003;56:6–9.

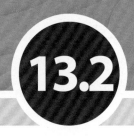

Karin A. Fox • Christopher Ian Cassady

"The eye sees only what the mind has prepared it to comprehend."
—Henri Bergson

INTRODUCTION

The human placenta is a unique, multifunctional organ. It is the only organ that exists temporarily; functions to invade; allows fetal oxygenation, respiration, nutrient transport, and waste clearance; and then is permanently shed, unlike the skin or blood, the cells of which regenerate to replace senescent cells. The human placenta is hemochorial in structure. Invasion of extravillous trophoblast cells into the primed maternal endometrial decidual endometrium is essential for normal implantation.[1] The decidual spiral arteries are remodeled to bathe the chorionic epithelium in maternal blood directly. The regulation of implantation and invasion is highly complex and is only now beginning to be understood. Insufficient placental invasion has been identified as a potential mechanism in recurrent pregnancy loss and preeclampsia.

Overinvasion, in which trophoblast cells breach past the endometrium and invade directly into myometrium, prevents timely placental separation after delivery. Such is the case in placenta accreta spectrum (PAS) disorders, in which the usual fibrinoid layer that develops and separates the placenta from myometrial cells is absent and the rests of chorionic villi invade to various depths. The most superficial cases are called *placenta accreta. Placenta increta* refers to cases in which villi reach deeply into the myometrium, and in cases of *placenta percreta*, placental tissue breaks through the outer serosa and sometimes invades surrounding tissues such as the bladder, bowel, or parametrium. The degree of abnormal involvement can vary widely, and foci of accreta, increta, and percreta can be identified within a single uteroplacental specimen. Forceful removal of a placenta with PAS causes tearing of highly vascular placental villi or the myometrium itself or both, leading to life-threatening hemorrhage.

Early clinical classification of the spectrum was introduced by Aaberg and Reid in 1945.[2] Many terms have been used to describe this heterogeneous disease process, including placental attachment disorder (PAD), morbidly adherent placenta (MAP), and abnormally invasive placenta (AIP). The terms PAD and MAP describe cases in which the placenta merely attaches more tenaciously to the uterus, as with retained placenta or placenta accreta, but do not reflect the invasive nature of increta or percreta. AIP clearly describes the nature of deeper invasive pathology but neglects the former categories. For this reason, a term that most accurately captures the variable presentation of the entire disease process, the PAS, is currently favored.[3–5]

Incidence: The reported incidence of PAS ranges widely. This is in part due to inconsistent definitions used to identify cases[3] and differences in risk factor patterns among study populations.[3] A population-based study from the United Kingdom estimates that PAS occurs in 1.7 of 10,000 maternities.[3] In the United States, estimates range from 1 in 533[4] to 1 in 731 live births.[5] In the most comprehensive systematic review and meta-analysis of the literature to date, Jauniaux et al. identified 22 retrospective studies and 7 prospective studies that included 7001 cases of PAS out of 5,719,992 births.[6] The pooled incidence was 0.17%, ranging from 0.01% to 1.1% of all births. What is clear and consistent among studies is that the incidence is increasing worldwide, concomitant with the rise in the rates of cesarean delivery.[6–8]

Embryology/Pathogenesis: Normal placental implantation relies upon the ability of the developing embryo to attach and then invade into primed maternal endometrial decidua. Disruption of the normal maternal decidual layer allows invasion into and beyond myometrial layers. The exact pathophysiological mechanisms underlying abnormal placental implantation are still relatively poorly understood, largely because study of human placentation has historically relied upon inference and deduction from animal models, which do not exactly mimic human physiology; the analysis of human placental tissues obtained at the time of delivery, which likely does not reflect placental structure and function during implantation; and evaluation of first-trimester placental tissue. The last is problematic because first-trimester tissue can only be obtained with risk to an ongoing pregnancy, after spontaneous abortion (by nature pathological), or after elective termination, a practice that, in many countries, is highly controversial and restricted.

Early investigators postulated various potential mechanisms that might cause decidual disruption sufficient to lead to pathological placental invasion, including hormonal influences and scarring due to aggressive manual removal of the placenta and/or surgical interventions, such as curettage and cesarean delivery. Mounting epidemiological evidence supports the scar disruption hypothesis, specifically the strong association of cesarean section (C-section) with PAS in a subsequent pregnancy. Most cesarean deliveries are performed using a low transverse uterine incision, which explains why placenta previa is the second most common risk associated with PAS. Ultrasound (US) research has described early low and cesarean scar implantation with progression to the PAS.[9,10] Newer research provides insight into the mechanisms at work in establishing this spectrum. These include an abnormal interaction between normally invading extravillous trophoblast cells with maternal decidual natural killer cell regulatory signaling, disrupting the balance between initial extravillous trophoblast invasion and the "stop" signal that normally occurs once invasion is sufficient.[11] Scars, devoid of decidual epithelium, lack this normal regulation and allow trophoblasts to reach deeper myometrial layers. In addition, lack of decidua may induce dysregulation of vascular remodeling regulators, leading to the hypervascularization encountered in PAS.[12] These phenomena may explain the rare cases of placenta accreta identified in nulliparous women with no history of prior intrauterine procedures but who have a placenta previa; the cervix is often poorly decidualized and composed, to a greater extent, of fibrous stroma and connective tissue than the highly muscular uterine wall, making it theoretically more at risk for dysregulation. A complete list of clinical risk factors is presented in Table 13.2-1.

TABLE 13.2-1	Risk Factors Associated with the Placenta Accreta Spectrum

RISK FACTORS

Previous cesarean deliveries, especially multiple

Placenta previa

In vitro fertilization, especially with cryopreserved
    embryos

Asherman syndrome

Endometrial ablation

Uterine fibroids

Myomectomy transecting into the endometrial cavity

Smoking

Advanced maternal age

Prior pelvic irradiation

Uterine anomalies, especially with a history of resection/
    repair

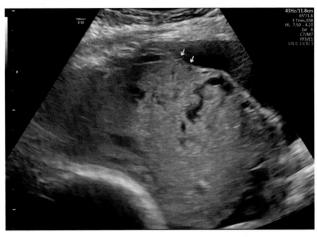

FIGURE 13.2-1: Irregular lacunae. Two-dimensional grayscale US shows placenta lacunae appearing as the dark, irregularly shaped areas within the otherwise gray placenta, giving it a "moth-eaten" appearance. In this image, the transition to loss of the hypoechoic zone and thinning of the myometrium is also seen (*arrows*).

IMAGING

Imaging performed to assess for PAS disorders is not the diagnostic gold standard, even though reference to "antenatal diagnosis" is commonly used. Rather, antenatal imaging is more analogous to screening, whereby antenatal imaging is used to estimate the likelihood of risk for the PAS but does not firmly establish the diagnosis. Both US and magnetic resonance imaging (MRI) of the placenta are associated with inherent false-positive and false-negative rates, which vary depending on the quality of imaging and the experience of the operators performing and interpreting the examinations. Final diagnosis of accreta, increta, or percreta is confirmed at the time of delivery based on clinical and/or histopathological findings. Before imaging, eliciting a thorough history is critical to assess *a priori* risk. It is important to be able to identify abnormal placental imaging using visual signs alone, and the use of checklists helps alert providers to look more closely at images in patients with increased risk. This is not meant to discourage a thorough review in all patients but rather to "cue" the mind for what one might miss if not primed.

Ultrasound

US is widely available, relatively inexpensive, rapid, reliable, and noninvasive, all of which make it an ideal first-line imaging modality in antenatal screening for PAS. US has an excellent safety record in pregnancy, and signs have been identified that are highly useful in identifying PAS disorders, especially when imaging is performed by experienced operators.[13] The sensitivity and specificity can be higher than 90% in specialty centers with extensive experience in diagnosis and management of PAS; however, independent, multicenter studies including both community and referral centers from the United States[5] and the United Kingdom[14] indicate that only about 50% of cases of PAS are identified prior to delivery, suggesting either that the placenta is often inadequately interrogated or that a wide variability of experience exists in recognition of imaging findings.[15]

PAS may be suspected in the first trimester if a low and offset implantation is seen (such as a cesarean scar implantation),[16]

occasionally with small placental lacunae.[17] More commonly, however, PAS is identified at the time of the second-trimester anatomy survey, and sometimes only confirmed later with referral to a subspecialist.

Members of an ad hoc international expert group in PAS published recommended guidelines specifically aimed at standardization of imaging and imaging reporting[18]; the International Society for Abnormally Invasive Placenta (IS-AIP, previously the European Working Group for AIP) proposed standardized US descriptors of PAS.[19] Use of additional, locally available imaging tools such as color three-dimensional (3D) Doppler and MRI is reasonable when needed, but for the purposes of standardization, US investigation as listed in the pro forma is recommended at a minimum. This functional checklist includes elements to identify key clinical risk factors and recommends standardized reporting of US findings. Antenatal staging, analogous to that utilized in oncology, has been proposed using multiple different scoring systems[20]; however, the most recently proposed prenatal US staging system[21] utilizes the nomenclature PAS0, PAS1, PAS2, and PAS3, with increasing numbers as depth of invasion increases. This system is somewhat similar to the clinical classification system proposed by both the IS-AIP and the *Federation Internationale Gynecologie et Obstetrique* (FIGO) for staging at the time of delivery based on clinical and/or histopathology findings (Table 13.2-2). Surgical times, estimated blood loss, intensive care unit (ICU) admission, and surgical complications of the bladder and bowel correlate positively with higher antenatal US PAS stages. Common to many studies evaluating the sensitivity and specificity of US markers of PAS is that both increase with the number of findings that are found concomitantly. Reliance upon a single marker in isolation, especially in low-risk pregnancies, increases the risk of false-positive findings.[22]

Ultrasound Markers

- *Irregular lacunae:* Lacunae describe hypoechoic (dark) voids seen within the placenta on US (Fig. 13.2-1). The sensitivity and specificity of irregular placental lacunae for the detection of PAS have been estimated at 77% (95% confidence

TABLE 13.2-2	FIGO Classification of Placenta Accreta Spectrum Disorders	
GRADE	**CLINICAL CRITERIA**	**HISTOLOGICAL CRITERIA**
Grade 1 (placenta accreta)	• At vaginal delivery: No placental separation with oxytocin and gentle controlled cord traction • At laparotomy: Same as above. Macroscopically, the uterus shows no obvious distension over the placental bed (placental "bulge"), no placental tissue is seen invading through the surface of the uterus, and there are no or minimal superficial vascular changes.	• Microscopic evaluation of the placental bed samples from a hysterectomy specimen shows extended areas of absent decidua between villous tissue and myometrium, with placental villi attached directly to the superficial myometrium. • The diagnosis cannot be made on just-delivered placental tissue nor on random biopsies of the placental bed.
Grade 2 (placenta increta)	At laparotomy: • Abnormal macroscopic findings over the placental bed: bluish/purple coloring, distension present (placental "bulge") • Increased vascularity around the placental bed (dense tangled bed of vessels or multiple vessels running parallel craniocaudally in the uterine serosa). • No placental tissue seen to be invading through the surface of the uterus. • Gentle cord traction results in the uterus being pulled inwards without separation of the placenta (the "dimple" sign).	Hysterectomy specimen or partial myometrial resection of the increta area shows placental villi within the muscular fibers and sometimes in the lumen of the deep uterine vasculature.
Grade 3 (placenta percreta)		
Grade 3a (limited to uterine serosa)	At laparotomy: • Abnormal macroscopic findings on uterine surface (as above) and placental tissue seen to be invading through the surface of the uterus (serosa). • No invasion into any other organ, including the posterior wall of the bladder (a clear surgical plane can be identified between the bladder and the uterus).	Hysterectomy specimen shows villous tissue within or breaching the uterine serosa.
Grade 3b (with urinary bladder invasion)	At laparotomy • Same as grade 3a. • Placental villi are seen to be invading into the bladder, but no other organs. • Clear surgical plane cannot be identified between the bladder and the uterus.	Hysterectomy specimen shows villous tissue breaching the uterine serosa and invading the bladder wall tissue or urothelium.
Grade 3c (with invasion of other pelvic organs/tissues)	At laparotomy • Same as grade 3a. • Placental villi are seen to be invading into the broad ligament, vaginal wall, pelvic sidewall, or any other pelvic organ (and/or invasion of bladder).	Hysterectomy specimen shows villous tissue breaching the uterine serosa and invading pelvic tissues/organs.

From Jauniaux E, Ayres-de-Campos D, Langhoff-Roos J, et al.; FIGO Placenta Accreta Diagnosis and Management Expert Consensus Panel. FIGO classification for the clinical diagnosis of placenta accreta spectrum disorders. *Int J Gynaecol Obstet*. 2019;146(1):20–24; Jauniaux E, Hussein AM, Fox KA, et al. New evidence-based diagnostic and management strategies for placenta accreta spectrum disorders. *Best Pract Res Clin Obstet Gynaecol*. 2019;61:75–88.

interval [CI], 70.1 to 83.1) and 95% (95% CI, 94.1 to 95.8), respectively.[23] Irregular lacunae are often described as giving the placenta a "moth-eaten" appearance. This finding is one of the most commonly recognized findings associated with PAS; however, it is not always present and may be present in normal placentas. Small, round, or ovoid hypoechoic spaces may be seen near the center of increasingly defined cotyledons, in the third trimester, and irregular, large hypoechoic areas may be seen in cases of intraplacental hemorrhage or chronic abruption. In such cases, the echogenicity of the lacunar areas may appear more heterogeneous than in cases with PAS, in which swirling turbulent flow may be seen within the lacunae during real-time grayscale or color Doppler modes. Using pulsed-wave Doppler ultrasonography, high-velocity flow within the lacunae (>15 cm/s) for detection of PAS has a sensitivity of 73% and a specificity of 86%.[24]

- *Loss of the hypoechoic zone*: In the normal case, a fine, hypoechoic (dark) space is visible between the placenta and the myometrium on 2D grayscale imaging. The finding of loss of this line for detection of PAS has a sensitivity of 66% (95% CI, 58.3 to 73.6) and specificity of 98% (95% CI, 94.9 to 96.5).[23] This space is easy to obliterate, especially if too much pressure is applied with the probe. It is useful in cases in which one suspects loss of the zone to use the highest resolution possible at the uteroplacental interface and then gently apply and release pressure on the probe. If the interface is normal, this space appears once pressure from the probe is released. Loss of the hypoechoic zone has been reported to have the highest false-positive rate, if used as a single marker. However, if a clear hypoechoic space can be seen throughout the uteroplacental interface, the negative predictive value is high.
- *Loss of integrity of the hyperechoic (bright) bladder line* (Fig. 13.2-2): Sonographic signs of bladder wall interruption

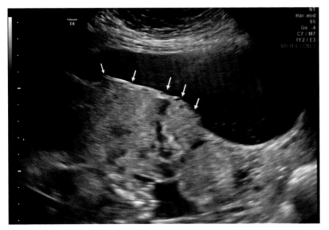

FIGURE 13.2-2: Longitudinal view of the uterine bladder interface on two-dimensional grayscale US. In this image, the normally white, thick, smooth bladder line has a "dot-dashed" or interrupted appearance, and a distinct exophytic placental mass can be seen pushing toward the bladder.

have been described as focal bulging, exophytic masses, and a "dot-dashed" or interrupted appearance of the normally echobright bladder wall. The "dot-dashed" appearance likely represents bridging vessels coursing from placenta toward bladder, seen in cross section. For this marker, the sensitivity is approximately 49.7% (95% CI, 41.4 to 58.0), and the specificity is 99.8% (95% CI, 99.5 to 99.8).[23]

- *Exophytic masses/bulging* (Fig. 13.2-2): Bulging of an exophytic placental mass indicates that a portion of placental tissue is seen beyond the usual confines of the myometrial serosa, most commonly toward the bladder, though, depending on the site and extent of PAS, this finding may be seen along the parametria, particularly in transverse lateral sweeps, and less commonly at the serosal interface superior to the bladder dome.
- *Color Doppler ultrasonography* (Fig. 13.2-3): Color Doppler ultrasonography may be useful to identify neovascularization, bridging vessels running perpendicular to the bladder line/myometrium, and vessels originating within the parametrium and either feeding into or lying in precariously close proximity to placental tissue. Color Doppler ultrasonography is not universally available in some settings and is, therefore, not considered a part of mandatory screening,[18] yet it may be useful where available. "Hypervascularity" is often cited as a finding in cases of PAS, though there is no clear definition of "normal" vascularity of the already highly vascular gravid uterus and placenta; therefore, this finding remains subjective. Misinterpretation may result from lack of care in optimizing Doppler settings (see section "Image Optimization").[13]
- *3D ultrasonography* (Fig. 13.2-3) is not available everywhere; however, although not a part of the standard evaluation as described by FIGO and the IS-AIP, it has been shown to have a very high sensitivity and specificity when used by experienced imaging providers.[25]

Image Optimization

Antenatal identification is possible only if the placenta is interrogated along its entire surface and at optimal settings. There is

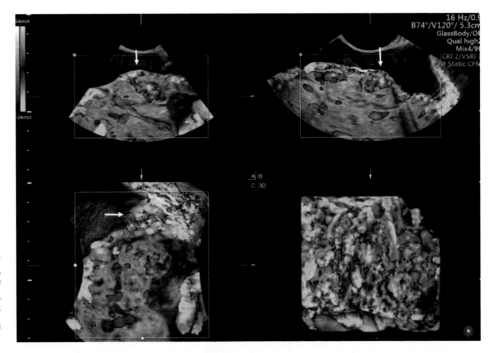

FIGURE 13.2-3: Three-dimensional color Doppler. In this US, color Doppler is used to render a 3D image (lower right corner) of the same placenta seen in Figure 2. Note the large area of confluence of Doppler signal, suggestive of placenta percreta (white arrow).

evidence that PAS is more difficult to identify antenatally when the placenta is not low lying or behind the bladder, and especially when it is posterior, as portions of the interface may be shadowed by overlying fetal parts.[26] Herein, we discuss techniques to optimize US imaging.

- *Fill the bladder:* Assessment of the interface between the lower uterine segment (LUS) and bladder requires a full bladder (200 to 300 mL), and the importance of this cannot be overstated.[27] It may be necessary to ask patients not to void prior to imaging or provide adequate hydration to allow the bladder to fill while imaging the fetus and prior to interrogating the placenta. When the bladder is relatively empty and the wall lax, a low-lying placenta may falsely appear to "bulge" toward the bladder, or, conversely, exophytic masses into the bladder and hypervascularity with bridging vessels may be difficult to see. Patient and probe positioning are equally important in the proper evaluation of the normally hyperechoic, smooth bladder line. When the probe is oriented in the sagittal plane over the LUS/bladder, the curvature of the LUS causes the lowermost portion of the uterovesicular interface to lie parallel to the sound beam, resulting in dropout of a significant portion of the image (Fig. 13.2-4A). This artifact can be addressed by placing the patient in Trendelenburg (head down) position while simultaneously decreasing the angle of the probe such that the probe handle is nearly parallel to the patient's thighs. The angle between the bladder line and the probe then becomes more perpendicularly oriented to the sound beam, and the interface can be seen much more clearly and completely (Fig. 13.2-4B). In some cases, transvaginal ultrasonography may be necessary to evaluate the cervix and lowermost portion of the bladder completely.

- *Obtain ultrasound sweeps:* Use cine-clips or sweeps of the placenta to evaluate the entire uteroplacental interface and topography. Simply reviewing still images is insufficient, and small or focal areas of involvement can be missed easily. We recommend performing sweeps in the sagittal plane from right to left, and in the transverse plane from low to high in the midline and again along the parametrium on each side to assess for lateral placental invasion. These clips can be done first in grayscale mode and repeated with the addition of color Doppler examination. While viewing the sweeps, a subtle bulge or myometrial defect may be perceptible when

an area of previously present myometrium disappears, or when the contour of the uterine surface changes. Color Doppler interrogation can sometimes help identify the close proximity of placental tissue to large feeding vessels and hypertrophied uterine vasculature or neovascularization within the parametrium.

- *Ensure adequate depth, angle width, and focus:* 3D US rendering involves a process of acquisition and reconstruction based on highly complex mathematical formulae built into the US imaging software. The quality of 3D image acquisition depends first on the quality of the acquired 2D images used to reconstruct the image in 3D format, both for still renderings and for real-time use.[28] By obtaining clear 2D images from which to start 3D sweeps, optimizing image depth and focus, one will improve 3D images significantly. Widening the sweep angle for the 3D acquisition will allow evaluation of a greater surface area but may also allow for greater motion artifact if either the mother or fetus moves during the acquisition.

- *Optimize color Doppler interrogation settings:* Because individual factors such as patient body mass index (BMI), placental depth, and variations among US machines may influence the results of 3D color Doppler ultrasonography, it is critical to individualize gain settings in a manner that uses the patient's unique anatomy as the control. This may be done with an individualized "sub-noise gain" (SNG) setting.[29] The technique to obtain an individualized SNG Doppler setting is simple and does not rely upon proprietary US manufacturer settings. One should increase the gain until artifactual noise is present (i.e., there is power Doppler signal scattered throughout the whole image) and then slowly reduce the gain to a level in which the scatter and the artifact have disappeared and only the vascular flow is seen.

Magnetic Resonance Imaging

MRI has been used with increased frequency in recent years, noting that the sensitivity and specificity profiles of MRI in the diagnosis of PAS are comparable to US.[30–32] However, its precise role in the management of the patient at risk is openly debated.[26,33,34] There are a variety of proposed algorithms for imaging evaluation, ranging from US-only protocols to those in which MRI is used in every patient, for surgical planning.[35] Most have reserved the additional use of MRI for cases in which US has limitations in

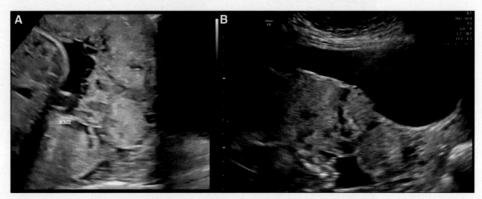

FIGURE 13.2-4: Two-dimensional grayscale sagittal US of the uterovesical interface. **Panel A:** The probe is held perpendicular to the abdomen. Note that the bladder line is parallel to the beam, and there is significant signal dropout. **Panel B:** The same placenta imaged with the patient in Trendelenburg position, with the probe angled, such that the handle is nearly parallel to the patient's legs. Note that the bladder line is now more perpendicular to the beam and is clearly visible.

providing all of the information either for a diagnosis or to plan the safest delivery.[34,36,37] These have been cases, for example, in which there is posterior previa, marked maternal obesity, or a clinical/imaging discordance.

If MRI is used, it is best performed between 24 and 30 weeks of gestation.[38,39] Sequence acquisition is in planes orthogonal to the patient with a moderately full bladder, with additional angled imaging orthogonal to the placenta as indicated. A phased-array surface coil will maximize signal. Sequence choices follow fetal sequence parameters, but with generally thicker slices, and include T2 single-shot fast spin echo (SSFSE) and steady-state free precession (SSFP) imaging in three planes, with a T1 gradient echo (GRE) or Dixon sequence at least in sagittal plane. Some advocate high-resolution angled imaging orthogonal to the cervix as appropriate for surgical planning, akin to evaluation for malignancy.[30] Diffusion-weighted imaging has been suggested to be helpful in some cases to define the placental–myometrial interface,[40] but, in one small study, was not shown to be reliable.[41] Because, in the United States, gadolinium is categorized as a pregnancy class C medication, its use in pregnancy is controversial; therefore, contrast-enhanced imaging is typically avoided, except in certain circumstances.[42,43]

Placental tissue that clearly breaches the uterine wall into the extrauterine space on MRI is highly specific for placenta percreta. MR findings in less invasive but equally morbid cases reflect the altered structure and pathology of the abnormally adherent placenta within the uterine wall. Suggestive findings include the following:

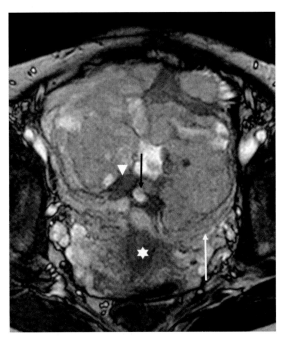

FIGURE 13.2-5: Axial SSFP MRI demonstrating many features of high-grade placenta accreta spectrum (PAS): previa; asymmetric myometrial and serosal bulge at the dorsal left (*white arrow*); large intraparenchymal vessels, including just at the os (*black arrow*); thick black band dividing the placenta into two (*white arrowhead*); marked heterogeneity. White star indicates the cervical canal.

- *Altered uterine contour:* Two kinds of bulging are distinguished, although they often occur together. The more common use of the term applies when the configuration no longer conforms to the typical "upside-down pear" shape that is symmetrically expected in the normal gravid uterus, or, in other words, when there is serosal-surface contour asymmetry or *external* bulge (Fig. 13.2-5). This finding is highly associated with PAS but is not pathognomonic, particularly because foci of uterine scarring, such as at a C-section site, can be thinned and weakened even if there is no true abnormal placental attachment. The second use of the term is associated with an asymmetric interface between the placental margin and the uterine wall; the placenta *internally* "bulges" into the myometrium, with or without external bulge. This finding can be accompanied by loss of clear visualization of the T2 low signal fine demarcation between the placenta and the myometrium, or focal interruption of the myometrial line, which corresponds to the US finding of loss of the retroplacental clear space. One should be cautious about overreliance on this finding in isolation, just as on US.[44] Uterine thinning and less conspicuity of this line with increasing gestational age, especially at a level of prior surgery, is expected.
- *Asymmetric vascularity:* There are two principal considerations when assessing for abnormal vascularity: Are there asymmetrically distributed or enlarged abnormal vessels on the uterine surface, and/or are there any abnormally enlarged vascular spaces inside the placenta? The first recognizes that there can be abnormal perfusion to sites of placental invasion, including collateral vessels from the mesentery, the bladder wall, or the parametrium to the serosal surface of the uterus.[45,46] (Fig. 13.2-6) The second describes abnormally enlarged vessels completely surrounded by placental tissue (as opposed to those on the placental surface) that measure 6 mm

or greater.[47] These are best recognized when comparing the change in signal in these foci of flow between T2 SSFSE (dark blood) and T2 SSFP (bright blood) sequences. They are highly associated with PAS. An interesting observation of association between PAS and lesser cervical venous plexus distension than is typically expected has been suggested.[48]

- *Distortion of adjacent viscera:* If there is percreta, there may be imaging evidence of mass effect on, tethering of, or frank invasion into adjacent anatomy, including the bladder (commonly, as invasion associated with LUS C-section scars is classic), bowel, mesentery, adnexa, or cervix.[49,50] Both the "India-ink" (bladder) and "shaggy-dog" (parametrium) signs describe the loss of the sharp low-signal demarcation of the normal uterine serosal surface.[45,51] T1 sagittal imaging is especially helpful when there is enough intrapelvic fat to define the mesodermal space between the bladder and the uterus; focal loss of visualization of the fat can be a strong clue to percreta even when the bladder lumen is unaffected, and vice versa, preservation of the fat line here is reassuring (Fig. 13.2-7). Low-signal artifact on T1 imaging from a prior C-section is a common finding and helpful for localization. Because the placenta is abnormally attached in PAS, and typically to the LUS given the site of most uterine surgeries, adhesion has a high association with placenta previa. Placental tissue inside the cervical canal, termed the "placental protrusion sign," is meant to be indicative of PAS.[38]
- *Placental signal and contour changes:* Heterogeneity to the placental signal is typical but nonspecific and should not be used as a diagnostic feature in isolation. The degree of heterogeneity may attract attention, however.[52] Much of the literature has focused on the presence of T2 low-signal "black bands,"[52,53] though, perhaps surprisingly, there is no standard

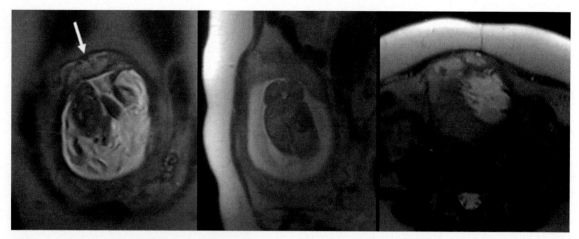

FIGURE 13.2-6: Coronal, sagittal, and axial SSFSE MRI. The patient had a history of multiple uterine interventions, including dilation and curettage (D&C). Not all PAS is at the lower uterine segment; note the focal bulge and breach of the serosa at the fundal ventral right. Note the small cluster of asymmetrically enlarged serosal vessels (*white arrow*). The patient developed acute abdominal pain and, at surgery, had uterine rupture.

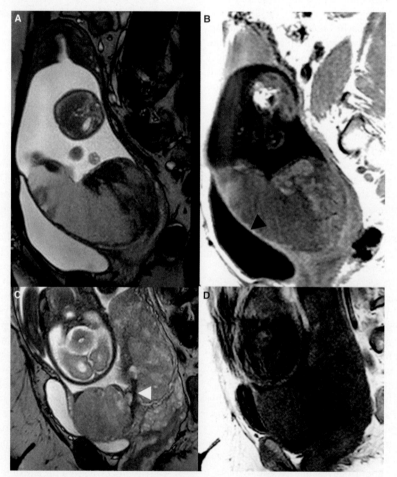

FIGURE 13.2-7: Sagittal T2 SSFP and GRE T1 images **(A, B)**. There is extensive dark signal deposition through this placenta previa, but despite extending from the decidual to the amniotic surfaces, there is no associated retraction, and on the T1 sequence, this signal is bright, consistent with blood product. When there has been previous surgery, as is typical at the lower uterine segment, there are often small foci of low-signal residual artifacts that can help localize the surgical site (not shown). Preservation of fat between the bladder and the uterus can help to exclude visceral invasion (*black arrowhead*). Compare with sagittal T2 SSFP and GRE T1 images in a case of PAS with true pathological black bands causing retraction and loss of the fat between bladder and uterus (**C, D;** *white arrowhead*).

definition of what constitutes an abnormal band nor is there complete agreement on the pathology, although this is often attributed to fibrin.[54] To increase specificity, these bands probably need to be of a minimum length, such as 2 cm,[55] based from the decidual side of the placenta and variably extending to the amniotic surface; when they do, they often cause a retraction that makes the placenta appear bilobed (the "placental recess")[56] (Fig. 13.2-5). The association of black bands with PAS is high and typically is the single finding with highest sensitivity in detection of invasion across its spectrum.[32,45] In addition to an acquired abnormal bilobed placental contour, some authors have noted irregular rather than smooth tapering of placental edges in higher association with PAS.[49] T1 imaging can aid in distinguishing between hemorrhage and true black bands as necessary.

Multiple studies suggest that signal heterogeneity, myometrial thinning, and focal interruption of the myometrium (internal bulge) have lower specificity than the findings of serosal (external) bulge, abnormal intraplacental or serosal vessels, or dark intraplacental bands. Some consider the combination of intraplacental dark bands and focal interruption of the myometrium with any other positive MR sign diagnostic of PAS.[57]

Prognosis and Management: PAS carries a high risk for severe maternal morbidity and mortality, most commonly due to hemorrhage, sequelae of massive blood transfusion, and/or injury to or involvement of nearby structures such as the urinary tract.[6,13] Management of PAS can be classified as surgical or conservative. Surgical management usually refers to planned hysterectomy at the time of delivery, which is definitive. Conservative management has been used to describe a range of treatment modalities, from focal surgical resection of affected myometrium with uterine reconstruction, through hysteroscopic resection of invading placenta, to simply ligating the umbilical cord as close to the placental insertion as possible and leaving the placenta in situ until it is expelled or resorbed or until indications for hysterectomy arise. Chemotherapy may be used adjunctively. Both surgical and

conservative management of PAS carry significant risks. Specifically, cesarean hysterectomy is often complex, associated with hemorrhage, urinary tract injury, and loss of fertility; and conservative management is associated with delayed hemorrhage, disseminated intravascular coagulation (DIC), infection, or uterine rupture in subsequent pregnancies.[58] Large case series of patients who were managed conservatively show a considerably high fertility rate, ranging between 83% and 89%.[59,60]

The risk of maternal mortality in PAS has declined markedly from 4% to 7%, reported near the turn of the 21st century,[4] to as low as 0.05% in a recent large review and meta-analysis.[6] The rates of major complications and maternal death are disproportionately higher in low-resource settings.[6] Morbidity and mortality are significantly lower when women with PAS are managed by experienced teams[61,62] and when PAS is diagnosed prior to delivery, which permits care management planning and appropriate referral.

Recurrence: The recurrence of PAS obviously does not exist with classic surgical therapy by hysterectomy. It does, however, become relevant for patient counseling when conservative management is considered. The recurrence rate for PAS after conservative therapy, when results of all types of treatment have been combined, has been reported to be nearly 20% and is as high as almost 29% in one series.[22,59,63] For occult (or focal) accreta, defined as myometrial invasion seen only histologically and clinically separable from the uterus at surgery, there is report of an increased risk for retained placenta and recurrent occult accreta in subsequent pregnancies.[64]

Differential Diagnosis: Adenomyosis has been reported to mimic PAS on both US and MR examinations, specifically with lacunae, asymmetric uterine bulging, loss of the myometrial line/thinning, and atypical vascularity.[65] A so-called "myometrial window," in which the scar site from prior surgery is stretched so thin by uterine expansion that placenta can be seen through it on direct inspection, also can show focal bulge and thinning, making these findings less specific for PAS (Fig. 13.2-8). Neither of these differential diagnoses has been reported with abnormal

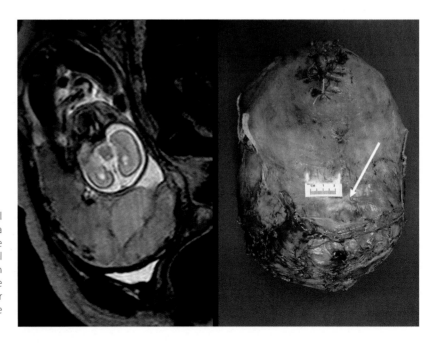

FIGURE 13.2-8: Sagittal T2 SSFSE MRI and coronal gross pathological specimen in a patient with a myometrial window. There is a large broad-based bulge that distorts the lower uterine segment out of its typical "inverted pear" configuration, but little else to confirm abnormal invasion. White arrow directs attention to the purplish placenta seen transversely across the lower uterus, where the cesarean section scar has become transparently thin.

black bands or enlarged intraplacental vessels on MRI. Subacute hemorrhage may mimic black bands on T2 MR imaging but is typically bright on T1 sequences and more parallel than perpendicular to the placental long axis. Because the heterogeneity of the normally aging placenta can occasionally offer a concerning appearance, MRI performed after 30 weeks should be interpreted with caution in the absence of other signs of PAS. One should be aware that "marginal sinus" placental previa in which the placenta does not cover the cervical os may not have the same association with PAS as classic previa.[66]

CONCLUSIONS

Antenatal detection of PAS is the cornerstone on which patient referral, delivery planning, and clinical management depend. Standardization of terminology, imaging protocols, and reporting are essential to moving forward with meaningful data for future collaborative studies, meta-analyses, and tracking of epidemiological trends. Improvements in technology and novel imaging approaches continue to enhance our imaging ability, but these cannot replace fundamental working knowledge of the strengths and limitations of each imaging modality. By improving our ability to identify PAS accurately antenatally, we empower the providers managing clinical and surgical care and thereby save lives.

REFERENCES

1. Franczyk M, Lopucki M, Stachowicz N, et al. Extracellular matrix proteins in healthy and retained placentas, comparing hemochorial and synepitheliochorial placentas. *Placenta*. 2017;50:19–24.
2. Aaberg ME, Reid DE. Manual removal of the placenta: a policy of treatment. *Am J Obstet Gynecol*. 1945;47(3):368–377.
3. Fitzpatrick KE, Sellers S, Spark P, et al. Incidence and risk factors for placenta accreta/increta/percreta in the UK: a national case-control study. *PLoS One*. 2012;7(12):e52893.
4. Publications Committee, Society of Maternal-Fetal Medicine, Belfort MA. Placenta accreta. *Am J Obstet Gynecol*. 2010;203(5):430–439.
5. Bailit JL, Grobman WA, Rice MM, et al. Morbidly adherent placenta treatments and outcomes. *Obstet Gynecol*. 2015;125(3):683–689.
6. Jauniaux E, Bunce C, Grønbeck L, et al. Prevalence and main outcomes of placenta accreta spectrum: a systematic review and metaanalysis. *Am J Obstet Gynecol*. 2019;221(3):208–218.
7. Wu S, Kocherginsky M, Hibbard JU. Abnormal placentation: twenty-year analysis. *Am J Obstet Gynecol*. 2005;192(5):1458–1461.
8. Clark SL, Koonings PP, Phelan JP. Placenta previa/accreta and prior cesarean section. *Obstet Gynecol*. 1985;66(1):89–92.
9. Timor-Tritsch IE, Monteagudo A, Cali G, et al. Cesarean scar pregnancy and early placenta accreta share common histology. *Ultrasound Obstet Gynecol*. 2014;43(4):383–395.
10. Timor-Tritsch IE, Monteagudo A, Cali G, et al. Cesarean scar pregnancy is a precursor of morbidly adherent placenta. *Ultrasound Obstet Gynecol*. 2014;44(3):346–353.
11. Hu Y, Dutz JP, MacCalman CD, et al. Decidual NK cells alter in vitro first trimester extravillous cytotrophoblast migration: a role for IFN-gamma. *J Immunol*. 2006;177(12):8522–8530.
12. Duzyj CM, Buhimschi IA, Laky CA, et al. Extravillous trophoblast invasion in placenta accreta is associated with differential local expression of angiogenic and growth factors: a cross-sectional study. *BJOG*. 2018;125(11):1441–1448.
13. Jauniaux E, Bhide A, Kennedy A, et al. FIGO consensus guidelines on placenta accreta spectrum disorders: Prenatal diagnosis and screening. *Int J Gynaecol Obstet*. 2018;140(3):274–280.
14. Fitzpatrick KE, Sellers S, Spark P, et al. The management and outcomes of placenta accreta, increta, and percreta in the UK: a population-based descriptive study. *BJOG*. 2014;121(1):62–70; discussion 70–71.
15. Silver RM, Fox KA, Barton JR, et al. Center of excellence for placenta accreta. *Am J Obstet Gynecol*. 2015;212(5):561–568.
16. Rac MW, Moschos E, Wells CE, et al. Sonographic findings of morbidly adherent placenta in the first trimester. *J Ultrasound Med*. 2016;35(2):263–269.
17. Ballas J, Pretorius D, Hull AD, et al. Identifying sonographic markers for placenta accreta in the first trimester. *J Ultrasound Med*. 2012;31(11):1835–1841.
18. Alfirevic Z, Tang AW, Collins SL, et al. Pro forma for ultrasound reporting in suspected abnormally invasive placenta (AIP): an international consensus. *Ultrasound Obstet Gynecol*. 2016;47(3):276–278.
19. Collins SL, Ashcroft A, Braun T, et al. Proposal for standardized ultrasound descriptors of abnormally invasive placenta (AIP). *Ultrasound Obstet Gynecol*. 2016;47(3):271–275.
20. Rac MW, Dashe JS, Wells CE, et al. Ultrasound predictors of placental invasion: the Placenta Accreta Index. *Am J Obstet Gynecol*. 2015;212(3):343.e1–e7.
21. Cali G, Forlani F, Lees C, et al. Prenatal ultrasound staging system for placenta accreta spectrum disorders. *Ultrasound Obstet Gynecol*. 2019;53(6):752–760.
22. Philips J, Gurganus M, DeShields S, et al. Prevalence of sonographic markers of placenta accreta spectrum in low-risk pregnancies. *Am J Perinatol*. 2019;36(8):733–780.
23. D'Antonio F, Iacovella C, Bhide A. Prenatal identification of invasive placentation using ultrasound: systematic review and meta-analysis. *Ultrasound Obstet Gynecol*. 2013;42(5):509–517.
24. Cali G, Giambanco L, Puccio G, et al. Morbidly adherent placenta: evaluation of ultrasound diagnostic criteria and differentiation of placenta accreta from percreta. *Ultrasound Obstet Gynecol*. 2013;41(4):406–412.
25. Collins SL, Stevenson GN, Al-Khan A, et al. Three-dimensional power doppler ultrasonography for diagnosing abnormally invasive placenta and quantifying the risk. *Obstet Gynecol*. 2015;126(3):645–653.
26. Budorick NE, Figueroa R, Vizcarra M, et al. Another look at ultrasound and magnetic resonance imaging for diagnosis of placenta accreta. *J Matern Fetal Neonatal Med*. 2017;30(20):2422–2427.
27. Maynard H, Zamudio S, Jauniaux E, et al. The importance of bladder volume in the ultrasound diagnosis of placenta accreta spectrum disorders. *Int J Gynaecol Obstet*. 2018;140(3):332–337.
28. Huang Q, Zeng Z. A Review on real-time 3D ultrasound imaging technology. *Biomed Res Int*. 2017;2017:6027029.
29. Collins SL, Stevenson GN, Noble JA, et al. Influence of power Doppler gain setting on Virtual Organ Computer-aided AnaLysis indices in vivo: can use of the individual sub-noise gain level optimize information? *Ultrasound Obstet Gynecol*. 2012;40(1):75–80.
30. D'Antonio F, Iacovella C, Palacios-Jaraquemada J, et al. Prenatal identification of invasive placentation using magnetic resonance imaging: systematic review and meta-analysis. *Ultrasound Obstet Gynecol*. 2014;44(1):8–16.
31. Meng X, Xie L, Song W. Comparing the diagnostic value of ultrasound and magnetic resonance imaging for placenta accreta: a systematic review and meta-analysis. *Ultrasound Med Biol*. 2013;39(11):1958–1965.
32. Familiari A, Liberati M, Lim P, et al. Diagnostic accuracy of magnetic resonance imaging in detecting the severity of abnormal invasive placenta: a systematic review and meta-analysis. *Acta Obstet Gynecol Scand*. 2018;97(5):507–520.
33. Einerson BD, Rodriguez CE, Kennedy AM, et al. Magnetic resonance imaging is often misleading when used as an adjunct to ultrasound in the management of placenta accreta spectrum disorders. *Am J Obstet Gynecol*. 2018;218(6):618 e1–e7.
34. Matsubara S, Takahashi H, Takei Y. Magnetic resonance imaging for diagnosis of placenta accreta spectrum disorders: still useful for real-world practice. *Am J Obstet Gynecol*. 2018;219(3):312–313.
35. Palacios-Jaraquemada JM. Diagnosis and management of placenta accreta. *Best Pract Res Clin Obstet Gynaecol*. 2008;22(6):1133–1148.
36. Dwyer BK, Belogolovkin V, Tran L, et al. Prenatal diagnosis of placenta accreta: sonography or magnetic resonance imaging? *J Ultrasound Med*. 2008;27(9):1275–1281.
37. American College of Obstetricians and Gynecologists. ACOG Practice Bulletin: Clinical Management Guidelines for Obstetrician-Gynecologists Number 76, October 2006: postpartum hemorrhage. *Obstet Gynecol*. 2006;108(4):1039–1047.
38. Ueno Y, Kitajima K, Kawakami F, et al. Novel MRI for diagnosis of invasive placenta praevia: evaluation of findings for 65 patients using clinical and histopathological correlations. *Eur Radiol*. 2014;24(4):881–888.
39. Horowitz JM, Berggruen S, McCarthy RJ, et al. When timing is everything: are placental MRI examinations performed before 24 weeks' gestational age reliable? *AJR Am J Roentgenol*. 2015;205(3):685–692.
40. Morita S, Ueno E, Fujimura M, et al. Feasibility of diffusion-weighted MRI for defining placental invasion. *J Magn Reson Imaging*. 2009;30(3):666–671.
41. Sannananja B, Ellermeier A, Hippe DS, et al. Utility of diffusion-weighted MR imaging in the diagnosis of placenta accreta spectrum abnormality. *Abdom Radiol (NY)*. 2018;43(11):3147–3156.
42. Millischer AE, Deloison B, Silvera S, et al. Dynamic contrast enhanced MRI of the placenta: a tool for prenatal diagnosis of placenta accreta? *Placenta*. 2017;53:40–47.
43. Millischer AE, Salomon LJ, Porcher R, et al. Magnetic resonance imaging for abnormally invasive placenta: the added value of intravenous gadolinium injection. *BJOG*. 2017;124(1):88–95.
44. Comstock CH, Love JJ, Bronsteen RA, et al. Sonographic detection of placenta accreta in the second and third trimesters of pregnancy. *Am J Obstet Gynecol*. 2004;190(4):1135–1140.
45. Goergen SK, Posma E, Wrede D, et al. Interobserver agreement and diagnostic performance of individual MRI criteria for diagnosis of placental adhesion disorders. *Clin Radiol*. 2018;73(10):908.e1–e9.
46. Chen X, Shan R, Zhao L, et al. Invasive placenta previa: placental bulge with distorted uterine outline and uterine serosal hypervascularity at 1.5T MRI—useful features for differentiating placenta percreta from placenta accreta. *Eur Radiol*. 2018;28(2):708–717.
47. Derman AY, Nikac V, Haberman S, et al. MRI of placenta accreta: a new imaging perspective. *AJR Am J Roentgenol*. 2011;197(6):1514–1521.

48. Ishibashi H, Miyamoto M, Shinnmoto H, et al. Cervical varicosities may predict placenta accreta in posterior placenta previa: a magnetic resonance imaging study. *Arch Gynecol Obstet.* 2017;296(4):731–736.

49. Bourgioti C, Zafeiropoulou K, Fotopoulos S, et al. MRI features predictive of invasive placenta with extrauterine spread in high-risk gravid patients: a prospective evaluation. *AJR Am J Roentgenol.* 2018;211(3):701–711.

50. Bourgioti C, Zafeiropoulou K, Fotopoulos S, et al. MRI prognosticators for adverse maternal and neonatal clinical outcome in patients at high risk for placenta accreta spectrum (PAS) disorders. *J Magn Reson Imaging.* 2019;50(2):602–618.

51. Kumar I, Verma A, Jain S, et al. Chemical shift artifact on steady-state MRI sequences for detection of vesical wall invasion in placenta percreta. *J Obstet Gynaecol India.* 2016;66(2):101–106.

52. Lax A, Prince MR, Mennitt KW, et al. The value of specific MRI features in the evaluation of suspected placental invasion. *Magn Reson Imaging.* 2007;25(1):87–93.

53. Alamo L, Anaye A, Rey J, et al. Detection of suspected placental invasion by MRI: do the results depend on observer' experience? *Eur J Radiol.* 2013;82(2):e51–e57.

54. Rahaim NS, Whitby EH. The MRI features of placental adhesion disorder and their diagnostic significance: systematic review. *Clin Radiol.* 2015;70(9):917–925.

55. Ueno Y, Maeda T, Tanaka U, et al. Evaluation of interobserver variability and diagnostic performance of developed MRI-based radiological scoring system for invasive placenta previa. *J Magn Reson Imaging.* 2016;44(3):573–583.

56. Sato T, Mori N, Hasegawa O, et al. Placental recess accompanied by a T2 dark band: a new finding for diagnosing placental invasion. *Abdom Radiol (NY).* 2017;42(8):2146–2153.

57. Maurea S, Romeo V, Mainenti PP, et al. Diagnostic accuracy of magnetic resonance imaging in assessing placental adhesion disorder in patients with placenta previa: correlation with histological findings. *Eur J Radiol.* 2018;106:77–84.

58. Fox KA, Shamshirsaz AA, Carusi D, et al. Conservative management of morbidly adherent placenta: expert review. *Am J Obstet Gynecol.* 2015;213(6):755–760.

59. Sentilhes L, Kayem G, Ambroselli C, et al. Fertility and pregnancy outcomes following conservative treatment for placenta accreta. *Hum Reprod.* 2010;25(11):2803–2810.

60. Alanis M, Hurst BS, Marshburn PB, et al. Conservative management of placenta increta with selective arterial embolization preserves future fertility and results in a favorable outcome in subsequent pregnancies. *Fertil Steril.* 2006;86(5):1514.e3–e7.

61. Shamshirsaz AA, Fox KA, Salmanian B, et al. Maternal morbidity in patients with morbidly adherent placenta treated with and without a standardized multidisciplinary approach. *Am J Obstet Gynecol.* 2015;212(2):218.e1–e9.

62. Tikkanen M, Paavonen J, Loukovaara M, et al. Antenatal diagnosis of placenta accreta leads to reduced blood loss. *Acta Obstet Gynecol Scand.* 2011;90(10):1140–1146.

63. Cunningham KM, Anwar A, Lindow SW. The recurrence risk of placenta accrete following uterine conservative management. *J Neonatal-Perinatal Med.* 2015;8:293–296.

64. Mullen C, Battarbee A, Ernst LM, et al. Occult placenta accrete: risk factors, adverse obstetrical outcomes, and recurrence in subsequent pregnancies. *Am J Perinat.* 2019;36:472–475.

65. Tongsong T, Khunamornpong S, Sirikunalai P, et al. Adenomyosis in pregnancy mimicking morbidly adherent placenta. *BMJ Case Rep.* 2014;2014.

66. Ishibashi H, Miyamoto M, Soyama H, et al. Marginal sinus placenta previa is a different entity in placenta previa: a retrospective study using magnetic resonance imaging. *Taiwan J Obstet Gynecol.* 2018;57(4):532–535.

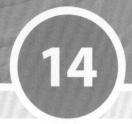

14 Ultrasound Imaging of the Uterine Cervix

Edgar Hernandez-Andrade • Lami Yeo • Anderson J. Lo • Sonia S. Hassan • Roberto Romero

The uterine cervix plays a central role in the maintenance of pregnancy. During most of normal gestation, the cervix remains firm and closed despite uterine distension and a progressive increase in fetal size. At the end of pregnancy and during labor, the cervix softens, shortens, and dilates to allow delivery of the fetus. Labor, delivery, and the postpartum period are accompanied by dramatic changes in the uterine cervix.[1–13] Early activation of parturition can often be visualized in the form of a prematurely shortened cervix. Cervical disorders have been implicated in common obstetrical complications, for example, "cervical insufficiency,"[14] preterm labor and delivery,[15–18] and prolonged latent phase of labor.[19] Progress has been made toward decreasing the rate of preterm birth with the use of progestogens.[20–24] Yet, preterm parturition is a syndrome with many etiologies, and further investigation is needed. It is well established that a sonographic short cervix is the most powerful predictor of spontaneous preterm birth.[15–18,25–41]

Preterm birth is the leading cause of perinatal morbidity and infant mortality worldwide.[42] The prevalence of preterm birth is approximately 11%[43] and it is implicated in up to 75% of perinatal deaths.[44] The consequences of preterm birth may include respiratory distress syndrome (RDS),[45] necrotizing enterocolitis,[46] neonatal sepsis,[47] cerebral palsy,[48] cognitive disability,[49] and neonatal death.[50] Approximately 500,000 neonates are born preterm annually in the United States,[51] but the rate of preterm deliveries increases annually.[51] From 2016 to 2017, late preterm births increased from 7.09% to 7.17%, whereas early preterm deliveries remained stable in 2.8% of all deliveries. The rate of early and late preterm deliveries is significantly higher in women older than 35 years (early, 3.1%; late, 8.1%) and in women older than 40 years (early, 4.3%; late, 10.4%).[51]

This chapter focuses on the following topics: (1) the role of sonographic evaluation of the cervix in the prediction and prevention of preterm birth, (2) possible etiologies of a short cervix, (3) therapeutic options for women with a short cervix, and (4) novel imaging modalities for cervix evaluation.

SONOGRAPHIC EVALUATION OF THE CERVIX IN THE PREDICTION AND PREVENTION OF PRETERM BIRTH

The Role of the Cervix in Pregnancy and Parturition

We have proposed that parturition has a common terminal pathway characterized by increased myometrial contractility, cervical ripening, and membrane/decidual activation.[52] These processes are required for both term and preterm parturition (Fig. 14.1). Normal labor at term is characterized by coordinated activation of the three processes, while premature activation is observed in patients presenting with preterm labor and progressive cervical dilation that lead to preterm delivery (Fig. 14.2).[53] Premature cervical ripening may lead to different clinical conditions ranging from midtrimester abortion,

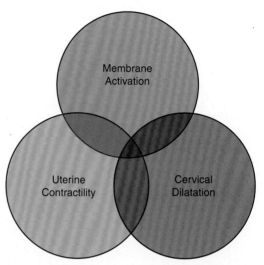

FIGURE 14.1: Uterine components of the common pathway of parturition.[53] (Republished with permission of Walter de Gruyter & Co., from Romero R, Yeo L, Miranda J, et al. A blueprint for the prevention of preterm birth: vaginal progesterone in women with a short cervix. *J Perinat Med.* 2013;41(1):27–44; permission conveyed through Copyright Clearance Center, Inc.)

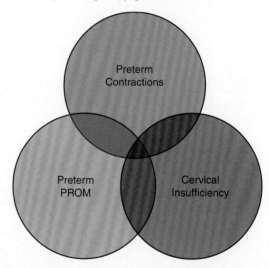

FIGURE 14.2: Clinical manifestations of preterm activation of the common pathway of parturition.[53] (Republished with permission of Walter de Gruyter & Co., from Romero R, Yeo L, Miranda J, et al. A blueprint for the prevention of preterm birth: vaginal progesterone in women with a short cervix. *J Perinat Med.* 2013;41(1):27–44; permission conveyed through Copyright Clearance Center, Inc.)

preterm labor with or without preterm delivery, and precipitous labor at term.

Importantly, sonographic cervical length is more informative than a history of previous preterm birth in predicting preterm birth.[15–18,25–41,54,55] Sonographic cervical length is not a screening test for spontaneous preterm delivery as only a few patients who will experience a spontaneous preterm birth develop a short cervix in the midtrimester of pregnancy. However, sonographic cervical length is a method for risk assessment of spontaneous preterm delivery. Its importance derives from the observation that patients with a short cervix might benefit from preventive treatment to reduce the rate of preterm delivery.[21–24,54,56–58]

Sonographic Evaluation of the Cervix: Which Method Should Be Used to Examine the Cervix?

The cervix can be evaluated by ultrasound using a transabdominal (Fig. 14.3), transvaginal, or transperineal approach (Fig. 14.4). The transvaginal technique (Fig. 14.5) is the preferred method for optimal assessment of the cervix given the limitations of image acquisition by the other two approaches. Transabdominal sonography requires a full bladder for adequate visualization of the cervix; as a result, bladder distension can compress and artificially lengthen the cervix.[26,59,60]

By contrast, transvaginal ultrasound does not require a distended bladder. Indeed, this situation may even falsely depict a shortened cervix as having a greater length. The cervical length measurement is longer (by 5.2 mm, on average) when assessed by transabdominal ultrasound as compared to transvaginal ultrasound.[26] Furthermore, transabdominal ultrasound has been reported to fail in detecting a short cervix in 57% of the cases.[61] The transperineal technique, introduced prior to the development of the transvaginal transducer, can be used when a transvaginal transducer is not available. This approach does not require a full bladder,[62–67] yet the presence of air in the vagina or from bowel gas may obscure the images. One study using transperineal ultrasound reported that a clear image of the cervix could not be obtained in 30% of patients at midtrimester nor in 19% of patients in the third trimester of pregnancy.[67] Therefore, transvaginal ultrasound is the recommended technique for evaluation of the uterine cervix in pregnancy.

Technique

Patients are asked to empty their bladder before undergoing transvaginal ultrasound. During the procedure, the patient lies in the supine position with flexed knees and hips. The probe is covered with an appropriate and clean sheath. Gel is placed

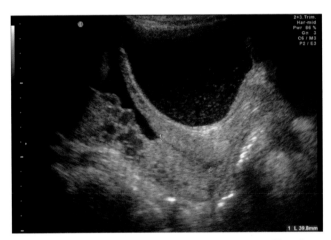

FIGURE 14.3: Transabdominal measurement of the cervical length.

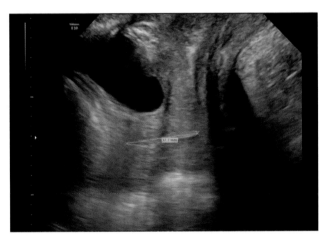

FIGURE 14.4: Transperineal measurement of the cervical length.

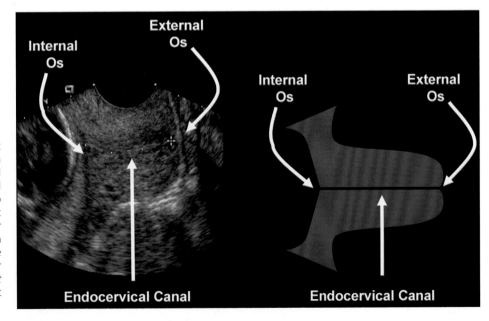

FIGURE 14.5: Transvaginal sonographic appearance of a normal uterine cervix with a clear visualization of the internal cervical os, the external os and the endocervical canal. (Reprinted from Gomez R, Galasso M, Romero R, et al. Ultrasonographic examination of the uterine cervix is better than cervical digital examination as a predictor of the likelihood of premature delivery in patients with preterm labor and intact membranes. *Am J Obstet Gynecol*. 1994;171(4):956–964. Copyright © 1994 Elsevier. With permission.)

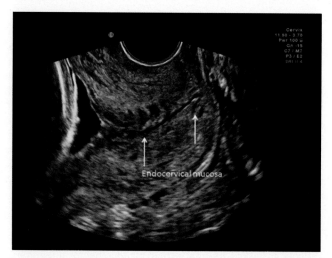

FIGURE 14.6: Endocervical mucosa observed around the endocervical canal.

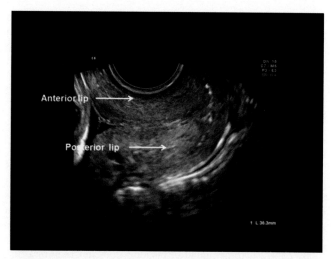

FIGURE 14.7: Excessive pressure applied with the ultrasound probe.

between the transducer and the cover as well as on the surface sheath. The operator introduces the vaginal probe into the anterior fornix until a midline sagittal view of the cervix and lower uterine segment can be visualized. The images of the internal os, external os, cervical canal, and endocervical mucosa should be clearly identifiable (Figs 14.5 and 14.6).

The endocervical mucosa is used to define the upper edge of the cervix; otherwise, the cervical length may erroneously include part of the lower uterine segment (Fig. 14.6).

Excessive pressure with the probe may elongate the cervix (Fig. 14.7).

To avoid this pitfall, the ultrasound probe is slowly withdrawn until the image blurs, and pressure is subsequently reapplied to restore the image. This aspect can further be adjusted by confirming equal cervical width and equal density of the anterior and posterior lips of the cervix[68,69] (Fig. 14.8).

Specific recommendations for the standardization of each cervical examination within the ultrasound unit can improve the quality of image acquisition (Fig. 14.8).[69] The following criteria may be used to capture each image of the cervix:

- Flat internal os or isosceles triangle
- Entire length of the cervical canal
- Symmetrical image of the external os
- Equal size and density of the anterior and posterior lips of the cervix

The cervical length is measured on three separate images. The optimal time for examination ranges from 5 to 10 minutes. It should be noted that if the duration of the examination is too short and the patient presents with dynamic cervical changes during the examination, the cervical length may not represent the true length of the cervix. This result may account for some observations in which patients seem to gain cervical length over time. The contours of the anterior and posterior lips of the cervix are usually clearly defined. For clinical purposes, the shortest cervical length is reported, provided that the image is adequate.

When the cervical canal is curved, the cervical length can be determined by tracing along the canal or by adding the sum of two straight sections. From a prospective study performed in 301 women at 23 weeks of gestation, To et al.[70] concluded that the question of whether to measure the cervix as a straight line or along the cervical canal might not have any clinical significance given that a short cervix (<16 mm) is always straight. Indeed, from a practical point of view, a short cervix is virtually always straight (Fig. 14.9).

Although a cervical examination may appear to be a simple procedure to the experienced sonographer, certain patients may present significant challenges; therefore, several potential pitfalls should be avoided: (1) excessive probe pressure (result: a falsely long measurement; Fig. 14.7); (2) short examination time (result: miss true cervical shortening); (3) failure to recognize a poorly developed lower uterine segment (result: a falsely long measurement); (4) unequal

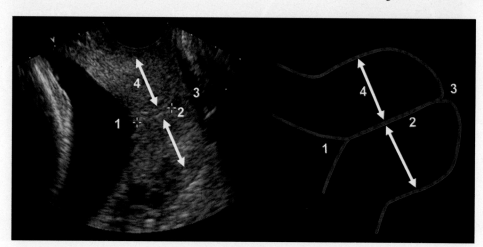

FIGURE 14.8: Clear visualization of (1) the internal cervical os, (2) the endocervical canal, (3) the external cervical os, and (4) similar thickness of the anterior and posterior cervical lips.

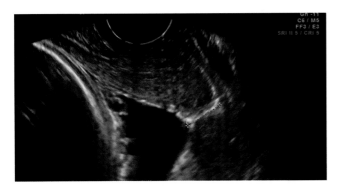

FIGURE 14.9: Short cervix: a) 13.7 mm length; the endocervical canal is a straight line.

size and density of the anterior and posterior lips (Fig. 14.7); and (5) poor visualization of the cervix and of the endocervical canal (Fig. 14.10). An unusual orientation or a retroverted uterus might also pose a challenge in measuring the cervical length.[71]

Ultrasound Probe Disinfection

Disinfection of the ultrasound probe after each examination is mandatory. The American Institute of Ultrasound in Medicine (AIUM) suggests routine high-level usage of disinfection as internal transducers can carry a variety of pathogens, including the human papillomavirus (HPV). High-level disinfectants may include glutaraldehyde, hydrogen peroxide, and phenol-phenolate sodium, among others.[72]

First-Trimester Cervical Sonography for Risk Assessment

The identification of a short cervix, and thus a patient at risk for preterm birth early in pregnancy, allows for more timely follow up and treatment (if such an intervention is proven) prior to the typical midgestation cervical length examination. The accurate measurement of cervical length in the first trimester can be technically difficult as the lower uterine segment may not be distended and can appear to be part of the cervix (Fig. 14.11). Several authors have evaluated the use of first-trimester cervical length to predict preterm birth.[73–79]

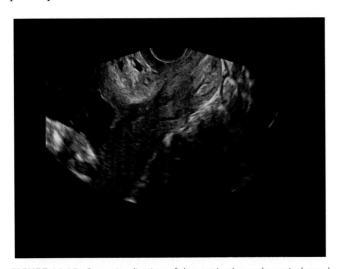

FIGURE 14.10: Poor visualization of the cervix; the endocervical canal and the internal and external cervical os are not clearly defined.

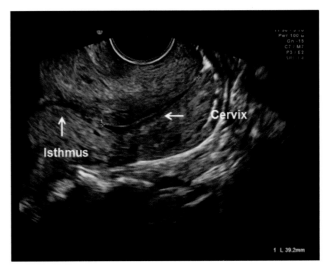

FIGURE 14.11: Cervicoisthmic complex in the first trimester of pregnancy. Only the cervical length should be measured.

Greco et al.[79] reported a shorter endocervical length at 11+0 to 13+6 weeks of gestation in women who delivered at less than 34 weeks than in those who delivered at greater than or equal to 34 weeks of gestation. The same group reported that sonographic cervical length at 11+0 to 13+6 weeks of gestation in combination with maternal characteristics such as ethnicity and obstetrical history can predict 55% of preterm deliveries less than 34 weeks with a false-positive rate of 10%.[77–79] Sananes et al.[80] reported that the isthmus adds about 14 mm to the cervicoisthmic complex and that shortening of the isthmus in the first trimester of pregnancy is the factor that provides the prediction of preterm delivery.

Conversely, several studies concluded that cervical length obtained by a first-trimester ultrasound does not reliably predict preterm birth.[73–75] Parra-Cordero et al.[81] evaluated 3,480 low-risk pregnant women at 11+0 to 13+6 weeks of gestation to identify predictors of preterm delivery at less than 34 weeks of gestation. The authors reported no differences in cervical length between women who underwent preterm delivery at less than 34 weeks and women who delivered at greater than or equal to 34 weeks of gestation. Cervical length did not indicate a significant predictive value for preterm delivery.

Nevertheless, a short cervix detected in the first trimester of pregnancy might be useful in defining a population as high risk for a midtrimester loss. Papastefanou et al.[82] reported that women who experienced a midtrimester loss had a significantly shorter cervix at 11 to 14 weeks than did women continuing with a pregnancy at greater than 24 weeks of gestation. Similarly, Wulff et al.[83] reported that a cervical length less than 25 mm at 11 to 14 weeks of gestation increased by nine-fold the risk of a short cervix in the second trimester of pregnancy. Therefore, women with a short cervix in the first trimester should be considered as high risk for a midtrimester loss and should be followed up closely until delivery.

Midtrimester Cervical Sonography for Preterm Birth Risk Assessment

The optimal gestational age to examine the cervix for preterm birth risk assessment is in the midtrimester of pregnancy. The predictive value of cervical length is greater at 18 to 25 weeks when compared to an earlier stage of gestation (i.e., <18 weeks).[17,18,73–79] Furthermore, effective interventions have been demonstrated in trials that evaluated the uterine cervix at 18 to 25 weeks of gestation.[22–24]

Predicting Preterm Birth

Cervical length is generally stable in nulliparous and multiparous women between 18 and 30 weeks of gestation with an uncomplicated pregnancy, showing a progressive (although not substantial) shortening in the third trimester of pregnancy.[15,25,27,84–87] Cervical sonography has been used to assess the risk of preterm birth in three groups: (1) asymptomatic low-risk patients, (2) asymptomatic patients with risk factors for preterm birth and/or a previous midtrimester loss, and (3) patients presenting with symptoms of preterm labor. This section highlights some of the studies that have contributed to establishing the value of cervical sonography in the risk assessment for spontaneous preterm birth. Emerging strategies for risk assessment are also discussed.

Cervical Length for the Prediction of Preterm Delivery

Low-Risk, Asymptomatic Patients

Andersen et al.[15] performed one of the first studies to evaluate the relationship between a sonographic short cervix and the risk of spontaneous preterm birth. A cohort of 113 women was evaluated by transabdominal and transvaginal sonography together with digital assessment of the cervix before 30 weeks of gestation. The patient population, which had an overall prematurity rate of 15%, was not separated into low-risk and high-risk categories. The authors reported that a cervical length less than 39 mm was associated with a 25% risk of preterm delivery, while a cervical length greater than or equal to 39 mm indicated a lower risk of preterm birth (6.7%).[15] Furthermore, the risk of spontaneous preterm birth was inversely related to the cervical length. These findings have been confirmed by other investigators, both in low-risk[15,17,18,25,27–32,35,37,39,41,87–91] and in high-risk asymptomatic patients.[33,36,38,40,68,92–94] Table 14.1 describes the details of some of the studies with adequate information to allow for the calculation of diagnostic indices and predictive values of the cervical length measurement.

In a prospective cohort study, Iams et al.[29] evaluated the cervix with transvaginal ultrasound at 24 weeks and at 28 weeks in 2,915 patients to estimate the risk of preterm delivery at less than 35 weeks of gestation. The authors reported an exponential increase in the relative risk (RR) of preterm delivery as the cervical length shortened (Fig. 14.12). This study confirmed the results of Andersen et al.,[15] indicating that a short cervix increases the risk of preterm delivery, while the risk is reduced as the cervical length increases.[29] Our group evaluated 6,877 women at 14 to 24 weeks of gestation and reported odds ratios (OR) for preterm delivery at less than or equal to 32 weeks of gestation; OR, 29.3 (95% confidence interval [CI], 11.3 to 75.8) for cervical length less than or equal to 10 mm; OR, 24.3 (95% CI, 12.9 to 45.9) for cervical length less than or equal to 15 mm; OR, 18.3 (95% CI, 10.8 to 31.0) for cervical length less than or equal to 20 mm; OR, 13.4 (95% CI, 8.8 to 20.6) for cervical length less than or equal to 25 mm; and OR, 3.2 (95% CI, 2.4 to 4.4) for cervical length less than or equal to 30 mm. Forty-seven percent (47.6%) of patients with a cervical length less than or equal to 15 mm underwent preterm delivery at less than or equal to 32 weeks of gestation.[18]

Heath et al.[17] reported that a cervical length less than or equal to 15 mm at 23 weeks of gestation was observed in 58% of women who delivered at less than or equal to 32 weeks and in

86% of women who delivered at less than or equal to 28 weeks of gestation in a population of 2,567 pregnant women. The authors also reported that patients of Afro-Caribbean origin with a history of preterm birth, low maternal age (<20 years), and low body mass index had a shorter cervix than did pregnant women without such risk factors. Logistic regression analysis showed that a transvaginal sonographic (TVS) short cervix was the best predictor of preterm birth (≤32 weeks of gestation).[17] A history of preterm delivery and African-American ethnicity were also associated with the occurrence of spontaneous preterm birth, although the OR was considerably lower than that of a short cervix.

Several studies have confirmed and extended the observations of Andersen et al.[15] in asymptomatic patients at low risk for preterm delivery.[15,17,18,25,27,29–32,34–37,39,41,84,89–91,95-99] Although studies that evaluated the prediction of a short cervix for preterm birth are difficult to compare directly given the differences in study design (i.e., gestational age at cervical length measurement and assessed outcomes), the available data consistently show that the shorter the cervical length measurement, the higher the risk for preterm birth. The high positive predictive value of a short cervix (nearly 50% for spontaneous preterm birth at less than 32 weeks with a cervical length ≤15 mm) has justified trials of intervention (progesterone, cerclage, and pessary to prevent preterm birth).[22–24,54,56–58] Nevertheless, a considerable number of patients who deliver at less than 32 weeks of gestation will not present with a sonographic short cervix in the midtrimester; hence, a cervical length measured by ultrasound is not a screening tool but rather a method for risk assessment.

Cervical Length at Midtrimester and Risk of Cesarean Delivery

Smith et al.[100] reported the prediction of cesarean delivery by measurement of cervical length during the midtrimester (22 to 23 weeks of gestation). The authors hypothesized that a long cervix in midgestation would be associated with an increased risk of cesarean delivery during labor at term. After excluding 1,345 women having a prelabor cesarean delivery, the authors included 27,472 primiparous women reaching term pregnancy. A total of 5,542 women underwent cesarean delivery. Cervical length was categorized as quartile one (16 to 30 mm), quartile two (31 to 35 mm), quartile three (36 to 39 mm), and quartile four (40 to 67 mm). The prevalence of cesarean section was 16% (quartile one); 18.4% (quartile two); 21.7% (quartile three); and 25.7% (quartile four); $P < 0.001$ for trend. Rates of cesarean delivery started to rise at a cervical length of 25 mm and plateaued at a cervical length of 50 mm. Therefore, the authors concluded that a longer cervical length at midgestation is an independent predictor of the risk of cesarean delivery at term in primiparous women.

Maternal Factors Associated with Cervical Length

Maternal factors have been reported to affect the prediction of preterm delivery by cervical length. Rosenbloom et al.[101] evaluated 13,508 pregnant women—43% of whom were nulliparous—undergoing transvaginal ultrasound for cervical length measurement at 17 to 23 weeks of gestation. They observed that cervical length was more predictive of preterm delivery in nulliparous women than in multiparous women at any cervical length threshold used to define a short cervix (10 mm, 15 mm, 20 mm, or 25 mm). Palatnik et al.[102] reported the effect of maternal characteristics in the cervical length in 18,100 pregnant women at 18 to 24 weeks of gestation. Maternal body mass

TABLE 14.1 Diagnostic Indices of Sonographic Cervical Length in Low-Risk Asymptomatic Pregnant Women According to Different Cervical Length Cutoffs

AUTHOR, YEAR (STUDIED CASES)	IDENTIFIED AT (wk)	PRETERM DELIVERY (wk; PREVALENCE %)	SENSITIVITY (%)	SPECIFICITY (%)	POSITIVE PREDICTIVE VALUE (%)	NEGATIVE PREDICTIVE VALUE (%)
Cervical Length ≤15 mm						
Heath et al. (1998) (n = 2,702)	23	≤32 (1.5)	58	99	52	99
Hassan et al. (2000) (n = 6,877)	14–24	≤32 (3.6)	8	99	47	97
Cervical Length ≤20 mm						
Iams et al. (1996) (n = 2,915)	24	<35 (4)	23	97	26	97
Orzechowski et al. (2016) (n = 1,569)	18–24	<37 (3.2)	20	99	20	96
Cervical Length ≤25 mm						
Taipale et al. (1998) (n = 3,694)	18–22	<37 (2)	6	100	39	99
Cervical Length ≤30 mm						
Antsaklis et al. (2011) (n = 1,113)	11–14	<37 (8.5)	4.1	99	20	80
Cervical Length ≤35 mm						
Tongsong et al. (1995) (n = 730)	29–30	<37 (12)	66	62	20	93
Cervical Length ≤39 mm						
Andersen et al. (1990) (n = 113)	<30	<37 (15)	76	59	25	93

Reproduced with permission of McGraw-Hill Education, from Gervasi MT, Romero R, Maymon E, et al. Ultrasound examination of the uterine cervix during pregnancy. In: Fleischer AC, Manning FA, Jeanty P, et al., eds. *Sonography in Obstetrics and Gynecology: Principles and Practice.* 6th ed. New York, NY: McGraw-Hill; 2001:821–841; permission conveyed through Copyright Clearance Center, Inc.

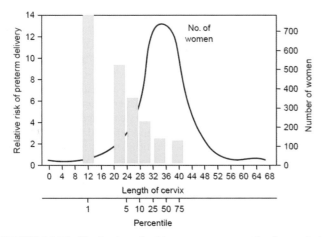

FIGURE 14.12: Distribution of subjects among percentiles for cervical length measured by transvaginal ultrasonography at 24 weeks of gestation (*solid line*) and relative risk of spontaneous preterm delivery before 35 weeks of gestation according to percentiles for cervical length (*bars*). (From Iams JD, Goldenberg RL, Meis PJ, et al. The length of the cervix and the risk of spontaneous premature delivery. *N Engl J Med.* 1996;334(9):567–573. Copyright © 1996 Massachusetts Medical Society. Reprinted with permission from Massachusetts)

index had a significant effect on the length of the cervix: as the body mass index increased, the cervix was measurably longer. Nevertheless, no significant differences among women with different body mass indices were observed for the definition of the 10th percentile of cervical length, meaning that the definition of a short cervix should be the same for all. The association between increased body mass index and longer cervical length has also been reported by Venkatesh et al.[103] Buck et al.[104] reported differences in the cervical length of women with diverse ethnic origins. Black women had a higher incidence of a short cervix (≤25 mm) than non-Hispanic White women when evaluated in the second trimester of pregnancy. In a study performed in the Netherlands,[105] maternal factors were evaluated for their impact on cervical length. The authors reported that maternal weight, parity, and ethnic origin had an impact on cervical length. Women with higher weight, who were multiparous, and of Caucasian origin had a longer cervical length than did nulliparous women, Black women, or women with reduced weight. They also noted that body mass index was associated with cervical length but only for the effect of weight, as differences in maternal height did not affect cervical length. The lack of a significant effect of maternal height on cervical length has also been corroborated by other groups.[78,106]

Celik et al.[55] reported the use of an individualized risk assessment for the prediction of preterm birth. The authors performed a large, prospective observational study of more than 58,000 patients. Transvaginal (TVS) cervical length screening was performed between 20^{+0} and 24^{+6} weeks of gestation. Using logistic regression analysis, adjusted ORs were calculated for spontaneous delivery at less than 28 weeks (extreme), at 28 to 30 weeks (early), at 31 to 33 weeks (moderate), and at 34 to 36 weeks (mild). The authors concluded that cervical length was the best predictor of spontaneous preterm birth. The risk estimation was improved by the addition of obstetric history but not by any maternal characteristics or other interactions. The detection rates of extreme, early, moderate, and mild spontaneous preterm birth, by combining the obstetric history and cervical length, were 80.6%, 58.5%, 53.0%, and 28.6%, respectively, with a 10% screen-positive rate.[55] This model provides for a higher detection rate than does obstetric history or cervical length alone; it also allows for population-based screening, which may have great value in a setting of potential effective interventions. In conclusion, cervical length and the definition of a short cervix can be influenced by maternal parity, ethnic origin, history of previous preterm delivery, and maternal weight.

High-Risk Singleton Gestations

Several authors evaluated the utility of cervical length in assessing the risk of preterm birth in women with a history of preterm birth, an excisional cervical procedure, a known uterine anomaly, or a history of second-trimester dilation and evacuation procedure.[33,38,84,92,94,107-114]

Guzman et al.[33] evaluated 469 high-risk patients between 15 and 24 weeks of gestation. High risk was defined by any of the following: a history of spontaneous preterm birth at less than 37 weeks of gestation, prior midtrimester loss, more than two terminations of pregnancy, cone biopsy, uterine malformation, previous cerclage, and exposure to diethylstilbestrol (DES). Transvaginal cervical sonography and transfundal uterine pressure were performed, and the shortest cervical length, funnel width, funnel length, and cervical index were recorded serially. The results showed that cervical length was the best parameter in the prediction of preterm birth in high-risk women. Owen et al.[38] reported an observational study comprised of 183 patients with a history of spontaneous preterm birth at less than 32 weeks of gestation. Patients were enrolled between 16 and 19 weeks of gestation and followed up every 2 weeks until 24 weeks of gestation. Forty-eight (26%) women delivered at less than 35 weeks of gestation. A short cervix (≤25 mm) at the first scan was associated with an RR of 3.3 (95% CI, 2.1 to 5.0) for spontaneous preterm birth (<35 weeks of gestation). The sensitivity, specificity, and positive predictive values were 19%, 98%, and 75%, respectively. After adjustment for cervical length, neither funneling nor dynamic shortening was an independent predictor of spontaneous preterm birth. A systematic review of 14 studies evaluating the use of sonographic cervical length to predict preterm birth in a high-risk population demonstrated that patients with a history of spontaneous preterm delivery presenting a cervical length less than 25 mm at less than 20 weeks of gestation had a positive likelihood ratio (LR) of 4.31 (95% CI, 3.08 to 6.01), and when observed at 20 to 24 weeks, a positive LR of 2.78 (95% CI, 2.22 to 3.49) for preterm delivery at less than 35 weeks.[112,115] The number of previous preterm deliveries seems to not add a cumulative effect on the predictive value of the cervical length.[111] A sonographic short cervix is also predictive of preterm birth in other high-risk populations, that is, patients with uterine anomalies,[93] in those with multiple prior-induced abortions,[94] or in women

after surgery for cervical intraepithelial neoplasia.[116,117] Crane et al. evaluated 35 pregnant women with a bicornuate uterus at 16 to 30 weeks of gestation matched by gestational age with 122 pregnant women with a normal uterus. The authors reported a higher frequency of preterm delivery at less than or equal to 35 weeks (8.6% vs. 0.8%) and a shorter cervical length (34.6 mm vs. 43.2 mm) in women with a bicornuate uterus as compared to women with a normal uterus. A cervical length of less than or equal to 30 mm in women with a bicornuate uterus had a 37.5% positive predictive value for preterm delivery at less than 35 weeks of gestation.[118]

Cervical Insufficiency

The hypothesis that cervical competence or sufficiency represents a spectrum has been analyzed by Parikh and Mehta,[119] who used digital examination of the cervix to assess sufficiency. The authors, however, concluded that degrees of cervical competence did not exist. By contrast, Iams et al.,[28] using sonographic examination of the cervix, demonstrated that cervical sufficiency/insufficiency is a continuum; the authors reported a strong relationship between cervical length and previous obstetrical history. This relationship was nearly linear, and patients with a typical history of an "insufficient" cervix did not constitute a separate group from those who delivered preterm.[28] Similar results have been reported by Guzman et al.[120] Collectively, these studies suggest that there is a relationship between a history of preterm delivery and the cervical length in a subsequent pregnancy. Considering that patients with a short cervix are at increased risk for a midtrimester pregnancy loss (clinically referred to as "cervical insufficiency") or a spontaneous preterm delivery with either intact membranes or rupture of membranes,[15-18,25-30,33,34,36-41,89-92,120] a short cervix can be considered as the expression of a spectrum of cervical diseases or abnormal function (Figure 14.14). It is noteworthy that some women with a short cervix have an adverse pregnancy outcome, while others have an uncomplicated term delivery.[120-124] Indeed, approximately 50% of women with a cervix less than or equal to 15 mm deliver after 32 weeks of gestation,[17,18] indicating that cervical length may be only one of the factors determining the degree of cervical strength and that a short cervix should not be equated with "cervical insufficiency."

Cervical Shortening

Some studies suggest that the rate of change in cervical length can be associated with spontaneous preterm birth at less than 36 weeks of gestation among women with a sonographic short cervix less than 25 mm.[125] Moroz et al. evaluated 2,695 women with a singleton gestation from the general obstetric population using transvaginal ultrasound for cervical length at 24 weeks of gestation (range, 21 to 28 weeks) and repeated the evaluation at 28 weeks (range, 25 to 33 weeks) of gestation.[125] The change in cervical length between 24 and 28 weeks was the primary variable of interest. The rate of change was calculated by dividing the difference in cervical length by the number of days between measurements. The relationships between change in cervical length, average daily change in cervical length, and spontaneous preterm birth before 36 weeks of gestation were evaluated using logistic regression. Among women with a sonographic short cervix (<25 mm), the results demonstrated that a shortening in cervical length between the two visits was significantly associated with a higher probability of spontaneous preterm birth occurring at less than 36 weeks of gestation. The authors reported a 3% increase in the risk of preterm delivery for every millimeter of cervical shortening between 24 and 28 weeks of gestation.

Several other groups have evaluated repeated measurements in the second trimester and the rate of change in cervical length associated with the risk of preterm birth in high- and low-risk patients.[33,125–130] Guzman et al.[33] reported serial changes in cervical length in high-risk women between 15 and 24 weeks of gestation. The rate of change in women who did not develop cervical insufficiency was nonsignificant, while those women destined to develop a cervix less than 20 mm in length, defined as "insufficient," had a significant rate of cervical length change of −5.2 mm per week. The serial evaluation of cervical length in women found to have a short cervix, measuring less than or equal to 25 mm on an initial scan between 16 and 28 weeks of gestation, demonstrated that women whose cervix had undergone further shortening by the second measurement delivered at an earlier gestational age (36^{+4} vs. 38^{+2} weeks, days of gestation, $P = 0.031$).[127] These data collectively indicate that cervical shortening is part of the activation of the parturition process. This shortening occurs as a continuum, and subsequent cervical length measurements in women at risk may help differentiate between those with a short cervix who will deliver at term and those who will have a preterm delivery. Moroz and Simhan[125] reported differences in cervical length between 24 and 28 weeks in a cohort of women from the general obstetric population. Within the group of women with an initial cervical length less than or equal to 25 mm, additional shortening was associated with an increased risk of preterm birth. The authors also suggested a lower risk of preterm birth in women with an initially identified short cervix if the cervix remained stable or increased in length. As the interval for a repeat examination reported in the literature varies from 1 to 8 weeks,[127] the optimal timing of a repeat measurement and how clinical management should be adjusted are yet to be determined.

Carvalho et al.[74] reported on the utility of serial cervical length measurements obtained at 11 to 14 weeks and at 22 to 24 weeks of gestation in an unselected group of pregnant women. The authors found that cervical length at 11 to 14 weeks was not significantly different between women who delivered preterm and those who delivered at term, but that cervical length assessments obtained in the second trimester of pregnancy were predictive of preterm delivery. The cases of cervical shortening that occurred between the first and second examinations were more pronounced in the group of women who delivered preterm. Ozdemir et al.[131] subsequently confirmed the observation of a more rapid cervical change between the first and second trimesters in women destined to deliver preterm.

Conversely, other groups have reported that the rate of cervical shortening does not significantly improve the prediction of preterm delivery as compared to only a single cervical length measurement. Conde-Agudelo et al.[132] reported the results of a systematic review and meta-analysis of the predictive value of cervical shortening. The authors included seven studies comprising a total of 3,374 pregnant women with a singleton gestation and another eight studies including 1,024 women with a twin pregnancy. They indicated that changes in cervical length occurring over time had a low predictive accuracy for preterm delivery at less than 35 weeks and at less than 37 weeks of gestation. The authors concluded that a single measurement of the cervical length at 18 to 24 weeks of gestation seems to be a better test of predicting preterm delivery as compared to changes in cervical length occurring as gestation progresses. Similar results were reported by Esplin et al.,[133] who prospectively evaluated 9,410 women for whom two ultrasound examinations were performed at least 4 weeks apart to estimate the rate of cervical shortening, and to predict preterm delivery at less than 37 weeks of gestation. The

authors could not find an additional value of repeated cervical length examinations to that obtained from a single measurement. Subramanian et al.[134] estimated the length of the cervix and the subsequent probability of shortening, reporting that a cervical length greater than or equal to 39 mm will be very unlikely to show shortening within 2 weeks of measurement; thus, a less strict follow-up should be considered for this subset of patients. In practice, most algorithms for the management of patients at risk for preterm birth include serial ultrasound evaluation of the uterine cervix; however, there is no consensus on the time interval between measurements, the patient population requiring serial ultrasound evaluation, and whether serial evaluations improve pregnancy outcomes.

Cervical Insufficiency and Eradication of Intra-amniotic Infection/Inflammation

Recent studies have shown that administration of broad-spectrum antibiotics is effective in eradicating intra-amniotic infection/inflammation in selected women with a singleton pregnancy who presented with cervical insufficiency. This condition was defined as (1) painless cervical dilatation of greater than 1 cm between 16.0 and 27.9 weeks of gestation, (2) intact membranes, and (3) absence of uterine contractions.[135] Among these patients, 52% had intra-amniotic infection, defined as a positive amniotic fluid culture or a positive polymerase chain reaction (PCR) assay for *Ureaplasma* spp., whereas intra-amniotic inflammation was defined as an elevated amniotic fluid interleukin (IL)-6 concentration (>2.6 ng/mL). Intra-amniotic inflammation, isolation of microorganisms by amniotic fluid culture, or detection of *Ureaplasma* nucleic acids was an indication for antibiotic administration. The authors used a combination of ceftriaxone 1 g (intravenous) every 24 hours, clarithromycin 500 mg (oral) every 12 hours, and metronidazole (intravenous) 500 mg every 8 hours. Metronidazole was administered for a maximum of 4 weeks. The decision to use and discontinue antibiotics and tocolytics was left to the discretion of the treating clinicians given the lack of uniformity among them. The authors reported that 44 women fulfilled the inclusion criteria and had at least one amniocentesis, 28 patients had intra-amniotic infection/inflammation, and 22 received a combination of antibiotics (2 with infection/20 with inflammation). Among the 22 patients receiving treatment, 6 delivered within 1 week of amniocentesis and 16 remained pregnant for more than 1 week. A second amniocentesis was offered and performed in 75% (12/16) of patients; in 75% (9/12) of this group, there was evidence of resolution of intra-amniotic infection or intra-amniotic inflammation. Of the four patients who did not have a follow-up amniocentesis, all delivered after 34 weeks of gestation (two of them at term). Thus, treatment success occurred in 59% (13/22) of patients with cervical insufficiency and intra-amniotic infection/inflammation who received the antibiotic regimen; such neonates had no short-term morbidity. These results suggest that among women with proven intra-amniotic infection/inflammation in the setting of preterm labor with intact membranes or cervical insufficiency, antibiotics may help to prolong pregnancy and improve short-term neonatal outcomes through the eradication of intra-amniotic infection/inflammation.

Cervical Length and Induction of Labor

Eduard Bishop et al.[136] proposed a method to evaluate the cervix before induction of labor. A digital examination of the cervix was performed to assess effacement and dilation as well as fetal head location. The results showed that patients whose cervix was 3 cm dilated and 60% effaced and with the fetal head in station −1 or lower were favorable for labor induction.

The Bishop score is the most frequently used clinical parameter to evaluate the cervix before and during labor in term or preterm pregnancies. Currently, an evaluation of the cervix by transvaginal ultrasound has been proposed to identify women with higher/lower probability of a successful induction of labor. Park et al.[137] reported that assessment of cervical length by transvaginal ultrasound reduced the need for preinduction medication with prostaglandins as compared to clinical assessment by the Bishop score (Table 14.2). The authors evaluated 150 women with a term pregnancy admitted for induction of labor who were randomly assigned either to the Bishop score or a transvaginal measurement of cervical length. The results indicate that the use of cervical length prior to induction of labor can reduce the need for prostaglandin administration by approximately 50% without adversely affecting the outcome of induction of labor as compared to the Bishop score. Pandis et al.[138] reported the Bishop score and cervical length in 240 women with a term pregnancy admitted for labor induction. Logistic regression analysis showed that cervical length, Bishop score, and parity were significantly associated with delivery within 24 hours of admission. The prediction of successful induction of labor by cervical length measurement was better than that of the Bishop score (cervical length sensitivity 87%; Bishop score sensitivity 58%). The best cutoff value to predict delivery within 24 hours was a cervical length of 28 mm (sensitivity 87%, specificity 71%) as compared to the Bishop score (sensitivity 58%, specificity 77%). The authors also showed that the interval between labor induction and delivery increased as the cervix lengthened and the Bishop score decreased. Brik et al.[139] also compared the predictive performance of cervical length and the Bishop score for failed induction of labor in term pregnancies. Of 245 women, 16 had a failed induction of labor defined as not achieving 3 to 4 cm dilation after 12 hours of oxytocin administration and regular and intense uterine contractions. In the group with failed induction of labor, the mean cervical length was 30.9 mm as compared to 23.9 mm in the group with a successful induction of labor ($P = 0.001$). A cervical length of 28 mm best predicted nonsuccessful induction of labor indicated by 83% sensitivity, 67% specificity, 13.7% positive predictive value, 98% negative predictive value, and a positive LR of 2.3 (95% CI, 1.7 to 3.1). The authors reported that a shorter cervical length was associated with a shorter induction-to-delivery interval and a reduced duration of the second stage of labor. Similar results were reported by Pereira et al.,[140] who showed that cervical length was predictive of vaginal delivery and of a shorter induction-to-delivery interval (Fig. 14.13).

In conclusion, there is a strong body of evidence showing that cervical length is a good predictor of a successful induction of labor, for estimation of the induction-to-delivery interval, and of vaginal delivery.[141]

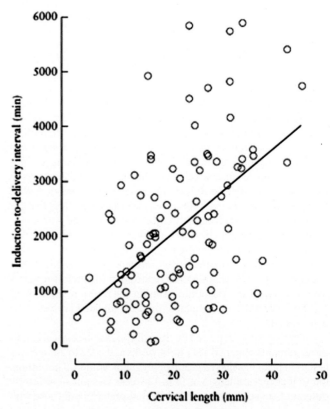

FIGURE 14.13: Plot of induction-to-delivery interval against cervical length in 99 women with singleton pregnancy undergoing preinduction ultrasound assessment. (From Pereira S, Frick AP, Poon LC, et al. Successful induction of labor: prediction by preinduction cervical length, angle of progression and cervical elastography. *Ultrasound Obstet Gynecol.* 2014;44(4):468–475. Copyright © 2014 ISUOG. Reprinted by permission of John Wiley & Sons, Inc.)

TABLE 14.2	The Bishop Score			
	SCORE			
CERVIX	**0**	**1**	**2**	**3**
Position	Posterior	Intermediate	Anterior	
Consistency	Firm	Medium	Soft	
Effacement	0%–30%	40%–50%	60%–70%	>80%
Dilation	0	1–2	3–4	≥5
Fetal station	−3	−3	−1	+1, +2

Cervical Length in Multiple Gestations

Twin Pregnancies

Twin gestations occur in 1% of all pregnancies and are at increased risk of preterm birth. Several studies of twin pregnancies have examined the value of transvaginal sonography for the prediction of preterm delivery and reported an increased risk in patients with a sonographic short cervix.[142-158] The median cervical length in women with a twin pregnancy at 23 weeks of gestation is similar to that of a singleton pregnancy (36 mm).[150] However, a greater proportion of women with a twin pregnancy have a cervical length less than or equal to 25 mm (12.9%) when compared to women with a singleton pregnancy (8.4%).[150] The same holds true for patients with a cervical length less than or equal to 15 mm (4.5% of twin pregnancies) versus 1.5% of singleton pregnancies. One study of twin pregnancies indicated that the sensitivity of a short cervix (≤25 mm) at 23 weeks of gestation in predicting spontaneous preterm delivery at 28, 30, 32, and 34 weeks of pregnancy was 100%, 80%, 47%, and 35%, respectively.[147] The rate of spontaneous delivery at less than or equal to 32 weeks of gestation increases exponentially as the cervical length decreases when measured at 23 weeks of gestation. The risk of preterm delivery for patients with a cervical length less than or equal to 25 mm in a twin pregnancy is similar to the risk in a singleton pregnancy for those with a cervical length less than or equal to 15 mm (52%).[17,18] Thus, the cervical length required in a twin gestation to provide assurance against the occurrence of preterm delivery is greater than that in a singleton gestation. Approximately 95% of twin gestations among patients with a cervical length greater than or equal to 35 mm deliver at greater than 34 weeks of gestation.[146]

Conde-Agudelo et al.[159] reported the results of a systematic review and meta-analysis of the predictive test accuracy for cervical length in asymptomatic twin pregnancies. A cervical length less than or equal to 20 mm at 20 to 24 weeks of gestation had a pooled positive LR of 10.1 and a negative LR of 0.64 to predict preterm birth at less than 32 weeks (Table 14.3). A cervical length less than or equal to 25 mm at 20 to 24 weeks of gestation had a pooled positive LR of 9.6 to predict preterm birth at less than 28 weeks. A study reported by Melamed et al.[160] included 441 women with a twin pregnancy for whom cervical length was measured every 2 to 3 weeks from 14 to 18 weeks to 28 to 32 weeks of gestation. The authors divided the periods of analysis as 18^{+0} to 21^{+6}, 22^{+0} to 24^{+6}, 25^{+0} to 27^{+6}, and 28^{+0} to 32^{+0} weeks and reported that a cervical length less than the 10th percentile was significantly associated with preterm delivery at each gestational period. The authors also reported that the degree of cervical shortening between the different periods of analysis was predictive of preterm delivery. Kindinger et al.[161] reported an individual patient-level meta-analysis to determine the prediction of preterm birth in twin pregnancies by cervical length. The authors included 4,409 women with a twin pregnancy and showed that cervical length and gestational age at examination were significant predictors of spontaneous preterm delivery: the earlier in gestation a short cervix was found, the higher the risk of

TABLE 14.3   Prediction of Spontaneous Preterm Birth by Cervical Length at 20 to 24 Weeks of Gestation in Asymptomatic Women with a Twin Pregnancy

PRETERM BIRTH (wk)	CERVICAL LENGTH CUTOFF (mm)	N	SENSITIVITY (%, 95% CI)	SPECIFICITY (%, 95% CI)	LR POSITIVE (95% CI)	LR NEGATIVE (95% CI)
<28	20	591	35 (14–62)	93 (91–95)	5.2 (2.6–10.6)	0.69 (0.49–1.01)
	25	637	64 (41–83)	93 (91–95)	9.6 (5.8–14.8)	0.4 (0.23–0.68)
	35	637	82 (60–95)	66 (62–69)	2.4 (1.9–3.0)	0.28 (0.11–0.67)
<32	20	1955	39 (31–48)	96 (95–97)	10.1 (7.4–13.9)	0.64 (0.55–0.73)
	25	2036	54 (45–62)	91 (90–92)	6.0 (4.8–7.4)	0.51 (0.43–0.61)
	30	1812	65 (56–74)	78 (76–80)	3.0 (2.5–3.5)	0.45 (0.35–0.57)
	35	1889	81 (73–87)	58 (56–61)	1.9 (1.7–2.2)	0.33 (0.23–0.48)
<34	20	1760	29 (23–35)	97 (96–98)	9.0 (6.1–12.7)	0.74 (0.68–0.8)
	25	1987	40 (38–46)	93 (92–94)	5.8 (4.5–7.2)	0.64 (0.58–0.71)
	30	2014	56 (50–62)	81 (79–83)	3.0 (2.6–3.4)	0.55 (0.48–0.63)
	35	1884	79 (74–84)	60 (57–62)	2.0 (1.8–2.2)	0.35 (0.27–0.44)
≤37	25	434	21 (15–27)	95 (92–98)	4.4 (2.4–8.2)	0.83 (0.75–0.92)
	30	218	29 (18–43)	91 (86–95)	3.4 (1.6–6.7)	0.78 (0.65–0.92)
	35	134	56 (43–68)	63 (50–74)	1.5 (1.0–2.2)	0.71 (0.51–0.98)

Reprinted from Conde-Agudelo A, Romero R. Prediction of preterm birth in twin gestations using biophysical and biochemical tests. *Am J Obstet Gynecol.* 2014;211(6): 583–595. Copyright © 2014 Elsevier. With permission.

early preterm delivery. The authors concluded that measurement of cervical length in twin pregnancies might be initiated before 18 weeks of gestation.

Conversely, Hester et al.[162] evaluated 178 women with a twin pregnancy and reported that cervical length measured at 16 to 20 weeks was not a good predictor of preterm delivery at less than 34 weeks of gestation. Pagani et al.[163] measured the cervical length of 940 women with a twin pregnancy at 18 to 23 weeks of gestation to predict preterm delivery at less than 32 weeks of gestation. The authors reported a poor prediction with an area under the ROC curve of 0.65. Fox et al.[164] reported the utility of a repeat cervical examination 2 to 6 weeks after obtaining a baseline examination at 18 to 24 weeks of gestation. Among twin pregnancies for which the cervical length decreased by 20% or more, there was an increased risk of preterm birth, even in the setting of a normal cervical length (36.8% rate of preterm birth at <34 weeks vs. 12.9% with a stable examination, $P = 0.018$).

A cutoff value less than or equal to 25 mm has been proposed for the risk assessment of preterm birth in twin pregnancies.[154,156] Roman et al.[165] evaluated 580 women with a twin pregnancy at 18 to 23^{+6} weeks of gestation; among this population, 405 were dichorionic and 175 were monochorionic-diamniotic twin pregnancies. The authors reported shorter cervices in women with monochorionic twins, and that the prediction of preterm delivery was higher for monochorionic pregnancies as compared to dichorionic pregnancies. Another study assessed the utility of preoperative sonographic cervical length measurement to predict preterm birth in 137 cases of twin-to-twin transfusion syndrome that had undergone endoscopic laser coagulation of placental anastomoses at less than 26 weeks of gestation.[155] The prevalence of delivery at less than 34 weeks was 74% in patients with a cervical length less than 30 mm. In addition, logistic regression analysis identified cervical length less than 30 mm (OR, 3.53; 95% CI, 1.55 to 8.03) and multiparity (OR, 2.27; 95% CI, 1.09 to 4.74) as independent risk factors for preterm birth occurring at less than 34 weeks of gestation.[155] Sonographic cervical length is predictive of preterm birth in twin gestations within 7 days of the date of the ultrasound scan.[154] In a study of 87 twin pregnancies presenting with preterm labor, 80% (4/5) of patients with a cervical length of 1 to 5 mm and 24% (15/61) with cervical length of 6-25 mm delivered within 7 days, in contrast to 0% (0 of 21) of patients with a cervical length greater than 25 mm.[154] The available data suggests that cervical length is a good predictor of preterm delivery in twin pregnancies, either dichorionic or monochorionic, when measured at midgestation. In general, in twin pregnancies, a cervical length less than or equal to 25 mm has a sensitivity of 40%, specificity of 93%, and a positive LR of 5.8 (95% CI, 4.5 to 7.2) for preterm delivery at less than 34 weeks of gestation and a sensitivity of 64%, specificity of 93%, positive LR of 9.6 (95% CI, 5.8 to 14.8) for preterm delivery at less than 28 weeks of gestation.

Triplet Pregnancies

Cervical length is predictive of preterm delivery in triplet gestations. The sensitivity, specificity, positive predictive value, and negative predictive value of a short cervical length measured between 21 and 24 weeks of gestation are 86%, 79%, 40%, and 97%, respectively; and when measured between 25 and 28 weeks of gestation, they are 100%, 57%, 18%, and 100%, respectively.[123,166] A short cervix identifies triplet pregnancies at risk for preterm birth, and when compared to similar cervical length measurements in a singleton pregnancy, the risk of preterm delivery in a triplet pregnancy is higher.[123,166]

Pils et al.[167] performed a longitudinal study in 78 women with a triplet pregnancy; 55 (70.5%) cases presented as trichorionic, 22 (28.2%) as dichorionic-triamniotic, and 1 (1.3%) as monochorionic-triamniotic. The authors measured the cervical length in all women every 2 weeks from 16 to 30 weeks of gestation. They reported a stable cervical length between 16 and 22 weeks of gestation with a median length of 37 mm and a fast rate of cervical shortening after 22 weeks of gestation. When the cervical lengths were compared between women who delivered at less than 32 weeks of gestation and those who delivered at greater than or equal to 32 weeks of gestation, no differences were observed at 16 weeks of gestation; however, at 22 weeks, women who delivered preterm had a median cervical length of 33 mm, which decreased to 21 mm at 24 weeks. The authors reported that a reduction in cervical length of 10 mm occurring between 22 and 24 weeks of gestation was predictive of preterm delivery at less than 32 weeks with a sensitivity of 54%, a specificity of 94%, a positive predictive value of 78%, and a negative predictive value of 85%. The authors reported that chorionicity had no influence on the predictive performance of cervical length. Similar results on the predictive value of cervical shortening were reported by Rosen et al.,[168] who noted that the rate of shortening was more pronounced in women with a triple pregnancy who delivered at less than 32 weeks of gestation. The same group reported a more progressive rate of cervical shortening in triplet than in twin pregnancies.[169]

The value of a single cervical length measurement in triplet pregnancies was evaluated by Fichera et al.[170] The authors studied 120 triplet pregnancies at 20 to 24 weeks of gestation and reported that women who delivered at less than 28 weeks of gestation had a cervical length less than 15 mm more frequently than do women who delivered at greater than or equal to 28 weeks of gestation. Similarly, women who delivered at less than 32 weeks of gestation more frequently presented a cervical length less than 20 mm than women who delivered at greater than or equal to 32 weeks of gestation. However, logistic regression analysis indicated that a single cervical length measurement at 20 weeks of gestation was not a significant predictor for preterm delivery at less than 32 weeks in triplet pregnancies; the area under the ROC curve for preterm delivery at less than 32 weeks of gestation was 0.42.

The identification of patients at risk for preterm birth with a triplet gestation may be improved by implementing the combination of cervical length and fetal fibronectin (fFN). In a retrospective study, Fox et al.[171] evaluated the combination of fFN and cervical length as predictors of preterm birth in triplet pregnancies. A historical cohort of 39 consecutive women with a triplet pregnancy, managed in one maternal–fetal medicine practice from 2005 to 2011, was included in this study. A positive fFN was significantly associated with spontaneous preterm birth at less than 28, 30, 32, and 34 weeks of gestation, while a sonographic short cervix was significantly associated with spontaneous preterm birth at less than 32 weeks of gestation. Combined screening of fFN and cervical length in asymptomatic triplet pregnancies was associated with a high likelihood of spontaneous preterm birth at all gestational ages. For example, a positive fFN test result and a short cervix together had a sensitivity of 62.5%, a specificity of 90%, a positive predictive value of 62.5%, and a negative predictive value of 90% for the prediction of spontaneous preterm birth at less than 32 weeks of gestation. The authors proposed that the combination of fFN and cervical length assessment in the screening of asymptomatic triplet pregnancies is particularly useful in predicting spontaneous preterm birth.

Cervical Examination in Patients Presenting with Preterm Labor

Sonographic examination of the cervix in patients presenting with preterm labor can contribute to the risk assessment for preterm delivery as nearly 47% of these patients deliver at term.[172]

Gomez et al.[173] reported the diagnostic performance of cervical length evaluated with transvaginal ultrasound and digital examination of the cervix to predict preterm delivery. The authors included 59 women with a singleton gestation admitted due to the diagnosis of preterm labor and intact membranes with a cervical dilatation less than 3 cm. Cervical effacement was qualitatively estimated by digital examination and reported as a percentage. Transvaginal ultrasound was performed and two parameters were evaluated: cervical length and cervical funneling. Preterm delivery was considered as that occurring at less than 37 weeks of gestation. The results of the sonographic examination of the cervix were not available to clinicians. The prevalence of preterm delivery was 37.3% (22/59). The authors reported that the combination of cervical length and funneling had a sensitivity of 76%, specificity of 94%, positive predictive value of 89%, and RR of 6.4 (95% CI, 2.8 to 14.7) for preterm delivery. Cervical length alone less than or equal to 18 mm had 73% sensitivity, 78% specificity, 67% positive predictive value, and RR of 3.9 (95% CI, 1.8 to 8.5) for preterm delivery at less than 37 weeks. In univariate logistic regression analysis, cervical length, funneling, and gestational age at admission were significantly associated with preterm delivery, but not cervical dilatation or cervical effacement. No correlation between cervical length estimated by ultrasound and cervical effacement by digital examination was observed.

Iams et al.[16] reported the results of cervical assessment in 48 singleton and 12 twin pregnancies presenting with preterm labor. Cervical length assessment indicated that all patients with a cervical length greater than 30 mm delivered at term. The high negative predictive value for preterm birth associated with a long cervix provides important clinical information in symptomatic patients.[16,173–187] The observation that a sonographic short cervix is a powerful predictor of preterm birth in patients presenting with symptoms of preterm labor has been confirmed and extended in several other studies. Maia et al.[188] evaluated 126 women with clinical signs suggestive of preterm labor and reported that a cervical length less than or equal to 15 mm had a sensitivity of 77% and a specificity of 77% for delivery within 7 days of the ultrasound scan. The clinical value of cervical length measurement was reported in a systematic review and meta-analysis comprising 287 women with a singleton gestation and threatened preterm labor.[189] Patients were randomly allocated into two groups: cervical length measurement or no cervical length measurement. If the cervical length was above the threshold (i.e., 15 mm, 20 mm, or 25 mm), as defined by the authors, then after conservative management and improvement of clinical signs, the patient was discharged; however, if the patient had a short cervix, tocolytics and steroids were administered. In the group with no cervical length evaluation, women were treated at the physician's discretion with tocolysis and steroids. The results showed that women who underwent cervical length measurement had a lower rate of spontaneous preterm birth at less than 37 weeks of gestation and a longer gestational age at delivery, mainly attributable to optimized clinical management based on cervical length and clinical signs. Palacio et al.[190] reported a randomized controlled trial based on admissions of women presenting with threatened preterm labor who had a cervical length measurement. Women were randomized to two groups: group 1, the cervical length was reported to clinicians; and group 2, results of the cervical length measurement were not reported. In the physician-informed group, there was a significant reduction in days of hospitalization; however, no reduction in the rate of preterm delivery was observed.

Similar results were reported by Alfirevic et al.[184] in a randomized controlled trial that comprised 41 pregnant women with threatened preterm labor. Patients underwent a sonographic evaluation of the cervix or received treatment (tocolytics and steroids; [control group]), according to the physician's criteria. Treatment was provided among patients in the ultrasound group if the cervical length was less than 15 mm. A higher proportion of patients in the control group received steroid treatment despite remaining undelivered for more than 1 week when compared to those undergoing cervical length measurement (90% [18/20] vs. 14% [3/21]; RR, 0.16; (95% CI, 0.05 to 0.39)). In addition, there was a significant difference in the duration of hospital stay between the two groups (median [range]; 0 hours [0 to 24] in the group undergoing cervical length measurement vs. 24 hours [0 to 67] in women managed according to the physician's clinical criteria; $P < 0.0001$).[184]

Table 14.4 summarizes the results of specific studies published to date that evaluated the use of sonographic cervical length in patients presenting with preterm labor. Although the studies utilized different cervical length cutoff values, gestational ages, and patient populations, there is agreement that the shorter the cervix in preterm labor, the higher the risk for preterm delivery.

Cervical Length and the Likelihood of Intra-amniotic Infection/Inflammation

Patients presenting with preterm labor and a short cervix are also at an increased risk for intrauterine infection/inflammation. Gomez et al.[193] reported a study of 401 pregnant women presenting with preterm labor and cervical dilation less than or equal to 3 cm (as assessed by digital examination). All patients underwent a transabdominal amniocentesis. The prevalence of microbial invasion of the amniotic cavity (MIAC) was 7% (28/401). Patients with a short cervix (<15 mm) had a higher rate of MIAC (26.3%; 15/57) than those with a cervical length greater than or equal to 15 mm (3.8%: 13/344; $P < 0.05$). Women with a cervical length less than 15 mm had a higher prevalence of preterm delivery at less than 35 weeks (66.7%; 38/57) than did women with a cervical length greater than or equal to 15 mm (13.5%: 44/327; $P < 0.01$). Furthermore, the rate of infection was higher in patients presenting at less than or equal to 30 weeks with a cervical length less than 15 mm when compared to those whose cervix measured greater than or equal to 15 mm (43% [9/21] vs. 3.9% [3/76], $P < 0.05$). The authors provided an estimated risk of MIAC in patients presenting with preterm labor according to gestational age and cervical length (Table 14.5).

In summary, cervical sonography is a powerful method used to assess the risk of preterm delivery in patients presenting with preterm labor. Clinicians and patients can be reassured by the finding of a long cervix and therefore avoid unnecessary interventions. Patients in preterm labor who are diagnosed with a short cervix are at increased risk for intra-amniotic infection/inflammation as well as a higher rate of preterm delivery; thus, they may benefit from a targeted intervention (i.e., antibiotic and/or steroid administration and transfer to a center with a neonatal intensive care unit [NICU]). Further investigation into the most efficacious algorithm of management for these patients is still necessary.

TABLE 14.4 Measurement of Cervical Length by Transvaginal Ultrasound in Women with Symptoms of Preterm Labor

REFERENCE	YEAR	N	GESTATION (wk)	CL	PTD	PREVALENCE OF OUTCOME (%)	SENS (%)	SPEC (%)	PPV (%)	LR+	LR−
Murakawa et al.[174]	1993	32	18–37	<20	<37	34	27	100	100	nc	0.7 (0.51–1.04)
Iams et al.[16]	1994	60	24–35	<30	<36	40	100	44	55	1.8 (1.3–2.4)	nc
Gomez et al.[173]	1994	59	20–35	≤18	<36	37	72	78	67	3.3 (1.7–6.5)	0.4 (0.2–0.7)
Rizzo et al.[175]	1996	108	24–36	≤20	<37	43	68	79	71	3.2 (1.9–5.4)	0.4 (0.3–0.6)
Rozenberg et al.[191]	1997	76	24–34	≤26	<37	26	75	73	50	2.8 (1.7–4.6)	0.3 (0.2–0.7)
Tsoi et al.[179]	2005	510	24–33 6/7	≤15	<35	14.9	71.1	90.6	56.8	7.6 (5.4–10.4)	0.3 (0.2–0.4)
Daskalakis et al.[181]	2005	172	24–34	<20	<34	37	56	96	90	15 (5.7–40.7)	0.5 (0.3–0.6)
Palacio et al.[186]	2007	116	24–31 6/7	<20	<34	10.3	16.7	92	20	2.1 (0.6–9.9)	0.8 (0.7–1.2)
Eroglu et al.[185]	2007	51	24–35	<25	<35	19.6	60	92.7	66.7	8.2 (2.6–32.8)	0.4 (0.2–0.8)
Schmitz et al.[187]	2008	395	24–31 6/7	≤30	within 7 days	8.1	94	42	12	1.6 (1.4–1.8)	0.2 (0.04–0.6)
Hiersch et al.[192]	2016	792	29.2 (SD 2.7)	<25	<34	6.6	44.2	80.7	13.9	2.2 (1.6–3.1)	0.7 (0.54–0.9)
Maia et al.[188]	2019	95	25–34	≤15	within 7days	13.7	77	78	35.7	3.5 (2.1–5.8)	0.3 (0.1–0.8)

CL; cervical length cutoff; *LR+,* likelihood ratio positive; *LR−,* likelihood ratio negative; *nc,* not calculated; *PPV,* positive predictive value; *PTD,* preterm delivery; *SD,* standard deviation; *Sens,* sensitivity; *Spec,* specificity.

TABLE 14.5 Risk of Microbial Invasion of the Amniotic Cavity (MIAC) According to Cervical Length and Gestational Age at Cervical Length Measurement

CERVICAL LENGTH (mm)	GESTATIONAL AGE (wk) AT EXAMINATION			
	<35	<32	<30	<28
<15	26.3% (15/57)	33.3% (10/30)	42.9% (9/21)	45.5% (5/11)
15–29	5.5% (10/183)	4.8% (4/84)	6.3% (2/32)	11.8% (2/17)
>30	1.9% (3/161)	2.5% (2/79)	2.3% (1/44)	0% (0/24)
Prevalence of MIAC	7.0% (28/401)	8.3% (16/193)	12.4% (12/97)	13.5% (7/52)

Reprinted from Gomez R, Romero R, Nien JK, et al. A short cervix in women with preterm labor and intact membranes: a risk factor for microbial invasion of the amniotic cavity. *Am J Obstet Gynecol.* 2005;192(3):678–689. Copyright © 2005 Elsevier. With permission.

Cervical Length and Fetal Fibronectin for the Prediction of Preterm Birth

A screening test that detects the presence of fFN in the cervicovaginal fluid has been used in conjunction with sonographic cervical length measurement to identify patients at risk for preterm delivery. Gomez et al.[194] reported the use of sonographic cervical length and the fFN test to predict spontaneous preterm delivery within 48 hours, 7 days, and 14 days of admission as well as delivery occurring at less than 32 weeks and at less than 35 weeks of gestation. A cervical length less than 15 mm was the most powerful predictor of preterm birth within 48 hours (OR, 9.7; $P < 0.05$). Both cervical length and fFN test results were predictive of preterm birth within 7 and 14 days of admission.

When fFN test results were added to a cervical length cutoff less than 30 mm, there was significant improvement in the prediction of preterm delivery.[194]

A systematic review demonstrated improved accuracy in predicting preterm labor and preterm birth using the combination of fFN testing and ultrasound assessment of cervical length, as compared to the traditional clinical method of digital cervical examination.[195] The authors reported that classic clinical criteria correctly identified 30.2% of women presenting with symptoms of preterm labor who delivered preterm at less than 37 weeks of gestation. The combination of fFN testing and ultrasound assessment of cervical length had a modest positive predictive value of 49.4% for preterm birth occurring at less than 37 weeks of gestation. The diagnostic accuracy of the combination of fFN testing with sonographic cervical length assessment was significantly higher when predicting risk of preterm birth within a short period of time (<7 days) and at an earlier gestational age (<28 weeks). Using the combined method, the sensitivity for delivery at less than 7 days was 71.4% with a negative predictive value of 98.9%. Thus, the combined screening approach of sonographic cervical length assessment with fFN sampling may be useful in predicting short-term risk and may be used to guide acute management of patients presenting with symptoms of preterm labor. Kyozuka et al.[196] studied 285 pregnant women who presented with uterine contractions, abdominal pain, or cervical changes (determined by digital examination) at 21 to 24 weeks of gestation. The authors reported that a cervical length less than 15 mm and an fFN greater than or equal to 200 ng/mL were highly predictive of delivery at less than 28 weeks of gestation.

Quantitative Fetal Fibronectin

Brujin et al.[197] performed a multicenter study in women with a singleton pregnancy, intact membranes, and symptoms of preterm labor at 24 to 34 weeks of gestation (≥3 contractions per 30 minutes, vaginal blood loss, or abdominal or back pain). The authors aimed to compare the sensitivities of the quantitative to qualitative fFN testing to predict spontaneous preterm birth within 7 days of study entry. Exclusion criteria included (1) administration of tocolytic treatment for more than 18 hours, (2) cervical dilation greater than 3 cm, and (3) iatrogenic delivery within 7 days of study entry for hypertensive disorders, fetal distress, or other reasons for immediate delivery. For qualitative assessment of fFN, a 50 ng/mL cutoff value was used to define a result as positive or negative. To obtain risk stratification for the quantitative fFN test, thresholds of 10, 50, 200, and 500 ng/mL were predefined before analysis, and cervical length measurements were allocated into separate groups of less than 15 mm, 15 to 29 mm, and 30 to 50 mm. A total of 455 women fulfilled the inclusion criteria, showing a mean gestational age at inclusion of 29 weeks; 11% (n = 48) had a delivery within 7 days of inclusion. The majority of women (n = 258) had an fFN result of less than 50 ng/mL; among them, only five (1.9%) had a spontaneous delivery within 7 days. Further results indicated that 197 women had an fFN greater than or equal to 50 ng/mL, and 43 women (29%) had a spontaneous delivery within 7 days. Stratification of quantitative fFN testing showed

that the prevalence of spontaneous delivery within 7 days was higher in women with an fFN test result greater than or equal to 500 ng/mL (14/37, 38%) as compared to women with an fFN test result of 50 to 199 ng/mL (9/76, 12%). The combination of quantitative fFN testing and cervical length showed that among women with a cervical length greater than 30 mm (n = 82) only two (one with an fFN result >500 ng/mL) had a spontaneous delivery within 7 days. The prevalence of spontaneous preterm delivery within 7 days of study entry among women with a cervical length 15 to 29 mm (n = 270) differed according to the quantitative fFN: (1) fFN of less than 50 ng/mL had a prevalence of 2.4% (4/164); (2) fFN of 50 to 199 ng/mL had a prevalence of 9% (4/45); (3) fFN of 200 to 499 ng/mL had a prevalence of 16% (7/44); and (4) fFN greater than or equal to 500 ng/mL had a prevalence of 18% (3/17). The prevalence of spontaneous delivery within 7 days among women with a cervical length less than 15 mm also varied according to the fFN concentration: women having an fFN less than 10 ng/mL had a prevalence of 5% (1/19), while those having an fFN greater than or equal to 500 ng/mL had a 64.3% prevalence (9/14) (Table 14.6). Univariable logistic regression analysis showed that (1) a positive qualitative fFN test was associated with a higher risk of preterm birth within 7 days (OR, 11; 95% CI, 4.7 to 27); (2) a quantitative fFN concentration increased the OR for spontaneous delivery within 7 days by 1.006 per ng/mL (95% CI, 1.005 to 1.008); and (3) a longer cervix was associated with a lower risk of preterm birth within 7 days (OR, 0.90 per mm; 95% CI, 0.86 to 0.94). The ROC curves showed the following predictive values: quantitative fFN alone, area under the curve (AUC) = 0.82 (95% CI, 0.76 to 0.89); cervical length measurement and quantitative fFN, AUC = 0.84 (95% CI, 0.78 to 0.89); and cervical length measurement and qualitative fFN, AUC = 0.83 (95% CI, 0.77 to 0.88). The authors also reported that the positive predictive value of fFN increased from 30% to 37% as compared to qualitative fFN. The combination of cervical length and quantitative fFN testing provides a better estimation of the risk of delivery within 7 days than does using a qualitative fFN test alone. The authors concluded that quantification of fFN provides additional information on risk stratification of the risk of preterm birth.

In a study from Australia, Nguyen et al.[198] evaluated 367 women with a singleton pregnancy admitted for threatened preterm labor between 22 and 33[+6] weeks of gestation. The authors estimated the cervical length and performed a quantitative fFN test for prediction of spontaneous delivery within 2 weeks of study inclusion (n = 11). The authors reported that women who

TABLE 14.6 **Risk Stratification of Preterm Birth (PTB) within 7 Days with the Use of Quantitative Fetal Fibronectin in Combination with Cervical Length (CL; n = 455)**

| CL groups, mm | QUANTITATIVE FETAL FIBRONECTIN GROUPS | | | | | |
	<10 ng/mL	10–49 ng/mL	50–199 ng/mL	200–499 ng/mL	>500 ng/mL	Total
<15	19 (1 PTB, 5%)	18 (1 PTB, 6%)	19 (5 PTB, 26%)	33 (13 PTB, 39%)	14 (9 PTB, 64%)	103 (29 PTB, 28%)
15–29	78 (2 PTB, 3%)	86 (1 PTB, 1%)	45 (4 PTB, 9%)	44 (7 PTB, 16%)	17 (3 PTB, 18%)	270 (17 PTB, 6%)
30–50	37 (0 PTB)	20 (0 PTB)	12 (0 PTB)	7 (0 PTB)	6 (2 PTB, 33%)	82 (2 PTB, 2%)
Total	134 (3 PTB, 2%)	124 (2 PTB, 2%)	76 (9 PTB, 12%)	84 (20 PTB, 24%)	37 (14 PTB, 38%)	455 (48 PTB, 11%)

Reprinted from Bruijn MM, Kamphuis EI, Hoesli IM, et al. The predictive value of quantitative fibronectin testing in combination with cervical length measurement in symptomatic women. *Am J Obstet Gynecol.* 2016;215(6):793.e1–793.e8. Copyright © 2016 Elsevier. With permission.

delivered within 14 days had a higher mean fFN compared to women who delivered after 14 days (214 ng/mL vs. 26 ng/mL, respectively; $P < 0.001$). The rates of spontaneous preterm birth within 14 days also increased progressively with increased fFN concentrations from 0.8% (2/251), 2.7% (2/74), 2.9% (1/34) to 42.9% (6/14) for fFN values of 0 to 9 ng/mL, 10 to 49 ng/mL, 50 to 199 ng/mL and greater than 200 ng/mL, respectively. The RR of spontaneous preterm birth within 14 days relative to the lowest fFN category of 0 to 9 ng/mL also increased as the fFN concentration increased: fFN of 10 to 49 ng/mL (RR, 3.4; 95% CI, 0.5 to 23.7; $P < 0.2$); fFN of 50 to 199 ng/mL (RR, 3.7; 95% CI, 0.3 to 39.6; $P < 0.3$); and fFN greater than 200 ng/mL (RR, 53.8; 95% CI, 11.9 to 242.8; $P < 0.0001$). Similar results have been reported by other studies.[196,199]

Shen et al.[200] reported evidence of a longer interval to delivery in a cohort of women with symptomatic preterm labor who had fFN testing as part of triage evaluation. The authors classified the patients into four groups based on the use of cervical length measurement and fFN positive testing as (1) fFN only; (2) transvaginal ultrasound only; (3) both fFN and transvaginal ultrasound; and (4) neither fFN nor transvaginal ultrasound. In this cohort, 6.7% of patients had an fFN test only, while 3.2% had both fFN testing and transvaginal ultrasound; the average time to delivery was 31.2 days and 31.4 days, respectively. In comparison, those who did not have an fFN test had an average time to delivery of 16.3 days (transvaginal ultrasound only) and 12.1 days (neither fFN test nor transvaginal ultrasound).

In women with Müllerian congenital anomalies evaluated at 16 to 24 weeks of gestation, quantitative fFN testing showed a higher AUC for prediction of preterm delivery than did cervical length. Ridout et al.[201] evaluated 319 pregnant women presenting with congenital uterine anomalies, that is, a unicornuate ($n = 27$, 9%), a didelphic ($n = 34$, 11%), a bicornuate ($n = 189$, 59%), a septate ($n = 56$, 18%), or an arcuate ($n = 13$, 4%) uterus. The authors reported a rate of spontaneous preterm birth according to the type of uterine anomaly: unicornuate, 27% (7/26); didelphic, 20% (6/30); bicornuate, 9% (13/143); septate, 13% (6/48); and arcuate, 10% (1/10). It is noteworthy that 80% of patients who had a preterm delivery did not present a short cervix at 16 to 24 weeks of gestation. The AUC of cervical length for preterm delivery at less than 34 weeks of gestation was 0.56 (95% CI, 0.48 to 0.64), and for preterm delivery at less than 37 weeks, it was 0.59 (95% CI, 0.55 to 0.64). Quantitative

fFN had an AUC of 0.63 (95% CI, 0.49 to 0.77) for preterm delivery at less than 34 weeks, and for preterm delivery at less than 37 weeks of gestation, the AUC was 0.58 (95% CI, 0.49 to 0.68).

ETIOLOGIES OF A SONOGRAPHIC SHORT CERVIX

A short cervix often develops as the cervix ripens. However, not all short cervices are ripe; hence, many women with a short cervix deliver at term. We proposed that a short cervix is syndromic in nature and can be caused by multiple etiologies[52,202] such as (1) the loss of connective tissue after a cervical conization,[203–206] or a loop electrosurgical excision procedure (LEEP)[207,208]; (2) a congenital disorder, for example, cervical hypoplasia; (3) after exposure to DES[204,209–211]; (4) an intra-amniotic infection/inflammation[193,212,213]; (5) an alteration in progesterone action[214]; and/or (6) a cervical disorder that manifests itself as premature cervical dilation. Each of these causes can be affected by genetic or environmental factors, and more than one mechanism of disease may be present in a particular patient (Fig. 14.14). The possibility of novel and yet undiscovered mechanisms of disease that play a role must also be considered.

Pregnancy History

Several authors have documented a relationship between a previous obstetrical history of preterm birth and cervical length.[28,120] Iams et al.[28] evaluated the cervical length in patients with (1) a previous history of "cervical insufficiency"; (2) a previous preterm delivery at less than 26 weeks of gestation; (3) a previous preterm delivery between 27 and 32 weeks of gestation; (4) a previous preterm delivery between 33 and 35 weeks of gestation; and (5) a control group of women with no history of previous preterm delivery. A strong relationship was established between cervical length in the index pregnancy and previous obstetric history. Similar results were reported by Guzman et al.,[120] who described a strong relationship between previous obstetrical history and cervical length in the subsequent pregnancy. Specifically, the authors observed that the frequency of a short cervix (cervical length <20 mm), or progressive shortening of the cervix to a length of less than 20 mm, was associated with the gestational age at delivery in the previous pregnancy; thus, the earlier the previous preterm delivery, the earlier a short cervix was found in a subsequent pregnancy.[120] Collectively, these studies

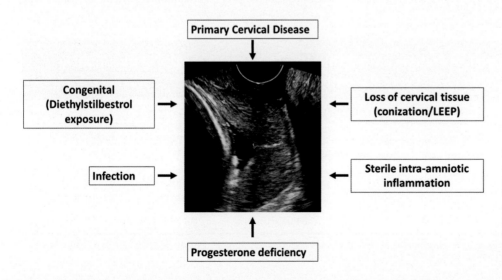

Primary Cervical Disease

Congenital (Diethylstilbestrol exposure)

Infection

Loss of cervical tissue (conization/LEEP)

Sterile intra-amniotic inflammation

Progesterone deficiency

FIGURE 14.14: The syndromic nature of a short cervix (Republished with permission of Walter de Gruyter & Co., from Romero R, Yeo L, Miranda J, et al. A blueprint for the prevention of preterm birth: vaginal progesterone in women with a short cervix. *J Perinat Med.* 2013;41(1):27–44; permission conveyed through Copyright Clearance Center, Inc.).

suggest a relationship between a history of preterm delivery and the development of a short cervix in a subsequent pregnancy. A short cervical length in the subsequent pregnancy may reflect the result of genetic and environmental factors predisposing to preterm delivery, which can express themselves as changes in the cervical structure.

Is There a Molecular Basis for Sonographic Shortening?

We demonstrated that sonographic cervical shortening prior to the onset of labor is associated with changes in the transcriptome of the human uterine cervix.[13] A study was performed in 19 pregnant women at term, but not in labor, with a ripe cervix (Bishop score >5), in which the sonographic cervical length was measured, and cervical biopsies were obtained. Changes in the transcriptome of the uterine cervix were evaluated as a function of each centimeter decrease in cervical length. Microarray analysis, pathway analysis, and quantitative real-time PCR analysis were employed. Cervical length shortening was associated with the (1) differential expression of 687 genes; (2) enrichment of 54 biological processes, 22 molecular functions, and 9 pathways; and (3) downregulation of bone morphogenetic protein-7 (BMP-7), claudin-1, integrin beta-6, endometrial progesterone-induced protein (EPIP), and messenger ribonucleic acid (mRNA). Changes in expression included genes involved in epithelial cell function, signal transduction, and epithelial-mesenchymal transition. The biological processes, molecular functions, and pathway analyses further demonstrated respective roles for the inflammatory response, the immune system response, transmembrane receptor activity, and pathways involved in antigen processing and presentation in cervical shortening at term.

Recently, Tarca et al.[215] reported the amniotic fluid inflammatory-related protein (IRP) network ($n = 33$ proteins) in 223 pregnant women with a short cervix who underwent a transabdominal amniocentesis. The time periods when the amniocentesis was performed were divided as follows: 16^{+5} to 22^{+1}, 22^{+2} to 26^{+1}, and 26^{+2} to 31^{+5} weeks of gestation. The authors reported that the concentration of most of the IRPs increased as the cervix shortened. At 16^{+5} to 22^{+1} weeks, the concentration of the majority of inflammatory proteins was higher in women who delivered preterm at less than 32 weeks of gestation; IL-8, macrophage inflammatory protein (MIP)-1, IL-6, and IL-10 showed the largest changes in concentration. At 22^{+2} to 26^{+1} weeks, changes were of a lesser magnitude, and IL-8, IL-6, and MIP-1 were the three proteins with the highest concentrations in women presenting with spontaneous preterm delivery at less than 32 weeks of gestation. The association between a short cervix and increased concentrations of inflammatory proteins measured in amniotic fluid or in cervical/vaginal secretions has also been reported by another group of investigators.[216]

Sundtoft et al.[217] analyzed the results of cervical biopsies obtained 1 year or more after a pregnancy in the following groups of women: (1) history of normal delivery (n=55), (2) history of cervical insufficiency (n=27; resulting from an extreme preterm delivery and/or a late spontaneous abortion), and (3) history of a short cervix (n=10; cervical length <5th percentile). The authors reported a lower concentration of cervical collagen in women with cervical insufficiency as compared to the control group of women with a normal pregnancy. They also showed that women with a short cervix had a significantly lower concentration of collagen (62.1%) as compared to women with a normal cervical length (67.8%; $P = 0.02$).

A Sonographic Short Cervix is a Clinical Manifestation of Intra-amniotic Infection and/or Intra-amniotic Inflammation

Premature cervical ripening in response to a pathologic stimulus, such as infection, may result in a sonographic short cervix. Gray et al.[218] reported that all women with a positive amniotic fluid culture for *Ureaplasma urealyticum* at the time of genetic amniocentesis delivered a preterm neonate with histological evidence of chorioamnionitis. This study, however, did not contain information about cervical length. Our group established that 9% (5/57) of asymptomatic women in the midtrimester with a cervical length less than or equal to 25 mm without cervical dilation had microbiologically proven intra-amniotic infection.[213] The isolated microorganisms included *Ureaplasma urealyticum* and *Fusobacterium*. Patients with amniotic fluid cultures positive for *Ureaplasma urealyticum* received intravenous antibiotics (azithromycin) for 7 days and underwent a test-of-cure amniocentesis. Three of the four patients had a negative amniocentesis result, thus demonstrating eradication of *Ureaplasma urealyticum*, and they subsequently delivered at term. Kiefer et al.[219] reported an association between a cervical length less than or equal to 5 mm in the midtrimester and increased amniotic fluid concentrations of inflammatory cytokines such as monocyte chemotactic protein-1 (MCP-1) and IL-6. In a subsequent study of 44 patients in the midtrimester with a cervical length less than or equal to 25 mm, in which those with intra-amniotic infection and/or preterm labor were not excluded, amniotic fluid MCP-1 was predictive for spontaneous preterm delivery.[220] Vaisbuch et al.[221] reported that intra-amniotic inflammation (defined as an amniotic fluid matrix metalloproteinase-8 concentration greater than 23 ng/mL) was present in 22.2% of asymptomatic patients (10/45) with a cervical length less than or equal to 15 mm in the midtrimester of pregnancy, an occurrence associated with adverse pregnancy outcome. Indeed, women with intra-amniotic inflammation had a shorter median diagnosis-to-delivery interval than those without this condition. Furthermore, 40% of patients with intra-amniotic inflammation delivered within 1 week of the amniocentesis.

Previous studies have indicated that up to 50% of patients presenting with painless cervical dilation at less than 24 weeks of gestation have a positive amniotic fluid culture for microorganisms.[212,222] In these cases, infection can be a cause of premature cervical dilation or may be secondary to the prolonged exposure of chorioamniotic membranes to the microbial flora present in the lower genital tract.[212] Jung et al.[223] reported a prevalence of 22.2% (16/72) of intra-amniotic infection/inflammation in 72 women with cervical insufficiency (determined by painless cervical dilatation or a short cervix ≤15 mm). They also showed that women with intra-amniotic infection/inflammation had a higher prevalence of preterm delivery at less than or equal to 34 weeks of gestation than do women with cervical insufficiency but without intra-amniotic infection/inflammation.

A high concentration of amniotic fluid IL-6 (≥2.6 ng/mL) without evidence of microorganisms either by cultivation or molecular analysis is known as sterile inflammation. Romero et al.[224] studied amniotic fluid samples obtained by amniocentesis from 231 women with a short cervix. The presence of microorganisms was observed in 2.2% (5/231), whereas sterile inflammation was observed in 10.4% (24/231) of the patients. Women with a short cervix and sterile inflammation had a higher rate of preterm delivery at less than 34 weeks of gestation as compared to patients with no intra-amniotic infection/inflammation.

ADDITIONAL PARAMETERS TO ASSESS THE RISK OF PRETERM BIRTH DURING TRANSVAGINAL SONOGRAPHY

Parameters other than cervical length are often noted during transvaginal ultrasound to assess a patient's risk for preterm birth. These factors include the presence or absence of a funnel, evidence of dynamic cervical changes, and the presence of amniotic fluid "sludge." While the presence or absence of a funnel and dynamic changes do not increase the predictive value of preterm birth beyond that provided by cervical length alone, the detection of amniotic fluid sludge has been found to be useful in the risk assessment for preterm birth.[225,226]

Amniotic Fluid "Sludge"

Particulate matter in the amniotic fluid is present in about 4% of pregnancies during transvaginal ultrasound in the first and early second trimesters.[227] The prevalence of this sonographic finding increases with gestational age, reaching 88% by 35 weeks.[228] Particulate matter in the first two trimesters of pregnancy has been associated with intra-amniotic bleeding[229–231] and acrania-anencephaly sequence when observed in women with a high concentration of maternal serum alpha-fetoprotein.[232,233] By contrast, in the last trimester of pregnancy, particulate matter and "echogenic amniotic fluid" have been attributed to the presence of vernix caseosa and/or meconium[234–237] and with a lecithin-sphingomyelin ratio indicative of lung maturity.[238,239] Congenital anomalies associated with particulate matter in the amniotic fluid include harlequin ichthyosis[240] and epidermolysis bullosa letalis.[241] Amniotic fluid sludge is defined as hyperechogenic dense aggregates of particulate matter in the amniotic fluid, often seen in close proximity to the internal cervical os during a TVS examination of the cervix[242] (Fig. 14.15). On microscopic examination, amniotic fluid sludge consists of a combination of epithelial cells, neutrophils, and bacteria, forming microbial biofilms (Fig.14.17). When visualized grossly, such material resembles pus. Amniotic fluid sludge is an independent risk factor for histological chorioamnionitis and MIAC in patients with spontaneous preterm labor and intact membranes. Moreover, the presence of sludge in asymptomatic women in the midtrimester of pregnancy increases the risk of preterm prelabor rupture of membranes (PROM) and spontaneous preterm delivery.[243]

The first description of amniotic fluid sludge, originating from patients in preterm labor, was reported by Espinoza et al.[242] in 84 patients with preterm labor and intact membranes; 22.6% (19/84) of them had amniotic fluid sludge. Patients with

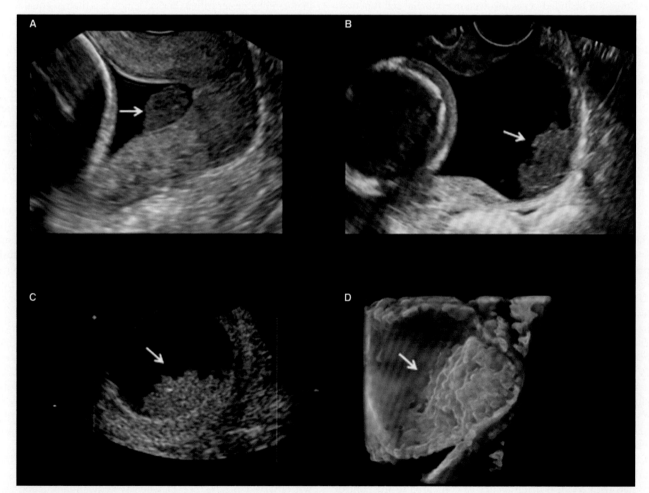

FIGURE 14.15: Transvaginal sonographic images of three patients with a short cervix and amniotic fluid sludge. The arrows illustrate the presence of dense aggregates of particulate matter in close proximity to the internal cervical os; **A:** Short cervix and amniotic fluid sludge; **B:** no-measurable cervix and amniotic fluid sludge; **C:** three dimensional ultrasound image obtained from a gestation with no-measurable cervix, bulging membranes, and amniotic fluid sludge; **D:** rendered image of the irregular surface of the amniotic fluid sludge.

TABLE 14.7	Diagnostic Indices and Predictive Value of Amniotic Fluid Sludge						
OUTCOME VARIABLE	PREVALENCE % (NUMBER)	SENSITIVITY %	SPECIFICITY %	PPV %	NPV %	LR (+)	LR (−)
Positive amniotic fluid cultures	12.1 (7/58)	86	76	33	98	3.3	0.19
Histological chorioamnionitis	32.9 (25/76)	56	92	78	81	7.1	0.48
Spontaneous delivery within 48 hours	13.6 (8/59)	75	84	43	96	4.8	0.30
Spontaneous delivery within 7 days	28.8 (17/59)	59	90	71	84	6.2	0.46

LR, likelihood ratio; *NPV*, negative predictive value; *PPV*, positive predictive value..
From Espinoza J, Gonçalves LF, Romero R, et al. The prevalence and clinical significance of amniotic fluid sludge in patients with preterm labor and intact membranes. *Ultrasound Obstet Gynecol.* 2005;25(4):346–352.

amniotic fluid sludge had higher frequencies of a positive amniotic fluid culture and histological chorioamnionitis as well as a higher rate of spontaneous preterm delivery within 48 hours, 7 days from examination, less than 32 weeks of gestation (75% [9/12] vs. 25.8% [8/31], P = 0.005), and less than 35 weeks of gestation (92.9% [13/14] vs. 37.8% [17/45], P < 0.001) than those without amniotic fluid sludge. Stepwise logistic regression analysis indicated that the presence of sludge was an independent factor associated with the likelihood of spontaneous delivery within 48 hours and 7 days from examination but not less than 32 weeks or less than 35 weeks of gestation. The diagnostic indices for amniotic fluid sludge are presented in Table 14.7.

Survival analysis demonstrated that patients with amniotic fluid sludge had a shorter examination-to-delivery interval compared to those without sludge (sludge median: 1 day [interquartile range: 1 to 5 days] vs. no sludge median: 33 days [interquartile range: 18 to 58 days]; P < 0.001) (Fig. 14.16). These results indicate that amniotic fluid sludge observed during transvaginal examination of the cervix is a risk factor for MIAC, histological chorioamnionitis, and preterm delivery.[242]

The presence of amniotic fluid sludge on transvaginal examination in asymptomatic patients is also associated with delivery within 14 days of an ultrasound examination and with preterm delivery at less than 32 weeks and at less than 34 weeks of gestation.[243-246] Bujold et al.[243] reported a retrospective study of 89 women at 18 to 32 weeks who were considered as high risk for preterm delivery. Logistic regression analysis revealed that a cervical length less than 25 mm and the presence of light or dense amniotic fluid sludge were independent predictors of delivery within 14 days and less than 34 weeks of gestation. In a retrospective case control study, Kusanovic et al.[244] included 281 patients with (n = 66) or without (n = 215) amniotic fluid sludge at 13 to 29 weeks of gestation. Amniotic fluid sludge was identified as an independent risk factor for the following outcomes: spontaneous preterm delivery at less than 28, at less than 32, and at less than 35 weeks of gestation, preterm PROM, MIAC, and histological chorioamnionitis. The prevalence of amniotic fluid sludge was 23.5% among patients considered as high risk for preterm birth

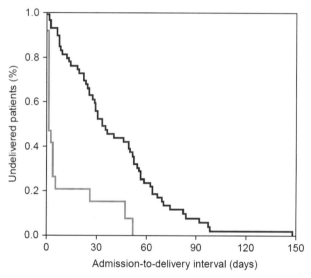

FIGURE 14.16: Results of survival analysis in patients in preterm labor with and without the presence of amniotic fluid sludge. Patients with amniotic fluid sludge (*blue line*) had a shorter examination-to-delivery interval compared with those without sludge (*red line*). (From Espinoza J, Goncalves LF, Romero R, et al. The prevalence and clinical significance of amniotic fluid sludge in patients with preterm labor and intact membranes. *Ultrasound Obstet Gynecol.* 2005;25(4):346–352. Copyright © 2005 ISUOG. Adapted by permission of John Wiley & Sons, Inc.)

based upon the presence of one or more of the following factors: a history of spontaneous preterm delivery, previous midtrimester loss, a short cervix (<25 mm), Müllerian duct anomalies, and a history of cervix cone biopsy.

Several microorganisms have been reported in the amniotic fluid of women with amniotic fluid sludge, i.e., *Ureaplasma* spp., *Mycoplasma hominis, Fusobacterium nucleatum, Peptostreptococcus* spp., Group B *Streptococcus, Gardnerella vaginalis, Acinetobacter* spp., *Streptococcus mutans, Aspergillus flavus,* and

Staphylococcus warneri.[226,247–249] Recently, Kusanovic et al.[250] reported the presence of *Candida albicans* in a sample of amniotic fluid sludge obtained by transabdominal amniocentesis in a patient with a short cervix and an intrauterine device. Amniotic fluid sludge represents a biofilm.[225,226] This finding was confirmed in a sample of sludge obtained from a patient at 28 weeks of gestation with spontaneous labor and clinical chorioamnionitis by transvaginal amniotomy under ultrasound guidance. Grossly, the sludge had a "puslike" appearance, and the Gram stain showed Gram-positive bacteria. The amniotic fluid culture was positive for *S. mutans*, *M. hominis*, and *A. flavus*. Of interest, the results of the amniocentesis performed at the time of admission for preterm labor were negative for intra-amniotic infection.[225,226] Amniotic fluid sludge should be considered as a sign of MIAC. The clinical significance of this finding relates to the challenges of diagnosis and treatment, as the formation of amniotic fluid sludge might protect the microorganisms against the maternal inflammatory response and from the action of antibiotics (Fig. 14.17). The presence of amniotic fluid sludge in women at risk for preterm delivery reinforces the need for an amniocentesis to confirm intra-amniotic infection/inflammation. The sample of amniotic fluid should be obtained near the location of the amniotic fluid sludge, as the protective action of the biofilm might prevent identification of microorganisms in amniotic fluid samples obtained distantly from the amniotic fluid sludge.

Antibiotic Treatment for Women with Amniotic Fluid Sludge

Women with amniotic fluid sludge can be treated with antibiotics due to the association with intrauterine infection/inflammation. Dinglas et al.[251] reported resolution of amniotic fluid sludge in a patient diagnosed at 18 weeks of gestation with a short cervix (18 mm) and amniotic fluid sludge. The patient had a history of three previous second-trimester losses at 19, 22, and 16 weeks of gestation with confirmatory histological chorioamnionitis. The patient was treated with antibiotics (metronidazole, azithromycin, and amoxicillin) and cerclage. Follow-up ultrasound evaluation showed resolution of amniotic fluid sludge. The patient had a normal term delivery at 37 weeks and delivered a neonate with normal birthweight. Hatanaka et al.[252] compared two historical groups of patients diagnosed with amniotic fluid sludge in the

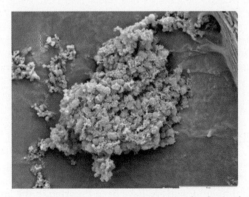

FIGURE 14.17: Scanning electron micrograph of a flock of amniotic fluid sludge. Bacterial cells and the exopolymeric matrix material that constitute a biofilm are shown. (Reprinted from Romero R, Schaudinn C, Kusanovic JP, et al. Detection of a microbial biofilm in intraamniotic infection. *Am J Obstet Gynecol*. 2008;198(1):135.e1–135.e5. Copyright © 2008 Elsevier. With permission.)

midtrimester of pregnancy. The first group ($n = 22$) did not receive treatment with antibiotics, whereas the second group ($n = 64$) received treatment with antibiotics. Patients were further classified into two groups: high risk (cervical length ≤25 mm; Müllerian malformations; history of preterm delivery, late miscarriages, or cervical conization) and low risk (without any of these characteristics). Patients at high risk received intravenous clindamycin (600 mg/8 hours) and cefazolin (1 g/8 hours) for 5 days, followed by oral treatment of the same antibiotics for another 5 days. Women at low risk received oral clindamycin (300 mg/6 hours) and cephalexin (500 mg/6 hours) for 7 days. The results of this study showed that high-risk women receiving intravenous antibiotics had a reduction in the prevalence of preterm delivery at less than 34 weeks of gestation (13.2% vs. 38.5%; $P = 0.047$) as compared to low-risk women treated with oral antibiotics. When all women were evaluated, those receiving antibiotics had newborns with significantly higher birthweight than did women receiving no antibiotics despite a similar gestational age at delivery. In a study including 245 women evaluated with transvaginal ultrasound at 15 to 24 weeks of gestation, 29 of them had amniotic fluid sludge (11.8%).[253] All patients with sludge received clindamycin, while 16 of them additionally received cefoperazone/sulbactam and 8 received amoxicillin/clavulanate for 5 days. After 2 weeks of treatment with cefoperazone/sulbactam, amniotic fluid sludge was no longer present in the ultrasound scans, and the prevalence of preterm delivery was lower in these women than in those treated with amoxicillin/clavulanate. Despite these encouraging results, the optimal antibiotics treatment in women with amniotic fluid sludge has yet to be determined.

THERAPEUTIC OPTIONS FOR WOMEN WITH A SHORT CERVIX

Vaginal Progesterone

There is substantial evidence to support the use of vaginal progesterone for the prevention of preterm birth in patients with a sonographic short cervix regardless of pregnancy history.[254,255] Fonseca et al.[22] reported a randomized, double-blind, placebo-controlled trial in which women with a short cervix (≤15 mm), measured between 20 and 25 weeks of gestation, were allocated to a daily vaginal administration of 200 mg of micronized progesterone or a placebo (safflower oil) from 24^{+0} to 33^{+6} weeks of gestation. The frequency of spontaneous preterm delivery at less than 34 weeks (primary end point for the trial) was significantly lower in the progesterone group than that in the placebo group (19.2% [24/125] vs. 34.4% [43/125]; $P = 0.007$). A secondary analysis of this trial indicated that among women without a history of preterm delivery at less than 34 weeks of gestation, the incidence of preterm birth was significantly lower in women receiving progesterone than in those allocated to placebo (17.9% [20/112] vs. 31.2% [34/109]; RR, 0.57; 95% CI, 0.35 to 0.93; $P = 0.03$). The trial was not designed to test whether progesterone administration could reduce neonatal morbidity, and such a reduction was not observed.[22]

DeFranco et al.[21] reported a secondary analysis of the effect of vaginal progesterone on pregnancy outcome (preterm birth and infant outcome) as a function of cervical length less than 30 mm and less than 28 mm. For patients with a cervical length less than 30 mm, there was a trend for a longer randomization-to-delivery interval in women receiving progesterone than that for those receiving placebo (Wilcoxon $P = 0.043$; log-rank $P = 0.057$). However, no differences in the frequency of preterm delivery at less than 32 weeks were observed. Patients with a cervical length less than 28 mm who received vaginal progesterone had a lower rate of spontaneous preterm delivery at less than 32 weeks of gestation, although the prevalence of preterm delivery at less than 35 weeks and at less than 37 weeks did not differ among women receiving progesterone or placebo. Of note, the frequency of NICU admission and duration of NICU stay were lower in women with a short cervix (<30 mm and <28 mm) who received vaginal progesterone. This analysis provided the first evidence that vaginal progesterone administration may improve infant outcome. However, these conclusions were considered tentative as they were derived from a secondary analysis, which was intended to be hypothesis generating[21]; thus, further investigation was necessary.

Hassan et al.[23] performed a multicenter, randomized, double-blind, placebo-controlled trial (PREGNANT trial) evaluating the efficacy of vaginal progesterone gel (90 mg daily) for the prevention of preterm delivery in patients with a sonographic short cervix (10 to 20 mm) between 19^{+0} and 23^{+6} weeks of gestation regardless of pregnancy history. A total of 465 patients were randomized to receive 90 mg of vaginal progesterone gel or placebo beginning at 20^{+0} to 23^{+6} weeks until 36^{+6} weeks of gestation or rupture of membranes or delivery, whichever occurred first. The study demonstrated a significant 45% reduction in the risk of preterm delivery at less than 33 weeks of gestation in the group treated with vaginal progesterone when compared to those receiving a placebo. There was also a significant reduction in the risk of preterm delivery at less than 28 weeks and at less than 35 weeks of gestation (50% and 38%, respectively). Most notably, there was a significant decrease in the risk of neonatal RDS (61%), any neonatal morbidity/mortality (43%), and low birthweight less than 1,500 g (53%).

Romero et al.[255] reported the results of an individual patient data meta-analysis of 974 women with a singleton pregnancy and a short cervix (cervical length ≤25 mm) in the midtrimester of pregnancy. All patients had been enrolled in five randomized controlled trials comparing vaginal progesterone treatment versus placebo for preventing preterm birth. Vaginal progesterone was administered to 498 women and 476 received placebo. Treatment with vaginal progesterone was associated with a significant reduction in the risk of preterm birth at less than 33 weeks of gestation (RR, 0.62; 95% CI, 0.47 to 0.81; $P = 0.0006$) as compared to placebo. Subgroup analysis showed that vaginal progesterone significantly reduced the risk of preterm delivery at less than 28 weeks (RR, 0.67; 95% CI, 0.45 to 0.99; $P = 0.04$), at less than 30 weeks (RR, 0.70; 95% CI, 0.49 to 0.98; $P = 0.04$), at less than 32 weeks (RR, 0.64; 95% CI, 0.48 to 0.86; $P = 0.003$), at less than 34 weeks (RR, 0.65; 95% CI, 0.51 to 0.83; $P = 0.0006$), and at less than 36 weeks (RR, 0.80; 95% CI, 0.67 to 0.97; $P = 0.02$) of gestation as compared to placebo administration. Vaginal progesterone treatment in patients with a cervical length less than or equal to 25 mm was also associated with a significant reduction in neonatal morbidity caused by RDS (RR, 0.47; 95% CI, 0.27 to 0.81; $P = 0.007$), composite neonatal morbidity and mortality (RR, 0.59; 95% CI, 0.38 to 0.91; $P = 0.02$), NICU admission (RR, 0.68; 95% CI, 0.53 to 0.88; $P = 0.003$), and birthweight less than 1,500 g (RR, 0.62; 95% CI, 0.44 to 0.86; $P = 0.004$).

Progesterone in Women with a History of Preterm Delivery and a Short Cervix

In women with a history of preterm delivery and a short cervix, Conde-Agudelo et al.[256] reported that vaginal progesterone is as effective as cervical cerclage in reducing the rate of preterm

delivery. The authors reported the results of an indirect comparison meta-analysis comprised of 10 studies and a total of 769 women with a singleton pregnancy, a history of preterm delivery, and a short cervix (≤25 mm). Five studies compared vaginal progesterone versus placebo, and the remaining five compared cerclage versus no cerclage. Direct comparisons showed that vaginal progesterone reduced the risk of preterm birth at less than 35 weeks of gestation (RR, 0.68; 95% CI, 0.50 to 0.93) and at less than 32 weeks of gestation (RR, 0.60; 95% CI, 0.39 to 0.92), neonatal sepsis (RR, 0.38; 95% CI, 0.15 to 0.96), composite neonatal morbidity (RR, 0.29; 95% CI, 0.11 to 0.81), composite perinatal morbidity and mortality (RR, 0.43; 95% CI, 0.20 to 0.94), and admission to the NICU (RR, 0.46; 95% CI, 0.30 to 0.70) as compared to women receiving placebo. Cervical cerclage also showed a significant reduction in preterm delivery at less than 37 weeks (RR, 0.70; 95% CI, 0.58 to 0.83), at less than 35 weeks (RR, 0.70; 95% CI, 0.55 to 0.89), at less than 32 weeks (RR, 0.66; 95% CI, 0.48 to 0.91), and at less than 28 weeks of gestation (RR, 0.64; 95% CI, 0.43 to 0.96), composite perinatal morbidity and mortality (RR, 0.64; 95% CI, 0.45 to 0.91), and birthweight less than 1,500 g (RR, 0.64; 95% CI, 0.45 to 0.90) as compared to women without cerclage. Adjusted indirect comparison meta-analyses showed no significant differences between vaginal progesterone and cerclage in preventing preterm birth at less than 35 weeks of gestation. There were no significant differences between vaginal progesterone and cerclage for any of the secondary outcomes. The authors concluded that vaginal progesterone and cerclage are equally effective in preventing preterm birth and improving perinatal outcomes in women with a singleton gestation, previous spontaneous preterm birth, and a midtrimester sonographic short cervix.

Progesterone in Women with a Twin Pregnancy and a Short Cervix

In twin pregnancies, Romero et al.[257] reported the results of a meta-analysis of individual patient data. A total of 303 women with a twin pregnancy and a cervical length less than or equal to 25 mm in the midtrimester of pregnancy were assigned to treatment with either vaginal progesterone ($n = 159$) or placebo ($n = 144$). Women treated with vaginal progesterone had a significantly lower risk of preterm delivery at less than 33 weeks of gestation (RR, 0.69; 95% CI, 0.51 to 0.93; $P = 0.01$) and at less than 35 weeks of gestation (RR, 0.83; 95% CI, 0.69 to 0.99) than did women receiving placebo. Twin neonates from women treated with vaginal progesterone showed a lower risk of RDS (RR, 0.70; 95% CI, 0.56 to 0.89), perinatal death (RR, 0.58; 95% CI, 0.39 to 0.84), composite neonatal morbidity/mortality (RR, 0.61; 95% CI, 0.34 to 0.98), and a need for mechanical ventilation (RR, 0.54; 95% CI, 0.36 to 0.81) than did women receiving placebo. The authors concluded that the administration of vaginal progesterone to asymptomatic women with a twin gestation and a midtrimester sonographic short cervix significantly reduces the risk of preterm birth at less than 33 weeks of gestation by 31% and of neonatal death by 47%. Based on this evidence, we recommend vaginal progesterone treatment for pregnant women with either a singleton or a twin pregnancy and a sonographic short cervix (≤25 mm), regardless of pregnancy history. The individual data meta-analysis showed that the number of patients needed to treat with vaginal progesterone is 12 to prevent one case of preterm birth at less than 35 weeks of gestation, and the number is 18 to prevent one case of RDS.[255] The administration of vaginal progesterone has not been related to adverse maternal outcomes and complications.

Cost-Effectiveness of Vaginal Progesterone

There is evidence to support the role of universal transvaginal cervical length screening in the identification of patients at risk for preterm delivery.[258-262] The policy of universal cervical length screening and treatment with vaginal progesterone based on the identification of a midtrimester short cervix is in compliance with the general principles that the World Health Organization (WHO) outlined as the basis of an effective screening test.[261-266] Werner et al.[267] developed a decision analysis model to compare the cost-effectiveness of two strategies intended to identify a pregnancy at risk for preterm birth in an otherwise low-risk singleton pregnancy. The two models specified were (1) no routine cervical length screening and (2) a single routine transvaginal cervical length; patients with a short cervix were offered vaginal progesterone treatment. The results of the decision analysis model predicted that routine cervical length screening when coupled with the use of vaginal progesterone treatment has a potential savings of $19,603,380 for every 100,000 women screened using ultrasound. Furthermore, universal TVS cervical length screening and vaginal progesterone administration for women with a short cervix is a cost-effective intervention to prevent preterm birth and associated morbidity and mortality regardless of the cutoff value (≤15 mm, ≤20 mm, ≤25 mm, 10 to 20 mm or 10 to 30 mm[268-271]) used to define a short cervix in the decision and economic analyses.

In a clinical opinion, Conde-Agudelo et al.[265] estimated that 303,613 women with a singleton gestation and a cervical length less than or equal to 25 mm could have been identified in the United States if universal TVS cervical length screening had been implemented. Based on the results of an individual patient data meta-analysis,[24] if all of the women with a cervical length less than or equal to 25 mm had received vaginal progesterone, then 30,545 preterm births (<34 weeks of gestation) and 17,433 cases of major neonatal morbidity or mortality could have been prevented. The authors noted, given that the rate of preterm birth at less than 34 weeks among singleton gestations was 2.72% (n = 103,228),[272] the implementation of universal TVS cervical length screening and treatment with vaginal progesterone could contribute to a decrease of 30% (30,545/103,228) in the rate of preterm birth occurring at less than 34 weeks of gestation in the United States. Finally, universal TVS screening for a short cervix and treatment with vaginal progesterone appears to be a relevant public health strategy when compared to universal screening for maternal group B streptococcal colonization and intrapartum antibiotic prophylaxis.[265]

17-Alpha Hydroxyprogesterone Caproate

The use of 17-alpha-hydroxyprogesterone caproate (17-OHPC), a synthetic progestogen, has been proposed to prevent recurrent preterm birth in patients with a history of spontaneous singleton preterm birth. This potential benefit is largely based on a single randomized controlled trial. In 2003, Meis et al.[273] reported a significant reduction in the rate of recurrent preterm birth at less than or equal to 37 weeks of gestation among women who received a weekly injection of 17-OHPC compared to a placebo group. However, the results of this study raised questions about the true efficacy of 17-OHPC. Keirse et al.[274] suggested that this demonstrable difference may be attributed to the unexpectedly high rate of preterm birth in the placebo group (54.9%; 84/153), given that the rate of preterm birth in the 17-OHPC group (36.3%; 111/306) was similar to the 34.6%

(106/306) rate of recurrent preterm birth in a similar population of a previous Maternal-Fetal Medicine Network Study.[275] Notably, the U.S. Food and Drug Administration (FDA) approval of 17-OHPC for prevention of preterm birth in women with a history of preterm delivery fell under Subpart H of the Code of Federal Regulations, because the decision was made on the basis of one clinical trial using a surrogate endpoint (delivery at <37 weeks of gestation), and further confirmatory study was required. The confirmatory study, named the PROLONG (Progestin's Role in Optimizing Neonatal Gestation) trial, a multicenter, multinational, placebo-controlled, randomized clinical trial, was designed to assess the safety and efficacy of 17-OHPC in reducing the risks of preterm birth and neonatal morbidity/mortality in women with a singleton gestation and a prior singleton spontaneous preterm birth.[276] The PROLONG trial did not demonstrate a statistically significant difference between treatment with 17-OHPC or placebo for the two co-primary outcomes: 1) frequency of preterm delivery at less than 35 weeks of gestation (17-OHPC-treated group, 11.0% vs. placebo 11.5%; RR = 0.95 [95% CI: 0.71-1.26]); and 2) neonatal morbidity composite index (17-OHPC-treated group, 5.6% vs. placebo 5.0%, RR = 0.95 [95% CI: 0.68-1.61]). There was also no statistically significant difference in the safety outcome of fetal/early infant death (17-OHPC-treated group, 1.7% vs. placebo 1.9%, RR = 0.87 [95% CI: 0.4-1.81]).[277]

Other studies have also shown that intramuscular injections of 17-OHPC are not effective in preventing spontaneous delivery in women with a sonographic short cervix. A multicenter randomized controlled study (SCAN trial) performed by Grobman et al.[278] failed to demonstrate a significant improvement in the prevention of preterm delivery in nulliparous patients with a short cervix (cervical length <30 mm) who received a weekly administration of intramuscular 17-OHPC. The subgroup analysis of patients with a cervical length less than 15 mm did not result in a significant reduction in preterm delivery. In the study by Meis et al.,[20] weekly administration of 17-OHPC was given to women with previous spontaneous preterm birth. However, the cervical length was not evaluated; therefore, a common clinical challenge occurs when a patient with a prior spontaneous preterm birth receives weekly 17-OHPC and is found to have a short cervix. Another clinical challenge is the potential additive effect of cerclage placement in patients receiving 17-OHPC who subsequently develop a short cervix. A secondary analysis of a large randomized trial investigating the use of ultrasound-indicated cerclage for the prevention of preterm birth in high-risk women demonstrated that cerclage did not provide additional benefit for the prevention of recurrent preterm birth in women with a subsequent short cervix who had received at least one dose of 17-OHPC.[279,280] Winer et al.[281] reported a multicenter, open-label, randomized, controlled clinical trial comprised of asymptomatic women with a singleton pregnancy, a history of previous preterm birth, and a short cervix (≤25 mm) to evaluate the efficacy of 17-OHPC in prolonging pregnancy. After the inclusion of 105 patients, the trial was stopped due to the lack of efficacy of 17-OHPC in prolonging pregnancy. The rate of preterm delivery at less than 37 weeks (45% vs. 44%, P > 0.99), at less than 34 weeks (24% vs. 30%, P = 0.51), and at less than 32 weeks of gestation (14% vs. 20%, P = 0.44) was similar in patients treated with 17-OHPC and those in the control group. The authors concluded that 17-OHPC did not prolong pregnancy in women with a singleton gestation, a sonographic short cervix, and a prior history of preterm delivery. Jarde et al.[282] reported the results of a systematic review and meta-analysis comparing vaginal progesterone, oral progesterone, 17-OHPC, cerclage, and pessary in preventing preterm delivery at less than 34 weeks of gestation. The study included 40 trials and 11,311 women with a singleton pregnancy at risk for preterm delivery. Of all available treatments, only vaginal progesterone consistently reduced the rate of preterm birth at less than 34 weeks of gestation (OR, 0.43; 95% CI, 0.2 to 0.81) and at less than 37 weeks of gestation (OR, 0.51; 95% CI, 0.34 to 0.74) and the rate of neonatal morbidity (OR, 0.41; 95% CI, 0.2 to 0.83). The authors concluded that vaginal progesterone was the only intervention consistently showing a reduction in the prevalence of preterm birth.

Summary of Recommendations and Facts Regarding the Use of Progesterone for the Prevention of Preterm Birth

1. Universal cervical length screening and vaginal progesterone treatment (90 mg of vaginal gel or 200 mg of micronized vaginal suppositories) for patients with a cervical length less than or equal to 25 mm is clinically effective and cost-effective in the prevention of preterm birth.
2. Women with a sonographic short cervix less than or equal to 25 mm diagnosed in the midtrimester of pregnancy should be offered daily vaginal progesterone treatment until 37 weeks of gestation or until the onset of preterm labor.
3. Weekly injections of 17-OHPC are not effective for the prevention of preterm delivery in patients with a sonographic short cervix.
4. Patients with a midtrimester short cervix less than or equal to 25 mm and previous history of spontaneous preterm delivery can be offered either vaginal progesterone or cervical cerclage. Treatment choice should be based upon consideration of the risks of both treatments and patient/clinician preferences. An amniocentesis for the evaluation of subclinical intra-amniotic infection/inflammation is recommended especially prior to the placement of a cervical cerclage.
5. Vaginal progesterone reduces the rate of preterm delivery and neonatal morbidity in pregnant women with a twin gestation and a short cervix (≤25 mm).

Cervical Cerclage

The clinical value of cervical cerclage has been the subject of many observational and randomized clinical trials[56,283–286] and several systematic reviews.[58,287,288] The evidence suggests the following conclusions:

1. Cervical cerclage is a therapeutic option in women with a sonographic short cervix and a history of preterm delivery for the prevention of subsequent preterm birth (Figs. 14.18 to 14.20).[54,287–290]
2. Cervical cerclage in women with a sonographic short cervix and no history of preterm delivery does not reduce the rate of preterm birth.[286]
3. The role of prophylactic cerclage in high-risk patients without a sonographic short cervix for the prevention of preterm delivery/midtrimester abortion (by history) is unclear. While the largest trial done prior to the introduction of ultrasound evaluation of the cervix suggested a modest beneficial effect, other trials and systematic reviews[291–295]

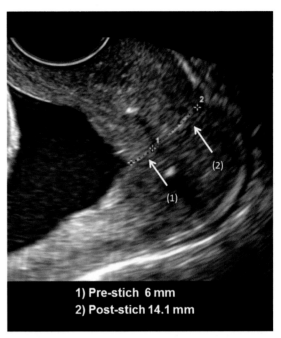

1) Pre-stich 6 mm
2) Post-stich 14.1 mm

FIGURE 14.18: Cervical length (CL) after cerclage: (1) CL precerclage (6 mm); (2) CL postcerclage (14.1 mm); total CL = 20.1 mm

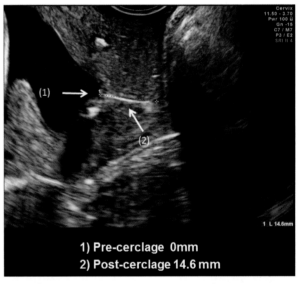

1) Pre-cerclage 0mm
2) Post-cerclage 14.6 mm

FIGURE 14.19: Shortening of cervical length after cerclage: cervical length = 14.6 mm: (1) precerclage (0 mm); (2) postcerclage (14.6 mm).

prior to the use of ultrasound indicated that the evidence of effectiveness is either weak or nonexistent. In patients at risk for preterm delivery, serial sonographic examination of the cervix followed by cerclage in those with a short cervix is a reasonable alternative to prophylactic placement of a cerclage based on uncontrolled studies.[54,296,297]

Prognostic Value of Cervical Length Measurement after Cerclage Placement

Measurement of cervical length after cerclage can identify patients who have an increased risk of preterm birth.[298,299] Andersen et al.[300] evaluated 32 women who underwent cerclage placement at 10 to 36 weeks of gestation upon diagnosis of an

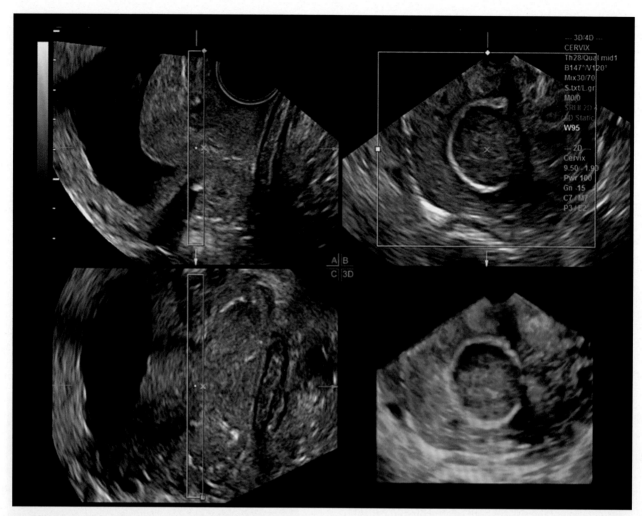

FIGURE 14.20: 3D rendered image of a cervical cerclage.

incompetent cervix; this group was characterized by a history of repeated midtrimester pregnancy loss and/or cervical dilation determined by digital examination. The authors reported that women with a cervical length less than or equal to 10 mm measured above (from the internal cervical os to the cerclage) the cerclage placement, evaluated before 30 weeks of gestation, had a higher prevalence (50% [6/12] vs. 5%, [1/20]; $P = 0.003$) and a higher risk (RR, 5.8; 95% CI, 1.8 to 18.9) of preterm birth at less than 34 weeks of gestation than did women with a cervical length greater than 10 mm. Guzman et al.[301] reported the results of cervical length assessment, performed after emergency cerclage placement, in a cohort of 29 women who underwent emergency cerclage placement at a median gestational age of 21 weeks (range 16 to 26 weeks). The results showed that a cervical length less than 10 mm above the cerclage, measured within 48 hours of placement, had a sensitivity of 85.7%, a specificity of 66.7%, a positive predictive value of 70.6%, and a negative predictive value of 83% for preterm birth at less than 36 weeks of gestation. In a retrospective cohort study of 179 women who had a cerclage placed due to a previous history of preterm birth, a midtrimester loss, or a cervical surgery (knife cone biopsy/large loop excision), and a short cervix (≤25 mm), Cook et al.[302] reported that the cervical length measured 14 days after cerclage placement correlated with the risk of preterm birth at less than 34 weeks and at less than 37 weeks of gestation. The authors

suggested the following recommendations for cervical length measurement after cerclage:

- Empty bladder
- Ultrasound probe inserted into the anterior fornix of the vagina
- Sagittal long-axis view of the cervical canal
- Avoidance of applying excessive pressure on the cervix
- Cervical length measured from the internal os to the cervical suture (above cerclage) and from the cervical suture to the external cervical os (below cerclage [cervical height])
- At least three measurements, using the shortest for analysis

Among women with a cervical height at less than or equal to 10 mm, the RR for preterm birth at less than 34 weeks of gestation was 1.85 (95% CI, 1.14 to 2.99; $P = 0.0155$) and for preterm birth at less than 37 weeks of gestation was 2.37 (95% CI, 1.45 to 3.87; $P = 0.0005$) as compared to women with a cervical height greater than 10 mm. Further, among women with a total cervical length less than or equal to 25 mm after cerclage placement, the authors reported the RR for preterm birth at less than 34 weeks as 1.46 (95% CI, 1.05 to 2.02; $P = 0.03$) and for preterm delivery at less than 37 weeks as 1.40 (95% CI, 1.01 to 1.93; $P = 0.04$) as compared to those with a cervical length greater than 25 mm.[302] Song et al.[303] evaluated 52 women who underwent cervical cerclage due to a history of advanced cervical dilation and/or bulging membranes through the external os in the second trimester, a history of conization, a history of cervical pregnancy, or a history of preterm delivery before 28 weeks of gestation. The cervical length was measured after cerclage placement in the operating room. The authors reported that a cervical length of 25 mm after cerclage had an AUC of 0.71 (95% CI, 0.56 to 0.87; $P = 0.03$) with a sensitivity of 91.0% and a specificity of 30.0% for preterm delivery less than 32 weeks of gestation.

Further, Pils et al.[304] evaluated 88 women who underwent cerclage placement at 16 to 18 weeks of gestation due to a history of previous preterm birth or second-trimester miscarriage; 56 of them had a short cervix less than or equal to 25 mm. The cervix was evaluated at (median) 4 days (range 3 to 6 days) after cerclage placement. In women with a history of a previous pregnancy loss and a short cervix, a cervical length less than or equal to 20 mm, measured 4 days after cerclage placement, had an area under the ROC curve of 0.87, a sensitivity of 84.2%, a specificity of 83.8%, a positive predictive value of 72%, and a negative predictive value of 91.2% for preterm delivery at less than 35 weeks of gestation.

Cerclage in Women with a Short Cervix and No History of Preterm Delivery

Berghella et al.[305] reported a systemic review and meta-analysis on the effect of cerclage placement in women with a short cervix and no history of preterm delivery. Five studies and 419 asymptomatic women with a short cervix at midgestation were included. The results showed no differences in the prevalence of preterm delivery at less than 28 weeks, at less than 32 weeks, at less than 34 weeks, and at less than 35 weeks of gestation between women treated with cerclage as compared to women with expectant management. When subgroups of cervical length were compared, the authors reported a significant reduction in preterm delivery at less than 35 weeks of gestation in women with a cervical length less than 10 mm treated with cerclage. However, given the low quality of the evidence and the effect of multiple comparisons, these results might not constitute robust evidence indicating that cerclage reduces the risk of preterm delivery in asymptomatic women with a cervical length less than 10 mm and no history of preterm delivery.[306]

Cerclage in Women with a Twin Gestation

The American College of Obstetricians and Gynecologists[307] and the Society for Maternal-Fetal Medicine[308] both recommend against the use of cerclage in women with a twin gestation and a short cervix. This recommendation was based largely on the 2005 meta-analysis of randomized controlled trials that assessed whether cerclage prevents preterm birth in women with a short cervical length. Although this meta-analysis was not designed for twin gestations, among the 49 twin pregnancies in the study, cerclage for a short cervix measuring less than 25 mm was associated with an increased risk for preterm birth before 35 weeks of gestation (RR 2.15, 95% CI 1.15 to 4.01).[309] In 2015, Saccone et al. reported an individual patient data meta-analysis of randomized trials of women with a twin pregnancy and a cervical length less than 25 mm before 24 weeks of gestation.[310] Eligible women were randomized to cerclage versus no cerclage (control). After adjusting for prior preterm birth and gestational age at randomization, the authors found no statistically significant differences in the primary outcome of preterm birth at less than 34 weeks (adjusted odds ratio 1.17, 95% CI 0.23 to 3.79).

In a Letter to the Editor, Roman et al. highlighted the paucity of randomized controlled trials evaluating cerclage in women with a twin gestation and a short cervix since the publication of the 2005 meta-analysis.[311] Instead, there have been several retrospective studies suggesting that the management of twin pregnancies with a short cervix is an unresolved topic. In a retrospective cohort study of 140 women, Roman et al. reported that the use of cerclage in asymptomatic twin pregnancies with transvaginal cervical length less than or equal to 25 mm between 16 and 24 weeks of gestation was not associated with decreased rates of preterm birth compared to that in controls.[312] However, among those patients with a cervical length less than 15 mm who were managed with cerclage, there was a significantly prolonged interval to delivery of almost 4 additional weeks, a significant reduction of 49% in the rate of spontaneous preterm birth occurring at less than 34 weeks of gestation, and a significant reduction of 58% in the rate of admission to the NICU, as compared to controls.

In a recent publication, Li et al. reported the results of a systematic review and meta-analysis of both randomized controlled trials and cohort studies comparing women with a twin pregnancy who received cerclage versus no cerclage.[313] The authors reported that cerclage placement for cervical length less than 15 mm was associated with significant pregnancy prolongation by a mean difference of 3.89 weeks and a significant reduction in preterm birth at less than 37, less than 34, and less than 32 weeks of gestation, compared to that in the control group. Further, cerclage placement for cervical dilation greater than 10 mm was associated with significant pregnancy prolongation by a mean difference of 6.78 weeks and a significant reduction in preterm birth at less than 34, less than 32, less than 28, and less than 24 weeks of gestation, compared to that in the control group. In this study, cerclage placement was not beneficial for twin pregnancies with a cervical length greater than 15 mm. The authors concluded that cerclage placement is beneficial in twin pregnancies with a cervical length less than 15 mm or a dilated cervix greater than 10 mm.

In response to the meta-analysis reported by Li et al.,[313] Sanchez-Ramos underscored the fact that the conclusions supporting the benefit of cerclage were based solely on data from three retrospective studies rather than on data from randomized controlled trials.[314] From these three cohort studies, Sanchez-Ramos highlighted the differences in clinical characteristics among those who received cerclage placement and those who did not: (1) proportion who had undergone assisted reproductive technologies, (2) race, (3) rate of previous preterm birth, and (4) the use of supplemental vaginal progesterone. Moreover, the results of the separately analyzed randomized controlled trials indicated that cerclage placement was associated with an increased risk of preterm birth and adverse perinatal outcome.

The data from randomized controlled trials are limited and, in combination with cohort studies, still do not provide enough evidence to make a strong recommendation in the management of asymptomatic women with a twin gestation and a short cervical length. Therefore, many authors involved in these studies have highlighted the need for additional randomized controlled trials to assess this issue.

Cerclage versus Vaginal Progesterone

There are no prospective randomized trials that directly compare vaginal progesterone and cervical cerclage for the prevention of preterm birth in women with a short cervix in the

| TABLE 14.8 Direct Comparisons between Vaginal Progesterone and Placebo, and Cerclage and No Cerclage, and Indirect Comparison between Vaginal Progesterone and Cerclage in Women with a Short Cervix and History of Previous Preterm Delivery for Prediction of Preterm Birth and Perinatal Mortality |

	VAGINAL PROGESTERONE VS. PLACEBO			CERCLAGE VS. NO CERCLAGE			VAGINAL PROGESTERONE VS. CERCLAGE	
	VAGINAL PROGESTERONE	PLACEBO	RELATIVE RISK (95% CI)	CERCLAGE	NO CERCLAGE	RELATIVE RISK (95% CI)	RELATIVE RISK (95% CI)	P VALUE
Preterm birth <35 weeks	22/58 (38%)	31/55 (56%)	0.64 (0.42–0.98)	28/80 (35%)	43/74 (58%)	0.59 (0.42–0.83)	1.09 (0.63–1.87)	0.87
Preterm birth <32 weeks	18/58 (31%)	23/55 (42%)	0.69 (0.42–1.14)	18/80 (23%)	33/74 (45%)	0.50 (0.32–0.78)	1.38 (0.71–2.69)	0.54
Perinatal mortality	2/58 (3%)	5/55 (9%)	0.39 (0.10–1.51)	11/80 (14%)	16/74 (22%)	0.59 (0.31–1.14)	0.66 (0.15–2.98)	0.67

Reprinted from Conde-Agudelo A, Romero R, Da Fonseca E, et al. Vaginal progesterone is as effective as cervical cerclage to prevent preterm birth in women with a singleton gestation, previous spontaneous preterm birth, and a short cervix: updated indirect comparison meta-analysis. *Am J Obstet Gynecol.* 2018;219(1):10–25. Copyright © 2018 Elsevier. With permission.

midtrimester and previous preterm birth. The previously described study of Conde-Agudelo et al.[58] on the indirect comparison between vaginal progesterone and cerclage showed that vaginal progesterone is as effective as cerclage in reducing the rate of preterm delivery in women with a previous history of preterm delivery and a short cervix (Table 14.8). Furthermore, vaginal progesterone seems to have a greater impact on reducing neonatal morbidity compared to cerclage placement. Nevertheless, even though both interventions appear to be effective, cerclage has inherent risks that are greater than vaginal progesterone; thus, a discussion and consideration of treatment should include the risks associated with each treatment (surgical vs. medical) as well as costs and patient/clinician preferences.

Cervical Pessary

Cervical pessaries have been proposed as an alternative method to reduce the prevalence of preterm delivery in woman with a short cervix.[315,316] Goya et al.[57] reported an open-label randomized controlled study (PECEP [Pesario Cervical para Evitar Prematuridad] trial) in women with a midtrimester short cervix less than or equal to 25 mm treated with a pessary placement versus women receiving expectant management (Fig. 14.21). The authors reported a significant 78% reduction in the prevalence of spontaneous preterm delivery at less than 34 weeks of gestation in patients who received a pessary when compared to those in the control group. This reduction in preterm birth suggests that cervical pessary placement may be effective. However, given the high preterm delivery rate of 27% at less than 34 weeks of gestation in the expectant management group, some have raised concerns regarding the generalizability of this treatment. Another multicenter open-label randomized noninferiority trial done in Spain compared cervical pessary and vaginal progesterone for the prevention of preterm delivery at less than 34 weeks of gestation in women with a short cervix at midgestation. The study included 27 hospitals and 254 patients (127 treated with pessary and 119 with vaginal

progesterone). The authors reported that cervical pessary was not inferior to vaginal progesterone in reducing the prevalence of preterm delivery at less than 34 weeks of gestation.[317]

On the contrary, Hui et al.[318] reported the results of a randomized trial including 108 asymptomatic women with a singleton pregnancy and a short cervix less than or equal to 25 mm at midgestation. Patients were randomized to pessary versus expectant management. The authors did not find a significant reduction in preterm birth between the groups (5.5% treated with pessary vs. 9.4% with expectant management). Nicolaides et al.[319] conducted a multicenter randomized controlled trial in asymptomatic women at 20 to 24 weeks of gestation with a short cervix less than or equal to 25 mm; 465 participants received a vaginal pessary and 467 received expectant management. All pregnant women with a cervical length less than 15 mm received vaginal progesterone. There was no difference in the rate of preterm delivery at less than 34 weeks of gestation or in neonatal morbidity between women treated with pessary placement and those managed expectantly. The authors reported an increased incidence in vaginal discharge in women treated with pessary. Saccone et al.[320] performed a systematic review and meta-analysis, including the three randomized trials comparing pessary placement to expectant management for the prevention of preterm delivery[322] in asymptomatic women with a singleton pregnancy and a short cervix. A total of 1,420 women were included in the analysis. The results showed no significant reduction in the prevalence of preterm birth at less than 34 weeks, at less than 32 weeks, and at less than 28 weeks of gestation in women treated with a cervical pessary. No reduction in neonatal morbidity was observed. The use of a vaginal pessary was associated with a higher prevalence of vaginal discharge.

A recent systematic review and meta-analysis was published by Conde-Agudelo et al. aiming to evaluate the efficiency and safety of cervical pessary for preventing preterm delivery at less than 34

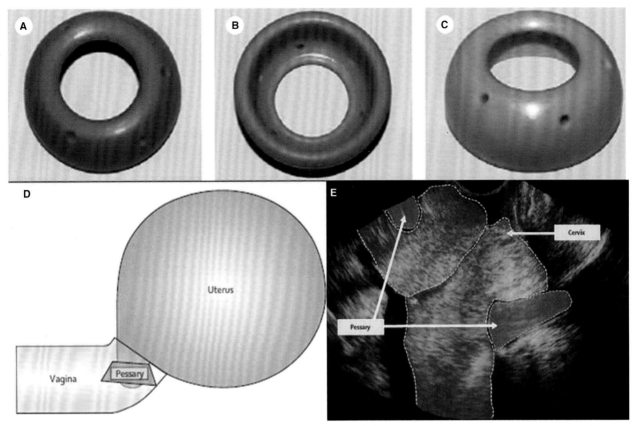

FIGURE 14.21: Cervical pessary: **A:** inner diameter; **B:** outer diameter; **C:** lateral view. **D:** The smaller diameter of the pessary is fitted around the cervix and the larger diameter faces the pelvic floor, thus rotating the cervix to the posterior vaginal wall and correcting the cervical angle; **E:** ultrasound visualization of cervical length in women with a cervical pessary. (Reprinted from Goya M, Pratcorona L, Merced C, et al. Cervical pessary in pregnant women with a short cervix (PECEP): an open-label randomised controlled trial. Lancet. 2012;379(9828):1800–1806. Copyright © 2012 Elsevier. With permission; and From Goya M, Pratcorona L, Higueras T, et al. Sonographic cervical length measurement in pregnant women with a cervical pessary. *Ultrasound Obstet Gynecol.* 2011;38(2):205–209. Copyright © 2011 ISUOG. Reprinted by permission of John Wiley & Sons, Inc.)[336]

weeks of gestation in women with a short cervix.[321] The systematic review included 12 studies: 8 comparing pessary versus no pessary in singleton pregnancies; 2 comparing pessary versus no pessary in multiple pregnancies; and 2 comparing pessary versus vaginal progesterone. The results showed that in women with either a singleton or a twin pregnancy and a short cervix (≤25 mm), the use of a pessary did not reduce the rate of preterm delivery at less than 34 weeks when compared to women not using a pessary (singleton pregnancies: RR, 1.05 [95% CI, 0.79 to 1.41]; twin pregnancies; [RR 0.72; 95% CI, 0.25 to 2.06]). As secondary outcomes, a vaginal pessary did not reduce the rate of preterm delivery at less than 37, less than 32, and less than 28 weeks of gestation or the rate of neonatal complications when compared to women not receiving a pessary. Two studies showed no differences in the rate of preterm delivery at less than 34 weeks between cervical pessary and vaginal progesterone; however, these studies were based on very low-quality evidence. The rate of pessary removal ranged from 0.5% to 51.7% in singleton pregnancies and from 2.9% to 69.6% in twin pregnancies as a result of preterm labor with no response to tocolytic treatment, active vaginal bleeding, preterm prelabor rupture of the membranes, severe patient discomfort, and patient request. The authors concluded that the available evidence does not support the use of cervical pessary to prevent preterm delivery in singleton or twin pregnancies with a short cervix.

The STOPPIT (Study of Progesterone for the Prevention of Preterm Birth in Twins) 2 open-label randomized trial from the United Kingdom and Belgium included 503 women with a twin pregnancy at 18[+0] and 20[+6] weeks of gestation whose cervical length was less than or equal to 35 mm; these patients were randomized either to cervical Arabin pessary and standard care or to standard care only.[322] The results showed no difference in the rate of preterm delivery at less than 34 weeks between the groups and no difference in the prevalence of neonatal outcomes, including stillbirth, neonatal death, periventricular leukomalacia, early respiratory morbidity, intraventricular hemorrhage, necrotizing enterocolitis, or proven sepsis. The authors concluded that the cervical Arabin pessary is ineffective in the prevention of preterm birth in women with a twin pregnancy and a short cervix.

Cervical Length Measurement after Pessary Placement

Goya et al.[323] reported a new TVS technique for visualization of cervical length after pessary placement. The ultrasound probe is placed in the space between the pessary and the posterior vaginal wall, if possible, touching the external cervical os or the anterior cervical lip (Fig. 14.21D). The authors compared the agreement of cervical length measurements obtained by this new technique to cervical length measurements obtained using the standard transvaginal and the transperineal sonography techniques in 48 women who had pessary placement due to a short cervix less than or equal to 25 mm (Fig. 14.22).

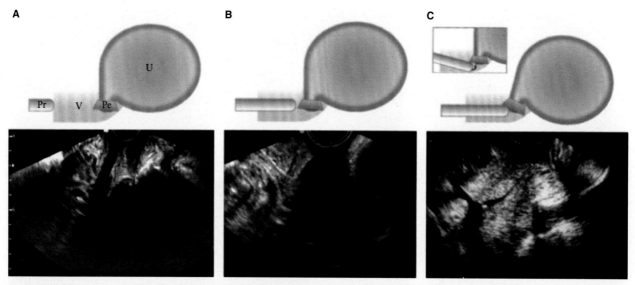

FIGURE 14.22: Ultrasound evaluation of the cervical length using **(A)** transperineal ultrasound **(B)** transvaginal ultrasound with the probe in the anterior fornix (standard approach), and **(C)** the new transvaginal measurement approach with the probe just inside the pessary. *Pe*, pessary; *Pr*, probe; *U*, uterus; *V*, vagina. (From Goya M, Pratcorona L, Higueras T, et al. Sonographic cervical length measurement in pregnant women with a cervical pessary. *Ultrasound Obstet Gynecol.* 2011;38(2):205–209. Copyright © 2011 ISUOG. Reprinted by permission of John Wiley & Sons, Inc.)

The results showed lower interobserver differences using the new transvaginal technique as compared to the standard transvaginal or the transperineal sonography techniques. The interobserver correlation coefficients were as follows: 0.97 (95% CI, 0.95 to 0.98) for the new transvaginal technique, 0.65 (95% CI, 0.44 to 0.79) for the standard transvaginal technique, and 0.58 (95% CI, 0.34 to 0.75) for the transperineal technique. A Bland–Altman analysis showed a mean difference between operators of −0.01 (95% limits of agreement [LA], −2.57 to 2.55 mm) for the new transvaginal technique; −0.23 (95% LA, −10.90 to 10.44 mm) for the standard transvaginal technique; and −0.99 (95% LA, −13.23 to 11.25 mm) for the transperineal technique. The authors concluded that the new transvaginal technique may be helpful in monitoring the cervical length during pregnancy in patients carrying a cervical pessary.[323]

In a retrospective cohort study of 35 patients who had pessary placement after measurement of a short cervix less than or equal to 25 mm, Bolanos et al.[324] reported a significant increase in cervical length from 12.4 mm at the time of pessary placement (gestational age 24 weeks) to 19.2 mm ($P < 0.001$) measured 1 week after pessary placement. The same authors reported no significant differences in cervical length in subsequent evaluations at 26 weeks (17.8 mm) and at 28 weeks (16 mm; $P = 0.148$).

In another study, the PECEP trial comprising 380 asymptomatic women with a short cervix (≤25 mm), 190 of them were managed with pessary and 190 with expectant management, Mendoza et al.[325] reported a significantly longer cervix (21.5 mm) after pessary placement than that in women managed expectantly (15.4 mm; $P < 0.0001$), despite both groups having a similar cervical length of 19.0 mm at randomization. Nevertheless, an increment in cervical length after pessary placement did not significantly correlate with an increase in gestational age at delivery ($r = 0.4$; 95% CI, 0.3 to 0.5). The authors reported that, after pessary, women delivering at less than 28 weeks and at less than 34 weeks of gestation had a higher prevalence of cervical

shortening. The same research group further reported that the median cervical length increased by 4.5 mm immediately after pessary insertion among asymptomatic women with a short cervix.[326] Although these studies demonstrated increased cervical length after cervical pessary placement, the clinical significance and the prognostic value of cervical length measurements after pessary placement warrant further investigation.

ALTERNATIVE IMAGING MODALITIES FOR CERVICAL EVALUATION

Although a short cervix is a powerful risk factor for preterm delivery, the assessment of cervical length alone still provides a low prediction for preterm delivery. Emerging imaging modalities that seek to evaluate different characteristics of the cervix, such as "softness" or "firmness" and tissue organization, might contribute to improved detection of women at risk of preterm delivery.

Ultrasound Elastography

Ultrasound-derived elastography has been applied to evaluate tissue elasticity, that is, softness or firmness. Two main modalities have been applied in the evaluation of the cervix: (1) strain elastography and (2) shear-wave elastography (SWE).[327]

Strain Elastography

Strain elastography is a qualitative or semiquantitative estimation of tissue displacement that can be related to the softness/firmness of tissues.[327–329] Strain images are generated by motion induced by the ultrasound transducer or caused by the physiological movement of tissues. Strain elastography generates a color map (Elastogram) based on the differences in strain within tissues (Fig. 14.23). The data are subjectively analyzed by the operator based on the color content (qualitative) or by a semiquantitative approach using a reference material to compare the displacement of the tissue; strain is then expressed as a ratio. Strain can also be estimated by averaging the displacement (rest-motion) of all the tissues included in a region of interest.[329] The main challenge of strain elastography is the standardization of the mechanical compression needed to create tissue displacement.[330] Several groups reported an association between increased cervical strain and preterm delivery.[331–337] Our group observed that increased/reduced strain in the internal cervical os evaluated at 16 to 24 weeks of gestation is related to a higher or lower risk of preterm delivery at less than 34 weeks of gestation, respectively, as compared to women with normal strain values in the cervix.[334]

Shear-Wave Elastography

SWE estimates tissue elasticity by quantifying the velocity of propagation of an acoustic radiation force impulse (ARFI). The ARFI is generated by the ultrasound system and propagates within the tissues as shear waves. Depending on the softness/firmness of the tissue, the velocity of propagation will be slower or faster, respectively.[338] The ultrasound system tracks the velocity of propagation of the shear waves using ultrafast ultrasound emission. Data are presented either as velocity (meters/second) or as pressure (Kilopascals).[339,340] A low velocity of propagation is associated with soft tissues, and an increased velocity with stiff tissues. SWE also creates a color map based on the velocities of propagation of the shear waves within a region of interest (Fig. 14.24).[341] SWE provides a more reproducible, reliable estimation of the elastic properties of the cervix than does strain elastography. A reduced or an increased shear-wave velocity in the internal cervical os at 18 to 24 weeks of gestation is related to a soft or a stiff cervix and thus to an increased or a decreased risk for preterm delivery (Table 14.9), respectively, as compared to women with normal shear-wave

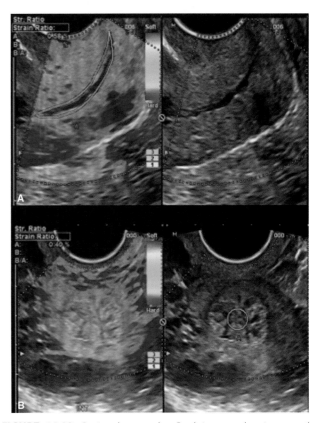

FIGURE 14.23: Strain elastography. Dual images showing, on the right side, the gray scale images of **(A)** sagittal plane of the cervix; **(B)** cross-sectional plane of the internal cervical os. On the left side, the superimposed color elastograms are shown. The color bar shows increased strain (*soft tissue*) in red color and reduced strain (*stiff tissue*) in blue color. The endocervical canal is delineated in the two images: (a) sagittal endocervical strain 0.58%; (b) internal cervical os strain 0.40%. Strain represents the averaged displacement within the region of interest.

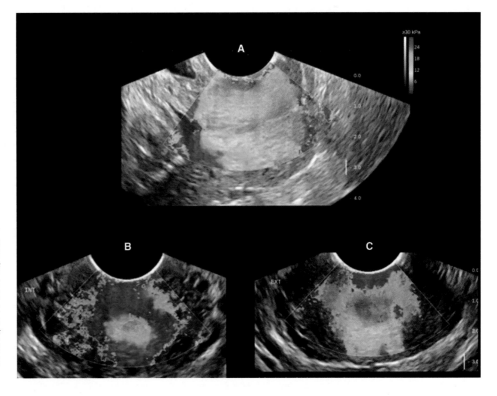

FIGURE 14.24: Shear-wave elastography of the cervix: **(A)** sagittal plane; **(B)** cross-sectional plane of the internal cervical os; **(C)** cross-sectional image of the external cervical os. The color bar shows in yellow to red color reduced velocity of propagation of the acoustic radiation impulse (*soft tissue*), and in green-blue color, increased velocity of propagation (*stiff tissue*). The internal cervical os is stiffer than is the external cervical os.

velocity in the internal os.[341] SWE is an independent factor to estimate the risk of preterm delivery and can also be used in women with a short cervix to identify those with a higher or lower risk of preterm delivery. Nevertheless, the use of elastography in clinical practice is not routine. Future research is needed to confirm that the changes in strain elastography and SWE correlate with changes in cervical remodeling and to evaluate the best use of this technology in risk assessment for preterm birth.

Acoustic Attenuation

Cervical tissue hydration increases as a function of cervical ripening and of advancing gestational age.[1-4,342] Acoustic attenuation, the loss of energy as an ultrasonic wave propagates through tissue, has been noted to be related to tissue stiffness, collagen concentration, and water concentration.[343] Forty women underwent transvaginal ultrasound that utilized a system allowing access to radiofrequency image data. Radiofrequency data were analyzed by implementing an attenuation coefficient derived from a tissue phantom. Regression analysis revealed that attenuation of the ultrasound signals by the cervical tissue was predictive of the exam-to-delivery interval (β = 0.43; P = 0.011). Interestingly, two pregnant women who participated in the study had a short cervical length in the midtrimester but moderate or high attenuation values, indicating an unripened cervix. Both women delivered at more than 34 weeks of gestation and remained pregnant for at least 11 weeks after the cervical length measurement. A limitation of the attenuation technique is the high variation between subjects in selecting the optimal regions of interest for evaluation. Furthermore, cervical tissue is nonhomogeneous, which may limit the application of an attenuation algorithm that relies on tissue homogeneity.[344] McFarlin et al.[345] evaluated 67 pregnant women at five time points during pregnancy from 17 to 39 weeks of gestation. Ultrasound attenuation was analyzed comparing the attenuation of the ultrasound signals obtained in different regions of the cervix with an attenuation value obtained from a tissue-mimicking reference phantom

(attenuation coefficient) using the same ultrasound settings. The results showed that the attenuation coefficient was lower at 17 to 19 weeks among women who delivered preterm at less than 37 weeks of gestation than that observed in women with a term delivery. The authors reported changes in cervical attenuation before changes were observed in cervical length.

Quantitative Analysis of Cervical Texture

This novel technique characterizes microstructural changes of the uterine cervix by analyzing speckle patterns. Quantitative analysis of cervical texture computes the distribution of binary patterns in the circular neighborhood of each pixel. Ultrasound images are obtained by following a specific protocol for image acquisition. Baños et al.[346] evaluated 310 pregnant women at 19 to 24 weeks of gestation: 283 delivered at term and 27 delivered at less than 37 weeks of gestation. The authors reported a total of 18 different speckle patterns in the cervix of patients delivering at term; variance from these specific patterns was associated with an increased risk of preterm delivery. Texture analysis seems to be independent of cervical length, showing a significant prediction of preterm delivery < 37 weeks when evaluated between 19 and 24[+6] weeks of gestation.

CONCLUSION

A large body of literature has examined the nature of cervical change during pregnancy in both human and animal studies. Cervical disease is one of the etiologies of the preterm parturition syndrome. The success of available treatments, such as progesterone or cerclage placement, requires the adequate identification of women with cervical disease. Treatment with progesterone or cerclage may benefit some patients who have a primary cervical condition and are in the reversible phase of parturition. It is clear that obstetrical history is insufficient to identify such patients; thus, cervical sonography represents an important tool for the identification of patients with premature cervical ripening. Further

TABLE 14.9 Shear-Wave Speed (SWS, m/s) in the Internal and the External Cervical Os at 18 to 24 Weeks of Gestation

GESTATIONAL WEEK	INTERNAL CERVICAL OS					EXTERNAL CERVICAL OS				
	10TH	25TH	50TH	75TH	95TH	10TH	25TH	50TH	75TH	95TH
18 (n = 90)	1.97	2.60	3.29*	3.99	4.62	1.41	1.91	2.46	3.02	3.52
19 (n = 88)	1.88	2.48	3.14*	3.81	4.41	1.38	1.84	2.36	2.88	3.35
20 (n = 107)	1.79	2.36	3.00*	3.64	4.21	1.35	1.78	2.27	2.75	3.19
21 (n = 99)	1.71	2.26	2.87*	3.48	4.02	1.32	1.72	2.18	2.63	3.04
22 (n = 85)	1.64	2.16	2.74*	3.33	3.85	1.29	1.67	2.10	2.52	2.91
23 (n = 61)	1.57	2.07	2.63*	3.19	3.69	1.26	1.62	2.02	2.42	2.78
24 (n = 98)	1.50	1.98	2.52*	3.06	3.54	1.24	1.58	1.95	2.33	2.67

*p = 0.001 as compared to the mean SWS in the external cervical os.
n, number of patients per week.
From Hernandez-Andrade E, Maymon E, Luewan S, et al. A soft cervix, categorized by shear-wave elastography, in women with short or with normal cervical length at 18–24 weeks is associated with a higher prevalence of spontaneous preterm delivery. J Perinat Med. 2018;46:489–501.

research, for example, on the biochemical characteristics of a short cervix in preterm gestation, may contribute to the differentiation of patients with a short cervix who will deliver before 37 weeks from those who will deliver at term as well as patients who may benefit from cerclage placement or progesterone therapy.

An important challenge is the development of a model to improve the prediction of spontaneous preterm birth. The following outstanding questions remain:

1. Can serum markers provide further individualized risk assessment for preterm delivery when combined with cervical length?
2. Does noninvasive assessment of collagen content provide prognostic information? (Quantitative ultrasonic tissue characterization of the cervix)
3. Do Doppler velocimetry and/or cervical gland evaluation have predictive value for preterm delivery?

ACKNOWLEDGMENTS

This research was supported, in part, by the Perinatology Research Branch, Division of Obstetrics and Maternal-Fetal Medicine, Division of Intramural Research, *Eunice Kennedy Shriver* National Institute of Child Health and Human Development, National Institutes of Health, U.S. Department of Health and Human Services (NICHD/NIH/DHHS); and, in part, with Federal funds from NICHD/NIH/DHHS under Contract No. HHSN275201300006C. This work is based on several review articles and chapters published previously by the authors in other publications. We thank Maureen McGerty and Andrea Bernard, (Wayne State University) for their critical reading(s) of the manuscript and/or editorial support.

REFERENCES

1. Maillot KV, Zimmermann BK. The solubility of collagen of the uterine cervix during pregnancy and labour. *Arch Gynakol.* 1976;220:275–280.
2. Kleissl HP, van der Rest M, Naftolin F, et al. Collagen changes in the human uterine cervix at parturition. *Am J Obstet Gynecol.* 1978;130:748–753.
3. Junqueira LC, Zugaib M, Montes GS, et al. Morphologic and histochemical evidence for the occurrence of collagenolysis and for the role of neutrophilic polymorphonuclear leukocytes during cervical dilation. *Am J Obstet Gynecol.* 1980;138:273–281.
4. Rajabi MR, Dodge GR, Solomon S, et al. Immunochemical and immunohistochemical evidence of estrogen-mediated collagenolysis as a mechanism of cervical dilatation in the guinea pig at parturition. *Endocrinology.* 1991;128:371–378.
5. Osmers RG, Blaser J, Kuhn W, et al. Interleukin-8 synthesis and the onset of labor. *Obstet Gynecol.* 1995;86:223–229.
6. Osman I, Young A, Ledingham MA, et al. Leukocyte density and pro-inflammatory cytokine expression in human fetal membranes, decidua, cervix and myometrium before and during labour at term. *Mol Hum Reprod.* 2003;9:41–45.
7. Sakamoto Y, Moran P, Searle RF, et al. Interleukin-8 is involved in cervical dilatation but not in prelabour cervical ripening. *Clin Exp Immunol.* 2004;138:151–157.
8. Word RA, Landrum CP, Timmons BC, et al. Transgene insertion on mouse chromosome 6 impairs function of the uterine cervix and causes failure of parturition. *Biol Reprod.* 2005;73:1046–1056.
9. Hassan SS, Romero R, Haddad R, et al. The transcriptome of the uterine cervix before and after spontaneous term parturition. *Am J Obstet Gynecol.* 2006;195:778–786.
10. Hassan SS, Romero R, Tarca AL, et al. Signature pathways identified from gene expression profiles in the human uterine cervix before and after spontaneous term parturition. *Am J Obstet Gynecol.* 2007;197:250.e1–250.e7.
11. Hassan SS, Romero R, Tarca AL, et al. The transcriptome of cervical ripening in human pregnancy before the onset of labor at term: identification of novel molecular functions involved in this process. *J Matern Fetal Neonatal Med.* 2009;22:1183–1193.
12. Hassan SS, Romero R, Pineles B, et al. MicroRNA expression profiling of the human uterine cervix after term labor and delivery. *Am J Obstet Gynecol.* 2010;202:80.e1–80.e8.
13. Hassan SS, Romero R, Tarca AL, et al. The molecular basis for sonographic cervical shortening at term: identification of differentially expressed genes and the epithelial-mesenchymal transition as a function of cervical length. *Am J Obstet Gynecol.* 2010;203:472.e1–472.e14.
14. Romero R, Espinoza J, Erez O, et al. The role of cervical cerclage in obstetric practice: can the patient who could benefit from this procedure be identified? *Am J Obstet Gynecol.* 2006;194:1–9.
15. Andersen HF, Nugent CE, Wanty SD, et al. Prediction of risk for preterm delivery by ultrasonographic measurement of cervical length. *Am J Obstet Gynecol.* 1990;163:859–867.
16. Iams JD, Paraskos J, Landon MB, et al. Cervical sonography in preterm labor. *Obstet Gynecol.* 1994;84:40–46.
17. Heath VC, Southall TR, Souka AP, et al. Cervical length at 23 weeks of gestation: prediction of spontaneous preterm delivery. *Ultrasound Obstet Gynecol.* 1998;12:312–317.
18. Hassan SS, Romero R, Berry SM, et al. Patients with an ultrasonographic cervical length < or =15 mm have nearly a 50% risk of early spontaneous preterm delivery. *Am J Obstet Gynecol.* 2000;182:1458–1467.
19. Huszar G, Naftolin F. The myometrium and uterine cervix in normal and preterm labor. *N Engl J Med.* 1984;311:571–581.
20. Meis PJ, Klebanoff M, Thom E, et al.; National Institute of Child Health and Human Development Maternal-Fetal Medicine Units Network. Prevention of recurrent preterm delivery by 17 alpha-hydroxyprogesterone caproate. *N Engl J Med.* 2003;348:2379–2385.
21. DeFranco EA, O'Brien JM, Adair CD, et al. Vaginal progesterone is associated with a decrease in risk for early preterm birth and improved neonatal outcome in women with a short cervix: a secondary analysis from a randomized, double-blind, placebo-controlled trial. *Ultrasound Obstet Gynecol.* 2007;30:697–705.
22. Fonseca EB, Celik E, Parra M, et al. Progesterone and the risk of preterm birth among women with a short cervix. *N Engl J Med.* 2007;357:462–469.
23. Hassan SS, Romero R, Vidyadhari D, et al. Vaginal progesterone reduces the rate of preterm birth in women with a sonographic short cervix: a multicenter, randomized, double-blind, placebo-controlled trial. *Ultrasound Obstet Gynecol.* 2011;38:18–31.
24. Romero R, Nicolaides K, Conde-Agudelo A, et al. Vaginal progesterone in women with an asymptomatic sonographic short cervix in the midtrimester decreases preterm delivery and neonatal morbidity: a systematic review and meta-analysis of individual patient data. *Am J Obstet Gynecol.* 2012;206:124.e1–e19.
25. Kushnir O, Vigil DA, Izquierdo L, et al. Vaginal ultrasonographic assessment of cervical length changes during normal pregnancy. *Am J Obstet Gynecol.* 1990;162:991–993.
26. Andersen HF. Transvaginal and transabdominal ultrasonography of the uterine cervix during pregnancy. *J Clin Ultrasound.* 1991;19:77–83.
27. Okitsu O, Mimura T, Nakayama T, et al. Early prediction of preterm delivery by transvaginal ultrasonography. *Ultrasound Obstet Gynecol.* 1992;2:402–409.
28. Iams JD, Johnson FF, Sonek J, et al. Cervical competence as a continuum: a study of ultrasonographic cervical length and obstetric performance. *Am J Obstet Gynecol.* 1995;172:1097–1103; discussion 1104–1096.
29. Iams JD, Goldenberg RL, Meis PJ, et al. The length of the cervix and the risk of spontaneous premature delivery. National Institute of Child Health and Human Development Maternal Fetal Medicine Unit Network. *N Engl J Med.* 1996;334:567–572.
30. Hasegawa I, Tanaka K, Takahashi K, et al. Transvaginal ultrasonographic cervical assessment for the prediction of preterm delivery. *J Matern Fetal Med.* 1996;5:305–309.
31. Berghella V, Kuhlman K, Weiner S, et al. Cervical funneling: sonographic criteria predictive of preterm delivery. *Ultrasound Obstet Gynecol.* 1997;10:161–166.
32. Goldenberg RL, Iams JD, Mercer BM, et al. The preterm prediction study: the value of new vs standard risk factors in predicting early and all spontaneous preterm births. NICHD MFMU Network. *Am J Public Health.* 1998;88:233–238.
33. Guzman ER, Mellon C, Vintzileos AM, et al. Longitudinal assessment of endocervical canal length between 15 and 24 weeks' gestation in women at risk for pregnancy loss or preterm birth. *Obstet Gynecol.* 1998;92:31–37.
34. Taipale P, Hiilesmaa V. Sonographic measurement of uterine cervix at 18–22 weeks' gestation and the risk of preterm delivery. *Obstet Gynecol.* 1998;92:902–907.
35. Watson WJ, Stevens D, Welter S, et al. Observations on the sonographic measurement of cervical length and the risk of premature birth. *J Matern Fetal Med.* 1999;8:17–19.
36. Andrews WW, Copper R, Hauth JC, et al. Second-trimester cervical ultrasound: associations with increased risk for recurrent early spontaneous delivery. *Obstet Gynecol.* 2000;95:222–226.
37. Hibbard JU, Tart M, Moawad AH. Cervical length at 16–22 weeks' gestation and risk for preterm delivery. *Obstet Gynecol.* 2000;96:972–978.
38. Owen J, Yost N, Berghella V, et al.; National Institute of Child Health and Human Development, Maternal-Fetal Medicine Units Network. Mid-trimester endovaginal sonography in women at high risk for spontaneous preterm birth. *JAMA.* 2001;286:1340–1348.
39. To MS, Skentou C, Liao AW, et al. Cervical length and funneling at 23 weeks of gestation in the prediction of spontaneous early preterm delivery. *Ultrasound Obstet Gynecol.* 2001;18:200–203.
40. Durnwald CP, Walker H, Lundy JC, et al. Rates of recurrent preterm birth by obstetrical history and cervical length. *Am J Obstet Gynecol.* 2005;193:1170–1174.
41. Matijevic R, Grgic O, Vasilj O. Is sonographic assessment of cervical length better than digital examination in screening for preterm delivery in a low-risk population? *Acta Obstet Gynecol Scand.* 2006;85:1342–1347.
42. Behrman RE, Butler AS, eds. *Preterm Birth: Causes, Consequences, and Prevention.* Washington, DC: National Academies Press; 2007.

43. Frey HA, Klebanoff MA. The epidemiology, etiology, and costs of preterm birth. *Semin Fetal Neonatal Med.* 2016;21:68–73.
44. Ananth CV, Vintzileos AM. Epidemiology of preterm birth and its clinical subtypes. *J Matern Fetal Neonatal Med.* 2006;19:773–782.
45. Moss TJ. Respiratory consequences of preterm birth. *Clin Exp Pharmacol Physiol.* 2006;33:280–284.
46. Rose AT, Patel RM. A critical analysis of risk factors for necrotizing enterocolitis. *Semin Fetal Neonatal Med.* 2018;23:374–379.
47. Collins A, Weitkamp JH, Wynn JL. Why are preterm newborns at increased risk of infection? *Arch Dis Child Fetal Neonatal Ed.* 2018;103:F391–F394.
48. Stavsky M, Mor O, Mastrolia SA, et al. Cerebral palsy-trends in epidemiology and recent development in prenatal mechanisms of disease, treatment, and prevention. *Front Pediatr.* 2017;5:21.
49. Pascal A, Govaert P, Oostra A, et al. Neurodevelopmental outcome in very preterm and very-low-birthweight infants born over the past decade: a meta-analytic review. *Dev Med Child Neurol.* 2018;60:342–355.
50. Bos AF, Roze E. Neurodevelopmental outcome in preterm infants. *Dev Med Child Neurol.* 2011;53(suppl 4):35–39.
51. Martin JA, Hamilton BE, Osterman MJK. Births in the United States, 2017. *NCHS Data Brief.* 2018:1–8.
52. Romero R, Espinoza J, Kusanovic JP, et al. The preterm parturition syndrome. *BJOG.* 2006;113(suppl 3):17–42.
53. Romero R, Yeo L, Miranda J, et al. A blueprint for the prevention of preterm birth: vaginal progesterone in women with a short cervix. *J Perinat Med.* 2013;41:27–44.
54. Althuisius SM, Dekker GA, Hummel P, et al. Final results of the Cervical Incompetence Prevention Randomized Cerclage Trial (CIPRACT): therapeutic cerclage with bed rest versus bed rest alone. *Am J Obstet Gynecol.* 2001;185:1106–1112.
55. Celik E, To M, Gajewska K, et al. Cervical length and obstetric history predict spontaneous preterm birth: development and validation of a model to provide individualized risk assessment. *Ultrasound Obstet Gynecol.* 2008;31:549–554.
56. Owen J, Hankins G, Iams JD, et al. Multicenter randomized trial of cerclage for preterm birth prevention in high-risk women with shortened midtrimester cervical length. *Am J Obstet Gynecol.* 2009;201:375.e1–375.e8.
57. Goya M, Pratcorona L, Merced C, et al. Cervical pessary in pregnant women with a short cervix (PECEP): an open-label randomised controlled trial. *Lancet.* 2012;379:1800–1806.
58. Conde-Agudelo A, Romero R, Nicolaides K, et al. Vaginal progesterone vs. cervical cerclage for the prevention of preterm birth in women with a sonographic short cervix, previous preterm birth, and singleton gestation: a systematic review and indirect comparison metaanalysis. *Am J Obstet Gynecol.* 2013;208:42.e1–42.e2.e18.
59. Mason GC, Maresh MJ. Alterations in bladder volume and the ultrasound appearance of the cervix. *Br J Obstet Gynaecol.* 1990;97:457–458.
60. To MS, Skentou C, Cicero S, et al. Cervical assessment at the routine 23-weeks' scan: problems with transabdominal sonography. *Ultrasound Obstet Gynecol.* 2000;15:292–296.
61. Hernandez-Andrade E, Romero R, Ahn H, et al. Transabdominal evaluation of uterine cervical length during pregnancy fails to identify a substantial number of women with a short cervix. *J Matern Fetal Neonatal Med.* 2012;25:1682–1689.
62. Jeanty P, d'Alton M, Romero R, et al. Perineal scanning. *Am J Perinatol.* 1986;3:289–295.
63. Zilianti M, Azuaga A, Calderon F, et al. Monitoring the effacement of the uterine cervix by transperineal sonography: a new perspective. *J Ultrasound Med.* 1995;14:719–724.
64. Cicero S, Skentou C, Souka A, et al. Cervical length at 22–24 weeks of gestation: comparison of transvaginal and transperineal-translabial ultrasonography. *Ultrasound Obstet Gynecol.* 2001;17:335–340.
65. Hertzberg BS, Livingston E, DeLong DM, et al. Ultrasonographic evaluation of the cervix: transperineal versus endovaginal imaging. *J Ultrasound Med.* 2001;20:1071–1078.
66. Yazici G, Yildiz A, Tiras MB, et al. Comparison of transperineal and transvaginal sonography in predicting preterm delivery. *J Clin Ultrasound.* 2004;32:225–230.
67. Meijer-Hoogeveen M, Stoutenbeek P, Visser GH. Transperineal versus transvaginal sonographic cervical length measurement in second- and third-trimester pregnancies. *Ultrasound Obstet Gynecol.* 2008;32:657–662.
68. Sonek JD, Iams JD, Blumenfeld M, et al. Measurement of cervical length in pregnancy: comparison between vaginal ultrasonography and digital examination. *Obstet Gynecol.* 1990;76:172–175.
69. Burger M, Weber-Rossler T, Willmann M. Measurement of the pregnant cervix by transvaginal sonography: an interobserver study and new standards to improve the interobserver variability. *Ultrasound Obstet Gynecol.* 1997;9:188–193.
70. To MS, Skentou C, Chan C, et al. Cervical assessment at the routine 23-week scan: standardizing techniques. *Ultrasound Obstet Gynecol.* 2001;17:217–219.
71. Yost NP, Bloom SL, Twickler DM, et al. Pitfalls in ultrasonic cervical length measurement for predicting preterm birth. *Obstet Gynecol.* 1999;93:510–516.
72. AIUM. Guidelines for Cleaning and Preparing External- and Internal-Use Ultrasound Transducers Between Patients, Safe Handling, and Use of Ultrasound Coupling Gel. Official Statement; www.aium.org 2018.
73. Berghella V, Talucci M, Desai A. Does transvaginal sonographic measurement of cervical length before 14 weeks predict preterm delivery in high-risk pregnancies? *Ultrasound Obstet Gynecol.* 2003;21:140–144.
74. Carvalho MH, Bittar RE, Brizot ML, et al. Cervical length at 11–14 weeks' and 22–24 weeks' gestation evaluated by transvaginal sonography, and gestational age at delivery. *Ultrasound Obstet Gynecol.* 2003;21:135–139.
75. Conoscenti G, Meir YJ, D'Ottavio G, et al. Does cervical length at 13–15 weeks' gestation predict preterm delivery in an unselected population? *Ultrasound Obstet Gynecol.* 2003;21:128–134.
76. Antsaklis P, Daskalakis G, Pilalis A, et al. The role of cervical length measurement at 11–14 weeks for the prediction of preterm delivery. *J Matern Fetal Neonatal Med.* 2011;24:465–470.
77. Greco E, Lange A, Ushakov F, et al. Prediction of spontaneous preterm delivery from endocervical length at 11 to 13 weeks. *Prenat Diagn.* 2011;31:84–89.
78. Souka AP, Papastefanou I, Michalitsi V, et al. Cervical length changes from the first to second trimester of pregnancy, and prediction of preterm birth by first-trimester sonographic cervical measurement. *J Ultrasound Med.* 2011;30:997–1002.
79. Greco E, Gupta R, Syngelaki A, et al. First-trimester screening for spontaneous preterm delivery with maternal characteristics and cervical length. *Fetal Diagn Ther.* 2012;31:154–161.
80. Sananes N, Schuller E, Gaudineau A, et al. What is predictive of preterm delivery in the first trimester: isthmus or cervical length? *Prenat Diagn.* 2013;33:894–898.
81. Parra-Cordero M, Sepulveda-Martinez A, Rencoret G, et al. Is there a role for cervical assessment and uterine artery Doppler in the first trimester of pregnancy as a screening test for spontaneous preterm delivery? *Ultrasound Obstet Gynecol.* 2014;43:291–296.
82. Papastefanou I, Kavalakis I, Pilalis A, et al. First trimester cervical length is associated with mid-trimester loss. *J Matern Fetal Neonatal Med.* 2016;29:51–54.
83. Wulff CB, Rode L, Rosthoj S, et al. Transvaginal sonographic cervical length in first and second trimesters in a low-risk population: a prospective study. *Ultrasound Obstet Gynecol.* 2018;51:604–613.
84. Zorzoli A, Soliani A, Perra M, et al. Cervical changes throughout pregnancy as assessed by transvaginal sonography. *Obstet Gynecol.* 1994;84:960–964.
85. Cook CM, Ellwood DA. A longitudinal study of the cervix in pregnancy using transvaginal ultrasound. *Br J Obstet Gynaecol.* 1996;103:16–18.
86. Bergelin I, Valentin L. Patterns of normal change in cervical length and width during pregnancy in nulliparous women: a prospective, longitudinal ultrasound study. *Ultrasound Obstet Gynecol.* 2001;18:217–222.
87. Theron G, Schabort C, Norman K, et al. Centile charts of cervical length between 18 and 32 weeks of gestation. *Int J Gynaecol Obstet.* 2008;103:144–148.
88. Riley L, Frigoletto FD Jr., Benacerraf BR. The implications of sonographically identified cervical changes in patients not necessarily at risk for preterm birth. *J Ultrasound Med.* 1992;11:75–79.
89. Tongsong T, Kamprapanth P, Srisomboon J, et al. Single transvaginal sonographic measurement of cervical length early in the third trimester as a predictor of preterm delivery. *Obstet Gynecol.* 1995;86:184–187.
90. de Carvalho MH, Bittar RE, Brizot Mde L, et al. Prediction of preterm delivery in the second trimester. *Obstet Gynecol.* 2005;105:532–536.
91. Leung TN, Pang MW, Leung TY, et al. Cervical length at 18–22 weeks of gestation for prediction of spontaneous preterm delivery in Hong Kong Chinese women. *Ultrasound Obstet Gynecol.* 2005;26:713–717.
92. Owen J, Yost N, Berghella V, et al. Can shortened midtrimester cervical length predict very early spontaneous preterm birth? *Am J Obstet Gynecol.* 2004;191:298–303.
93. Airoldi J, Berghella V, Sehdev H, et al. Transvaginal ultrasonography of the cervix to predict preterm birth in women with uterine anomalies. *Obstet Gynecol.* 2005;106:553–556.
94. Visintine J, Berghella V, Henning D, et al. Cervical length for prediction of preterm birth in women with multiple prior induced abortions. *Ultrasound Obstet Gynecol.* 2008;31:198–200.
95. Orzechowski KM, Boelig RC, Berghella V. Cervical length screening in asymptomatic women at high risk and low risk for spontaneous preterm birth. *Clin Obstet Gynecol.* 2016;59:241–251.
96. Rozenberg P, Gillet A, Ville Y. Transvaginal sonographic examination of the cervix in asymptomatic pregnant women: review of the literature. *Ultrasound Obstet Gynecol.* 2002;19:302–311.
97. Welsh A, Nicolaides K. Cervical screening for preterm delivery. *Curr Opin Obstet Gynecol.* 2002;14:195–202.
98. Erasmus I, Nicolaou E, van Gelderen CJ, et al. Cervical length at 23 weeks' gestation—relation to demographic characteristics and previous obstetric history in South African women. *S Afr Med J.* 2005;95:691–695.
99. Souka AP, Papastefanou I, Pilalis A, et al. Implementation of universal screening for preterm delivery by mid-trimester cervical-length measurement. *Ultrasound Obstet Gynecol.* 2019;53:396–401.
100. Smith GC, Celik E, To M, et al. Cervical length at mid-pregnancy and the risk of primary cesarean delivery. *N Engl J Med.* 2008;358:1346–1353.
101. Rosenbloom JI, Raghuraman N, Temming LA, et al. Predictive value of midtrimester universal cervical length screening based on parity. *J Ultrasound Med.* 2019. doi:10.1002/jum.15091.
102. Palatnik A, Miller ES, Son M, et al. Association among maternal obesity, cervical length, and preterm birth. *Am J Perinatol.* 2017;34:471–479.
103. Venkatesh KK, Cantonwine DE, Zera C, et al. Is there an association between body mass index and cervical length? Implications for obesity and cervical length management in pregnancy. *Am J Perinatol.* 2017;34:568–575.

104. Buck JN, Orzechowski KM, Berghella V. Racial disparities in cervical length for prediction of preterm birth in a low risk population. *J Matern Fetal Neonatal Med.* 2017;30:1851–1854.

105. van der Ven AJ, van Os MA, Kleinrouweler CE, et al. Is cervical length associated with maternal characteristics? *Eur J Obstet Gynecol Reprod Biol.* 2015;188:12–16.

106. Gagel CK, Rafael TJ, Berghella V. Is short stature associated with short cervical length? *Am J Perinatol.* 2010;27:691–695.

107. Cook CM, Ellwood DA. The cervix as a predictor of preterm delivery in "at-risk" women. *Ultrasound Obstet Gynecol.* 2000;15:109–113.

108. Mercer BM, Goldenberg RL, Meis PJ, et al. The Preterm Prediction Study: prediction of preterm premature rupture of membranes through clinical findings and ancillary testing. The National Institute of Child Health and Human Development Maternal-Fetal Medicine Units Network. *Am J Obstet Gynecol.* 2000;183:738–745.

109. Odibo AO, Berghella V, Reddy U, et al. Does transvaginal ultrasound of the cervix predict preterm premature rupture of membranes in a high-risk population? *Ultrasound Obstet Gynecol.* 2001;18:223–227.

110. Kishida T, Yamada H, Furuta I, et al. Increased levels of interleukin-6 in cervical secretions and assessment of the uterine cervix by transvaginal ultrasonography predict preterm premature rupture of the membranes. *Fetal Diagn Ther.* 2003;18:98–104.

111. Yost NP, Owen J, Berghella V, et al.; National Institute of Child Health and Human Development Maternal-Fetal Medicine Units Network. Number and gestational age of prior preterm births does not modify the predictive value of a short cervix. *Am J Obstet Gynecol.* 2004;191:241–246.

112. Crane JM, Hutchens D. Transvaginal sonographic measurement of cervical length to predict preterm birth in asymptomatic women at increased risk: a systematic review. *Ultrasound Obstet Gynecol.* 2008;31:579–587.

113. Vaisbuch E, Romero R, Erez O, et al. Clinical significance of early (<20 weeks) vs. late (20–24 weeks) detection of sonographic short cervix in asymptomatic women in the mid-trimester. *Ultrasound Obstet Gynecol.* 2010;36:471–481.

114. Poon LC, Savvas M, Zamblera D, et al. Large loop excision of transformation zone and cervical length in the prediction of spontaneous preterm delivery. *BJOG.* 2012;119:692–698.

115. Crane JM, Hutchens D. Transvaginal ultrasonographic measurement of cervical length in asymptomatic high-risk women with a short cervical length in the previous pregnancy. *Ultrasound Obstet Gynecol.* 2011;38:38–43.

116. Pils S, Eppel W, Seemann R, et al. Sequential cervical length screening in pregnancies after loop excision of the transformation zone conisation: a retrospective analysis. *BJOG.* 2014;121:457–462.

117. Hughes K, Kane SC, Araujo Junior E, et al. Cervical length as a predictor for spontaneous preterm birth in high-risk singleton pregnancy: current knowledge. *Ultrasound Obstet Gynecol.* 2016;48:7–15.

118. Crane J, Scott H, Stewart A, et al. Transvaginal ultrasonography to predict preterm birth in women with bicornuate or didelphus uterus. *J Matern Fetal Neonatal Med.* 2012;25:1960–1964.

119. Parikh MN, Mehta AC. Internal cervical os during the second half of pregnancy. *J Obstet Gynaecol Br Emp.* 1961;68:818–821.

120. Guzman ER, Mellon R, Vintzileos AM, et al. Relationship between endocervical canal length between 15–24 weeks gestation and obstetric history. *J Matern Fetal Med.* 1998;7:269–272.

121. Guzman ER, Pisatowski DM, Vintzileos AM, et al. A comparison of ultrasonographically detected cervical changes in response to transfundal pressure, coughing, and standing in predicting cervical incompetence. *Am J Obstet Gynecol.* 1997;177:660–665.

122. Guzman ER, Vintzileos AM, McLean DA, et al. The natural history of a positive response to transfundal pressure in women at risk for cervical incompetence. *Am J Obstet Gynecol.* 1997;176:634–638.

123. To MS, Skentou C, Cicero S, et al. Cervical length at 23 weeks in triplets: prediction of spontaneous preterm delivery. *Ultrasound Obstet Gynecol.* 2000;16:515–518.

124. Macdonald R, Smith P, Vyas S. Cervical incompetence: the use of transvaginal sonography to provide an objective diagnosis. *Ultrasound Obstet Gynecol.* 2001;18:211–216.

125. Moroz LA, Simhan HN. Rate of sonographic cervical shortening and the risk of spontaneous preterm birth. *Am J Obstet Gynecol.* 2012;206:234.e1–234.e5.

126. Dilek TU, Yazici G, Gurbuz A, et al. Progressive cervical length changes versus single cervical length measurement by transvaginal ultrasound for prediction of preterm delivery. *Gynecol Obstet Invest.* 2007;64:175–179.

127. Fox NS, Jean-Pierre C, Predanic M, et al. Short cervix: is a follow-up measurement useful? *Ultrasound Obstet Gynecol.* 2007;29:44–46.

128. Hofmeister C, Brizot Mde L, Liao A, et al. Two-stage transvaginal cervical length screening for preterm birth in twin pregnancies. *J Perinat Med.* 2010;38:479–484.

129. Crane JM, Hutchens D. Follow-up cervical length in asymptomatic high-risk women and the risk of spontaneous preterm birth. *J Perinatol.* 2011;31:318–323.

130. Iams JD, Cebrik D, Lynch C, et al. The rate of cervical change and the phenotype of spontaneous preterm birth. *Am J Obstet Gynecol.* 2011;205:130.e1–130.e6.

131. Ozdemir I, Demirci F, Yucel O, et al. Ultrasonographic cervical length measurement at 10–14 and 20–24 weeks gestation and the risk of preterm delivery. *Eur J Obstet Gynecol Reprod Biol.* 2007;130:176–179.

132. Conde-Agudelo A, Romero R. Predictive accuracy of changes in transvaginal sonographic cervical length over time for preterm birth: a systematic review and metaanalysis. *Am J Obstet Gynecol.* 2015;213:789–801.

133. Esplin MS, Elovitz MA, Iams JD, et al. Predictive accuracy of serial transvaginal cervical lengths and quantitative vaginal fetal fibronectin levels for spontaneous preterm birth among nulliparous women. *JAMA.* 2017;317:1047–1056.

134. Subramaniam A, Harper LM, Szychowski JM, et al. Predictive value of initial cervical length for subsequent cervical length shortening in women with a prior preterm birth. *Am J Perinatol.* 2016;33:350–355.

135. Oh KJ, Romero R, Park JY, et al. Evidence that antibiotic administration is effective in the treatment of a subset of patients with intra-amniotic infection/inflammation presenting with cervical insufficiency. *Am J Obstet Gynecol.* 2019;221:140.e1–140.e18.

136. Bishop EH. Elective induction of labor. *Obstet Gynecol.* 1955;5:519–527.

137. Park KH, Kim SN, Lee SY, et al. Comparison between sonographic cervical length and Bishop score in preinduction cervical assessment: a randomized trial. *Ultrasound Obstet Gynecol.* 2011;38:198–204.

138. Pandis GK, Papageorghiou AT, Ramanathan VG, et al. Preinduction sonographic measurement of cervical length in the prediction of successful induction of labor. *Ultrasound Obstet Gynecol.* 2001;18:623–628.

139. Brik M, Mateos S, Fernandez-Buhigas I, et al. Sonographical predictive markers of failure of induction of labour in term pregnancy. *J Obstet Gynaecol.* 2017;37:179–184.

140. Pereira S, Frick AP, Poon LC, et al. Successful induction of labor: prediction by preinduction cervical length, angle of progression and cervical elastography. *Ultrasound Obstet Gynecol.* 2014;44:468–475.

141. Gabriel R, Darnaud T, Chalot F, et al. Transvaginal sonography of the uterine cervix prior to labor induction. *Ultrasound Obstet Gynecol.* 2002;19:254–257.

142. Michaels WH, Schreiber FR, Padgett RJ, et al. Ultrasound surveillance of the cervix in twin gestations: management of cervical incompetency. *Obstet Gynecol.* 1991;78:739–744.

143. Kushnir O, Izquierdo LA, Smith JF, et al. Transvaginal sonographic measurement of cervical length. Evaluation of twin pregnancies. *J Reprod Med.* 1995;40:380–382.

144. Goldenberg RL, Iams JD, Miodovnik M, et al. The preterm prediction study: risk factors in twin gestations. National Institute of Child Health and Human Development Maternal-Fetal Medicine Units Network. *Am J Obstet Gynecol.* 1996;175:1047–1053.

145. Crane JM, Van den Hof M, Armson BA, et al. Transvaginal ultrasound in the prediction of preterm delivery: singleton and twin gestations. *Obstet Gynecol.* 1997;90:357–363.

146. Imseis HM, Albert TA, Iams JD. Identifying twin gestations at low risk for preterm birth with a transvaginal ultrasonographic cervical measurement at 24 to 26 weeks' gestation. *Am J Obstet Gynecol.* 1997;177:1149–1155.

147. Souka AP, Heath V, Flint S, et al. Cervical length at 23 weeks in twins in predicting spontaneous preterm delivery. *Obstet Gynecol.* 1999;94:450–454.

148. Guzman ER, Walters C, O'Reilly-Green C, et al. Use of cervical ultrasonography in prediction of spontaneous preterm birth in twin gestations. *Am J Obstet Gynecol.* 2000;183:1103–1107.

149. Yang JH, Kuhlman K, Daly S, et al. Prediction of preterm birth by second trimester cervical sonography in twin pregnancies. *Ultrasound Obstet Gynecol.* 2000;15:288–291.

150. Skentou C, Souka AP, To MS, et al. Prediction of preterm delivery in twins by cervical assessment at 23 weeks. *Ultrasound Obstet Gynecol.* 2001;17:7–10.

151. Soriano D, Weisz B, Seidman DS, et al. The role of sonographic assessment of cervical length in the prediction of preterm birth in primigravidae with twin gestation conceived after infertility treatment. *Acta Obstet Gynecol Scand.* 2002;81:39–43.

152. Vayssiere C, Favre R, Audibert F, et al. Cervical length and funneling at 22 and 27 weeks to predict spontaneous birth before 32 weeks in twin pregnancies: a French prospective multicenter study. *Am J Obstet Gynecol.* 2002;187:1596–1604.

153. Bergelin I, Valentin L. Cervical changes in twin pregnancies observed by transvaginal ultrasound during the latter half of pregnancy: a longitudinal, observational study. *Ultrasound Obstet Gynecol.* 2003;21:556–563.

154. Fuchs I, Tsoi E, Henrich W, et al. Sonographic measurement of cervical length in twin pregnancies in threatened preterm labor. *Ultrasound Obstet Gynecol.* 2004;23:42–45.

155. Robyr R, Boulvain M, Lewi L, et al. Cervical length as a prognostic factor for preterm delivery in twin-to-twin transfusion syndrome treated by fetoscopic laser coagulation of chorionic plate anastomoses. *Ultrasound Obstet Gynecol.* 2005;25:37–41.

156. Sperling L, Kiil C, Larsen LU, et al. How to identify twins at low risk of spontaneous preterm delivery. *Ultrasound Obstet Gynecol.* 2005;26:138–144.

157. Vayssiere C, Favre R, Audibert F, et al., Research Group in Obstetrics and Gynecology. Cervical assessment at 22 and 27 weeks for the prediction of spontaneous birth before 34 weeks in twin pregnancies: is transvaginal sonography more accurate than digital examination? *Ultrasound Obstet Gynecol.* 2005;26:707–712.

158. Fuchs F, Senat MV. Multiple gestations and preterm birth. *Semin Fetal Neonatal Med.* 2016;21:113–120.

159. Conde-Agudelo A, Romero R, Hassan SS, et al. Transvaginal sonographic cervical length for the prediction of spontaneous preterm birth in twin pregnancies: a systematic review and metaanalysis. *Am J Obstet Gynecol.* 2010;203:128.e1–128.e2.

160. Melamed N, Pittini A, Hiersch L, et al. Do serial measurements of cervical length improve the prediction of preterm birth in asymptomatic women with twin gestations? *Am J Obstet Gynecol.* 2016;215:616.e1–616.e4.

161. Kindinger LM, Poon LC, Cacciatore S, et al. The effect of gestational age and cervical length measurements in the prediction of spontaneous preterm birth in twin pregnancies: an individual patient level meta-analysis. *BJOG.* 2016;123:877–884.

162. Hester AE, Ankumah NE, Chauhan SP, et al. Twin transvaginal cervical length at 16–20 weeks and prediction of preterm birth. *J Matern Fetal Neonatal Med.* 2019;32:550–554.

163. Pagani G, Stagnati V, Fichera A, et al. Cervical length at mid-gestation in screening for preterm birth in twin pregnancy. *Ultrasound Obstet Gynecol.* 2016;48:56–60.

164. Fox NS, Rebarber A, Klauser CK, et al. Prediction of spontaneous preterm birth in asymptomatic twin pregnancies using the change in cervical length over time. *Am J Obstet Gynecol.* 2010;202:155.e1–155.e4.

165. Roman A, Saccone G, Dude CM, et al. Midtrimester transvaginal ultrasound cervical length screening for spontaneous preterm birth in diamniotic twin pregnancies according to chorionicity. *Eur J Obstet Gynecol Reprod Biol.* 2018;229:57–63.

166. Ramin KD, Ogburn PL Jr., Mulholland TA, et al. Ultrasonographic assessment of cervical length in triplet pregnancies. *Am J Obstet Gynecol.* 1999;180:1442–1445.

167. Pils S, Springer S, Wehrmann V, et al. Cervical length dynamics in triplet pregnancies: a retrospective cohort study. *Arch Gynecol Obstet.* 2017;296:191–198.

168. Rosen H, Hiersch L, Freeman H, et al. The role of serial measurements of cervical length in asymptomatic women with triplet pregnancy. *J Matern Fetal Neonatal Med.* 2018;31:713–719.

169. Hiersch L, Rosen H, Okby R, et al. The greater risk of preterm birth in triplets is mirrored by a more rapid cervical shortening along gestation. *Am J Obstet Gynecol.* 2016;215:357.e1–357.e6.

170. Fichera A, Pagani G, Stagnati V, et al. Cervical-length measurement in mid-gestation to predict spontaneous preterm birth in asymptomatic triplet pregnancy. *Ultrasound Obstet Gynecol.* 2018;51:614–620.

171. Fox NS, Rebarber A, Roman AS, et al. Combined fetal fibronectin and cervical length and spontaneous preterm birth in asymptomatic triplet pregnancies. *J Matern Fetal Neonatal Med.* 2012;25:2308–2311.

172. King JF, Grant A, Keirse MJ, et al. Beta-mimetics in preterm labour: an overview of the randomized controlled trials. *Br J Obstet Gynaecol.* 1988;95:211–222.

173. Gomez R, Galasso M, Romero R, et al. Ultrasonographic examination of the uterine cervix is better than cervical digital examination as a predictor of the likelihood of premature delivery in patients with preterm labor and intact membranes. *Am J Obstet Gynecol.* 1994;171:956–964.

174. Murakawa H, Utumi T, Hasegawa I, et al. Evaluation of threatened preterm delivery by transvaginal ultrasonographic measurement of cervical length. *Obstet Gynecol.* 1993;82:829–832.

175. Rizzo G, Capponi A, Arduini D, et al. The value of fetal fibronectin in cervical and vaginal secretions and of ultrasonographic examination of the uterine cervix in predicting premature delivery for patients with preterm labor and intact membranes. *Am J Obstet Gynecol.* 1996;175:1146–1151.

176. Tsoi E, Akmal S, Rane S, et al. Ultrasound assessment of cervical length in threatened preterm labor. *Ultrasound Obstet Gynecol.* 2003;21:552–555.

177. Fuchs IB, Henrich W, Osthues K, et al. Sonographic cervical length in singleton pregnancies with intact membranes presenting with threatened preterm labor. *Ultrasound Obstet Gynecol.* 2004;24:554–557.

178. Sanin-Blair J, Palacio M, Delgado J, et al. Impact of ultrasound cervical length assessment on duration of hospital stay in the clinical management of threatened preterm labor. *Ultrasound Obstet Gynecol.* 2004;24:756–760.

179. Tsoi E, Fuchs IB, Rane S, et al. Sonographic measurement of cervical length in threatened preterm labor in singleton pregnancies with intact membranes. *Ultrasound Obstet Gynecol.* 2005;25:353–356.

180. Botsis D, Papagianni V, Vitoratos N, et al. Prediction of preterm delivery by sonographic estimation of cervical length. *Biol Neonate.* 2005;88:42–45.

181. Daskalakis G, Thomakos N, Hatziioannou L, et al. Cervical assessment in women with threatened preterm labor. *J Matern. Fetal Neonatal Med.* 2005;17:309–312.

182. Botsis D, Makrakis E, Papagianni V, et al. The value of cervical length and plasma proMMP-9 levels for the prediction of preterm delivery in pregnant women presenting with threatened preterm labor. *Eur J Obstet Gynecol Reprod Biol.* 2006;128:108–112.

183. Tsoi E, Akmal S, Geerts L, et al. Sonographic measurement of cervical length and fetal fibronectin testing in threatened preterm labor. *Ultrasound Obstet Gynecol.* 2006;27:368–372.

184. Alfirevic Z, Allen-Coward H, Molina F, et al. Targeted therapy for threatened preterm labor based on sonographic measurement of the cervical length: a randomized controlled trial. *Ultrasound Obstet Gynecol.* 2007;29:47–50.

185. Eroglu D, Yanik F, Oktem M, et al. Prediction of preterm delivery among women with threatened preterm labor. *Gynecol Obstet Invest.* 2007;64:109–116.

186. Palacio M, Sanin-Blair J, Sanchez M, et al. The use of a variable cut-off value of cervical length in women admitted for preterm labor before and after 32 weeks. *Ultrasound Obstet Gynecol.* 2007;29:421–426.

187. Schmitz T, Kayem G, Maillard F, et al. Selective use of sonographic cervical length measurement for predicting imminent preterm delivery in women with preterm labor and intact membranes. *Ultrasound Obstet Gynecol.* 2008;31:421–426.

188. Maia MC, Nomura R, Mendonca F, et al. Is cervical length evaluated by transvaginal ultrasonography helpful in detecting true preterm labor? *J Matern Fetal Neonatal Med.* 2019:1–7.

189. Berghella V, Palacio M, Ness A, et al. Cervical length screening for prevention of preterm birth in singleton pregnancy with threatened preterm labor: systematic review and meta-analysis of randomized controlled trials using individual patient-level data. *Ultrasound Obstet Gynecol.* 2017;49:322–329.

190. Palacio M, Caradeux J, Sanchez M, et al. Uterine Cervical Length Measurement to Reduce Length of Stay in Patients Admitted for Threatened Preterm Labor: A Randomized Trial. *Fetal Diagn Ther.* 2018;43:184–190.

191. Rozenberg P, Goffinet F, Malagrida L, et al. Evaluating the risk of preterm delivery: a comparison of fetal fibronectin and transvaginal ultrasonographic measurement of cervical length. *Am J Obstet Gynecol.* 1997;176:196–199.

192. Hiersch L, Melamed N, Aviram A, et al. Role of cervical length measurement for preterm delivery prediction in women with threatened preterm labor and cervical dilatation. *J Ultrasound Med.* 2016;35:2631–2640.

193. Gomez R, Romero R, Nien JK, et al. A short cervix in women with preterm labor and intact membranes: a risk factor for microbial invasion of the amniotic cavity. *Am J Obstet Gynecol.* 2005;192:678–689.

194. Gomez R, Romero R, Medina L, et al. Cervicovaginal fibronectin improves the prediction of preterm delivery based on sonographic cervical length in patients with preterm uterine contractions and intact membranes. *Am J Obstet Gynecol.* 2005;192:350–359.

195. DeFranco EA, Lewis DF, Odibo AO. Improving the screening accuracy for preterm labor: is the combination of fetal fibronectin and cervical length in symptomatic patients a useful predictor of preterm birth? A systematic review. *Am J Obstet Gynecol.* 2013;208:233.e1–233.e6.

196. Kyozuka H, Murata T, Sato T, et al. Utility of cervical length and quantitative fetal fibronectin for predicting spontaneous preterm delivery among symptomatic nulliparous women. *Int J Gynaecol Obstet.* 2019;145:331–336.

197. Bruijn MM, Kamphuis EI, Hoesli IM, et al. The predictive value of quantitative fibronectin testing in combination with cervical length measurement in symptomatic women. *Am J Obstet Gynecol.* 2016;215:793.e1–793.e8.

198. Nguyen AD, Liu CZ, Lehner C, et al. The efficacy of quantitative fetal fibronectin in predicting spontaneous preterm birth in symptomatic women: a retrospective cohort study. *Aust N Z J Obstet Gynaecol.* 2019;59(5):656–661.

199. Centra M, Coata G, Picchiassi E, et al. Evaluation of quantitative fFn test in predicting the risk of preterm birth. *J Perinat Med.* 2017;45:91–98.

200. Shen XP, Sullivan E, Troeger K, Sciacione A. Utilization of TVUS and fFN screening, antenatal steroids use and risk of preterm delivery. *Obstet Gynecol.* 2018;131:895.

201. Ridout AE, Ibeto L, Ross G, et al. Cervical length and quantitative fetal fibronectin in the prediction of spontaneous preterm birth in asymptomatic women with congenital uterine anomaly. *Am J Obstet Gynecol.* 2019;221(4):341.e1–341.e9.

202. Romero R, Dey SK, Fisher SJ. Preterm labor: one syndrome, many causes. *Science.* 2014;345:760–765.

203. Kristensen J, Langhoff-Roos J, Wittrup M, et al. Cervical conization and preterm delivery/low birth weight. A systematic review of the literature. *Acta Obstet Gynecol Scand.* 1993;72:640–644.

204. Levine RU, Berkowitz KM. Conservative management and pregnancy outcome in diethylstilbestrol-exposed women with and without gross genital tract abnormalities. *Am J Obstet Gynecol.* 1993;169:1125–1129.

205. Romero R. Prenatal Medicine: the child is the father of the man. *Prenat Neonetal Med.* 1996;1:8–11.

206. Raio L, Ghezzi F, Di Naro E, et al. Duration of pregnancy after carbon dioxide laser conization of the cervix: influence of cone height. *Obstet Gynecol.* 1997;90:978–982.

207. Jakobsson M, Gissler M, Paavonen J, et al. Loop electrosurgical excision procedure and the risk for preterm birth. *Obstet Gynecol.* 2009;114:504–510.

208. Noehr B, Jensen A, Frederiksen K, et al. Depth of cervical cone removed by loop electrosurgical excision procedure and subsequent risk of spontaneous preterm delivery. *Obstet Gynecol.* 2009;114:1232–1238.

209. Craig CJ. Congenital abnormalities of the uterus and foetal wastage. *S Afr Med J.* 1973;47:2000–2005.

210. Mangan CE, Borow L, Burtnett-Rubin MM, et al. Pregnancy outcome in 98 women exposed to diethylstilbestrol in utero, their mothers, and unexposed siblings. *Obstet Gynecol.* 1982;59:315–319.

211. Ludmir J, Landon MB, Gabbe SG, et al. Management of the diethylstilbestrol-exposed pregnant patient: a prospective study. *Am J Obstet Gynecol.* 1987;157:665–669.

212. Romero R, Gonzalez R, Sepulveda W, et al. Infection and labor. VIII. Microbial invasion of the amniotic cavity in patients with suspected cervical incompetence: prevalence and clinical significance. *Am J Obstet Gynecol.* 1992;167:1086–1091.

213. Hassan S, Romero R, Hendler I, et al. A sonographic short cervix as the only clinical manifestation of intra-amniotic infection. *J Perinat Med.* 2006;34:13–19.

214. Stys SJ, Clewell WH, Meschia G. Changes in cervical compliance at parturition independent of uterine activity. *Am J Obstet Gynecol.* 1978;130:414–418.

215. Tarca AL, Fitzgerald W, Chaemsaithong P, et al. The cytokine network in women with an asymptomatic short cervix and the risk of preterm delivery. *Am J Reprod Immunol.* 2017;78(3).

216. Raiche E, Ouellet A, Berthiaume M, et al. Short and inflamed cervix predicts spontaneous preterm birth (COLIBRI study). *J Matern Fetal Neonatal Med.* 2014;27:1015–1019.

217. Sundtoft I, Langhoff-Roos J, Sandager P, et al. Cervical collagen is reduced in non-pregnant women with a history of cervical insufficiency and a short cervix. *Acta Obstet Gynecol Scand.* 2017;96:984–990.

218. Gray DJ, Robinson HB, Malone J, et al. Adverse outcome in pregnancy following amniotic fluid isolation of Ureaplasma urealyticum. *Prenat Diagn.* 1992;12:111–117.

219. Kiefer DG, Keeler SM, Rust OA, et al. Is midtrimester short cervix a sign of intraamniotic inflammation? *Am J Obstet Gynecol.* 2009;200:374–375.

220. Keeler SM, Kiefer DG, Rust OA, et al. Comprehensive amniotic fluid cytokine profile evaluation in women with a short cervix: which cytokine(s) correlates best with outcome? *Am J Obstet Gynecol.* 2009;201:276.e1–276.e6.

221. Vaisbuch E, Hassan SS, Mazaki-Tovi S, et al. Patients with an asymptomatic short cervix (<or=15 mm) have a high rate of subclinical intraamniotic inflammation: implications for patient counseling. *Am J Obstet Gynecol.* 2010;202:433–438.

222. Mays JK, Figueroa R, Shah J, et al. Amniocentesis for selection before rescue cerclage. *Obstet Gynecol.* 2000;95:652–655.

223. Jung EY, Park KH, Lee SY, et al. Non-invasive prediction of intra-amniotic infection and/or inflammation in patients with cervical insufficiency or an asymptomatic short cervix (≤15 mm). *Arch Gynecol Obstet.* 2015;292:579–587.

224. Romero R, Miranda J, Chaiworapongsa T, et al. Sterile intra-amniotic inflammation in asymptomatic patients with a sonographic short cervix: prevalence and clinical significance. *J Matern Fetal Neonatal Med.* 2015;28:1343–1359.

225. Romero R, Kusanovic JP, Espinoza J, et al. What is amniotic fluid "sludge?" *Ultrasound Obstet Gynecol.* 2007;30:793–798.

226. Romero R, Schaudinn C, Kusanovic JP, et al. Detection of a microbial biofilm in intraamniotic infection. *Am J Obstet Gynecol.* 2008;198:135.e1–e5.

227. Zimmer EZ, Bronshtein M. Ultrasonic features of intra-amniotic "unidentified debris" at 14–16 weeks' gestation. *Ultrasound Obstet Gynecol.* 1996;7:178–181.

228. Parulekar SG. Ultrasonographic demonstration of floating particles in amniotic fluid. *J Ultrasound Med.* 1983;2:107–110.

229. Sepulveda W, Reid R, Nicolaidis P, et al. Second-trimester echogenic bowel and intraamniotic bleeding: association between fetal bowel echogenicity and amniotic fluid spectrophotometry at 410 nm. *Am J Obstet Gynecol.* 1996;174:839–842.

230. Vengalil S, Santolaya-Forgas J, Meyer W, et al. Ultrasonically dense amniotic fluid in early pregnancy in asymptomatic women without vaginal bleeding. A report of two cases. *J Reprod Med.* 1998;43:462–464.

231. Tskitishvili E, Tomimatsu T, Kanagawa T, et al. Amniotic fluid "sludge" detected in patients with subchorionic hematoma: a report of two cases. *Ultrasound Obstet Gynecol.* 2009;33:484–486.

232. Cafici D, Sepulveda W. First-trimester echogenic amniotic fluid in the acrania-anencephaly sequence. *J Ultrasound Med.* 2003;22:1075–1079; quiz 1080–1071.

233. Hallak M, Zador IE, Garcia EM, et al. Ultrasound-detected free-floating particles in amniotic fluid: correlation with maternal serum alpha-fetoprotein. *Fetal Diagn Ther.* 1993;8:402–406.

234. Benacerraf BR, Gatter MA, Ginsburgh F. Ultrasound diagnosis of meconium-stained amniotic fluid. *Am J Obstet Gynecol.* 1984;149:570–572.

235. DeVore GR, Platt LD. Ultrasound appearance of particulate matter in amniotic cavity: vernix or meconium? *J Clin Ultrasound.* 1986;14:229–230.

236. Sepulveda WH, Quiroz VH. Sonographic detection of echogenic amniotic fluid and its clinical significance. *J Perinat Med.* 1989;17:333–335.

237. Sherer DM, Abramowicz JS, Smith SA, et al. Sonographically homogeneous echogenic amniotic fluid in detecting meconium-stained amniotic fluid. *Obstet Gynecol.* 1991;78:819–822.

238. Gross TL, Wolfson RN, Kuhnert PM, et al. Sonographically detected free-floating particles in amniotic fluid predict a mature lecithin-sphingomyelin ratio. *J Clin Ultrasound.* 1985;13:405–409.

239. Mullin TJ, Gross TL, Wolfson RN. Ultrasound screening for free-floating particles and fetal lung maturity. *Obstet Gynecol.* 1985;66:50–54.

240. Vohra N, Rochelson B, Smith-Levitin M. Three-dimensional sonographic findings in congenital (harlequin) ichthyosis. *J Ultrasound Med.* 2003;22:737–739.

241. Dolan CR, Smith LT, Sybert VP. Prenatal detection of epidermolysis bullosa letalis with pyloric atresia in a fetus by abnormal ultrasound and elevated alpha-fetoprotein. *Am J Med Genet.* 1993;47:395–400.

242. Espinoza J, Goncalves LF, Romero R, et al. The prevalence and clinical significance of amniotic fluid "sludge" in patients with preterm labor and intact membranes. *Ultrasound Obstet Gynecol.* 2005;25:346–352.

243. Bujold E, Pasquier JC, Simoneau J, et al. Intra-amniotic sludge, short cervix, and risk of preterm delivery. *J Obstet Gynaecol Can.* 2006;28:198–202.

244. Kusanovic JP, Espinoza J, Romero R, et al. Clinical significance of the presence of amniotic fluid "sludge" in asymptomatic patients at high risk for spontaneous preterm delivery. *Ultrasound Obstet Gynecol.* 2007;30:706–714.

245. Himaya E, Rhalmi N, Girard M, et al. Midtrimester intra-amniotic sludge and the risk of spontaneous preterm birth. *Am J Perinatol.* 2011;28:815–820.

246. Ventura W, Nazario C, Ingar J, et al. Risk of impending preterm delivery associated with the presence of amniotic fluid sludge in women in preterm labor with intact membranes. *Fetal Diagn Ther.* 2011;30:116–121.

247. Gauthier S, Tetu A, Himaya E, et al. The origin of Fusobacterium nucleatum involved in intra-amniotic infection and preterm birth. *J Matern Fetal Neonatal Med.* 2011;24:1329–1332.

248. Rhalmi N, Himaya E, Girard M, et al. Intra-amniotic sludge in a woman with asymptomatic cervical dilatation. *J Obstet Gynaecol Can.* 2011;33:1201.

249. Paules C, Moreno E, Gonzales A, et al. Amniotic fluid sludge as a marker of intra-amniotic infection and histological chorioamnionitis in cervical insufficiency: a report of four cases and literature review. *J Matern Fetal Neonatal Med.* 2016;29:2681–2684.

250. Kusanovic JP, Romero R, Martinovic C, et al. Transabdominal collection of amniotic fluid "sludge" and identification of Candida albicans intra-amniotic infection. *J Matern Fetal Neonatal Med.* 2018;31:1279–1284.

251. Dinglas C, Chavez M, Vintzileos A. Resolution of intra-amniotic sludge after antibiotic administration in a patient with short cervix and recurrent mid-trimester loss. *Am J Obstet Gynecol.* 2019;221:159.

252. Hatanaka AR, Franca MS, Hamamoto T, et al. Antibiotic treatment for patients with amniotic fluid "sludge" to prevent spontaneous preterm birth: a historically controlled observational study. *Acta Obstet Gynecol Scand.* 2019;98:1157–1163.

253. Pustotina O. Effects of antibiotic therapy in women with the amniotic fluid "sludge" at 15–24 weeks of gestation on pregnancy outcomes. *J Matern Fetal Neonatal Med.* 2019:1–12.

254. Romero R, Nicolaides KH, Conde-Agudelo A, et al. Vaginal progesterone decreases preterm birth ≤34 weeks of gestation in women with a singleton pregnancy and a short cervix: an updated meta-analysis including data from the OPPTIMUM study. *Ultrasound Obstet Gynecol.* 2016;48:308–317.

255. Romero R, Conde-Agudelo A, Da Fonseca E, et al. Vaginal progesterone for preventing preterm birth and adverse perinatal outcomes in singleton gestations with a short cervix: a meta-analysis of individual patient data. *Am J Obstet Gynecol.* 2018;218:161–180.

256. Conde-Agudelo A, Romero R, Da Fonseca E, et al. Vaginal progesterone is as effective as cervical cerclage to prevent preterm birth in women with a singleton gestation, previous spontaneous preterm birth, and a short cervix: updated indirect comparison meta-analysis. *Am J Obstet Gynecol.* 2018;219:10–25.

257. Romero R, Conde-Agudelo A, El-Refaie W, et al. Vaginal progesterone decreases preterm birth and neonatal morbidity and mortality in women with a twin gestation and a short cervix: an updated meta-analysis of individual patient data. *Ultrasound Obstet Gynecol.* 2017;49:303–314.

258. Cahill AG, Odibo AO, Caughey AB, et al. Universal cervical length screening and treatment with vaginal progesterone to prevent preterm birth: a decision and economic analysis. *Am J Obstet Gynecol.* 2010;202:548.e1–548.e8.

259. Campbell S. Universal cervical-length screening and vaginal progesterone prevents early preterm births, reduces neonatal morbidity and is cost saving: doing nothing is no longer an option. *Ultrasound Obstet Gynecol.* 2011;38:1–9.

260. Werner EF, Han CS, Pettker CM, et al. Universal cervical-length screening to prevent preterm birth: a cost-effectiveness analysis. *Ultrasound Obstet Gynecol.* 2011;38:32–37.

261. Berghella V. Universal cervical length screening for prediction and prevention of preterm birth. *Obstet Gynecol Surv.* 2012;67:653–658.

262. Combs CA. Vaginal progesterone for asymptomatic cervical shortening and the case for universal screening of cervical length. *Am J Obstet Gynecol.* 2012;206:101–103.

263. Miller ES, Grobman WA. Cost-effectiveness of transabdominal ultrasound for cervical length screening for preterm birth prevention. *Am J Obstet Gynecol.* 2013;209:546.e1–546.e6.

264. Jungner G, Wilson JMG. Principles and practice of screening for disease. *Public Health Papers.* 1968:34.

265. Conde-Agudelo A, Romero R. Vaginal progesterone to prevent preterm birth in pregnant women with a sonographic short cervix: clinical and public health implications. *Am J Obstet Gynecol.* 2016;214:235–242.

266. Brown S, Mozurkewich E. Cost analysis of universal cervical length screening and progesterone therapy in remote populations. *Am J Obstet Gynecol.* 2014;210(suppl 1):S201.

267. Werner EF, Hamel MS, Orzechowski K, et al. Cost-effectiveness of transvaginal ultrasound cervical length screening in singletons without a prior preterm birth: an update. *Am J Obstet Gynecol.* 2015;213:554.e1–554.e6.

268. Fonseca EB, Nishikawa AM, Paladini L, et al. Cervical assessment with progesterone in the prevention of preterm birth: a strategy based on cost-effectiveness. *Value Health.* 2014;17:A510.

269. Eke A, Buras A, Woo J, et al. Vaginal progesterone versus cervical cerclage for the prevention of preterm births in women with a sonographically short cervix; a cost effectiveness and decision analysis. *Am J Obstet Gynecol.* 2015;212:S367–S368.

270. Pizzi LT, Seligman NS, Baxter JK, et al. Cost and cost effectiveness of vaginal progesterone gel in reducing preterm birth: an economic analysis of the PREGNANT trial. *Pharmacoeconomics.* 2014;32:467–478.

271. Page J, Emerson J, Cahill A, et al. The impact of cervical length on the cost-effectiveness of vaginal progesterone as a preterm birth intervention. *Am J Obstet Gynecol.* 2013;208(suppl 1):S66.

272. Martin JA, Hamilton BE, Osterman MJ, et al. Births: final data for 2013. *Natl Vital Stat Rep.* 2015;64:1–65.

273. Meis PJ, Klebanoff M, Thom E, et al. Prevention of recurrent preterm delivery by 17 alpha-hydroxyprogesterone caproate. *N Engl J Med.* 2003;348:2379–2385.

274. Keirse MJ. Progesterone and preterm: seventy years of "deja vu" or "still to be seen"? *Birth.* 2004;31:230–235.

275. Iams JD, Newman RB, Thom EA, et al. Frequency of uterine contractions and the risk of spontaneous preterm delivery. *N Engl J Med.* 2002;346:250–255.
276. Blackwell SC, Gyamfi-Bannerman C, Biggio JR Jr., et al. PROLONG clinical study protocol: hydroxyprogesterone caproate to reduce recurrent preterm birth. *Am J Perinatol.* 2018;35:1228–1234.
277. AMAG Pharmaceuticals. Results from the PROLONG trial evaluating hydroxy-progesterone caproate injection. *Media Contact.* 2019:2–6.
278. Grobman WA, Thom EA, Spong CY, et al.; Eunice Kennedy Shriver National Institute of Child H, Human Development Maternal-Fetal Medicine Units N. 17 alpha-hydroxyprogesterone caproate to prevent prematurity in nulliparas with cervical length less than 30 mm. *Am J Obstet Gynecol.* 2012;207:390.e1–390.e8.
279. O'Brien JM. The safety of progesterone and 17-hydroxyprogesterone caproate administration for the prevention of preterm birth: an evidence-based assessment. *Am J Perinatol.* 2012;29:665–672.
280. Szychowski JM, Berghella V, Owen J, et al.; Vaginal Ultrasound Trial Consortium. Cerclage for the prevention of preterm birth in high risk women receiving intramuscular 17-alpha-hydroxyprogesterone caproate. *J Matern Fetal Neonatal Med.* 2012;25:2686–2689.
281. Winer N, Bretelle F, Senat MV, et al. 17 alpha-hydroxyprogesterone caproate does not prolong pregnancy or reduce the rate of preterm birth in women at high risk for preterm delivery and a short cervix: a randomized controlled trial. *Am J Obstet Gynecol.* 2015;212:485.e1–485.e10.
282. Jarde A, Lutsiv O, Beyene J, et al. Vaginal progesterone, oral progesterone, 17-OHPC, cerclage, and pessary for preventing preterm birth in at-risk singleton pregnancies: an updated systematic review and network meta-analysis. *BJOG.* 2019;126:556–567.
283. Hassan SS, Romero R, Maymon E, et al. Does cervical cerclage prevent preterm delivery in patients with a short cervix? *Am J Obstet Gynecol.* 2001;184:1325–1329.
284. Althuisius SM, Dekker GA, Hummel P, et al.; Cervical Incompetence Prevention Randomized Cerclage Trial. Cervical incompetence prevention randomized cerclage trial: emergency cerclage with bed rest versus bed rest alone. *Am J Obstet Gynecol.* 2003;189:907–910.
285. Berghella V, Odibo AO, Tolosa JE. Cerclage for prevention of preterm birth in women with a short cervix found on transvaginal ultrasound examination: a randomized trial. *Am J Obstet Gynecol.* 2004;191:1311–1317.
286. To MS, Alfirevic Z, Heath VC, et al. Cervical cerclage for prevention of preterm delivery in women with short cervix: randomised controlled trial. *Lancet.* 2004;363:1849–1853.
287. Berghella V, Rafael TJ, Szychowski JM, et al. Cerclage for short cervix on ultrasonography in women with singleton gestations and previous preterm birth: a meta-analysis. *Obstet Gynecol.* 2011;117:663–671.
288. American College of Obstetricians and Gynecologists; Committee on Practice Bulletins—Obstetrics. ACOG practice bulletin no. 127: management of preterm labor. *Obstet Gynecol.* 2012;119:1308–1317.
289. Society for Maternal-Fetal Medicine Publications Committee, with assistance of Vincenzo Berghella. Progesterone and preterm birth prevention: translating clinical trials data into clinical practice. Am J Obstet Gynecol. 2012;206:376–386.
290. Final report of the Medical Research Council/Royal College of Obstetricians and Gynaecologists multicentre randomised trial of cervical cerclage. MRC/RCOG Working Party on Cervical Cerclage. Br J Obstet Gynaecol. 1993;100:516–523.
291. Lazar P, Gueguen S, Dreyfus J, et al. Multicentred controlled trial of cervical cerclage in women at moderate risk of preterm delivery. *Br J Obstet Gynaecol.* 1984;91:731–735.
292. Rush RW, Isaacs S, McPherson K, et al. A randomized controlled trial of cervical cerclage in women at high risk of spontaneous preterm delivery. *Br J Obstet Gynaecol.* 1984;91:724–730.
293. Guzman ER, Forster JK, Vintzileos AM, et al. Pregnancy outcomes in women treated with elective versus ultrasound-indicated cervical cerclage. *Ultrasound Obstet Gynecol.* 1998;12:323–327.
294. Novy MJ, Gupta A, Wothe DD, et al. Cervical cerclage in the second trimester of pregnancy: a historical cohort study. *Am J Obstet Gynecol.* 2001;184:1447–1454.
295. Simcox R, Seed PT, Bennett P, et al. A randomized controlled trial of cervical scanning vs history to determine cerclage in women at high risk of preterm birth (CIRCLE trial). *Am J Obstet Gynecol.* 2009;200:623.e1–623.e6.
296. Berghella V, Mackeen AD. Cervical length screening with ultrasound-indicated cerclage compared with history-indicated cerclage for prevention of preterm birth: a meta-analysis. *Obstet Gynecol.* 2011;118:148–155.
297. Higgins SP, Kornman LH, Bell RJ, et al. Cervical surveillance as an alternative to elective cervical cerclage for pregnancy management of suspected cervical incompetence. *Aust N Z J Obstet Gynaecol.* 2004;44:228–232.
298. Fox R, Holmes R, James M, et al. Serial transvaginal ultrasonography following McDonald cerclage and repeat suture insertion. *Aust N Z J Obstet Gynaecol.* 1998;38:27–30.
299. Dijkstra K, Funai EF, O'Neill L, et al. Change in cervical length after cerclage as a predictor of preterm delivery. *Obstet Gynecol.* 2000;96:346–350.
300. Andersen HF, Karimi A, Sakala EP, et al. Prediction of cervical cerclage outcome by endovaginal ultrasonography. *Am J Obstet Gynecol.* 1994;171:1102–1106.
301. Guzman ER, Houlihan C, Vintzileos A, et al. The significance of transvaginal ultrasonographic evaluation of the cervix in women treated with emergency cerclage. Am J Obstet Gynecol. 1996;175:471–476.
302. Cook JR, Chatfield S, Chandiramani M, et al. Cerclage position, cervical length and preterm delivery in women undergoing ultrasound indicated cervical cerclage: a retrospective cohort study. *PLoS One.* 2017;12:e0178072.
303. Song RK, Cha HH, Shin MY, et al. Post-cerclage ultrasonographic cervical length can predict preterm delivery in elective cervical cerclage patients. *Obstet Gynecol Sci.* 2016;59:17–23.
304. Pils S, Eppel W, Promberger R, et al. The predictive value of sequential cervical length screening in singleton pregnancies after cerclage: a retrospective cohort study. *BMC Pregnancy Childbirth.* 2016;16:79.
305. Berghella V, Ciardulli A, Rust OA, et al. Cerclage for sonographic short cervix in singleton gestations without prior spontaneous preterm birth: systematic review and meta-analysis of randomized controlled trials using individual patient-level data. *Ultrasound Obstet Gynecol.* 2017;50:569–577.
306. Romero R, Conde-Agudelo A, Nicolaides KH. There is insufficient evidence to claim that cerclage is the treatment of choice for patients with a cervical length <10 mm. *Am J Obstet Gynecol.* 2018;219:213–215.
307. ACOG Practice Bulletin No 142: Cerclage for the management of cervical insufficiency. *Obstet Gynecol.* 2014;123 (2 pt 1): 372–379.
308. Society for Maternal Fetal Medicine. Fifteen things physicians and patients should question. Choosing Wisely. www.smfm.org.
309. Berghella V, Odibo AO, To MS. Cerclage for short cervix on ultrasonography: meta-analysis of trials using individual patient-level data. *Obstet Gynecol.* 2005;106:181–189.
310. Saccone G, Rust O, Althuisius S, et al. Cerclage for short cervix in twin pregnancies: systematic review and meta-analysis of randomized trials using individual patient-level data. *Acta Obstet Gynecol Scand.* 2015;94:352–358.
311. Roman A, Berghella V. Cerclage in twin pregnancies with short cervical length: more level 1 data are needed. *Am J Obstet Gynecol.* 2020. doi:10.1016/j.ajog.2020.01.048.
312. Roman A, Rochelson B, Fox N, et al. Efficacy of ultrasound-indicated cerclage in twin pregnancies. *Am J Obstet Gynecol.* 2015;212:788.e1–788.e6.
313. Li C, Shen J, Hua K. Cerclage for women with twin pregnancies: a systematic review and metaanalysis. *Am J Obstet Gynecol.* 2019;220:543–547.
314. Sanchez-Ramos L. The placement of a cerclage in patients with twin pregnancies and a short cervix is associated with increased risk of preterm birth and adverse perinatal outcome. *Am J Obstet Gynecol.* 2020;222:194–196.
315. Newcomer J. Pessaries for the treatment of incompetent cervix and premature delivery. *Obstet Gynecol Surv.* 2000;55:443–448.
316. Arabin B, Halbesma JR, Vork F, et al. Is treatment with vaginal pessaries an option in patients with a sonographically detected short cervix? *J Perinat Med.* 2003;31:122–133.
317. Cruz-Melguizo S, San-Frutos L, Martinez-Payo C, et al. Cervical pessary compared with vaginal progesterone for preventing early preterm birth: a randomized controlled trial. Obstet Gynecol. 2018;132:907–915.
318. Hui SY, Chor CM, Lau TK, et al. Cerclage pessary for preventing preterm birth in women with a singleton pregnancy and a short cervix at 20 to 24 weeks: a randomized controlled trial. Am J Perinatol. 2013;30:283–288.
319. Nicolaides KH, Syngelaki A, Poon LC, et al. A randomized trial of a cervical pessary to prevent preterm singleton birth. N Engl J Med. 2016;374:1044–1052.
320. Saccone G, Ciardulli A, Xodo S, et al. Cervical pessary for preventing preterm birth in singleton pregnancies with short cervical length: a systematic review and meta-analysis. J Matern Fetal Neonatal Med. 2017;30:1535–1543.
321. Conde-Agudelo A, Romero R, Nicolaides KH. Cervical pessary to prevent preterm birth in asymptomatic high-risk women; a systematic review and meta-analysis. Am J Obstet Gynecol. 2020. doi:10.1016/j.ajog.2019.12.266.
322. Norman JE, Norrie J, Maclennan G, Cooper D, et al. Open randomised trial of the (Arabin) pessary to prevent preterm birth in twin pregnancy with health economics and acceptability: STOPPIT-2 a study protocol. BMJ Open. 2018;8(12):e026430.
323. Goya M, Pratcorona L, Higueras T, et al. Sonographic cervical length measurement in pregnant women with a cervical pessary. Ultrasound Obstet Gynecol. 2011;38:205–209.
324. Bolanos R, Childress KS, Flick A, et al. The effect of vaginal pessary on cervical length in pregnant women with a short cervix. Am J Obstet Gynecol. 2014;210(suppl 1):S383–S384.
325. Mendoza M, Goya M, Gascon A, et al. Modification of cervical length after cervical pessary insertion: correlation weeks of gestation. J Matern Fetal Neonatal Med. 2017;30:1596–1601.
326. Mendoza Cobaleda M, Ribera I, Maiz N, et al. Cervical modifications after pessary placement in singleton pregnancies with maternal short cervical length: 2D and 3D ultrasound evaluation. Acta Obstet Gynecol Scand. 2019;98(11):1442–1449.
327. Bamber J, Cosgrove D, Dietrich CF, et al. EFSUMB guidelines and recommendations on the clinical use of ultrasound elastography. Part 1: Basic principles and technology. Ultraschall Med. 2013;34:169–184.
328. Ophir J, Cespedes I, Ponnekanti H, et al. Elastography: a quantitative method for imaging the elasticity of biological tissues. Ultrason Imaging. 1991;13:111–134.
329. Ophir J, Alam SK, Garra B, et al. Elastography: ultrasonic estimation and imaging of the elastic properties of tissues. Proc Inst Mech Eng H. 1999;213:203–233.
330. Fruscalzo A, Mazza E, Feltovich H, et al. Cervical elastography during pregnancy: a critical review of current approaches with a focus on controversies and limitations. J Med Ultrason (2001). 2016;43:493–504.
331. Hernandez-Andrade E, Hassan SS, Ahn H, et al. Evaluation of cervical stiffness during pregnancy using semiquantitative ultrasound elastography. Ultrasound Obstet Gynecol. 2013;41:152–161.

332. Köbbing K, Fruscalzo A, Hammer K, et al. Quantitative elastography of the uterine cervix as a predictor of preterm delivery. *J Perinatol.* 2014;34:774–780.

333. Woźniak S, Czuczwar P, Szkodziak P, et al. Elastography in predicting preterm delivery in asymptomatic, low-risk women: a prospective observational study. *BMC Pregnancy Childbirth.* 2014;14:238.

334. Hernandez-Andrade E, Romero R, Korzeniewski SJ, et al. Cervical strain determined by ultrasound elastography and its association with spontaneous preterm delivery. *J Perinat Med.* 2014;42:159–169.

335. von Schöning D, Fischer T, von Tucher E, et al. Cervical sonoelastography for improving prediction of preterm birth compared with cervical length measurement and fetal fibronectin test. *J Perinat Med.* 2015;43:531–536.

336. Woźniak S, Czuczwar P, Szkodziak P, et al. Elastography for predicting preterm delivery in patients with short cervical length at 18–22 weeks of gestation: a prospective observational study. *Ginekol Pol.* 2015;86:442–447.

337. Oturina V, Hammer K, Möllers M, et al. Assessment of cervical elastography strain pattern and its association with preterm birth. *J Perinat Med.* 2017;45(8): 925–932.

338. Ozturk A, Grajo JR, Dhyani M, et al. Principles of ultrasound elastography. *Abdom Radiol (NY).* 2018;43:773–785.

339. Taljanovic MS, Gimber LH, Becker GW, et al. Shear-wave elastography: basic physics and musculoskeletal applications. *Radiographics.* 2017;37:855–870.

340. Nowicki A, Dobruch-Sobczak K. Introduction to ultrasound elastography. *J Ultrason.* 2016;16:113–124.

341. Hernandez-Andrade E, Maymon E, Luewan S, et al. A soft cervix, categorized by shear-wave elastography, in women with short or with normal cervical length at 18-24 weeks is associated with a higher prevalence of spontaneous preterm delivery. *J Perinat Med.* 2018;46:489–501.

342. Leppert PC. Anatomy and physiology of cervical ripening. *Clin Obstet Gynecol.* 1995;38:267–279.

343. Feltovich H, Hall TJ, Berghella V. Beyond cervical length: emerging technologies for assessing the pregnant cervix. *Am J Obstet Gynecol.* 2012;207:345–354.

344. Guerrero QW, Feltovich H, Rosado-Mendez IM, et al. Anisotropy and spatial heterogeneity in quantitative ultrasound parameters: relevance to the study of the human cervix. *Ultrasound Med Biol.* 2018;44:1493–1503.

345. McFarlin BL, Kumar V, Bigelow TA, et al. Beyond cervical length: a pilot study of ultrasonic attenuation for early detection of preterm birth risk. *Ultrasound Med Biol.* 2015;41:3023–3029.

346. Baños N, Perez-Moreno A, Julia C, et al. Quantitative analysis of cervical texture by ultrasound in mid-pregnancy and association with spontaneous preterm birth. *Ultrasound Obstet Gynecol.* 2018;51:637–643.

15 Multiple Gestation

Mourina Habli

Multiple gestations, of which 98% are twins, are associated with a higher risk of morbidity and mortality than singleton pregnancies. During the past three decades, the rate of twin births has skyrocketed, increasing by 70% from 1980 to 2004.[1] After 2005, this rate slowed to 0.5% annually, and in 2011, the rate actually declined by 1% from the previous year.[1] According to the Centers for Disease Control and Prevention, 33 of every 1,000 births are twin deliveries. In 2011, this totaled 131,269 twins births.[1] Increases in twin births are largely attributed to two factors: delayed childbearing and the increased use of assisted reproductive technology (ART), which includes fertility drugs to superovulate the ovaries and the transfer of multiple embryos. Compared with younger mothers, spontaneously conceived pregnancies in older mothers are prone to twinning because of the different actions of follicle-stimulating hormones.[2] Multiple gestations are a well-known possibility in ART.[3] The use of more selective procedures, such as single-embryo transfer, can decrease the risk of twinning,[4] whereas other procedures that decrease the risk of higher multiples actually contribute to more twin gestations.[5] A spontaneously conceived infant has a 1 in 90 chance of being a twin and a tiny chance of being triplet or more.[6] However, an ART infant has 20 to 30 times more likelihood of being a twin and a 400-fold increased risk of triplets. In a recent U.S. review, 47% of ART infants were multiple gestations compared with 3.3% of all births.[7] In that review, 43% of ART pregnancies were twins versus 3.3% of all births, and 3.6% of ART infants were triplets or higher order multiples compared with 0.2% of all infants.[7] Through regulation, European countries have been able to reduce multiple gestations with ART to a rate of 22.7%, whereas the United States, owing to lack of regulation, has been unable to reduce the number below 32%.[6]

In this chapter, the management and outcomes for twin pregnancies, the unique challenges in prenatal screening and diagnosis, the importance of early diagnosis of chorionicity, prenatal genetic testing, and maternal and fetal complications are discussed. The outcomes of twin pregnancies are largely based on chorionicity, with complication rates lower in dichorionic twins and higher in monochorionic twins. Given the higher infant mortality, with twins being five times more likely to die in infancy than a singleton,[8] and higher maternal risks, including death,[9] this chapter reviews contemporary strategies of care for the mother and twins.

IMAGING

Ultrasonography has been the imaging modality of choice for diagnosing fetal anomalies for decades. It is relatively inexpensive, has real-time capability, and is considered safe, making it the standard in the evaluation of the fetus.[10] However, ultrasound (US) performance depends highly on the skill and experience of the sonographer, resulting in detection rates of abnormalities that vary from 13% to 82%.[10,11] The sensitivity and specificity of US depend on the fetal position, presence of oligohydramnios, degree of ossification, and maternal body habitus.[10,11]

Recently, magnetic resonance imaging (MRI) has emerged as a technique to image fetuses when US findings are inconclusive. Several authors agree that MRI is as good as US in prenatal diagnosis and in some cases superior, particularly for defining intracranial anatomy. When US is inconclusive, MRI has been effective in defining both the type of acardiac twinning and the extent of conjoined twins. MRI will likely be utilized more in the future and in conjunction with US to aid when diagnosis by US is not definitive and when maternal habitus is not conducive to US. Several studies have shown that a higher detection rates is achieved by MRI for abnormalities of the central nervous system (CNS), thorax, abdomen, and skeleton[12] and that additional anatomical information can be provided in 45% of cases.[13] In a more recent case series of complicated multifetal pregnancies, MRI was superior to US in 64% of cases.[14] Improved diagnosis occurred mainly in CNS abnormalities, abdominal organs, and conjoined twin. In this case series, diagnosis as well as counseling and management were affected.

EMBRYOLOGY OF TWINNING/ PLACENTATION/AMNION

The embryology of twinning is fascinating. Timing of cell division by 1 day earlier or later greatly affects the twin outcome. In a normally developing pregnancy, the placenta (or chorion) develops on day 3. Although most sources agree on the timing of embryogenesis, there are several hypotheses that explain why twinning occurs. From a genetics standpoint, a portion of dizygotic twins can be linked to dominant inheritance on chromosome 3.[15-17]

Zygosity

Twins can be either monozygotic (identical) or dizygotic (fraternal) (Fig. 15.1).

Definition/Incidence
Monozygotic twins, approximately one-third of twin gestations, result from ovulation and fertilization of single oocyte and subsequent division of the zygote into two fetuses with either monochorionic or dichorionic "fused" placentation (Fig. 15.2). During embryogenesis, dichorionic–diamniotic twins split on days 2 to 3, monochorionic–diamniotic twinning occurs between days 3 and 7, monochorionic–monoamniotic twinning occurs from days 7 to 14, and conjoined twinning occurs between days 14 and 15.[18] The incidence of monozygotic birth is fairly constant, accounting for 1 in 330 of spontaneous live births, or about 1 in 160 babies.[19-21] Of these, 70% are concordant healthy monozygotic twins, and 30% are dizygotic[19-21] (Fig. 15.3). Monozygotic twins have increased risks of complications, such as twin-reversed arterial perfusion (TRAP) syndrome, conjoined twins, and twin-to-twin transfusion.

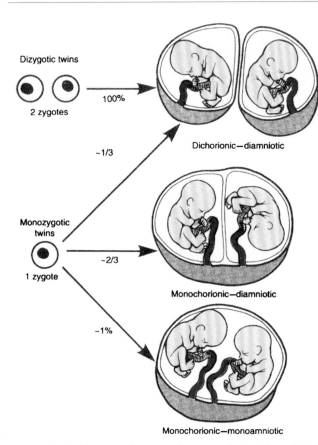

FIGURE 15.1: Monozygotic versus dizygotic twins. All dizygotic twins have dichorionic–diamniotic placentation. Monozygotic twins may form dichorionic–diamniotic, monochorionic–diamniotic, or monochorionic–monoamniotic placentation.

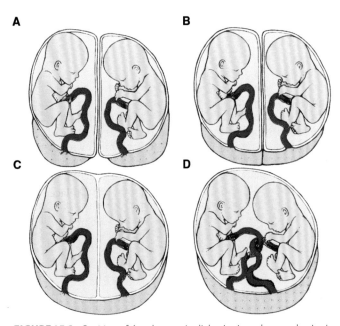

FIGURE 15.2: Position of the placenta in dichorionic and monochorionic placentation. **A:** Dichorionic–diamniotic placentation with two separate placentas. **B:** Dichorionic–diamniotic placentation with a fused placenta. **C:** Monochorionic–diamniotic placentation with a single placenta. **D:** Monochorionic–monoamniotic placentation with a single placenta.

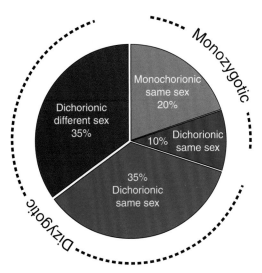

FIGURE 15.3: Frequency of dichorionic and monochorionic placentation with regard to zygosity and fetal sex.

Dizygotic twins represent two-thirds of twin gestations and occur from ovulation and fertilization of two oocytes (see Fig. 15.1), almost always resulting in a dichorionic placentation (see Fig. 15.2). Dizygotic twinning is a type of superfecundation in which more than one fertilized egg is present in the uterus. The spontaneous prevalence of live-born dizygotic twinning in North America and Britain is 1 in 100 births,[20] but incidence varies widely by region (see Fig. 15.3). Hereditary tendency may increase the risk three times that of normal population.

Diagnosis

Zygosity can be determined by placentation or biochemical testing such as blood types, enzyme polymorphisms, and human leukocyte antigen (HLA) types.[22–25] Regarding placentation, a monochorionic placenta is monozygotic until proven otherwise. On the other hand, DNA typing is considered the most useful and reliable way of defining zygosity.[26] However, because 70% of monozygotic twins share vascular placental connections, DNA in blood cells may appear to be identical even if the twin pair is genetically or epigenetically discordant.[25,26]

Classification

Twins can be classified clinically via chorionicity or genetically based on zygosity. Controversy persists on whether outcomes of twin gestations are best assessed by zygosity or chorionicity. In the United Kingdom, a prospective observational study was conducted to compare fetal outcome based on chorionicity or zygosity. Carroll et al. used umbilical cord blood with microsatellite markers and placenta histology to determine zygosity and chorionicity, respectively. Carroll et al.[27] reported that fetal outcomes in twin pregnancies are better predicted by chorionicity rather than zygosity. They also reported misclassification between genetic testing and clinical diagnosis of chorionicity. Similarly, Spiegler et al.[28] reported significantly higher rates of clinical misclassification in monozygotic twins when compared with dizygotic twins (37% and 11%, respectively). Several studies have reported perinatal outcomes based on both clinical and genetic zygosities (Table 15.1).[28,29] When defining outcomes based on chorionicity, monochorionic–monoamniotic pregnancies have the highest

TABLE 15.1	Perinatal Outcomes in Multiple Gestation Based on Zygosity							
AUTHOR, YEAR, COUNTRY	STUDY DESIGN	SAMPLE SIZE (n CASES)	CONTROL CASES (n)	ZYGOSITY CLINICAL AND GENETIC	PRETERM DELIVERY MONO VS. DI	INTRAUTERINE INFECTION MONO VS. DI	CESAREAN MONO VS. DI	COMMENTS
Spiegler, 2012, Germany	Case–control study	165 twins 87 (monozygotic) 78 (dizygotic)	2,535 singletons	Yes	44% vs. 46% (P > 0.05)	20% vs. 33% (P = 0.012)	94% vs. 92% (P > 0.05)	Neonatal outcomes as respiratory or brain abnormalities no difference among groups.
Gao, 2011, China	Retrospective study	295 twins 70 (monozygotic) 225 (dizygotic)	NA	Yes				Monozygosity was a risk factor for FGR (OR was 1.747, 95% CI, 1.164–2.621). Dizygosity was a preventive factor for FGR (OR was 0.815, 95% CI, 0.685–0.971).

CI, confidence interval; FGR, fetal growth restriction; OR, odds ratio.

mortality rate at 50%, followed by monochorionic–diamniotic at 26% and dichorionic–diamniotic pregnancies at 9%.

Determining Chorionicity

Early sonographic documentation of the number of placentas, or chorionicity, is important for optimal management of twin gestations. Evaluating the number of sacs and amniotic membrane also provides clues to chorionicity. In a dichorionic gestation, the amniotic membrane is thick as it is composed of two layers of amnion and two interposed layers of chorion. In monochorionic twins, the membrane is thin, composed only of amnions from each gestational sac. As the pregnancy continues, images of the placenta, sacs, and membranes become more difficult to obtain.[30–32] Some authors have reported that the chorionicity, fetuses, and amnions can be documented by 5, 6, and 8 weeks, respectively.[33] Most attest that accuracy is highest if the assessment of chorionicity is undertaken before 14 weeks' gestation.[34] In a study of 131 twin pregnancies, Stenhouse et al.[34] reported US sensitivity of 77% for monochorionicity and 90% for dichorionicity after 14 weeks, whereas 99% accuracy was achieved for both groups before 14 weeks. With a composite of second-trimester US markers (i.e., number of placentas, fetal phenotype, membrane thickness, and twin-peak sign), the sensitivity and specificity for correct identification of monochorionic pregnancies is reported at 91.7% and 97.3%, respectively.[35] Sometimes, there are cases of twin pregnancies where chorionicity can be difficult to determine. In these mothers, the pregnancy can be diagnosed as dichorionic without other US parameters if the fetuses *differ in sex*.[33] Providers are cautioned against diagnosing a dichorionic pregnancy based on visualization of two placentas, especially

during the second and third trimesters, because the "second" placenta could represent a succenturiate lobe.[33] When chorionicity cannot be determined even with available diagnostics, the provider should consider sending the placenta to pathology after delivery.

Diagnosis
Imaging
Before 10 Weeks
Markers for chorionicity include the number of gestational sacs, amniotic sacs within chorionic cavity, and yolk sacs. A strong relationship exists between the number of gestational sacs and chorionicity. Two gestational sacs and two embryo poles with fetal cardiac activity are suggestive of a dichorionic twin pregnancy, whereas one sac with two embryo poles is most consistent with monochorionicity (Fig. 15.4).[36] The use of transvaginal US is helpful before 10 weeks to identify the number of amniotic sacs. Similarly, the number of yolk sacs may help in the diagnosis of amnionicity: For example, two yolk sacs are suggestive of a diamniotic pregnancy (Fig. 15.5).[37] When these findings are no longer present after 10 weeks, later sonographic findings become standard.

After 10 Weeks
Lambda sign: The lambda sign is a histological feature of dichorionicity, representing extension of placental tissue into the base of the intertwine membrane (Fig. 15.6). The presence of a lambda or twin-peak sign is diagnostic of a dichorionic pregnancy (Fig. 15.7).[33] The lambda sign, which refers to the shape of the lateral edges of the membranes, was first described by Bessis and Papernik[35] in 1981 and later by Finberg[38] in 1992. In the second

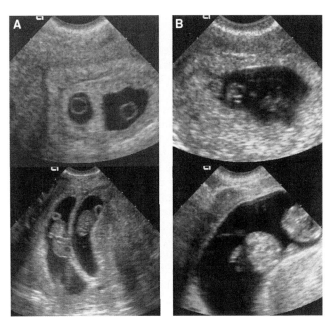

FIGURE 15.4: Dichorionic and monochorionic twins. First-trimester examples of dichorionic **(A)** and monochorionic **(B)** twin gestations. Note the thick separating membranes of dichorionic placentation.

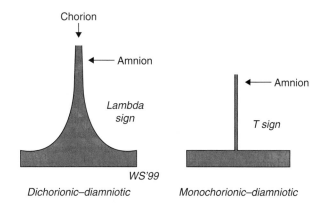

FIGURE 15.6: Schematic illustrating the lambda, or twin-peak, and T signs observed in dichorionic and monochorionic twin pregnancies, respectively. In a dichorionic pregnancy with fused placentas, both the amnions and the chorions reflect away from the placental surface, creating a potential space into which villi can grow. This is called the lambda or twin-peak sign. Monochorionic–diamniotic pregnancies have a single layer of continuous chorion, limiting villous growth. This is called the T sign.

trimester, the twin-peak sign becomes more difficult to visualize and disappears in about 7% of dichorionic pregnancies between 16 and 20 weeks.[39–41] Therefore, the absence of this sign in the second or third trimester cannot exclude dichorionicity.[39]

T sign: In contrast, monochorionic placentation is characterized as a single placental mass and a thin separating membrane, which is optimally detected when the membrane is oriented perpendicular to the US beam (see Fig. 15.6). This membrane intersects the placental junction with a "T" sign (Fig. 15.8). Although the T sign generally indicates a monochorionic-diamniotic pregnancy,[33] other instances can occur when this sign is not diagnostic. For example, as a dichorionic pregnancy progresses, the hallmark lambda sign may not be visible and can simulate a T configuration. This reiterates the importance of early US diagnosis of chorionicity.

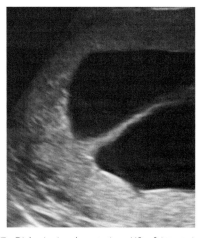

FIGURE 15.7: Dichorionic placentation. US of intertwin membrane–placental junction in a dichorionic twin gestation shows extension of the placental tissue into the base of the intertwin membrane (the lambda sign).

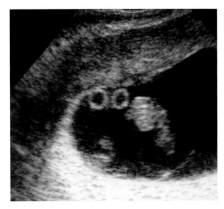

FIGURE 15.5: Monochorionic–diamniotic placentation with two yolk sacs. US of a monochorionic twin pregnancy in which there was difficulty in identification of the intertwin membrane shows two discrete yolk sacs, confirming a diamniotic gestation.

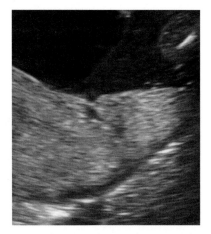

FIGURE 15.8: Monochorionic placentation. Transabdominal US of a monochorionic twin pregnancy shows the absence of the lambda sign and the presence of the T sign with the intertwin membrane abruptly joining the placental surface with no intervening chorion.

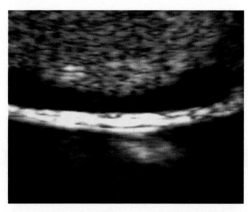

FIGURE 15.9: Dichorionic twin. In this US of a section of intertwin membrane in a dichorionic twin pregnancy, the intertwin membrane is thick and echogenic, and three layers are seen, confirming dichorionicity.

Thickness of intertwin membrane: Several authors have measured the thickness of the intertwin membrane as a tool for diagnosing chorionicity.[33] In 1989, Winn et al.[42] reported that during second trimester, the mean thickness of the intertwin membrane was 2.4 mm for dichorionic pregnancies and 1.4 mm for monochorionic pregnancies, with an accuracy in predicting monochorionic or dichorionic twinning of 82% and 95%, respectively. Clinically, however, this has been difficult to apply as while the mean for dichorionic and monochorionic pregnancies differs, these dimensions can overlap for each type of placentation. Because it is not universally applicable, this measurement is not routinely used in clinical practice. In general, an intertwin membrane thickness of more than 2 mm indicates dichorionicity with a positive predictive value of 95%, whereas a thickness ≤2 mm indicates monochorionicity with a positive predictive value of 90% (Fig. 15.9).[32] On fetal MRI, differences in membrane thickness may also provide clues to chronicity (Fig. 15.10).

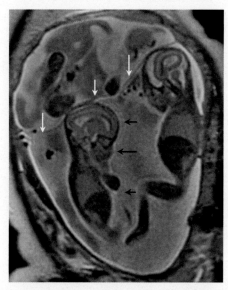

FIGURE 15.10: Membranes on fetal MRI. Coronal SSFSE T2 image in a dichorionic–triamniotic triplet gestation. The membrane separating the chorions is thick (*white arrows*) versus that separating the twins that share a placenta (*black arrows*).

Layers of intertwin membrane: In the second trimester, the number of membranes may be counted to determine chorionicity, and if there are more than 2, then dichorionicity is strongly suggested (see Fig. 15.9).[33,43] This technique requires high-powered US technology that is not routinely available in clinical practice. Using this technique, researchers noted that visualization of four membranes indicated a dichorionic pregnancy and two membranes a monochorionic pregnancy.

Prenatal Diagnosis: Prenatal diagnosis evolved tremendously in the past century in response to increasing pregnancies with higher maternal ages and thus an associated increased risk of Down syndrome. Prenatal diagnosis shifted from a risk assessment based solely on the mother's age (i.e., medical history) to a quantitative risk assessment that evolved from the measurement of maternal alpha-fetoprotein (AFP) to that of human chorionic gonadotropin (hCG) levels later during that decade.[44] In the 1990s, nuchal translucency (NT) was introduced as another first-trimester screening tool.[45] In 1997, Lo et al.[46] revolutionized prenatal screening and diagnosis with their discovery of cell-free fetal DNA (cff DNA), which is now commercially available. Each of these diagnostic markers has been validated first in singletons and then extrapolated to include twins and other higher order multiples. Twin and multiple gestations present unique challenges in prenatal screening and diagnosis. Monitoring of a twin pregnancy via US is more complicated than that of a singleton pregnancy. Chorionicity determination is very essential in any twin pregnancy. Counseling, antenatal care, and US monitoring are all based on the type of twin pregnancy. In uncomplicated dichorionic and monochorionic pregnancies, US monitoring essentially starts as early as 10 weeks (Fig. 15.11).

MULTIPLE GESTATIONS AND CONGENITAL MALFORMATION

For any given defect, the pregnancy may be concordant or discordant in terms of the presence, type, and severity of the abnormality. However, the majority (80% to 90%) of structural defects are discordant, regardless of zygosity.

Rustico et al.[47] recently described structural anomalies in 312 twin pregnancy. Ninety percent of major structural anomalies affected one and 10% affected multiple systems. Median gestational age at diagnosis was 19.1 weeks. The most frequent single-system anomalies involved the nervous and circulatory systems. In total, 72 (46%) anomalous twins and 116 (74%) normal co-twins were delivered at a median gestational age of 34.6 weeks. Neonatal/infant death of the anomalous twin occurred in 14%, with an overall survival rate of 32%. Surviving anomalous twins underwent major surgery in 44%. The authors concluded that the outcome for the anomalous twin is generally poor, while the survival rate for the normal co-twin was 71%, with a favorable overall prognosis.

Incidence

The overall prevalence of structural defects is 1.2 to 2.0 times higher in fetuses from twin pregnancies compared with singletons, with most of the excess risk due to increased rates in monochorionic twins.[48] Monozygotic twins have two to three times higher rates of congenital anomalies than singletons or dizygotic twins. The rate per fetus in dizygotic twins is probably

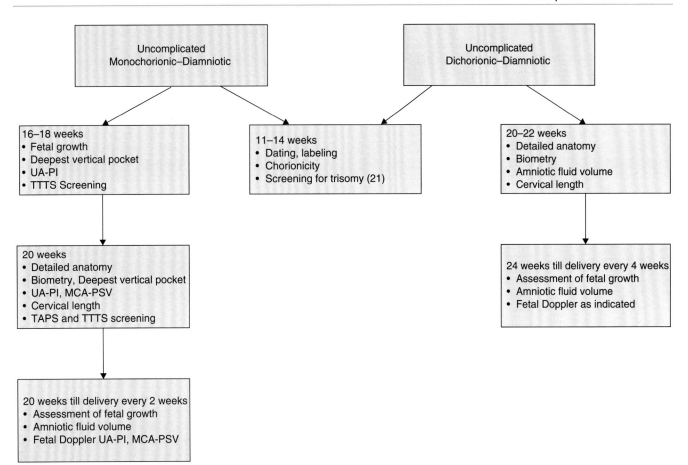

FIGURE 15.11: Flowchart for monitoring uncomplicated monochorionic–diamniotic and dichorionic–diamniotic pregnancies. *MCA*, middle cerebral artery; *PSV*, peak systolic velocity; *PI*, pulsatility index; *TAPS*, twin anemia–polycythemia sequence; *TTTS*, twin-to-twin transfusion syndrome; *UA*, umbilical artery.

the same as that in singletons, whereas it is two to three times higher in monozygotic twins.

In around 1 in 25 dichorionic, 1 in 15 monochorionic-diamniotic, and 1 in 6 monoamniotic twin pregnancies, there is a major congenital anomaly that typically affects only one twin.[49,50] Abnormalities associated with twins include neural tube defects, anterior abdominal wall defects, facial clefts, brain abnormalities, cardiac defects, and gastrointestinal anomalies. Therefore, screening cardiac assessment should be performed, including laterality, situs and four-chamber, ventricular outflow tract, and aortic arch views.[51]

Pathogenesis/Risk

Zygosity, rather than chorionicity, determines the risk of chromosomal abnormalities and whether the fetuses may be concordant or discordant for the anomaly. In dizygotic pregnancies, each twin has an independent risk for aneuploidy with the maternal age-related risk for chromosomal abnormalities for each twin being the same as in singleton pregnancies. Therefore, the chance of at least one fetus in a dizygotic twin gestation being affected by a chromosomal defect is twice as high as in singleton pregnancies (if zygosity is unknown, multiply singleton risk by 5/3). For these twins, the pregnancy-specific risk is based on the sum of the individual risk estimates for each fetus. In monozygotic twins, the

risk for chromosomal abnormalities in each fetus is the same as in singleton pregnancies.[52]

Given the higher rates of congenital abnormalities in twins and also higher order pregnancies, understanding how multiples affect the sensitivity and specificity of the various prenatal screening and diagnostic tests is crucial. Clinicians should consider that although there are prenatal diagnostic options for twins and multiple gestations, screening accuracy is lower than that for a single pregnancy.[53]

Risk for fetal aneuploidy is associated with *advancing maternal age*.[54] In patients with singletons, advanced maternal age is defined as older than 35 years on the expected date of delivery.[55] This designation is applied to women with a singleton or monochorionic twins. However, defining advanced maternal age is far more complex in women with dizygotic twins, triplets, and high-order multiples. In dizygotic twins, the risk of one fetus having an aneuploidy is twice that for a woman of the same age with a singleton.[56]

Diagnosis

First-Trimester Screening
Ultrasound: In a retrospective study to evaluate the accuracy of antenatal US in the detection of fetal anomalies in 245 twin pregnancies, Edwards et al.[55] reported overall prevalence rates

of 4.9%. Antepartum US had a sensitivity of 88% and a specificity of 100% for the detection of anomalies in these patients, with a positive predictive value of 100% and a negative predictive value of 99%. Despite these findings, data are insufficient to make recommendations about frequency of anatomical US in multiple gestations.

Nuchal tranlucency (NT) is a noninvasive US technique that can be used between 11.0 and 13.6 weeks to detect aneuploidy. Although biochemical results vary according to the number of gestations, gestational age, and other factors, NT is an effective choice because it provides direct visualization of the embryo.[55,57] Screening can be technically challenging in multiple gestations; however, if the nuchal region is visible for each fetus, the test can be effective. In evaluating NT in 448 twin pregnancies (both dichorionic and monochorionic), Sebire et al.[58] reported that 7.3% of normal fetuses had an elevated NT above the 95th percentile. In 88.4% of twin pregnancies, both fetuses had a normal NT. The overall sensitivity of 88% was comparable with the singleton detection rate. The screen false-positive rate was higher in monochorionic twins at 8.4% than in dichorionic twins at 5.4%. In multiples, risk assessment using first-trimester methods can be calculated for each fetus or for the entire pregnancy. In monochorionic twins, each fetus has the same risk of being affected with Down syndrome. Thus, a single risk estimate for the duration of pregnancy is based on the average of the NT measurements. Each fetus in a dichorionic twin pregnancy is treated as a separate individual, and the risk for each fetus is calculated using published NT values for singletons.[59,60]

Another interesting application of NT in monochorionic twins is the ability to predict twin-to-twin transfusion syndrome (TTTS).[61,62] An NT threshold at the 95th percentile had a positive and a negative predictive value of 43% and 91%, respectively.[61] Discordance in NT of ≥20% is found in around 25% of monochorionic twins, with the risk of early intrauterine demise or development of severe TTTS in this group being more than 30%.[62]

Biochemical Markers

Pregnancy-Associated Placental Protein A: One screening tool for aneuploidy is the pregnancy-associated placental protein A (PAPP-A), a molecule that is secreted by the placenta. In singleton pregnancies, low levels of PAPP-A occur in fetuses with Down syndrome. However, compared with singleton pregnancies, PAPP-A levels are nearly double in normal twin pregnancies.[63] The magnitude of the value depends on chorionicity, such that PAPP-A is higher in dichorionic than in monochorionic twins.[64] In general, maternal analyte levels can be adjusted for twin pregnancy; however, the detection rate for Down syndrome is lower than that in singleton pregnancy (e.g., 93% detection in monochorionic twins, 78% detection in dichorionic twins, and 95% detection in singletons).[65] In addition, maternal analyte levels for Down syndrome screening in twin pregnancy may be affected by early loss of one embryo of a triplet gestation.[66,67]

Beta-Human Chorionic Gonadotropin: It is a hormone that is also secreted from the placental trophoblast. Compared with singletons, beta-hCG levels are approximately double in twins compared with singletons.[63] Similar to PAPP-A, the levels of beta-hCG are lower in monochorionic than that in dichorionic pregnancies.[64] These values are also affected by the mode of conception, whether spontaneous or ART.

Combined Screening Using Ultrasound and Serum Analyte: In singletons, first-trimester combined screening, which includes maternal age, NT, and maternal serum-free beta-hCG and PAPP-A levels, has been shown to detect approximately 82% of cases of Down syndrome, with a 5% false-positive rate.[68] Wald et al.[60] reported the detection with a 5% false-positive rate for Down syndrome in monochorionic, dichorionic, and all twins as 73%, 68%, and 69% for NT alone and 84%, 70%, and 72% for combined tests, respectively. The accuracy of combined testing in the detection of Down syndrome approximated to singleton rates.

Karyotyping/Invasive Procedures: Screening detection rates for twin pregnancies are estimated to be 15% less than for singleton pregnancies.[63] This can be explained at least in part as being due to the chemicals produced by the chromosomally normal fetus and abnormal fetus being averaged; thus, a total reported number may cause a normal test result. For these reasons, both fetuses of a dizygotic pair should undergo karyotyping unlike monozygotic twins.

Chorionic villus sampling: Chorionic villus sampling is a diagnostic test performed at 10 to 12 weeks of gestation to obtain placental cells for prenatal diagnosis. The procedure can be performed transcervically or transabdominally. Before samples are collected, a US is obtained to confirm the number of placentas and fetuses and determine chorionicity. In a transcervical technique, the patient is prepped, a sterile speculum is placed, and a small catheter is placed through the cervix under direct US visualization to obtain chorionic villi. Although some surgeons prefer biopsy forceps rather than a catheter under negative pressure, either technique can be used. In an abdominal approach, the abdomen is prepped, and a needle is inserted through the abdominal wall into the placenta, cells are aspirated, and then the needle is withdrawn. Only one chorionic villus sample is traditionally needed for monochorionic pregnancies. However, there are case reports of genetically discordant monochorionic twins, and thus two samples can be required. For dichorionic pregnancies, two separate placental samples are needed. If access to both placentas can be achieved via a transcervical approach without contamination, one could choose this method. However, if the second placenta is not accessible through a cervical approach, sampling in this twin pregnancy may be achieved using both cervical and abdominal approaches.

As with any invasive procedure, there are risks and benefits associated with chorionic villus sampling. Many patients opt for this test because it can be performed earlier than an amniocentesis. Reported complications of chorionic villus sampling include placental mosaicism, bleeding, infection, maternal–fetal hemorrhage, limb reduction defects, insufficient sample for analysis, and oromandibular hypogenesis.[69-71] Moreover, any Rh-negative patient should receive RhoGAM to prevent isoimmunization.

Second-Trimester Screening

Ultrasound/Magnetic Resonance Imaging: US in discordant twins can define multiple anomalies, which may provide clues to chromosomal anomaly or genetic syndrome (Fig. 15.12A). MRI is sometimes utilized to exclude additional anomalies (Fig. 15.12B) and confirm diagnosis, particularly in the case of complicated monochorionic gestations (Fig. 15.13).

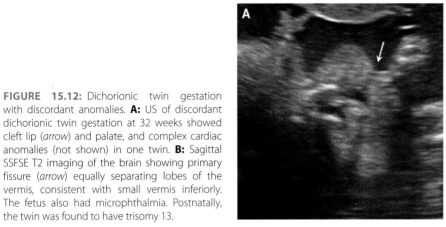
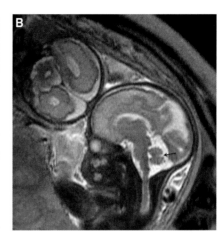

FIGURE 15.12: Dichorionic twin gestation with discordant anomalies. **A:** US of discordant dichorionic twin gestation at 32 weeks showed cleft lip (*arrow*) and palate, and complex cardiac anomalies (not shown) in one twin. **B:** Sagittal SSFSE T2 imaging of the brain showing primary fissure (*arrow*) equally separating lobes of the vermis, consistent with small vermis inferiorly. The fetus also had microphthalmia. Postnatally, the twin was found to have trisomy 13.

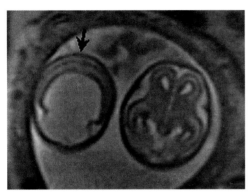

FIGURE 15.13: Discordant monochorionic twins axial SSFSE T2 imaging in an 18-week monochorionic gestation with twin-to-twin transfusion syndrome. One twin with alobar holoprosencephaly (*arrow*). Fetal MRI confirmed normal brain in the co-twin.

Biochemical Markers: In singletons, the second-trimester quad test that combines maternal age with second-trimester serum AFP, beta-hCG, unconjugated estriol, and inhibin-A detects approximately 75% of cases of Down syndrome with a 5% false-positive rate.[72] Many medical centers do not routinely offer this quad screening to patients with multiple fetuses owing to the paucity of data related to the efficacy of second-trimester maternal serum screening for aneuploidy in twins. In addition, reports in the literature reflect the inconsistencies in both sensitivity and detection rates of these analytes and the difficulty in interpreting the variability. On average, maternal serum biochemical markers are twice as high in twins as in singletons of the same gestational age.[73] Muller et al.[74] evaluated second-trimester maternal serum screening for Down syndrome in 3,292 twin pregnancies and reported that median AFP levels were similar between dichorionic and monochorionic twins and that free beta-hCG levels were higher in monochorionic pregnancies. Rates for Down syndrome detection and screen positivity, respectively, were 27.3% and 6.6% using maternal age alone, 54.5% and 24.6% using maternal age corrected for chorionicity, 54.5% and 7.75% using AFP and free beta-hCG divided by 2, 54.5% and 8.05% using median values observed from the global twin population, and 54.5% and 7.75% using median values specific to monochorionic and dichorionic twins. The authors concluded that maternal serum screening is better than maternal age alone but still yields low detection rates. In another study[75] of second-trimester serum screening, high false-positive rates led to an 18.3% amniocentesis rate for twins versus 7.5% rate in singletons. Thus, first-trimester US screening has been suggested to be favored for the detection of Down syndrome.

Cell-Free Fetal DNA: In 1997, Dr. Lo and his coworkers discovered cff DNA, an innovation that revolutionized prenatal screening. Cff DNA is released into the maternal bloodstream after placental cells undergo apoptosis.[71] It constitutes approximately 10% of the total DNA in maternal plasma and is rapidly cleared from maternal blood, within 2 hours of delivery.[76,77] The half-life of fetal DNA is short at approximately 16 minutes, but it has recently been found that the entire fetal genome, in the form of cell-free DNA (cfDNA), is present in maternal blood.[78] Cff DNA has been demonstrated as early as prior to the seventh week of gestation.[79] Therefore, cff DNA has become the focus of research for the development of noninvasive prenatal testing (NIPT).

Of the several types, including digital polymerase chain reaction (PCR), massively parallel DNA sequencing (MPS) of the whole genome, and target sequencing of the selected genomic loci on the chromosome of interest, utilized for NIPT for the detection of Down syndrome, the primary methods applied in the United States, Asia, and parts of Europe are MPS and target sequencing.[80] The first approach, MPS, uses the whole genome and requires sequencing of many millions of DNA fragments to generate sufficient reads to detect differences in the level of chromosome 21, which constitutes 1.5% of sequenced fragments. The second alternative targets sequencing the select genomic loci on the chromosome of interest, for example, chromosome 21 for NIPT for the detection of Down syndrome.[81–87] In a series of validation studies in singletons, the MPS technique demonstrated high accuracy with sensitivity rates between 79% and 100%, and less than 1% false-positive rates for diagnosis of Down syndrome[88–90]; 97% to 100% for trisomy 18[89–91]; and 75% to 79% for trisomy 13.[90,91] Of note, cfDNA should be timed appropriately, typically after the ninth week.

In twin pregnancies, Huang et al.[92] reported the use of cff DNA in 189 twin pregnancies, with sensitivity and specificity using maternal plasma sequencing for fetal trisomy 21 being both 100% and for fetal trisomy 18 at 50% and 100%, respectively. This study further supported that sequencing-based NIPT of trisomy 21 in twin pregnancies could be achieved with a high accuracy. Furthermore, in a recent meta-analysis, Gil et al.[92a] showed that the performance of cfDNA testing for trisomy 21 in a twin pregnancy is similar to that reported in a singleton pregnancy and is superior to that of the first-trimester combined test or second-trimester biochemical testing. However, the number of cases of trisomies 18 and 13 was too small for accurate assessment of the predictive performance with the cfDNA test.

Karyotype/Invasive Procedures

Amniocentesis: Amniocentesis is the gold standard for prenatal diagnosis. The procedure is typically performed in the second trimester to obtain amniotic fluid for genetic analysis by a needle inserted through a prepped abdominal wall under continuous US guidance. Complications of amniocentesis include infection, bleeding, and maternal–fetal hemorrhage. As in chorionic villus sampling, an Rh-negative patient should receive Rhogam. Like most procedures, amniocentesis in twins presents unique diagnostic challenges. After correctly identifying placental location and the intended twin to be tested first, the needle is inserted into the amniotic sac of the first twin, followed by injection of indigo carmine before removing the needle. Methylene blue should not be used because of the risk of atresia of the fetal small bowel, staining of the skin, and methemoglobinemia in the infant. Next, the needle is inserted into the second twin's amniotic sac. If the fluid aspirated appears blue tinged, the first sac is reentered and the physician should remove the needle and try again.[94–96]

The American Congress of Obstetricians and Gynecologists (ACOG) reports the procedure-related loss rate from 1 per 300 to 500 performed.[97] Several studies agree that the loss rate for twins exceeds this, but by what extent is controversial. Loss rates have approximated 1%[98] in some studies, but others were inconclusive because of the heterogeneity of the populations studied and inconsistencies in the definition of procedure-related loss.[53]

Management

Management of the pregnancy is individualized and mainly expectant or termination. Selective termination is relatively safe in dichorionic twins but can be fraught with danger in monochorionic gestations, putting both twins at risk for demise.

Recurrence Risk

Recurrence risk is dependent on the type of genetic transmission.

PRETERM DELIVERY

Definition/Incidence

Preterm delivery, defined as delivery before 37.0 weeks' gestation, affects approximately 12% of singleton births in the United States[1] and approximately 11% worldwide.[99] Over half of twin deliveries occur before 37.0 weeks, and about one-tenth of twin deliveries before 32 weeks.[1] Preterm delivery is the most significant cause of morbidity and mortality in twin gestations.

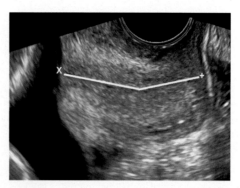

FIGURE 15.14: US of normal cervix with equal thickness of anterior and posterior cervical lips. *X* marks the internal cervical os; + marks the external cervical os; the echodense line connecting the two points is the endocervical canal.

Pathogenesis

It is not surprising that multiple gestations are at risk for preterm labor, given greater uterine distention, which can initiate labor and cause earlier cervical changes.

Diagnosis/Surveillance

Sonographic measurement of cervical length (Fig. 15.14) and biochemical testing of fetal fibronectin are the two main screening tools used to predict preterm birth (PTB). However, recently, Bergalla et al.[93] reported in a Cochrane database report that there are limited data on the effects of knowing the cervical length, measured by US, for preventing PTBs, which preclude us from drawing any conclusions for women with asymptomatic twin or singleton pregnancies, singleton pregnancies with preterm premature rupture of membranes (PPROM), or other populations and clinical scenarios. Limited evidence suggests that knowledge of transvaginal US-measured cervical length, used to inform the management of women with singleton pregnancies and symptoms of preterm labor, appears to only prolong pregnancy by about 4 days over a group of women in which the cervical length had not been measured or studied. Ongoing research in this topic is essential (see Chapter 14).

Imaging

A shortened cervical length (Fig. 15.15) indicates a higher risk of preterm delivery for twin pregnancies. Among 464 twin pregnancies seen for routine care, Skentou et al.[100] found that the median cervical length at 23 weeks was 36 mm. The rate of spontaneous delivery before 33 weeks was inversely related to cervical length at 23 weeks. It increased gradually from approximately 2.5% at 60 mm to 5% at 40 mm, and to 12% at 25 mm, and exponentially below this length to 17% at 20 mm and to 80% at 8 mm (Fig. 15.16). A meta-analysis of studies that measured cervical length by transvaginal US to predict spontaneous PTB in twin pregnancies found that the test was most useful when performed in asymptomatic women at 20 to 24 weeks of gestation.[101] In establishing a cutoff of 20 mm, the authors found that the positive likelihood ratios for PTB were 5.2 and 10.1, respectively, in the 35% of pregnancies delivered before 28 weeks and 39% before 32 weeks.[101] The usefulness of screening cervical length is limited by high frequency of short cervices in women not at imminent risk of delivery and by the lack of

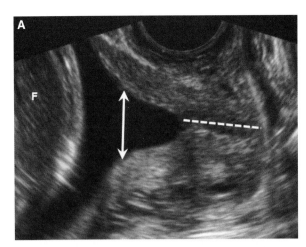

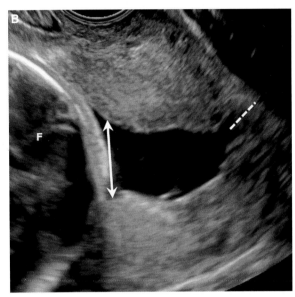

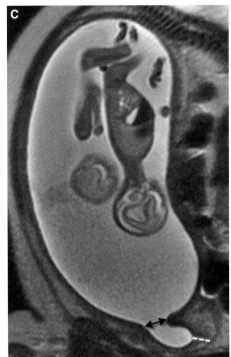

FIGURE 15.15: Shortened cervix by US and MRI. **A:** A transvaginal scan at 23 weeks in twin pregnancy showing dilatation and funneling of the internal cervical os (*line with end arrows*). The closed cervical length (*dotted line*) measures 2.5 cm with funneling cervix, with walls of funnel in a Y-shaped configuration. *F*, fetus. **B:** Transvaginal US with nearly completely effaced cervix, with U-shaped funnel. Same annotations in **A**. **C:** MRI of U-shaped funneling and shortened cervical length. The *black arrows* show internal os, and *dotted lines* show shortened closed cervix.

effective interventions to prevent PTB. Consequently, universal screening in this population is controversial because there are no known treatments. Despite this disagreement, at our institution when imaging a twin pregnancy with a cervical length less than 25 mm, the mom is evaluated for signs of PTB and may require additional therapy if surgery is contemplated.

In contrast, for women with signs and symptoms of preterm labor between 23 and 33 weeks, cervical length was a better predictor of preterm delivery than funneling or digital examination.[102] In symptomatic twin pregnancies, Crane et al.[102] found rates of delivery were 44% for cervical lengths less than 15 mm as compared with no delivery within a week if cervical length was more than 25 mm.

Biochemical

Fetal fibronectin is a protein found between the fetal sac and the uterine lining that can be used to predict PTB in both singleton and twin pregnancies. In the largest prospective study of 147 women expecting twins, fibronectin testing was done at 2-week intervals between weeks 24 and 30.[103] Using fibronectin levels at gestational week 28, Goldenberg et al.[103] reported deliveries prior to 32 weeks in 30% of women with a positive test (≥50 ng/mL) and 4% of women with a negative result. Although these data

support the feasibility of fibronectin in predicting preterm twin birth, this testing is not routinely performed in asymptomatic twin pregnancies in the absence of other prematurity risk factors.

Management/Prevention

Progesterone has been the biggest advancement in the prevention of PTB in singleton pregnancies for women with a history of preterm delivery. However, this therapy does not extrapolate to twin gestations.[104] Furthermore, in a meta-analysis, Sotiriadis et al.[104] reported that progesterone used for the prevention of preterm delivery in twin pregnancy was associated with increased rates of perinatal death. At this time, there are no effective methods of preventing preterm delivery in twins, even with a history of a preterm delivery.[105]

For women who have a short cervix, vaginal progesterone results are promising but do not reach statistical significance in reducing preterm twin birth.[106] Similarly, intramuscular injection of 17 hydroxyprogesterone does not reduce the risk for twin pregnancies complicated with a shortened cervix.[107] Although cerclage has proven beneficial in preventing PTB in singleton gestations for women with a history of preterm delivery and short cervix, this benefit does not appear to be true for twin gestations.

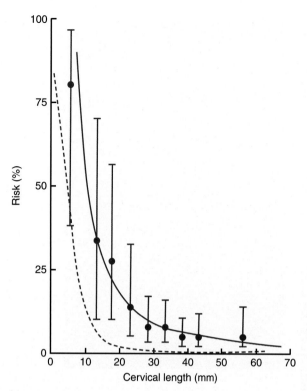

FIGURE 15.16: Risk of preterm delivery before 33 weeks' gestation compared with closed cervical length at 23 weeks in twin pregnancies. The rate of spontaneous delivery before 33 weeks is inversely related to cervical length measured at 23 weeks. It increased gradually from approximately 2.5% at 6 cm to 5% at 4 cm, and 12% at 2.5 cm. (Adapted from Skentou C, Souka AP, To MSW, et al. Prediction of preterm delivery in twins by cervical assessment at 23 weeks. *Ultrasound Obstet Gynecol.* 2001;17:7–10.)

In fact, a 2005 meta-analysis shows a higher incidence of PTB in twin gestations with cerclage.[108]

Recently, Dang et al.[109] published randomized clinical trial comparing Arabin pessary to vaginal progesterone for the prevention of PTB in women with twin pregnancies and a short cervix defined as less than 38 mm. The authors reported that there is no significant difference in rate of PTB at less than 34 weeks of gestation in women in the pessary 16% or progesterone group (400-mg vaginal progesterone) 22%. However, the use of pessary significantly reduced the composite of poor perinatal outcomes (19% vs. 27%). In women with cervical length of 28 mm or less (25th percentile), pessary significantly reduced the PTB rate at less than 34 weeks of gestation from 46% to 21% and significantly improved the composite of poor perinatal outcomes. Therefore, further studies are needed to report outcome in this subpopulation of twin pregnancies complicated with short cervix less than 28 mm. In addition, there has been a report of cervical incompetence treated with a cerclage and pessary[110] in a monochorionic–monoamniotic twin pregnancy. Some authors have also proposed pessaries to prevent PTB in severe TTTS treated by laser.[111] However, the use of pessary in preventing PTB in twins remains unclear.

Unfortunately, no intervention has been shown to improve outcomes in twins when the mother's US has identified a short cervix or there is a history of preterm delivery.[112] Since higher rates of preterm delivery occur in twins conceived by ART than those conceived naturally, the most effective strategy against morbidity and mortality associated with preterm delivery is the prevention of multiple gestations in the ART setting.

FETAL DEATH

Single intrauterine fetal death (sIUFD) in multiple gestation pregnancies occurs in roughly 3.7% to 6.8% of twin pregnancies.[113–115] In 2006, a systematic review of 19 studies demonstrated that the increased risk of death of a co-surviving twin after the death of one twin was 12% for monochorionic pregnancies and 4% for dichorionic pregnancies. The odds ratio (OR) for monochorionic co-twin intrauterine death (IUD) was six times that of dichorionic twins.[116] Moreover, the studies reinforced that fetal death can occur at any time.

Single-Twin Gestation Demise Before 14 Weeks (Vanishing Twin Syndrome)

This syndrome usually occurs in the first trimester with the identification of a single fetus weeks after confirmation and diagnosis of any twin pregnancy (Fig. 15.17). The true incidence of vanishing twins is unknown but may be as high as 29%.[117] In vanishing twin syndrome, outcomes based on chorionicity are yet unknown. As for long-term outcome, Anand et al.[118] reported no developmental delays in children up to age 1 when comparing surviving twins from a vanishing twin pregnancy and children from singleton pregnancies.[118]

Single-Twin Demise After 14 Weeks

Incidence

The overall incidence of single-twin death after 20 weeks of pregnancy is estimated between 2.6% and 6.2%.[119]

Pathogenesis

In primarily *monochorionic* twins, the morbidity and mortality in the surviving twin has been explained by two theories: transchorionic embolization and coagulopathy or transient hemodynamic fluctuations between the twins. In the first theory, passage of thrombotic materials from the dead twin occurs along the placental vascular anastomoses, resulting in disseminated

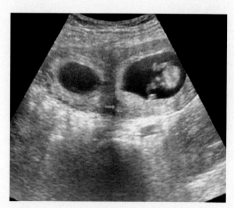

FIGURE 15.17: Vanishing twin syndrome in dichorionic pregnancy. A transvaginal scan at 9 weeks showing dichorionic twin pregnancy with thick separation (*green arrow*). Left sac is empty (representing vanishing twin), and right sac shows an embryonic pole.

intravascular coagulopathy in the initially healthy surviving twin.[117] The resulting disseminated intravascular coagulopathy may result in infarcts and cystic degenerative changes in the survivor's renal, pulmonary, hepatic, splenic, and neurological organs.[120] However, data has demonstrated normal coagulation in the surviving twin after IUD of the co-twin, refuting this hypothesis.[121]

The alternative theory is based on rapid and profound hemodynamic alteration that occurs when one twin dies. Specifically, an acute shift of blood from the surviving twin flows into the dead fetus along the superficial anastomotic channels.[121,122] There has been *in utero* demonstration of severe fetal anemia in the surviving twin after death of co-twin, thus supporting this hypothesis.[121,123]

Etiology

The multiple causes for fetal death in twin pregnancy include fetal chromosomal or congenital malformations, and maternal diseases (e.g., diabetes, placenta diseases). Twin pregnancies complicated by a fetal death are at increased risk for both preterm delivery and death of the co-twin.

Diagnosis/Surveillance

Imaging: Regardless of chorionicity, management after a single fetal death is challenging. Expert opinions recommend US assessment of fetal growth every 2 to 4 weeks. In some cases of single fetal death in a multifetal pregnancy, prenatal US can detect intracranial abnormalities in the surviving twin.[124] Patten et al.[125] have demonstrated that a normal initial scan cannot rule out damage and that sonographic evidence of intracranial abnormalities in the surviving twin may manifest as early as 7 days after the death of its co-twin. Structural abnormalities observed in survivors include neural tube defects, optic nerve hypoplasia, hypoxic–ischemic lesions of the white matter, multicystic encephalomalacia, microcephaly, hydranencephaly, porencephaly, hemorrhagic lesions (Fig. 15.18A), posthemorrhagic hydrocephalus, bilateral renal cortical necrosis, unilateral absence of

a kidney, gastrointestinal tract atresia, gastroschisis, hemifacial microsomia, and aplasia cutis of the scalp, trunk, or limbs.[126] Sonographic scan might be complemented with MRI.[127]

Fetal MRI may show positive restricted diffusion and edema days following the cotwin demise. Imaging in the first weeks may demonstrate early volume loss and encephalomalacia. However, some believe that, the best timing for MRI is at 32 weeks or later, when white matter is developed and minor (yet clinically important) lesions in the white matter can be visualized.

Three patterns of brain pathology have been described in the surviving twin.[117] First, hypoxic–ischemic lesions of white matter usually occur in the area supplied by the middle cerebral artery, which may evolve to porencephaly, multicystic encephalomalacia, microcephaly, and hydranencephaly (Fig. 15.18B). Second, hemorrhagic lesions, either isolated or in combination with ischemic lesions, may lead to posthemorrhagic hydrocephalus (Fig. 15.18C). Third, anomalies secondary to a vascular disturbance can occur, including neural tube defects, limb reduction anomalies, and optic nerve hypoplasia. In a recent study, fetal MRI demonstrated more ischemic lesions that spared the brainstem and cerebellum and were more commonly nonhemorrhagic versus hemorrhagic (83% vs. 17%).[128] Less commonly detected nonfocal lesions included periventricular leukomalacia and generalized and posterior encephalomalacia. When including imaging prenatal and postnatal, significant cerebral injury has been reported in over than 25% of surviving co-twins.[129]

Prognosis

Timing of fetal death and chorionicity are important factors that impact management, counseling, and short- and long-term outcomes. In studies examining neurological outcome after one fetal death in twin pregnancies,[117] reports noted rates of cerebral palsy were 6.3% in surviving twins and 1.8% higher in monozygotic twin pregnancies. Nelson and Ellenberg[130] also reported an increased rate of nonfebrile seizures in the surviving twin (5%) after fetal death versus 0.8% when

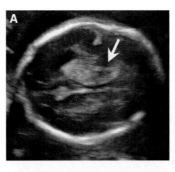
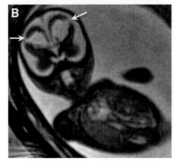
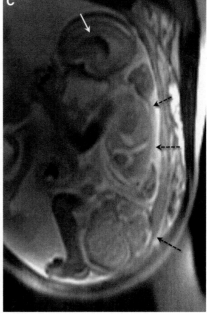

FIGURE 15.18: Twin demise in three different monochorionic pregnancies with intracranial injury in the surviving twin. **A:** Axial cranial US of surviving twin demonstrating heterogeneous echogenicity of the choroid, suggestive of hemorrhage (*arrow*). **B:** Coronal SSFP MRI in a monochorionic gestation at 21 weeks, 3 weeks after demise of co-twin showing moderate ventriculomegaly and areas of porencephaly/multicystic encephalomalacia (*arrows*) in the surviving twin. Fetus sent for MRI as US demonstrated increasing ventricular dilatation. **C:** Monochorionic twin gestation at 20 weeks with recent demise of co-twin (*dotted arrows*). The SSFSE T2 image demonstrating a large germinal matrix hemorrhage in the surviving twin (*solid arrow*).

both twins survive. In terms of IQ testing, no significant differences have been observed between survivors after their co-twin's death and surviving twins.[130] However, recently, Mackie et al.[131] in a meta-analysis to determine the prognosis of the surviving co-twin following spontaneous sIUFD reported the following. In monochorionic twins with sIUFD at less than 28 weeks' gestation, there was significantly increased rate of co-twin intrauterine fetal death (OR 2.31) and neonatal death (OR 2.84) compared with when the sIUFD occurred at more than 28 weeks' gestation. Neonatal death in monochorionic twins was significantly higher if the pregnancy was complicated by fetal growth restriction (OR 4.83) or PTB (OR 4.95). Abnormal antenatal brain imaging was reported in 20.0% of surviving monochorionic co-twins.

Management
Several factors impact management and outcome of the surviving co-twin, including chorionicity, gestational age at time of fetal death, and maternal and placental diseases.

Monochorionic
Previable Pregnancy (<24 Weeks): Because of the lack of predictive investigation on long-term outcome at this gestational age, regardless of chronicity, most patients are managed conservatively during that period. Despite sparse data, some patients consider termination as another treatment option.[132]

Viable Pregnancy (≥24 Weeks): The prevalence of monochorionic twinning in the presence of a single fetal death ranges from 50% to 70%.[133] Fetal death increases 1% to 2% per week in monochorionic gestations after 32 weeks.[134] The surviving twin faces increased risk of fetal and neonatal morbidity and mortality, most often fetal death, neurological morbidities, and prematurity. In a 2006 meta-analysis[116] that assessed the risk of co-twin mortality and neurological morbidity following the death of one twin after 14 weeks' gestation, researchers reported a 12% risk of death and 18% neurological abnormality for the monochorionic surviving twin.

Timing of Delivery: Based on the 2011 National Institute of Child Health and Human Development (NICHD) workshop, the proceedings recommended delivery if fetal death occurs at or after 34 weeks and considering delivery in cases before 34 weeks based on concurrent maternal and fetal conditions.[134]

Dichorionic: In the presence of single fetal death, the main risk in the surviving dichorionic–diamniotic twin is preterm delivery. In 2006, a meta-analysis[116] reported an estimated risk of both iatrogenic and spontaneous preterm deliveries after single fetal death as being 68% and 57% in monochorionic and dichorionic pregnancies, respectively. Based on the NICHD workshop, management strategy for dichorionic–diamniotic twin pregnancies is directed similarly to monochorionic–diamniotic twin pregnancies.[134] However, expert opinion recommends a conservative approach for dichorionic–diamniotic twin pregnancies that includes regular fetal and maternal surveillance and delivery between 37 and 38 weeks.[134] The mode of delivery should be based on the obstetrical indications for either vaginal birth or cesarean section. For maternal monitoring after fetal death, Rh-negative women should undergo a Kleihauer test and regular blood pressure monitoring because of the increased risk of preeclampsia.[114]

FETAL GROWTH ABNORMALITIES

Incidence
Patients with multifetal pregnancies are at risk for growth abnormalities, along with their associated increased risks of obstetric complications, and perinatal morbidity and mortality.[127]

Pathogenesis/Etiology
Growth discordance can occur secondary to multiple known risk factors classified as fetal (monochorionic, infections), placental (placenta previa, abruption, velamentous cord insertion), and maternal (maternal age >30 years, nulliparity, tobacco use, no prenatal care).[135]

Diagnosis/Surveillance

Normal Growth
The normal fetal growth trajectory of a twin gestation diverges around 8 weeks, slowing to a rate lower than for singletons.[136–138] This rate persists until 30 to 32 weeks, at which time a second diversion in slower growth occurs. The slower growth rate in twins has been attributed to placental crowding and the more frequent anomalous umbilical cord insertion (Fig. 15.19). These findings have led to an emerging paradigm, explaining that events early in twin gestation, perhaps at the time of conception, play a critical role in determining intrauterine growth trajectories and size at birth. The ACOG technical bulletin on assessment of growth suggests that centers should use growth tables derived from twin gestations.[136] However, most studies of twin growth curves are derived from a small sample size and do not take into account chorionicity, race, or sex or represent singleton curves applied to multiple gestation.[137,138]

Growth Discordance
In trying to improve the assessment of fetal weight in multiple gestations, several investigators have focused on individual biometric parameters. For example, an abdominal circumference ratio of less than 0.93 has a 3.8 likelihood ratio for twin 25% discordant weight, and a higher head circumference/abdominal circumference has increased rates of adverse pregnancy outcome. Another important assessment is growth discordance, with studies showing an association between significant differences in twin birth weights and increased mortality and morbidity.[139–142]

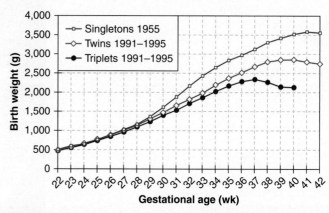

FIGURE 15.19: The 50th percentile of birth weight for gestational age was approximately similar among singletons, twins, and triplets before 28 weeks of gestation.

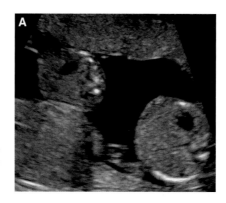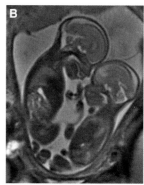

FIGURE 15.20: Growth discordance in twin pregnancies. **A:** US manifestation of abdominal circumference discordant size in a monochorionic–diamniotic twin pregnancy. **B:** MRI showing discordant size in monochorionic–diamniotic pregnancy.

Growth discordance is defined as estimated fetal weight (EFW) of larger twin—EFW of smaller twin/EFW of larger twin ×100. The ACOG considers growth discordance from 15% to 25% as significant (Fig. 15.20). Growth discordance more than 20% occurs in 16% of twin pairs and more than 30% occurs in 5% of twin gestations, regardless of chronicity.[135]

Most patients with twin pregnancies undergo several US assessments beginning in the early first trimester. Regardless of chronicity, first-trimester US cannot predict growth discordance. However, Lewi et al.[143] reported that monochorionic twin pregnancies with early-onset discordance (i.e., difference in crown–rump length at ≥90th percentile) had higher rates of adverse pregnancy outcomes and fetal death compared with those with late-onset discordance in the second trimester (i.e., EFW difference >20%). However, there are few published studies to indicate how often routine reassessment should be done in twin pregnancies in such instances.

In general, US scans in monochorionic twin pregnancies are performed every 2 weeks, starting at 16 to 18 weeks, to better ascertain early evidence of TTTS. This is followed by an anatomy comprehensive US between 18 and 22 weeks.[144] In contrast, US scans in dichorionic twin pregnancies are recommended every 3 to 4 weeks[144] (see Fig. 15.11). Fetal surveillance should be increased when there is either growth restriction observed in one twin or significant growth discordance. Available data show no benefit for routine surveillance by umbilical artery Doppler waveforms in twin pregnancies, regardless of chorionicity, unless there is a complication such as fetal growth restriction.

Prognosis

Several factors may increase adverse pregnancy outcomes in twin pregnancies, regardless of chorionicity. Discordance of more than 20% compared with the presenting twin and a delivery interval less than 15 minutes and between 15 and 30 minutes (1.3 and 2.3 times, respectively) have been implicated as risk factors for adverse perinatal outcome.[135] D'Antonio et al.[145] recently published a systematic and meta-analysis review including 22 studies with 10,877 twins to explore the strength of association between birth weight discordance and perinatal mortality in twin pregnancy. The secondary aim was to ascertain the contribution of gestational age and growth restriction in predicting mortality in growth-discordant twins. The findings of this systematic review showed that both dichorionic and monochorionic twin pregnancies with fetal growth discordance were generally at higher risk of IUD but not of neonatal demise, compared with pregnancies with birth weight-concordant twins. The risk of IUD in discordant twins was higher when at least one fetus was small for gestational age, whereas it was not increased when considering only appropriate for gestational age twins. When comparing the smaller twin with the larger twin, the risk of IUD was usually higher in the smaller twin than in the larger twin in dichorionic pregnancies; whereas in monochorionic pregnancies, there was an increased risk of perinatal neonatal death in the smaller twin versus the larger twin for a birth weight discrepancy ≥20%. However, because of the lack of consensus definition about growth discordance in twin pregnancy based on chorionicity, controversial and conflicting results persist regarding perinatal morbidity and mortality.

Management

Data are too limited to establish optimal timing for delivery of twin pregnancies complicated with growth discordance. Experts suggest that in the absence of clinical indications for delivery after 34 weeks, delivery for monochorionic twins is recommended at 36 to 37 weeks and for dichorionic gestations at 37 to 38 weeks to avoid late-preterm delivery complications.[134]

Recommendations for mode of delivery are based mainly on presenting twin and weight difference relative to the presenting twin.[146] The ACOG recommends cesarean delivery if the presenting twin is nonvertex or breech extraction of the second twin is required, even if the presenting twin is vertex. If the presenting twin is vertex, the possible route for delivery includes vaginal, planned cesarean, or combined delivery (vaginal delivery for twin A and emergency cesarean for twin B).[136] However, combined delivery is a relatively low occurrence, in only 4% of twin gestations, regardless of weight discordance.[147]

Recurrence

This is controversial and not well documented.

TWIN-TO-TWIN TRANSFUSION SYNDROME

Almost all monochorionic twins share a single placenta with intertwin vascular anastomoses that allows blood to transfer from one fetus to the other and vice versa.[148] Unbalanced net intertwin blood transfusion may lead to various complications; the best known of these is twin to twin transfusion syndrome (TTTS).[49]

Incidence

TTTS is a chronic form of fetofetal transfusion that affects approximately 9% of monochorionic twins.[142]

Pathogenesis/Etiology

TTTS is a complex and dynamic pathological condition that involves placental intertwin vascular anastomoses, unequal

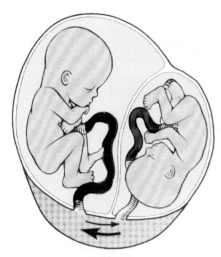

FIGURE 15.21: Monochorionic gestation with twin-to-twin transfusion syndrome. The recipient twin is larger and in a polyhydramniotic sac. The donor twin is smaller and in an oligohydramniotic sac.

and type of anastomoses present, the exchange of blood may be either balanced or unbalanced. Pregnancies with TTTS tend to have fewer anastomoses, particularly of the arterio-venous type than those without TTTS. Based on pathological examination and/or fetoscopic studies, the percentage of each of the three types of vascular anastomoses ranges from 20% to 90%.[150,151]

The relationship of vascular anastomoses and perinatal outcome in monochorionic twins and TTTS has been reported in several studies. In a retrospective study of placental angioarchitecture in relation to survival in monochorionic twins, fetal survival was higher in pregnancies with artery–artery anastomoses than in those with vein–vein anastomoses.[152,153] In addition to placental vascular changes in TTTS, the unbalanced blood shunting from donor to recipient has been reported to cause hormonal, hemodynamic, and biochemical fetal changes. Vasoactive hormonal changes include an increase in vasopressin, endothelin 1 (ET-1),[154] and natriuretic peptides, mainly atrial natriuretic peptide (ANP) and brain natriuretic peptide (BNP) in the recipient, which are likely contributing factors in worsening hypervolemia, polyuria, and polyhydramnios.

Diagnosis and Staging

Imaging

First-Trimester Ultrasound: NT is a marker utilized as an early first-trimester predictor for developing TTTS. The presence of an increased NT greater than 95th percentile for gestational age assessed between 11.0 and 13.6 weeks in at least one of the fetuses predicted the development of severe TTTS with a sensitivity of 0.32, a specificity of 0.88, and a positive likelihood ratio of 1.45.[155] Another US marker is folding of the intertwin membrane, which reflects a decreased amount of amniotic fluid in one sac. In a prospective study of 83 monochorionic-diamniotic pregnancies that presented for routine NT screening, Sebire et al.[156] reported that 52% of those with membrane folding developed severe TTTS.

Second-Trimester Imaging

Ultrasound: *The main diagnostic criterion for TTTS is the presence of oligohydramnios in the donor twin and polyhydramnios in the recipient twin* (Fig. 15.23).[49] Diagnosis of TTTS is one of exclusion based on US findings. Although not all of the following

placental sharing, fetal humoral, biochemical and functional changes, and fetal hemodynamic imbalance (Fig. 15.21). This fetal hemodynamic imbalance creates a hydrostatic difference between the recipient and the donor twins manifested as hyperdynamic, hypervolemic recipient state and hypovolemic, hypodynamic donor state.[49] Due to these volume imbalances, the recipient twin is at risk for cardiac dysfunction, while the donor twin may experience placental insufficiency and growth restriction. These changes appear to be responsible for the progression and outcome of this syndrome. Almost all monochorionic twins are believed to have intertwin vascular anastomoses.[149]

These anastomoses can be either direct and superficial between the twins' umbilical cord branch vessels on the chorionic plate surface or deep, in which case the arterial vessels from one twin's cord pierce the chorionic plate to supply a placental cotyledon that is drained by the venous system of its co-twin (Fig. 15.22). Considering the type of anastomoses, vascular communications between the recipient and the donor twin may be from artery to artery, from vein to vein, or from artery to vein within a placental cotyledon. Depending on the number

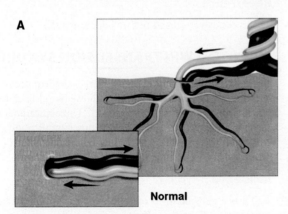
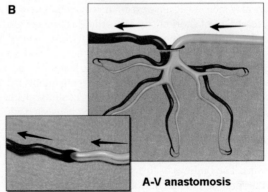

A Normal   **B** A-V anastomosis

FIGURE 15.22: Placental anastomoses. Schematic representation of placental vessels showing the artery depicted in *blue* and the vein in *red*. *Arrows* indicate the direction of blood flow. The *superimposed drawing*, at the lower left of each diagram, shows the vascular structures as viewed from the fetal surface of the placenta. **A:** Normal artery and vein pair emanating from and returning to the fetal cord insertion site. **B:** Arteriovenous (*A-V*) anastomosis. As shown, the artery and vein each travel unaccompanied along the placental surface and traverse a common, shared foramen to perfuse the placenta. (Reproduced with permission from Machin GA, Feldstein VA, Van Gemert MJC, et al. Doppler sonographic demonstrations of arteriovenous anastomosis in monochorionic twin gestation. *Ultrasound Obstet Gynecol.* 2000;16:214–217.)

TABLE 15.2   Twin-to-Twin Transfusion Features

FEATURES	DONOR TWIN	RECIPIENT TWIN
Size	Small	Large
Fluid	Oligohydramnios	Polyhydramnios
Bladder	Small to absent	Normal to distended
Umbilical cord	Small to normal	Normal to enlarged
Blood volume	Hypodynamic hypovolemia	Hyperdynamic hypervolemia
Cardiac dysfunction	Normal with minimal changes	Normal to abnormal
Doppler changes	Normal to abnormal	Normal to abnormal
Complications	Stuck twin, intrauterine growth restriction, hydrops, death	Cardiac dysfunction, hydrops, death

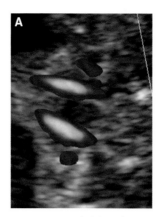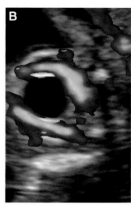

FIGURE 15.24: Bladder discrepancy in twin-to-twin transfusion syndrome. **A:** A donor twin in monochorionic pregnancy with TTTS showing small bladder. **B:** Recipient twin demonstrated large and cycling bladder in same pregnancy.

sonographic criteria are necessary for a diagnosis of TTTS, these findings are suggestive of disorder (Table 15.2):

1. Monochorionicity
2. Discrepancy in amniotic fluid between the amniotic sacs with polyhydramnios of one twin (largest vertical pocket >8 cm) and oligohydramnios of the other (largest vertical pocket <2 cm). In conjunction, the bladders are often discrepant with the donor's small or absent and recipient's large and constantly cycling (Fig. 15.24).
3. Discrepancy in size of the umbilical cords (Fig. 15.25)
4. The presence of cardiac dysfunction in the polyhydramniotic twin (Fig. 15.26)
5. Characteristically abnormal umbilical artery, umbilical vein or ductus venosus Doppler velocimetry (Fig. 15.27)
6. Less specifically, significant growth discordance of often ≥20% (see Fig. 15.20).

Abnormal Doppler waveform is defined as at least one of the following: absent/reverse end-diastolic flow (A/REDF) in the umbilical artery, reverse flow in the ductus venosus, or pulsatile

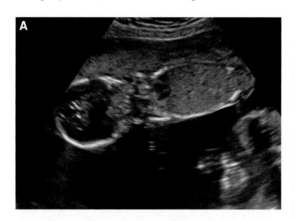

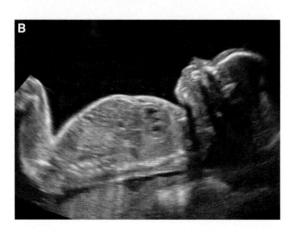

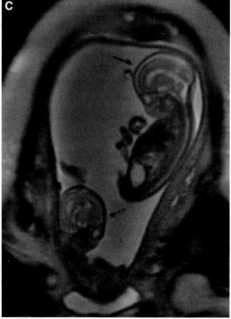

FIGURE 15.23: Twin-to-twin transfusion syndrome. **A:** Oligohydramnios in donor sac stuck to the uterine wall. **B:** Polyhydramnios in recipient sac. **C:** Fetal MRI showing decreased fluid around the donor (*dotted arrow*), stuck to the wall of the myometrium, and increased fluid around the recipient (*solid arrow*).

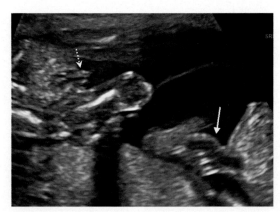
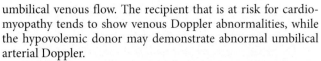

FIGURE 15.25: Axial US of both donor and recipient abdominal cord insertions. Notice small cord (*dotted arrow*) for the donor due to diminished flow. The recipient cord is large (*solid arrow*). Edema of the cord can be present.

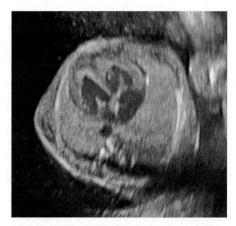

FIGURE 15.26: Recipient twin with twin-to-twin transfusion syndrome cardiomyopathy. The heart is enlarged, and there is biventricular hypertrophy.

umbilical venous flow. The recipient that is at risk for cardiomyopathy tends to show venous Doppler abnormalities, while the hypovolemic donor may demonstrate abnormal umbilical arterial Doppler.

In European centers, the gestational age is taken into consideration with polyhydramnios consisting of a deepest vertical pocket of more than 8 cm before 20 weeks of gestation and more than 10 cm after 20 weeks.[49] Recently, Khalil suggested a modified diagnostic criteria for TTTS prior to 18 weeks' gestation,[157] given that a new study,[158] which investigated the amniotic fluid volume in monochorionic twins from the first trimester until delivery, found that a deepest vertical pocket of 6 cm represented the 90th centile and 7 cm was the 97.5th centile from 16 to 17 weeks of gestation. Consequently, a deepest vertical pocket

of 6 cm before 18 weeks of gestation may be a more sensitive cutoff than one of 8 cm.

Of note, TTTS is less common in monochorionic-monoamniotic twin pregnancies (prevalence 6%),[50] owing to close umbilical cord insertions and plenty of anastomoses between the two placental shares that allow for more balanced flow between the two twins. When TTTS is present in a monoamniotic twin pregnancy, US will demonstrate polyhydramnios in the common amniotic sac and discrepancy in fetal bladder filling.

There are at least four staging systems available to define TTTS. The Quintero staging was the first and others have built on this initial grading. However, the Quintero is still the most commonly utilized by imaging centers.

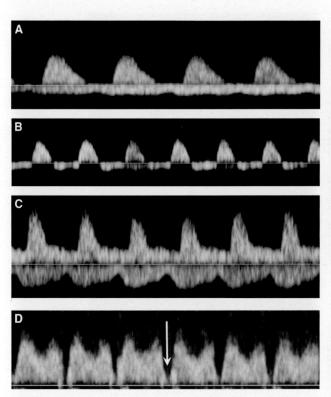
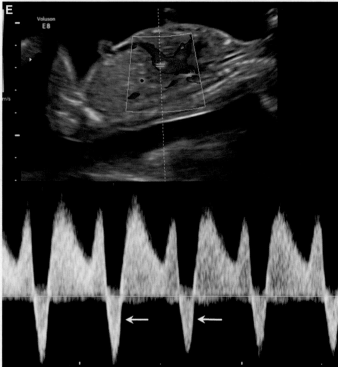

FIGURE 15.27: Twin-to-twin transfusion syndrome with abnormal Doppler studies. Absent end-diastolic flow in umbilical artery (typically donor) **(A)**; reversed end-diastolic flow of umbilical artery (typically donor) **(B)**; pulsatile umbilical vein (typically recipient) **(C)**; absent "a" wave (*arrow*) of ductus venosus (typically recipient) **(D)**; and reversed "a" wave (*arrows*) of ductus venosus (typically recipient) **(E)**.

Quintero Stages

I. Oligohydramnios-polyhydramnios sequence
II. No bladder in donor
III. Doppler abnormalities in either twin (A/REDF umbilical artery, pulsatile umbilical vein, reversed a wave ductus venosus)
IV. Hydrops in either twin
V. Demise of one or both twins

The Cincinnati staging system is described in Table 15.3.[159]

The Children's Hospital of Philadelphia (CHOP) system scores based on (1) ventricular function, (2) valve function, (3) venous Doppler, (4) great vessel findings, and (5) donor twin umbilical artery Doppler.

The cardiovascular profile scoring system (CVPS) utilizes (1) hydrops fetalis, (2) venous and arterial Doppler abnormalities, and (3) cardiac function.[159]

Some of these staging systems include recipient echocardiographic changes (CVPS, CHOP, and Cincinnati system).[159] Cardiovascular compromise occurs in most recipient twins, is a major cause of death for these fetuses, and contributes to morbidity and mortality in the donor co-twin.[160] The most common recipient cardiovascular abnormalities in TTTS are unilateral or bilateral ventricular hypertrophy (18% to 49%), increased cardiothoracic ratio as high as 47%, ventricular dilation (17% to 31%), tricuspid regurgitation (35% to 52%), and mitral regurgitation (13% to 15%).[160–162] These abnormalities are more common with advanced stages of disease. In addition, several cases of acquired pulmonary atresia/stenosis with intact ventricular septum have been described in the recipient twin.[160,163]

Magnetic Resonance Imaging: Given the risk for cerebral injury, fetal MRI is utilized in some centers to exclude neurological sequelae of the syndrome. The prenatal incidence of cerebral abnormalities in TTTS is reported at 8%.[164] Kline-Fath et al., in a recent review of 270 twin gestations, noted cerebral pathology in 12% of pregnancies with TTTS, again showing that 7% to 8% are related to ischemic and hemorrhagic pathology.[165] Quarello et al.[164] reported that in 22 cases of TTTS complicated with CNS abnormalities, fetal MRI was discordant from US in 45% of cases. Similarly, Kline-Fath et al.,[166] in a retrospective chart review of 25 fetal MRI examinations in TTTS, reported additional findings when compared with US consisting of renal collecting system dilation in 63% of recipients, lung lesions in 4% (Fig. 15.28), cerebral

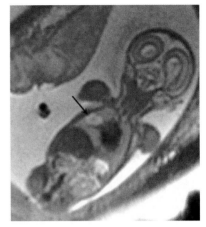

FIGURE 15.28: Lung lesion in twin-to-twin transfusion syndrome. Coronal SSFSE T2 image demonstrating a small T2 hyperintense lesion (*arrow*) in the right midlung of a recipient. The lesion was not delineated via US.

TABLE 15.3 Cincinnati Staging System

STAGE	DONOR	RECIPIENT	RECIPIENT CARDIOMYOPATHY
I	Oligohydramnios (DVP < 2 cm)	Polyhydramnios (DVP > 8 cm)	No
II	Absent bladder	Bladder seen	No
III	Abnormal Doppler	Abnormal Doppler	None
IIIa			Mild
IIIb			Moderate
IIIc			Severe
IV	Hydrops	Hydrops	
V	Death	Death	
Variables/cardiomyopathy	Mild	Moderate	Severe
AV regurgitation	Mild	Moderate	Severe
RV/LV thickness	>+2 Z-score	>3+ Z-score	>4+ Z-score
MPI Normal RV MPI is 0.32 ± 0.08 Normal LV MPI is 0.33 ± 0.05	>+2 Z-score	>3+ Z-score	Severe biventricular dysfunction

AV, atrioventricular valve; MPI, myocardial performance index; RV/LV, right ventricular/left ventricular.

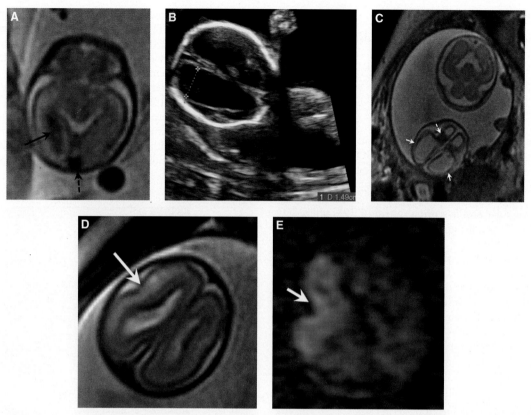

FIGURE 15.29: Brain findings in twin-to-twin transfusion syndrome. **A:** Axial SSFSE T2 MRI showing hemorrhage along the germinal matrix (*solid arrow*) and enlarged venous sinuses (*dotted arrow*). **B:** Axial US demonstrating ventriculomegaly in donor twin. **C:** Axial SSFSE T2 MRI of the same fetus in B demonstrating extensive cerebral parenchymal thinning (*solid arrows*) and abnormal decreased signal in the basal ganglia (dotted arrow) consistent with severe encephaloclastic event. **D:** Axial SSFSE T2 in a recipient twin showing abnormal bright signal (*arrow*) in the anatomic area of the right middle cerebral artery. **E:** Diffusion imaging of the same fetus in D confirming restricted diffusion (*arrow*) consistent with acute ischemia. The fetal cerebral US was normal.

ischemia or hemorrhage in 8% (Fig. 15.29), and cerebral venous sinus dilation in 13%. A higher incidence of congenital anomalies of the donor brain was also detected. In addition, thinning of the cerebral brain mantle and cerebellar volume loss is noted in the hypovolemic donor.[165,167] Recipient twins are more likely to develop germinal matrix hemorrhages, possibly related to venous hypertension in the presence of cardiac disease.[165] Thus, despite the need for further studies, fetal MRI may be helpful in TTTS for screening of brain lesions and may be an important component in counseling prior to intervention.

Differential Diagnosis

The differential diagnosis of TTTS includes uteroplacental insufficiency, growth disturbances caused by abnormal cord insertions, discordant manifestation of intrauterine infection, premature rupture of membranes (PPROM) of one twin, and discordant chromosomal or structural anomalies of one twin.[168,169]

Prognosis

Short-Term Outcome

In the absence of therapy, the perinatal mortality rate is high at 60% to 100%. With therapy, typically laser photocoagulation, survival is significantly improved, being 64% to 68% for both twins.[159]

The reported miscarriage rate ranges between 3.5% and 17%, 1% and 13% PPROM less than 24 weeks, 5% and 9.8% PPROM more than 24 weeks with a preterm labor (<33 weeks) rate of 27% to 44%.[170-175] Recently, Gijtenbeek et al.[156a] published a systematic and meta-analysis to investigate fetal echocardiographic parameters preoperatively in prediction of fetal death in TTTS. The authors reported that recipient twins have an increased risk of demise in case of preoperative A/REDF in the umbilical artery, absent or reversed a-wave in the ductus venosus, or a middle cerebral artery peak systolic velocity (MCA-PSV) more than 1.5 multiples of the median (MoM). In donors, only A/REDF in the umbilical artery and absent or reversed a-wave in the ductus venosus were associated with IUFD. No association was found between donor IUFD and preoperative myocardial performance index. The authors concluded that ongoing research in this field is recommended.

Despite improved survival after fetoscopic laser treatment, neonates of TTTS pregnancies, compared with non-TTTS monochorionic gestations, still suffer severe neonatal morbidities secondary to prematurity and TTTS-related conditions. Furthermore, TTTS neonates in neonatal intensive care unit have a 4.8% to 7% rate of acute renal failure, 3% to 4% rate of necrotizing enterocolitis, and 27% to 62% rate of respiratory distress syndrome with 4% to 34% prevalence of intraventricular hemorrhage grades 3 to 4. There are also some reported cases of persistent pulmonary hypertension (3%) in pregnancies complicated with TTTS. This wide range in frequency of neonatal morbidity is mainly because of inadequate sample size, different outcome measure definitions, different centers' experience, and diverse treatment modalities between centers.[170–176]

Long-Term Outcome

Neurodevelopmental Outcome: In multifetal pregnancies, the risk of developing white matter necrosis in monochorionic twin pregnancy is 10-fold as compared with that in dichorionic twin pregnancies (33% vs. 3%).[177] In TTTS, the reported incidence of neurological developmental abnormalities ranges between 7% and 16% after laser photocoagulation.[178] Furthermore, Merhar et al.[179] did a prospective study of 22 premature TTTS cases with prenatal brain injury. The authors reported that postnatal brain injury correlated with severity of Quintero stage but not gestational age at delivery or birth weight. However, Lopriore et al.[180] have published a detailed neurological, mental, and psychomotor follow-up of 115 laser-treated TTTS survivors at 2 years of age corrected for prematurity. The incidence of neurodevelopmental impairment is 17%, with etiologies including cerebral palsy, mental developmental delay, psychomotor developmental delay, and deafness. Perinatal factors, including gestational age at delivery and Apgar score, correlate with adverse outcome.

Cardiovascular Outcome: There has been a paucity of information concerning the long-term cardiovascular implications of TTTS. Herberg et al.[181] reported long-term cardiac function in a prospective study of 89 survivors (38 donor and 51 recipient) at 21 months of age after fetoscopic laser photocoagulation for 73 cases of severe TTTS pregnancies. The authors noted an 11.2% incidence of structural heart disease and, specifically, a 7.8% pulmonary stenosis rate, which is higher than the general population. Eighty-seven percent of the survivors demonstrated a normal cardiac examination. Despite the high rate and severity of prenatal cardiac impairment in recipients, systolic or diastolic ventricular function completely normalized over the long term.

Management

Numerous treatments for TTTS have been proposed, including selective feticide, cord coagulation, sectio parva (removing one fetus), placental bloodletting, maternal digitalis, maternal indomethacin, serial amnioreduction, microseptostomy of the intertwin membrane, and non–selective or selective fetoscopic laser photocoagulation (non-SFLP or SFLP). Microseptostomy has fallen out of favor, given the possibility of creating a monoamniotic gestation with risk for cord entanglement. Selective cord coagulation is center dependent but may be considered when a twin is irretrievably compromised. For decades in the United States, serial amnioreduction was the most prevalent therapy for TTTS. However, in the past decade, SFLP has become more widely accepted and is the primary treatment offered in many centers today.

Amnioreduction

Amnioreduction was used initially for maternal comfort and as a means to control polyhydramnios in the hope of prolonging the pregnancy until the risk of extreme prematurity lessened. In addition, amnioreduction has been shown to improve uteroplacental blood flow, likely by reducing intra-amniotic pressure from polyhydramnios. In a review of 26 reports dating from the 1930s of 252 fetuses, Moise[182] found an overall survival of 49% in twins treated with amnioreduction. In more recent series with more consistently aggressive serial amnioreduction to normalize amniotic fluid volumes, survival ranged from as low as 37% to as high as 83%.[183,184]

Fetoscopic Laser Photocoagulation

The first therapy for TTTS that attempted to treat the anatomic basis for the syndrome was reported by De Lia et al.,[185] who described non-SFLP of all vessels crossing the intertwin membrane. Today, SFLP, laser of only vascular anastomoses across the intertwin membrane, is the standard of care for TTTS between 18 and 26 weeks with Quintero stage II and higher. The turning point in its usage was the 2004 Eurofetus multicenter randomized controlled trial that compared serial amnioreduction with SFLP in 142 women with monochorionic–diamniotic twins and TTTS between January 1999 and March 2002.[186] The laser therapy group, compared with the amnioreduction group, reached a significantly higher gestational age at delivery (mean 33 weeks vs. 29 weeks) and had increased survival of at least one fetus to 28 days of age (76% vs. 56%). Although postnatal follow-up was only 6 months in duration, the laser therapy group showed improved neurological outcomes with decreased risk of periventricular leukomalacia (6% vs. 14%) and a higher likelihood of being free of neurological complications at 6 months of age (52% vs. 31%).[186]

Few studies have addressed laser complications in TTTS pregnancies. In a retrospective study of 175 TTTS pregnancies treated with laser, Yamamoto et al.[187] reported that the most frequent complication was PPROM, which occurred in 28% of the cases. Twelve percent developed PROM in the first 3 weeks after laser, with the remaining 17% occurred thereafter. The entry of the trocar, which was transplacental in 48 (27%) cases, was not associated with adverse outcome.

Few case series have reported late complications of laser photocoagulation, including monoamniotic gestation, amniotic band syndrome, ischemic limb, and bowel atresia related to vascular accidents. However, these complications can also occur in monochorionic twins without TTTS. All laser-treated cases should be followed closely with weekly US surveillance to detect any late complications.

In a large cohort of 151 cases, Robyr et al.[188] demonstrated that progression of the disease occurred in 14% of cases, while another 13% had reversal of TTTS, with the recipient behaving like the donor and vice versa. In addition, twin anemia–polycythemia sequence (TAPS) has been reported in up to 13% of cases following TTTS. In a 2008 report of early and late complication rates in a cohort of 139 consecutively treated cases with SFLP from the Fetal Care Center of Cincinnati, Habli et al.[171] noted progression or persistence of TTTS in only 2 (1.4%) cases and TAPS in 3 (2.2%) cases. The low rate of complications was suggested to be due to infrequent missed vascular connections in the presence of a stringent mapping protocol used by this group during SFLP. Based on this, the consensus that all vascular anastomoses should be ablated during the fetoscopic laser procedure was reached. However, this raises the question whether all connecting vessels can be identified and coagulated.

It has been reported that after standard fetoscopic laser technique, patent anastomoses can be seen in up to one-third of the placentas.[189,190] Therefore, a new laser method, called the "Solomon" technique, has been developed. After identifying and coagulating the anastomoses, a thin line is drawn with the laser from one placental edge to the other connecting the laser dots.

The rationale of this method is to ablate the entire vascular equator and minimize the risk of residual anastomoses that are not visible by naked eye. In a recent randomized controlled trial, the standard selective laser method was compared with the Solomon technique.[191] In all, 274 women were randomly assigned, of whom 139 were treated with the Solomon technique and 135 received standard treatment. The new technique has been associated with a significant reduction of recurrent TTTS and postlaser TAPS. Concerns remain whether lasering of healthy placental tissue between the anastomoses is justified, given the resultant increased placental injury.

TWIN ANEMIA–POLYCYTHEMIA SEQUENCE

In 2007, Lopriore et al.[192] reported a new form of chronic fetofetal transfusion termed twin anemia–polycythemia sequence (TAPS). TAPS is characterized by large intertwin hemoglobin (Hb) differences without signs of TTTS (oligopoly sequence) in monochorionic pregnancies.[192]

Incidence

The incidence of TAPS varies according to definition, type, and diagnostic criteria, such as whether it is antenatal only or both antenatal and postnatal. TAPS can occur spontaneously or postlaser for TTTS. The spontaneous form complicates 3% to 5% of monochorionic twin pregnancies,[49,193] whereas the postlaser form occurs in 2% to 13% of TTTS cases.[171,188] In a report on late complications of 101 TTTS cases treated with fetoscopic laser surgery, Robyr et al.[188] found a 13% incidence of postlaser TAPS, whereas Habli et al.[171] reported a lower than 2% incidence.

Pathogenesis

The pathogenesis of TAPS is based on a unique placental angioarchitecture characterized by the presence of only few arteriovenous (AV) vascular anastomoses. These minuscule anastomoses allow for a slow transfusion of blood from the donor to the recipient, leading gradually to highly discordant

Hb levels without hormonal imbalance.[194] In addition to very few and small unidirectional AV anastomoses, twins with TAPS have less arterio-arterial anastomoses, 11% cited in cases of spontaneous TAPS.[195] Importantly, the diameter of these arterio-arterial anastomoses are very small.[196,197] In comparison, the incidence of artery–artery anastomoses in uncomplicated monochorionic pregnancies and TTTS pregnancies is 80% and 25%, respectively.[196,197]

Several studies report different placental angioarchitecture based on the type of TAPS, spontaneous versus postlaser. Recently, in a placental injection study of 43 monochorionic twin pregnancies complicated by spontaneous TAPS ($N = 16$) and postlaser TAPS ($n = 27$), Villiers et al.[196] noted that all 43 had AV anastomosis and nearly 96% had AV anastomosis with small diameter localized at placental margins. As compared with twins with postlaser TAPS, spontaneous TAPS had a higher number of anastomosis (4 vs. 2) with increased arterio-arterial anastomosis (18% vs. 14%). Velamentous or marginal cord insertion was found in 43% and 57% of spontaneous and postlaser TAPS, respectively.[196]

The pathogenesis of absent oligo-polyhydramnios sequelae in TAPS is likely related to very slow intertwin blood transfusion, allowing for more time for hemodynamic compensatory mechanisms to take place.[195]

Diagnosis

Ultrasound

Given that TAPS has just recently been described, uniform criteria are yet to be clearly established. Diagnosis is based on antenatal findings or postnatal findings or both.

Antenatal diagnosis of TAPS can be defined by both grayscale and Doppler findings. In TAPS, there is absence of oligopoly sequence, and there is an increased peak systolic velocity (PSV) in the middle cerebral artery (MCA) in the donor twin, suggestive of fetal anemia and a decreased MCA-PSV in the recipient twin, suggestive of polycythemia. Robyr et al.[188] proposed the use of an MCA-PSV more than 1.5 MoM for the donor twin and less than 0.8 MoM in the recipient (Fig. 15.30). None of these criteria are validated despite their use by most physicians.

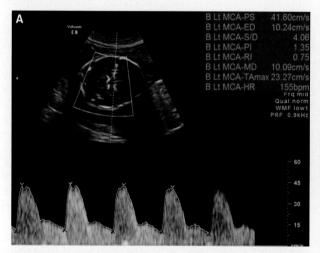
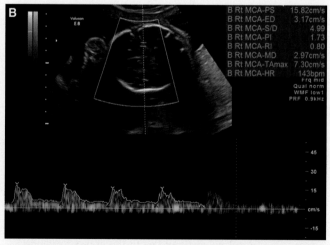

FIGURE 15.30: Twin anemia–polycythemia sequence. Monochorionic–diamniotic twin pregnancy with postlaser TAPS. **A:** Middle cerebral artery peak systolic velocity Doppler of donor twin is more than 1.5 multiples of the median (MoM). **B:** Doppler in the recipient with less than 0.8 MoM. *ED*, end-diastolic; *HR*, heart rate; *PI*, pulsatility index; *RI*, resistance index; *S/D*, systolic/diastolic.

Recently, Tollenaar et al.[198] published a retrospective cohort of monochorionic twin pregnancies complicated with postnatal TAPS to investigate the diagnostic accuracy of delta MCA-PSV more than 0.5 MoM and to compare its predictive value with that of the current MCA-PSV cutoff values of more than 1.5 MoM in the donor and less than 1.0 MoM in the recipient, for the diagnosis of TAPS in monochorionic twin pregnancy. The authors reported that delta MCA-PSV more than 0.5 MoM has a greater diagnostic accuracy for predicting TAPS compared to the current MCA-PSV cutoff criteria. The authors therefore propose a new antenatal classification system for TAPS (Table 15.4).

Postnatal criteria include intertwin Hb difference more than 8.0 g/dL *with* at least one of the following: reticulocyte count ratio more than 1.7 or a placenta with only small (diameter <1 mm) vascular anastomoses at pathological examination.

Magnetic Resonance Imaging
Fetuses with TAPS are at risk for brain injury; therefore, sequential US and/or fetal MRI may be considered. A recent study utilizing sequential prenatal US and MRI after laser therapy for TTTS notes that cerebral abnormalities can be detected in slightly less than 3% of patients, and this risk for brain injury correlates with incomplete surgery for TTTS or development of TAPS.[199] In several case reports, evidence of MRI changes in the anemic fetus was manifested by numerous large cysts in the basal ganglia, bilateral white matter injury, multiple microhemorrhages, and parenchymal hemorrhage in the right occipital lobe.[200] These findings were seen in both postlaser and spontaneous TAPS.[201]

Differential Diagnosis

The differential diagnosis of TAPS includes uteroplacental insufficiency, discordant manifestation of intrauterine infection, and any cause of fetal anemia.

Prognosis

Perinatal outcome in TAPS is not well known but has varied from mild hematological complications to severe cerebral injury and perinatal death.[202] Perinatal survival rates vary depending on treatment but are cited from 50% to 100%, with the average gestational age at diagnosis ranging from 19 to 24 weeks and delivery from 28 to 34 weeks.[203]

Data are sparse for short- and long-term neurological outcomes. In a case–control study of twins with TAPS paired with two monochorionic twin pairs without TAPS, Lopriore et al.[202] found no differences in risk of severe cerebral injury among groups; however, long-term outcomes were not reported. In a large multicenter study of long-term follow-up for 212 TTTS pregnancies treated with laser surgery, 16 (4%) pregnancies were affected by TAPS, of which four were treated with intrauterine transfusion.[204] Perinatal survival was 75% for the postlaser surgery TAPS cases. In all 12 surviving TAPS infants, evaluation at 2 years of age, which included a Bayley developmental test, showed that none of these infants had long-term neurodevelopmental impairment. In conclusion, cerebral injury in TAPS cases, treated with or without intrauterine transfusion, may be less common than initially thought. Therefore, large multicenter follow-up studies are needed.

TABLE 15.4 Previous and Proposed Classification and Therapy for Twin Anemia–Polycythemia Sequence

STAGING	PREVIOUS	PROPOSED	THERAPY
1	MCA-PSV donor > 1.5 MoM MCA-PSV recipient < 1 MoM No fetal compromise	Delta MCA-PSV > 0.5 MoM No fetal compromise	Expectant management
2	MCA-PSV donor > 1.7 MoM MCA-PSV recipient < 0.8 MoM No fetal compromise	Delta MCA-PSV > 0.7 MoM No fetal compromise	Expectant management vs. laser and/or IUT if <28 wk Expected management vs. IUT if >28 wk Consider delivery based on gestational age and clinical status
3	MCA-PSV like stage 1 or 2 Cardiac compromise donor	Delta MCA-PSV like stage 1 or 2 Cardiac compromise donor	Laser and/or IUT if <28 wk IUT if >28 wk Consider delivery based on gestational age and clinical status
4	Hydrops donor	Hydrops donor	Laser and/or IUT if <28 wk IUT if >28 wk Consider delivery based on gestational age and clinical status
5	Demise one or both fetuses	Demise one or both fetuses	

IUT, intrauterine transfusion; MCA, middle cerebral artery; PSV, peak systolic velocity.
Adapted from Tollenaar LSA, Lopriore E, Middeldorp JM, et al. Improved prediction of twin anemia-polycythemia sequence by delta middle cerebral artery peak systolic velocity: new antenatal classification system. *Ultrasound Obstet Gynecol.* 2019;53:788–793.

Management

The treatment options by case reports and small series include expectant management, induction of labor, selective feticide, fetoscopic laser surgery, or intrauterine transfusion. Intrauterine transfusion is considered to be a temporary option, most commonly to treat the anemic donor. Potentially, transfusing the donor may worsen the polycythemia in the other twin. Choosing which modality is the best treatment is difficult, given the limited experience in both the intravenous and/or the intraperitoneal transfusion in TAPS cases. Spontaneous resolution of antenatal TAPS has also been reported.

Recently, Tollenaar et al.[198] suggested a treatment algorithm based on TAPS staging system. Expectant management for stages 1 and 2 TAPS at any gestational age and nonprogressive TAPS and more than 28 weeks' gestational age; laser therapy for stage ≥ 2 TAPS and less than 28 weeks; intrauterine transfusion for stage ≥ 3 TAPS or stage 2 with progression and 28 to 32 weeks' gestational age; and delivery for stage ≥ 3 TAPS or stage 2 with progression and more than 32 weeks' gestational age.

Recurrence

Risk of recurrence is unknown.

TWIN-REVERSED ARTERIAL PERFUSION

Acardiac anomaly or twin-reversed arterial perfusion (TRAP) refers to a complication unique to monochorionic twins. The lack of a well-formed cardiac structure is found in one fetus (acardiac), which is abnormally perfused by a structurally normal cotwin (pump twin) through a superficial artery-to-artery placental anastomosis (Fig. 15.31). This anomaly can be recognized antenatally from the first trimester, and a range of *in utero* interventions have been attempted.[205–207]

Incidence

TRAP sequence affects around 1 in 35,000 to 40,000 pregnancies, representing around 1% of monochorionic twins.[205–207]

Pathogenesis

Two conditions are necessary for TRAP development. First, abnormal cardiac embryogenesis occurs between 8 and 12 weeks in one of the two twins of a monochorionic pregnancy.[208] Second, a specific abnormal placental angioarchitecture defined by an arterio-arterial and a veno-venous intertwin anastomosis supports

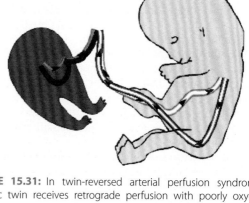

FIGURE 15.31: In twin-reversed arterial perfusion syndrome, the acardiac twin receives retrograde perfusion with poorly oxygenated blood.

the development of an abnormal twin (acardiac twin).[208–210] Furthermore, heterokaryotypic monozygotism, such as aneuploidy, which arises after splitting of the fertilized ovum, has been discussed as a possible etiological factor in TRAP.[211]

In acardiac twin development, all organs are affected, resulting in variable presentation and size. Most commonly, acardiac twins are acephalic with absent upper extremities, as deoxygenated blood from the umbilical artery preferentially supplies the lower rather than the upper part of the body. Other structures that are often absent include the heart (<20% of fetuses have identifiable cardiac tissue), pancreas, lungs, liver, and small intestines (Fig. 15.32). A two-vessel cord is found in more than two-thirds of cases.[212] Because of the lack of communication between the lymphatic and the vascular systems, the acardiac twin frequently develops severe subcutaneous edema and lymphatic abnormality, which can significantly increase the size of the fetus and further distort the abnormal anatomy.

A detailed classification system of the acardiac twin had been suggested on the basis of morphology (Table 15.5). The simplest classification system of acardiac twins differentiates between two types: pseudoacardius, with evidence of a rudimentary cardiac structure, and holoacardius, without cardiac structure present. These classifications do not correlate with outcome.

Diagnosis

Ultrasound

Common features in TRAP are described in Table 15.6. The prenatal diagnosis of acardiac twins should be suspected when a

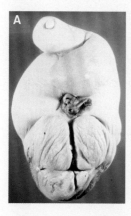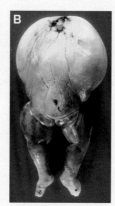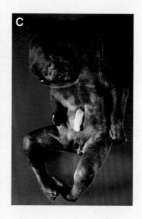

FIGURE 15.32: Acardiac twins in twin-reversed arterial perfusion. **A–C:** Pathological photographs showing variable development of acardiac twins.

TABLE 15.5	Description of Acardiac Twins
MALFORMATION	**DESCRIPTION**
Acephalus	No cephalic structure present
Anceps	Some cranial structure or neural tissue present
Acormus	Cephalic structure but no truncal structures
Amorphus	No distinguishable rostral-to-caudal structure

TABLE 15.6	Features Associated with Acardiac Twin
Biometric discordance between the twins
Absence of identifiable cardiac pulsation in one twin
Due to preferential arterial perfusion of lower body, poor definition of the head, trunk, and upper extremities and usually deformed lower extremities
Marked and diffuse subcutaneous edema and abnormal cystic areas in the upper part of the body of the affected twin
An abnormal two-vessel cord is found in more than two-thirds of cases

grossly malformed fetus is seen in the setting of a monochorionic twin pregnancy[213,214] (Fig. 15.33). The diagnosis is further established by retrograde flow of the umbilical artery by color Doppler US. Specifically, arterial blood flows toward rather than away from the acardiac twin and in a caudal-to-cranial direction in the abdominal aorta (Fig. 15.34).[215]

Although the pump twin is structurally normal in most cases, associated anomalies reported include prune belly, renal agenesis and dysplasia, renal tubular dysgenesis, anal atresia, gastroschisis, and pulmonary artery calcification.[216] Further karyotyping of the pump twin should be offered because as many as 9% of pump twins have an abnormal karyotype, including monosomy, trisomy, deletions, mosaicism, and polyploidy.[212]

Magnetic Resonance Imaging

Fetal MRI has been used to evaluate complications in TRAP syndrome. Guimaraes et al.[217] reported fetal MRI findings in 35 cases diagnosed with TRAP. The authors reported 91% correct diagnosis by US. However, fetal MRI identified 14% associated abnormalities in the pump twin not related to cardiac etiology, including 3% with brain ischemia (Fig. 15.35).[217] Despite this, MRI is considered an adjunct to fetal US, and further studies are needed.

Differential Diagnosis

Fetal death in a monochorionic twin pregnancy, teratoma, or other mass arising from the placenta or umbilical cord may mimic an acardiac twin.

Prognosis

As the acardiac twin depends on the pump twin for growth, the healthy pump twin's survival is threatened by the risk of congestive heart failure, polyhydramnios, intrauterine fetal death,

PPROM, and preterm labor and delivery. The primary contributors of perinatal death for the pump twin in TRAP are congestive heart failure and preterm delivery. Perinatal mortality of the pump twin ranges from 35% to 55%.[208,209]

In attempting to improve outcome and define optimal management of TRAP, several authors reported prenatal prognostic factors that affect pump twin outcome. Moore et al.[209] reported the percentage of pump twin weight as a prognostic factor. The authors developed a regression model to estimate acardiac twin weight as follows: weight (g) = 1.21 × length (cm)^2 − (1.66 × length [cm]) (Fig. 15.36A), with the length of the parabiotic twin representing the longest linear dimension. They reported that if the ratio exceeded 70%, the incidence of preterm delivery was 90%, polyhydramnios was 40%, and pump twin congestive heart failure was 30%, whereas if a ratio was less than 70%, rates were 75%, 30%, and 10%, respectively.

Some have used Doppler US of the umbilical artery to determine impact on the pump twin. In analyzing the ratio of the umbilical artery pulsatility index between the acardiac and the pump twins, Brassard et al.[218] noted a low acardiac pulsatility index. This value represented a high diastolic velocity in the acardiac twin compared with the lower diastolic flow and higher pulsatility index of the pump twin, which correlated with poor prognosis because it reflected substantial flow into the acardiac twin. Dashe et al.[219] noted that pump twin outcomes varied by differences in resistance index between the twins. Resistance index difference of less than 0.05 was associated with poor outcome, whereas more than 0.2 resulted in favorable outcomes.

In a 2013 retrospective chart review, Oliver et al.[220] correlated sonographic findings associated with the pump twin's adverse outcome with acardiac twin mass size using the formula of

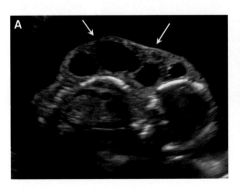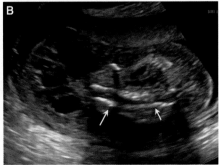

FIGURE 15.33: Acardiac twins in twin-reversed arterial perfusion. **A:** Acardiac twin with cranium and fairly well-defined body. Note large complex lymphatic malformation (*arrows*). **B:** Different acardiac twin with absent cranium but remnants of spine (*arrows*) and also large associated lymphatic abnormality.

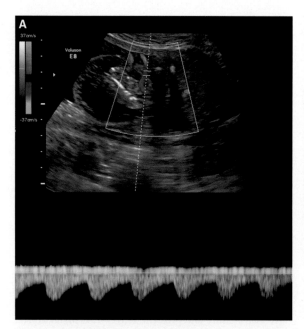

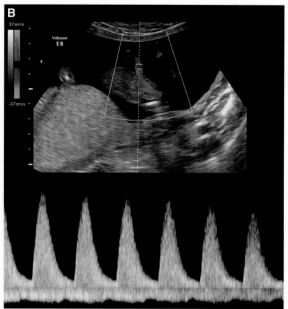

FIGURE 15.34: Doppler in twin-reversed arterial perfusion. **A:** Reverse flow on Doppler image in acardiac twin: Arterial flow going in (*under the baseline*) and venous flow going out (*above the baseline*). **B:** Normal umbilical artery Doppler flow in pump twin.

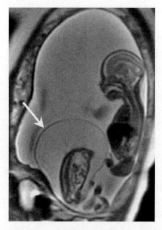

FIGURE 15.35: Fetal MRI in twin-reversed arterial perfusion. Coronal SSFSE T2 image demonstrating hydropic acardiac *twin* (*arrow*) and pump twin.

a prolate ellipsoid (Fig. 15.36B). Acardiac twin mass, which was estimated by summing body and extremity volumes, was calculated using the equation (width × height × length × 0.523). The total volume was then converted to mass by assuming that soft-tissue density was similar to water (1 g/mL). After the volume was converted, a percentage of the acardiac to pump twin (i.e., acardiac/pump twin weight ratio) was obtained. Two groups were classified: acardiac/pump twin weight ratio that was either greater than 70% or less than 70%. The authors reported that acardiac twin size exceeding 70% of the pump twin weight correlated with an increased risk of pump twin compromise if using the prolate ellipsoid formula ($P = 0.002$) but not the sonographic Moore method ($P = 0.09$).

To further assess the impact of the acardiac twin on the cardiovascular status of the pump twin, two-dimensional US can detect physical signs of early cardiovascular deterioration of the pump twin, specifically polyhydramnios, cardiomegaly, and pericardial effusion. Fetal echocardiography can also assess cardiac function

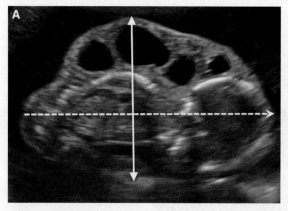

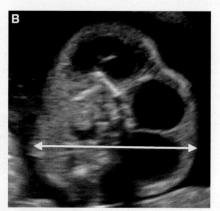

FIGURE 15.36: Acardiac measurements. **A:** The total length (*dotted line*) of the acardiac twin used in Moore regression formula to assess estimated weight of acardiac twin: weight (g) = 1.21 × length (cm)^2 − (1.66 × length [cm]). Anteroposterior (AP) dimension (*solid line with arrows*) is obtained for the Oliver technique. **B:** Transverse dimension of the acardiac twin. Orthogonal measurement of acardiac twin including hydropic tissues for Oliver technique (length, AP, and transverse).

and provide evidence of congestive heart failure by comparing with cardiac output appropriate for gestational age. Color Doppler US should be used to look for tricuspid regurgitation, reverse flow in the ductus venosus, pulsation in the umbilical vein, and high peak velocity of middle cerebral artery flow secondary to fetal anemia. The presence of any one of these US features predicts a poor prognosis.

Management

The goal of treating acardiac anomaly is to maximize the likelihood of term delivery and survival of the pump twin in a safe and effective manner. The goal of surgery is to interrupt the vascularization of the acardiac twin. There are several techniques described that include US-guided fetal cord ligation or compression,[221] bipolar coagulation, laser coagulation, trans-section with harmonic US scalpel,[222] thermocoagulation,[223] and radiofrequency ablation (RFA).[224]

RFA is becoming more popular as a safe and reliable treatment method for TRAP. In a systematic review of the literature reporting seven studies using RFA as treatment choice for TRAP sequence, Cabassa et al.[225] found a total of 85 TRAP cases that included twin and triplets (n = 3) who underwent RFA. Average gestational ages were 18.6 weeks at the time of the procedure and 36.4 weeks at delivery. Neonatal survival rate of the pump twin was 85%. In this review, the rate of preterm delivery/PPROM less than 37 weeks was 28%; fetal death 3.5%; and maternal complications, mainly thermal injury at grounding pads, 2.4%. Neonatal survival rates for cord coagulation ranged between 70% and 80%, comparable to RFA, but were associated with higher rate of preterm delivery (58%).

Other fetoscopic techniques, such as intrafetal laser therapy, have been proposed to prevent the demise of the pump twin. Pagani et al.[226] in 2013 reported outcome data for intrafetal laser therapy of TRAP by systemic review and meta-analysis of 11 studies. Pagani et al. included 51 cases consisting of 5 triplets (dichorionic–triamniotic) and 46 twins (monochorionic). Average gestational age was 17.2 weeks at the time of the procedure, with delivery at 37 weeks and neonatal survival of 82%. Rates of preterm birth were 7% at less than 32 weeks, 21% at less than 34 weeks, and 40% at less than 37 weeks. Rates of adverse pregnancy outcome (i.e., intrauterine death or preterm birth before 37 weeks) were related to gestational age at the procedure, with a significantly lower rate at 19% when treatment was undertaken before 16 weeks compared with 66% for pregnancies treated ≥16 weeks. These findings suggest that intrafetal laser therapy could be a good and safe option when performed before 16 weeks.

MONOCHORIONIC–MONOAMNIOTIC TWIN

Monochorionic–monoamniotic twin pregnancies have a single placenta and sac, and occur after splitting of single blastocyst on days 8 to 13 postfertilization.[227] Although the umbilical cords typically insert close to one another (within 6 cm of each other) and are generally located centrally, one-third are either marginal or velamentous.[228] Intertwin vascular anastomoses are always present, but twin-to-twin transfusion is less common than in monochorionic–diamniotic twins.[229]

Incidence

Monoamniotic twin pregnancies occur in 1% of monozygotic twin pregnancies.[227]

Diagnosis

Rodis et al.[230] defined the criteria for diagnosis of monoamniotic twin pregnancies as one placenta, same-sex fetuses, adequate fluid around both fetuses, and the absence of a dividing

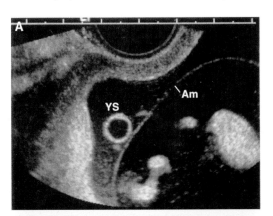
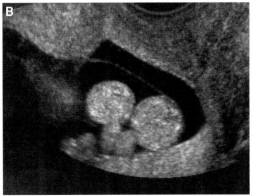
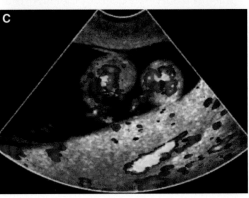

FIGURE 15.37: Monoamniotic gestation with single yolk sac at 10.5 weeks. **A:** Yolk sac (*YS*) and single amnion (*Am*). **B:** Two adjacent fetuses are nearly touching. **C:** Color-flow Doppler image showing two adjacent umbilical cords. (Courtesy of Gerald Mulligan, MD.)

membrane (Fig. 15.37). However, a first-trimester transvaginal US that shows one sac and two embryo poles before 8 weeks is not always diagnostic of monochorionic-monoamniotic twin. Several reported cases actually turned out to be triplets or diamniotic–dichorionic twins. Thus, late first-trimester and early second-trimester US are recommended for accurate diagnosis. Cord entanglement is diagnostic for a monochorionic–monoamniotic twin pregnancy.

Prognosis

Monoamniotic twin pregnancies suffer from a high perinatal mortality rate that ranges from 10% to 47%, malformation rate of 10%, and cord entanglement up to 70%.[231,232] Cause of death is typically attributed to cord entanglement (50%), with other etiologies including premature deliveries, intrauterine growth restriction, and congenital anomalies. In a Japanese study, the prospective risk of fetal death was 13.9% for women who reached gestational week 22. This rate gradually decreased to the range of 4.5% to 8.0% between gestational weeks 30.0 and 36.0.[233] Most studies show, however, that fetal loss can occur after 32 weeks in monoamniotic twin gestations.

TTTS can also occur in monochorionic–monoamniotic twin pregnancies, although its incidence has been reported to be 2.4 to 2.7 times lower than in monochorionic–diamniotic twin gestation. Recently, Murgano et al.[234] published a systematic review and meta-analysis to report outcome of TTTS in monoamniotic twins. The authors report the following. In cases not undergoing intervention, miscarriage occurred in 10.7% of fetuses, while the incidence of intrauterine demise (IUD), neonatal and perinatal death was 24.3%, 13.5%, and 32.4% respectively. Rate of preterm birth complicated 54.0% of these pregnancies. In cases treated by laser surgery, the incidence of miscarriage, IUD, neonatal and perinatal death was 19.6%, 27.4%, 7.4%, and 35.9% respectively. The incidence of preterm birth less than 32 weeks of gestation was 64.9%. In cases treated with amniodrainage, the incidence of IUD, neonatal and perinatal death was 30.3%, 19.1%, and 35.9%, respectively. Preterm birth complicated 78.1% of cases.

Management

Antepartum management of a monoamniotic twin pregnancy is challenging. These patients should be offered first-trimester screening, an anatomy scan between 18 and 20 weeks, and fetal echocardiography because of the increased risk of congenital malformation. Prenatal fetal surveillance and delivery early in the third trimester are indicated because of the high rate of perinatal mortality, often due to cord entanglement.

Data from observational studies to define the value of intensive fetal monitoring are insufficient but suggest that inpatient monitoring provided a better perinatal outcome. In a retrospective study of 87 monochorionic–monoamniotic twin pregnancies ≥24 weeks' gestation with two surviving fetuses, Heyborne et al.[235] reported that 43 patients were hospitalized electively (mean 26.5 weeks) and 28 were hospitalized for specific indications (mean 30.1 weeks). No fetal deaths occurred in the 43 hospitalized patients who were monitored for at least 2 hours daily, whereas 13 intrauterine fetal deaths occurred in 8 of 16 outpatients monitored one to three times weekly. Compared with indicated admissions, the authors found elective inpatient management achieved a lower rate of composite neonatal morbidity

(29% vs. 50%), significant improvement in birth weight (3,750 g vs. 3,470 g), higher gestational age at delivery (33 weeks vs. 31 weeks), and no difference in NICU days.

D'Antonio et al.[236] published a systematic review to quantify the rate of perinatal mortality in monochorionic–monoamniotic twin pregnancies, according to gestational age, and to ascertain the incidence of mortality in pregnancies managed as inpatients compared with those managed as outpatients. Twenty-five studies (1,628 nonanomalous twins reaching 24 weeks of gestation) were included. Single and double IUDs occurred in 2.5% and 3.8% of cases, respectively. IUD occurred in 4.3% of twins at 24 to 30 weeks, in 1.0% at 31 to 32 weeks, and in 2.2% at 33 to 34 weeks of gestation, while there was no case of IUD, either single or double, from 35 weeks of gestation. In monochorionic–monoamniotic twin pregnancies managed mainly as inpatients, the incidence of IUD was 3.0%, while the corresponding figure for those managed mainly as outpatients was 7.4%. Finally, 37.8% of these pregnancies were delivered before the scheduled time, due mainly to spontaneous preterm labor or abnormal cardiotocographic findings.

Timing of delivery is not well established for monochorionic–monoamniotic twin pregnancies of uncertain or precarious fetal status. In view of risk of sudden death after 32 weeks, which some cite as 5% to 10%, the recommended delivery is cesarean section between 32 and 34 weeks after administration of steroids for fetal lung maturity.[134]

CORD ENTANGLEMENT

High rates of perinatal loss in monochorionic–monoamniotic twin pregnancies are mostly attributed to cord entanglement and cord knotting.[237]

Incidence

Current prevalence of umbilical cord entanglement is estimated between 70% and 91% of cases at birth, with 22% sonographically diagnosed.[235,238]

Diagnosis

Although 2D color and power Doppler sonography are usually most helpful for prenatal diagnosis of cord entanglement (Fig. 15.38A, B), this method does not easily visualize the exact location or continuity of the cord or define spatial relationships related to cord entanglement, twin pairs, and placenta as effectively as 3D US. When imaging twins, MRI can also define cord entanglement (Fig. 15.38C).

Another indirect sonographic diagnosis of cord entanglement can be achieved by Doppler flow velocimetry. This method reflects hemodynamic alterations in the fetal–placental circulation secondary to narrowing of the umbilical vessels involved in cord entanglement. These Doppler findings include high blood velocity in the umbilical vein,[239,240] a notch in the umbilical artery waveform,[241] or persistent absent end-diastolic flow (Fig. 15.39).[242]

Prognosis/Management

A systematic review and meta-analysis[243] of 114 monochorionic–monoamniotic twin pregnancies with cord entanglement reported overall survival at birth at 89%. In this study, 11% perinatal deaths occurred, of which 65% resulted *in utero* and 35%

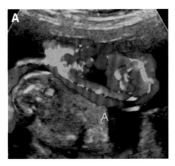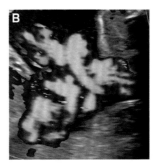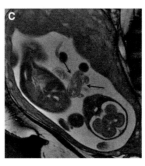

FIGURE 15.38: Cord entanglement. **A:** Color Doppler of monochorionic–monoamniotic twin pregnancy with cord entanglement. **B:** Power Doppler flow studies confirming cord entanglement. **C:** MRI of monochorionic–monoamniotic twin pregnancy with cord entanglement (*arrows*).

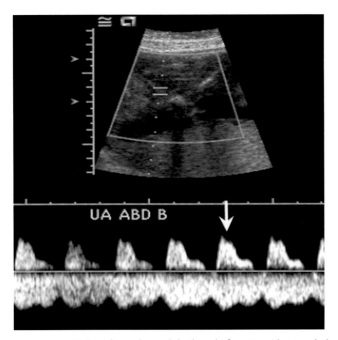

FIGURE 15.39: Doppler in the umbilical cord of a twin with a tangled cord. Notch in the umbilical artery denoted with *arrow*. There is also absent end-diastolic flow in the umbilical artery and a pulsatile waveform in the umbilical vein.

neonatal. Gestational age at fetal death ranged between 14 and 33 weeks. Thus, no consensus was reached in this review about the optimal antenatal management of these patients. At Cincinnati Fetal Care Center, delivery is planned between 32 and 34 weeks, unless abnormal umbilical artery Doppler is found.

CONJOINED TWINS

The most striking anomaly, conjoined twins, occurs when monozygotic twins fail to separate into two individuals.[244] The extent of conjunction ranges from a simple joining of ectodermal tissues to an extreme case of one twin contained within the other.

Incidence

The incidence ranges from 1 in 50,000 to 100,000 live births with a female-to-male ratio of 3:1.[244]

Pathogenesis/Etiology

Conjoined twins have been reported to arise at around 12 or 13 days postconception from a single blastocyst that had undergone incomplete division of the embryonic cell mass at one pole or at the point between the poles.[245] More recently, embryological studies of conjoined twinning have indicated that this developmental anomaly could originate from the secondary union of two separate embryonic discs.[245] Thus, two hypotheses exist on the origin of conjoined twins: the fission theory, in which a fertilized ovum divides incompletely, and the fusion theory, explaining secondary fusion of two originally distinct monovular embryos. The recent finding of a monochorionic–diamniotic conjoined twin pregnancy may further contribute to the fusion theory.[245,246] Others are in favor of the fission theory, maintained by the observation that the incidence of mirror imaging is higher in conjoined twins than that in monozygotic twins.[246,247]

Diagnosis

Conjoined twins are classified by the site of their most prominent union, which is ventral or dorsal in 87% and 13%, respectively (Fig. 15.40).[248] The abnormality is named with the suffix -pagus, which means fixed (Table 15.7).

The diagnosis of conjoined twins is often made on a prenatal US scan as early as gestation week 12. Prior to that time, false positives may occur in monoamniotic twins due to less fetal movement allowing for separation. Typical features include a fixed position of the fetal heads, an inability to detect separate bodies or skin contours, umbilical cord with three or more vessels, and the lack of separating membranes.[244]

Detailed ultrasonography, MRI, and echocardiography should be performed at 18 to 20 weeks to characterize the anatomy and the structure and function of the heart or hearts (Figs. 15.41 and 15.42). Each twin should be labeled appropriately and evaluated separately for detailed examination of shared and isolated organs. Malformations in nonshared organs are often present and complicate management. Doppler US provides another tool to assess prognosis of vital organs, especially the liver and heart (see Fig. 15.41B), which may be shared between the twins. MRI in conjoined twins (Figs. 15.41 and 15.42) can provide accurate diagnosis of shared and separate organs and other associated anomalies that are essential in prognosis, counseling, and management. 3D US and 3D MRI with printing software are helpful in understanding anatomy, especially when surgical intervention is contemplated.

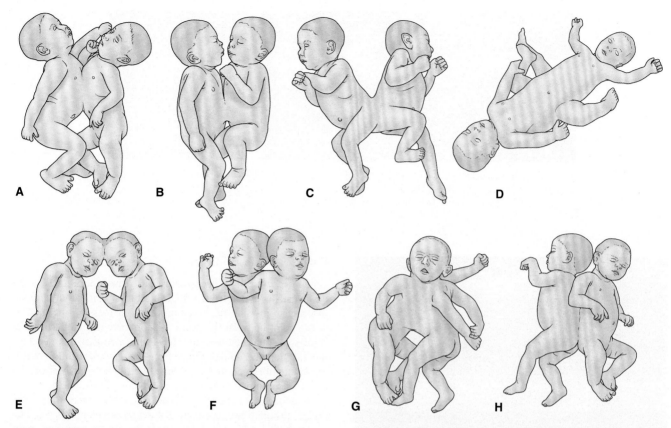

FIGURE 15.40: Different types of conjoined twins: thoracopagus **(A)**, omphalopagus **(B)**, pygopagus **(C)**, ischiopagus **(D)**, craniopagus **(E)**, parapagus **(F)**, cephalopagus **(G)**, and rachipagus **(H)**.

Prognosis/Management

Little is known about the antenatal natural history of conjoined twins. Around 20% to 40% of conjoined twins are stillborn, and more than half of those born alive die during the neonatal period before any surgical procedure can be attempted.[249] Overall, the prognosis depends on the type of fusion and presence of associated structural defects. As soon as the diagnosis of conjoined twins is made, management of the pregnancy begins. Elective termination is usually offered if severe deformities are anticipated or when there is a cardiac or cerebral fusion in which separation is not possible.[244] If the pregnancy is continued, elective cesarean delivery is planned at a center where appropriate obstetric, neonatal, and pediatric surgical facilities are available.

TABLE 15.7	Conjoined Twin Classification Based on Union Distribution	
TYPE	**AREA OF UNION**	**PERCENTAGE/VIABILITY**
Cephalopagus	Head-to-umbilicus fusion	11%, nonviable and nonseparable
Thoracopagus	Thorax-to-umbilicus fusion	19%, nonviable and nonseparable
Omphalopagus	At the umbilicus	18%, viable and separable
Ischiopagus	Lower abdomen and pelvis	11%, viable and separable
Parapagus	Pelvis and variable trunk	28%, viable but unlikely separable
Dorsal		Less frequent, viable but unlikely separable
Craniopagus	Brain	5%, viable but unlikely separable
Rachiopagus	Vertebral column	2%, viable but unlikely separable
Pygopagus	Sacrum	6%, viable but unlikely separable

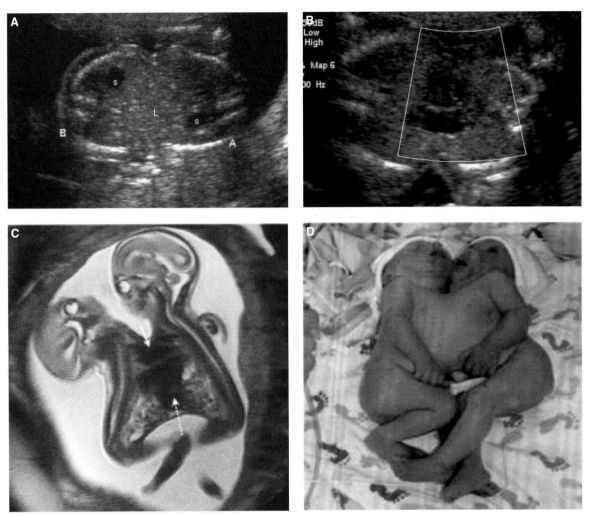

FIGURE 15.41: Conjoined thoracopagus twins at 20 weeks. **A:** On axial US, a single liver (*L*) is identified in the midline. Note two stomachs (*s*). Letters A and B represent twins. **B:** Color Doppler demonstrating a single heart shared between the two twins. **C:** T2 SSFSE MRI confirming single heart (*solid arrow*) and fused liver (*dotted arrow*). **D:** Color photo of the twins at birth.

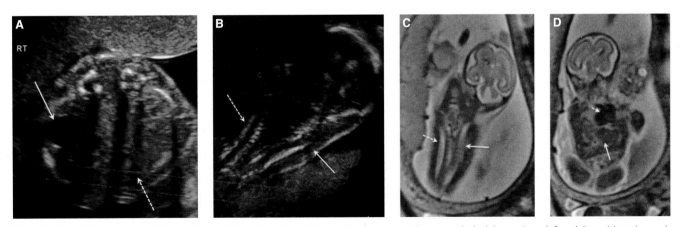

FIGURE 15.42: Parapagus conjoined twins at 22 weeks. **A:** Axial US showing a single stomach (*solid arrow*) and fused liver (*dotted arrow*). **B:** Two spines side by side are identified (*solid and dotted arrow*). **C:** Coronal T2 MRI confirming separate spinal canals (*solid and dotted arrows*). **D:** Coronal T2 MRI through anterior chest and abdomen demonstrating fused heart (*dotted arrow*) and single liver (*solid arrow*).

ACKNOWLEDGMENT

The author thanks Dr. Rachel Sinky for the help she provided as regards the introduction of this chapter.

REFERENCES

1. Martin JA, Hamilton BE, Ventura SJ, et al. Births: final data for 2010. *Natl Vital Stat Rep.* 2012;61(1):1–72.
2. Lambalk CB, Boomsma DI, DeBoer L, et al. Increased levels and pulsatility of follicle-stimulating hormone in mothers of hereditary dizygotic twins. *J Clin Endocrinol Metab.* 1998;83:481–486.
3. Ananth CV, Chauhan SP. Epidemiology of twinning in developed countries. *Semin Perinatol.* 2012;36(3):156–161.
4. Dickey RP. The relative contribution of assisted reproductive technologies and ovulation induction to multiple births in the United States 5 years after the Society for Assisted Reproductive Technology/American Society for Reproductive Medicine recommendation to limit the number of embryos transferred. *Fertil Steril.* 2007;88(6):1554–1561.
5. Chauhan SP, Scardo JA, Hayes E, et al. Twins: prevalence, problems and preterm births. *Am J Obstet Gynecol.* 2010;203:305–315.
6. Velikonja U. The cost of multiple gestation pregnancies in assisted reproduction. *Harv J Law Gend.* 2009;32:462–504.
7. Sunderam S, Kissin D, Flowers L, et al. Assisted reproductive technology surveillance—United States 2009. *MMWR Morb Mortal Wkly Rep.* 2012; 61(SS7):1–23.
8. Mathews TJ, MacDorman MF. Infant mortality statistics from the 2008 period linked birth/infant death data set. *Natl Vital Stat Rep.* 2012;60(5):1–28.
9. Kinzler WL, Ananth CV, Vintzileos AM. Medical and economic effects of twin gestations. *J Soc Gynecol Invest.* 2000;7(6):321–327.
10. Chasen ST, Chervenak FA. What is the relationship between the universal use of ultrasound, the rate of detection of twins, and outcome differences? *Clin Obstet Gynecol.* 1998;41:66–77.
11. Sherer DM. Is less intensive fetal surveillance of dichorionic twin gestations justified? *Ultrasound Obstet Gynecol.* 2000;15:167–173.
12. Vimercati A, Greco P, Vera L, et al. The diagnostic role of in-utero magnetic resonance imaging. *J Perinat Med.* 1999;27:303–308.
13. Bekkar M, van Vught JM. The role of magnetic resonance imaging in the prenatal diagnosis of fetal anomalies. *Eur J Obstet Gynecol Reprod Biol.* 2001;96:173–178.
14. Bekiesinska-Figatowska M, Herman-Sucharska I, Romaniuk-Doroszewska A, et al. Diagnostic problems in case of twin pregnancies: US vs. MRI study. *J Perinat Med.* 2013;41(5):535–541.
15. Lewis CM, Healy SC, Martin NG. Genetic contribution to dizygotic twinning. *Am J Med Genet.* 1996;61:237–246.
16. Meulemans WJ, Lewis CM, Boomsma DI, et al. Genetic modeling of dizygotic twinning in pedigrees of spontaneous dizygotic twins. *Am J Med Genet.* 1996;61:258–263.
17. Busjahn A, Knoblauch H, Faulhaber H-D, et al. A region on chromosome 3 is linked to dizygotic twinning. *Nat Genet.* 2000;26:398–399.
18. Hall JG. Twinning. *Lancet.* 2003;362(9385):735–743.
19. Nylander PPS. Frequency of multiple births. In: MacGillivray I, Nylander PPS, Corney G, eds. *Human Multiple Reproduction.* London, England: WB Saunders; 1975:87–98.
20. Kiely JL, Kiely B. Epidemiological trends in multiple births in the United States, 1971–1998. *Twin Res.* 2001;4:131–133.
21. Murphy M, Hey K. Twinning rates. *Lancet.* 1997;349:1398–1399.
22. Benirschke K. Accurate recording of twin placentation: a plea to the obstetrician. *Obstet Gynecol.* 1961;18:334–347.
23. Benirschke K, Kim CK. Multiple pregnancy 1. *N Engl J Med.* 1973;288:1276–1284.
24. Benirschke K, Kim CK. Multiple pregnancy 2. *N Engl J Med.* 1973;288:1329–1336.
25. Burn J, Corney G. Zygosity determination and the types of twinning. In: MacGillivray I, Campbell DM, Thompson B, eds. *Twinning and Twins.* Chichester, England: John Wiley and Sons; 1988:7–25.
26. Machin GA, Keith LG, Bamforth F. *An Atlas of Multiple Pregnancy: Biology and Pathology.* New York, NY: Parthenon; 1999.
27. Carroll SG, Tyfield L, Reeve L, et al. Is zygosity or chorionicity the main determinant of fetal outcome in twin pregnancies? *Am J Obstet Gynecol.* 2005;193(3 pt 1):757.
28. Spiegler J, Härtel C, Schulz L, et al; German Neonatal Network (GNN). Causes of delivery and outcomes of very preterm twins stratified to zygosity. *Twin Res Hum Genet.* 2012;15(4):532–536.
29. Gao Y, He Z, Luo Y, et al. Selective and non-selective intrauterine growth restriction in twin pregnancies: high-risk factors and perinatal outcome. *Arch Gynecol Obstet.* 2012;285(4):973–978.
30. Monteagudo A, Timor-Tritsch IE, Sharma S. Early and simple determination of chorionic and amniotic type in multiple gestation in the first 14 weeks by high frequency transvaginal ultrasonography. *Am J Obstet Gynecol.* 1994;170:824–829.
31. Hill LM, Chenevey P, Hecker J, et al. Sonographic determination of first trimester twin chorionicity and amnionicity. *J Clin Ultrasound.* 1996;24:305–308.
32. Sepulveda W, Sebire NJ, Hughes K, et al. The lambda sign at 10–14 weeks of gestations as a predictor of chorionicity in twin pregnancies. *Ultrasound Obstet Gynecol.* 1996;7:421–423.
33. Shetty A, Smith AP. The sonographic diagnosis of chorionicity. *Prenat Diagn.* 2005;25(9):735–739.
34. Stenhouse E, Hardwick C, Maharaj S, et al. Chorionicity determination in twin pregnancies: how accurate are we? *Ultrasound Obstet Gynecol.* 2002;19:350–352.
35. Bessis R, Papernik E. Echographic imagery of amniotic membranes in twin pregnancies. In: Gedda L, Parisi P, eds. *Twin Research 3: Twin Biology and Multiple Pregnancy.* New York, NY: Alan R Liss; 1981:183–187.
36. Monteagudo A, Roman AS. Ultrasound in multiple gestations: twins and other multifetal pregnancies. *Clin Perinatol.* 2005;32:329–354, vi.
37. Bromley B, Benacerraf B. Using the number of yolk sacs to determine amnionicity in early first trimester monochorionic twins. *J Ultrasound Med.* 1995;14:415–419.
38. Finberg HJ. The twin peak sign: reliable evidence of dichorionic twinning. *J Ultrasound Med.* 1992;11:571–577.
39. Scardo JA, Ellings JM, Newman RB. Prospective determination of chorionicity, amnionicity, and zygosity in twin gestations. *Am J Obstet Gynecol.* 1995;173:1376–1380.
40. Sepulveda W. Chorionicity determination in twin pregnancies: double trouble. *Ultrasound Obstet Gynecol.* 1997;10:79–81.
41. Chervenak FA, Skupski DW, Romero R, et al. How accurate is fetal biometry in the assessment of fetal age? *Am J Obstet Gynecol.* 1998;178:678–687.
42. Winn HN, Gabrielli S, Reece EA, et al. Ultrasonographic criteria for the prenatal diagnosis of placental chorionicity in twin gestations. *Am J Obstet Gynecol.* 1989;161:1540–1542.
43. D'Alton ME, Dudley DK. The ultrasonographic prediction of chorionicity in twin gestation. *Am J Obstet Gynecol.* 1989;160:557–561.
44. Powell KH, Grudzinskas JG. Screening for Down syndrome in the first trimester. *Reprod Fertil Dev.* 1995;7(6):1413–1417.
45. Jackson M, Rose NC. Diagnosis and management of fetal nuchal translucency. *Semin Roentgenol.* 1998;33(4):333–338.
46. Lo YM, Corbetta N, Chamberlain PF, et al. Presence of fetal DNA in maternal plasma and serum. *Lancet.* 1997;350(9076):485–487.
47. Rustico MA, Lanna M, Faiola S, et al. Major discordant structural anomalies in monochorionic twins: spectrum and outcomes. *Twin Res Hum Genet.* 2018;21(6):546-555. doi:10.1017/thg.2018.58.
48. Baldwin VJ. Anomalous development of twins. In: Baldwin VJ, ed. *Pathology of Multiple Pregnancy.* New York, NY: Springer-Verlag; 1994:169–197.
49. Lewi L, Jani J, Blickstein I, et al. The outcome of monochorionic diamniotic twin gestations in the era of invasive fetal therapy: a prospective cohort study. *Am J Obstet Gynecol.* 2008;199:514–518.
50. Baxi LV, Walsh CA. Monoamniotic twins in contemporary practice: a single center study of perinatal outcomes. *J Matern Fetal Neonatal Med.* 2010;23:506–510.
51. International Society of Ultrasound in Obstetrics and Gynecology, Carvalho JS, Allan LD, Chaoui R, et al. ISUOG Practice Guidelines (updated): sonographic screening examination of the fetal heart. *Ultrasound Obstet Gynecol.* 2013;41:348–359.
52. Jenkins TM, Wapner RJ. The challenge of prenatal diagnosis in twin pregnancies. *Curr Opin Obstet Gynecol.* 2000;12(2):87–92.
53. Vink J, Wapner R, D'Alton ME. Prenatal diagnosis in twin gestations. *Semin Perinatol.* 2012;36(3):169–174.
54. Cleary-Goldman J, Malone FD, Vidaver J, et al. Impact of maternal age on obstetric outcome. *Obstet Gynecol.* 2005;105:983–990.
55. Edwards MS, Ellings JM, Newman RB, et al. Predictive value of antepartum ultrasound examination for anomalies in twin gestations. *Ultrasound Obstet Gynecol.* 1995;6(1):43–49.
56. Nicolaides KH. Screening for fetal chromosomal abnormalities: need to change the rules. *Ultrasound Obstet Gynecol.* 1994;4:353–354.
57. Sebire NJ, Noble PL, Psarra A, et al. Fetal karyotyping in twin pregnancies: selection of technique by measurement of fetal nuchal translucency. *Br J Obstet Gynaecol.* 1996;103:887–880.
58. Sebire NJ, Snijders RJ, Hughes K, et al. Screening for trisomy 21 in twin pregnancies by maternal age and fetal nuchal translucency thickness at 10–14 weeks of gestation. *Br J Obstet Gynaecol.* 1996;103:999–1003.
59. Maymon R, Jauniaux E, Herman A. Down's syndrome screening in twin pregnancies by nuchal translucency measurement current concept. *Minerva Ginecol.* 2002;54:211–215.
60. Wald NJ, Rish S, Hackshaw AK. Combining nuchal translucency and serum markers in prenatal screening for Down syndrome in twin pregnancies. *Prenat Diagn.* 2003;23:588–592.
61. Sebire NJ, D'Ercole C, Hughes K, et al. Increased nuchal translucency thickness at 10–14 weeks of gestation as a predictor of severe twin-to-twin transfusion syndrome. *Ultrasound Obstet Gynecol.* 1997;10:86–89.
62. Kagan KO, Gazzoni A, Sepulveda-Gonzalez G, et al. Discordance in nuchal translucency that thickness in the prediction of severe twin-to-twin transfusion syndrome. *Ultrasound Obstet Gynecol.* 2007;29:527–532.
63. Bush MC, Malone FD. Down syndrome screening in twins. *Clin Perinatol.* 2005;32:373–386, vi.
64. Linskens IH, Spreeuwenberg MD, Blankenstein MA, et al. Early first-trimester free beta-hCG and PAPP-A serum distributions in monochorionic and dichorionic twins. *Prenat Diagn.* 2009;29:74–78.
65. Wald NJ, Rish S. Prenatal screening for Down syndrome and neural tube defects in twin pregnancies. *Prenat Diagn.* 2005;25(9):740.
66. Spencer K, Staboulidou I, Nicolaides KH. First trimester aneuploidy screening in the presence of a vanishing twin: implications for maternal serum markers. *Prenat Diagn.* 2010;30(3):235.

67. Chasen ST, Perni SC, Predanic M, et al. Does a "vanishing twin" affect first-trimester biochemistry in Down syndrome risk assessment? *Am J Obstet Gynecol.* 2006;195(1):236.

68. Malone FD, D'Alton ME; Society for Maternal-Fetal Medicine. First-trimester sonographic screening for Down syndrome. *Obstet Gynecol.* 2003;102:1066–1079.

69. Olney RS, Khoury MJ, Alo CJ, et al. Increased risk for transverse digital deficiency after chorionic villus sampling: results of the United States Multistate Case-Control Study, 1988–1992. *Teratology.* 1995;51(1):20.

70. Firth HV, Boyd PA, Chamberlain PF, et al. Analysis of limb reduction defects in babies exposed to chorionic villus sampling. *Lancet.* 1994;343:1069–1071.

71. Van der Zee DC, Bax KM, Vermeij-Keers C. Maternoembryonic transfusion and congenital malformations. *Prenat Diagn.* 1997;17:59–69.

72. Wald NJ, Huttly WJ, Hackshaw AK. Antenatal screening for Down's syndrome with the quadruple test. *Lancet.* 2003;361:835–836.

73. Graham G, Simpson LL. Diagnosis and management of obstetrical complications unique to multiple gestations. *Clin Obstet Gynecol.* 2004;47:163–180.

74. Muller F, Dreux S, Dupoizat H, et al. Second-trimester Down syndrome maternal serum screening in twin pregnancies: impact of chorionicity. *Prenat Diagn.* 2001;23:331–335.

75. Lo YM, Lo ES, Watson N, et al. Two-way cell traffic between mother and fetus: biologic and clinical implications. *Blood.* 1996;88(11):4390–4395.

76. Lun FM, Chiu RW, Allen Chan KC, et al. Microfluidics digital PCR reveals a higher than expected fraction of fetal DNA in maternal plasma. *Clin Chem.* 2008;54:1664–1672.

77. Lo YM, Zhang J, Leung TN, et al. Rapid clearance of fetal DNA from maternal plasma. *Am J Hum Genet.* 1999;64:218–224.

78. Lo YM, Chan KC, Sun H, et al. Maternal plasma DNA sequencing reveals the genome-wide genetic and mutational profile of the fetus. *Sci Transl Med.* 2010;2:61.

79. Devaney SA, Palomaki GE, Scott JA, et al. Noninvasive fetal sex determination using cell-free fetal DNA: a systematic review and meta-analysis. *JAMA.* 2011;306(6):627–636.

80. Boon EM, Faas BH. Benefits and limitations of whole genome versus targeted approaches for noninvasive prenatal testing for fetal aneuploidies. *Prenat Diagn.* 2013;33:563–568.

81. Sparks AB, Wang ET, Struble CA, et al. Selective analysis of cell-free DNA in maternal blood for evaluation of fetal trisomy. *Prenat Diagn.* 2012;32:3–9.

82. Sparks AB, Struble CA, Wang ET, et al. Non-invasive prenatal detection and selective analysis of cell-free DNA obtained from maternal blood: evaluation for trisomy 21 and trisomy 18. *Am J Obstet Gynecol.* 2012;206:319.e1–319.e9.

83. Ashoor G, Syngelaki A, Wagner M, et al. Chromosome-selective sequencing of maternal plasma cell-free DNA for first-trimester detection of trisomy 21 and trisomy 18. *Am J Obstet Gynecol.* 2012;206:322.e1–322.e5.

84. Norton E, Brar H, Weiss J, et al. Non-Invasive Chromosomal Evaluation (NICE) Study: results of a multicenter prospective cohort study for detection of fetal trisomy 21 and trisomy 18. *Am J Obstet Gynecol.* 2012;207:137.e1–137.e8.

85. Nicolaides KH, Syngelaki A, Ashoor G, et al. Non-invasive prenatal testing for fetal trisomies in a routinely screened first-trimester population. *Am J Obstet Gynecol.* 2012;207:374.e1–374.e6.

86. Zimmermann B, Hill M, Gemelos G, et al. Non-invasive prenatal aneuploidy testing of chromosomes 13, 18, 21, X, and Y, using targeted sequencing of polymorphic loci. *Prenat Diagn.* 2012;32:1233–1241.

87. Nicolaides H, Syngelaki A, Gil M, et al. Validation of targeted sequencing of single-nucleotide polymorphisms for non-invasive prenatal detection of aneuploidy of chromosomes 13, 18, 21, X, and Y. *Prenat Diagn.* 2013;33:575–579.

88. Garfield SS, Armstrong SO. Clinical and cost consequences of incorporating a novel non-invasive prenatal test into the diagnostic pathway for fetal trisomies. *J Manag Care Med.* 2012;15:34–41.

89. Song K, Musci TJ, Caughey AB. Clinical utility and cost of non-invasive prenatal testing with cfDNA analysis in high-risk women based on a US population. *J Matern Fetal Neonatal Med.* 2013;26:1180–1185.

90. Ohno M, Caughey AB. The role of noninvasive prenatal testing as a diagnostic versus a screening tool—a cost-effectiveness analysis. *Prenat Diagn.* 2013;33:630–635.

91. Cuckle H, Benn P, Pergament E. Maternal cfDNA screening for Down syndrome—a cost sensitivity analysis. *Prenat Diagn.* 2013;33:636–642.

92. Huang X, Zheng J, Chen M, et al. Noninvasive prenatal testing of trisomies 21 and 18 by massively parallel sequencing of maternal plasma DNA in twin pregnancies. *Prenat Diagn.* 2014;34:335–340.

92a. Gil MM, Galeva S, Jani J, Konstantinidou L, Akolekar R, Plana MN, Nicolaides KH. *Ultrasound Obstet Gynecol.* 2019 Jun;53(6):734–742.

93. Berghella V, Saccone G. Cervical assessment by ultrasound for preventing preterm delivery. *Cochrane Database Syst Rev.* 2019;(9):CD007235. doi:10.1002/14651858. CD007235.pub4.

94. Weisz B, Rodeck CH. Invasive diagnostic procedures in twin pregnancies. *Prenat Diagn.* 2005;25:751–758.

95. Jeanty P, Shah D, Roussis P. Single-needle insertion in twin amniocentesis. *J Ultrasound Med.* 1990;9:511–517.

96. Van Vugt JM, Nieuwint A, van Geijn HP. Single-needle insertion: an alternative technique for early second-trimester genetic twin amniocentesis. *Fetal Diagn Ther.* 1995;10:178–181.

97. ACOG practice bulletin No 88. *Obstetrics and Gynecology.* 2007; 110 (6):1459–1467.

98. Agarwal K, Alfirevic Z. Pregnancy loss after chorionic villus sampling and genetic amniocentesis in twin pregnancies: a systematic review. *Ultrasound Obstet Gynecol.* 2012;40:128–134.

99. WHO. March of Dimes, Partnership for Maternal, Newborn & Child Health, Save the Children. Born Too Soon: The Global Action Report on Preterm Birth. www.who.int/maternal_child_adolescent/documents/born_too_soon/en/. Accessed May 4, 2012.

100. Skentou C, Souka AP, To MS, et al. Prediction of preterm delivery in twins by cervical assessment at 23 weeks. *Ultrasound Obstet Gynecol.* 2001;17(1):7–10.

101. Conde-Agudelo A, Romero R, Hassan SS, et al. Transvaginal sonographic cervical length for the prediction of spontaneous preterm birth in twin pregnancies: a systematic review and metaanalysis. *Am J Obstet Gynecol.* 2010;203(2):128.e1.

102. Crane JM, Van den Hof M, Armson BA, et al. Transvaginal ultrasound in the prediction of preterm delivery: singleton and twin gestations. *Obstet Gynecol.* 1997;90:357–363.

103. Goldenberg RL, Iams JD, Miodovnik M, et al. The preterm prediction study: risk factors in twin gestations. National Institute of Child Health and Human Development Maternal-Fetal Medicine Units Network. *Am J Obstet Gynecol.* 1996;175(4 pt 1):1047.

104. Sotiriadis A, Papatheodorou S, Makrydimas G. Perinatal outcome in women treated with progesterone for the prevention of preterm birth: a meta-analysis. *Ultrasound Obstet Gynecol.* 2012;40(3):257–266.

105. Durnwald CP. 17 OHPC for prevention of preterm birth in twins: back to the drawing board? *Am J Obstet Gynecol.* 2013;208(3):167–168.

106. Romero R, Nicolaides K, Conde-Agudelo A, et al. Vaginal progesterone in women with an asymptomatic sonographic short cervix in the midtrimester decreases preterm delivery and neonatal morbidity: a systematic review and metaanalysis of individual patient data. *Am J Obstet Gynecol.* 2012;206(2):124.e1–124.e19.

107. Senat MV, Porcher R, Winer N, et al; Groupe de Recherche en Obstétrique et Gynécologie. Prevention of preterm delivery by 17 alpha-hydroxyprogesterone caproate in asymptomatic twin pregnancies with a short cervix: a randomized controlled trial. *Am J Obstet Gynecol.* 2013;208(3):194.e1–194.e8.

108. Berghella V, Odibo AO, To MS, et al. Cerclage for short cervix on ultrasonography: meta-analysis of trials using individual patient-level data. *Obstet Gynecol.* 2005;106(1):181–189.

109. Dang VQ, Nguyen LK, Pham TD, et al. Pessary compared with vaginal progesterone for the prevention of preterm birth in women with twin pregnancies and cervical length less than 38 mm: a randomized controlled trial. *Obstet Gynecol.* 2019;133(3):459-467. doi:10.1097/AOG.0000000000003136.

110. Kosińska-Kaczyńska K, Szymusik I, Bomba-Opoń D, et al. Effective treatment of cervical incompetence in a monochorionic monoamniotic twin pregnancy with a rescue cervical cerclage and pessary—a case report and review of the literature. *Ginekol Pol.* 2012;83(12):946–949.

111. Carreras E, Arévalo S, Bello-Muñoz JC, et al. Arabin cervical pessary to prevent preterm birth in severe twin-to-twin transfusion syndrome treated by laser surgery. *Prenat Diagn.* 2012;32(12):1181–1185.

112. Prevention and prediction of preterm birth. Number 130 October 2012. Replaces Practice Bulletin Number 31, October 2001 and Committee Opinion No. 419, October 2008.

113. Enbom JA. Twin pregnancy with intrauterine death of one twin. *Am J Obstet Gynecol.* 1985;152:424–429.

114. Kilby MD, Govind A, O'Brien PM. Outcome of twin pregnancies complicated by a single intrauterine death: a comparison with viable twin pregnancies. *Obstet Gynecol.* 1994;84:107–109.

115. Woo HH, Sin SY, Tang LC. Single foetal death in twin pregnancies: review of the maternal and neonatal outcomes and management. *Hong Kong Med J.* 2000;6:293–300.

116. Ong SS, Zamora J, Khan KS, et al. Prognosis for the co-twin following single-twin death: a systematic review. *BJOG.* 2006;113:992–998.

117. Murphy KW. Intrauterine death in a twin: implications for the survivor. In: Ward RH, Whittle M, eds. *Multiple Pregnancy.* London, England: RCOG Press; 1995:218–230.

118. Anand D, Platt MJ, Pharoah POD. Comparative development of surviving co-twins of vanishing twin conceptions, twins and singletons. *Twin Res Hum Genet.* 2007;10:210–215.

119. Carlson NJ, Towers CV. Multiple gestation complicated by the death of one fetus. *Obstet Gynecol.* 1989;73:685–689.

120. Cleary-Goldman J, D'Alton M. Management of single fetal demise in a multiple gestation. *Obstet Gynecol Surv.* 2004;59:285–298.

121. Okamura K, Murotsuki J, Tanigawara S, et al. Funipuncture for evaluation of hematologic and coagulation indices in the surviving twin following co-twin's death. *Obstet Gynecol.* 1994;83:975–978.

122. Fusi L, McParland P, Fisk N, et al. Acute twin-twin transfusion: a possible mechanism for brain-damaged survivors after intrauterine death of a monochorionic twin. *Obstet Gynecol.* 1991;78(3 pt 2):517–520.

123. Nicolini U, Pisoni MP, Cela E, et al. Fetal blood sampling immediately before and within 24 hours of death in monochorionic twin pregnancies complicated by single intrauterine death. *Am J Obstet Gynecol.* 1998;179(3 pt 1):800–803.

124. Jelin AC, Norton ME, Bartha AI, et al. Intracranial magnetic resonance imaging findings in the surviving fetus after spontaneous monochorionic co-twin demise. *Am J Obstet Gynecol.* 2008;199(4):398.e1–398.e5.

125. Patten RM, Mack LA, Nyberg DA, et al. Twin embolization syndrome: prenatal sonographic detection and significance. *Radiology.* 1989;173:685–689.

126. Karl WM. Intrauterine death in a twin: implications for the survivor. In: Ward RH, Whittle M, eds. *Multiple Pregnancy.* London, England: RCOG Press; 1995:218–230.

127. De Laveaucoupet J, Audibert F, Guis F, et al. Fetal magnetic resonance imaging (MRI) of ischemic brain injury. *Prenat Diagn.* 2001;21:729–736.

128. Conte G, Righini A, Griffiths PD, et al. Brain-injured survivors of monochorionic twin pregnancies complicated by single intrauterine death: MR

findings in a multicenter study. *Radiology*. 2018;288(2):582–590. doi:10.1148/radiol.2018171267.

129. van Klink JM, van Steenis A, Steggerda SJ, et al. Single fetal demise in monochorionic pregnancies: incidence and patterns of cerebral injury. *Ultrasound Obstet Gynecol*. 2015;45(3):294-300. doi:10.1002/uog.14722.

130. Nelson KB, Ellenberg JH. Childhood neurological disorders in twins. *Paediatr Perinat Epidemiol*. 1995;9:135–145.

131. Mackie FL, Rigby A, Morris RK, et al. Prognosis of the co-twin following spontaneous single intrauterine fetal death in twin pregnancies: a systematic review and meta-analysis. *BJOG*. 2019;126(5):569-578. doi:10.1111/1471-0528.15530.

132. Ong S, Zamora J, Khan K, et al. Single twin demise; consequences to the survivor. In: Kilby MD, Baker P, Critchley H, eds. *Multiple Pregnancy*. London, England: RCOG Press; 2006.

133. Santema JG, Swaak AM, Wallenburg HC. Expectant management of twin pregnancy with single fetal death. *Br J Obstet Gynaecol*. 1995;102:26–30.

134. Spong CY, Mercer BM, D'alton M, et al. Timing of indicated late-preterm and early-term birth. *Obstet Gynecol*. 2011;118(2 pt 1):323–333.

135. Miller J, Chauhan SP, Abuhamad AZ. Discordant twins: diagnosis, evaluation and management. *Am J Obstet Gynecol*. 2012;206(1):10–20.

136. American College of Obstetricians and Gynecologists. *Multiple Gestation: Complicated Twin, Triplet, and High-Order Multifetal Pregnancy*. Washington, DC: American College of Obstetricians and Gynecologists; 2004. ACOG practice bulletin no 56.

137. Caravello JW, Chauhan SP, Morrison JC, et al. Sonographic examination does not predict growth discordance accurately. *Obstet Gynecol*. 1997;89:529–533.

138. Grobman WA, Parilla BV. Positive predictive value of suspected growth aberration in twin gestations. *Am J Obstet Gynecol*. 1999;181:1139–1141.

139. Alam Machado Rde C, Brizot Mde L, Liao AW, et al. Early neonatal morbidity and mortality in growth-discordant twins. *Acta Obstet Gynecol Scand*. 2009;88:167–171.

140. Kato N, Matsuda T. The relationship between birthweight discordance and perinatal mortality of one of the twins in a twin pair. *Twin Res Hum Genet*. 2006;9:292–297.

141. Branum AM, Schoendorf KC. The effect of birth weight discordance on twin neonatal mortality. *Obstet Gynecol*. 2003;101:570–574.

142. Hollier LM, McIntire DD, Leveno KJ. Outcome of twin pregnancies according to intrapair birth weight differences. *Obstet Gynecol*. 1999;94:1006–1010.

143. Lewi L, Gucciardo L, Huber A, et al. Clinical outcome and placental characteristics of mono chorionic diamniotic twin pairs with early- and late-onset discordant growth. *Am J Obstet Gynecol*. 2008;199:511.e1–511.e7.

144. Barrett J, Bocking A. Management of twin pregnancies. SOGC consensus statement: part 1, no 91, July 2000. *J Soc Obstet Gynaecol Can*. 2000;22:519–529.

145. D'Antonio F, Odibo AO, Prefumo F, et al. Weight discordance and perinatal mortality in twin pregnancy: systematic review and meta-analysis. *Ultrasound Obstet Gynecol*. 2018;52:11–23. doi:10.1002/uog.18966.

146. Chervenak FA, Johnson RE, Youcha S, et al. Intrapartum management of twin gestation. *Obstet Gynecol*. 1985;65:119–124.

147. Persad VL, Baskett TF, O'Connell CM, et al. Combined vaginal-cesarean delivery of twin pregnancies. *Obstet Gynecol*. 2001;8:1032–1037.

148. Robertson EG, Neer KJ. Placental injection studies in twin gestation. *Am J Obstet Gynecol*. 1983;147:170–174.

149. Denbow ML, Cox P, Taylor M, et al. Placental angioarchitecture in monochorionic twin pregnancies: relationship to fetal growth, fetofetal transfusion syndrome, and pregnancy outcome. *Am J Obstet Gynecol*. 2000;182:417–426.

150. Umur A, van Gemert MJ, Nikkels PG. Monochorionic twins and twin-twin transfusion syndrome: the protective role of arterio-arterial anastomoses. *Placenta*. 2002;23:201–209.

151. Crombleholme TM, Shera D, Lee H, et al. A prospective, randomized, multicenter trial of amnioreduction vs selective fetoscopic laser photocoagulation for the treatment of severe twin-twin transfusion syndrome. *Am J Obstet Gynecol*. 2007;197:396.e1–396.e9.

152. De Paepe ME, Burke S, Luks FI, et al. Demonstration of placental vascular anatomy in monochorionic twin gestations. *Pediatr Dev Pathol*. 2002;5:37–44.

153. Bajoria R, Wee LY, Anwar S, et al. Outcome of twin pregnancies complicated by single intrauterine death in relation to vascular anatomy of the monochorionic placenta. *Hum Reprod*. 1999;14(8):2124–2130.

154. Cameron VA, Ellmers LJ. Minireview: natriuretic peptides during development of the fetal heart and circulation. *Endocrinology*. 2003;144(6):2191–2194.

155. Sebire NJ, Souka A, Skentou H, et al. Early prediction of severe twin-to-twin transfusion syndrome. *Hum Reprod*. 2000;15(9):2008–2010.

156a. Gijtenbeek M, Eschbach SJ, Middeldorp JM, et al. The value of echocardiography and Doppler in the prediction of fetal demise after laser coagulation for TTTS: A systematic review and meta-analysis. *Prenat Diagn*. 2019 Sep;39(10):838–847. doi: 10.1002/pd.5511.

156. Sebire NJ, D'Ercole C, Carvelho M, et al. Inter-twin membrane folding in monochorionic pregnancies. *Ultrasound Obstet Gynecol*. 1998;11(5):324–327.

157. Khalil A. Modified diagnostic criteria for twin-to-twin transfusion syndrome prior to 18 weeks' gestation: time to change? *Ultrasound Obstet Gynecol*. 2017;49:804–805.

158. Dekoninck P, Deprest J, Lewi P, et al. Gestational age-specific reference ranges for amniotic fluid assessment in monochorionic diamniotic twin pregnancies. *Ultrasound Obstet Gynecol*. 2013;41:649–652.

159. Habli M, Lim FY, Crombleholme T. Twin-to-twin transfusion syndrome: a comprehensive update. *Clin Perinatol*. 2009;36(2):391–416.

160. Barrea C, Alkazaleh F, Ryan G, et al. Prenatal cardiovascular manifestations in the twin-to-twin transfusion syndrome recipients and the impact of therapeutic amnioreduction. *Am J Obstet Gynecol*. 2005;192:892–902.

161. Sueters M, Middeldorp JM, Vandenbussche FP, et al. The effect of fetoscopic laser therapy on fetal cardiac size in twin-twin transfusion syndrome. *Ultrasound Obstet Gynecol*. 2008;31(2):158–163.

162. Habli M, Michelfelder E, Livingston J, et al. Acute effects of selective fetoscopic laser photocoagulation on recipient cardiac function in twin-twin transfusion syndrome. *Am J Obstet Gynecol*. 2008;199(4):412.e1–412.e6.

163. Lougheed J, Sinclair BG, Fung KFK, et al. Acquired right ventricular outflow tract obstruction in the recipient twin in twin-twin transfusion syndrome. *J Am Coll Cardiol*. 2001;38:1533–1538.

164. Quarello E, Molho M, Ville Y. Incidence, mechanisms, and patterns of fetal cerebral lesions in twin-to-twin transfusion syndrome. *J Matern Fetal Neonatal Med*. 2007;20(8):589–597.

165. Kline-Fath, et al. TTTS and cerebral pathology: a comparison of fetal MRI and ultrasound, SPR International Society for Pediatric Radiology Meeting, Chicago Illinois, May 2016.

166. Kline-Fath BM, Calvo-Garcia MA, O'Hara SM, et al. Twin-twin transfusion syndrome: cerebral ischemia is not the only fetal MR imaging finding. *Pediatr Radiol*. 2007;37(1):47–56.

167. Tarui T, Khwaja O, Estroff J, et al. Altered fetal cerebral and cerebellar development in twin-twin transfusion syndrome. *AJNR Am J Neuroradiol*. 2012;33:1121–1126.

168. Brennan JN, Diwan RV, Rosen MG, et al. Fetofetal transfusion syndrome: prenatal ultrasonographic diagnosis. *Radiology*. 1982;143(2):535–536.

169. Uotila J, Tammela O. Acute intrapartum fetoplacental transfusion in monochorionic twin pregnancy. *Obstet Gynecol*. 1999;5:819–821.

170. Umur A, van Gemert MJ, Nikkels PG. Monoamniotic-versus diamniotic–monochorionic twin placentas: anastomoses and twin-twin transfusion syndrome. *Am J Obstet Gynecol*. 2003;189:1325–1329.

171. Habli M, Bombrys A, Lewis D, et al. Incidence of complications in twin-twin transfusion syndrome after selective fetoscopic laser photocoagulation: a single-center experience. *Am J Obstet Gynecol*. 2009;201(4):417.

172. Duncombe GJ, Dickinson JE, Evans SF. Perinatal characteristics and outcomes of pregnancies complicated by twin-twin transfusion syndrome. *Obstet Gynecol*. 2003;101(6):1190–1196.

173. Lopriore E, Sueters M, Middeldorp JM, et al. Neonatal outcome in twin-to-twin transfusion syndrome treated with fetoscopic laser occlusion of vascular anastomoses. *J Pediatr*. 2005;147(5):597–602.

174. Lutfi S, Allen VM, Fahey J, et al. Twin-twin transfusion syndrome: a population-based study. *Obstet Gynecol*. 2004;104(6):1289–1297. Erratum in: *Obstet Gynecol*. 2005;105(2):451.

175. Acosta-Rojas R, Becker J, Munoz-Abellana B, et al; for the Catalunya and Balears Monochorionic Network. Twin chorionicity and the risk of adverse perinatal outcome. *Int J Gynaecol Obstet*. 2007;96(2):98–102.

176. Lenclen R, Paupe A, Ciarlo G, et al. Neonatal outcome in preterm monochorionic twins with twin-to-twin transfusion syndrome after intrauterine treatment with amnioreduction or fetoscopic laser surgery: comparison with dichorionic twins. *Am J Obstet Gynecol*. 2007;196(5):450.e1–450.e7.

177. Bejar R, Vigliocco G, Gramajo H, et al. Antenatal origin of neurologic damage in newborn infants, II: multiple gestations. *Am J Obstet Gynecol*. 1990;162(5):1230–1236.

178. Graef C, Ellenrieder B, Hecher K, et al. Long-term neurodevelopmental outcome of 167 children after intrauterine laser treatment for severe twin–twin transfusion syndrome. *Am J Obstet Gynecol*. 2006;194:303–308.

179. Merhar SL, Kline-Fath BM, Meinzen-Derr J, et al. Fetal and postnatal brain MRI in premature infants with twin-twin transfusion syndrome. *J Perinatol*. 2013;33(2):112–118.

180. Lopriore E, Nagel HT, Vandenbussche FP, et al. Long-term neurodevelopmental outcome in twin-to-twin transfusion syndrome. *Am J Obstet Gynecol*. 2003;189:1314–1319.

181. Herberg U, Gross W, Bartmann P, et al. Long term cardiac follow up of severe twin to twin transfusion syndrome after intrauterine laser coagulation. *Heart*. 2006;92(1):95–100.

182. Moise KJ Jr. Polyhydramnios: problems and treatment. *Semin Perinatol*. 1993; 17:197–209.

183. Rodestal A, Thomassen PA. Acute polyhydramnios in twin pregnancy. A retrospective study with special reference to therapeutic amniocentesis. *Acta Obstet Gynecol Scand*. 1990;69:297–300.

184. Mari G, Roberts A, Detti L, et al. Perinatal morbidity and mortality rates in severe twin-twin transfusion syndrome: results of the International Amnioreduction Registry. *Am J Obstet Gynecol*. 2001;185:708–715.

185. De Lia JE, Cruikshank DP, Keye WR Jr. Fetoscopic neodymium: YAG laser occlusion of placental vessels in severe twin-twin transfusion syndrome. *Obstet Gynecol*. 1990;75:1046–1053.

186. Senat MV, Deprest J, Boulvain M, et al. Endoscopic laser surgery versus serial amnioreduction for severe twin-to-twin transfusion syndrome. *N Engl J Med*. 2004;351(2):136–144.

187. Yamamoto M, El Murr L, Robyr R, et al. Incidence and impact of perioperative complications in 175 fetoscopy-guided laser coagulations of chorionic plate anastomoses in fetofetal transfusion syndrome before 26 weeks of gestation. *Am J Obstet Gynecol*. 2005;193(3 pt 2):1110–1116.

188. Robyr R, Lewi L, Salomon LJ, et al. Prevalence and management of late fetal complications following successful selective laser coagulation of chorionic plate anastomoses in twin-to-twin transfusion syndrome. *Am J Obstet Gynecol*. 2006;194(3):796.

189. Lewi L, Jani J, Cannie M, et al. Intertwin anastomoses in monochorionic placentas after fetoscopic laser coagulation for twin-to-twin transfusion syndrome: is there more than meets the eye? *Am J Obstet Gynecol.* 2006;194:790–795.

190. Lopriore E, Middeldorp JM, Oepkes D, et al. Residual anastomoses after fetoscopic laser surgery in twin-to-twin transfusion syndrome: frequency, associated risks and outcome. *Placenta.* 2007;28:204–208.

191. Slaghekke F, Lopriore E, Lewi L, et al. Fetoscopic laser coagulation of the vascular equator versus selective coagulation for twin-to-twin transfusion syndrome: an open-label randomised controlled trial. *Lancet.* 2014;383:2144–2151.

192. Lopriore E, Middeldorp JM, Oepkes D, et al. Twin anemia-polycythemia sequence in two monochorionic twin pairs without oligo-polyhydramnios sequence. *Placenta.* 2007;28:47–51.

193. Lopriore E, Slaghekke F, Middeldorp JM, et al. Residual anastomoses in twin-to-twin transfusion syndrome treated with selective fetoscopic laser surgery: localization, size, and consequences. *Am J Obstet Gynecol.* 2009;201:66.e1–66.e4.

194. Van den Wijngaard JP, Lewi L, Lopriore E, et al. Modeling severely discordant hematocrits and normal amniotic fluids after incomplete laser therapy in twin-to-twin transfusion syndrome. *Placenta.* 2007;28:611–615.

195. Lopriore E, Deprest J, Slaghekke F, et al. Placental characteristics in monochorionic twins with and without twin anemia-polycythemia sequence. *Obstet Gynecol.* 2008;112:753–758.

196. De Villiers S, Slaghekke F, Middeldorp JM, et al. Arterio-arterial vascular anastomoses in monochorionic twin placentas with and without twin anemia-polycythemia sequence. Placenta. 2012;33(3):227–229.

197. De Villiers SF, Slaghekke F, Middeldorp JM, et al. Placental characteristics in monochorionic twins with spontaneous versus post-laser twin anemia-polycythemia sequence. *Placenta.* 2013;34(5):456–459.

198. Tollenaar LSA, Lopriore E, Middeldorp JM, et al. Improved prediction of twin anemia–polycythemia sequence by delta middle cerebral artery peak systolic velocity: new antenatal classification system. *Ultrasound Obstet Gynecol.* 2019;53. doi:10.1002/uog.20096.

199. Stirnemann J, Chalouhi G, Essaoui M, et al. Fetal brain imaging following Glaser surgery in twin to twin surgery. *BJOG.* 2018;125(9):1186-1191.

200. Genova L, Slaghekke F, Klumper FJ, et al. Management of twin anemia-polycythemia sequence using intrauterine blood transfusion for the donor and partial exchange transfusion for the recipient. *Fetal Diagn Ther.* 2013;34:121–126. doi:10.1159/000346413.

201. Lopriore E, Slaghekke F, Kersbergen K, et al. Severe cerebral injury in a recipient with twin anemia-polycythemia sequence. *Ultrasound Obstet Gynecol.* 2013;41(6):702–706.

202. Lopriore E, Slaghekke F, Oepkes D, et al. Clinical outcome in neonates with twin anemia-polycythemia sequence. *Am J Obstet Gynecol.* 2010;203(1):54.e1–54.e5.

203. Slaghekke F, Kist WJ, Oepkes D, et al. Twin anemia-polycythemia sequence: diagnostic criteria, classification, perinatal management and outcome. *Fetal Diagn Ther.* 2010;27(4):181–190.

204. Lopriore E, Ortibus E, Acosta-Rojas R, et al. Risk factors for neurodevelopment impairment in twin-twin transfusion syndrome treated with fetoscopic laser surgery. *Obstet Gynecol.* 2009;113(2 pt 1):361–366.

205. Chmait RH, Quintero RA. Operative fetoscopy in complicated monochorionic twins: current status and future direction. *Curr Opin Obstet Gynecol.* 2008; 20:169–174.

206. Jelin E, Hirose S, Rand L, et al. Perinatal outcome of conservative management versus fetal intervention for twin reversed arterial perfusion sequence with a small acardiac twin. *Fetal Diagn Ther.* 2010;27:138–141.

207. Sebire NJ. Anomalous development in twins (including monozygotic duplication). In: Kilby M, Baker P, Critchley H, et al, eds. *Multiple Pregnancy.* London, England: RCOG Press; 2006:59–88.

208. De Groot R, Van Den Wijngaard JP, Umur A, et al. Modeling acardiac twin pregnancies. *Ann N Y Acad Sci.* 2007;1101:235–249.

209. Moore TR, Gale S, Benirschke K. Perinatal outcome of forty nine pregnancies complicated by acardiac twinning. *Am J Obstet Gynecol.* 1990;163:907–912.

210. Van Allen MI, Smith DW, Shepard TH. Twin reversed arterial perfusion (TRAP) sequence: a study of 14 twin pregnancies with acardius. *Semin Perinatol.* 1983;7:285–293.

211. Chaliha C, Schwarzler P, Booker M, et al. Trisomy 2 in an acardiac twin in a triplet in-vitro fertilization pregnancy. *Hum Reprod.* 1999;14:1378–1380.

212. Healey MG. Acardia: predictive risk factors for the co-twin's survival. *Teratology.* 1994;50:205–213.

213. Sepulveda WH, Quiroz VH, Giuliano A, et al. Prenatal ultrasonographic diagnosis of acardiac twin. *J Perinat Med.* 1993;21:241–246.

214. Sebire NJ, Sepulveda W, Jeanty P, et al. Multiple gestations. In: Nyberg DA, McGahan JP, Pretorius DH, et al, eds. *Diagnostic Imaging of Fetal Anomalies.* Philadelphia, PA: Lippincott Williams & Wilkins; 2003:777–813.

215. Fouron JC, Leduc L, Grignon A, et al. Importance of meticulous ultrasonographic investigation of the acardiac twin. *J Ultrasound Med.* 1994;14:1001–1004.

216. Buntinx IM, Bourgeois N, Buytaert PM, et al. Acardiac amorphous twin with prune belly sequence in the co-twin. *Am J Med Genet.* 1991;39:453–457.

217. Guimaraes CV, Kline-Fath BM, Linam LE, et al. MRI findings in multifetal pregnancies complicated by twin reversed arterial perfusion sequence (TRAP). *Pediatr Radiol.* 2011;41(6):694–701.

218. Brassard M, Fouron JC, Leduc L, et al. Prognostic markers in twin pregnancies with an acardiac fetus. *Obstet Gynecol.* 1999;94:409–414.

219. Dashe JS, Fernandez CO, Twickler DM. Utility of Doppler velocimetry in predicting outcome in twin reversed-arterial perfusion sequence. *Am J Obstet Gynecol.* 2001;185:135–139.

220. Oliver ER, Coleman BG, Goff DA, et al. Twin reversed arterial perfusion sequence: a new method of parabiotic twin mass estimation correlated with pump twin compromise. *J Ultrasound Med.* 2013;32(12):2115–2123.

221. Gallot D, Laurichesse H, Lemery D. Selective feticide in monochorionic twin pregnancies by ultrasound-guided umbilical cord occlusion. *Ultrasound Obstet Gynecol.* 2003;22:484–488.

222. Lopoo JB, Paek PW, Maichin GA, et al. Cord ultrasonic transection procedure for selective termination of a monochorionic twin. *Fetal Diagn Ther.* 2000; 15:177–179.

223. Rodeck C, Deans A, Jauniaux E. Thermocoagulation for the early treatment of pregnancy with an acardiac twin. *N Engl J Med.* 1998;339:1293–1295.

224. Tsao K, Feldstein VA, Albanese CT, et al. Selective reduction of acardiac twin by radiofrequency ablation. *Am J Obstet Gynecol.* 2002;187:635–640.

225. Cabassa P, Fichera A, Prefumo F, et al. The use of radiofrequency in the treatment of twin reversed arterial perfusion sequence: a case series and review of the literature. *Eur J Obstet Gynecol Reprod Biol.* 2013;166(2):127–132.

226. Pagani G, D'Antonio F, Khalil A, et al. Intrafetal laser treatment for twin reversed arterial perfusion sequence: cohort study and meta-analysis. *Ultrasound Obstet Gynecol.* 2013;42(1):6–14.

227. Pauls F. Monoamniotic twin pregnancy: a review of the world literature and a report of two new cases. *Can Med Assoc J.* 1969;100:254–256.

228. Baldwin V. Twinning mechanisms and zygosity determination. In: *Pathology of Multiple Gestation.* New York, NY: Springer-Verlag; 1994:201.

229. Bajoria R. Abundant vascular anastomoses in monoamniotic versus diamniotic monochorionic placentas. *Am J Obstet Gynecol.* 1998;179(3 pt 1):788.

230. Rodis JF, Vintzileos AM, Campbell WA, et al. Antenatal diagnosis and management of monoamniotic twins. *Am J Obstet Gynecol.* 1987;157:1255–1257.

231. Lumme RH, Saarikoski SV. Monoamniotic twin pregnancy. *Acta Genet Med Gemellol (Roma).* 1986;35:99–105.

232. Allen VM, Windrin R, Barrett J, et al. Management of monoamniotic twin pregnancies: a case series and systemic review of the literature. *BJOG.* 2001;108:931.

233. Morikawa M, Yamada T, Yamada T, et al. Prospective risk of intrauterine fetal death in monoamniotic twin pregnancies. *Twin Res Hum Genet.* 2012;15(4):522–526.

234. Murgano D, Khalil A, Prefumo F, et al. Outcome of twin-to-twin transfusion syndrome in monochorionic monoamniotic twin pregnancies: a systematic review and meta-analysis. *Ultrasound Obstet Gynecol.* 2019. doi:10.1002/uog.21889.

235. Heyborne KD, Porreco RP, Garite TJ, et al; for the Obstetrix/Pediatrix Research Study Group. Improved perinatal survival of monoamniotic twins with intensive inpatient monitoring. *Am J Obstet Gynecol.* 2005;192(1):96.

236. D'Antonio F, Odibo A, Berghella V, et al. Perinatal mortality, timing of delivery and prenatal management of monoamniotic twin pregnancy: systematic review and meta-analysis. *Ultrasound Obstet Gynecol.* 2019;53:166–174. doi:10.1002/uog.20100.

237. Hack KE, Derks JB, Schaap AH, et al. Perinatal outcome of monoamniotic twin pregnancies. *Obstet Gynecol.* 2009;113:353–360.

238. Dias T, Mahsud-Dornan S, Bhide A, et al. Cord entanglement and perinatal outcome in monoamniotic twin pregnancies. *Ultrasound Obstet Gynecol.* 2010;35:201–204.

239. Belfort MA, Moise KJ Jr, Kirshon B, et al. The use of color flow Doppler ultrasonography to diagnose umbilical cord entanglement in monoamniotic twin gestations. *Am J Obstet Gynecol.* 1993;168(2):601.

240. Gembruch U, Baschat AA. True knot of the umbilical cord: transient constrictive effect to umbilical venous blood flow demonstrated by Doppler sonography. *Ultrasound Obstet Gynecol.* 1996;8(1):53.

241. Abuhamad AZ, Mari G, Copel JA, et al. Umbilical artery flow velocity waveforms in monoamniotic twins with cord entanglement. *Obstet Gynecol.* 1995;86(4 pt 2):674.

242. Rosemond RL, Hinds NE. Persistent abnormal umbilical cord Doppler velocimetry in a monoamniotic twin with cord entanglement. *J Ultrasound Med.* 1998;17(5):337.

243. Rossi AC, Prefumo F. Impact of cord entanglement on perinatal outcome of monoamniotic twins: a systematic review of the literature. *Ultrasound Obstet Gynecol.* 2013;41(2):131–135.

244. Spitz L, Kiely EM. Conjoined twins. *JAMA.* 2003;289(10):130.

245. Spencer R. Theoretical and analytical embryology of conjoined twins, part I: embryogenesis. *Clin Anat.* 2000;13:36–53.

246. Destephano CC, Meena M, Brown DL, et al. Sonographic diagnosis of conjoined diamniotic monochorionic twins. *Am J Obstet Gynecol.* 2010;203(6):e4–e6.

247. Kaufman MH. The embryology of conjoined twins. *Childs Nerv Syst.* 2004;20:508–525.

248. Spencer R. Anatomic description of conjoined twins: a plea for standardized terminology. *J Pediatr Surg.* 1996;31(7):941.

249. Harper RG, Kenigsberg K, Sia CG, et al. Xiphopagus conjoined twins: a 300-year review of the obstetric, morphopathologic, neonatal, and surgical parameters. *Am J Obstet Gynecol.* 1980;137:617.

Salma A. Nassef • Sarah Mayes Huguenard • Ignatia B. Van den Veyver

Birth defects occur in 3% to 5% of the general population and can be caused by environmental factors, such as maternal diabetes or by genetic defects, often as a phenotypic feature of a complex developmental syndrome.[1,2] Chromosomal abnormalities affect about 1:150 live births, but are more common early in pregnancy, because aneuploidy is an important cause of pregnancy loss.[3] Thus, depending on the circumstances, genetic evaluation offered to pregnant women includes a variable combination of parental carrier screening, different iterations of maternal screening for aneuploidy, and/or diagnostic genetic testing for chromosomal abnormalities or other genetic disorders.[4,5]

Carrier screening may be offered preconceptionally or prenatally to determine the parental carrier status for autosomal recessive and X-linked disorders using an ethnicity-based limited panel or using larger expanded pan-ethnic panels.[6–9] While each disorder is rare, the cumulative detection rate of expanded carrier screening panels is significant. Yet, many genetic disorders are *de novo* or involve larger chromosomal abnormalities and are not identifiable through carrier screening.

All pregnant women are offered a combination of genetic screening and testing alongside prenatal ultrasound imaging to detect fetal structural and growth abnormalities and to identify fetuses at increased risk for common aneuploidies; trisomies 21, 13, and 18; or other chromosomal abnormalities and genetic conditions. Although the risk of these trisomies increases with maternal age, women of all ages can have affected pregnancies. When fetal structural abnormalities are detected by ultrasound, genetic diagnostic testing should be offered.[4] This is usually performed by chorionic villus sampling (CVS) or amniocentesis, and rarely by other procedures such as percutaneous umbilical cord blood sampling (PUBS). Chromosomal microarray analysis (CMA) is the recommended first-line genetic test when there are fetal structural anomalies.[4,10–12]

GENETIC SCREENING AND TESTING OFFERED TO REPRODUCTIVE AGE AND PREGNANT WOMEN

Carrier Screening for Recessive Disorders

Carrier screening focuses on identifying carrier parents of selected autosomal recessive and X-linked conditions. Most carriers do not have a family history of these conditions, making carrier screening useful in all populations. There is a wide variation in the conditions for which carrier screening is offered. The traditional approach consists of testing with small limited panels that include more common serious recessive or X-linked conditions with onset in infancy or childhood and are associated with a significant health impact or a reduced lifespan, which often have a higher prevalence in certain ethnic groups for which specific ethnicity-based carrier screening panels are developed.[13] Both the American College of Obstetrics and Gynecology (ACOG) and the American College of Medical Genetics and Genomics (ACMG) have issued guidance on which conditions should be

included in these targeted panels[6,13] (Table 16.1). The second approach is pan-ethnic expanded carrier screening using gene panels for a much larger number of conditions that are offered to all patients, irrespective of their ethnic background. These panels are variable in content and can include from approximately 100 to several hundreds of genes.[14,15] The likelihood of identifying carriers increases as panels get larger. With panels of approximately 150 to 200 genes, nearly 50% of individuals screen positive, but this increases to 2 to 3 pathogenic variants each in greater than 80% of screened individuals when genes for greater than 400 disorders are sequenced.[16] Carrier couples for recessive disorders and female carriers for X-linked conditions are detected about 1.5% to 3% of the time depending on the size of the panel. The ACOG recently stated that both targeted (ethnicity-based) and expanded carrier screening are acceptable strategies.[7]

The two most commonly used laboratory methods are genotyping and sequence analysis. With genotyping, a limited set of well-described genetic variants associated with the conditions are analyzed; but with sequencing, the entire coding region of each gene on the panel is sequenced to identify all pathogenic or likely pathogenic variants. In addition, the number of included inherited conditions varies between different panels. Carrier screening of (prospective) parents can be done sequentially or simultaneously. With sequential carrier screening, one parent is screened first, and the other parent is only tested if the initially tested parent has positive results. In simultaneous carrier screening, both parents undergo carrier screening at the same time and results are compared. This is often the preferred method in the prenatal setting because it allows more rapid information on risk for the fetus.

Patients must be informed during pretest counseling and result disclosure of the benefits and limitations of carrier screening.[8] A negative carrier screening result significantly reduces but does not eliminate carrier risk for the covered conditions on the panel, and there is always, albeit much lower, a residual risk. Not all genetic diseases, for example, those with multifactorial or polygenic inheritance or caused by new (*de novo*) mutations in offspring, can be assessed by carrier screening. Some conditions can be caused by more than one gene or by different types of mutations affecting the included gene, not all of which may be covered in the panel (e.g., microdeletions). It is important that health providers are familiar with the content and limitations of the carrier screening panels they offer to patients.

When there is a family history of a genetic condition and the disease-causing genetic variant(s) in the affected individual are known, targeted carrier testing for the known variant(s) in parents and other at-risk family members should be offered, but it can be complemented by carrier screening for other disorders. Finally, although not the intended use for parental carrier screening, it has occasionally been successfully utilized when ultrasound detects fetal anomalies likely associated with a recessive condition and patients declined diagnostic testing by amniocentesis or CVS. For example, carrier screening can detect parental carrier status for autosomal recessive polycystic

TABLE 16.1   Carrier Frequencies for Common Recessive Conditions by Ethnicity

DISEASE NAME	ETHNICITY AND CARRIER FREQUENCY	GENE
Alpha thalassemia	Southeast Asian (1 in 7)	HBA1/HBA2
Autosomal recessive polycystic kidney disease	General population (1 in 50)	PKHD1
Beta thalassemia	Middle Eastern (1 in 5) African American (1 in 10) Southeast Asian (1 in 30)	HBB
Bloom syndrome	Ashkenazi Jewish (1 in 107)	BLM
Canavan disease	Ashkenazi Jewish (1 in 41)	ASPA
21-Hydroxylase deficiency congenital adrenal hyperplasia	General population (1 in 60)	CYP21A2
Cystic fibrosis	Ashkenazi Jewish (1 in 25) Caucasian (1 in 25) Hispanic (1 in 46) African American (1 in 65) Asian (1 in 90)	CFTR
Familial dysautonomia	Ashkenazi Jewish (1 in 34)	ELP1
Family hyperinsulinism	Finnish (1 in 29) Ashkenazi Jewish (1 in 52)	ABCC8
Fanconi anemia, type C	Ashkenazi Jewish (1 in 98)	FANCC
Fragile X	General population (1 in 180)	FMR1
Galactosemia	African American (1 in 78) Caucasian (1 in 108) Ashkenazi Jewish (1 in 172)	GALT
Gaucher disease	Ashkenazi Jewish (1 in 18)	GBA
Glycogen storage disease type 1A	Ashkenazi Jewish (1 in 71)	G6PC
Joubert syndrome	Ashkenazi Jewish (1 in 93)	TMEM216
Maple syrup urine disease type 1A	Mennonite (1 in 10)	BCKDHA
Maple syrup urine disease type 1B	Ashkenazi Jewish (1 in 97)	BCKDHB
Mucolipidosis IV	Ashkenazi Jewish (1 in 119)	MCOLN1
Niemann–Pick disease type A	Ashkenazi Jewish (1 in 115)	SMPD1
Phenylketonuria (PKU)	Caucasian (1 in 40) Ashkenazi Jewish (1 in 55)	PAH
Sickle cell anemia	African American (1 in 12)	HBB
Smith–Lemli–Opitz syndrome	Ashkenazi Jewish (1 in 36) Caucasian (1 in 50)	DHCR7
Spinal muscular atrophy	Caucasian (1 in 47) Asian (1 in 59) Ashkenazi Jewish (1 in 67) Hispanic (1 in 68) African American (1 in 72)	SMN1
Tay–Sachs disease	French Canadian/Cajun (1 in 13) Ashkenazi Jewish (1 in 27)	HEXA

Adapted by permission from Nature: Gross SJ, Pletcher BA, Monaghan KG. Carrier screening in individuals of Ashkenazi Jewish descent. *Genet Med.* 2008;10(1):54–56. Copyright © 2008 Springer Nature.

TABLE 16.2   Detection Rates for Down Syndrome in the First Trimester (5% FPR)

Maternal age only	30%
Maternal age + free β-hCG	60%
Maternal age + nuchal translucency	70%
Maternal age + nuchal translucency + free β-hCG + PAPP-A	90%
Maternal age + nuchal translucency + nasal bone + free β-hCG + PAPP-A	97%

β-hCG, β-human chorionic gonadotropin; FPR, false-positive rate; PAPP-A, pregnancy-associated plasma protein A.
From Nicolaides KH. Screening for chromosomal defects. *Ultrasound Obstet Gynecol.* 2003;21(4):313–321. Copyright © 2003 ISUOG. Adapted by permission of John Wiley & Sons, Inc.

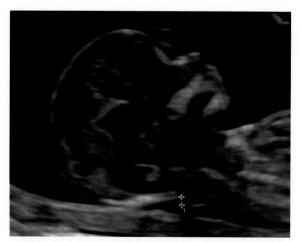

FIGURE 16.1: Normal nuchal translucency.

kidney disease when polycystic kidneys are detected on second-trimester ultrasound. Identifying carrier couples in this way can also narrow the differential diagnosis and help focus targeted prenatal diagnostic testing.

Maternal Serum Analyte-Based Screening for Fetal Aneuploidy in the First and Second Trimester

Healthcare providers rely on *a priori* risk estimates along with family history and clinical circumstances, including ultrasound findings, to select the most appropriate genetic screen or test to offer to pregnant women. Maternal serum screening identifies pregnancies at increased risk for genetic conditions. It does not diagnose or rule out these conditions, but adjusts the *a priori* risk upward or downward, allowing women to make better informed decisions about invasive diagnostic testing.

The first introduced multiple marker–based prenatal genetic screening algorithms were for common aneuploidies that can affect live borns. These provide a risk score that is based on a combination of maternal age, levels of maternal serum analytes, and, in the first trimester, the nuchal translucency (NT) measurement (Table 16.2).[5,17,18] The type of maternal screening that can be offered depends on the gestational age. Screening is offered in either the first or second trimester for trisomy 21 (Down syndrome), which has an incidence of 1:700 live borns, and trisomy 18 (Edwards syndrome) which affects 1:7,000 newborns. Some first-trimester screening algorithms also provide risk estimates for trisomy 13 (Patau syndrome), which has an incidence of 1:16,000 newborns. Accurate dating of the pregnancy is required for reliable

interpretation of first- and second-trimester serum screening, because the serum analyte levels (and, in the first trimester, the NT measurement) vary with gestational age.

First-trimester screening is performed between 10 weeks 0 days and 13 weeks 6 days of gestation, when the ultrasound-measured crown-rump length is between 38 to 45 mm and 84 mm. Combined first-trimester screening incorporates a standardized measurement of fetal NT in the fetal sagittal plane by a trained and "NT-certified" sonography provider who enrolls in ongoing quality review of NT measurement (Fig. 16.1). The NT measurement, expressed in multiples of the median (MoM) for gestational age, is combined with maternal age, gestational age, and maternal serum levels in MoMs of free β human chorionic gonadotropin or hCG and pregnancy-associated plasma protein A to estimate the risks for trisomies 21 and 18. Some laboratories will calculate a combined risk for trisomies 18 and 13. A positive combined first-trimester screening result indicates that the risk of one of those aneuploidies exceeds a laboratory-determined threshold (Table 16.3).[5] Its sensitivity to identify pregnancies with trisomy 21 is approximately 85% to 90% for a 5% screen-positive rate. The sensitivity to identify pregnancies with trisomy 18 is greater than 90%.[5,18,19] Similar numbers have been reported for trisomy 13.

The NT measurement alone can adjust the genetic risk in pregnancy. An increased NT (>3 mm or >99th percentile for gestational age) is also by itself associated with an increased risk of chromosome abnormalities with a 64% to 70% detection rate for a 5% screen-positive rate. An increased NT is also associated with an increased risk of many other conditions, the most important ones being other chromosomal abnormalities (trisomies 13, 18, and 45,X or Turner syndrome), congenital

TABLE 16.3   First-Trimester Screening (10 to 13 weeks 6 days)

	PAPP-A	FREE β-HCG	NT	RISK CUTOFF	DETECTION
Down syndrome	↓	↑	↑	>1:270	85%–90%
Trisomy 18	↓	↓	↑	>1:100	90%–95%
Trisomy 13	↓	↓	↑	>1:100	90%–95%

β-hCG, β-human chorionic gonadotropin; NT, nuchal translucency; PAPP-A, pregnancy-associated plasma protein A.

TABLE 16.4 Select Conditions Associated with Increased Nuchal Translucency

Aneuploidy (trisomy 21, 18, 13, 45X)

Triploidy

Cardiac defects

Noonan syndrome

Skeletal dysplasia

Fetal akinesia

Renal anomalies

Genitourinary abnormalities

Congenital diaphragmatic hernia

Abdominal wall defect

Adapted from Hyett J, Perdu M, Sharland G, et al. Using fetal nuchal translucency to screen for major congenital cardiac defects at 10–14 weeks of gestation: population based cohort study. *BMJ*. 1999;318(7176):81–85, and Souka AP, Snijders RJ, Novakov A, et al. Defects and syndromes in chromosomally normal fetuses with increased nuchal translucency thickness at 10–14 weeks of gestation. *Ultrasound Obstet Gynecol*. 1998;11(6):391–400.

heart defects, Noonan syndrome, skeletal dysplasias, abdominal wall defects, congenital diaphragmatic hernia, and renal or other genitourinary abnormalities (Table 16.4).[5,20–23] When none of these are found, it can still be a normal variant with a favorable outcome. Thus, if an increased NT measurement is identified and no aneuploidy is detected with diagnostic testing, a targeted second-trimester ultrasound examination, dedicated fetal echocardiogram, and genetic testing for Noonan syndrome should be offered. Another ultrasound marker included in first-trimester aneuploidy screening algorithms is the evaluation of the fetal nasal bone.[24,25] An absent nasal bone in the first trimester is associated with an increased risk of Down syndrome in the fetus but can also be seen in unaffected fetuses and is influenced by ethnicity. While the primary goal of combined first-trimester screening is to detect pregnancies at increased risk for trisomies 21 or 18, its results may secondarily provide information about the risk of adverse pregnancy outcomes. A very low level of pregnancy-associated plasma protein A carries an increased risk of fetal growth restriction and preterm birth.[26,27]

The second-trimester serum analyte screening is most commonly done as a quadruple screen, performed between 15 and 22 weeks and uses an algorithm that incorporates maternal age, gestational age, ethnicity, and maternal serum levels of hCG, unconjugated estriol, dimeric inhibin A and maternal serum alpha-fetoprotein (MSAFP) reported in MoMs for the gestational age. One laboratory in the United States offers a penta screen that includes hyperglycosylated hCG, but its superiority over other screens has not been fully determined. The second-trimester multiple marker screen provides risk estimates for trisomies 21 and 18, but not for trisomy 13 (Table 16.5).[5] The MSAFP levels by themselves also correlate with the risk of fetal open neural tube defects (ONTDs) or open abdominal wall defects (OAWDs). A positive result indicates that the risk of that condition exceeds a laboratory-determined cutoff for the screened conditions; 1:270 for trisomy 21 and 1:100 for trisomy 18. The sensitivity of a second-trimester screen for trisomy 21 is approximately 81% for a 5% screen-positive rate and for trisomy 18 is 60% to 70%. Only MSAFP is used to assess the risk primarily for ONTD (and secondarily OAWD) and can be used as a stand-alone test in the second trimester for this purpose, for example, for those women who had first-trimester combined screening or cell-free DNA-based aneuploidy screening. MSAFP is elevated in ONTD and OAWD and the cutoff is usually set at 2.5 MoM or greater than 1:250 risk. An elevated MSAFP is an indication to offer a targeted ultrasound to evaluate for ONTD, OAWD, and other structural anomalies (Table 16.6).[28] When after full evaluation, the MSAFP is unexplained, it is associated with an increased risk of adverse pregnancy outcomes, such as fetal growth restriction and low birth weight, preterm delivery, stillbirth, placental abnormalities, and preeclampsia.[5] Additional monitoring of these pregnancies should be considered. Other explanations for an elevated MSAFP include multiple gestation, inaccurate gestational age, placental bleeds, and fetal protein loss associated with renal disease, for example, the rare congenital Finnish nephrosis.[29] Congenital Finnish nephrosis is a lethal autosomal recessive condition associated with very elevated MSAFP (>10 MoM) and elevated amniotic fluid alpha-fetoprotein with normal acetylcholinesterase levels.

Different combinations of first- and second-trimester screening that improve the sensitivity and specificity can be offered. In integrated screening, the woman undergoes both first- and second-trimester screening, but the results are provided only after the second-trimester screening step. Serum-integrated screening is the same, but without the NT measurement. In sequential screening, women in the highest risk category after the first-trimester screen are offered a

TABLE 16.5 Second-Trimester Screening (15–22 weeks)

	AFP	HCG	UE3	DIA	RISK CUTOFF	DETECTION
Down syndrome	↓	↑	↓	↑	>1:270	70%–80%
Trisomy 18	↓	↓	↓		>1:100	60%–70%
ONTD	↑				>2.5 MoM > 1 in 250	80%–85%

AFP, alpha-fetoprotein; DIA, dimeric inhibin A; hCG, human chorionic gonadotropin; MoM, multiples of the median; ONTD, open neural tube defect; uE3; unconjugated estriol.

TABLE 16.6   Select Conditions Associated with Elevated Maternal Serum Alpha-Fetoprotein

NTD

Twin gestations

Placental bleeds

Abdominal wall defects (gastroschisis) (5–8 MoM)

Kidney abnormalities

Diaphragmatic hernia

Congenital Finnish nephrosis (>10 MoM)

Anencephaly

Low birth weight

Preeclampsia

Prematurity

Stillbirth

MoM, multiples of the median; NTD, neural tube defect.
Adapted from Milunsky A, Jick SS, Bruell CL, et al. Predictive values, relative risks, and overall benefits of high and low maternal serum alpha-fetoprotein screening in singleton pregnancies: new epidemiologic data. *Am J Obstet Gynecol.* 1989;161(2): 291–297. Copyright © 1989 Elsevier. With permission.

diagnostic procedure, but all other women are offered the second-trimester screen to better estimate their risk from the combined results. In contingent screening, women at highest risk are offered diagnostic testing after the first trimester, and women at the lowest risk can discontinue screening, but only the "intermediate risk" group is offered second-trimester screening. While these approaches increase the performance of the serum analyte screening, they are limited by the requirement for women to return for the second phase of screening and the delay in reporting of the screening result for a subgroup of women after the first trimester.

Cell-free DNA Screening for Fetal Aneuploidy

Since the discovery of circulating fetal cell-free DNA (cfDNA) in maternal blood in 1997,[30] and subsequent demonstration in 2008 that cfDNA analysis can be used to determine if there is fetal aneuploidy,[31,32] the test was technically and clinically validated for the common fetal aneuploidies (trisomies 21, 13, and 18), first in women at high risk and then in women at average risk.[33–42] This was followed by rapid development and introduction into the clinic of commercially offered cfDNA-based tests to identify pregnancies at increased risk for these fetal aneuploidies and gender determination. These tests are known and marketed as noninvasive prenatal testing or noninvasive prenatal screening. The circulating fetal cfDNA consists of short DNA fragments of less than 200 nucleotides derived from apoptotic trophoblast cells. These cfDNA fragments are mixed with maternal cfDNA fragments, which make up the bulk of the circulating cfDNA.

The ratio of fetal cfDNA fragments over maternal cfDNA fragments, referred to as fetal fraction, is about 5% to 20% after 10 weeks' gestation, but can be lower or higher. Most laboratories offer cfDNA screening after 10 weeks' gestation. Before that time, the fetal fraction is often too low to achieve reliable results. Traditional cfDNA screening tests include evaluation of chromosomes 21, 18, 13, X, and Y for aneuploidy and can also provide information about the fetal gender.

The sensitivity, specificity, and false-positive and false-negative rates are often used to describe the performance of cfDNA screening. However, the best metric to evaluate its clinical performance for the analyzed aneuploidies are the positive predictive value (PPV), which determines the likelihood that a positive (increased risk) result is a true positive and identifies an affected fetus, and the negative predictive value (NPV), which determines the likelihood that a negative (low risk) result is a true negative and identifies an unaffected fetus. Importantly, the PPV and NPV depend on the prevalence of the condition. Overall, cfDNA-based tests perform best for trisomy 21 with a detection rate of approximately 99.2% and false-positive rate 0.09%, but the detection rates are lower and false-positive rates are higher for trisomy 18 (96.3% and 0.13%), trisomy 13 (91.0% and 0.13%), and sex chromosome aneuploidies (93.0% and 0.14%), including monosomy X (90.3% and 0.23%) (Table 16.7).[43,44] Those numbers were mostly obtained from studies in a high-risk population,[43] where the PPV for common aneuploidies is higher. They also do not take into account the small numbers of samples where no results could be obtained, which is around 1% or higher, depending on the type of cfDNA assay. The PPVs of cfDNA screening are lower in low- to average-risk women,[38,42,45–50] but better than those of the standard multiple marker serum screening algorithms.[44] All positive cfDNA screen results should be followed up with diagnostic testing.

A number of factors affect the clinical performance of cfDNA screening and can cause unreportable or abnormal results that are best addressed in pre- and posttest counseling.[5,51] Because the fetal cfDNA originates from the placenta, aneuploidy detected by cfDNA screening could be mosaic and confined to the placenta in

TABLE 16.7   Prenatal Cell-free DNA Screening

CHROMOSOME	DETECTION RATE (%)	FALSE-POSITIVE RATE
Trisomy 21	99.2	0.09
Trisomy 18	96.3	0.13
Trisomy 13	91.0	0.13
Monosomy X	90.3	0.23
Other SCA	93.0	0.14
Twin pregnancy trisomy 21	93.7	0.23

cfDNA, cell-free DNA; SCA, sex chromosome aneuploidy.
From Gil MM, Quezada MS, Revello R, et al. Analysis of cell-free DNA in maternal blood in screening for fetal aneuploidies: updated meta-analysis. *Ultrasound Obstet Gynecol.* 2015;45(3):249–266. Copyright © 2015 ISUOG. Adapted by permission of John Wiley & Sons, Inc.

a small fraction of tested samples.[52] Mosaicism is more common for trisomy 13 and SCAs than it is for trisomies 21 or 18. Low fetal fraction, which is primarily influenced by early gestational age and maternal obesity, is an important cause of unreportable results. Low fetal fraction by itself increases the risk of aneuploidy. Other reasons for unreportable or atypical findings include maternal conditions, such as low-level maternal mosaicism for Turner syndrome (45,X) that can be constitutional or somatically acquired with age, maternal benign copy number variants (CNVs) that interfere with the bioinformatics algorithms used in the assay, uterine fibroids, or prior organ transplants. In rare cases, cfDNA screening may incidentally identify maternal cancer.[53,54] Expanded cfDNA screening tests include evaluation for specific microdeletions known to be associated with human developmental disorders,[55] such as the 22q11.2 deletion[56] (DiGeorge syndrome) which is associated with heart defects, cleft palate, learning differences, and other less frequent features.[57] More recently, laboratories have also begun exploring cfDNA screening for rarer autosomal trisomies and CNVs (deletions and duplications) across the genome.[58,59] One commercial laboratory offers a cfDNA screen that includes deletions greater than 7 megabases (Mb) across the genome.[60] These more expanded cfDNA screening assays have not been thoroughly validated and have low PPVs.[5,61,62] When fetal structural defects are noted on ultrasound imaging and patients decline amniocentesis or CVS for diagnostic genetic testing after genetic counseling, this form of genome-wide cfDNA screening can be considered, but the PPVs and NPVs of CNV detection by cfDNA screening are far less favorable than they are for common aneuploidy and many false positives have been reported.

Noninvasive Genetic Screening and Testing for Fetal Single-Gene Defects

Applications of cfDNA testing have also moved beyond common aneuploidies and microdeletions to test and screen for mutations responsible for single-gene disorders associated with structural fetal anomalies or significant developmental disability or disease.[63] In fact, fetal gender testing in women at risk for X-linked disorders or testing for the presence of the Rhesus D gene in pregnancies of Rh-negative women at risk for Rhesus hemolytic disease were some of the earliest demonstrations of the possibilities for noninvasive testing by cfDNA analysis.[30,64] Several laboratories have optimized cfDNA-based tests for small groups of conditions, such as skeletal dysplasias that are often caused by *de novo* or paternally inherited dominant mutations (e.g., osteogenesis imperfecta, thanatophoric dysplasia, achondroplasia, etc.).[63,65,66] Because these mutations are not present in the mother, their detection in cfDNA analysis can only come from the pregnancy. Such noninvasive testing is already offered clinically in certain countries. Approaches for recessive disorders, where the mother is a carrier, are more complex, but tests for conditions like cystic fibrosis, congenital adrenal hyperplasia, spinal muscular atrophy, and sickle cell diseases or thalassemias are also being developed and validated.[63,67–70]

In the United States, two commercial laboratories now offer a test that can screen for paternally inherited or *de novo* pathogenic and likely pathogenic variants in 30 genes implicated in skeletal dysplasias, Noonan spectrum disorders, and other disorders frequently seen in fetuses and newborns with congenital abnormalities or developmental genetic syndromes. While these are not yet standard of care, early data with this test indicates high sensitivity and specificity.[71] This test requires both maternal and paternal blood samples at the time of collection and cannot be performed if the mother carries the mutation. Like cfDNA screening for aneuploidy, all positive results from the 30-gene panel should be followed with diagnostic testing, such as CVS or amniocentesis.

Practical Approach to Reproductive and Prenatal Genetic Screening and Testing in Pregnancies at Average Risk

It is important that all women of reproductive age are asked about their personal and family history of genetic disorders that could affect their health or increase their risk of transmitting a genetic disorder to their children. In addition, all reproductive age women should be informed about genetic screening and testing options available to them before and during pregnancy, preferentially before they are pregnant. Carrier screening can be offered anytime, but when done in the preconception period, more time and options are available to address individual risks. Professional guidelines agree that both ethnicity-based and expanded screening are currently considered acceptable options, but women should be counseled about benefits and pitfalls of each. Pregnant women should be offered genetic evaluation for fetal chromosomal abnormalities that takes into account their age and other risk factors. The risk for trisomies 21, 13, and 18 increases with age, but all women have a 1% to 1.7% risk for clinically significant CNVs. Thus, amniocentesis or CVS with genetic testing is an option available to all women. For those who choose not to have these procedures, the earliest noninvasive screening option is cfDNA screening at 10 weeks' gestation. While this was initially reserved for women at high risk for aneuploidy (e.g., due to advanced maternal age), it can be offered to all women with appropriate counseling. cfDNA screening for CNVs and rare autosomal trisomies has not been optimally validated. Between 10 and 13 weeks 6 days, they can be offered first-trimester serum screening and NT measurement, which is still considered an acceptable and cost-effective screen for common aneuploidies. Women who present later for prenatal care can be offered second-trimester multiple marker screening or cfDNA screening, which can be done at any time in pregnancy. Diagnostic testing (usually amniocentesis) should be offered to all women who have a positive result on any noninvasive screening test and as the first-line test when fetal congenital anomalies are detected. If women decline amniocentesis or CVS, cfDNA screening can be offered as an alternative, but limitations must be included in counseling.

PRENATAL GENETIC DIAGNOSIS FOR PREGNANCIES COMPLICATED BY ABNORMAL ULTRASOUND FINDINGS

General Approach to the Patient with Structural Abnormalities Detected on Prenatal Ultrasound

Prenatal diagnosis is available through CVS, amniocentesis, and, more rarely, PUBS or any other procedure that provides direct access to fetal samples.

Chorionic Villus Sampling and Amniocentesis

For CVS, typically performed between gestational weeks 10 and 14, a small amount (30 to 40 mg) of placental villi is obtained either

TABLE 16.8	Diagnostic Testing		
PROCEDURE	GESTATIONAL AGE	RISK	CONSIDERATIONS
CVS	11w–13w6d	1 in 355 (0.28%)	Mosaicism (<1%) Maternal cell contamination (<1%) Spotting and cramping
Amniocentesis	15w+	1 in 900 (0.11%)	Amniotic fluid leakage Spotting and cramping
PUBS	15w+	1 in 100 to 1 in 33 (1%–3%)	May be used for assessment of fetal infections and hematologic indications

CVS, chorionic villus sampling; PUBS, percutaneous umbilical cord blood sampling.

transabdominally or transcervically, dependent on the location of the placenta. The procedure-related risk of CVS is estimated to be 1 in 455.[4,72] Amniocentesis is typically performed after 16 weeks' gestation and involves obtaining about 20 mL or more of amniotic fluid, which contains fetal cells. The procedure-related risk of amniocentesis is estimated to be 1 in 900.[72] Other common complications of both procedures include temporary cramping, bleeding, infection, membrane rupture, or leakage of fluid (amniocentesis only).[4] PUBS may be utilized to obtain fetal cells from an umbilical vein if amniocentesis is impossible, for example, in cases of anhydramnios. Genetic testing can be performed on the sample obtained from these procedures. Rarely, patients may undergo procedures such as bladder shunt placement, or drainage of cysts or pleural effusions. Material retrieved at these procedures can also be used as a source of fetal cells or DNA if no other options are available, although the yield can be variable. The common risks and considerations associated with diagnostic testing options are listed in Table 16.8.

Fluorescence In Situ Hybridization, Karyotype Analysis and Chromosomal Microarray Analysis

A number of different genetic tests can be done on fetal samples obtained through prenatally diagnostic procedures. The choice of which tests or combination of tests is used depends on the indication for testing and the desire for a fast result.

A karyotype analysis requires cell culture to generate the metaphase spreads of dividing cells and typically takes 2 weeks to obtain results (Table 16.9).[73] The metaphases are visualized and aligned under the microscope (Fig. 16.2A) to assess cells for aneuploidy (full and mosaic trisomies, monosomies, and triploidy) and structural chromosomal abnormalities. These include unbalanced structural chromosomal abnormalities (deletions and duplications and unbalanced translocations) and balanced translocations and inversions. A karyotype cannot detect rearrangements that are smaller than 5 to 10 Mb, and often closer to 10 Mb on prenatal karyotypes from CVS and amniocytes. This is significantly lower than that of a chromosomal microarray. Usually, metaphases from approximately 20 cells are imaged and scored, unless mosaicism—where only a proportion of the cells have an abnormal karyotype—is present; then more cells are analyzed. When the possibility of a mosaic finding is considered, providers should inform the laboratory so that more cells can be evaluated. Mosaicism is more common with CVS than with amniotic fluid analysis, because there is a 1% to 2% risk of confined placental mosaicism.[73,74] In confined placental mosaicism, a mosaic cell line is present only in the placenta and not in the fetus. When mosaicism is discovered in a CVS sample, a follow-up amniocentesis may be required to test if it is also present in the fetus. Mosaicism can also be an acquired artefact during cell culture in the laboratory.

When there is a need for a fast result (within 48 to 72 hours) for aneuploidy of chromosomes 21, 18, 13, X or Y, a fluorescence in situ hybridization (FISH) test that specifically targets these chromosomes is sometimes ordered.[73] FISH can be performed on cultured and uncultured cells. The DNA in the cells is exposed to fluorescently labeled short DNA probes that bind to complementary sequences in the DNA (in this case, to unique sequences if chromosomes 21, 13, 18, X and Y; Fig. 16.2B). FISH results for aneuploidy are consistent with karyotype results in 98% of cases. Thus, it is recommended that if FISH testing is ordered, a karyotype or CMA is also performed for final confirmation. Another application is "locus-specific FISH" with probes that can detect deletions or duplications of specific regions that may be associated with genetic deletion or duplication syndromes. This application requires prior knowledge of which deletion or duplication syndrome to expect and has largely been replaced by CMA.

For CMA, the DNA from the patient (amniotic fluid or CVS sample) is sheared into small fragments, fluorescently labeled and hybridized to small oligonucleotide fragments of DNA that are aligned on a DNA array. The hybridization

TABLE 16.9	Turnaround Time for Prenatal Testing
TEST	TURNAROUND TIME
Karyotype	2 wk
CMA	7–14 d
FISH	24–48 h
Whole exome trio	3+ wk
Single-gene testing	3 wk
Panel testing	Variable

CMA, chromosomal microarray analysis; FISH, fluorescence in situ hybridization.

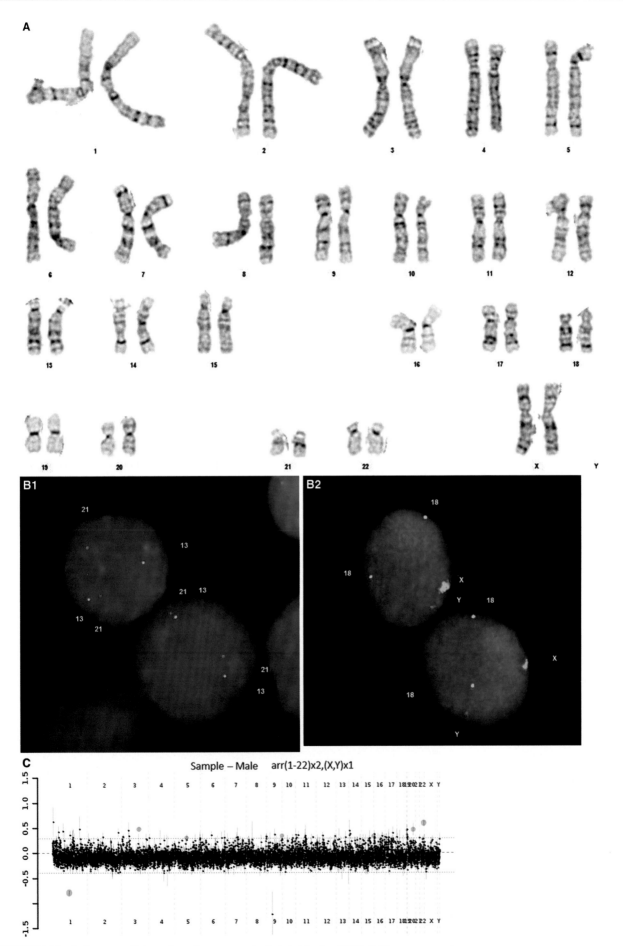

FIGURE 16.2: **A:** Karyotype. **B:** Interphase fluorescence *in situ* hybridization (FISH). **C:** Chromosome microarray.

pattern is compared to that of a reference DNA to look for missing or extra fragments in the patient's DNA (Fig. 16.2C). CMA analysis can identify any condition that is caused by an unbalanced chromosomal rearrangement, resulting in a CNV in specific regions of the DNA. These include aneuploidy and unbalanced translocations and (micro)deletions and (micro) duplications. The resolution of CMA varies by the platform used, but is significantly higher than that of a karyotype, down to 50 to 100 kilobases (kb), with some platforms down to a single exon resolution. The results of a large multicenter trial and other studies investigating the benefits of CMA for prenatal diagnosis indicate that CMA identifies clinically relevant copy number changes, not seen by karyotype, in 6% to 7% of fetuses with ultrasound anomalies (Table 16.10) and in 1% to 1.7% of fetuses with a normal ultrasound examination and a normal karyotype that were tested for other indications.[10,12,75,76] This has led the ACOG to recommend that

CMA should be offered as first-line diagnostic testing when a fetus has been diagnosed with one or more major structural abnormalities.[4] Additional benefits of CMA over karyotyping are the ability to do the test using DNA directly extracted from the amniotic fluid or CVS sample, without the need for cell culture. This reduces the turnaround time, which is about 7 to 14 days total, and allows diagnoses to be performed on samples with poor or failed cell growth, for example, in cases of fetal demise. Although the clinical diagnostic rate of CMA is superior to that of a karyotype, it has some limitations or complexities that must be addressed in pretest counseling. One is that CMA can yield variants of uncertain significance in 1% of cases.[11] These are CNVs for which the clinical implication is uncertain because either the associated condition is not fully penetrant in all individuals who have the CNV, or the CNV includes genes for which it is uncertain that an extra or missing copy will cause disease. Another is the possibility for CMA to detect incidental findings unrelated to the fetal phenotype.[11] Finally, CMA cannot detect balanced chromosomal abnormalities, but those cause a very small proportion of the chromosomal abnormalities that cause fetal congenital anomalies.

Gene Panels

When CMA, karyotype, or FISH does not provide a diagnosis, and in cases where the fetal phenotype or the family history indicates an increased risk of a single-gene disorder, specific testing for known familial mutations, multigene panel testing, or exome sequencing is also available. In these cases, it is recommended that testing is guided by multidisciplinary expertise that includes a healthcare professional with prenatal medical genetics expertise.[77,78] These sequencing tests have a slower turnaround time, typically around 3 weeks. Gene-specific panels are available prenatally when a diagnostic testing sample, such as amniotic fluid or chorionic villi, is available and a condition that could be caused by a pathogenic variant in one of a number of different genes that have been associated with a category of conditions with overlapping presentations is suspected.[79] The size, composition, and detection rates of gene panels vary by laboratory. Many laboratories utilize gene sequencing and may also include deletion/duplication analysis for specific genes, depending on the frequency of specific types of mutations in each gene. Gene panels may be designed to diagnose a particular condition; for example, Noonan syndrome, which is caused by a mutation in 1 of at least 13 genes. If Noonan syndrome is suspected on the basis of ultrasound findings, such a Noonan panel may be considered.[22,23] Other laboratories may curate gene panels for specific ultrasound findings. For example, when there are bowed femurs on ultrasound, which can be seen in a variety of skeletal dysplasias, a skeletal dysplasia panel may be considered.[80] It is important to note that unless a particular single-gene condition is strongly suspected, CMA is recommended prior to considering single-gene testing when there are abnormal ultrasound findings.

Exome Sequencing

Exome sequencing (ES) has been introduced prenatally to diagnose single-gene conditions. Prenatal diagnostic ES involves sequencing the majority of the exons, or coding regions, in the genes of the fetus. In a prenatal setting, it is often performed as a trio, in which parental DNA is sequenced in parallel with that of the fetus to

TABLE 16.10 Chromosomal Microarray Analysis Detection Rate by Ultrasound Anomaly	
ULTRASOUND FINDING	PERCENTAGE WITH SIGNIFICANT CMA FINDING FOLLOWING NORMAL KARYOTYPE
Structural abnormalities in multiple systems	10
Structural abnormalities in multiple systems + nonstructural anomalies	8.3
Structural abnormality(ies) in a single system:	
CNS	7.1
Heart	3.1
Facial features	4.3
Respiratory	6.3
Gastrointestinal	11.1
Body wall	7.7
Genitourinary	4.3
Musculoskeletal	9.1
Neck and/or body fluids	3.9
Polyhydramnios or oligohydramnios, isolated	11
Multiple nonstructural abnormalities	2

CMA, chromosomal microarray analysis; CNS, central nervous system.
From Shaffer LG, Dabell MP, Fisher AJ, et al. Experience with microarray-based comparative genomic hybridization for prenatal diagnosis in over 5000 pregnancies. *Prenat Diagn.* 2012;32(10):976–985. Copyright © 2012 John Wiley & Sons, Ltd. Adapted by permission of John Wiley & Sons, Inc.

aid with interpretation of the fetal data. Multiple reports of cases and case series have highlighted the benefit of ES for challenging clinical prenatal phenotypes. In pregnancies where CMA and karyotype do not explain the fetal phenotype, the detection rate of pathogenic and likely pathogenic variants by ES varies between 6% and greater than 80%, with higher rates for specific conditions such as skeletal dysplasias.[77] Series from commercial laboratories where more selected cases are sequenced, show a detection rate greater than 35%.[79,81] Two recent larger studies that included less selected cases with abnormal ultrasound findings and normal karyotype and CMA showed a detection rate of 8% to 13%.[82,83] All reports indicate higher detection rates with multiple congenital anomalies than with single anomalies. Prenatal ES is most useful when the list of possible differential diagnoses based on ultrasound findings is long or nonspecific. Prenatal ES may incidentally identify unrelated genetic conditions in the fetus and parents, including carrier status for recessive conditions or variants of uncertain significance. Laboratories may offer the ability for couples to opt-in or opt-out of receiving certain types of secondary findings not related to the reason for which the testing was ordered. Standardized laboratory and clinical guidelines for reporting secondary findings and variants of uncertain significance do not include prenatal samples, but general recommendations are that reports should focus on pathogenic and likely pathogenic findings that are directly related to the fetal phenotype or that are indicative of a serious childhood disorder. While it is recognized that more research is needed to fully address the clinical utility of prenatal ES, it can be offered prenatally in selected cases under guidance of a multidisciplinary team that includes experts in prenatal genetics.[78] In the future, genome sequencing, which includes sequencing of introns, or noncoding regions of the genome, may become available prenatally.

COMMON CONDITIONS AND ASSOCIATED ULTRASOUND FINDINGS

Chromosome Aneuploidy

The most common chromosomal aneuploidies seen in live borns that can be associated with structural congenital anomalies detectable on prenatal ultrasound are trisomies 21, 13, and 18; Turner syndrome or monosomy X; and, rarer, triploidy. Other sexual chromosomal aneuploidies 47,XXY (Klinefelter syndrome),

47,XYY, and 47,XXX are also relatively common, but not usually associated with prenatally detectable congenital anomalies. All pregnant women should be offered screening and testing for aneuploidy. The presence of soft markers on ultrasound associated with fetal trisomies can further refine the risk estimates for these aneuploidies when interpreted in the context of the screening results. The likelihood ratios for specific aneuploidies vary by study, and data from a meta-analysis are listed in Table 16.11.[84,85] When major structural birth defects suggestive of aneuploidy are present, diagnostic testing should always be offered. A fetal echocardiogram is recommended when chromosome aneuploidy is prenatally suspected or confirmed. The common defects associated with trisomies 21, 18, and 13 and with Turner syndrome are listed in Table 16.12.[86]

Trisomy 21

Trisomy 21 (Down syndrome; 1:700) is the most common aneuploidy in live births. Second-trimester ultrasound can identify soft signs for Down syndrome, such as absent or short nasal bone, thickened nuchal fold, dilatation of the renal pelvis, intracardiac echogenic foci, echogenic bowel, and short femurs and humeri.[84,87] Occasionally, ultrasound may also detect sandal gap toes that are characteristic of Down syndrome. Ultrasound can also detect fetal abnormalities associated with an increased risk for Down syndrome, including cystic hygroma, ventriculomegaly, and congenital heart defects. Ultrasound detects soft markers or fetal abnormalities in at least 77% of pregnancies affected with Down syndrome.[88] If ultrasound detects structural anomalies, diagnostic testing should be offered.

Trisomy 18

Trisomy 18 (Edwards syndrome) affects 1:7,000 live births. Along with increased NT, choroid plexus cysts and ventriculomegaly are associated with an increased risk of trisomy 18. Second-trimester ultrasound may detect abnormalities associated with trisomy 18 such as congenital heart defects, clenched hands, cleft lip and/or palate, rocker bottom feet, clubfeet (talipes equinovarus) (Fig. 16.3), microcephaly, dolichocephaly, and micrognathia.[89] Ultrasound detects fetal abnormalities in greater than 90% of pregnancies affected with trisomy 18 and if these soft signs or structural anomalies are found, diagnostic testing should be offered.

TABLE 16.11	Soft Markers and Aneuploidy Likelihood Ratios	
SOFT SIGN	**ASSOCIATED CONDITION(S)**	**ANEUPLOIDY LIKELIHOOD RATIO (OVERALL)**
Intracardiac echogenic focus	Down syndrome	5.83
Echogenic bowel	Down syndrome, cystic fibrosis	11.44
Pyelectasis	Down syndrome	7.63
Thickened nuchal fold	Down syndrome	23.3
Short humerus	Down syndrome	4.81
Short femur	Down syndrome	3.72
Choroid plexus cysts	Trisomy 18	8.6

From Agathokleous M, Chaveeva P, Poon LC, et al. Meta-analysis of second-trimester markers for trisomy 21. *Ultrasound Obstet Gynecol.* 2013;41(3):247–261. Copyright © 2012 ISUOG. Adapted by permission of John Wiley & Sons, Inc.

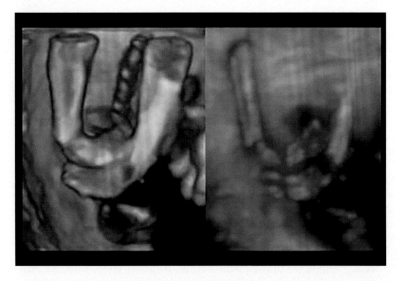

FIGURE 16.3: Clubbed feet (21 weeks 5 days). Three-dimensional ultrasound demonstrates bilateral clubbed feet by surface rendering *(left panel)* and for skeletal structures using maximum intensity projection *(right panel)*.

TABLE 16.12   Ultrasound Findings in Common Aneuploidies

COMMON ANEUPLOIDIES	INCI-DENCE	COMMON SOFT SIGNS	COMMON ULTRASOUND FINDINGS/DEFECTS
Trisomy 21	1 in 700	Absent nasal bone, thickened nuchal fold, dilation of the renal pelvis, intracardiac echogenic foci, echogenic bowel	Cystic hygroma, short femurs and humeri, ventriculomegaly, congenital heart defects (VSD and endocardial cushion defects)
Trisomy 18	1 in 7,000	Choroid plexus cysts, increased nuchal translucency	Congenital heart defects, ventriculomegaly, clenched hands, cleft lip and/or palate, rocker bottom feet, clubfeet (talipes equinovarus), microcephaly, dolichocephaly, micrognathia
Trisomy 13	1 in 16,000	Increased nuchal translucency	CNS anomalies (holoprosencephaly, agenesis of the corpus callosum, microcephaly), midline facial defects (cyclopia, proboscis, midline cleft lip), cardiac anomalies, genitourinary anomalies, limb anomalies, and abdominal wall defects (omphalocele)
Turner syndrome	1 in 2,500	Increased nuchal translucency	Cystic hygroma, congenital heart defects (coarctation), hydrops

CNS, central nervous system; VSD, ventricular septal defect.
Adapted from Griffin DK. The incidence, origin, and etiology of aneuploidy. *Int Rev Cytol.* 1996;167:263–296. Copyright © 1996 Elsevier. With permission.

Trisomy 13

Trisomy 13, also known as Patau syndrome, occurs in approximately 1 in 16,000 live births. Ultrasound detects fetal abnormalities in greater than 90% of pregnancies affected with trisomy 13. Characteristic ultrasound findings on second-trimester ultrasound may include brain defects (specifically holoprosencephaly [Fig. 16.4], agenesis of the corpus callosum, and microcephaly), midline facial defects (cyclopia, proboscis, midline cleft lip), cardiac anomalies, genitourinary anomalies, limb anomalies, and abdominal wall defects (omphalocele). In the first trimester, an increased NT or cystic hygroma may be noted.[89] If these structural anomalies are found, diagnostic testing should be offered.

Turner Syndrome

Turner syndrome, 45,X or monosomy X, affects 1:2,500 female live births. Increased NT and cystic hygroma are associated with

Turner syndrome. Turner syndrome is associated with a high risk of miscarriage, particularly in the first trimester. Fetal hydrops is a common precursor to miscarriage in fetuses with Turner syndrome. Turner syndrome is associated with an increased risk of heart defects. Turner syndrome is also associated with renal malformations, including horseshoe kidney.[89] If structural anomalies are found, diagnostic testing should be offered.

Triploidy

In triploidy, there is an entire extra haploid set of chromosomes, resulting in a 69,XXX, 69,XXY, or 69,XYY karyotype. Triploidy occurs in 1% to 3% of recognized conceptions, but almost all triploid pregnancies are lost as first-trimester miscarriages or second-trimester fetal demises. In diandric triploidy, the extra set of chromosomes is paternally derived either through dispermic fertilization, from fertilization with a diploid sperm, or with a haploid sperm that duplicates its genome. These pregnancies

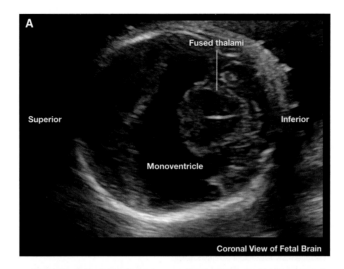

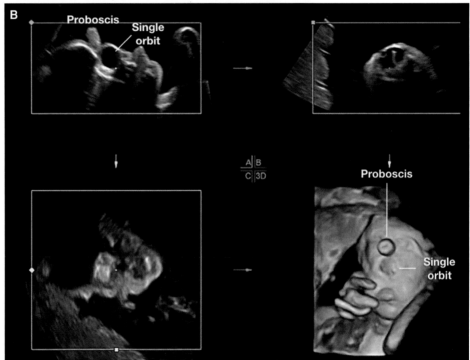

FIGURE 16.4: Holoprosencephaly (32 weeks 1 day). Failure of the embryonic forebrain to separate normally will lead to a single ventricle with partially or entirely fused thalami. The most severe form of this serious condition is often found with facial defects including cyclops and either a missing nose or a nose appendage located above the orbit. 3D ultrasonography confirms the presence of a single orbit and proboscis **(B)**.

are characterized by large partial molar placentas. In digynic triploidy, the extra set of chromosomes is maternally inherited and thought to be derived from a diploid oocyte or duplication of the haploid oocyte genome. All of these events are believed to be sporadic and thus the recurrence risk is estimated to be less than 1%. Triploid fetuses are often severely growth restricted but with a larger head relative to the body size and can have multiple congenital anomalies including heart defects, brain anomalies, cystic kidneys, neural tube defects, and hydrops.[89]

Other Common Genetic Conditions with Typical Ultrasound Findings

Autosomal Recessive Polycystic Kidney Disease

Autosomal Recessive Polycystic Kidney Disease (ARPKD) is caused by biallelic mutations in the gene *PKHD1* and affects 1 in 10,000 to 1 in 40,000 individuals. Typical ultrasound findings are very large kidneys that appear echogenic because of the presence of multiple small cysts (Fig. 16.5). Because the kidneys do not produce urine, there is anhydramnios and the urinary bladder cannot be visualized. Newborns do not survive due to pulmonary hyperplasia and present with typical features of Potter sequence.[90] Diagnostic testing for ARPKD by gene analysis is available but may require a placental biopsy due to the lack of amniotic fluid. When this is not possible, or parents decline the diagnostic procedure, parental carrier screening of both parents can be offered. Infants with this severe presentation of ARPKD often die soon after delivery, and confirmation of the diagnosis, preferentially by genetic testing or alternatively by pathological analysis, is important, as the condition is autosomal recessive and has a recurrence risk of 25% or 1:4 with each subsequent pregnancy.

Cystic Fibrosis

Cystic Fibrosis (CF), caused by mutations in the gene *CFTR*, is the most common autosomal recessive condition in individuals

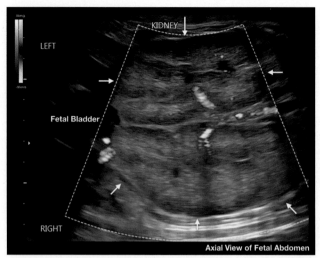

FIGURE 16.5: Infantile polycystic kidney disease (34 weeks). Enlarged and echogenic kidneys *(arrows)* are typical of an autosomal recessive form of polycystic kidney disease. The color Doppler signals demonstrate the presence of two renal arteries. Unfortunately, anhydramnios from poor renal function is often associated with fetal growth restriction and pulmonary hypoplasia.

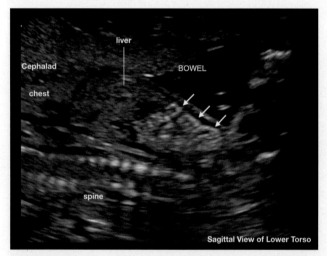

FIGURE 16.6: Echogenic bowel (21 weeks). The ultrasound gain was turned down to the lowest "dark" setting at which the fetal bone still appeared white. The diagnosis of echogenic bowel can be made if the bowel has similar echogenicity after this gain adjustment *(arrows)*.

with northern European ancestry and affects approximately 1 in 3,200 in this population. CF causes pulmonary disease, pancreatic insufficiency, malnutrition, and male infertility resulting from congenital absence of the vas deferens. CF is diagnosed in approximately 6.7% of fetuses with echogenic bowel (Fig. 16.6) caused by meconium impaction.[91] Thus, identification of echogenic bowel and/or dilated bowel on ultrasound warrants an evaluation of CF by diagnostic testing and carrier screening of both parents, which can also be pursued if amniocentesis is declined.

Cornelia de Lange Syndrome

Cornelia de Lange Syndrome (CdLS) is caused by mutations in the *NIPBL, RAD21, SMC3, HDAC8,* or *SMC1A* genes and can be inherited either in an autosomal dominant or in an X-linked manner. CdLS is characterized by growth retardation, upper limb

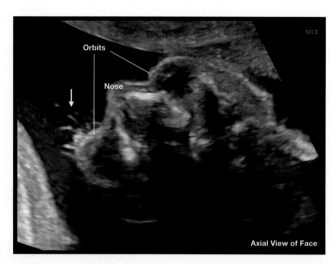

FIGURE 16.7: Cornelia de Lange syndrome (30 weeks 3 days). Micrognathia is more typically identified with prenatal imaging of fetuses with Cornelia de Lange syndrome, although this affected fetus had characteristically long eyelashes *(arrow)* as well.

reduction defects, oligodactyly, cardiac septal defects, hirsutism including long eyelashes, which can all be seen on ultrasound examinations.[92,93] The typical CdLS profile consisting of micrognathia, prominent upper lip, depressed nasal bridge, and anteverted nares can also be noted on prenatal ultrasound (Fig. 16.7). CdLS is associated with prenatal-onset symmetric slow growth (<fifth percentile); however, this is often not noted until the second or third trimester. Other features include autism, intellectual disability, gastrointestinal dysfunction, hearing loss, myopia, and cryptorchidism. An increased NT in the first trimester is sometimes associated with CdLS. A low maternal serum PAPP-A in the first and second trimester is also associated with CdLS.[93] When CdLS is suspected, diagnostic testing via CVS or amniocentesis with a panel of genes that can be mutated in CdLS is necessary to confirm the diagnosis. The cfDNA screening panel for 30 single-gene conditions also includes several CdLS genes.

L1 Syndrome

L1 syndrome describes a spectrum of conditions including hydrocephalus with aqueductal stenosis, agenesis of the corpus callosum, and/or spastic paraplegia. L1 syndrome is inherited in an X-linked manner and is caused by mutations in the gene *L1CAM*. As such, L1 syndrome should be considered when hydrocephalus is identified in a male fetus. Affected fetuses may develop hydrocephalus in the second or third trimester of pregnancy. Adducted thumbs may also be visible on ultrasound in affected fetuses.[94] Diagnostic testing for L1 syndrome may be performed through CVS or amniocentesis. Carrier screening for *L1CAM* for the mother also identifies at-risk pregnancies.

22q11.2 Deletion Syndrome

22q11.2 deletion syndrome (22q11.2DS), also known as DiGeorge syndrome or velocardiofacial syndrome, is caused by a deletion of variable size on chromosome 22. The 22q11.2DS is a variable condition most commonly associated with congenital heart defects, palatal abnormalities, characteristic facial features, learning disabilities, and immune deficiency, among other findings. The most common finding on prenatal ultrasound is a congenital heart defect, including VSD, tetralogy of Fallot interrupted aortic arch, or truncus arteriosus (Fig. 16.8). Skeletal

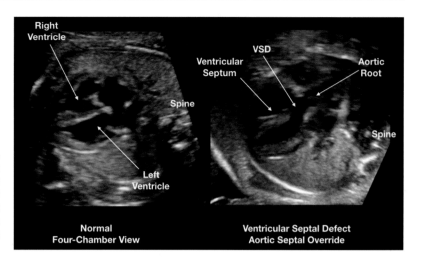

FIGURE 16.8: Tetralogy of Fallot (second trimester). Transverse views of the chest indicate an unremarkable cardiac four-chamber view *(left image)*. However, a more anterior image slice *(right image)* indicates the presence of a large ventricular septal defect (VSD) with an aortic root that overrides the ventricular septum. Narrowing of the pulmonary artery can be a later finding during a pregnancy with tetralogy of Fallot.

abnormalities, including scoliosis with or without vertebral anomalies, clubbed feet, polydactyly, and craniosynostosis can also be seen prenatally in a fetus with 22q11.2DS. Ultrasound detection of cleft lip and/or palate, central nervous system anomalies such as polymicrogyria and tethered cord, congenital diaphragmatic hernia, umbilical or inguinal hernia, tracheoesophageal fistula, esophageal atresia, or renal anomalies also warrant an evaluation for 22q11.L1 yndrome.[57] A CVS or amniocentesis with CMA is the best test to diagnose 22q11.2DS, although deletions in 22q11.2 can be detected through FISH. The majority of prenatally detected of 22q11.2DS are *de novo*, but 7% are inherited, and parental testing is recommended when a prenatal diagnosis is made.[95] Because up to 25% of individuals with 22q11.2DS develop psychiatric disease, including schizophrenia, the complexity of genetic counseling is increased when an affected parent is incidentally discovered after diagnosis of an affected pregnancy.

Congenital Adrenal Hyperplasia

Congenital adrenal hyperplasia (CAH) encompasses several autosomal recessive disorders, all of which involve a deficiency or relative defect in cortisol synthesis, aldosterone synthesis, or both that results in some degree of cortisol deficiency, aldosterone deficiency, or both.[96] The most common cause of CAH is 21-hydroxylase deficiency, accounting for approximately 90% of cases, which is caused by mutations in the *CYP21A2* gene. Classic CAH has a prevalence of 1 in 15,000 live births and is divided into a simple virilizing form and a salt-wasting form. The virilization of a female fetus can cause ambiguous genitalia on prenatal ultrasound. 11-beta-Hydroxylase deficiency accounts for 5% to 8% of all CAH cases. Diagnostic testing for CAH may be performed through CVS or amniocentesis. Carrier screening is now available on some panels and may be used to identify at-risk pregnancies. Recently, a noninvasive cfDNA-based test has been developed to determine not only gender but also mutations status of the fetus.[69] In pregnancies at risk for classic CAH with a female fetus, maternal dexamethasone treatment has been shown to be effective in preventing or mitigating virilization or masculinization of the genitalia of affected fetuses with classical CAH. It must be initiated before 9 weeks' gestation in order to avert labial fusion, but clitoromegaly will be mitigated even if started later. This treatment has become more controversial and it is now recommended only within a research protocol.[96]

Skeletal Dysplasia

Skeletal dysplasias are a complex group of conditions of bone and cartilage development. To date, over 350 distinct disorders have been identified, many of which can be detected in the prenatal period. Diagnosis of a specific skeletal dysplasia is challenging *in utero* because there is frequent overlap in characteristic features (short long bones, bowed bones, small chest cavity) identified on ultrasound between the different types.[97] Single-gene or panel testing can diagnose skeletal dysplasias prenatally and can be obtained only through CVS or amniocentesis. cfDNA screening for single-gene conditions also includes a select number of autosomal dominant skeletal dysplasias but is not comprehensive or diagnostic. Fetal MRI may be recommended when skeletal dysplasia is suspected, especially in cases where a specific diagnosis has not been made or lethality is being determined. The most common types of skeletal dysplasias and their features are summarized in Table 16.13. Osteogenesis imperfecta (OI), caused primarily by autosomal dominant mutations in *COL1A1* and *COL1A2* genes, has many subtypes, ranging from a perinatal lethal form to a mildly affected form that typically escapes detection on prenatal ultrasound. Common features of OI include skeletal deformities, frequent fractures, blue sclerae, hearing loss, and joint hypermobility, and, in some, dentinogenesis imperfecta (Fig. 16.9). Second-trimester ultrasound findings associated with OI include multiple fractures, leading to very short or bowed long bones, beaded appearance of ribs, demineralized skull, and growth restriction.

Achondroplasia is the most common form of disproportionate short stature, present in 1 in 15,000 to 1 in 40,000 live births. It is caused by autosomal dominant mutations in *FGFR3* and over 80% of individuals with achondroplasia have a *de novo* gene mutation. Achondroplasia is characterized by short stature with rhizomelic shortening of upper and lower limb long bones, a large head, and characteristic facial features with frontal bossing and midface hypoplasia. Characteristic ultrasound findings include rhizomelic shortening of long bones, small chest, large head, and, sometimes, polyhydramnios, but do not usually present until the third trimester.[98]

Thanatophoric dysplasia (TD) is a lethal condition with a prevalence of 1 in 20,000 that is caused by a different sporadic *de novo* dominant mutation in *FGFR3*. In the first trimester, shortening of the long bones and an increased NT can be seen.[99] In the second trimester, characteristic features may include growth restriction (< centile), platyspondyly, ventriculomegaly,

TABLE 16.13   Common Ultrasound Findings in Select Skeletal Dysplasias

SKELETAL DYSPLASIA	INHERITANCE	INCIDENCE	GENE	COMMON ULTRASOUND FINDINGS
Osteogenesis imperfecta (OI)	AD/AR	1 in 15,000	COL1A1 and COL1A2	Multiple fractures, short or bowed long bones, demineralized skull, growth restriction
Achondroplasia	AD	1 in 15,000–40,000	FGFR3	Short limbs, small chest, macrocephaly, polyhydramnios
Thanatophoric dysplasia	AD	1 in 20,000	FGFR3	Growth restriction (<fifth centile), platyspondyly, ventriculomegaly, a narrow chest cavity with short ribs, polyhydramnios, bowed femurs ("telephone receiver"), cloverleaf skull (typically in type II), macrocephaly
Campomelic dysplasia	AD	1 in 40,000–80,000	SOX9	Ambiguous genitalia (female appearance XY karyotype), macrocephaly, 11 pairs of ribs, short bowed limbs, clubfeet, scapular hypoplasia
Diastrophic dysplasia	AR	1 in 100,000	SLC26A2	Short limbs, polyhydramnios, radially deviated thumbs (hitchhiker thumbs), clubfeet, small thorax

AD, autosomal dominant; AR, autosomal recessive.

a very narrow chest cavity with short ribs, polyhydramnios, bowed femurs ("telephone receiver" typically seen in TD type I), cloverleaf skull (typically in TD type II), and macrocephaly.[100]

Campomelic dysplasia is a skeletal dysplasia with a prevalence of 1 in 40,000 to 1 in 80,000 caused by usually sporadic dominant mutations in the SOX9 gene. It is characterized by shortening and bowing of long bones (especially femurs and ulna), clubfeet, laryngotracheomalacia with respiratory compromise, small chest with hypoplastic scapulae and ambiguous or normal female genitalia with an XY karyotype, distinctive facial features, Pierre Robin sequence with cleft palate, many of which are visible on second-trimester ultrasound examinations.[101]

Finally, diastrophic dysplasia is a rare (1:100,000) autosomal recessive condition caused by mutations in the SLC26A2 gene. Characteristic features include disproportionate short stature, cleft palate, club foot, progressive scoliosis, limited joint mobility, "hitchhiker thumbs," and "cauliflower deformity" of the ear. Intelligence in individuals with diastrophic dysplasia is normal and there is a wide variation in the phenotype. On second-trimester ultrasound, short limbs, polyhydramnios, radially deviated thumbs (hitchhiker thumbs), club foot, and a small thorax may be noted.[102]

Other Common Ultrasound Findings

Spina Bifida
Spina bifida is a type of ONTD that occurs in approximately every 1 in 500 pregnancies (Fig. 16.10). Spina bifida is often a multifactorial condition, caused by a combination of small genetic factors and small environmental factors, such as lack of folic acid and maternal diabetes. However, identification of spina bifida on ultrasound in the presence of additional anomalies may warrant further evaluation for a syndromic etiology of spina bifida. Trisomies 13 and 18 and triploidy are also associated with spina bifida. Spina bifida can be screened for using MSAFP in the second trimester of pregnancy or using amniotic fluid alpha-fetoprotein and high-resolution ultrasound is very sensitive for detection of spina bifida.[103]

Omphalocele and Gastroschisis
Omphalocele and gastroschisis are the two most common fetal abdominal wall defects caused by an abnormal opening in the abdominal wall and can be detected by ultrasound as early as 12 to 14 weeks' gestation. Omphalocele occurs in 1.86 per every 10,000 live births and consists of a membrane-covered sac including the fetal intestines and sometimes the liver (Fig. 16.11). Regardless of the etiology, up to 80% of fetuses with omphalocele have associated structural anomalies.

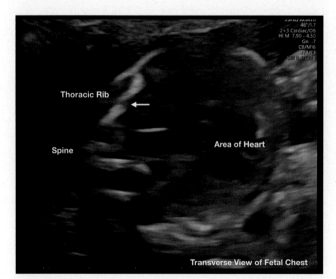

FIGURE 16.9: Rib fracture (21 weeks 3 days). Oblique view of the fetal chest demonstrates a discontinuous rib, consistent with a bony fracture (arrow) found with osteogenesis imperfecta.

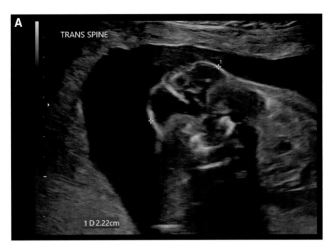
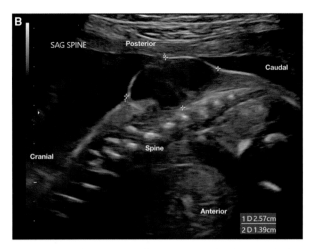

FIGURE 16.10: Spina bifida (21 weeks 5 days). Transverse view of the lumbar spine reveals the presence of a meningomyelocele sac with disrupted vertebral elements *(left)*. Sagittal view of the lumbosacral spine reveals another view of a meningomyelocele sac *(right)*.

Omphalocele is associated with trisomies 18 and 13, and less commonly with Down syndrome, Turner syndrome, and triploidy. The imprinting disorder, Beckwith Wiedemann syndrome (BWS), is the cause for up to 20% of omphaloceles. CVS or amniocentesis can be performed to assess for BWS through DNA methylation studies of imprinting center 1 and imprinting center 2, uniparental disomy testing, sequence analysis with deletion/duplication analysis of the *CDKN1C* gene, and CMA.[104] Amniotic fluid provides a more reliable sample for methylation studies than does CVS. Assessment of additional ultrasound anomalies can guide whether testing for additional genetic syndromes is indicated. Gastroschisis is a protrusion of the fetal bowel outside the abdominal wall and occurs in 4.49 per 10,000 live births (Fig. 16.12). Gastroschisis should be considered when MSAFP is elevated. Although associated gastrointestinal anomalies and problems are found in up to 25% of cases of gastroschisis, extraintestinal abnormalities are rare. In the absence of additional anomalies, further genetic screening based on the presence of gastroschisis alone is not indicated, as gastroschisis is largely considered to occur sporadically.

Cystic Hygroma

Cystic hygromas are multiloculated fluid-filled sacs that result from blockage of the lymphatic system drainage (Fig. 16.13). Cystic hygromas are present in approximately 1 in 100 fetuses and are associated with an increased risk of structural abnormalities, including cardiac and skeletal defects. Over 50% of fetuses with cystic hygromas have aneuploidy, most commonly trisomy 21 and Turner syndrome, but also trisomies 18 and 13.[105] Chromosomal microdeletions and microduplications may also cause a cystic hygroma and can be evaluated through CMA on diagnostic testing.[106] Numerous single-gene conditions, including skeletal dysplasias and lysosomal storage diseases, have been associated with cystic hygroma. One of the more common single-gene conditions is Noonan syndrome, which is a dominant condition caused by mutations in 1 of at least 13 genes. If chromosome abnormalities have been ruled out, Noonan syndrome panel testing on CVS or amniotic fluid is appropriate. Single-gene cfDNA screening has the ability to screen for some types of Noonan syndrome if diagnostic testing is not possible.[107]

SUMMARY

Creating individualized prenatal genetic screening and testing plans for a patient is often a multidisciplinary effort. Considerations include turnaround time, cost, insurance coverage, and informed consent. Timely return of results maximizes patient autonomy and access to pregnancy decision options, including termination in accordance with local laws and regulations. Shorter turnaround times will increase the utility of diagnostic testing, even with declining numbers of diagnostic procedures due to changing practices in prenatal screening. Cost and reimbursement are significant factors that can influence individual decisions about which testing to pursue. All patients undergoing genetic evaluation should provide informed consent prior to testing. The information provided during the informed consent process must include benefits, risks, and limitations of the selected screening or diagnostic test. In addition, a discussion about the potential to detect incidental findings in the fetus

FIGURE 16.11: Omphalocele (20 weeks 4 days). Unlike gastroschisis, the extruded abdominal viscera are surrounded by a thin membrane *(arrows)*.

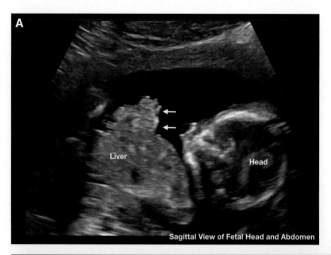

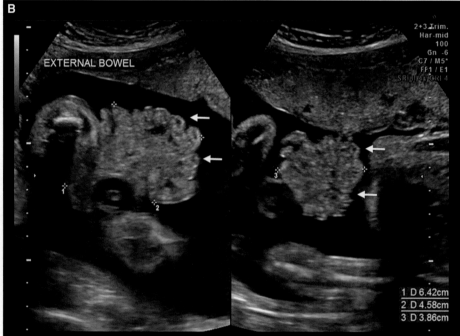

FIGURE 16.12: Gastroschisis (15 weeks 2 days). There is no membrane covering the exteriorized bowel. Exteriorized free loops of bowel are visualized just anterior to the fetal abdominal wall *(arrows)*.

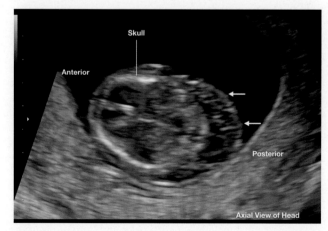

FIGURE 16.13: Cystic hygroma (12 weeks). Cystic hygromas most commonly affect the back of the head/neck *(arrows)* but can occur in other areas, including the axilla, retroperitoneum, limbs, and mediastinum.

and the parents, as well as variants of uncertain significance should be included where appropriate. Genetic counselors and other genetics health professionals may be consulted to discuss these nuances. If prenatal screening and/or diagnostic testing is declined in the prenatal period, postnatal evaluation should be considered and coordinated shortly after delivery.

REFERENCES

1. Heron M. Deaths: leading causes for 2016. *Natl Vital Stat Rep.* 2018;67(6):1–77.
2. Centers for Disease Control and Prevention. Update on overall prevalence of major birth defects—Atlanta, Georgia, 1978–2005. *MMWR Morb Mortal Wkly Rep.* 2008;57(1):1–5.
3. McKinlay Gardner RJ, Amor DJ. *Gardner and Sutherland's Chromosome Abnormalities and Genetic Counseling.* New York, NY: Oxford University Press; 2018.
4. American College of Obstetrics and Gynecology Practice Bulletin No. 162 Summary: prenatal diagnostic testing for genetic disorders. *Obstet Gynecol.* 2016;127(5):976–978.
5. American College of Obstetrics and Gynecology Practice Bulletin No. 163 Summary: screening for fetal aneuploidy. *Obstet Gynecol.* 2016;127(5):979–981.

6. ACOG Committee on Genetics. Committee opinion 691: carrier screening for genetic conditions. *Obstet Gynecol.* 2017;129:e41–e55.

7. ACOG Committee on Genetics. Committee opinion 690: carrier screening in the age of genomic medicine. *Obstet Gynecol.* 2017;129:e35–e40.

8. Gregg AR, Edwards JG. Prenatal genetic carrier screening in the genomic age. *Semin Perinatol.* 2018;42(5):303–306.

9. Haque IS, Lazarin GA, Wapner RJ. Prenatal carrier screening. *JAMA.* 2016;316(24):2675–2676.

10. Wapner RJ, Martin CL, Levy B, et al. Chromosomal microarray versus karyotyping for prenatal diagnosis. *N Engl J Med.* 2012;367(23):2175–2184.

11. Wou K, Levy B, Wapner RJ. Chromosomal microarrays for the prenatal detection of microdeletions and microduplications. *Clin Lab Med.* 2016;36(2):261–276.

12. Hillman SC, McMullan DJ, Hall G, et al. Use of prenatal chromosomal microarray: prospective cohort study and systematic review and meta-analysis. *Ultrasound Obstet Gynecol.* 2013;41(6):610–620.

13. Gross SJ, Pletcher BA, Monaghan KG; Professional Practice and Guidelines Committee. Carrier screening in individuals of Ashkenazi Jewish descent. *Genet Med.* 2008;10(1):54–56.

14. Chokoshvili D, Vears DF, Borry P. Growing complexity of (expanded) carrier screening: direct-to-consumer, physician-mediated, and clinic-based offers. *Best Pract Res Clin Obstet Gynaecol.* 2017;44:57–67.

15. Lazarin GA, Goldberg JD. Current controversies in traditional and expanded carrier screening. *Curr Opin Obstetr Gynecol.* 2016;28(2):136–141.

16. Bell CJ, Dinwiddie DL, Miller NA, et al. Carrier testing for severe childhood recessive diseases by next-generation sequencing. *Sci Transl Med.* 2011;3(65):65ra4.

17. Nicolaides KH. Screening for chromosomal defects. *Ultrasound Obstet Gynecol.* 2003;21(4):313–321.

18. Malone FD, Canick JA, Ball RH, et al. First-trimester or second-trimester screening, or both, for Down's syndrome. *N Engl J Med.* 2005;353(19):2001–2011.

19. Wapner R, Thom E, Simpson JL, et al. First-trimester screening for trisomies 21 and 18. *N Engl J Med.* 2003;349(15):1405–1413.

20. Souka AP, Von Kaisenberg CS, Hyett JA, et al. Increased nuchal translucency with normal karyotype. *Am J Obstet Gynecol.* 2005;192(4):1005–1021.

21. Hyett J, Perdu M, Sharland G, et al. Using fetal nuchal translucency to screen for major congenital cardiac defects at 10–14 weeks of gestation: population based cohort study. *BMJ.* 1999;318(7176):81–85.

22. Pergament E, Alamillo C, Sak K, et al. Genetic assessment following increased nuchal translucency and normal karyotype. *Prenat Diagn.* 2011;31(3):307–310.

23. Ali MM, Chasen ST, Norton ME. Testing for Noonan syndrome after increased nuchal translucency. *Prenat Diagn.* 2017;37(8):750–753.

24. Rosen T, D'Alton ME, Platt LD, et al. First-trimester ultrasound assessment of the nasal bone to screen for aneuploidy. *Obstet Gynecol.* 2007;110(2 pt 1):399–404.

25. Sonek J, Nicolaides K. Additional first-trimester ultrasound markers. *Clin Lab Med.* 2010;30(3):573–592.

26. Smith GC, Stenhouse EJ, Crossley JA, et al. Early pregnancy levels of pregnancy-associated plasma protein a and the risk of intrauterine growth restriction, premature birth, preeclampsia, and stillbirth. *J Clin Endocrinol Metab.* 2002;87(4):1762–1767.

27. Goetzl L, Krantz D, Group NBs. Low first-trimester PAPP-A identifies pregnancies requiring IUGR screening. *Am J Obstet Gynecol.* 2004;189(6):S215.

28. Milunsky A, Jick SS, Bruell CL, et al. Predictive values, relative risks, and overall benefits of high and low maternal serum alpha-fetoprotein screening in singleton pregnancies: new epidemiologic data. *Am J Obstet Gynecol.* 1989;161(2):291–297.

29. Rose NC, Peters SB, Tomaszewski JE, et al. Prenatal characteristics of congenital nephrosis: results of a survey. *J Matern Fetal Med.* 1997;6(3):164–167.

30. Lo YM, Corbetta N, Chamberlain PF, et al. Presence of fetal DNA in maternal plasma and serum. *Lancet.* 1997;350(9076):485–487.

31. Fan HC, Blumenfeld YJ, Chitkara U, et al. Noninvasive diagnosis of fetal aneuploidy by shotgun sequencing DNA from maternal blood. *Proc Natl Acad Sci U S A.* 2008;105(42):16266–16271.

32. Chiu RW, Chan KC, Gao Y, et al. Noninvasive prenatal diagnosis of fetal chromosomal aneuploidy by massively parallel genomic sequencing of DNA in maternal plasma. *Proc Natl Acad Sci U S A.* 2008;105(51):20458–20463.

33. Chiu RW, Akolekar R, Zheng YW, et al. Non-invasive prenatal assessment of trisomy 21 by multiplexed maternal plasma DNA sequencing: large scale validity study. *BMJ.* 2011;342:c7401.

34. Palomaki GE, Kloza EM, Lambert-Messerlian GM, et al. DNA sequencing of maternal plasma to detect Down syndrome: an international clinical validation study. *Genet Med.* 2011;13(11):913–920.

35. Palomaki GE, Deciu C, Kloza EM, et al. DNA sequencing of maternal plasma reliably identifies trisomy 18 and trisomy 13 as well as Down syndrome: an international collaborative study. *Genet Med.* 2012;14(3):296–305.

36. Bianchi DW, Platt LD, Goldberg JD, et al. Genome-wide fetal aneuploidy detection by maternal plasma DNA sequencing. *Obstet Gynecol.* 2012;119(5):890–901.

37. Liang D, Lv W, Wang H, et al. Non-invasive prenatal testing of fetal whole chromosome aneuploidy by massively parallel sequencing. *Prenat Diagn.* 2013;33(5):409–415.

38. Song Y, Liu C, Qi H, et al. Noninvasive prenatal testing of fetal aneuploidies by massively parallel sequencing in a prospective Chinese population. *Prenat Diagn.* 2013;33(7):700–706.

39. Mazloom AR, Dzakula Z, Oeth P, et al. Noninvasive prenatal detection of sex chromosomal aneuploidies by sequencing circulating cell-free DNA from maternal plasma. *Prenat Diagn.* 2013;33(6):591–597.

40. Stumm M, Entezami M, Haug K, et al. Diagnostic accuracy of random massively parallel sequencing for non-invasive prenatal detection of common autosomal aneuploidies: a collaborative study in Europe. *Prenat Diagn.* 2014;34(2):185–191.

41. Porreco RP, Garite TJ, Maurel K, et al. Noninvasive prenatal screening for fetal trisomies 21, 18, 13 and the common sex chromosome aneuploidies from maternal blood using massively parallel genomic sequencing of DNA. *Am J Obstet Gynecol.* 2014;211(4):365.e1–365.e12.

42. Bianchi DW, Parker RL, Wentworth J, et al. DNA sequencing versus standard prenatal aneuploidy screening. *N Engl J Med.* 2014;370(9):799–808.

43. Gil MD, Quezada MS, Bregant B, et al. Cell-free DNA analysis for trisomy risk assessment in first-trimester twin pregnancies. *Fetal Diagn Therap.* 2014;35(3):204–211.

44. Benn P, Borrell A, Chiu RW, et al. Position statement from the Chromosome Abnormality Screening Committee on behalf of the Board of the International Society for Prenatal Diagnosis. *Prenat Diagn.* 2015;35(8):725–734.

45. Nicolaides KH, Syngelaki A, Ashoor G, et al. Noninvasive prenatal testing for fetal trisomies in a routinely screened first-trimester population. *Am J Obstet Gynecol.* 2012;207(5):374.e1–374.e6.

46. Norton ME, Jacobsson B, Swamy GK, et al. Cell-free DNA analysis for noninvasive examination of trisomy. *N Engl J Med.* 2015;372(17):1589–1597.

47. Pergament E, Cuckle H, Zimmermann B, et al. Single-nucleotide polymorphism-based noninvasive prenatal screening in a high-risk and low-risk cohort. *Obstet Gynecol.* 2014;124(2 pt 1):210–218.

48. Dan S, Wang W, Ren J, et al. Clinical application of massively parallel sequencing-based prenatal noninvasive fetal trisomy test for trisomies 21 and 18 in 11,105 pregnancies with mixed risk factors. *Prenat Diagn.* 2012;32(13):1225–1232.

49. Dar P, Curnow KJ, Gross SJ, et al. Clinical experience and follow-up with large scale single-nucleotide polymorphism-based noninvasive prenatal aneuploidy testing. *Am J Obstet Gynecol.* 2014;211(5):527.e1–527.e17.

50. Zhang H, Gao Y, Jiang F, et al. Non-invasive prenatal testing for trisomies 21, 18 and 13: clinical experience from 146,958 pregnancies. *Ultrasound Obstet Gynecol.* 2015;45(5):530–538.

51. Gray KJ, Wilkins-Haug LE. Have we done our last amniocentesis? Updates on cell-free DNA for Down syndrome screening. *Pediatr Radiol.* 2018;48(4):461–470.

52. Grati FR. Implications of feto-placental mosaicism on cell-free DNA testing: a review of a common biological phenomenon. *Ultrasound Obstet Gynecol.* 2016;48(4):415–423.

53. Bianchi DW, Chudova D, Sehnert AJ, et al. Noninvasive prenatal testing and incidental detection of occult maternal malignancies. *JAMA.* 2015;314(2):162–169.

54. Bianchi DW. Cherchez la femme: maternal incidental findings can explain discordant prenatal cell-free DNA sequencing results. *Genet Med.* 2017;20(9):910–917.

55. Martin K, Iyengar S, Kalyan A, et al. Clinical experience with a single-nucleotide polymorphism-based noninvasive prenatal test for five clinically significant microdeletions. *Clin Genet.* 2017;93(2):293–300.

56. Grati FR, Gross SJ. Noninvasive screening by cell-free DNA for 22q11.2 deletion: benefits, limitations, and challenges. *Prenat Diagn.* 2019;39(2):70–80.

57. McDonald-McGinn DM, Sullivan KE, Marino B, et al. 22q11.2 deletion syndrome. *Nat Rev Dis Primers.* 2015;1:15071.

58. Pescia G, Guex N, Iseli C, et al. Cell-free DNA testing of an extended range of chromosomal anomalies: clinical experience with 6,388 consecutive cases. *Genet Med.* 2017;19(2):169–175.

59. Pertile MD, Halks-Miller M, Flowers N, et al. Rare autosomal trisomies, revealed by maternal plasma DNA sequencing, suggest increased risk of feto-placental disease. *Sci Transl Med.* 2017;9(405):1-11.

60. Lefkowitz RB, Tynan JA, Liu T, et al. Clinical validation of a non-invasive prenatal test for genome-wide detection of fetal copy number variants. *Am J Obstet Gynecol.* 2016;215(2):227.e1–227.e16.

61. Petersen AK, Cheung SW, Smith JL, et al. Positive predictive value estimates for cell-free noninvasive prenatal screening from data of a large referral genetic diagnostic laboratory. *Am J Obstet Gynecol.* 2017;217(6):691.e1–691.e6.

62. Schwartz S, Kohan M, Pasion R, et al. Clinical experience of laboratory follow-up with non-invasive prenatal testing using cell-free DNA and positive microdeletion results in 349 cases. *Prenat Diagn.* 2018; 38(3):210–218.

63. Hayward J, Chitty LS. Beyond screening for chromosomal abnormalities: advances in non-invasive diagnosis of single gene disorders and fetal exome sequencing. *Semin Fetal Neonatal Med.* 2018;23(2):94–101.

64. Lo YM, Hjelm NM, Fidler C, et al. Prenatal diagnosis of fetal RhD status by molecular analysis of maternal plasma. *N Engl J Med.* 1998;339(24):1734–1738.

65. Drury S, Mason S, McKay F, et al. Implementing non-invasive prenatal diagnosis (NIPD) in a National Health Service Laboratory; from dominant to recessive disorders. *Adv Exp Med Biol.* 2016;924:71–75.

66. Chitty LS, Mason S, Barrett AN, et al. Non-invasive prenatal diagnosis of achondroplasia and thanatophoric dysplasia: next-generation sequencing allows for a safer, more accurate, and comprehensive approach. *Prenat Diagn.* 2015;35(7):656–662.

67. Hill M, Twiss P, Verhoef TI, et al. Non-invasive prenatal diagnosis for cystic fibrosis: detection of paternal mutations, exploration of patient preferences and cost analysis. *Prenat Diagn.* 2015;35(10):950–958.

68. Parks M, Court S, Bowns B, et al. Non-invasive prenatal diagnosis of spinal muscular atrophy by relative haplotype dosage. *Eur J Hum Genet.* 2017;25(4):416–422.

69. New MI, Tong YK, Yuen T, et al. Noninvasive prenatal diagnosis of congenital adrenal hyperplasia using cell-free fetal DNA in maternal plasma. *J Clin Endocrinol Metab.* 2014;99(6):E1022–E1030.

70. Xiong L, Barrett AN, Hua R, et al. Non-invasive prenatal testing for fetal inheritance of maternal beta-thalassaemia mutations using targeted sequencing and relative mutation dosage: a feasibility study. *BJOG.* 2018;125(4):461–468.

71. Zhang J, Li J, Saucier JB, et al. Non-invasive prenatal sequencing for multiple Mendelian monogenic disorders using circulating cell-free fetal DNA. *Nat Med.* 2019;25(3):439–447.

72. Eddleman KA, Malone FD, Sullivan L, et al. Pregnancy loss rates after midtrimester amniocentesis. *Obstet Gynecol.* 2006;108(5):1067–1072.

73. Mennuti MT. Cytogenetics: part 1, general concepts and aneuploid conditions. In: Norton ME, Kuller JA, Dugoff L, eds. *Perinatal Genetics.* St. Louis, Missouri: Elsevier; 2019:27–38.

74. Grati FR, Malvestiti F, Branca L, Agrati C, Maggi F, Simoni G. Chromosomal mosaicism in the fetoplacental unit. *Best Pract Res Clin Obstet Gynaecol.* 2017;42:39–52.

75. Shaffer LG, Dabell MP, Fisher AJ, et al. Experience with microarray-based comparative genomic hybridization for prenatal diagnosis in over 5000 pregnancies. *Prenat Diagn.* 2012;32(10):976–985.

76. Breman A, Pursley AN, Hixson P, et al. Prenatal chromosomal microarray analysis in a diagnostic laboratory; experience with >1000 cases and review of the literature. *Prenat Diagn.* 2012;32(4):351–361.

77. Best S, Wou K, Vora N, et al. Promises, pitfalls and practicalities of prenatal whole exome sequencing. *Prenat Diagn.* 2018;38(1):10–19.

78. Joint Position Statement from the International Society for Prenatal Diagnosis (ISPD), the Society for Maternal Fetal Medicine (SMFM), and the Perinatal Quality Foundation (PQF) on the use of genome-wide sequencing for fetal diagnosis. *Prenat Diagn.* 2018;38(1):6–9.

79. Normand EA, Van den Veyver IB. Next-generation sequencing for gene panels and clinical exomes. In: Leung PCK, Qiao J, eds. *Human Reproductive and Prenatal Genetics.* London: Academic Press; 2019:554–575.

80. Chandler N, Best S, Hayward J, et al. Rapid prenatal diagnosis using targeted exome sequencing: a cohort study to assess feasibility and potential impact on prenatal counseling and pregnancy management. *Genet Med.* 2018;20(11):1430–1437.

81. Normand EA, Braxton A, Nassef S, et al. Clinical exome sequencing for fetuses with ultrasound abnormalities and a suspected Mendelian disorder. *Genome Med.* 2018;10(1):74.

82. Lord J, McMullan DJ, Eberhardt RY, et al. Prenatal exome sequencing analysis in fetal structural anomalies detected by ultrasonography (PAGE): a cohort study. *Lancet.* 2019;393(10173):747–757.

83. Petrovski S, Aggarwal V, Giordano JL, et al. Whole-exome sequencing in the evaluation of fetal structural anomalies: a prospective cohort study. *Lancet.* 2019;393(10173):758–767.

84. Agathokleous M, Chaveeva P, Poon LC, et al. Meta-analysis of second-trimester markers for trisomy 21. *Ultrasound Obstet Gynecol.* 2013;41(3):247–261.

85. Aagaard-Tillery KM, Malone FD, Nyberg DA, et al. Role of second-trimester genetic sonography after Down syndrome screening. *Obstet Gynecol.* 2009;114(6):1189–1196.

86. Griffin DK. The incidence, origin, and etiology of aneuploidy. *Int Rev Cytol.* 1996;167:263–296.

87. Rao R, Platt LD. Ultrasound screening: status of markers and efficacy of screening for structural abnormalities. *Semin Perinatol.* 2016;40(1):67–78.

88. Moreno-Cid M, Tenias Burillo JM, Rubio-Lorente A, et al. Systematic review of the clinical prediction rules for the calculation of the risk of Down syndrome based on ultrasound findings in the second trimester of pregnancy. *Prenat Diagn.* 2014;34(3):265–272.

89. Donnenfeld AE, Mennuti MT. Sonographic findings in fetuses with common chromosome abnormalities. *Clin Obstet Gynecol.* 1988;31(1):80–96.

90. Zerres K, Rudnik-Schoneborn S, Deget F, et al. Autosomal recessive polycystic kidney disease in 115 children: clinical presentation, course and influence of gender. Arbeitsgemeinschaft fur Padiatrische, Nephrologie. *Acta Paediatr.* 1996;85(4):437–445.

91. Bosco AF, Norton ME, Lieberman E. Predicting the risk of cystic fibrosis with echogenic fetal bowel and one cystic fibrosis mutation. *Obstet Gynecol.* 1999;94(6):1020–1023.

92. Avagliano L, Bulfamante GP, Massa V. Cornelia de Lange syndrome: to diagnose or not to diagnose in utero? *Birth Defects Res.* 2017;109(10):771–777.

93. Clark DM, Sherer I, Deardorff MA, et al. Identification of a prenatal profile of Cornelia de Lange syndrome (CdLS): a review of 53 CdLS pregnancies. *Am J Med Genet A.* 2012;158A(8):1848–1856.

94. Senat MV, Bernard JP, Delezoide A, et al. Prenatal diagnosis of hydrocephalus-stenosis of the aqueduct of Sylvius by ultrasound in the first trimester of pregnancy. Report of two cases. *Prenat Diagn.* 2001;21(13):1129–1132.

95. Bassett AS, McDonald-McGinn DM, Devriendt K, et al. Practical guidelines for managing patients with 22q11.2 deletion syndrome. *J Pediatr.* 2011;159(2):332–339.e1.

96. Speiser PW, Arlt W, Auchus RJ, et al. Congenital adrenal hyperplasia due to steroid 21-hydroxylase deficiency: an endocrine society clinical practice guideline. *J Clin Endocrinol Metab.* 2018;103(11):4043–4088.

97. Pajkrt E, Chitty LS. A sonographic approach to the prenatal diagnosis of skeletal dysplasias. *Prenat Diagn.* 2019;39(9):701–719. doi:10.1002/pd.5501.

98. Hatzaki A, Sifakis S, Apostolopoulou D, et al. FGFR3 related skeletal dysplasias diagnosed prenatally by ultrasonography and molecular analysis: presentation of 17 cases. *Am J Med Genet A.* 2011;155A(10):2426–2435.

99. Tonni G, Azzoni D, Ventura A, et al. Thanatophoric dysplasia type I associated with increased nuchal translucency in the first trimester: early prenatal diagnosis using combined ultrasonography and molecular biology. *Fetal Pediatr Pathol.* 2010;29(5):314–322.

100. Martinez-Frias ML, Egues X, Puras A, et al. Thanatophoric dysplasia type II with encephalocele and semilobar holoprosencephaly: insights into its pathogenesis. *Am J Med Genet A.* 2011;155A(1):197–202.

101. Gentilin B, Forzano F, Bedeschi MF, et al. Phenotype of five cases of prenatally diagnosed campomelic dysplasia harboring novel mutations of the SOX9 gene. *Ultrasound Obstet Gynecol.* 2010;36(3):315–323.

102. Tongsong T, Wanapirak C, Sirichotiyakul S, et al. Prenatal sonographic diagnosis of diastrophic dwarfism. *J Clin Ultrasound.* 2002;30(2):103–105.

103. Sepulveda W, Corral E, Ayala C, et al. Chromosomal abnormalities in fetuses with open neural tube defects: prenatal identification with ultrasound. *Ultrasound Obstet Gynecol.* 2004;23(4):352–356.

104. Weksberg R, Shuman C, Smith AC. Beckwith-Wiedemann syndrome. *Am J Med Genet C Semin Med Genet.* 2005;137C(1):12–23.

105. Kharrat R, Yamamoto M, Roume J, et al. Karyotype and outcome of fetuses diagnosed with cystic hygroma in the first trimester in relation to nuchal translucency thickness. *Prenat Diagn.* 2006;26(4):369–372.

106. Grande M, Jansen FA, Blumenfeld YJ, et al. Genomic microarray in fetuses with increased nuchal translucency and normal karyotype: a systematic review and meta-analysis. *Ultrasound Obstet Gynecol.* 2015;46(6):650–658.

107. Myers A, Bernstein JA, Brennan ML, et al. Perinatal features of the RASopathies: Noonan syndrome, cardiofaciocutaneous syndrome and Costello syndrome. *Am J Med Genet A.* 2014;164A(11):2814–2821.

CENTRAL NERVOUS SYSTEM

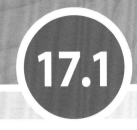

17.1 Supratentorial Anomalies

Beth M. Kline-Fath

INTRODUCTION

The central nervous system (CNS) is frequently abnormal in the fetus. Up to 1 of 100 neonates are born with a CNS anomaly.[1] CNS malformations vary from minor with little symptomatology to extremely complex, causing high morbidity and mortality. Prenatal diagnosis is essential to guide counseling and direct pregnancy decisions, including continuation, mode of delivery, and perinatal and postnatal care.

In this chapter, brain malformations are listed in the order of expected embryonic insult. However, classification can be difficult, given that it is sometimes not possible to identify the timing of the anomaly and the primary event is often linked to other pathologies, making it challenging to stage the embryonic event. Since many structures in the brain are developing at the same time, it is not unusual for multiple malformations to occur simultaneously, limiting the ability to classify an anomaly as primary. CNS disorders can also be of different severity, probably because of inherited and environmental factors, so they are best described individually unless known to be syndromic. Importantly, when imaging the fetal brain, it is imperative that all extracranial areas are evaluated. When one organ is abnormal, often many body parts are involved. Having an understanding of all anomalies may give clues to an underlying genetic syndrome, which can have significant impact on fetal outcome.

EMBRYOLOGY/PATHOPHYSIOLOGY

The embryology of the brain is covered in detail in normal imaging of the fetal brain. The stages of development are provided in Table 9.2 in Chapter 9. Human development is dependent on correct chromosomal complement and organization. Environmental factors can have an adverse, disruptive effect on the embryo or fetus. Common teratogens include drugs, radiation, and infection. Maternal conditions, especially type I diabetes mellitus, often have an impact on genetic or acquired defects in the fetus. Mechanical disruptions can result from trauma, vascular, amniotic, or extraneous effects.

IMAGING TECHNIQUES

Ultrasound (US) has significant advantages over other imaging. There is no radiation, images have high anatomical resolution, real-time capabilities allow for dynamic assessment of the fetus, and color Doppler provides excellent interrogation of blood flow. Three-dimensional (3D) imaging enhances fetal neurosonology by allowing for multiplanar reformats. US is sensitive at detecting the vast majority of primary CNS anomalies through careful examination of the cranium and spine.[2] With 2D and 3D techniques, neurosonography examinations have been reported to provide a diagnosis in 83.7% of studies in which a CNS abnormality is present.[3] Inadequacies of the technique include small field of view, limited soft-tissue contrast, and loss in cerebral detail in the near field due to reverberation artifact. In addition, fetal head position, maternal body habitus, oligohydramnios, and ossification of the fetal skull can degrade cerebral detail. Importantly, US is dependent on the ability of the person to correctly display anatomy and the skill of the reader to diagnose the abnormality.[4]

Fetal magnetic resonance imaging (MRI) is an excellent adjunct to prenatal US. It has multiple advantages, including large field of view that allows for evaluation of the fetus in multiple planes and high soft-tissue contrast and resolution, both of which allow for depiction of the complex normal and abnormal maturation of the developing brain. Neuronal migration, gyration, sulcation, and myelination are accurately depicted. MRI does not suffer from acoustic shadowing of the fetal skull. The posterior fossa, brainstem, and corpus callosum can be easily evaluated, and injury from hemorrhage and ischemia is accurately defined. Multiple authors have demonstrated that prenatal MRI is a valuable adjunct to US in the evaluation of fetal brain.[1,4–8] Levine et al. found that MRI changed diagnosis in 32% of US detected fetal brain abnormalities, counseling in 50%, and patient management in 19%.[6] Griffith recently demonstrated that in fetuses with abnormal US and brain malformations, MRI provided additional diagnostic information in 50%, changed prognostic information in 20%, and changed clinical management in more than one-third.[7]

There are, however, limitations to this technique. Fetal MRI is not widely available and high in cost. The study is also operator dependent, and imaging can be suboptimum in the presence of significant fetal and maternal motion and claustrophobia. Imaging early in gestation can be difficult to interpret and less diagnostic because of primitive brain architecture. This may have significant implications if termination of pregnancy is being considered. At this time, restricted sequences and coils are available. Higher MRI techniques, such as spectroscopy, functional and diffusion tractography, are difficult as longer acquisition times are required.

VENTRICULOMEGALY

Ventriculomegaly (VM) is a descriptive term indicating the presence of excess cerebrospinal fluid (CSF) in the ventricles of the brain. Hydrocephalus is present when there is increased CSF pressure in the ventricles, usually in association with increased head circumference (HC). VM can be isolated (IVM) or associated with other anomalies (AVM). It is important to recognize VM because it is often an indicator of an underlying CNS defect.

Incidence: The incidence for fetal VM ranges from 0.3 to 2.5 cases per 1,000 births.[9–11] It is the most common CNS anomaly identified by prenatal sonography.[12–14] Lateral ventricular enlargement represents the tip of the iceberg in fetal CNS imaging, being sensitive for the detection of a wide variety of fetal CNS abnormalities.[15] Reportedly, about 60% of cases with VM have associated anomalies.[10,16,17] IVM is cited in approximately 40% of cases, with an incidence of 0.4 to 0.9 per 1,000.[10,17]

Pathogenesis: The pathophysiology underlying the dynamics of normal and abnormal CSF flow is still incompletely understood. The major portion of the CSF is produced by the choroid plexus in the lateral and, to a lesser extent, third and fourth ventricles.[18] Normal CSF flow is from the lateral ventricles, through the foramen of Monroe into the third ventricle, and then by way of the aqueduct of Sylvius to the fourth ventricle, out the foramen of Magendie and Luschka into the subarachnoid space (Fig. 9.5 in Chapter 9). The major pathway for CSF reabsorption postnatal is via arachnoid granulations into the blood capillaries, which then drain to the cerebral venous sinuses. Minor CSF absorption also occurs via the lymphatic system at the level of cribriform plate and nasal submucosa, the interstitial and perivascular space, and the choroid plexus via capillaries to the vein of Galen.[18,19] In the immature brain, it is favored that the minor pathways are the primary route for CSF reabsorption as the arachnoid granulations are not developed prenatal.[19]

The mechanisms for development of VM are varied (Table 17.1-1). The two main categories of VM are *obstructive* with hydrocephalus or *nonobstructive* due to pathology resulting in decreased cerebral volume or abnormal development of the parenchyma. With hydrocephalus, there are two obstructive types that lead to imbalance between production and resorption of CSF: *noncommunicating* and *communicating*. *Noncommunicating* VM does not allow for communication between the ventricular system and the subarachnoid space, and thus the obstruction is internal to the ventricular system, as in maldevelopment of the aqueduct of Sylvius, or external to the ventricular system, such as in Chiari II malformation. *Communicating* obstructive VM is rare in the fetus but occurs when there is abnormal absorption of the CSF by the cerebral venous sinuses or lymphatics.[20] Rarely, increased CSF production can cause nonobstructive hydrocephalus in the presence of a choroid plexus papilloma. Nonobstructive VM is typically related to ex vacuo dilatation secondary to brain injury, chromosomal/genetic disorders, or malformations in neuronal development.

The natural history of VM can be difficult to predict and is often complex. Prenatal, the dilatation can resolve, stabilize, or progress. In the presence of obstructive VM, in which there is increased pressure, there is potential for progressive brain injury. If hydrocephalus develops, impairment is dependent on the age of onset, magnitude and duration of VM, and primary areas affected, most commonly the periventricular white matter.[21] Secondary changes due to hydrocephalus include neuronal injury due to axonal disconnection and ischemia with consequential gliosis and neuroinflammation, and abnormal CSF and blood flow dynamics resulting in altered metabolism and toxin accumulation.[21]

Etiology: There are multiple mechanisms responsible for the development of VM. Therefore, the etiologies are extensive. The most common include congenital CNS malformations, genetic disorders, obstructive masses or structural anomalies, developmental anomalies due to infectious or metabolic processes,

TABLE 17.1-1 Mechanisms for Development of Ventriculomegaly

OBSTRUCTIVE

Noncommunicating

Intrinsic—Ventricular
- Aqueductal stenosis
- Posterior fossa malformation
- Posthemorrhagic obstruction
- Postinfectious obstruction

Extrinsic—Parenchymal or Mass
- Tumor or arachnoid cyst
- Hemorrhage or edema
- Malformation (Chiari II)

Communicating
- Lack of resorption of CSF by venous sinuses

NONOBSTRUCTIVE

Overproduction of CSF
- Choroid plexus lesion

Malformation of Cerebral Development
- Holoprosencephaly
- Lissencephaly/schizencephaly
- Agenesis of corpus callosum
- Disorder of proliferation and neuronal migration
- Disorder of organogenesis
- Genetic etiology
  - Trisomies 13, 18, and 21, and many others

Destructive Ex Vacuo Dilatation
- Vascular
- Infection
- Ischemic

CSF, cerebrospinal fluid.
Modified from Levine D, Feldman HA, Kazam Tannus JF, et al. Frequency and cause of disagreements in diagnoses for fetuses referred for ventriculomegaly. *Radiology*. 2008;247:515–527.

intraventricular hemorrhage, and ex vacuo dilatation due to an encephaloclastic event.[21] When VM is not isolated, the most common underlying brain anomalies cited in the fetus are aqueductal stenosis (30% to 40%), Chiari II malformation (15% to 30%), dysgenesis of the corpus callosum (20% to 30%), and posterior fossa abnormalities (7% to 10%).[10,16,22]

Diagnosis: When VM is identified, a detailed prenatal US should be performed. Fetal MRI is helpful, especially in the verification of the diagnosis and depiction of associated anomalies. Fetal echocardiography, karyotype with chromosomal microarray, and TORCH screening is highly recommended.[23] In the presence of intracranial hemorrhage, a fetomaternal alloimmune thrombocytopenia (FAT) screen for anti–human platelet antigen (HPA) antibodies may be considered.[20,24]

Ultrasound: The fourth ventricle can be detected earliest on sonograms at 9 menstrual weeks, initially a large anechoic ellipsoid structure compared with the total brain.[15] After brief visibility, the fourth ventricle becomes small. The third ventricle is identified slightly later and demonstrates adult slit-like linear hypoechoic configuration, lying between the thalami.[15] The lateral ventricles are apparent, being large and globular at 13 to 14 menstrual weeks, but change dramatically over time to achieve an adult-like configuration due to the development of the corpus callosum, basal ganglia, periventricular white matter, and frontal and occipital lobes.[15] Although the volume of the ventricles increases with gestational age (GA), the CSF spaces of the lateral ventricles become less conspicuous during the pregnancy. The choroid plexus can be a helpful landmark, extending from the foramen of Monroe to fill the posterior horn of a normal lateral ventricle.[15]

Normal technique and measurements of the lateral ventricles are imperative to avoid false-negative and false-positive diagnosis of VM. The atrium of the lateral ventricle is preferred as a measurable landmark, since the size and configuration is essentially stable during the second and the third trimesters, in contrast to the frontal horn, which changes in configuration with GA.[25-27] In addition, since the trigone and occipital horn are typically the first areas to dilate in VM, this area of investigation is most important in the diagnosis.[25,26] As the wall of the atrium is perpendicular to the beam in the axial plane, it can be easily identified. The measurement is obtained by placing calipers in the largest part of the lateral ventricles inside the echogenic interface defining the lateral ventricular walls (Fig. 17.1-1).[15,27] Care must be taken to obtain the measurement on a true transventricular plane at the level of the glomus of the choroid.[28] Since the choroid plexus fills the ventricular atrium with only 1 to 2 mm of CSF separating the choroid from the adjacent lateral ventricular wall, the choroid can be utilized as a marker for the most distant ventricular wall.[15,26]

Measurements are subject to error because of off-axis image plane, angled measurement, or improper choice of ventricular boundary.[29] In an attempt to decrease these possible deficiencies, it has been further suggested that the axial view should be strictly assessed by demonstrating that the proximal and distal calvarial margins are equidistant and that anterior landmarks include the cavum septi pellucidi (CSP) or fornix and posterior landmark, the fluid-filled V shape of the ambient cistern (Fig. 17.1-2).

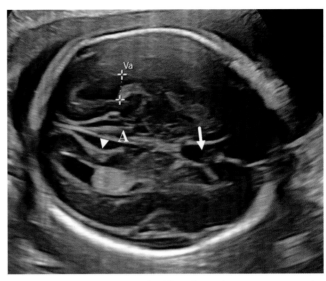

FIGURE 17.1-2: Transventricular US with atrial measurement at the level of the cavum septum pellucidum (*arrow*), ambient (*A*) cistern, and parieto-occipital sulcus (*arrowhead*).

The measurement should be opposite the internal parieto-occipital sulcus and placed at the junction of the ventricular lumen and wall perpendicular to the inner and outer border of the ventricle.[29]

The normal mean diameter of the atrium of the lateral ventricle midgestation is 7.6 ± 0.6 mm from 14 to 38 weeks with excellent interobserver reliability.[25] The atrial width of one or both ventricles >10 mm is more than 2.5 to 4 standard deviation (SD) above the mean and is thus considered VM midgestation irrespective of gender.[12,25-27] The ventricle wall should be smooth without irregularity or nodularity. Ventricle asymmetry ≥ 2 mm without dilatation can be present physiologically as a normal variant.[30,31]

When the ventricle enlarges, the choroid hangs in a dependent location and separates from the nondependent wall. This appearance of a "dangling choroid" will often provide clues to the presence of VM (Fig. 17.1-3).[32] VM can also be diagnosed

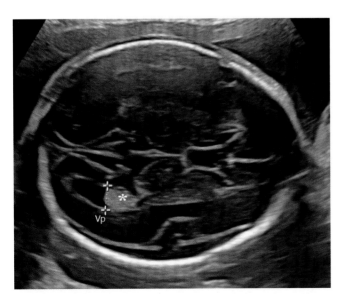

FIGURE 17.1-1: US measurements of the atrium of the lateral ventricles in a 23-week fetus. Note echogenic choroid plexus (*asterisk*). Ventricular measurements are also obtained inside the echogenic interface.

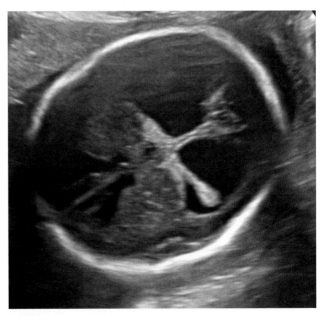

FIGURE 17.1-3: Axial US transventricular view with dangling choroid in a 27-week fetus with ventriculomegaly secondary to aqueduct stenosis.

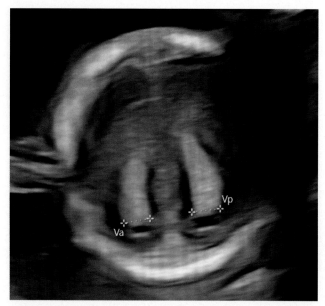

FIGURE 17.1-4: Coronal US through the fetal brain demonstrating bilateral atria and echogenic choroid in a 22-week fetus.

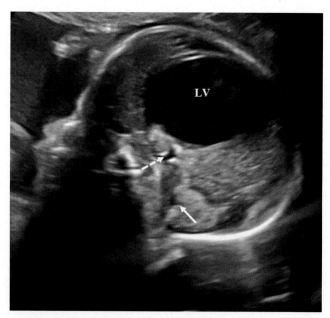

FIGURE 17.1-5: Sagittal US in a 27-week fetus with aqueduct stenosis. There is severe lateral ventriculomegaly (LV). The third (dotted arrow) is mildly enlarged, and the fourth (solid arrow) is normal.

when there is choroid plexus separation from the medial ventricular wall of >3 mm.[33] In the past, borderline or mild VM has been defined as atrial measurements of 10 to 15 mm, and severe VM when atrial width is >15 mm. Recently, VM has been further segregated such that mild represents measurements between 10 and 12 mm, moderate >12 to 15 mm, and severe >15 mm.[20,34]

Limitations of the technique include visualization of only one lateral ventricle in the distal hemisphere because of near-field artifacts. Angled views through the brain may be helpful to overcome this shortcoming.[35] In addition, it can be difficult to visualize the entire ventricle because of fetal position or calvarial ossification. If the true transverse axial plane cannot be obtained, then a coronal image at the level of the atria should be utilized for the measurement (Fig. 17.1-4).[27]

Sensitivity of diagnosis is controversial. Previous studies have reported a sensitivity of 88% to 93.5% in the presence of a ventricular dilatation greater than 10 mm.[36] However, before 24 weeks, the sensitivity drops to 35%.[9] In fact, one study noted that only 57% of cases of severe VM were diagnosed prior to 24 weeks.[35] False-positive diagnosis has been reported between 10% and 33%, with the most common disagreement being in the diagnosis of mild VM.[4,37,38] Causes for the false-positive prenatal diagnosis include regression of VM during fetal life, measurement variability, and difference in criteria with regard to the presence of VM close to 10 mm.[4,20]

Although diagnosis of lateral VM is extremely important, the third and fourth ventricles should also be closely assessed as they may provide clues to the underlying diagnosis. Enlarged third and fourth ventricles are documented when the transverse dimensions are ≥3.5 and ≥4.8 mm, respectively.[10] These measurements may be possible on routine axial imaging, but a complete neurosonographic examination should include both coronal and sagittal views through the fetal brain (Fig. 17.1-5).[39,40] A midsagittal image can be very helpful with a positive predictive value of 93%, improving detection of anomalies of the posterior fossa and corpus callosum.[41] If these planes are difficult to perform, transvaginal, and/or 3D

imaging can assist with fetal anatomy.[39–41] Transvaginal imaging, especially if the head is in cephalic positioning, uses the fetal fontanelles as an acoustic window allowing for visualization of both hemispheres and ventricles without artifact related to fetal skull or maternal obesity.[42]

It is very important to determine whether the VM is isolated or associated with other CNS or non-CNS anomalies. Evaluation of the morphology and borders of the lateral ventricle can provide important clues. In the presence of angular lateral ventricles, a neural tube defect should be sought. With a pattern of colpocephaly, agenesis of the corpus callosum (ACC) may be suggested.[43] Asymmetric or unilateral ventriculomegaly (UVM) should raise the suspicion for an underlying encephaloclastic/vascular pathology.[44] Evaluation of the ventricular wall for increased echogenicity, thickening or irregularity should be performed to exclude hemorrhage or periventricular heterotopia. Internal ventricular debris, fluid–fluid level, or enlargement of a heterogeneous choroid plexus would indicate hemorrhage. Septation of the ventricles raises the suspicion of infection. The parenchyma, Sylvian fissure, and gyration pattern should be assessed. The septum pellucidum and extra-axial spaces should be closely examined, as in obstructive hydrocephalus, these structures may be absent.[44] Head circumference and biparietal diameter (BPD) should be obtained to evaluate for volume loss versus hydrocephalus; however, early in gestation, these measurements may not be helpful. Finally, the entire fetus should be evaluated for extra-CNS anomalies. Most studies indicate that it matters little whether the associated anomaly is CNS or of another organ system in predicting an unfavorable outcome.[15] Although a high-quality US is essential, even in the most experienced hands, anomalies can be difficult to detect on US with a false-negative rate reported between 10% and 40%.[14,15,33]

Magnetic Resonance Imaging: Fetal MRI is an excellent adjunct to US. Aside from the technical limitations of US, some anomalies in cortical migration, hemorrhage, and parenchymal injury have been noted to be too subtle to be defined by US.[45]

In fetuses with VM, diagnostic accuracy of US has been shown to be approximately 90% and fetal MRI 99%; however, MRI changed the prognosis in 23% and had a significant effect on clinical management in approximately 26% of cases imaged by both modalities.[46] As fetal outcome is dependent on identifying cause and separating IVM from AVM, additional imaging with MRI should be considered in the presence of sonographic diagnosis of VM.

On MRI, precise measurements of the lateral, third, and fourth ventricles can be defined (Chapter 9). Some authors have found that measurements of the lateral ventricles on MRI are slightly larger than on US by an average of 0.6 mm.[4] However, most conclude that there is a 90% agreement between the atrial dimensions on US when compared with MRI.[47] Rarely, measurements defined as VM on US are found to be normal on fetal MRI.[47] Overall, in the presence of VM, there is excellent agreement between US and MRI.[48]

With MRI, many prefer measuring the lateral ventricles on a coronal image containing choroid and parallel to the brainstem, as it is more reliable than the axial.[10] On a coronal plane, the lateral ventricles should measure <10 mm and third ventricle <4 mm. On sagittal imaging, CSF should be present in the aqueduct of Sylvius and the fourth ventricle should measure <7 mm.[10]

An organized approach in evaluation of the fetal brain is recommended. Working from inside to out by evaluating the ventricles, germinal matrix, brain parenchyma, sulcation, extra-axial spaces, and, finally, vascular structures, calvarium and face, is my typical approach. Below 20 weeks, the ventricles demonstrate a primitive configuration, and up to approximately 24 weeks, the occipital horns are mildly disproportionate to the frontal horns (see Chapter 9).[49] If the ventricles are angular, a neural tube defect is almost always present.[43,49] Colpocephaly, marked dilatation of the posterior horn with abnormal frontal horns, should raise concern for a corpus callosum abnormality (Fig. 17.1-24C).[43,49] Septations would support infection. The septum pellucidum should be present after 18 weeks. The third ventricle should be small and slit like.

The germinal matrix should be symmetric and of appropriate size for GA. The ventricular wall should be evaluated for irregularity, thickening, or nodularity that would suggest heterotopia. T1 imaging and gradient echo are helpful to confirm hemorrhage. Cystic lesions in the germinal matrix suggest insult. Parenchymal lamination pattern and sulcation should be appropriate for GA. Diffusion imaging is essential to exclude ischemia. Measurements of the fronto-occipital diameter and BPD and evaluation of the subarachnoid spaces may be clues to hydrocephalus or volume loss.

Midline anatomy is important and includes the corpus callosum, aqueduct of Sylvius, brainstem, fourth ventricle, and vermis. A midline sagittal image of the fetal brain is therefore imperative. Parenchymal signal and sulcation of the vermis and cerebellar hemispheres should be correlated with GA. Extra-axial spaces (especially the cisterna magna) and vascular structures examined. Calvarial configuration and facial structures evaluated for clues to syndromes. Biometry of the vermis, cerebellum, and brainstem should be performed.

Fetal MRI in the presence of VM has been shown to demonstrate a higher percentage of associated anomalies (43%) versus US (32%).[50] However, it is important to remember that migrational abnormalities may not be apparent early in gestation, especially below 20 weeks when the brain is primitive in its development. Cortical brain development advances significantly

after 20 weeks, which allows for better detection of anomalies. Previous work has not shown any advantage at detecting additional abnormalities by delaying fetal MRI to 30 to 32 weeks versus typical 20 to 24 weeks imaging.[47] However, it should be remembered that there is often a lag in development of the sulci and gyri when a fetus has VM or other CNS abnormalities, and therefore, delayed imaging may be considered on a case-to-case basis.[51]

Associated Anomalies: VM is often the tip of the iceberg, representing the first and only sign of associated multisystem fetal abnormalities.[25,28] Associated anomalies are present in 70% to 85% of fetuses with VM, and 60% of those malformations may be extracranial.[22]

There is a clear relationship between the degree of VM and the risk of other brain abnormalities.[52] Severe VM is 10 times more likely to be associated with a brain anomaly than mild or moderate VM.[52]

The overall frequency of chromosomal anomalies in the presence of VM has been quoted from 2% to 29%.[35,53] The incidence of chromosomal anomalies is strongly related to the presence of multisystem malformations.[53] In a fetus with AVM, chromosomal anomalies are higher at 25% to 36%, whereas in IVM, the risk falls to 3% to 6%.[20,22,54]

Differential Diagnosis: Misinterpretation of the anechoic brain can sometimes result in incorrect atrial measurements, leading to the false diagnosis of VM. A cystic lesion, such as arachnoid or dermoid cyst, or an enlarged extra-axial fluid space can be misinterpreted as VM.

Prognosis: Review of the literature suggests that fetal VM is not associated with outcome in a simple or consistent way. VM has many causes and can evolve during gestation. Therefore, counseling should always be performed with a certain degree of caution.[54] Although significant research has been performed in an attempt to improve counseling, one should review the literature carefully. There are variations in outcome and standards between many studies, and this, unfortunately, is because of small sample sizes, variable techniques in the evaluation of VM, variable ages at assessment of development, and lack of standardized methods to assess development. Therefore, prognosticators of outcome are sometimes inconsistent.

The prognosis of VM overall has been stated to be guarded with mortality of 70% to 80% and only half of surviving children developing normally.[15,55] When attempting to determine which VM cases will have a worse outcome, there is agreement in the literature that some factors can guide prognosis.

There is a positive correlation with the degree of VM, survival, and neurodevelopmental delay.[16,17] Survival greater than 24 months in fetuses with IVM is noted to be 98% with mild, 80% with moderate, and 33.3% with severe VM.[34] In those that survive with isolated VM, in the presence of mild VM, normal outcome has been noted in 93% versus 75% in those with moderate VM and 62.5% in those with severe VM.[34]

The cause of VM plays an important role in the prognosis for the fetus.[22] The presence of associated intracranial and extracranial malformations decreases the likelihood of a good outcome.[16,17,55] There is a 56% increased morbidity and mortality in AVM versus 6% with IVM.[56] Neurological delay in IVM ranges from 9% to 36% as compared to 84% with AVM.[57]

The association of chromosomal abnormality is another negative prognostic indicator.[22] In the presence of VM due to chromosomal/genetic defects, a normal outcome is present in 28% of cases with severe VM and 87% in fetus with VM between 10 and 15 mm.[20] Those cases in which VM is associated with viral infection tend to have poor outcomes.[23]

Most confirm that progression of VM *in utero* is a poor prognosticator, with 80% demonstrating neurodevelopmental delay.[10,16] In a review of nearly 300 cases of IVM, 29% resolved, 57% stabilized, and 14% progressed.[58] When VM improves or resolves, 70% to 80% of fetuses have a good outcome.[20] Stable or nonprogressive IVM also tends to have a favorable prognosis.[16]

Multiple debated patterns have been described. The early appearance of the VM in pregnancy is controversial but has been associated with a poor prognosis.[10,23,59] It is favored that UVM has a better outcome than bilateral VM.[10,59] Asymmetrical VM has been most commonly described with severe VM, which tends to have a worse prognosis.[16,54,60] Controversial data suggest that a male fetus with VM has a better outcome than female.[10,20]

Management: Prenatal counseling is complex and challenging, but having knowledge of the degree of VM, associated anomalies, cause whether structural, chromosomal, or infectious and progression will improve discussion.[61] Depending on GA at identification, management options include termination or expectant management at delivery.[62] Previous intervention with intrauterine CSF diversion utilizing ventriculo-amniotic shunts were unfavorable, but there is a renewed interest in shunting and third ventriculostomies that have yet become standard fetal care.[61] Counseling should be directed toward known findings and potential outcomes. If continuation of the pregnancy is decided, repeat US should be obtained to assess changes in VM and evaluate for additional anomalies.[62] Most fetuses with VM have normal head size, but cesarean delivery is recommended for those fetuses with enlarged cranium.[62] In this case, delivery must be delayed until the fetus is mature enough to survive. Dilemma occurs in the presence of progressive hydrocephalus, as increasing ventricular dilatation can result in brain damage.[62] The current recommendation is early shunt placement after induced delivery as soon as lung maturity permits.[54]

Postnatal treatment is directed toward cause. In cases of VM due to cerebral malformation or destruction, no surgical intervention is typically warranted. Neurological consultation and directed neurodevelopmental therapy should be considered to improve outcome. In the presence of open neural tube defect or hydrocephalus, surgical intervention is typically necessary. With increased intracranial pressure, ventricular peritoneal shunt is the first line of therapy.

Recurrence: Recurrence risk depends on the etiology. The overall recurrence risk for VM without associated anomalies is less than 4%.[61,63] In the presence of a genetic syndrome, the risk may increase.

Mild, Moderate, and Unilateral Ventriculomegaly

In the literature, there is lack of standardization in the terms mild and borderline VM. In the past, mild or borderline VM has been described as lateral ventricular dilatation between 10 and 15 mm and a choroid lateral ventricular separation of greater than or equal to 3 mm and less than or equal to 8 mm. However, more recently, VM has been further refined into borderline or mild VM when lateral ventricle dilatation is between 10 and 12 mm and moderate when dilatation is noted between greater than 12

and 15 mm. Given these differences in terminology, this section sometimes group outcomes for VM combining both mild and moderate VM.

Incidence: Mild-to-moderate bilateral VM (10 to 15 mm) represents 15% to 20% of all VM cases, with a prevalence of 0.7% to 1% of pregnancies, being more common in males.[14,15,56,64] Unilateral VM (UVM) has been reported to be rare in some literature, present in 0.07% of pregnancies, though more recent studies suggest that UVM is more common than bilateral VM, being present in up to 50% of VM cases.[64–66]

Pathogenesis: Mild-to-moderate IVM is overall less well defined, probably because it can be a dynamic process *in utero*.[58] The head circumference is usually normal, and the VM is typically not associated with increased intracranial pressure. Mild-to-moderate IVM may resolve in 41%, remain stable in 43%, and progress in 16%.[57] Progression in UVM is only cited in 5% of cases.[66] Postnatally, regression of VM has been described in a significant number of fetuses with bilateral VM and UVM.[67]

Etiology: Mild or borderline IVM (10 to 12 mm) as a pathology can be a diagnostic dilemma, given that prior research suggests that it may represent a variation of normal.[25,52] US studies have shown that atrial diameters above 10 mm can include fetuses that are healthy.[68] Salomon et al. noted that a ventricular width greater than 10 mm can be found in 1% of normal fetuses throughout gestation.[12] In the third trimester, the mean diameter of the lateral ventricles has been found slightly larger, with upper range at 10.2 mm, representing 2 SD at term.[12] Another study demonstrated that the 95% confidence interval exceeded 10 mm from 34 weeks to term.[26,69]

In addition, studies have found that the lateral ventricles are larger in boys than those in girls, with a difference of approximately 0.4 to 0.6 mm.[10,68,70] Because of the difference in gender ventricular size, 0.28% of males and 0.06% of healthy girls will have measurements equal to or above 10 mm atrial size.[68] In support of these findings, some authors have shown that the rate of male fetuses with ventricular size <12 mm is higher than that of females and correlates with a good prognosis, probably because of inclusion of normal fetuses.[59,71] In addition, mild VM and UVM have also been noted in large for GA fetuses and thus may represent normal dimensions for size.[72,73]

However, these and other authors still support that the 10-mm value should be maintained regardless of gender.[68,70,74] Mild and moderate VM are seen in the presence of CNS anomalies, chromosomal aberrations, and infection; therefore, systematic referral and evaluation for every degree of VM is warranted, regardless of size.[75]

Both mild and moderate VM can be associated with major and minor CNS anomalies.[76] In an overall review of 176 cases of VM, additional brain abnormalities were diagnosed in approximately 11% of mild VM and 24% of case of moderate VM.[34] Increase in each millimeter in ventricular diameter increases the risk for major and minor CNS anomalies, especially in the presence of moderate VM; however, symmetric VM in both mild and moderate cases also increases the risk for associated CNS malformation.[76] The incidence of additional CNS and non-CNS sonographic anomalies identified in fetuses with mild-to-moderate VM is <50%.[77]

Chromosomal anomalies in association with mild-to-moderate VM are reported between 3% and 12.6%, with mean of 9%.[58] The majority of fetuses with mild-to-moderate VM and abnormal karyotype will have additional sonographic abnormalities.[58] With IVM between 10 and 15 mm, positive chromosomal anomaly is defined in 3% to 5%, and in mild IVM, aneuploidy is detected in 3%.[24,60,72]

Fetal infection, most commonly due to toxoplasmosis or cytomegalovirus (CMV), is found in 1% to 5% of cases of mild-to-moderate VM.[75,78] If the VM is isolated and between 10 and 15 mm and between 10 and 12 mm, positive infection is 1.5% and 0.4%, respectively.[24,60,72] Cerebral VM is one of the more common prenatal US abnormalities in fetuses with CMV, present in 18% of cases, half of which are isolated.[24]

UVM has been hypothesized to result from atresia, maldevelopment, or obstruction of the foramen of Monroe or unilateral volume loss in the adjacent hemisphere.[73] UVM has also demonstrated a higher incidence in males or fetuses with birth weight of >90 percentile and may represent a normal variant when mild and nonprogressive.[65,73] However, up to 24% may have additional anomalies.[66] In addition, UVM in isolation has been found to have positive infectious titers in approximately 8% of cases.[66]

Diagnosis: Genetic testing with karyotype and possible microarray and TORCH screening should be considered.

Ultrasound: When VM is identified, the opposite ventricle should be evaluated to exclude UVM (Fig. 17.1-6). Detailed neurosonography with multiplanar imaging should be obtained to exclude additional anomalies.[24] Transvaginal with high-resolution probe usually results in the greatest detail. However, if this is not possible, 3D imaging should be attempted.[24] The false-negative rate in detection of anomalies with IVM is equivalent to 11%.[56] IVM is a diagnosis of exclusion.

As progression is possible and 13% of anomalies are detected on sequential US, follow-up US examination is suggested.[24] At least one additional detailed US should be performed between 28 and 34 weeks to search for other cerebral and extracerebral anomalies.[24] Some advocate for monthly US to determine whether the ventricles return to normal, remain stable, or progress.[78]

Magnetic Resonance Imaging: Performing fetal MRI in the presence of mild-to-moderate VM remains controversial, though many

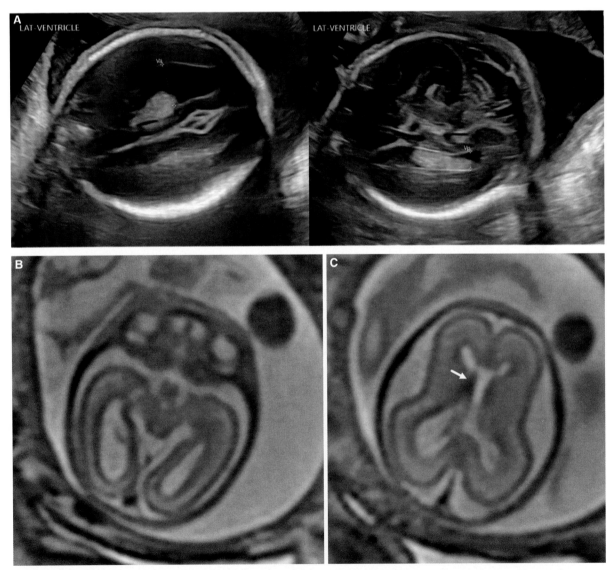

FIGURE 17.1-6: Unilateral ventriculomegaly in a fetus at 22 weeks' gestation. **A:** Axial US of both right and left ventricles demonstrating asymmetric enlargement of the right lateral ventricle. **B:** Axial T2 MRI from same fetus demonstrating asymmetric ventricles. **C:** Axial T2 MRI at level of the basal ganglia with right germinal matrix hemorrhage (*arrow*) as source for mild asymmetric ventriculomegaly.

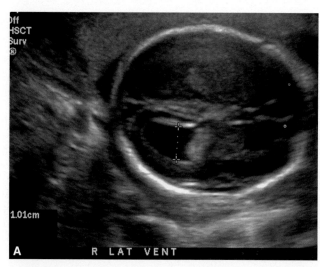 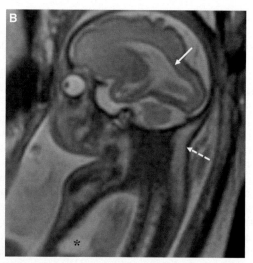

FIGURE 17.1-7: Fetus at 29 weeks diagnosed with trisomy 21. **A:** Axial US demonstrating mild ventriculomegaly. **B:** Sagittal T2 MRI of the same fetus demonstrating mild lateral VM (*white arrow*), but also moderate pleural effusion (*black asterisk*) and nuchal thickening (*dotted white arrow*).

support MRI when there is suspicion of a cerebral anomaly or in the case of moderate VM or AVM (Fig. 17.1-7). At our institution, fetal MRI is utilized routinely in the presence of any grade of VM.

However, the argument against routine MRI in mild-to-moderate VM is that a dedicated neurosonogram with operator expertise may detect many anomalies noted by fetal MRI.[64] Furthermore, fetal MRI is also only as good as the imaging and the skill of the reader.[64] Despite these important facts, it is known that MRI is more sensitive to pathologies, such as ischemia, hemorrhage, lamination abnormalities, white matter tract formation, and cortical development compared to US.[64] In a recent study in which a dedicated neurosonogram diagnosed fetuses with mild-to-moderate VM, the authors noted that fetal MRI provided additional information in 5% of cases, lower than previous studies, but still supporting that early MRI had excellent performance when identifying additional CNS anomalies.[79] A recent study with regard to isolated UVM noted that fetal MRI also detected additional findings in 5% of case.[66] MRI performed in the presence of mild IVM provided information that modified obstetric management in 6% of cases and was reassuring to families in the presence of isolation.[80] However, the contribution of fetal MRI in cases of mild IVM remains debated.[81]

There is also no consensus on the optimal time for imaging; but MRI after 25 weeks or third trimester has been suggested to have better detection of anomalies, such as cortical, white matter, and intracranial hemorrhage.[79]

Associated Anomalies: The rate of associated anomalies in mild-to-moderate VM ranged between 10% and 76%, with an average of 41%.[9,56] Those with mild VM had a lower rate of associated anomalies than those with moderate VM.

Differential Diagnosis: False-positive diagnosis may occur with incorrect imaging plane, incorrect placement of calipers, and differences in measurement interpretation for the presence of VM.

Prognosis: Outcome in mild-to-moderate VM is dependent on the presence of associated anomalies, genetic/chromosomal anomalies, or positive titers. Being able to prove that VM is isolated is important for prognosis. Moderate VM, when compared

with mild VM, is more likely to demonstrate associated anomalies, 56% versus 6%.[24,56] Mild-to-moderate IVM has a reported survival of 85%, with normal outcome in 85%.[55] In those with mild-to-moderate AVM, perinatal or early childhood death increased to an average of 37%.[82] Fetuses with mild-to-moderate IVM have abnormal neurological outcome in 10% to 20%, while those with AVM are abnormal in up to 40% to 50%.[1,56]

Most believe that the degree of VM is also an important prognosticator, although a recent study notes that size may not be a factor when predicting outcome in IVM.[83] Prior research has cited neurodevelopmental delay being an average of 14% to 17% when the IVM is moderate versus 3% to 11.8% when mild.[9] Another study demonstrated approximately 6% neurodevelopmental delay in children diagnosed with mild IVM.[84] These numbers have also been supported by a study that utilized fetal MRI, in which mild IVM had 94% excellent outcome and those with moderate IVM had 85% good outcome.[59]

The overall risk of neurological sequelae in stable VM is significantly lower than in progressive VM.[55,56,60] Sixteen percent of fetuses with mild-to-moderate VM have progression, and the neurodevelopmental outcome is worse, 44% versus 7% without progression.[24] There is also a higher incidence of chromosomal anomalies in progressive VM, 22% compared to 1% without progression.[24] Cases of mild-to-moderate IVM that resolve before birth tend to have a normal outcome.

Because males have a more generous ventricular size, mild IVM is more commonly depicted in males.[56] In support of normal larger ventricles in males, some have found that the risk for abnormal outcome in male fetuses with IVM and normal karyotype is 5% versus 23% for female.[56,71,83] However, several studies have demonstrated that there is no difference in outcome when comparing male and female fetuses.[24,59] Signorelli et al.[84] have shown that all cases of mild VM had a normal outcome up to 10 years after birth. Therefore, some believe that mild IVM may be a variation of normal.[72,84,85]

There is a controversy in the literature as to whether UVM has a better prognosis than bilateral VM.[59,72] In a review of 366 cases, 97% had normal development with UVM versus 90% with mild bilateral IVM.[82] Another study reported developmental delay in mild bilateral IVM and unilateral as being very similar at 6% and

7.4%, respectively.[24] However, it is important to understand that UVM follows the same rules as bilateral VM in determining outcome. Although many believe UVM tends to be benign as it is less likely to have a clinically significant associated anomaly, there is still a 3% risk for chromosomal aberration, 8% risk for infection, and 6% to 15% risk for neurodevelopmental delay.[31,66,86]

Finally, sometimes although the diagnosis of IVM is made, the VM is in fact not really isolated.[24] In the presence of IVM via prenatal sonography, postnatal imaging has shown a 7% prevalence of undiagnosed findings.[87] Even with prenatal workup and fetal MRI, additional anomalies can be discovered at birth, including white matter signal abnormalities, which may not be detected until after birth, some of which were not visible on MRI until 1 year of age.[59] Neonates with prenatal mild VM have higher cortical volume and reduced white matter volume, suggesting altered cortical development and either delayed or abnormal white matter development.[88] Bloom found a significant linear relationship between ventricle width and decreased mental development index.[89] Fetuses with mild VM and postnatal neurological follow-up showed abnormal, mostly motor disabilities in 12% to 28% of cases and intellective retardation in 5%.[24,90] In addition, studies have demonstrated that up to one-third of cases of moderate IVM have additional findings detected later in pregnancy or postnatally that had a negative impact on neurological outcome.[68] Therefore, IVM may not be normal, and the physiological development of the brain should be taken into account.

Management: Counseling should be performed after all testing has been obtained with knowledge of associated anomalies, genetic abnormalities, and positive infection titers. In the presence of mild IVM, survival is high 93% to 98% and normal neurological development >90% and in isolated UVM normal neurological development in >92%; therefore, counseling should note that outcome is favorable.[77] In moderate IVM, survival is between 80% and 97%, and likelihood of normal neurodevelopment is 75% and 93%; thus, counseling should reinforce that outcome is likely favorable, but there is increased risk of neurodevelopmental disabilities. In the presence of associated abnormalities, prognosis depends on the specific abnormality.[77]

Most cases of mild-to-moderate VM can be delivered vaginally as the head is not macrocephalic. Postnatal management includes confirming the diagnosis and checking for associated disorders that were not detected prenatally. Follow-up should continue until development is established as normal. If delay occurs, neurological consultation and therapeutic intervention should be considered as this can improve outcome.[73] MRI, especially after 1 year of life, may be helpful to evaluate for white matter lesions.[59,88]

Recurrence: Recurrence is rare in isolation but is dependent on the cause and the presence of a genetic or chromosomal aberration.

Severe Ventriculomegaly/Aqueduct Stenosis

Incidence: The birth prevalence of severe VM is 0.3 to 1.5 per 1,000 pregnancies.[91,92] The overall incidence of severe hydrocephalus not associated with Chiari II malformation is 0.2 to 2.1 per 1,000 births.[93] Aqueduct stenosis (AS) is a common cause for fetal VM, accounting for 30% to 40% of cases.[22] X-linked hydrocephalus or hydrocephalus due to stenosis of the aqueduct of Sylvius (HSAS) is the most common hereditary hydrocephalus with an incidence of 1 in 30,000, accounting for 5% to 10% of primary idiopathic hydrocephalus in newborn males.[94]

Pathogenesis: Severe VM may occur due to a malformation in development (such as ACC) or volume loss after an insult (hydranencephaly). However, hydrocephalus is typically the etiology of severe fetal VM, being secondary to a structural or extrinsic obstructive lesion, genetic syndrome, or unknown cause in the presence of communicating hydrocephalus.[95]

AS is the most common cause for hydrocephalus in the fetus and has many etiologies.[22] In the presence of complete aqueduct obstruction/atresia, anomalies of the diencephalon, mesencephalon, brainstem, and/or rhombencephalon often coincide.[96-98] Diencephalosynapsis is present when there is fusion of the thalami and third ventricular atresia, and in mesencephalosynapsis, there is fusion of the colliculi. Both of these entities will cause fetal hydrocephalus. Diencephalic–mesencephalic dysplasia, defined by a poorly defined junction between the diencephalon and the mesencephalon, is likely rare but present in high association with moderate-to-severe obstructive lateral VM.[98] When present, the dysplasia is often associated with a small kinked brainstem and cerebellar vermian hypoplasia.[98] These findings share phenotypic features with *L1CAM*- and *L1CAM*-like syndromes and overlap with findings seen in congenital muscular dystrophies (CMDs) and tubulinopathies, which are also a cause for fetal AS.[98,99]

Rhombencephalosynapsis (RES), which is fusion of the cerebellar hemispheres in conjunction with complete or partial absence of the cerebellar vermis, is identified frequently in fetuses with AS.[100,101] In the presence of AS and no other major anomalies, 50% of fetuses will have RES, most having complete absence of the vermis.[101] In a pathological case series of fetuses with hydrocephalus and AS but absent *L1* mutation, approximately 30% were found to have RES.[94] Conversely in patients with RES, up to 50% of cases have associated AS.[100] The anomaly is believed to be related to a defect in dorsal midline signaling, leading to malformation of the brainstem and cerebellum.[100] The correlation makes sense as both the aqueduct and the vermis originate embryonically from the mesencephalon.

In the absence of aqueduct atresia, there is evidence that AS may occur secondarily due to early fetal hydrocephalus. In the presence of massive lateral ventricular enlargement, the midbrain may be compressed laterally, resulting in aqueductal narrowing.[102] Others suggest that the aqueduct may inherently become narrowed, particularly at the superior colliculus or intercollicular sulcus. In some cases, the aqueduct can be "forked," with branching dorsal and ventral channels.[22] Less commonly, a web can develop along the most inferior recess of the aqueduct.

Acquired AS has many etiologies, including infection, bleeding, or other pathologies, that may incite gliosis and then obliterate the aqueduct.[22] AS may result in rapidly evolving VM in late pregnancy or slowly progressive ventricular dilatation after diagnosis in the second trimester.[97] A more benign pattern is possible in that the VM is stable or even resolves.[97]

In the presence of AS, increased intracranial pressure occurs. When hydrocephalus develops, there is pressure on the developing brain from the ventricular system, but there is also uterine amniotic pressure restraining the expansion of the overlying skull.[11] This increased pressure causes alteration in neuronal proliferation, migration, and delayed maturation.[103] With pressure in the ventricles, there is flattening of the ependyma and interruption of the CSF–brain–barrier with ependymal rupture, edema in the periventricular white matter, and axonal swelling. Ventricular rupture can lead to the formation of diverticula that are lined with pia matter and separated from the subarachnoid space. In the late phase, destruction of nerve fibers, demyelination, gliosis, and volume loss in the white matter and corpus callosum occur.[62]

Etiology: Multiple congenital malformations are responsible for severe VM. Tully et al. categorizes the common causes for hydrocephalus into five groups: Chiari II/myelomeningoceles, AS, posterior fossa crowding or obstruction, cyst or encephaloceles, and communicating hydrocephalus.[104]

Genetic syndromes associated with AS and hydrocephalus are listed in Table 17.1-2, with the most common being the *L1CAM* gene on chromosome Xq28.[93,94] The *L1* gene is related to a wide variety of phenotypes, now known as the *L1* syndrome. This syndrome can result in severe hydrocephalus and death in HSAS but with milder outcomes in MASA (mental retardation, aphasia, spastic paraplegia, adducted thumbs) syndrome, SPG1 (X-linked complicated hereditary spastic paraplegia type 1), and X-lined agenesis of corpus callosum.[94] The gene responsible encodes a neural cell adhesion molecule *L1*, which is involved in neuronal migration, fasciculation, outgrowth, and regeneration. *L1* is also essential for the formation of the pyramids and corticospinal tracts. The mutation primarily affects males, but females are carriers and have a 5% risk for mild manifestations of the disorder.[105] Most cases pathologically have stenosis of the aqueduct, though in the absence of stenosis, it is likely that the aqueduct is narrowed by lateral ventricular compression rather than primary maldevelopment.[94,106]

Acquired causes of VM are multifactorial. Intracranial hemorrhage predisposes to aqueduct obstruction or communicating hydrocephalus. Congenital hydrocephalus is noted at a higher rate in male fetuses, primogeniture, older maternal age, maternal insulin-dependent diabetes, maternal alcohol abuse, and lower social class of the father.[106] Certain maternal medications increase the risk for fetal hydrocephalus and include misoprostol, metronidazole, antidepressants, and isotretinoin.[95] Infection, mainly TORCH, is also a source for severe VM.[20]

Encephaloclastic insults can present as ex vacuo dilatation of the ventricles secondary to severe parenchymal brain loss. In the presence of porencephaly, genetic mutations of the *COL4A1* should be considered.

Diagnosis: In the presence of severe VM, it is important to perform karyotype and infectious testing for TORCH. If HSAS is suspected, screening should be performed for *L1CAM* gene mutations, as the detection rate can be as high as 41%.[94] Microarray testing may also be considered to evaluate for other genetic disorders, particularly the tubulinopathies and CMDs.

Ultrasound: When severe VM is noted, there is typically a mild-to-moderately dilated third ventricle with disruption of the septum pellucidum (Fig. 17.1-8A, B). Measurements are usually not necessary to define the lateral VM, but can be useful to monitor the progression of ventricular dilatation. The third ventricle should be identified, and adjacent thalami closely examined. If the third is not seen and thalami fused, a diagnosis of diencephalosynapsis should be considered. In the presence of the third dilated, the thalami are typically separated, supporting primary aqueduct obstruction.[96]

TABLE 17.1-2   Syndromes Associated with Aqueduct Obstruction

CONDITION	MAJOR CLINICAL	MAJOR IMAGING	GENES	INHERITANCE
HSAS	Adducted thumbs Male	Agenesis CS tracts Abnormal corpus callosum Hypoplastic/ Z brainstem	*L1CAM*	X- linked
Fried syndrome		Basal ganglia calcification	*AP1S2*	X- linked

Alpha-Dystroglycanopathies
  Walker–Warburg
  Muscle–eye–brain
  Fukyama
	Eye findings
	Cleft lip/palate
		Cobblestone lissencephaly
		Z shaped brainstem
		Cerebellar dysplasia/cyst
		Vermian hypoplasia
		Pontine cleft
		Cephalocele
			POMT1 and POMT2,
			POMGNT1 and POMGNT2
			FKTN, FKRP
			LARGE, ISPD
			B3GALNT2, B3NGT1
			B4GAT1,DAG1
			TMEM5
				AR

Tubulinopathy		Dysmorphic basal ganglia Lissencephaly/dysgyria Abnormal corpus callosum Hypoplastic/Z brainstem	*TUBA1A* *TUBA8* *TUBB2B and TUBB2A* *TUBB3, TUBB* *TUBG1*	AD/Sporadic
VACTERL	VACTERL features	Possible RES	*FANCB*	X- linked/Sporadic

HSAS, hydrocephalus due to stenosis of the aqueduct Sylvius; *AR*, autosomal recessive; *AD*, autosomal dominant; *RES*, rhomboencephalosynapsis; *CS*, corticospinal.
Modified from Tully HM, Dobyns WB. Infantile hydrocephalus: a review of epidemiology, classification and causes. *Eur J Med Genet.* 2014;57(8):359–368. Copyright © 2014 Elsevier Masson SAS. With permission.

The aqueduct may be difficult to define, but if visualized, the obstructed area is depicted as an echogenic line without lumen.[96] The fourth ventricle should be normal in size in AS. However, a diamond-like configuration of the fourth ventricle in the presence of a small transverse cerebellar diameter should raise suspicion for RES (Fig. 17.1-8B)

An obstructive pattern is suggested when there is increase in cephalic biometry, rupture of the septum pellucidum leaflets, reduction in pericerebral spaces, and a dilated suprapineal recess.[97,107] At 18 to 20 weeks, the subarachnoid spaces are large, and with increasing gestation, there is progressive decrease in their size. In the presence of severe VM, the supratentorial parenchyma may be compressed between the skull and the dilated ventricles (Fig. 17.1-9A). With increasing ventricular dilatation, disruption of the cortical mantle can occur due to damage from the intraventricular pressure.[11] Evaluation of the brain and extracranial structures is essential to exclude other anomalies. A search of the hands for adducted thumbs in a male fetus may support HSAS (Fig. 17.1-10).

Magnetic Resonance Imaging: On fetal MRI, the aqueduct of Sylvius is well depicted. With obstruction to CSF flow, there can be complete or partial obliteration of the CSF space in the aqueduct (Fig. 17.1-8C).[101] The tectum may be deformed or thickened (Fig. 17.1-9B). The lateral and third ventricles are dilated. If the third ventricle is absent, diencephalosynapsis should be considered. Fetal MRI is accurate at detecting AS, with typical findings related to hydrocephalus, including enlarged inferior third ventricular recess.[108]

Ventricular disruption may be depicted in the posterior mesial aspects of the brain, the location of the choroidal fissure, and weakest part of the ventricular wall (Fig. 17.1-9C).[102] This results in a focal ventricular diverticulum and thinning of the adjacent brain parenchymal mantle, which is lined with white matter, and are thus not consistent with schizencephaly. In a review of fetuses with AS, ventricular rupture can be present in up to 60% of cases, with further risk for new rupture in the presence of increase in lateral ventricular growth.[109] With hydrocephalus, there is loss of septal leaflets, and the corpus callosum is displaced, severely stretched, or partially absent with progressive volume reduction, which corresponds significantly with increase in ventricular rupture.[109] White matter volume loss is present in all cases, and sulcation delayed in over 50%.[109] The subarachnoid spaces may be normal, but progressively decrease with increase in GA.[109] The posterior fossa may be small owing to mass effect, and there is a risk for cerebellar ectopia and Chiari I anomaly in 27% and 6%, respectively.[109] Utilizing MRI and US, accurate diagnosis of severe IVM is possible.[110]

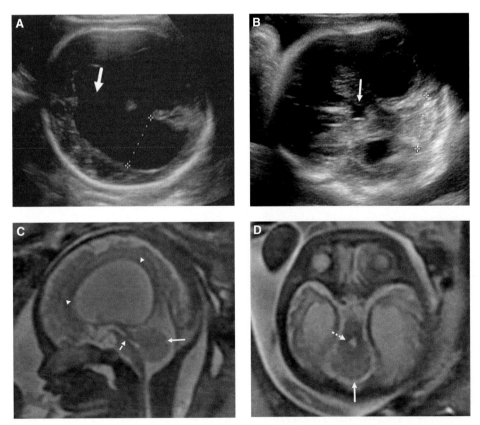

FIGURE 17.1-8: Fetus at 36 weeks with AS and RES. **A:** Axial US demonstrating severe ventriculomegaly with atrium measuring 34 mm and septum pellucidum absent (*arrow*). **B:** Axial US demonstrating dilated third ventricle (*arrow*). The cerebellum measured small, appropriate for a 28-week fetus. Notice the continuous foliation of the superior cerebellum. **C:** Sagittal T2 MRI demonstrating obstruction of the aqueduct of Sylvius distally (*dashed arrow*). Notice that the vermis does not appear normal as the deepest fissure is the horizontal fissure (*solid arrow*), typical for the cerebellar hemispheres. The corpus callosum is thin (*arrowheads*) due to the hydrocephalus. **D:** Axial T2 MRI confirms the absence of cerebellar vermis with continuous foliation across midline (*solid arrow*) consistent with fusion of the cerebellar hemispheres in RES. Notice diamond-shaped fourth ventricle (*dotted arrow*).

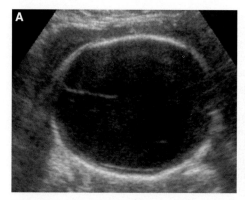
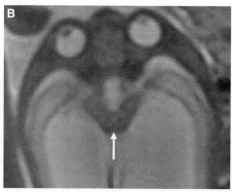
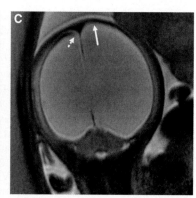

FIGURE 17.1-9: Fetus at 34 weeks with AS secondary to TORCH. **A:** Axial US demonstrating severely dilated ventricles and subtle suggestion of brain parenchyma compressed along the calvarium. It would be difficult to exclude hydranencephaly. **B:** Axial T2 MRI demonstrating heart-shaped midbrain and deformity of tectum (*arrow*), typical of AS. **C:** Coronal T2 MRI demonstrates ventricular rupture of the left lateral ventricle with destruction of adjacent brain parenchyma (*solid arrow*). The ventricular wall is ballooned on the right with thinning of the adjacent brain (*dotted arrow*). The sulcation is significantly delayed for age 34 weeks.

RES is present in high association with fetal AS; therefore, the vermis should be closely evaluated and the primary fissure identified.[101] Clues to RES include diamond-shaped fourth ventricle, absent or small vermis, and fusion of dentate nuclei and cerebellar hemispheres (Fig. 17.1-8D). However, given the limitation in imaging sequences, partial RES is often difficult to confirm prenatal and may be better detected after birth.[101] Brain biometry is extremely important and may provide insight to other anomalies, such as RES. In RES, the transcerebellar diameter is significantly smaller, anterior to posterior pons is decreased, and brain and bone BPD increased.[101] RES can be associated with other malformations, including diencephalosynapsis and Gomez-Lopez-Hernández syndrome, a disorder with parietal/temporal alopecia, possible trigeminal anesthesia, and towering skull due to craniosynostosis.[100] RES is also seen in VACTERL patients; therefore, imaging of the entire fetus is important.[100]

Other anomalies, such as mesencephalic-diencephalic dysplasia and kinked brainstem, may be present, which should raise the suspicion for CMDs, tubulinopathy, and *L1CAM* mutations (Fig. 17.1-11A, B).[98,99] In CMDs or α-dystroglycanopathies, the spectrum is wide, but common findings include cobblestone lissencephaly, white matter changes, polymicrogyria, cerebellar cysts, and orbital anomalies with muscle weakness/hypotonia. The tubulinopathies, particularly genes such as *TUBA1A*, may have similar findings with lissencephaly and polymicrogyria present; however, differentiation may be possible, given dysmorphic appearance of the basal ganglia with absence of the anterior limb of the internal capsule and germinolytic cysts at the caudothalamic groove (Fig. 17.1-11C).[99,111] In the presence of HSAS, hydrocephalus is noted in 100%, stenosis of the aqueduct in 90%, corpus callosum agenesis/hypoplasia in 68%, absence/hypoplasia of the pyramidal tract in 98%, and adducted thumbs in 88%.[94] Fetuses with *L1* mutation will have five or six of these anomalies in 75% of cases; therefore, genetic testing is highly recommended when at least three or four findings are identified.[94] The highest positive predictive findings for HSAS are adducted thumbs; whereas the highest sensitivity is identification of corticospinal tract abnormalities.[94]

Associated Anomalies: Associated abnormalities have been diagnosed in 50% to 65% of severe VM.[14,91,106] Structural anomalies are noted in 43%, the most common being that of the CNS.[91] Chromosomal anomalies are reported between 3% and 15%, and there is a high association with genetic syndromes.[9,91,95] The rate of associated infection in severe VM is 10% to 20%.[14]

Differential Diagnosis: Severe VM is not a diagnostic difficulty, but defining the cause is a differential with multiple etiologies, both common and rare. Hydranencephaly may mimic hydrocephalus, but lack of cerebral parenchyma in the distribution of the anterior circulation is diagnostic. Holoprosencephaly (HPE) is best separated by lack of an interhemispheric fissure.

Prognosis: Children with hydrocephalus of variable causes can eat by mouth in 87%, walk independently in 72% after 2 years of age, require physical therapy in 17%, and with epilepsy in 18%.[104] Neurodevelopmental outcome is, however, worse for those with AS.[104] In the presence of AS, overall mortality is 40%, perinatal mortality of 16% to 23%, and of those who survive, only 10% have normal development.[91,112] Patients with HSAS

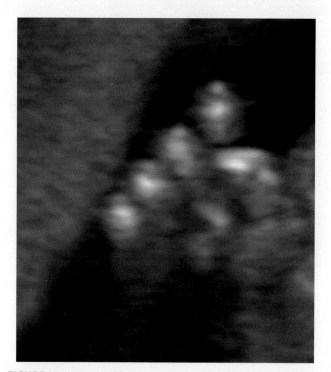

FIGURE 17.1-10: US of fetus at 23 weeks with adducted thumb, aqueduct stenosis (AS), and *L1CAM* mutation.

have variable clinical symptomatology.[113] Some die *in utero* or early infancy. If a child with HSAS survives, severe mental retardation and spastic diplegia are often present; however, affected patients may live into adulthood.[105,113]

Prognosis has been shown to depend on age at diagnosis as progressive increased intracranial pressure can result in further insult to the brain.[106,114] The presence of additional anomalies, karyotype abnormality, and *in utero* progression of VM results in a negative outcome.[106] When additional anomalies are present, only 23.5% are noted to survive, and only 15% of the survivors are normal, with the majority having cerebral palsy, seizures, and impaired motor capabilities.[16,22] However, in the presence of severe IVM, there is a survival rate of 88%, and of those who survive, no disability is observed in 42%, mild-to-moderate delays in 18%, and severe disability in 40%.[115]

Management: In the presence of AS or severe VM, termination may be considered, depending on the severity of dilatation and presence of associated anomalies. As it is known that progressive injury can occur to the brain over time, in the past, decompression of the ventricular system was attempted by performing cephalocentesis and/or the placement of *in utero* shunts.[62,116] However, the ventriculo-amniotic shunts, due to high pressure in the amniotic cavity, sometimes did not allow for drainage of fetal CSF, and the catheters often migrated or obstructed.[100] The main problem, more importantly, became overall case selection as many of the fetuses treated had associated anomalies. Because of controversial results and the inability to define a group of fetuses that would benefit, the procedure was mostly abandoned in 1986.[116] With improved understanding of the natural history of the disease *in utero* and improved shunt technology, revisitation of the intervention is being entertained.

Most fetuses with enlarged cranium require delivery by cesarean section. Postnatally, the majority of infants require ventricular shunting. In the presence of RES, likely due to complete aqueduct

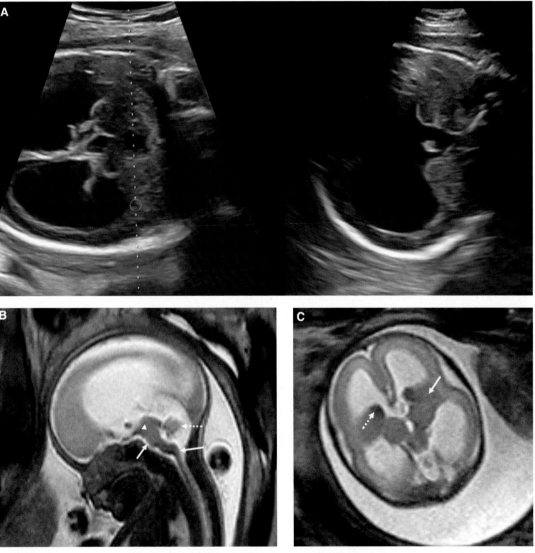

FIGURE 17.1-11: Fetus at 28 weeks diagnosed with *TUBA1A* mutation. **A:** Biplane axial and coronal US demonstrating severe lateral and third ventriculomegaly. **B:** Sagittal T2 MRI demonstrating lack of CSF in the proximal aqueduct (*arrowhead*) and kinked appearance of the brainstem (*solid arrows*). There is also mild vermian hypoplasia (*dotted arrow*). **C:** Axial T2 MRI showing prominence of the ganglionic eminence (*dotted arrow*) with globular poorly defined basal ganglia structures (*solid arrow*) due to lack of development of the anterior internal capsule.

obstruction, early neonatal shunting and feeding assistance are typically required.[101]

Recurrence: The recurrence risk for sporadic cases is 0.5% to 4%.[80] However, in the presence of HSAS, the risk of recurrence is 50% in a male fetus and, in the case of a girl, 50% risk for carrier with low (<5%) risk for manifesting clinical features.[105]

DISORDERS OF VENTRAL INDUCTION

Holoprosencephaly

Holoprosencephaly (HPE) is a complex congenital malformation of the brain and face in which there is impaired or incomplete cleavage of the prosencephalon.

Incidence: HPE is considered the most frequent CNS defect in humans, occurring at a prevalence of 1:250 conceptions.[117] However, as only 3% of fetuses with HPE survive to delivery, the incidence decreases to 1 in 10,000 to 20,000 live newborns.[117] There is a female preponderance, being 3:1 in the alobar type.[117,118]

Pathogenesis: Ventral induction results in the formation of the prosencephalon, followed by separation and development of midline structures. HPE occurs due to failed cleavage of the embryonic prosencephalon in the first 4 weeks of embryogenesis. The primary disorder results from lack of migration of the prechordal mesoderm, which is responsible for induction of ventral forebrain, nasofrontal process, and median facial structures.[119] With the lack of migration, Sonic Hedgehog (*SHH*) gene, which normally signals from the prechordal plate to initiate a cascade to induce appropriate cleavage of the forebrain and eyefield into paired right and left structures, does not occur. HPE represents a defect in dorsoventral patterning, beginning in the area of the hypothalamus but contiguous

along cortex, striatum, midline ventricles, thalamus, and mesencephalon.[120]

HPE is subdivided based on the site and degree of failed cleavage; however, no precise boundaries are present, and intermediate cases may occur.[121,122] Classically, DeMyer divided HPE into three subcategories from severe to mild: alobar, semilobar, and lobar.[123] Of the three classic forms, alobar is the most frequent type, occurring between 40% and 75% of cases, with semilobar second, followed by lobar.[117] However, it is now accepted that HPE represents a wide spectrum of lesions and also includes a more severe defect known as aprosencephaly-atelencephaly and milder forms known as middle interhemispheric fusion, septopreoptic fusion, and microform (Fig. 17.1-12).[120,124] In the following discussion, the types of HPE are described from most severe to mild.

Aprosencephaly and atelencephaly are rare disorders. Aprosencephaly is complete absence of both telencephalon and diencephalon structures, and atelencephaly is the absence of telencephalon structures but presence of some differentiated diencephalic structures, both conditions in the presence of abnormal or normally developed hindbrain.[124] The cause is likely heterogeneous, but the pathology results in destruction of the primordia before growth and patterning of the prosencephalon.[124]

In classic HPE, the ventral forebrain or embryonic floor plate, in the region of the hypothalamus and subcallosal cortex, is most severely affected. Common possible associated midline anomalies include undivided hypothalamus and thalami, undivided deep gray structures, absent or dysgenetic corpus callosum, absent septum pellucidum, and absent or hypoplastic olfactory bulbs and tracts, and optic bulbs and tracts (Table 17.1-3).

In *alobar* HPE, there is a single midline forebrain ventricle and cerebral holosphere with absent midline structures and thalamic fusion. The monoventricle is continuous with a cyst (dorsal cyst), hypothesized to represent remnant third ventricle, velum

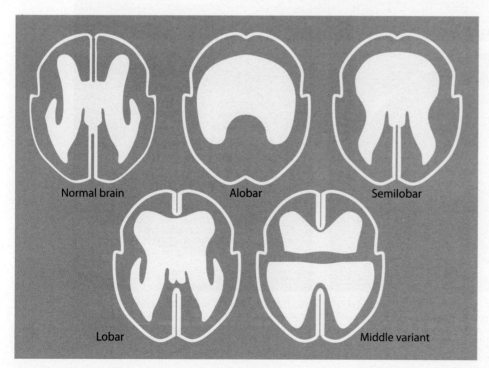

Normal brain   Alobar   Semilobar

Lobar   Middle variant

FIGURE 17.1-12: Diagram of the four major types of holoprosencephaly. (From Volpe P, Campobasso G, De Robertis V, et al. Disorders of prosencephalic development. *Prenatal Diagnosis.* 2009;29(4): 340–354. Copyright © 2009 John Wiley & Sons, Ltd. Modified by permission of John Wiley & Sons, Inc.)

TABLE 17.1-3   Findings in Holoprosencephaly

TYPES	ALOBAR	SEMILOBAR	LOBAR	MIH	SEPTOPREOPTIC
IHF/falx absent	All	Anterior	Hypoplastic anterior	Midportion	Deep
Cerebral nonseparation	All	Frontal	Basal frontal/cingulate	Posterior frontal/anterior parietal	Preoptic/subcallosal
Lateral ventricles	Single	Absent anterior	Rudimentary anterior	Fused midlateral	N/small
		Rudimentary occipital	Normal posterior	N/hypoplastic anterior	frontal
Dorsal cyst	Yes	Variable	Rare	Present 25%	No
Third ventricle	Absent	Small	Present	Present	N
Septum pellucidum	Absent	Absent	Absent/hypoplastic	Absent/hypoplastic	N/hypoplastic/absent
Thalami	Fused	Partial fusion	Divided	Fused 30%–50%	N
Deep gray	Fused	Partial/caudate	Variable	Caudate fused	N
Corpus callosum absent	All	Rostrum, genu, body	Rostrum, genu	Body	Rostrum/genu
Hypothalamus	Fused	Often fused	Likely fused	Separated	Anterior fused
Hippocampal fornix	Fused	Often fused	Fused	Separated	N
Olfactory bulbs and neurohypophysis	Absent	Absent/hypoplastic	Absent/hypoplastic/N	N	N
Optic tracts	N/fused/absent	Absent/hypoplastic	Present	Present	N
Sylvian fissures	Absent	Anterior medial	Anterior medial	Connected over midline	N
Cortical dysplasia/heterotopia	Broad gyri	Occasional broad gyri	Rare midline/frontal	Very common	N
Cerebral vasculature	No ACA MCA Rete vessels	Azygos ACA	Azygos ACA	Azygos ACA	N/azygos ACA
Craniofacial	Severe/mild	Severe/mild	Mild	Hypertelorism	Mild

N, normal; ACA, anterior cerebral artery; MCA, middle cerebral artery; IHF, interhemispheric fissure.
Modified from Hahn JS, Plawner LL. Evaluation and management of children with holoprosencephaly. *Pediatr Neurol.* 2004;31(2):79–88. Copyright © 2004 Elsevier. With permission.

interpositum, or primitive prosencephalic vesicle, demarcated from the ventricular cavity by ridge of cerebral tissue representing hippocampal fornix.[125,126]

In *semilobar*, the defect is localized anteriorly with some posterior interhemispheric fissure, rudimentary lateral ventricles but absent frontal horns, partial fusion of thalami, and variable corpus callosum, usually splenium. Basal ganglia are not completely separated, and there is lack of a normal Sylvian (telencephalic) fissure.[124]

The *lobar* type has noncleavage of the frontal basal lobes and separation of most of the cerebral hemisphere, rudimentary frontal horns, and absent anterior corpus callosum. There is continuity of the cingular cortex crossing midline at the bottom of the interhemispheric fissure.

In the *middle interhemispheric variant (MIH) or syntelencephaly*, there is a defect of the dorsal mesenchyme or the roof plate, resulting in failure of separation of the posterior frontal and parietal lobes with the poles of the frontal and occipital well separated.[127,128] The genu and splenium of the corpus callosum are present, but the body is poorly defined. The Sylvian fissure is abnormal, vertically oriented, and often connected with contralateral side over the vertex.

Septopreoptic HPE is a very mild variation with noncleavage of the septal, subcallosal, and/or preoptic area with no or minimal fusion of the frontal neocortex.[124] An absent or hypoplastic rostrum and hypoplastic genu of the corpus callosum is often present.

Classification is not well defined in less severe ends of the phenotypic spectrum, which include absent olfactory tracts and bulbs (arrhinencephaly), absent septum pellucidum, and hypopituitarism.[124,129]

In addition, with recent molecular data, it has been found that the HPE phenotypic spectrum is very large, including a *microform* variety, encompassing facial malformation such as cleft lip or single median incisor but normal brain.[129] Despite normal brain midline anatomy, some patients affected by microform type may have microcephaly and/or intellectual disability.[130]

HPE is associated with a number of midline anomalies of the face (Table 17.1-4).[123,131,132] There is an 80% correlation with the severity of the HPE and the extent of the facial malformation; thus, in these cases, the "face may predict the brain."[129,133] However, in 10% to 20% of cases, there is no clear correlation between face and brain anomaly subtypes.[117] A*lobar* HPE is highly associated with severe facial abnormalities, such as cyclopia, *semilobar* with premaxillary agenesis, cleft lip or palate, and mild ocular findings, and *lobar* HPE with mild midface malformations, such as pyriform sinus stenosis and choanal atresia. In *MIH*, the face is typically normal or with hypertelorism.

Etiology: Genetic, environmental, multifactorial, and unknown causes appear to be involved in the development of HPE (Table 17.1-5).[117] Chromosomal anomalies account for 25% to 50% of HPE cases.[131,134] The most common association is trisomy 13, representing 75% of cases, followed by triploidy at 20% and trisomy 18 at 1% to 2%.[135] The incidence of chromosomal abnormalities is strongly related to the presence of multisystem anomalies.[136] About 18% to 25% of HPE are syndromic with a single-gene mutation.[122,133] Aprosencephaly/atelencephaly is

also typically sporadic with heterogeneous causes but has also been described in XK aprosencephaly syndrome.[124]

The nonsyndromic or isolated HPE can be inherited autosomal dominant, autosomal recessive, X-linked inheritance, and sporadic.[130,135] In the cases with normal karyotype, genetic mutations have been identified in at least 25% of cases.[130] To date, at least 18 genes and mutations thereof have been shown to cause HPE.[130] The main genes described in HPE include *SHH*, *ZIC2*, *SIX3*, *TGIF*, and *GLI2*, with the most common found at testing for HPE being *SHH*, *ZIC2*, and *SIX3*.[130,137]

Many of the genes in HPE are linked to *SHH* signal networks. *SHH* mutations are detected in 6% of cases of HPE, being the most common gene mutation.[130] The second most common HPE gene is *ZIC2*, which is associated with variable CNS malformations, including syntelencephaly and mild facial anomalies.[129,132] This gene may have a role in editing the response to *SHH* protein signaling but affects the roof plate and dorsal brain structures.[132] New genes associated with HPE have been found important in fibroblast growth factor and ciliary pathways.[130] However, the mutations are always heterozygous, and there is extreme variability in phenotypic outcome, with a similar gene mutation resulting in severe HPE in one person and others apparently normal. Given the variability of expression, it may be that HPE is due to interactions of multiple genetic mutations.[130]

The most common environmental factors that increase the risk for HPE include maternal diabetes and ethanol exposure.[138] Infants of diabetic mothers have a 1% risk (200-fold increase) for HPE.[134] About 10% of individuals with HPE have defects in cholesterol biosynthesis, as cholesterol is required for activation of the *SHH* molecule.[122,134] Infection (especially CMV) and twin

TABLE 17.1-4   Facial Anomalies in Association with Holoprosencephaly

FACIAL DEFECT	FEATURES/ASSOCIATIONS	BRAIN HPE
Cyclopia	Single eye, arhinia, possible proboscis	Alobar
Synophthalmia	Partially fused eyes in single-eye fissure	Alobar
Anophthalmia/microphthalmia	Absent or small eye	Alobar or semilobar
Ahrinia	Absent nose	Alobar or semilobar
Ethmocephaly	Hypotelorism proboscis between eyes	Alobar or semilobar
Cebocephaly	Hypotelorism, single nostril	Alobar or semilobar
Median cleft lip/palate (premaxillary agenesis)	Hypotelorism, flat nose	Alobar or semilobar
Bilateral cleft lip	Philtrum–premaxilla anlage	Alobar/semilobar/lobar
Hypotelorism		All types/microform
Hypertelorism		All types/microform
Eye abnormalities	Iris or retinal coloboma	All types/microform
Flat nose		All types/microform
Mild palate	Lateral cleft, high arch, bifid uvula	All types/microform
Single central incisor	Hypoplasia pyriform aperture	All types/microform

Modified from Dubourg C, Bendavid C, Pasquier L, et al. Holoprosencephaly. *Orphanet J Rare Dis.* 2007;2:1–14. http://creativecommons.org/licenses/by/2.0. Copyright © 2007 Dubourg et al; licensee BioMed Central Ltd.

TABLE 17.1-5 Causes and Conditions Associated with Holoprosencephaly

CHROMOSOMAL

Trisomy 13

Trisomy 18

Triploidy

Trisomy 21

Rare trisomies 22 and 16

Deletions, duplications, unbalanced aberrations
13q deletion
18p deletion
Partial monosomy 14q

SYNDROMIC—MONOGENETIC

Autosomal Dominant

Dysgnathia complex

Pallister-Hall

CHARGE syndrome

Kallmann syndrome

Rubinstein–Taybi

Thanatophoric dysplasia type II

Hartsfield syndrome (HPE, cleft lip/palate, and ectrodactyly)

Steinfeld syndrome (HPE, renal, reduction limb defects, heart disease)

Culler–Jones syndrome (HPE, hypopituitarism, postaxial polydactyly)

Agnathia-otocephaly complex (agnathia, microstomia, ventro-medial ear, HPE)

X-linked

Aicardi

Ectrodactyly

Fetal hypokinesia/akinesia

SYNDROMIC—MONOGENETIC (continued)

Autosomal Recessive

Spinocerebellar ataxia

Ivemark (heterotaxy)

Lambotte syndrome (HPE, microcephaly, growth restriction, facial anomalies)

Meckel–Gruber syndrome

Genoa (HPE and craniosynostosis)

Hydrolethalus (hydrocephalus, absent midline structures, micrognathia, polydactyl, defective lung lobulation)

Pseudotrisomy 13 (HPE, polydactyly syndrome)

Smith–Lemli–Opitz

XK aprosencephaly (aprosencephaly, limb anomalies, hypoplastic genitalia)

NONSYNDROMIC

Familial

Inherited autosomal dominant

Gene mutations, such as *SHH* or *ZIC2*

ENVIRONMENTAL

Retinoic acid

Ethyl alcohol

Salicylates

Estrogen/progestin

Anticonvulsants

CMV

Rubella

Toxoplasma

Maternal diabetes

Maternal hypocholesterolemia

Modified from Simon EM, Barkovich AJ. Holoprosencephaly: new concepts. *Magn Reson Imaging Clin N Am.* 2001;9(1):149–164. Copyright © 2001 Elsevier. With permission.

gestations are also reported in HPE.[131] Despite these known associations, 75% of HPE have no known chromosomal abnormality or molecular basis, and therefore, a "multiple hit" from both environment and genetics is likely.[121]

Diagnosis: When HPE is identified, karyotype should always be performed. If karyotype is normal, genetic counseling with molecular testing may be considered. Prenatal history, detailed family history, and focused examination of the parents may help identify microforms of HPE.[122,134] A search for additional anomalies with US, MRI, and echocardiogram should be performed.

Ultrasound: Transabdominal or transvaginal US can confirm severe HPE as early as 10 weeks.[121,125] Coronal and axial imaging of the brain should be performed to verify noncleavage

of hemispheres and thalami and lack of interhemispheric fissure. In *atelencephaly*, a noncleaved deep gray matter mass is typically present with little delineation of remaining cerebral parenchyma (Fig. 17.1-13A). A helpful marker of *alobar* HPE is the featureless configuration of the monoventricle and dorsal cyst lacking occipital, temporal, and frontal horns (Fig. 17.1-14).[125] The choroid is prominent at this age, and the absence of the normal choroidal "butterfly" configuration may also be a helpful clue.[139]

In the second trimester after 18 weeks gestation when the cavum septum pellucidum (CSP) is normally present, interrogation of this structure is imperative as it is absent in most forms of HPE and can direct imaging and diagnosis.

In *alobar HPE*, there is usually no difficulty in diagnosis with US. There is complete lack of cleavage of the cerebral hemispheres, absence of midline structures, and fusion of basal

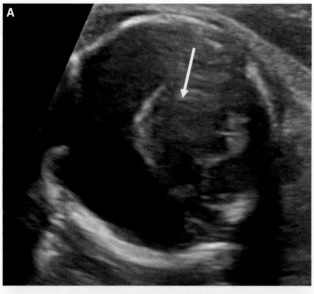

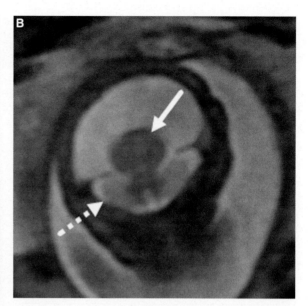

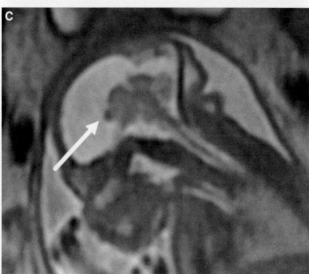

FIGURE 17.1-13: Atelencephaly in a fetus at 27 weeks. **A:** Axial US demonstrating little cerebral tissue but fused deep gray matter structures (*arrow*). **B:** Coronal T2 MRI demonstrating noncleaved mass of supratentorial parenchyma (*solid arrow*) with normal cerebellum (*dotted arrow*). **C:** Sagittal T2 MRI again demonstrating amorphous supratentorial parenchyma (*solid arrow*) with high torcula and small but normally formed posterior fossa structures.

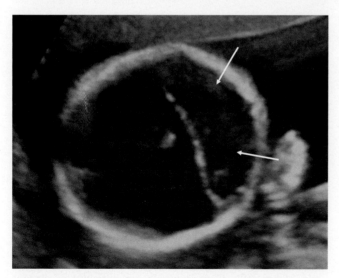

FIGURE 17.1-14: Axial US demonstrating large monoventricle and pancake mantle of brain anteriorly (*arrows*) in a fetus with alobar holoprosencephaly.

ganglia and thalami with a monoventricle. Depending on the amount of cortex, the prosencephalon may encircle the cyst, appearing as a ball, may partially cover the cyst mimicking a cup or be displaced rostrally, assuming the shape of a pancake (Fig. 17.1-15A).[140] Single azygos anterior cerebral artery may be present, and there may be lack of visualization of anterior and middle cerebral arteries, replaced by a network of anomalous vessels. Severe facial malformations are often present.

Defining lesser grades of HPE can be technically more difficult to differentiate from other anomalies by US, especially those with absent septum pellucidum.[134,141] If there is absent cleavage of anterior hemisphere with single anterior ventricle, cleavage of the posterior hemispheres with rudimentary occipital horns, partial falx, and incomplete fusion of the thalami, the diagnosis of *semilobar HPE* should be considered (Fig. 17.1-16A, B).[125,142] Sometimes, a dorsal cyst may be present when thalamic fusion is present.

In *lobar* HPE, a midcoronal US image demonstrates absence of the CSP and central fusion of the frontal horns, appearing as a boxlike-squared shape with flattened roof in communication with the third ventricle (Fig. 17.1-17A, B). The absence of the

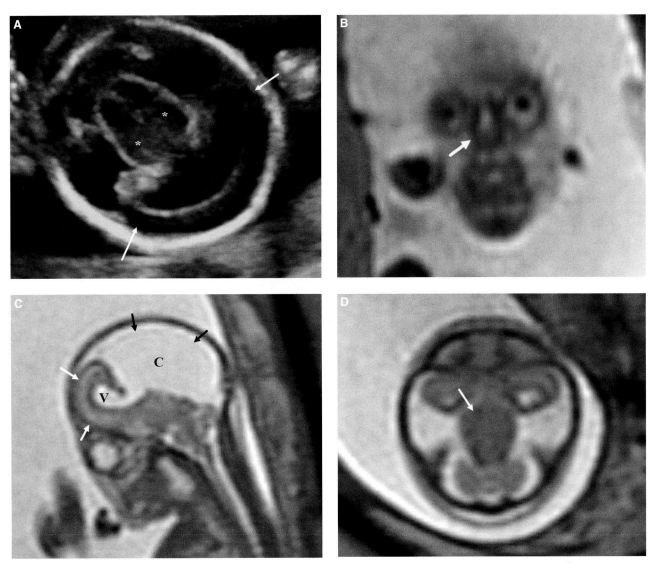

FIGURE 17.1-15: Fetus at 21 weeks with alobar holoprosencephaly. **A:** Axial US demonstrating distorted choroid plexus and cuplike brain (*arrows*). The thalami (*asterisks*) are not separated. **B:** Coronal T2 MRI demonstrating hypotelorism and single nostril (*arrow*). **C:** Sagittal MRI demonstrating cuplike noncleaved cerebral mantle (*white arrows*) and monoventricle *(V)* contiguous with dorsal cyst (C). *Black arrows* denote the wall of the cyst. **D:** Axial MRI demonstrating lack of cleavage of deep gray nuclei, thalami, and midbrain (*arrow*).

falx can be difficult to identify via US. However, the presence of an echogenic rounded structure variably identified within the third ventricle, representing fused fornices traveling from the anterior to posterior commissure, may help secure diagnosis.[143] An additional sonographic sign on midsagittal view is known as the "snake under the skull," representing a single (azygos) anterior cerebral artery displaced by the abnormal bridging inferior frontal tissue.[144]

In *syntelencephaly*, mild-to-moderate VM without CSP is common, but basal ganglia and thalami are normal (Fig. 17.1-18A). Fusion of hemispheres posterior frontal and anterior parietal across the convexity can confirm this variant of HPE (Fig. 17.1-18B).

US is limited in diagnosing the HPE type, being inconsistent in 41% of cases.[118] Prenatal diagnosis detection rate of HPE by US has been noted to be as high as 71% but also as low as 22%.[131,140]

Early diagnosis of facial abnormalities may assist in confirmation of HPE. Sonographic assessment of the fetal face, especially midline structures, is imperative.[145] The orbits should always be

visualized and measured to exclude hypotelorism. The nose, lip, palate, and maxilla (attention for solitary central incisor) should be interrogated. 3D/4D imaging is extremely helpful in further depiction of these anomalies and facilitates parent's understanding of the abnormality (Fig. 17.1-19).[146]

Growth restriction is found in over 50% of fetuses with HPE.[118] Microcephaly is noted in 75% of classic HPE and 50% with syntelencephaly.[122] As the pregnancy progresses, macrocephaly can develop because of disturbances in CSF dynamics.[136] Dorsal cysts can be seen in all classic forms of HPE and syntelencephaly, but is most common in the fetus with alobar HPE. In the presence of severely nonseparated thalami, cyst, and monoventricle, hydrocephalus may develop because of blockage at the third ventricle and aqueduct of Sylvius.[122,147] Exclusion of extracranial anomalies is imperative. In HPE, there is a high incidence of polyhydramnios.[119]

Magnetic Resonance Imaging: It is important to define the grade of HPE, as the image predicts the postnatal function. MRI has a major role in diagnosing HPE, given that the technique

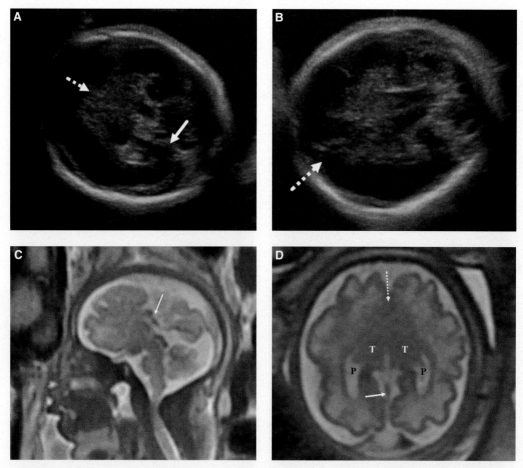

FIGURE 17.1-16: Fetus at 34 weeks with semilobar holoprosencephaly. **A:** Axial US demonstrating falx posteriorly (*solid arrow*). There is poor separation of the brain tissue anteriorly (*dotted arrow*). **B:** More inferior axial image verifies lack of cleavage of the anterior hemisphere (*dotted arrow*) and partial separation of thalami. **C:** Sagittal MRI demonstrating lack of cleavage of cerebral hemispheres anterior and small splenium of the corpus callosum (*arrow*). **D:** Axial T2 MRI demonstrating separation of hemispheres posteriorly (*solid arrow*). The posterior (*P*) horns of the lateral ventricles are normal, but frontal horns and septum pellucidum absent owing to lack of cleavage of the anterior hemispheres across midline (*dotted arrow*). The thalami (*T*) are partially separated, and there is lack of cleavage of the deep gray nuclei.

can identify all forms of HPE by demonstrating areas of cerebral nonseparation, abnormalities of the corpus callosum, and deep gray matter fusion.[148] In addition, MRI may help define subtle but significant facial anomalies and associated brainstem and cerebellar anomalies not visualized by US (Fig. 17.1-15D).[148] Of note, it is not always possible to separate the spectrum of HPE into subcategories, especially in the presence of limited size of the brain and imaging sequences when performing fetal MRI.[148,149]

In the presence of *aprosencephaly* or *atelencephaly*, the rudimentary prosencephalic tissue will be defined as amorphous uncleaved tissue in the midline in the absence of a monoventricle (Fig. 17.1-13B, C).[149] The brainstem and cerebellum are present but torcula elevated.

In the classic forms of HPE, the severity of noncleavage of the cerebral hemispheres (grade) correlates with the severity of nonseparation of the deep gray nuclei.[150] The hypothalamus and caudate nuclei, 99% and 96%, respectively, are the most commonly nonseparated deep gray structures.[122,151] The thalami are noncleaved in 67% of HPE, and the degree of thalamic fusion correlates strongly with the presence of dorsal cyst.[120,140] In most

forms of HPE, except syntelencephaly, there is a low incidence of sulcation or cortical migrational abnormalities, with broad gyri being seen in severe forms, absent Sylvian fissures in alobar, vertical wide Sylvian fissures in semilobar and lobar, and, rarely, cortical abnormalities medial frontal in lobar HPE.[152]

MRI is not typically necessary to diagnose *alobar* HPE, but noncleaved cerebral mass; monoventricle, almost always in continuity with a dorsal cyst; and absence of septum pellucidum, corpus callosum, olfactory bulb/tracts, Sylvian, and interhemispheric fissure are well delineated (Fig. 17.1-15C). The holosphere will have broad gyri with the configuration of a ball, cup, or pancake, depending on the coverage of the ventricle. A high percentage will show nonseparation of the mesencephalon and diencephalon, and 11% will demonstrate a single deep gray nuclear mass, replacing basal ganglia, thalami, and midbrain (Fig. 17.1-15D).[140] There may be either microcephaly or macrocephaly, due to obstructed CSF flow. Cerebral vascular abnormalities are possible but may be difficult to characterize on fetal MRI.[149] Facial anomalies are often severe.

In *semilobar HPE*, there is nonseparation anteriorly with absent anterior interhemispheric fissure, presence of falx

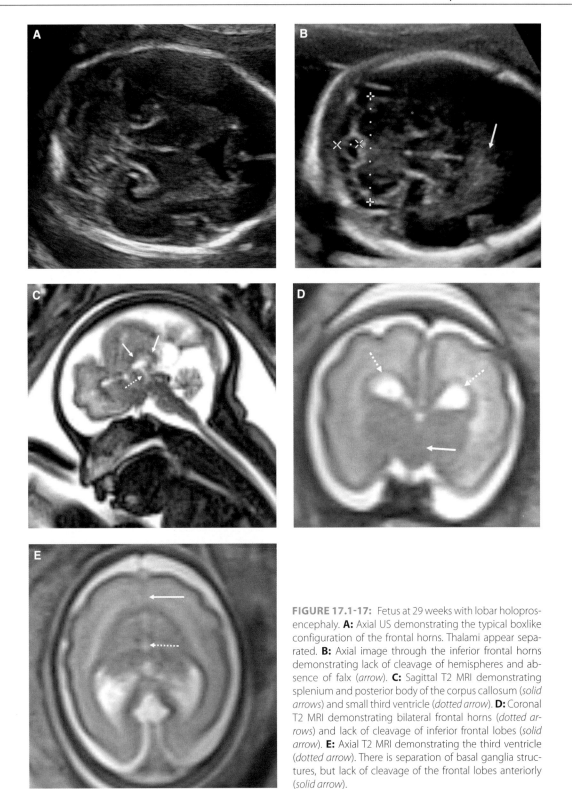

FIGURE 17.1-17: Fetus at 29 weeks with lobar holoprosencephaly. **A:** Axial US demonstrating the typical boxlike configuration of the frontal horns. Thalami appear separated. **B:** Axial image through the inferior frontal horns demonstrating lack of cleavage of hemispheres and absence of falx (*arrow*). **C:** Sagittal T2 MRI demonstrating splenium and posterior body of the corpus callosum (*solid arrows*) and small third ventricle (*dotted arrow*). **D:** Coronal T2 MRI demonstrating bilateral frontal horns (*dotted arrows*) and lack of cleavage of inferior frontal lobes (*solid arrow*). **E:** Axial T2 MRI demonstrating the third ventricle (*dotted arrow*). There is separation of basal ganglia structures, but lack of cleavage of the frontal lobes anteriorly (*solid arrow*).

posteriorly, and partial cleavage of the thalami. The splenium and varying posterior body of the corpus callosum are present, the deep gray is variably separated, but hypothalami are not separated.[149] The septum pellucidum is absent with poor formation of the frontal horns (Fig. 17.1-16C, D). Noncleaved frontal lobes are small, Sylvian fissures are fused to frontal lobes

anterior medial, and azygos artery is present.[149] Less severe craniofacial defects are present.

If the third ventricle is present, thalami are separate, and anterior inferior frontal noncleavage is identified in conjunction with some frontal horn formation and splenium/posterior body corpus callosum noted, then HPE variant is considered *lobar*

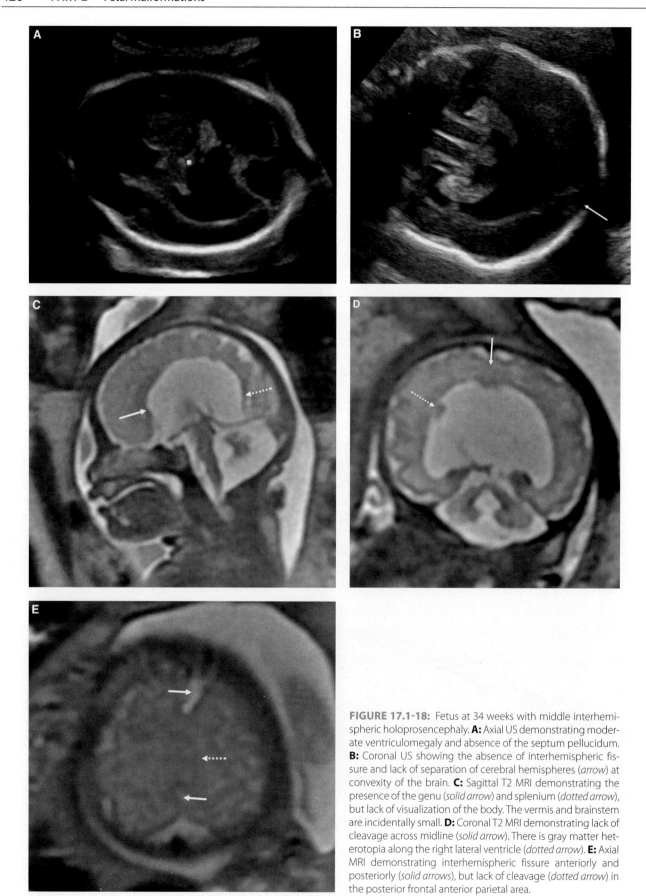

FIGURE 17.1-18: Fetus at 34 weeks with middle interhemispheric holoprosencephaly. **A:** Axial US demonstrating moderate ventriculomegaly and absence of the septum pellucidum. **B:** Coronal US showing the absence of interhemispheric fissure and lack of separation of cerebral hemispheres (*arrow*) at convexity of the brain. **C:** Sagittal T2 MRI demonstrating the presence of the genu (*solid arrow*) and splenium (*dotted arrow*), but lack of visualization of the body. The vermis and brainstem are incidentally small. **D:** Coronal T2 MRI demonstrating lack of cleavage across midline (*solid arrow*). There is gray matter heterotopia along the right lateral ventricle (*dotted arrow*). **E:** Axial MRI demonstrating interhemispheric fissure anteriorly and posteriorly (*solid arrows*), but lack of cleavage (*dotted arrow*) in the posterior frontal anterior parietal area.

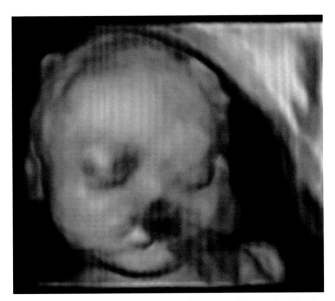

FIGURE 17.1-19: Three-dimensional reformat in a fetus with alobar holoprosencephaly and median cleft lip and palate and absent nose.

(Fig. 17.1-17C, D). In general, more than half of the volume of the frontal lobes should be separated to be considered lobar HPE.[149] Frontal horns are small or absent with septum pellucidum dysplastic or absent but third ventricle present. Fusion of the fornices in lobar HPE is better depicted on MRI than on US.[121] Basal ganglia and thalami are normal, but hypothalami not separated, which may be difficult to detect via fetal MRI.[148] Azygos artery is often present, and, rarely, midline subcortical heterotopia and associated syntelencephaly are noted.[149]

In *syntelencephaly*, the Sylvian fissures are vertical and are connected across the midline vertex of the brain due to lack of separation of the posterior frontal lobe from the anterior parietal lobe (Fig. 17.1-18C–E). Abnormal cortex extending across midline may appear "seam like."[149] There is lack of visualization of the body of the corpus callosum and absence of the septum pellucidum with normal hypothalamus and lentiform nuclei but variably separated caudate and thalami. The third ventricle is formed

but may be contiguous with a dorsal cyst in 25% to 40% of cases, correlating with thalamic nonseparation (Fig. 17.1-20A, B).[149] Two-thirds have subcortical heterotopic gray or cortical dysplasia and often an azygos anterior cerebral artery (Fig. 17.1-18D).[152] Significant craniofacial defects are not described, with the most common finding being hypertelorism.[122]

In *septopreoptic HPE*, there is noncleavage in the septal (subcallosal) or preoptic region, which is demonstrated by abnormal tissue thickening along the anterior wall of the third ventricle (Fig. 17.1-21A, B).[153] The septum pellucidum may be dysplastic but usually present, fornix is dysplastic or thickened, corpus callosum may be thickened or hypoplastic missing rostrum with less hypoplasia genu, and azygos artery is usually present.[153,154] Basal ganglia are normal, but thalami and hypothalami may appear nonseparated. Craniofacial defects include congenital nasal pyriform aperture stenosis and single median maxillary central incisor. However, due to fetal size and limited resolution of the technique, the abnormal tissue along the third ventricle and corpus callosum anomalies may be difficult to reliably detect.[149] In addition, overdiagnosis can occur prior to 28-30 weeks as the third ventricular walls are apposed till this age.

Associated Anomalies: In 93% of cases of HPE, there are abnormalities of the CNS, including migration disorders, displaced hippocampi, and fusion of basal ganglia, which are considered part of the HPE phenotype.[124] Some degree of midbrain noncleavage is noted in 27%, often in association with aqueduct abnormalities that result in hydrocephalus. Endocrine disorders, most commonly related to the pituitary, are present in HPE. Posterior pituitary dysfunction manifesting as diabetes insipidus is the most frequent association.[155]

About 55% of nonsyndromic HPE have multiple congenital defects.[117] HPE is typically associated with other anomalies of the CNS, heart, skeleton, and gastrointestinal tract.[121] Of the CNS, HPE has higher association with neural tube defects, posterior fossa abnormalities, and rhomboencephalosynapsis.[124,156] Of noncraniofacial anomalies, 24% of HPE cases can demonstrate genitourinary defects, 8% postaxial polydactyly, 5% vertebral anomalies, 4% limb reduction, and 4% transposition of the great arteries.[117] Rarely, HPE is seen in the presence of heterotaxy syndromes.[154]

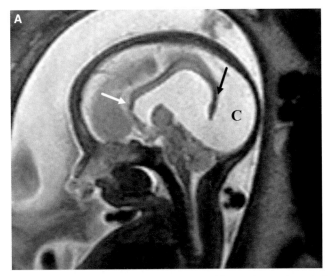
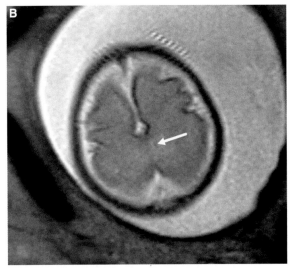

FIGURE 17.1-20: Fetus at 28 weeks with middle interhemispheric holoprosencephaly and dorsal cyst. **A:** Sagittal MRI demonstrating the presence of genu (*white arrow*) and splenium (*black arrow*), but missing body. Note large dorsal cyst (*C*). This fetus also had a large cleft lip and palate. **B:** Axial MRI demonstrating lack of cleavage posterior frontal and anterior parietal area (*arrow*).

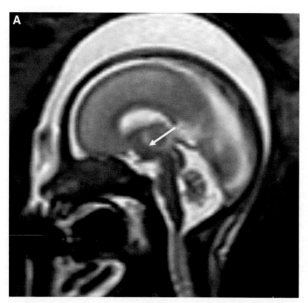
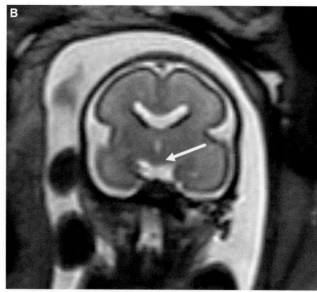

FIGURE 17.1-21: Fetus at 28 weeks with septopreoptic holoprosencephaly. **A:** Sagittal MRI demonstrating abnormal parenchyma (*arrow*) along the anterior aspect of the third ventricle. Notice that the brainstem and vermis are small. **B:** Coronal MRI demonstrating noncleaved tissue (*arrow*) septopreoptic area and also absent septum pellucidum.

Differential Diagnosis: The main differential includes hydrocephalus, hydranencephaly, midline cerebral defects such as agenesis of the corpus callosum (ACC), and septo-optic dysplasia (SOD). Hydrocephalus can be differentiated by demonstrating persistence of the interhemispheric fissure, distinct separate ventricles, and splaying of the thalami. In hydranencephaly, thin cerebral cortex, partially present or deviated falx, and lack of fused thalami are noted. ACC with interhemispheric cyst is best discriminated by normal cleavage of the brain. SOD is differentiated from lobar HPE by identifying normally developed interhemispheric fissure between the anterior hemispheres.

Prognosis: There is a natural loss of fetuses with HPE, being as high as 40%, mostly during the first trimester.[131] Postnatal, there is a direct correlation with the severity of HPE and presence of genetic disorders and outcome.[122] The prognosis at birth is much worse for those with severe facial disorders and cytogenetic anomalies, with only 2% surviving beyond 1 year, compared with 30% to 54% with normal karyotype.[122] In those with normal karyotype, an inverse relationship between survival and severity of HPE and facial anomalies is noted.[121] Most with alobar HPE will not survive beyond infancy, with 89% perinatal mortality rate.[121] Those with milder forms can survive into childhood and beyond and may only have mild cognitive impairment.[122]

Children with HPE have multiple neurological problems, including mental retardation, motor dysfunction, seizure disorder, and endocrine abnormalities. Motor dysfunction including hypotonia, dystonia, and spasticity are present in all types of HPE, with the classic forms only having involuntary movements.[122] The severity of the brain malformation and the higher degree of nonseparation of gray nuclei correlate with the severity of developmental delay and neurological deficit.[129,147] Children with alobar and semilobar have profound impairments, though some with semilobar HPE understand language and communicate with movements or augmented devices.[157] Lobar and syntelencephaly variants may have intellectual disability and behavior problems requiring special education.[157] Approximately 50% of HPE survivors will develop seizure, but only

25% will have chronic epilepsy.[129,147] Fifteen percent will require shunting to treat hydrocephalus.[157]

Feeding problems are common, and the severity of dysfunction correlates with the grade of HPE.[121,129] Seventy-five percent of children with classic HPE (excluding syntelencephaly) have diabetes insipidus, correlating with the degree of hypothalamic nonseparation rather than defects of the pituitary gland.[122,147] This can lead to severe dehydration, electrolyte imbalance, and seizures. Anterior pituitary abnormalities causing growth hormone deficiency and central hypothyroidism may occur, but less commonly.[157] Dysautonomic dysfunction can also be present with instability of temperature, heart, and/or respiratory rate.[129] Frequent causes of demise include infection, dehydration due to uncontrolled diabetes insipidus, intractable seizures, and brainstem malfunction.[158]

Management: Folic acid supplements have been found to have a protective effect; therefore, supplementation 3 months prior to conception is recommended.[157] After diagnosis, genetic counseling is imperative and karyotype and HPE genetic panels, which test for microdeletions and single-gene disorders, should be performed. In the presence of severe HPE, elective termination of the pregnancy may be considered. Cesarean delivery should be considered only for maternal indications in the absence of fetal macrocephaly.

After birth, treatment is based on symptoms and usually requires a multidisciplinary approach. Medical management should focus on endocrine dysfunction, motor and developmental impairments, respiratory issues, seizures, and hydrocephalus. Feeding difficulties are common in neonates with HPE, and about two-thirds of those with lobar and semilobar HPE require gastrostomy tubes.[129] Neurological management is not specific but may require anticonvulsive, physical, and occupational therapies. Surgery is typically performed early to treat hydrocephalus and typically after 1 year of age for cleft lip and/or palate.[129,134]

Recurrence: HPE has a higher recurrence risk than other major malformations, being 6% to 20% after an isolated case in a fetus with normal karyotype and no syndrome.[131,159] If inherited, the risk is 50% in the dominant form or 25% with recessive transmission.[134] Overall risk to the subsequent child with dominant transmission is 37% HPE, 27% HPE microform, and 36% normal phenotype.[160]

COMMISSURES/MIDLINE

Agenesis of the Corpus Callosum

The corpus callosum may be completely absent (agenesis), partially lacking (hypogenesis), globally or partially thin (hypoplastic), hump shaped (dysplastic), or globally thickened (hyperplastic). Agenesis of the corpus callosum (ACC) can also be associated with meningeal dysplasias, such as interhemispheric cysts and lipomas.

Incidence: ACC or hypoplasia of the corpus callosum is reported in 1.8 per 10,000 live births and is seen in approximately 13% of cases referred for VM.[161,162] There is a male preponderance.[162] With regard to race, the order of risk is higher for blacks, then whites, and finally Asian descent.[162] Prenatal complete ACC (cACC) is more commonly diagnosed when compared to partial ACC (pACC).[163] ACC is isolated in approximately 25% to 30% of cases, with the remaining associated with other cerebral or extracranial anomalies.[161,164]

Pathogenesis: The corpus callosum is the largest and most significant of the five midline forebrain commissures, composed of axons that facilitate communication between the cerebral hemispheres. It contains five sections, anterior to posterior: rostrum, genu, body, isthmus, and splenium (see Fig. 9.25 in Chapter 9). The corpus callosum arises from the lamina terminalis, originates in the area of the massa commisuralis between 7 and 20 weeks of gestation, and reaches adult size by 2 years of age (see section "Normal Corpus Callosum" in Chapter 9).

There are many factors that may result in its absence, with three possible mechanisms described: missing or defective development of the massa commisuralis, failure of the axons to form in the cerebral cortex, or inhibited cellular migration due to the absence of normal chemical attractants or repellants or an interhemispheric lesion. It is suspected that cACC is a primary embryological disorder with failure of development of the termina laminalis or massa commisuralis, whereas pACC is a malformation or destructive event in which there is partial absence of the commissural plate or lack of normal growth.[165,166] Hypoplasia is likely secondary to a developmental error or insult later in fetal development.

If the axons develop but are unable to cross the midline because of the absence of the massa commisuralis or a lesion in the interhemispheric space, large heterotopic axons that were destined to cross the corpus callosum lie parallel to the interhemispheric fissure along the medial walls of the lateral ventricles, forming the bundles of Probst. If there is a defect in the commissural axons or their parent cell bodies fail to form in the cerebral cortex, the commissures are absent, Probst bundles are absent, and white matter volume is decreased.[167] If the corpus callosum is partially absent, the posterior aspect is usually deficient. ACC is primary when it is the main pathology; however, it can be secondary if it is due to destructive events or when associated with other major malformations, such as encephaloceles and HPE.[167]

In the presence of ACC, there is distortion of the intracranial architecture. The cingulate gyrus remains everted, and the sulci

of the medial brain extend into the third ventricle, creating a radial or sunburst pattern.[168] When callosal bundles of Probst are present, the lateral ventricles, especially in the frontal area, have a crescentic "steer-horn" appearance.[168] The third ventricle is large and high riding, communicating with the interhemispheric fissure (Fig. 17.1-22). The foramen of Monroe is enlarged. White matter volume loss is nearly uniform, likely representing a primary dysplasia or hypogenesis. In the case of complete absence, the lateral ventricles maintain a straight parallel configuration, with focal dilatation of the temporal, atrial, and occipital horn due to hypogenetic and loose white matter tracts.[169] This ventricular dilatation posteriorly is known as colpocephaly. Abnormalities of the anterior and hippocampal commissures, either being absent or abnormal in size, are common.[170] The hippocampal formations are often incompletely rotated.[169] Malformations in cortical development and delay in sulcation are common, with gray matter heterotopias identified in approximately 29% of cases.[170]

Meningeal dysplasias include cysts and lipomas. Interhemispheric cysts are associated with ACC in 14% to 30% of cases.[170] The cyst can communicate with the ventricles (*type 1*) or lack ventricular continuity (*type 2*). Type 1 lesions represent a single ventricular diverticulation of CSF, which is not typically associated with hemispheric malformations.[166,171] In *type 2* cysts, multilocular complex cysts are present, and these children are more likely to be born with hydrocephalus. Associated brain malformations are more common with type 2, and in the presence of hemispheric asymmetry and polymicrogyria, Aicardi syndrome should be considered.

Up to 3% of patients with ACC will have interhemispheric lipomas.[170] Pericallosal lipomas are favored to develop due to abnormal resorption of the meninx primitiva, which then results in abnormal development of the corpus callosum.[172] Two types are described: the *tubulonodular*, which develop earlier and are round, measuring >2 cm, and the *curvilinear*, which is thin and elongated, measuring <1 cm in diameter. The tubulonodular type is seen with major, usually anterior callosal malformations, and they often have internal calcification and

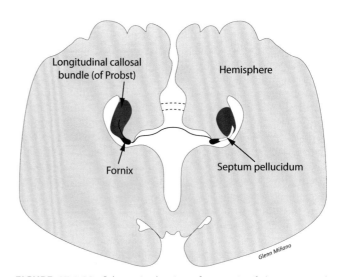

FIGURE 17.1-22: Schematic drawing of agenesis of the corpus callosum. The lateral ventricles demonstrate a crescentic shape due to the presence of Probst bundles. The third ventricle is large, extending upward into the interhemispheric fissure. The cingulate gyri are everted, and sulci do not form.

may be associated with frontofacial anomalies. The curvilinear is overall more common, typically posterior along the corpus callosum with less severe callosal abnormalities.[166,172,173] Goldenhar, frontonasal dysgenesis, and trisomies have been associated with ACC with lipoma.[172,173]

Etiology: There are innumerable causes of ACC, including chromosomal, genetic, infectious, vascular, inborn errors of metabolism, or toxic causes (Table 17.1-6), but the etiology is unknown in more than 50% of defined cases.[174] For 30% to 45% of individuals with cACC and pACC, the cause is chromosomal (10% to 20%) or genetic syndromes (16% to 35%).[175] The most common chromosomal anomalies are trisomies 18, 13, and 21 and mosaic 8.[176] In the presence of additional structural abnormalities and/or advanced maternal age, ACC is seen at a higher frequency with chromosomal disorders.[162] In isolated cases, abnormal karyotype is noted in 4.8% of cACC and 7.5% of pACC.[177]

There are more than 200 syndromes in which ACC is a known association.[176] A well-known disorder with ACC is Aicardi syndrome. This X-linked dominant condition seen primarily in females and in males with Klinefelter syndrome (XXY) is due to a balanced translocation of the X chromosome and is characterized by infantile spasms, ACC, and chorioretinal lacunae. The presence of ACC with polymicrogyria; periventricular heterotopia; cysts of the choroid plexus and posterior fossa, pineal, and/or interhemispheric region; microphthalmia; asymmetry of the hemispheres; and abnormal electroencephalogram (EEG) is highly suggestive of Aicardi syndrome.[178] In the presence of cortical malformation and ACC, tubulinopathy should also be considered.

Metabolic disorders, fetal infections, or *in utero* exposure to teratogens, such as fetal alcohol syndrome and maternal diabetes, have been described with ACC. Infants born prematurely have an almost fourfold higher prevalence.[162]

Diagnosis: Fetal karyotype should be performed to exclude chromosomal anomaly. Directed genetic panels, exome and whole-genome sequencing should be considered.

Ultrasound: In the first trimester, US at 11 to 14 weeks can provide clues to the presence of ACC. Normal anatomy of the pericallosal arteries on the sagittal plane demonstrates the vessels arising from the anterior cerebral arteries to curve posteriorly following the normal anatomy of the corpus callosum.[179] Lack of visualization of the normal pericallosal artery raises the suspicion of ACC (Fig. 17.1-23A, B).[179] With ACC, the midbrain diameter is typically increased and falx diameter decreased, yielding a high midbrain-to-falx diameter ratio.[180] Visualization of the pericallosal artery and a midbrain-to-falx ratio of <95% or 0.79 has, respectively, a 98% and 100% sensitivity in diagnosis of the presence of the corpus callosum.[181]

In the second trimester, the diagnosis of a callosal abnormality is typically suggested by the presence of mild-to-moderate VM and abnormality of the septum pellucidum.[182] Direct visualization of the corpus callosum is best via coronal or sagittal imaging but can be difficult prior to 22 weeks (Fig. 17.1-24).[183] The sensitivity in identifying ACC by direct visualization is variable in the literature, ranging from 28% to 85%.[184] 3D reformats of axial images in the sagittal plane are helpful, or in the presence of a cephalic fetus, transvaginal US can increase visualization.

TABLE 17.1-6   Common Etiologies for Agenesis of Corpus Callosum

GENETIC DISORDERS

Consistently Associated with ACC

Aicardi syndrome—chorioretinal lacunae, infantile spasms

Andermann syndrome—peripheral neuropathy, dementia

Acrocallosal syndrome—hallux duplication, polydactyly, craniofacial

Calloso-genital dysplasia—coloboma, amenorrhea

Shapiro syndrome—ataxia, drowsiness

CRASH/L1CAM—hydrocephalus, adducted thumbs

Inconsistently Associated with ACC

Meckel–Gruber—encephalocele, polydactyly, polycystic kidneys

Rubinstein-Taybi—broad thumbs and great toes, microcephaly

Sotos syndrome—physical overgrowth, craniofacial

Fryns—congenital diaphragmatic hernia, pulmonary hypoplasia, craniofacial changes

Tubulinopathy

INBORN ERRORS OF METABOLISM

Glutaric aciduria type 2

Neonatal adrenoleukodystrophy

Nonketotic hyperglycinemia

Pyruvate dehydrogenase deficiency

CHROMOSOMAL DISORDERS

Trisomies 18, 13, 21 and 8

TERATOGENS

Fetal alcohol syndrome

Cocaine

Data from Bedeschi MF, Bonaglia MC, Grasso R, et al. Agenesis of corpus callosum: clinical and genetic study in 63 young patients. *Pediatr Neurol*. 2006;34(3):186–193.

When the corpus callosum cannot be directly visualized, high suspicion for the diagnosis is via indirect signs (Fig. 17.1-25). The indirect signs of ACC include the following[182,183,185]:

- Absent septum pellucidum identified as early as 17 to 18 weeks
- VM with disproportionate dilatation of the occipital horns, creating a teardrop configuration (colpocephaly)
- Increased distension of the interhemispheric fissure with separation of the lateral ventricles and both medial and lateral walls aligned parallel to the midline
- Concave appearance of the medial, especially anterior horns of the lateral ventricles, due to protrusion of the cingulate gyrus and Probst bundles
- Upward displacement of a variably dilated third ventricle
- Radial arrangement of medial cerebral sulci
- Abnormal appearance of the pericallosal artery

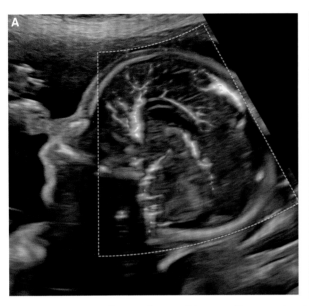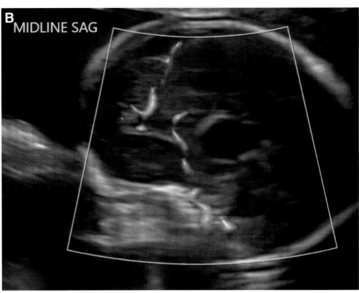

FIGURE 17.1-23: **A:** Fetus with normal corpus callosum and pericallosal artery anatomy. **B:** Fetus with agenesis of the corpus callosum and lack of normal curvature of the pericallosal artery. (Courtesy of HaiThuy Nguyen, MD.)

However, these indirect findings may be absent early in the second trimester, with colpocephaly often not apparent until 26 weeks and radial arrangement of the medial sulci until third trimester.[183]

Although the septum pellucidum is absent in cACC, in pACC, it is often abnormally shaped and short and wide.[186] Fetuses with a normal corpus callosum have a length-to-width ratio of the septum pellucidum of >1.5 in the second half of

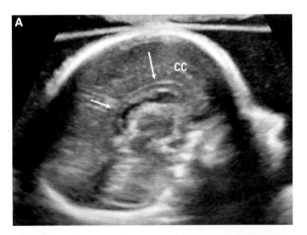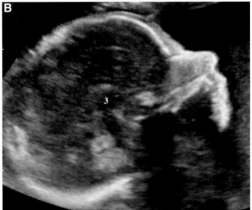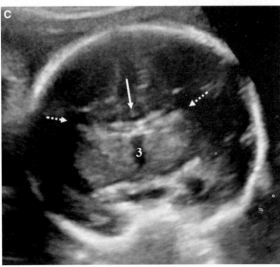

FIGURE 17.1-24: Twin gestation at 30 weeks, one with agenesis of the corpus callosum. **A:** Sagittal US in twin with normal corpus callosum (*arrows*). **B:** Sagittal US in twin with agenesis of the corpus callosum showing absent corpus callosum and prominent third (*3*) ventricle. **C:** Coronal US demonstrating typical findings of ACC, including crescentic frontal horns (*dotted arrows*), lack of corpus callosum across midline (*solid arrow*), and enlarged third (*3*) ventricle.

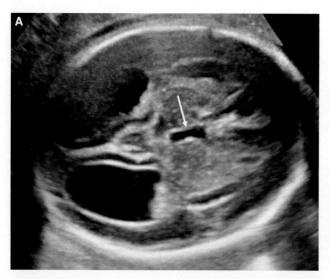
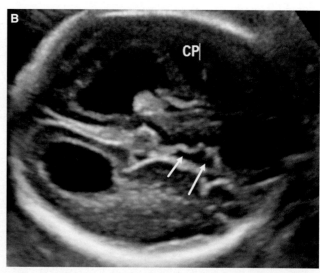

FIGURE 17.1-25: Indirect signs of agenesis of the corpus callosum. **A:** Axial US demonstrating colpocephaly and dilatation of the third ventricle (*arrow*). No septum pellucidum was identified. **B:** Axial US through dilated posterior ventricular horns with prominent interhemispheric fluid (*arrows*). *CP,* choroid plexus.

gestation. Most fetuses with pACC have decreased septum pellucidum ratio, which can be utilized to assist in diagnosis.[186] An important pitfall in sonography is that in pACC or cACC, dysplastic or displaced leaflets of the septum pellucidum and fornix may simulate a normal cavum, and therefore, direct visualization of the corpus callosum with sagittal imaging in conjunction with pericallosal color Doppler may be required.[187,188] However, using expert sonography with 3D reformation and comparison with normative callosal values, hypogenesis and hypoplasia can be diagnosed.[189]

In the presence of interhemispheric cyst, the third ventricle can be mildly dilated or significantly enlarged. The cyst may be simple and communicate with the third or lateral ventricles (Fig. 17.1-26A) or may be complex multilocular without

ventricular communication (Fig. 17.1-27A). Lipomas are nodular or curvilinear echogenic masses within the pericallosal sulcus.[190] The larger, usually tubulonodular lipomas are more easily detected as echogenic masses, which can have spiculated margins with or without extension into the frontal horns or the choroid plexus (Fig. 17.1-28A).[172,173] Curvilinear are smaller, and since early hypoechoic brown fat is replaced over time by echogenic white fat, the lipoma is often not seen in the second trimester. Clues to its presence would be short, thick, or dysgenetic corpus callosum, with improved visualization of the lipoma as the lesion grows in the third trimester.[173,190]

In a recent study when a dedicated neurosonogram was performed, particularly with transvaginal and sagittal views, there is a high consistency of 91% between US and fetal MRI in the diagnosis of corpus callosum anomalies.[163] Another study found that

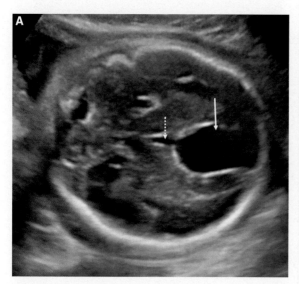
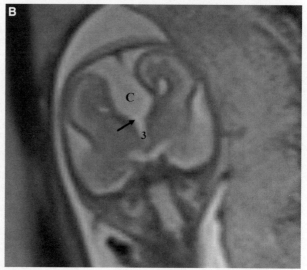

FIGURE 17.1-26: Type I interhemispheric cyst in a 20-week fetus with agenesis of the corpus callosum. **A:** Coronal oblique US demonstrating simple interhemispheric cyst (*solid arrow*) in continuity with the third ventricle (*dotted arrow*). **B:** Coronal T2 MRI verifies cyst *(C)* and confirms communication (*arrow*) with the third *(3)* ventricle.

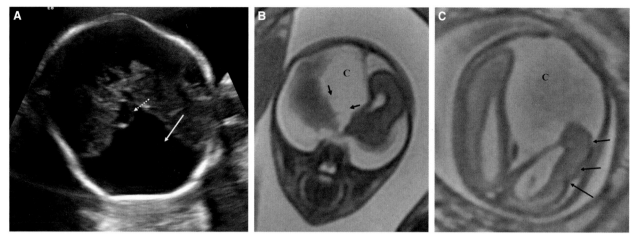

FIGURE 17.1-27: Fetus at 23 weeks with agenesis of the corpus callosum and type II interhemispheric cyst. **A:** Axial US demonstrating a large interhemispheric cyst (*solid arrow*) with septation (*dotted arrow*) midline. **B:** Coronal MRI SSFP demonstrating small septated areas (*arrows*) deep in the interhemispheric cyst *(C)*. No communication with ventricular system was noted. **C:** Axial T2 image demonstrating large cyst *(C)*. The left hemisphere is small with abnormal cortical lobulation (*arrows*) consistent with migrational abnormality.

both US and MRI can accurately classify type of corpus callosum abnormality; however, a third-trimester MRI detected additional anomalies in 15% of cases.[191]

Magnetic Resonance Imaging: Fetal MRI is useful in evaluation of the corpus callosum and has high sensitivity in confirming the presence or absence of the structure and identification of associated anomalies.[184] A recent comparative study showed diagnostic accuracy for detecting corpus callosum deficiency with US at 34% and for MRI 94%, with MRI having a significant effect on clinical management in 44%.[192] In prior studies, fetal MRI has identified an intact corpus callosum in about 20% of cases referred for ACC.[193] MRI has also been shown to identify additional brain anomalies, especially migration anomalies, in 63% to 93% fetuses with ACC that were not apparent on US (Fig. 17.1-29).[193,194]

Prenatal MRI can depict the common intracranial direct and indirect signs that are present with this pathology (Fig. 17.1-30). However, one must remember that the rostrum is difficult to define in greater than 50% of cases and that the flexion of the genu is frequently poorly seen in early gestation.[195] Hypoplasia of the

corpus callosum, often seen in conjunction with volume loss, may be difficult to detect, given the thin caliber of the normal fetal corpus callosum.

Sulcation delay likely represents white matter dysgenesis but often is associated with good neurodevelopmental outcome. In fact, sulcation delay is seen at a high frequency in fetuses with ACC in the third trimester, likely because of failed commiseration and not because of additional brain malformations.[196] As noted in postnatal studies, the hippocampus is underdeveloped and smaller in fetuses with cACC and pACC.[197] In addition, with isolated ACC, other commissures may be absent, though most cases demonstrate the presence of the anterior commissure and approximately half with a hippocampal commissure with or without rudimentary body of the corpus callosum.[198]

If delay in sulcation is excluded, only 69% of ACC cases have additional anomalies via fetal MRI.[196] Associated malformations detected on fetal MRI include cortical developmental defects (40%), cerebellar malformations (30%), interhemispheric cysts (20%), and microcephaly (9%).[164] Cortical dysplasias, commonly polymicrogyria in the frontal

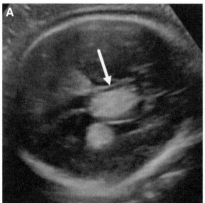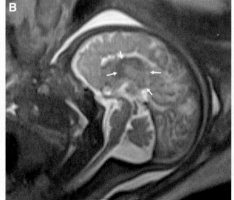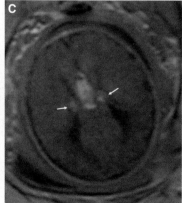

FIGURE 17.1-28: Agenesis of the corpus callosum and tubulonodular lipoma of a fetus at 35 weeks. **A:** Axial US demonstrating echogenic midline mass (*arrow*) with prominent choroid plexus. **B:** Sagittal T2 MRI demonstrating ACC with heterogeneous hypointense (*arrows*) mass in the midline. **C:** Axial T1 MRI demonstrating hyperintense mass in midline and small nodules extending into the choroid (*arrows*).

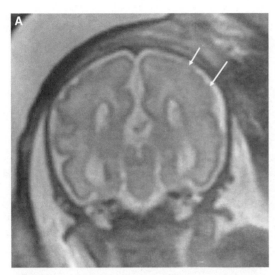
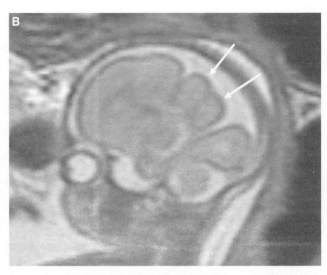

FIGURE 17.1-29: Migrational anomaly in two fetuses with ACC. **A:** Fetus at 30 weeks. Coronal T2 MRI demonstrating irregularity and poor gray white differentiation left parietal area (*arrows*) consistent with polymicrogyria. Compare with the opposite normal right side. **B:** Sagittal MRI in fetus at 24 weeks with ACC and abnormal broad gyri and deep sulci (*arrows*) right parietal.

lobes, are more frequently seen in cACC rather than pACC.[164] Approximately 33% have disorders of the brainstem, often in conjunction with cerebellar pathology (Fig. 17.1-31).[194] Severe VM with corpus callosum deficiency is commonly associated with multiple malformations, while mild-to-moderate VM is more likely to be isolated.[164]

MRI can also define characteristics and extent of associated interhemispheric cysts and lipomas. In type 1, the cysts are isointense to CSF and communicate with the ventricle (Fig. 17.1-27B), whereas type 2 cysts present as multiple cysts demonstrating higher signal than CSF on T1 and heterogeneous signal on T2 imaging and do not communicate with the ventricular system (Fig. 17.1-28B, C). Tubulonodular lipomas due to size will demonstrate typical hyperintense signal on T1 and hypointense signal on T2 and may extend into the choroid plexus (Fig. 17.1-29B, C). However, curvilinear lipomas are

thinner and are often T1 isointense on prenatal MRI, likely due to size and brown fat content, and therefore may be better seen on postnatal MRI when they are T1 hyperintense.[190,199]

In the presence of focal abnormal sulcation morphology, 42% of cases of ACC on prenatal MRI have been found to be associated with multiple brain anomalies and a syndrome.[194] In 25% of ACC cases, additional findings identified by fetal MRI led to a diagnosis of a specific disorder or syndrome.[193] Fetal US and MRI are helpful in suggesting the diagnosis of Aicardi by evaluating for choroid plexus cysts, microphthalmia, asymmetric hemispheres, and cortical malformations (Fig. 17.1-32). In 10% of ACC cases, destructive changes may suggest acquired injury.[194]

Associated Anomalies: Both intracranial and extracranial anomalies are seen in corpus callosum disorders (Table 17.1-7).

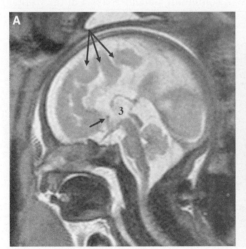
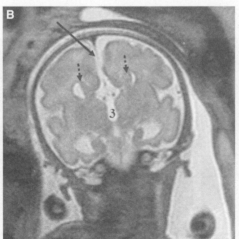
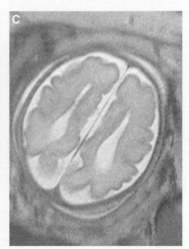

FIGURE 17.1-30: MRI of fetus at 30 weeks with agenesis of the corpus callosum. **A:** Sagittal MRI showing the absence of the corpus callosum and missing hippocampal commissure and fornix. Anterior commissure is present (*arrow*). Notice radial arrangement of gyri (*converging arrows*) and prominent third *(3)* ventricle. **B:** Coronal MRI demonstrating prominent the third *(3)* ventricle and interhemispheric fluid (*arrow*). Probst bundles are noted (*dotted arrows*) adjacent to crescentic frontal horns. No cavum septum pellucidum. Hippocampi are incompletely rotated. **C:** Axial MRI demonstrating parallel configuration of the lateral ventricles consistent with colpocephaly.

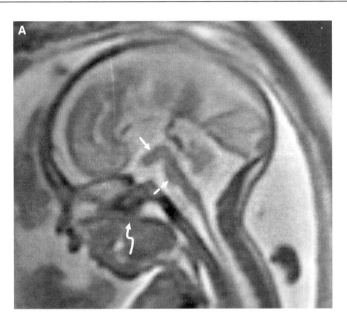
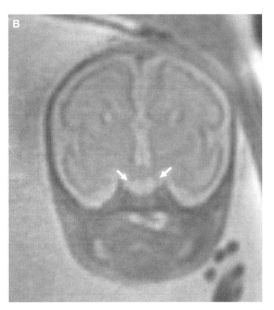

FIGURE 17.1-31: Fetus at 30 weeks with agenesis of the corpus callosum and epignathus. **A:** Sagittal T2 image showing ACC with small brainstem (*dotted arrow*). Cerebellar vermis also measured small. The hypothalamus is thick (*arrow*). There is heterogeneous tissue in the area of the palate (*curved arrow*). **B:** Coronal T2 image demonstrating two infundibula (*arrows*) consistent with duplicated pituitary.

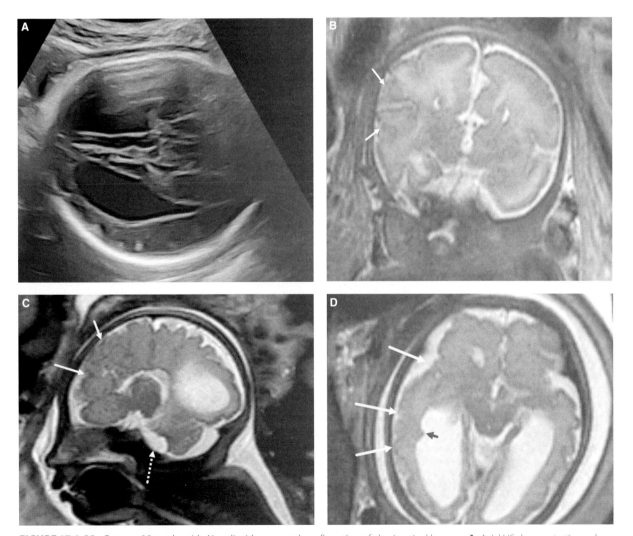

FIGURE 17.1-32: Fetus at 35 weeks with Aicardi with postnatal confirmation of chorioretinal lacunae. **A:** Axial US demonstrating colpocephaly and parallel ventricles consistent with agenesis of the corpus callosum. **B:** Coronal MRI demonstrating irregularity of the cortex, especially in the Sylvian fissure area, (*arrows*) consistent with polymicrogyria. **C:** Sagittal MRI again showing abnormal irregular cortex (*white arrows*) consistent with polymicrogyria. There is also a cyst in the posterior fossa (*dotted arrow*). **D:** Axial MRI demonstrating gray matter heterotopia (*black arrow*) and polymicrogyria (*white arrows*).

TABLE 17.1-7   CNS and Extra-CNS Abnormalities with Agenesis of Corpus Callosum

CNS ABNORMALITIES	EXTRA-CNS ABNORMALITIES
Periventricular nodular heterotopia	Craniofacial
Pachygyria	Skeletal
Hypothalamic, pituitary, and optic hypoplasia	Cardiac
Polymicrogyria	Ocular
Dandy–Walker malformation	Genital
Cerebellar vermis agenesis	Renal
Pontine hypoplasia	

Data from Bedeschi MF, Bonaglia MC, Grasso R, et al. Agenesis of corpus callosum: clinical and genetic study in 63 young patients. *Pediatr Neurol.* 2006;34(3):186–193.

Associated brain malformations are noted in nearly 50% of cases, which include disorders of neuronal organization, posterior fossa malformations, and neural tube defects.[161,162,200] Extra-CNS anomalies are present in approximately 65% of ACC patients.[175] Common organ systems include eye (88%), skull (64%), craniofacial (50%), and cardiac (34%).[200]

Differential Diagnosis: ACC should be differentiated from other causes of VM. In the presence of ACC with an interhemispheric cyst, differential would include enlarged CSP et vergae, arachnoid cyst, porencephaly, ventricular rupture in obstructive hydrocephalus, and vein of Galen malformation. Interhemispheric cysts may be confused with the dorsal sac of HPE, but the morphology of the separated frontal horns aids in differentiation. Hydrocephalus and ventricular rupture, particularly in fetuses with AS, may also mimic ACC with interhemispheric cyst. In the presence of a lipoma, differential diagnosis includes hemorrhage or rare tumor such as craniopharyngioma or choroid plexus papilloma.

Prognosis: Outcome is dependent on multiple factors, including the presence of microcephaly, genetic abnormality, and/or associated anomalies.[174] In the presence of ACC with syndrome or chromosomal abnormalities, the outcome is typically poor.[165] Children with Aicardi have significant developmental delay, seizures, and shortened life span, with survival of 76% at 6 years and 40% at 14 years, demise most commonly due to respiratory infection.[178]

A main determinant in adverse outcome is the presence of associated CNS anomalies.[176] Children with ACC and associated migrational disorder are more likely to have moderate-to-severe developmental delay.[200] It is controversial whether pACC versus cACC has better outcome, and it may be that it is more dependent on the presence of additional anomalies.[200] When reviewing all patients with ACC, moderate-to-severe developmental delay is described in 80%, epilepsy in 35% to 45.8%, cerebral palsy in 37.5%, microcephaly in 33.3%, and visual and hearing defects and behavioral disorders in many.[174,201] However, a recent study of school-aged children noted 50% with intellectual, academic, executive social, or behavioral difficulties and 20% functioning at a level equivalent with typical children.[202]

In isolated ACC, a normal neurodevelopmental outcome may be possible. A recent systemic review noted that isolated cACC confirmed at birth had normal outcome in 76%, with borderline-to-moderate impairment in 16% and severe disabilities in 8%.[177] Epilepsy was noted in 6.8% and abnormal language in 8%. Prenatal isolated pACC confirmed at birth had normal development in 71%, mild-to-moderate impairment 15%, and severe disabilities 12.5%. Epilepsy was found in 16% and coordination and language abnormal in 12%.[177] However, even though a prenatal diagnosis of isolated ACC is provided, risk of additional anomalies detected after birth is 5% in cACC and 15% in pACC.[176] Also, some individuals with isolated ACC have deficits in expressive language, which affect the social and behavioral domain, that may place them in the spectrum of autism, attention deficit disorder, and schizophrenia. These disorders usually do not become evident until preteenage years.[176]

In ACC with interhemispheric cyst, seizures are noted in less than half of patients.[203] It has been suggested that type 1 cysts tend to have more developmental delay and neurological deficits than type 2; however, outcome is likely dependent on associated anomalies and the development of hydrocephalus.[171,203] In the presence of associated lipoma, neurological status is variable, depending on the type of lipoma, associated callosal anomalies, and other malformations. Overall, 50% of children with ACC and lipoma have seizures and psychological disorders.[172]

Management: Diagnosis should be performed at a center with expertise in separating isolated versus nonisolated cases and with available genetic testing and counseling. At birth, evaluation for extracerebral malformations should be performed to exclude underlying genetic syndrome. If no other abnormalities are detected and the ACC is isolated, close clinical follow-up is suggested. If anomalies are present, postnatal MRI and evaluation by a multidisciplinary team, including neonatologists, neuroradiologists, neurologist, and geneticist, is indicated. Comorbidities, including epilepsy and feeding problems, should be addressed.

Recurrence: In most cases of ACC, recurrence is moderately increased at 5% to 10%.[204] If the etiology is syndromic, recurrence is dependent on the type of transmission. Risk is high in a family with previous child diagnosed with Aicardi syndrome.

Septo-optic Dysplasia

Septo-optic dysplasia (SOD), also known as hypoplastic optic nerve syndrome or De Morsier syndrome (described pathology in 1959), is a disorder of midline anomalies that include a triad of findings of complete or partial absence of the septum pellucidum, optic nerve hypoplasia, and hypothalamic–pituitary abnormalities.

Incidence: SOD is fairly rare, with an incidence of 1.9 to 2.5 per 100,000 live births, with equal prevalence in males and females.[205] The disorder is noted at a higher incidence when there is bleeding early in pregnancy, low socioeconomic status, and/or in children born to younger mothers.[205,206]

Pathogenesis: The septum pellucidum is intimately associated with the corpus callosum and is also formed from the lamina terminalis. The structure is bounded by the corpus callosum anteriorly and superiorly and by the fornix inferiorly and posteriorly. The septum pellucidum forms the medial border of the frontal horns of the lateral ventricles, the posterior margin defined by the foramen Monroe. Each leaflet from lateral to medial has a ventricular ependymal lining, thin layer of gray matter, thin layer of white matter, and inner pial layer.

SOD is a heterogeneous condition with pathogenesis uncertain.[207] Many support that SOD is due to a vascular disruption sequence.[208,209] As the optic nerve develops at the seventh week and septum pellucidum between 15 and 21 weeks, differences in timing would make a developmental anomaly related to ventral induction unlikely.[209] In addition, given that the structures affected in SOD are in close proximity and the common association with porencephalic/schizencephalic defects, a vascular etiology may better explain SOD.[209]

The phenotype of SOD is variable, with the diagnosis obtained by identifying two or more of the triad of findings. Usually, the diagnosis is confirmed postnatal by imaging and ophthalmology when hypoplasia of the optic discs is present in conjunction with partial or complete absence of the septum pellucidum. Pituitary dysfunction is often in association with structural abnormalities, such as ectopic or absent posterior pituitary, truncated or absent infundibulum, and hypoplastic anterior lobe.

Approximately 30% to 41% of patients have the triad of findings, approximately 65% have hypopituitarism, and 60% to 75% demonstrate absent septum.[207,208,210] About 75% to 100% of patients with SOD have optic nerve hypoplasia (gold standard for the diagnosis), which may be unilateral (12%) or more commonly bilateral (88%).[207,210] SOD can also be associated with absence, hypogenesis, or hypoplasia of the corpus callosum.[211]

Two distinct groups of SOD are noted. One group has complete or partial absence of the septum pellucidum in conjunction with malformations of cortical development, usually polymicrogyria, schizencephaly and gray matter heterotopia.[210] The term "SOD-plus" is sometimes utilized to describe these complex cases and is seen in up to greater than 75% of those affected.[210,212] The second group has complete absence of the septum, hypoplasia of the cerebral white matter, normal cortex, and often pituitary dysfunction.[213] These findings overlap with HPE, possibly representing a milder form of lobar HPE.

Finally, as more fetal imaging is being performed, it has been discovered that there are cases where the septum pellucidum is absent but there are no associated pituitary or optic nerve anomalies, and these cases can be isolated postnatal and likely should not be designated SOD.[214–216]

Etiology: SOD is primarily sporadic with the etiology likely multifactorial. Environmental factors that may result in intrauterine vascular disruption include viral infections, teratogens such as exposure to alcohol or drugs, maternal diabetes, antiepileptic drugs, and quinidine.[207,208,217] Genetic abnormalities have been found in 1% of SOD.[218] Rare autosomal recessive and dominant familial cases have been cited.[5] A gene found to cause SOD, documented in familial cases, is the *HESX1*, which is produced by tissue adjacent to the developing prosencephalon and is suggested to be important for proper induction of the forebrain and midline.[207] The *HESX1* gene is also one of the earliest markers of the pituitary primordium and may explain the associated hypopituitarism. *SOX2* and *SOX3* genes are also necessary for development of the pituitary, and these genes have been implicated in pituitary anomalies seen in SOD.[207,219] Many other genes recently

cited in association with SOD include *OTX2, PROKR2, FGF1,* and *FGF8*.[218]

Diagnosis

Ultrasound: On US, the leaves of the septum pellucidum and interposed cavum can be visualized sonographically as a rectangular or triangular fluid-filled space between the frontal horns in 100% of normal fetuses from at least 18 to 37 weeks.[220] At midgestation, however, if only axial imaging is obtained, an artifact created by US beam crossing can mimic the septum pellucidum and result in misdiagnosis.[221] Two other causes of false positive include an enlarged cavum with displaced leaflets laterally and imaging slightly below the plane of the septum pellucidum in which the columns of the fornix, defined as two hypoechoic tubular structures separated by three echogenic interfaces, can be misinterpreted as the cavum (Fig. 17.1-33).[222] Coronal and sagittal planes either 2D or 3D should be attempted. Transvaginal imaging may also prove helpful.

On US, the absence of the septum pellucidum can be diagnosed after 20 weeks and causes the frontal horns to appear fused and squared (Fig. 17.1-34).[212,223] Mild-to-moderate VM may be present, likely because of white matter volume loss. Cortical defects in the brain parenchyma, especially bilateral and frontal extending from the lateral ventricles to the arachnoid space, are typical findings of open-lipped schizencephaly (Fig. 17.1-35A).

3D axial reconstruction of the brain at the level of the circle of Willis can be helpful in confirming normal pituitary tissue and evaluating the optic nerve/tracts.[224,225] Although measurement of the optic tract can be difficult to obtain, recent US data have shown a linear increase in optic tract diameter with GA, which may be helpful in determining the presence of optic nerve hypoplasia.[225] In addition, utilizing normal values of the optic chiasm on coronal 2D transvaginal imaging has been described in diagnosis of optic nerve hypoplasia in SOD.[226]

Magnetic Resonance Imaging: MRI has been shown to be 100% accurate when identifying absence of the septum pellucidum, whereas US has been noted to detect only 70% of cases.[227] On MRI, excellent thin sagittal midline and coronal views are important.

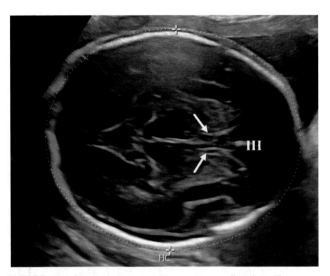

FIGURE 17.1-33: Fornices mimicking septum pellucidum. The *arrows* point to the fornices. *IH,* interhemispheric fissure.

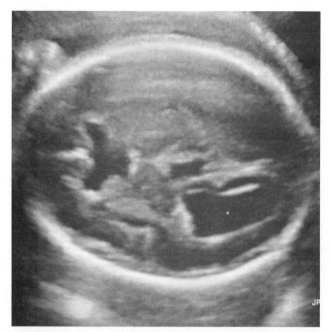

FIGURE 17.1-34: Axial US in fetus at 30 weeks with septo-optic dysplasia. Note the absence of the septum pellucidum, squared frontal horns, and mild ventriculomegaly.

Similar to US, when the septum pellucidum is absent, the frontal horns will appear square, bat wing, or boxlike (Fig. 17.1-36A). There is usually low position of the fornices, which may be fused, and associated with mild dilatation of the suprasellar cistern and anterior recess of the third ventricle (Fig. 17.1-36B).[228] In the presence of severe hypoplasia of the optic nerves, the imaging may be suggestive, but optic nerve hypoplasia is usually difficult to diagnose prenatally, owing to the small size of the nerve, slice thickness, and fetal imaging technique.[227] Clinical postnatal ophthalmological examination

remains the standard reference. The pituitary gland can be identified on T2 and T1 imaging. In the fetus, both the anterior and the posterior lobes are hyperintense on T1 sequences; therefore, no distinction is typically possible between the anterior and the posterior lobes, unless the posterior is ectopic.[224] Cortical malformations, especially schizencephaly, usually in the frontal lobe area, should be excluded (Fig. 17.1-35B).

Associated Anomalies: Up to 75% of patients with SOD have associated brain anomalies, the most common being bilateral polymicrogyria (33%) and schizencephaly (24%), followed by cortical heterotopias (12%).[217] Ectopic pituitary is noted in 18%.[217] Anterior falx dysplasia (48%), fusion of the fornices (60%), and thinning or absence of the corpus callosum (30%) are often present.[217,218] Incomplete hippocampal inversion is noted in 42%. Olfactory bulb and/or sulcus hypoplasia are typically bilateral and present in over one-third of patients with SOD.[217] Midbrain and hindbrain anomalies can be present in 55% of patients, with the most common being hypoplasia of the pons, medulla, and vermis.[218] Hypertrophy of the tectum may result in AS and hydrocephalus.[218]

Dysmorphic features, especially of the head (macrocephaly/microcephaly) and face, are often noted.[211] Ocular abnormalities in addition to optic nerve hypoplasia include coloboma, anophthalmia, and microphthalmia[218] Genital anomalies and delayed skeletal maturation are usually attributed to pituitary dysfunction.[211] Limb abnormalities such as constriction rings, syndactyly, and reduction deformity of the digits are not uncommonly described.[208,219]

Differential Diagnosis: The absence of the septum pellucidum is associated with various malformations, including HPE, ACC, and encephaloceles.[228] Fusion of the hemispheres and basal ganglia, especially in the presence of facial anomalies, supports the diagnosis of HPE. However, some cases of lobar HPE overlap and may be difficult to separate from SOD. In ACC, typical findings should be sought, including separated ventricles, colpocephaly,

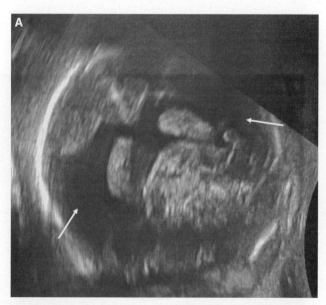
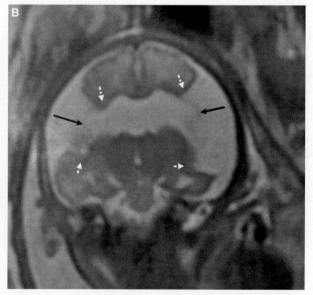

FIGURE 17.1-35: Fetus at 36 weeks with septo-optic dysplasia with bilateral open-lipped schizencephaly. **A:** Axial oblique US demonstrating the absence of the septum pellucidum and large bilateral frontal defects (*black arrows*). **B:** Coronal T2 MRI demonstrating open-lipped schizencephaly defects (*black arrows*) lined with gray matter (*dotted arrow*). Notice the absence of the septum pellucidum. This fetus would be considered in the spectrum of SOD-plus.

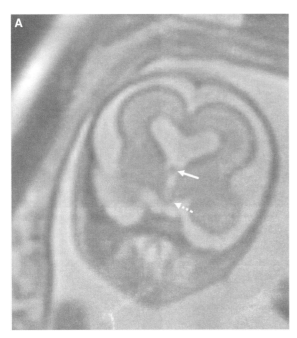 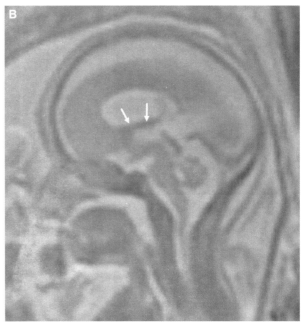

FIGURE 17.1-36: Fetus at 23 weeks with septo-optic dysplasia. **A:** Coronal T2 MRI demonstrating the absence of the septum pellucidum. The fornix is fused (*solid arrow*). The optic nerves are identified (*dotted arrow*), but it is difficult to exclude hypoplasia. **B:** Sagittal T2 image from same fetus again demonstrating low position of fused fornix (*arrows*). No pituitary abnormality was detected despite T1 imaging. The morphology in this fetus may be considered to be in the spectrum of lobar holoprosencephaly. Note also the absence of the secondary palate.

and radial array of medial sulci. Disruption of the septum can occur because of hydrocephalus from AS or Chiari malformations and in an encephaloclastic event, such as hydranencephaly and porencephaly.

Prognosis: In the presence of isolated absence of septum, greater than 75% have positive developmental outcomes, with 75% to 80% retaining the diagnosis of isolated absence of the septum pellucidum and the remaining showing findings within the spectrum of SOD.[214–216]

The outcome for patients diagnosed with SOD ranges from mild-to-severe endocrine and neurological dysfunction, with greater than 75% showing deficits.[210] Patients with complete absence of the septum pellucidum have worse neurological and developmental outcome than those with partial absence. Those with isolated optic nerve findings have good developmental prognosis.[229] However, in the presence of hemisphere abnormalities and posterior pituitary ectopia, the prognosis is more guarded.[229]

Endocrine abnormalities are variable, and 22% with abnormal septum and normal pituitary have endocrine dysfunction, versus 25% with normal septum and abnormal pituitary, and 56% with abnormal septum and pituitary. Overall, in 50% to 90% of patients with SOD, there is associated early or delayed hypothalamic–pituitary dysfunction, usually manifesting at a mean age of 4 to 5 years as growth retardation secondary to low levels of growth hormone and thyroid-stimulating hormone.[223,230] Diabetes insipidus and hypoglycemia are less commonly associated.[207,230]

Visual symptoms include normal vision, decreased acuity, or nystagmus. Neurological deficits range from global retardation (55% to 78%) to focal deficits such as epilepsy (22%) or hemiparesis.[219,230] In addition, over half have behavioral disorders, nearly one-third diagnosed with autism.[219]

Management: Prenatal management includes possible termination of the pregnancy or no alteration of standard obstetrical care.[212] Low maternal serum and urinary estriol levels can suggest fetal adrenal insufficiency and aid in the diagnosis of SOD.[223] There is an increased risk for prematurity may result seen in nearly 20% of pregnancies, which would support closer prenatal evaluation.[205]

Delivery should take place in a hospital where timely endocrine evaluation is possible.[216] Early recognition of growth hormone deficiency, pituitary dysfunction including hypopituitarism and diabetes insipidus, and hypothyroidism is important; therefore, testing should be performed in the first 3 days of life.[216] Hypopituitarism is a serious problem, and failure to recognize carries a risk of adrenal crisis, hypoglycemia, and death. Given the possibility for later development of hormonal deficiencies, long-term follow-up is necessary.[219] Ophthalmological evaluation to exclude optic nerve hypoplasia in the first month of life is reasonable.[216] Postnatal imaging and neurological consultation is important in the presence of seizures or neurological delay.

Recurrence: Most cases are sporadic, with low recurrence risk at 2% to 3%.[231] The risk may be increased in the presence of familial transmission.

Diencephalic–Mesencephalic Junction Dysplasia

Incidence: Diencephalic–mesencephalic junction dysplasia (DMJD) is likely rare. True incidence is unknown, but in a recent study of patients with brain malformations, 3% had DMJD.[232]

Pathogenesis: The diencephalic–mesencephalic junction is also known as the isthmic organizer and is responsible for signaling centers that result in correct regionalization of the forebrain, mesencephalon, and hindbrain. Fibroblast growth factor

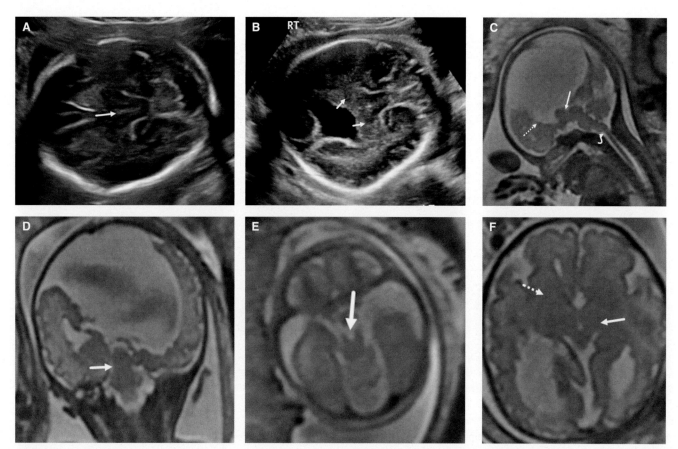

FIGURE 17.1-37: Diencephalic–mesencephalic junction dysplasia in a 30-week fetus. **A:** Axial US at the level of the midbrain demonstrating a deep cleft (*arrow*). **B:** Coronal oblique US demonstrating lack of separation of the midbrain and thalami (*arrows*). **C:** Sagittal MRI demonstrating that the interthalamic adhesions are ventrally placed and enlarged (*solid arrow*). There is aqueduct obstruction with small pons, rhomboencephalosynapsis, and kink at the cervicomedullary junction (*curved arrow*). The corpus callosum is partially agenetic (*dotted arrow*). **D:** Coronal MRI showing fusion between the midbrain and the thalami (*arrow*). Notice severe lateral ventriculomegaly in the presence of the third ventricle and aqueduct obstruction. **E:** Axial MRI at the level of the midbrain demonstrating a deep ventral cleft (*arrow*) with butterfly appearance. **F:** Axial MRI at the level of the deep gray nuclei demonstrating small thalamus (*solid arrow*) and basal ganglia (*dotted arrow*).

8 (*FGF8*) is likely the main isthmic organizer signaling molecule.[233] *FGF8* regulates anterior to posterior positioning of the diencephalon and mesencephalon through the genes engrailed (*EN1*) and Paired box transcription factors (*PAX6* and *PAX2*). Overexpression or underexpression of these genes may result in abnormal positioning due to loss of diencephalon and gain in mesencephalon or vice versa.[234] Combined loss of *EN2/EN3* and *FGF8* results in fusion of the forebrain and hindbrain.[233]

Two types of DMJD are described. In *type A*, there is nonseparation of the midbrain and hypothalamus, resulting an enlargement and abnormal contour of the dorsoventral midbrain on axial imaging. Many of these patients will also have a midbrain ventral cleft. Thalamic hypoplasia and basal ganglia abnormalities are common, ranging from bilateral agenesis of the putamen and globus pallidus, marked hypoplasia, or dysmorphic fused basal ganglia. *Type B* manifests as incomplete cleavage of the thalamus and midbrain on sagittal images, with bands/tissue extending from the interthalamic adhesion to the midbrain.[232] However, in most articles, patients described with DMJD have imaging findings containing malformations of hypothalamus, thalamus, and midbrain, thus encompassing both types.

Etiology: The etiology of DMJD is unknown but likely genetic. At this time, the only known genetic association is biallelic mutations in the nonclustered protocadherin-12 (*PCDH12*) gene. The gene results in brainstem malformations and abnormalities of the white matter tract, likely due to defects in neurite growth.[235] Tubulinopathies, *L1CAM*, and CMDs may manifest with DMJD.

Diagnosis

Ultrasound: Prenatal US diagnosis of DMJD has not been reported. However, close examination of the third ventricle that can extend into the midbrain as a cleft may provide clues to the diagnosis (Fig. 17.1-37A).[96] In addition, evaluation of thalamic and midbrain continuity on coronal or sagittal plane should raise suspicion (Fig. 17.1-37B). 3D US or transvaginal neurosonography should be considered to increase posterior fossa detail.

Magnetic Resonance Imaging: In DMJD, on fetal MRI, there is poor definition of the diencephalon–mesencephalon junction on sagittal and coronal imaging (Fig. 17.1-37C, D). With fusion of the midbrain and thalami, the interthalamic adhesion is enlarged and displaced ventrally.[98] The midbrain appears decreased in anterior to posterior on axial imaging, but is enlarged dorsoventral. A ventral cleft in the midbrain is contiguous with the third ventricle, with a characteristic butterfly sign on axial imaging (Fig. 17.1-37E).[233,98] Fetal cases to date have all been associated with AS and triventricular VM. Pontine hypoplasia and small cerebellar vermis with variable kinking brainstem, especially bulbo-medullary junction, are noted in 90% (Fig. 17.1-37C).[98] Callosal abnormalities are frequent. The thalamus and basal ganglia may be small (Fig. 17.1-37F). Many of the fetal cases have *L1CAM*-like features.

Associated Anomalies: Patients are typically microcephalic and with white matter tract anomalies.[233] In general and for both types, VM with reduced white matter, hydrocephalus especially in the presence of obstruction of the third ventricle, and gray matter heterotopia are noted. Corpus callosum anomalies and small/absent anterior commissure are frequently present.[232] In *type A*, basal ganglia anomalies are common, and abnormal course of the corticospinal tracts may be seen.[232] Dysmorphic facial features include low-set ears, prominent nasal bridge, long flat philtrum, and thin upper lip.[235]

Differential Diagnosis: The interthalamic adhesion is normal and seen in 80% of patients. The location is variable but typically anterior upper quadrant of the third ventricle.[232] Only 1% of normal cases have location of the interthalamic adhesion in the posterior inferior quadrant of the third ventricle.[232]

Prognosis: Patients have typically global developmental delay with severe cognitive impairment, hypotonia, spasticity, and seizures.[235] Speech and gait disturbances and autistic features are also common.[235,232] *Type A* patients have more severe deficits than *type B*. In *type A*, all are severely neurologically impaired with spastic tetra paresis and dystonic/dyskinetic movement. Hypothalamic dysfunction manifests as unexplained fevers, vasomotor instability, and sleeping disorders. Seizures and dysphasia are noted in slightly less than half. In *type B*, patients are less neurologically impaired, most with mild developmental delay, possible tonic–clonic seizures, and unilateral hemiparesis.

Management: Prenatal management includes possible termination of the pregnancy or no alteration of standard obstetrical care. Genetic testing and consultation is encouraged. Ventricular shunting will likely be required in the presence of the third ventricle and aqueduct obstruction.

Recurrence: Risk of recurrence is unknown but is likely dependent on genetic cause.

DISORDERS OF CORTICAL DEVELOPMENT

Cortical disorders are classified by the pattern of development, which includes the overlapping phases of radial cell progenitor formation and neurogenesis, proliferation, differentiation, migration, and organization including postmigratory differentiation and connectivity (Table 17.1-8). In humans, radial cell progenitor formation and neurogenesis results in basic cell type and then proliferation takes place from 5 to 6 weeks in the ventricular zone after the neural tube is complete. Neuron and glial cells arise from neuroblast precursors, primarily to about 15 to 20 weeks (finished 30 weeks) through approximately 35 divisions. Differentiation of the neurons and glial cells into a refined cell type is followed by migration between 6 and 7 weeks to 20 and 24 weeks. Cortical organization starts at 22 weeks and continues until 2 years of age. Organization includes postmigratory differentiation and connectivity with axons, dendrites, and synapse with neurotransmitters to other areas of the brain.

TABLE 17.1-8 Disorders of Cortical CNS Formation

Neurogenesis	Abnormal	Hemimegalencephaly Tuberous sclerosis
Proliferation	Decreased	Microcephaly/simplified gyral pattern
	Increased	Macrocephaly/megalencephaly
Differentiation	Abnormal	CNS tumors
Migration	Undermigration	Lissencephaly Gray matter heterotopia
	Overmigration	Cobblestone lissencephaly
Organization	Deranged	Polymicrogyria Schizencephaly Porencephaly Hydranencephaly

CNS, central nervous system.

This next section is separated into disorders of neurogenesis, differentiation, migration, and organization. Organization abnormalities in this chapter include polymicrogyria and schizencephaly, with varied causes such as genetic abnormalities and ischemic or hemorrhagic insult. With increasing knowledge with regard to embryonic pathology due to genetic interactions, it is becoming evident that destructive insults such as porencephaly and hydranencephaly are also likely best reflected in the continuum of cortical organization abnormalities that overlap with polymicrogyria and schizencephaly, reflecting time of insult to the brain, etiology, and severity of insult. Therefore, destructive insults are now included in the cortical organization section, representing postmigrational disruption.

In addition, it should be stressed that disorders of cortical development often present with multiple coexisting anomalies of neuronal transition. In these instances, the cortical disorder is described by the earliest disturbed developmental process.[236] Pathology related to cortical development is often caused by lack of normal gene expression, production of an abnormal gene, or interruption of gene function via infection or ischemia.[237] Unfortunately, the etiology is unknown in about 50% of cases.[236]

Disorders of Neurogenesis

Hemimegalencephaly/Dysplastic Megalencephaly

Hemimegalencephaly (HME), dysplastic megalencephaly (DM), and focal cortical dysplasia (FCD) are within a spectrum of diseases known as mTORopathies, which result in dysmorphic and disorganized cortex with intractable seizures. Terminology is dependent on the variable brain involvement, with localized being FCD type II, parts of the brain DM, and cerebral hemispheric HME. It is uncommon to diagnose FCD prenatal; therefore, this section emphasizes HME and DM.

Incidence: HME is a rare sporadic disorder. It is cited in 1 to 3 cases per 1,000 epileptic children and is equal in sex distribution.[238,239]

Pathogenesis: HME and DM are hamartomatous brain malformations characterized by overdevelopment and enlargement of all or part of one cerebral hemisphere (Fig. 17.1-38). In this disorder, cells are altered in their growth, migration, and/or differentiation with disorganization of the tissue architecture, such that there is an abnormal gyral pattern in the affected hemisphere that may manifest as agyria, pachygyria, polygyria, and polymicrogyria.

Pathogenesis likely occurs after the neural plate stage due to a mutation in the mammalian target of rapamycin (mTOR) pathway in the dorsal cerebral progenitors. The cells with mutation have a relative proliferative advantage over other cells.[240] In HME/DM/FCD, there is a primary disturbance in cellular neurogenesis and growth, with secondary effects being disturbed cell migration and organization.[238,241] It is interesting that HME and FCD are along a continuum in the same mutation in the dorsal telencephalic progenitors.[240] The timing of the mutation likely results in the pathology, with earlier mutations in larger number of cells resulting in HME whereas later mutations in smaller cell numbers causing FCD.[240] Microscopically, in all these disorders, the cells are immature or abnormal with mixed lineage and disturbed morphology, and there is a complete disorganization of the cytoarchitecture and loss of normal lamination with giant immature neurons and glial cells within the cortex and white matter.[238,241] Bizarre glial cells or balloon cells, myelination delay, and white matter gliosis have been described postnatally.

Etiology: HME, DM, and FCD are due to *de novo* somatic mutations in the components of the phosphatidylinositol 3-kinase (P13K)-AKT mTOR pathway.[240,242] Mutations of genes, which influence mTOR function including *AKT1*, *AKT3*, *PIK3CA*, *PIK3R2*, *PTEN*, *DEPDC5*, *TSC2*, and *MTOR*, are critical for regulation of cellular proliferation, size, and metabolism.[240,242] The most common mutated gene seen in HME is the *PIK3CA*.[243]

HME is isolated in approximately 53% to 66% of cases. In the remaining, it is seen in conjunction with neurocutaneous syndromes, including epidermal nevus, Proteus, CLOVES (congenital lipomatous overgrowth, vascular malformations, epidermal nevi, and skeletal/spinal anomalies) syndrome, hypomelanosis of Ito, Klippel–Weber–Trenaunay, neurofibromatosis type 1, and tuberous sclerosis.[238,239] In these syndromes, hemicorporal hypertrophy may be present. Total HME is a rare form described in the presence of ipsilateral enlargement of the cerebral hemisphere, brainstem, and cerebellum.[244]

Megalencephaly with polymicrogyria can be seen in two syndromes, both also with disturbances in the mTOR pathway with mutations of *PIK3CA* or *AKT3*.[245] Megalencephaly-capillary malformation syndrome is associated with capillary malformations of the face, limbs, and trunk; focal or segmental body overgrowth; and syndactyly or polydactyly. Megalencephaly–polymicrogyria–polydactyly–hydrocephalus syndrome has postaxial polydactyl in up to half.[245] *PTEN* mutations are also associated with hamartomatous syndromes, including Cowden syndrome, Bannayan–Riley–Ruvalcaba syndrome, and Lhermitte–Duclos syndrome.

Diagnosis

Ultrasound: Prenatal diagnosis should be suspected in the presence of UVM, with the most commonly dilated area being the posterior horn of the lateral ventricle (Fig. 17.1-39A). The head circumference is increased, usually in the 90th percentile. In conjunction, midline shift, usually in the occipital area, is noted due to asymmetry of the cerebral hemispheres.[246] 3D multiplanar reconstruction may be helpful in detecting subtle asymmetry and additional segmental overgrowth.[247,248] Sometimes, especially with 3D and transvaginal imaging, abnormal sulcation and cortical thickening along the affected hemisphere can be noted (Fig. 17.1-39B). Detection of hemicorpal overgrowth and vascular malformation should raise the suspicion for HME.

Magnetic Resonance Imaging: The enlarged hemisphere will have deformity of the lateral ventricle with diffuse dilatation and/or straightening or collapse of the frontal horn and/or disproportionate dilatation of the occipital horn (colpocephaly) (Fig. 17.1-39C, D).[244] The midline is straight or displaced contralaterally, especially in the occipital area. The white matter may be increased in volume and may demonstrate abnormal decreased signal because of heterotopia, gliosis, or abnormal myelination (Fig. 17.1-39D).[249] Sulcation is abnormal for GA, demonstrating cortex with too many lobulations or not enough, which later will manifest as polymicrogyria, pachygyria, and agyria. The dysplastic gray and white matter is typically heterogeneous, demonstrating increased and decreased T1 and T2 signals, respectively.[250] There is typically loss of

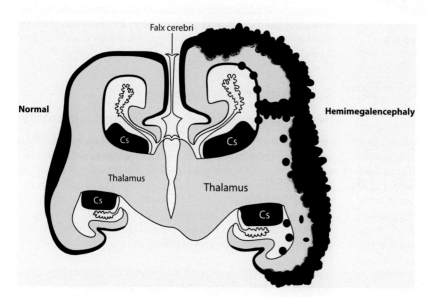

FIGURE 17.1-38: Hemimegalencephaly of the left hemisphere showing overgrowth with abnormal migration of gray matter throughout the hemisphere.

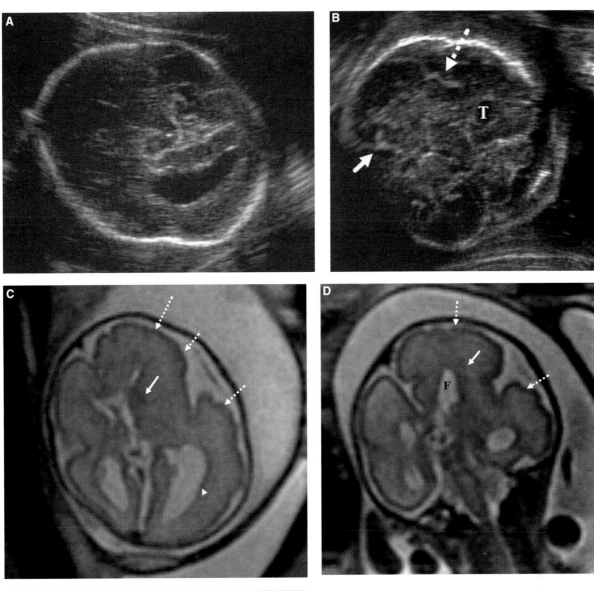

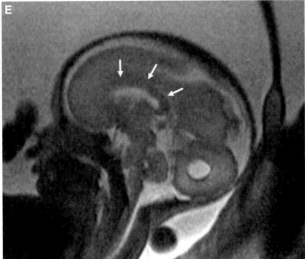

FIGURE 17.1-39: Hemimegalencephaly in a 29-week fetus diagnosed with Klippel–Weber–Trenaunay. **A:** Axial US demonstrating mild unilateral dilatation of the left lateral ventricle. Note slight shift of the left occipital lobe across midline. Head circumference was increased. **B:** Coronal US demonstrating subtle asymmetry of sizes of the hemisphere with left larger than right and shift of midline falx (*solid arrow*). The left temporal horn *(T)* is prominent. *Dotted arrow* denotes subtle lobulation along the cortex. **C:** Axial T2 MRI demonstrating enlargement of the left hemisphere and dilated occipital horn. Note nodularity (*arrowhead*) along ventricle consistent with heterotopia. The cortex (*dotted arrows*) demonstrates abnormal sulcation (compared with normal opposite side). Note the enlarged germinal matrix (*solid arrow*). **D:** Coronal image demonstrating straightened frontal *(F)* horn with abnormal dark signal (*solid arrow*) in the white matter consistent with disorganized neurons. There is abnormal sulcation with blurring of normal gray white interface (*dotted arrows*). **E:** Sagittal T2 demonstrating thickening of the corpus callosum (*arrows*).

normal fetal brain layering and blurring of gray white matter interfaces.[244,251] The corpus callosum, particularly on the affected side, may be thick (Fig. 17.1-39E).[244] Restricted diffusion can be present, likely owing to increased cellularity in the affected hemisphere.[251]

In the presence of a milder case, the distribution may be primarily lobar. In 40% of cases of HME, enlarged deep and/or superficial veins can be seen along the enlarged hemisphere (Fig. 17.1-40).[244,252] The ipsilateral cerebellar hemisphere can be enlarged in 47%, although only 7% will demonstrate ipsilateral brainstem hypertrophy. Abnormal folia of the cerebellum may be identified bilaterally.[252] In 26% of cases, ipsilateral olfactory and, in 3%, optic nerve enlargement can accompany HME.[252] The opposite hemisphere may be smaller than normal and distorted due to midline shift.

Associated Anomalies: Of the neurocutaneous syndromes, epidermal nevus syndrome is the most commonly associated and typically presents with linear nevus, sebaceous nevus, facial lipoma, and hypertrophy, typically on the affected hemispheric side.[253] Rarely, abnormal vascular shunting over the enlarged hemisphere can lead to congestive heart failure.[249]

Differential Diagnosis: The main differential is cerebral hemisphere enlargement due to tumor or hemorrhage. Shift of midline anatomy also may be related to volume loss in one hemisphere.

Prognosis: Symptoms are similar in the isolated and syndromic children.[253] The worse developmental outcome has been correlated with the most severe cerebral asymmetry.[242,249-252] Those with severe HME are at risk of mortality in the first year of life.[244] However, most patients demonstrate developmental delay, psychomotor deficits, progressive hemiparesis, and intractable

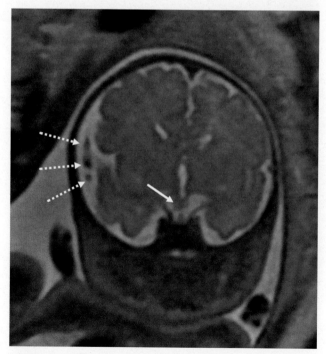

FIGURE 17.1-40: Coronal MRI of a case of right hemimegalencephaly of a fetus at 34 weeks. Notice prominent extra-axial space along the abnormal right hemisphere with large dilated veins (*dotted arrows*). The right optic chiasm is also enlarged (*solid arrow*).

seizures.[238] The marked hyperexcitability of the dysplastic cortex results in catastrophic epilepsy, with seizures typically beginning in the first 6 months of life.[246] It has been found that the earlier the onset of seizures, the more severe motor and intellectual deficit in children with HME.[253]

Management: Therapy is directed toward seizure control. Although anticonvulsant drug therapy may be utilized in mild cases, the most common treatment option is surgery, though some recent literature suggests endovascular embolic hemispherectomy may also be a strategy for seizure management. In the past, anatomical total or partial hemispherectomy was performed, but at a high morbidity secondary to development of hydrocephalus, intracranial hematomas, and infection.[238,239] Because of fewer complications, the most common surgical approach is now a functional hemispherectomy, a technique that involves disrupting internal capsule and corona radiata with resection and interruption of the mesial temporal structures, section of the corpus callosum, and frontal horizontal fibers.[250] After surgery, approximately 60% to 85% of children have control of their seizures.[242,250] With control of the seizures, there is improved intellectual and physical development.[246,250a]

While most advocate surgical intervention as early as possible to preserve neurological development, future therapies may be medical via drugs that inhibit mTOR activity (rapamycin and everolimus), which potentially could prevent or decrease epilepsy in these disorders.[240,243]

Recurrence: HME is mostly sporadic with low recurrence risk.

Tuberous Sclerosis

Tuberous Sclerosis (TS), or Bourneville disease, is an mTORopathy and the second most common phakomatosis after neurofibromatosis type 1. TS represents a complex characterized by the formation of benign hamartomas and low-grade neoplasms in multiple organ systems, most notably the brain, heart, kidneys, and skin.

Incidence: The incidence of TS is 1 in 10,000, and prevalence is 1 per 6,000 to 10,000 live births.[254] The disorder occurs equally in all races and both genders.

Pathogenesis: TS is characterized by widespread development of hamartomas in many different tissues, owing to a disorder of cell lineage. TS is similar to HME, but has pathologically more cellular and nuclear pleomorphism and a potential for neoplastic formation.[241] Almost all patients with TS have cutaneous stigmata, with the most common and earliest being multiple hypopigmented macules known as ash-leaf spots. Adenoma sebaceum, a misnomer, is present in 70% of TS patients, representing angiofibromas on the malar region of the face.[255]

Brain lesions include subependymal nodules and cortical tubers, seen in infants in 93% and 88%, respectively.[256] Less common lesions include white matter abnormalities and subependymal giant cell astrocytomas.[256] Prenatal, the most common lesions detected are cortical tubers and subependymal nodules, diagnosed second half of the second trimester to third trimesters.[257] Tubers are hamartomas that exhibit disorganized cortical lamination with atypical giant astrocytes, maloriented neurons, and bizarre giant cells. Subependymal nodules represent dysplastic astrocytic and neuronal cells. White matter lesions are heterotopic neuronal and glial elements arrested in migration. Subependymal giant cell tumors develop in 10% to 15% of all patients with TS but are rare prenatal.[258]

Cardiac rhabdomyomas are the most common cardiac tumors prenatally, with 70% to 90% associated with TS.[259,260] Rhabdomyomas usually present during the second or third trimester and are the most common fetal finding in TS.[256] There is increased risk for TS whether there is single or multiple cardiac tumors; however, multiple tumors are a strong predictor of TS.[260]

The most common renal findings in TS are angiomyolipomas, which are tumors composed of abnormal blood vessels, smooth muscle, and fat. These tumors are rare prenatal, usually developing during childhood and adolescence.[261] Renal cysts are not as common as angiomyolipomas in TS but have been detected prenatal and may be seen in the presence of polycystic kidney disease.[262]

Etiology: TS is caused by pathogenic mutations of either the *TSC1* or the *TSC2* gene located on chromosomes 9q34 and 16p13, respectively.[258] The gene products hamartin (*TSC1*) and tuberin (*TSC2*) act as tumor suppressors by negative feedback of the mTOR kinase cascade, whose activity is important in regulating cell growth and proliferation. In familial cases, transmission is autosomal dominant with variable expression and incomplete penetrance. However, approximately 70% to 80% of TS cases are sporadic, resulting from *de novo* genetic mutations.[258,263] *TSC2* mutations are more common, lead to a more severe phenotype, and tend to be spontaneous, while the *TSC1* are less common and more likely to be familial.[255] Polycystic kidney disease is sometimes associated with TS as the gene responsible for this disorder lies adjacent to the *TSC2* gene.[258]

Diagnosis: Genetic testing for the *TSC1* and *TSC2* genes from amniotic fluid or chorionic villus sampling can be definitive in about 80% of mutations.[254] However, because of genetic heterogeneity, testing can have a false-negative rate of 10% to 25%.[264]

Clinical diagnosis of TS requires identification of two major or one major and at least two minor features in the complex (Table 17.1-9).[264] A normal genetic result does not exclude TS or have effect on the clinical diagnostic criteria needed to diagnose TS.[264] Fetal echocardiography, US, and MRI are recommended to identify anomalies within the TS complex.

Ultrasound: About 80% of fetuses with TS have rhabdomyomas, presenting as early as 15 weeks, but typically after 24 weeks.[265,266] Rhabdomyomas are primarily round, homogeneous echogenic intraluminal and sometimes intramural masses, often located in more than one cardiac chamber but usually along ventricular walls or septum (Fig. 17.1-41A).[263] Most grow slowly, with only 15% causing cardiac complications.[260]

Brain lesions are often inconspicuous on prenatal US. If identifiable, subependymal nodules present as echogenic masses along the lateral ventricular wall or a cortical tuber as a focal area of echogenicity in the brain parenchyma (Fig. 17.1-41B).[267] Renal masses are rarely detected prenatally but include cysts, multiple cysts as in polycystic kidney disease, or focal smooth echogenic lesions in the renal cortex, consistent with angiomyolipomas (Fig. 17.1-41C).[262]

Magnetic Resonance Imaging: On prenatal MRI, cortical tubers and subependymal nodules are the most common CNS lesions

TABLE 17.1-9 Criteria for Diagnosis of Tuberous Sclerosis	
MAJOR FEATURES	**MINOR FEATURES**
Hypomelanotic macules (≥3, at least 5 mm)	"Confetti" skin lesions
Angiofibromas (≥3) or fibrous cephalic plaque	Dental enamel pits (>3)
Ungual fibromas (≥2)	Intraoral fibromas (≥2)
Shagreen patch	Retinal achromic patch
Multiple retinal hamartomas	Multiple renal cysts
Cortical dysplasias (cortical tubers and cerebral white matter radial migration lines)	Nonrenal hamartoma
Subependymal nodules	
Subependymal giant cell astrocytoma	
Cardiac rhabdomyoma	
Lymphangiomyomatosis	
Angiomyolipomas (≥2)	
DIAGNOSIS	
Definitive: two major or one major plus ≥ two minor	
Possible: Either one major or ≥ two minor	

detected with an incidence of 33% to 62%.[258] Other TS lesions, including white matter abnormalities and subependymal astrocytomas, are less frequent. Prenatal imaging is limited by spatial resolution, and small subtle lesions can be missed.[268] However, both T1 and T2 imaging are important as T1 signal abnormality may be more easily detected.[268]

In the fetus, the tubers are present in the cortex and/or subcortical white matter of primarily the supratentorial brain and demonstrate wedge-shaped or banded areas of increased T1 and decreased T2 signal, opposite of a myelinated child or adult (Fig. 17.1-41D, E).[268,269] Subependymal nodules, when present, dot the ependymal surface of the lateral ventricles, especially near the caudate and foramen Monroe, and are isointense to gray matter, being T1 hyperintense and T2 hypointense (Fig. 17.1-41C, F).[268,269] It is important to verify these lesions in two anatomical planes as motion artifact can mimic a lesion. Given the lower signal-to-noise ratio for fetal MRI sequences, lesions may be too subtle to be detected and probably are similar to lower diagnosis of gray matter heterotopia. Ninety percent of subependymal lesions do mineralize, but prenatal identification is unlikely as most do not calcify until 1 year of age.[258,265] Subependymal giant cell astrocytomas are rare prenatally but, when present, typically arise near the foramen of Monroe, measure greater than 5 mm, grow, and can obstruct the ventricular system.[258]

Associated rhabdomyomas are isointense to cardiac muscle on T1 and T2 images (Fig. 17.1-41G). Renal lesions may be

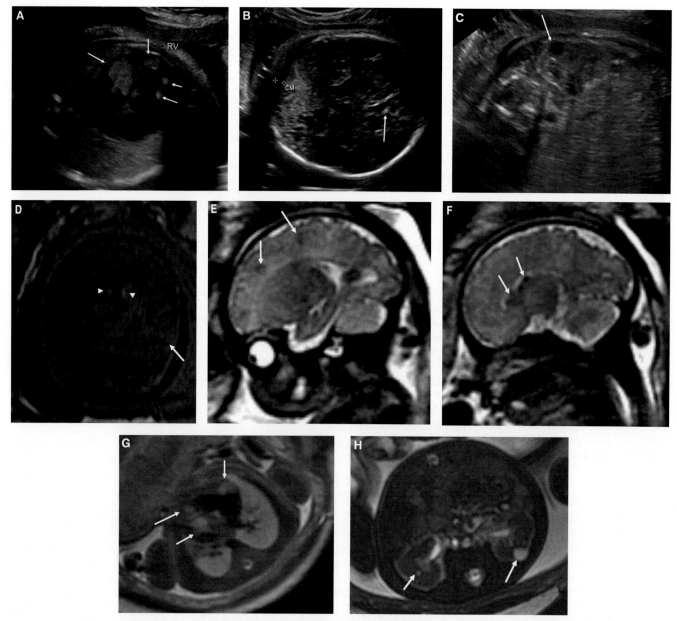

FIGURE 17.1-41: Tuberous sclerosis in a fetus at 35 weeks. **A:** Axial US demonstrating multiple homogeneous echogenic masses in the right ventricle and large mass in the left ventricle (*arrows*). **B:** Axial cranial image showing the area of the foramen Monroe with questionable nodularity (*arrow*). **C:** Axial US of the left kidney demonstrating the presence of a cyst (*arrow*). **D:** Axial T1 MRI in the fetal brain demonstrating a band of T1 signal in the left hemisphere consistent with parenchymal tuber (*dotted arrow*). Also note small hyperintense lesions at the foramen of Monroe (*solid arrows*) consistent with small subependymal tubers. **E:** Sagittal T2 MRI showing focal areas of dark signal (*arrows*) consistent with tubers. **F:** Sagittal T2 demonstrating dark round nodules (*arrows*) near the foramen of Monroe consistent with subependymal tubers. **G:** Axial T2 showing T2 hyperintense masses in the left and right ventricles (*arrows*) consistent with rhabdomyomas. **H:** Axial SSFP MRI through the kidneys confirms left renal cyst (*arrow*) but also defines an additional small right renal lesion (*arrow*).

heterogeneous but typically follow cystic characteristics, being T1 hypointense and T2 hyperintense (Fig. 17.1-41H).

Associated Anomalies: Retinal hamartomas occur in 40% to 50% of patients, with one-third bilateral.[270] Hamartomatous gastrointestinal polyps and oral gingival fibromas can develop. Patients with TS are at increased risk for arterial aneurysms, including aorta, peripheral, and intracranial. Pulmonary manifestations are present in 1% to 26% of patients, with the most common being lymphangiomyomatosis.[270] Sclerotic and cystic bone lesions and ungual fibromas adjacent to or underneath the nail bed are sometimes noted.

Differential Diagnosis: In the presence of a cardiac mass, the most common differential is a fibroma that is typically solitary and T2 hypointense and can be seen with orofacial abnormalities and Gorlin syndrome. Intracranial lesions, especially when solitary, should be differentiated from subacute hemorrhage, tumor, congenital infection, ischemia, or cortical dysplasia of other cause. When lesions are defined along the ventricle, germinal matrix hemorrhage or gray matter heterotopia should be considered.

Prognosis: Cardiac rhabdomyomas tend to increase in size *in utero* up to 32 weeks and regress after delivery, with 80% resolving in infancy or early childhood.[263,271] In the presence of a large lesion >3 cm, fetal dysrhythmia and/or compromised fetal cardiac function due to tumor obstruction, prenatal medication, early delivery, and/or surgery may be indicated. Preterm delivery in TS is as high as 35%, and cesarean delivery is reported at 33%.[271] However, most cardiac tumors are well tolerated, with only a 4% to 6% risk of fetal demise.[263] Negative neonatal outcome predictors include tumor size, arrhythmias, and fetal hydrops.[266]

The clinical triad of TS (epilepsy, mental retardation, and facial angiofibromas) is actually noted in only 30% to 40% of patients.[258] The most common cause of morbidity is neurological, with seizures in 70% to 90%, mental retardation in 50% to 70%, and developmental delay, behavioral problems, and autism in 25% to 50%.[258,272] Postnatally, there is a correlation between number, size, and volume of cerebral lesions and neurodevelopmental outcome.[273] However, utilizing these variables prenatal is not possible, given lower resolution in fetal imaging and the possibility of lesions developing later in pregnancy and postnatal.[259] Early onset of seizures, especially infantile spasms, has also been found to result in greater impairment in intellectual development.[273,274] Diagnosis of TS before the onset of seizures, particularly prenatal, can decrease epilepsy and result in better neurological outcomes due to early medical therapies.[273]

TS-associated renal disease also increases the risk of perinatal complications, including renal failure, polyhydramnios, and oligohydramnios. Postnatally, renal complications are the most common cause of death, with 10% developing renal failure or hypertension.[258] Angiomyolipomas that are present in 60% to 80% of TS patients are benign but can cause morbidity in about 10% of cases because of catastrophic hemorrhage, either spontaneous or in the presence of minimal trauma.[255] Polycystic renal disease is noted in 5% of TS patients and confers a worse prognosis.[258] Renal carcinomas are seen in 2% to 3% of patients.[258] In female postmenarchal patients, lymphangiomyomatosis of the lung can develop due to smooth muscle cell metastases, with 5% progressing to end-stage lung disease.[258]

Management: Diagnosis, screening of family members, and appropriate counseling are indicated. Termination may be considered. Close surveillance during the pregnancy is warranted. In the presence of a complicating rhabdomyoma, early delivery may be necessary.

Postnatally, brain and abdominal imaging should assess for neoplasm, complicating renal tumors, and vascular malformations, including aneurysms. Monitoring for seizure activity should be performed via EEG and with close clinical evaluation. Early preventative seizure therapy with agents such as vigabatrin before the onset may decrease the severity of seizures and improve developmental outcome.[274] mTOR inhibitors (rapamycin or everolimus) should also be considered early, especially for refractory seizures.[273,274] Surgical resection of dysplastic lesions is recommended after failure of two antiepileptic drugs.[274]

Ketogenic diet may decrease mTOR activation. mTOR inhibitors also cause regression of giant cell astrocytomas and may be helpful in the treatment of rhabdomyomas, angiomyolipomas, and lymphangiomyomatosis.[255,270] Embolization of symptomatic or large angiomyolipomas may be necessary.

Recurrence: The recurrence risk of an unaffected parent having a child with TS is 2% to 3%.[265] In the presence of an affected parent, transmission is 50%.

Disorders of Cellular Multiplication/Proliferation

Microcephaly

Synonyms: Microcephaly vera, true microcephaly, radial microbrain, microcephaly with simplified gyral pattern, oligogyria, and microlissencephaly.

Microcephaly implies a small head size, whereas micrencephaly represents a small brain. Microcephaly is diagnosed when head circumference (HC) measurements are less than 3 standard deviation (SD) below the mean for gestational age (GA).

Incidence: Utilizing less than 3 SD below the mean for GA as true microcephaly, prevalence is estimated 1.5 to 7.4 per 10,000 births with significant regional and ethnic variation.[275,276] Higher occurrence is noted with parental consanguinity. Microcephaly may present prenatally; however, a significant number of cases develop postnatal.

Pathogenesis: Microcephaly results from multiple pathologies and is typically categorized by the time of the insult.[236] The premigrational category includes multiple genetic disorders, which result in either decreased cell production or increased programmed cell death in the germinal zones. Some also utilize the terminology of primary or congenital microcephaly for this group, as these cases present fetal or early neonatal. Postmigrational microcephaly is related to decreased brain growth late in gestation or early postnatal and is also termed secondary or progressive microcephaly. Most of these cases are due to brain injury from ischemia, infection, inborn errors of metabolism, and teratogens with some related to genetic disorders. The isolated genetic microcephaly is typically primary, whereas the syndromic can be diagnosed prenatally or postnatally.

In primary or congenital microcephaly, the brain may have a well-preserved gyral pattern or abnormal gyral pattern.[277] Most manifest as alterations in gyral patterning and cortical surface area associated with changes in size of the corpus callosum. Some, though, will have cortical malformations.[278] Microcephaly without extracerebral malformation in the presence of a small architecturally normal brain and normal gyral pattern is known as true microcephaly or microcephaly vera. Microcephaly with simplified gyral pattern is likely in the continuum of true microcephaly, demonstrating reduced gyri, shallow sulci, normal cortical architecture, and normal or reduced thickness cortex. There is a strong correlation between the degree of microcephaly and the presence of a simplified gyral pattern and white matter volume loss.[279] Microlissencephaly or lissencephaly type III is utilized to describe a brain with abnormal gyration and thickened cortex in the presence of severe microcephaly and is described further in the section on lissencephaly.

Etiology: The cause of microcephaly is heterogeneous, being chromosomal or syndromic, related to errors of metabolism, infections, disruptive events, or teratogens. In a recent study including both primary and secondary microcephaly, 31% were found to be genetic, 27% perinatal brain injuries, and 41% unknown (Table 17.1-10).[280] Excluding holoprosencephaly, in a group of fetuses with primary microcephaly, 28% were shown to have abnormal fetal karyotype, 24% genetic syndrome, 28% with complex anomalies, and 20% isolated.[281] The etiology of primary microcephaly may be detected in only 57%.[282]

The key genes responsible for primary microcephaly are those that affect pathways that are important for neurogenesis and cell replication. Genes that modulate cell progression and checkpoint regulation, mitotic-spindle formation, centrosome duplication and maturation, and formation of microtubules are critical for normal proliferation (Table 17.1-10).[278] Some genetic disorders, however, result in secondary or postmigrational microcephalies, including Rett syndrome, pontocerebellar hypoplasia, and Angelman syndrome.[278] Many new loci are being identified; the most common mode of transmission being autosomal recessive.[283] It has been estimated that 20% to 35% of idiopathic microcephaly is hereditary.[284] Genetic associations with microcephaly cannot be completely listed here, as more than 600 associations are described in online Mendelian inheritance in man (OMIM).

Diagnosis: In addition to US and MRI, infectious workup and genetic testing with rapid aneuploidy detection and microarray are recommended.

Ultrasound: Most concur that fetal microcephaly should only be diagnosed when the HC is smaller than 3 SD below the gestational mean.[276,285] Research has found that there is no deficit in neuropsychological outcome with isolated microcephaly with HC −2 to 3 SD below the mean.[286] A biparietal diameter (BPD) and fronto-occipital diameter −3 SD below the mean has also been utilized but can be falsely positive in the presence of calvarial deformity.[287] Because more than half of fetuses with microcephaly are small for GA, the majority of HC/abdominal circumference and one-third of HC-to-femur length ratios are situated within normal range.[281,282,288] In addition, prenatal diagnosis may be challenging, particularly in the second trimester, as head measurements may be normal until the third trimester, usually after 27 to 28 weeks.[287,289]

Sonographic findings that may be helpful include small frontal lobes, sloping forehead, enlarged subarachnoid spaces, and VM due to neuronal loss (Fig. 17.1-42A, B).[290,291] Frontal lobe dimensions in the plane of the BPD from the posterior margin of the cavum septum pellucidum to the inner midline fetal skull can identify small frontal lobes and help diagnose microcephaly.[292] Sometimes, fetuses with microcephaly have narrow sutures and closed fontanelles, providing restricted visibility. However, the brain should be imaged through available windows to exclude abnormal morphology, calcification, and hemorrhage. Poor visualization or smaller caliber of the anterior cerebral circulation when compared with the posterior circulation on Doppler may be helpful.[291] Most cases of microcephaly (83%) are complex; therefore, associated anomalies should be excluded.[281]

Some have suggested that prenatal US is more accurate in detecting the absence of microcephaly than its true presence.[293] US at less than 3 SD has a relatively poor predictive value for postnatal confirmed microcephaly, being 67% resulting in 43% false positive.[288] Higher SD, being less than 4 or 5 SD from the mean and third-trimester imaging, can improve positive predictive value.[285,288,293] However, the main problem is the difference in technique between prenatal and postnatal measurements, which prevent accurate prediction and standards in microcephaly.[288]

Magnetic Resonance Imaging: MRI has the advantage of better depiction of the brain with measurements that are representative of the cerebrum rather than the calvarium. Because of this, US and MRI biometry are not well correlated, but with depiction of the brain, fetal MRI can aid in confirming the diagnosis of microcephaly in the presence of small HC via US.[294]

In microcephaly, decreased fronto-occipital diameter and BPD should be present (Fig. 17.1-42C). In the presence of simplified gyral pattern, MRI early in pregnancy can be diagnostically difficult. Delayed sulcation can be detected after 26

TABLE 17.1-10 Causes of Primary Microcephaly

GENETIC

Chromosomal Aberrations, Microdeletions, and Duplications

Common genes: *MCPH1, CENPJ, CDK5RAP2, ASPM, WDR62, NED1, TUBA1A, TUBB2B, TUBB3, TUBG1, LIS1, DCX, DYNC1H, KIF5C*

Trisomies 11, 13, 21, 22

Pallister-Killian, tetrasomy 12p

Microdeletion 22q11

Klinefelter syndrome

Triple X

Mosaics

Monogenetic Microcephaly

Autosomal recessive microcephaly

Autosomal dominant microcephaly

X-linked chromosomal microcephaly

Cornelia de Lange

Aicardi-Goutières syndrome

Cockayne syndrome

Seckel syndrome

Cohen syndrome

Mowat-Wilson syndrome

Rett syndrome (*FOXG1*)

Angelman syndrome (*UBE3A*)

Pontocerebellar hypoplasia (*CASK, TSEN54, TSEN2, TSEN34, RATS2*)

METABOLIC

Serine biosynthesis, sterol biosynthesis, mitochondriopathy, and congenital disorders of glycosylation

ENVIRONMENTAL

Disruptive: Vascular, hypoxic–ischemic, intrauterine twin death

Infection: TORCH, Zika, varicella, syphilis, human immunodeficiency

Teratogens: Alcohol, cocaine, antiepileptic drugs, lead or mercury, radiation

Maternal disease: Hyperphenylalaninemia, anorexia, diabetes

Placenta insufficiency

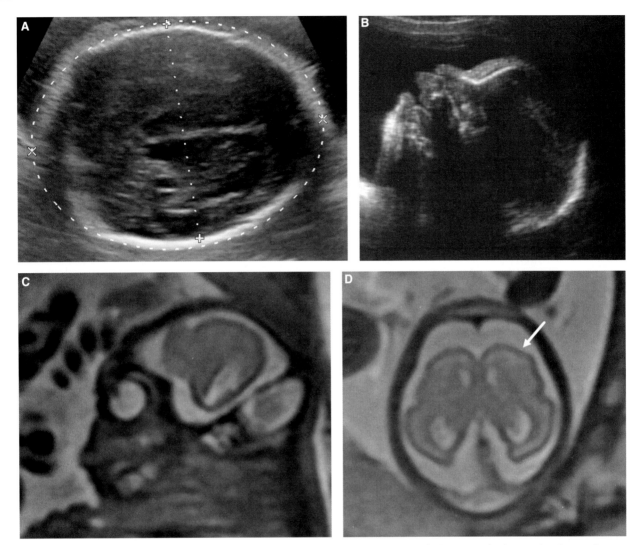

FIGURE 17.1-42: Fetus with microcephaly and simplified gyral pattern at 30 weeks. **A:** Axial US at 30 weeks showing head circumference (calipers). Head circumference measured appropriate for 25 weeks, 3 standard deviation below the mean for age. **B:** Sagittal US demonstrating small head with regard to face and sloping forehead. **C:** Sagittal T2 MRI showing small brain and prominent face. There is little sulcation along the hemisphere. **D:** Axial T2 MRI showing small brain and large extra-axial fluid spaces. Only a few sulci are present, and those identified are very shallow (*arrow*).

weeks, but confirmation may require imaging after 30 weeks.[295] MRI may identify wide and shallow primary and secondary sulci, especially in the frontal lobes, and absent tertiary fissures (Fig. 17.1-42D).[296,297] The cortex is usually thin (normal 3 to 4 mm), but, in some cases, can be thick. There is also usually white matter volume loss and mild-to-moderate ventricular dilatation with obliquity of the lateral ventricles. The corpus callosum, brainstem, and cerebellum can be abnormal. Cortical migrational defects should be excluded.

In the tubulinopathies, lissencephaly, simplified gyral pattern, pachygyria, and polymicrogyria can be present. The hallmark signs, though, are dysmorphic basal ganglia, present in 75% of cases, agenesis of corpus callosum in 40% and severe cerebellar hypoplasia/dysplasia in nearly 80%.[298]

Associated Anomalies: Microcephaly is often associated with other cortical malformations, including agyria, pachygyria, polymicrogyria, and gray matter heterotopia. Agenesis/hypogenesis of corpus callosum, delayed myelination, and dysplasia/hypoplasia

of the cerebellum and brainstem may be present.[277,283] In Cohen syndrome, a thick corpus callosum is present with microcephaly.

Extracranial anomalies are frequent in the presence of microcephaly and include ophthalmological disorders (30%), cleft palate (13%), cardiac (14%), renal (13%), skeletal system (13%), and gastrointestinal tract (9%) anomalies.[280]

Differential Diagnosis: Holoprosencephaly and lissencephaly have abnormal gyral pattern and often present with microcephaly. Microcephaly can also be seen in conjunction with encephaloceles and craniosynostosis.

Prognosis: Prenatal HC between 2 and 3 SD below may not correspond with microcephaly postnatal.[286,289] An occipitofrontal circumference of more than 2 SD below the mean in the past has been considered microcephaly postnatal; however, this value includes 2% of normal individuals with normal cognitive outcome. Evaluation of family HC should be considered as small head size may be a normal developmental variant.[277]

A recent study of microcephaly diagnosed prenatal and postnatal found that 65% have intellectual impairment and greater than 40% with epilepsy.[280] Neurodevelopmental outcome depends on the etiology of smaller brain volume.[275] Microcephaly in the presence of abnormal karyotype or intrauterine infection has a poor outcome.[290] Severity of mental delay is also related to the severity of microcephaly, with median IQ decreasing linearly with HC, primarily in those less than 3 to 4 SD below the mean.[275,286,299]

An isolated, nonprogressive, and moderate decrease in fetal HC can be associated with favorable outcome.[275] Children with microcephaly and preserved gyral pattern demonstrate mild delay in early development, some difficultly with feeding, and limited language skills.[277,283] Those with a simplified or abnormal gyral pattern have a more severe clinical course, including poor feeding, severe developmental delay, intractable epilepsy, and early death.[283] Perinatal mortality for children with microcephaly has been quoted as high as 70%.[281]

Management: Microcephaly is not treatable. Evaluation of family HC is important as similar small head in the fetus may be a developmental variant. Genetic testing should be performed. Termination of the pregnancy may be considered, depending on chromosomal studies and associated anomalies; however, delayed third-trimester diagnosis may limit possibility. Should the pregnancy be terminated, fetal autopsy or postmortem MRI should be offered.[275] Postnatally, children with mild microcephaly usually require special schooling, intensive speech therapy, and early psychomotor support.[295] Children with more severe microcephalies require anticonvulsive therapy and nasogastric tube feeding.[295]

Recurrence: Recurrence risk is 25% in the presence of primary microcephaly.[283]

Macrocephaly/Megalencephaly

Macrocephaly is noted when head circumference (HC) is above 95th to 98th percentile or more than 2 SD above the mean. Megalencephaly indicates a large brain with weight or volume greater than 98th percentile or ≥2 SD above the mean.

Incidence: Limited data quote isolated macrocephaly in 0.5% of the population.[300]

Pathogenesis: Isolated or benign macrocephaly is typically associated with enlarged subarachnoid spaces and is favored to be related to a disorder in absorption of the CSF.[301] Megalencephaly occurs because of increased neuronal and glial cell proliferation and/or faulty apoptosis. Most cases do not become apparent until the last trimester of pregnancy or postnatal.[302]

Etiology: Benign familial macrocephaly that results in enlarged extra-axial fluid spaces accounts for approximately 50% of the cases and is transmitted autosomal dominant.[303] Rarely, glutaric aciduria, an inborn error in metabolism, may present with enlarged spaces and fetal macrocephaly.[304] Macrocephaly may be also related to chromosomal microdeletions.[302]

Megalencephaly may be associated with over 200 genetic syndromes, many of which are difficult to diagnose prenatally.[302,303] Many of the genetic disorders that cause megalencephaly affect the mTOR pathway, such as *PTEN* and *PI3K/ART* genetic mutations, and the *TSC1* and *TSC2* genes resulting in TS. Common groups of genetic disorders with enlarged head size include those listed below.[305,306]

Overgrowth syndromes include Sotos, Weaver, Simpson-Golabi–Behmel, and Beckwith–Wiedemann.

RASopathies are genetic disorders caused by mutations in genes of the *Ras-MAPK* pathway transmitted autosomal dominant. These may have brain overgrowth and cutaneous abnormalities and include Noonan, LEOPARD (Noonan with multiple lentigines), Costello, Neurofibromatosis type 1 (NF1), Cardiofaciocutaneous, and Legius syndrome.[306]

mTOR-Related Genetic Disorders

PTEN (phosphatase and tensin homolog deleted on chromosome TEN) provides an enzyme that regulates cell division and thus acts as a tumor suppressor. Mutations are inherited or acquired and are usually associated with cutaneous (hamartomas) findings and include Bannayan–Riley–Ruvalcaba, Cowden syndrome, Lhermitte-Duclos, and macrocephaly with associated autism disorder.

Mutations in PI3K-ART pathway are due to de novo mutations during embryogenesis.[245] *PI3K-ART* pathway is integral to brain growth and development, regulating cell proliferation, metabolism, survival, and apoptosis. The two syndromes most described with this mutation pathway include megalencephaly-capillary malformation polymicrogyria (MCAP) and megalencephaly-polydactyly-polymicorgyria hydrocephalus syndrome (MPPH), both which may have perisylvian polymicrogyria.

- PIK3CA-related overgrowth spectrum disorders (also known as PROs)
  - *MCAP*, in addition to vascular lesions, may have asymmetric brain (hemimegalencephaly) and segmental body overgrowth (hemihypertrophy).
  - *Congenital lipomatous overgrowth, vascular malformation and epidermal nevi (CLOVES)* resulting in macrodactyly, focal adipose overgrowth, epidermal nevi, and facial infiltrating lipomatosis.[245]
  - *Macrodactyly, hemihyperplasia multiple lipomatosis (HHML)*
  - *Fibroadipose overgrowth (FAO)*
- ART related
  - *MPPH* with brain development symmetric and variable VM or hydrocephalus may be present.
  - *Proteus syndrome* with overgrowth of bones, skin, and other tissue, often asymmetrically and with abnormal blood vessel and fat proliferation
  - *Lipodystrophy syndrome hypoglycemia*

Diagnosis

Ultrasound: Most fetuses with macrocephaly have a normal second-trimester HC, and diagnosis is not made until late in the pregnancy or postnatal.[302] In those with isolated macrocephaly, enlarged extra-axial spaces are common (Fig. 17.1-43A).[301] Fetuses with larger HC and associated anomalies due to underlying syndromes will tend to be identified earlier (28 weeks) versus those with isolated macrocephaly (32 weeks) (Fig. 17.1-44A).[302] Syndromes diagnosed prenatally, such as MCAP, may demonstrate segmental body overgrowth and/or hemihypertrophy. Most fetuses with macrocephaly will be large for GA.[301]

However, enlarged fetal HC has low specificity, with only 67% of children diagnosed prenatally having large HC postnatally.[300] Some of this variation is technical, related to limitations in accuracy of HC, but also inconsistencies between prenatal and postnatal-derived HC growth curves.[300]

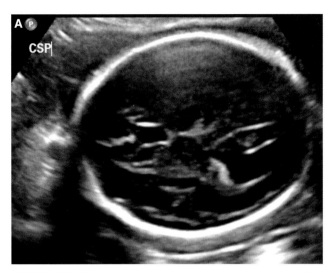
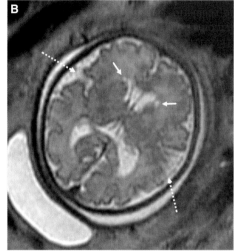

FIGURE 17.1-43: Macrocephaly of unknown origin in a fetus at 36 weeks. **A:** Head circumference on US was at 3 standard deviation above the mean. **B:** MRI biparietal and fronto-occipital dimensions were increased. Axial T2 image demonstrates enlarged extra-axial fluid spaces (*dotted arrows*) and mild asymmetric left lateral ventricular dilatation. Also note bilateral connatal cysts (*solid arrows*).

Magnetic Resonance Imaging: Increased brain and/or bone biometry for GA is present. Mild VM and enlarged extra-axial fluid spaces are often present and, in isolation, are common for benign macrocephaly (Fig. 17.1-43B).[302] In the presence of additional white matter signal abnormality and significantly enlarged Sylvian fissures, glutaric aciduria type 1 should be considered.[304]

In syndromic cases, frontal bossing, callosal anomalies, including thick corpus callosum, VM, enlargement of germinal matrix, and cortical migrational abnormalities may be present (Fig. 17.1-44B, C). A thick corpus callosum has been linked to enlarged white matter and can be seen in syndromes such as NF1 and MCAP.[307]

Associated Anomalies: Macrocephaly is present in the overgrowth syndromes, many of which are at increased risk for brain, heart, limb, and spine anomalies.[303] Fragile X is also an overgrowth syndrome in white males with facial abnormalities.[305]

Cutaneous abnormalities are present in the *PTEN* and *PI3K-ART* mutations and RASopathies. Some RASopathies have relative macrocephaly, macrosomia, lymphatic, cardiac, and renal anomalies.[305,306] Other RASopathies such as NF1 and Legius

syndrome (similar to NF 1) may have nerve sheath tumors.[305] *PI3K-ART* mutations often present with polydactyly, which is postaxial in MPPH and MCAP, though MCAP has higher incidence of syndactyly.[305]

Differential Diagnosis: In the presence of enlarged extra-axial fluid spaces, subdural collections or cerebral atrophy should be excluded. Disproportionate head size due to intrauterine growth restriction should also be considered. Macrocephaly may be secondary to other pathologies, including hydrocephalus, triploidy, and intracranial neoplasms.

Prognosis: Prognosis is dependent on associated anomalies, etiology, and head size.[302] Prenatal HC between 2 and 3 SD above the mean is typically isolated and has a good outcome, while an HC >3 SD is more likely to be syndromic with developmental delay.[300,302]

Children with isolated, particularly familial, macrocephaly usually have normal intelligence, with enlarged CSF spaces normalizing by 3 to 4 years of age.[300,301] Macrocephaly in the presence of a syndrome is often associated with abnormal development. In children with overgrowth syndromes, there is increased risk for solid and hematologic neoplasms.[303]

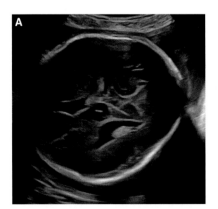
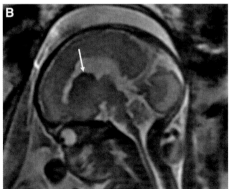
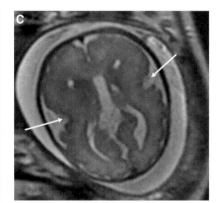

FIGURE 17.1-44: Megalencephaly in a fetus at 27 weeks with polymicrogyria. **A:** Head circumference measured appropriate for a 37-week gestation fetus but no ventriculomegaly detected. **B:** Sagittal MRI demonstrating enlarged brain with thick ganglionic eminences (*arrow*) **C:** Axial MRI showing irregularity in the perisylvian area consistent with polymicrogyria. Findings suspect for a *PI3K-ART* mutation.

Management: Prenatal evaluation should include family history and parental/sibling HC measurements to evaluate for benign familial macrocephaly. Amniocentesis for karyotype and microarray may be considered. Postnatal imaging and evaluation by appropriate pediatrician and clinical geneticist is suggested, especially when there is increased risk for neoplasm.

Recurrence: Type of genetic transmission guides recurrence risk.

Disorders of Cellular Differentiation

Central Nervous System Tumors

Tumors are uncommon prenatally, described primarily through case reports. There is considerable overlap of fetal neoplasms with congenital brain tumors, defined as a tumor presenting within 60 days after birth.

Incidence: The overall incidence of perinatal brain tumors ranges 1.4 to 3.6 per 100,000.[308] Fetal intracranial tumors are very rare, accounting for approximately 0.5% to 1.9% of intracranial tumors in childhood.[309] Brain tumors represent only 10% of all antenatal tumors.[310]

Pathogenesis: The pathogenesis for fetal intracranial neoplasms is unknown. These "congenital tumors" have a different pathophysiology than typical pediatric neoplasms. Normal embryonic cells have a high mitotic rate like neoplasms. Fetal tumor development is believed to be due to lack of normal cellular differentiation and maturation of these embryonic cells. In the presence of high mitotic activity, it is not surprising that many of these lesions, whether benign or malignant, grow rapidly and reach enormous proportions.

Unlike pediatric tumors, fetal masses tend to be supratentorial, either cerebral hemisphere, suprasellar, or pineal; however, the epicenter of many is undetermined because of the size and extent.[310,311] Fetal tumors often cause demise because of their size and location, inhibiting normal organ development. Large tumors may result in cardiovascular compromise and hydrops.

Etiology: Fetal tumors are different in prevalence, location, and histological and biological behaviors when compared to pediatric intracranial neoplasms (Table 17.1-11). The most common fetal intracranial tumor is a teratoma, a germ cell tumor.[309] This is followed by astrocytomas, chorid plexus papillomas (CPPs), craniopharyngiomas, and embryonal tumors.[310] Neuronal–glial tumors are infrequent prenatally, being more commonly identified in the first year of life.[312] Ependymal and meningeal tumors are rare.

Of note, tumor classification has changed, with the most recent update being the World Health Organization (WHO) in 2016 in which molecular parameters are now included.[313] Embryonal tumors, which are tumors with multilayered rosettes, previously known as primitive neuroectodermal tumor (PNET), medulloblastoma, and atypical teratoid/rhabdoid tumor (ATRT), are now grouped together.[313]

Teratomas represent 33% to 50% of congenital brain tumors. These tumors originate from abnormal development of pluripotent cells of three germ layers and immature neuroglial elements, can be benign or malignant, and often arise along the midline.[314] There are several forms described: **large** replacing all intracranial contents, **small** with hydrocephalus, or as **bulky** lesions with

TABLE 17.1-11 Types of Fetal Brain Tumors, Prevalence, and Location[309,310]

TYPE	PREVALENCE (%)	LOCATION
Teratoma	30–50	Cerebral hemisphere, suprasellar, pineal
Astrocytoma	25	Cerebral hemisphere, basal nuclei
Choroid plexus papilloma	5	Intraventricular
Craniopharyngioma	2–5	Suprasellar
Embryonal tumor	Uncommon	Cerebral hemisphere, cerebellum
Ependymal	Rare	Ventricular
Meningeal	Rare	Extra-axial

extension into orbit, oropharynx, or neck.[309] Because many are very large, it is difficult to identify site of origin, but greater than two-thirds are supratentorial, and when determined, most are in cerebral hemispheres, third or lateral ventricles, and the pineal region.[314] The lesions are complex, containing solid and cystic areas with or without calcification.

Astrocytomas are composed of astrocytes of varying degrees of differentiation, from low grade to high grade. Unlike pediatric-aged tumors, fetal astrocytomas are found supratentorial rather than posterior fossa.[309,312] Glioblastomas (malignant/high-grade astrocytoma) represent greater than 50% of fetal astrocytomas and are found in the cerebral hemisphere and basal nuclei.[309,312] These tumors often involve more than one lobe.[314] Hemorrhage and rapid growth are common findings. Subependymal giant cell astrocytomas in TS are the second most common followed by low-grade astrocytomas.[312] Hamartomas, which are benign tumors of heterotopic normal tissue usually hypothalamic or intraventricular, can be detected prenatally, particularly in the presence of syndromes.

Choroid plexus tumors are intraventricular tumors arising from the choroid plexus epithelium, representing 5% of perinatal tumors.[315] CPPs are grade I by WHO, atypical grade II, and carcinomas are grade III. CPPs are benign, and the most common prenatal, followed by choroid plexus carcinomas and then atypical type.[315] These lesions are nodular, cauliflower-like lesions typically in the lateral, less likely third or fourth ventricle. CPPs have slow growth but can block drainage of CSF. The tumor is vascular and secretes CSF and therefore can cause rapid onset hydrocephalus.

Craniopharyngiomas represent 2% to 5% of congenital tumors.[316] These suprasellar masses are epithelial tumors that arise from Rathke pouch, an ectodermal diverticulum important for development of the pituitary gland. Tumors are usually heterogeneous, frequently containing calcification.

Embryonal tumors, including PNET, medulloblastoma, and ATRT, demonstrate undifferentiated or poorly differentiated neuroepithelial cells, with divergent differentiation of neuronal, astrocytic, and ependymal cells.[314] The most common congenital tumors in this group are the medulloblastomas and ATRT. Congenital medulloblastomas tend to be supratentorial, rather than arising from the vermis.[314] ATRT can arise intra-axial or extra-axial, on histopathology contain rhabdoid cells, and are noted in the presence of mutation or loss of the *INI1/hSNF5* gene locus at chromosome 22q11.2.[314] PNET has been removed in terminology with new classification related to amplification of the C19 MC region on chromosome 19, now diagnosed embryonal tumor with multilayered rosettes.[313] All embryonal tumors are aggressive, grow rapidly, and metastasize early to the CSF and meninges. Extensive hemorrhage, cyst formation, necrosis, and calcification in a very large mass are common.

Neuronal and mixed neuronal–glial tumors include desmoplastic infantile astrocytomas (DIAs) and desmoplastic infantile gangliomas (DIGs), which are low-grade large intracranial cystic tumors that involve superficial cortex and leptomeninges, attached to the dura by a desmoplastic reaction.[314] Most are supratentorial, involve more than one lobe, and commonly present frontal or parietal.[314]

Ependymal lesions arise from the ependymal cells lining the ventricles or spinal cord central canal. Most are very cellular and primitive prenatal, with common histology ependymoblastoma. These lesions also metastasize to the CSF pathways and tend to have extensive necrosis with location in the lateral and fourth ventricles.

Meningeal are extra-axial benign or malignant mesenchymal tumors arising from the meninges of primarily the middle and less likely anterior or posterior cranial fossa.

Diagnosis

Ultrasound: Fetal tumors typically present in the third trimester of pregnancy, with 60% diagnosed later than 30 weeks' gestation.[317] If a tumor is diagnosed before 22 weeks, teratoma or hamartoma is typically the diagnosis.[318] Astrocytoma and glioblastoma are usually detected after 32 weeks.[318]

US may be obtained because of a sudden increase in maternal uterine size. Polyhydramnios, owing to decreased fetal swallowing, is a typical presenting sign.[319] Initial imaging findings include macrocephaly and intracranial mass followed by hydrocephalus (Table 17.1-12) (Fig. 17.1-45A). Masses, in general, displace midline structures and distort normal anatomy.

TABLE 17.1-12 Prenatal Imaging Findings in Brain Tumors[309,310]

Macrocephaly	58%
Intracranial mass	58%
Hydrocephalus	52%
Intrauterine death	35%
Mass filling intracranial cavity	21%
Brain replaced by tumor	21%
Hydramnios	12%
Cephalopelvic disproportion	11%
Breech	10%
Hemorrhage	8%
Fetal hydrops	6.5%

In the presence of an enormous lesion, it may not be possible to identify normal cerebrum, midline structures, or ventricles (Fig. 17.1-45B, C).[308]

Most fetal tumors are supratentorial and have a heterogeneous US pattern. Evaluation for calcification is extremely helpful, being present in the most common tumor, a teratoma. The differential though would include craniopharyngioma and embryonal tumors, such as ATRT. Cystic or necrotic areas in the tumor are also common with teratoma, but may be present in many other lesions such as craniopharyngioma, astrocytomas/glial tumors, embryonal, and ependymal mass. Teratomas can be a primarily cystic lesion and would be the most likely diagnosis, but the uncommon DIA/DIG should be considered.[320]

Location may help with diagnosis (Table 17.1-11). A homogeneous vascular echogenic lesion, especially intraventricular with hydrocephalus, would support CPP (Fig. 17.1-46A).[321]

Doppler typically demonstrates vascularization in a mass, although a minor amount may show no Doppler signal, and thus,

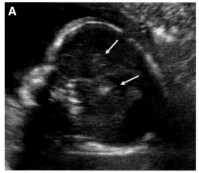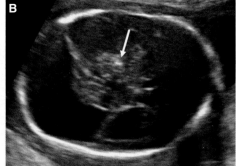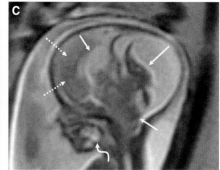

FIGURE 17.1-45: Fetus at 21 weeks with intracranial teratoma. **A:** Sagittal US demonstrating macrocephaly and heterogeneous mass, replacing most of the brain (*arrows*). **B:** Axial US showing a heterogeneous mass with echogenic area (*arrow*) that shadowed consistent with calcification. **C:** Sagittal T2 MRI of primarily isointense mass containing cystic area anteriorly. The lesion is present in both the supratentorial and the infratentorial locations (*solid arrows*), replacing most of the normal brain. Small normal brain anteriorly (*dotted arrow*). Fetus also had a sacrococcygeal teratoma, and cystic lesion at the base of the tongue (*curved arrow*) confirmed to be a teratoma.

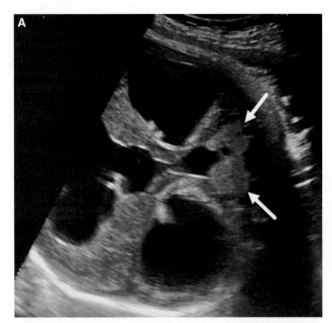
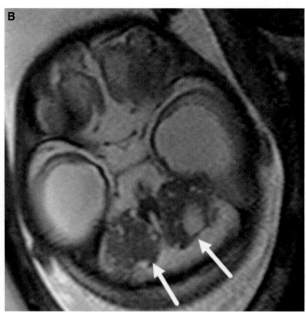

FIGURE 17.1-46: Fetus with choroid plexus papilloma. **A:** Axial US demonstrating severe lateral and third ventricular dilatation with bilobed echogenic mass (*arrows*) filling the fourth ventricle. **B:** Axial T2 MRI in same fetus showing heterogeneous primarily T2 hypointense bilobed mass (*arrows*) in the fourth ventricle. Notice severe ventriculomegaly of temporal horns. (Courtesy of Chris Cassady, MD.)

it can be difficult to exclude hematoma.[321] In the presence of large tumors, especially teratomas, high-output cardiac failure and hydrops may develop due to arteriovenous shunting.

The overall accuracy in diagnosis of cell type by US is approximately 57%.[320]

Magnetic Resonance Imaging: MRI is ideally suited in the evaluation of fetal tumors and can confirm diagnosis. The internal architecture and extension of the tumor are better assessed by MRI than US.[321] Identification of tumor location and presence of additional lesions may help in definition of cell type.

Most fetal tumors are heterogeneous, being isointense on T1 images and hyperintense on T2 images.[321] CPPs are lobular homogeneous iso-hyperintense on T1 and hypointense on T2 imaging (Fig. 17.1-46B). The solid tissue in embryonal tumors and ependymomas may be T1 isointense and T2 hypointense due to high cellularity (Fig. 17.1-47A, B). The presence of hemorrhage, which is described in 3% to 18% of intracranial masses, is most commonly observed in glioblastoma and embryonal neoplasms.[308] Hemorrhage can be detected on T1 sequences as bright signal and gradient echo images with susceptibility artifact (Fig. 17.1-47C).[322] Punctate dark areas on T2, bright areas on T1, or susceptibility artifact on gradient echo may define foci of calcification. Diffusion-weighted imaging is often positive in the presence of an embryonal neoplasm and may be helpful in identification of metastasis (Fig. 17.1-47D).[322]

Associated Anomalies: Most tumors are present in isolation. Approximately 12.5% of fetal brain tumors have associated anomalies.[311] Teratomas and craniopharyngiomas can have associated abnormalities of the head or face, with cleft lip or palate being the most frequent.[308,318]

CPPs may be associated with Aicardi syndrome and Li-Fraumeni syndrome, which also has a higher association with embryonal and astrocytic tumors.[315,316] Other familial syndromes that have higher incidence of tumors include NF1 (optic glioma/astrocytoma), NF2 (schwannoma, meningioma,

astrocytoma, ependymoma), TS (giant cell astrocytoma), and von Hippel-Lindau (hemangioblastomas). Hypothalamic hamartoma may suggest Pallister-Hall syndrome (polydactyly, dysplastic nails, bifid epiglottis, imperforate anus, renal and pituitary anomalies) or oral-facial-digital syndrome type 1.

Differential Diagnosis: Many intracranial masses are missed as they mimic common pathologies such as hemorrhage and hydrocephalus. In the presence of hemorrhage, Doppler shows no flow. MRI may be helpful to exclude mass with or without hemorrhage. Primarily cystic tumors can mimic infarct, porencephaly, arachnoid cyst, or interhemispheric cysts. Other benign lesions to include in the differential are lipomas, intracranial hemangiomas, and vascular malformations. Lipomas are well-defined midline homogeneous echogenic masses often in association with agenesis of corpus callosum. Hemangiomas are typically extra-axial and appear as a highly vascularized echogenic lesion. Rarely, *fetus in fetu* may present as an intracranial mass.

Prognosis: A fetus with a brain tumor has a poor prognosis.[309] Approximately 35% are stillborn. Overall survival rate is only 15%. Those who survive to birth, die shortly thereafter, with survival rate of 28%.[308] Prognosis worsens with increasing tumor size and decreasing GA at diagnosis.[309,317]

Intracranial teratomas, glioblastomas, and embryonal tumors have the lowest survival rate of brain tumors (6% to 8%).[309] A fetus with meningeal tumor has survival rate of 17%, craniopharyngiomas 23%, and those with astrocytoma approximately 20% to 90%, higher usually in the presence of low-grade lesions.[312] CPPs have the best outcome with survival at 40% to 80%.[311] In those cases in which the tumor is resected postnatal, overall survival is approximately 67%.[309]

Management: Prenatal imaging to identify the site and size of the lesion allows for an obstetric plan of management. In teratomas, high levels of alpha-fetoprotein may be detected in the fetal serum or amniotic fluid but is not diagnostic. Many

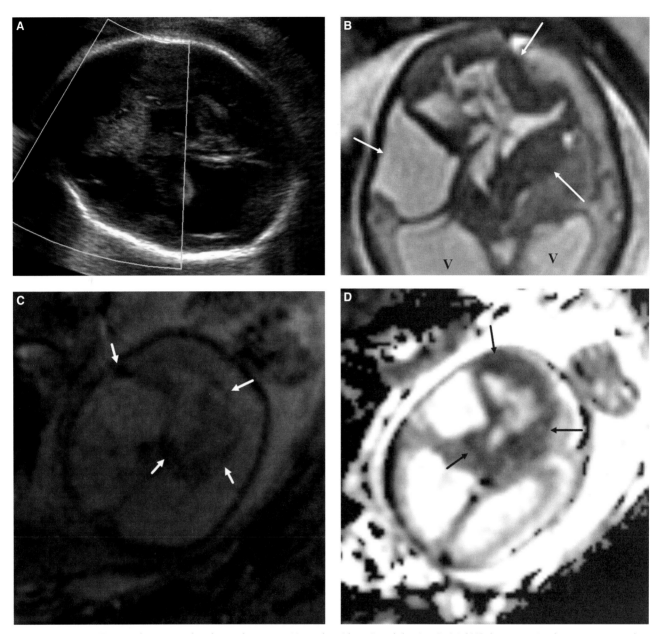

FIGURE 17.1-47: Fetus with suspected embryonal tumor at 33 weeks with perinatal demise. **A:** Axial US demonstrating heterogeneous echogenic mass with internal blood flow centered in frontal lobe distorting anatomy. Ultrasound 1 month prior was normal. **B:** Axial T2 MRI demonstrating a large heterogeneous solid and cystic lesion centered in frontal lobe (*arrows*). Note rind of tissue that demonstrates hypointense T2 signal. There is bilateral obstructive ventriculomegaly (*V*). **C:** Gradient echo axial image demonstrating multiple areas of susceptibility artifact (*arrows*), suggesting hemorrhage and/or calcification. **D:** Restricted diffusion (*arrows*) is noted as dark signal on the apparent diffusion coefficient map. Findings support a high-grade cellular lesion.

times, the imaging is nonspecific, and histological diagnosis is obtained after birth. With hydrocephalus, cephalocentesis may be repeated to decrease mass effect on the developing brain.[319] Early delivery, at or even before 34 weeks, may be considered.[319] In the presence of a large mass, cranial decompression or cephalocentesis may be required for vaginal delivery, but most believe C-section should be performed to prevent dystocia.[311,319] Postnatal treatment may be solely supportive care. In the presence of hydrocephalus, a shunt is indicated. Surgical resection of the primary tumor, followed by chemotherapy, is typical therapy. Radiation is contraindicated because of side effects on normal brain development. Survivors often have significant psychomotor deficits.[310,311]

Recurrence: Most are sporadic, except in the case of familial or genetic predisposition.[317]

Disorders of Cellular Migration

Gray matter heterotopia

Incidence: Prevalence in the general population is unknown, but gray matter heterotopias have been described to occur in 11% to 20% of patients with epilepsy.[323]

Pathogenesis: Gray matter heterotopias are normal neurons present in an abnormal location, usually situated anywhere from the

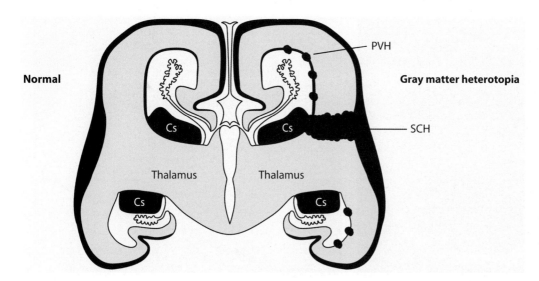

FIGURE 17.1-48: Types of gray matter heterotopia. *PVH*, periventricular heterotopia; *SCH*, subcortical heterotopia.

subependymal surface to the cerebral cortex (Fig. 17.1-48). Research suggests that periventricular nodular heterotopia (PVH) likely is due to a disruption in the neuroependyma, related to membrane gaps and impaired adhesion of the postmitotic neurons to the radial glial cells, thus impairing migration from the germinal matrix.[324]

PVH is the most common form of gray matter heterotopia. Histologically, the nodules show rudimentary lamination, similar to that in the cortex. The heterotopia is located adjacent to the ventricular wall, within the ventricular zone, usually along the trigone or occipital horns of the lateral ventricles.[325] PVH may be nodular or laminar and are commonly described as focal, unilateral, bilateral focal, or bilateral diffuse.[326] PVH is often grouped as

- **Classic bilateral PVH:** symmetric nodules of gray matter lining ventricles, especially frontal horns and body
- **Bilateral posterior or asymmetrical PVH:** bilateral nodules of gray matter restricted to trigones, temporal and occipital lobes or asymmetric bilateral on both sides
- **Unilateral PVH:** unilateral single or continuous nodule of gray matter

Subcortical heterotopia, also due to premature arrest of neurons, is less common but has many appearances. Some are transmantle, composed of linear columns of neurons continuous from the ependymal surface to cortex. Others may be nodular, curvilinear, or mixed, often solely present in the subcortical white matter.[327] Subcortical heterotopia can present as a small, large, sublobar, or regional mass in an otherwise normal hemisphere.

Etiology: Genetic and nongenetic causes for gray matter heterotopia include single-gene disorders, chromosomal anomalies, and disruptive events.[324] Unilateral or sparsely scattered PVH is typically sporadic. Bilateral PVH is present in 54% of cases, and in this group, genetic syndromes and associated intracranial anomalies are more likely.[328]

As research progresses, new genetic variants associated with PVH are being discovered, with molecular cytogenetic abnormalities being found in up to 36% of cases of PVH.[329] The most common genetic association with PVH is an X-linked dominant mutation of the *FLNA* gene localized at the Xq28 loci.[330] Lack of production of the encoding filamin protein arrests neuronal

migration. Since the disorder is X-linked, the phenotype in males results in death or severe neurological deficit, whereas females are only mildly affected.[330] *FLNA* genetic mutations may be present in up to 49% of all patients with PVH, and as high as 93% of females with PVH.[328] *FLNA* mutations in women are found in 80% to 100% of familial cases and sporadic in 20% to 30% of cases.[331]

Females with this disorder typically show classic bilateral PVH with symmetric continuous heterotopia along the walls of the lateral ventricles, sparing the temporal horns. These patients may also have a mega cistern magna and cerebellar hypoplasia.[325] Cardiovascular defects including patent ductus arteriosus, valvular disorders, coarctation of aorta, and ascending aorta aneurysm are known associations.[325] *FLNA* mutations are also described in patients with Ehlers–Danlos syndrome and otopalatodigital syndrome.[328]

A rare autosomal recessive defect in the *ARFGEF2* gene is characterized by microcephaly and delayed myelination with PVH.[329] Other genetic disorders associations include 7q11.23 (Williams syndrome), deletion 6p25 usually with white matter abnormalities, 1p36 monosomy with agenesis of corpus callosum, 6q terminal deletion, 5q14.3–q15, and duplication of 5p15 with anterior PVH.[323,332]

Gray matter heterotopia is often seen in association with other CNS malformations and present in up to 19% of cases of agenesis of corpus callosum and 30% of fetuses with Chiari II malformation.[323,333] With posterior (temporal and occipital) distributed PVH, anomalies are more common, including cerebellar dysgenesis, corpus callosum abnormalities, under-rotated hippocampus, and temporal lobe dysgenesis.[324,332]

Diagnosis

Ultrasound: PVH tends to be underdiagnosed, with targeted neurosonography missing 36% detected by MRI.[323] When detected, US typically identifies the anomaly in the third trimester at an average of 29 weeks' gestation.[331] PVH can be identified as irregular ventricular margins and/or hyperechoic or intermediate echogenic bands or nodules, sometimes bulging along the ventricle surface or in periventricular area (Fig. 17.1-49A).[323,334] Dedicated axial and coronal images of the ventricles allow for improved detection.[323] In a recent review, the two major US findings in PVH were not identification of the heterotopia but

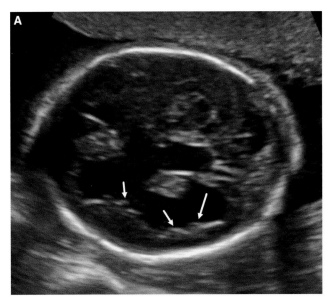
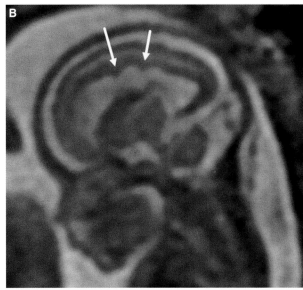

FIGURE 17.1-49: Fetus at 20 weeks with agenesis of the corpus callosum and suspected Aicardi. **A:** Axial US demonstrating echogenic irregularity (*arrows*) along the wall of the ventricle suspect for gray matter heterotopia. **B:** Sagittal MRI demonstrating irregularity along the wall of the ventricle (*arrows*) consistent with periventricular heterotopia.

VM associated with dysmorphic squared–shaped frontal horns in 60% and posterior fossa anomalies in 73%, most common in the diffuse form of PVH.[331]

Magnetic Resonance Imaging: Most cases of gray matter heterotopia are detected on a fetal MRI being performed for another indication. On MRI, PVH appears as round or oval nodules, which are isointense to the cortex, being dark on T2 (Fig. 17.1-49B). The nodules are typically within the wall of the ventricle, projecting into the ventricle and/or periventricular area.[325] Mild ventricular dilatation, thinning of the overlying cortex, and shallow sulci may be present.

Fetal MRI can define two different groups of heterotopia, with the easiest and most commonly diagnosed prenatally being the diffuse form, often associated with mega cisterna magna and high association with *FLNA* mutations.[331] Nondiffuse types can be identified, with 60% of these cases noted in the presence of additional cortical malformations.[331] The most common associated malformations described on fetal MRI are polymicrogyria and microcephaly.[331]

Fetal MRI has been stated to be only 67% sensitive for detection of heterotopia, but has 100% specificity when the abnormality is verified on two imaging planes.[335] Another study also suggested limited ability to diagnose PVH, detected prospectively only in 40% of fetuses with Chiari II malformation.[333] The detection of heterotopia, especially less than 24 weeks, is often difficult in view of the small size of heterotopia and fetal brain, similar signal to the germinal matrix and artifact due to motion.[335]

Subcortical heterotopia will show gray matter signal extending from the ventricular surface to the cortex or manifest as a focal mass in the white matter (Fig. 17.1-50). The overlying cortex tends to be thin and deficient in sulcation, and the affected area of the brain is small.[326] If large, blood vessels and prominent undulations with CSF signal can be seen in the ectopic gray tissue.

Associated Anomalies: In the presence of bilateral frontal PVH, most patient are females with *FLNA* mutations and arachnoid cysts and cardiac disorder.[336] Asymmetrical bilateral PVH is more likely to have additional abnormalities, including hippocampal and cerebellar abnormalities.[336] Other intracranial anomalies are common with PVH and include pachygyria, polymicrogyria, agenesis of corpus callosum, Chiari II malformation, posterior fossa anomalies, schizencephaly, encephaloceles, and metabolic disorders such as Zellweger.[325,326] Limb and frontonasal disorders can be seen with PVH.[328] Subcortical heterotopia is often associated with areas of polymicrogyria and dysgenesis of the corpus callosum in greater than 70%.[236,326]

Differential Diagnosis: The normal germinal matrix, especially the area of the ganglionic eminences, is prominent early in gestation and should not be confused with nodular heterotopia. Motion artifact may also falsely simulate nodularity on fetal MRI. In addition, in the presence of VM, stretching of the ependyma/subependyma may mimic nodularity along the germinal matrix.[333]

Differential for PVH includes tuberous sclerosis (TS) and early subacute subependymal hemorrhage. Nodules from TS appear similar to PVH; however, family history and the presence of cardiac or renal findings may help differentiate. Subacute hemorrhage usually occurs in the presence of intraventricular hemorrhage and VM and will evolve over time. Subcortical heterotopia should be differentiated from tumor or schizencephaly, which demonstrates a central cleft.

Prognosis: In the presence of associated anomalies, the outcome is worse for both PVH and subcortical heterotopia, with developmental delay of variable severity and early seizure onset.[324,325] Males with X-linked PVH have a worse prognosis than females, with high incidence of neurodevelopmental disorders and seizures.[325,326] Cognition deficit are less likely in the unilateral focal PVH group than those with bilateral asymmetrical PVH.[324,326] Interestingly, though, the majority of patients with *FLNA* mutations and symmetric PVH have normal psychomotor and normal or slightly impaired intelligence.[330,336] In some patients with PVH, the lesion is incidental, as no symptoms are present. Overall, 20% to 60% of patients with PVH have disorders of cognition.[326]

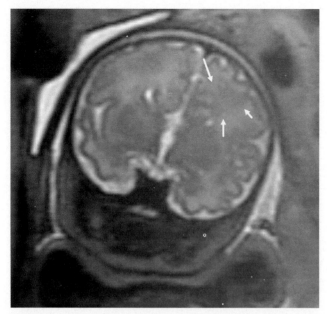

FIGURE 17.1-50: Fetus at 35 weeks with agenesis of the corpus callosum and proven subcortical heterotopia. Coronal T2 image demonstrates a wedge shaped band of gray matter signal (*arrows*) extending from the ventricular surface to the cortex.

Approximately 80% to 90% of patients with PVH develop epilepsy, which can begin at any age but usually in the second decade of life.[324,325,332] In patients with *FLNA* mutations, seizures occur in the second or third decade, which may delay medical surveillance of associated cardiovascular complications.[330,336]

Nearly all patients with subcortical heterotopia develop seizures in the second decade of life.[326] Variable motor and intellectual deficiencies occur, depending on the site and size of the lesion.[326]

Management: With epilepsy, treatment with antiepileptic drugs is the first line of therapy. Localization of the epileptogenic area is complex as the PVH may be active and engage overlying cortex.[332] If seizures are refractory, surgical resection of the epileptogenic focus may be considered.[326]

Recurrence: Recurrence is dependent on whether the lesion is sporadic or associated with a genetic disorder. In *FLNA* mutation, the disorder is X-linked autosomal dominant, with 50% transmission to a female offspring and 100% to male.

Lissencephaly (Classic or Type 1 LIssencephaly)/Agyria, Pachygyria, Dysgryia, and Subcortical Band Hetertopia

Agyria represents a thick cortex with lack of gyri, also consistent with complete lissencephaly (LIS). Broad, shallow, and flat gyri with thickened cortex are diagnostic of pachygyria and are often present in incomplete forms of LIS. Dysgyria represents an abnormal sulcal pattern that does not fit aforementioned, often seen in the tubulinopathies consisting of intermediate between pachygyria and polymicrogyria. Subcortical band heterotopia represents a band of heterotopic gray matter beneath the cortex, separated by a thin layer of white matter. Microlissencephaly represents LIS

in association with a small brain, <3 SD below the mean. Often, there is a combination of these anomalies.[337]

Incidence: The estimated incidence of classic LIS or type I LIS is 1.2 per 100,000 births.[135]

Pathogenesis: LIS is a severe malformation of the fetal brain that occurs because of impaired neuronal migration during the third to fourth month of gestation.[338] The prime defect is a genetic flaw that results in disruption of normal neural migration.[135] The classic genetic disorders in LIS are related to dysfunction of microtubules, a major component of the neuronal cytoskeleton and essential for almost all cellular processes, including cell division, motility, and intracellular organization.[332] Microtubules are composed of α and β tubulins that bind to a γ tubulin ring and regulate neuronal migration but also cell division and axon guidance. Microtubule-associated proteins (MAPs) enable microtubules to participate in many of these functions. The genetic disorders of the tubulins and MAPs are now grouped under the term tubulinopathies, as all these genes affect microtubule function. Recent classification of LIS includes the classic LIS caused by mutations of tubulin genes or MAPs (*LIS1, DCX, KIF5C, KIF2A,* and *DYNC1H1*).[332] Variant LIS is caused by genetic mutations of *ARX* or the Reelin pathway, also important in neurogenesis and neuronal migration.[332]

A normal brain contains six cortical layers. In classic LIS, the lack of normal migration results in two or four cortical layers. The tubulin genetic defects, especially *TUBA1A* and *TUBB2B*, may result in a two- or four-layer pattern. The *MAP* genes, with most common being *LIS1*, give rise to a four-layer pattern in which the cortex is abnormally thick as the cells arrested lie in disorganized radial columns.[339] On histology, the two most superficial layers, a cell dense marginal zone and superficial cortical gray zone, are formed by normal neuronal migration early in gestation. The third layer is cell sparse, with only a few dysplastic neurons. The fourth layer is densely cellular with radial orientated neurons, lacking lamination (Fig. 17.1-51). Because axonal and dendritic connections do not develop, the subcortical white matter is thin and lacks gray white matter interdigitation.[339]

In subcortical band heterotopia, normal cortical and subcortical white matter architecture is present with a band of heterotopic columnar neurons.[340] LIS and subcortical band heterotopia can be diffuse or partial and may demonstrate a gradient being more anterior, posterior, or temporal. The classic LIS is divided into six grades based on the severity of the malformation, grade I being the most severe (Table 17.1-13).[332]

In the variant form of LIS, the cortex is only slightly thick, there is an anterior to posterior gradient, variable lack of sulcation, and no cell-sparse zone. *ARX* mutations have agenesis of the corpus callosum (ACC) and small dysplastic basal ganglia and Reelin pathway disorders cerebellar hypoplasia and hippocampal hypoplasia/dysplasia.[332] *ARX* mutations have been described to have a three-layer cortex, with thick outer molecular, middle pyramidal layer and expanded third layer with no myelinated axons.[332,337]

Etiology: Multiple genes have been associated with LIS (Table 17.1-14).[337] The topography of the malformation is dependent on the gene that is affected. Cortical morphology, gradient, and thickness vary, and many are associated with noncortical malformations, with cerebellar hypoplasia being the most common association.[337]

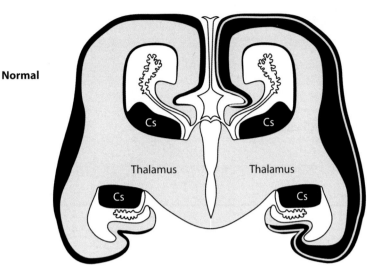

Normal

Lissencephaly type I

Thalamus   Thalamus

FIGURE 17.1-51: Diagram of the layered pattern in classic four-layer lissencephaly type I.

LIS may be isolated or associated with a syndrome. The first diagnosed case of LIS was in a case of Miller–Dieker syndrome, due to *de novo* chromosomal deletion at 17p13.3 causing mutation of the *LIS1* and *YWHAE* genes. Miller–Dieker syndrome is seen in the presence of severe classic LIS and facial dysmorphism consisting of prominent forehead, bitemporal hollowing, short upturned nose, thickened upper lip, low-set ears, and small jaw. Other less common anomalies include cardiac and genitourinary, omphalocele, and duodenal atresia.

Baraitser–Winter syndrome is characterized by pachygyria, trigonocephaly, shallow orbits, ptosis, and colobomas and is due to mutations of *ACTG1* and *ACTB*, cytoplasmic actins necessary for cell growth and migration.[340,341] X-linked LIS with abnormal genitalia (XLAG) is associated with *ARX* mutation, resulting in temporal predominant thin LIS; is phenotypically more severe in males than in females; and is seen in association with abnormal genitalia, facial dysmorphism, ACC, and often hypoplastic basal ganglia.[337]

However, the majority of cases, approximately 80%, are considered isolated classic LIS.[337] The most common pattern is partial agyria–pachygyria with posterior gradient, almost all by mutations of the *LIS1* gene.[337] The second most common is posterior prominent pachygyria, followed by tubulinopathy dysgyria and diffuse agyria with or without cerebellar hypoplasia. *LIS1* (65%) and *DCX* (12%) account for approximately 77% of isolated LIS, and *TUBA1A* a small percent, all commonly due to *de novo* mutations.[342] *TUBA1A* accounts for 30% of cases of LIS with cerebellar hypoplasia.[341] *DCX* is associated with 90% of cases of subcortical band heterotopia.[343]

The *LIS1* gene mutation is present equally in both males and females, with gyral abnormalities more severe posteriorly, demonstrating agyria parieto-occipital and pachygyria frontal and temporal.[340,344] Almost all posterior gradient LIS are associated with mutation of *LIS1* or the less common tubulin genes.[337]

The *DCX* gene is present on the X chromosome and affects the anterior aspect of the brain more than the posterior; in males, it causes LIS, whereas in females, a milder phenotype with subcortical band heterotopia is noted.[345] Mutations of the *DCX* and actin isoforms (*ACTB* and *ACTG1*) cause most of the thick cortex anterior predominant LIS.

Tubulinopathies encompass a wide spectrum of tubulin-related genes. Mutations can result in undermigration as well as overmigration of cells.[229] Disorders of these genes result in many brain anomalies, including microcephaly, LIS, pachygyria, dysgyria, subcortical band heterotopia, anomalies of white matter tracts, corticospinal tracts, and cranial nerves and malformations of the midbrain and hindbrain.[229] Common noncortical findings in tubulinopathies include basal ganglia dysgenesis (fused striatum due to impaired formation of anterior limb of internal capsule), complete or partial absence of corpus callosum, tectal hyperplasia, brainstem hypoplasia or dysgenesis, and cerebellar, often vermian hypoplasia.[337] The spectrum of LIS is wide, with the tubulinopathies ranging from microlissencephaly to classic LIS to dysgyria.

In subcortical band heterotopia, *DCX* is the most common genetic mutation, presenting with anterior predominant partial or diffuse thick and thin band heterotopia. Posterior partial band heterotopia is due to *LIS1* mutations in 30%, but tubulinopathies are increasingly found to be the etiology.[332]

The most severe LIS is present in male with *DCX*, *LIS1* (most often with *YWHAE* deletion), *TUBA1A*, *TUBB2B*, and *CDK5* mutations.[337]

TABLE 17.1-13	Grading of Classic Lissencephaly
GRADE AND GRADIENT	**IMAGING**
1 a = p	Complete agyria
2 p > a or a > p	Diffuse agyria with few undulations frontal/occipital poles
3 p > a or a > p	Mixed agyria and pachygyria
4 p > a or a > p	Diffuse pachygyria or mixed pachygyria and normal/simplified pattern
5 a > p	Mixed pachygyria and subcortical band heterotopia
6 p > a or a > p	Subcortical band heterotopia only

a, anterior location of malformations, *p*, posterior location.
From DiDonato N, Chiari S, Mirzaa GM, et al. Lissencephaly: expanded imaging and clinical classification. *Am J Med Genet.* 2017;173A:1473–1488.

TABLE 17.1-14 **Genes and Syndromes in Association with Lissencephaly Type Based on Imaging**

IMAGING	GRADIENT	GENES
Classic Thick Lissencephaly		
AG *with cerebellar hypoplasia (thin or thick AG)*	*DIF*	*LIS1-YWHAE/***MDS**, *DCX* *TUBA1A, TUBB2B, CDK5*
AG-PG (mixed)	*PA*	*LIS1, TUBA1A*
PG *With noncortical malformations[a]*	*PA*	*LIS1, DYNC1H1, TUBG1* *TUBA1A, TUBB2B, DYNC1H1*
AG-PG	*AP*	*DCX*
PG *With noncortical malformations[a]* *Band*	*AP*	*DCX, ACTB, DYNC1H1, ACTG1, KIFSC,* **BWS** *KIFSC* *ACTB, ACTG1, DCX*
Thin Undulating Lissencephaly		
PG *With cerebellar hypoplasia* *With normal cerebellum*	*AP*	 *RELN, VLDLR* *CRADD*
PG with ACC, abnormal WM	*TL*	*ARX,* **XLAG**
Microlissencephaly		
MLIS with cerebellar hypoplasia	*DIF*	*TUBA1A*
MLIS with MOPD1	*DIF*	*RNU4ATAC*
MLIS Barth type		
Tubulinopathy-Related Dysgyria		
DG	*PA*	*TUBA1A, TUBB2B, DYNC1H1, TUBB, TUBB3, TUBAB*
DG	*AP*	*KIF5C*
Subcortical Band Heterotopia		
SBH (thick or thin band)	*DIF*	*DCX*
SBH partial (thick or thin band)	*PA*	*LIS1, LIS1-YWHAE mosaic, TUBA1A, TUBG1*
SBH partial (thick or thin band)[a]	*AP*	*DCX, KIF2A*

[a]Noncortical malformations include agenesis of corpus callosum (ACC), dysplastic basal ganglia, tectal hyperplasia, and cerebellar hypoplasia with or without dysplasia.
DIF, diffuse; *PA,* posterior to anterior; *AP,* anterior to posterior; *TL,* temporal; *MDS,* Miller–Dieker syndrome; *BWS,* Baraitser–Winter syndrome; *XLAG,* X-linked LIS with abnormal genitalia; *MOPD1,* microcephalic osteodysplastic primordial dwarfism type 1; *AG,* agyria; *PG,* pachygyria; *DG,* dysgyria; *MLIS,* microlissencephaly, SBH, subcortical band heterotopia.
From DiDonato N, Chiari S, Mirzaa GM, et al. Lissencephaly: expanded imaging and clinical classification. *Am J Med Genet.* 2017;173A:1473–1488.

In the variant LIS group, *ARX* causes ACC, dysplastic basal ganglia and an X-linked LIS and therefore is phenotypically more severe in males than in females. Reelin genes, *RELN* and *VLDLR,* cause thin LIS with anterior gradient in association with severe cerebellar and hippocampal hypoplasia/dysplasia and often brainstem abnormalities.[337,135] In the differential though with thin LIS, diffuse agyria and cerebellar hypoplasia are genes *TUBA1A, TUBB2B,* and *CDK5.*[337]

Diagnosis: When there is a concern for LIS, karyotype is suggested, as fluorescence in situ hybridization (FISH) analysis of 17p13.3 deletions and sequencing for abnormalities of the *LIS1* and *DCX* genes and tubulinopathies can be diagnostic.

Ultrasound: Severe forms of LIS are easier to detect than milder incomplete forms.[346] Agyria/pachygyria can be suggested as early as 23 to 24 weeks when there is a smooth, thick cerebral surface with absence of parieto-occipital and calcarine fissure and wide Sylvian fissures due to abnormal opercular formation.[346] After 28 weeks, in the presence of a smooth brain, diagnosis of LIS can be confirmed (Fig. 17.1-52A).[346] 3D imaging may demonstrate sulci better than 2D.[347]

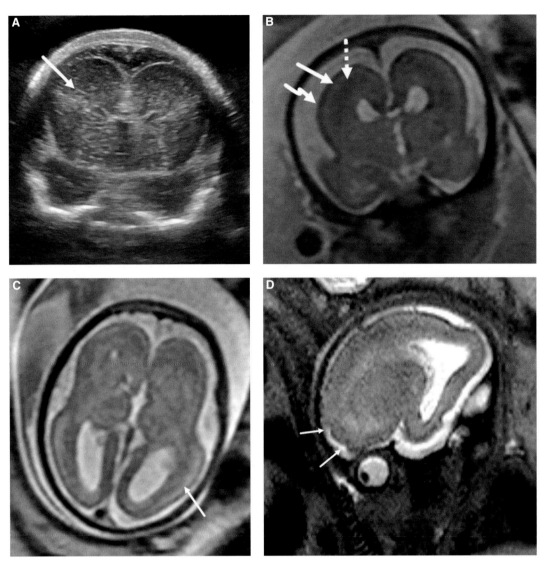

FIGURE 17.1-52: Multiple fetuses with lissencephaly. **A:** Fetus at 36 weeks' gestation with classic type I LIS. Coronal US demonstrates abnormal smooth appearance of the cortex. There is increased echogenicity in the area of the intermediate zone (*arrow*). **B:** Coronal T2 MRI in the same fetus demonstrating thin peripheral cortex (*curved arrow*), cell-sparse zone (*solid arrow*), and deep thick disorganized neurons (*dotted arrow*). Notice abnormal smooth architecture of the brain for gestational age. (Courtesy of Dorothy Bulas, MD.) **C:** Axial MRI in a different fetus at 31 weeks with classic LIS. Notice smooth brain with figure-8 appearance and prominent cell-sparse zone posterior (*arrow*). **D:** Fetus at 35 weeks with mild ventriculomegaly and agyria posterior but shallow sulci consistent with pachygyria anterior (*arrows*).

Lamination of the fetal brain can normally be detected as early as 17 weeks, present to 28 weeks' gestation, and disappearing by 34 weeks.[348] The subplate should be anechoic, and the intermediate zone homogeneously more echogenic.[348] When LIS is present, no laminar pattern, prominent increased echogenicity in the intermediate zone representing thick disorganized neurons, or persistence of lamination pattern after 33 weeks can be noted.[348] Mild VM and enlarged subarachnoid spaces are often present (Fig. 17.1-53A).[338,349] Immature sulcation with wide and thick gyri is typical.[349]

In the presence of other intracranial and extracranial findings, a diagnosis of Miller–Dieker syndrome may be suggested. The most common findings that should raise suspicion of Miller–Dieker syndrome are polyhydramnios (66%), intrauterine growth restriction (62%), and VM (59%).[345] US diagnosis for MDS has been noted to be as high as 41% prenatal, mostly the third trimester.[345]

Magnetic Resonance Imaging: Postnatal, agyria is considered when sulci are >3 cm apart, pachygyria 1.5 to 3 cm, and dysgyria with a mix of pachygyria and polymicrogyria separated by shallow sulci with smooth gray white border. These findings do not readily apply in the fetus, especially at early gestational ages. After birth, normal cortical thickness is 3 to 4 mm, and in LIS, the thickness is either mildly increased at 5 to 10 mm or classically thick at 10 to 20 mm.[337,340] Unfortunately, cortical thickness changes are also not described prenatal.

Diagnosis of LIS in the fetus relies on detecting absence of normal sulcation. Early in gestation, mild VM, especially colpocephaly, is often present owing to lack of development of the calcarine sulcus.[350] Large temporal horns likely represent arrest in hippocampal maturation and invagination.[350] At 23 to 24 weeks, absence of normal parieto-occipital and calcarine sulcus with wide Sylvian fissures may suggest LIS.[346] However, these findings are nonspecific. False positives must be entertained as fetuses can have delay in sulcation for many reasons beyond LIS.[351]

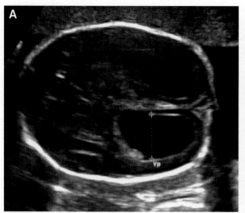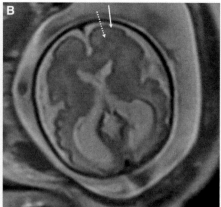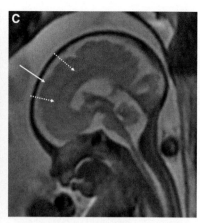

FIGURE 17.1-53: Fetus at 33 weeks with confirmed pachygyria and band heterotopia. **A:** Axial US demonstrating moderate ventriculomegaly. **B:** Axial T2 MRI showing abnormal lack of sulci (*solid arrows*) in the frontal lobes bilaterally. Notice dark band of signal in the white matter (*dotted arrow*), which is abnormal for gestational age and represented band heterotopia postnatal. **C:** Sagittal MRI again demonstrating band of heterotopia (*dotted arrows*) with shallow sulci anterior hemisphere (*solid arrow*).

In conjunction with abnormal sulcation, a fetus with LIS may have some degree of cortical thickening with visualization of the abnormal layered pattern of classic LIS (Fig. 17.1-52B). Between 20 and 28 weeks, this may be a problem as the band of hyperintense T2 signal, which represents the cell-sparse layer, may be difficult to differentiate from the normal subplate. A figure-8 configuration of the brain is often described postnatal and is due to lack of development of the Sylvian fissures, also known as opercular dysplasia (Fig. 17.1-52C). However, prior to 20 weeks, the normal fetal brain is smooth with a figure-8 configuration. Cavitations in the ganglionic eminences, especially in conjunction with abnormality of the corpus callosum, have been described and may raise suspicion.[352] MRI may also detect associated anomalies of the basal ganglia, brainstem, and cerebellum. However, as described above, most cases of LIS cannot be diagnosed until after 28 weeks, and serial MRI may be needed to confirm the pathology.[351]

In the third trimester, MRI is more likely to detect LIS and subcortical band heterotopia.[346] In agyria–pachygyria, the brain is relatively smooth, and the cortex may develop an element of thickness with a smooth gray white matter junction and shallow sulci in the primitive pattern of the primary fissures (Fig. 17.1-52D) With subcortical band heterotopia, there is a ribbon of abnormal gray matter separated from the normal cortex by white matter. The band tends to be more pronounced and focal than the dark signal of the intermediate zone present from 20 to 28 weeks. Beyond 28 weeks, a band of gray matter signal in the white matter is diagnostic of neuronal heterotopia (Fig. 17.1-53B, C).

Associated Anomalies: Associated intracranial anomalies are common. The cerebellum, brainstem, basal ganglia and corpus callosum are often abnormal. Extracerebral anomalies may point to the diagnosis of Miller–Dieker syndrome and other genetic disorders.

Differential Diagnosis: Understanding normal brain development is imperative as early in gestation the brain is smooth, and this should not be interpreted as LIS. Diagnosis of delayed sulcation should not be considered until after 20 weeks, and it must be remembered that there can be a 2-week difference in visualization of a normal fissure. In the presence of other intracranial anomalies, sulcation may be delayed more than 2 weeks owing to

the primary CNS abnormality. Abnormal operculization of the Sylvian fissure does not necessarily support a migration abnormality as it may be related to extracortical factors and can be a normal variant, particularly when only the anterior portion is abnormal.[353]

Prognosis: The severity of the malformation usually correlates with clinical outcome, with agyria manifesting severe neurodevelopmental deficits, pachygyria intermediate, and subcortical band heterotopia mild described in Table 17.1-15.[337] Exceptions

TABLE 17.1-15	Clinical Severity of Lissencephaly	
GRADE	**IMAGING**	**OUTCOME**
Mild	*Partial SBH* *Diffuse thin SBH* *Partial PG* *Isolated thin or undulating LIS*	Borderline-to-moderate ID Variable seizures Survival adulthood expected
Moderate	*Diffuse thick SBH* *Mixed PG-SBH* *Diffuse PG*	Moderate-to-severe ID Severe language impairment Seizures often poorly controlled Life expectancy reduced though many survive to adulthood
Severe	*Mixed PG-AG* *Diffuse AG* *AG and cerebellar hypoplasia*	Profound ID Poorly controlled seizures Short survival 50% mortality by 10 years with normal cerebellum Higher mortality with cerebellar hypoplasia

SBH, subcortical band heterotopia; *ID*, intellectual disability; *PG*, pachygyria; *AG*, agyria, LIS, lissencephaly.
From DiDonato N, Chiari S, Mirzaa GM, et al. Lissencephaly: expanded imaging and clinical classification. *Am J Med Genet.* 2017;173A:1473–1488.

occur in the presence of significant epilepsy, which lowers overall neurodevelopment.[337]

Newborns have hypotonia, poor feeding, and often transient elevations in bilirubin. The head circumference tends to be normal at birth, but is small by 1 year of age. Seizures develop by 6 months in more than 90% of children, and infantile spasms are seen in 80%.[340] With the onset of infantile spasms, there is a rapid decline in function. Children have poor control of their airway and gastroesophageal reflux, predisposing to aspiration pneumonia, the most common cause for demise. In children with Miller–Dieker syndrome, death is typically in the first 2 years.[340]

Management: Delayed prenatal US and MRI in the third trimester may be necessary to confirm diagnosis. Termination may be considered but may not be possible, depending on time of diagnosis. With knowledge of the anomaly, decisions can be made with regard to the site of delivery and management/support at the time of birth. Genetic counseling is indicated both prenatal and postnatal. Parental testing should be considered as up to 20% of fetuses with Miller–Dieker syndrome will inherit the genetic deletion from a parent.[338] In X-linked LIS, genetic testing may be performed in the mother to exclude inherited mutation. Discussion of prognosis with decisions on limitations of care should be communicated.

Most children with LIS require feeding via enteric or gastrostomy tubes. Aggressive management of seizures is imperative to prevent rapid decline in function.[340]

Recurrence: Most cases of isolated LIS and Miller–Dieker syndrome (80% *de novo*) are sporadic, and the risk of recurrence is negligible.[340,345] If a female carries a defective *DCX* and has a mild phenotype, risk can be increased to 50%. Also, when one parent has balanced translocation of *LIS1* gene, recurrence risk increases to 10% to 15%.[351]

Cobblestone Lissencephaly (Type II Lissencephaly; Alpha-Dystroglycanopathy; Congenital Muscular Dystrophy; Cerebro-ocular Dysgenesis; Walker–Warburg Syndrome)

Incidence: Cobblestone or type II lissencephaly (CLIS) is rare with unknown worldwide distribution.[354]

Pathogenesis: CLIS results in disorders of the brain, muscle, and eye due to abnormal linkage of the basement membrane to muscle cells or radial glia transporting migrating neurons.[332]

For normal neuronal migration, a normal interaction must occur between the radial glial cells and the outermost pial–glial membrane known as the glia limitans.[355] In CLIS, the neurons move too far past the glia limitans into the subpial space. Pathologically, this is caused by impaired linkage of the radial glia to the pial basement membrane, leading to a disruption of the pial barrier, with resultant absence of normal cortical plate lamination and neuroglial ectopia in the subarachnoid space (Fig. 17.1-54).[236,355] The cerebellum is affected similar to the supratentorial brain; however, in the cerebellum, there is disrupted adhesion of the developing granule cells to the pial basement membrane.[355] The phenotype depends on the glia limitans gap size and amount of linkage with radial glia cells.[278] Small gaps result in nearly normal cortex with small surface bumps, intermediate gaps with imaging findings of polymicrogyria (PMG), and large gaps as smooth cortical surface, similar to CLIS (Fig. 17.1-55).[278]

Congenital muscular dystrophies (CMDs) are a group of heterogeneous disorders, some primarily affecting muscle and others with muscle and CNS involvement.[356] In those with CNS abnormalities, the genetic mutations of CLIS affect the glia limitans. The most common group, the α-dystroglycanopathies, results in hypoglycosylation of alpha-dystroglycan. Alpha-dystroglycan is a glycoprotein that binds cells to the extracellular

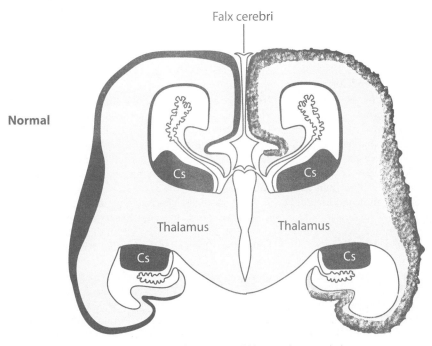

FIGURE 17.1-54: Diagram of imaging findings in cobblestone lissencephaly.

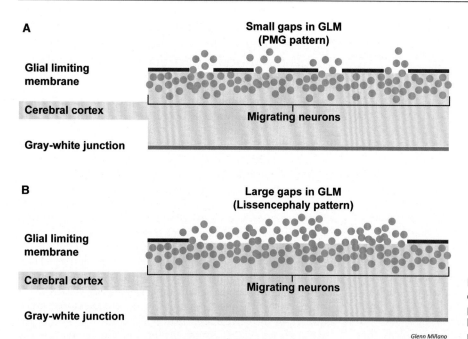

A

**Small gaps in GLM
(PMG pattern)**

Glial limiting
membrane

Cerebral cortex

Migrating neurons

Gray-white junction

B

**Large gaps in GLM
(Lissencephaly pattern)**

Glial limiting
membrane

Cerebral cortex

Migrating neurons

Gray-white junction

Glenn Miñano

FIGURE 17.1-55: Diagram of pathogenesis of glial limitans with small gaps resulting in a polymicrogyria pattern **(A)** and larger gaps cobblestone lissencephaly **(B)**. *GLM*, glial-limiting membrane; *PMG*, polymicrogyria.

matrix. The glycosylation-deficient glycoprotein on the radial glial and muscle fiber endfeet results in defective formation of the basement membrane of the brain, muscle, and retina.[236] Mutations of the laminins, receptors for alpha-dystroglycan on the glia limitans, and *GPR56* on the radial glia endfeet and its collagen receptors (*COL4A1*) result in a similar defect.[332]

Etiology: Multiple genes, many inherited autosomal recessive, have been linked to CLIS. Alpha-dystroglycanopathies include *POMT1, POMT2, FKTN, FKRP, LARGE, POMGNT1, ISPD, GTDC3, TMEM5, POMK, B4GAT1,* and *B3GALNT2.*[135,236] Basement membrane genes include *LAMB1, LAMB2, LAMC3, SRD5A3,* and *COL4A1.*[278] Clinical phenotypes vary widely and do not necessarily correlate well with genetic defect.[332]

The CLISs include Walker–Warburg syndrome (WWS), muscle–eye–brain (MEB) disease (initially described in the Finnish), and Fukuyama muscular dystrophy (FMD) (described in Japanese descent). The most common and severe phenotype is WWS, also known as *h*ydrocephalus, *a*gryia, and *r*etinal *d*ysplasia with or without *e*ncephalocele (HARD+E).[338,357] WWS has been associated with multiple identified and many yet unknown genetic abnormalities. The syndrome is typically caused by *POMT2, POMT2, FRKP,* and fukutin genes, but only 10% to 20% of cases have been diagnosed with these genetic markers.[354]

Diagnosis of WWS includes CLIS, cerebellar malformation, retinal malformation, and muscular dystrophy (Table 17.1-16).[338,358] VM may be present with or without hydrocephalus. Brainstem abnormalities are common and include fused colliculi, small pons, and dysmorphic mesencephalon with a dorsal pontomedullary kink and ventral cervicomedullary kink that is characteristic of primitive hindbrain morphology.[359] Ocular abnormalities may or may not be present and include microphthalmia, anterior and posterior segment anomalies, persistent fetal vasculature, retinal dysplasia, retinal detachment, coloboma, and optic nerve hypoplasia.[357] Muscle changes often do not occur till late fetal period or postnatal.

The brain malformations of WWS are most severe, followed by MEB and finally, FMD on the milder end of the spectrum.[360] MEB

disease findings are similar to WWS, with eye findings milder, including progressive myopia and retinal detachment.[354,360] In FMD, frontal or occipital temporal CLIS, cerebellar PMG and hypogenesis, often in the presence of subcortical cerebellar cysts and simple myopia, are noted.[361,360] Mutations in the *ADGRG1* (*GPR56*) gene cause bilateral frontoparietal PMG, seen in conjunction with myelination abnormalities and dysplasia of the brainstem and cerebellum that overlap with CLIS. In addition, *COL4A1* (collagen IV disorders) is also expressed in the muscles, kidney, and eye, and may be part of the CLIS phenotype, presenting with pontocerebellar volume loss, cataracts, or other eye abnormalities.

Diagnosis: Amniocentesis with DNA analysis, particularly of the *POMT1* gene, may be performed.

Ultrasound: In the presence of VM and abnormalities of the posterior fossa, CLIS should be considered for prenatal diagnosis.[338,362] On US, a recent study has described that CLIS can be identified as a thick outer echogenic band in place of the normal thin echogenic interface of cortex with the subarachnoid space (Fig. 17.1-56A).[363] Abnormal thick echogenicity can be apparent along the cerebrum, cerebellum, and brainstem. In addition, small pericerebral spaces, particularly interhemispheric, are also present.[363] These findings in association with a kinked brainstem are pathognomonic of CLIS and can be detected as early as 14 weeks when the brainstem should normally have a straight configuration.[363]

VM has been cited as the most common finding, noted in 90% of cases, followed by cerebellar abnormalities in 33% (Fig. 17.1-56B).[338,362] Previous studies have shown that smooth brain, cerebellar and retinal malformations may be visualized by US in only 25% of cases.[362] Sulcation abnormalities are difficult to diagnose prior to 24 weeks, and this may be even more problematic in the presence of VM, which effaces subarachnoid spaces.[359,362] US may show loss of normal brain parenchymal lamination and/or a thin smooth cortex.[348,349] Transvaginal and 3D imaging may help in evaluation, allowing for better detail of the corpus callosum and posterior fossa.[359,362] Ocular anomalies may be present, such as bilateral echogenic lenses and/or conical structures within the globe apex toward the retina representing primary hyperplastic vitreous with retinal detachment (Fig. 17.1-56C).[357]

Magnetic Resonance Imaging: On MRI, the supratentorial brain may be smooth, but may demonstrate a pebbled appearance of PMG (Fig. 17.1-56D).[338] The normal pattern of lamination is absent.[364] There is irregular gray white matter interface, and the white matter can demonstrate increased T2 signal due to edema or dysmyelination.[360]

The cerebellum, especially vermis, is usually hypoplastic with abnormal foliation.[361] An enlarged superior cerebellar cistern is commonly present, and cerebellar cysts may be noted.[365] The most helpful finding in this pathology is brainstem hypoplasia with a dorsal kink at the pontomesencephalic junction and ventral in the cervicomedullary area, resulting in Z-shaped configuration (Fig. 17.1-56E).[338,361] The pons may have a central cleft. The tectum may be thick, and aqueductal stenosis can be present, which is often the cause for the VM. The extra-axial fluid spaces are small owing to neuronal and glial heterotopia.[360] Ocular abnormalities can also be detected (Fig. 17.1-56F).[338]

Associated Anomalies: Intracranial anomalies of the brainstem, cerebellum, white matter, and corpus callosum are common. Encephaloceles are often present in WWS.[355] Associated extracranial anomalies are listed in Table 17.1-16.

TABLE 17.1-16   Findings of Walker–Warburg Syndrome
Common
Widespread agyria, pachygyria, polymicrogyria
Ventriculomegaly
Cerebellar hypoplasia and dysplasia, especially vermis
Occipital encephalocele
Abnormal brainstem, Z-shaped
Heterotopias
Aqueduct stenosis
Abnormalities of the corpus callosum
Disorganized myelination
Eye abnormalities
Muscular disease
Less Common
Cleft lip
Microtia
Clubfoot
Renal dysplasia
Genital abnormalities
Intrauterine growth retardation

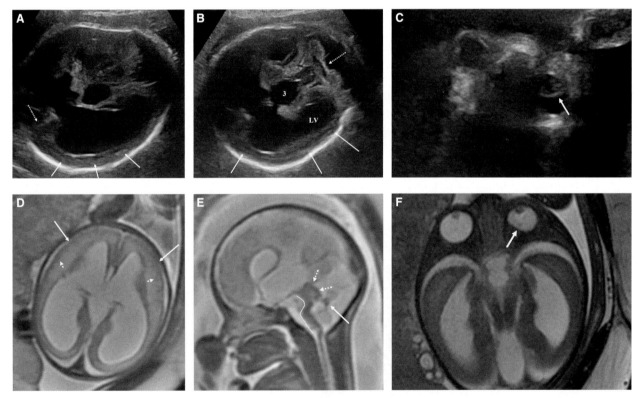

FIGURE 17.1-56: Fetus at 33 weeks with Walker–Warburg syndrome. **A:** Axial US demonstrating a band of echogenicity along the periphery of the brain (*solid arrow*). There is lack of subarachnoid space, particularly along the interhemispheric fissure (*dotted arrow*). **B:** Axial US demonstrating moderately severe lateral *(LV)* and third *(3)* ventriculomegaly. The visualized cortex is smooth (*solid arrows*). The cerebellar vermis is small (*dashed arrow*). **C:** Left globe demonstrating abnormal echogenic tissue extending vertically through the orbit consistent with primary hyperplastic vitreous (*arrow*). **D:** Axial T2 MRI demonstrating smooth mildly irregular cortex (*solid arrows*) with irregular nodular interface with white matter (*dashed arrows*). The white matter appears hyperintense. The lateral ventricles are enlarged. **E:** Sagittal T2 MRI demonstrating the Z- or cobra-shaped configuration of the brainstem (*curved line*). The tecum is thick (*dotted arrows*), and vermis is dysgenetic (*solid arrow*). **F:** Axial SSFP MRI demonstrating small left globe with abnormal tissue (*arrow*) extending from the lens to the retina.

Differential Diagnosis: A kinked brainstem can also be seen in cases of *L1CAM* mutations and tubulinopathies. Tubulinopathies may be differentiated by dysplastic basal ganglia. *L1CAM* mutations are in males, and adducted thumbs could provide clue to diagnosis. Congenital infection and rare metabolic disorders may mimic findings of the CLIS. Classic LIS will also demonstrate abnormal sulcation but a thick smooth cortex.

Prognosis: Children with WWS never reach any developmental milestones; have severe hypotonia, ocular abnormalities, muscle weakness, and occasional seizures; and usually die in the first year of life because of respiratory illness.[354] MEB is less severe, and children with FMD, although typically with severe mental retardation, can live to 4 to 6 years of age, usually with progressive myopathy.[360]

Management: With family history of WWS, US in the early second trimester demonstrating kinked brainstem, VM, and decreased pericerebral spaces may direct genetic testing.[366] Termination of pregnancy may be considered. Laboratory testing will demonstrate elevated creatine kinase and a muscular dystrophy characterized by hypoglycosylation of alpha-dystroglycan.[354] No specific treatment is available, and management is supportive. Control of seizures with medication, shunting for hydrocephalus, and surgical repair of encephalocele may be required.

Recurrence: Most forms are autosomal recessive, with a 25% risk for recurrence.[354]

Disorders of Cellular Organization

Polymicrogyria

Incidence: The incidence of polymicrogyria (PMG) is unknown; however, it is one of the most common brain malformations, accounting for approximately 20% of all anomalies of cortical development.[367]

Pathogenesis: PMG is a malformation in which there is abnormal cortical lamination and folding pattern, resulting in excessive number of small gyri. Imaging findings in PMG overlap with those of cobblestone lissencephaly (CLIS). However, not all disorders with multiple small gyri are consistent with true PMG.

PMG is heterogeneous in histology and cause, with a pathogenesis still incompletely understood. It is likely that PMG is a common endpoint of many etiologies, occurring at particular times in cortical development. Some have stated that PMG may not represent a cell migration disorder but rather a postmigration disorder in cortical development.[368]

Recent pathological studies have found that over 80% of cases of PMG are associated with prenatal damage of the glia limitans, resulting in adherent thickened leptomeninges invaded by neural or glial cells overlying the neural cortex (Fig. 17.1-55).[369–371] The cortical surface with arachnoid, pial cells, basement membrane, radial glial/astrocytic endfeet, and Cajal–Retzius cells regulates neurogenesis, cell migration, and positioning, and disruption in their organization is likely to be the primary cause of PMG. Abnormality of the glia limitans is present in 90% of acquired PMG and nearly 70% of genetic forms.[369] However, as it is not present in all cases, other factors including inflammatory response by macrophages, microglia, and glial cells may play a role in PMG development.[371] PMG can result in two-, four-, or six-layer lamination and sometimes fusion of the cortical layers. The most cited fusion is the molecular layer that in the past was felt to be a hallmark finding of this malformation.[368,370] However, fusion and number of cortical layers are highly variable and are not reliable for definition of PMG.[370]

In PMG, numerous 2- to 3-mm gyri, some separated by shallow sulci, with excessive cortical folding, and abnormal cortical cellular architecture are present (Fig. 17.1-57). PMG may be bilateral, unilateral, focal, multifocal, or diffuse. There is a strong tendency for PMG to develop in the Sylvian fissures, seen in up to 61% of patients.[372] Other common patterns include generalized (13%), frontal (5%), and parasagittal parieto-occipital (3%).[372] Asymmetric involvement, with 80% right dominance, is frequently associated with deletions of chromosome 2q11.2. The medial surface of the brain is rarely involved.[332] In PMG, other malformations are commonly present, particularly white matter heterotopia, seen in up to 60% of cases.[369]

Etiology: The etiology of PMG is varied. Cytotoxic, hypoperfusion, or genetic disturbances are possible etiologies for PMG (Table 17.1-17).[373]

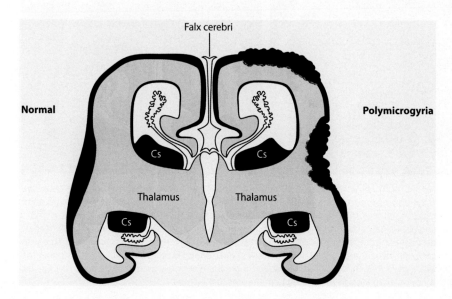

FIGURE 17.1-57: Diagram of polymicrogyria.

TABLE 17.1-17   Causes of Polymicrogyria

ETIOLOGIES	PMG DISTRIBUTION
Postinsult	
Infection: *CMV, toxoplasmosis, parvovirus, Zika, syphilis, varicella-zoster*	Variable
Toxins: *Fetal alcohol, maternal drug ingestion*	Variable
Hypoxic–ischemic: *monochorionic twins(including co-twin demise and twin-to-twin transfusion syndrome), maternal hypotension*	Variable
Trauma	Variable
Malformations with PMG	
Schizencephaly	In, along defect, variable
Septo-optic dysplasia	Variable
Periventricular nodular heterotopia	Variable
Genetic	
Chromosomal/Multiple genes	
Velocardiofacial/DiGeorge syndrome—deletion of chromosome 22q11	Perisylvian—unilateral or bilateral
Deletion of 1p36	Perisylvian—unilateral or bilateral
Bilateral perisylvian PMG—X-linked, autosomal recessive or dominant at Xq28	Bilateral perisylvian PMG
Bilateral frontoparietal PMG—Autosomal recessive at 16q12.2–21	Bilateral frontoparietal
Autosomal recessive	Generalized
Aicardi—X-linked	Variable—multifocal
Ehlers–Danlos	Perisylvian and frontal
Kabuki makeup (facial dysmorphisms, digital anomalies, skeletal, microcephaly)	Perisylvian
Thanatophoric dysplasia (skeletal dysplasia, hypoplastic lungs)	Temporal
Adams–Oliver (defects of scalp and cranium and limbs)	Variable
Delleman (oculocerebral–cutaneous syndrome)	Frontal
Meckel–Gruber/Joubert syndrome/orofacial–digital syndrome 1	Variable/frontal and parietal
Pena–Shokeir (arthrogryposis, IUGR, pulmonary hypoplasia)	Variable/perisylvian
Single Genes	
Tubulinopathies	Bilateral, asymmetric, perisylvian, frontal, parietal
mTORopathies (*PIK3-AKT*) *Megalencephaly-capillary malformation PMG (MCAP) syndrome* *Megalencephaly-PMG-polydactyly-hydrocephalus (MPPH) syndrome*	Variable though often perisylvian with Megalencephaly
Cobblestone lissencephalies/ CMDs	Variable
RAB3GAP (Micro-Warburg-microcephaly, cataracts, hypoplasia corpus callosum), *DYNC1H1, EOMES, TBR2, NDE1, WDR62*	Variable with microcephaly
OCLN1/pseudo-TORCH	Variable with band-like calcification
COL18A1/Knobloch (eye and occipital skull defects)	Frontal
COL4A1	Schizencephaly
NHEJ1, ARX	Variable with heterotopia
EML1	Overlying ribbon-like heterotopia
GPSM2 (Cudley-McCollough syndrome—hearing loss, hydrocephalus, ACC)	Parasagittal frontal
PAX6 (absence of anterior commissure and pineal, cerebellar hypoplasia)	Unilateral
Metabolic	
Peroxisomal disorders—Zellweger (white matter dysmyelination, facial dysmorphism, stippled epiphyses, renal cyst, biliary dysgenesis)	Generalized/perisylvian/perirolandic
Mitochondrial—Leigh and pyruvate dehydrogenase deficiency (neurodegeneration, ocular)	Variable
Neonatal adrenoleukodystrophy	Variable

ACC, agenesis of corpus callosum, PMG, polymicrogyria, IUGR, intrauterine growth restriction

Given common watershed perisylvian distribution and the presence of laminar necrosis, PMG has been hypothesized to arise secondary to an arterial ischemic event during the second trimester.[370] However, numerous prenatal insults, including infection (CMV being the most common), monochorionic twin pathology, and maternal trauma can cause PMG.[236,374,375] Cytotoxic and hypoperfusion injuries typically result in asymmetrical or focal PMG and likely occur later in cortical development.[376] Bilateral PMG is favored to represent an early insult, which may be sporadic, but should raise suspicion for genetic abnormalities.

Perisylvian PMG (unilateral and bilateral) can be seen in chromosomal aneuploidies. The most common abnormality is deletion of chromosome 22q11.2, (velocardiofacial or DiGeorge syndrome), which include cardiac defects, parathyroid hypoplasia, facial dysmorphism, thymus hypoplasia, and, possibly, microcephaly.[356] The second most common chromosomal deletion with PMG is 1p36, which is associated with neurodevelopmental delay, dysmorphic facial features, and, possibly, microcephaly.[367] Multiple syndromes are associated with PMG, as noted in Table 17.1-17.

A high number of single-gene disorders have been found to cause PMG. Big categories include the mTORopathies (PI3K-AKT-MTOR), tubulinopathies, dystroglycanopathies, and other causes of CLIS.[367] Mutations in the ADGRG1 (formerly GPR56) gene cause bilateral frontoparietal PMG and other imaging findings that overlap with CLIS.[367]

Multiple metabolic disorders are reported with PMG, including nonketotic hyperglycinemia, fumaric aciduria, glutaric academia type II, maple syrup urine disease, histinemia, and mitochondrial disorders including pyruvate dehydrogenase deficiency.[367] Zellweger syndrome or cerebrohepatorenal syndrome is the most common metabolic cause of PMG.[367] It is a peroxisomal metabolic disorder caused by a defect of the PEX gene family, transmitted autosomal recessive. In Zellweger, PMG and pachygyria in the perisylvian and perirolandic region occur.[377] Germinolytic cysts, severe hypomyelination, hepatosplenomegaly due to hepatic dysfunction, and renal cystic disease help diagnose this syndrome.[377,378]

Diagnosis: Infectious workup should be performed. Comprehensive genetic testing with chromosomal microarray, exome sequencing, and PMG gene panel may be considered. Parental consanguinity may suggest an autosomal recessive disorder.[367] PEX gene molecular testing or biochemical testing for very long-chain fatty acids in the amniotic fluid may be considered if there is concern for Zellweger.[378]

Knowledge of head size is important when performing US and MRI. In the presence of macrocephaly, PI3K-AKT-MTOR disorders should be considered.[367] With microcephaly and fetal brain disruption, consider NDE1-related LIS and WDR62. Microcephaly and complex brain malformations include the differential of pseudo-TORCH, RAB18 deficiency, and tubulinopathies. Normal head or lower normal is seen in 50% of cases, but would include 22q11.2 and 1p36 deletions.[367]

Ultrasound: Five percent of patients with PMG will present with abnormal US, usually microcephaly (50%) or associated malformations.[372] Dysmorphic features of the face or extremities suggesting arthryogryposis, should raise suspicion for perisylvian PMG.

PMG may be suggested in the presence of premature sulci or abnormal overfolded sulci and gyri, overdeveloped often with

respect to the gestational age (GA) (Fig. 17.1-58).[349,379] Hyperechogenicity of the cerebral cortex has also been described, representing subcortical necrosis or the excessive infolding (Figs. 17.1-59A and 17.1-60A).[375,380] Enlargement of the subarachnoid space overlying the PMG is often present.[379] Measuring the Sylvian fissure on a coronal image obtained transvaginal and demonstrating a high angle for GA are strong support for migrational disorder.[381] PMG is often diagnosed later in pregnancy, though it is easier in the second trimester than later in the third due to development of the secondary sulci.[372,379]

Magnetic Resonance Imaging: PMG typically leads to accelerated development in gyration with patterns including multiple irregular small bulging and invaginating areas, presence of a major sulcus not yet expected for GA, sawtooth pattern, or single to multiple bumps (Figs. 17.1-59B and 17.1-61A).[382,383] There is burring and reduced thickness in the subplate and intermediate zone in 80% of cases (Fig. 17.1-61B).[383] Infrequently, PMG may cause delay in sulcation with irregularity or invaginations in areas unexpected for GA (Fig. 17.1-60B, C). Volume loss and enlarged subarachnoid spaces have been described.[379,384] Venous anomalies in the area of abnormal gyration are present in more than half of cases.[384] Early in gestation, detection may be more difficult, especially less than 24 weeks, but attention to the normal signal of the cortical ribbon, presence of sulci that are not expected for GA, and irregular surface of the brain should raise suspicion.[335] Fetal MRI has an overall 85% sensitivity and 100% specificity in detection of PMG.[335]

Associated Anomalies: PMG may be isolated but is more commonly associated with other intracranial pathologies, such as schizencephaly, septo-optic dysplasia, periventricular/subcortical heterotopia, and agenesis of corpus callosum.[385] Imaging findings of encephaloclastic insult may be present. Genetic and chromosomal syndromes that are associated with PMG often present with additional intracranial and extracranial anomalies.

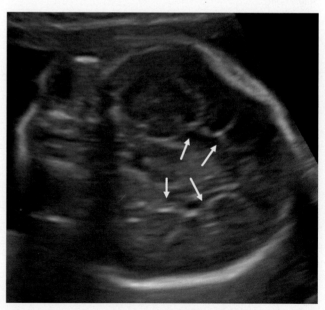

FIGURE 17.1-58: Polymicrogyria in thanatophoric dysplasia at 21 weeks. Axial US demonstrating abnormal advanced sulci along the bilateral medial temporal lobes (*arrows*).

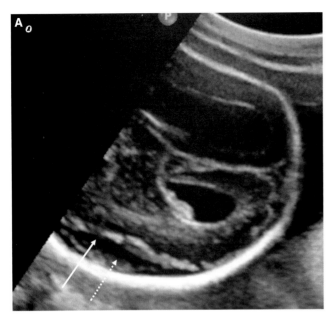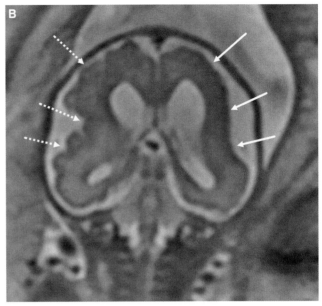

FIGURE 17.1-59: Polymicrogyria in a fetus at 27 weeks. **A:** Axial US demonstrating increased echogenicity and irregularity of the cortex (*solid arrows*) and enlarged extra-axial fluid space (*dotted arrows*). **B:** Coronal T2 MRI demonstrating multiple small lobulations along the right hemisphere (*dotted arrows*) and sawtooth pattern along the left (*solid arrows*). Notice loss of gray white differentiation and lamination with reduced thickness of the brain parenchyma in the left hemisphere.

Differential Diagnosis: Normal sulcation anatomy should not be confused with PMG. CLIS may have a bumpy cortical contour but should be distinguished by associated posterior fossa anomalies. Schizencephaly is often associated with PMG, but is defined by a central cleft. Pachygyria and lissencephaly may be considered but have reduced cortical folding and thick cortex postnatal. Encephaloclastic insults such as hemorrhage and ischemia may mimic cortical ribbon abnormalities.

Prognosis: Outcome depends on the location and extent of the PMG and the presence of associated anomalies.[383,386] The most common complications are epilepsy (78%), global developmental delay (70%), and spasticity (51%).[372] Seizures usually begin second half of the first decade in approximately 65%.[332]

Patients with extensive patterns of PMG present at an earlier age than those with restricted or unilateral forms.[332,372] Bilateral or diffuse PMG or PMG of more than half of a single hemisphere are poor prognostic factors, with these children having moderate-to-severe developmental delay and significant motor dysfunction.[383]

Sporadic cases of bilateral perisylvian PMG have 100% oropharyngeal dysfunction and dysarthria, epilepsy in 80% to 90%, mental retardation in 50% to 80%, and sometimes congenital arthrogryposis.[383] Familial perisylvian PMG tends to be less symptomatic.[356] Frontoparietal PMG has developmental delay, mild spastic quadriparesis, impaired language, disconjugate gaze, cerebellar signs, and epilepsy.[383] Zellweger has a poor prognosis, with death in the first month of life.[378]

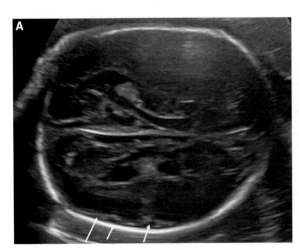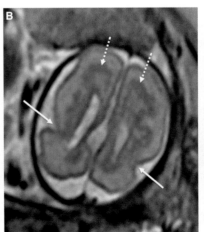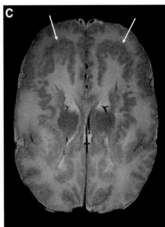

FIGURE 17.1-60: Polymicrogyria and band heterotopia in a fetus at 28 weeks. **A:** Axial US demonstrating abnormal increased echogenicity and irregularity of the cortex. **B:** Axial MRI demonstrating an overall delay in sulcation for gestational age, but abnormal invaginations bilateral parietal area (*solid arrows*) in association with band of gray matter signal within deep white matter (*dotted arrows*). **C:** Postnatal T2 MRI demonstrating diffuse polymicrogyria, even in the area of subcortical band heterotopia (*arrows*). Child was found to have a mutation in the *DOK7* gene.

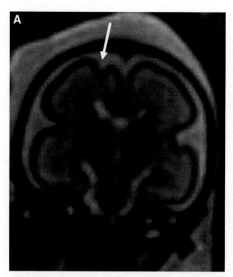
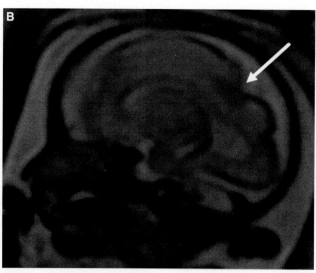

FIGURE 17.1-61: Polymicrogyria in two fetuses. **A:** Fetus at 24 weeks with abnormal bump (*arrow*) focally within the right frontal cortex. **B:** Fetus at 28 weeks with arthrogryposis and focal irregular invagination in the right parietal cortex (*arrow*) in association with blurring and reduced volume in the subplate and intermediate zone. Postnatally, the child was proven to have perisylvian syndrome.

Management: Depending on the severity of the defect and associated anomalies, termination of the pregnancy may be considered. Postnatal therapy is primarily supportive and includes treatment of epilepsy and physical therapy for neurological deficits.

Recurrence: In the sporadic form, there is no risk of recurrence. In genetic forms, the recurrence is dependent on the type of the transmission, which may be autosomal recessive, dominant, or X-linked.[367]

Schizencephaly

Schizencephaly (SZ), also known as agenetic porencephaly or true porencephaly, represents a transcerebral cleft with a pial ependymal seam, defined as a cleft lined by gray matter from the ependymal lining of the ventricles to the pial covering of the cortex.[387]

Incidence: Prevalence is approximately 1.5 in 100,000 births.[388,389] There is a high association with young maternal age.[388,389]

Pathogenesis: SZ may be considered a variant of polymicrogyria (PMG) but is likely in the spectrum of porencephaly, both postmigrational and likely acquired.[332,390] SZ occurs when there is injury of the entire thickness of the hemisphere. Pathologically, there may be a primary insult to the germinal matrix, failure in induction of neuronal migration, or focal ischemic necrosis with destruction of the radial glial fibers during neuronal migration.[388,391,392] Evidence suggests that SZ is a vascular disruptive process, likely before 24 weeks' gestation.[388,389] As the perisylvian area is typically abnormal, many believe that SZ may represent a small vessel insult in the watershed zone. Since PMG, SZ, and porencephaly can result from similar events, it is likely that PMG and SZ reflect differences in the severity of injury and SZ and porencephaly difference in the time of insult.[278,390]

SZ may be bilateral, unilateral, symmetrical, asymmetrical, small, or large. Two types of SZ are described (Fig. 17.1-62). Type I represents a cleft that is closed with gray matter lined lips in contact with each other. Type II is an open defect with CSF separating the gray matter lined clefts.[387] Some would include a dysplastic

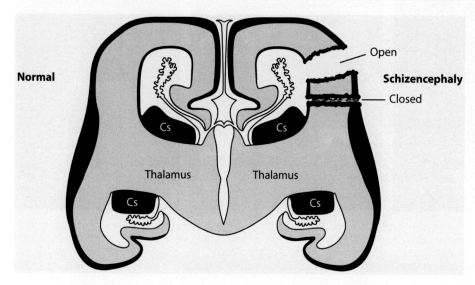

FIGURE 17.1-62: Diagram of types of schizencephaly.

gray matter column extending from the ependyma to the pia without a CSF cleft as SZ, overlapping with extreme transmantle heterotopia.[393]

In the fetus, SZ will be closed in approximately 45% of cases and open in 55%. Unilateral is slightly more common, present in 64%, and bilateral in 36%.[393] Postnatally, approximately 49% of SZ are bilateral, 51% unilateral, and 83% are open lipped with remaining fused.[392] The most common location by far is the perisylvian cortex, especially posterior region.[278] SZ can also be in the frontal area with temporal and parietal less likely and occipital least.[392] Approximately 66% of SZ cases are associated with other CNS anomalies. PMG is noted lining the cleft in nearly half of the cases, within cortex surrounding the cleft in nearly all cases, and present in the ipsilateral hemisphere in two-thirds of cases.[278,388] When SZ is unilateral, PMG is noted in the contralateral hemisphere in the same location in one-third of cases.[278]

Etiology: The causes for SZ are heterogeneous, but of those cited, most are acquired. SZ is seen in association with young maternal age, absence of prenatal care, and alcohol use. Over half can be attributed to a vascular disruptive event *in utero*, including infection, teratogen, hypoperfusion injury in twins, inherited thrombophilia, or trauma in the first or second trimester.[388]

Familial cases are reported.[394] Adams–Oliver syndrome with limb reduction and encephaloclastic changes in the brain, Aicardi, Arima, Delleman, Galloway–Mowat, microdactyly, and ectrodactyly syndromes are described in association.[388,393] Others genes associated with SZ include *EMX2*, *SHH*, and *SIX3*.[373] *COL4A1* is important for collagen in the basement membranes in the brain, muscle, eye, and kidney. A defect in the gene results in capillary fragility with propensity for hemorrhage. Mutations of *COL4A1* have been identified in many cases of fetal SZ.[373,395] As collagen type IV disorders cause both porencephaly and SZ, it is likely that the timing of the hemorrhage dictates the pathology, with earlier insult resulting in SZ and later porencephaly.

Diagnosis

Ultrasound: There are no US reports of SZ prior to 20 weeks, with most cases identified after 28 weeks' gestation.[389,396] It is suggested that the damaging process in SZ may occur early in pregnancy, possibly as a focal hemorrhage, that continues to evolve into SZ, not apparent until later gestation.[389,397,398] Therefore, it is possible that an early second-trimester scan will miss the abnormality.[389]

VM is often the first sign detected.[398] Wide clefts of CSF communicating between the lateral ventricles and subarachnoid spaces should raise suspicion (Fig. 17.1-63A).[349,399] Small open- or closed-lipped cleft SZ can be more difficult to detect with antenatal US but may be suggested in the presence of parallel echogenic tissue extending from the lateral ventricle to extra-axial fluid space (Fig. 17.1-64A).[398] 3D and transvaginal imaging may prove helpful in characterizing the cleft.[397,400] Transvaginal imaging of the Sylvian fissure with increased or asymmetric Sylvian fissure angle may also provide clues to diagnosis.[381]

Linear echogenic structures in the white matter may represent normal veins or fetal white matter tracts, so care should be taken not to misinterpret them falsely as clefts.[397] In addition, the inability to demonstrate gyration anomalies of SZ and detail lost due to near-field reverberation may lower the diagnostic sensitivity of transabdominal US in SZ.[401]

Magnetic Resonance Imaging: Gray matter lining a cleft extending from the ventricular surface to the subarachnoid space is necessary for diagnosing SZ (Fig. 17.1-63B).[391,399] A fine membrane, likely representing remnant of the pia mater or ependyma, can sometimes be detected (Fig. 17.1-63C).[396] A CSF signal-tented area may also be identified, extending from the wall of the ventricle, pointing to the defect (Fig. 17.1-64B).[394] Steady-state free precession imaging is excellent at defining edges of CSF and soft tissue and may be helpful in verifying the CSF cleft.[399] Gradient echo may demonstrate hemosiderin staining along the defect, seen in as high as 83% (Fig. 17.1-65).[396]

Most clefts identified in the prenatal time are open lipped; however, nearly 50% will close postnatally.[396] Sensitivity in detection of SZ on fetal MRI has been cited at 100% sensitivity and 99% specificity.[335] Small fetal head size is noted in more than 50% of cases, with approximately one-third being below the third percentile.[393] Anomalies can be detected, which include the absence or partial absence of the septal leaflets or corpus callosum.[398]

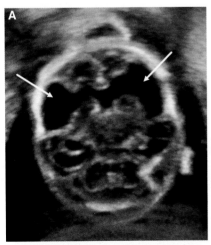 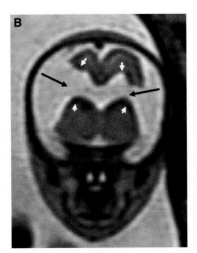 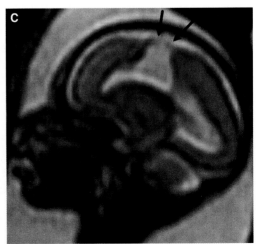

FIGURE 17.1-63: Axial image of fetus at 23 weeks with septo-optic dysplasia and open-lipped schizencephaly. **A:** Coronal US showing the absence of the septum pellucidum, and large bilateral frontal defects (*arrows*) proved to represent open-lipped schizencephaly. **B:** Coronal MRI demonstrating open-lipped schizencephaly defects (*black arrows*) lined with gray matter (*white arrows*). Notice the absence of the septum pellucidum. **C:** Sagittal T2 image of open-lipped defect with thin membrane (*arrows*).

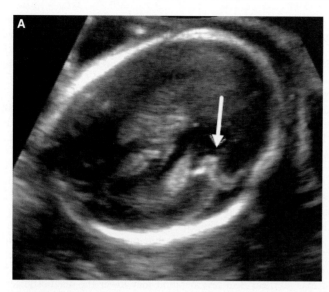
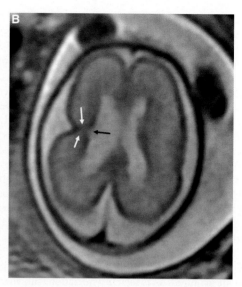

FIGURE 17.1-64: Fetus at 22 weeks with closed-lipped schizencephaly. **A:** Axial US demonstrating parallel echogenic lines (*arrow*) extending from ventricular to extra-axial fluid space. **B:** Axial MRI showing the closed defect lined with gray matter (*white arrows*). Notice tenting or nipple (*black arrow*) extending from the ventricle.

PMG tends not to be detected in the cleft prenatally, and PMG and nodular heterotopia outside the area of SZ are not commonly defined prenatally.[396] Optic hypoplasia is very limited in diagnosis prenatally, owing to lower resolution limits of fetal MRI.[396]

Cerebellar clefts may be identified prenatally.[402] Some of these clefts extend from the cerebellar surface to the fourth ventricle, often in association with loss of normal architecture, maloriented cerebellar foliation, and irregular gray white matter junction (Fig. 17.1-66). These clefts likely have similar pathogenesis to SZ.[402]

Associated Anomalies: Approximately two-thirds of patients with SZ will have additional anomalies.[393] Microcephaly is present in approximately 40% to 50% of cases.[393] SZ is often associated with PMG (66%), nodular heterotopia (50%), thin or absent corpus callosum (42%), white matter volume loss, white matter signal abnormalities (20%), optic nerve hypoplasia (20% to 30%), and absence of the septum pellucidum (50% to 70%).[388,392,393,403] The septum pellucidum is usually absent when the defect is bilateral, open lipped, or in the frontal lobe.[403] VM is seen in 70% of cases and is more likely to be associated with open defects.[392,400] Posterior fossa anomalies are also reported.[399] SZ can be associated with other extracranial vascular insults, including amniotic band, arthrogryposis, gastroschisis, and cleft palate and lip.[388]

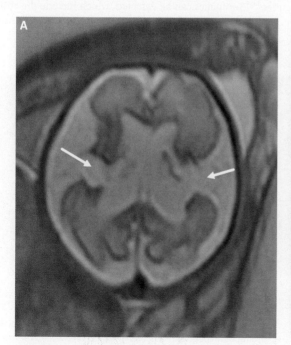
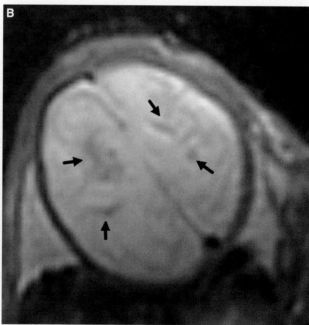

FIGURE 17.1-65: Fetus at 32 weeks with bilateral open-lipped schizencephaly. **A:** Axial T2 MRI demonstrating the gray matter lined open clefts (*arrows*). **B:** Gradient echo imaging demonstrating susceptibility artifact along the margins of the cleft (*arrows*).

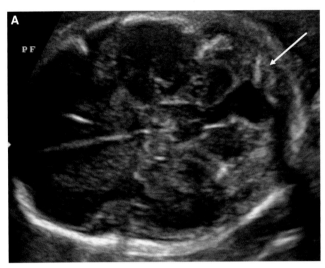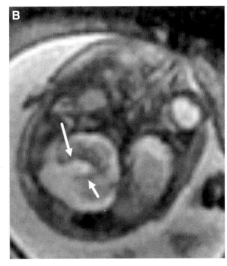

FIGURE 17.1-66: Cerebellar cleft in a fetus at 24 weeks. **A:** Axial US demonstrating a prominent cerebrospinal fluid defect in the cerebellum with mild increased echogenicity of the parenchyma along the defect (*arrow*). Vermian abnormality was questioned. **B:** Axial T2 MRI showing gray matter (*arrows*) lined defect through right cerebellar hemisphere. Fetus also had a closed-lipped schizencephaly in the occipital lobe (not shown).

Differential Diagnosis: Porencephaly should be considered but is lined by white matter instead of gray matter. Glioependymal cysts, arachnoid cysts, and areas of cystic encephalomalacia may mimic a defect but have normal surrounding parenchyma or white matter. In the presence of large open defects, hydranencephaly and holoprosencephaly can be excluded by detection of normal basal ganglia structures and midline falx.

Prognosis: The size and location of the SZ and, more importantly, associated cerebral anomalies should be noted as bilateral SZ, with presence of open clefts and additional anomalies having adverse effect on outcome.[391,393] Motor dysfunction tends to correspond to clefts in the frontal lobe. Prenatal diagnosed cases tend to be bilateral, often associated with other CNS anomalies such as the absence of the septum pellucidum and have a more guarded prognosis.[394] However, when counseling, it should be remembered that an apparently open cleft prenatal may become closed postnatal.[396,397]

Most patients with SZ have neurological impairments in motor (90%) and cognition (77%).[404] Patients with bilateral SZ have severe developmental delay with language impairment and spastic quadriparesis. Children with unilateral SZ experience variable hemiplegia and mild intellectual deficiencies, likely due to the plasticity of the brain at the time of injury.[391] Bilateral clefts, motor impairment, microcephaly, and corpus callosum agenesis are strongly associated with higher neurodevelopmental impairment.[404]

Seizures occur in 68% to 81% of patients with SZ.[404,405] Surprisingly, seizures are more common in unilateral SZ than bilateral, but bilateral SZ is more likely to present earlier in life with seizures and be more severe.[405]

Management: When counseling, it is important to remember that clefts that appear open prenatally may be closed on postnatal imaging. Termination of the pregnancy may be discussed. Management is supportive with therapy directed toward seizure control and rehabilitation of motor deficits.

Recurrence: No increased risk of recurrence is known in the absence of familial history or known syndrome.

Porencephaly

Porencephaly represents a cavitary fluid-filled area within the brain that usually communicates with the ventricles or subarachnoid spaces or both.

Incidence: Porencephaly is found in 1 per 9,000 births.[406]

Pathogenesis: Porencephaly is a cystic lesion replacing cerebral substance, which is smooth and lacks adjacent glial reaction. The inciting event occurs typically before 27 weeks, prior to the acquisition of a mature astroglial response.[407] Porencephaly and schizencephaly (SZ) likely arise from similar injuries, both being postmigrational disorders with the timing of injury dictating the imaging appearance. When the insult occurs beyond 24 weeks, porencephaly develops, whereas when the insult is less than 24 weeks, SZ arises. Therefore, both disorders affect cellular organization at different stages in development.[390,408]

Two types of porencephaly have been described. Type I or encephaloclastic porencephaly is the most common. These cases are usually related to a venous medullary infarct or less likely, an arterial insult.[409,410] Type II or developmental porencephaly is believed to arise from a primary defect in the germinal matrix and abnormal migration of neurons.[411]

Etiology: Porencephaly typically is acquired due to an intraparenchymal hemorrhage between 24 and 32 weeks secondary to medullary vein thrombosis in the presence of a germinal matrix/intraventricular hemorrhage.[412]

Genetic causes are rare but are being increasingly identified. There is a single-case report of tubulinopathy presenting with porencephaly.[413] Hereditary porencephaly with hemiplegia has been described in families, usually presenting with frontal porencephaly, hemiparesis, and seizures.[409,414] However, the collagen IV disorders, related to defects in the *COL4A1* and *COL4A2* genes, are the most commonly associated genetic disorders known to cause sporadic and hereditary (autosomal dominant) porencephaly. These genes are also associated with HANAC syndrome (hereditary angiopathy with nephropathy, aneurysm, and muscle cramps).[390]

COL4A1 and *COL4A2* genes are expressed in the basement membrane of the brain, heart, muscle, kidney, and eyes and play a key role in endothelial cell proliferation and neovascularization.[415] In the presence of a mutation, vascular membrane vulnerability leads to small vessel fragility, causing hemorrhage or ischemia that can then evolve into SZ and/or porencephaly.[416] The disorder has a wide phenotype and can have multiple associated abnormalities, including small vessel disease of the eye and cataracts, additional brain findings of diffuse periventricular white matter injury, polymicrogyria, focal cortical dysplasia, pontocerebellar atrophy and basal ganglia/white matter calcifications, nephropathy, angiopathy including aneurysms, muscle cramps with elevated creatine kinase levels, and hemolytic anemia.[390,408,415] In a recent study of patients with porencephaly and/or SZ, greater than 20% were found to have mutations of *COL4A1*, with the majority of cases resulting in porencephaly.[390]

Diagnosis

Ultrasound: Initially, an echogenic clot is identified periventricular arising from the germinal matrix. As the clot retracts, the hyperechoic area is replaced by a lesion that is centrally anechoic but with a peripheral echogenic border. Up to 6 weeks later, the area of porencephaly becomes completely anechoic and usually communicates with the lateral ventricle (Fig. 17.1-67A).[412] Coronal and sagittal imaging is often helpful. Sometimes, the septum pellucidum may be partially or completely absent.[412] The cleft of the porencephalic cavity is chronically lined by white matter and, therefore when mature, should not have an echogenic lining. Asymmetrical enlargement of the lateral ventricle with midline shift to the affected side is common.[412] There is no blood flow within the lesion.[411] Microcephaly or macrocephaly may be present.

Magnetic Resonance Imaging: Porencephaly appears as a defined area of CSF signal on T1 and T2 images, which extends from the white matter typically in continuity with the ventricle (Fig. 17.1-67B). MRI will often demonstrate evolving hemorrhage or hemosiderin staining along the defect (Fig. 17.1-67C).[406] Volume loss is typically noted in the associated hemisphere.

Associated Anomalies: In the presence of a genetic disorder, especially the collagen type IV disorders, other intracranial and extracranial anomalies may be noted. Hippocampal and amygdala volume loss are often present.[417]

Differential Diagnosis: The main differential diagnosis is SZ. In SZ, the malformation extends from the ventricle to the subarachnoid space and is lined by gray matter. Porencephaly is lined by white matter. In addition, SZ is often bilateral, whereas porencephaly tends to be unilateral. Small lesions may be confused with subependymal or connatal cysts or cystic periventricular injury. If the lesion abuts the subarachnoid space, an arachnoid cyst may be considered, though these lesions demonstrate mass effect and are extra-axial; whereas porencephaly is intra-axial and is usually associated with volume loss.

Prognosis: Outcome is related to the underlying etiology, timing of the insult, lesion size, and location.[412] Neurological deficits are typical.[410] The child may have spastic hemiparesis or quadriparesis and infantile spasms.[409] Many children with porencephaly suffer from epilepsy and cognitive deficits. Seizures tend to correlate with abnormalities in the temporal lobes, rather than the porencephalic defect.[417]

Management: Epilepsy is treated with antiepileptic drugs, though some children may become refractory to the drugs and require surgical resection.[406]

Recurrence: In the absence of a genetic syndrome, the risk of recurrence is low.

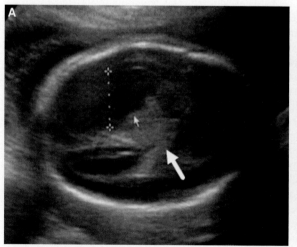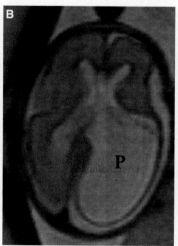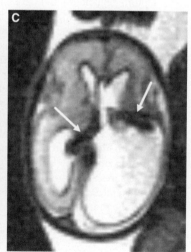

FIGURE 17.1-67: Fetus at 26 weeks with diagnosis of porencephaly. **A:** Axial US demonstrating asymmetric severe dilatation (calipers and *small arrow*) posterior horn of the left lateral ventricle. Echogenic area adjacent is consistent with hemorrhage (*long white arrow*) **B:** Axial T2 MRI demonstrating posterior horn of the lateral ventricle contiguous with porencephalic *(P)* cyst replacing most of the left posterior hemisphere. **C:** Gradient echo axial image demonstrating susceptibility artifact *(arrows)* consistent with hemosiderin staining along the defect.

Hydranencephaly

Hydranencephaly is characterized by complete or near-complete absence of cerebral cortex, primarily in the area of the anterior circulation.

Incidence: Nearly all cases of hydranencephaly are sporadic, with an incidence of approximately 1 in 5,000 continuing pregnancies or 1 in 10,000 births.[418,419]

Pathogenesis: In hydranencephaly, pathologically, there is a liquefaction necrosis and resorption of most of the cerebral brain. There is complete or near-complete absence of the cerebral cortex in the location of the anterior circulation, with most of the brain replaced by large CSF collections. Cortical layers are not present, and the empty CSF spaces are covered by leptomeninges, connective tissue, and a layer of ectopic glioneuronal tissue.[409] The occipital and small portions of the frontal and temporal lobes are often present because of collateral flow from the posterior circulations.[420] The basal ganglia and thalami are hypoplastic but present. The cerebellum and brainstem are intact but are often hypoplastic. Rarely, cerebellar hemisphere liquefaction has been noted.[419] The choroid plexus is present but freely floating, as the lateral ventricles are destroyed. The falx is usually present but may be partially or completely absent. Hydrocephalus may develop due to aqueduct stenosis or poor CSF absorption.[409]

The most commonly proposed mechanism for hydranencephaly is bilateral occlusion of the supraclinoid internal carotid arteries probably between late first to second trimester, after the brain and ventricles have been formed but before glial response is present.[421,422] However, since normal and hypoplastic anterior cerebral circulation has been detected in some hydranencephaly cases, it has also been hypothesized that the disorder may be due to a nonspecific devastating hypoperfusion, thromboembolic or vascular insult in the area of the anterior circulation, which then leads to diffuse extensive intracranial hemorrhage and necrosis.[422–424]

Etiology: In most cases, the etiology is unknown. Numerous prenatal cases have been described in association with monochorionic twin gestations, fetal infection, ischemia, hemorrhage, thrombophilia, or vasculopathies.[423,424] Young maternal age and exposure to toxins such as cocaine, smoking, estrogens, sodium valproate, carbon monoxide, or butane gas have also been cited.[425] Infrequently, hydranencephaly has been noted in conjunction with chromosomal aberrations, including trisomy 13 and triploidy.[422,426]

Fowler syndrome, also known as proliferative vasculopathy and hydranencephaly–hydrocephaly or encephaloclastic proliferative vasculopathy, is a genetic syndrome associated with the *FLVCR2* gene. This gene is important for regulation of cell growth and calcium metabolism and essential for normal proliferation and motility of vascular endothelial cells.[427] The mutation results in a glomeruloid vascular proliferation, which impedes development of the neocortex during the first trimester at the time of vascular invasion of the cerebral mantle.[409] The result is ischemic lesions and progressive destruction of the nervous tissue, uniformly involving the cerebral mantle, deep gray matter, brainstem, cerebellum, and spinal cord.[427] Brain injury most commonly presents as hydrocephalus, though hydranencephaly is also possible.[428] The syndrome has an autosomal recessive inheritance.[428,429]

Diagnosis

Ultrasound: Diagnosis of hydranencephaly has been described in both early and late gestations, but is usually detected between 12 and 30 weeks.[420,430] In hydranencephaly, a cerebral falx, although at times partially or rarely absent, is typically identified, and though the supratentorial brain is abnormal, there is usually a brainstem and cerebellum with measurements small owing to hypoplasia.[430,431] The US appearance is dependent on etiology and the stage of evolution. In the phase of vascular insult, homogeneous hyperechoic or diffuse uniform low-level echogenic material may replace the supratentorial brain, and no ventricles or cortical structures can be defined. The abnormal echotexture likely represents liquefied brain and hemorrhage (Fig. 17.1-68).[431] In the second phase, the echogenic material becomes more hypoechoic with identification of falx and thalami. The final phase demonstrates anechoic fluid surrounding the thalami and midbrain, absence of cortical tissue, and enlargement of the CSF spaces (Fig. 17.1-69A, B).[423,430] The head size may be normal, large or small, depending on the development of hydrocephalus. Color Doppler of the circle of Willis is often normal.[431] Usually, polyhydramnios is present because of lack of fetal swallowing.

In Fowler syndrome, fetal akinesia deformation sequence may be detected in the first trimester. In conjunction with hydrocephalus or hydranencephaly, there is often arthrogryposis, pterygia, cystic hygroma, and polyhydramnios.[423,428,429,432] Calcification and necrosis of the white matter, basal ganglia, brainstem, and cerebellum may be present (Fig. 17.1-70A).[428]

Magnetic Resonance Imaging: There is complete or near-complete absence of the cerebral hemispheres with remnants of occipital, temporal, and frontal lobes and basal ganglia and preservation of the thalami, brainstem, and cerebellum (Fig. 17.1-69C, D).[433] Hemorrhage may be detected

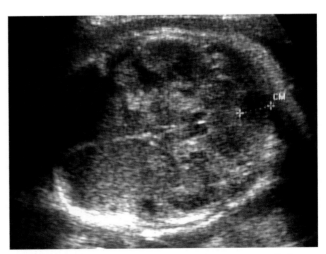

FIGURE 17.1-68: Fetus with early findings of hydranencephaly at 24 weeks. The supratentorial brain demonstrates diffuse low-level echogenicity on axial US.

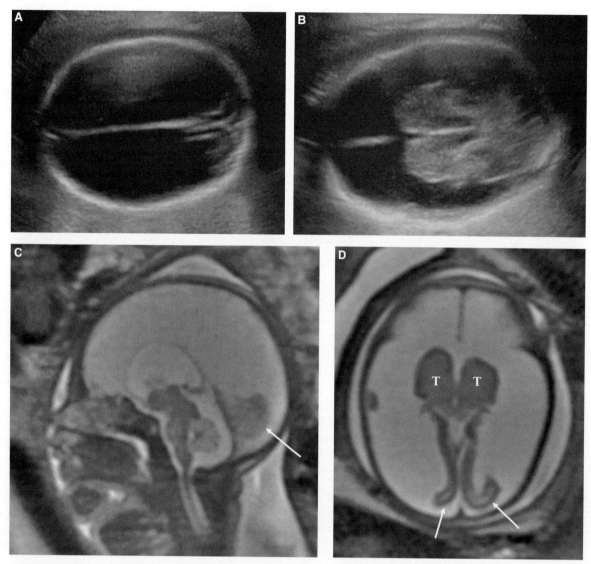

FIGURE 17.1-69: Fetus at 25 weeks with hydranencephaly. **A:** Axial US demonstrating persistence of the falx, but lack of visualization of normal brain parenchyma. **B:** Axial US showing the presence of thalami and posterior fossa structures. **C:** Sagittal T2 MRI showing lack of supratentorial brain other than small remnants of the occipital lobe (*arrow*). The posterior fossa anatomy is normal. **D:** Axial MRI demonstrating the absence of brain parenchyma in the area supplied by the anterior circulation. Small occipital lobes are present (*arrows*), and thalami (*T*) are small but present.

by high signal on T1, dark signal on T2, or susceptibility artifact on gradient echo images. If there is severe cerebellar volume loss, small brainstem, and associated calcifications, the differential of Fowler syndrome should be entertained (Fig. 17.1-70B).[427]

Associated Anomalies: With Fowler syndrome, additional anomalies may be apparent, particularly arthrogyposis.

Differential Diagnosis: In hydranencephaly, the presence of the falx is important in differentiation from holoprosencephaly, which demonstrates nonseparated tissue, especially in the frontal lobe region. Facial abnormalities in holoprosencephaly may also help secure the diagnosis. Hydrocephalus should also be considered, but the presence of cerebral tissue, though sometimes quite thin, should help differentiate. Severe porencephaly or large schizencephaly may be in the differential, but these cases can be distinguished by areas of preserved supratentorial brain. *COL4A1*

genetic mutations may also present with encephalomalacia that can simulate hydranencephaly.[425]

Prognosis: Although rare, cases of prolonged survival have been recorded. Prognosis is typically poor with reduced life expectancy, most being either stillborn or dying within the first few weeks of life.[418] Severe retardation is uniform among survivors.[418,434] Survival is possible but complicated by spastic quadriplegia, impossibility of oral feeding, respiratory infections, and episodic dysthermoregulation.[409,425] Some consciousness, mainly auditory, may be present.[409] Seizures are common, and pituitary dysfunction can occur. Fowler syndrome is usually lethal.[429,432]

Management: Termination of pregnancy may be discussed given poor outcome. At birth, supportive care such as drugs for seizures and intervention for nutrition may be provided. Some children with hydranencephaly develop hydrocephalus, and

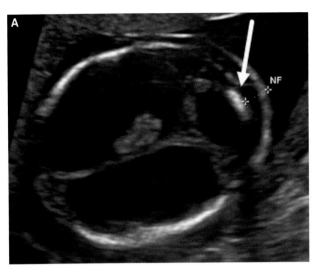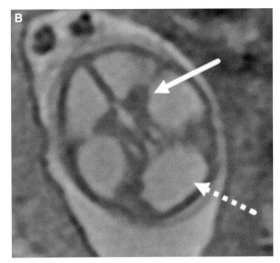

FIGURE 17.1-70: Fetus with Fowler syndrome at 21 weeks. **A:** Axial US demonstrating severe parenchymal volume loss supratentorial and infratentorial with lack of normal cerebellum and echogenic shadowing structure consistent with calcification (*arrow*). **B:** Axial MRI showing cystic replacement of the brain both supratentorial and infratentorial (*dotted arrow*) with remnant parenchyma in area of basal ganglia and thalami (*solid arrow*).

although ventriculoperitoneal shunting has been typically performed, more recently, choroid plexus coagulation with or without endoscopic third ventriculostomy has proven effective.[425]

Recurrence: In the absence of genetic anomalies, the recurrence risk is negligible. In the presence of Fowler syndrome, there is a 25% risk for recurrence.[427]

DESTRUCTIVE DISORDERS THAT MAY AFFECT CELLULAR MIGRATION/POSTMIGRATION

Subependymal Cyst (Germinolytic or Psudocyst)

Incidence: Subependymal cysts (SCs) are found in 0.5% to 5% of all neonates, being more common in the preterm.[435–437] The prevalence of *in utero* SCs is not known, but they are described less frequently in the fetal literature.[438]

Pathogenesis: Histologically, SCs are pseudocysts, given that the cavities lack an epithelial wall and are instead limited by a pseudocapsule aggregate of germinal cells and glial tissue encircling fluid containing macrophages with rare iron staining.[439] Two types are suggested, one of which is congenital and the other germinolytic due to injury.[440] The congenital is believed to be due to regression of remnant germinal matrix, as an acellular area exists between the germinal zone and the ependyma, which may normally become cystic with growth of the fetus.[435,436] However, the more commonly entertained etiology is that SCs develop from prenatal lysis of undifferentiated germinal matrix cells, likely due to ischemia, inflammation, or hemorrhage.[435,437,440] It is not surprising that these cysts are found most commonly at the caudothalamic groove, inferior frontal by caudate nucleus, or, rarely, adjacent to the temporal/atrial horn, representing areas of the ganglionic eminences that persist late in gestation.[435,437] When a SC is found in other areas, it may suggest an earlier insult.[441] Prenatal SCs are more common bilateral, in greater than 75%.[442] Neonatal SCs are bilateral in 49% of cases, but can be unilateral, simple, or complex; however, when unilateral, the left side tends to be more common.[437]

Etiology: SCs are often isolated, being idiopathic in etiology in greater than 70% of cases[443] However, SCs can be caused by vascular disorders; toxic exposures, including cocaine abuse, infection, most notably rubella, Zika, and CMV; and metabolic or chromosomal anomalies. Up to 63% of cases of SCs will have a positive antenatal history predisposing the fetus to hypoperfusion injury.[437] The incidence for infection and SC is as high as 35%, though mean is 13%.[435,442] Chromosomal abnormalities associated with SC include deletions that impair neuronal migration.[435] Associated genetic disorders include Aicardi-Goutières transmitted autosomal recessive, with imaging that mimics a viral infection. Metabolic disorders described with SCs include Zellweger, mitochondrial, Canavans, pyruvate dehydrogenase deficiency, congenital disorders of glycosylation, organic aciduria, and holocarboxylase synthetase deficiency.[435,438]

Simple SCs are found in up to 50% of cases as isolated cysts and are often bilateral and symmetrical in the common locations.[435] In the presence of bilateral simple SCs, there is still a 20% to 25% chance of the cysts being related to a congenital infection or genetic anomaly. A single cyst has a lower risk for injury.[444] Atypical SCs have ill-defined borders, square morphology and are irregular, multilocular, large, along uncommon areas of the ventricle, or different in echotexture or signal from CSF and are very suggestive of an insult.[441,445] Atypical cysts, cysts with great axis >9 mm and cysts located adjacent to the occipital or temporal horns or posterior to caudothalamic notch, raise suspicion for underlying pathology.[443] In the presence of other CNS abnormalities, an underlying etiology is also more likely.[443]

Diagnosis

Ultrasound: SCs may be seen as early as 12 weeks.[438] However, most are detected in the third trimester.[438] Unilateral SCs tend to be smaller than bilateral and present on the left side.[443] Most SCs are simple, anechoic, well-defined cavities adjacent to the frontal horns, often with a tear-shaped configuration on sagittal imaging (Fig. 17.1-71A).[435] The cyst may become increased in echotexture, mimicking hemorrhage.[438] With evolution, SCs can be multiseptated and may increase in size (Fig. 17.1-72).[438] However, greater than 85% remain stable or decrease in size with increasing gestational age.[442]

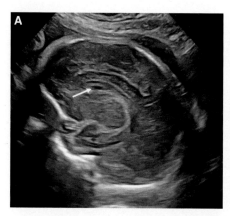 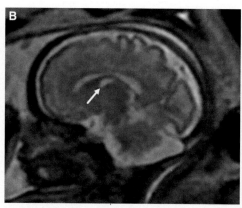 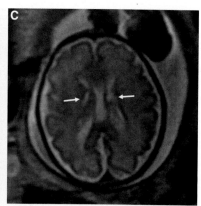

FIGURE 17.1-71: Fetus at 31 weeks with bilateral subependymal pseudocysts. **A:** Sagittal US demonstrating teardrop cystic structures at the caudothalamic groove (*arrow*). **B:** Sagittal MRI demonstrating cyst at the caudothalamic groove. **C:** Axial MRI demonstrating small bilateral cysts (*arrows*) adjacent to the caudate heads.

Magnetic Resonance Imaging: Simple SCs are high signal on T2 imaging and low signal on T1 sequences, usually present below the external angle of the ventricle near caudate or posterior to the foramen of Monroe at the caudothalamic groove (Fig. 17.1-71B–D).[435,440] Typical cysts demonstrate well-defined margins and oval shape with height smaller than anterior to posterior dimension.[443] If the wall of the cyst is very thin or the lesion is less than 5 mm, the cyst may not be apparent.[436] SSFP or heavily T2 imaging may be considered in the presence of an US abnormality.

Atypical cysts have ill-defined margins and square shape with increased height.[443] The cysts may be multilocular and complex, and hemorrhage may be suggested by high T1 signal, low T2 signal, and susceptibility artifact on gradient echo imaging. Atypical cysts may be present in association with other anomalies, including mild or moderately dilated or asymmetric lateral ventricles or T2 hyperintense signal in the white matter.[446] MRI may define 10% to 30% of SCs not identified on US and is helpful to confirm the topography of the cyst and exclude additional cerebral pathology.[438,443,446]

Associated Anomalies: Associated anomalies depend on etiology, though many SCs are isolated.

Differential Diagnosis: SCs should be differentiated from choroid plexus cysts that are intraventricular in location. There are three additional cystic lesions that can lie by the ventricle: coarctation, cystic white matter disease, and porencephaly (Fig. 17.1-73). Coarctation of the lateral ventricle (also known as connatal or frontal horn cysts) manifests as a cystic area anterior to the foramen of Monroe and adjacent to the superolateral margin of the body and frontal horn of the lateral ventricles (Fig. 17.1-43). These cystic areas represent approximation of the walls of the ventricle and are a normal variant.[440] Injury in the white matter may become cystic and simulate a SC. However, cystic degeneration in the white matter is above the angle of the ventricle, whereas a SC is below.[440] A porencephalic cyst typically communicates with the ventricle and extends into the adjacent white matter.

Prognosis: Isolated SCs are overall associated with normal neurodevelopment.[437,442,443] When isolated, 93.5% of SCs regress spontaneously within 1 to 12 months after birth.[441,442]

Atypical cysts, larger in size and atypical location, are more guarded in outcome, usually dependent on the etiology and associated anomalies.[435,438,443] Cysts in the temporal

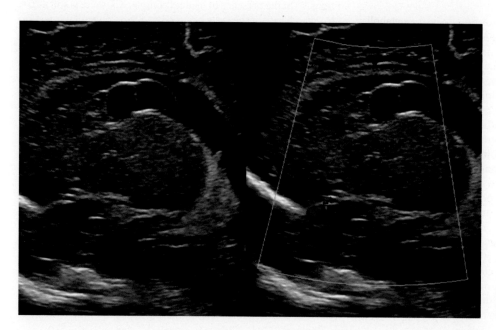

FIGURE 17.1-72: Neonatal ultrasound showing complex cysts at the caudothalamic groove. The child had positive cytomegalovirus titers.

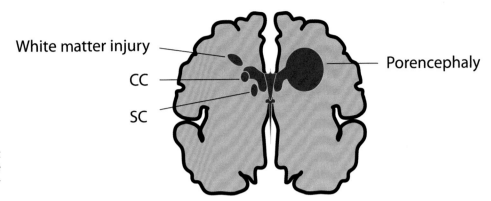

FIGURE 17.1-73: Diagram of different types of cysts and their locations: white matter injury, coarctation cyst (CC), sub-ependymal cyst (SC), and porencephaly.

and occipital horns have a higher association with CMV infection.[446] In the presence of a history of intrauterine growth restriction, fetal infection, malformation, and chromosomal anomaly, or if the cyst does not resolve postnatally, there is a higher risk of neurodevelopmental impairment, 50% with positive CMV titer.[437,441] Prior studies have suggested that bilateral or multilocular cysts are at higher risk for infection or genetic abnormalities; however, other studies do not support these associations.[387,443] A recent review with follow-up of children with SCs to ages between 5 and 15 years demonstrated developmental delay, particularly with attention deficit disorder and autism, in approximately 5% cases, being more common in the presence of multiple SCs.[447]

Management: Infection titers or genetic testing may be considered based on the presence of associated anomalies. If the lesion is isolated, no intervention is necessary.

Recurrence: There is no risk of recurrence for isolated SCs.

Inborn Errors in Metabolism

This section is not meant to review all possible types of errors in metabolism but to highlight those that may present with prenatal brain findings.

Incidence: Prenatal incidence of inborn errors in metabolism (IEM) with brain dysgenesis is not known. Limited knowledge is provided by case reports in the literature.

Pathogenesis: The IEM presenting in the fetus are related to severe errors in metabolic pathways that are not compensated by maternal or placental metabolism.

Etiology: The entities listed below are the most commonly cited IEM resulting in fetal brain dysgenesis. Abnormalities of folic acid and its association with neural tube defects will not be emphasized.

Pyruvate Dehydrogenase Deficiency (PDHD) and **pyruvate carboxylase deficiency (PCD)** are caused by genetic mutations of the pyruvate pathway, leading to primary lactic acidosis.[448] *De novo* mutations of *PDHE1* lead to X-linked form of PDHD that is symptomatic in males and heterozygous in females.[449] PCD is not diagnosed as commonly prenatal when compared to PDHD.[448]

Smith–Lemli–Opitz syndrome (SLOS) is caused by a defect in the enzyme 7-dehydrocholesteral reductase, involved in cholesterol biosynthesis, causing low levels of cholesterol but high levels of 7-dehydrocholesterol. The disorder is autosomal recessive. Multiple anomalies of the face, limbs, heart, lungs, kidney, brain, and genitalia are identified and discussed in chapter 30. SLOS can be associated with holoprosencephaly, reported in approximately 1% of cases.[450]

Glutaric aciduria type 1 (GA1) is transmitted autosomal recessive and results in a defect in glutaryl-CoA dehydrogenase enzyme, necessary for degradation of amino acids, which when abnormal leads to accumulation of glutaric acid and its derivatives in urine, blood, and CSF.

Congenital disorders of glycosylation type 1a (CDG1a) results from mutation in the *PMM2* gene, coding for enzyme phosphomannomutase. The glycosylation defect results in reduced availability of GDP-mannose as a substrate in the endoplasmic reticulum.

Mitochondrial disorders (MD) result in abnormalities of the respiratory chain, causing defective oxidative phosphorylation that results in tissue energy deficiency, especially in those areas requiring high energy such as the brain, muscle, and heart. These disorders rarely present *in utero*, with antenatal diagnosis in only 7% of all cases and with brain findings in only 1%.[451] Inheritance is autosomal recessive, dominant, and X-linked.[449]

Maternal phenylketonuria (mPK) is transmitted autosomal recessive and is due to deficiency of phenylalanine hydroxylase, an enzyme necessary for hydroxylation of phenylalanine to tyrosine. Phenylalanine maternal levels greater than 20 mg/dL have teratogenic effects during pregnancy with direct effect on the oligodendroglia, impairing intrauterine myelination.

Zellweger syndrome (ZS), also known as cerebrohepatorenal syndrome, is a peroxisomal biogenesis disorder transmitted autosomal recessive, primarily associated with the *PEX* gene, leading to deficiency of multiple peroxisomal enzymes that are necessary for metabolism of branched chain and very long-chain fatty acids, ether lipids, polyamines, amino acids, and glyoxylate.

Nonketotic Hyperglycinemia (NKH) is an autosomal recessive disorder that causes a defect in the glycine cleavage system, resulting in a large accumulation of glycine in all body tissues.

Cerebral dysmorphism in these IEMs can occur at any stage of brain development, though most prenatal cases are discovered in the second and third trimesters. The pathogenesis for cerebral malformation in IEM is likely complex, occurring via many different pathways listed below[449,452]:

Accumulation of neurotoxic intermediaries: glycine in NKH and phenylalanine in mPK

Defects in cell respiration and energy metabolism: PDHD and MDs affect aerobic metabolism, which increases during neuronal proliferation, differentiation, and migration.

Abnormalities of cell signaling pathways: SLOS results in low cholesterol, a metabollite necessary for normal development of cell membranes and function of *SHH* gene.

Interrelationships in subcellular organelle function: ZS causes disturbance in peroxisomal function affecting cholesterol biosynthesis, particularly in the mitochondria. Cholesterol is important in the cell membranes, and deficiency may prevent anchoring of receptors and diffusion of molecules critical for axonal guidance.

Neuroplasticity of the CNS: responsible for the final pathology after the disturbance

Diagnosis: Diagnostic testing should be considered in the presence of imaging that suggests IEM, in the context of consanguinity and/or history of *in utero* fetal death or unexplained neonatal death.[448,453] SLOS may be diagnosed by maternal serum and urinary dihydroxysteroid ratios in a fetus with anomalies. Amniocentesis or chorionic villus sampling for biochemical and molecular genetic testing should be considered. PDHD and NKH can be diagnosed by enzyme assays and molecular studies on cultured amniotic cells. ZS relies on prenatal identification of very long-chain fatty acids and plasmalogen synthesis or molecular testing for the *PEX* gene. CDG1a can be diagnosed on demonstration of hypoglycosylation of serum proteins using isoelectric focusing transferrin. Prenatal diagnosis is typically not possible for MDs as the abnormal enzyme activity may be tissue specific, not present in amniotic cells, and expression is also time dependent during fetal life.[449]

Imaging/Associated Anomalies

Ultrasound/Magnetic Resonance Imaging: Findings in IEM are nonspecific and usually are noted until the second and third trimesters. However, in the presence of ventriculomegaly (VM), subependymal cysts, and disorders of the corpus callosum, a metabolic process should be highly considered (Fig. 17.1-74A, B). US is excellent at excluding intracranial calcification. Biometrics are essential to exclude intrauterine growth restriction (IUGR), microcephaly, and macrocephaly. MRI is extremely helpful in evaluation of the corpus callosum, parenchymal signal, gyration, and posterior fossa structures. Table 17.1-18 provides a list of the most common IEM and associated imaging findings.[449]

In this section, each disorder is described with common prenatal CNS and non-CNS findings.

PDHD commonly presents with VM, gyration abnormalities (delayed more common than abnormal), ventricular septations, subependymal cysts, periventricular cysts, anomalies of the corpus callosum, and small pons (Fig. 17.1-75A–D).[448] Less frequent findings include cerebellar hypoplasia, IUGR, and hyperintense signal in the white matter. Although postnatal studies have shown elevated lactate on MR spectroscopy at 1.33 PPM, this was not possible on a fetal trial, probably due to placental maternal circulation efficiently removing excess lactate.[454] **PCD deficiency** is more likely to have macrocephaly with subependymal cysts, hemorrhage and VM.[448]

SLOS on prenatal imaging demonstrates IUGR and nuchal edema. CNS anomalies include microcephaly, hypoplasia of frontal lobes, holoprosencephaly, callosal dysgenesis, and cerebellar hypoplasia. Other organs abnormalities are often present and include limb anomalies, ambiguous or hypoplastic genitalia, and renal pathology such as agenesis, cysts, and hydronephrosis.

GA1 is highly suggested in the presence of macrocrania, abnormal operculization of the Sylvian fissure, VM, germinolytic cysts, and enlarged pericerebral spaces with possible subdural effusions/hematomas.[304] Frontotemporal volume loss and atrophy of the caudate and putamen may be visible on MRI.[449]

CDG1a should be considered in the presence of cerebellar hypoplasia and fetal akinesia. Sometimes, nonimmune hydrops, hyperechoic kidneys, and cardiomyopathy may be detected.

MDs may cause both brain dysplasia and disruption. Imaging findings are varied and include VM, ventricular and parenchymal hemorrhages, porencephalic cysts, cerebellar hypoplasia, agenesis of corpus callosum, periventricular cyst, and malformations

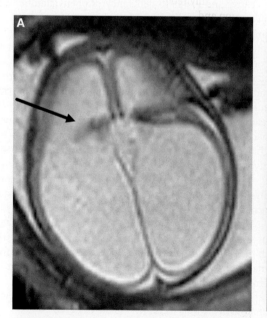
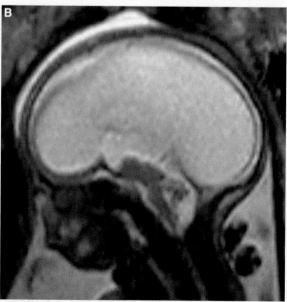

FIGURE 17.1-74: Fetus at 28 weeks diagnosed with aqueduct stenosis but postnatal was found to have pyruvate dehydrogenase deficiency. **A:** Axial MRI demonstrating severe ventriculomegaly, thin cerebral parenchyma, and relatively little tissue in the area of the basal ganglia and thalami (*arrow*). **B:** Sagittal MRI demonstrating no significant corpus callosum tissue.

TABLE 17.1-18 Inborn Errors of Metabolism and Imaging Findings

IMAGING FINDINGS	ERROR OF METABOLISM
Intrauterine growth retardation	Nonspecific, frequently disorders of energy metabolism
Fetal akinesia/hypokinesia	ZS, CDG1a
Microcephaly	mPK, PDHD, PCD, MD
Macrocephaly	GA1, PCD, MD
Midline prosencephalon/holoprosencephaly	SLOS
Callosal abnormalities	NKH, PDHD, MD, mPK, ZS, CDG1a, sulfite oxidase and molybdenum cofactor deficiency
Posterior fossa abnormalities	CDG1a, MD
Disruptive events	MD, PDHD, PCD
Cerebral atrophy and calcification	MD
Subdural effusions	GA1
Stroke, encephaloclastic	MD, PDHD, sulfite oxidase deficiency
Malformations of cortical development	ZS, PDHD, SLOS
Subependymal cysts	PDHD, PCD, MD, ZS, GA1

ZS, Zellweger syndrome; *MD*, mitochondrial disorder; *PDHD*, pyruvate dehydrogenase deficiency; *PCD*, pyruvate carboxylase; *GA1*, glutaric acidura type 1; *SLOS*, Smith–Lemli–Opitz syndrome; *mPK*, maternal phenylketonuria; *NKH*, nonketotic hyperglycemia.

of cortical development including polymicrogyria and in familial forms with intracerebral calcifications. Diagnosis should be suggested when multiple organ malformations without common embryological origin are noted. These anomalies include cardiac disorders, renal and gastrointestinal defects, VACTERL association, arthrogryposis, and IUGR.[451]

Maternal phenylketonuria causes microcephaly, dysgenetic corpus callosum, and delay in myelination. Congenital heart defects and IUGR are common.

ZS may initially be associated with increased nuchal translucency. Brain malformations include cortical malformations of the perisylvian and perirolandic regions (perirolandic and occipital pachygyria, frontal and perisylvian polymicrogyria), hypomyelination, VM, and subependymal cysts (Fig. 17.1-76A, B).[378] Heterotopias, focal band or cerebellar, and corpus callosum anomalies are described. Fetal hypokinesia, renal cysts, and hepatosplenomegaly may be noted. In addition, craniofacial dysmorphism with prominent forehead, hypoplastic supraorbital ridges, broad nasal bridge, hypertelorism, deformed ear lobes, dysplasia olfactory bulbs, optic atrophy, glaucoma, and cataracts are commonly present. Other non-CNS findings, including echogenic kidneys and stippling of epiphysis, are diagnostic.[453]

NKH may be first suggested by hypoplasia of the corpus callosum, though cortical malformations, colpocephaly, and cerebellar hypoplasia are also possible.[450] MR spectroscopy detection of glycine in the fetus has not been described in the literature.

Differential Diagnosis: The differential is wide including chromosomal or genetic syndromes and environmental factors such as exposure to infection or toxic substance including diabetes, drugs, or alcohol. Hypoxic–ischemic insults should also be included in the differential, especially in the presence of monochorionic twins. In the differential for glutaric aciduria, bilateral arachnoid cysts can simulate frontotemporal hypoplasia.[450]

Prognosis: Infants with **PDHD** have lactic acidosis and encephalopathy at birth with progressive neurological deterioration and seizures resulting in death typically in infancy or childhood.[455]

GA1 causes significant neurological disability with hypotonia, dystonia, and encephalopathy in conjunction with febrile illness. Survivors often have dystonic movements, seizures, and developmental delay.

CDG1a patients have mental retardation and hypotonia.

If **MD** presents prenatally, the neonatal course is typically fatal with fulminant lactic acidosis and multiorgan failure.[449]

ZS causes severe mental retardation and usually death in the first year of life.[449]

Neonates with **NKH** present with lethargy, hypotonia, and myoclonic jerks progressing to apnea and often death. Those who regain respiration develop intractable seizures and profound mental retardation.[449]

Management: In the presence of mPK, phenylalanine levels should be monitored and controlled with a phenylalanine-restricted diet. Some forms of PDHD are thiamin responsive. Lactic acidosis may also be treated with ketogenic diet and use of dichloroacetate, improving outcome.[449,455] Multidisciplinary approach is typically required to provide medical support. Genetic consultation and testing is recommended.

Recurrence: IEM are often inherited, many with 25% risk of recurrence.[450]

Infection

This section covers infections that may be detected by imaging in the fetus. Those that present in the perinatal time will not be emphasized.

Incidence: True incidence for all forms of intrauterine infection is not known. In most places in the world, congenital cytomegalovirus (CMV) is the most common cause of intrauterine viral infection due to near elimination of rubella infection after compulsory immunization in developed countries.[456] In the United States, 0.0.5% to 1% of pregnancies are infected with CMV and approximately 4,000 infants per year are born with congenital disease.[456,457] Table 17.1-19 provides etiologies and incidence of common infectious agents that may present intrauterine.[456]

Pathogenesis: Infection in the fetus may occur via two routes, either ascending from the cervix or transplacental via the maternal circulatory system.

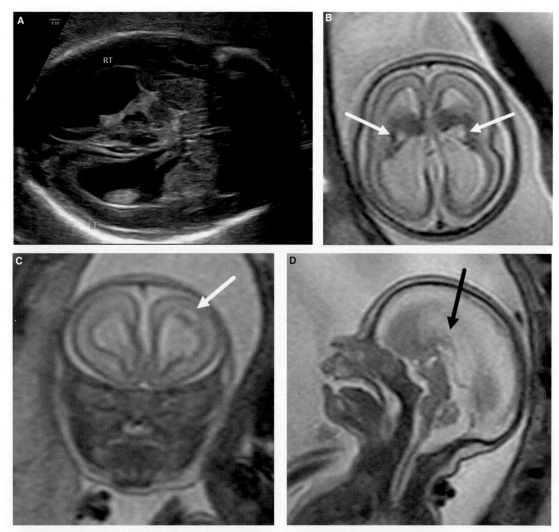

FIGURE 17.1-75: Fetus imaged at 19 weeks diagnosed with pyruvate dehydrogenase deficiency. **A:** Axial US demonstrating moderate ventriculomegaly. **B:** Axial MRI demonstrating prominent ganglionic eminences containing subependymal (germinolytic) cysts (*arrows*). **C:** Coronal MRI demonstrating a subtle periventricular cyst (*arrow*). **D:** Sagittal MRI showing dysgenetic corpus callosum, horizontal in configuration and diffusely thin (*arrow*). (Courtesy of Carolina Guimaraes, MD and Chris Cassady, MD.)

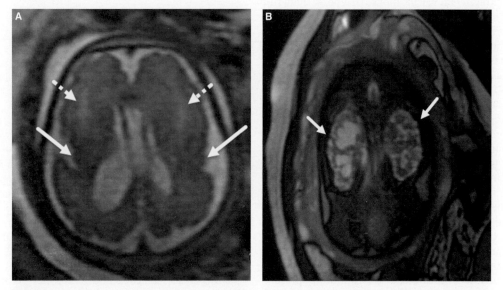

FIGURE 17.1-76: Fetus at 35 weeks diagnosed postmortem with Zellwegers syndrome. **A:** Axial MRI demonstrating areas of irregularity and nodularity along the high perisylvian/perirolandic area (*solid arrows*) consistent with polymicrogyria. Hyperintense signal in frontal white matter is also noted (*dotted arrow*). **B:** Coronal MRI through the kidneys demonstrate multiple peripheral renal cysts (arrows). Images courtesy of Jennifer Kucera, MD.

Bacterial infection may ascend from the cervix to the amniotic fluid, resulting in chorioamnionitis, often in the presence of prolonged rupture of membranes. Common infectious organisms include *Mycoplasma, Streptococcus hominis, Fusobacterium, Gardnerella vaginalis, Escherichia coli,* and *Candida albicans.*[458] In the presence of chorioamnionitis, fetuses are at risk for intraventricular hemorrhage and periventricular leukomalacia, incited by fetal inflammation and hypoxia.[458]

The infectious agents that will be stressed in this section are due to pathogens that cross the placenta from the maternal circulatory system. Consequences for the fetus are dependent on the infectious agent, immune status of the pregnant mother, and timing of the infection.[459] With maternal infection, viremia, parasitemia, or spirochetemia seeds the placenta. Placental inflammation leads to vasculitis and placental insufficiency, which may lead to fetal death, stillbirth, or intrauterine growth restriction (IUGR).[456] Placental infection and disruption of the maternal–fetal barrier causes release of the agent to the fetus with replication in target organs and damage to fetal tissues, including the brain.[456] Many infectious agents are neurotropic, meaning that they tend to or preferentially attack the nervous system. These pathogens can enter the CNS via a variety of pathways such as infected peripheral neurons, endothelial cells, or migration of infected inflammatory cells. The injury to the fetal brain is the result of pathogen-specific endotoxins and the host's inflammatory response at the time of the infection. The infectious agent may attach to neural progenitor cells, resulting in decrease in cortical neuron numbers and decreased brain mass, a primary cause for microcephaly.[457,460] Infection in the first or early second trimester can attack the germinal matrix, which results in disruption of normal neuronal development, initiating migration abnormalities, cortical disorganization, and altered white matter myelination.[461] In addition, inflammatory response and vasculitis leads to destruction of neurons via apoptosis and tissue loss due to increase microglial cells and/or cystic degeneration.[457] Dystrophic calcification is present in many infections, attributed to pathogen-induced necrosis of neural tissue.

Etiology: TORCH, an acronym for *Toxoplasma gondii,* **O**ther being syphilis, congenital **R**ubella, **C**ytomegalovirus (CMV), and **H**erpesvirus, was invented to remind clinicians of the most common infectious agents that produce similar presentations including insult on the developing CNS.[456] The "other" category has now increased to include varicella-zoster virus, lymphocytic choriomeningitis virus, parvovirus B19, human immunodeficiency virus (HIV), and Zika virus. HIV, by yet unknown mechanisms, can infect the fetus through the placenta, though, with medical therapy, this mode of vertical transmission has decreased significantly. Rare infections that have occasionally been associated with congenital infection include Chagas disease via protozoan *Trypanosoma cruzi,* with findings similar to toxoplasmosis, and Venezuelan equine and West Nile virus.[459]

Most of the common offending organisms are viruses. The exceptions are *Toxoplasma gondii* and Chagas, both due to parasites, and syphilis a spirochete. Each organism is transmitted differently, and although the mother is infected, she may or may not be symptomatic from the illness. Many pathogens attack as a primary illness, though some may occur with reactivation of the infectious agent from a prior exposure. In CMV, toxoplasmosis, herpes, and syphilis, primary or reactivation

maternal illness is possible. However, importantly, infection rate in the fetus is generally higher when the maternal illness is primary.[457,459,461] In addition, although varicella can reactivate with shingles, it is surprisingly not associated with congenital varicella syndrome.[459]

Most of the time, the fetus is unaffected by the pathogen, with overall low percentage of congenital disease or syndrome at birth. In general, when the disease or syndrome is present, infection earlier in pregnancy results in more severe brain pathology. However, it is interesting that many of the pathogens have higher rates of infection in advanced gestation, likely related to placental cell susceptibility[457] Table 17.1-19 provides information with regard to these differences.[456]

CMV infection incites brain injury when the virus seeds to the choroid plexus and replicates in the ependyma, germinal matrix, neurons, glial cells, and capillary endothelium causing meningoencephalitis.[457] Neuronal differentiation has been found to be delayed, inhibited, or to occur prematurely.[460] Involvement in the germinal matrix causes disorders of neuronal migration, and capillary involvement causes thrombosis and brain ischemia. CMV is the most studied pathogen that clearly demonstrates the trend that early infection results in more devastating fetal brain findings. In the first and early second trimesters, infection leads to microcephaly, lissencephaly, ventriculomegaly (VM), periventricular calcification, and cerebellar hypoplasia. Infection at 18 to 24 weeks results in cerebellar hypoplasia and migrational abnormalities such as polymicrogyria and schizencephaly, and third trimester injury is manifested as delayed myelination/white matter abnormality and low brain volume, but normal gyral pattern.[461]

Toxoplasmosis is asymptomatic in 80% of immune competent hosts, but infection results in a parasite septicemia.[457] Cerebral inflammation is primary periventricular and periaqueductal with lymphocytes and plasma cells in response to the parasite causing necrosis of the infected and adjacent unaffected cells. Vasculitis causes tissue necrosis.

Syphilis infection causes fetal spirochetemia to all organs. Intrauterine manifestations are rare, with acute findings presenting at 3 to 6 months of age with syphilitic leptomeningitis that can result in hydrocephalus and infarcts.

Rubella is transmitted blood-placental during maternal viremia, with highest risk of congenital defects when infection occurs in the first 10 weeks of gestation.[457] Severe brain damage, leptomeningitis, parenchymal, perivascular and periventricular tissue necrosis, and subarachnoid hemorrhage are noted.

Herpes and varicella are both herpesviruses. Herpes infects sensory nerves and remains lifelong as a latent virus in the dorsal root ganglia. However, herpes rarely causes intrauterine infection, with most common route of infection perinatal from contact of the fetus with infected genital tract.[461] Varicella rarely causes congenital infection as the transmission rate is low, and cases have decreased with vaccine introduction. Both viruses commonly result in parenchymal destruction, VM, hydrocephalus, and, possibly polymicrogyria and cerebellar hypoplasia.

Lymphocytic choriomeningitis virus replicates preferentially in the meninges, choroid plexus, and ependyma.[461] Hydrocephalus develops in more than half of these cases due to ependymitis obstructing cerebral aqueduct.

Parvovirus B19 infects the bone marrow and fetal liver and results in fetal anemia due to direct suppression of erythroid

TABLE 17.1-19   Intrauterine Infections: Transmission and Incidence

INFECTION	PATHOGEN	TRANSMISSION BY INFECTED	ANNUAL INCIDENCE (PER 1,000 LIVE BIRTHS)	PERCENT WITH CONGENITAL DISEASE AT BIRTH	RISK OF TRANSMISSION
Cytomegalo-virus	Herpes family virus	Saliva, urine, semen, cervical secretions, caregivers for children higher risk	2.9–10	10–15%	Higher primary than recurrent Increases with advancing gestational age
Toxoplasmosis	Parasite *Toxoplasma gondii*	Primarily cats to soil to human by ingested water or foods or undercooked foods	0.1–1	10%	Increases with advancing gestational age
Syphilis	Spirochete *Treponema pallidum*	Human oral, anal, vaginal secretions	0.1	Rare, most acute findings at 3–5 mo age	High for primary and lower for secondary infection
Rubella	Ribovirus	Respiratory secretions	0–1	Rare due to vaccine	90% from 1 to 12 wk 20% 16–20th wk Low later gestation
Herpes	Herpesvirus	Mucosal surfaces and skin breaks	0.001–0.003	5–10% Most perinatal exposure	Greatest primary rather than reactivation
Varicella	Herpesvirus	Mucosal surfaces and skin breaks	<0.01	Rare due to vaccine	Highest second trimester 2% risk 13–20 wk
Lymphocytic choriomeningitis	Arenavirus	Rodent borne to human via infected aerosols or fomites	Unknown but rare	Rare	
Parvovirus B19	Parvoviridae virus	Respiratory secretions or hand-to-mouth contact	Variable time and country	26% requiring transfusion	High viral load
Human immunodeficiency virus	Retrovirus	Sexual transmission, contaminated blood/needles	Infrequent with medicine	<2%	High viral load, chorioamnionitis, preterm delivery
Zika	Flavivirus	Bite from infected Aedes mosquito or sexual transmission	Variable times and country	10%	Any time during pregnancy

precursors in early stages of hematopoiesis. Severe fetal anemia may lead to high-output cardiac failure and in the presence of also myocarditis, hypoxic–ischemic encephalopathy. However, direct damage to the brain via virus is also suspected as DNA for the virus has been found in multiple cells, including microglial, endothelial, and multinucleated giant.[462] Brain injury is seen in approximately 26% of cases requiring intrauterine transfusion, and typically in the presence of high viral load.[462]

Zika virus is both neurotropic and gliotropic but preferentially targets neural progenitor cells. Neuronal proliferation, migration, and differentiation are disrupted by meningoencephalitis, slowing development *in utero* and postnatal.[461] It can infect the fetus any time through pregnancy, though greatest sequelae result from first-trimester infection with the most common endpoint being microcephaly.

Most infections intrauterine will present with systemic signs in the neonatal period, which include jaundice, hepatomegaly, splenomegaly, rash, IUGR, microcephaly, hydrocephalus, or chorioretinitis.[456] However, not all intrauterine infections cause systemic findings, being uncommon in rubella and infrequent in varicella, lymphocytic choriomeningitis virus, and Zika.[459] In addition, hydrops and intrauterine demise is not as likely in Zika as compared to other infections.[463]

Diagnosis: Suspicion for infection may be raised by maternal findings of fever or rash. During acute infection, laboratory confirmation is only possible when clinical symptoms are present.[460] Most viruses can be detected in the amniotic fluid via polymerase chain reaction (PCR). In CMV, a 6- to 8-week window exists between infection and detection in the amniotic fluid or 20 to 21 weeks' gestation and is best when combined with culture.[460] Fluid is typically obtained at 18 week for toxoplasmosis.[460] PCR testing is possible for Zika virus.

Imaging: Brain imaging findings in congenital infections overlap significantly. VM due to neuronal destruction or migrational defect is common (Table 17.1-20). However, some imaging findings may point to a certain pathogen:

Intracranial calcifications are common, and their appearance and location may be clues. CMV is typically periventricular and thick and irregular (Fig. 17.1-77A–D). Toxoplasmosis is nodular and diffuse, and Zika demonstrates coarse calcification at the gray white junction.[463]

Microcephaly is caused by infections in about 20% of case, with most common being Zika (Fig. 17.1-78), followed by CMV, toxoplasmosis, rubella, herpes, and syphilis.[463] First-trimester infection and microcephaly in Zika is present in up to 13% with congenital infection.[463]

Migrational disorders are most common in CMV (Fig. 17.1-77E–G), less extensive in Zika, and more infrequent lymphocytic choriomeningitis virus, though parvovirus B19 and varicella may cause polymicrogyria.[463]

Encephaloclastic lesions are common in infection with toxoplasmosis, syphilis, rubella, herpes, varicella, parvovirus B19, and HIV. Toxoplasmosis, syphilis, and lymphocytic choriomeningitis virus are more likely to result in hydrocephalus.

Cerebellar volume loss and hemorrhage should raise suspicion for parvovirus B19.[462]

Hydrocephalus is more likely to occur in infections with toxoplasmosis, syphilis, and lymphocytic choriomeningitis virus.

White matter signal with temporal lobe cysts is highly suggestive of CMV (Fig. 17.1-79).

Brainstem and spinal cord abnormalities are common in Zika virus syndrome, rather unique in this group of disorders. Arthrogryposis can also occur with Zika due to the spinal cord injury, though sometimes can be seen with CMV, rubella, and varicella virus.[463]

Ultrasound: Suspicion for infection may be first raised during US by the presence of fetal growth restriction, abnormal amniotic fluid volume, intrahepatic calcifications, hyperechogenic bowel, and fluid in the abdomen, around the heart or lungs, leading to hydrops.[464] Placentomegaly may be seen. Anemia may occur secondary to infection; therefore, middle cerebral artery (MCA) Doppler should be considered.[457]

Sonographic brain findings may not be apparent in the second trimester.[465] The most common finding is VM, which in conjunction with small head size should raise suspicion for infection; however, VM and microcephaly may not be detected until after 30 weeks' gestation/advanced fetal age.[465] Increased periventricular echogenicity that correlates with ventriculitis and leukoencephalopathy may be more difficult to identify in the third trimester.[465] US is helpful in identification of calcifications, often punctate or coarse. Calcifications intrauterine do not typically demonstrate shadowing and may be best appreciated via transvaginal technique.[465] Lenticulostriate and thalamic (also known as candlestick sign) echogenicity may be a clue for fetal infection. Subependymal cysts are known association, though US is limited in detection of those in the temporal lobe. Intraventricular synechiae result from fusion of periventricular cysts and separation of ependyma from germinal matrix, usually present in the occipital but sometimes temporal

horn and are highly suggestive of CMV.[465] Cortical malformations can be diagnosed if early, abnormal, overfolded small, or delay sulcation is noted. Hypoplastic corpus callosum or cerebellum, parenchymal cysts, and hemorrhage may be noted.[465] Enlarged cisterna magna is often present.[464,466] The presence of two or more findings should raise suspicion for infection, especially CMV.[466]

Magnetic Resonance Imaging: Fetal MRI has a higher detection of polar temporal cysts, micrencephaly, cortical malformations, and cerebellar hypoplasia than US, providing additional information in 50% of cases.[467] Imaging later in pregnancy can show additional findings in up to 40% of cases.[467] However, fetal brain MRI can be normal with postnatal imaging demonstrating signs of infection, particularly calcifications.[468] It is important to remember to perform susceptibility imaging for identification of calcification when there is concern for a congenital infection.

MRI allows for excellent depiction of both white matter and cortical abnormalities. More acute findings include T2 hyperintense white matter signal with loss of the lamination pattern and diffuse or focal necrosis, present in approximately 17.5% of cases.[468] In CMV infection, white matter signal is predominately noted in the temporal and parietal areas, with posterior involvement commonly sparing periventricular and subcortical white matter.[461] Diffusion in white matter signal in CMV demonstrates increased apparent diffusion coefficient (ADC) value, but there are overall low ADC values detected in CMV infected fetuses when compared to controls.[469,470] However, neither of these findings correlate with changes in neurocognitive outcome.[469,470]

Chronic findings include VM (80%, often unilateral), loss of volume, parenchymal cyst (37%), subependymal cyst, intraventricular synechia, calcifications, malformations of development such as polymicrogyria (13%), delay in cortical development and cerebellar hypoplasia (5% to 50%).[467,468] Brain malformations of the corpus callosum and posterior fossa are present in 22% of cases. Subependymal cysts in the anterior temporal lobes are common in CMV. Hydrocephalus may develop in many infections, especially toxoplasmosis. Brainstem and spinal cord hypoplasia should be assessed, especially when Zika infection is possible.

Associated Anomalies: Associated non-CNS anomalies with intrauterine infection are covered in chapter 31. Ocular findings are common and include chorioretinitis, cataracts, optic atrophy, and microphthalmia. Chorioretinitis occurs in 90% with lymphocytic choriomeningitis virus, 75% with toxoplasmosis, 50% varicella, and 10% to 20% with CMV. Eighty percentage of congenital rubella patients have cataracts, retinopathy, or microphthalmia. Cataracts are also present in varicella, herpes, and lymphocytic choriomeningitis virus, but uncommon in CMV and toxoplasmosis.[463] Sensorineural hearing loss is prominent in congenital rubella, CMV, and toxoplasmosis. However, in the presence of congenital heart defects such as patent ductus arteriosus, congenital rubella should be considered.

Differential Diagnosis: There is a group of rare genetic disorders known as the *type 1 interferonopathies* that cause cerebral and basal ganglia calcifications, gyral simplification, microcephaly, hepatomegaly, thrombocytopenia, and leukoencephalopathy that mimic congenital infections.[471] The most

TABLE 17.1-20   Intrauterine Infections: Imaging and Testing

PATHOGEN	BRAIN	CALCIFICATIONS	EXTRACRANIAL FETAL IMAGING FINDINGS	DIAGNOSTIC PCR/OTHER	TESTING SEROLOGY
CMV	Migrational, white matter signal, periventricular cysts temporal, subependymal cysts, cerebellar hypoplasia	**Thick/Irregular** periventricular, basal ganglia, other	Microphthalmia, HSM	Urine, Serum, AF	Specific I-IgM
Toxoplasmosis	Hydrocephalus parenchymal destruction, volume loss	**Nodules** diffuse, periventricular or basal ganglia	Microphthalmia, HSM	CSF, serum, AF	Specific I-IgM
Syphilis	Cerebral infarction, hydrocephalus		HSM	Placenta/umbilical cord spirochetes	Serum/CSF VDRL
Rubella	VM, myelination abnormalities, patchy frontal periventricular signal Total brain destruction and microcephaly	Periventricular and basal ganglia	Heart defects, cataracts (80%), glaucoma, microphthalmia, clubfoot	Urine, throat	Specific I-IgM
Herpes	VM, microcephaly, encephalomalacia	Periventricular, thalamic, basal ganglia, cerebral cortex	Microphthalmia, cataracts, hydrops	Serum, CSF, vesicles, AF	PCR
Varicella	Lobar parenchymal destruction, basal ganglia necrosis, cerebellar hypoplasia, polymicrogyria, hydrocephalus		Microphthalmia, cataracts, limb hypoplasia, gastrointestinal anomalies	CSF, AF	Specific I-IgM
LCM	Hydrocephalus due to cerebral aqueduct obstruction, migrational, cerebellar hypoplasia, microcephaly	Periventricular, ependymal, and parenchymal	Cataracts	CSF, AF	Specific I-IgM
Parvovirus B19	Hydrocephalus, cerebellar hemorrhage/hypoplasia, polymicrogyria		Hydrops, anemia	Serum, AF	Specific I- or M-IgM
HIV	Atrophy, infarct	Basal ganglia, white matter, cerebral cortex	HSM, craniofacial dysmorphism	HIV nucleic acid amplification tests	PCR based
Zika	Microcephaly, VM, volume loss including brainstem and spinal cord, subependymal cysts -occipital horns, migrational, cerebellar, and vermian hypoplasia, abnormal corpus callosum, white matter signal abnormality	**Coarse** gray–white matter junction, especially frontal and parietal lobes, thalamus, basal ganglia, cortex, periventricular, brainstem	Arthrogryposis, microphthalmia, cataracts, redundant posterior scalp skin folding	Urine, Serum, AF Examine placenta	Specific I- or M-IgM and PRNT serum

PCR, polymerase chain reaction; *PRNT*, plaque reduction neutralization test; *I*, infant; *M*, maternal; *AF*, amniotic fluid; *VM*, ventriculomegaly; *HSM*, hepatosplenomegaly; *IgM*, immunoglobulin M; *CMV*, Cytomegalovirus, *LCM*, Lymphocytic choriomeningitis, *HIV*, human immunodeficiency virus.

commonly known is Aicardi-Goutières; however, Cree encephalitis, microcephaly intracranial calcification syndrome, and pseudo-TORCH or Baraitser-Reardon syndrome are all postulated to be closely related autosomal recessive conditions characterized by increased interferon alpha (INF-α) in the CSF, also interestingly raised in infections including TORCH and autoimmune conditions such as lupus. Mutations in multiple genes such as *TREX 1*, *RNASEH2A*, *RNASEH2C*, *SAMJD1*, *ADAR*, and *IFIH1* are noted in patients affected.[472] Clinical presentation at birth suggests an infectious etiology with CSF lymphocytosis; however, extensive testing for infection is negative.

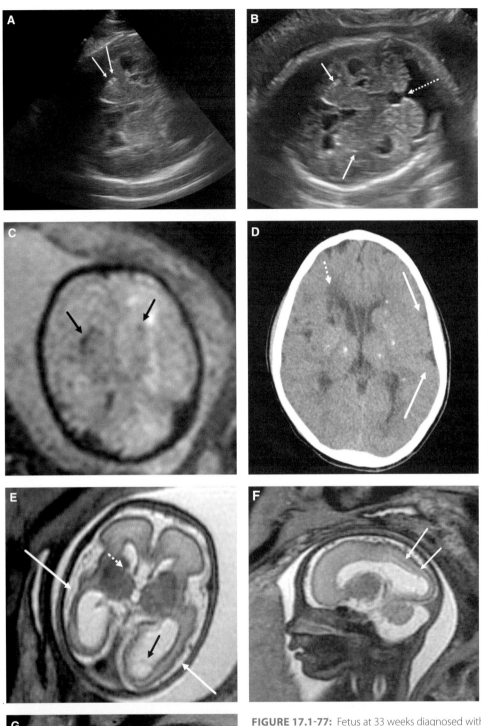

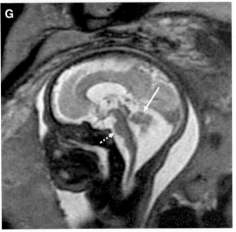

FIGURE 17.1-77: Fetus at 33 weeks diagnosed with cytomegalovirus infection. **A:** Axial US demonstrating echogenic foci in area of basal ganglia consistent with calcifications (*arrows*). **B:** Axial US demonstrating bilateral echogenic foci (*solid arrows*) consistent with calcification. Mild ventriculomegaly and inferior vermian hypoplasia are also noted (*dotted arrow*). Fetus also had microcephaly and elevated peak systolic velocity in the middle cerebral artery. **C:** Axial gradient echo MRI showing susceptibility artifact (*arrows*) in areas of basal ganglia calcification. **D:** Axial postnatal computed tomography demonstrating calcification in the basal ganglia and periventricular white matter. Notice abnormal sulcation left hemisphere (*solid arrows*) and abnormal low attenuation right frontal white matter (*dotted arrow*). **E:** Axial fetal MRI demonstrating abnormal sulcation with irregular bumpy contour of cortex (*white arrows*) consistent with polymicrogyria. There is small subependymal cyst (*dotted arrow*) and intraventricular septation (*black arrow*). **F:** Sagittal MRI demonstrating a dark band of signal (*arrow*) in the central white matter consistent with band heterotopia. **G:** Sagittal MRI demonstrating vermian hypoplasia (*solid arrow*) and small brainstem (*dotted arrow*).

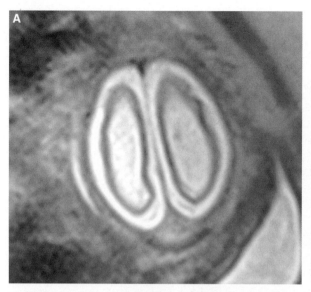
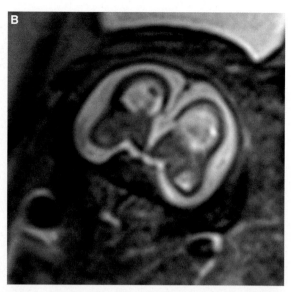

FIGURE 17.1-78: A 25-week fetus with microcephaly and proven Zika virus infection. **A:** Axial MRI demonstrating thin supratentorial mantle. **B:** Coronal MRI shows again thin cerebral mantle with secondary ventriculomegaly. Brain measurements were markedly low for gestational age. (Courtesy of Dorothy Bulas, MD.)

Metabolic disorders may also be considered in the differential, particularly Cockayne syndrome which may present with basal ganglia calcification, white matter signal abnormality, and volume loss. *COL4A1* genetic mutations can also cause intracranial calcifications and parenchymal destruction.

Prognosis: Although fetal infection may resolve without affecting the fetus, spontaneous abortion, intrauterine demise, and stillbirth can occur.[456] Infants surviving infection are at high risk for cerebral palsy, deafness, visual dysfunction, epilepsy, and developmental delay or mental retardation.[456] In general, infection, particularly before week 20, is associated with more severe neurodevelopmental abnormalities.[456]

Intracranial calcifications increase the risk of adverse outcome.[456] The presence of microcephaly and/or imaging of intracranial anomalies, such as migration disorders, carries a severe neurodevelopment prognosis and higher risk for hearing loss.[465,473] Brain volumes are decreased in fetuses with CMV, and specifically lower cerebellar volumes correlate with lower neurodevelopmental outcomes.[474] Temporal cysts in CMV have been associated with 55% hearing loss and 25% neurological impairment.[473] Periventricular cysts, lenticulostriate echodensities, and abnormal T2 hyperintense white matter signal likely carry a better prognosis.[465,467,473]

Hearing loss is most common in fetuses with CMV, toxoplasmosis, congenital rubella, and Zika. CMV and toxoplasmosis

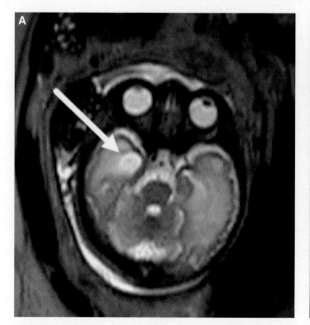
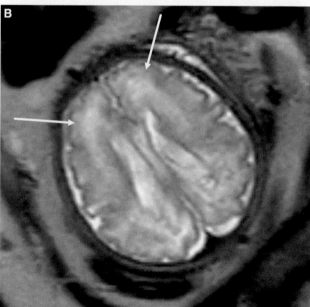

FIGURE 17.1-79: Fetus at 35 weeks with congenital cytomegalovirus infection. **A:** Axial MRI demonstrating cystic structure (*arrow*) in the right temporal lobe. **B:** Axial MRI demonstrating abnormal hyperintense T2 signal within the supratentorial white matter (*arrows*). No cortical malformations were detected.

will exhibit these findings in 70% to 75% of cases. Many fetuses infected with CMV are asymptomatic, though, postnatally, 10% to 15% develop symptoms of CMV during the first year and 25% hearing loss by age 2.[470] Other infections such as congenital rubella and toxoplasmosis may have delayed hearing loss and mental deficits after appearing uninfected.[467] In addition, the full spectrum of Zika virus is still being investigated as microcephaly may evolve late in gestation and after birth, and CNS abnormalities are being found in previously denoted asymptomatic fetuses.[475,476]

Management: Immunization prevents congenital rubella. Congenital syphilis can be prevented with penicillin when infection is diagnosed. CMV can be avoided with simple hygienic measures and avoiding contact with young children's saliva and urine.[459] Toxoplasmosis may be diminished by recommending that pregnant women not clean cat litter boxes and ensuring meats are properly cooked, and lymphocytic choriomeningitis virus by evading contact with mice, hamsters, or excretions. Zika can be prevented by avoiding travel to endemic areas and sexual contact with men who have traveled to endemic regions in the preceding 6 months.[459] Vertical transmission of HIV has significantly decreased with antiretroviral medication, neonatal postexposure prophylaxis, delivery by C-section, and discouragement of breastfeeding.

Upon diagnosis of maternal infection, monthly US may be reasonable. Parvovirus B19 diagnosis requires close monitoring for 10 weeks with MCA Doppler, and if anemia develops, umbilical blood cord sampling and transfusion should be performed.[463]

Treatment for toxoplasmosis in the first trimester with spiramycin and early second with pyrimethamine and sulfadiazine and leucovorin in the late second and third trimesters are beneficial.[459] After birth, antiviral medications can be helpful for some pathogen exposures. Acyclovir may decrease herpes or varicella virus. Ganciclovir therapy in the first 30 days postnatal or valganciclovir for 6 months in severely symptomatic CMV exposed patients is associated with improved hearing and neurodevelopmental outcomes.[459]

Infants with congenital infection should have periodic ophthalmological examinations and auditory brainstem evoked response testing to identify sensorineural hearing loss.[459] Shunting of obstructive hydrocephalus improves neurological outcome.

Recurrence: In viruses with potential reactivation, pregnancies of mothers who are seropositive may have slight increased risk.[464] Otherwise, congenital infections are sporadic or at highest risk in areas or times of infestation. Mimics such as Aicardi-Goutières are likely autosomal recessive with 25% risk of recurrence.

Hypoxic–Ischemic Injury/Fetal Stroke

Incidence: The incidence of perinatal stroke, defined as injury between 28 weeks' gestation and 28 days postnatal, is reported to occur in 1 in 4,000 live births.[477] The incidence of fetal intracranial hemorrhage and stroke is not clearly known but has been suggested in 1 per 10,000 pregnancies.[478] Fetal intracranial hemorrhage alone has an estimated incidence of 0.6 to 1 per 1,000 cases.[479] Many children remain undiagnosed perinatally as symptomatology is not evident until the first year of life.[477]

Pathogenesis: During intrauterine life, the fetus is exposed to a low oxygen environment that is supplemented by higher heart rate, higher hemoglobin concentration, and large surface area for gas exchange in the placenta.[480] When hypoxia occurs, the fetus tries to compensate and maintain oxygenation by changing hematological and hemodynamic parameters, especially increased erythropoiesis and cardiac output that is directed to the brain and heart at the expense of other organs such as the kidneys and gut.[480] In addition, in the acute phase, other compensatory changes include biophysical, metabolic, and endocrine. In the chronic form of hypoxia, the fetus does not demonstrate normal growth, and although not fully understood, deficiency in nutrients and endocrine changes are common drivers.[480]

The placenta is a transient organ that is extremely important in fetal development and has nutritional, endocrine, immunological, and protective barrier properties. Low oxygen is required for normal placental formation and normal regulation in cellular differentiation, immune defense, and tissue repair. Placental pathology is closely linked to fetal hypoxic ischemia.[480] Neurological impairment and cerebral palsy have been shown to be highly correlated with large fetal placental vascular lesions, such as fetal thrombotic vasculopathy, chronic villitis with obliterative fetal vasculopathy, chorioamnionitis with severe fetal vasculitis, and meconium-associated fetal vascular necrosis.[481]

In the fetal brain, hypoxia results in differential neurogenesis, impaired neuronal migration and neurotransmitter expression, and induces changes in genes.[480] In the presence of hypoxia, multiple cells types produce and release hypoxia-inducible factor (HIF-1α) that mediates cellular response to the low oxygen, increasing vascularization to ischemic areas.[480] In addition, hypoxia affects the rapamycin complex (mTOR) pathways and elevates levels of cortisol, both of which have an impact on cell growth, proliferation, and metabolism.[480] The fetal cerebrovasculature exposed to hypoxia is less reactive and slower to respond to changes in blood pressure, blood gases, and other stimuli. The severity, type, and distribution of the injury depend on numerous factors, such as the duration and intensity of the hypoperfusion and the time (fetal gestational age).[480] In contrast to the neonate, an acute response to hypoxia in the fetus is not common. The fetus can sustain longer periods of hypoperfusion and hypotension before developing injury due to high cardiac and neural tolerance, given that the cells contain higher glycogen stores that facilitate anaerobic metabolism.[482] Most fetal hypoxic injuries are chronic and are associated with intrauterine growth restriction (IUGR) or small for gestational age (SGA) infants commonly in conjunction with placental insufficiency.[482] Sometimes, chronic imaging findings or a combination of acute and chronic insults may be observed.[483,484]

Injury in the fetal brain may be due to hemorrhage, ischemia, or thrombosis. Hemorrhage can occur anywhere in the fetal brain: germinal matrix (GMH), ventricles, choroid plexus, intraparenchymal, subarachnoid, or subdural spaces. Approximately 80% to 90% of fetal hemorrhagic injuries are intra-axial, and the remaining 20% extra-axial hemorrhage.[485,486] In the presence of intracranial hemorrhage, nearly 90% are supratentorial, and the remaining infratentorial.[477] The GMH is most common type, representing two-thirds of fetal intracranial hemorrhage, with the rest being non-GMH locations.[478,487]

Ischemic and hemorrhagic parenchymal injuries are often mixed as after ischemia, reperfusion of a lesion may result in hemorrhage. In addition, it is known that venous hypertension is more commonly associated with hemorrhagic pathology. Arterial stroke and basal ganglia, cortex, and white matter ischemia are less common in the fetus due to greater resistance of neurons and also the infrequent acute *in utero* event.[484] In the chronic phase, endpoint reflects the complexity of the ischemia with factors such as the severity of the event, the time of hypoxia during brain development, and the inflammatory response. A wide spectrum of imaging pathologies can be seen, including subependymal cysts, ventriculomegaly (VM), porencephaly, schizencephaly, polymicrogyria, cystic encephalomalacia, and hydranencephaly.[488]

Etiology: In the majority of cases of fetal stroke, there is no identified cause.[477] Etiology of fetal stroke may be detected in 20% to 45% of cases, with many associations listed in Table 17.1-21.[477,485] Inciting causes for fetal hypoxia can be separated by sight of origin: preplacental, uteroplacental, and postplacental.[480] In the fetus, hypoxic injury is typically asymptomatic and is rarely recognized unless imaging is performed for maternal or fetal concerns. In general, most cases of fetal stroke present during the late second and third trimesters as an incidental finding after a normal second-trimester anatomical scan.[489]

Preplacental is typically linked to maternal cause, being either exposure to environment creating low oxygen or due to maternal respiratory, cardiovascular, metabolic, or hematological disorders.[480] The most frequently identified factors are hematological or maternal trauma.[477,485]

Of those with a cause, hemorrhage due to fetal alloimmune thrombocytopenia (FAT) has been cited in up to 15% of cases.[485] FAT occurs in 1 to 2 of 50,000 pregnancies, can affect the first born child, and results from maternal–fetal platelet antigen incompatibility, the most common of the greater than 30 known being HPA-1a incompatibility, present in 75% to 90% Caucasians.[490,491,492] Fetal platelets carrying specific paternal-derived antigens gain access to the maternal system through the placenta, causing alloimmunization. After sensitization, maternal immunoglobulin G (IgG) platelet-specific antibody is produced, which then crosses the placenta and results in fetal platelet destruction. The risk of intracranial hemorrhage with this disorder is 10% to 30%, with 80% occurring antenatal during the second and third trimesters.[488,490–492]

Uteroplacental hypoxia results from placental insufficiency and includes deficient implantation, impaired vascular remodeling, and other factors that result in reduction of maternal–fetal surface area for exchanges.[480] Placental thrombosis or vasculopathy in the presence of infection is noted in 11% of case.[486] Inflammation via chorioamnionitis is also a common cause for ischemia, being present in 95% of preterm deliveries and 10% of infants born after 33 to 36 weeks.[482]

Monochorionic twins are covered in detail in chapter 15; however, the presence of vascular anastomosis in this type of multiple gestations significantly increases the risk for brain injury.[493] Intrauterine hypoxia, venous hypertension, and fetal anemia may result in antenatal brain injury in twin-to-twin transfusion.[485,486] Other monochorionic pathologies such as twin anemia polycythemia, twin reversed arterial perfusion syndrome, and single twin demise also increase risk. Single twin demise especially has a high risk for fetal stroke due to hypoperfusion and hypovolemia injury.[488]

Postplacental causes are due to mechanical obstruction of the umbilical vessels and fetal malformations/diseases. Fetal causes include cardiac anomalies, cardiac dysfunction, polycythemia, and large vascular disorders. Fetal anemia is believed to cause ischemia and hemorrhage by disruption of vessels due to hyperdynamic circulation. Metabolic disorders can be the source in as high as 22% of cases, postulated to cause chronic ischemia due to metabolite depletion in the germinal matrix.[486]

Diagnosis

Ultrasound: US criteria for fetal hypoxia include IUGR; abnormal Doppler findings, especially umbilical artery and cerebral; and later a poor biophysical profile score that reflects abnormalities in fetal heart rate, amniotic fluid volume, fetal breathing, gross body movements, and fetal tone.[493] Imaging may be initiated by decreased fetal movements and low amniotic fluid.[494] Fetal heart changes including smooth baseline variability and late decelerations with sinusoidal pattern may represent the first sign of brain injury.[477,495]

In the presence of fetal hypoxia, Doppler of the uterine arteries can show diastolic notching.[480] Doppler of the umbilical artery will often demonstrate decreased, absent, or reversed end-diastolic flow. Reduced cerebroplacental ratio below 1, measured by the ratio of the middle cerebral artery (MCA) to umbilical artery resistance index, suggests redistribution of flow to the brain or brain sparing.[480] In some cases, fetal anemia may be detected by elevated peak systolic velocity in the MCA.[477] Increased resistance in the MCA may be a sign of increase in intracranial pressure related to a hemorrhage.[490] Absent or reversed diastolic flow in the MCA has been associated with poor outcome.[495–497]

On US, VM is the most common finding, present in 55% of patients. The detection of intracranial hemorrhage ranges from 22% to 64%, with the higher percentage being in a directed neurosonology examination.[487]

Magnetic Resonance Imaging: MRI is valuable to confirm the presence of hemorrhage or ischemia and to evaluate for parenchymal abnormalities that may not be apparent via US.[498] On fetal MRI, hemorrhage is variable signal but typically hyperintense T1 and hypointense T2 signal. With diffusion, acute ischemia can be detected. MRI has been shown to be more accurate and/or provides additional information after US in approximately 30% to 55% of cases.[487,489] In addition, MRI clarifies parenchymal involvement, possibly providing clues to the timing of the hemorrhage and cause of injury, and often detects higher grade of hemorrhage than suspected via US.[489]

In utero hypoxia tends to depict chronic imaging finding of injury (67%) rather than acute (33%).[484] MRI may define cerebral abnormalities in up to 67% of cases of hypoxic–ischemic injury. The most common findings are ventricular dilatation (77%), hemorrhage (15%), or brain destruction (35%).[484] Hemorrhagic injury is typically identified in the germinal matrix.[488] T1, gradient echo, and/or susceptibility-weighted imaging and diffusion are essential when imaging the fetal brain.

Germinal Matrix Hemorrhage

Between 24 and 32 weeks, the germinal matrix is highly proliferative and metabolically active and contains a thin multilayer, highly vascular network that is particularly sensitive to variations in blood pressure, hypoxia, acidosis, and anoxia. A germinal matrix hemorrhage (GMH) occurs due to hypoxia and sudden changes in the cerebral blood pressure, which then cause bleeding in the fragile premature capillary bed, likely due to a hypoperfusion–reperfusion cycle.[477] Rupture of the ependyma may then result in intraventricular hemorrhage.

A modified grading system denoted by Burstein and Papile can be used to stage fetal germinal matrix injuries (Fig. 17.1-80, Table 17.1-22).[477,485,499] Most cases are bilateral or left hemispheric, and when detected, the majority (70% to 85%) are grade III and grade IV.[489] GMH is rarely detected prior to 23 weeks,

TABLE 17.1-21	Predisposing Factors and Patterns of Fetal Stroke	
LOCATION	**PATTERNS OF NEUROIMAGING**
Preplacental/Maternal	
Bleeding Disorders Maternal–fetal alloimmune thrombocytopenia Idiopathic thrombocytopenia purpura Von Willebrand disease Rh alloimmunization	Germinal matrix hemorrhage ± venous infarct Intraparenchymal hemorrhage Subdural and subarachnoid hemorrhage
Vitamin K deficiency	Intraparenchymal hemorrhage Subdural hemorrhage
Drugs including warfarin, cholestyramine, and antiepileptic medications	Subdural hemorrhage Germinal matrix hemorrhage ± venous infarct
Toxic exposure alcohol, cocaine, carbon monoxide	Intraparenchymal hemorrhage Schizencephaly Porencephaly
Trauma and Iatrogenic trauma related to amniocentesis, cordocentesis, blood sampling	Germinal matrix hemorrhage ± venous infarct Subdural hemorrhage
Hypoxia related to maternal illness Stroke, hemorrhage, diabetic ketoacidosis, seizure, preeclampsia, carbon monoxide, febrile illness, or cardiac arrest	Germinal matrix hemorrhage ± venous infarct Porencephaly
Cholestasis of pregnancy	Nonspecific brain injury
Uteroplacental	
Placental hemorrhage/thrombosis	Arterial ischemic stroke ± hemorrhage Germinal matrix hemorrhage ± venous infarct
Monochorionic pathologies Twin-to-twin transfusion syndrome Twin anemia polycythemia syndrome Single twin demise Severe IUGR Twin reversed arterial perfusion syndrome	Arterial ischemic stroke ± hemorrhage Intraparenchymal hemorrhage Germinal matrix hemorrhage ± venous infarct Subdural hemorrhage Polymicrogyria and schizencephaly Microcephaly
Chorioamnionitis/prolonged rupture of membranes	Intraparenchymal hemorrhage Ischemia ± hemorrhage
Placenta previa	Germinal matrix hemorrhage ± venous infarct
Abruptio placenta	Germinal matrix hemorrhage ± venous infarct Arterial ischemic stroke ± hemorrhage
Postplacental/Fetal	
Cord accident	Germinal matrix hemorrhage ± venous infarct Arterial ischemic stroke ± hemorrhage
Fetal anemia/Hematological Alloimmune thrombocytopenia Fetal Rhesus Congenital factor V or X deficiency Von Willebrand disease Protein C deficiency	Infratentorial hemorrhage Subdural hemorrhage Germinal matrix hemorrhage ± venous infarct
Fetal cardiac	Arterial ischemic stroke ± hemorrhage
COL4A1, COL4A2 mutations	Schizencephaly Porencephaly Germinal matrix hemorrhage ± venous infarct Infratentorial hemorrhage
GATA1 mutations	Intraparenchymal hemorrhage
Metabolic disorders—mitochondrial, pyruvate carboxylase deficiency, nonketotic hyperglycemia, amino acid metabolism, and peroxisomal disorders	Germinal matrix hemorrhage ± venous infarct
Infection—TORCH and parvovirus B19	Intraparenchymal ischemia + hemorrhage Infratentorial hemorrhage
Space-occupying lesions—tumors and cysts	Usually secondary to lesion

IUGR, intrauterine growth restriction.

with average age at presentation of 28 weeks.[487] This is dissimilar to other sites of hemorrhage, which typically present earlier, usually at average of 22 weeks.[487]

Periventricular hemorrhagic infarction or grade IV occurs secondary to a venous infarct that develops if a large intraventricular hemorrhage compresses or obstructs terminal veins along the surface of the ventricle.[500] Hydrocephalus may develop if the intraventricular hemorrhage incites an inflammatory ependymitis or obstructs the aqueduct of Sylvius or fourth ventricle with clot.

Cerebellar hemorrhage has also been described prenatal and is likely the result of GMH in the cells of the external granular layer or fourth ventricle.[501] The insult makes sense as this is when the cells from the external granular layer start migrating to the internal granule layer, a time of intense angiogenesis stimulated by metabolic needs of the new cell population making immature vessels prone to hemorrhage.[501,502] Cause is unknown, though fetal infection, fetal distress, IUGR, placental thrombotic vasculopathy, maternal thrombophilia or septic shock, and anemia/hydrops have been cited.[501]

Chronic parenchymal changes after insult include migrational anomalies such as polymicrogyria and schizencephaly, described earlier in this chapter. Before 20 to 26 weeks, insults in the brain result in parenchymal necrosis without gliosis, with the most common appearance being porencephaly. After 26 weeks, there is astrocyte proliferation, which will result in glial septated cavities, known as cystic encephalomalacia. Later in gestation, the insult will usually result in pure gliosis with no cyst.[407]

Ultrasound: Most cases of intracranial hemorrhage are detected between 26 and 33 weeks, but some have been described as early as 20 weeks.[495] Intracranial hemorrhage appears different depending on the time of imaging after the initial insult. Acutely in the first 3 to 8 days, the clot is hyperechoic (Fig. 17.1-81A). If there is significant intraventricular component, the choroid plexus may appear large and irregular.[498] Choroid plexus is not present anterior to the foramen of Monro, and therefore in the presence of echogenic tissue in the frontal horns, hemorrhage should be suspected.[498] After 3 to 8 days, the liquefying clot appears heterogeneous in echotexture, often with an external echogenic lining and an internal echolucent core (Fig. 17.1-81B). From 7 to 28 days, the clot has completely liquefied, begins to decrease in size, and appears as a cystic and/or with layering debris (Fig. 17.1-81C).[495] Unilateral hemorrhage is more likely to occur in the left than right hemisphere, possibly because of less

TABLE 17.1-22 Burstein and Papile Modified Grading System to Stage Fetal Germinal Matrix Injuries[485,499]

GRADE	DESCRIPTION
I	Subependymal hemorrhage
II	Intraventricular hemorrhage, filling less than 50% of the ventricle with ventricle size 15 mm or less
III	Intraventricular, filling more than 50% of the ventricle with ventriculomegaly >15 mm
IV	I–III with intraparenchymal periventricular hemorrhage

susceptibility of right hemisphere vessels to hypoperfusion.[477] Echogenicity of the ventricular wall due to ventriculitis may be noted (Fig. 17.1-81D). With complete resolution, the brain and ventricles may be normal.[495] Sometimes, a transient VM occurs, which resolves over time as the blood products degrade, relieving obstruction at the foramen of Monroe.[485] In grades III and IV, ventricular dilatation is more likely to persist.[503] VM has been detected in as high as 60%, and some may progress to hydrocephalus due to aqueductal stenosis or ventricular obstruction.[485,486] However, it has been reported that only a minority of cases result in obstructive hydrocephalus in the fetus.[487]

Intraparenchymal hemorrhage (IPH) is seen acutely as a densely echogenic mass, frequently extending from the subependymal layer of the ventricle (Fig. 17.1-81E).[485] As the clot degrades, these lesions often become hypoechoic and then evolve into a porencephalic cyst.[485] Cerebellar hemorrhages have similar imaging, and clues to the presence include an irregular cerebellum and obliterated cistern magna (Fig. 17.1-81F).[406] Because of limited contrast resolution of US in solid tissues, small clots within the cerebral and cerebellar parenchyma may be missed.[406]

Magnetic Resonance Imaging: The appearance of hemorrhage changes on MRI with age of the clot; however, evolving MRI signal changes for hemorrhage have not been studied in the fetus. In general, acute hemorrhage is intermediate on T1 and hypointense on T2, subacute blood is hyperintense on T1 and hypointense on T2, and chronic hemorrhage is heterogeneous

Grade I

Grade II

Grade III

Grade IV

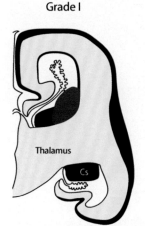 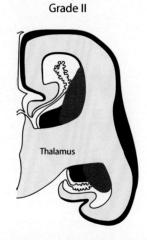 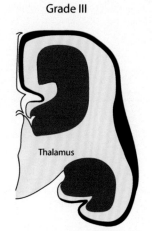 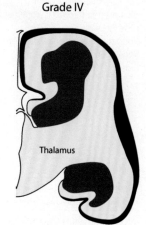

FIGURE 17.1-80: The grades of germinal matrix hemorrhage in the fetus.

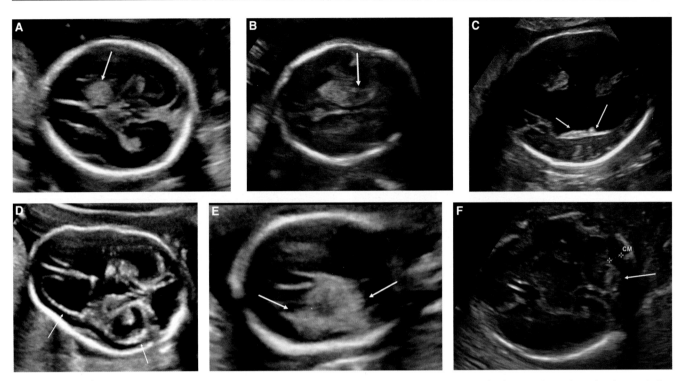

FIGURE 17.1-81: US of multiple fetuses with intracranial hemorrhage. **A:** Axial image demonstrating a round echogenic lesion (*arrow*) in the caudothalamic groove area consistent with an acute germinal matrix hemorrhage. **B:** Evolving subacute hemorrhage depicted by a large heterogeneous choroid with internal echolucent area (*arrow*). **C:** Axial US of subacute hemorrhage with significant ventriculomegaly and layering echogenic blood products (*arrow*). **D:** Axial image in a fetus diagnosed previously with bilateral grade III hemorrhages. There is significant ventriculomegaly and residual layering blood in the lateral ventricle (*arrows*). Increased echogenicity of the ependymal surface is consistent with ventriculitis. **E:** Axial view of focal hemorrhage in the cerebrum (*arrows*). **F:** Axial view of posterior fossa demonstrating abnormal echogenicity (*arrow*) in the left cerebellum proven to represent hemorrhage. Calipers denote cisterna magna *(CM)*.

but with areas of hypointense signal on T1 and hyperintense T2 (Fig. 17.1-82A, B). The grade of GMH is defined by identifying hemorrhage along the ventricular wall, intraventricular, or parenchymal (Fig. 17.1-83).[477,483] As hemorrhage has the same signal as the germinal matrix, utilizing symmetry of the brain and knowledge of normal is important. Hemorrhages tend to be larger and more irregular than the germinal matrix, often associated with ventricular dilatation. T1 imaging, gradient echo, and/or susceptibility-weighted imaging can aid in detecting hemorrhage (Fig. 17.1-82C).[483] MRI is more accurate than US with regard to grading GMHs and is more sensitive in the detection of either acute or small ischemic lesions.[477,486] In the presence of VM, evaluation of the aqueduct is important to exclude obstruction.[504]

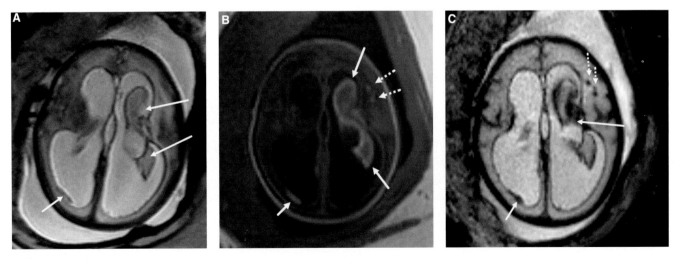

FIGURE 17.1-82: Germinal matrix hemorrhage and white matter injury in a fetus at 31 weeks. **A:** Axial T2 MRI demonstrating heterogeneous hypointense material (*arrows*) in the lateral ventricles, left greater than right in the presence of ventriculomegaly. Notice abnormal hyperintense signal in the frontal periventricular white matter. **B:** Axial T1 MRI confirms hemorrhage demonstrating hyperintense signal in the ventricles (*solid arrows*). Note also high signal in the adjacent white matter (*dotted arrows*) consistent with hemorrhagic white matter injury. **C:** Axial susceptibility imaging showing artifact in the hemorrhages in the ventricles (*solid arrows*) and in the adjacent frontal white matter (*dotted arrows*).

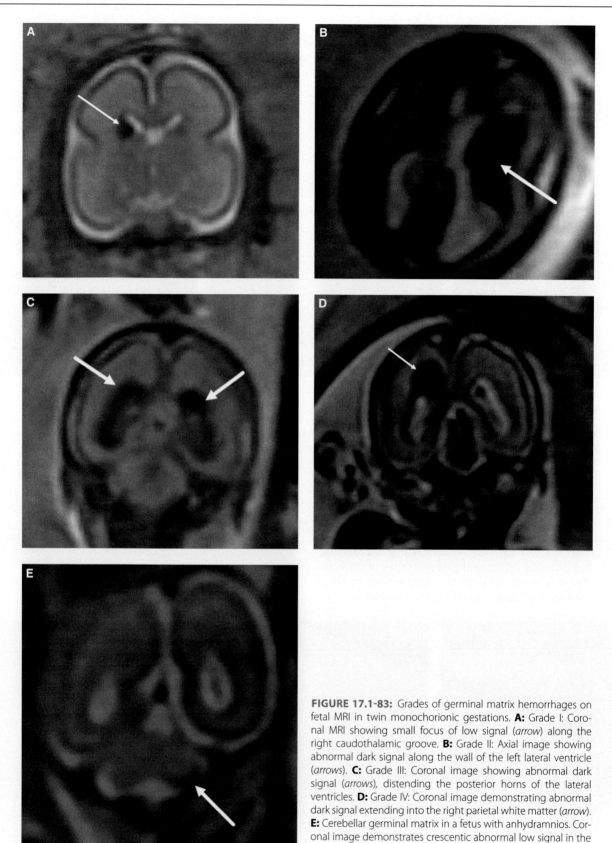

FIGURE 17.1-83: Grades of germinal matrix hemorrhages on fetal MRI in twin monochorionic gestations. **A:** Grade I: Coronal MRI showing small focus of low signal (*arrow*) along the right caudothalamic groove. **B:** Grade II: Axial image showing abnormal dark signal along the wall of the left lateral ventricle (*arrows*). **C:** Grade III: Coronal image showing abnormal dark signal (*arrows*), distending the posterior horns of the lateral ventricles. **D:** Grade IV: Coronal image demonstrating abnormal dark signal extending into the right parietal white matter (*arrow*). **E:** Cerebellar germinal matrix in a fetus with anhydramnios. Coronal image demonstrates crescentic abnormal low signal in the left cerebellum peripherally (*arrow*).

IPH demonstrates similar signal changes to the GMH but may show adjacent edema that is manifested as T2 hyperintensity. Hemorrhage and edema may be transient and resolve. In the cerebellum, most of the hemorrhages are caudal and peripheral portion of the hemispheres (bilateral or unilateral) and are detected incidentally before 26 weeks' gestation (20 to 30 weeks). The vermis is often involved, and evolution of the hemorrhage often leads to malformation of the cerebellar folia or sometimes a cleft.[501]

Chronic changes of volume loss, which include unilateral or bilateral large, sometimes distorted ventricles with enlarged subarachnoid spaces, can be noted when injury is permanent. Irregularity of the ventricular wall or premature loss of the germinal matrix is consistent with germinal matrix injury.[504] Parenchymal defects, some appearing cystic or septated, can develop (Fig. 17.1-84). Subependymal cysts may be seen. Laminar necrosis refers to selective destruction of distinct cortical layers, being most susceptible beginning at 28 weeks. Calcification with laminar necrosis appears as a linear cortical signal abnormality that is hyperintense on T1 and hypointense on gradient echo imaging.[504] The corpus callosum may be thin or deficient. The sulcation is often abnormal, with polymicrogyria developing in 2% of hypoxia cases.[407]

Intraparenchymal Hemorrhage (unrelated to GMH)
Imaging findings of IPH are similar to those previously described. However, certain disorders are highly associated with IPH, the most common being alloimmune thrombocytopenia, parvovirus B19, and genetic mutations. In fetal alloimmune thrombocytopenia, the majority of brain injuries in the fetus are in the presence of very low platelet count.[484,488] Two genetic mutations cause IPH. *COL4A1* is typically autosomal dominant and causes small vessel disease with stroke and eye abnormalities. *GATA1* is responsible for differentiation of blood cells, the mutation, an X-linked disorder seen in males, causes anemia and thrombocytopenia, which may lead to fatal hydrops, hemochromatosis, and/or intracranial hemorrhage.[505]

Extra-axial Hemorrhage
Subdural and, less commonly, epidural hemorrhage have been described in the fetus, occurring most commonly over the cerebral convexity but also in the posterior fossa.[496] Subdural hemorrhages typically develop from tearing of loose draining veins and are seen more commonly in the third trimester. Epidural and subdural hemorrhages tend to be related to maternal trauma, maternal coagulopathy including vitamin K deficiency, fetal vascular anomaly or infection.[479,496,497,406] The most common causes cited are maternal trauma and use of warfarin.[450] A significant number, approximately 47%, will not have an identifiable cause.[479]

Ultrasound: Subdural hematomas (SDHs) appear as echogenic, heterogeneous, or hypoechoic collections along the cerebral hemisphere or less commonly posterior fossa and displace the brain parenchyma away from the calvarium (Fig. 17.1-85A).[490,497,506] Imaging findings described on a prenatal US findings in the presence of SDH include abnormal intracranial echogenicity (42%), lateral VM (38%), presence of intracranial mass (31%), macrocephaly (24%), midline deviation of the falx (20%), and intracranial fluid collection (10%). Other findings that may be noted include reversed diastolic flow (11%) and/or elevated peak systolic flow (2%) in the MCA, echogenic bowel (4%), and hydrops (2%).[507] With organization of the clot, there may be echogenic layering debris in a cyst, an echogenic rim, or development of new collections over time.[506] Cerebral edema may result in acoustic enhancement adjacent to the collection.[507]

Magnetic Resonance Imaging: MRI can detect up to 42% of cases of SDH not suggested by US.[479] This technique is excellent at defining extra-axial hemorrhage in the subdural or epidural space, and susceptibility imaging is helpful in reinforcing hemorrhagic products (Fig. 17.1-85B, C). Even small collections of hemorrhage are easily identified.[506] MRI also can depict mass effect and injury to the adjacent brain (Fig. 17.1-85D, E).

White Matter Injury/Parenchymal Ischemia
White matter injury typically occurs in fetuses less than 32 weeks' gestation. The pathogenesis is suggested to be due to incomplete development of the vascular supply in the white matter, lack of regulation in blood flow early in gestation, and immaturity of the oligodendrocyte cell, especially when exposed to glutamate. In the presence of hypoxia, subsequent cell death results in release of glutamate.[508] Microglial cells present in the white matter aggravate the process with inflammatory cytokines. Astrocytes attempt to repair the injury and reduce glutamate, however this subsequently leads to cell membrane swelling and cytotoxic edema. Eventually, there is lysis of the cell membrane and increase in water in the extracellular space with loss of blood–brain barrier and vasogenic edema.

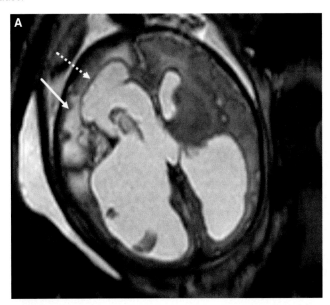
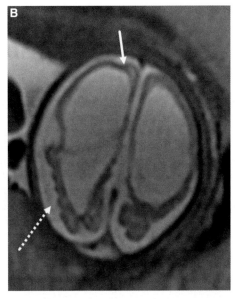

FIGURE 17.1-84: Chronic changes with resolution of hemorrhage and ischemia. **A:** Fetus at 26 weeks with germinal matrix hemorrhage and evolving porencephaly (*dotted arrow*) and cystic encephalomalacia (*solid arrow*). **B:** Fetus at 31 weeks with enlarged ventricles, enlarged subarachnoid spaces (*dotted arrow*), and thin cerebral mantle (*solid arrow*) consistent with volume loss following hypoxic–ischemic injury. Notice nodularity of posterior hemispheres suspicious for polymicrogyria.

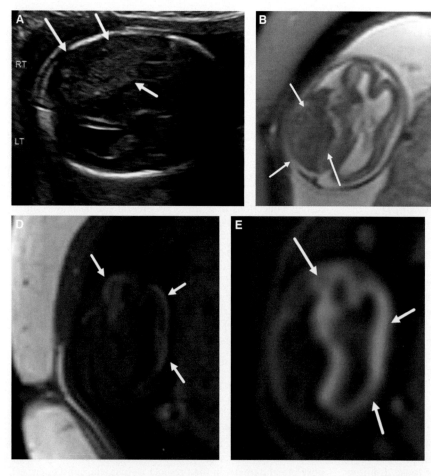

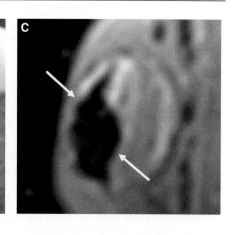

FIGURE 17.1-85: Subdural hemorrhage in a fetus at 20 weeks with congenital cytomegalovirus and maternal preeclampsia. **A:** Axial US demonstrating a heterogeneous hyperechoic collection along the right hemisphere (*arrows*). **B:** Axial MRI demonstrating a T2 hypointense collection (*arrows*) with mass effect on the adjacent brain. **C:** Susceptibility imaging showing intense artifact (*arrows*) consistent with hemorrhage. **D:** T1 axial MRI demonstrating abnormal hyperintense signal in the cortex consistent with laminar necrosis (*arrows*). **E:** Axial diffusion imaging demonstrating restricted diffusion throughout the cerebral hemispheres (*arrows*).

Ischemic infarcts have rarely been noted in the fetus, with most occurring secondary to abnormalities of the MCA or venous thrombosis.[508] This type of injury can be seen in monochorionic twins, placenta emboli, and maternal cocaine abuse.[488]

Ultrasound: Acute white matter injury is more difficult to detect on US but can be suggested in the presence of periventricular echodensities that result in loss of normal brain parenchymal lamination.[509] If followed up over greater than 2 weeks, cystic areas may become apparent in the periventricular white matter.[490] Chronic imaging findings are more likely to be detected, including VM and cystic encephalomalacia.

Magnetic Resonance Imaging: In the fetus, white matter injury is different than postnatal. Some cases show increased T2 and decreased T1 signal in the subcortical white matter rather than increased T1 and decreased T2 in the periventricular area (Fig. 17.1-86).[484] Injury in the white matter will cause loss of normal laminar pattern, especially in the intermediate zone.[483] Sometimes, these lesions are harder to detect on fetal MRI due to lower signal-to-noise ratio and the high-water content of the brain. In general, MRI is more accurate in the detection of small focal lesions than diffuse white matter abnormalities.[407] In some cases, diffusion imaging may be helpful by identifying restricted diffusion, though care should be made to ensure delineation from the normal germinal matrix.[504] In the presence of vasogenic edema and astrogliosis, the ADC value is increased, which may help confirm white matter injury.[508]

Parenchymal ischemic lesions cause edema, which tends to be hypointense T1 and hyperintense on T2, usually with loss of the normal lamination pattern of the brain (Fig. 17.1-87A).[504]

In the presence of acute ischemia, restricted diffusion is noted as high signal on the diffusion image and low on the ADC map (Fig. 17.1-87B).[504] Acute response in the fetal brain is not common, so many of these areas of signal abnormality will not show diffusion restriction.[484] Proton spectroscopy may have a role in the future for evaluation of ischemic lesions, although it is technically more difficult in the fetus and normal fetal lactate levels are not yet standardized.[484,504]

Associated Anomalies: Extracerebral findings may be seen in the presence of hypoxic–ischemic disease. The most common is IUGR.[504] Infection and ischemia may affect the kidneys, liver, and heart. Fetal hydrops may be present. Evaluation of the placenta may yield important clues to the cause of intracranial injury.

Differential Diagnosis: Tumor should be considered in the presence of a heterogeneous echogenic mass, but unlike a hemorrhage, which decreases in size, a tumor will remain stable or grow. Lipomas in association with agenesis of the corpus callosum may mimic hemorrhage. Motion CSF artifact can cause a swirling area of decreased T2 signal in the ventricles also simulating hemorrhage.

In late stages, hemorrhage liquefies and appears cystic. Differential would include cystic lesions such as choroid plexus, glioependymal, or arachnoid cyst and, if in the posterior fossa, malformations of Blake pouch or enlarged cisterna magna.

Prognosis: Neurodevelopmental outcome can range from normal to neurologic deficits, such as seizure, mental retardation, psychomotor delays, and cerebral palsy. Extreme cases may result in fetal or neonatal death.[477] Prognosis is dependent on the

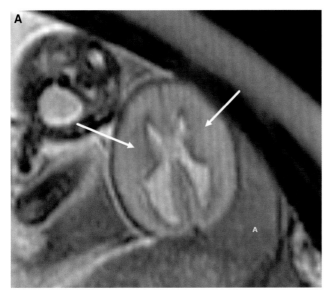
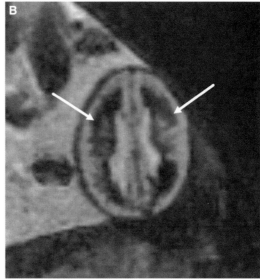

FIGURE 17.1-86: Twin-to-twin transfusion syndrome and donor twin at 21 weeks with white matter injury. **A:** Axial T2 MRI demonstrating abnormal hyperintense T2 signal in the white matter (*arrows*) with loss of the normal five layer lamination pattern. **B:** Axial susceptibility imaging in the same fetus showing artifact (*arrows*) consistent with diffuse hemorrhagic white matter injury.

etiology, associated anomalies, and extent and location of the hemorrhage.[489] In prenatally diagnosed large intracranial hemorrhages, 40% to 55% of fetuses die *in utero* or within the first month of life, though some series have shown survival as high as 87%.[485,486,489] Among survivors, approximately 45% to 50% can be expected to be neurologically normal, although in studies with high survival, this rate decreases to 29%.[485,489]

If a GMH is detected, perinatal mortality and neurological outcome are dependent on the grade of injury.[485,489] Lower grade of GMH and those bleeds that disappear are associated with a better outcome.[477] Grade III–IV hemorrhages are associated with a worse prognosis, with outcome in grade III demise 5% and severe deficit 32%, whereas grade IV demise in 17% and severe impairment in

60%.[477,489] Intrauterine progression of a bleed is associated with a worse neurological outcome.[477] Up to 60% of surviving infants will develop hydrocephalus requiring CSF diversion.[486] Those fetuses with cerebellar GMH are at high risk for impaired motor and cognitive development, especially if the vermis is involved.[502]

IPH in the presence of alloimmune thrombocytopenia represents a high risk of perinatal death (35% to 48%) and severe neurological deficit (80%).[510] Cases of non-GMH have been suggested to have higher intrauterine demise (58%) versus those with GMH (4%).[487]

Subdural hemorrhage may be fatal or may resolve completely without therapy, though some require surgical intervention.[506] Approximately 32% of fetuses with SDH will die *in utero* or during neonatal period, with normal neurological outcome in 58%

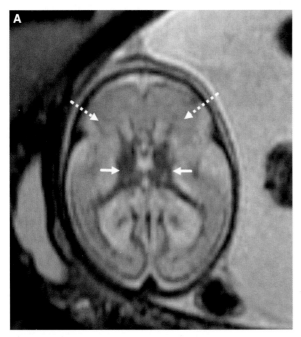
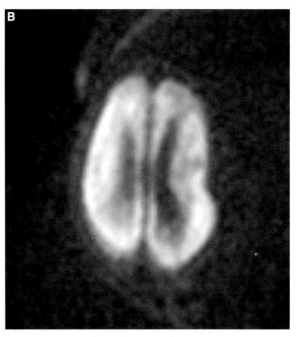

FIGURE 17.1-87: Severe hypoxic–ischemic injury in recipient twin secondary to twin-to-twin transfusion syndrome. **A:** Axial T2 MRI demonstrating abnormal hyperintense signal in the white matter (*dotted arrows*) with loss of normal lamination and the basal ganglia also demonstrated abnormal dark T2 signal (*solid arrows*) similar to ischemic disease in the newborn. **B:** Axial diffusion image showing diffuse hyperintense signal consistent with ischemia.

of the survivors.[479] It is interesting that the 42% with impaired neurological function have often developed SDH without known etiology.[479] Poor prognosis is more likely if the subdural is in the presence of hydrocephalus, cerebral infarction, or cerebral atrophy, leading to microcephaly.[507]

White matter injury may lead to significant neurological deficits, but prognosis is dependent on the extent and persistent area of abnormality.[406] Associated anomalies or genetic syndromes have a more guarded outcome.[477]

Management: Depending on the severity of the lesion, termination or supportive care may be solely provided.[485] In the presence of a subdural collection or large hematoma, close monitoring intrauterine is recommended to check for increase in bleeding, hydrocephalus, or hydrops secondary to fetal anemia. Maternal history of Crohn disease, eating disorder, hyperemesis, or drug usage that may increase risk for vitamin K deficiency should direct testing and supplementation with vitamin K as required.

Laboratory testing for fetal platelet disorder may be considered. Treatment of alloimmune thrombocytopenia is debatable.[485] If the fetus is positive for alloimmune thrombocytopenia, maternal therapy with high-dose intravenous immunoglobulin weekly and oral corticosteroids is typically recommended.[490,492] Although transfusion for thrombocytopenia has previously been primary therapy, recent evidence suggests immunoglobulins with or without steroids may prevent hemorrhage as immune-mediated mechanisms may disrupt angiogenesis and endothelial function.[488] For nonresponders, fetal blood sampling and platelet transfusion may still be necessary; however, these invasive procedures do carry a risk of fetal loss.[492]

The optimum mode of delivery is uncertain and likely case dependent.[485] Elective C-section may be considered in the presence of thrombocytopenia to prevent intracranial hemorrhage during labor and delivery.[492]

Some infants require postnatal surgical evacuation of hematoma.[506] In those children who develop hydrocephalus, ventricular shunting may be required. Neurological consultation is typically advised.

Recurrence: The risk of recurrence is low, being between 3% and 5%.[485] With a history of alloimmune thrombocytopenia, the recurrence risk is 75% to 100%, with increased severity of symptoms with sequential pregnancies.[490,507] Genetic disorders such as COL4A1 and GATA1 can have increased risk of recurrence.

DISORDERS OF CHOROID, LEPTOMENINGEAL, NEUROEPITHELIAL, AND VASCULAR DIFFERENTIATION

Choroid Plexus Cyst

Incidence: Choroid plexus cysts (CPCs) occur in about 0.18% to 3.6% of routine midgestation USs.[511,512]

Pathogenesis/Etiology: The choroid plexus first appears as a lobulated protrusion of ependymal epithelium, accompanied by mesenchyme and pia mater in the sixth week of gestation. In the eighth week, the choroid plexus becomes wavy because of formation of capillary loops, and in the ninth week, the choroid produces CSF.[513] Loose mesenchyme stroma, scattered islets of

nucleated blood cells, and poorly defined vascular walls become accentuated by spaces and cysts from 9 to 16 weeks. From 17 to 28 weeks, the loose mesenchymal stroma decreases with increase in connective tissue fibers and fully formed vascular walls. After 29 weeks, the choroid plexus contains a mature vascular stroma.

The CPC is actually a pseudocyst with a wall of interconnecting angiomatous irregular capillaries.[513] CPCs are believed to occur in the mesenchymal stroma when CSF is entrapped between the intervillous clefts, hypothesized to develop when there is failure in transformation of the lobulated embryonal capillaries into the wavy fetal pattern.[513] Most cysts form from 13 to 18 weeks when the choroid plexus proliferates. The cysts then regress by week 28 when proliferation of vascular walls and reduction in mesenchymal stroma occur. Approximately 95% of CPCs disappear by 26 and 28 weeks' gestation, usually within 2 months of time of diagnosis.[514,515]

Diagnosis

Ultrasound: The glomus, a focal thickened bulge along the posterior choroid, develops after 13 weeks and is the most common site for a CPC.[514] A CPC is an echolucent, well-circumscribed structure surrounded by echogenic choroid plexus (Fig. 17.1-88A). A true CPC can be diagnosed when the cyst measures 2.5 mm before 22 weeks and at least 2 mm thereafter.[516] CPCs may be multiple or bilateral, can contain septations, and protrude into the ventricle (Fig. 17.1-88B). Approximately 86% are detected in the second trimester in isolation as an incidental finding.[517] However, when a CPC is identified, a careful anatomical survey with attention to heart, brain, and hands should be performed.[518]

Magnetic Resonance Imaging: In the presence of the typical subcentimeter lesion, MRI provides no added advantage, and in fact, most CPCs are not well visualized by MRI. With larger lesions, especially in the presence of complicating factors such as ventriculomegaly, MRI can confirm diagnosis of CPC by defining a CSF signal lesion within choroid, evaluating mass effect, and excluding other differentials.[519] In a high-risk pregnancy with CPC or in the presence of multiple other anomalies, MRI is often performed to confirm and define other abnormalities, which may support the presence of a genetic syndrome.

Associated Anomalies: About 1% of infants with isolated CPCs will have an underlying chromosomal abnormality, the most common being trisomy 18 followed by trisomy 21.[517] Others have suggested that CPCs may also be associated with congenital heart disease and hydronephrosis.[520]

Differential Diagnosis: Before 22 weeks, the choroid plexus is heterogeneous, and small anechoic areas measuring <2 mm can mimic a cyst.[516] Partial volume averaging of the striatum and choroid with mild ventriculomegaly may falsely suggest CPC.[516] Choroid plexus papillomas are differentiated by solid nature and color Doppler flow. Subacute intraventricular clot adherent to choroid plexus may be difficult to discern from CPC in the absence of other findings. Other intraventricular cysts in the differential include colloid, glioependymal, or neuroepithelial cysts, which demonstrate a true epithelial wall.

Prognosis: Most CPCs are incidental and isolated without progression after birth.[519] Studies have shown that fetuses with isolated CPC and normal karyotype have normal neurocognitive development postnatal.[511,521] In general, if the cyst is isolated, the

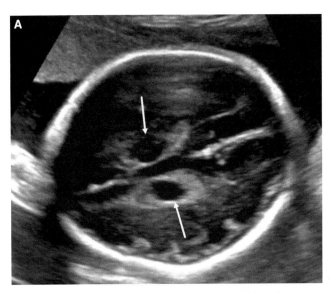
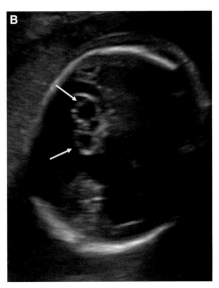

FIGURE 17.1-88: Choroid plexus cyst. **A:** Axial US of bilateral cysts (*arrows*) in the choroid of the lateral ventricles in an otherwise normal fetus. **B:** Axial US demonstrating multiple complex choroid cysts (*arrows*) in a fetus with suspected Aicardi.

risk for aneuploidy is low at 0.9% to 6.7%; therefore, other factors such as baseline risk should be considered.[517,522,523]

However, in approximately 14% of cases, additional anomalies are noted, which raises the risk to as high as 48% for aneuploidy.[517,518] The possibility for aneuploidy in the presence of bilateral and complex CPCs is controversial; therefore, targeted scan for other markers should be performed.[522,524] A large CPC in excess of 10 mm has been suggested to increase risk.[522]

In the presence of a large CPC, space-occupying effects can cause obstructive hydrocephalus and/or injury to adjacent tissue that may manifest postnatal as focal neurological deficits or seizure.[519]

Management: Perinatal surveillance is warranted. Counseling is indicated as increased parental anxiety often occurs.[511] In the presence of CPC and associated anomalies, advanced maternal age, abnormal triple screen analysis, or cell-free DNA, most recommend genetic counseling with amniocentesis or chorionic villus sampling as risk for aneuploidy is 1:3.[516–518,525] Although controversial, most concur that testing should not be performed in the presence of an isolated CPC as the likelihood of trisomy 18 is low.[523,526] Postnatally, nearly all CPCs resolve, and no further therapy is required. Persistence of a large cyst is extremely rare but could require neurosurgical decompression with fenestration or shunt if size causes obstruction of the ventricular system.[519]

Recurrence: Most CPCs are incidental and sporadic.

Arachnoid Cysts

Incidence: Arachnoid cysts (ACs) represent 1% of all intracranial masses in newborns.[527]

Pathogenesis/Etiology: ACs are related to abnormal development of the leptomeninges. The outer layer represents the arachnoid web and inner layer pia, with the intervening space filled by fine trabeculae. The most accepted theory for development of an AC is that early first trimester, at the time of evolution of the meninges, there is an abnormal localized splitting of cell layers in the area between the arachnoid and the pia, allowing for distension of a potential space with CSF. The wall of the AC is usually composed of a thick layer of collagen and hyperplastic arachnoid cells; however, suprasellar cysts may also contain neuroglial elements.[528]

The congenital AC does not typically communicate with the subarachnoid space, whereas a secondary or acquired AC, which develops because of CSF entrapment within arachnoid adhesions following *in utero* hemorrhage, infection, or trauma, is usually patent with the subarachnoid space. Some cysts enlarge, and this is hypothesized to be due to active secretion of CSF from the cyst membrane, osmotic gradients caused by higher protein in the cyst fluid, or cyst communicating with the subarachnoid space via ball-valve mechanism.[528]

Intracranial ACs vary in size and location. In the fetus, the majority of ACs are supratentorial (63%), followed by infratentorial (22%), and finally along the incisura (15%).[527,529] Although, in children, most supratentorial ACs are located in the Sylvian fissure or middle cranial fossa, in the fetus, the most common location is interhemispheric, followed by skull base, suprasellar, and hemispheric.[527–530]

Diagnosis

Ultrasound: Most cysts are diagnosed in the second or third trimester, rarely before a GA of 20 weeks.[527,530,531] ACs are present in the extra-axial fluid space and are unilocular and uniformly sonolucent (Fig. 17.1-89A). An AC will have thin regular walls and posterior acoustic enhancement. The lesion should be devoid of blood flow on color Doppler. Septation within the cyst is possible. A thorough search for additional anomalies with special attention to the corpus callosum is indicated.[530,532] The ventricles and cerebral parenchyma should be assessed for enlargement and mass effect, respectively.[527] Approximately 20% to 25% of cysts can cause ventriculomegaly with risk for hydrocephalus.[531] 3D US may be helpful to define the nature of the cyst.[532] US has an accuracy of greater than 85% in detection of ACs.[531]

Magnetic Resonance Imaging: MRI is helpful in confirming diagnosis by identifying the extra-axial location and CSF signal intensity (Fig. 17.1-89B) and in excluding associated anomalies. MRI can also define the extent of the cyst, compression of adjacent structures, communication with the ventricle, and other associated anomalies, especially of the corpus callosum.[529,533] The technique is helpful in excluding other intracranial cysts that may mimic an AC. In a recent study, MRI changed the US diagnosis of AC to other anomalies in 8% of cases.[531]

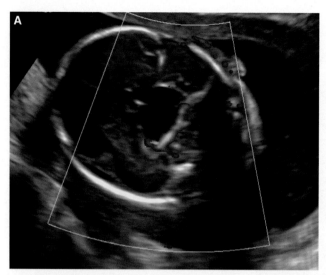
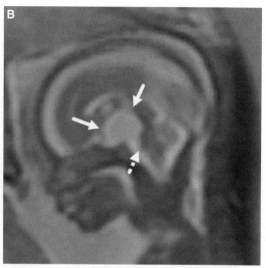

FIGURE 17.1-89: Suprasellar arachnoid cyst in a fetus at 21 weeks. **A:** Axial Color Doppler US demonstrating a sonolucent lesion posterior to the frontal lobes with absence of internal color flow. **B:** Sagittal MRI in the same fetus demonstrating a suprasellar cystic lesion (*solid arrows*) with thin peripheral wall. There is mass effect on the adjacent pons (*dotted arrow*). The cyst continued to grow, and postnatal, the child had fenestration of the cyst with good outcome.

Associated Anomalies: ACs are commonly isolated but can be seen with chromosomal abnormalities in approximately 6% of cases, usually in the presence of additional anomalies.[527,534] Common associated findings include ventriculomegaly and, in the presence of interhemispheric cyst, abnormalities of the corpus callosum.[534] Syndromes such as Aicardi and Chudley–McCullough should be considered. Prenatal suprasellar cysts have been seen in association with hypothalamic hamartomas, representing ectopic benign neural tissue that image as a gray matter mass along the floor of the third ventricle.[535] Sometimes, ACs are noted in the presence of metabolic diseases such as glutaric aciduria Type 1.[532]

Differential Diagnosis: Other "cystic" lesions that should be included in the differential are porencephaly, schizencephaly, cystic neoplasms, subacute intracranial hemorrhage, choroid plexus cyst, and vein of Galen anomalies. In the presence of porencephaly, the lesion typically communicates with the ventricle, and in schizencephaly, clefts are lined by gray matter. In both, volume loss, not mass effect, should be present. Cystic neoplasms typically have associated solid tissue. Vein of Galen is documented in the presence of color flow on Doppler. Enlargement of the Sylvian fissures in glutaric aciduria may mimic bilateral ACs. Lesions that may be difficult to separate from AC include glioependymal, neuroepithelial, or colloid cysts (usually in third ventricle).

Enlargement of the septum pellucidum and vergae may mimic an interhemispheric cyst. A prominent cavum velum interpositum is a developmental variant that appears midline as a triangular CSF space below the splenium of the corpus callous, dorsal to the tectum, and bound laterally by the internal cerebral veins.[536] These cysts are benign, will regress in nearly 25%, and have negligible adverse neurodevelopmental outcome.[534]

Differential for cysts in the posterior fossa includes mega cisterna magna, Blake pouch cyst, malformations with retrocerebellar cyst, and dural venous malformations.

Prognosis: Prognosis is dependent on the presence of other malformations, the rate of cyst growth, and the progression of ventriculomegaly.[531] Early age at diagnosis, growth of the cyst *in utero*, and a size of more than 15 mm are unfavorable factors.[537]

In general, fetal/neonatal ACs have a higher risk for growth than the adult population. Cysts increase in volume in 20% to 28% of fetuses and children; however, cyst volume and location do not necessarily determine clinical outcome, with some large lesions being asymptomatic.[527,529,534] Hydrocephalus has been shown to occur in approximately 17% to 25%.[529,530,534] Hydrocephalus is more likely to occur with midline ACs, including interhemispheric, incisural (quadrigeminal), or suprasellar cysts, which obstruct the aqueduct or third ventricle.[529] Suprasellar ACs also have an increased risk for visual disturbances and pituitary dysfunction.[538]

Approximately 28% to 35% (or higher) of ACs will require postnatal intervention either because of hydrocephalus or due to symptoms from mass effect.[529,534,538] There is a slightly higher risk for subdural hematoma with head trauma, which is thought to be due to tearing of vulnerable bridging veins by the lesions.[538] Overall, though, an AC without associated chromosomal or structural anomaly has a favorable outcome. Normal behavior, neurological development, and intelligence are noted in 80% to 88% of cases.[529,531]

Management: Serial prenatal US should be performed to assess for cyst growth and/or hydrocephalus.[527] Close postnatal imaging is indicated due to higher risk for enlarging cyst and secondary complications. In the presence of symptoms from significant mass effect and/or hydrocephalus, favored therapy is endoscopic cyst fenestration either cystoventriculostomy or cystocisternostomy.[527,528] Most do not support shunting of the cyst due to higher risk for secondary complications, including CSF overdrainage.[538]

Recurrence: Most are isolated without risk for recurrence.

Cyst of Septum Pellucidum

Incidence: Cysts of the cavum septum pellucidum (CSP) are rare, with an incidence of 0.04%.[539]

Pathogenesis/Etiology: The septum pellucidum is related to the development of the commissures, with the leaflets containing glial, neuronal, and ependymal cells. The space between the leaflets, or the cavum, does not communicate with the ventricles. In 85% of cases, the CSP will disappear in the first 3 to 6 months after birth; however, a persistent normal CSP is noted in 15% to 20% of children and adults.[539]

Abnormal dilatation of the CSP has been attributed to a one-way valve mechanism allowing CSF flow into the cavum.[540] CSP cysts have been associated with hemorrhage or inflammation from trauma or infection and have been hypothesized to be a sign of cerebral dysgenesis. However, it is less likely that fluid secreted by migrated ependymal cells within the septal leaflets result in this pathology.[540,541] Cysts of the CSP tend to be more common in males and are typically associated with a cavum vergae cyst.[542] Increase in intracranial pressure may develop because of obstruction of the interventricular foramina, and the cyst can compress adjacent structures such as the hypothalamus, septal nuclei, and subependymal and internal cerebral veins.[539]

Ultrasound: A CSP greater than 1 cm in width is considered abnormal at any gestational age.[543,544] Most cysts of the septum pellucidum range in width from 2 to 5 cm, cause lateral bowing of the septal leaflets with collapse of the frontal horns, and extend posteriorly into vergae, to the splenium of the corpus callosum.[545] US will show a dilated CSF cavity, measuring greater than 1 cm, above the thalami and anterior to the third ventricle in the anatomical location of the septum pellucidum (Fig. 17.1-90A).[546]

Magnetic Resonance Imaging: A CSP cyst appears as a CSF signal space greater than 10 mm between the lateral ventricles with different degrees of bowing of the cyst wall, sometimes collapsing the frontal horns (Fig. 17.1-90B).[543] The lateral ventricles appear more parallel, and VM may occur owing to obstruction of the foramen of Monroe.[539,543]

Associated Anomalies: Cysts of the CSP are typically not associated with intracranial anomalies other than ventriculomegaly.[547]

Differential Diagnosis: Differential for a cyst of the CSP includes a large third ventricle; vein of Galen malformation; interhemispheric cyst; epidermoid, arachnoid, or neuroglial cyst; and an enlarged cavum velum interpositum. A predominately cystic tumor could also mimic a CSP cyst.

Prognosis: Asymptomatic cysts of the CSP are assumed to communicate with the subarachnoid space, while symptomatic are noncommunicating.[542] Some cysts will resolve spontaneously due to rupture into the lateral or third ventricles.[539,547] Symptomatic CSP cysts can cause partial obstruction of the intraventricular foramina and venous congestion, resulting in intracranial hypertension; clinical signs including headaches, nausea, and vomiting; and also sudden collapse with loss of consciousness.[542] Hydrocephalus occurs in up to 32%, more likely under 5 years of age.[539] Compression of optic pathway may lead to visual symptoms, and mass effect on the hypothalamoseptal area may cause bizarre behavior, memory loss, disturbed sleep, eating disorder, hypothermia, and developmental delay, more common in children than adults.[542] Children with CSP cysts have focal deficit in 23%, seizures in 10%, and mental status changes in 42%.[539]

Management: Serial prenatal US should be performed when the cavum measures larger than 10mm to assess for increase in size of the cyst and ventricles. Symptoms may not be clear, but treatment is usually considered when there is ventricular

obstruction or significant clinical signs related to compression of adjacent structures.[539] Neuroendoscopic cyst fenestration is therapy of choice because of high success and low complication rate.[539,542]

Recurrence: Most are isolated without risk for recurrence.

Glioependymal/Neuroglial Cyst (Choroidal, Epithelial, Ependymal)

Incidence: Glioependymal cysts (GECs) are uncommon, representing fewer than 1% of all intracranial cysts.[548]

Pathogenesis/Etiology: The ventricle is lined with ependyma, but in some areas, the ependyma is covered by the tela choroidea, an area with invaginated pial vessels that will form the choroid plexus. It is favored that GECs originate from the wall of the neural tube with tela choroidea or in displaced intraparenchymal tissue for unknown reason. On histology, the GEC typically demonstrates an inner ependymal layer, middle glial, and outer connective tissue.[549] The wall of the cyst is always lined with neuroglial cells, but the complexing terminology is based on histology, reflecting variable neural, glial, ependymal, and choroidal cells. These cysts can be identified anywhere in the neuroaxis, usually over the cerebral hemisphere but also intraparenchymal and intraventricular.[549,550] In the fetus, most case reports describe the cyst in the interhemispheric fissure, often in conjunction with agenesis of the corpus callosum.[550-553] GECs have been seen in association with ischemic or hemorrhagic insults.[552] Progressive growth of the cysts can occur, likely due to secretory activity of ependymal cells.[549]

Diagnosis
Ultrasound: GECs are sonolucent but may be septated or multilocular (Fig. 17.1-91A).[551] The lesion can cause mass effect and, when interhemispheric, is usually associated with agenesis of the corpus callosum. Additional anomalies should be excluded.

Magnetic Resonance Imaging: The cystic lesion is often similar to CSF but can be slightly hyperintense to CSF on T1 imaging and hypointense on T2 imaging owing to high-protein content.[550,552] The lesion may be unilocular, multilocular, or septated (Fig. 17.1-91B). Since these lesions can occur intra-axial or extra-axial, the GEC may or may not communicate with the ventricular system.[551] MRI allows for depiction of anatomy of the lesion, mass effect, and exclusion of associated anomalies.

Associated Anomalies: When present with agenesis of the corpus callosum, other anomalies including heterotopic gray matter, cerebellar hypoplasia, and polymicrogyria should be excluded.[550] When present in the posterior fossa, GEC can cause obstructive hydrocephalus.[554]

Differential Diagnosis: GEC can only be differentiated from an arachnoid cyst and choroid plexus cyst by histology. Dorsal cysts in holoprosencephaly, porencephaly, hydranencephaly, cystic encephalomalacia, dermoids, epidermoids, and other cystic tumors should be considered.

Prognosis: There is a good prognosis for an isolated appropriately treated GEC.[551,552] A more guarded prognosis may be seen in the presence of associated anomalies.[552]

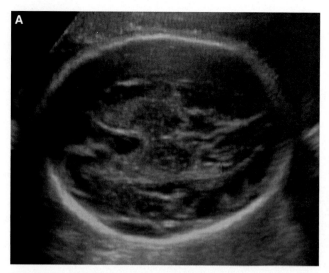
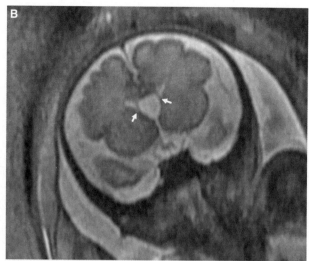

FIGURE 17.1-90: Fetus referred at 31 weeks due to concern for agenesis of corpus callosum but found to have cyst of the septum pellucidum. **A:** Axial US showing a prominent cavum septum pellucidum that measured 11 mm. **B:** Coronal MRI in the same fetus demonstrating enlarged cavum with lateral bowing of the septal leaflets (*arrows*).

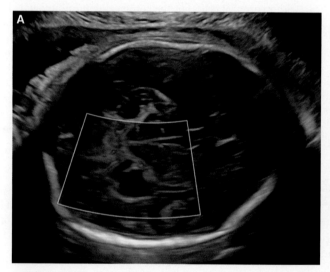
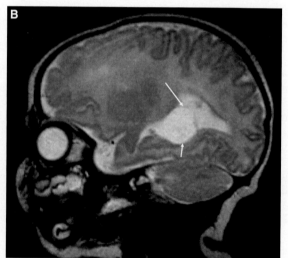

FIGURE 17.1-91: Neuroglial cyst in fetus at 34 weeks. **A:** Axial color Doppler US demonstrating avascular lobular cystic area adjacent to the temporal horn. **B:** Postnatal Sagittal MRI showing lobulated T2 hyperintense lesion (*arrow*) along the wall of the temporal horn.

Management: Ideal treatment for a GEC will depend on cyst location.[549] As the cyst not uncommonly recurs due to cellular components in the wall that produce CSF, complete resection is favored.[552,553] Other therapies include fenestration, shunting, and partial resection.[549]

Recurrence: There is no known increased risk for recurrence.

VASCULAR ANOMALIES

Arteriovenous Malformations/Vein of Galen

Incidence: Most arteriovenous malformations (AVMs) in the fetus are vein of Galen malformations (VGMs), representing less than 1% of intracranial AVMs but 30% of all pediatric vascular malformations.[555,556]

Pathogenesis: Early in embryology, a primitive sinusoidal vascular network is present with direct connections between the arteries and the veins. If there is error in normal differentiation of these vascular

connections, the arteries and veins remain in direct communication, resulting in an AVM. As AVMs have no intervening capillaries between the artery and the vein, high-flow AV shunting develops that can secondarily result in cardiac failure and brain injury.

A "vein of Galen malformation" is a misnomer as the defect is not truly of the vein of Galen. In VGMs, there is a persistent communication of the primitive choroidal arterial system and the *median prosencephalic vein of Markowski*.[555] During the fifth week, choroidal and quadrigeminal arteries develop. On the roof of the diencephalon, between 6 and 11 weeks, the lateral choroid plexus expands and is drained via choroidal veins into a central primitive vein known as the median prosencephalic vein. In the 12th week, the vein regresses, with a dorsal remnant persisting as the vein of Galen. The straight sinus, developing from fusion of multiple small tentorial veins, appears on the 50th day and drains the lateral choroid plexus.

A VGM is hypothesized to occur due to lack of involution of the prosencephalic vein because of early occlusion or lack of formation of the straight sinus or in the presence of continuous elevated blood flow through persistent abnormal communications between the choroidal arteries and the median prosencephalic vein. Mutations in genetic pathways are recently being found to also have an impact on development of this malformation.

Not surprisingly, choroidal arteries, especially the posterior choroidal, are the most common arterial feeders in VGM.[557] This is followed by subependymal perforators of the posterior cerebral arteries and thalamoperforators.[558] Often, branches of the pericallosal artery, vessels arising from the anterior cerebral and an important supply for the choroid plexus in the third ventricle, also supply the VGM.[557] In approximately half of neonates, a persistent limbic arterial arch, which connects the cortical branches of the anterior choroidal artery with the posterior cerebral artery via the pericallosal artery, is noted.[559] Supply from the middle cerebral artery is uncommon. Transmesencephalic branches directly from the basilar artery can supply an AVM; however, in their presence, the AVM is not a true VGM but rather indicative of a tectal not choroidal malformation.[558]

In a VGM, the median prosencephalic vein is arterialized, thick walled, and dilated due to high turbulent flow from either direct or indirect AV connections. The abnormal angioarchitecture of the VGM prevents normal development of the intracranial venous drainage, resulting in persistence of other embryological venous sinuses, most commonly the occipital, marginal and falcine sinus, which extends from the vein of Galen to the sagittal sinus and ascends in the falx cerebri. In over half of cases, the straight sinus is absent or thrombosed, and sometimes there is lack of continuity of the VGM with the deep cerebral veins. Maturation of the jugular bulbs occurs perinatal and postnatal, and in the presence of a VGM, the maturation process, which includes remodeling of torcula, regression of occipital and marginal sinus, and development of jugular bulbs, may not occur.[558] Occlusions and stenosis of the venous channels can evolve, especially the jugular bulbs and sigmoid sinuses, which can improve cardiac function by decreasing overload but at the expense of increase in venous pressure.[558] Anterior venous collateral drainage

through the petrous, cavernous, thalamic, lateral mesencephalic, facial, and ophthalmic veins may develop.

Potential complications of VGM include heart failure, hydrocephalus, and brain injury. In the presence of an AVM, increased blood to the heart results in progressive heart failure, which, when severe, will cause fetal hydrops. As the pacchionian granulations do not function until after the first few months of life, CSF must be absorbed at least partly by medullary veins. Because of the AV shunt and particularly if stenosis of veins develop, venous hypertension increases, which then causes CSF malabsorption, leading to communicating hydrocephalus.[558] Obstructive hydrocephalus may also develop due to compression of the aqueduct via mass effect from the VGM.

Cerebral maturation is dependent on normal blood flow and a normal venous system. Intracranial venous hypertension likely in conjunction with cerebrovascular steal in the presence of cardiac dysfunction results in brain injury, which is typically manifested as subcortical white matter calcification, white matter lesions, and diffuse brain destruction (melting brain), especially with subependymal atrophy (occipital) and ex vacuo ventricular dilatation.[558]

VGMs are usually classified by fistula angioarchitecture. The *choroidal type* is a primitive shunt in the velum interpositum with multiple bilateral feeding arteries that converge on the anterior wall of prosencephalic vein (Fig. 17.1-92).[557,558] The most common feeding arteries are the choroidal, pericallosal, and thalamoperforators. This type of VGM leads to a more severe pathology, presenting earlier in life, often with cardiac failure. The *mural type* is better tolerated and is defined by a single or few feeding arteries, typically collicular and posterior choroidal, that insert laterally into the wall of the dilated vein. Sometimes, the malformation may be a combination of both types.

Etiology: VGMs are sporadic and rare, which has limited genetic understanding. However, recent studies have shown that

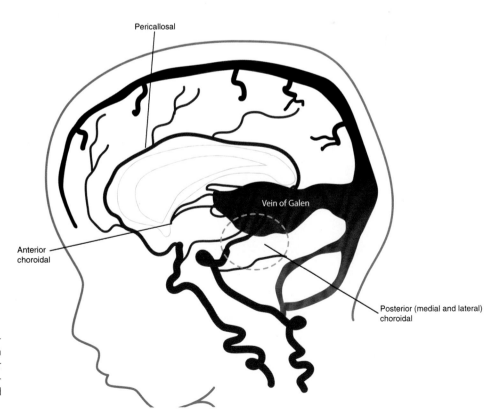

FIGURE 17.1-92: Diagram of choroidal type vein of Galen malformation with feeding vessels from the anterior choroidal, posterior choroidal, and pericallosal vessels forming the so-called limbic arterial arch.

Pericallosal

Vein of Galen

Anterior choroidal

Posterior (medial and lateral) choroidal

genomics play a role in development of this vascular malformation, with 30% of VGM cases due to mutations in the chromatin modifier and Ephrin genes.[560] The chromatin modifier genes (*KMT2D, SMARCA2, SIRT1,* and *KAT6A*) are essential for neuronal and vascular development and have been described in 8% of cases of VGM.[560,561] Ephrin signaling genes, including *EPHRINB2* and *EPHB4,* are responsible for approximately 16% of inherited VGM. *EPHB4,* in 7% of VGM patients, is a bona fide risk gene for VGM, given that it directly disrupts the vein of Galen precursor.[560,561] *RASA1* works downstream with *EPHB4* to ensure normal vascular development and is also implicated in VGMs. The *RASA1* gene mutation is also a cause for capillary malformations and other AVMs, which have been recently noted in patients with VGMs.[560,561] Given the inherited variability and incomplete penetrance and expression, it is likely that there is a two-hit mechanism at work, where phenotypic expression relies on an inherited mutation and also a mutation in other alleles.[560] Variability may also depend on environmental modifiers that are yet unknown.[560]

Diagnosis

Ultrasound: VGMs are typically identified in the third trimester, less frequently in the second trimester.[562] Diagnosis relies on visualization of a hypoechogenic, less likely heterogeneous lesion with central color Doppler in the midline posterior recess of the third ventricle (Fig. 17.1-93A, B).[555] Doppler will demonstrate bidirectional turbulent flow with very pulsatile "arterialized" veins and high diastolic arterial waveforms (Fig. 17.1-94A, B).[563] If only normal venous Doppler is obtained in the VGM, the dilatation may be related to varicosity or other type of AVM. The sagittal sinus or persistent falcine sinus is often dilated.[563] On 2D US, it can sometimes be difficult to precisely identify the feeders or exclude a parenchymal AVM that drains via the vein of Galen.[556] However, power Doppler, especially with 3D reconstruction, can provide very detailed anatomy of the complex angioarchitecture, allowing for depiction of the feeding arteries and venous anatomy (Fig. 17.1-95A, B).[563–565] Limitations of 3D include poor resolution and difficulty in differentiating veins from arteries.[564]

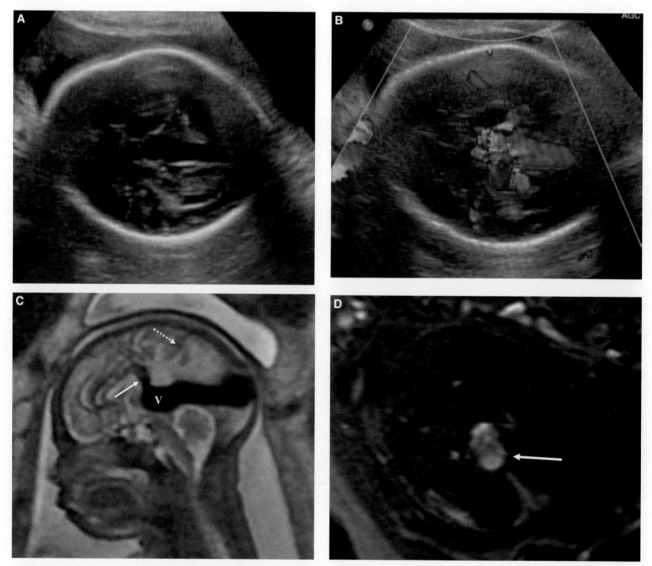

FIGURE 17.1-93: Fetus at 33 weeks with vein of Galen malformation. **A:** Axial US demonstrating a tubular hypoechoic lesion posterior to the third ventricle. **B:** With color, the tubular area demonstrates flow. There is a tangle of vessels and turbulent flow along the anterior aspect of the vein. **C:** Sagittal T2 MRI demonstrating the feeding vessels from the pericallosal artery (*solid arrow*) into *persistent prosencephalic vein (V)*. There is partial visualization of a persistent falcine sinus (*dotted arrow*). The brain was normal in this fetus. **D:** Axial two-dimensional magnetic resonance angiography demonstrating large prosencephalic vein (*arrow*) and small feeding vessels anteriorly.

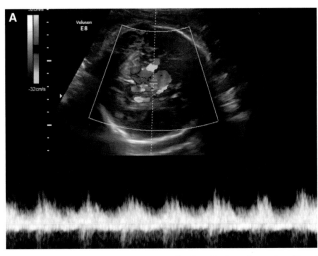
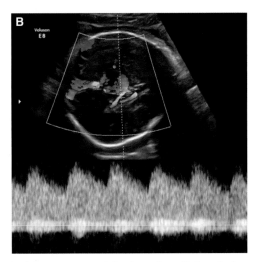

FIGURE 17.1-94: Doppler in a vein of Galen. **A:** Doppler in the dilated vein demonstrates arterialized waveform. **B:** Doppler in a feeding artery shows high diastolic flow.

Since brain injury is a known complication, close evaluation for calcification, hemorrhage, abnormal parenchymal echogenicity, volume loss, and ventriculomegaly should be performed (Fig. 17.1-96A).[566] Clues to heart failure include cardiomegaly, tricuspid valve insufficiency, dilated inferior vena cava, retrograde aortic diastolic flow, and tachycardia (>200 bpm).[558,566] Enlarged neck vessels, especially the jugular veins, are pathognomonic and can be seen in approximately one-third of cases (Fig. 17.1-96B).[562,566] Elevated cardiac output may be measured and has been suggested to correlate with the magnitude of AV shunt.[567] Polyhydramnios, pericardial and pleural effusion, edema, and ascites consistent with hydrops carry a poor prognosis, reflecting intractable high flow.[555,566]

Magnetic Resonance Imaging: Fetal MRI can aid in confirmation of a VGM and help exclude other AV anomalies or intracranial lesions that can mimic a VGM (Figs. 17.1-93C and 17.1-95C). MRI can identify flow void in pathological vessels and

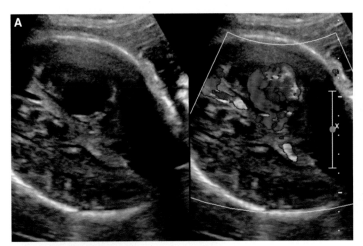
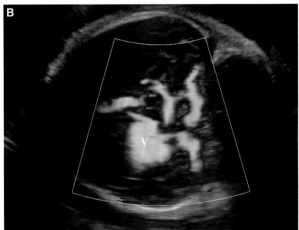
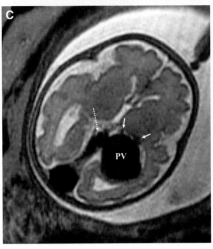

FIGURE 17.1-95: Fetus at 33 weeks with arteriovenous fistula. **A:** Axial US and color Doppler shows a round hypoechoic lesion in the left choroidal fissure that demonstrates turbulent color flow. **B:** Power Doppler of the same fetus demonstrating the feeding arteries extending to the large choroidal fissure vein *(V)*. **C:** Axial MRI showing multiple feeding arteries *(sold arrows)* extending to a large perimesencephalic dilated vein *(PV)*. The vein of Galen is mildly dilated, acting as secondary drainage *(dotted arrow)*. No brain injury was identified.

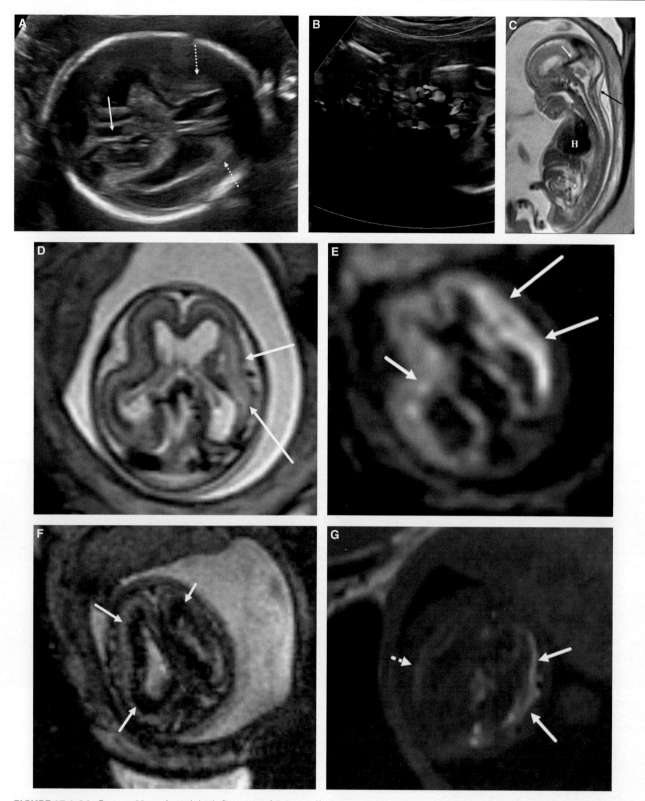

FIGURE 17.1-96: Fetus at 22 weeks with high-flow vein of Galen malformation. **A:** Axial US demonstrating VGM (*solid arrow*) and dilatation of lateral ventricles concerning for parenchymal volume loss. The brain parenchyma is increased in echogenicity (*dotted arrows*), also suggesting injury. **B:** Coronal color Doppler demonstrating enlarged jugular veins supporting high-grade arteriovenous (AV) shunting. **C:** Sagittal MRI of the fetus showing large prosencephalic vein (*white arrow*) draining to falcine sinus. The heart (*H*) is large, and nuchal soft-tissue edema (*black arrow*) is present. **D:** Axial T2 showing loss of normal lamination and hyperintense T2 signal (*arrows*) in the left hemisphere. **E:** Axial diffusion showing restricted diffusion in the left hemisphere and, to lesser extent, right hemisphere (*arrows*). **F:** Axial susceptibility imaging showing abnormal pronounced dark signal *(arrows)* along the ventricles, consistent with hemorrhage and/or calcification. **G:** Axial T1 image of similar level showing abnormal hyperintense signal along the left hemisphere (*solid arrows*) consistent with calcification/laminar necrosis. Subtle abnormal signal is seen the right hemisphere *(dotted arrows).*

can verify the size of the AVM, which may demonstrate flow void or heterogeneous signal due to turbulence.[568] Magnetic resonance angiography, especially 2D time of flight (TOF), which is shorter in scan time than 3D TOF, may be helpful in defining the vascular anatomy of the malformation (Fig. 17.1-93D).[569]

However, MRI is mostly valued in its ability to detect brain injury, important for counseling and directed therapy. MRI is superior at evaluating for cerebral injury, which may manifest as ventriculomegaly, polymicrogyria, cortical thickening, porencephaly, schizencephaly, periventricular injury, and intraparenchymal edema or hemorrhage (Fig. 17.1-96C, D).[555,570] Diffusion imaging may provide information about acute ischemia (Fig. 17.1-96E). T1 and echo planar imaging (EPI) or susceptibility-weighted imaging are important to exclude acute hemorrhage and/or calcification (Fig. 17.1-96F, G).

Associated Anomalies: VGMs are not associated with chromosomal anomalies. However, in families with VGM, 68% have cutaneous capillary malformations or other vascular lesions.[560] Autosomal dominant syndromes such as capillary malformation—AVM types 1 and 2 and hereditary hemorrhagic telangiectasia types 1 and 2—have been associated with VGMs.[560]

Differential Diagnosis: Although the majority of AVMs in the fetus are VGMs, also described antenatally are dural sinus malformations (DSMs) and pial arteriovenous fistulas (AVFs). DSMs are rare, more common in males, and represent persistence of an embryonic sinus with or without AV shunt in the wall of a dural lake (see section "Dural Venous Malformation").[571,572] Pial AVFs are typically supratentorial with peripheral pial or cortical feeding arteries draining into an ectatic vein. The pial AVFs may secondarily dilate the vein of Galen. Both DSMs and pial AVFs can result in high-output cardiomegaly and brain injury.[571–573]

Varicose dilatation of the vein of Galen may occur in the absence of AVM. This type of enlargement is associated with heart disease or vascular anomalies that cause venous hypertension.[555] The falcine sinus can be a normal variant or be seen in the presence of an atretic encephalocele. Other differentials for avascular masses include arachnoid cyst, glioependymal cyst, porencephaly, choroid plexus cyst or intracranial hematoma. Masses that are vascular without a nidus include choroid plexus papilloma, pineal tumor, and hemangioma.

Prognosis: Fetuses with prenatal diagnosis of VGM and cardiac failure, hydrops, or cerebral injury have a poor outcome.[555,558] These fetuses at birth typically suffer from severe irreversible multiorgan failure.[558] The number and size of the arterial feeders and the size of the draining vein reflect the severity of shunt and have implications for outcome.[555,566] Those with isolated VGM and mural type have a more favorable prognosis.

Utilizing US variables, a VGM grayscale 3D rendered volume (craniocaudal, laterolateral, and anteroposterior dimensions of the VGM using ellipsoid formula) of the dilated vein $\geq$ 20,000 mm^3 and tricuspid regurgitation are predictors of poor outcome.[556] Progression in brain lesions is possible over the weeks prior to delivery in greater than 10% of cases, especially in the presence of tricuspid regurgitation and a VGM 3D volume of greater than 40,000 mm^3.[556]

In cases with prenatal diagnosis, overall mortality of VGM has been reported at 22% to 25%, with normal neurological outcome in 67%.[557,574] However, another review suggested a much higher perinatal death rate of 54%.[555] In this study, 32% of prenatally diagnosed VGM were alive and well, whereas 14% were alive with mental retardation. Without embolization, mortality in

VGM is as high as 90%. With embolization, 82% of patients are cured, with outcomes recorded at 5% to 10% demise, 20% to 26% moderate-to-severe disability, and 66% to 74% neurologically and developmentally intact.[558,575]

Management: Rarely, mirror syndrome can develop; therefore, close fetal and maternal monitoring is warranted.[576] In the future, in the presence of known mutation in the *ephrinB2-EphB4-RAS1*, fetuses may be treated with drugs such as rapamycin, which are chemical inhibitors of the PI3K-TORC1 pathway. In the presence of Ephrin gene *RAS* mutations, the mTOR pathway activity is increased, and animal models treated with inhibitors have shown promise in reversing cerebrovascular mutation effects.[560,561] As patient selection for therapy is usually dependent on the severity of heart failure and degree of brain injury, counseling with this knowledge may include discussion of termination or comfort care at birth.[557,558]

Antenatal diagnosis is usually not an indication for early delivery or C-section.[558] Delivery should be performed at a tertiary center with neurosurgical, cardiovascular, and interventional radiology expertise. At birth, cardiac failure can worsen after delivery because of removal of the low-resistance placenta, facilitating more flow through the foramen ovale. Medical therapy is directed toward cardiac dysfunction and includes administration of diuretics to decrease preload. The other main goal is to address feeding so that weight gain occurs in the first few months. MRI of the brain should be obtained to assess the degree of brain injury.

In a VGM, clinical and laboratory evaluation regarding cardiac, cerebral, respiratory, renal, and liver function are utilized in a scoring system (Bicêtre) to determine need and timing for therapy (Table 17.1-23). A score of 8 and below is a decision not to treat and that between 8 and 12 is considered an emergency endovascular intervention.[559] In the presence of cardiac decompensation or with development of hydrocephalus, immediate embolization therapy is warranted to decrease AV shunt and reverse venous hypertension.[558,577] Ventriculoperitoneal shunt is avoided as it shifts pressure gradient to the sagittal sinus and leads to dilatation of the VGM, progressive white matter loss and calcification, and, possibly, subdural collections and slit-like ventricles.[575] If the patient is stable and neonatal score is between 13 and 20, it is preferable to delay intervention till 5 to 6 months of age.[575]

The first line of therapy for VGM is embolization, usually transarterial, with the transvenous route being utilized as a second choice because of higher morbidity.[558,577] Surgical treatment is dangerous, difficult, and often incomplete. The goal of therapy is not always to obliterate the AVM but to balance therapy to allow the brain to mature and develop normally by either improving cardiac status or preventing the development of neurological symptoms.[558] Several sessions of embolization may be required to safely treat, either completely or incompletely, the vascular anastomosis. Spontaneous thrombosis can occur rarely in VGM (2.5%) and is typically associated with 50% neurological impairment.[558,559] Complications from the lesion and/or therapy include hemorrhage, stroke, and continued brain injury, which can lead to neurological deficits and seizures. Macrocrania and hydrocephalus that do not respond to therapy are managed with endoscopic ventriculostomy or shunting.[559] With therapy, venous thrombosis and cerebellar tonsillar herniation due to venous congestion can occur.

Pial AVFs have the same complications as VGM.[571–573] Pial AVFs, in contradistinction to VGMs, are treated with embolotherapy at birth to prevent brain injury.[573]

Recurrence: In familial cases, transmission is autosomal dominant. In sporadic cases, there is no cited increased risk of recurrence.

TABLE 17.1-23   Bicêtre Neonatal Evaluation Score

POINTS	CARDIAC FUNCTION	CEREBRAL FUNCTION	RESPIRATORY FUNCTION	HEPATIC FUNCTION	RENAL FUNCTION
5	Normal	Normal	Normal	—	—
4	Overload, no medical treatment	Subclinical isolated EEG abnormalities	Tachypnea, finishes bottle	—	—
3	Failure, stable with medical treatment	Nonconvulsive intermittent neurological signs	Tachypnea, does not finish bottle	No hepatomegaly, normal function	Normal
2	Failure, not stable with medical treatment	Isolated convulsion	Assisted ventilation, normal saturation $FiO_2 < 25\%$	Hepatomegaly, normal function	Transient anuria
1	Ventilation necessary	Seizures	Assisted ventilation, normal saturation $FiO_2 > 25\%$	Moderate or transient hepatic insufficiency	Unstable diuresis with treatment
0	Resistant to medical treatment	Permanent neurological signs	Assisted ventilation, desaturation	Abnormal coagulation, elevated enzymes	Anuria

Maximal score = 5 (cardiac) + 5 (cerebral) + 5 (respiratory) + 3 (hepatic) + 3 (renal) = 21.
From Lasjaunias PL, Chng SM, Sachet M, et al. The management of vein of Galen aneurysmal malformation. *Neurosurgery*. 2006;59(suppl 3):184–194. Copyright © 2006 by the Congress of Neurological Surgeons. Reproduced by permission of Oxford University Press.

Dural Venous Sinus Malformation

Incidence: Dural venous sinus malformations (DSMs) are rare, representing less than 2% of vascular malformations.[578]

Pathogenesis: The dural venous sinuses run between the two layers of dura mater and are endothelial lined channels that lack muscular walls and venous valves. During the third gestational month, the venous and galenic sinuses begin to develop. The sagittal sinus forms via fusion of bilateral marginal sinuses, which initially are separate, draining into each respective transverse sinus. From the fourth to fifth months, there is ballooning of the occipital sinus, and from the fourth to sixth months, the lateral then medial transverse and sometimes the posterior sagittal sinus enlarge.[579] This dilatation is believed to occur due to increased venous flow from rapidly growing cerebral hemispheres. In the sixth fetal month, with fusion of the marginal sinuses, the venous confluence or torcula develops with its many variations in anatomy. In the seventh month, the ballooning of the sinuses resolves. The venous drainage further develops after birth as a result of additional differentiation of the jugular and cavernous sinuses.[580]

The etiology of a DSM is not known, but ectasia of the venous sinus is a described variant in development. Given this information, some have hypothesized that a DSM occurs due to persistent dilatation of the venous sinus after the time of expected balloon reduction, potentially due to disorganized development, venous hypertension, and/or arteriovenous (AV) shunting.[581,582] Disorganized development is possible, especially if genetically driven, and since venous thrombosis causes venous hypertension, it may play a part in venous dilatation. However, because venous enlargement is not normally detected on fetal imaging, the recently described, likely best theory is that a DSM is the sequela of a prior dural AV fistula (AVF) that leads to remodeling of the sinus, turbulent, and stagnant flow with occlusion of the fistula, followed by progressive thrombosis and involution of the DSM.[583]

The two possible inciting factors, AVFs and venous thrombosis, are not uncommonly seen in association with prenatal DSM. The dural AVFs are less described, noted in up to one-third of cases, and may develop due to disturbed flow within the sinus and elevated venous pressure.[581,583,584] AV shunting in a DSM typically takes place in the venous wall, fed by multiple vessels being commonly distal branches of the middle cerebral artery. These AV shunts are usually characterized by low flow but rarely may cause systemic hemodynamic complications and/or disruption in the venous drainage, resulting in venous thrombosis and intracranial venous hypertension.[585]

The second commonly described lesion in DSMs is venous thrombosis, which likely develops due to altered low-velocity flow within the dilated sinus, immaturity of venous channels, and venous hypertension.[580,584] Thrombosis is present in a high percentage of DSMs (likely >80%).[583] Most cases of thrombosis on prenatal imaging are in the area of the torcular Herophili or venous confluence and resolve spontaneously in conjunction with decrease in ectasia of the sinus, likely due to the presence of multiple anastomotic channels.[584,586] However, when there are limited anastomoses, extension of the clot into the cerebral veins, or spontaneous thrombosis of a giant sinus, cerebral ischemia, hemorrhage, and ventriculomegaly can occur.[580,584] DSMs with thrombus, though, commonly result in maturation of the sinus with a favorable outcome.[585]

DSMs have been classified into two types: midline giant pouches involving the torcula, transverse sinuses, and posterior sagittal sinus with slow flow AV shunts, and lateral, involving the jugular bulbs, that can have high-flow sigmoid sinus AVF.[571] Midline DSMs are generally stated to carry a worse prognosis, and lateral a more benign/good prognosis. Prenatally, the midline type is common, but the previously discussed poor outcome does not seem to apply to fetuses with DSM, as discussed in the following prognosis section.

Etiology: Thrombosis of the torcular Herophili in a DSM is the most common cause of fetal intracranial venous thrombosis.[587] At this time, the etiology of DSMs is not known. DSMs are not associated with known genetic mutations, chromosomal defects, thombophilic conditions, or environmental exposures.[587] Unlike the neonate in which common causes for thrombosis include prothrombotic states such as dehydration, shock, hypoxia, polycythemia, leukemia, and congenital deficiency of anticoagulants, these factors have not been implicated in prenatal DSM and thrombosis.[586,588]

Diagnosis

Ultrasound: DSMs tend to be detected in the second trimester, as early as 18 weeks but typically around 24 to 26 weeks' gestation.[578,584,589] Imaging will demonstrate a dilated venous lake, almost always in the area of the torcular Herophili, though ectasia may also extend into the transverse or posterior sagittal sinus or rarely solely involve the superior sagittal sinus.[582,587] US typically demonstrates a well-defined triangular or rounded anechoic collection above the cerebellum between the cerebral hemispheres. When imaged, most DSMs contain an echogenic structure within the hypoechoic area, consistent with acute clot (Fig. 17.1-97A).[578,588–590] 2D with 3D and transvaginal imaging may be helpful to define clot location.[588] Imaging findings are variable, depending on the size and stage of the thrombus.[580,584] As the clot matures, the lesion becomes more heterogeneous with concentric rings (Fig. 17.1-98A).[580,588] Most clots show a slow and late decrease in size. There may be recanalization of the clot, best depicted on color Doppler before birth.[586]

Color Doppler is excellent at assessing the intracranial venous system with a more continuous waveform noted in vein of Galen and straight sinus, whereas triphasic pulsatile flow is normally noted in the transverse and sagittal.[591] Due to low-flow velocity, color Doppler, in most cases of DSM, with or without dural thrombus, confirms lack of blood flow centrally even in the presence of AV shunting (Fig. 17.1-97B).[584,588,592] Flow around thrombus is rarely apparent on color Doppler.[590] Pulsatile venous flow before thrombus development has been described.[585] In some cases of AV shunting, high-velocity arterial flow may be identified along the periphery of the dilated veins.[485,588,593] If arterialization of the malformation occurs, the most likely source are branches of the middle cerebral artery.[589]

The brain should be evaluated for hemorrhage, infarct, and ventriculomegaly. Macrocrania may develop in the presence of venous hypertension. Serial US and color Doppler at intervals of 4 weeks should be obtained to monitor head biometry and decreasing thrombus size.

Magnetic Resonance Imaging: MRI is useful in the evaluation of DSMs because it is able to confirm venous sinus pathology, identify the presence and age of thrombus, exclude other masses, and define the presence or absence of brain injury.[584] The dilated venous sinus on MRI appears as a well-defined rounded or triangular area of T2 and T1 intermediate signal in the extra-axial space, conforming to a dilated venous confluence with variable extension into other dural sinuses (Figs. 17.1-97C, D and 17.1-98B, C).[578,584] Eccentric clot is usually identified in the abnormal venous sinus appearing decreased T2 signal but isointense T1 when acute (<3 days) and with T1 hyperintensity in the subacute phase (<10 days) (Fig. 17.1-97E).[584,586,587,588] With progression, the signal becomes more heterogeneous, often with central T2 hyperintensity and peripheral hypointensity.[580,589] On diffusion imaging, the intralesional thrombus can demonstrate hyperintense diffusion signal and dark ADC (Fig. 17.1-97F).[594] MRI does well at defining the location, size, number, and extent of thrombi.[586]

With a DSM, there is usually mass effect and displacement of adjacent brain, especially in the posterior fossa or posterior cerebral hemispheres. MRI is extremely helpful to exclude brain parenchymal findings, including infarction, hemorrhage, or gyration abnormalities such as polymicrogyria (Fig. 17.1-97G).[586] Diffusion imaging can also assist in exclusion of brain ischemia.[584,594]

After diagnosis, follow-up MRI may be considered to exclude development of intraparenchymal hemorrhage or infarction and monitor resolution of the thrombus.[584,586]

Associated Anomalies: Edema and parenchymal hemorrhages may occur due to venous infarctions. Hydrocephalus may also develop in the presence of venous hypertension. Rarely, a DSM with AVF may cause cardiac failure and hydrops.

Differential Diagnosis: VGMs demonstrate an oblong midline lesion with turbulent flow and, when thrombosed, may mimic a DSM with clot. Other differentials would include tumors, cystic lesions such as arachnoid, glioependymal or dermoid cysts, and malformations of the posterior fossa. Tumors are heterogeneous intraparenchymal lesions, whereas cysts tend to be fluid attenuated in the extra-axial space. Subdural or large intraparenchymal hematomas and venous thrombosis in the absence of a DSM may also be considered in the differential.

Prognosis: DSMs with venous thrombosis have a good outcome. This is likely because the fetus is less sensitive to hemodynamic changes and more conducive to collateral drainage.[578] Review of cases in the literature shows no neurocognitive sequelae in up to 75% to 90% of antenatal detected cases and survival in 80% to 90%.[578,582–584,571,588] In general, there is better outcome for fetal detected DSM than those discovered postnatally.[583] Despite overall favorable prognosis, review of prenatal cases demonstrate termination of pregnancy in 21% of cases.[582]

The natural history of the DSM is for 97% to undergo spontaneous resolution, though in 13% of cases, there is often an increase in size first.[583] Resolution of the DSM can occur prior to birth in 50% of cases.[587] If there is a normal brain, absence of AVF, decrease in size of dilated sinus, progressive clot, and/or the DSM undergoes spontaneous regression *in utero*, a favorable outcome has been noted.[578,580,583,588] Associated cerebral findings such as ventriculomegaly, especially progressing to hydrocephalus; parenchymal injury; deep venous thrombosis (internal cerebral veins); signs of cardiac decompensation; DSM arterialization; and need for intervention are unfavorable prognostic factors.[578,583,585] A fetus with these complications may have intrauterine or postnatal demise or neurological deficits.

Management: Counseling with regard to good prognosis is important, though some families may consider termination. Management should include monthly US with color Doppler to evaluate for AV shunting and ventricular enlargement. MRI is also helpful to evaluate the size of DSM, presence of clot, and new brain injury. Vaginal delivery does not seem to be contraindicated with normal head size.[585,589] After birth, the child should be evaluated for complications, including cardiac failure, anemia, and coagulopathy, with appropriate medical management.[581] Imaging should include an MRI and MR venogram to assess venous ectasia, thrombus, and brain parenchymal injury. Expected outcome is spontaneous resolution of the DSM.[578,583] An arteriogram, usually at 4 to 5 months of age, is indicated if spontaneous resolution has not occurred or there are signs for arterialization.[583,586] Surgery is not advised because of risk of bleeding and the high likelihood of spontaneous regression.[595] Endovascular embolization is the therapy of choice, which is typically performed in the setting of a dural AVF, increase in ventricular caliber, and signs of congestive heart failure.[589,]

Recurrence: DSM and associated thrombosis are sporadic conditions with no known risk for recurrence.[586]

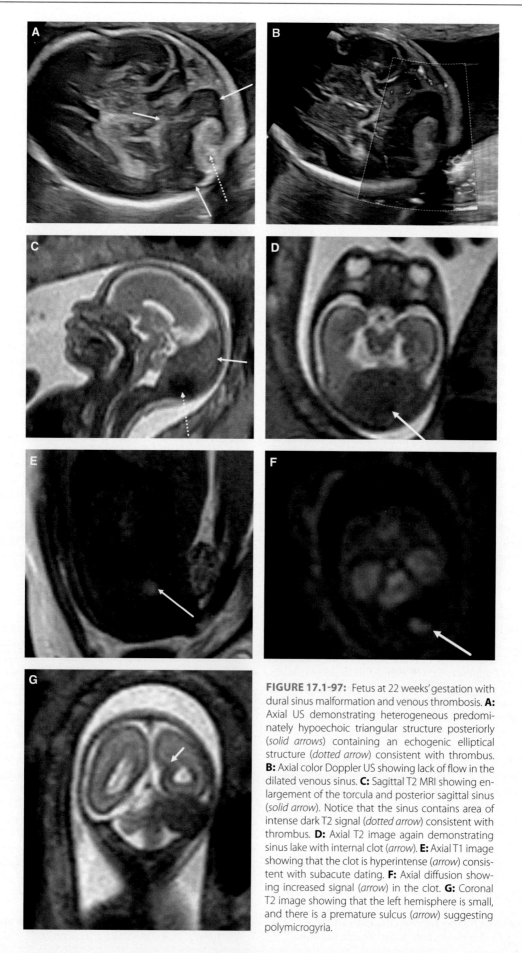

FIGURE 17.1-97: Fetus at 22 weeks' gestation with dural sinus malformation and venous thrombosis. **A:** Axial US demonstrating heterogeneous predominately hypoechoic triangular structure posteriorly (*solid arrows*) containing an echogenic elliptical structure (*dotted arrow*) consistent with thrombus. **B:** Axial color Doppler US showing lack of flow in the dilated venous sinus. **C:** Sagittal T2 MRI showing enlargement of the torcula and posterior sagittal sinus (*solid arrow*). Notice that the sinus contains area of intense dark T2 signal (*dotted arrow*) consistent with thrombus. **D:** Axial T2 image again demonstrating sinus lake with internal clot (*arrow*). **E:** Axial T1 image showing that the clot is hyperintense (*arrow*) consistent with subacute dating. **F:** Axial diffusion showing increased signal (*arrow*) in the clot. **G:** Coronal T2 image showing that the left hemisphere is small, and there is a premature sulcus (*arrow*) suggesting polymicrogyria.

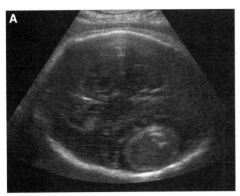
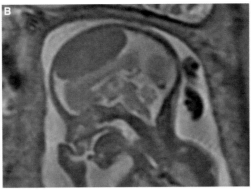
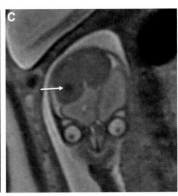

FIGURE 17.1-98: Fetus at 22 weeks with dural venous sinus malformation and clot. **A:** Axial US demonstrating echogenic area containing concentric rings consistent with clot. **B:** Sagittal T2 image of the same fetus showing abnormal enlargement and isointense signal of the anterior sagittal sinus. **C:** Coronal T2 image showing a focal area of decreased T2 signal (arrow) in the dilated vein corresponding to the echogenic clot seen in **A**. Note mass effect on the adjacent frontal lobe. The child did well postnatally, with spontaneous resolution of the defect.

REFERENCES

1. Huisman TA. Fetal magnetic resonance imaging of the brain: is ventriculomegaly the tip of the syndromal iceberg? *Semin Ultrasound CT MR.* 2011;32:491–509.
2. Nyberg DA. Recommendations for obstetric sonography in the evaluation of the fetal cranium. *Radiology.* 1989;172:309–311.
3. Paladini D, Quarantelli M, Sglavo G, et al. Accuracy of neurosonography and MRI in Clinical Management of Fetuses referred with central nervous system abnormalities. *Ultrasound Obstet Gynecol.* 2014;44:188–196.
4. Levine D, Feldman HA, Tannus JF, et al. Frequency and cause of disagreements in diagnoses for fetuses referred for ventriculomegaly. *Radiology.* 2008;247:515–527.
5. Whitby EH, Paley MN, Sprigg A, et al. Comparison of ultrasound and magnetic resonance imaging in 100 singleton pregnancies with suspected brain abnormalities. *BJOG.* 2004;111:784–792.
6. Levine D, Barnes PD, Robertson RR, et al. Fast MR imaging of fetal central nervous system abnormalities. *Radiology.* 2003;229:51–61.
7. Griffiths PD, Bradburn M, Campbell MJ, et al. Use of MRI in the diagnosis of fetal brain abnormalities in utero (MERIDIAN); a multicenter, prospective cohort study. *Lancet.* 2017;389:538–546.
8. Simon EM, Goldstein RB, Coakley FV, et al. Fast MR imaging of fetal CNS anomalies in utero. *AJNR Am J Neuroradiol.* 2000;21:1688–1698.
9. D'Addario V, Rossi AC. Neuroimaging of ventriculomegaly in the fetal period. *Semin Fetal Neonatal Med.* 2012;17:310–318.
10. Garel C, Luton D, Oury JF, et al. Ventricular dilatations. *Childs Nerv Syst.* 2003;19:517–523.
11. Zimmerman RA, Bilaniuk LT. Magnetic resonance evaluation of fetal ventriculomegaly-associated congenital malformations and lesions. *Semin Fetal Neonatal Med.* 2005;10:429–443.
12. Salomon LJ, Bernard JP, Ville Y. Reference ranges for fetal ventricular width: a non-normal approach. *Ultrasound Obstet Gynecol.* 2007;30:61–66.
13. Achiron R, Schimmel M, Achiron A, et al. Fetal mild idiopathic lateral ventriculomegaly: is there a correlation with fetal trisomy? *Ultrasound Obstet Gynecol.* 1993;3:89–92.
14. Goldstein RB, Pidus AS, Filly RA, et al. Mild lateral cerebral ventricular dilatation in utero: clinical significance and prognosis. *Radiology.* 1990;176:237–242.
15. Filly RA, Goldstein RB, Callen PW. Fetal ventricle: importance in routine obstetric sonography. *Radiology.* 1991;181:1–7.
16. Weichert J, Hartge D, Krapp M, et al. Prevalence, characteristics and perinatal outcome of fetal ventriculomegaly in 29,000 pregnancies followed at a single institution. *Fetal Diagn Ther.* 2010;27:142–148.
17. Kumar M, Garg N, Hasija A, et al. Two year postnatal outcome of 263 cases of fetal ventriculomegaly. *J Matern Fetal Neonatal Med.* 2018:1–7.
18. Brodbelt A, Stoodley M. CSF pathways: a review. *Br J Neurosurg.* 2007;21:510–520.
19. Oi S, Di Rocco C. Proposal of "evolution theory in cerebrospinal fluid dynamics" and minor pathway hydrocephalus in developing immature brain. *Childs Nerv Syst.* 2006;22:662–669.
20. Gaglioti P, Oberto M, Todros T. The significance of fetal ventriculomegaly: etiology, short- and long-term outcomes. *Prenat Diagn.* 2009;29:381–388.
21. McAllister JP 2nd. Pathophysiology of congenital and neonatal hydrocephalus. *Semin Fetal Neonatal Med.* 2012;17:285–294.
22. D'Addario V, Pinto V, Di Cagno L, et al. Sonographic diagnosis of fetal cerebral ventriculomegaly: an update. *J Matern Fetal Neonatal Med.* 2007;20:7–14.
23. Yamaski M, Nonaka M, Bamba Y, et al. Diagnosis, treatment, and long-term outcomes of fetal hydrocephalus. *Semin Fetal Neonatal Med.* 2012;17:330–335.
24. Melchiorre K, Bhide A, Gika AD, et al. Counseling in isolated mild fetal ventriculomegaly. *Ultrasound Obstet Gynecol.* 2009;34:212–224.
25. Cardoza JD, Goldstein RB, Filly RA. Exclusion of fetal ventriculomegaly with a single measurement: the width of the lateral ventricular atrium. *Radiology.* 1988;169:711–714.
26. Alagappan R, Browning PD, Laorr A, et al. Distal lateral ventricular atrium: re-evaluation of normal range. *Radiology.* 1994;193:405–408.
27. Paladini D, Malinger G, Monteagudo A, et al. Sonographic examination of the fetal central nervous system: guidelines for performing the "basic examination" and the "fetal neurosonogram." *Ultrasound Obstet Gynecol.* 2007;29:109–116.
28. Heiserman J, Filly RA, Goldstein RB. Effect of measurement errors on sonographic evaluation of ventriculomegaly. *J Ultrasound Med.* 1991;10:121–124.
29. Guibaud L. Fetal cerebral ventricular measurement and ventriculomegaly: time for procedure standardization. *Ultrasound Obstet Gynecol.* 2009;34:127–130.
30. Meyer R, Bar-Yosef O, Barzilay E, et al. Neurodevelopmental outcome of fetal isolated ventricular asymmetry without dilatation: a cohort study. *Ultasound Obstet Gynecol.* 2018;52:467–472.
31. Sadan S, Malinger G, Schweiger A, et al. Neuropsychological outcome of children with asymmetric ventricles or unilateral mild ventriculomegaly identified in utero. *BJOG.* 2007;114:596–602.
32. Cardoza JD, Filly RA, Podrasky AE. The dangling choroid plexus: a sonographic observation of value in excluding ventriculomegaly. *Am J Roentgenol.* 1988;151:767–770.
33. Hertzberg BS, Lile R, Foosaner DE, et al. Choroid plexus-ventricular wall separation in fetuses with normal-sized cerebral ventricles at sonography: postnatal outcome. *AJR Am J Roentgenol.* 1994;163:405–410.
34. Gaglioti P, Danelon D, Bontempo S, et al. Fetal cerebral ventriculomegaly: outcome in 176 cases. *Ultrasound Obstet Gynecol.* 2005;25:372–377.
35. Mahony BS, Nyberg DA, Hirsch JH, et al. Mild idiopathic lateral cerebral ventricular dilatation in utero: sonographic evaluation. *Radiology.* 1988;169:715–721.
36. Grandjean H, Larroque D, Levi S. The performance of routine ultrasonographic screening of pregnancies in the Eurofetus study. *Am J Obstet Gynecol.* 1999;181:446–454.
37. Martinez-Zamora MA, Borrell A, Borobio V, et al. False positives in the prenatal ultrasound screening of fetal structural anomalies. *Prenat Diagn.* 2007;27:18–22.
38. Richmond S, Atkins J. A population-based study of the prenatal diagnosis of congenital malformation over 16 years. *BJOG.* 2005;112:1349–1357.
39. Timor-Tritsch IE, Monteagudo A. Transvaginal fetal neurosonography: standardization of the planes and sections by anatomic landmarks. *Ultrasound Obstet Gynecol.* 1996;8:42–47.
40. Malinger G, Ben-Sira L, Lev D, et al. Fetal brain imaging: a comparison between magnetic resonance imaging and dedicated neurosonography. *Ultrasound Obstet Gynecol.* 2004;23:333–340.
41. D'Addario V, Pinto V, Di Cagno L, et al. The midsagittal view of the fetal brain: a useful landmark in recognizing the cause of fetal cerebral ventriculomegaly. *J Perinatal Med.* 2005;33:423–427.
42. Monteagudo A, Timor-Tritsch IE, Moomjy M. Nomograms of the fetal lateral ventricles using transvaginal sonography. *J Ultrasound Med.* 1993;5:265–269.
43. Rickard S, Morris J, Paley M, et al. In utero magnetic resonance of the non-isolated ventriculomegaly: does ventricular size or morphology reflect pathology. *Clin Radiol.* 2006;61:844–853.
44. Guibaud L, Lacalm A. Etiological diagnostic tools to elucidate "isolated" ventriculomegaly. *Ultrasound Obstet Gynecol.* 2015;46:1–11.
45. Li Y, Estroff JA, Mehta TS, et al. Ultrasound and MRI of fetuses with ventriculomegaly: can cortical development be used to predict postnatal outcome. *AJR Am J Roentgenol.* 2011;196:1457–1467.
46. Griffiths PD, Brackley K, Bradburn M, et al. Anatomic subgroups analysis of the MERIDIAN cohort: ventriculomgely. *Ultrasound Obstet Gynecol.* 2017;50:736–744.
47. Griffith PD, Morris JE, Mason G, et al. Fetuses with ventriculomegaly diagnosed in the second trimester of pregnancy by in utero MR imaging: what happens in the third trimester? *Am J Neuroradiol.* 2011;32:474–480.
48. Perlman S, Shashar D, Hoffman C, et al. Prenatal diagnosis of fetal ventriculomegaly: agreement between fetal brain ultrasonography and MR imaging. *AJNR.* 2014;35:1214–1218.

49. Levine D, Trop I, Mehta TS, et al. MR imaging appearance of fetal cerebral ventricular morphology. *Radiology.* 2002;223:652–660.

50. Manganaro L, Savelli S, Francioso A, et al. Role of fetal MRI in the diagnosis of cerebral ventriculomegaly assessed by ultrasonography. *Radiol Med.* 2009;114:1013–1023.

51. Levine D, Barnes PD. Cortical maturation in normal and abnormal fetuses as assessed with prenatal MR imaging. *Radiology.* 1999;210:751–758.

52. Griffiths PD, Reeves MJ, Morris JE, et al. A prospective study of fetuses with isolated ventriculomegaly investigated by antenatal sonography and in utero MR imaging. *AJNR Am J Neuroradiol.* 2010;31:106–111.

53. Nicolaides KH, Berry S, Snijders RJM, et al. Fetal lateral cerebral ventriculomegaly: associated malformations and chromosomal defects. *Fetal Diagn Ther.* 1990;5:5–14.

54. Lee SB, Hong SH, Wang KY, et al. Fetal ventriculomegaly: prognosis in cases in which prenatal neurosurgical consultation was sought. *J Neurosurg.* 2006;105:265–270.

55. Quahba J, Luton D, Vuillard E, et al. Prenatal isolated mild ventriculomegaly: outcome in 167 cases. *BJOG.* 2006;113:1072–1079.

56. Vergani P, Locatelli A, Strobelt N, et al. Clinical outcome of mild fetal ventriculomegaly. *Am J Obstet Gynecol.* 1998;178:218–222.

57. Parilla BV, Endres LK, Dinsmoor MJ, et al. In utero progression of mild fetal ventriculomegaly. *Int J Gynaecol Obstet.* 2006;93:106–109.

58. Kelly EN, Allen VM, Seaward G, et al. Mild ventriculomegaly in the fetus, natural history, associated findings and outcome of isolated mild ventriculomegaly: a literature review. *Prenat Diagn.* 2001;21:697–700.

59. Falip C, Blanc N, Maes E, et al. Postnatal clinical and imaging follow-up of infants with prenatal isolated mild ventriculomegaly: a series of 101 cases. *Pediatr Radiol.* 2007;37:981–989.

60. Devaseelan P, Cardwell C, Bell B, et al. Prognosis of isolated mild to moderate fetal cerebral ventriculomegaly: a systematic review. *J Perinat Med.* 2010;38:401–409.

61. Pisapia JM, Sinha S, Zarnow DM, et al. Fetal ventriculomegaly: diagnosis, treatment, and future directions. *Childs Nerv Syst.* 2017;33:1113–1123.

62. Davis GH. Fetal hydrocephalus. *Clin Perinatol.* 2003;30:531–539.

63. Chervenak FA, Berkowitz RL, Romero R, et al. The diagnosis of fetal hydrocephalus. *Am J Obstet Gynecol.* 1983;147:703–716.

64. Prayer D, Paladini D, Deprest J. Current controversies in prenatal diagnosis 1: should MRI be performed on all fetuses with mild ventriculomegaly? *Prenat Diagn.* 2019;39:331–338.

65. Kinzler WL, Smulian JC, McLean DA, et al. Outcome of prenatally diagnosed mild unilateral cerebral ventriculomegaly. *J Ultrasound Med.* 2001;20:257–262.

66. Scala C, Familiari A, Pinas A, et al. Perinatal and long term outcomes in fetuses diagnosed with isolated unilateral ventriculomegaly: systemic review and meta-analysis. *Ultrasound Obstet Gynecol.* 2017;49:450–459.

67. Perlman S, Bar-Yosef O, Jacobson JM. Natural history of fetal isolated ventriculomegaly: comparison between pre-and post-natal imaging. *J Matern Fetal Neonatal Med.* 2018;31(13);1762–1767.

68. Patel MD, Goldstein RB, Tung S, et al. Fetal cerebral ventricular atrium: difference in size according to sex. *Radiology.* 1995;194:713–715.

69. Snijders RJM, Nicolaides KH. Fetal biometry at 14–40 weeks' gestation. *Ultrasound Obstet Gynecol.* 1994;4:34–48.

70. Nadel AS, Benacerraf BR. Lateral ventricular atrium: larger in male than female fetuses. *Int J Gynaecol Obstet.* 1995;51:123–126.

71. Patel MD, Filly AL, Hersh DR, et al. Isolated mild fetal cerebral ventriculomegaly: clinical course and outcome. *Radiology.* 1994;192:759–764.

72. Pilu G, Falco P, Gabrielli S, et al. The clinical significance of fetal isolated cerebral borderline ventriculomegaly: report of 31 cases and review of the literature. *Ultrasound Obstet Gynecol.* 1999;14:320–326.

73. Senat MV, Bernard JP, Schwarzler P, et al. Prenatal diagnosis and follow-up of 14 cases of unilateral ventriculomegaly. *Ultrasound Obstet Gynecol.* 1999;14:327–332.

74. Almog B, Gamzu R, Achiron R, et al. Fetal lateral ventricular width: what should be its upper limit? A prospective cohort study and reanalysis of the current and previous data. *J Ultrasound Med.* 2003;22:39–43.

75. Lavongtheung A, Jedraszak G, Naepels P, et al. Should isolated fetal ventriculomegaly measured below 12 mm be viewed as a variant of the norm? Results of a 5 year experience in prenatal referral center. *J Matern Fetal Neonatal Med.* 2018;31(17):2325–2335.

76. Barzilay E, Bar-Yosef O, Dorembus S, et al. Fetal brain anomalies associated with ventriculomegaly or asymmetry: an MRI-Based study. *AJNR.* 2017;38:371–375.

77. Society for maternal–Fetal Medicine (SMFM), Fox NS, Monteagudo A, Kuller JA, et al. Mild fetal ventriculomegaly: diagnosis, evalution and management. 2018;219(1):B2–B9.

78. Wyldes M, Watkinson M. Isolated mild fetal ventriculomegaly. *Arch Dis Child Fetal Neonatal ED.* 2004;89:F9–F13.

79. Di Mascio D, Sileo FG, Khalil A, et al. Systemic review and meta-analysis on the role of prenatal magnetic resonance imaging in the era of fetal neurosonography: mild and moderate ventriculomegaly. *Ultasound Obstet Gynecol.* 2018;54(2).

80. Salomon LJ, Ouahba J, Delezoide AL, et al. Third-trimester fetal MRI in isolated 10- to 12-mm ventriculomegaly: is it worth it? *BJOG.* 2006;113:942–947.

81. Parazzini C, Righini A, Doneda C, et al. Is fetal magnetic resonance imaging indicated when ultrasound isolated mild ventriculomegaly is present in pregnancies with no risk factors. *Prenat Diagn.* 2012;32:752–757.

82. Wax JR, Bookman L, Cartin A, et al. Mild fetal cerebral ventriculomegaly: diagnosis, clinical associations, and outcomes. *Obstet Gynecol Surv.* 2003;58:407–414.

83. Bar-Yosef O, Barzilay E, Darembus S, et al. Neurodevelopmental outcome of isolated ventriculomegaly: a prospective cohort study. *Prenat Diagn.* 2017;37:764–768.

84. Signorelli M, Tiberti A, Valseriath D, et al. Width of the fetal lateral ventricular atrium between 10 and 12 mm: a simple variation of the norm? *Ultrasound Obstet Gynecol.* 2004;23:14–18.

85. Leitner Y, Stolar O, Rotstein M, et al. The neurocognitive outcome of mild isolated fetal ventriculomegaly verified by prenatal magnetic resonance imaging. *Am J Obstet Gynecol.* 2009;201:215.e1–215.e6.

86. Lipitz S, Yagel S, Malinger G, et al. Outcome of fetuses with isolated borderline unilateral ventriculomegaly diagnosed at mid-gestation. *Ultrasound Obstet Gynecol.* 1998;12:23–26.

87. Pagani G, Thilaganathan B, Prefumo F. Neruodevelopmental outcome in isolated mild fetal ventriculomgegaly: systematic review and meta-anaalysis. *Ultrasound Obstet Gynecol.* 2014;44:254–260.

88. Gilmore JH, Smith LC, Wolfe HM, et al. Prenatal mild ventriculomegaly predicts abnormal development of the neonatal brain. *Biol Psychiatry.* 2008;64:1069–1076.

89. Bloom SL, Bloom DD, Dellanebbia C, et al. The developmental outcome of children with antenatal mild isolated ventriculomegaly. *Obstet Gynecol.* 1997;90:93–97.

90. Gomez-Arriaga P, Herraiz I, Puente JM, et al. Mid-term neurodevelopmental outcome in isolated mild ventriculomegaly diagnosed in fetal life. *Fetal Diagn Ther.* 2012;31:12–18.

91. Verhagen WI, Bartels RH, Fransen E, et al. Familial congenital hydrocephalus and aqueduct stenosis with probably autosomal dominant inheritance and variable expression. *J Neurol Sci.* 1998;158:101–105.

92. Kenwrick S, Jouet M, Donnai D. X-linked hydrocephalus and MASA syndrome. *J Med Genet.* 1996;33:59–65.

93. Weller S, Gartner J. Genetic and clinical aspects of X-linked hydrocephalus (L1 disease): mutations in the L1CAM gene. *Hum Mutat.* 2001;18:1–12.

94. Adle-Biassette H, Saugier-Veber P, Fallet-Bianco C, et al. Neuropathological review of 138 cases genetically tested for X-linked hydrocephalus: evidence for closely related clinical entities of unknown molecular bases. *Acta Neuropathol.* 2013;126:427–442.

95. Tully HM, Dobyns WB. Infantile hydrocephalus: a review of epidemiology, classification and causes. *Eur J Med Genet.* 2014;57:359–368.

96. Cagneaux M, Vasiljevic A, Massoud M, et al. Severe second trimester obstructive ventriculomegaly related to disorders of diencephalic, mesencephalic and rhombencephalic differentiation. *Ultrasound Obstet Gynecol.* 2013;42:596–602.

97. Rault E, Lacalm A, Massoud M, et al. The many faces of prenatal imaging diagnosis of primitive aqueduct obstruction. *Eur J Paediatr Neurol.* 2018;22:910–918.

98. Severino M, Righini A, Tortora D, et al. MR Imaging diagnosis of diencephalic-mesencephalic junction dysplasia in fetuses with developmental ventriculomegaly. *AJNR.* 2017;38:1643–1646.

99. Amir T, Poretti A, Boltshauser E, et al. Differential diagnosis of ventriculomegaly and brainstem kinking on fetal MRI. *Brain Dev.* 2016;38:103–108.

100. Ishak GE, Dempsey JC, Shaw DWW, et al. Rhombencephalosynapsis: a hindbrain malformation associated with incomplete separation of midbrain and forebrain hydrocephalus and a broad spectrum of severity. *Brain.* 2012;135:1370–1386.

101. Kline-Fath BM, Arroyo MS, Calvo-Garcia MA, et al. Prenatal aqueduct stenosis: association with rhomboencephalosynapsis and neonatal outcome. *Prenat Diagn.* 2018;38:1028–1034.

102. Humphreys P, Muzumdar DP, Sly LE, et al. Focal cerebral mantle disruption in fetal hydrocephalus. *Pediatr Neurol.* 2007;36:236–243.

103. Oi S, Honda U, Hidaka M, et al. Intrauterine high resolution magnetic resonance imaging in fetal hydrocephalus and prenatal estimation of postnatal outcomes with "perspective classification." *J Neurosurg.* 1998;88:685–694.

104. Tully HM, Ishak GE, Rue TC, et al. 236 children with developmental hydrocephalus: causes and clinical consequences. *J Child Neurol.* 2016;31(3):309–320.

105. Schrander-Stumpel C, Fryns JP. Congenital hydrocephalus: nosology and guidelines for clinical approach and genetic counseling. *Eur J Pediatr.* 1998;157:355–362.

106. Varadi V, Csecsei K, Szeifert GT, et al. Prenatal diagnosis of X linked hydrocephalus without aqueductal stenosis. *J Med Genet.* 1987;24:207–209.

107. Azzi C, Giaconia MB, Lacalm A, et al. Dilatation of the supra-pineal recess on prenatal imaging: early clue for obstructive ventriculomegaly downstream of the third ventricle. *Prenat Diagn.* 2014;43:394–401.

108. Heaphy-Henult KJ, Guimaraes CV, Mehollin-Ray AR, et al. Congenital aqueductal stenosis: findings at fetal MRI that accurately predict a postnatal diagnosis. *AJNR.* 2018;39:942–948.

109. Kline-Fath BM, Arroyo MS, Calvo-Garcia MA, et al. Congenital aqueduct stenosis: progressive brain findings in utero to birth in the presence of severe hydrocephalus. *Prenat Diagn.* 2018;38:706–712.

110. Emery SP, Hogge A, Hill LM. Accuracy of prenatal diagnosis of isolated aqueductal stenosis. *Prenat Diagn.* 2015;35:319–324.

111. Driver AM, Pitstick AL, Mayhew CN, et al. A de novo missense mutation in TUBA1A results in reduced neural progenitor survival and differentiation. *Biorxiv.* 2017. doi:10.1101/201814.

112. Levitsky DB, Mack LA, Nyberg DA, et al. Fetal aqueductal stenosis diagnosed sonographically: how grave is the prognosis? *AJR Am J Roentgenol.* 1995;164:725–730.

113. Holmes LB, Nash A, ZuRhein GM, et al. X-linked aqueductal stenosis: clinical and neuropathological findings in two families. *Pediatrics.* 1973;51:697–704.

114. Kennelly MM, Cooley SM, McFarland PJ. Natural history of apparently isolated severe fetal ventriculomegaly: perinatal survival and neurodevelopmental outcomes. *Prenat Diagn.* 2009;29:1135–1140.

115. Carta S, Kealin Agten A, Belcaro C, et al. Outcome of fetuses with prenatal diagnosis of isolated severe bilateral ventriculomegaly: systemic review and meta-analysis. *Ultrasound Obstet Gynecol.* 2018;52:165–173.

116. Cavalheiro S, Fernandes Moron A, Zymberg ST, et al. Fetal hydrocephalus—prenatal treatment. *Childs Nerv Syst.* 2003;19:561–573.

117. Orioli IM, Castilla EE. Epidemiology of holoprosencephaly: prevalence and risk factors. *Am J Med Genet C Semin Med Genet.* 2010;154C:13–21.

118. Wenghoefer M, Ettema AM, Sina F, et al. Prenatal ultrasound diagnosis in 51 cases of holoprosencephaly: craniofacial anatomy, associated malformations, and genetics. *Cleft Palate Craniofac J.* 2010;47:15–21.

119. Joo GJ, Beke A, Papp C, et al. Prenatal diagnosis, phenotypic and obstetric characteristics of holoprosencephaly. *Fetal Diagn Ther.* 2005;20:161–166.

120. Simon EM, Barkovich AJ. Holoprosencephaly: new concepts. *Magn Reson Imaging Clin N Am.* 2001;9:149–164.

121. Volpe P, Campobasso G, De Robertis V, et al. Disorders of prosencephalic development. *Prenat Diagn.* 2009;29:340–354.

122. Hahn JS, Plawner LL. Evaluation and management of children with holoprosencephaly. *Pediatr Neurol.* 2004;31:79–88.

123. DeMyer W, Zeman W, Palmer CG. The face predicts the brain: diagnostic significance of median facial anomalies for holoprosencephaly (arhinencephaly). *Pediatrics.* 1964;34:256–263.

124. Fallet-Bianco C. Neuropathy of holoprosencephaly. *Am J Med Genetic.* 2018;178C:214–228.

125. Nyberg DA, Mack LA, Bronstein A, et al. Holoprosencephaly: prenatal sonographic diagnosis. *AJR Am J Roentgenol.* 1987;149:1051–1058.

126. Filly RA, Chinn DH, Callen PW. Alobar holoprosencephaly: ultrasonographic prenatal diagnosis. *Radiology.* 1984;151:455–459.

127. Barkovich AJ, Quint DJ. Middle interhemispheric fusion: an unusual variant of holoprosencephaly. *AJNR Am J Neuroradiol.* 1993;14:431–440.

128. Simon EM, Hevner RF, Pinter JD, et al. The middle interphemispheric variant of holoprosencephaly. *AJNR Am J Neuroradiol.* 2002;23:151–155.

129. Dubourg C, Bendavid C, Pasquier L, et al. Holoprosencephaly. *Orphanet J Rare Dis.* 2007;2:1–14.

130. Dubourg C, Kim A, Watrin E, et al. Recent advances in understanding inheritance of holoprosencephaly. *Am J Med Genet.* 2018;178C:258–269.

131. Bullen PJ, Rankin JM, Robson SC. Investigation of the epidemiology and prenatal diagnosis of holoprosencephaly in the north of England. *Am J Obstet Gynecol.* 2001;184:1256–1262.

132. Yamada S. Embryonic holoprosencephaly: pathology and phenotypic variability. *Congenit Anom.* 2006;46:164–171.

133. Johnson CY, Rasmussen SA. Non-genetic risk factors for holoprosencephaly. *Am J Med Genet C Semin Med Genet.* 2010;154C:73–85.

134. Solomon BD, Gropman A, Muenke M. Holoprosencephaly overview. In: Pagon RA, Adam MP, Bird TD, et al, eds. *GeneReviews™* [Internet]. Seattle, WA: University of Washington; 1993–2013, December 27, 2000. [Updated November 3, 2011].

135. Huang J, Wah IY, Pooh RK, et al. Molecular genetics in fetal neurology. *Semin Fetal Neonatal Med.* 2012;17:341–346.

136. Berry SM, Gosden C, Snijders RJM, et al. Fetal holoprosencephaly: associated malformations and chromosomal defects. *Fetal Diagn Ther.* 1990;5:92–99.

137. Kruszka P, Martinez AF, Muenke M. Molecular testing in holoprosencephaly. *Am J Med Genet.* 2018;178C;187–193.

138. Ginblat Y, Lipinski RJ. A forebrain undivided: unleashing model organisms to solve mysteries of holoprosencephaly. *Dev Dynam.* 2019. doi:10.1002/dvdy.41.

139. Sepulveda W, Dezerega V, Be C. First-trimester sonographic diagnosis of holoprosencephaly: value of the "Butterfly" sign. *J Ultrasound Med.* 2004;23:761–765.

140. Hahn JS, Barnes PD. Neuroimaging advances in holoprosencephaly: refining the spectrum of the midline malformation. *Am J Med Genet C Semin Med Genet.* 2010;154C:120–132.

141. Pilu G, Sandri F, Perolo A, et al. Prenatal diagnosis of lobar holoprosencephaly. *Ultrasound Obstet Gynecol.* 1992;2:88–94.

142. Cayea PD, Balcar I, Alberti O Jr, et al. Prenatal diagnosis of semilobar holoprosencephaly. *AJR Am J Roentgenol.* 1984;142:401–402.

143. Pilu G, Ambrosetto P, Sandri F, et al. Intraventricular fused fornices: a specific sign of fetal lobar holoprosencephaly. *Ultrasound Obstet Gynecol.* 1994;4:65–67.

144. Bernard JP, Drummond CL, Zaarour P, et al. A new clue to the prenatal diagnosis of lobar holoprosencephaly: the abnormal pathway of the anterior cerebral artery crawling under the skull. *Ultrasound Obstet Gynecol.* 2002;19:605–607.

145. McGahan JP, Nyberg DA, Mack LA. Sonography of facial features of alobar and semilobar holoprosencephaly. *AJR Am J Roetgenol.* 1990;154:143–148.

146. Chen CP, Shih JC, Hsu CY, et al. Prenatal three-dimensional/four-dimensional sonographic demonstration of facial dysmorphisms associated with holoprosencephaly. *J Clin Ultrasound.* 2005;33:312–318.

147. Plawner LL, Delgado MR, Miller VS, et al. Neuroanatomy of holoprosencephaly as predictor of function, beyond the face predicting the brain. *Neurology.* 2002;59:1058–1066.

148. Griffith PD, Jarvis D. In utero MR imaging of fetal holoprosencephaly: a structured approach to diagnosis and classification. *AJNR.* 2016;37:536–543.

149. Kousa YA, du Plessis AJ, Vezina G. Prenatal diagnosis of holoprosencephaly. *Am J Med Genet.* 2018;178(2):206–213.

150. Hahn JS, Barkovich AJ, Stashinko EE, et al. Factor analysis of neuroanatomical and clinical characteristics of holoprosencephaly. *Brain Dev.* 2006;28:413–419.

151. Simon EM, Hevner R, Pinter JD, et al. Assessment of the deep gray nuclei in holoprosencephaly. *AJNR Am J Neuroradiol.* 2000;21:1955–1961.

152. Barkovich AJ, Simon EM, Clegg NJ, et al. Analysis of the cerebral cortex in holoprosencephaly with attention to the Sylvian fissures. *AJNR Am J Neuroradiol.* 2002;23:143–150.

153. Hahn JS, Barnes PD, Clegg NJ, et al. Septopreoptic holoprosencephaly: a mild subtype associated with midline craniofacial anomalies. *AJNR Am J Neuroradiol.* 2010;31:1596–1601.

154. Koob M, Weingertner AS, Gasser B, et al. Thick corpus callosum: a clue to the diagnosis of fetal septopreoptic holoprosencephaly? *Pediatr Radiol.* 2012;42:886–890.

155. Martinez AF, Kruszka PS, Muenke M. Extracephalic manifestations of nonchromosomal, nonsyndromic holoprosencephaly. *Am J Med Genet.* 2018;178(2);246–257.

156. Cohen MM Jr. Holoprosencephaly: clinical, anatomic and molecular dimensions. *Birth Defects Res A Clin Mol Teratol.* 2006;76:658–673.

157. Weiss K, Kruszka PS, Levey I, et al. Holoprosencephaly from conception to adulthood. *Am J Med Genet.* 2018;178(2):122–127.

158. Raam MS, Solomon BD, Muenke M. Holoprosencephaly: a guide to diagnosis and clinical management. *Indian Pediatr.* 2011;48:457–466.

159. David AL, Gowda V, Turnbull C, et al. The risk of recurrence of holoprosencephaly in euploid fetuses. *Obstet Gynecol.* 2007;110:658–662.

160. Dill P, Poretti A, Boltshauser E, et al. Fetal magnetic resonance imaging in midline malformations of the central nervous system and review of the literature. *J Neuroradiol.* 2009;36:138–146.

161. Li Y, Estroff JA, Khwaja O, et al. Callosal dysgenesis in fetuses with ventriculomegaly: levels of agreement between imaging modalities and postnatal outcome. *Ultrasound Obstet Gynecol.* 2012;40:522–529.

162. Glass HC, Shaw GM, Ma C, et al. Agenesis of the corpus callosum in California 1983–2003: a population-based study. *Am J Med Genet.* 2008;146A:2495–2500.

163. Turkyilmaz G, Sarac Sivrikoz TS, Erturk E, et al. Utilization of neurosonography for evaluation of corpus callosum malformations in the era of fetal magnetic resonance imaging. *J Obstet Gynaecol Res.* 2019;45(8):1472–1478.

164. Manganaro L, Bernard S, De Vito C, et al. Role of fetal MRI in the evaluation of isolated and non0isolated corpus callosum dysgenesis: results of a cross-sectional study. *Prenat Diagn.* 2017;37:244–252.

165. Vasudevan C, McKechnie L, Levene M. Long-term outcome of antenatally diagnosed agenesis of the corpus callosum and cerebellar malformations. *Semin Fetal Neonatal Med.* 2012;17:292–300.

166. Raybaud C. The corpus callosum, the other great forebrain commissures, and the septum pellucidum: anatomy, development and malformation. *Neuroradiology.* 2010;52:447–477.

167. Dobyns WB. Absence makes the search grow longer. *Am J Hum Genet.* 1996;58:7–16.

168. Barkovich AJ, Norman D. Anomalies of the corpus callosum: correlation with further anomalies of the brain. *AJR Am J Roentgenol.* 1988;151:171–179.

169. Atlas SW, Zimmerman RA, Bilaniuk LT, et al. Corpus callosum and limbic system: neuroanatomic MR evaluation of developmental anomalies. *Radiology.* 1986;160:355–362.

170. Hetts SW, Sherr EH, Chao S, et al. Anomalies of the corpus callosum: an MR analysis of the phenotypic spectrum of associated malformations. *AJR Am J Roentgenol.* 2006;187:1343–1348.

171. Barkovich AJ, Simon EM, Walsh CA. Callosal agenesis with cyst: a better understanding and new classification. *Neurology.* 2001;56:220–227.

172. Ickowitz V, Eurin D, Rypens F, et al. Prenatal diagnosis and postnatal follow-up of pericallosal lipoma: report of seven new cases. *AJNR Am J Neuroradiol.* 2001;22:767–772.

173. Shinar S, Lerman-Sagie T, Echevarria Telleria M, et al. Fetal pericallosal lipomas-Clues to diagnosis in the second trimester. *Eur J Paediatr Neurol.* 2018;22:929–934.

174. Shevell MI. Clinical and diagnostic profile of agenesis of the corpus callosum. *J Child Neurol.* 2002;17:895–899.

175. Bedeschi MF, Bonaglia MC, Grasso R, et al. Agenesis of the corpus callosum: clinical and genetic study in 63 young patients. *Pediatr Neurol.* 2006;34:186–193.

176. Leombroni M, Khalil A, Liberati M, et al. Fetal midline anomalies: diagnosis and counselling Part 1: corpus acallosum anomalies. *Eur J Paediatr Neurol.* 2018;22:951–962.

177. E'Antonio F, Pagani G, Familiari A, et al. Outcomes associated with isolated agenesis of the corpus callosum: a meta-analysis. *Pediatrics.* 2018;138(3).

178. Aicardi J. Aicardi syndrome. *Brain Dev.* 2005;27:164–171.

179. Diaz-Guerrero L, Giugni-Chalbaud G, Sosa-Olavarria A. Assessment of pericallosal arteries by color Doppler ultrasonography at 11–14 weeks: an early marker of fetal corpus callosum development in normal fetuses and agenesis in cases with chromosomal anomalies. *Fetal Diagn Ther.* 2013;34:85–89.

180. Lachmann R, Sodre D, Barmpas M, et al. Midbrain and falx in fetuses with absent corpus callosum at 11–13 weeks. *Fetal Diagn Ther.* 2013;33:41–46.

181. Kalayci H, Tarim E, Ozdemir H, et al. Is the presence of corpus callosum predictable in the first trimmest? *J Obstet Gynaecol.* 2018;38(3):310–315.

182. Pilu G, Sandri F, Perolo A, et al. Sonography of fetal agenesis of the corpus callosum: a survey of 35 cases. *Ultrasound Obstet Gynecol.* 1993;3:318–329.

183. Bennett GL, Bromley B, Benacerraf BR. Agenesis of the corpus callosum: prenatal detection usually is not possible before 22 weeks of gestation. *Radiology.* 1996;199:447–450.

184. Manfredi R, Tognolini A, Bruno C, et al. Agenesis of the corpus callosum in fetuses with mild ventriculomegaly: role of MR imaging. *Radiol Med.* 2010;115:301–312.

185. Bertino RE, Nyberg DA, Cyr DR, et al. Prenatal diagnosis of agenesis of the corpus callosum. *J Ultrasound Med.* 1988;7:251–260.

186. Karl K, Esser T, Heling KS, et al. Cavum septi pellucidi (CSP) ratio: a marker for partial agenesis of the fetal corpus callosum. *Ultrasound Obstet Gynecol.* 2017;50:336–341.

187. Volpe P, Paladini D, Resta M, et al. Characteristics, associations and outcome of partial agenesis of the corpus callosum in the fetus. *Ultrasound Obstet Gynecol.* 2006;27:509–516.

188. Griffiiths PD, Batty R, Connolly DAJ, et al. Effects of failed commissuration on the septum pellucidum and fornix: implications for fetal imaging. *Neuroradiology.* 2009;51:347–356.

189. Ghi T, Carletti A, Contro E, et al. Prenatal diagnosis and outcome of partial agenesis and hypoplasia of the corpus callosum. *Ultrasound Obstet Gynecol.* 2010;35:35–41.

190. Atallah A, Lacalm A, Massoud M, et al. Prenatal diagnosis of pericallosal curvilinear lipoma: specific imaging pattern and diagnostic pitfalls. *Ultrasound Obstet Gynecol.* 2018;51:269–273.

191. Santirocco M, Rodo C, Illescas T, et al. Accuracy of prenatal ultrasound in the diagnosis of corpus callosum anomalies. *J Matern Fetal Neonatal Med.* 2019:1–6. doi:10.1080/14767058.2019.1609931.

192. Griffith PD, Brackley K, Bradburn M, et al. Anatomical subgroup analysis of the MERIDIAN cohort: failed commissuration. *Ultrasound Obstet Gynecology.* 2017;50:753–760.

193. Glenn OA, Goldstein RB, Li KC, et al. Fetal magnetic resonance imaging in the evaluation of fetuses referred for sonographically suspected abnormalities of the corpus callosum. *J Ultrasound Med.* 2005;24:791–804.

194. Tang PH, Bartha AI, Norton ME, et al. Agenesis of the corpus callosum: an MR imaging analysis of associated abnormalities in the fetus. *AJNR Am J Neuroradiol.* 2009;30:257–263.

195. Herreld JH, Bhore R, Chason DP, et al. Corpus callosum length by gestational age as evaluated by fetal MR imaging. *AJNR Am J Neuroradiol.* 2011;32:490–494.

196. Warren DJ, Connolly DJA, Griffiths PD. Assessment of sulcation of the fetal brain in cases of isolated agenesis of the corpus callosum using in utero MR imaging. *AJNR Am J Neuroradiol.* 2010;31:1085–1090.

197. Knezović V, Kasprian G, Štajduhar A, et al. Underdevelopment of the human hippocampus in callosal agenesis: an in vivo fetal MRI study. *AJNR Am J Neuroradiol.* 2019;40:576–581.

198. Cesaretti C, Nanni M, Ghi T, et al. Variability of forebrain commissures in callosal agenesis: a prenatal MR imaging study. *AJNR Am J Neuroradiol.* 2016;37:521–527.

199. Chougar L, Blondiaux E, Moutard ML, et al. Variability of T1 weighted signal intensity of pericallosal lipomas in the fetus. *Pediatr Radiol.* 2018;48:383–391.

200. Romaniello R, Marelli S, Giorda R, et al. Clinical characterization, genetics and long term follow-up of a large cohort of patients with agenesis of the corpus callosum. *J Child Neurol.* 2017;32(1):60–71.

201. Moes P, Schilmoeller K, Schmilmoeller G. Physical, motor, sensory and developmental features associated with agenesis of the corpus callosum. *Child Care Health Dev.* 2009;35:656–672.

202. Siffredi V, Anderson V, McEilroy A, et al. A neuropsychological profile for agenesis of the corpus callosum? Cognitive, academic, executive, social and behavioral function in school-age children. *J Int Neurosychol Soc.* 2018;24:445–455.

203. Uccella S, Accogli A, Tortora D, et al. Dissecting the neurological phenotype in children with callosal agenesis, interhemispheric cysts and malformations of cortical development. *J Neurol.* 2019;266:1167–1181.

204. Blum A, André M, Droullé P, et al. Prenatal echographic diagnosis of corpus callosum agenesis. *Genet Couns.* 1990;38(2):115–126.

205. Garne E, Rissmann A, Addor MC, et al. Epidemiology of septo-optic dysplasia with focus on prevalence and maternal age—A Eurocat study. *Eur J Med Genet.* 2018;61:483–488.

206. Atapattu N, Ainsworth J, Willshaw H, et al. Septo-optic dysplasia: antenatal risk factors and clinical features in a regional study. *Horm Res Paediatr.* 2012;78: 81–87.

207. Kelberman D, Dattani MT. Septo-optic dysplasia—novel insights into the aetiology. *Horm Res.* 2008;69:257–265.

208. Stevens CA, Dobyns WB. Septo-optic dysplasia and amniotic bands: further evidence for a vascular pathogenesis. *Am J Med Genet.* 2004;125A:12–16.

209. Lubinsky MS. Hypothesis: Septo-Optic Dysplasia is a vascular disruption sequence. *Am J Med Genet.* 1997;69:235–236.

210. Alt D, Shevell M, Poulin C, et al. Clinical and radiologic spectrum of septo-optic dysplasia: review of 17 cases. *J Child Neurol.* 2017;32(9):797–803.

211. Polizzi A, Pavone P, Iannetti P, et al. Septo-optic dysplasia complex: a heterogeneous malformation syndrome. *Pediatr Neurol.* 2006;34:66–71.

212. Leonhardt EE, Tann-Sinn PA. Septo-optic dysplasia: a neurosonographic review. *J Diagn Med Sonogr.* 2005;21:479–486.

213. Barkovich AJ, Fram EK, Norman D. Sept-optic dysplasia: MR imaging. *Radiology.* 1989;171:189–192.

214. Malinger G, Lev D, Oren M, et al. Non-visualization of the cavum septi pellucidi is not synonymous with agenesis of the corpus callosum. *Ultrasound Obstet Gynecol.* 2012;40:165–170.

215. Pilliod RA, Pettersson DR, Gibson T, et al. Diagnositc accuracy and clinical outcomes associated with prenatal diagnosis of fetal absent cavum septi pellucidi. *Prenat Diagn.* 2018;38:395–401.

216. Vawter-Lee M, Wasserman H, Thomas CW, et al. Outcome of isolated absent septum pellucidum diagnosed by fetal magnetic resonance imaging scan. *J Child Neurol.* 2018;33(11):693–699.

217. Benson JC, Nascene D, Truwit C, et al. Septo-optic dysplasia: assessment of associated findings with special attention to the olfactory sulci and tracts. *Clin Neuroradiol.* 2019;29(3):505–513.

218. Severino M, Allegri A, Pistorio A, et al. Midbrain-hindbrain involvement in septo-optic dysplasia. *AJNR Am J Neuroradiol.* 2014;35:1586–1592.

219. McCabe MJ, Alatzoglou KS, Dattani MT. Septo-optic dysplasia and other midline defects: the role of transcription factors: HESX1 and beyond. *Best Pract Res Clin Endocrinol Metab.* 2011;25:115–124.

220. Falco P, Gabrielli S, Visentin A, et al. Transabdominal sonography of the cavum septum pellucidum in normal fetuses in the second and third trimesters of pregnancy. *Ultrasound Obstet Gynecol.* 2000;16:549–553.

221. Pilu G, Tani G, Carletti A, et al. Difficult early sonographic diagnosis of absence of the fetal septum pellucidum. *Ultrasound Obstet Gynecol.* 2005;25:70–72.

222. Callen PW, Callen AL, Glenn OA, et al. Columns of the fornix, not be mistaken for the cavum septi pellucidi on prenatal sonography. *J Ultrasound Med.* 2008;27:25–31.

223. Lepinard C, Coutant R, Boussion F, et al. Prenatal diagnosis of absence of the septum pellucidum associated with septo-optic dysplaia. *Ultrasound Obstet Gynecol.* 2005;25:73–75.

224. Katorza E, Bault JP, Gilboa Y, et al. Prenatal visualization of the pituitary gland using 2- and 3-dimensional sonography: comparison to prenatal magnetic resonance imaging. *J Ultrasound Med.* 2012;31:1675–1680.

225. Bault JP, Salomon LJ, Guibaud L, et al. Role of three-dimensional ultrasound measurement of the optic tract in fetuses with agenesis of the septum pellucidum. *Ultrasound Obstet Gynecol.* 2011;37:570–575.

226. Viñals F, Ruiz P, Correa F, et al. Two-dimensional visualization and measurement of fetal optic chiasm: improving counseling for antenatal diagnosis of agenesis of the septum pellucidum. *Ultrasound Obstet Gynecol.* 2016;48:733–738.

227. Li Y, Sansgiri R, Estroff JA, et al. Outcome of fetuses with cerebral ventriculomegaly and septum pellucidum leaflet abnormalities. *AJR Am J Roentgenol.* 2011;196:W83–W92.

228. Barkovich AJ, Norman D. Absence of the septum pellucidum: a useful sign in the diagnosis of congenital brain malformations. *AJR Am J Roentgenol.* 1989;152:353–360.

229. Belhocine O, Andre C, Kalifa G, et al. Does asymptomatic septal agenesis exist? A review of 34 cases. *Pediatr Radiol.* 2005;35:410–418.

230. Antonini SRR, Filho AG, Elias LLK, et al. Cerebral midline developmental anomalies: endocrine, neuroradiographic and ophthalmological features. *J Pediatr Endocrinol Metab.* 2002;15:1525–1530.

231. Wales JK, Quarrell OW. Evidence for possible Mendelian inheritance of septo-optic dysplasia. *Acta Paediatr.* 1996;85:391–392.

232. Severino M, Tortora D, Pistorio A, et al. Expanding the spectrum of congenital anomalies of the diencephalic—mesencephalic junction. *Neuroradiology.* 2016;58:33–44.

233. Zaki MS, Saleem SN, Dobyns WB, et al. Diencephalic-mesencephalic junction dysplasia: a novel recessive brain malformation. *Brain.* 2012;135:2416–2427.

234. Barkovich AJ, Millen KJ, Dobyns WB. A developmental and genetic classification for midbrain-hindbrain malformations. *Brain.* 2009;132:3199–3230.

235. Guemez-Gamboa A, Calglayna AO, Stanley V, et al. Loss of Protocadherin-12 leads to diencephalic mesencephalic junction dysplasia syndrome. *Ann Neurol.* 2018;84:646–655.

236. Barkovich AJ, Guerrini R, Kuzniecky RI, et al. A developmental and genetic classification for malformations of cortical development: update 2012. *Brain.* 2012;135(5):1348–1369.

237. Razek AAKA, Kandell AY, Elsorogy LG, et al. Disorders of cortical formation: MR imaging features. *AJNR Am J Neuroradiol.* 2009;30:4–11.

238. Manoranjan B, Provias JP. Hemimegalencephaly: a fetal case with neuropathological confirmation and review of the literature. *Acta Neuropathol.* 2010;120:117–130.

239. Tinkle BT, Schorry EK, Franz DN, et al. Epidemiology of hemimegalencephaly: a case series and review. *Am J Med Genet A.* 2005;139(3):204–211.

240. D'Gama AM, Woodworth MB, Hossain AA, et al. Somatic mutations activating the mTOR pathoway in dorsal telencephalic progenitors cause a continuum of cortical dysplasias. *Cell Rep.* 2017;21:3743–3766.

241. Flores-Sarnat L, Sarnat HB, Davila-Gutierrez G, et al. Hemimegalencephaly, part 2: neuropathology suggests a disorder of cellular lineage. *J Child Neurol.* 2003;18:776–785.

242. Baek ST, Gibbs EM, Gleeson JG, et al. Hemimegalencephaly, a paradigm for somatic postzygotic neurodevelopmental disorders. *Curr Opin Neurol.* 2013;26:122–127.

243. Mirzaa GM, Campbell CD, Solovieff N, et al. Association of MTOR mutations with developmental brain disorders, including megalencephaly, focal cortical dysplasia, and pigmentary mosaicism. *JAMA Neurol.* 2016;73(7):836–845.

244. Flores-Sarnat L. Hemimegalencephaly, part I: genetic, clinical and imaging aspects. *J Child Neurol.* 2002;17:373–384.

245. Shrot S, Hwang M, Stafstrom CE, et al. Dysplasia and overgrowth: magnetic resonance imaging of pediatric brain abnormalities secondary to alterations in the mechanistic target of rapamycin pathway. *Neuroradiology.* 2018;60:137–150.

246. Alvarez RM, Garcia-Diaz L, Marquez J, et al. Hemimegalencephaly: prenatal diagnosis and outcome. *Fetal Diagn Ther.* 2011;30:234–238.

247. Hafner E, Bock W, Zoder G, et al. Prenatal diagnosis of unilateral megalencephaly by 2D and 3D ultrasound: a case report. *Prenat Diagn.* 1999;19:159–162.

248. Resit Asolgu M, Higgs A, Esin S, et al. The importance of prenatal 3-dimensional sonography in a case of a segmental overgrowth syndrome with unclear chromosomal microarray results. *J Clin Ultrasound.* 2018;46:351–354.

249. Barkovich AJ, Chuang SH. Unilateral megalencephaly: correlation of MR imaging and pathologic characteristics. *AJNR Am J Neuroradiol.* 1990;11:523–531.

250. Di Rocco C, Battaglia D, Pietrini D, et al. Hemimegalencephaly: clinical implications and surgical treatment. *Childs Nerv Syst.* 2006;22:852–866.

250a. Oluigbo C, Pearl MS, Tsuchida TN, et al. "Endovascular embolic hemispherectomy": a strategy for the initial management of catastrophic holohemispheric epilepsy in the neonate. *Childs Nerv Syst.* 2017;33(3):521–527. doi:10.1007/s00381-016-3289-6.

251. Williams F, Griffith PD. The diagnosis of hemimegalencephaly using in utero MRI. *Clin Radiol.* 2014;69:e291–e297.

252. Sato N, Yagishita A, Oba H, et al. Hemimegalencephaly: a study of abnormalities occurring outside the involved hemisphere. *AJNR Am J Neuroradiol.* 2007;28:678–682.

253. Sasaki M, Hashimoto T, Furushima W, et al. Clinical aspects of hemimegalencephaly by means of a nationwide survey. *J Child Neurol.* 2005;20:337–341.

254. Milunsky A, Ito M, Maher TA, et al. Prenatal molecular diagnosis of tuberous sclerosis complex. *Am J Obstet Gynecol.* 2009;200:321.e1–321.e6.

255. Baskin HJ Jr. The pathogenesis and imaging of the tuberous sclerosis complex. *Pediatr Radiol.* 2008;38:936–952.

256. Gusman M, Servaes S, Feygin T, et al. Multimodal imaging in the prenatal diagnosis of tuberous sclerosis complex. *Case Rep Pediatr.* 2012;2012:925646.

257. Wortmann SB, Reimer A, Creemers JWT, et al. Prenatal diagnosis of cerebral lesions in Tuberous sclerosis complex. Case report and review of the literature. *Eur J Paediatr Neurol.* 2008;12:123–126.

258. Curatolo P, Bombardieri R, Jozwiak S. Tuberous sclerosis. *Lancet.* 2008;372:657–668.

259. Saada J, Rabia SH, Fermont L, et al. Prenatal diagnosis of cardiac rhabdomyomas: incidence of associated cerebral lesions of tuberous sclerosis complex. *Ultrasound Obstet Gynecol.* 2009;34:155–159.

260. Chen J, Wang J, Sun H, et al. Fetal cardiac tumor: echocardiography, clinical outcome and genetic analysis in 53 cases. *Ultrasound Obstet Gynecol.* 2019;54:103–109.

261. Gedikbasi A, Oztarhan K, Ulker V, et al. Prenatal sonographic diagnosis of tuberous sclerosis complex. *J Clin Ultrasound.* 2011;39:427–430.

262. Zhang YX, Meng H, Zhong DR, et al. Cardiac rhabdomyoma and renal cyst in a fetus: early onset of tuberous sclerosis with renal cystic disease. *J Ultrasound Med.* 2008;27:979–982.

263. Bader RS, Chitayat D, Kelly E, et al. Fetal rhabdomyoma: prenatal diagnosis, clinical outcome, and incidence of associated tuberous sclerosis complex. *J Pediatr.* 2003;143:620–624.

264. Northrup H, Krueger DA. Tuberous Sclerosis Complex diagnostic criteria update: recommendations of the 2012 International Tuberous Sclerosis Complex Consensus Conference. *Pediatr Neurol.* 2013;49:243–254.

265. Muhler MR, Rake A, Schwabe M, et al. Value of fetal cerebral MRI in sonographically proven cardiac rhabdomyoma. *Pediatr Radiol.* 2007;37:467–474.

266. Chao AS, Chao A, Wang TH, et al. Outcome of antenatally diagnosed cardiac rhabdomyoma: case series and a meta-analysis. *Ultrasound Obstet Gynecol.* 2008;31:289–295.

267. Sgro M, Barozzimo T, Toi A, et al. Prenatal detection of cerebral lesions in a fetus with tuberous sclerosis. *Ultrasound Obstet Gynecol.* 1999;14:356–359.

268. Sonigo P, Elmaleh A, Fermont L, et al. Prenatal MRI diagnosis of fetal cerebral tuberous sclerosis. *Pediatr Radiol.* 1996;26:1–4.

269. Baron Y, Barkovich A. MR imaging of tuberous sclerosis in neonates and young infants. *AJNR Am J Neuroradiol.* 1999;20:907–916.

270. Rosser T, Panigrahy A, McClintock W. The diverse clinical manifestations of tuberous sclerosis complex: a review. *Semin Pediatr Neurol.* 2006;13:27–36.

271. King JA, Stamilio DM. Maternal and fetal Tuberous sclerosis complicating pregnancy: a case report and overview of the literature. *Am J Perinatol.* 2005;22(2):103–108.

272. Chung CWT, Lawson JA, Sarkozy V, et al. Early detection of Tuberous sclerosis complex: an opportunity for improved neurodevelopmental outcome. *Pediatr Neurol.* 2017;76:20–26.

273. Jansen FE, Vincken KL, Algra A, et al. Cognitive impairment in tuberous sclerosis complex is a multifactorial condition. *Neurology.* 2008;70:916–923.

274. Curatolo P, Nabbout R, Lagae L, et al. Management of epilepsy associated with tuberous sclerosis complex: updated clinical recommendations. *Eur J Pediatr Neurol.* 2018;22:738–748.

275. De Bie I, Boucoiran I. No. 380-Investigation and management of prenatally identified microcephaly. *J Obstet Gynaecol Can.* 2019;380;855–861.

276. Gelber SE, Grumebau A, Chervenak FA. Prenatal screening for microcephaly: an update after three decase. *J Perinat Med.* 2017;45(2):167–170.

277. Sztriha L, Dawodu A, Gururaj A, et al. Microcephaly associated with abnormal gyral pattern. *Neuropediatrics.* 2004;35:346–352.

278. Desidan RS, Barkovich AJ. Malformations of cortical development. *Ann Neurol.* 2016;80:797–810.

279. Adachi Y, Poduri A, Kawaguch A, et al. Congenital microcephaly with a simplified gyral pattern: associated findings and their significance. *AJNR Am J Neuroradiol.* 2011;32:1123–1129.

280. Von Der Hagen M, Pivarcsi M, Liebe J, et al. Diagnostic approach to microcephaly in childhood: a two center study and review of the literature. *Dev Med Child Neurol.* 2014;56:732–741.

281. Den Hollander NS, Wessel MW, Los FJ, et al. Congenital microcephaly detected by prenatal ultrasound: genetic aspects and clinical significance. *Ultrasound Obstet Gynecol.* 2000;15:282–287.

282. Dahlgren L, Wilson RD. Prenatally diagnosed microcephaly: a review of etiologies. *Fetal Diagn Ther.* 2001;16:323–326.

283. Dobyns WB. Primary microcephaly: new approaches for an old disorder. *Am J Med Genet.* 2002;112:315–317.

284. Jaffe M, Tirosh E, Oren S. The dilemma in prenatal diagnosis of idiopathic microcephaly. *Dev Med Child Neurol.* 1987;29:187–189.

285. Society for Maternal-Fetal Medicine Publications Committee. Ultrasound screening for fetal microcephaly following Zika virus exposure. *Am J Obstet Gynecol.* 2016;214(6):B2–B4.

286. Stoler-Poria S, Lev D, Schweiger A, et al. Developmental outcome of the isolated fetal microcephaly. *Ultrasound Obstet Gynecol.* 2010;36:154–158.

287. Bromley B, Benacerraf BR. Difficulties in the prenatal diagnosis of microcephaly. *J Ultrasound Med.* 1995;14:303–305.

288. Leibovitz Z, Daniel-Spiegel E, Malinger G, et al. Prediction of microcephaly at birth using three reference ranges for fetal head circumference: can we improve prenatal diagnosis? *Ultrasound Obstet Gynecol.* 2016;47:586–592.

289. Malinger G, Lerman-Sagie T, Watemberg N, et al. A normal second-trimester ultrasound does not exclude intracranial structural pathology. *Ultrasound Obstet Gynecol.* 2002;20:51–56.

290. Malinger G, Lev D, Lerman-Sagie T. Assessment of fetal intracranial pathologies first demonstrated late in pregnancy: cell proliferation disorders [review]. *Reprod Biol Endocrinol.* 2003;14(1):110.

291. Pilu G, Falco P, Milano V, et al. Prenatal diagnosis of microcephaly assisted by vaginal sonography and power Doppler. *Ultrasound Obstet Gynecol.* 1998; 11:357–360.

292. Persutte WH, Coury A, Hobbins JC. Correlation of fetal frontal lobe transcerebellar diameter measurements: the utility of a new prenatal sonographic technique. *Ultrasound Obstet Gynecol.* 1997;10:94–97.

293. Chibueze EC, Parsons AJQ, da Silva Lopes K, et al. Diagnostic accuracy of ultrasound scanning for prenatal microcephaly in the context of Zika virus infection: a systematic review and meta-analysis. *Sci Rep.* 2017;7:2310.

294. Yaniv G, Katorza E, Tsehmaister Abitbol V, et al. Discrepancy in fetal head biometry between ultrasound and MRI in suspected microcephalic fetuses. *Acta Radiol.* 2017;58(12):1519–1527.

295. Verloes A. Microcephalia vera and microcephaly with simplified gyral pattern. *Orphanet Encyclopedia.* 2004;1–5. http://www.orpha.net/data/patho/GB/uk-MVMSG.pdf.

296. Tao G, Yew DT. Magnetic resonance imaging of fetal brain abnormalities. *Neuroembryol Aging.* 2008;5:49–55.

297. Fogliarini C, Chaumoitre K, Chapon F, et al. Assessment of cortical maturation with prenatal MRI, part II: abnormalities of cortical maturation. *Eur Radiol.* 2005;15:1781–1789.

298. Bahi Buisson N, Poirier K, Fourniol F, et al. The wide spectrum of tubulinopathies: what are the key features for the diagnosis? *Brain.* 2014;137:1676–1700.

299. Abuelo D. Microcephaly syndromes. *Semin Pediatr Neurol.* 2007;14:118–127.

300. Biran-Gol Y, Malinger G, Cohen H, et al. Developmental outcome of isolated fetal macrocephaly. *Ultrasound Obstet Gynecol.* 2010;36:147–153.

301. Baron J, Mastrolia A, Shelef I, et al. Fetal wide subarachnoid space and its outcome in cases of macrocephaly without ventriculomegaly. *J Matern Fetal Neonatal Med.* 2018:1–191.

302. Malinger G, Lev D, Ben-Sira L, et al. Can syndromic macrocephaly be diagnosed in utero? *Ultrasound Obstet Gynecol.* 2011;37:72–81.

303. Toi A, Chitayat D, Blaser S. Abnormalities of the foetal cerebral cortex. *Prenat Diagn.* 2009;29:355–371.

304. Mallerio C, Marignier S, Roth P, et al. Prenatal cerebral ultrasound and MRI findings in glutaric aciduria Type 1: a de novo case. *Ultrasound Obstet Gynecol.* 2008;31:712–714.

305. Williams CA. Macrocephaly syndromes. In: Stalker HJ, ed. *RC Philips Research and Education Unit Newsletter.* 2008;20(1). http://www.peds.ufl.edu/divisions/genetics/newsletters/macrocephaly.pdf.

306. Myers A, Bernstein JA, Brennan ML. Perinatal features of the RASopathies: noonan syndrome, cardiofaciocutaneous syndrome and Costello syndrome. *Am J Med Genet A.* 2014;164A(11):2814–2821.

307. Lerman-Sagie T, Ben-Sira L, Achiron R, et al. Thick fetal corpus callosum: an ominous gin? *Ultra Obstet Gynecol.* 2009;34:55–61.

308. Isaacs H Jr. I: perinatal brain tumors: a review of 250 cases. *Pediatr Neurol.* 2002;27:249–261.

309. Isaacs H Jr. Fetal brain tumors: a review of 154 cases. *Am J Perinatol.* 2009;26: 453–466.

310. Woodward PJ, Sohaey R, Kennedy A, et al. From the archives of the AFIP: a comprehensive review of fetal tumors with pathologic correlation. *Radiographics.* 2005;25:215–242.

311. Schlembach D, Bornemann A, Rupprecht T, et al. Fetal intracranial tumors detected by ultrasound: a report of two cases and review of the literature. *Ultrasound Obstet Gynecol.* 1999;14:407–418.

312. Isaacs H. Perinatal (fetal and neonatal) astrocytoma: a review. *Childs Nerv Syst.* 2016; 32:2086–2096.

313. Louis DN, Perry A, Reifenberger G, et al. The 2016 World Health Organization classification of tumors of the central nervous sytem: a summary. *Acta Neuropathol.* 2016;131(6):803–820.

314. Shekdar DV, Simon Schwartz E. Brain tumors in the neonate. *Neuroimag Clin N Am.* 2017;27:69–83.

315. Crawford JR, Hart I. Perinatal (fetal and neonatal) choroid plexus tumors: a review. *Child's Nervous System.* 2019;35:937–944.

316. Milan HJ, Junior EA, Cavalheiro S, et al. Fetal brain tumors: prenatal diagnosis by ultrasound and magnetic resonance imaging. *World J Radiol.* 2015;28:17–21.

317. Rickert CH. Neuropathology and prognosis of foetal brain tumours. *Acta Neuropathol.* 1999;98:567–576.

318. Sugimoto M, Kurishima C, Satoshi M, et al. Congenital brain tumor within the first 2 months of life. *Pediatr Neonatol.* 2015;56:369–375.

319. Cavalheiro S, Moron AF, Hisaba W, et al. Fetal brain tumors. *Childs Nerv Syst.* 2003;19:529–536.

320. D'Addario V, Pinto V, Meo F, et al. The specificity of ultrasound in the detection of fetal intracranial tumors. *J Perinat Med.* 1998;26:480–485.

321. Cassart M, Bosson N, Garel C, et al. Fetal intracranial tumors: a review of 27 cases. *Eur Radiol.* 2008;18:2060–2066.

322. Vazquez E, Castellote A, Mayolas N, et al. Congenital tumours involving the head, neck and central nervous system. *Pediatr Radiol.* 2009;39:1158–1172.

323. Bloundiaux E, Sileo C, Nahama-Allouche C, et al. Periventricular nodular heterotopia on prenatal ultrasound and magnetic resonance imaging. *Ultrasound Obstet Gynecol.* 2013;42:149–155.

324. Gonzalez G, Vedolin L, Barry B, et al. Location of periventricular nodular heterotopia is related to the malformation phenotype on MRI. *AJNR Am J Neuroradiol.* 2013;34:877–889.

325. Manganaro L, Saldari M, Bernardo S, et al. Bilateral subependymal heterotopia, ventriculomegaly and cerebellar asymmetry: fetal MRI findings of a rare association of brain anomalieis. *J Radiol Case Rep.* 2013;7:38–45.

326. Barkovich AJ, Kuzniecky RI. Gray matter heterotopia. *Neurology.* 2000;55:1603–1608.

327. Barkovich AJ. Morphologic characteristics of subcortical heterotopia: MR imaging study. *AJNR Am J Neuroradiol.* 2000;21:290–295.

328. Parrini E, Ramazzotti A, Dobyns WB, et al. Periventricular heterotopia: phenotypic heterogeneity and correlation with Filamin A mutations. *Brain.* 2006;129:1892–1906.

329. Cellini E, Vetro A, Conti V, et al. Multiple genomic copy number variants associated with periventricular nodular heterotopia indicate extreme genetic heterogeneity. *Eur J Human Genet.* 2019;27:909–918.

330. Poussaint TY, Fox JW, Dobyns WB, et al. Periventricular nodular heterotopia in patients with filamin-1 gene mutations: neuroimaging findings. *Pediatr Radiol.* 2000;30:748–755.

331. Deloison B, Sonigo P, Millischer-Bellaiche AE, et al. Prenatally diagnosed periventricular nodular heterotopia: further delineation of the imaging phenotype and outcome. *Eur J Med Genet.* 2018;61:773–782.

332. Barkovich AJ, Dobyns WB, Guerrini R. Malformations of cortical development and epilepsy. *Cold Spring Harb Perspect Med.* 2015;5:a022392.

333. Nagaraj UD, Peiro JL, Bierbrauer KS, et al. Evaluation of subependymal gray matter heterotopias on fetal MRI. *AJNR Am J Neuroradiol.* 2016;37:720–725.

334. Mitchell LA, Simon EM, Filly RA, et al. Antenatal diagnosis of subependymal heterotopia. *AJNR Am J Neuroradiol.* 2000;21:296–300.

335. Glenn OA, Cuneo AA, Barkovich AJ, et al. Malformations of cortical development: diagnostic accuracy of fetal MR imaging. *Radiology.* 2012;263:843–855.

336. Liu W, Yan B, Xiao J, et al. Sporadic periventricular nodular heterotopia: classification, phenotype and correlation with Filamin A mutations. *Epilepsy Res.* 2017;133:33–40.

337. DiDonato N, Chiari S, Mirzaa GM, et al. Lissencephaly: expanded imaging and clinical classification. *Am J Med Genet A.* 2017;173(6):1473–1488.

338. Ghai S, Fong KW, Toi A, et al. Prenatal US and MR imaging findings of lissencephaly: review of fetal cerebral sulcal development. *Radiographics.* 2006;26:389–405.

339. Barkovich AJ, Chuang SH, Norman D. MR of neuronal migration anomalies. *AJR Am J Roentgenol.* 1988;150:179–187.

340. Dobyns WB, Das S. *LIS1-associated lissencephaly/subcortical band heterotopia.* In: Pagon RA, Adam MP, Bird TD, et al, eds. *GeneReviews* [Internet]. Seattle, WA: University of Washington; 1993–2014.

341. Fry AE, Cushion TD, Pilz DT. The genetics of lissencephaly. *Am J Med Genet Part C Semin Med Genet.* 2014;166C:198–210.

342. Guerrini R, Dobyns WB, Barkovich AJ. Abnormal development of the human cerebral cortex: genetics, functional consequences and treatment options. *Trends Neurosci.* 2088;31(3):154–162.

343. Haverfield EV, Whited AJ, Petras KS, et al. Intragenic deletions and duplications of the LIS1 and DCX genes: a major disease-causing mechanism in lissencephaly and subcortical band heterotopia. *Eur J Hum Genet.* 2009;17:911–918.

344. Abdel Razek AA, Kandell AY, Elsorogy LG, et al. Disorders of cortical formation: MR imaging features. *AJNR Am J Neuroradiol.* 2009;30:4–11.

345. Chen CP, Chang TY, Guo WY, et al. Chromosome 17p13.3 deletion syndrome: aCGH characterization, prenatal findings and diagnosis, and literature review. *Gene.* 2013;532:152–159.

346. Fong KW, Ghai S, Toi A, et al. Prenatal ultrasound findings of lissencephaly associated with Miller-Dieker syndrome and comparison with pre- and postnatal magnetic resonance imaging. *Ultrasound Obstet Gynecol.* 2004;24:716–723.

347. Rolo LC, Araujo E Jr, Nardozza LMM, et al. Development of fetal brain sulci and gyri: assessment through two and three-dimensional ultrasound and magnetic resonance imaging. *Arch Gynecol Obstet.* 2011;283:149–158.

348. Pugash D, Hendson G, Dunham CP, et al. Sonographic assessment of normal and abnormal patterns of fetal cerebral lamination. *Ultrasound Obstet Gynecol.* 2012;40:642–651.

349. Malinger G, Kidron D, Schreiber L, et al. Prenatal diagnosis of malformations of cortical development by dedicated neurosonography. *Ultrasound Obstet Gynecol.* 2007;29:178–191.

350. Barkovich AJ, Koch TK, Carrol CL. The spectrum of lissencephaly: report of ten patients analyzed by magnetic resonance imaging. *Ann Neurol.* 1991;30:139–146.

351. Williams F, Griffiths PD. In utero MR imaging in fetuses at high risk of lissencephaly. *Br J Radiol.* 2017;90(1072):20160902.

352. Righini A, Frassoni C, Inverardi F, et al. Bilateral cavitations of ganglionic eminence: a fetal MR imaging sign of halted brain development. *AJNR Am J Neuroradiol.* 2013;34:1841–1845.

353. Guibaud L, Selleret L, Larroche JC, et al. Abnormal Sylvian fissure on prenatal cerebral imaging: significance and correlation with neuropathological and postnatal data. *Ultrasound Obstet Gynecol.* 2008;32:50–60.

354. Vajsar J, Schacter H. Walker-Warburg syndrome. *Orphanet J Rare Dis.* 2006;1:29–33.

355. Devisme L, Bouchet C, Gonzales M, et al. Cobblestone lissencephaly: neuropathological subtypes and correlations with genes of dystroglycanopathies. *Brain.* 2012;135:469–482.

356. Barkovich AJ. Magnetic resonance imaging: role in the understanding of cerebral malformations. *Brain Dev.* 2002;24:2–12.

357. Brasseur-Daudruy M, Vivier PH, Ickowicz V, et al. Walker-Warburg syndrome diagnosed by findings of typical ocular abnormalities on prenatal ultrasound. *Pediatr Radiol.* 2012;42:488–490.

358. Dobyns WB, Pagon RA, Armstrong D, et al. Diagnostic criteria for Walker-Warburg syndrome. *Am J Med Genet.* 1989;32:195–210.

359. Stroustrup Smith A, Levine D, Barnes PD, et al. Magnetic resonance imaging of the kinked fetal brain stem, a sign of severe dysgenesis. *J Ultrasound Med.* 2005;24:1697–1709.

360. Pabuscu Y, Baulakbasy N, Kocaoglu M, et al. Walker-Warburg syndrome variant. *Comput Med Imaging Graph.* 2002;26:453–458.

361. Barkovich AJ. Neuroimaging manifestations and classification of congenital muscular dystrophies. *AJNR Am J Neuroradiol.* 1998;19:1389–1396.

362. Low ASC, Lee SL, Tan AS, et al. Difficulties with prenatal diagnosis of the Walker-Warburg syndrome. *Acta Radiol.* 2005;46:645–651.

363. Lacalm A, Nadaud B, Massoud M, et al. Prenatal diagnosis of cobblestone lissencephaly associated with Walker-Warburg syndrome based on a specific sonographic pattern. *Ultrasound Obstet Gynecol.* 2016;47:117–122.

364. Widjaja E, Geibprasert S, Blaser S, et al. Abnormal fetal cerebral laminar organization in cobblestone complex as seen on post-mortem MRI and DTI. *Pediatr Radiol.* 2009;39:860–864.

365. Strigini F, Valleriani A, Cecchi M, et al. Prenatal ultrasound and magnetic resonance imaging features in a fetus with Walker-Warburg syndrome [letter]. *Ultrasound Obstet Gynecol.* 2009;33:363–368.

366. Monteagudo A, Alayon A, Mayberry P. Walker-Warburg syndrome: case report and review of the literature. *J Ultrasound Med.* 2001;20:419–426.

367. Stutterd CA, Dobyns WB, Jansen A, et al. Polymicrogyria overview. Gene Reviews [internet]. 2018.

368. Judkins AR, Martinz D, Ferreira P, et al. Polymicrogyria includes fusion of the molecular layer and decreased neuronal populations, but normal cortical laminar organization. *J Neuropath Exp Neurol.* 2011;70(6):438–443.

369. Jansen AC, Robitaille Y, Honavar M, et al. The histopathology of polymicrogyria: a series of 71 brain autopsy studies. *Dev Med Child Neuro.* 2016;58:39–48.

370. Squier W, Jansen A. Polymicrogyria: pathology, fetal origins and mechanisms. *Acta Neuropathol Commun.* 2014;2:80.

371. Diamandis P, Chitayat D, Toi A, et al. The pathology of incipient polymicrogyria. *Brain Dev.* 2017;39:23–39.

372. Leventer RJ, Jansen A, Pilz DT, et al. Clinical and imaging heterogeneity of polymicrogyria: a study of 328 patients. *Brain.* 2010;133:1415–1427.

373. Stutterd CA, Leventer RJ. Polymicrogyria: a common and heterogeneous malformation of cortical development. *Am J Med Genet C Semin Med Genet.* 2014;166C:227–239.

374. Glenn OA, Norton ME, Goldstein RB, et al. Prenatal diagnosis of polymicrogyria by fetal magnetic resonance imaging in monochorionic co-twin death. *J Ultrasound Med.* 2005;24:711–716.

375. Simonazzi G, Segata M, Ghi T, et al. Accurate neurosonographic prediction of a brain injury in the surviving fetus after the death of a monochorionic co-twin. *Ultrasound Obstet Gynecol.* 2006;27:517–521.

376. Jansen A, Andermann E. Genetics of polymicrogyria syndromes. *J Med Genet.* 2005;42:369–378.

377. Barkovich AJ, Peck WW. MR of Zellweger syndrome. *AJNR Am J Neuroradiol.* 1997;18:1163–1170.

378. Mochel F, Grebille AG, Benachi A, et al. Contribution of fetal MR imaging in the prenatal diagnosis of Zellweger syndrome. *AJNR Am J Neuroradiol.* 2006;27:333–336.

379. Dhombres F, Nahama-Allouche C, Gelot A, et al. Prenatal ultrasonographic diagnosis of polymicrogyria. *Ultrasound Obstet Gynecol.* 2008;32:951–954.

380. Delle Urban LA, Righini A, Rustico M, et al. Prenatal ultrasound detection of bilateral focal polymicrogyria. *Prenat Diagn.* 2004;24:808–811.

381. Pooh RK, Machida M, Nakamura T, et al. Increased sylvian fissure angle as early sonographic sign of malformation of cortical development. *Ultrasound Obstet Gynecol.* 2019;54:199–206.

382. Righini A, Parazzini C, Doneda C, et al. Early formative stage of human focal cortical gyration anomalies: fetal MRI. *AJR Am J Roentgenol.* 2012;198:439–447.

383. Righini A, Zirpoli S, Mrakic F, et al. Early prenatal MR imaging diagnosis of polymicrogyria. *AJNR Am J Neuroradiol.* 2004;25:343–346.

384. Hayashi N, Tsutsumi Y, Barkovich AJ. Polymicrogyria without porencephaly/schizencephaly. MRI analysis of the spectrum and the prevalence of macroscopic finding in the clinical population. *Neuroradiology.* 2002;44:647–655.

385. Barkovich AJ. Current concepts of polymicrogyria. *Neuroradiology.* 2010;52:479–487.

386. Barkovich AJ, Hevner R, Guerrini R. Syndromes of bilateral symmetrical polymicrogyria. *AJNR Am J Neuroradiol.* 1999;20:1814–1821.

387. Yakovlev PI, Wadsworth RC. Schizencephalies: a study of the congenital clefts in the cerebral mantle, II: clefts with hydrocephalus and lips separated. *J Neuropathol Exp Neurol.* 1946;5(3):169–206.

388. Curry CJ, Lammer EJ, Nelson V, et al. Schizencephaly: heterogeneous etiologies in a population of 4 million California births. *Am J Med Genet A.* 2005;137(2):181–189.

389. Howe DT, Rankin J, Draper ES. Schizencephaly prevalence, prenatal diagnosis and clues to etiology: a register-based study. *Ultrasound Obstet Gynecol.* 2012;39:75–82.

390. Yoneda Y, Haginoya K, Mitsuhio K, et al. Phenotypic spectrum of COL4A1 mutations: porencephaly to schizencephaly. *Ann Neurol.* 2013;73(1):48–57.

391. Barkovich AJ, Kjos BO. Schizencephaly: correlation of clinical findings with MR characteristics. *AJNR Am J Neuroradiol.* 1992;13:85–94.

392. Hayashi N, Tsutsumi Y, Barkovich AJ. Morphological features and associated anomalies of schizencephaly in the clinical population: detailed analysis of MR images. *Neuroradiology*. 2002;44:418–427.

393. Griffiths PD. Schizencephaly revisited. *Neuroradiology*. 2018;60:945–960.

394. Oh KY, Kennedy AM, Frias AE Jr, et al. Fetal schizencephaly: pre- and post-natal imaging with a review of the clinical manifestations. *Radiographics*. 2005;25:647–657.

395. Khalid R, Krishnan P, Andres K, et al. COL4A1 and fetal vascular origins of schizencephaly. *Neurology*. 2018;90:232–234.

396. Nabavizadeh SA, Zarnow D, Bilaniuk LT, et al. Correlation of prenatal and post-natal MRI findings in schizencephaly. *AJNR Am J Neuroradiol*. 2014;35(7):1418–1424. doi:10.3174/ajnr.A3872.

397. Lee W, Comstock CH, Kazmierczak C, et al. Prenatal diagnostic challenges and pitfalls for schizencephaly. *J Ultrasound Med*. 2009;28:1379–1384.

398. Denis D, Maugey-Laulom B, Carles D, et al. Prenatal diagnosis of schizencephaly by fetal magnetic resonance imaging. *Fetal Diagn Ther*. 2001;16:354–359.

399. Edris F, Kielar A, Fung KFK, et al. Ultrasound and MRI in the antenatal diagnosis of schizencephaly. *J Obstet Gynaecol Can*. 2005;27:864–868.

400. Rios LTM Jr, Araujo E, Nardozza LMM, et al. Prenatal and postnatal schizencephaly findings by 2D and 3D ultrasound: pictorial essay. *J Clin Imaging Sci*. 2012;2:30.

401. Kutuk MS, Gorkem SB, Bayram A, et al. Prenatal diagnosis and postnatal outcome of schizencephaly. *J Child Neurol*. 2015;30(10):1388–1394.

402. Poretti A, Leventer RJ, Cowan FM, et al. Cerebellar cleft: a form of prenatal cerebellar disruption. *Neuropediatrics*. 2008;39:106–112.

403. Raybaud C, Girard N, Levrier O, et al. Schizencephaly: correlation between the lobar topography of the cleft(s) and absence of the septum pellucidum. *Childs Nerv Syst*. 2001;17:217–222.

404. Braga VL, da Costa MDS, Riera R, et al. Schizencephaly: a review of 734 patients. *Pediatr Neurol*. 2018;86:23–29.

405. Hung JH, Shen SH, Guo WY, et al. Prenatal diagnosis of schizencephaly with septo-optic dysplasia by ultrasound and magnetic resonance imaging. *J Obstet Gynaecol Res*. 2008;34:674–679.

406. Lituania M, Passamonti U. Prenatal ultrasound: brain. In: Raybaud C, Paolo TD, Rossi A, eds. *Pediatric Neuroradiology*. Heidelberg, Germany: Springer Berlin; 2005:1157–1218.

407. Garel C, Delezoide AL, Elmaleh-Berges M, et al. Contribution of fetal MR imaging in the evaluation of cerebral ischemic lesions. *AJNR Am J Neuroradiol*. 2004;25:1563–1568.

408. Cavallin M, Mine M, Philbert M, et al. Further refinement of COL4A1 and COL4A2 related cortical malformations. *Eur J Med Genet*. 2018;61:765–772.

409. Govaert P. Prenatal stroke. *Semin Fetal Neonatal Med*. 2009;14:250–266.

410. Grant EG, Kerner M, Schellinger D, et al. Evolution of porencephalic cysts from intraparenchymal hemorrhage in neonates: sonographic evidence. *AJR Am J Roentgenol*. 1982;138:467–470.

411. Gul A, Gungorduk K, Yildirm G, et al. Prenatal diagnosis of porencephaly secondary to maternal carbon monoxide poisoning. *Arch Gynecol Obstet*. 2009;279:697–700.

412. Eiler KM, Kuller JA. Fetal porencephaly: a review of the etiology, diagnosis and prognosis. *Obstet Gynecol Surv*. 1995;50:684–687.

413. Sato T, Kato M, Moriyama K, et al. A case of tubulinopathy presenting with porencephaly caused by a novel missense mutation in the TUBA1A gene. *Brain Dev*. 2018;40:819–823.

414. Berg RA, Aleck KA, Kaplan AM. Familial porencephaly. *Arch Neurol*. 1983;40:567–569.

415. Sato Y, Shibasaki J, Aida N, et al. Novel COL4A1 mutation in a fetus with early prenatal onset of schizencephaly. *Hum Genome Var*. 2018;5:4.

416. Vitale G, Pichiecchio A, Ormitti F, et al. Cortical malformations and COL4A1 mutation: three new cases. *Eur J Paediatr Neurol*. 2019; 23:410–417.

417. Ho SS, Kuzniecky RI, Gilliam F, et al. Congenital porencephaly: MR features and relationship to hippocampal sclerosis. *AJNR Am J Neuroradiol*. 1998;19:135–141.

418. Quek YW, Su PH, Tsao TF, et al. Hydranencephaly associated with interruption of bilateral internal carotid arteries. *Pediatr Neonatol*. 2008;49:43–47.

419. Taori KB, Sargar KM, Disawal A, et al. Hydranencephaly associated with cerebellar involvement and bilateral microphthalmia and colobomas. *Pediatr Radiol*. 2011;41:270–273.

420. Byers BD, Barth WH, Stewart TL, et al. Ultrasound and MRI appearance and evolution of hydranencephaly in utero. *J Reprod Med*. 2005;50:53–56.

421. Myers RE. Brain pathology following fetal vascular occlusion: an experimental study. *Invest Ophthalmol*. 1969;8:41–50.

422. Cecchetto G, Milanese L, Giordano R, et al. Looking at the missing brain: hydranencephaly case series and literature review. *Pediatr Neurol*. 2013;48:152–158.

423. Greene MF, Benacerraf B, Crawford JM. Hydranencephaly: US appearance during in utero evolution. *Radiology*. 1985;156:779–780.

424. Edmondson SR, Hallak M, Carpenter RJ Jr, et al. Evolution of hydranencephaly following intracerebral hemorrhage. *Obstet Gynecol*. 1992;79:870–871.

425. Pavone P, Pratico AD, Vitaliti G, et al. Hydranencephaly: cerebral spinal fluid instead of cerebral mantles. *Italian J Pediatr*. 2014;40:79.

426. Dixon A. Hydranencephaly. *Radiography*. 1998;54:12–13.

427. Kline-Fath BM, Merrow AC Jr, Calvo-Garcia MA, et al. Fowler Syndrome and fetal MRI findings: a genetic disorder mimicking hydranencephaly/hydrocephalus. *Pediatr Radiol*. 2018;48(7):1032–1034.

428. Williams D, Patel C, Fallet-Bianco C, et al. Fowler syndrome: a clinical, radiological, and pathological study of 14 cases. *Am J Med Genet A*. 2010;152A:153–160.

429. Laurichesse-Delmas H, Beaufrere AM, Martin A, et al. First-trimester features of Fowler syndrome (hydrocephaly-hydranencephaly proliferative vasculopathy). *Ultrasound Obstet Gynecol*. 2002;20:612–615.

430. Lam YH, Tang HY. Serial sonographic features of a fetus with hydranencephaly from 11 weeks to term. *Ultrasound Obstet Gynecol*. 2000;16:77–79.

431. Sepulveda W, Cortes-Yepes H, Wong AE, et al. Prenatal sonography in hydranencephaly, findings during the early stages of disease. *J Ultrasound Med*. 2012;31:799–804.

432. Usta IM, AbuMusa AA, Khoury NG, et al. Early ultrasonographic changes in Fowler syndrome features and review of the literature. *Prenat Diagn*. 2005;25:1019–1023.

433. Aguirre Vila-Coro A, Dominguez R. Intrauterine diagnosis of hydranencephaly by magnetic resonance. *Magn Reson Imaging*. 1989;7:105–107.

434. Merker B. Editorial: life expectancy in hydranencephaly. *Clin Neurol Neurosurg*. 2008;110:213–214.

435. Bats AS, Molho M, Senat MV, et al. Subependymal pseudocysts in the fetal brain: prenatal diagnosis of two cases and review of the literature. *Ultrasound Obstet Gynecol*. 2002;20:502–505.

436. Malinger G, Lev D, Sira LB, et al. Congenital periventricular pseudocysts: prenatal sonographic appearance and clinical implications. *Ultrasound Obstet Gynecol*. 2002;20:447–451.

437. Cevey-Macherel M, Forcada M, Bickle Graz M, et al. Neurodevelopment outcome of newborns with cerebral subependymal pseudocysts at 18 and 46 months: a prospective study. *Arch Dis Child*. 2013;98:497–502.

438. Correa F, Lara C, Carreras E, et al. Evolution of fetal subependymal cysts throughout gestation. *Fetal Diagn Ther*. 2013;34:127–130.

439. Shackelford GD, Fulling KH, Glasier CM. Cysts of the subependymal germinal matrix: sonographic demonstration with pathologic correlation. *Radiology*. 1983;149:117–121.

440. Epelman M, Daneman A, Blaser SI, et al. Differential diagnosis of intracranial cystic lesions at head US: correlation with CT and MR imaging. *Radiographics*. 2006;26:173–196.

441. Makhoul IR, Zmora O, Tamir A, et al. Congenital subependymal pseudocysts: own data and meta-analysis of the literature. *Isr Med Assoc J*. 2001;3:178–183.

442. Yang M, Jiang Y, Chen Q, et al. Prenatal diagnosis and prognosis of isolated subependymal cysts: a retrospective cohort study. *Prenat Diagn*. 2017;37:1322–1326.

443. Esteban H, Blondiaux E, Audureau E, et al. Prenatal features of isolated subependymal pseudocysts associated with adverse pregnancy outcome. *Ultrasound Obstet Gynecol*. 2015;46:678–687.

444. Fernandez Alvarez JR, Arness PN, Gandhi RS, et al. Diagnostic value of subependymal pseudocysts and choroid plexus cysts on neonatal cerebral ultrasound: a meta-analysis. *Arch Dis Child Fetal Neonatal Ed*. 2009;94:F443–F446.

445. Larcos G, Gruenewald SM, Lui K. Neonatal subependymal cysts detected by sonography: prevalence, sonographic findings, and clinical significance. *AJR Am J Roentgenol*. 1994;162:953–956.

446. Cooper S, Bar-Yosef O, Berkenstadt M, et al. Prenatal evaluation, imaging features and neurodevelopmental outcome of prenatally diagnosed periventricular pseudocysts. *AJRN Am J Neuroradiol*. 2016;37:2382–2388.

447. Chang H, Tsai CM, Hou CY, et al. Multiple subependymal pseudocyst in neonates play a role in later attention deficit hyperactivity and autistic spectrum disorder. *J Formos Med Assoc*. 2019;118:692–169.

448. Egloff C, de Pecoulas AE, Mechler C, et al. Prenatal sonographic description of fetuses affected by pyruvate dehydrogenase or pyruvate carboxylase deficiency. *Prenat Diagn*. 2018;38:607–616.

449. Prasad AN, Malinger G, Lerman-Sagie T. Primary disorders of metabolism and disturbed fetal brain development. *Clin Perinatol*. 2009;36:621–638.

450. Nissenkorn A, Michelson M, Ben-Zeev B, et al. Inborn errors of metabolims. A cause of abnormal brain development. *Neurology*. 2001;45:1265–1272.

451. Von Kleist-Retzow JC, Cormer-Daire V, Viot G, et al. Antenatal manifestations of mitochondrial respiratory chain deficiency. *J Pediatr*. 2003;143(2):208–212.

452. Prasad AN, Bunzeluck K, Prasad C, et al. Agenesis of the corpus callosum and cerebral anomalies in inborn errors of metabolism. *Congenit Anom*. 2007;47:125–135.

453. Guibaud L, Collardeau-Frachon S, Lacalm A, et al. Antenatal manifestations of inborn errors of metabolism: prenatal imaging findings. *J Inherit Metab Dis*. 2017;40:103–112.

454. Robinson JN, Norwitz ER, Mulkern R, et al. Prenatal diagnosis of pyruvate dehydrogenase deficiency using magnetic resonance imaging. *Prenat Diagn*. 2001;21:1053–1056.

455. Natarajan N, Tully HM, Chapman T. Prenatal presentation of pyruvate dehydrogenase complex deficiency. *Pediatr Radiol*. 2016;46(9):1354–1357.

456. Bale JF. Fetal infections and brain development. *Clin Perinatolog*. 2009; 36:639–653.

457. Frenkel LD, Gomez F, Sabahi F. The pathogenesis of microcephaly resulting from congenital infections: why is my baby's head so small? *Eur J Clin Micorbiol Infect Dis*. 2019;47:209–226.

458. Paton MCB, McDonald CA, Alilison BJ, et al. Perinatal brain injury as a consequence of preterm birth and intrauterine inflammation: designing target stem cell therapies. *Front Neurosci*. 2017;11:200.

459. Ostrander B, Bale JR. Congenital and perinatal infections. *Handb Clin Neurol*. 2019;162:133–153.

460. Devakumar D, Bamfor A, Ferreira MU, et al. Infectious causes of microcephaly: epidemiology, pathogenesis, diagnosis and management. *Lancet Infect Dis*. 2018;18(1):e1–e13.

461. Neuberger I, Garcia J, Meyers M, et al. Imaging of congenital central nervous system infections. *Pediatr Radiol*. 2018;48:513–523.

462. Maissonneuve E, Garel C, Friszer S, et al. Fetal brain injury associated with Parvovirus B19 congenital infection requiring intrauterine transfusion. *Fetal Diagn Ther*. 2019;46:1–11.

463. Levine D, Jani JC, Castro-Aragon I, et al. How does imaging of congenital Zika compare with imaging of other TORCH infections? *Radiology.* 2017;285(3):744–761.

464. Dogan Y, Yuksel A, Kalelioglus IH, et al. Intracranial ultrasound abnormalities and fetal cytomegalovirus infection: report of 8 cases and review of the literature. *Fetal Diagn Ther.* 2010;39:141–149.

465. Malinger G, Lev D, Lerman-Sagie T. Imaging of fetal cytomegalovirus infection. *Fetal Diagn Ther.* 2011;29:117–126.

466. Malinger G, Lev D, Zahalka N, et al. Fetal cystomegalovirus infection of the brain: the spectrum of sonographic findings. *AJNR.* 2003;24:28–32.

467. Doneda C, Parazzini C, Righini A, et al. Early cerebral lesions in cytomegalovirus infection: prenatal MR imaging. *Radiology.* 2010;255(2):613–621.

468. Barkovich Aj, Girad N. Fetal brain infections. *Childs Nerv Syst.* 2003;19:501–507.

469. Katorza E, Strauss G, Cohen R, et al. Apparent diffusion coefficient levels and neurodevelopmental outcome in fetuses with brain MR imagin white matter hyperintense signal. *AJNR Am J Neuroradiol.* 2018;39(10):1926–1931.

470. Kotovich D, Guedalia JSB, Hoffman C, et al. Apparent diffusion coefficient value cahges and clinical correlation in 90 cases of cytomegalovirus-infected fetuses with unremarkable feteal MRI results. *AJNR Am J Neuroradiol.* 2017;28(7):1443–1448.

471. Stephenson JBP. Aicardi-Goutieres syndrome. *Eur J Paediatr Neurol.* 2008;12:355–358.

472. Crow YJ. Type 1 interferonopathies: Mendelian type 1 interferon up-regulation. *Curr Opin Immunol.* 2015;32:7–12.

473. Cannie MM, Devlieger R, Leyder M, et al. Congenital cytomegalovirus infection: contribution and best timing of prenatal MR imaging. *Eur Radiol.* 2016;26:3760–3769.

474. Grinber A, Katorza E, Hoggman D, et al. Volumetric MRI study of the brain in fetuses with intrauterine cytomegalovirus infection and its correlation to neurodevelopmental outcome. *AJNR Am J Neuroradiol.* 2019;40(2):353–358.

475. Cortes MS, Rivera AM, Yepez M, et al Clinical assessment and brain findings in a cohort of mothers, fetuses and infants infected with Zika virus. *Am J Obstet Gynecol.* 2018;129(4):440.e1–440.e36.

476. Mulkey SB, Bulas DI, Vezina G. Sequential neuroimaging of the fetus and newborn with in utero Zika virus exposure. *JAMA Pediatr.* 2019;173(3):52–59.

477. Elchalal U, Yagel S, Gomori JM, et al. Fetal intracranial hemorrhage (fetal stroke): does grade matter. *Ultrasound Obstet Gynecol.* 2005;26:233–243.

478. Vergani P, Strobelt N, Locatelli A, et al. Clinical significance of fetal intracranial hemorrhage. *Am J Obstet Gynecol.* 1996;175:536–543.

479. Cheung KW, Tan LN, Seto MTY, et al. Prenatal diagnosis, management and outcome of fetal subdural haematoma: a case report and systematic review. *Fetal Diag Ther.* 2019;46(5):1–11.

480. Fajersztajn L, Veras MM. Review article hypoxia: from placental development to fetal programming. *Birth Defects Res.* 2017;109:1377–1385.

481. Redline RW. Severe fetal placental vascular lesions in term infants with neurologic impairment. *Am J Obstet Gynecol.* 2005;192:452–457.

482. Dhillon SK, Lear CA, Galinsky R, et al. The fetus at the tipping point: modifying the outcome of fetal asphyxia. *J Physio.* 2018;23:5571–5592.

483. Brunel H, Girard N, Confort-Gouny S, et al. Fetal brain injury. *J Neuroradiol.* 2004;31:123–137.

484. Girard N, Gire C, Sigaudy S, et al. MR imaging of acquired fetal brain disorders. *Childs Nerv Syst.* 2003;19:490–500.

485. Ghi T, Simonazzi G, Perolo A, et al. Outcome of antenatally diagnosed intracranial hemorrhage: case series and review of the literature. *Ultrasound Obstet Gynecol.* 2003;21:121–130.

486. Ozduman K, Pober BR, Barnes P, et al. Fetal stroke. *Pediatr Neurol.* 2004;30:151–162.

487. Sanopo L, Whitehead MT, Bulas DI, et al. Fetal intracranial hemorrhage: role of fetal MRI. *Prenatal Diagn.* 2017;37:827–836.

488. Kirkham FJ, Zafeiriou D, Howe D, et al. Fetal stroke and cerebrovascular disease advances in understanding from lenticulostriate and venous imaging, alloimmune thrombocytopaenia and monochorionic twins. *Eur J Paediatr Neurol.* 2018;22:989–1005.

489. Adiego B, Martínez-Ten PM, Bermejo C, et al. Fetal intracranial hemorrhage. Prenatal diagnosis and postnatal outcomes. *J Matern Fetal Neonatal Med.* 2019;32(1):21–30.

490. Sherer DM, Anyaebunam A, Onyeije C. Antepartum fetal intracranial hemorrhage, predisposing factors and prenatal sonography: a review. *Am J Perinatol.* 1998;15:431–441.

491. Sharif I, Kuban K. Prenatal intracranial hemorrhage and neurologic complications in alloimmune thrombocytopenia. *J Child Neurol.* 2001;16:838–842.

492. Zdravic D, Yougbare I, Vadasz B, et al. Fetal and neonatal alloimmune thrombocytopenia. *Semin Fetal Neonatal Med.* 2016;21:19–27.

493. Dubinsky T, Lau M, Powell F, et al. Predicting poor neonatal outcome: a comparative study of noninvasive antenatal testing methods. *AJR Am J Roentgenol.* 1997;168:827–831.

494. de Laveaucoupet J, Audibert F, Guis F, et al. Fetal magnetic resonance imaging (MRI) of ischemic brain injury. *Prenat Diagn.* 2001;21:729–736.

495. Huang YF, Chen WC, Tseng JJ, et al. Fetal intracranial hemorrhage (fetal stroke): report of four antenatally diagnosed cases and review of the literature. *Taiwan J Obstet Gynecol.* 2006;45:135–141.

496. Muench MV, Zheng M, Bilica PM, et al. Prenatal diagnosis of a fetal epidural hematoma using 2- and 3-dimensional sonography and magnetic resonance imaging. *J Ultrasound Med.* 2008;27:1369–1373.

497. De Spirlet M, Goffinet F, Philippe HJ, et al. Prenatal diagnosis of a subdual hematoma associated with reverse flow in the middle cerebral artery: case report and literature review. *Ultrasound Obstet Gynecol.* 2000;16:72–76.

498. Hines N, Mehta T, Romero J, et al. What is the clinical importance of echogenic material in the fetal frontal horns? *J Ultrasound Med.* 2009;28:1629–1637.

499. Burstein J, Papile LA, Burstein R. Intraventricular hemorrhage and hydrocephalus in premature newborns: a prospective study with CT. *AJR Am J Roentgenol.* 1979;132:621–635.

500. Groothuis AMC, de Kleine MJK, Guid Oei S. Intraventricular haemorrhage in utero: a case report and review of the literature. *Eur J Obstet Gynecol Reprod Biol.* 2000;89:207–211.

501. Martino F, Malova M, Cesaretti C, et al. Prenatal MR imaging features of isolated cerebellar haemorrhagic lesions. *Eur Radiol.* 2016;26:2685–2696.

502. Hayashi M, Poretti A, Gorra M, et al Prenatal cerebellar hemorrhage: fetal and postnatal neuroimaging findings and postnatal outcome. *Pediatr Neurol.* 2015;52:529–534.

503. Fleischer AC, Hutchison AA, Bundy AL, et al. Serial sonography of posthemorrhagic ventricular dilatation and porencephaly after intracranial hemorrhage in the preterm neonate. *AJNR Am J Neuroradiol.* 1983;4:971–975.

504. Prayer D, Brugger PC, Kasprian G, et al. MRI of fetal acquired brain lesions. *Eur J Radiol.* 2006;57:233–249.

505. Bouchghoul H, Quelin C, Loget P, et al. Fetal cerebral hemorrhage due to X-linked GATA1 gene mutation. *Prenat Diagn.* 2018;38:772–778.

506. Folkerth RD, McLaughlin ME, Levine D. Organizing posterior fossa hematomas simulating developmental cysts on prenatal imaging, report of three cases. *J Ultrasound Med.* 2001;20:1233–1240.

507. Rios LTM, Araujo E Jr, Nardozza LMM, et al. Hidden maternal autoimmune thrombocytopenia complicated by fetal subdural hematoma, case report and review of the literature. *Childs Nerv Syst.* 2012;28:1113–1116.

508. Guimiot F, Garel C, Fallet-Bianco C, et al. Contribution of diffusion-weighted imaging in the evaluation of diffuse white matter ischemic lesions in fetuses: correlation with fetopathologic findings. *AJNR Am J Neuroradiol.* 2008;29: 110–115.

509. Strigini FAL, Cioni G, Canapicchi R, et al. Fetal intracranial hemorrhage: is minor maternal trauma a possible pathogenetic factor? *Ultrasound Obstet Gynecol.* 2001;18:335–342.

510. Winkelhorst D, Kamphuis MM, Steggerda SJ, et al. Perinatal outcome and long term neurodevelopment after intracranial haemorrhage due to fetal and neonatal alloimmune thrombocytopenia. *Fetal Diagn Ther.* 2019;45:184–191.

511. DiPietro JA, Cristofalo EA, Voegtline KM, et al. Isolated prenatal choroid plexus cysts do not affect child development. *Prenat Diagn.* 2011;31:745–749.

512. Achiron R, Barkai G, Katznelson BM, et al. Fetal lateral ventricle choroid plexus cysts: the dilemma of amniocentesis. *Obstet Gynecol.* 1991;78:815–818.

513. Kraus I, Jirasek JE. Some observations of the structure of the choroid plexus and its cysts. *Prenat Diagn.* 2002;22:1223–1228.

514. Zafar HM, Ankola A, Coleman B. Ultrasound pitfalls and artifacts related to six common fetal findings. *Ultrasound Q.* 2012;28:105–124.

515. Yhoshu E, Mahajan JK, Singh UB. Choroid plexus cysts—antenatal course and postnatal outcome in a tertiary hospital in North India. *Childs Nerv Syst.* 2018;24:2449–2453.

516. Turner SR, Samei E, Hertzberg BS, et al. Sonography of fetal choroid plexus cysts. *J Ultrasound Med.* 2003;22:1219–1227.

517. Morcos CL, Platt LD, Carlson DE, et al. The isolated choroid plexus cyst. *Obstet Gynecol.* 1998;92:232–236.

518. Sullivan A, Giudice T, Vavelidis F, et al. Choroid plexus cysts: is biochemical testing a valuable adjunct to targeted ultrasonography. *Am J Obstet Gynecol.* 1999;181:260–265.

519. Becker S, Niemann G, Schoning M, et al. Clinically significant persistence and enlargement of an antenatally diagnosed isolated choroid plexus cyst. *Ultrasound Obstet Gynecol.* 2002;20:620–622.

520. Norton KI, Rai B, Desai AT, et al. Prevalence of choroid plexus cysts in term and near-term infants with congenital heart disease. *AJR Am J Roentgenol.* 2011;196:W326–W329.

521. Bernier FP, Crawford SG, Dewey D. Developmental outcome of children who had choroid plexus cysts detected prenatally. *Prenat Diagn.* 2005;25:322–326.

522. Lopez JA, Reich D. Choroid plexus cysts. *J Am Board Fam Med.* 2006;19:422–425.

523. Ghidini A, Strobelt N, Locatelli A, et al. Isolated fetal choroid plexus cysts: role of ultrasonography in establishment of the risk of trisomy 18. *Am J Obstet Gynecol.* 2000;812:972–977.

524. Zhang S, Lei C, Wu J, et al A retrospective study of cytogenetic results from amniotic fluid in 5328 fetuses with abnormal obstetric sonographic findings. *J Ultrasound Med.* 2017;46:1809–1817.

525. Gupta JK, Cave M, Lilford RJ, et al. Clinical significance of fetal choroid plexus cysts. *Lancet.* 1995;346:724–729.

526. Reinsch RC. Choroid plexus cysts—association with trisomy: prospective review of 16,059 patients. *Am J Obstet Gynecol.* 1997;176:1381–1383.

527. Chen CP. Prenatal diagnosis of arachnoid cysts. *Taiwan J Obstet Gynecol.* 2007;46:187–198.

528. Pradilla G, Jallo G. Arachnoid cysts: case series and review of the literature. *Neurosurg Focus.* 2007;22:1–4.

529. Pierre-Kahn A, Hanlo P, Sonigo P, et al. The contribution of prenatal diagnosis to the understanding of malformative intracranial cysts: state of the art. *Childs Nerv Syst.* 2000;16:618–626.

530. Pilu G, Falco P, Perolo A, et al. Differential diagnosis and outcome of fetal intracranial hypoechoic lesions: report of 21 cases. *Ultrasound Obstet Gynecol.* 1997;9:229–236.

531. Yin L, Yang Z, Pan Q, et al. Sonographic diagnosis and prognosis of fetal arachnoid cysts. *J Clin Ultrasound*. 2018;46:96–102.

532. Gedikbasi A, Palabiyik F, Oztarhan A, et al. Prenatal diagnosis of a suprasellar arachnoid cyst with 2- and 3-dimensional sonography and fetal magnetic resonance imaging: difficulties in management and review of the literature. *J Ultrasound Med*. 2010;29:1487–1493.

533. Blaicher W, Prayer D, Kuhle S, et al. Combined prenatal ultrasound and magnetic resonance imaging in two fetuses with suspected arachnoid cysts. *Ultrasound Obstet Gynecol*. 2001;18:166–168.

534. Youssef A, D'Antonio F, Khalil A, et al. Outcome of fetuses with supratentorial extra-axial intracranial cysts: a systematic review. *Fetal Diagn Ther*. 2016;40:1–12.

535. Booth TN, Timmons C, Shapiro K, et al. Pre- and postnatal MR imaging of hypothalamic hamartomas associated with arachnoid cysts. *AJNR Am J Neuroradiol*. 2004;25:1283–1285.

536. Blasi I, Henrich W, Argento C, et al. Prenatal diagnosis of a cavum veli interpositi. *J Ultrasound Med*. 2009;28:683–687.

537. Barjot P, von Theobald P, Refahi N, et al. Diagnosis of arachnoid cysts on prenatal ultrasound. *Fetal Diagn Ther*. 1999;14:306–309.

538. Hayward R. Postnatal management and outcome for fetal-diagnosed intra-cerebral cystic masses and tumours. *Prenat Diagn*. 2009;29:396–401.

539. Borha A, Ponte KF, Emery E. Cavum septum pellucidum cyst in children: a case-based update. *Childs Nerv Syst*. 2012;28:813–819.

540. Kojder K. Clinical and radiological characteristics of the cyst of the septum pellucidum in endoscopically treated patients. *Pom J Life Sci*. 2015;61:12–33.

541. Scoffings DJ, Kurian KM. Congenital and acquired lesions of the septum pellucidum. *Clin Radiol*. 2008;63:210–219.

542. Krejčí T, Vacek P, Krejčí O, et al. Symptomatic cysts of the cavum epti pollucidi, cavum vergae and cavum veli interpositi: a retrospective duocentric study of 10 patients. *Clin Neurol Neurosurg*. 2019;185:105494.

543. Sarwar M. The septum pellucidum: normal and abnormal. *AJNR Am J Neuroradiol*. 1989;10:989–1005.

544. Mott SH, Bodensteiner JB, Allan WC. The cavum septi pellucidi in term and preterm newborn infants. *J Child Neurol*. 1992;7:35–38.

545. Hicdonmez T, Suslu HT, Butuc R, et al. Treatment of a large and symptomatic septum pellicidum cyst with endoscopic fenestration in a child: case report and review of the literature. *Clin Neurol Neurosurg*. 2012;114:1052–1056.

546. Bronshtein M, Weiner Z. Prenatal diagnosis of dilated cava septi pellucidi et vergae: associated anomalies, differential diagnosis, and pregnancy outcome. *Obstet Gynecol*. 1992;80:838–842.

547. Vergani P, Locatelli A, Piccoli MG, et al. Ultrasonographic differential diagnosis of fetal intracranial interhemispheric cysts. *Am J Obstet Gynecol*. 1999;180:423–428.

548. Osborn AG, Preece MT. Intracranial cysts: radiologic-pathologic correlation and imaging approach. *Radiology*. 2006;239:650–664.

549. Robles LA, Paez J, Auala D, et al. Intracranial glioependymal (neuroglial) cysts: a systemic review. *Acta Neurochir (Wien)*. 2018;160:1439–1449.

550. Tange Y, Aoki A, Mori K, et al. Interhemispheric glioependymal cyst associated with agenesis of the corpus callosum, case report. *Neurol Med Chir (Tokyo)*. 2000;40:536–542.

551. Moriyama E, Nishida A, Sonobe H. Interhemispheric multilocated ependymal cyst with dysgenesis of the corpus callosum: a case in a preterm fetus. *Childs Nerv Syst*. 2007;23:807–813.

552. Muhler MR, Hartmann C, Werner W, et al. Fetal MRI demonstrates glioependymal cyst in a case of sonographic unilateral ventriculomegaly. *Pediatr Radiol*. 2007;37:391–395.

553. Uematsu Y, Kubo K, Nishibayashi T, et al. Interhemispheric neuroepithelial cyst associated with agenesis of the corpus callosum. *Pediatr Neurosurg*. 2000;33:31–36.

554. Pelkey TJ, Ferguson JE, Veille JC, et al. Giant glioependymal cyst resembling holoprosencephaly on prenatal ultrasound: case report and review of the literature. *Ultrasound Obstet Gynecol*. 1997;9:200–203.

555. Deloison B, Chalouhi GE, Sonigo P, et al. Hidden mortality of prenatally diagnosed vein of Galen aneurysmal malformation: retrospective study and review of the literature. *Ultrasound Obstet Gynecol*. 2012;40:652–658.

556. Paladini D, Deloison B, Rossi A, et al. Vein of Galen aneurysmal malformation in the fetus: retrospective analysis of perinatal prognostic indicators in a two-center series of 49 cases. *Ultrasound Obstet Gynecol*. 2017;50:192–199.

557. Brunelle F. Arteriovenous malformation of the vein of Galen malformation in children. *Pediatr Radiol*. 1997;27:501–513.

558. Alvarez H, Garcia Monaco R, Rodesch G, et al. Vein of Galen aneurysmal malformation. *Neuroimaging Clin N Am*. 2007;17:189–206.

559. Lasjaunias PL, Chng SM, Sachet M, et al. The management of Vein of Galen aneurysmal malformation. *Neurosurgery*. 2006;59(5)(suppl 3):S184–S194.

560. Duran D, Zeng X, Jin SC, et al. Mutations in chromatin modifier and Ephrin signaling genes in vein of Galen malformation. *Neuron*. 2019;101:429–443.

561. Zeng X, Hunt A, Jin SC, et al. EphrinB2-EphB4-RASA1 signaling in human cerebrovascular development and disease. *Trends Mol Med*. 2019;25(4):265–286.

562. Sepulveda W, Platt CC, Fisk NM. Prenatal diagnosis of cerebral arteriovenous malformation using color Doppler ultrasonography: case report and review of the literature. *Ultrasound Obstet Gynecol*. 1995;6:282–286.

563. Heling KS, Chaoui R, Bollmann R. Prenatal diagnosis of an aneurysm of the vein of Galen with three-dimensional color power angiography. *Ultrasound Obstet Gynecol*. 2000;15:333–336.

564. Ruano R, Benachi A, Aubry MC, et al. Perinatal three-dimensional color power Doppler ultrasonography of vein of Galen of aneurysms. *J Ultrasound Med*. 2003;22:1357–1362.

565. Lee TH, Shih JC, Peng SSF, et al. Prenatal depiction of angioarchitecture of an aneurysm of the vein of Galen with three-dimensional color power angiography. *Ultrasound Obstet Gynecol*. 2000;15:337–340.

566. Yuval Y, Lerner A, Lipitz S, et al. Prenatal diagnosis of vein of Galen aneurysmal malformation: report of two cases with proposal for prognostic indices. *Prenat Diagn*. 1997;17:972–977.

567. Patermoster DM, Manganelli F, Moroder W, et al. Prenatal diagnosis of vein of Galen aneurysmal malformations. *Fetal Diagn Ther*. 2003;18:408–411.

568. Kosla K, Majos M, Polguj M, et al. Prenatal diagnosis of a vein of Galen aneurysmal malformation with MR imaging, report of two cases. *Pol J Radiol*. 2013;78:88–92.

569. Kurihara N, Tokieda K, Ikeda K, et al. Prenatal MR findings in a case of aneurysm of the vein of Galen. *Pediatr Radiol*. 2001;31:160–162.

570. Heuer GG, Gabel B, Beslow LA, et al. Diagnosis and treatment of vein of Galen aneurysmal malformations. *Childs Nerv Syst*. 2010;26:879–887.

571. Barbosa M, Mahadevan J, Weon YC, et al. Dural sinus malformations (DSM) with giant lakes, in neonates and infants, review of 30 consecutive cases. *Interv Neuroradiol*. 2003;9:407–424.

572. Komiyama M, Ishiguro T, Kitano S, et al. Serial antenatal sonographic observation of cerebral dural sinus malformation. *AJNR Am J Neuroradiol*. 2004;25:1446–1448.

573. Garel C, Azarian M, Lasajaunias P, et al. Pial arteriovenous fistulas: dilemmas in prenatal diagnosis, counseling and postnatal treatment. Report of three cases. *Ultrasound Obstet Gynecol*. 2005;26:293–296.

574. Rodesch G, Hui F, Alvarez H, et al. Prognosis of antenatally diagnosed vein of Galen aneurysmal malformations. *Childs Nerv Syst*. 1994;10:79–83.

575. Berenstein A, Paramasivam S, Sorscher M, et al. Vein of Galen aneurysmal malformation: advance in management and endovascular treatment. *Neurosurgery*. 2019;84 (2):469–478.

576. Kush ML, Weiner CP, Harman CR, et al. Lethal progression of a fetal intracranial arteriovenous malformation. *J Ultrasound Med*. 2003;22:645–648.

577. Mitchell PJ, Rosenfeld JV, Dargaville P, et al. Endovascular management of vein of Galen aneurysmal malformations presenting in the neonatal period. *AJNR Am J Neuroradiol*. 2001;22:1403–1409.

578. Rayssiguier R, Dumont C, Flunker S, et al. Thrombosis of the torcular herophili: diagnosis, prenatal management and outcome. *Prenat Diagn*. 2014;34: 1168–1175.

579. Okudera T, Peng Huang Y, Ohta T, et al. Development of posterior fossa dural sinuses, emissary veins, and jugular bulb: morphological and radiologic study. *AJNR Am J Neuroradiol*. 1994;15:1871–1883.

580. Merzoug V, Flunder S, Drissi C, et al. Dural sinus malformation (DSM) in fetuses: diagnostic value of prenatal MRI and follow-up. *Eur Radiol*. 2008;18:692–699.

581. Pandey V, Dummula K, Parimi P. Antenatal thrombosis of torcular herophili presenting with anemia, consumption coagulopathy and high-output cardiac failure in a preterm infant. *J Perinatol*. 2013;32:728–730.

582. Xia W, Hu D, Xiao P, et al. Dural sinus malformation imaging in the fetus: based on the 4 cases and literature review. *J Stroke Cerebrovasc Dis*. 2018;27(4): 1068–1076.

583. Yang E, Storey A, Olson HE, et al. Imaging features and prognostic factors in fetal and postnatal torcular dural sinus malformations, part II: synthesis of the literature and patient management. *J Neurointerv Surg*. 2018;10:471–475.

584. Fanou EM, Reeves MJ, Howe DT, et al. In utero magnetic resonance imaging for diagnosis of dural venous sinus ectasia with thrombosis in the fetus. *Pediatr Radiol*. 2013;43:1591–1598.

585. Legendre G, Picone O, Levaillant JM, et al. Prenatal diagnosis of a spontaneous dural sinus thrombosis. *Prenat Diagn*. 2009;29:808–813.

586. Laurichesse-Delmas H, Winer N, Gallot D, et al. Prenatal diagnosis of thrombosis of the dural sinuses: report of six cases, review of the literature and suggested management. *Ultrasound Obstet Gynecol*. 2008;32:188–198.

587. Corral E, Stecher X, Malinger G, et al. Thrombosis of the torcular herophili in the fetus: a series of eight cases. *Prenat Diagn*. 2014;34:1176–1181.

588. Has R, Esmer AC, Kalelioglu I, et al. Prenatal diagnosis of torcular herophili thrombosis, report of two cases and review of the literature. *J Ultrasound Med*. 2013;32:2205–2211.

589. Yang E, Storey A, Olson HE, et al. Imaging features and prognostic factors in fetal and postnatal torcular dural sinus malformations, part I: review of experience at Boston Children's Hospital. *J Neurointerv Surg*. 2018;10:467–470.

590. Grange G, LeTohic A, Merzoug V, et al. Prenatal demonstration of afferent vessels and progressive thrombosis in a torcular malformation. *Prenat Diagn*. 2007;27:670–673.

591. Laurichesse-Delmas H, Grimaud O, Moscoso G, et al. Color Doppler study of the venous circulation in the fetal brain and hemodynamic study of the cerebral transverse sinus. *Ultrasound Obstet Gynecol*. 1999;13:34–42.

592. Visentin A, Falco P, Pilu G, et al. Prenatal diagnosis of thrombosis of the dural sinuses with real-time and color Doppler ultrasound. *Ultrasound Obstet Gynecol*. 2001;17:322–325.

593. Rossi A, De Biasio P, Scarso E, et al. Prenatal MR imaging of dural sinus malformation: a case report. *Prenat Diagn*. 2006;26:11–16.

594. Ebert M, Esenkaya A, Huisman T, et al. Multimodality, anatomical and diffusion weighted fetal imaging of a spontaneously thrombosing congenital dural sinus malformation. *Neuropediatrics*. 2012;43:279–282.

595. Jenny B, Zerah M, Swift D, et al. Giant dural venous sinus ectasia in neonates, report of four cases. *J Neurosurg Pediatr*. 2010;5:523–528.

INTRODUCTION

Evaluation of the posterior fossa is an essential part of routine fetal sonography, as defined by guidelines from the American College of Radiology, American Institute of Ultrasound in Medicine, and American College of Obstetricians and Gynecologists, and also the Society of Obstetricians and Gynaecologists of Canada and Canadian Association of Radiologists, which state that views of the cerebellum and cisterna magna should be specifically included.[1-3] Normal measurements of the cisterna magna (between 2 and 11 mm) and ventricular atrium (<10 mm) confer a very high negative predictive value ($P < 0.005\%$) for abnormal CNS and spinal cord development.[4]

When an abnormality is found, however, there are a variety of pathologies that can look similar and even identical by standard axial ultrasonography, including Dandy–Walker continuum (DWC) and other vermian hypoplasia syndromes, mega cisterna magna, persistent Blake pouch, and posterior fossa arachnoid cyst. Differentiation is difficult, and although direct sagittal and coronal views of the posterior fossa are possible,[5-8] they can often be technically difficult. For this reason, in the past considerable attention has been paid to the more readily obtained axial sonographic views, and while most of the aforementioned disorders can be demonstrated, so can a variety of false-positive vermian pathologies.[9-11] For example, imaging the posterior fossa in the semicoronal plane can give a false appearance of an enlarged cisterna magna or even partial vermian agenesis.[12]

The advent of three-dimensional ultrasound (US) and fetal magnetic resonance imaging (MRI) has provided new tools in the imaging armamentarium that is proving to be extremely useful in difficult cases, because those orthogonal views are more readily obtainable, and because other limitations of ultrasonography such as maternal obesity, fetal skull ossification, and oligohydramnios can frequently be overcome by MRI. These newer techniques, therefore, allow additional further assessment of the fourth ventricle, brainstem, cisterna magna, and cerebellum that was not previously possible.

Important Embryology Milestones

At around 8 to 10 weeks' gestation, a focal dilatation of the neural tube is seen in the dorsal aspect of the developing hindbrain, which is the rhombencephalic vesicle, the predecessor to the fourth ventricle (Fig. 17.2-1A, B). At this level in the brainstem, which is known as the open medulla, the two alar laminae do not touch in the midline dorsally, and the gap is bridged by a layer of tela choroidea,[13] known as the area membranacea, which forms the roof of the rhombencephalic vesicle (Fig. 17.2-1C). The hindbrain develops a kink, known as the dorsal pontine flexure, which causes a transverse crease to form in the area membranacea, dividing it into anterior (rostral) and posterior (caudal) membranous areas (Fig. 17.2-2A, B). The cerebellum

develops from the rhombic lips at the cranial end of the area membranacea, and the vermis and cerebellum grow exophytically, inferiorly, and laterally to cover it. Because of its thinness, this layer of tela choroidea has until recently been nonresoluble by in vivo imaging, thus giving the false impression that the fourth ventricle is initially open to the developing subarachnoid space and then appears to close owing to caudal growth of the overlying vermis.[14,15] This developmental appearance is, therefore, often referred to in the literature as "closure" of the fourth ventricle. This process is usually complete by around 18 weeks' gestation; however, physiological variation may give the appearance that the vermis is incomplete at the time of initial midtrimester assessment.[16]

The vermis does not completely cover the roof of the fourth ventricle, and a part of the posterior membranous area evaginates beneath the vermis into the overlying meninx primitiva.[17,18] This evagination occurs through a space that is delimited by the vermis superiorly, nucleus gracilis inferiorly, and the developing cerebellar hemispheres laterally, also known in the mature state as the cerebellar vallecula (Fig. 17.2-2C). This evagination was first described in 1900s and is known as Blake pouch,[13] and where it constricts to pass through the cerebellar vallecula, it is known as Blake metapore (Fig. 17.2-2D, E). Normal linear echoes (the cisterna magna septa), which are typically seen in the fetal and neonatal cisterna magna and which are most often described as bridging arachnoid septations,[19] have recently been shown to represent the walls of Blake pouch, a normal and persistent structure in the posterior fossa. The cisterna magna septa or Blake pouch walls are a potential marker for normal development (Fig. 17.2-3).[18]

The future cisterna magna, therefore, forms in two compartments, a mesial compartment between the cisterna magna septa, which is derived from the rhombencephalic vesicle (Blake pouch), and compartments lateral to the cisterna magna septa that develop through cavitation of the meninx primitiva overlying the surface of the brain, forming the subarachnoid space proper.

Blake pouch usually, but not always, fenestrates to a variable degree[13,20] down to the obex (the inferior recess of the fourth ventricle), leading to communication between the mesial ventricular–derived compartment and the true subarachnoid space of the cisterna magna. Fenestration and disappearance of Blake pouch thus leaves an opening at Blake metapore,[18,20,21] which is the predecessor to the foramen of Magendie, allowing free communication between the fourth ventricle and the cisterna magna. Imaging the posterior fossa in the semicoronal plane will show this normal opening,[14,18,22] but can give a false appearance of partial vermian agenesis[12] (Fig. 17.2-4). This error can be avoided by making sure that the cavum septum pellucidum is included in the image, thus ensuring that the scan plane is truly axial or modified axial. Thus, the foramen of Magendie does not demarcate the actual junction between the fourth ventricle and the true subarachnoid space of the cisterna magna. A *small* communication beneath the vermis, between the fourth ventricle and the "cisterna

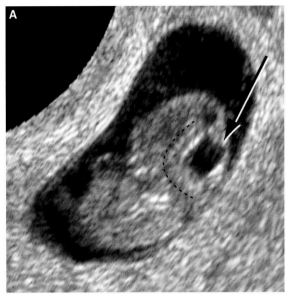
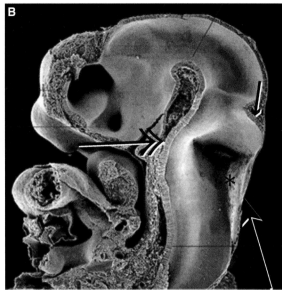
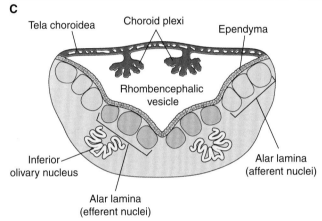

FIGURE 17.2-1: Embryology of the posterior fossa. **A:** Sagittal sonogram of the cranial end of the fetal pole at 8 to 10 weeks' gestation demonstrating the rhombencephalic vesicle *(long arrow)* and the dorsal pontine flexure *(dotted line)*. **B:** Electron micrograph of the embryo. Rhombencephalic vesicle *(asterisk)*, rhombic lips *(small arrow)*, rhombencephalic roof *(long arrow)*, and dorsal flexure of pons *(double arrow)*. **C:** Diagram of section through open medulla. The roof of the rhombencephalic vesicle comprises tela choroidea, which comprises an inner layer of ependyma continuous with the lining of the neural tube, outer layer of pia-arachnoid continuous with over the surface of the brain, and intervening attenuated neuroglial tissue. (**A**, from Robinson AJ, Goldstein R. The cisterna magna septa: vestigial remnants of Blake's pouch and a potential new marker for normal development of the rhombencephalon. *J Ultrasound Med.* 2007;26:83–95, with permission of the American Institute of Ultrasound in Medicine. **B, C**, reprinted with permission from Sadler TW. Langman's Essential Medical Embryology. Baltimore, MD: Lippincott Williams & Wilkins; 2005.)

magna," often shown in the literature by sonography[14,15,18,22,23] and sometimes subsequently "confirmed" on midsagittal images, is, therefore, the normal Blake metapore. Unfortunately, it is often wrongly ascribed to "Dandy–Walker variant" (vide infra).

In the literature, the phrase "a posterior fossa cyst communicating with the fourth ventricle" is often used to describe cystic malformations of the posterior fossa; however, this is actually a description of the normal anatomy. What is abnormal is the size of the posterior fossa "cyst," not the fact that it communicates with the fourth ventricle. The Dandy–Walker "cyst" is in fact Blake pouch, which expands to fill the subarachnoid space of the cisterna magna.[18] The cisterna magna septa are not typically seen in cystic malformations of the posterior fossa[24] because as Blake pouch expands, its walls, that is the septa, are displaced laterally and can become indistinguishable from the walls of the cisterna magna, although often the true subarachnoid space of the cisterna magna is still visible very laterally beyond the septa. Additionally seen in the literature is the description of the fourth ventricle "widely communicating with the cisterna magna." Again, it is not actually the cisterna magna with which the fourth ventricle is in communication; it is in communication with Blake pouch, which, in turn, is itself contained within the cisterna magna.

CYSTIC ANOMALIES

Blake Pouch Cyst and Persistent Blake Pouch

Incidence: This is a rare diagnosis. The largest study to date of all posterior fossa collections (including Blake pouch cyst, mega cisterna magna, DWC, and posterior fossa arachnoid cysts) had a total of 105 fetuses over a 10-year period in two referral centers for prenatal diagnosis.[25]

Embryology and Genetics: In persistent Blake pouch (Fig. 17.2-5), there is thought to be inadequate fenestration of both Blake pouch and the foramen of Luschka, leading to imbalance of cerebrospinal fluid (CSF) egress into the subarachnoid space of the cisterna magna with consequent dilatation of the fourth ventricle.[21] Although the pouch communicates freely with the fourth ventricle, there is a failure of communication between the pouch and the perimedullary subarachnoid spaces.[20,26] Unfortunately, the consequent elevation of the vermis often leads to the false-positive diagnosis of inferior vermian hypoplasia (vide infra). This explains why there has historically been poor correlation of US and autopsy findings in apparent cystic malformations of the posterior fossa.[11]

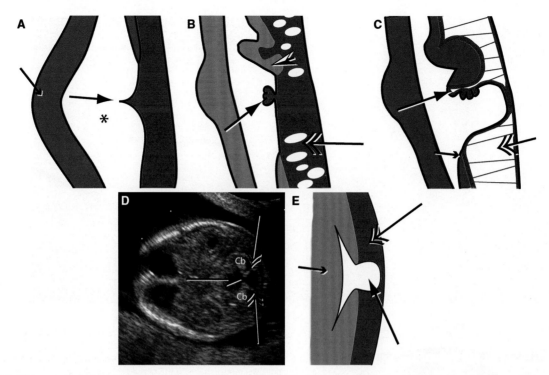

FIGURE 17.2-2: Blake pouch. **A:** Diagrammatic representation demonstrating the formation of the dorsal pontine flexure *(white tipped arrow)* and the consequent crease that develops in the roof of the rhombencephalic vesicle *(solid black arrow)*. The vesicle *(asterisk)* is the predecessor to the fourth ventricle. **B:** Choroid plexus forms as the wedge of meninx primitiva within the transverse crease becomes vascularized *(long arrow)*. The overlying meninx primitiva starts to cavitate *(double arrow)*. Cerebellum starts to develop in area membranacea anterior *(short arrow)*. **C:** The posterior membranous area evaginates below the developing vermis *(long arrow)* and the nucleus gracilis *(short arrow)*. Coalescence of the cavities within the meninx primitiva leads to development of the subarachnoid space, which is trabeculated in random planes by multiple pia-arachnoid septations *(double arrow)*. **D:** Axial fetal sonogram at 13 weeks' gestation demonstrating Blake pouch evaginating into the cavitating meninx primitiva, between the developing cerebellar hemispheres *(Cb)*. The walls of the pouch are visible as linear echoes *(double arrows)*. Blake metapore *(single arrow)* is the predecessor of the foramen of Magendie. **E:** Diagrammatic representation showing the meninx primitiva *(double arrow)*, Blake pouch *(long arrow)*, and tegmentum of the brainstem *(short arrow)*. (**A–D**, from Robinson AJ, Goldstein R. The cisterna magna septa: vestigial remnants of Blake's pouch and a potential new marker for normal development of the rhombencephalon. *J Ultrasound Med.* 2007;26:83–95, with permission of the American Institute of Ultrasound in Medicine. **E**, from Robinson AJ. Inferior vermian hypoplasia: preconception, misconception. *Ultrasound Obstet Gynecol.* 2014;43:123–136, with permission of John Wiley & Sons Ltd.)

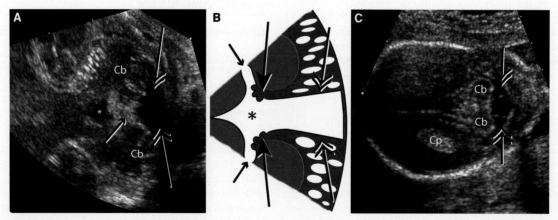

FIGURE 17.2-3: Development of the fourth ventricle. **A:** Above vallecula, the fourth ventricle *(asterisk)* and septa *(double arrows)* are separated by the inferior vermis *(small arrow)*. **B:** Diagrammatic representation demonstrating the relationship between the fourth ventricle *(asterisk)* and the space between the septa *(double arrows)*. The foramen of Luschka *(short arrows)* forms at the lateral recesses of the fourth ventricle. Lateral caudal extensions of the choroid plexus form on each side *(long arrows)*. **C:** Semicoronal fetal sonogram at 20 weeks' gestation. The cerebrospinal fluid (CSF) between the septa *(double arrows)* is completely anechoic because it forms as an evagination of the neural tube, whereas the CSF lateral to the septa is slightly echogenic because it forms through cavitation of the meninx primitiva. *Cb,* cerebellar hemispheres; *Cp,* choroid plexus of the lateral ventricle. (From Robinson AJ, Goldstein R. The cisterna magna septa: vestigial remnants of Blake's pouch and a potential new marker for normal development of the rhombencephalon. *J Ultrasound Med.* 2007;26:83–95, with permission of the American Institute of Ultrasound in Medicine.)

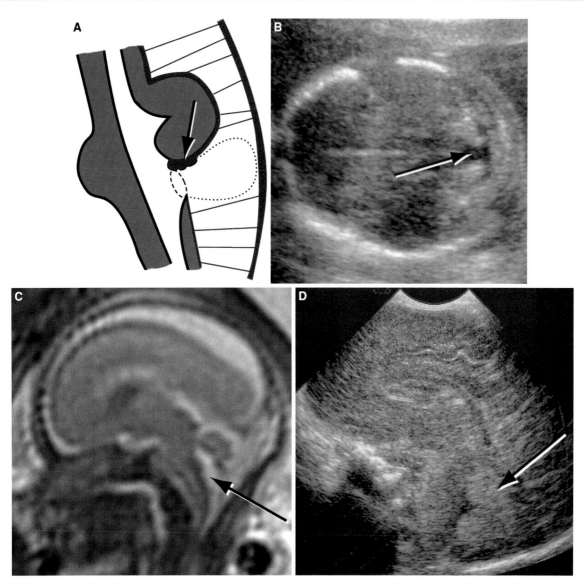

FIGURE 17.2-4: Imaging of the fourth ventricle. **A:** Once Blake pouch fenestrates, its neck or Blake metapore *(dashed oval)* becomes the foramen of Magendie. The choroid plexus in the roof of the fourth ventricle *(short arrow)* now appears to be "in the cisterna magna." **B:** On sonography at 19 weeks, fetus having an apparently normal vermis was seen superiorly (not shown). Modified axial sonogram in the same fetus demonstrating normal appearances of the communication between the fourth ventricle and the subarachnoid space *(arrow)*, in keeping with the foramen of Magendie. **C:** Sagittal fetal MRI at 21 weeks' gestation in the same fetus showing a small "defect" *(arrow)* gap between the inferior vermis and the brainstem. **D:** Postnatal sagittal sonography on day 1 of life demonstrates an apparently complete vermis *(arrow)*, with no evidence of an increased tegmento-vermian angle. This baby had normal development at 2 years of age. (**A**, from Robinson AJ, Goldstein R. The cisterna magna septa: vestigial remnants of Blake's pouch and a potential new marker for normal development of the rhombencephalon. *J Ultrasound Med.* 2007;26:83–95, with permission of the American Institute of Ultrasound in Medicine. **B–D**, reprinted with permission from Robinson AJ, Blaser S, Toi A, et al. The fetal cerebellar vermis: assessment for abnormal development by ultrasonography and magnetic resonance imaging. *Ultrasound Q.* 2007;23(3):211–223.)

Etiology and Pathogenesis: The *lateral* recesses of the rhomb-encephalic vesicle are in direct contact with the developing sub-arachnoid space and fenestrate to form the foramen of Luschka. If fenestration of Blake pouch/metapore does not occur, it is the later fenestration of the foramen of Luschka that leads to equili-bration of CSF between the ventricular system and the subarach-noid space,[27] and therefore in lower species, where it is normal for Blake pouch not to fenestrate, the foramen of Luschka is cor-respondingly larger than in humans. In humans, therefore, the foramen of Luschka is not large enough to compensate for the lack of fenestration of Blake pouch at the foramen of Magendie,

so equilibration of CSF might only be achieved with the ven-tricles persistently enlarged.[28] Even at the foramen of Luschka, the degree of fenestration can be variable.[29] The variable degrees of fenestration at both Blake pouch/metaphor or Magendie and the foramen of Luschka and the balance of CSF production and egress into the subarachnoid space probably explain why out-ward bowing of the cisterna magna septa is often normally seen giving the impression of a posterior fossa cyst[19] (Fig. 17.2-6), which subsequently may resolve as fenestration progresses, depending on the degree and timing of fenestration.[25] In one study, Blake pouch cyst was seen to resolve by 26 weeks,[30] which

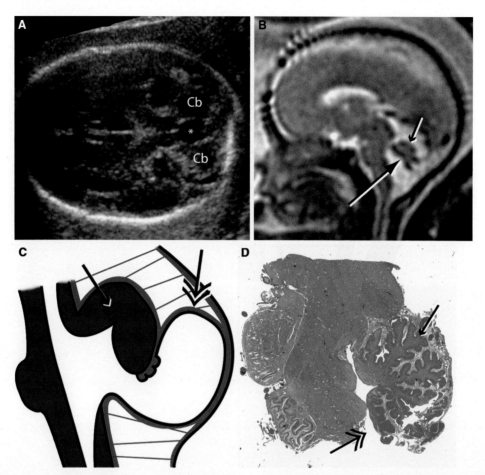

FIGURE 17.2-5: Blake pouch cyst. **A:** Modified axial fetal sonogram at 23 weeks' gestation demonstrating a distended and misshapen fourth ventricle *(asterisk)* with mass effect on the adjacent cerebellar hemispheres *(Cb)*. **B:** Sagittal fetal MRI of the same fetus demonstrating that the vermis is morphologically normal; its craniocaudal diameter was gestation appropriate, and the major landmarks comprising the primary fissure *(short arrow)* and fastigial point *(long arrow)* are present. **C:** Diagrammatic representation of Blake pouch cyst. In this condition, there is inadequate fenestration of the pouch *(double arrow)* and coexistent inadequate fenestration of the foramen of Luschka, leading to elevation of the vermis *(short arrow)* and hydrocephalus. **D:** Histopathological specimen of the same fetus showing that the vermis *(short arrow)* is normal and that the pouch *(double arrow)* has decompressed. (**A, D**, reprinted with permission from Robinson AJ, Blaser S, Toi A, et al. The fetal cerebellar vermis: assessment for abnormal development by ultrasonography and magnetic resonance imaging. *Ultrasound Q.* 2007;23(3):211–223; **C**, from Robinson AJ, Goldstein RG. The cisterna magna septaVa vestigial remnant of Blake's pouch and a potential new marker for normal development of the rhombencephalon. *J Ultrasound Med.* 2007;26(1):83–95. Copyright © 2016 by the American Institute of Ultrasound in Medicine. Reprinted by permission of John Wiley & Sons, Inc.)

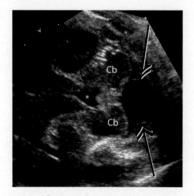

FIGURE 17.2-6: Modified axial neonatal sonogram at 24 weeks' gestation demonstrating outward bowing of the cisterna magna septa *(double arrows)*, giving the impression of a posterior fossa cyst. Position of the fourth ventricle *(asterisk)* and cerebellar hemispheres *(Cb)*. (From Robinson AJ, Goldstein R. The cisterna magna septa: vestigial remnants of Blake's pouch and a potential new marker for normal development of the rhombencephalon. *J Ultrasound Med.* 2007;26:83–95, with permission of the American Institute of Ultrasound in Medicine.)

corresponds exactly with the timing of opening of the foramen of Luschka by another author.[31]

It has also been indicated by several cases in the literature that persistent Blake pouch phenotype can be acquired if the balance of CSF egress is upset by the presence of fetal intraventricular hemorrhage[25,28,32] and fetal infection,[33–35] which result in tetra-ventricular dilatation and enlargement of the "cisterna magna" (Blake pouch). Presumably, the obstruction occurs through a process of cortico-pial hemosiderosis or debris within the ventricular system, causing obstruction of the fenestrations in both the foramen of Luschka and Blake pouch, in much the same way as can be demonstrated postnatally[36] (Fig. 17.2-7), recognizing that depending on the nature and timing of the insult, injury to the brain parenchyma itself can also occur because of endotoxins, free radicals, and inflammatory cytokines.[37–39] Consequently, a compensated Blake pouch cyst may never be diagnosed even in adults until such a precipitating event tips the balance of CSF egress in favor of hydrocephalus, at which time the patient becomes symptomatic.

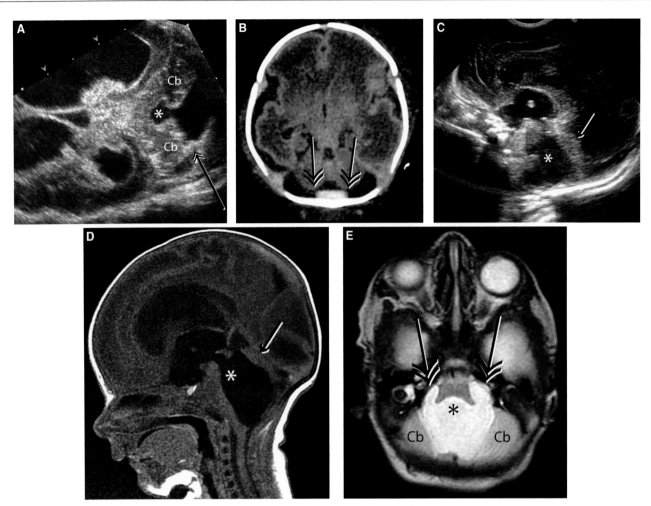

FIGURE 17.2-7: Acquired Blake pouch phenotype. **A:** Axial neonatal sonogram at 31 weeks' gestation. There is blood apparently "within the cisterna magna" *(double arrow)* with hydrocephalus. Position of the fourth ventricle *(asterisk)* and cerebellar hemispheres *(Cb)*. Closer inspection shows that the blood is limited in its lateral extent; the more dependent subarachnoid space over the cerebellar hemisphere does not contain blood but is slightly more echogenic because of the pia-arachnoid trabeculations. **B:** Axial neonatal computed tomography in a different patient again showing blood "within the cisterna magna." Closer inspection shows that the blood is limited in its lateral extent by invisible walls *(double arrows)* and is most likely contained within Blake pouch. **C:** Sagittal US in a neonate postintraventricular hemorrhage showing fourth ventricular dilatation *(asterisk)* and an abnormal (compressed) vermis *(arrow)* similar in appearance to Dandy–Walker continuum. **D:** Sagittal MRI in the same neonate. The vermis is elevated *(arrow)* by the distended Blake pouch, and there is wide communication with the fourth ventricle *(asterisk)*. **E:** Axial MRI in the same neonate demonstrating a distended Blake pouch and the fourth ventricle *(asterisk)*. The *Cb* are displaced laterally. It also appears as though the fenestrae at the foramen of Luschka are also blocked, causing their evagination *(double arrows)* into the perimedullary subarachnoid space. **(A, B**, from Robinson AJ, Goldstein R. The cisterna magna septa: vestigial remnants of Blake's pouch and a potential new marker for normal development of the rhombencephalon. *J Ultrasound Med.* 2007;26:83–95, with permission of the American Institute of Ultrasound in Medicine.)

Diagnosis: The wall of Blake pouch can be seen by US, but with more difficulty by MRI. The Blake pouch elevates/rotates the vermis away from the brainstem. This has been described as an increased tegmento-vermian angle (vide infra).[15] Importantly, the vermis is intrinsically normal; that is, this is an isolated abnormality of the posterior membranous area, and there is no associated abnormality of the anterior membranous area structures (vermis). Thus, the essential task is to ensure that the vermis is normal. The problem is our ability to distinguish an isolated persistent Blake pouch from vermian hypoplasia (vide infra), which have different outcomes.

Differential Diagnosis: Other causes of cystic malformations of the posterior fossa include vermian hypoplasia (Dandy-Walker continuum), mega cisterna magna, and posterior fossa arachnoid cyst.

Prognosis: Isolated elevation/rotation of the vermis due to a persistent Blake pouch does not necessarily indicate an adverse outcome.[14,18,40–46] In one study, one-third of cases of Blake pouch cyst or mega cisterna magna underwent spontaneous resolution in utero, and 90% of survivors with no associated anomalies had normal developmental outcome at 1 to 5 years once the initial referral misdiagnosis of vermian hypoplasia had been excluded.[25] Resolution on follow-up imaging during the third trimester or later should support Blake pouch as the likely cause.[47,48]

In another large retrospective study of 19 cases of Blake pouch cyst, associated anomalies were seen in 8 cases, 5 being congenital heart disease. There were 8 terminations and two neonatal deaths. Of the nine survivors, one had trisomy 21, and the other eight were neurodevelopmentally normal, although one developed obstructive hydrocephalus.[30]

In adults with Blake pouch cyst, after ventricular shunting, subtotal or total re-expansion of the cerebellar hemispheres and vermis can be seen. Sometimes, these structures may appear to be hypoplastic because of mass effect of the cyst; however, there is actually no intrinsic hypoplasia, and these patients are neurologically normal.[27]

Management: Blake pouch cyst often regresses in utero.[25] Expectant management is indicated, provided vermian hypoplasia and other associated abnormalities can be excluded. If cyst persists postnatal, follow up may be indicated to exclude interval development of obstructive hydrocephalus.

Recurrence Risk: This is unknown. Full evaluation of any subsequent pregnancies is suggested.

Mega Cisterna Magna

Incidence: This is a rare diagnosis. The largest study to date of all posterior fossa collections (including Blake pouch cyst, mega cisterna magna, DWC, and posterior fossa arachnoid cysts) had a total of 105 fetuses over a 10-year period in two referral centers for prenatal diagnosis.[25]

Embryology and Genetics In mega cisterna magna, the vermis is fully formed, but fenestration of Blake pouch and the foramen of Luschka is mildly deficient, thus allowing sufficient CSF equilibration for Blake pouch to cause mild expansion of the cisterna magna, but not sufficient to cause elevation of the vermis or obstructive hydrocephalus.[18] In this sense, mega cisterna magna may be more accurately termed "mega Blake pouch" (Fig. 17.2-8). Partial fenestration would explain the communication seen

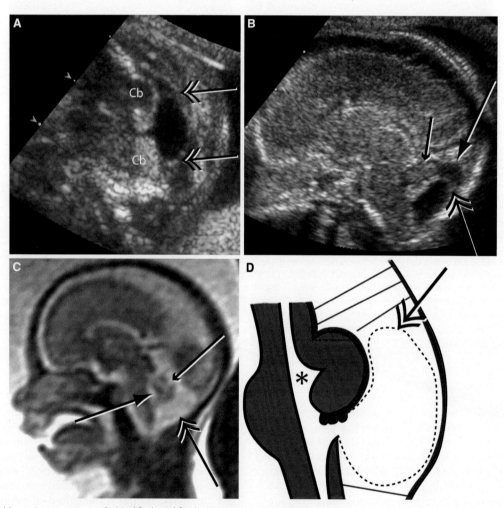

FIGURE 17.2-8: Mega cisterna magna. **A:** Modified axial fetal sonogram at 19 weeks' gestation showing a prominent "cisterna magna" with the septa displaced laterally *(double arrows)*. The cerebellar hemispheres *(Cb)* appear normal. **B:** Direct sagittal fetal sonogram of the same fetus demonstrating the anechoic cerebrospinal fluid (CSF) contained within Blake pouch *(double arrow)*, the echogenic true subarachnoid space below the falx cerebelli *(long arrow)*, and slight mass effect on the underside of the cerebellar vermis *(small arrow)*. **C:** Sagittal MRI of the same fetus showing that the vermis has the normal morphological features of the primary fissure *(long arrow)* and the fastigial point *(short arrow)*. The "cisterna magna" appears large *(double arrow)*, but the walls of Blake pouch are not resoluble. **D:** Diagrammatic representation of mega cisterna magna. In this condition, the pouch expands within the subarachnoid space of the cisterna magna *(double arrow)*, but later there is sufficient fenestration to allow communication with the fourth ventricle *(asterisk)* by contrast cisternography. (From Robinson AJ, Goldstein R. The cisterna magna septa: vestigial remnants of Blake's pouch and a potential new marker for normal development of the rhombencephalon. *J Ultrasound Med.* 2007;26:83–95, with permission of the American Institute of Ultrasound in Medicine.)

between the fourth ventricle and the subarachnoid space that can be demonstrated on cisternography.[21]

Etiology and Pathogenesis: Mega cisterna magna is thought to result from a defect of the posterior membranous area during embryogenesis.[21]

Diagnosis: Mega cisterna magna refers to an enlargement of the cisterna magna greater than 10 mm (see Fig. 17.2-8). The vermis should be intact and in a normal position, and the cerebellar hemispheres should be normal. No associated abnormalities should be present.

Differential Diagnosis: Other causes of cystic malformations of the posterior fossa include the vermian hypoplasia (DWC), persistent Blake pouch, and posterior fossa arachnoid cyst. This differential is further discussed in the section on Blake pouch cyst (vide supra).

The presence of subependymal nodular heterotopia should be excluded since there is a known association with retrocerebellar

cysts.[49,50] The main sonographic features are ventriculomegaly and a squared-off appearance to the lateral ventricle on coronal views. Additional features include irregular ventricular borders, callosal agenesis, polymicrogyria, and vermian hypoplasia. The constellation of nodular heterotopia, mega cisterna magna, and corpus callosum dysgenesis, more commonly seen in a female fetus, should prompt the diagnosis of X-linked bilateral subependymal nodular heterotopia and filamin A (*FLNA*) gene mutation (Fig. 17.2-9).[51–54] Subependymal nodular heterotopia may also sometimes be revealed in the mother, but most fetuses have a de novo mutation.

Prognosis: Mega cisterna magna often regresses in utero.[25] It is associated with overall normal cognitive function, but subjects may score inferior to controls on some parameters of memory and verbal fluency.[55]

Management: This often regresses in utero.[25] Expectant management is indicated, provided vermian hypoplasia and other associated abnormalities can be excluded.

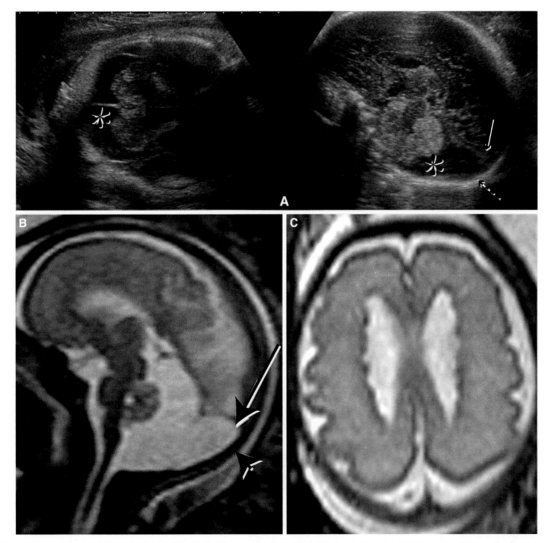

FIGURE 17.2-9: Ultrasonographic appearance of posterior fossa cyst at 35.5 weeks' gestation. **A:** Axial view at the level of the cerebellum. The retrocerebellar space (*asterisk*) is markedly enlarged. Midline sagittal view showing the posterior fossa cyst (*asterisk*), the elevation of the distal insertion of the tentorium (*plain arrow*), and the scalloping of the occipital vault (*dotted arrow*). **B:** T2 MRI midline sagittal slice. The mass effect on the inferior insertion of the tentorium (*arrow*) and the scalloping of the occipital vault (*arrowhead*) are well visible. **C:** T2 MRI (*axial view*) of fetus with periventricular nodular heterotopia demonstrating irregular lateral borders of the lateral ventricles.

Recurrence Risk: This is unknown. Full evaluation of any subsequent pregnancies is suggested.

Arachnoid Cyst

Incidence: This is a rare diagnosis. The largest study to date of all posterior fossa collections (including Blake pouch cyst, mega cisterna magna, DWC, and posterior fossa arachnoid cysts) had a total of 105 fetuses over a 10-year period in two referral centers for prenatal diagnosis.[25]

Embryology and Genetics: Embryologically, the pia-arachnoid is initially a solid condensation of mesenchyme over the brain, known as the meninx primitiva. Small fluid-filled cavities form within the meninx primitiva, which then coalesce to form a sponge-like network of cavities over the surface of the brain (Fig. 17.2-10). The inner membrane directly in contact with the surface of the brain is the pia mater, and the outer is the arachnoid mater. The subarachnoid space is, therefore, trabeculated by numerous pia-arachnoid septations,[19] making it diffusely echogenic by US compared with the CSF in the ventricular system. This relative echogenicity decreases throughout gestation as cavitation increases.[18]

Etiology and Pathogenesis: If coalescence is incomplete, a cavity may not communicate with its neighbors and remains isolated from the surrounding subarachnoid space.

Diagnosis: Because of its embryology, an arachnoid cyst, in contradistinction to a Blake pouch cyst, does not communicate with the fourth ventricle. Sometimes, a membrane can be seen separating the arachnoid cyst from the fourth ventricle. Because of the fact that it has to arise in the subarachnoid space, its continued enlargement can cause mass effect on the vermis and cerebellar hemispheres, but it does not elevate the vermis-like a Blake pouch cyst (Fig. 17.2-11).

Differential Diagnosis: Other causes of cystic malformations of the posterior fossa include vermian hypoplasia (DWC), persistent Blake pouch, and syndromes associated with cysts in the posterior fossa, such as Aicardi syndrome.

Prognosis: If not associated with brain insult or karyotype anomalies, these have an excellent prognosis. Most either stabilize or regress, and prenatal hydrocephalus is rare. Those who develop hydrocephalus postnatally tend not to have hydrocephalus prenatally, and therefore, postnatal surveillance is advised, especially in the first few months of life.[56,57]

Management: Neurosurgical consultation is advised because postnatal surveillance imaging and surgical intervention may be necessary.

Recurrence Risk: There is no recurrence risk.

CEREBELLO-VERMIAN ANOMALIES

Vermian Hypoplasia and Dandy–Walker Continuum

The DWC, the preferred nomenclature, includes classic Dandy–Walker malformation (DWM), Dandy–Walker variant, and, possibly, also mega cisterna magna and persistent Blake pouch cyst.[18,27]

Classic DWM comprises complete or partial vermian agenesis, cystic dilatation of the fourth ventricle, and enlargement of the posterior fossa with elevation of transverse sinus, tentorium, and torcula ("torcular-lambdoid inversion")[58] (Fig. 17.2-12). The problem with the nomenclature arises in that the vermis can be variably abnormal, the size of the fourth ventricle and retrocerebellar CSF inconsistent, and defining whether the tentorium is high enough to be inverted with regard to the lambdoid impossible by fetal imaging. In addition, some authors also include hydrocephalus[59]; however, hydrocephalus is a frequent complication of, but not actually a part of, the malformation[58] and is not usually present at birth.[60]

Dandy–Walker "variant" is a terminology that should probably be abandoned, possibly in favor of Dandy–Walker "continuum" or "complex"[61] as abnormalities of the posterior fossa remain unclear from a prognostic perspective and the term "continuum" more clearly refers to the variable degrees of vermian hypoplasia, fenestration of the fourth ventricular outlet foramen, and associated anomalies that are seen in these cases.[15,60] The term "inferior vermian hypoplasia" is growing in usage apparently as an alternative to the nomenclature "Dandy–Walker variant."[10,62–64] However, despite the confusing terminology, in the absence of a known genetic syndrome, it is probably more important for counseling to identify the anomalies present than to provide a "defined name."

Although still controversial, an attempt at summarization is demonstrated in Table 17.2-1.

Incidence: The reported incidence of DWM is 1 in 30,000.[60]

Embryology and Genetics: The DWC is associated with single-gene disorders such as Walker–Warburg syndrome, Meckel–Gruber syndrome, and chromosomal abnormalities.[65]

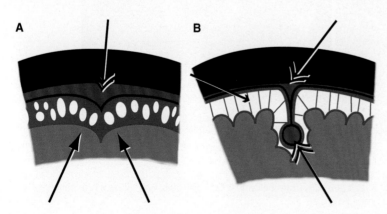

FIGURE 17.2-10: Development of subarachnoid space. **A:** The meninx primitiva starts to cavitate *(red with white bubbles)* and the lateral neural tissues overgrow the midline structures *(long arrows)* trapping a wedge of conjunctive tissue containing rich vascular plexi in the midline *(double arrow).* **B:** The rich vascular plexi coalesce to form the dural venous sinuses, for example, the superior sagittal sinus *(double superior arrow)* and inferior sagittal sinus *(inferior double arrow).* Subarachnoid space is single arrow. (From Robinson AJ, Goldstein R. The cisterna magna septa: vestigial remnants of Blake's pouch and a potential new marker for normal development of the rhombencephalon. *J Ultrasound Med.* 2007;26:83–95, with permission of the American Institute of Ultrasound in Medicine.)

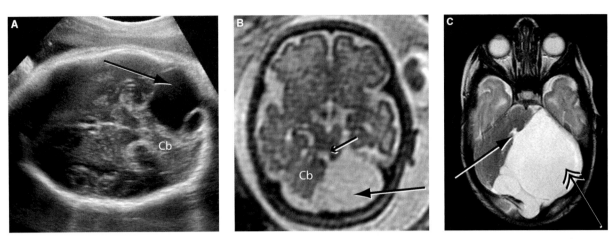

FIGURE 17.2-11: Arachnoid cyst. **A:** Modified axial US of a fetus showing a large cyst in the posterior fossa *(arrow)*. **B:** Axial fetal MRI of the same fetus demonstrating the cyst *(long arrow)* with displacement of the brainstem, fourth ventricle *(short arrow)*, and cerebellum *(Cb)*. **C:** Axial neonatal MRI of the same fetus demonstrating that the cyst *(double arrow)* and the fourth ventricle are definitely separated by a thin septum *(long arrow)*.

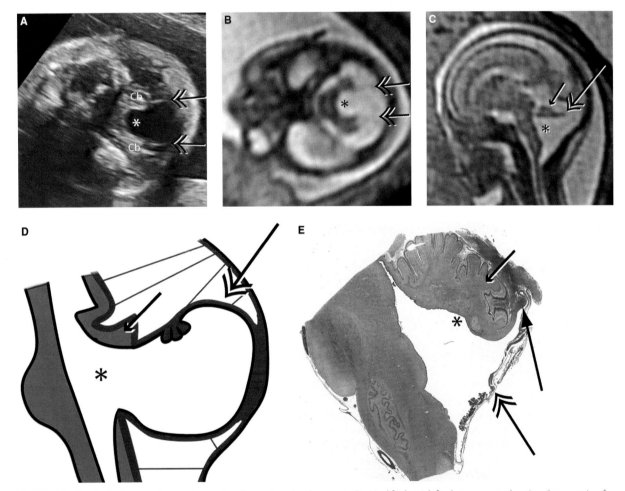

FIGURE 17.2-12: Dandy–Walker continuum/anomaly of vermian development. **A:** Modified axial fetal sonogram showing "a posterior fossa cyst communicating with the fourth ventricle." The cisterna magna septa (walls of Blake pouch) are displaced laterally *(double arrows)*. The pia-arachnoid trabeculations can be seen lateral to the septa. The space between the septa is continuous with the fourth ventricle *(asterisk)* where Cb is cerebellar hemisphere. **B:** Axial fetal MRI of the same fetus showing the cisterna magna septa *(double arrows)* and fourth ventricle *(asterisk)*. The septa are very rarely visible on fetal MRI. **C:** Sagittal fetal MRI of the same fetus showing the vermis *(small arrow)* is elevated by the distended Blake pouch. Displaced germinal matrix can be seen *(double arrow)* at the superior aspect of the pouch. There is wide communication between the pouch and the fourth ventricle *(asterisk)*. **D:** Diagrammatic representation of Dandy–Walker continuum. There is variable vermian hypoplasia *(small arrow)*, and variable fenestration of Blake pouch *(double arrow)* and the foramen of Luschka. Position of the fourth ventricle *(asterisk)*. **E:** Sagittal histopathological specimen of a different fetus, akin to Dandy–Walker continuum. It can be seen that there is mild vermian dysmorphology with deficient lobulation *(small arrow)* and a flattened fastigial point *(asterisk)*. Blake pouch *(double arrow)* is intact. The germinal matrix is displaced *(long arrow)*. (**C, D**, Reprinted from Robinson AJ, Blaser S, Toi A, et al. The fetal cerebellar vermis: assessment for abnormal development by ultrasonography and magnetic resonance imaging. *Ultrasound Q.* 2007;23(3):211–223. **E**, courtesy of William Halliday, Department of Pathology, Hospital for Sick Children, Toronto, Canada; from Robinson AJ. Inferior vermian hypoplasia: preconception, misconception. *Ultrasound Obstet Gynecol.* 2014;43:123–136, with permission of John Wiley & Sons Ltd.)

TABLE 17.2-1	Categorization of "Cystic" Posterior Fossa Malformations				
	VERMIS				
FINDINGS	**ROTATION/ ELEVATION**	**HYPOPLASIA**	**CISTERNA MAGNA SEPTA**	**CHOROID PLEXUS POSITION**	**DIAGNOSIS**
Enlarged Blake pouch, **enlarged** posterior fossa, elevated torcula (often hydrocephalus)	Yes—greater than 40°–45°	Yes—variable— may be severe	Invisible— apposed to side walls of cisterna magna	Inferior margin of Blake pouch	Vermian hypoplasia— a.k.a. Dandy–Walker *malformation*
Enlarged Blake pouch, **normal**-sized posterior fossa, normal torcula	Yes—usually between 30° and 45°	Yes—variable— intermediate	Invisible— apposed to side walls of cisterna magna	Inferior margin of Blake pouch	Vermian hypoplasia— a.k.a. Dandy–Walker *variant* or "inferior vermian hypoplasia"
Enlarged Blake pouch, **normal**-sized posterior fossa, normal torcula	Yes—mild to moderate (usually <30°)	**No**—may be misdiagnosed as "inferior vermian hypoplasia"	Visible—bowed laterally	Superior margin of Blake pouch	Blake pouch cyst— a.k.a. persistent Blake pouch
Enlarged Blake pouch, **enlarged** posterior fossa (cisterna magna >10 mm)	**No**	**No**	Visible—bowed laterally	Superior margin of Blake pouch	Mega cisterna magna (= mega Blake pouch)
True cyst that does *not* communicate with the fourth ventricle (not Blake pouch)	**No**	**No**—may have extrinsic compression	Normal—but may be distorted by mass effect	Superior margin of Blake pouch	Posterior fossa arachnoid cyst

Note: Dandy–Walker variant is a term seen in the literature that referred to cases that resembled classic Dandy–Walker malformation but did not have an enlarged posterior fossa, hydrocephalus, and was often seen with associated anomalies and syndromes. Inferior vermian hypoplasia is now the latest nomenclature in the literature for the spectrum of abnormalities between classic Dandy–Walker and Blake pouch cyst, although this terminology is also debatable, and simply "vermian hypoplasia" may be more appropriate until it can be demonstrated precisely which part of the vermis is deficient.
Reproduced from Robinson AJ. Inferior vermian hypoplasia: preconception, misconception. *Ultrasound Obstet Gynecol.* 2014;43:123–136, with permission of John Wiley & Sons Ltd.

Etiology and Pathogenesis: Classic DWM was initially described in infants with hydrocephalus and was thought to be the sequelae of atresia of the foramina of Luschka and Magendie[66–68]; however, current theories suggest that it is a more global developmental defect affecting the roof of the rhombencephalon,[18,61] leading to variable degrees of vermian hypoplasia, variable fenestration of the fourth ventricular outlet foramen, and variable associated anomalies.[60]

Current theories suggest that the spectrum of findings with respect to the posterior fossa "cyst" in DWC might result from two potential processes: either arrest of vermian development so it does not cover the fourth ventricle, or failure of adequate fenestration of the fourth ventricular outflow foramen, leading to an enlarged Blake pouch with secondary elevation and compression of the vermis. Often, these two processes are seen together as in classic DWM.

Diagnosis

Assessment for Presence of the Vermis Using Its Major Landmarks: Various biometric and morphological criteria for assessment of vermian hypoplasia have been described.[14,44,69] By 17.5 weeks, one should be able to identify whether the vermis is present by assessing for the major landmarks that should be present by this gestation, as determined by in vitro studies.

This includes whether the fastigial point is present and has a normal acute angle, or whether it is deficient (i.e., absent or obtuse angle) and whether the primary fissure is identifiable (Fig. 17.2-13).

Assessment of Vermian Maturity: Having determined that the vermis is present, one must evaluate its developmental maturity, because this has been demonstrated to correlate with prognosis.[40] In addition to the fastigial point and the primary fissure, we can assess for vermian lobulation, biometry including the craniocaudal diameter of the vermis and the relative growth of the anterior versus posterior lobes, and the tegmento-vermian angle.

Lobulation: By 21 weeks, the prepyramidal fissure can be seen between the tuber and the pyramis, and by 21 to 22 weeks, the preculminate fissure can be seen between the central lobule and the culmen. By 24 weeks, the secondary fissure can be seen between the pyramis and the uvula, and from 27 weeks, all the vermian lobules and fissures become visible (Fig. 17.2-14).[70–73] Therefore, prior to 24 weeks' gestation, a critical time in many jurisdictions with respect to considering termination of pregnancy, it can be difficult to determine whether vermian lobulation is complete because the declive, folium, and tuber

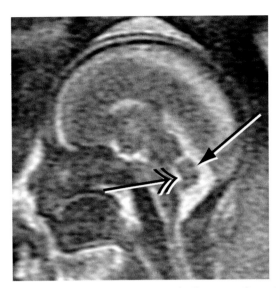

FIGURE 17.2-13: Primary fissure at 17.5 weeks. The primary fissure *(single arrow)* is the first major vermian fissure to appear and marks the boundary between the superior (anterior) and inferior (posterior) vermis. By MRI, it is seen as a high-signal indentation on the posterosuperior aspect of the vermis. The fastigial point *(double arrow)* is the posterosuperior recess of the fourth ventricle and should form an acute angle, giving it a diamond shape. (From Robinson AJ, Blaser S, Toi A, et al. The fetal cerebellar vermis: assessment for abnormal development by ultrasonography and magnetic resonance imaging. *Ultrasound Q.* 2007;23(3):211–223.)

are not normally separately distinguishable at that stage of development since they are the last to develop and differentiate. Also, all three are united by a single white matter core to the arbor vitae, whereas all the other named lobules have their own individual white matter cores (see Fig. 17.2-14F). Therefore, it will appear as if only seven out of nine lobules are present. MRI at 3 Tesla has potential to more confidently define vermian lobulation and exclude vermian hypoplasia.[74]

Biometry: The Craniocaudal and Anteroposterior Diameters and Surface Area of the Vermis: By 18 weeks, the fastigial point and primary fissure should always be visible. The declive is seen immediately below the primary fissure. A line can usually, therefore, be drawn through the fastigial point and declive (the fastigium-declive line). The craniocaudal diameter of the vermis should be measured perpendicular to this line, and this measurement is, therefore, independent of any tegmento-vermian angulation (Fig. 17.2-15B). According to this method of measurement,[71,75] growth of the craniocaudal diameter is linear, and this has been confirmed ultrasonographically. From this, we can predict expected craniocaudal diameter at any gestational age. Similar data have been derived for anteroposterior diameter, circumference, and surface area by both modalities.[7,8,76-82] The most contemporary data published include measurements of the craniocaudal diameter, anteroposterior diameter and surface area of the vermis and pons, and surface area of the brainstem

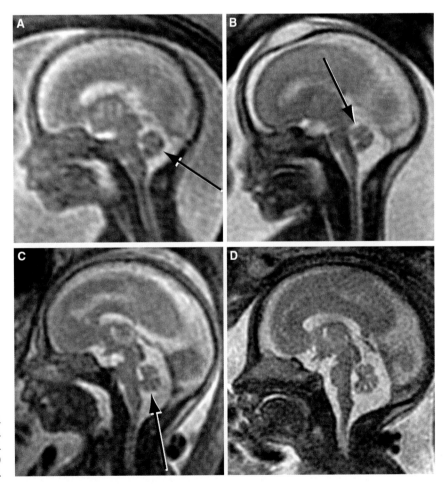

FIGURE 17.2-14: Fissures of the vermis. **A:** 21 weeks. Prepyramidal fissure *(arrow).* **B:** 21 to 22 weeks. Preculminate fissure *(arrow).* **C:** 24 weeks. Secondary (postpyramidal) fissure *(arrow).* **D:** 27 weeks. All lobules visible.

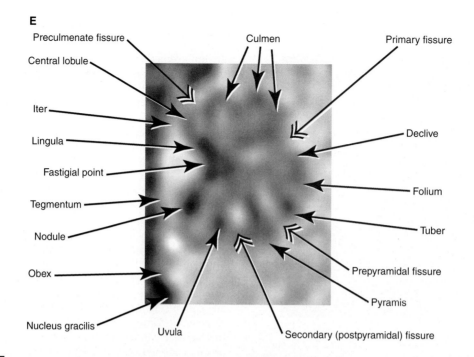

E

Preculmenate fissure

Central lobule

Iter

Lingula

Fastigial point

Tegmentum

Nodule

Obex

Nucleus gracilis

Culmen

Primary fissure

Declive

Folium

Tuber

Prepyramidal fissure

Pyramis

Uvula

Secondary (postpyramidal) fissure

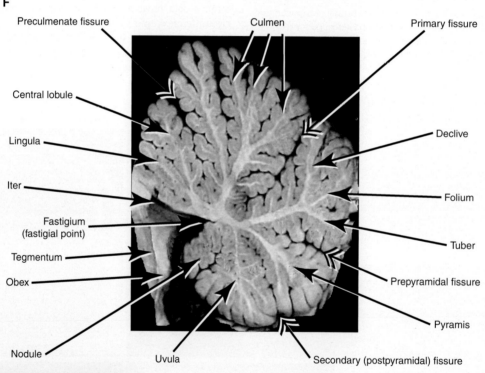

F

Preculmenate fissure

Central lobule

Lingula

Iter

Fastigium (fastigial point)

Tegmentum

Obex

Nodule

Culmen

Primary fissure

Declive

Folium

Tuber

Prepyramidal fissure

Pyramis

Uvula

Secondary (postpyramidal) fissure

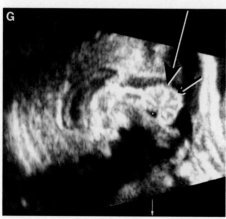

G

FIGURE 17.2-14: (*continued*) **E:** Detail of **D**. **F:** Detail of gross specimen for comparison. **G:** Three-dimensional midline sagittal US of the vermis at 25 weeks' gestation. The primary fissure (*long arrow*) as well as all the other fissures are visible. Note that the declive, folium, and tuber (*small arrow*) are barely differentiated. (**E**, reprinted from Robinson AJ, Blaser S, Toi A, et al. The fetal cerebellar vermis: assessment for abnormal development by ultrasonography and magnetic resonance imaging. *Ultrasound Q.* 2007;23(3):211–223. **F**, adapted with permission of Springer Nature Customer Service Center GmbH (SNCSC), from figure 9B in Duvernoy HM. *The Human Brainstem and Cerebellum.* Vienna, Austria: Springer Verlag; 1995;18–19. Copyright © 1995 Springer Nature. **G**, courtesy of Ants Toi, Department of Medical Imaging, University of Toronto, Canada; from Robinson AJ. Inferior vermian hypoplasia: preconception, misconception. *Ultrasound Obstet Gynecol.* 2014;43:123–136, with permission of John Wiley & Sons Ltd.)

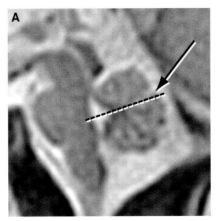
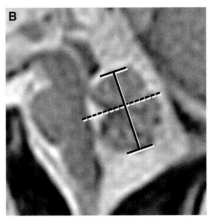

FIGURE 17.2-15: Vermian biometry (may also be done by ultrasound). **A:** Fastigial point-decline line (*dotted line*). The decline is the first lobule posterior to the primary fissure, seen as a low-signal focus (*arrow*). **B:** Craniocaudal diameter (perpendicular to fastigial point-decline line). (Reprinted with permission from Robinson AJ, Blaser S, Toi A, et al. The fetal cerebellar vermis: assessment for abnormal development by ultrasonography and magnetic resonance imaging. *Ultrasound Q.* 2007;23(3):211–223.)

by US (Table 20 in Appendix A1). Similar data by MRI are also provided (Tables 17.2-2 and 17.2-3).

The Ratio of Vermian Tissue Above and Below the Fastigial Point: A second measurement that can be made from the same fastigium-decline line is the relative growth of the superior and inferior lobes. Instead of measuring the entire vermis, it is measured above and below this line, and the values are compared (Fig. 17.2-15A). This is useful to determine whether the anterior or posterior lobes are primarily affected, for example, in cases of Joubert syndrome where the anterior lobe is typically smaller, or "inferior vermian hypoplasia" where the inferior vermis is smaller.

There should be linear and symmetrical growth of the vermis throughout gestation. The average height above and below the fastigial point should increase linearly, with average percentages above and below 47% and 53%, respectively, and no significant change in this ratio with gestational age.[71,75]

The Tegmento-Vermian Angle: The tegmento-vermian angle is a way of measuring "closure" of the fourth ventricle.[71,75] This angle is measured by drawing a line along the dorsal surface of the brainstem parallel to the tegmentum, which should transect the nucleus gracilis at the obex. A second line is drawn along the ventral surface of the vermis. The angle between them is the tegmento-vermian angle (Fig. 17.2-16A). The normal fetal tegmento-vermian angle is usually less than 18°, with average 2.5° + 2.3°, and a significantly elevated tegmento-vermian angle (>45° approximately) is typically associated with classic Dandy–Walker.[83–85] Angles in between are less clearly pathological, and the main differential is between Blake pouch cyst (normal vermis) and inferior vermian hypoplasia (Fig. 17.2-16B).

Utilizing these important measurements and landmarks, diagnosis of vermian and fourth ventricle anomalies can be obtained (Figs. 17.2-17 to 17.2-19).

Differential Diagnosis: Other causes of a cystic appearance of the posterior fossa are often confused with the more severe entities within DWC, particularly on axial sonographic images. Such appearances can be seen with persistent Blake pouch and mega cisterna magna (vide supra).[18] The latter can have normal outcomes; therefore, differentiation from true vermian pathology is imperative. Unfortunately, it is likely that literature, owing to the subtleties of distinguishing between Blake pouch cyst and a true inferior vermian hypoplasia, have included these two groups of patients together.

TABLE 17.2-2 Predicted Cerebellar Vermian Craniocaudal Diameter by Magnetic Resonance Imaging	
GESTATIONAL AGE (WK)	**MEAN DIAMETER (MM)**
14	4.6
15	5.3
16	6.1
17	6.8
18	7.5
19	8.3
20	9.0
21	9.7
22	10.4
23	11.2
24	11.9
25	12.6
26	13.4
27	14.1
28	14.8
29	15.6
30	16.3
31	17.0
32	17.7
33	18.5
34	19.2
35	19.9
36	20.7
37	21.4
38	22.1
39	22.9
40	23.6

Reproduced from Robinson AJ, Blaser S, Toi A, et al. The fetal cerebellar vermis: assessment for abnormal development by ultrasonography and magnetic resonance imaging. *Ultrasound Q.* 2007;23:211–223, permission of Wolters Kluwer Health.

TABLE 17.2-3   Cerebellovermian Biometry by Magnetic Resonance Imaging

	GESTATIONAL AGE (wk)												
	19	20	21	22	23	24	25	27/28	29/30	31/32	33	34/35	36/37
Transverse diameter of both cerebellar hemispheres (mm)	17	19.5	21.5	21.5	24	25	25	31.5	37	39	40	48.5	47.5
Anteroposterior diameter of the vermis (mm)	6	6.5	7	7	8	8	9.5	11.5	12.5	13	13	14.5	18.5
Height of the vermis (mm)	7.5	8.5	10	11	11	11	11.5	15.5	17	19	21	24	24

Reproduced from Triulzi F, Parazzini C, Righini A. MRI of fetal and neonatal cerebellar development. *Semin Fetal Neonatal Med.* 2005;10(5):411–420. Copyright © 2005 Elsevier. With permission.

One suggested useful landmark is that if the choroid plexus is in its normal position on the inferior surface of the vermis, then this is compatible with Blake pouch cyst, because it indicates that the anterior membranous area formed normally, whereas if the choroid plexus is on the inferior margin of the cyst, then it indicates that the anterior membranous area formed abnormally[21,42] and thus warrants further evaluation of the vermis.

Another suggested way of distinguishing between inferior vermian hypoplasia and persistent Blake pouch is the overall morphology of the fourth ventricle and Blake pouch. In true cerebellovermian pathology, the posterior fossa "cyst" appears either oval or trapezoidal with the walls of Blake pouch apposed to and indistinguishable from the peripheral margin of the posterior fossa on axial views, whereas in persistent Blake pouch, more of a keyhole (trefoil) shape is seen where the walls of the pouch may still be visible[22] (see Figs. 17.2-12, 17.2-17 to 17.2-19).

Prognosis: Specifically, of the three original morphological criteria for DWM (vermian dysgenesis, cystic dilatation of the fourth ventricle with enlargement of the posterior fossa, and elevation of the transverse sinus, tentorium, and torcula),[58] only vermian and regional cerebellar morphology has so far been demonstrated to correlate with prognosis.[40,87,88] Hydrocephalus is seen in 80% and, although also correlating with prognosis, was not part of the original criteria, and other associated abnormalities (see later) also have a much more significant prognostic value.

DWC is often associated with an abnormal karyotype in 29%[9,10]; CNS abnormalities in 50% to 70%, including ventriculomegaly, brainstem dysgenesis, callosal dysgenesis, migrational disorders, encephaloceles, and neural tube defects[60,65,89–93]; and in 47% with concurrent non-CNS anomalies,[9] including heart defects,[60,65,91,94] polydactyly and syndactyly,[60,91,95] and facial anomalies.[65,91] DWC with additional findings, especially brainstem dysgenesis, has an associated poorer outcome.[20,96] Seizures, hearing or visual difficulties, systemic abnormalities, and other CNS abnormalities are associated with poor intellectual development; the presence of two of these four risk factors identifies patients with borderline or lower intelligence 94% of the time.[97] In one meta-analysis of posterior fossa malformations, the overall rate of abnormal neurodevelopmental outcome in children with a prenatal diagnosis of DWM was 58.2%.[98]

The term "isolated inferior vermian hypoplasia" has been used to describe a subset in which there are no known underlying or associated abnormalities,[41,99,100] and this group generally has a better outcome.[101–106] However, it can be impossible to explain prenatally whether vermian hypoplasia is isolated, since associated abnormalities, genetic or chromosomal, may be undetectable.[107] In one study, 50% of Dandy–Walker and inferior vermian hypoplasia patients were abnormal even if the abnormality appeared to be isolated.[25] In another study, postnatal imaging and follow-up were normal in 6 of 19 cases of isolated inferior vermian hypoplasia, and those 13 with postnatal confirmation had good overall outcome with only mild developmental delays in a subset of infants.[41]

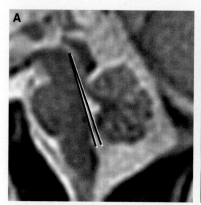
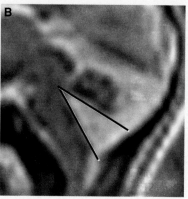

FIGURE 17.2-16: Construction of lines used to assess the tegmento-vermian angle (may also be done by ultrasound). **A:** Normal tegmento-vermian angle. **B:** Abnormal tegmento-vermian angle. (Reprinted with permission from Robinson AJ, Blaser S, Toi A, et al. The fetal cerebellar vermis: assessment for abnormal development by ultrasonography and magnetic resonance imaging. *Ultrasound Q.* 2007;23(3):211–223.)

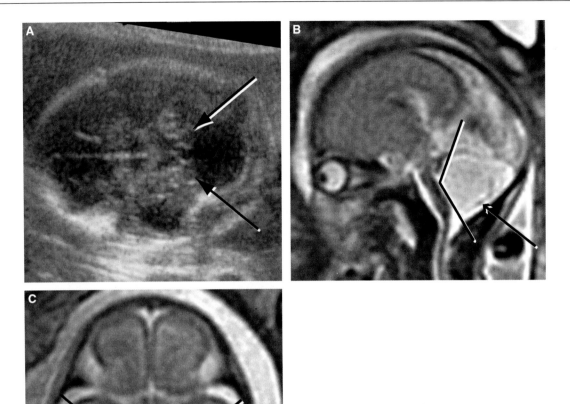

FIGURE 17.2-17: Cerebellar anomaly with abnormal tegmento-vermian angle. **A:** In this 22-week fetus, a large cystic posterior fossa is seen on axial sonography with small cerebellar hemispheres on either side of the midline *(arrows)*. No midline vermian tissue is identified. **B:** On sagittal MRI the tegmento-vermian angle is increased *(lines)* with the fourth ventricle uncovered *(arrow)*. The vermis is very small; there is no primary fissure or fastigial point, again in keeping with a primitive configuration. **C:** On axial MRI, the cerebellar hemispheres are small *(arrows)*. The ventricular system is dilated, resulting in large temporal horns. (Reprinted with permission from Robinson AJ, Blaser S, Toi A, et al. The fetal cerebellar vermis: assessment for abnormal development by ultrasonography and magnetic resonance imaging. *Ultrasound Q.* 2007;23(3):211–223.)

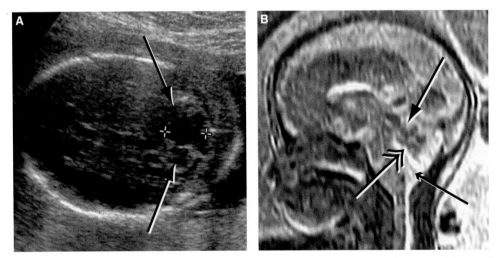

FIGURE 17.2-18: Vermian anomaly/Dandy–Walker continuum. **A:** In this 21-week fetus, there is a trapezoid shape to Blake pouch, and the cerebellar hemispheres *(arrows)* are larger than in the prior case. **B:** By fetal MRI, the tegmento-vermian angle is increased *(small arrow)*. The fastigial point is visible *(double arrow)*, and vermian lobulation is seen *(large arrow)*. Again, this would fall into the Dandy–Walker continuum, but this fetus had other facial, visceral, and skeletal anomalies. The autopsy diagnosis was Wolf–Hirschhorn syndrome, characterized by multiple congenital anomalies, including midline fusion defects, associated with a chromosomal deletion of the short arm of chromosome 4.[86] Thus even though the cerebellar hemispheres are larger and vermian morphology is better than in the prior case, the presence of associated abnormalities gives a worse prognosis. (Reprinted with permission from Robinson AJ, Blaser S, Toi A, et al. The fetal cerebellar vermis: assessment for abnormal development by ultrasonography and magnetic resonance imaging. *Ultrasound Q.* 2007;23(3):211–223)

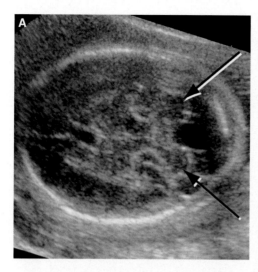
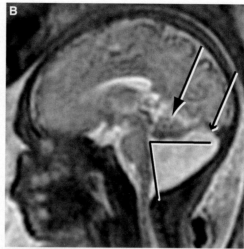
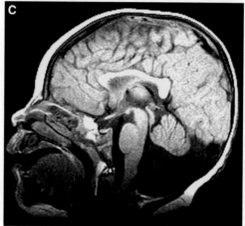

FIGURE 17.2-19: Vermian hypoplasia. **A:** In this fetus, at 34 weeks by axial sonography, the cerebellar hemispheres are approaching normal size *(arrows)*, and proportionally more midline vermian tissue is seen than in Figures 17.2-17 and 17.2-18. **B:** On sagittal MRI, the tegmento-vermian angle is increased *(lines)*, with elevation of the torcula *(small arrow)*. The vermis is less hypoplastic than in the previous examples, and the primary fissure is seen *(single arrow)*. The fastigial point is less flattened. **C:** Postnatal MRI at 8 months of age shows good vermian lobulation. (Reprinted with permission from Robinson AJ, Blaser S, Toi A, et al. The fetal cerebellar vermis: assessment for abnormal development by ultrasonography and magnetic resonance imaging. *Ultrasound Q.* 2007;23(3):211–223.)

Recurrence Risk: Because of the autosomal recessive nature of many of the causes of vermian hypoplasia, there is a 25% recurrence risk (Table 17.2-4).

Cerebellar Anomalies

Cerebellar Hemispheres

As previously mentioned, the cerebellar hemispheres develop from the rhombic lips on either side of the developing vermis, under the influence of the isthmic organizer and various genetic factors. The cerebellar hemispheres and the vermian lobules in the superior aspect of the posterior lobe comprise the neocerebellum. The neocerebellum is seen in mammals only and is largest in humans. Functionally, it is involved with complex motor tasks, cognitive function, and language. The transcerebellar diameter is, therefore, the primary method for assessment of growth in the fetus. Global (bilateral) cerebellar hypoplasia usually has a chromosomal or genetic etiology (Table 17.2-4).

Unilateral Cerebellar Hypoplasia

Unilateral cerebellar hypoplasia is seen in PHACES (posterior fossa malformation, segmental facial hemangioma, arterial anomalies, cardiac defects, eye abnormalities, sternal/ventral defect) syndrome, Moebius syndrome, neurofibromatosis type I, and COL4A1-associated disorders.[108–111]

PHACES syndrome is a rare neurocutaneous disorder, associated with unilateral cerebellar hypoplasia in 20%, more commonly the left. In the presence of unilateral cerebellar hypoplasia, the small cerebellum is displaced upwards by ipsilateral posterior fossa cyst communicating with an asymmetrically distended fourth ventricle. The upwardly rotated and deviated vermis forms an oblique configuration, resulting in a "tilted telephone receiver sign" on coronal plane through upper vermis (Fig. 17.2-20). Associated intracranial arterial variant anatomy and microphthalmia[112] may also be detected prenatally. The segmental hemangioma, being of the infantile type, would not, however, be detectable. Thus, because major criteria for diagnosis are absent in utero, the tilted telephone receiver sign should be considered diagnostic.

Other causes of unilateral cerebellar hypoplasia typically include clastic lesions (e.g., ischemia, infection) or unilateral arachnoid cyst and do not have the tilted telephone receiver sign. Evidence of clastic etiology includes hemorrhage, parenchymal calcifications and/or cysts, and irregular contour. Clastic lesions result in disruption (rather than a true malformation) of the normal cerebellar development, causing cerebellar clefts, disorderly alignment of the folia/fissures, irregular gray/white matter junction, and abnormal arborization of the white matter.[113,114]

Rhombencephalosynapsis

Rhombencephalosynapsis is a disorder in which the vermis is severely deficient and the cerebellar hemispheric folia are continuous across the midline (Fig. 17.2-21). The nomenclature

TABLE 17.2-4	Associations with Cerebellar Hypoplasia
ETIOLOGY	**DISORDER**
Chromosomal	45,X
	Trisomies 18, 13, 21, and 9
	Triploidy
	Unbalanced translocation
	Subtelomeric deletion
Genetic	
Congenital muscular dystrophies Lissencephalies	Walker–Warburg
	Muscle-eye brain
	Fukuyama
	RELN
	VLDRL
	TUBA1A
	TUBB2B
	TUBB3
Polymicrogyria	Tubulinopathies
	GPR56
Periventricular nodular heterotopia	FLNA
Ciliopathies (AR) *Confirmed*	Joubert syndrome
	Meckel–Gruber
	COACH
	CORS
	Arima (cerebro-oculo-hepato-renal)
	Oral-facial-digital syndrome
	Senior Loken
	Bardet–Biedl
	Leber congenital amaurosis
	Cogan-type congenital oculomotor apraxia
	Nephronophthisis
	Jeune (asphyxiating thoracic dystrophy)
	Ellis–van Creveld

ETIOLOGY	**DISORDER**
Suspected	Neural tube defects
	Polysyndactyly
	Callosal dysgenesis
	Congenital heart disease
Metabolic	Congenital disorders of glycosylation
	Opitz
	Mitochondrial disorders
	Infantile neuroaxonal dystrophy
Other	Aase–Smith arthrogryposis (AD)
	Ruvalcaba syndrome (AR)
	Aicardi syndrome (X-linked and XXY males)
	Fraser cryptophthalmos (AR)
	PHACES (associated with facial hemangioma)
	Klippel–Feil
	Cornelia de Lange
Teratogenic	Diabetes
	Alcohol
	Coumadin
	Isotretinoin
Infectious	CMV
	Rubella
Hemorrhagic	Intraventricular hemorrhage
	Cerebellar hemorrhage
Syndromic	Goldenhar
	Holoprosencephaly
Unknown	Cleft lip/palate
	Polymicrogyria
	Gray matter heterotopias

Reproduced and adapted from Robinson AJ. Inferior vermian hypoplasia: preconception, misconception. *Ultrasound Obstet Gynecol.* 2014;43:123–136, with permission.
AD, autosomal dominant; AR, autosomal recessive; CMV, cytomegalovirus; COACH, cerebellar vermis hypoplasia, oligophrenia, ataxia, coloboma, hepatic fibrosis; CORS, cerebro-oculo-renal syndrome; FLNA, filamin A; PHACES, posterior fossa malformation, segmental facial hemangioma, arterial anomalies, cardiac defects, eye abnormalities, sternal/ventral defect.

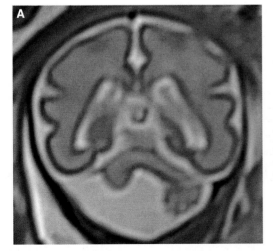
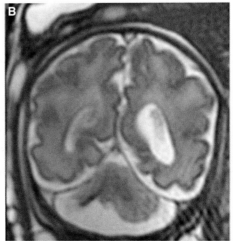

FIGURE 17.2-20: A: Coronal transcerebellar MRI of a fetus with unilateral cerebellar hypoplasia and PHACES demonstrating the "tilted telephone receiver" sign characterized by an upward displaced unilateral hypoplastic hemisphere; an asymmetric dilated fourth ventricle connecting to an ipsilateral retrocerebellar cyst; and a deviated vermis merging with a contralateral cerebellar peduncle, forming an elongated oblique connection between the hemispheres (the upward vermian rotation is not shown, seen only in sagittal plane). **B:** Coronal transcerebellar MRI of a fetus with unilateral cerebellar hypoplasia, but without PHACES. The "tilted telephone receiver" sign cannot be seen. Note abnormal hypointense signal suggestive of a hemorrhagic event on the surface of the affected cerebellar hemisphere.

does nothing to improve the understanding of the condition or cerebellar development in general. The etymology of "synapsis" is from Greek, meaning "fusion." Consequently, the description of the abnormalities seen in this condition includes "fusion" of the fastigial nuclei, "apposition" of deep cerebellar nuclei, "fusion" of the middle cerebellar peduncles, and folia "fused" across the midline. For this reason, it would probably be more accurate to rename rhombencephalosynapsis as holo*rhomb*encephaly, although "holo*pros*encephaly of the hindbrain" has also been suggested.[99] The frequent association of holo*pros*encephaly with rhombencephalosynapsis then becomes conceptually more logical.

In contradistinction to DWC, it is the anterior vermis that is usually absent, with the posterior vermis demonstrating variable deficiency, and, interestingly, the most inferior lobule, the nodulus, is typically preserved.[115]

Incidence: The incidence is rare.

Embryology and Genetics: The cerebellar primordium is a single but bilobed structure that is continuous across the midline, and the vermis grows from proliferation of the cerebellar primordium, not through fusion of the cerebellar hemispheres. The fact that, in rhombencephalosynapsis, the posterior vermis and most inferior lobule can sometimes be present in the absence of the anterior vermis[116] demonstrates that the posterior part of the vermis develops independently from its own primordium and not as a result of craniocaudal growth of a single midline primordium. This concept is backed up from experimental evidence, which shows that granule cells arising from the lateral upper rhombic lip migrate medially into the posterior cerebellum, whereas granule cells arising from the median upper rhombic lip are confined to an anterior cerebellar distribution.[117]

Rhombencephalosynapsis has been seen together with VACTERL-H association (vertebral, anorectal, cardiac, tracheoesophageal fistula, renal, limb, hydrocephalus), Gomez–Lopez–Hernandez syndrome[118–121] (trigeminal anesthesia,

bilateral temporal alopecia, short stature, mental retardation, midface hypoplasia, oxycephaly secondary to bilateral lambdoid suture synostosis, low-set ears, fifth finger clinodactyly), and polycystic kidney disease.[122]

Etiology and Pathogenesis: Although unknown, the association with holoprosencephaly is suggestive of defective dorsoventral patterning.[123]

Diagnosis: The key feature is that of the cerebellar folia crossing the midline from one cerebellar hemisphere to the other with no intervening vermis.[124] The normal dumbbell shape of the cerebellum on axial views is not present because the central "stem" of the dumbbell that represents the vermis is missing. There may be dorsal pointing of the fourth ventricle.

On midline sagittal views, the normal vermian landmarks cannot be seen. The craniocaudal diameter in the midline is larger than expected, because the normal vermis, which is absent in this condition, always has a smaller craniocaudal diameter than the adjacent cerebellar hemispheres (see Fig. 17.2-21).

Other midline structures may also be deficient, including the cavum septi pellucidi, corpus callosum, aqueduct of Sylvius leading to hydrocephalus, optic nerves, chiasm, tracts, posterior pituitary, quadrigeminal plate, or features of holoprosencephaly.[125]

Differential Diagnosis: Other forms of vermian hypoplasia are in the differential, although the continuous cerebellar folia without intervening vermis are a pathognomonic feature.

Prognosis: A wide range of clinical features have been reported,[126] and presentation correlates with the presence and degree of supratentorial abnormalities, most commonly in the spectrum of holoprosencephaly.

Clinical presentation after birth ranges from mild truncal ataxia and normal cognition to severe cerebral palsy with epilepsy and mental retardation. Most patients have some degree of

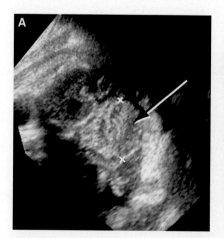 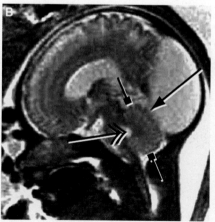 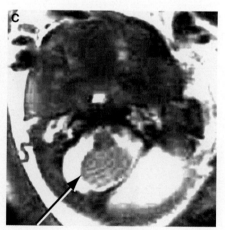

FIGURE 17.2-21: Rhombencephalosynapsis. **A:** In this fetus case at 30 weeks' gestation, axial sonography demonstrates an abnormal cerebellum with transverse folia that are seen to be continuous between the hemispheres across the midline *(arrow)*. The transcerebellar diameter was 3.02 cm, which would be normal for 26 weeks' gestational age. **B:** On sagittal MRI, the fastigial point is rounded off *(double arrow)* rather than triangular. There is no primary fissure *(single arrow)*. The craniocaudal diameter *(square calipers)* of the "vermis" is much larger than expected, because it is actually the "fused" cerebellar hemispheres that are being measured (see below for vermian craniocaudal diameter measurement). This could lead to false reassurance that the vermis is present. A large left-sided cerebrospinal fluid (CSF) collection is also present and included on the slightly off-axis sagittal image. **C:** On axial MRI, the cerebellar folia are again seen to be continuous across the midline *(arrow)*. (Courtesy of A. Michelle Fink, Department of Medical Imaging, Royal Children's Hospital, Melbourne, Australia; Reprinted with permission from Robinson AJ, Blaser S, Toi A, et al. The fetal cerebellar vermis: assessment for abnormal development by ultrasonography and magnetic resonance imaging. *Ultrasound Q.* 2007;23(3):211–223.)

cognitive dysfunction, often associated with attention deficit and hyperactivity. Motor milestones are often delayed.[123,127,128]

Management: Thorough evaluation for coexistent anomalies is necessary as these negatively impact prognosis. Presence of more severe forms of holoprosencephaly is incompatible with life.

Recurrence Risk: All cases are sporadic.

Joubert Syndrome and Related Disorders (Molar Tooth Malformations)

It has recently been shown that the molar tooth brainstem and cerebellar malformation is seen with many associated anomalies that encompass many syndromes, and these are collectively known as Joubert syndrome and related disorders (JSRD).[129–131] These disorders are unified by a common abnormality of ciliary function that in general are characterized by a combination of ocular, cerebral, hepatic, renal, and skeletal manifestations.

The classification of JSRD has recently been revised and divided into four distinct disorders[132]: Joubert syndrome, COACH (cerebellar vermis hypoplasia, oligophrenia, ataxia, coloboma, hepatic fibrosis) syndrome, CORS (cerebro-oculo-renal syndrome), and oculo-facial-digital syndrome type VI (OFDS-VI).

Incidence: Initially thought to be rare, but as our understanding expands around this group of conditions, it is apparent that many previously unclassified forms of vermian hypoplasia fall into the category of ciliopathies.

Embryology and Genetics: Most of the related syndromes seem to be the result of mutations to genes encoding ciliary proteins, which are important in a wide range of functions, including ciliogenesis, body axis formation, renal function, brain development, and ocular development.[133–136]

Etiology and Pathogenesis: It is at present unknown how the defective ciliary proteins have such wide-ranging effects, but they are known to play a role in normal cellular function in many cell types and are necessary for perceptory input such as sight, hearing, and smell.

Diagnosis: The classic finding is that of a "molar tooth" configuration of the mesencephalon, which can be demonstrated both sonographically[137] and by MRI.[15,138–141] This feature is seen on axial sections and is caused by thickened superior cerebellar peduncles (representing the roots of the molar tooth) and a deep interpeduncular cistern owing to the absence of decussation of the superior cerebellar peduncles.[142] The fourth ventricle has a bat-wing configuration and has a midline point posteriorly where the two cerebellar hemispheres touch each other in the midline. The vermis is abnormally lobulated (Fig. 17.2-22).

On sagittal views, the vermis is elevated, and the anterior lobe is generally the most hypoplastic. The fourth ventricle has a trapezoidal configuration. Often, partial volume effect from the adjacent cerebellar hemispheres that touch in the midline can give the false impression that the vermis is larger.

Associated retinopathy, hepatic fibrosis, renal cysts, polydactyly, facial clefting, hamartomas of the tuber cinereum, and tongue tumours[143] can help with the diagnosis; these may not be detectable antenatally.

Differential Diagnosis: Other forms of vermian hypoplasia should be considered, although the molar tooth configuration of the brainstem is a pathognomonic feature.

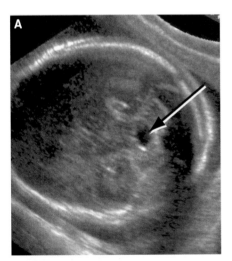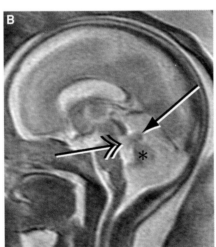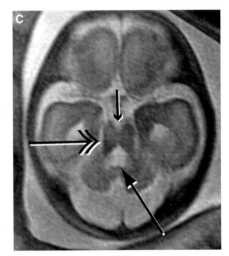

FIGURE 17.2-22: Molar tooth malformation. **A:** In this fetus at 20 weeks' gestation, axial sonography shows an enlarged cisterna magna measuring 15 mm in the standard anteroposterior direction. There is an abnormally shaped fourth ventricle *(arrow)*, which is rounded rather than the normal diamond shape. Some apparent tissue is seen to separate the fourth ventricle and cisterna magna, but this is actually the two cerebellar hemispheres touching in the midline. This has been referred to as the "buttocks" sign. **B:** On sagittal MRI, we see a small amount of midline tissue between the cerebellar hemispheres consistent with vermian tissue. On this view, most of what looks to be midline tissue is actually partial volume averaging of adjacent cerebellar hemispheres *(asterisk)*. The vermis is only the superior part, and there is no fastigial point *(double arrow)* or primary fissure *(single arrow)*. The roof of the fourth ventricle appears squared-off. **C:** On the axial MRI, there is a "molar tooth" shape to the brainstem because of thickened horizontally oriented superior cerebellar peduncles *(double arrow)* and a deep interpeduncular cistern *(small arrow)* secondary to nondecussation, and the fourth ventricle has an abnormal "batwing" shape *(large arrow)*. (**A**, courtesy of Dr. Phyllis Glanc, Department of Medical Imaging, Women's College Hospital, Toronto, Canada. **A–C**, reprinted with permission from Robinson AJ, Blaser S, Toi A, et al. The fetal cerebellar vermis: assessment for abnormal development by ultrasonography and magnetic resonance imaging. *Ultrasound Q.* 2007;23(3):211–223.)

Prognosis: Patients with the JSRD syndromes have hypotonia, ataxia, developmental delay (cognitive and motor), oculomotor apraxia, and the "molar tooth sign." Other features include episodic neonatal hyperpnea and rhythmic tongue protrusion, mental retardation, postaxial polydactyly, mild retinopathy, and polymicrogyria.[144]

Management: Genetic counseling is recommended. Infants and children with abnormal breathing may require stimulatory medications (e.g., caffeine), supplemental oxygen, mechanical support, or tracheostomy in rare cases. Other interventions may include speech therapy for oromotor dysfunction; occupational and physical therapy; educational support, including special programs for the visually impaired; and feedings by gastrostomy tube. Surgery may be required for polydactyly and symptomatic ptosis and/or strabismus. Nephronophthisis, end-stage renal disease, liver failure and/or fibrosis are treated with standard approaches.[145]

Recurrence Risk: Joubert is transmitted as an autosomal recessive, with recurrence risk of 25%.

BRAINSTEM ANOMALIES

Brainstem Hypoplasia and the Kinked or "Z-shaped" Brainstem

Embryology and Genetics: The cranial neural tube forms three primitive brain vesicles: the prosencephalon, mesencephalon, and rhombencephalon. The mesencephalon forms the midbrain. The rhombencephalon, which forms the caudal part of the brainstem, segments into eight rhombomeres, the most rostral pair of which form the future cerebellum. At around 5 weeks' gestation, the brainstem develops a posterior kink, known as the dorsal pontine flexure, which resolves into the normal mature configuration by 15 weeks' gestation.[146] In several conditions, the brainstem maintains this embryological configuration, and this is known as the kinked

or "Z-shaped" brainstem and generally carries a poor prognosis.[147] The three main differentials for this appearance are the congenital muscular dystrophies, tubulinopathy, and X-linked hydrocephalus (*L1CAM*)[148] (vide infra).

Differential Diagnosis: Severe brainstem and cerebellar anomalies include global brain malformations such as the congenital muscular dystrophies (α-dystroglycanopathies) and the similar-appearing tubulinopathies. In these conditions, the brainstem typically, but not always, retains its primitive dorsal pontine flexure seen in early embryogenesis, and may have a Z-shape.[147] It is difficult to differentiate tubulinopathy from congenital muscular dystrophy prenatally without genetic studies; however, in the latter, one would expect a normal head size and other features such as microphthalmia and occipital cephalocele (Fig. 17.2-23)[149] and, due to neuronal over-migration beyond the cortical surface, the subarachnoid space should be reduced and the layer of overmigrated neurons visible by both ultrasound and MRI (Fig. 17.2-24). In other forms of lissencephaly, the association of abnormal neuronal migration with abnormal axonal guidance, manifest as callosal dysgenesis, and should prompt the diagnosis of tubulinopathy (Figs. 17.2-25 and 17.2-26).[150,151] Additional findings of microcephaly and basal ganglia abnormalities may be helpful. In one study of tubulin-related (*TUBA1A, TUBB2B, TUBB3*) dysplasia, cerebellar abnormalities were seen in 86% of cases, with the postero-superior region of the cerebellar hemisphere most frequently affected, along with frequent brainstem involvement.[152]

The other differential of Z-shaped brainstem is x-linked hydrocephalus (*L1CAM*), which can also demonstrate callosal dysgenesis, however adducted thumbs are also a typical, but nonspecific, finding.[153]

Dorsal displacement of the brainstem can also be seen in tectocerebellar dysraphia.[154] characterized by posterior encephalocele with dorsal traction of the brainstem towards the occipital defect, vermian hypoplasia and "inversion" of the cerebellar hemispheres.

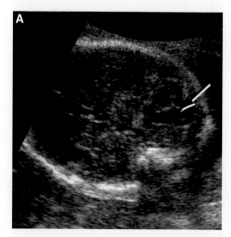 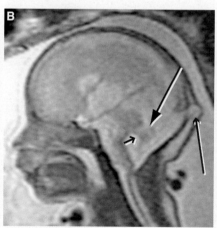 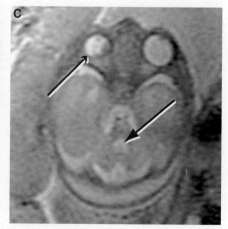

FIGURE 17.2-23: In this fetus at 28 weeks' gestation, axial sonography (**A**) shows a deficient vermis (*arrow*) apparently consistent with a Dandy–Walker variant. There was also asymmetric ventricular size (not shown). (**B**) On sagittal MRI, we see that the vermis is abnormally shaped with no fastigial point (*short arrow*) or primary fissure (*large arrow*). The fourth ventricle appears abnormally large, and an occipital cephalocele is seen (*small arrow*). The brainstem has a primitive configuration, retaining the embryonic dorsal pontine flexure giving it a "Z" shape. (**C**) On axial MRI, the fourth ventricle has lost its normal diamond shape (*arrow*), and one of the fetal eyes is small and distorted (*small arrow*). This is an example of congenital muscular dystrophy. The additional findings of occipital cephalocele and microphthalmia are consistent with Walker–Warburg phenotype; however, interestingly, this patient actually had a Fukutin gene mutation on postnatal genetic studies, a known but exceedingly rare variant cause of this condition. (Images courtesy of Beth Kline-Fath, MD.)

Pontocerebellar Hypoplasia

Incidence: Pontocerebellar hypoplasia (PCH) is very rare.[155]

Embryology and Genetics: PCH is a neurodegenerative process with early prenatal onset.[156] Changes typical of PCH include volume loss in the ventral pons and cerebellum and, to a lesser extent, cerebral cortex.[155] During gestation, especially third trimester and postnatal, there is progressive degeneration of the cerebellar cortex with loss of Purkinje cells, fragmentation of the dentate nuclei and often neuronal loss and degeneration of the inferior olivary nucleus.[155] Cerebellar hemispheres are typically more severely affected than the vermis. In the pons, there is progressive loss of ventral nuclei and transverse fibers.[155]

Etiology and Pathogenesis: Previously two classical types of pontocerebellar hypoplasia were described: type 1(PCH1) in which cases had accompanying spinal anterior horn disease with prenatal onset of contractures and polyhydramnios and type 2 (PCH2) with chorea and dyskinesia. Currently there are 11 subtypes of pontocerebellar hypoplasia described.[157] Many genes are now implicated and include *VRK1, EXOSC3, EXOSC8, SLC25A46, TSEN54, TSEN2, TSEN34, SEPSECS, VPS53, TSEN15, PCLO, RARS2, TOE1, CHMP1A, AMPD2, CLP1, TBC1D23*.[157] Inheritance is autosomal recessive. PCH2 is the most common type, and the most encountered gene mutation is TSEN54.[158]

Most of the genes responsible for PCH are essential for general protein synthesis and RNA transfer which are vital for maturing neurons.[155,158]

Diagnosis: Molecular genetic testing for known mutations in PCH may confirm diagnosis in the presence of positive family history. Prenatal diagnosis via US is often not possible in the first and second trimester as findings of volume loss manifested by decreased transverse cerebellar diameter are detected primarily in the third trimester, usually after 30 weeks' gestation.[156,159] Head circumference is typically normal prenatal since microcephaly tends to develop after birth.[159] Concern for PCH may be raised by intrauterine contractures, seizures, or development of polyhydramnios.

Fetal MRI may hold promise in earlier detection of the pontine and cerebellar volume loss as the technique allows excellent definition of brainstem hypoplasia and cerebellar pathology.[160] In addition, diffusion tensor imaging may be able to demonstrate absent crossing fibers at the level of the pons.[156] On postnatal MRI, the most common findings described in PCH are flat and severely reduced cerebellar hemispheres (dragonfly appearing) and small pons (Fig. 17.2-27).[158]

Differential Diagnosis: Brainstem abnormalities are often seen in conjunction with cerebellar hypoplasia/dysplasia as the

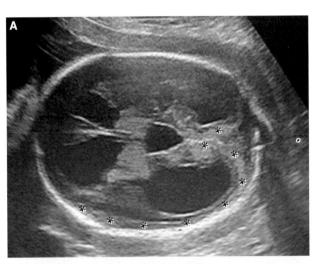
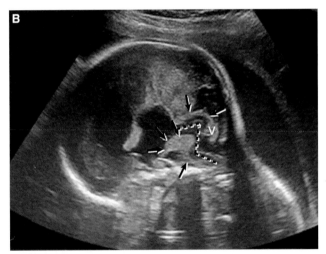
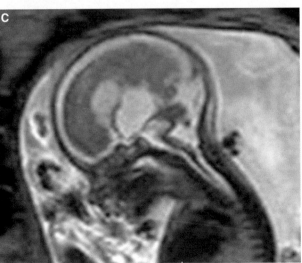

FIGURE 17.2-24: Congenital muscular dystrophy. Patient referred at 22 weeks' gestation for suspicion of obstructive ventriculomegaly, related to aqueduct stenosis and associated with an abnormal posterior fossa. Axial (**A**) supratentorial sonographic image showing an outer agyric echogenic band on the brain surface, associated with complete absence of pericerebral space *(asterisk)*. **B:** The sonographic midsagittal image showed a "Z"-shaped appearance of the brainstem *(dotted line)* that was surrounded by an echogenic band *(arrows)*, associated with a small vermis (*V*). **C:** Midsagittal MRI confirmed sonographic data, demonstrating a kinked brainstem. Overmigration was demonstrated retrospectively, as a band of hyperintensity anterior to mesencephalon and brainstem.

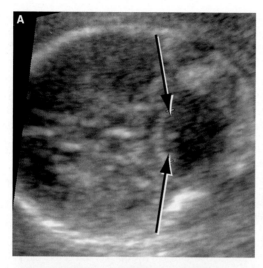
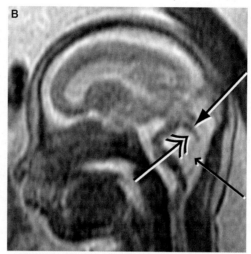
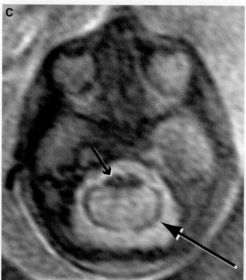

FIGURE 17.2-25: Tubulinopathy. **A:** In this fetus at 20 weeks' gestation, the axial sonogram shows a large posterior fossa cystic space and two tiny cerebellar hemispheres on either side of the midline *(arrows)*. Biometric measurements were abnormally small. **B:** On sagittal MRI, we see that the vermis is incomplete, and there is no fastigial point *(double arrow)* or primary fissure *(single arrow)*. The fourth ventricle is uncovered *(small arrow)*. There is a thin cerebral cortex with a prominent subarachnoid space, and the brainstem has a primitive "Z-shaped" configuration owing to a retained embryonic dorsal pontine flexure. There is complete agenesis of the corpus callosum that cannot be seen at all on this midline section. **C:** On axial MRI, there are shell-like cerebellar hemispheres *(arrow)* and a hypoplastic brainstem *(small arrow)*. (From Robinson AJ, Blaser S, Toi A, et al. The fetal cerebellar vermis: assessment for abnormal development by ultrasonography and magnetic resonance imaging. *Ultrasound Q.* 2007;23:211–223, with permission of Wolters Kluwer Health.)

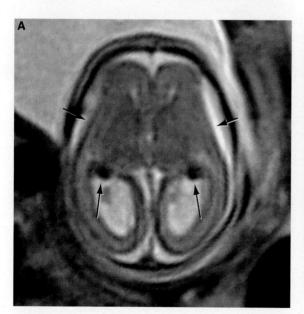
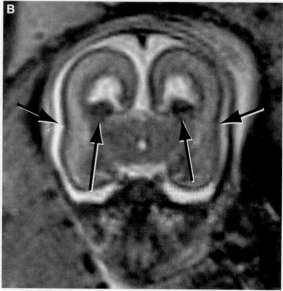

FIGURE 17.2-26: Tubulinopathy. In this fetus with cerebellar hypoplasia, axial (**A**) and coronal (**B**) MRI show a smooth brain surface with flat insula *(short arrows)* and abnormal prominence of the ganglionic eminences *(long arrows)* bilaterally. There is associated callosal agenesis clearly visible on the coronal view. In this particular case, there was no Z-shaped brainstem.

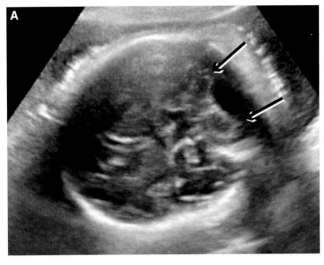

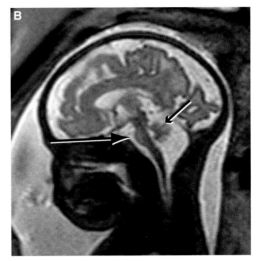

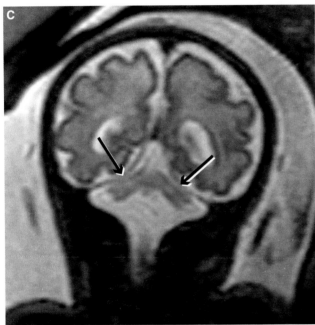

FIGURE 17.2-27: Pontocerebellar hypoplasia. **A:** Axial US demonstrating hypoplasia of the cerebellar hemispheres *(arrows)* with enlargement of the cisterna magna. **B:** Sagittal MRI demonstrating small pons *(long arrow)* and volume loss in the cerebellar vermis *(short arrow).* **C:** Coronal MRI demonstrating small bilateral cerebellar hemispheres *(arrows),* appearing like a dragonfly. (Images courtesy of Beth Kline-Fath.)

germinal matrix in the rhombic lips is responsible for the formation of the ventral pons.[161] Other disorders to consider often have a kinked brainstem and include the congenital muscular dystrophies, tubulinopathies, and *L1CAM* gene mutations. *RELN* and *VLDLR* mutations resulting in lissencephaly may have associated PCH.[157]

Prognosis: In all cases of PCH, children experience severe intellectual deficit, global developmental delay, swallowing problems, and seizures.[155] Most patients with PCH die during infancy or childhood due to primary respiratory insufficiency.[155,158]

Management: Termination of pregnancy may be considered if diagnosis can be confirmed. Management is primarily supportive after birth with nutrition obtained via gastrostomy tube.

Recurrence Risk: Most cases are transmitted autosomal recessive, with 25% risk of recurrence.

Pontine Tegmental Cap Dysplasia

Incidence: This is extremely rare, with only a few cases published in the prenatal literature and less than 50 postnatally.[162]

Embryology and Genetics: This is unknown, but thought to be due to a disorder of axonal guidance.

Etiology and Pathogenesis: Postulated to be due to failed neuronal connections, apoptosis, and false connections.[163]

Diagnosis: The classic finding is that of a characteristic elevation or bump of the tegmentum projecting into the fourth ventricle. There is severe hypoplasia of the middle and inferior cerebellar peduncles (Fig. 17.2-28).

Differential Diagnosis: The "cap" is a characteristic feature not seen in other brainstem dysplasias.

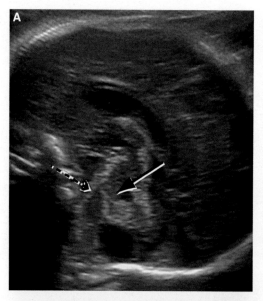

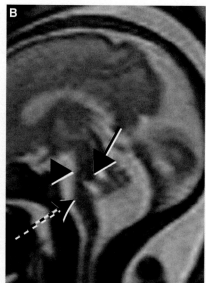

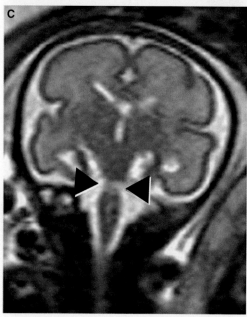

FIGURE 17.2-28: Pontine tegmental cap dysplasia. **A:** Prenatal ultrasonography at 28 weeks' gestation, midsagittal view of the cerebellum. The flat pons *(dashed arrow)* and the posterior pontine vaulted structure *(arrow)* protruding into the fourth ventricle are well visualized. The vermis is small, and its foliation is abnormal. Prenatal MRI at 28 weeks' gestation: T2 midline sagittal **(B)** and coronal **(C)** slices. The midline sagittal slice shows exactly the same abnormalities as ultrasonography. The mesencephalic isthmus is shortened *(black arrowhead)*, the pons is flat *(dashed arrow)*, and there is a posterior pontine vaulted structure *(arrow)*. The coronal view shows marked narrowing of the caudal pons *(black arrowheads)* due to absence of middle cerebellar peduncles.

Prognosis: This is associated with a poor outcome, with sensorimotor deficits in the cranial nerves V through IX, cerebellar hypoplasia, and other systemic abnormalities.

Management: Similar to PCH, termination of pregnancy may be considered. Postnatal management is primarily supportive.

Recurrence Risk: Sporadic with no recurrence risk.

Diencephalic-Mesencephalic Junction Dysplasia

Incidence: This is extremely rare, with only a single case series published in the prenatal literature.[164]

Embryology and Genetics: No causative genes have yet been linked, but possibly within the *L1CAM* and *L1*-like spectrum.

Etiology and Pathogenesis: Dorsoventral patterning defects with severe early neuronal dysgenesis.

Diagnosis: The classic finding is that of a poorly defined junction between the diencephalon and the mesencephalon, such that the thalami and midbrain appear fused on sagittal views, along with a deep ventral cleft in the midbrain, giving it a butterfly-like appearance on axial sections. Other associated features include callosal dysgenesis, mild kinking of the cervicomedullary junction, moderate brainstem kinking, an enlarged and ventrally located interthalamic adhesion, and poorly defined (stenotic) cerebral aqueduct with lateral and third ventriculomegaly (Fig. 17.2-29).

Differential Diagnosis: Other causes of developmental hydrocephalus include in particular X-linked hydrocephalus (*L1CAM*) and other conditions with a kinked brainstem (vide supra).

Prognosis: Clinical presentation includes severe cognitive impairment, postnatal progressive microcephaly, axial hypotonia, spastic tetraparesis, and seizures.[145]

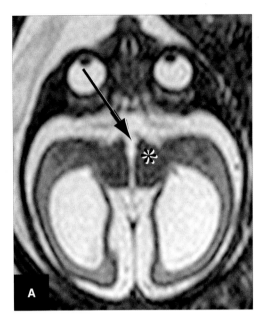
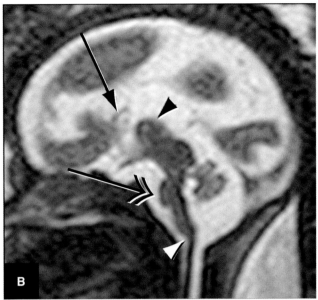

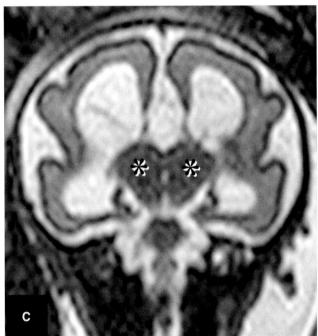

FIGURE 17.2-29: Diencephalic-mesencephalic junction dysplasia in a 28-week-old fetus. **A:** Axial T2 MRI reveals fusion of the hypothalamus and midbrain *(asterisk)*, enlargement of the dorsoventral axis of the midbrain, and a ventral midbrain cleft *(arrow)* resulting in a butterfly-like appearance. **B:** Sagittal T2 MRI demonstrates partial callosal agenesis *(black arrow)* associated with hypoplasia of the pons *(double arrow)* and vermis and mild kinking of the cervicomedullary junction *(white arrowhead)*. Note that the cerebral aqueduct is not visible. The interthalamic adhesion is enlarged and ventrally located *(black arrowhead)*. **C:** Coronal T2 MRI shows fusion between the midbrain and thalami *(asterisks)* as well as moderate supratentorial ventriculomegaly.

Management: Termination of pregnancy may be considered. Postnatal management is primarily supportive.

Recurrence Risk Sporadic with no recurrence risk.

ACKNOWLEDGMENTS

Portions of the text are reproduced from the following previous publications by the author:

1. Robinson AJ, Blaser S, Toi A, et al. The fetal cerebellar vermis: assessment for abnormal development by ultrasonography and magnetic resonance imaging. *Ultrasound Q.* 2007;23:211–223, with permission from Wolters Kluwer Health.
2. Robinson AJ, Goldstein R. The cisterna magna septa: vestigial remnants of Blake's pouch and a potential new marker for normal development of the rhombencephalon. *J Ultrasound Med.* 2007;26:83–95, with permission from the American Institute of Ultrasound in Medicine.
3. Robinson AJ. Inferior vermian hypoplasia: preconception, misconception. *Ultrasound Obstet Gynecol.* 2014;43:123–136, with permission from John Wiley and Sons Ltd.

REFERENCES

1. AIUM. *AIUM Practice Guideline for the Performance of an Antepartum Obstetric Ultrasound Examination.* Laurel, MD: American Institute of Ultrasound in Medicine; 2003. http://www.aium.org/publications/clinical/obstetrical.pdf. Accessed June 15, 2019.
2. SOGC. *SOGC Clinical Practice Guidelines. Antenatal Fetal Assessment.* No 90. Ottawa, ON, Canada: Society of Obstetricians and Gynaecologists of Canada; June 2000. http://www.sogc.org/guidelines/pdf/ps90.pdf.
3. CAR. *CAR Standards for Performing and Interpreting Diagnostic Antepartum Obstetric Ultrasound Examination.* Ottawa, ON, Canada: Canadian Association of Radiologists; September 2001. http://www.car.ca/ethics/standards/antepartum.htm.
4. Filly RA, Cardoza JD, Goldstein RB, et al. Detection of fetal central nervous system anomalies: a practical level of effort for a routine sonogram. *Radiology.* 1989;172:403–408.
5. Visentin A, Pilu G, Falco P, et al. The transfrontal view: a new approach to the visualization of the fetal midline cerebral structures. *J Ultrasound Med.* 2001;20:329–333.
6. Zalel Y, Seidman DS, Brand N, et al. The development of the fetal vermis: an in-vivo sonographic evaluation. *Ultrasound Obstet Gynecol.* 2002;19:136–139.

7. Achiron R, Kivilevitch Z, Lipitz S, et al. Development of the human fetal pons: in utero ultrasonographic study. *Ultrasound Obstet Gynecol.* 2004;24:506–510.

8. Malinger G, Ginath S, Lerman-Sagie T, et al. The fetal cerebellar vermis: normal development as shown by transvaginal ultrasound. *Prenat Diagn.* 2001;21:687–692.

9. Estroff JA, Scott MR, Benacerraf BR. Dandy-Walker variant: prenatal sonographic features and clinical outcome. *Radiology.* 1992;185:755–758.

10. Chang MC, Russell SA, Callen PW, et al. Sonographic detection of inferior vermian agenesis in Dandy-Walker malformations: prognostic implications. *Radiology.* 1994;193:765–770.

11. Carroll SG, Porter H, Abdel-Fattah S, et al. Correlation of prenatal ultrasound diagnosis and pathologic findings in fetal brain abnormalities. *Ultrasound Obstet Gynecol.* 2000;16:149–153.

12. Laing FC, Frates MC, Brown DL, et al. Sonography of the fetal posterior fossa: false appearance of mega-cisterna magna and Dandy-Walker variant. *Radiology.* 1994;192:247–251.

13. Blake JA. The roof and lateral recesses of the fourth ventricle considered morphologically and embryologically. *J Comp Neurol.* 1900;10:79–108.

14. Ben-Amin M, Perlitz Y, Peleg D. Transvaginal sonographic appearance of the cerebellar vermis at 14–16 weeks' gestation. *Ultrasound Obstet Gynecol.* 2002;19:208–209.

15. Robinson AJ, Blaser S, Toi A, et al. The fetal cerebellar vermis: assessment for abnormal development by ultrasonography and magnetic resonance imaging. *Ultrasound Q.* 2007;23:211–223.

16. Bromley B, Nadel AS, Pauker S, et al. Closure of the cerebellar vermis: evaluation with second trimester US. *Radiology.* 1994;193:761–763.

17. Strand RD, Barnes PD, Poussaint TY, et al. Cystic retrocerebellar malformations: unification of the Dandy-Walker complex and the Blake's pouch. *Pediatr Radiol.* 1993;23:258–260.

18. Robinson AJ, Goldstein R. The cisterna magna septa: vestigial remnants of Blake's pouch and a potential new marker for normal development of the rhombencephalon. *J Ultrasound Med.* 2007;26:83–95.

19. Knutzon RK, McGahan JP, Salamat MS, et al. Fetal cisterna magna septa: a normal anatomic finding. *Radiology.* 1991;180:799–801.

20. Raybaud C. Cystic malformations of the posterior fossa: abnormalities associated with the development of the roof of the fourth ventricle and adjacent meningeal structures. *J Neuroradiol.* 1982;9:103–133.

21. Tortori-Donati P, Fondelli MP, Rossi A, et al. Cystic malformations of the posterior cranial fossa originating from a defect of the posterior membranous area. Mega cisterna magna and persisting Blake's pouch: two separate entities. *Childs Nerv Syst.* 1996;12:303–308.

22. Phillips JJ, Mahony BS, Siebert JR, et al. Dandy-Walker malformation complex: correlation between ultrasonographic diagnosis and postmortem neuropathology. *Obstet Gynecol.* 2006;107:685–693.

23. Oh KY, Rassner UA, Frias AE Jr, et al. The fetal posterior fossa: clinical correlation of findings on prenatal ultrasound and fetal magnetic resonance imaging. *Ultrasound Q.* 2007;23:203–210.

24. Pretorius DH, Kallman CE, Grafe MR, et al. Linear echoes in the fetal cisterna magna. *J Ultrasound Med.* 1992;11:125–128.

25. Gandolfi Colleoni G, Contro E, Carletti A, et al. Prenatal diagnosis and outcome of fetal posterior fossa fluid collections. *Ultrasound Obstet Gynecol.* 2012;39:625–631.

26. Arai H, Sato K. Posterior fossa cysts: clinical, neuroradiological and surgical features. *Childs Nerv Syst.* 1991;7:156–164.

27. Calabro F, Arcuri T, Jinkins JR. Blake's pouch: an entity within the Dandy-Walker continuum. *Neuroradiology.* 2000;42:290–295.

28. Cornips EM, Overvliet GM, Weber JW, et al. The clinical spectrum of Blake's pouch cyst: report of six illustrative cases. *Childs Nerv Syst.* 2010;26:1057–1064.

29. ten Donkelaar HJ, Lammens M, Wesseling P, et al. Development and developmental disorders of the human cerebellum. *J Neurol.* 2003;250:1025–1036.

30. Paladini D, Quarantelli M, Pastore G, et al. Abnormal or delayed development of the posterior membranous area of the brain: anatomy, ultrasound diagnosis, natural history and outcome of Blake's pouch cyst in the fetus. *Ultrasound Obstet Gynecol.* 2012;39:279–287.

31. Brocklehurst G. The development of the human cerebrospinal fluid pathway with particular reference to the roof of the fourth ventricle. *J Anat.* 1969;105:467–475.

32. Pichiecchio A, Decio A, Di Perri C, Parazzini C, Rossi A, Signorini S. "Acquired" Dandy-Walker malformation and cerebellar hemorrhage: usefulness of serial MRI. *Eur J Paediatr Neurol.* 2016;20:188–191.

33. Malinger G, Lev D, Zahalka N, et al. Fetal cytomegalovirus infection of the brain: the spectrum of sonographic findings. *AJNR Am J Neuroradiol.* 2003;24:28–32.

34. Dogan Y, Yuksel A, Kalelioglu IH, et al. Intracranial ultrasound abnormalities and fetal cytomegalovirus infection: report of 8 cases and review of the literature. *Fetal Diagn Ther.* 2011;30:141–149.

35. Sanapo L, Wien M, Whitehead MT, et al. Fetal anemia, cerebellar hemorrhage and hypoplasia associated with congenital Parvovirus infection. *J Matern Fetal Neonatal Med.* 2017;30:1887–1890.

36. Shiohama T, Ando R, Fujii K, et al. An acquired form of Dandy-Walker malformation with enveloping hemosiderin deposits. *Case Rep Pediatr.* 2017;2017:3861608.

37. Tam EW, Ferriero DM, Xu D, et al. Cerebellar development in the preterm neonate: effect of supratentorial brain injury. *Pediatr Res.* 2009;66:102–106.

38. Volpe JJ. Neurobiology of periventricular leukomalacia in the premature infant. *Pediatr Res.* 2001;50:553–562.

39. Duncan JR, Cock ML, Scheerlinck JP, et al. White matter injury after repeated endotoxin exposure in the preterm ovine fetus. *Pediatr Res.* 2002;52:941–949.

40. Klein O, Pierre-Kahn A, Boddaert N, et al. Dandy-Walker malformation: prenatal diagnosis and prognosis. *Childs Nerv Syst.* 2003;19:484–489.

41. Limperopoulos C, Robertson RL, Estroff JA, et al. Diagnosis of inferior vermian hypoplasia by fetal magnetic resonance imaging: potential pitfalls and neurodevelopmental outcome. *Am J Obstet Gynecol.* 2006;194:1070–1076.

42. Nelson MD Jr, Maher K, Gilles FH. A different approach to cysts of the posterior fossa. *Pediatr Radiol.* 2004;34:720–732.

43. Zalel Y, Gilboa Y, Gabis L, et al. Rotation of the vermis as a cause of enlarged cisterna magna on prenatal imaging. *Ultrasound Obstet Gynecol.* 2006;27:490–493.

44. Triulzi F, Parazzini C, Righini A. Magnetic resonance imaging of fetal cerebellar development. *Cerebellum.* 2006;5:199–205.

45. Barkovich AJ, Kjos BO, Norman D, et al. Revised classification of posterior fossa cysts and cystlike malformations based on the results of multiplanar MR imaging. *AJR Am J Roentgenol.* 1989;153:1289–1300.

46. Wüest A, Surbek D, Wiest R, et al. Enlarged posterior fossa on prenatal imaging: differential diagnosis, associated anomalies and postnatal outcome. *Acta Obstet Gynecol Scand.* 2017;96:837–843.

47. Pinto J, Paladini D, Severino M, et al. Delayed rotation of the cerebellar vermis: a pitfall in early second-trimester fetal magnetic resonance imaging. *Ultrasound Obstet Gynecol.* 2016;48:121–124.

48. Ramaswamy S, Rangasami R, Suresh S, Suresh I. Spontaneous resolution of Blake's pouch cyst. *Radiol Case Rep.* 2015;8:877.

49. Blondiaux E, Sileo C, Nahama-Allouche C, et al. Periventricular nodular heterotopia on prenatal ultrasound and magnetic resonance imaging. *Ultrasound Obstet Gynecol.* 2013;42:149–155.

50. Bargalló N, Puerto B, De Juan C, Martinez-Crespo JM, Lourdes Olondo M. Hereditary subependymal heterotopia associated with mega cisterna magna: antenatal diagnosis with magnetic resonance imaging. *Ultrasound Obstet Gynecol.* 2002;20:86–89.

51. Teixeira SR, Blondiaux E, Cassart M, et al. Association of periventricular nodular heterotopia with posterior fossa cyst: a prenatal case series. *Prenat Diagn.* 2015;35:337–341.

52. Stoecklein S, Haberler C, Gruber G, et al. Bilateral periventricular nodular heterotopia detected on fetal and maternal MRI attributable to novel filamin A gene mutation. *Ultrasound Obstet Gynecol.* 2018;52:678–680.

53. Deloison B, Sonigo P, Millischer-Bellaiche AE, et al. Prenatally diagnosed periventricular nodular heterotopia: further delineation of the imaging phenotype and outcome. *Eur J Med Genet.* 2018;61:773–782.

54. Lange M, Kasper B, Bohring A, et al. 47 patients with *FLNA* associated periventricular nodular heterotopia. *Orphanet J Rare Dis.* 2015;15:134.

55. Zimmer EZ, Lowenstein L, Bronshtein M, et al. Clinical significance of isolated mega cisterna magna. *Arch Gynecol Obstet.* 2007;276:487–490.

56. Pierre-Kahn A, Sonigo P. Malformative intracranial cysts: diagnosis and outcome. *Childs Nerv Syst.* 2003;19:477–483.

57. Pierre-Kahn A, Hanlo P, Sonigo P, et al. The contribution of prenatal diagnosis to the understanding of malformative intracranial cysts: state of the art. *Childs Nerv Syst.* 2000;16:619–626.

58. Kollias SS, Ball WS Jr, Prenger EC. Cystic malformations of the posterior fossa: differential diagnosis clarified through embryologic analysis. *Radiographics.* 1993;13:1211–1231.

59. Bordarier C, Aicardi J. Dandy-Walker syndrome and agenesis of the cerebellar vermis: diagnostic problems and genetic counselling. *Dev Med Child Neurol.* 1990;32:285–294.

60. Hirsch JF, Pierre-Kahn A, Renier D, et al. The Dandy-Walker malformation: a review of 40 cases. *J Neurosurg.* 1984;61:515–522.

61. Barkovich AJ. *Pediatric Neuroimaging.* 3rd ed. Philadelphia, PA: Lippincott Williams & Wilkins; 2000:337–341.

62. Limperopoulos C, du Plessis AJ. Disorders of cerebellar growth and development. *Curr Opin Pediatr.* 2006;18:621–627.

63. Ko SF, Wang HS, Lui TN, et al. Neurocutaneous melanosis associated with inferior vermian hypoplasia: MR findings. *J Comput Assist Tomogr.* 1993;17:691–695.

64. Aynaci FM, Mocan H, Bahadir S, et al. A case of Menkes' syndrome associated with deafness and inferior cerebellar vermian hypoplasia. *Acta Paediatr.* 1997;86:121–123.

65. Murray JC, Johnson JA, Bird TD. Dandy-Walker malformation: etiologic heterogeneity and empiric recurrence risks. *Clin Genet.* 1985;28:272–283.

66. Dandy WE, Blackfan KD. Internal hydrocephalus: an experimental, clinical, and pathological study. *Am J Dis Child.* 1914;8:406–482.

67. Dandy WE. The diagnosis and treatment of hydrocephalus due to occlusion of the foramina of Magendie and Luschka. *Surg Gynecol Obstet.* 1921;32:112–124.

68. Taggart JK, Walker AE. Congenital atresias of the foramens of Luschka and Magendie. *Arch Neurol Psychiatr.* 1942;48:583–612.

69. Garel C. *MRI of the Fetal Brain: Normal Development and Cerebral Pathologies.* 2nd ed. Berlin, Germany: Springer-Verlag; 2004:30–31.

70. Adamsbaum C, Moutard ML, Andre C, et al. MR of the fetal posterior fossa. *Pediatr Radiol.* 2005;35:124–140.

71. Robinson AJ, Blaser S. In-utero MR imaging of developmental abnormalities of the fetal cerebellar vermis. In: Griffiths PD, Paley MNJ, Whitby EH, eds. *Imaging the Central Nervous System of the Fetus and Neonate.* New York, NY: Taylor & Francis; 2006.

72. Stazzone MM, Hubbard AM, Bilaniuk LT, et al. Ultrafast MR imaging of the normal posterior fossa in fetuses. *AJR Am J Roentgenol.* 2000;175:835–839.

73. Guibaud L. Practical approach to prenatal posterior fossa abnormalities using MR. *Pediatr Radiol.* 2004;34:700–711.

74. Kau T, Birnbacher R, Schwärzler P, Habernig S, Deutschmann H, Boltshauser E. Delayed fenestration of Blake's pouch with or without vermian hypoplasia: fetal MRI at 3 tesla versus 1.5 tesla. *Cerebellum Ataxias.* 2019;6:4.

75. Robinson AJ, Blaser S, Toi A, et al. MR imaging of the fetal cerebellar vermis in utero: description of some useful anatomical criteria for normal and abnormal development. In: *Radiological Society of North America Scientific Assembly and Annual Meeting Program.* Oak Brook, IL: Radiological Society of North America; 2003.

76. Smith PA, Johansson D, Tzannatos C, et al. Prenatal measurement of the fetal cerebellum and cisterna cerebellomedullaris by ultrasound. *Prenat Diagn.* 1986;6:133–141.

77. Chang CH, Chang FM, Yu CH, et al. Three-dimensional ultrasound in the assessment of fetal cerebellar transverse and antero-posterior diameters. *Ultrasound Med Biol.* 2000;26:175–182.

78. Garel C. *MR of the Fetal Brain: Normal Development and Cerebral Pathologies.* 2nd ed. (English translation). Berlin, Germany: Springer-Verlag; 2004:95.

79. Triulzi F, Parazzini C, Righini A. MR of fetal and neonatal cerebellar development. *Semin Fetal Neonatal Med.* 2005;10:411–420.

80. Bertucci E, Gindes L, Mazza V, et al. Vermian biometric parameters in the normal and abnormal fetal posterior fossa: three-dimensional sonographic study. *J Ultrasound Med.* 2011;30:1403–1410.

81. Tilea B, Alberti C, Adamsbaum C, et al. Cerebral biometry in fetal magnetic resonance imaging: new reference data. *Ultrasound Obstet Gynecol.* 2009;33:173–181.

82. Xie JX, You JH, Chen XK, et al. Three-dimensional sonographic minute structure analysis of fetal cerebellar vermis development and malformations: utilizing volume contrast imaging. *J Med Ultrason.* 2019;46:113–122.

83. Robinson AJ, Blaser S, Toi A, et al. MR imaging of the fetal cerebellar vermis in utero: criteria for abnormal development, with ultrasonographic and clinicopathologic correlation. *Pediatr Radiol.* 2004;32(Supplement 2):S135.

84. Volpe P, Contro E, De Musso F, et al. Brainstem-vermis and brainstem-tentorium angles allow accurate categorization of fetal upward rotation of cerebellar vermis. *Ultrasound Obstet Gynecol.* 2012;39:632–635.

85. Chapman T, Menashe SJ, Zare M, Alessio AM, Ishak GE. Establishment of normative values for the fetal posterior fossa by magnetic resonance imaging. *Prenat Diagn.* 2018;38:1035–1041.

86. Zollino M, Di Stefano C, Zampino G, et al. Genotype-phenotype correlations and clinical diagnostic criteria in Wolf-Hirschhorn syndrome. *Am J Med Genet.* 2000;94:254–261.

87. Boddaert N, Klein O, Ferguson N, et al. Intellectual prognosis of the Dandy-Walker malformation in children: the importance of vermian lobulation. *Neuroradiology.* 2003;45:320–324.

88. Bolduc ME, du Plessis AJ, Sullivan N, et al. Regional cerebellar volumes predict functional outcome in children with cerebellar malformations. *Cerebellum.* 2012;11:531–542.

89. Toi A. The fetal head and brain. In: Rumack CM, Wilson SR, Charbonneau JW, eds. *Diagnostic Ultrasound.* 3rd ed. St Louis, MS: Elsevier Mosby; 2005.

90. Sawaya R, McLaurin RL. Dandy-Walker syndrome: clinical analysis of 23 cases. *J Neurosurg.* 1981;55:89–98.

91. Nyberg DA, Cyr DR, Mack LA, et al. The Dandy-Walker malformation prenatal sonographic diagnosis and its clinical significance. *J Ultrasound Med.* 1988;7:65–71.

92. Cohen MM Jr, Lemire RJ. Syndromes with cephaloceles. *Teratology.* 1982;25:161–172.

93. Pilu G, Romero R, De Palma L, et al. Antenatal diagnosis and obstetric management of Dandy-Walker syndrome. *J Reprod Med.* 1986;31:1017–1022.

94. Olson GS, Halpe DC, Kaplan AM, et al. Dandy-Walker malformation and associated cardiac anomalies. *Childs Brain.* 1981;8:173–180.

95. Hart MN, Malamud N, Ellis WG. The Dandy-Walker syndrome: a clinicopathological study based on 28 cases. *Neurology.* 1972;22:771–780.

96. Blazer S, Berant M, Sujov PO, et al. Prenatal sonographic diagnosis of vermal agenesis. *Prenat Diagn.* 1997;17:907–911.

97. Bindal AK, Storrs BB, McLone DG. Management of the Dandy-Walker syndrome. *Pediatr Neurosurg.* 1990–1991;16:163–169.

98. D'Antonio F, Khalil A, Garel C, et al. Systematic review and meta-analysis of isolated posterior fossa malformations on prenatal imaging (part 2): neurodevelopmental outcome. *Ultrasound Obstet Gynecol.* 2016;48:28–37.

99. Alkan O, Kizilkilic O, Yildirim T. Malformations of the midbrain and hindbrain: a retrospective study and review of the literature. *Cerebellum.* 2009;8:355–365.

100. Keogan MT, DeAtkine AB, Hertzberg BS. Cerebellar vermian defects: antenatal sonographic appearance and clinical significance. *J Ultrasound Med.* 1994;13:607–611.

101. Fenichel GM, Phillips JA. Familial aplasia of the cerebellar vermis: possible X-linked dominant inheritance. *Arch Neurol.* 1989;46:582–583.

102. Imamura S, Tachi N, Oya K. Dominantly inherited early-onset non-progressive cerebellar ataxia syndrome. *Brain Dev.* 1993;15:372–376.

103. Sasaki-Adams D, Elbabaa SK, Jewells V, et al. The Dandy-Walker variant: a case series of 24 pediatric patients and evaluation of associated anomalies, incidence of hydrocephalus, and developmental outcomes. *J Neurosurg Pediatr.* 2008;2:194–199.

104. Long A, Moran P, Robson S. Outcome of fetal cerebral posterior fossa anomalies. *Prenat Diagn.* 2006;26:707–710.

105. Bolduc ME, Limperopoulos C. Neurodevelopmental outcomes in children with cerebellar malformations: a systematic review. *Dev Med Child Neurol.* 2009;51:256–267.

106. Patek KJ, Kline-Fath BM, Hopkin RJ, et al. Posterior fossa anomalies diagnosed with fetal MRI: associated anomalies and neurodevelopmental outcomes. *Prenat Diagn.* 2012;32:75–82.

107. Guibaud L, Larroque A, Ville D, et al. Prenatal diagnosis of "isolated" Dandy-Walker malformation: imaging findings and prenatal counselling. *Prenat Diagn.* 2012;32:185–193.

108. Poretti A, Boltshauser E, Doherty D. Cerebellar hypoplasia: differential diagnosis and diagnostic approach. *Am J Med Genet C Semin Med Genet.* 2014;166C(2):211–226.

109. Leibovitz Z, Guibaud L, Garel C, et al. The cerebellar "tilted telephone receiver sign" enables prenatal diagnosis of PHACES syndrome. *Eur J Paediatr Neurol.* 2018;22:900–909.

110. Benbir G, Kara S, Yalcinkaya BC, et al. Unilateral cerebellar hypoplasia with different clinical features. *Cerebellum.* 2011;10:49–60.

111. Bosemani T, Orman G, Boltshauser E, Tekes A, Huisman TAGM, Poretti A. Congenital abnormalities of the posterior fossa. *RadioGraphics.* 2015;35:200–220.

112. Fernández-Mayoralas DM, Recio-Rodríguez M, Fernández-Perrone AL, Jiménez-de-la-Peña M, Muñoz-Jareño N, Fernández-Jaén A. In utero diagnosis of PHACE syndrome by fetal magnetic resonance imaging (MRI). *J Child Neurol.* 2014;29:118–121.

113. Poretti A, Leventer RJ, Cowan FM, et al. Cerebellar cleft: a form of prenatal cerebellar disruption. *Neuropediatrics.* 2008;39:106–112.

114. Poretti A, Huisman TA, Cowan FM, et al. Cerebellar cleft: confirmation of the neuroimaging pattern. *Neuropediatrics.* 2009;40:228–233.

115. Utsunomiya H, Takano K, Ogasawara T, et al. Rhombencephalosynapsis: cerebellar embryogenesis. *AJNR Am J Neuroradiol.* 1998;19:547–549.

116. Pasquier L, Marcorelles P, Loget P, et al. Rhombencephalosynapsis and related anomalies: a neuropathological study of 40 fetal cases. *Acta Neuropathol.* 2009;117:185–200.

117. Sgaier SK, Millet S, Villanueva MP, et al. Morphogenetic and cellular movements that shape the mouse cerebellum; insights from genetic fate mapping. *Neuron.* 2005;45:27–40.

118. Tan TY, McGillivray G, Goergen SK, et al. Prenatal magnetic resonance imaging in Gomez-Lopez-Hernandez syndrome and review of the literature. *Am J Med Genet.* 2005;138A:369–373.

119. Brocks D, Irons M, Sadeghi-Najad A, et al. Gomez-Lopez-Hernandez syndrome: expansion of the phenotype. *Am J Med Genet.* 2000;94:405–408.

120. Gomez MR. Cerebellotrigeminal and focal dermal dysplasia: a newly recognized neurocutaneous syndrome. *Brain Dev.* 1979;1:253–256.

121. Gomy I, Heck B, Santos AC, et al. Two new Brazilian patients with Gomez-Lopez-Hernandez syndrome. *Am J Med Genet.* 2008;146A:649–657.

122. Elliott R, Harter DH. Rhombencephalosynapsis associated with autosomal dominant polycystic kidney disease Type 1. *J Neurosurg Pediatr.* 2008;2:435–437.

123. Barkovich AJ, Raybaud CA. Congenital malformations of the brain and skull. In: Barkovich AJ, ed. *Pediatric Neuroimaging.* Philadelphia, PA: Lippincott Williams & Wilkins; 2000:473–476.

124. Napolitano M, Righini A, Zirpoli S, et al. Prenatal magnetic resonance imaging of rhombencephalosynapsis and associated brain anomalies: report of 3 cases. *J Comput Assist Tomogr.* 2004;28:762–765.

125. Sergi C, Hentze S, Sohn C, et al. Telencephalosynapsis (synencephaly) and rhombencephalosynapsis with posterior fossa ventriculocele ("Dandy-Walker cyst"): an unusual aberrant syngenetic complex. *Brain Dev.* 1997;19:426–432.

126. Barkovich AJ. *Pediatric Neuroimaging.* 3rd ed. Philadelphia, PA: Lippincott Williams & Wilkins; 2000:346–350.

127. Toelle S, Yalcinkaya C, Kocer N, et al. Rhombencephalosynapsis: clinical findings and neuroimaging in 9 children. *Neuropediatrics.* 2002;33:209–214.

128. Poretti A, Alber FD, Bürki S, et al. Cognitive outcome in children with rhombencephalosynapsis. *Eur J Paediatr Neurol.* 2009;13:28–33.

129. Gleeson J, Keeler L, Parisi M, et al. Molar tooth sign of the midbrain-hindbrain junction: occurrence in multiple distinct syndromes. *Am J Med Genet A.* 2004;125A:125–134.

130. Satran D, Pierpont MEM, Dobyns WB. Cerebello-Oculo-Renal syndromes including Arima, Senior-Löken and COACH syndromes: more than just variants of Joubert syndrome. *Am J Med Genet.* 1999;86:459–469.

131. Louie CM, Gleeson JG. Genetic basis of Joubert syndrome and related disorders of cerebellar development. *Hum Mol Genet.* 2005;14:R235–R242.

132. Zaki MS, Abdel-Aleem A, Abdel-Salam GMH, et al. The molar tooth sign: a new Joubert syndrome and related cerebellar disorders classification system tested in Egyptian families. *Neurology.* 2008;70:556–565.

133. Badano JL, Mitsuma N, Beales PL, et al. The ciliopathies: an emerging class of human genetic disorders. *Annu Rev Genomics Hum Genet.* 2006;7:125–148.

134. Valente EM, Brancati F, Silhavy JL, et al. AHI1 gene mutations cause specific forms of Joubert syndrome-related disorders. *Ann Neurol.* 2006;59:527–534.

135. Valente EM, Silhavy JL, Brancati F, et al. Mutations in CEP290, which encodes a centrosomal protein, cause pleiotropic forms of Joubert syndrome. *Nat Genet.* 2006;38:623–625.

136. Cantagrel V, Silhavy J, Bielas S, et al. Mutations in the cilia gene ARL13B lead to the classical form of Joubert syndrome. *Am J Hum Genet.* 2008;83:170–179.

137. Pugash D, Oh T, Godwin K, et al. Sonographic "molar tooth" sign in the diagnosis of Joubert syndrome. *Ultrasound Obstet Gynecol.* 2011;38:598–602.

138. Saleem SN, Zaki MS. Role of MR imaging in prenatal diagnosis of pregnancies at risk for Joubert syndrome and related cerebellar disorders. *AJNR Am J Neuroradiol.* 2010;31:424–429.

139. Aslan H, Ulker V, Gulcan EM, et al. Prenatal diagnosis of Joubert syndrome: a case report. *Prenat Diagn.* 2002;22:13–16.

140. Doherty D, Glass IA, Siebert JR, et al. Prenatal diagnosis in pregnancies at risk for Joubert syndrome by ultrasound and MRI. *Prenat Diagn.* 2005;25:442–447.

141. Fluss J, Blaser S, Chitayat D, et al. Molar tooth sign in fetal brain magnetic resonance imaging leading to the prenatal diagnosis of Joubert syndrome and related disorders. *J Child Neurol.* 2006;21:320–324.

142. Widjaja E, Blaser S, Raybaud C. Diffusion tensor imaging of midline posterior fossa malformations. *Pediatr Radiol.* 2006;36:510–517.

143. Barkovich AJ, Raybaud CA. Congenital malformations of the brain and skull. In: Barkovich AJ, ed. *Pediatric Neuroimaging.* Philadelphia, PA: Lippincott Williams & Wilkins; 2000;481–483.

144. Joubert M, Eisenring JJ, Robb JP, et al. Familial agenesis of the cerebellar vermis: a syndrome of episodic hyperpnea, abnormal eye movements, ataxia, and retardation. *Neurology.* 1969;19:813–825.

145. Parisi M, Glass I. Joubert syndrome and related disorders: 2003 Jul 9 [Updated 2013 Apr 11]. In: Pagon RA, Adam MP, Bird TD, et al., eds. *GeneReviews™* [Internet]. Seattle, WA: University of Washington, Seattle; 1993–2014. Available from http://www.ncbi.nlm.nih.gov/books/NBK1325/.

146. Haratz KK, Lerman-Sagie T. Prenatal diagnosis of brainstem anomalies. *Eur J Paediatr Neurol.* 2018;22:1016–1026.

147. Smith AS, Levine D, Barnes PD, et al. Magnetic resonance imaging of the kinked fetal brain stem: a sign of severe dysgenesis. *J Ultrasound Med.* 2005;24:1697–1709.

148. Amir T, Poretti A, Boltshauser E, Huisman TA. Differential diagnosis of ventriculomegaly and brainstem kinking on fetal MRI. *Brain Dev.* 2016;38:103–108.

149. Barkovich AJ. *Pediatric Neuroimaging.* 3rd ed. Philadelphia, PA: Lippincott Williams & Wilkins; 2000:297–301.

150. Bahi-Buisson N, Poirier K, Fourniol F, et al. The wide spectrum of tubulinopathies: what are the key features for the diagnosis? *Brain.* 2014;137:1676–1700.

151. Wang H, Li S, Li S, et al. De novo mutated TUBB2B associated pachygyria diagnosed by medical exome sequencing and long-range PCR. *Fetal Pediatr Pathol.* 2019;38:63–71.

152. Romaniello R, Arrigoni F, Panzeri E, et al. Tubulin-related cerebellar dysplasia: definition of a distinct pattern of cerebellar malformation. *Eur Radiol.* 2017;27:5080–5092.

153. Timor-Tritsch IE, Monteagudo A, Haratz-Rubinstein N, Levine RU. Transvaginal sonographic detection of adducted thumbs, hydrocephalus, and agenesis of the corpus callosum at 22 postmenstrual weeks: the mass spectrum or L1 spectrum. A case report and review of the literature. *Prenat Diagn.* 1996;16(6):543–548.

154. Krishnamurthy S, Kapoor S, Sharma V, et al. Tectocerebellar dysraphia and occipital encephalocele: an unusual association with abdominal situs inversus and congenital heart disease. *Indian J Pediatr.* 2008;75:1178–1180.

155. Namavar Y, Barth P, Tien Poll-The B, Baas F. Classification, diagnosis and potential mechanisms in pontocerebellar hypoplasia. *Ophanet J Rare Dis.* 2001;6:1–50.

156. Graham J, Spencer A, Brinberg I, et al. Molecular and neuroimaging findings in pontocerebellar hypoplasia Type 2 (PCH2): is prenatal diagnosis possible? *Am J Med Genet.* 2010;152A:2268–2276.

157. van Dijk T, Baas F, Barth PG, et al. What's new in pontocerebellar hypoplasia? An update on genes and subtypes. *Orphanet J Rare Dis.* 2018;13:92.

158. Namavar Y, Barth P, Kasher P, et al. Clinical, neuroradiological and genetic findings in pontocerebellar hypoplasia. *Brain.* 2011;134:143–156.

159. Malinger G, Lev K, Lerman-Sagle T. The fetal cerebellum. Pitfalls in diagnosis and management. *Prenat Diagn.* 2009;29:372–380.

160. Tilea B, Delezoide A, Khung-Savatovshi S, et al. Comparison between magnetic resonance imaging and fetopathology in the evaluation of fetal posterior fossa non-cystic abnormalities. *Ultrasound Obstet Gynecol.* 2007;29:651–659.

161. Patel S, Barkovich A. Analysis and classification of cerebellar malformations. *Am J Neuroradiol.* 2002;23:1074–1087.

162. Blondiaux E, Valence S, Friszer S, et al. Prenatal imaging findings of pontine tegmental cap dysplasia: report of four cases. *Fetal Diagn Ther.* 2019;45:197–204.

163. Caan MW, Barth PG, Niermeijer JM, Majoie CB, Poll-The BT. Ectopic peripontine arcuate fibres, a novel finding in pontine tegmental cap dysplasia. *Eur J Paediatr Neurol.* 2014;18:434–438.

164. Severino M, Righini A, Tortora D, et al. MR imaging diagnosis of diencephalic-mesencephalic junction dysplasia in fetuses with developmental ventriculomegaly. *AJNR Am J Neuroradiol.* 2017;38:1643–1646.

Ashley James Robinson

EVALUATION

Sonographic assessment of the fetal eyes is not a requirement for routine prenatal sonography, according to the amalgamated guidelines from the American Institute of Ultrasound in Medicine (AIUM), American Congress of Obstetricians and Gynecologists (ACOG), American College of Radiology (ACR), Society of Maternal Fetal Medicine (SMFM), and Society of Radiologic Ultrasound (SRU).[1] Assessment of orbital biometry is a reasonable expectation as part of a detailed anatomy scan, particularly in the setting of suspected central nervous system (CNS) malformation. However, evaluation of the globe itself can be far more challenging.

Complete ocular evaluation comprises ocular biometry, assessment for the presence of the globes, and examination of the morphology of the lens, vitreous, and optic nerves.[2] There is a necessity for a working knowledge of ocular pathologies because syndromes involving the eyes can go unrecognized without a systematic approach.

Embryology

At 22 days' gestation, the optic vesicles start to develop as bilateral outpouchings from the inner wall of the forebrain. When the vesicles contact the surface ectoderm, this induces the lens placode, which then starts to invaginate into the optic vesicles that become the optic cups. By 5 to 7 weeks, the lens placode loses contact with the surface ectoderm to form the lens vesicle. Elongation of the cells within the lens vesicle fills the lumen of the lens vesicle to form the solid lens. With growth, the optic cups envelop the lens circumferentially to form the globe. The hyaloid artery, the primary supply of nutrients to the developing lens, is contained within the optic stalk, which extends from the optic disc through the vitreous humor to the lens. After the 10th week, the lens grows independent of blood supply and the hyaloid artery regresses, leaving a clear central zone, known as the hyaloid canal or Cloquet canal. Fetal eye movements can be seen from 14 weeks. The incidence, pattern, and frequency are increasingly being used in the evaluation of development of the fetal brainstem and functional networks.[3–7]

Imaging/Biometry

Growth charts for the fetal lens and orbit,[8–10] orbital total axial length (TAL),[11] eye volume,[12] as well as the measurements of binocular distance (BOD) and interocular distance (IOD) have been determined sonographically (Table 22A in Appendix A1).[13–15] The latter are measured according to the bony landmarks of the medial and lateral orbital walls. The orbital measurements are ideally made in the axial plane, with both orbits of equal and largest possible diameter.[16] The BOD is measured between the two malar margins, and the IOD between the two ethmoidal margins of the *bony orbits* (Fig. 18.1). These bony landmarks are difficult to see by fetal magnetic resonance imaging (MRI);

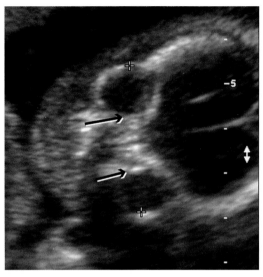

FIGURE 18.1: Orbital measurements by US. Transorbital view of the fetal face shows the measurement of the binocular distance (BOD) with the calipers on the malar margins of the orbit. The interocular distance (IOD) is measured between the two ethmoidal margins (*arrows*).

therefore, standard sonographic growth charts cannot accurately be applied to fetal MR studies.

On T2 MRI, the whole lens is low signal compared with the high signal of the vitreous. The BOD and IOD measurements can be made in any plane from true axial to true coronal, provided both eyes can be seen in the same image and have the most equal and largest possible transverse diameters. The BOD and IOD are, respectively, measured between the two malar or ethmoidal margins of each *vitreous* (Fig. 18.2). These measurements can be plotted against gestational age (Table 23A and 23B in Appendix A1).[2] Other available nomograms additionally include measurements of the orbital volume,[17] lens diameter and volume,[18,19] and anteroposterior diameter of the globe.[20] It has been noted that the globe is ellipsoid earlier in gestation. This is thought to be attributable to the presence of the hyaloid artery initially tethering the lens to the optic disc. With involution of the hyaloid artery, a process that starts at around 20 weeks' gestation and completes by around 30 weeks' gestation,[21] the globe is increased in anteroposterior diameter.[22]

ANOPHTHALMIA/MICROPHTHALMIA

Anophthalmia and microphthalmia can really only be differentiated pathologically. Anophthalmia is complete absence of the globe but in the presence of the ocular adnexa (eyelids, conjunctiva, and lacrimal apparatus). Microphthalmia, by definition, means small globe. It should be differentiated from cryptophthalmos, which is a failure of separation of the eyelids, which should occur by 24 weeks, but in the presence of normal

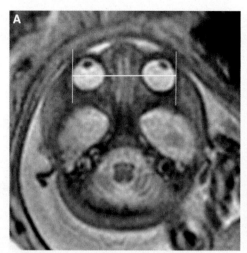 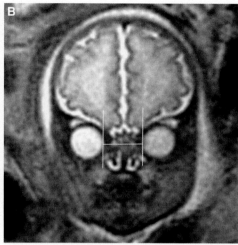

FIGURE 18.2: Orbital measurements by MRI. **A:** The binocular distance (BOD) is measured between the two malar margins of each high-signal vitreous. The measurements can be made in any plane orthogonal to the sagittal plane. **B:** The interocular distance (IOD) is measured in the coronal plane between the two orbital margins of each high-signal vitreous. (Reproduced by permission from Springer: Robinson AJ, Blaser S, Toi A, et al. Magnetic resonance imaging of the fetal eyes: morphologic and biometric assessment for abnormal development with ultrasonographic and clinicopathologic correlation. *Pediatr Radiol.* 2008;38(9):971–981. Copyright © 2008 Springer-Verlag.)

intraorbital contents. Cryptophthalmos is usually bilateral, and when it occurs with multiple other abnormalities, Fraser syndrome, which has an autosomal recessive inheritance, should be considered.

Incidence: Anophthalmia is seen in approximately 1 in 2,400 pregnancies.

Pathogenesis/Etiology: Primary anophthalmia/microphthalmia occurs when one or both eyes never form. It is usually associated with chromosomal abnormalities such as trisomy 13, genetic abnormalities such as CHARGE (colomba, heart defects, choanal atresia, growth retardation, genital, and ear abnormalities) syndrome (CHD7), incontinentia pigmenti (IKBKG), Norrie disease (NDP), SOX2-related eye disorders, Walker–Warburg syndrome (POMT1),[23-29] and over 180 syndromes.

In *secondary* anophthalmia/microphthalmia, the development of the eyes is initially normal but is disrupted by an insult. Etiologies include infection such as TORCH (toxoplasmosis, other, rubella, cytomegalovirus, and herpes), syphilis, Epstein–Barr virus (EBV), parvovirus, a vascular event (e.g., Goldenhar syndrome [oculo-auriculo-vertebral spectrum]), or a toxic or metabolic event, such as, low or high vitamin A, ethanol, and retinoic acid. Table 18.1 summarizes the ocular disorder and its primary and secondary causes.

Imaging: On ultrasound (US) and MRI, microphthalmia or anophthalmia may be present when the orbital diameter is below the 5th percentile.[16] Walker–Warburg syndrome, a type of congenital muscular dystrophy, comprises a Z-shaped brainstem on midline sagittal views, an occipital cephalocele, and ocular asymmetry (Fig. 18.3). Matthew–Wood syndrome, that is, Spear syndrome, comprises pulmonary agenesis, microphthalmia, and diaphragmatic defect (PMD) or pulmonary agenesis, diaphragmatic defect, anophthalmia, and cardiac anomalies (PDAC) (Fig. 18.4).[30] Aicardi syndrome is a rare genetic

TABLE 18.1	Ocular Abnormalities and Associations	
Anophthalmia/ Microphthalmia	Primary	Trisomy 13
		CHARGE syndrome Incontinentia pigmenti Norrie disease SOX2 Walker–Warburg syndrome
	Secondary	TORCH infections Syphilis EBV Parvovirus Goldenhar syndrome Hypervitaminosis A Hypovitaminosis A Ethanol Retinoic acid
Hypotelorism	Primary	Trisomy 13 Holoprosencephaly
	Secondary	Plagiocephaly Microcephaly
Hypertelorism	Primary	Median facial cleft syndrome Callosal dysgenesis
	Secondary	Frontal cephalocele Craniosynostosis

CHARGE, colomba, heart defects, choanal atresia, growth retardation, genital, and ear abnormalities; EBV, Epstein–Barr virus; TORCH, toxoplasmosis, other, rubella, cytomegalovirus, and herpes.

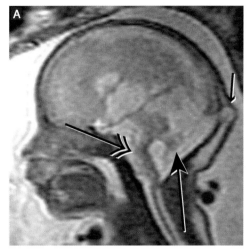
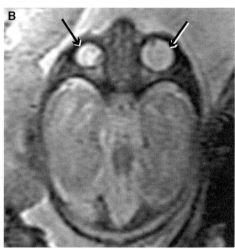

FIGURE 18.3: Walker–Warburg syndrome. **A:** Sagittal T2 MRI demonstrating Z-shaped brainstem (*double-headed arrow*), small vermis (*large arrow*), and occipital cephalocele (*small arrow*). **B:** Axial MRI showing asymmetric globes (*arrows*). (Reprinted with permission from Robinson AJ, Blaser S, Toi A, et al. The fetal cerebellar vermis: assessment for abnormal development by ultrasonography and magnetic resonance imaging. *Ultrasound Q.* 2007;23(3):211–223.)

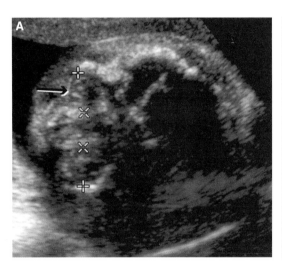
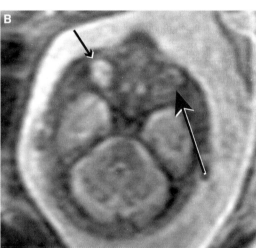
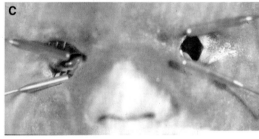

FIGURE 18.4: Matthew–Wood syndrome. **A:** US biometry was delayed, and there was an abnormal appearance to lens and globe, which appear echogenic (*arrow*). **B:** MRI demonstrating apparent anophthalmia (*large arrow*) and microphthalmia (*small arrow*). **C:** Postmortem showed absent globes. (Reproduced by permission from Springer: Robinson AJ, Blaser S, Toi A, et al. Magnetic resonance imaging of the fetal eyes: morphologic and biometric assessment for abnormal development with ultrasonographic and clinicopathologic correlation. *Pediatr Radiol.* 2008;38(9):971–981. Copyright © 2008 Springer-Verlag.)

malformation syndrome that can be diagnosed antenatally by the association of partial or complete absence of the corpus callosum, ocular abnormalities, and posterior fossa cyst (Fig. 18.5).

HYPOTELORISM

Pathogenesis/Etiology: The craniofacial skeleton is derived from both mesoderm and neural crest cells of the mesencephalon. Its development is intimately related to forebrain development and has a similar induction mechanism. For this reason, facial skeletal abnormalities are often associated with underlying cerebral malformations (the face predicts the brain[31]). Typically, the craniofacial abnormalities are actually secondary to a more

caudal expression of an abnormal genetic gradient that exists within the neural crest, and therefore, it is actually the brain abnormality that affects the development of the craniofacial skeleton; that is, the brain predicts the face (H. Sarnat, personal communication, 2012).

During normal embryological development, the opening for the eye forms during development of the face, when the paired nasal swellings on either side migrate medially and inferiorly and fuse with the midline frontal swelling to form the nose. If there is deficient forebrain development, with deficient development of the midline frontal swelling, the paired nasal swellings migrate more medially, and this results in *primary* hypotelorism. The corresponding underlying brain anomaly is often in the spectrum of

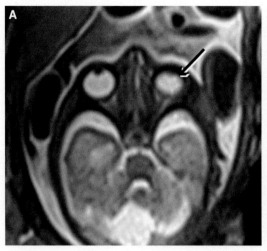
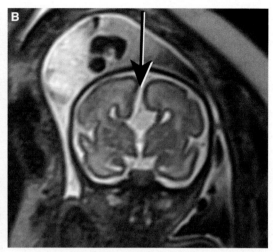

FIGURE 18.5: Aicardi syndrome. **A:** Axial MRI demonstrates unilateral microphthalmia (*arrow*). **B:** Coronal MRI shows callosal dysgenesis with "high-riding" third ventricle continuous with interhemispheric fissure (*arrow*).

holoprosencephaly,[16,32] with approximately 55% of cases associated with chromosomal abnormalities, most commonly trisomy 13.[13,16]

In *secondary* hypotelorism, the defect is most frequently the result of abnormalities of the bony skull, for example, microcephaly and plagiocephaly.[16]

Imaging: Hypotelorism is defined as an IOD below the 5th percentile on US and MRI.[16] Close inspection of the brain for imaging findings of holoprosencephaly is indicated (Fig. 18.6).

HYPERTELORISM

Pathogenesis/Etiology: In *primary* hypertelorism, the defect is due to deficient migration of the neural crest cells in the lamina terminalis of the prosencephalon. When this occurs, there is deficient formation of a structure known as the medial canthal

ligament, and the eyes stay in their early embryonic position on the side of the face similar to lesser mammals, fish, and birds (except owls). The deficient migration of neural crest cells also typically results in associated callosal dysgenesis. Hypertelorism can result from many chromosomal anomalies and genetic syndromes,[23] including median facial cleft syndrome, otherwise known as frontonasal dysplasia, which comprises hypertelorism, facial clefting, and callosal agenesis.

In *secondary* hypertelorism, the defect typically results from abnormalities of the skull; the most common being anterior cephalocele and craniosynostoses.[23,32,33] Although typically used to describe the appearance of the skull in type II thanatophoric dysplasia, the term "cloverleaf skull" has also been used to describe the dysmorphic appearance of the skull in craniosynostosis,[34,35] and several case reports have described the utility of fetal MRI in antenatal diagnosis.[36–38]

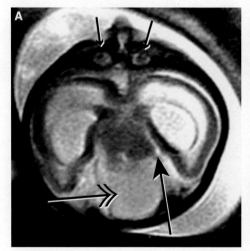
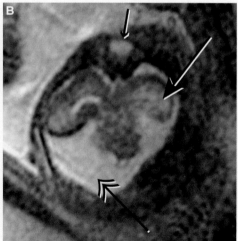

FIGURE 18.6: Holoprosencephaly. **A:** Axial MRI showing severe hypotelorism and microphthalmia (*small arrows*). There is a dorsal interhemispheric cyst (*double-headed arrow*), and the hippocampus touches the brainstem at the ambient cistern (*large arrow*), in keeping with lobar holoprosencephaly. **B:** Axial MRI showing a single small midline globe (*small arrow*). The hippocampus is not touching the brainstem (*large arrow*), and there is wide communication of the ambient cistern with the dorsal interhemispheric cyst (*double-headed arrow*), in keeping with alobar holoprosencephaly. (Reproduced by permission from Springer: Robinson AJ, Blaser S, Toi A, et al. Magnetic resonance imaging of the fetal eyes: morphologic and biometric assessment for abnormal development with ultrasonographic and clinicopathologic correlation. *Pediatr Radiol.* 2008;38(9):971–981. Copyright © 2008 Springer-Verlag.)

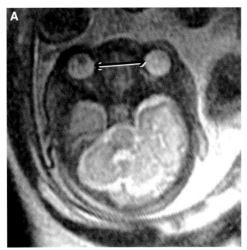
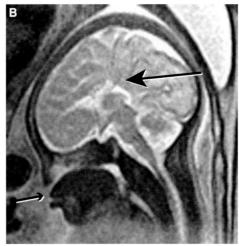

FIGURE 18.7: Frontonasal dysplasia **A:** Axial MRI showing hypertelorism (*double-headed arrow*). The binocular distance (BOD) and interocular distance (IOD) were both greater than the 95th centile for gestational age. **B:** Sagittal MRI shows absence of the corpus callosum (*large arrow*) and facial defect with absence of the hard palate separating the nasal and oral cavities with the tongue protruding through the defect (*small arrow*). (**A**, Reproduced by permission from Springer: Robinson AJ, Blaser S, Toi A, et al. Magnetic resonance imaging of the fetal eyes: morphologic and biometric assessment for abnormal development with ultrasonographic and clinicopathologic correlation. *Pediatr Radiol*. 2008;38(9):971–981. Copyright © 2008 Springer-Verlag.)

Imaging: Hypertelorism is defined as an IOD above the 95th percentile on US and MRI.[16] IOD may be the most reliable for making the diagnosis of hypertelorism, as by US this measurement is usually more than two standard deviations from the mean, whereas the BOD remains at the upper limit of normal.[16] In primary hypertelorism, other anomalies are commonly identified (Fig. 18.7). In the presence of craniosynostosis or cephaloceles, hypertelorism may be secondary (Fig. 18.8).

MORPHOLOGY OF THE LENS, VITREOUS, AND OPTIC NERVES

Cataract

Pathogenesis/Etiology: Cataracts represent clouding of the lens and are seen in a variety of metabolic, infectious, genetic,

and chromosomal abnormalities that affect the fetus, including toxoplasmosis; X-irradiation; in vitro fertilization; persistent hyperplastic primary vitreous; PHACES syndrome; Nance–Horan, Adams–Oliver, Walker–Warburg, and Neu–Laxova syndromes; rhizomelic chondrodysplasia punctata; trisomy 17 mosaicism; and trisomy 21.[26,39–50]

Imaging: By endovaginal US, the normal lens is visible by 14 weeks anteriorly within the globe as a thin echogenic rim with an anechoic center (Fig. 18.9A). Typically, however, the only reflection from the lens is from the surfaces perpendicular to the insonating beam, and it can, therefore, be difficult to visualize. On MRI, the normal lens is homogeneous low signal on T2 images compared with the high signal of the adjacent anterior chamber and vitreous (Fig. 18.9B). A cataract is seen as abnormal echogenicity by US (Fig. 18.9C) or abnormal signal on

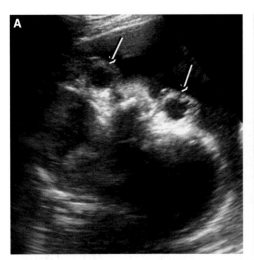
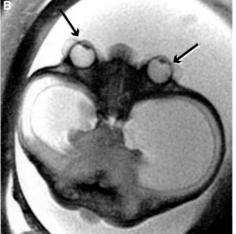
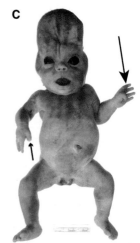

FIGURE 18.8: Craniosynostosis in Pfeiffer syndrome. **A:** Axial transorbital US showing severe hypertelorism and exorbitism (*arrows*). **B:** Fetal MRI demonstrates severe ventriculomegaly, exorbitism (*arrows*), and hypertelorism. **C:** Gross pathological specimen shows hypertelorism, broad thumbs (*small arrow*), and syndactyly (*long arrow*). (Reproduced by permission from Springer: Robinson AJ, Blaser S, Toi A, et al. Magnetic resonance imaging of the fetal eyes: morphologic and biometric assessment for abnormal development with ultrasonographic and clinicopathologic correlation. *Pediatr Radiol*. 2008;38(9):971–981. Copyright © 2008 Springer-Verlag.)

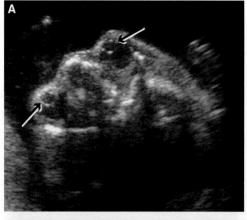

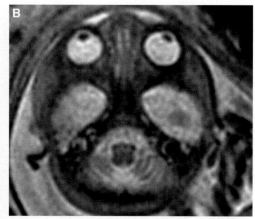

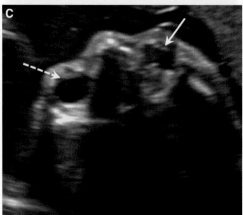

FIGURE 18.9: Normal lens and vitreous (**A**, **B**) and cataract (**C**). **A:** On US, the surfaces of the lenses are seen as faint curvilinear echoes in the anterior globe (*arrows*). **B:** MRI shows the whole lens is in low signal compared with the high signal of the vitreous. **C:** Axial US showing normal lens (*arrow*) in a small globe and echogenic lens (*dashed arrow*) in the opposite globe in this fetus with trisomy 13. (**A** and **B**, Reproduced by permission from Springer: Robinson AJ, Blaser S, Toi A, et al. Magnetic resonance imaging of the fetal eyes: morphologic and biometric assessment for abnormal development with ultrasonographic and clinicopathologic correlation. *Pediatr Radiol.* 2008;38(9):971–981. Copyright © 2008 Springer-Verlag.)

MRI in the position of the lens. Sometimes, it can be difficult to determine whether only the lens is abnormal. If the vitreous is also abnormal, then persistent hyperplastic primary vitreous and coloboma should be considered in the differential.

Persistent Hyperplastic Primary Vitreous

Pathogenesis/Etiology: Failure of involution of the hyaloid artery results in a spectrum of abnormalities known as persistent hyperplastic primary vitreous. The characteristic findings are a persistent hyaloid artery and a cone-shaped retrolental density. Other findings include a small irregular triangular-shaped lens with the apex pointing posteriorly and a shallow anterior chamber. Calcification is unusual. It is frequently seen with trisomy syndromes and other forms of abnormal brain development.[51,52]

Imaging: By US, the normal vitreous is hypoechoic, and on T2 MRI, it is high signal compared with the low signal of the lens. The hyaloid artery can be seen on US as an echogenic line bisecting the vitreous (Fig. 18.10A), which, during conversion of the primary vitreous to mature secondary vitreous, gradually becomes beaded as it involutes, a process which should be completed by 30 weeks' gestation.[21,53] Therefore, the hyaloid artery should not be identified via US past 30 weeks' gestation. The remnant channel through the vitreous is known as Cloquet canal. The normal hyaloid artery should not usually be detectable on MRI, and a corresponding abnormal low-signal linear plaque extending from the posterior part of the lens to the optic nerve head through the central vitreous in the position of Cloquet canal is considered to be pathological[2] (Fig. 18.10B–D).

Coloboma

Pathogenesis/Etiology: Coloboma is one of three types of excavation of the optic disc that can significantly impair visual function.[54] The other types, peripapillary staphyloma and morning glory disc, cannot be easily distinguished antenatally. Coloboma can be a unilateral or bilateral condition. During embryological development after the optic cup invaginates, it normally grows circumferentially to surround the lens vesicle and hyaloid artery, and once surrounded, the two sides close along the choroidal fissure to form the globe. If this envelopment is incomplete, the choroidal fissure stays open, resulting in a cleft anywhere along the length of the optic cup from the iris to the optic nerve.

In the majority of cases, coloboma is a feature of a syndrome; especially common associations are CHARGE and Aicardi syndrome.

Imaging: On US, associated ocular findings such as microphthalmia, an orbital cyst (outside the globe), or a persistent hyaloid artery may prompt the diagnosis (Fig. 18.11A). Because of the difficulties in depicting the posterior orbit sonographically, the diagnostic feature detectable antenatally is a deeply excavated optic disc on MRI (Fig. 18.11B, C).[55] Differential diagnosis includes persistent hyperplastic primary vitreous and cataract.

Optic Nerve Hypoplasia

Pathogenesis/Etiology: Optic nerve hypoplasia is usually sporadic and difficult to detect prenatally; however, it has

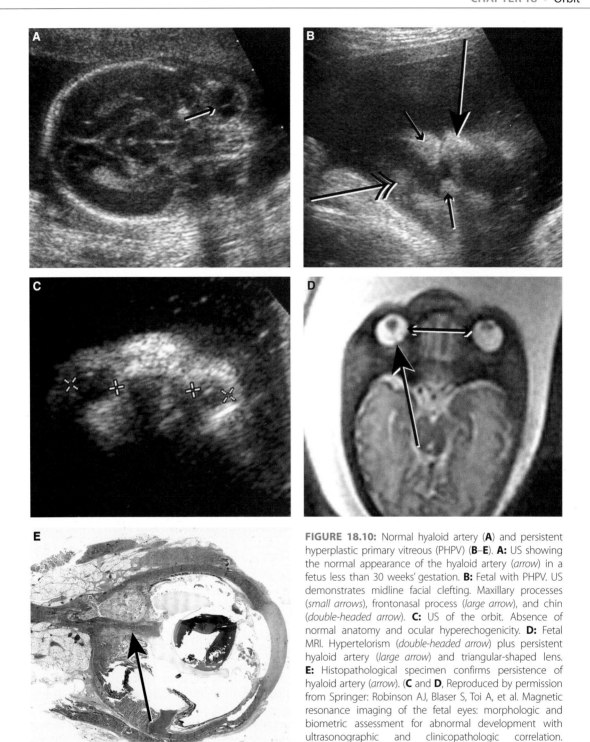

FIGURE 18.10: Normal hyaloid artery (**A**) and persistent hyperplastic primary vitreous (PHPV) (**B–E**). **A:** US showing the normal appearance of the hyaloid artery (*arrow*) in a fetus less than 30 weeks' gestation. **B:** Fetal with PHPV. US demonstrates midline facial clefting. Maxillary processes (*small arrows*), frontonasal process (*large arrow*), and chin (*double-headed arrow*). **C:** US of the orbit. Absence of normal anatomy and ocular hyperechogenicity. **D:** Fetal MRI. Hypertelorism (*double-headed arrow*) plus persistent hyaloid artery (*large arrow*) and triangular-shaped lens. **E:** Histopathological specimen confirms persistence of hyaloid artery (*arrow*). (**C** and **D**, Reproduced by permission from Springer: Robinson AJ, Blaser S, Toi A, et al. Magnetic resonance imaging of the fetal eyes: morphologic and biometric assessment for abnormal development with ultrasonographic and clinicopathologic correlation. Pediatr Radiol. 2008;38(9):971–981. Copyright © 2008 Springer-Verlag.)

a number of associations that can potentially be diagnosed intrauterine (Table 18.2). Evaluation of the optic nerves is usually necessary in the setting of absence of the cavum septi pellucidi, which can be an isolated finding or can be associated with severe neurological abnormalities such as holoprosencephaly or septo-optic dysplasia.[56]

Imaging: With US, optic tract hypoplasia can be assessed by fetal sonography,[57–59] by measurement of the transverse diameter

of the optic chiasm and optic nerves (Fig. 18.12A, B), and normal and abnormal growth of which has been described (Table 22E in Appendix A1).

The same anatomy can be assessed with some difficulty by fetal MRI[60]; however, a relatively crude assessment can be made by ensuring that the optic nerves are symmetric in size and approximately the same size as the adjacent carotid arteries and pituitary gland. The overall configuration is reminiscent of the Olympic rings (Fig. 18.12C).

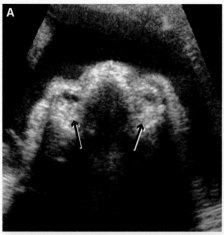

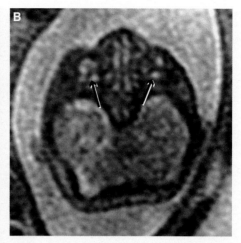

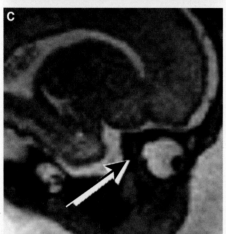

FIGURE 18.11: Coloboma. **A:** US demonstrating an abnormal echogenicity of the globes (*arrows*), but the lenses appear relatively normal. **B:** Axial MRI in the same fetus showing bilateral symmetrical abnormal globes with mixed low- and high-signal vitreous (*arrows*) and no definite lens structures. **C:** Parasagittal MRI through the globe showing deep excavation of the optic disc (*arrow*) in posterior coloboma in a different fetus. (**A** and **B**, Reproduced by permission from Springer: Robinson AJ, Blaser S, Toi A, et al. Magnetic resonance imaging of the fetal eyes: morphologic and biometric assessment for abnormal development with ultrasonographic and clinicopathologic correlation. *Pediatr Radiol.* 2008;38(9):971–981. Copyright © 2008 Springer-Verlag. **C**, reproduced from Righini A, Avagliano L, Doneda C, et al. Prenatal magnetic resonance imaging of optic nerve head coloboma. *Prenat Diagn.* 2008;28(3):242–246. Copyright © 2008 John Wiley & Sons, Ltd. Reprinted by permission of John Wiley & Sons, Inc.)

TABLE 18.2 Associations with Optic Nerve Hypoplasia
Aicardi syndrome
Anticonvulsants
CHARGE association
Congenital muscular dystrophy
Dominant inheritance
Duane retraction syndrome
Chromosome 5q distal deletion syndrome
Chromosome 6p partial deletion
Chromosome 7(q22–q34) and 7(q32–34) interstitial duplication
Chromosome 17 interstitial deletion
Ethanol toxicity
Frontonasal dysplasia
Goldenhar–Gorlin syndrome
Idiopathic growth hormone deficiency
Isotretinoin toxicity
Nevus sebaceous of Jadassohn
Maternal diabetes mellitus
Orbital hemangioma
Periventricular leukomalacia
Septo-optic dysplasia
Suprasellar teratoma
Valproic acid toxicity

CHARGE, coloboma, heart defects, choanal atresia, growth retardation, genital, and ear abnormalities.
Modified by permission from Nature: Dutton GN. Congenital disorders of the optic nerve: excavations and hypoplasia. *Eye (Lond).* 2004;18(11):1038–1048. Copyright © 2004 Nature Publishing Group.

ORBITAL ABNORMALITIES

Dacryocystocele

Incidence: The incidence on prenatal MRI studies has been reported between 0.7% and 2.7%, depending on definition, and only 50% of affected eyes are symptomatic postnatally.

Pathogenesis/Etiology: Congenital dacryocystocele is a distension of the nasolacrimal duct usually due to obstruction at its distal end at the valve of Hasner.

Imaging: Prenatal US and MRI can be used to make the diagnosis.[61,62] It is not expected to be seen prior to 24 weeks' gestation, because nasolacrimal duct canalization is incomplete, and even normal fluid-filled nasolacrimal ducts can be seen only by MRI after 24 weeks' gestation. Dacryocystoceles can also spontaneously resolve prior to delivery owing to rupture of the valve of Hasner[63,64] (Fig. 18.13).

Orbital Masses

Incidence: Orbital masses are sporadic and very uncommon and usually incidentally detected later in pregnancy, but most commonly detected postnatally.

Pathogenesis: The most common mass in the fetal head and neck is teratoma, and they can be large enough to interfere with labor and delivery. They can damage not only the globe because of mass effect but also the surrounding bony structures. They

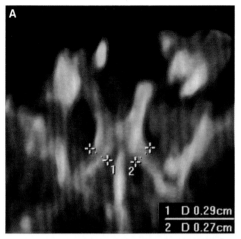

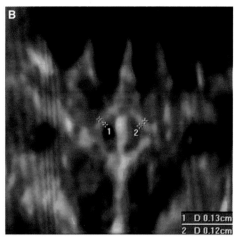

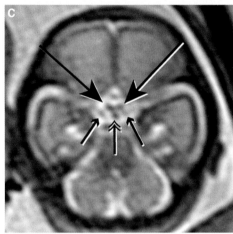

FIGURE 18.12: Normal optic nerves (**A**, **C**) and optic nerve hypoplasia/septo-optic dysplasia (SOD) (**B**). **A:** Measurement of optic tract diameter with US via transabdominal approach in a (normal) 28-week fetus. **B:** Hypoplastic optic tract in a 31-week fetus with agenesis of the septum pellucidum. **C:** "Olympic rings" sign on fetal MRI. Normal optic nerves (*large arrows*) and carotid arteries (*small arrows*). Pituitary stalk (*double-headed arrow*). (**A** and **B**, reproduced from Bault JP, Salomon LJ, Guibaud L, et al. Role of three-dimensional ultrasound measurement of the optic tract in fetuses with agenesis of the septum pellucidum. *Ultrasound Obstet Gynecol.* 2011;37(5):570–575. Copyright © 2011 ISUOG. Reprinted by permission of John Wiley & Sons, Inc.

may be detectable because of proptosis or via polyhydramnios by interfering with fetal swallowing.[65]

Imaging: The typical appearance of teratoma by US and MRI is a mixed solid and cystic mass with scattered amorphous calcifications.

Differential: The main differential is hemangioma, but other rarer tumors such as congenital fibrosarcoma and vascular malformations should also be considered.[66]

Management: Ideally, the eye should be preserved postnatally, but there is often secondary damage due to ocular exposure or optic nerve atrophy.[67]

ACKNOWLEDGMENT

Portions of this chapter are from Robinson AJ, Blaser S, Toi A, et al. Magnetic resonance imaging of the fetal eyes: morphologic and biometric assessment for abnormal development with ultrasonographic and clinicopathologic correlation. *Pediatr Radiol.* 2008;38:971–981, with permission of Springer-Verlag.

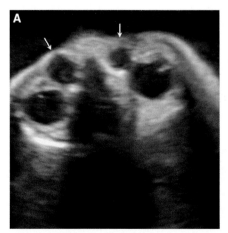

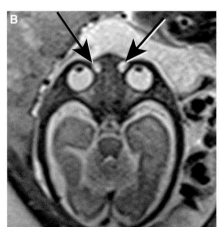

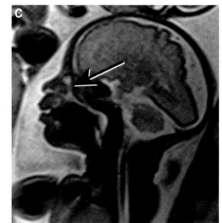

FIGURE 18.13: Dacryocystocele. **A:** Axial US demonstrating bilateral cysts (*arrows*) medial to the orbit consistent with bilateral dacryocystoceles. **B:** Fetal MRI showing bilateral cysts in the medial canthi (*arrows*). **C:** Fetal MRI showing dilated nasolacrimal duct (*arrow*).

REFERENCES

1. AIUM. AIUM-ACR-ACOG-SMFM-SRU practice parameter for the performance of standard diagnostic obstetric ultrasound examinations. https://www.aium.org/resources/guidelines/obstetric.pdf. Accessed June 15, 2019.

2. Robinson AJ, Blaser S, Toi A, et al. Magnetic resonance imaging of the fetal eyes: morphologic and biometric assessment for abnormal development with ultrasonographic and clinicopathologic correlation. *Pediatr Radiol.* 2008;38:971–981.

3. Inoue M, Koyanagi T, Nakahara H, et al. Functional development of human eye movement in utero assessed quantitatively with real-time ultrasound. *Am J Obstet Gynecol.* 1986;155:170–174.

4. Horimoto N, Hepper PG, Shahidullah S, et al. Fetal eye movements. *Ultrasound Obstet Gynecol.* 1993;3:362–369.

5. Chuang YM, Guo WY, Ho DM, et al. Skew ocular deviation: a catastrophic sign on MRI of fetal glioblastoma. *Childs Nerv Syst.* 2003;19:371–375.

6. Woitek R, Kasprian G, Lindner C, et al. Fetal eye movements on magnetic resonance imaging. *PLoS One.* 2013;8:e77439.

7. Schöpf V, Schlegl T, Jakab A, et al. The relationship between eye movement and vision develops before birth. *Front Hum Neurosci.* 2014;8:775.

8. Dilmen G, Köktener A, Turhan NO, et al. Growth of the fetal lens and orbit. *Int J Gynaecol Obstet.* 2002;76:267–271.

9. Goldstein I, Tamir A, Zimmer EZ, et al. Growth of the fetal orbit and lens in normal pregnancies. *Ultrasound Obstet Gynecol.* 1998;12:175–179.

10. Sukonpan K, Phupong V. A biometric study of the fetal orbit and lens in normal pregnancies. *J Clin Ultrasound.* 2009;37:69-74.

11. Feldman N, Melcer Y, Levinsohn-Tavor O, et al. Prenatal ultrasound charts of orbital total axial length measurement (TAL): a valuable data for correct fetal eye malformation assessment. *Prenat Diagn.* 2015;35:558–563.

12. Bojikian KD, de Moura CR, Tavares IM, et al. Fetal ocular measurements by three-dimensional ultrasound. *J AAPOS.* 2013;17:276–281.

13. Rosati P, Guariglia L. Early transvaginal fetal orbital measurements: a screening tool for aneuploidy? *J Ultrasound Med.* 2003;22:1201–1205.

14. Trout T, Budorick NE, Pretorius DH, et al. Significance of orbital measurements in the fetus. *J Ultrasound Med.* 1994;13:937–943.

15. Mayden KL, Tortora M, Berkowitz RL, et al. Orbital diameters: a new parameter for prenatal diagnosis and dating. *Am J Obstet Gynecol.* 1982;144:289–297.

16. Babcook C. The fetal face and neck. In: Callen P, ed. *Ultrasonography in Obstetrics and Gynecology.* Philadelphia, PA: WB Saunders; 2000:307–315.

17. Velasco-Annis C, Gholipour A, Afacan O, et al. Normative biometrics for fetal ocular growth using volumetric MRI reconstruction. *Prenat Diagn.* 2015;35:400–408.

18. Zhang Z, Lin X, Yu Q, et al. Fetal ocular development in the second trimester of pregnancy documented by 7.0 T postmortem magnetic resonance imaging. *PLoS One.* 2019;14:e0214939.

19. Paquette LB, Jackson HA, Tavare CJ, et al. In utero eye development documented by fetal MR imaging. *Am J Neuroradiol.* 2009;30:1787–1791.

20. Li XB, Kasprian G, Hodge JC, et al. Fetal ocular measurements by MRI. *Prenat Diagn.* 2010;30:1064–1071.

21. Birnholz JC, Farrell EE. Fetal hyaloid artery: timing of regression with US. *Radiology.* 1988;166:781–783.

22. Whitehead MT, Vezina G. Normal developmental globe morphology on fetal MR imaging. *AJNR Am J Neuroradiol.* 2016;37:1733–1737.

23. Robson CD, Barnewolt CE. MR imaging of fetal head and neck anomalies. *Neuroimaging Clin N Am.* 2004;14:273–291.

24. Berg C, Geipel A, Germer U, et al. Prenatal detection of Fraser syndrome without cryptophthalmos: case report and review of the literature. *Ultrasound Obstet Gynecol.* 2001;18:76–80.

25. Fryns JP, van Schoubroeck D, Vandenberghe K, et al. Diagnostic echographic findings in cryptophthalmos syndrome (Fraser syndrome). *Prenat Diagn.* 1997;17:582–584.

26. Bardakjian T, Weiss A, Schneider A. Anophthalmia/microphthalmia overview. NCBI. http://http://www.ncbi.nlm.nih.gov/books/NBK1378/. Accessed March 17, 2013.

27. Strigini F, Valleriani A, Cecchi M, et al. Prenatal ultrasound and magnetic resonance imaging features in a fetus with Walker-Warburg syndrome. *Ultrasound Obstet Gynecol.* 2009;33:363–365.

28. Castori M, Brancati F, Rinaldi R, et al. Antenatal presentation of the oculo-auriculo-vertebral spectrum (OAVS). *Am J Med Genet A.* 2006;140(14):1573–1579.

29. Mulvihill J, Sarkar A, Dixit A. Seeing the diagnosis on karyotype-SOX2 and eye development. *Ophthalmic Genet.* 2017;38:580–583.

30. Chitayat D, Sroka H, Keating S, et al. The PDAC syndrome (pulmonary hypoplasia/agenesis, diaphragmatic hernia/eventration, anophthalmia/microphthalmia, and cardiac defect) (Spear syndrome, Matthew-Wood syndrome): report of eight cases including a living child and further evidence for autosomal recessive inheritance. *Am J Med Genet A.* 2007;143:1268–1281.

31. Demyer W, Zeman W, Palmer CG. The face predicts the brain: diagnostic significance of median facial anomalies for holoprosencephaly (arrhinencephaly). *Pediatrics.* 1964;34:256–263.

32. Stroustrup A, Levine D. MR imaging of the fetal skull, face and neck. In: Levine D, ed. *Atlas of Fetal MRI.* Boca Raton, FL: Taylor & Francis; 2005:73–90.

33. Cohen MM Jr, Richieri-Costa A, Guion-Almeida ML, et al. Hypertelorism: interorbital growth, measurements, and pathogenetic considerations. *Int J Oral Maxillofac Surg.* 1995;24:387–395.

34. Nazzaro A, Della Monica M, Lonardo F, et al. Prenatal ultrasound diagnosis of a case of Pfeiffer syndrome without cloverleaf skull and review of the literature. *Prenat Diagn.* 2004;24:918–922.

35. David DJ, Cooter RD, Edwards TJ. Crouzon twins with cloverleaf skull malformations. *J Craniofac Surg.* 1991;2:56–60.

36. Tonni G, Panteghini M, Rossi A, et al. Craniosynostosis: prenatal diagnosis by means of ultrasound and SSSE-MRI: family series with report of neurodevelopmental outcome and review of the literature. *Arch Gynecol Obstet.* 2011;283:909–916.

37. Weber B, Schwabegger AH, Vodopiutz J, et al. Prenatal diagnosis of Apert syndrome with cloverleaf skull deformity using ultrasound, fetal magnetic resonance imaging and genetic analysis. *Fetal Diagn Ther.* 2010;27:51–56.

38. Itoh S, Nojima M, Yoshida K. Usefulness of magnetic resonance imaging for accurate diagnosis of Pfeiffer syndrome type II in utero. *Fetal Diagn Ther.* 2006;21:168–171.

39. Reches A, Yaron Y, Burdon K, et al. Prenatal detection of congenital bilateral cataract leading to the diagnosis of Nance-Horan syndrome in the extended family. *Prenat Diagn.* 2007;27:662–664.

40. Fayol L, Garcia P, Denis D, et al. Adams-Oliver syndrome associated with cutis marmorata telangiectatica congenita and congenital cataract: a case report. *Am J Perinatol.* 2006;23:197–200.

41. Başbuğ M, Serin IS, Ozçelik B, et al. Prenatal ultrasonographic diagnosis of rhizomelic chondrodysplasia punctata by detection of rhizomelic shortening and bilateral cataracts. *Fetal Diagn Ther.* 2005;20:171–174.

42. Terhal P, Sakkers R, Hochstenbach R, et al. Cerebellar hypoplasia, zonular cataract, and peripheral neuropathy in trisomy 17 mosaicism. *Am J Med Genet A.* 2004;130:410–414.

43. Vutova K, Peicheva Z, Popova A, et al. Congenital toxoplasmosis: eye manifestations in infants and children. *Ann Trop Paediatr.* 2002;22:213–218.

44. Cengiz B, Baxi L. Congenital cataract in triplet pregnancy after IVF with frozen embryos: prenatal diagnosis and management. *Fetal Diagn Ther.* 2001;16:234–236.

45. Romain M, Awoust J, Dugauquier C, et al. Prenatal ultrasound detection of congenital cataract in trisomy 21. *Prenat Diagn.* 1999;19:780–782.

46. Beinder EJ, Pfeiffer RA, Bornemann A, et al. Second-trimester diagnosis of fetal cataract in a fetus with Walker-Warburg syndrome. *Fetal Diagn Ther.* 1997;12:197–199.

47. Shapiro I, Borochowitz Z, Degani S, et al. Neu-Laxova syndrome: prenatal ultrasonographic diagnosis, clinical and pathological studies, and new manifestations. *Am J Med Genet.* 1992;43:602–605.

48. Brent RL. The effects of ionizing radiation, microwaves, and ultrasound on the developing embryo: clinical interpretations and applications of the data. *Curr Probl Pediatr.* 1984;14:1–87.

49. Drought A, Wimalasundera R, Holder S. Ultrasound diagnosis of bilateral cataracts in a fetus with possible cerebro-ocular congenital muscular dystrophy during the routine second trimester anomaly scan. *Ultrasound.* 2015;23:181–185.

50. Frieden IJ, Reese V, Cohen D. PHACE syndrome. The association of posterior fossa brain malformations, hemangiomas, arterial anomalies, coarctation of the aorta and cardiac defects, and eye abnormalities. *Arch Dermatol.* 1996;132:307–311.

51. Milic A, Blaser S, Robinson A, et al. Prenatal detection of microtia by MRI in a fetus with trisomy 22. *Pediatr Radiol.* 2006;36:706–710.

52. Ramji FG, Slovis TL, Baker JD. Orbital sonography in children. *Pediatr Radiol.* 1996;26:245–258.

53. Achiron R, Kreiser D, Achiron A. Axial growth of the fetal eye and evaluation of the hyaloid artery: in utero ultrasonographic study. *Prenat Diagn.* 2000;20:894–899.

54. Dutton GN. Congenital disorders of the optic nerve: excavations and hypoplasia. *Eye.* 2004;18:1038–1048.

55. Righini A, Avagliano L, Doneda C, et al. Prenatal magnetic resonance imaging of optic nerve head coloboma. *Prenat Diagn.* 2008;28:242–246.

56. Bault JP, Salomon LJ, Guibaud L, et al. Role of three-dimensional ultrasound measurement of the optic tract in fetuses with agenesis of the septum pellucidum. *Ultrasound Obstet Gynecol.* 2011;37:570–575.

57. Kusanovic J, Mittal P, Goncalves L, et al. 3D ultrasound evaluation of the fetal optic chiasma potential parameter for the differential diagnosis of developmental midline brain anomalies. *Ultrasound Obstet Gynecol.* 2005;26:311.

58. Bault JP. Prognostic value of fetal optic chiasm measurements in foetuses with septal agenesis. *Ultrasound Obstet Gynecol.* 2007;30:367–455.

59. Bault JP, Salomon LJ. Fetal optic chiasm measurements: reference range at 22–36 weeks of gestation. *Ultrasound Obstet Gynecol.* 2007;30:547–653.

60. Whitby E. In utero magnetic resonance imaging of developmental abnormalities of the fetal CNS. In: Griffiths P, Paley M, Whitby E, eds. *Imaging the Central Nervous System of the Fetus and Neonate.* New York, NY: Taylor & Francis; 2006:99–110.

61. Goldberg H, Sebire NJ, Holwell D, et al. Prenatal diagnosis of bilateral dacrocystoceles. *Ultrasound Obstet Gynecol.* 2000;15:448–449.

62. Davis WK, Mahony BS, Carroll BA, et al. Prenatal sonographic detection of benign dacrocystoceles (lacrimal duct cysts). *J Ultrasound Med.* 1987;6:461–465.

63. Yazici Z, Kline-Fath BM, Yazici B, et al. Congenital dacryocystocele: prenatal MRI findings. *Pediatr Radiol.* 2010;40:1868–1873.

64. Brugger PC, Weber M, Prayer D. Magnetic resonance imaging of the fetal efferent lacrimal pathways. *Eur Radiol.* 2010;20:1965–1973.

65. Smirniotopoulos JG, Chiechi MV. Teratomas, dermoids, and epidermoids of the head and neck. *Radiographics.* 1995;15:1437–1455.

66. Yoshida S, Kikuchi A, Naito S, et al. Giant hemangioma of the fetal neck, mimicking a teratoma. *J Obstet Gynaecol Res.* 2006;32:47–54.

67. Gnanaraj L, Skibell BC, Coret-Simon J, et al. Massive congenital orbital teratoma. *Ophthal Plast Reconstr Surg.* 2005;21:445–447.

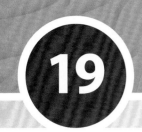

19 Face: Anomalies of Nose, Mouth, Lip and Tongue

Judy A. Estroff

Craniofacial abnormalities are among the most common human malformations (Table 19.1)[1] and may occur in isolation or associated with other anomalies, chromosomal aberrations, genetic and nongenetic syndromes, and physical- or toxin-induced injury. Identification of a craniofacial abnormality on fetal imaging should prompt a thorough search for abnormalities in all other organ systems. When associated with part of a syndrome of multiple anomalies, craniofacial defects are sometimes easier to identify sonographically than are more subtle abnormalities in other organs. After the face, the most frequently observed malformations are found in the cardiovascular, central nervous, and musculoskeletal systems.[2]

Facial abnormalities are important in and of themselves but may also herald an underlying problem, particularly a chromosome abnormality or syndromic condition (Table 19.2).[3] Therefore, it is important to evaluate the face when other anomalies are demonstrated and, conversely, to search for additional anomalies when facial abnormalities are evident.

Sonographic craniofacial evaluation has been technically feasible only since the early 1980s.[4,5] Reports of cohorts undergoing routine sonographic screening suggest that sensitivity for the detection of craniofacial anomalies, such as cleft lip and palate

TABLE 19.1 Examples of Most Common Craniofacial Anomalies

ANOMALY	PREVALENCE AT BIRTH PER 10,000
Cleft lip and/or palate	
Caucasian	10
Japanese	20
Native (North) American	36
African American population	3
Cleft palate	
Averaged across races	5
Craniosynostosis	3
Crouzon syndrome	0.4
Apert syndrome	0.15
Otomandibular anomalies	1.2
Treacher Collins syndrome	0.2
CHARGE association	1
Holoprosencephaly	1.2
Stickler syndrome	1
Fetal alcohol syndrome	2

Reprinted with permission from Shaw W. Global strategies to reduce the health care burden of craniofacial anomalies: report of WHO meetings on international collaborative research on craniofacial anomalies. *Cleft Palate Craniofac J.* 2004;41(3):238–243; Copyright © 2004 Allen Press Publishing Services.

TABLE 19.2 Common Craniofacial Syndromes

Trisomy 21 Down syndrome	Flat facial profile Upslanted palpebral fissures Small nose Small, dysplastic ears
Trisomy 13 Patau syndrome	Holoprosencephaly associated with midline facial anomalies, cyclopia, hypotelorism and clefts, scalp defects, microcephaly with sloping forehead, hypotelorism, microphthalmia with iris colobomas, dysplastic ears, premaxillary agenesis, cleft lip, micrognathia, cleft palate
Trisomy 18 Edward syndrome	Prominent occiput, bifrontal narrowing, low-set dysplastic ears, small mouth plus micrognathia
4p minus Wolf–Hirschhorn syndrome	Cleft lip/palate "Greek-warrior helmet" facies: prominent sloped forehead, hypertelorism, high-arched eyebrows, low-set ears with preauricular pit, short philtrum, downturned angles of the mouth, micrognathia, microphthalmia, and colobomas
5p minus Cri-du-chat syndrome	Round face, downslanting palpebral fissures, hypertelorism, low-set dysplastic and posteriorly rotated ears, downturned angles of mouth
Mosaic trisomy 8	Low-set dysplastic ears Micrognathia
22q11.2 deletion syndrome	Hypertelorism, low-set ears, micrognathia, cleft palate
Beckwith–Wiedemann syndrome	Macroglossia Abnormal ears, ear lobe creases Capillary hemangiomas over the forehead Coarse facial features
Campomelic dysplasia	Robin sequence, macrocephaly, large anterior fontanelle, flat nasal bridge, low-set ears, micrognathia, short neck
Stickler syndrome	Prominent eyes, midface hypoplasia, small nose, cataracts
Smith–Lemli–Opitz syndrome	Microcephaly, cleft palate, small anteverted nose, low-set ears, bifrontal narrowing, micrognathia
De Lange syndrome	Microbrachycephaly, excessive hair over the face, single eyebrow (synophrys), small anteverted nose, hairy dysplastic and low-set ears, long philtrum, thin upper lip, downturned angles of the mouth, micrognathia
Apert syndrome	Turribrachycephaly, hypertelorism with proptosis, beaked nose, low-set ears, high-arched cleft palate

Adapted from Suri M. Craniofacial syndromes. *Semin Fetal Neonatal Med.* 2005;10(3):243–257. Copyright © 2005 Elsevier. With permission.

559

(CLP), has historically been very low, under 20%.[6,7] Tertiary referral centers appear to have a significantly higher detection rate, as high as 88% for cleft lip (CL), but less than 73% for cleft palate (CP).[8–10] The detection rates have continued to improve.[9] This implies that although detection may be feasible, routine screening of the otherwise normal-appearing fetus may not always include complete evaluation of the fetal face and head.

The American Institute of Ultrasound and Medicine (AIUM) standard of 2003 did not include routine fetal face evaluation and only added this requirement to its guidelines for second- and third-trimester fetal sonography (US) in its revised statement in 2007, on the basis of the consensus that it is extremely important to demonstrate that evaluable craniofacial aspects of the fetus are normal or to characterize the abnormality in an anomalous fetus. The AIUM updated its guidelines in 2018.[11] Imaging of the fetal face in three planes, whenever possible, adds very little time and increases the likelihood of anomaly detection from 20% to 30% when only two planes are evaluated to nearly 90% when all the three planes are used and the anatomy is understood.[12] Especially in the era of high-resolution three-dimensional (3D) sonography, many craniofacial anomalies are detected when the sonographer attempts to take a keepsake 3D frontal or profile image of the fetus for the parents and notes an aberration.[13]

Fetal diagnosis of craniofacial anomalies, especially orofacial clefts, is even possible in the first trimester, at or before the time of first-trimester nuchal translucency measurement.[14–18] Timmerman et al.[19] found a strong association between increased nuchal translucency and orofacial clefts in chromosomally normal fetuses.

EMBRYOLOGY OF THE FACE

Facial morphology is established between weeks 4 and 10 after conception. Formation is based on the fusion of the midline frontonasal prominence (FNP) and three other paired prominences: maxillary processes (MXPs), lateral nasal processes (LNPs), and mandibular nasal processes (MNPs). These prominences are filled with neural crest cells. The FNP leads to the formation of the forehead, midline of the nose, philtrum, middle portion of the upper lip, and primary palate. The LNP gives rise to the nasal alae. The MXP forms the upper jaw, the sides of the face, the sides of the upper lip, and the secondary palate (Fig. 19.1).

The four branchial arches appear at 4 to 5 weeks of development and represent bars of mesenchymal tissue that are separated by clefts. They appear between days 22 and 29 and give rise to skeletal, visceral, arterial, muscular, and neurological components of the head and neck. At the end of week 4, the stomodeum (rudimentary mouth) forms in the center of the face and is surrounded by the first pair of branchial arches. Branchial arches have a mesenchymal core that is covered on the outside by ectoderm and on

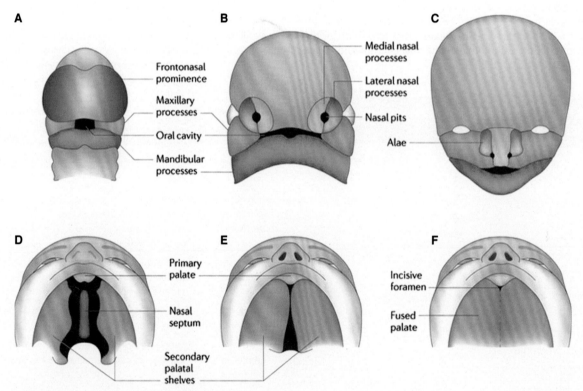

FIGURE 19.1: Embryological development of the face from 5 to 8 weeks. Schematic diagrams of the development of the lip and palate in humans. **A:** The developing frontonasal prominence, paired maxillary processes, and paired mandibular processes surround the primitive oral cavity by week 4 of embryonic development. **B:** By week 5, the nasal pits have formed, leading to the formation of the paired medial and lateral nasal processes. **C:** The medial nasal processes have merged with the maxillary processes to form the upper lip and primary palate by the end of week 6. The lateral nasal processes form the nasal alae. Similarly, the mandibular processes fuse to form the lower jaw. **D:** During week 6 of embryogenesis, the secondary palate develops as bilateral outgrowths from the maxillary processes, which grow vertically down the side of the tongue. **E:** Subsequently, the palatal shelves elevate to a horizontal position above the tongue, contact one another, and commence fusion. **F:** Fusion of the palatal shelves ultimately divides the oronasal space into separate oral and nasal cavities. (Reproduced with permission from Dixon MJ, Marazita ML, Beaty TH, et al. Cleft lip and palate: understanding genetic and environmental influences. *Nat Rev Genet.* 2011;12:167–178.)

the inside by epithelium (endodermal in origin). Branchial arches contain neural crest cells that contribute to the skeletal development of the face. The mesoderm develops into the muscles of the face and the neck. The first branchial arch gives rise to the maxilla and the mandible (including the premaxilla and zygoma) and part of the temporal bone.

The nasal placodes evaginate to form the nasal pits. The resulting ridges, the FNP, form the upper boundary of the stomodeum. Coming from the first branchial arch, the paired MXP forms the lateral boundaries of the stomodeum. The paired MNP (also from the first branchial arch) forms the caudal boundary. Between weeks 5 and 8, the MXP grows medially, obliterating the grooves between the nasal FNP and the MXP. The upper lip is formed by the fusion of the MXP and medial nasal prominences. The mandibular prominences (MNP) merge to form the lower lip, chin, and mandible.

The nose is formed by five prominences. The FNP forms the bridge of the nose, and the two medial nasal swellings that fuse together to form the intermaxillary segment are responsible in forming the crest, tip, and central portion and philtrum of the upper lip; the incisor teeth; and the front triangular portion of the palate (primary palate). The LNP forms the sides, or the alae. The secondary palate is formed by shelf-like outgrowth from the maxillary prominences. These palatine shelves appear in week 6 and ascend in week 7 in a horizontal position above the tongue, thus fusing to form the secondary palate. The triangular primary palate is separated from the secondary by the incisive foramen (see Fig. 19.1).

The partial or complete lack of fusion of one or both of the prominences with the medial nasal swellings and maxillary prominences results in a unilateral or bilateral CLP, which may involve the primary and/or secondary palate. A split in the primary palate occurs between the lateral incisors and the canine teeth and along the side of the upper lip in the paramedian position. If only the secondary palate is abnormal, a cleft behind the incisive foramen or bifid uvula may result. The rare median CL is caused by incomplete merging of the two medial nasal swellings, or intermaxillary segment, and is more often associated with severe congenital anomalies such as holoprosencephaly.

The primitive nasal cavity begins as a single chamber. The nasal septum has both a cartilaginous and a bony stage of development. At about 5 weeks, the septum forms anteriorly from the enlarging frontonasal process and continues to grow posteriorly until it meets with the horizontal palatine processes in the midline (see Fig. 19.1). Eventually, by week 9 or 10, the embryo has distinct and separate respiratory and digestive openings.

First branchial arch anomalies result from an insufficiency of neural crest cells. Malformations resulting from this defect include Treacher Collins syndrome (mandibulofacial dysostosis) and Robin sequence. Because neural crest cells also contribute to the formation of the aortic and pulmonary arteries, some first arch syndromes can be accompanied by congenital heart defects.[20]

TECHNIQUE FOR EXAMINATION

For those charged with the task of identifying and classifying fetal CL/P and other craniofacial anomalies, a comprehensive routine 2D and 3D sonographic (US) protocol should be in place and would ideally include the option for additional evaluation of the secondary palate and brain by fetal magnetic resonance imaging (MRI). The imager should have familiarity with craniofacial embryology and with the most common systems for classifying craniofacial anomalies (Table 19.3). There is great value in fostering a close and collaborative working relationship with regional craniofacial surgeons and their team and in understanding what these clinicians wish to know about the fetus to accurately counsel parents and prepare for postnatal evaluation and treatment.[21-24]

Ultrasound (US) can optimally demonstrate the external contour of the face when it is outlined by fluid (Fig. 19.2). Most imagers evaluate the fetal face subjectively using the following three orthogonal views (Table 19.4):

- **Coronal:** from the most superficial, "en face" view of the face, looking first at the soft tissues of the eyes, cheeks, nose, and mouth (Fig. 19.3A), from the outermost surface of the tip of the nose, then inward to deeper bony and soft-tissue structures of the nasal vomer, tooth-bearing bony alveolus, and tongue, and finally into the primary bony palate and orbits
- **Axial:** viewing the mandible, maxilla, tongue (Fig. 19.3B), tooth buds, and orbits
- **Sagittal:** evaluating the facial profile (Fig. 19.3C), including the nasal bridge, frontal bone, maxilla, mandible, and position of the tongue

Facial features can also be seen from a unique perspective using 3D sonography (Figs. 19.4 and 19.5), which is often helpful for clinicians and parents, but can be of limited use in the setting of oligohydramnios, fetal crowding, or unfavorable fetal position. 3D US often adds detail to the evaluation of fetal craniofacial malformations, including cleft lip, with or without cleft palate (CL/P).[13,25-27] Techniques using 3D US have been described to visualize the secondary palate, including the "3D reverse view" described by Campbell et al.[28] in 2005, the "flipped-face view" described by Platt et al.[29] in 2006, and the "oblique-face view" described by Pilu and Segata[30] in 2007. All of these views require software manipulation and add to the length of the study, although the patient may be discharged as these images are created. In expert hands, the manipulation may take only a few minutes. A study comparing the accuracy of reverse-, flipped-, and oblique-face methods for visualization of the hard and soft palate by Martinez-Ten et al. demonstrated accuracy of all three methods to visualize the upper lip and alveolar ridge (71%, 86%, and 100%, respectively). However, soft (secondary) palate involvement was diagnosed correctly in only one of seven fetuses in the flipped- and oblique-face views. The reverse-face view could not identify the secondary palate.[31]

Because of its unique display, 3D US aids parents and referring physicians to understanding the extent of the defects. Parental decisions may be affected in evaluation of CL/P, because they can view the abnormality on a recognizable image. 3D ultrasonographic imaging of fetal tooth buds can aid in the accurate classification of clefts,[13,30-32] but accurate detection of accompanying or isolated cleft secondary palate is often possible only by the addition of fetal MRI.

Fetal MRI has the potential to better visualize the palate as well as internal craniofacial, brain, and body anatomy. MRI is now routinely used to evaluate the fetal brain and chest and is increasingly being used to evaluate the fetal face.[33-36] Fetal MRI has an advantage over fetal sonography in its ability to demonstrate the secondary palate, which is mainly soft tissue (Fig. 19.6). Assessment of the secondary palate is limited on sonography because of the proximity of normal bony structures, which block US waves.

TABLE 19.3   Glossary of Craniofacial Terms

Aglossia	Absent tongue
Agnathia	Absent mandible
Ala or alar	Tissue comprising the lateral boundary of the nose
Alveolus/alveolar ridge/alveolar process/alveolar arches	Bony arches of the maxilla (upper jaw) and mandible (lower jaw) that contain teeth
Anotia	Absent ears
Canthus	Corner of the eyelids
Cebocephaly	Orbital hypotelorism associated with a single-nostril nose
Choanal atresia	Unilateral or bilateral obstruction of the posterior choanae of the nose
Coloboma	Congenital malformation of the eye, causing defects in the lens, iris, or retina
Columella	Fleshy lower margin of the nasal septum, between the nostrils; the strip of skin running from the tip of the nose to the upper lip, which separates the nostrils
Craniosynostosis	Premature closure of the skull sutures
Ethmoid bone	Bone between the eyes; forms upper part of nasal septum, sidewalls of eye socket
Exorbitism	Abnormal protrusion of the eyeball secondary to a shallow or small orbit
Frontal bone	Forehead, including brow and top of eye socket
Frenulum	Folds of mucous membrane connecting the inside of the lips to the gums, and the tongue to the floor of the mouth
Glabella	Bony part between the eyebrows
Globe	Eyeball
Glossoptosis	Downward and posterior displacement of the tongue
Glossopexy	Surgical anterior pexy of the tongue to prevent airway obstruction
Hypertelorism	Abnormally increased orbital distance
Hypotelorism	Abnormally decreased orbital distance
IOD (inner orbital distance)	Distance from inner to inner bony margins of the orbits
Incisive foramen	Opening in incisive fossa of the hard palate. Primary palate = anterior to incisive foramen. Secondary palate = posterior to incisive foramen
Macroglossia	Enlarged tongue
Macrostomia	Large or wide mouth
Malar	Cheekbone just below the eyes
Mandible	Lower jaw
Maxilla	Upper jaw
Microform cleft lip	Vermillion cutaneous notch less than 3 mm above the normal peak
Micrognathia	Having an unusually small upper or lower jaw
Microstomia	Small mouth
Microtia	Small ears
Midface retrusion	Posterior positioning and/or vertical shortening of the infraorbital and perialar regions. Increased concavity of the face
Mini-microform cleft lip	Disrupted vermillion–cutaneous junction without elevation of the bow peak
Minor-form cleft lip	Defect extending 3 mm or more above the normal Cupid's bow peak
Nasal bone	Bridge of the nose
Nares	Openings in the nasal cavity; nostrils
OOD (outer orbital distance)	Distance between bony margins of the outer lateral orbital walls
Otocephaly	Absent or hypoplastic mandible, microstomia, hypoglossia or aglossia, posteriorly rotated and low-set ears
Perpendicular plate of the ethmoid	Upper part of the nasal septum
Philtrum	Vertical groove in median portion of upper lip
Premaxilla	Front middle portion of the upper jaw containing front teeth (incisors)
Prolabium	Prominent central part of the upper lip overlying the premaxilla
Proptosis	Forward projection or displacement of the eyeball
Retrognathia	Posteriorly positioned lower jaw, set back from plane of the face
Robin sequence	Includes cleft soft palate, small mouth, micrognathia/retrognathia, and glossoptosis
Sphenoid bone	Central part of the cranial floor. Forms part of the floor and sidewalls of the eye socket
Submucous cleft palate	Cleft of the muscle layer of the soft palate with an intact layer of mucosa lying over the defect
Tissue band	Thin bridge of tissue connecting the lateral and medial sides of a cleft lip
Vermillion border	Pink/purple lip tissue outlining the upper lip; "Cupid's bow" of upper lip
Vomer	Back and bottom part of the nasal septum
Zygomatic arch	The cheekbone that connects to the temple, a continuation of the malar bone

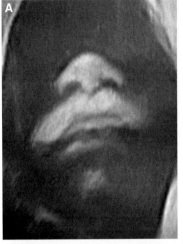
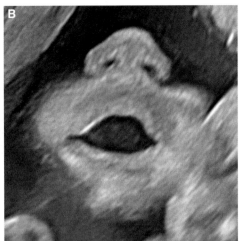
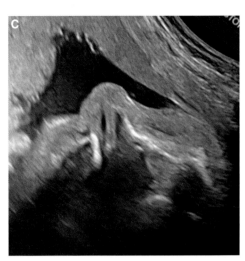
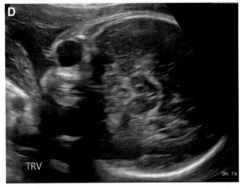

FIGURE 19.2: The normal fetal face in a 28-week fetus. **A:** Coronal 2D US of nose and vermillion border of the upper lip. **B:** Coronal 2D image with mouth open. **C:** Axial 2D image of nasal vomer and the tip of the nose. **D:** Axial 2D image of fetal eyelashes in a different 29-week fetus.

TABLE 19.4	Sonographic Protocol for Evaluation of Fetal Face and Neck: 2D and 3D in the Axial, Coronal, and Sagittal Planes
Skull and brain	Skull shape: normal, dolichocephalic, brachycephalic, unusual
	Sutures: open, no defects
	Normal underlying brain
	Measurements: normal head size compared with long bone and abdominal biometry for given gestational age (BPD/OFD/ HC vs. GA, AD, FL, HL)
	Skin around head: normal, thickened, mass
Face	Mouth: vermillion border intact
	Nares: symmetric, not flattened or cleft
	Vomer: straight, midline
	OOD/IOD, OD, orbital shape, symmetry: two orbits with normal size globes and normal interocular distance
	Maxilla: normal intact arc-shaped alveolus
	Mandible: normal intact arc-shaped alveolus
	Tongue: position, size
	Ears: size, shape, position
	Forehead: normal, sloped, bulging
	Midface: normal, retruded
	Chin: normal vs. small (micrognathia), retruded (retrognathia) or both
Neck and spine	Head position
	Length of spine, curvature
	Presence of nuchal cord, skin thickening
	Integrity of vertebrae, lamina, and spinous processes
	Position of trachea, thyroid, strap muscles
	Evaluate vallecula and pyriform sinuses, glottis, subglottic trachea, carina

AD, abdominal diameter; *BPD*, biparietal diameter; *FL*, femur length; *GA*, gestational age; *HC*, head circumference; *HL*, humeral length; *IOD*, inner orbital distance; *OD*, ocular diameter; *OFD*, occipitofrontal diameter; *OOD*, outer orbital distance.

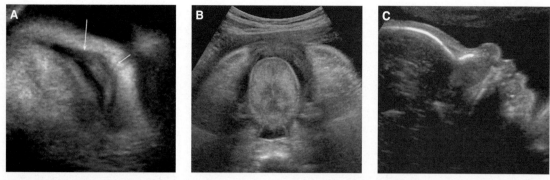

FIGURE 19.3: **A:** Normal lip. 2D sonogram of a normal fetal lip at 31 weeks showing the white roll, vermillion border (*long arrow*), and Cupid's bow (*short arrow*). **B:** Normal tongue. 2D sonogram of a normal fetal tongue in axial view at 36 weeks' gestation. **C:** Normal 2D sagittal face profile.

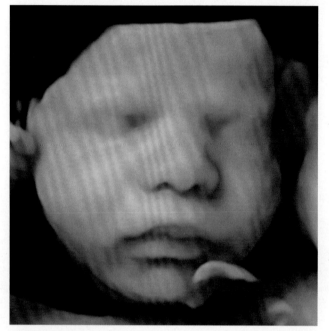

FIGURE 19.4: The normal fetal face. Three-dimensional sonogram at 32 weeks' gestation.

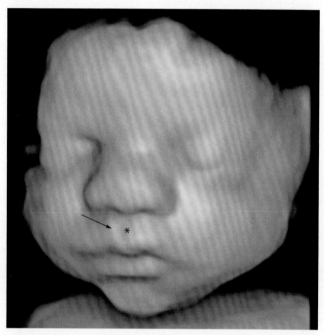

FIGURE 19.5: The normal fetal nose. Three-dimensional sonogram of a third-trimester fetus showing normal nasal structures: bridge, tip, nostrils, ala, alar base, philtral columns (*arrow*), and philtral dimple (*asterisk*).

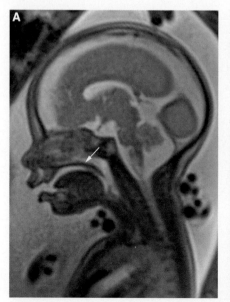

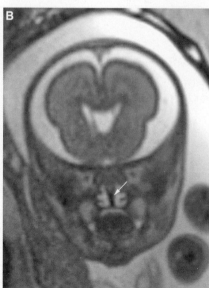

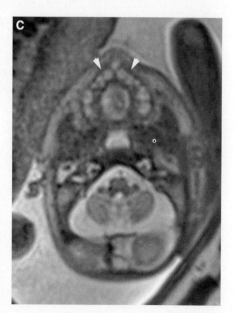

FIGURE 19.6: MRI of a 25-week fetus with normal palate. **A:** Sagittal plane shows secondary palate (*arrow*). **B:** Coronal plane shows vomer (*arrow*) and palatal shelves. **C:** Axial plane shows tooth-bearing alveolus (*arrowheads*) and ear anatomy.

Recent studies suggest a possible detection rate of over 90% for CP if MRI is used.

Nomograms for the proportions of the fetal face have been published, including frontomaxillary angle, nasal bone length, chin length, and tongue dimensions. Identification of tooth buds within the normal arc-shaped maxillary and mandibular alveoli is extremely helpful in assessing facial features and excluding facial clefts (Fig. 19.6C). Maxillary and mandibular shapes are readily assessed with 2D and 3D sonography as well as with fetal MRI. An abnormally shaped maxilla can be seen in various chromosomal anomalies, such as trisomy 21, in the setting of CL/P, and in many syndromes.[37]

Fetal nose evaluation is often subjective. However, normal biometric measurements for nasal bone width and length between 14 and 40 weeks are available, and there is a linear growth relationship between those measurements and gestational age.[38–40] Measurement of nasal bone length has been a standard part of the first-trimester (between 11 and 13 weeks) fetal sonogram (US), along with measurement of the nuchal translucency. A short or absent nasal bone raises the likelihood of trisomy 21. Very recent transition from imaging findings to routine first-trimester maternal serum screening by measurement of free fetal DNA has made first-trimester nasal bone measurement less important and has significantly reduced the use of second-trimester amniocentesis for advanced maternal age or the presence of "soft markers" for Down syndrome on sonography, including echogenic bowel, pyelectasis, and echogenic intracardiac focus.[41]

Evaluating fetal jaw position and morphology is also usually subjective. However, mandibular measurements may be obtained in several different ways. Chitty et al. advocate measuring the length of the mandibular rami and provide normative data between 12 and 28 weeks.[42]

The orbits (see Chapter 18, Fetal Eyes) are routinely assessed on sonography in an axial or a coronal view of the face, but are often seen to advantage on fetal MRI. Two equal-sized orbits should be present. The distance between the orbits (interorbital distance) should be slightly greater than the diameter of one globe. If these measurements are abnormal, the rest of the fetal face and body must be scrutinized because of the high number of associated systemic abnormalities.[43,44] It is important to note that MRI and US orbit nomograms are different and should not be interchanged.

Holoprosencephaly

De Meyer et al.[45] in 1964 pointed out that "The face predicts the brain." Certain facial anomalies predictably have associated brain anomalies, such as cyclopia with a proboscis seen in association with holoprosencephaly. Other facial anomalies seen in holoprosencephaly (Figs. 19.7 to 19.10) include cebocephaly, in which the eyes are close together and the nose has a single nostril; ethmocephaly, in which there is absence of the nose (arhinia) (Fig. 19.11) and a blind-ending tubular structure (proboscis) between the eyes (Fig. 19.12); or median CLP (Figs. 19.9 and 19.24).[46–51]

NOSE

The nose is well seen on fetal sonography (see Fig. 19.5) and is visible, but is often less well seen on fetal MRI. Contour anomalies of the nose can include asymmetry and flattening, as is seen in CL, especially in severe unilateral complete

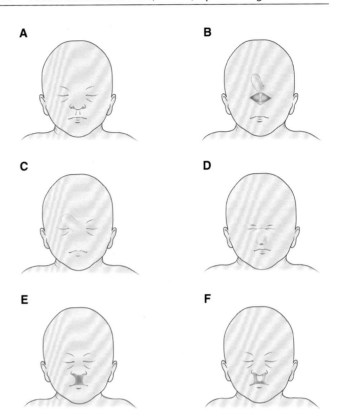

FIGURE 19.7: The many faces of holoprosencephaly: normal **(A)**, cyclopia **(B)**, ethmocephaly **(C)**, cebocephaly **(D)**, median cleft lip and palate **(E)**, and bilateral cleft lip and palate **(F)**.

CLP, frontonasal dysplasia, and arhinia. The nose may be abnormally prominent, as is seen when there is a nasal mass, such as a dermoid, frontal encephalocele, or a duplicated or supernumerary nostril (Fig. 19.13). The intermaxillary segment in bilateral CLP can be confused for a nasal mass. The normal regions of the nose include the bridge, nares, alae, and alar base.

Arhinia

Definition/Incidence: The absence of the nose, arhinia, is a rare anomaly with a poorly understood pathogenesis, likely occurring between weeks 3 and 10 of gestation.[52,53]

Pathogenesis/Etiology: The formation of the nose and sinuses is an intricate process that progresses through three distinct phases: the preskeletal phase, the chondrocranial stage, and the stage of ossification. In the preskeletal phase, mesenchymal swellings develop around the olfactory placodes. The primary nasal cavity appears at about 4 weeks, heralding the chondrocranial stage, in which the cartilaginous nasal framework develops. The bony structures of the nose and sinuses are well along in development by the end of the first trimester. Arhinia may develop from failure of the nasal epithelial plugs to reabsorb during the 13th to 15th weeks of gestation.

Imaging: In the fetus, arhinia can be suspected when on sonography, the imager cannot identify the nostrils or nasal bone, and the fetal profile shows severe midface flattening (Fig. 19.11). The upper lip can be mistaken for the nose. On fetal MRI, there will

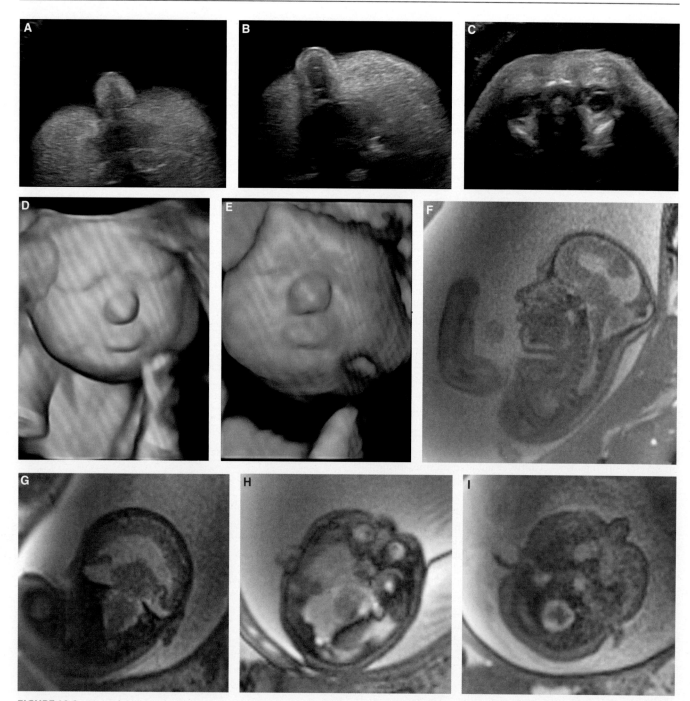

FIGURE 19.8: 32 week Fetus with trisomy 13 and holoprosencephaly. **A/B:** Two-dimensional sonography showing proboscis with single nostril and **C** with hypotelorism and microphthalmia. **D, E:** Three-dimensional sonography with similar findings. **F–I:** Fetal MRI demonstrating alobar holoprosencephaly and similar facial findings.

be absence of the nasal cavity and vomer. Multiple anomalies are associated with arhinia, including holoprosencephaly, CLP, and microphthalmia or anophthalmia.

Management: Infants who are born with arhinia have difficulty breathing and eating, as newborns are obligate nose-breathers. The condition is associated with CLP and anomalies affecting the eyes and brain, as well as anomalies related to chromosome 9. The diagnosis is obvious at birth, with an absent nose, hypoplastic maxilla, and a high-arched palate. Some reports indicate that the infant with arhinia can adapt to oral breathing, with nutritional support given directly into the stomach. If the child

survives, definitive repair is usually undertaken during the preschool years.[53]

Proboscis

Definition/Incidence: Proboscis lateralis, or congenital tubular nose, is a rare anomaly in which the external nose fails to develop on one side and is replaced by a small-caliber elephant trunk-like soft-tissue structure hanging from the inner canthus of the eye. It has no nasal cavity but may connect to deeper structures such as the dura or skull base. This peculiar abnormality is often associated with holoprosencephaly.

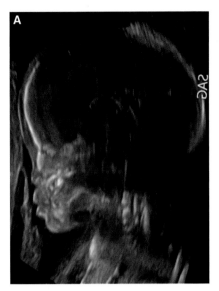
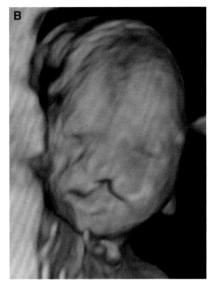

FIGURE 19.9: Fetus with holoprosencephaly and cleft lip. Two-dimensional **(A)** and three-dimensional **(B)** sonography of a 21-week 3-day fetus with a small nose, midline cleft lip, and holoprosencephaly.

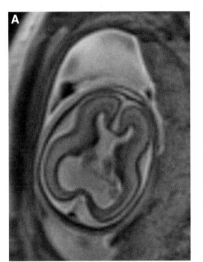
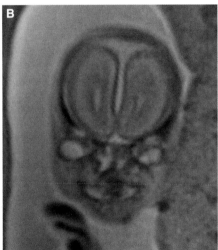
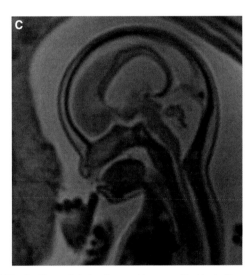

FIGURE 19.10: Fetus with 13q deletion and multiple anomalies. Axial, coronal, and sagittal MRI of a 20-week 1-day fetus with anomalies, including holoprosencephaly **(A)**, microphthalmia **(B)**, and cleft palate **(C)**.

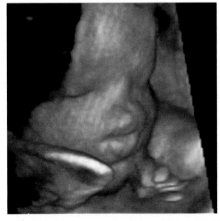

FIGURE 19.11: A 34-week gestation fetus with arhinia (absent nose) and microphthalmia. After birth, the diagnosis of Bosma arhinia syndrome was made.

Imaging: A proboscis appears as a soft-tissue protrusion in the middle of the face, usually between the eyes (Fig. 19.12). As it is fully formed of soft tissue, it is often seen best on sonography, especially early in gestation.

Management: Treatment involves excision of the proboscis at an early age and re-routing of the nasolacrimal duct.[53]

Frontonasal Dysplasia

Frontonasal dysplasia is a rare facial malformation associated with mutations in the *ALX* gene, causing abnormal skull formation (Fig. 19.14), leading to at least two of the following:

1. Ocular hypertelorism
2. Broad nose with a slit or cleft on one or both sides
3. No nasal tip

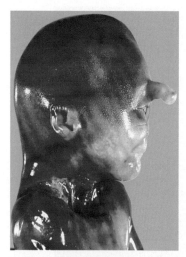

FIGURE 19.12: Proboscis. Pathological photograph of a fetus with proboscis and cyclopia.

4. Central cleft of the nose, upper lip, or palate
5. Anterior bifid cranium
6. Widow's peak hairline

It may also be associated with anomalies of the corpus callosum.[54]

Choanal Atresia

Definition/Incidence: Unilateral or bilateral obstruction of the posterior choanae of the nose occurs in approximately 1 in 7,000 to 1 in 8,000 live births. The condition occurs more often in females and on the right side.

Pathogenesis/Etiology: Choanal atresia is associated with other anomalies in up to 50% of cases, with the most common being the CHARGE syndrome (Fig. 19.15) (also see Chapter 21). The CHARGE syndrome occurs in approximately 1 in 10,000 to 1 in 15,000 births. CHARGE is an acronym for the following components: *c*oloboma; *h*eart (ASD, conotruncal lesions); *a*tresia, membranous or bony of the choanae; *r*etardation in growth and development; *g*enitourinary, involving undescended testes, microphallus, hydronephrosis; and *e*ar, involving external, middle, and inner ear defects.[53] The criteria for the diagnosis of CHARGE syndrome have been expanded to include any newborn with four major or three major and three minor criteria. Major criteria include coloboma, choanal atresia, external, middle or inner ear anomalies, and cranial nerve dysfunction. Minor criteria include genital hypoplasia, developmental delay, cardiovascular anomalies, short stature, cleft lip or palate, tracheoesophageal defects, and characteristic facial features.[3]

Imaging: On US, the nasal cavity is filled with fluid. On MRI, the posterionasal cavity is closed, either by bone or by soft tissue (Fig. 19.15B).

Prognosis/Management: Most choanal atresia is bony (90%). Bilateral choanal atresia is a neonatal emergency as the infant, an obligate nose-breather, presents with respiratory distress at rest, and relieved only by crying. Immediate treatment is by placement of an oral airway. Definitive treatment involves surgically creating new posterior choanae.[53] Isolated choanal atresia can

present as the only anomaly in otherwise normal fetuses or may be part of a syndrome.

Nasal Masses

Nasal masses are uncommon but are frequently seen in specialized pediatric centers and are often recognized in utero. The most common congenital nasal masses are nasal dermoids, nasopharyngeal teratomas, gliomas (Fig. 19.16), encephaloceles, and lacrimal duct cysts. Nasal duplication is a rare anomaly. Nasal dermoids and lacrimal duct cysts are benign, and most are treated fairly easily after birth. Teratomas, gliomas, and encephaloceles are much more concerning lesions as they often invade or distort adjacent tissues or craniofacial structures.

MOUTH AND LIP

Cleft Lip and/or Palate

Sonographic detection of facial clefts has been possible only since the early 1980s. Since then, advances in 2D, 3D, and 4D imaging have been startling, with continuous improvements in resolution and technique from year to year. It is now possible to detect even the most subtle surface anomalies, such as preauricular skin tags and microform incomplete CL, and to observe fetal facial expression and behavior.[26]

The value of detecting fetal craniofacial anomalies has been controversial, proponents arguing that fetal detection allows parents to prepare, both psychologically and practically, for the birth of a child with a facial anomaly, and that detection of a craniofacial anomaly allows the obstetric specialist the opportunity to search for other or associated anomalies and to refer the family to a craniofacial specialist. Opponents of fetal craniofacial screening argue that (1) facial clefts alone do not threaten fetal survival and (2) there is currently no practical fetal treatment and that (3) postnatal remedies are well established and have a very favorable outcome. However, both parents and specialists maintain that knowledge of the fetal anomaly is of great benefit and eases the transition into treatment after birth.[24]

Epidemiology/Incidence: CL/P is the most common congenital anomaly aside from congenital heart disease and occurs more frequently in aborted fetuses and stillborns than in live births. CL/P incidence is estimated at 1 in 500 to 1 in 1,000 live births.[1,4,15,32,55] The risk of genetic syndromes is increased if the alveolus or secondary palate is involved. There are racial differences in the incidence of clefts, with the highest in the Asian population (0.79 to 3.74/1,000), lower for Caucasians (0.91 to 2.7/1,000), and lowest for blacks (0.18 to 1.67/1,000). Males are more frequently affected than females for CL/P by approximately 1.4:1.0. Females more frequently have isolated CP. Males and females are equally affected by isolated CL.[56]

Pathogenesis/Types: Knowledge of normal embryology is important for understanding the pathogenesis of facial clefts. Nonfusion of the normal medial nasal swelling and maxillary prominence is the etiology for most CL/P. If the facial abnormality does not follow a normal embryological pattern, then an amniotic band syndrome should be considered.

The array of possible types of facial clefts is vast (Fig. 19.17). In a recent large series of 782 patients by Nagase et al., in Japan, the most frequent type of cleft was CLP (40.8%) (Fig. 19.18). CLP occurred more often in males; isolated CP

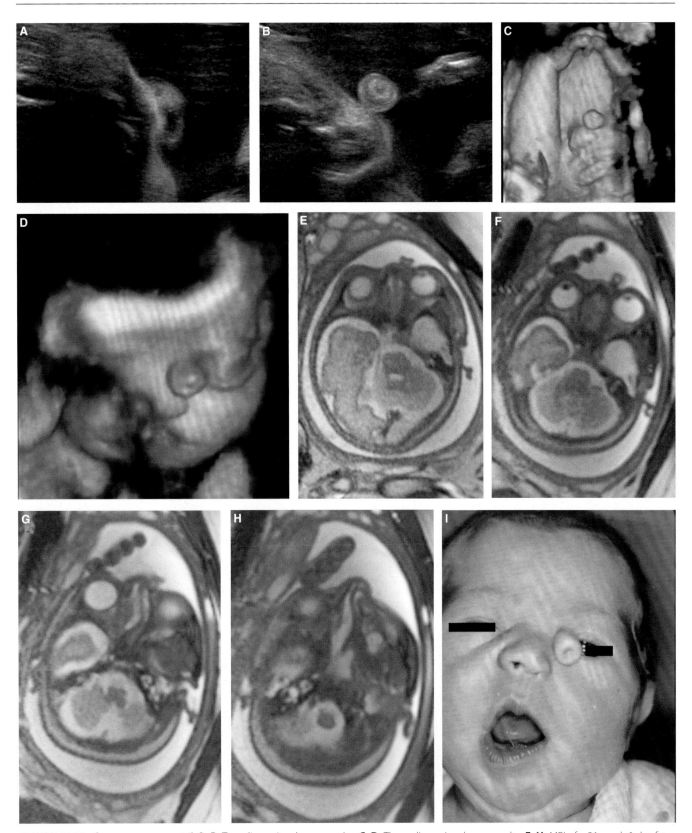

FIGURE 19.13: Supernumerary nostril. **A, B:** Two-dimensional sonography; **C, D:** Three-dimensional sonography; **E–H:** MRI of a 31-week 6-day fetus with a tubular mass medial to the left orbit, which represented a supernumerary nostril. The left nasal cavity and nostril are hypoplastic. **I:** Postnatal images of the same fetus.

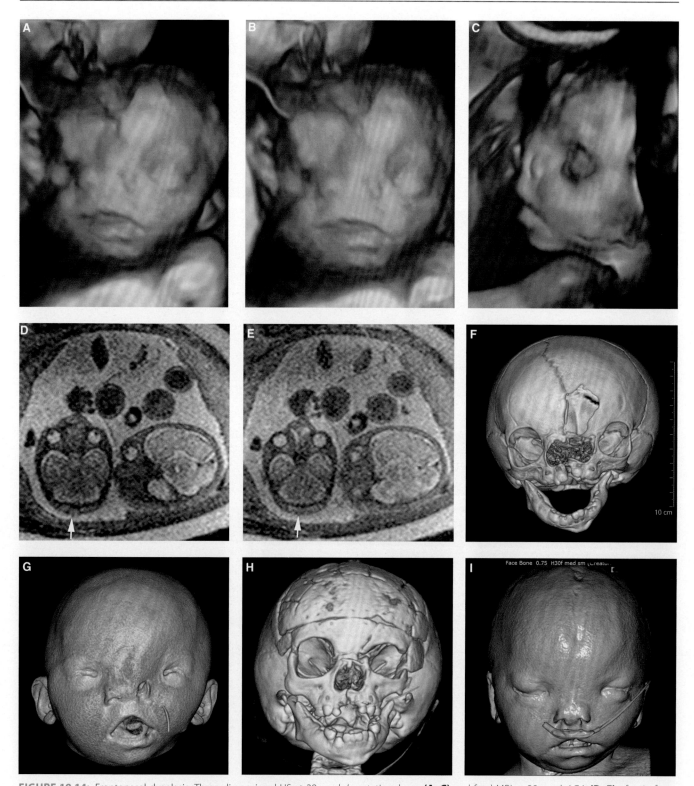

FIGURE 19.14: Frontonasal dysplasia. Three-dimensional US at 28 weeks' gestational age **(A–C)** and fetal MRI at 32 weeks' GA **(D, E)** of twin fetus A *(arrows)* with frontonasal dysplasia. The nose is wide and irregular, the nostrils are widely separated, and there is severe hypertelorism. Postnatal computed tomography images at 10 months before repair **(F, G)**, and at 21 months after surgical repair **(H, I)**.

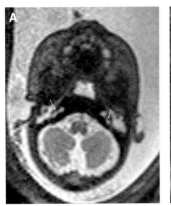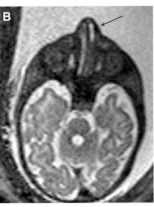

FIGURE 19.15: CHARGE syndrome. Fetal MRI at 34 weeks shows multiple anomalies in keeping with CHARGE syndrome, including bilateral inner ear anomalies (*arrows*) **(A)** and left choanal atresia (*black arrow*) **(B)**. The fetus also had left coloboma, esophageal atresia, and inferior vermian hypoplasia (not shown).

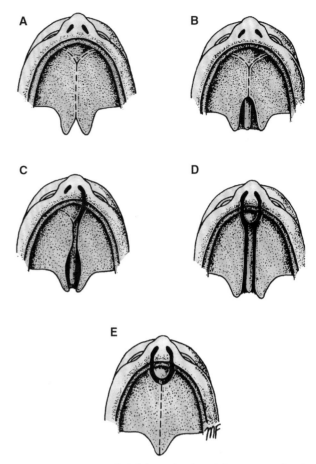

FIGURE 19.17: Types of cleft lip and palate. Inferior view of various types of cleft lip and palate. **A:** Bifid uvula. **B:** Cleft soft palate. **C:** Unilateral complete cleft lip and palate. **D:** Bilateral complete cleft lip and palate. **E:** Bilateral cleft lip. (Reprinted with permission from Snell RS. The head and neck. In: *Clinical Anatomy by Regions*. Philadelphia, PA: Wolters Kluwer Health/Lippincott Williams & Wilkins; 2011.)

occurred more often in females. CL (55.3%) and CLP (50.7%) occurred more often on the left side. A total of 44 cleft patterns were diagnosed, including nine patterns seen in only one patient each.[57] CL can be unilateral (Fig. 19.19) or bilateral, and each side can be completely cleft or incompletely cleft. If the cleft is bilateral, the sides may be symmetric or asymmetric (Fig. 19.20).

Mulliken defined three subgroups of incomplete CL and placed them in a spectrum termed "lesser-form" CL, depending on how far above the vermillion border of the lip they extend.[58] "Minor-form" cleft extends equal to or greater than 3 mm above the normal Cupid's bow peak; "microform" cleft has a notch less than 3 mm above the normal side; and "mini-microform" clefts have a discontinuity in the vermillion border (Fig. 19.21).

In patients with bilateral CL, there is also a wide variation in presentation. Bilateral symmetric complete CL with an uplifted, protruding premaxillary segment, is the most common (Figs. 19.22 and 19.23; see also Fig. 19.20). Bilateral symmetric incomplete CL is less common. In this form, there may be notches in the tooth-bearing maxillary alveolus, and the secondary palate is intact. The least common form of bilateral CL is complete or incomplete on the more severe side, and incomplete or lesser form on the contralateral side.[59]

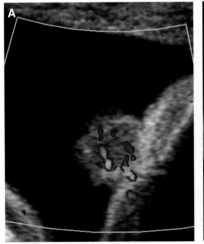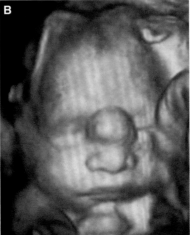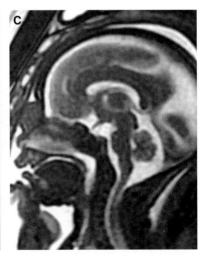

FIGURE 19.16: Nasal glioma. Fetal US **(A, B)** and MRI **(C)** at 28-week 5-day gestation showing vascular soft-tissue mass in the midline, above the bridge of the nose.

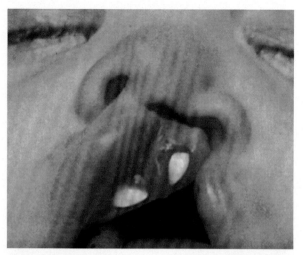

FIGURE 19.18: Unilateral cleft lip and palate. Infant at time of surgical repair showing unilateral cleft lip and palate with depression of nose on the side of cleft.

Median CLP occurs rarely, typically associated with other anomalies or syndromes such as holoprosencephaly (Fig. 19.24, See Fig. 19.9). Asymmetric or slash-like defects in the lip or palate should raise suspicion for amniotic band syndrome.

Imaging

Sonography: The ability to detect a CL is dependent on the technical resolution of the individual sonographic unit and on the knowledge and skill of the sonographer. In the early 1980s, the diagnosis was made by 2D US, which was supplemented by the additional capabilities of 3D technology in the late nineties, and 4D sonography in the decade following. 3D US technology, when optimal conditions are present (adequate amniotic fluid, favorable fetal position, and maternal habitus), is astonishingly detailed. The evolution of 4D US has allowed the evaluation of fetal behavior through the observation of fetal expressions. Using the intrinsic capability of 3D US, the imager can be certain when the rendered profile is midline, leading to increased accuracy and reproducibility of diagnoses such as micrognathia and midface hypoplasia (Fig. 19.25).[26]

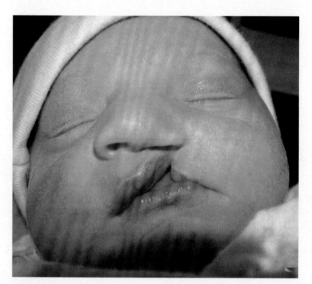

FIGURE 19.19: Incomplete cleft lip. Photograph of newborn with left unilateral incomplete cleft lip, intact alveolus, and secondary palate. Note the flattening and widening of the ipsilateral nostril and ala.

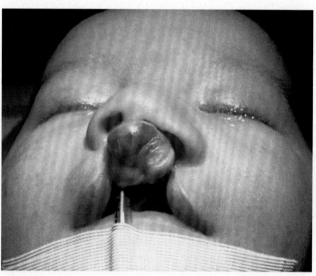

FIGURE 19.20: Bilateral cleft lip and palate with premaxillary protrusion. Photograph at time of surgical repair shows bilateral cleft lip and palate with prominent premaxillary protrusion.

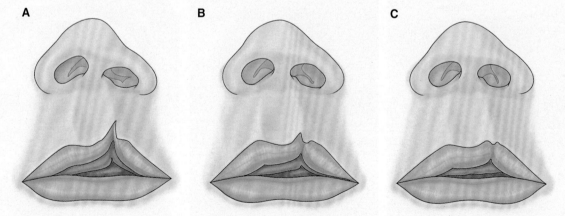

FIGURE 19.21: Lesser-form cleft lip. **A:** Minor-form cleft lip. **B:** Microform cleft lip. **C:** Mini-microform cleft lip. (Adapted with permission from Yuzuriha S, Mulliken JB. Minor-form, microform, and mini-microform cleft lip: anatomical features, operative techniques, and revisions. *Plast Reconstr Surg.* 2008;122(5):1485–1493.)

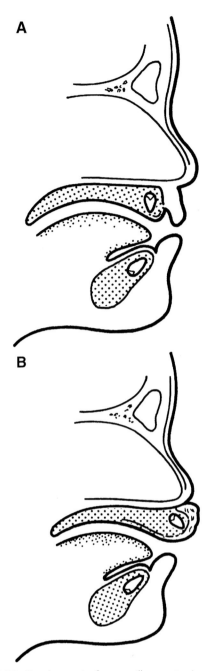

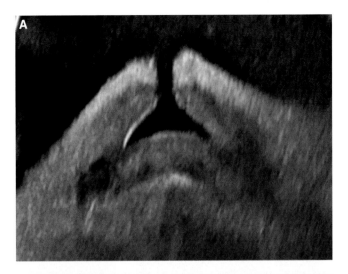

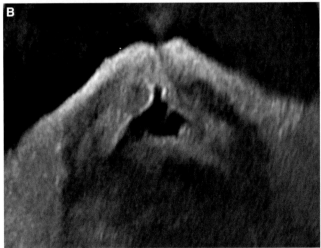

FIGURE 19.22: Development of premaxillary protrusion with bilateral cleft lip and palate. **A:** Normal sagittal view. **B:** Bilateral cleft lip and palate permits forward migration of the premaxillary segment.

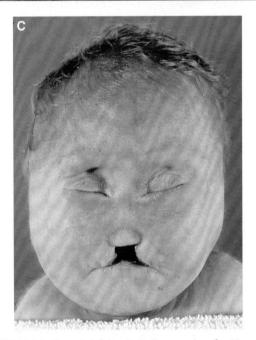

FIGURE 19.24: Central cleft lip. **A, B:** Sonography of a 28-week fetus with midline cleft lip. **C:** Postmortem photograph of a different infant with hypotelorism, holoprosencephaly, and a midline cleft lip and palate. (A, B images courtesy of Luis Goncalves MD, Director of Fetal Imaging, Phoenix Children's Hospital.)

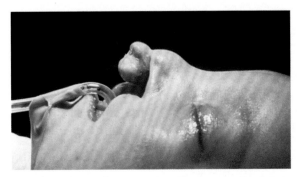

FIGURE 19.23: Premaxillary protrusion. Photograph of an infant with bilateral cleft lip and palate showing prominent premaxillary protrusion.

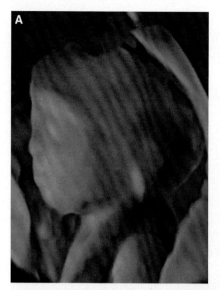
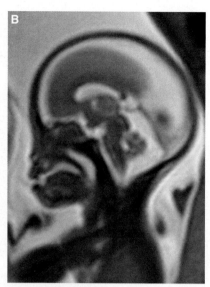
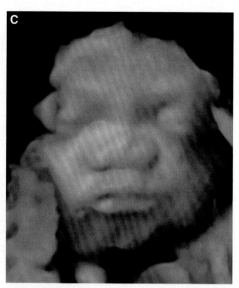

FIGURE 19.25: Midface hypoplasia. **A:** Sagittal 3D US of a 22-week fetus with midface hypoplasia. **B:** Sagittal MRI of a second 22-week fetus. **C:** 3D sonography of the second fetus at 30 weeks' gestation.

Although the major events in facial development have all occurred by 8 weeks' gestation, anomalies are difficult to see sonographically at that age. However, by the end of the first trimester, fortuitously corresponding to the ideal time point for first-trimester screening and measurement of the nuchal translucency, the fetal craniofacial structures are large enough to be evaluable in many patients.

In the first and second trimesters, evaluation by sonography involves both surface renderings and evaluation of deeper bony structures. Coronal and axial imaging are very helpful, and an axial view of the tooth-bearing aveolar ridge can determine whether a CP is present. Sonography is ideal for assessing the fetal lip and nose, and even subtle clefts of the lip can often be detected (Fig. 19.26). Although fetal MRI can be used for evaluation of the fetal lip, resolution of these tissues is better on US, especially in the second trimester. For evaluating the structures posterior to the lip, sonography may be exceptionally accurate for bone detail, if fetal position and amniotic fluid volume are favorable. Unilateral CLP is most common (Fig. 19.27). Bilateral CLP may be suggested by prominent echogenic soft tissue below the nose, representing the protuberant premaxillary segment (Fig. 19.28); sometimes, however, bilateral CLP is not associated with a protuberant premaxillary segment. Although there are secondary clues

to the presence of a CP on sonography, the secondary palate itself cannot easily or reliably be visualized (Table 19.5).

Clefts are more common in some populations than in others, and certain types of clefts are more common than others. Some specialized centers and practices have high rates of cleft detection on sonography, often using particular 2D- and 3D-enhanced views, which may not easily be transferable to screening practices.[60] A recent meta-analysis of cleft detection rate in 27 studies including both low- and high-risk populations showed rates of 9% to 100% for detection of CL without CP, 0% to 22% for CP only, and 0% to 73% for all clefts.[61]

Differing levels of expertise and use of a range of advanced and more basic or older US equipment likely led to this range of detection rates, but this variation may reflect the reality of contemporary screening. This study also pointed out that while 3D US did well in predicting CP in the presence of CL, 3D US is not reliable for the detection of isolated CP.

Most screening for CL and other anomalies takes place at centers relying on 2D sonography.[62–69] The routine use of 3D sonography for screening has not been validated, as it is time-consuming and not cost-effective. Analyzing 3D and 4D images as a primary screen often introduces artifacts that decrease the accuracy of cleft detection.[26,70–72]

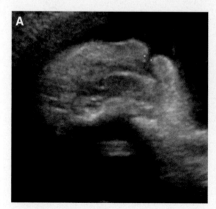
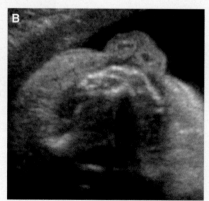
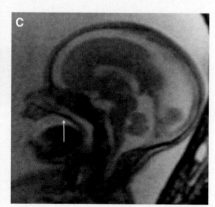

FIGURE 19.26: Microform cleft lip. A 26-week gestation fetus. **A:** Two-dimensional sonogram demonstrates a very small width cleft (*markers*) in the fetal lip. **B:** Intact maxillary alveolus. **C:** The secondary palate (*arrow*) was normal on MRI.

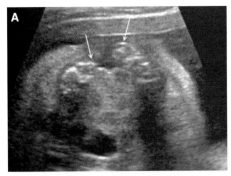
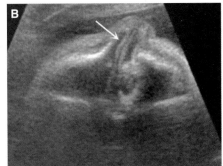
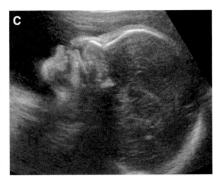

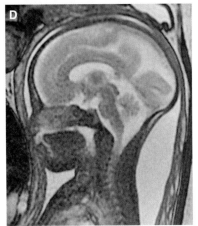
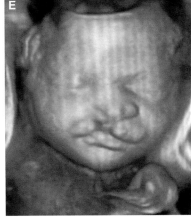

FIGURE 19.27: Unilateral complete cleft lip and palate. Fetus at 28 weeks' gestation. **A:** 2D sonogram showing interrupted axial view of alveolus (*arrows*). **B:** 2D sonogram showing deviation of the vomer (*arrow*) away from the cleft side. **C:** 2D sagittal sonogram showing midface hypoplasia and high tongue position *(T)*. **D:** Sagittal MRI of the same fetus showing absence of the secondary palate. **E:** 3D sonogram of a different fetus at 32-week 2-day showing left unilateral complete cleft lip and palate.

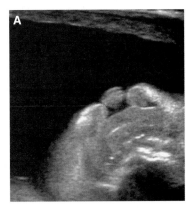
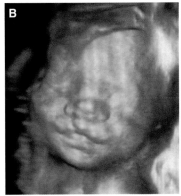

FIGURE 19.28: Bilateral incomplete cleft lip and intact palate. Two-dimensional **(A)** and three-dimensional **(B)** sonogram in a 22-week 5-day fetus with bilateral incomplete cleft lip and intact palate.

However, several authors have reported a higher sensitivity for facial clefts using various 3D sonographic techniques.[27,28,31,73–80] Even in the best of hands, the secondary palate cannot be well delineated on 2D or 3D sonography. In a study by Ramos et al.,[81] CP accuracy in the setting of CL ranged from 33% to 63%, and the specificity ranged from 84% to 95%. These authors concluded that their observed low sensitivity was mainly due to artifacts, shadowing, and suboptimal fetal position. In many studies, the sonographic detection rate for an isolated cleft secondary palate approaches 0%.[73,82]

Magnetic Resonance Imaging: Recent studies have confirmed the added value of fetal MRI to sonography in the detection of cleft secondary palate[83–97] in the setting of CL. Using T2 SSFSE and/or SSFP in the axial, coronal, and sagittal planes, excellent imaging of the lip and palate can be obtained. Although fetal MRI has limitations including excessive fetal motion and fetal crowding, the technique can usually detect deeper structures such as the

TABLE 19.5   Associated Signs of Cleft Palate in Presence of Cleft Lip on US and MRI

Axial/Coronal Views

Lips	Cleft
Nares	Flattened or deformed
Vomer	Deviated away from side of cleft; often midline if bilateral cleft lip and palate
Maxilla	Interrupted alveolus, wide gap
Orbits	Hypertelorism

Sagittal View

Profile	Midface retrusion
Position of tongue	High

MRI, magnetic resonance imaging; *US*, ultrasound.

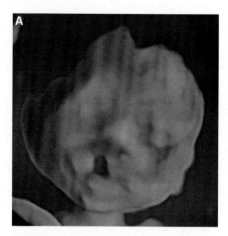
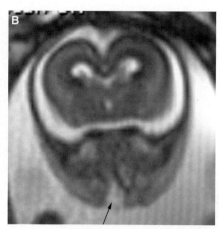
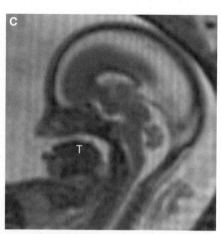

FIGURE 19.29: Unilateral complete cleft lip and palate. Three-dimensional ultrasound **(A)**, coronal **(B)**, and sagittal **(C)** fetal MRI in a 20-week fetus with unilateral complete right cleft lip and palate (*arrow*). *T*, tongue.

tooth-bearing alveolus, which is part of the primary palate; areas anterior to the incisive foramen; and anomalies of the secondary hard or soft palate, posterior to the incisive foramen (Figs. 19.29 and 19.30). In a series of 49 fetuses between 24 and 37 weeks' gestation with either a family history of cleft secondary palate or a facial cleft seen on screening sonography, the positive predictive value (PPV) of fetal MRI for the detection of cleft secondary palate was 96%, and the negative predictive value (NPV) was 80%.[87] Although isolated cleft secondary palate is often seen in the setting of other anomalies, such as micrognathia, fetal MRI may currently be the only way to accurately detect fetal cleft secondary palate when CL is not present (Fig. 19.31).

Numerous studies have all shown that additional information about fetal facial clefts can be obtained by fetal MRI. Manganaro et al.[90] studied 27 fetuses at a mean gestational age of 24 weeks. Descamps et al.[87] studied 49 fetuses between 24 and 37 weeks and found a PPV for palatal involvement of 96% and an NPV of 80% and noted that accuracy increased with experience during the study. A third study by Mailath-Pokorny et al.[89] in 34 Austrian women between 24 and 27 weeks' gestation also showed an advantage of MRI for evaluation of the fetal secondary palate.

Detection Rates: Detection rates vary depending on the type of cleft, and certain cleft types have more associated anomalies than do other cleft types. In a large series by Paterson et al.[98] in Scotland in 2010, isolated CL occurred in 20%; CL with cleft

alveolus was seen in 6%; CL, cleft alveolus, and CP were seen in 75%; and isolated CP was seen in 1%. In this series, detection rate was low overall (15%), but did improve over the 10 years of the study.

A large prospective series from Norway covering the period from 1987 to 2004 detected 101 facial clefts in fetuses or newborns in a population of 49,314 (incidence 1 in 500 to 1 in 1,000).[82] Isolated CL was detected prenatally in 4.5%, CLP in 43%, and CP alone in 0%. Associated anomalies were seen in 43% who had CLP and in 58% who had CP only. Twelve percent had chromosomal anomalies; 18% were part of a syndrome or sequence.

Another recent large series from Ireland studied 851 cases of facial clefts over 25 years from 1984 to 2008 in over 500,000 births.[99] In all, 483 (51%) had CLP; 413 (48.5%) had CP. This population differed somewhat from the other European populations in that mothers were older, abortions were less frequent, and the birth rate was high. The prevalence of all types of facial clefts was 16 per 10,000 births in this population over 25 years, which is similar to other studies.

In a study by Johnson et al.[100] in 2009, the frequencies for accurate prenatal diagnosis for CLP were as follows: CLP, 33.3%; CL only, 20.3%, and CP only, 0.3%, concluding that a prenatal diagnosis was made in only one-fifth of live-born infants with orofacial clefts. In this study, other factors were also at play, including the observation that higher income mothers were much more likely

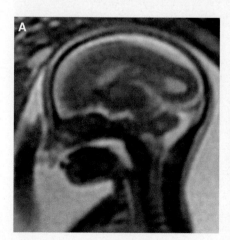
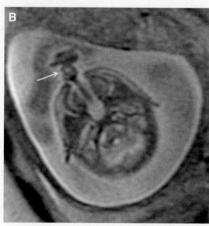

FIGURE 19.30: Bilateral complete cleft lip and palate. Sagittal **(A)** and axial **(B)** fetal MRI at 21 weeks' gestation showing absence of the secondary palate and two tooth buds (*arrow*) within the intermaxillary protrusion.

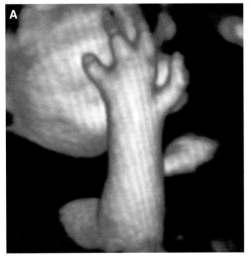
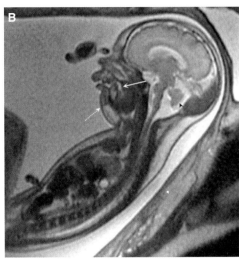

FIGURE 19.31: Cleft palate and micrognathia. Fetal images at 33 weeks' gestation. **A:** Three-dimensional fetal sonogram showing cleft hand and oligodactyly. **B:** Sagittal MRI showing micrognathia (*dotted arrow*) and cleft secondary palate (*arrow*). There is inferior vermian hypogenesis (*arrowhead*). The fetus also had congenital diaphragmatic hernia (not shown) and Robin sequence.

to receive a prenatal diagnosis than mothers with lower incomes. Other studies showed higher detection rates for clefts when they were accompanied by multiple other fetal malformations.

Associated Anomalies: Anomalies are present in 3% to 7% of all live births. Seventy-five percent of these involve the head, face, or neck. In a recent series of patients with CP alone or CLP,[2] 20% to 25% of associated malformations were also in the face, including:

- Nasal anomalies: bifid nose, frontonasal dysplasia, hypoplastic malar eminence, median cleft nose, and choanal atresia
- Ear anomalies: bifid ear lobe, ear pits, Mondini malformation, preauricular sinus or fistula, preauricular skin tags, or cysts
- Eye malformations: anterior segment dysgenesis, coloboma, congenital cataract, congenital eyelid fistula, hypertelorism, microphthalmia, and lacrimal duct atresia

A recent study in Minnesota found that congenital malformations are more frequently seen in CP without CL (38.7%) than in CLP (26.4%). Of the associated anomalies, 63.1% were chromosomal or syndromic, and 36.9% were nonchromosomal/syndromic.[2]

Although imagers, obstetricians, parents, and craniofacial surgeons all acknowledge that accurate detection of craniofacial anomalies is important so that prospective parents may be accurately counseled, there is no consensus about best imaging practices. A recent review of prenatal diagnosis and assessment of facial clefts by To[32] summarizes the current state of imaging and counseling, including the uses of sonography and MRI. This review discusses the increasing accuracy of CL detection because of new technology, accumulated expertise, and raised expectations for imagers. To, in his study, points out that in a prospective screening study in Norway between 1987 and 2004, the rate of detection of craniofacial clefts increased significantly from 34% in the first 8 years to 58% in the next 8 years.[82] Most cases (69%) were detected on routine US screening in the second trimester. In this study, associated anomalies were observed either before or after birth in 43% of infants with CLP and in 58% of those with isolated CP. Of those patients with associated anomalies, 12% had chromosomal aberrations, and 18% were part of a syndrome or sequence.[32]

Syndromic Associated Anomalies: There are more than 300 syndromes associated with orofacial clefts, affecting approximately 10% of all cases (Fig. 19.32).[56] Certain genetic loci are more frequently involved, including chromosomes 2p, 4p, 6p, 17q, 19q, and 22q. Some clefts are X-linked, autosomal dominant, or autosomal recessive. Syndromes associated with CL/P include Robin, Van der Woude, trisomy 21, Treacher Collins, Apert, Marfan, Turner, cleidocranial dysostosis, CATCH 22, velocardiofacial syndrome, frontonasal dysplasia, and 4p minus syndrome.[101]

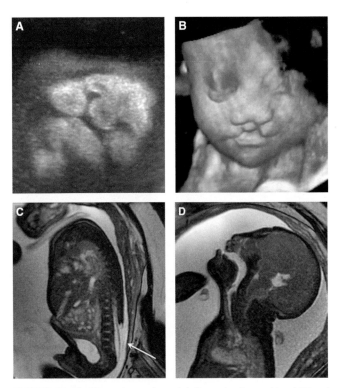

FIGURE 19.32: Bilateral complete cleft lip and palate, with additional anomalies. **A:** A 33-week fetal two-dimensional sonogram shows bilateral cleft lip. **B:** Three-dimensional sonogram of bilateral cleft lip. **C:** Sagittal fetal MRI showing associated open neural tube defect (*arrow*). **D:** Sagittal fetal MRI showing severe midface retrusion and cleft secondary palate.

Nonsyndromic Associated Anomalies: Nonsyndromic clefts may be secondary to genetic factors, such as a family history of CL; environmental factors such as smoking; exposure to certain drugs, such as retinoic acid and antiepileptic drugs; or lack of other factors such as folate.

Differential Diagnosis: It is possible for normal fetal facial structures, such as the philtrum, to simulate a CL. The umbilical cord overlying the lip could mimic a cleft. Amniotic bands, Tessier clefts, intracranial tumors, lip masses such as hemangiomas, or nasal masses could mimic a cleft.

Prognosis/Classification: There are more than 40 classification systems for CLP[102,103] (Table 19.6), and flowcharts are available for further definition (Fig. 19.33). In 1931, Veau[104] presented a widely accepted system for classifying oral clefts, consisting of four subtypes (Table 19.7 and Fig. 19.34).

Veau I: Cleft of the posterior soft palate
Veau II: Clefts of the soft and hard palate, posterior to the incisive foramen
Veau III: Complete unilateral CLP
Veau IV: Complete bilateral CLP

In 1971, Kernahan[105] improved upon existing earlier classification systems purely based on anatomy and suggested a pictorial representation using a "striped Y" diagram representing the lip, palate, and maxillary alveolus (Fig. 19.35). Kriens developed this classification system further using a right-to-left palindromic labeling system called **LAHSHAL** (*l*ip, *a*lveolus, *h*ard palate, *s*oft palate, *h*ard palate, *a*lveolus, *l*ip), which begins on the patient's right and moves to the left. This system, while complex, is excellent for accurate description in the hands of craniofacial surgeons and has been fairly widely adopted in international circles and by the large NIDCR-funded studies.[106] In 1976, Tessier[107] published a classification system for unusual facial clefts that do not easily fit into other categories and often involve complex clefts that extend from mouth to facial structures above the nose, such as the eyes

TABLE 19.6	Classification of Cleft Lip and Palate: Definitions
Cleft, lip/palate	Cleft of primary palate (anterior to incisive foramen) and secondary palate (posterior to incisive foramen)
Cleft lip and/or alveolus	Cleft of primary palate only (lip and/or alveolus) and intact secondary palate
Cleft palate	Cleft of secondary palate only (posterior to incisive foramen)
Atypical cleft	Examples include median, oblique, transverse/lateral clefts
Incomplete cleft lip	Labial cleft does not extend through nasal floor. Also with or without "notch" in alveolus, which does not extend through entire alveolus
Complete cleft lip/alveolus	Cleft involves entire lip and entire alveolus. No tissue connection between alar base, medial labial elements, or premaxilla
Tissue band	Small bridge of tissue between the two sides of complete cleft lip/alveolus, which has a vertical height of less than 5 mm
Microform	Tiny labial cleft or vertical notch

and forehead. Tessier clefts involve both superficial facial soft tissues and deeper bony structures (Figs. 19.36 and 19.37).

Following the guidance of our craniofacial surgeons, we use a combination of the modified Kernahan Y drawing, the Veau

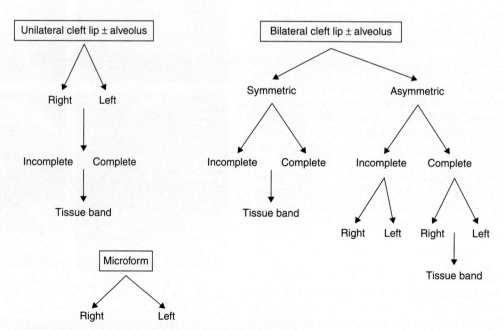

FIGURE 19.33: Flowchart for classification of cleft lip and alveolus.

TABLE 19.7	Cleft Palate: Veau Classification and Corresponding Modified Kernahan Y drawing	

VEAU CLASSIFICATION SHOWN IN FIGURE 19.34	DESCRIPTION AND CORRESPONDING Y DRAWING POSITION NUMBERS LABELED IN FIGURE 19.35
Type I	Cleft of the soft palate (#11)
Type II	Complete cleft secondary palate with both soft and hard palate involvement (#9–11)
Type III Greater segment = side opposite cleft Lesser segment = same side of cleft	Unilateral complete cleft lip and palate (right-sided cleft: #1–4 and #9–11; left-sided cleft: #5–8 and #9–11)
Type IV	Bilateral complete cleft lip and palate (#1–11)
Submucous cleft Location: Hard palate, soft palate	Cleft palate covered by mucosa. Features include bifid uvula, palatal muscle diastasis, midline blue mucosal lining, and notch in posterior hard palate

Modified by Mulliken, JB, data from Marrinan EM, LaBrie RA, Mulliken JB. Velopharyngeal function in nonsyndromic cleft palate: relevance of surgical technique, age at repair, and cleft type. *Cleft Palate Craniofac J.* 1998;35(2):95–100.

classification, and the Tessier system in classifying craniofacial clefts, with the goal of imager and surgeon understanding each other as accurately as possible and then presenting a precise description and prognosis for the anomaly to the prospective parents. Studies have shown that prepared parents deal more easily with the appearance of their newborn's face and with the subsequent series of surgeries predictably in store for the infant and child than those parents who discover the anomaly at birth.[21,24]

We have found the strength of the modified Kernahan Y classification to be the clarity of anatomic demarcation between the primary and the secondary palates by allowing the imager to comprehend the exact location and importance of the incisive foramen. The dividing point between the primary and the secondary palates, the incisive foramen, is represented symbolically at the junction of the limbs of the Y by a small circle, the incisive foramen (Fig. 19.35c). Anterior to the incisive foramen are the three distinct tissues of the primary palate: the lip, the bony tooth-bearing alveolus, and the area of the hard palate extending from the alveolus posteriorly to the incisive foramen. Posterior to the incisive foramen are the three segments of the secondary palate: two sections of hard palate posterior to the incisive foramen and the palatal shelves, and the most posterior tissues composing the entire soft palate ending in the uvula. The importance of understanding clefting of the primary and secondary palates cannot be overstated. If the secondary palate is cleft, the child will have significant issues with hearing and speech; if the secondary palate is *not* cleft, these serious problems do not occur.[23]

Understanding palatal embryology allows the imager to understand the common forms of both unilateral and bilateral CLP. Bilateral facial clefts may be suggested by the visualization of an anterior projection of the intermaxillary segment in combination with the nose, forming a mass that projects anteriorly and superiorly above the normal level of the lip, following embryological lines of fusion (see Figs. 19.28, 19.30, and 19.32). In bilateral facial clefts, the tooth-bearing maxillary alveolus is cleft between the lateral incisors and the canine teeth. This fact explains why there are often two tooth buds in the intermaxillary segment in complete bilateral CL.

Isolated cleft secondary palate without an associated CL is very difficult to detect on fetal sonography, but is readily detected on best-technique fetal MRI. Thin slices and cinegraphic imaging has increased CP detection. Most cases of isolated CP involve the secondary soft palate, but not the hard portions of the primary palate, Veau type II. There is a strong association of isolated cleft secondary palate with micrognathia and the Robin sequence (see Fig. 19.31). Indirect imaging features of isolated cleft secondary palate may include a small or nonvisualized fetal stomach and polyhydramnios, because of the fetus's difficulty in swallowing normally.

Management/Treatment: Infants with a cleft of the secondary palate, particularly those with Robin sequence, may have respiratory distress at birth; therefore, the airway must be secured. All infants with CLP will need assistance in feeding because they cannot generate adequate pressure during sucking and

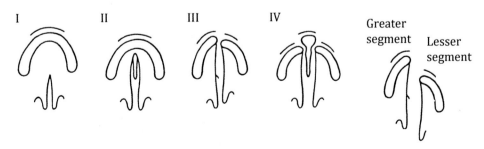

FIGURE 19.34: Veau classification of cleft palate. *I,* cleft soft palate; *II,* complete cleft secondary palate; *III,* unilateral complete cleft lip/palate; *IV,* bilateral cleft lip/palate. (Modified by Mulliken JB, data from Marrinan EM, LaBrie RA, Mulliken JB. Velopharyngeal function in nonsyndromic cleft palate: relevance of surgical technique, age at repair, and cleft type. *Cleft Palate Craniofac J.* 1998;35(2):95–100.)

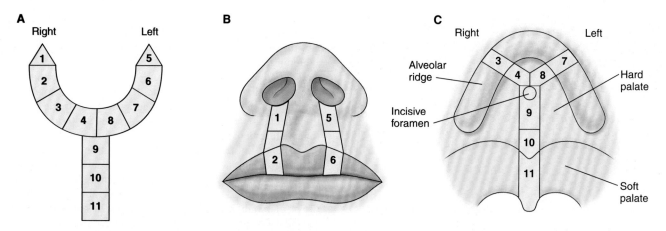

FIGURE 19.35: A–C: Modified Kernahan Y drawing. Algorithm for comprehensive characterization of cleft lip and palate. (Modified by Mulliken JB, reprinted with permission from Kernahan DA. The striped Y—a symbolic classification for cleft lip and palate. *Plast Reconstr Surg.* 1971;47(5):469–470.)

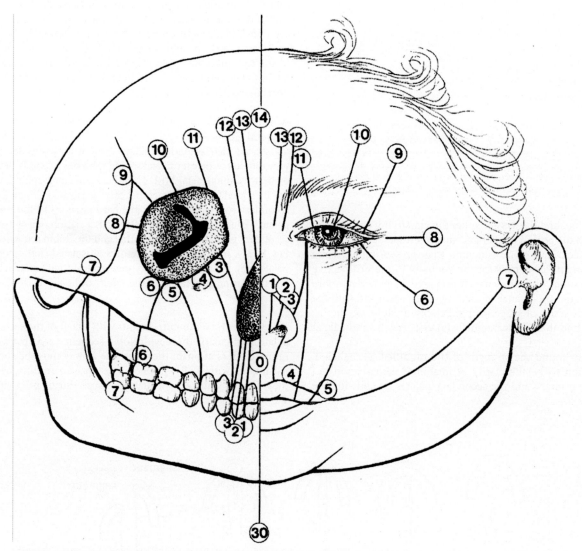

FIGURE 19.36: Classification of Tessier clefts. The left half (*right side of face*) depicts the various clefts relative to the skeletal landmarks, and the right half (*left side of face*) outlines the locations based on soft-tissue landmarks. Facial clefts = number 0 through number 7, and cranial clefts = number 8 through number 14. Mandibular midline facial cleft number 30 is also seen. (Reprinted with permission from Kawamoto H Jr, Bradley JP. Craniofacial clefts and hypertelorbitism. In: Thorne CH, Bartlett SP, Beasley RW, et al. *Grabb and Smith's Plastic Surgery.* 6th ed. Philadelphia, PA: Lippincott Williams & Wilkins; 2006.)

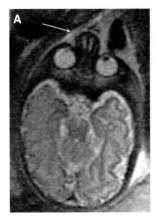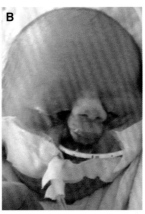

FIGURE 19.37: Tessier cleft. **A:** Fetal MRI at 35 weeks shows hypotelorism and an unusual configuration of the nose (*arrow*). **B:** Newborn photograph showing bilateral deep clefts of soft tissue and bone extending from the mouth to the eyes.

swallowing. Those with CP risk aspiration of liquids unless specialized nipples and bottle are used.[108] Unilateral CL is usually repaired in the first year of life. Dentofacial orthodontic appliances are often used before definitive surgery to bring the cleft segments closer together. The goal of all types of cleft surgery is nasolabial symmetry and repair of alveolar and palate deficiency. 3D photography is often used by the surgeon. CP repair is usually performed between 12 and 18 months of age, with the goal of attaining normal speech, hearing, dental occlusion, and facial and palatal growth. Staged repairs are then performed as needed in childhood and adolescence until skeletal maturity is

reached. The psychosocial journey can be difficult for both the child and the parents.

TONGUE

Fetal tongue evaluation is subjective, though tables exist for the normal size of the tongue between 14 and 26 weeks.[109] The fetal tongue is often well seen on sonography when fetal position is optimal and amniotic fluid is adequate (see Fig. 19.3B). It can also be seen on fetal MRI in all three planes and during real-time cine-mode imaging, especially if the fetus swallows during imaging (see Fig. 19.6A).[110]

Macroglossia

Incidence: There is a known association with trisomy 21, Beckwith–Wiedemann syndrome (BWS), and hypothyroidism. Adding up the incidences of trisomy 21, BWS, and hypothyroidism and the 1% of individuals with each of these conditions who have macroglossia, overall incidence is approximately 1 in 11,000 to 1 in 25,000 live births.[110]

Etiology/Management: Macroglossia may be congenital or acquired. Abnormal enlargement of the tongue may be because of overgrowth, as in BWS or Down syndrome, or due to the presence of benign or malignant tumors.[108] Masses known to involve the tongue include lymphatic malformations (Fig. 19.38), teratomas, and foregut duplication cysts (Fig. 19.39). An enlarged tongue may cause airway obstruction and prevent normal swallowing. Portions of the tongue can be surgically removed (glossectomy) to make the tongue fit properly into the closed oral cavity.

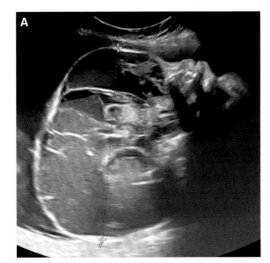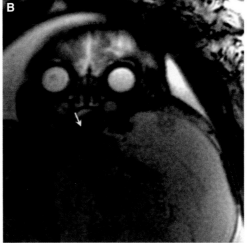

FIGURE 19.38: Lymphatic malformation invading tongue base. Third-trimester 34-week fetal sonograms **(A)** and MRI **(B)**, prior to EXIT delivery, showing very large, multiseptated fluid-filled mass (*markers*) that invades the face and tongue (*arrow*).

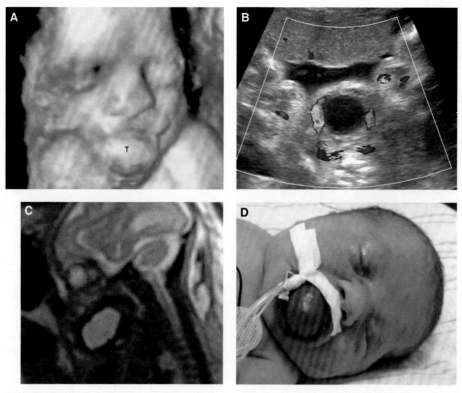

FIGURE 19.39: Macroglossia secondary to foregut duplication cyst of the tongue. **A:** Three-dimensional fetal sonogram at 28-week 5-day gestation showing macroglossia *(T)*. **B:** Color Doppler sonogram showing no flow in the cystic tongue mass. **C:** Sagittal fetal MRI of cystic tongue mass. **D:** Photograph of the newborn in the delivery room. After complete surgical resection, the pathological diagnosis was a gastrointestinal (GI) duplication cyst.

REFERENCES

1. Shaw W. Global strategies to reduce the health care burden of craniofacial anomalies: report of WHO meetings on international collaborative research on craniofacial anomalies. *Cleft Palate Craniofac J.* 2004;41:238–243.
2. Beriaghi S, Myers SL, Jensen SA, et al. Cleft lip and palate: association with other congenital malformations. *J Clin Pediatr Dent.* 2009;33:207–210.
3. Suri M. Craniofacial syndromes. *Semin Fetal Neonatal Med.* 2005;10:243–257.
4. Seeds JW. The routine or screening obstetrical ultrasound examination. *Clin Obstet Gynecol.* 1996;39:814–830.
5. Benacerraf BR, Frigoletto FD Jr, Bieber FR. The fetal face: ultrasound examination. *Radiology.* 1984;153:495–497.
6. Shaikh D, Mercer NS, Sohan K, et al. Prenatal diagnosis of cleft lip and palate. *Br J Plast Surg.* 2001;54:288–289.
7. Russell KA, Allen VM, MacDonald ME, et al. A population-based evaluation of antenatal diagnosis of orofacial clefts. *Cleft Palate Craniofac J.* 2008;45:148–153.
8. Vial Y, Tran C, Addor MC, et al. Screening for foetal malformations: performance of routine ultrasonography in the population of the Swiss Canton of Vaud. *Swiss Med Wkly.* 2001;131:490–494.
9. Fleurke-Rozema JH, van de Kamp K, Bakker MK, et al. Prevalence, diagnosis and outcome of cleft lip with or without cleft palate in The Netherlands. *Ultrasound Obstet Gynecol.* 2016;48(4):458–463.
10. Levaillant JM, Nicot R, Benouaiche L, et al. Prenatal diagnosis of cleft lip/palate: the surface rendered oro-palatal (SROP) view of the fetal lips and palate, a tool to improve information-sharing within the orofacial team and with the parents. *J Craniomaxillofac Surg.* 2016;44(7):835–842.
11. AIUM-ACR-ACOG-SMFM-SRU practice parameter for the performance of standard diagnostic obstetric ultrasound examinations. *J Ultrasound Med.* 2018;37(11):E13–E24.
12. Babcook CJ, McGahan JP, Chong BW, et al. Evaluation of fetal midface anatomy related to facial clefts: use of US. *Radiology.* 1996;201:113–118.
13. Rotten D, Levaillant JM. Prenatal diagnosis of facial clefts. In: Losee JE, Kirschner RE, eds. *Comprehensive Cleft Care.* New York, NY: McGraw-Hill Professional; 2008:44–70.
14. Gillham JC, Anand S, Bullen PJ. Antenatal detection of cleft lip with or without cleft palate: incidence of associated chromosomal and structural anomalies. *Ultrasound Obstet Gynecol.* 2009;34:410–415.
15. Tonni G, Grisolia G, Sepulveda W. Early prenatal diagnosis of orofacial clefts: evaluation of the retronasal triangle using a new three-dimensional reslicing technique. *Fetal Diagn Ther.* 2013;34:31–37.
16. Sepulveda W, Wong AE, Martinez-Ten P, et al. Retronasal triangle: a sonographic landmark for the screening of cleft palate in the first trimester. *Ultrasound Obstet Gynecol.* 2010;35:7–13.
17. Sepulveda W, Cafici D, Bartholomew J, et al. First-trimester assessment of the fetal palate: a novel application of the volume NT algorithm. *J Ultrasound Med.* 2012;31:1443–1448.
18. Martinez-Ten P, Adiego B, Illescas T, et al. First-trimester diagnosis of cleft lip and palate using three-dimensional ultrasound. *Ultrasound Obstet Gynecol.* 2012;40:40–46.
19. Timmerman E, Pajkrt E, Maas SM, et al. Enlarged nuchal translucency in chromosomally normal fetuses: strong association with orofacial clefts. *Ultrasound Obstet Gynecol.* 2010;36:427–432.
20. Rodriguez ED, Neligan PC, Losee JE. *Plastic Surgery: Craniofacial, Head and Neck Surgery and Pediatric Plastic Surgery.* Philadelphia, PA: Elsevier Saunders; 2012.
21. Mulliken JB. The changing faces of children with cleft lip and palate. *N Engl J Med.* 2004;351:745–747.
22. Mulliken JB. Microform cleft lip. In: Losee JE, Kirschner RE, eds. *Comprehensive Cleft Care.* New York, NY: McGraw-Hill Professional; 2008:273–283.
23. Mulliken JB, Benacerraf BR. Prenatal diagnosis of cleft lip: what the sonologist needs to tell the surgeon. *J Ultrasound Med.* 2001;20:1159–1164.
24. Costello BJ, Edwards SP, Clemens M. Fetal diagnosis and treatment of craniomaxillofacial anomalies. *J Oral Maxillofac Surg.* 2008;66:1985–1995.
25. Rotten D, Levaillant JM. Two- and three-dimensional sonographic assessment of the fetal face, 1: a systematic analysis of the normal face. *Ultrasound Obstet Gynecol.* 2004;23:224–231.
26. Kurjak A, Azumendi G, Andonotopo W, et al. Three- and four-dimensional ultrasonography for the structural and functional evaluation of the fetal face. *Am J Obstet Gynecol.* 2007;196:16–28.
27. Goncalves LF. Three-dimensional ultrasound of the fetus: how does it help? *Pediatr Radiol.* 2016;46(2):177–189.
28. Campbell S, Lees C, Moscoso G, et al. Ultrasound antenatal diagnosis of cleft palate by a new technique: the 3D "reverse face" view. *Ultrasound Obstet Gynecol.* 2005;25:12–18.
29. Platt LD, Devore GR, Pretorius DH. Improving cleft palate/cleft lip antenatal diagnosis by 3-dimensional sonography: the "flipped face" view. *J Ultrasound Med.* 2006;25:1423–1430.
30. Pilu G, Segata M. A novel technique for visualization of the normal and cleft fetal secondary palate: angled insonation and three-dimensional ultrasound. *Ultrasound Obstet Gynecol.* 2007;29:166–169.

31. Martinez-Ten P, Perez Pedregosa J, Santacruz B, et al. Three-dimensional ultrasound diagnosis of cleft palate: "reverse face", "flipped face" or "oblique face"—which method is best? *Ultrasound Obstet Gynecol.* 2009;33:399–406.

32. To WW. Prenatal diagnosis and assessment of facial clefts: where are we now? *Hong Kong Med J.* 2012;18:146–152.

33. Arangio P, Manganaro L, Pacifici A, et al. Importance of fetal MRI in evaluation of craniofacial deformities. *J Craniofac Surg.* 2013;24(3):773–776.

34. Bernardo S, Giancotti A, Antonelli A, et al. MRI and US in the evaluation of fetal anomalies: the need to work together. *Prenat Diagn.* 2017;37(13):1343–1349.

35. Nagarajan M, Sharbidre KG, Bhabad SH, et al. MR Imaging of the fetal face: comprehensive review. *Radiographics.* 2018;38(3):962–980.

36. Zugazaga Cortazar A, Martín Martínez C. Usefulness of magnetic resonance imaging in the prenatal study of malformations of the face and neck. *Radiologia.* 2012;54(5):387–400.

37. Ulm MR, Chalubinski K, Ulm C, et al. Sonographic depiction of fetal tooth germs. *Prenat Diagn.* 1995;15:368–372.

38. Guis F, Ville Y, Vincent Y, et al. Ultrasound evaluation of the length of the fetal nasal bones throughout gestation. *Ultrasound Obstet Gynecol.* 1995;5:304–307.

39. Pinette MG, Blackstone J, Pan Y, et al. Measurement of fetal nasal width by ultrasonography. *Am J Obstet Gynecol.* 1997;177:842–845.

40. Sonek JD, Cicero S, Neiger R, et al. Nasal bone assessment in prenatal screening for trisomy 21. *Am J Obstet Gynecol.* 2006;195:1219–1230.

41. Morain S, Greene MF, Mello MM. A new era in noninvasive prenatal testing. *N Engl J Med.* 2013;369:499–501.

42. Chitty LS, Campbell S, Altman DG. Measurement of the fetal mandible—feasibility and construction of a centile chart. *Prenat Diagn.* 1993;13:749–756.

43. Goldstein I, Tamir A, Zimmer EZ, et al. Growth of the fetal orbit and lens in normal pregnancies. *Ultrasound Obstet Gynecol.* 1998;12:175–179.

44. Robinson AJ, Blaser S, Toi A, et al. MRI of the fetal eyes: morphologic and biometric assessment for abnormal development with ultrasonographic and clinicopathologic correlation. *Pediatr Radiol.* 2008;38:971–981.

45. De Meyer W, Zeman W, Palmer CG. The face predicts the brain: diagnostic significance of median facial anomalies for holoprosencephaly (arhinencephaly). *Pediatrics.* 1964;34:256–263.

46. Bundy AL, Lidov H, Soliman M, et al. Antenatal sonographic diagnosis of cebocephaly. *J Ultrasound Med.* 1988;7:395–398.

47. Rolland M, Sarramon MF, Bloom MC. Astomia-agnathia-holoprosencephaly association: prenatal diagnosis of a new case. *Prenat Diagn.* 1991;11:199–203.

48. Greene MF, Benacerraf BR, Frigoletto FD Jr. Reliable criteria for the prenatal sonographic diagnosis of alobar holoprosencephaly. *Am J Obstet Gynecol.* 1987;156:687–689.

49. McGahan JP, Nyberg DA, Mack LA. Sonography of facial features of alobar and semilobar holoprosencephaly. *AJR Am J Roentgenol.* 1990;154:143–148.

50. Kousa YA, du Plessis AJ, Vezina G. Prenatal diagnosis of holoprosencephaly. *Am J Med Genet C Semin Med Genet.* 2018;178(2):206–213.

51. Măluțan AM, Dudea M, Ciortea R,, et al. Cyclopia and proboscis—the extreme end of holoprosencephaly. *Rom J Morphol Embryol.* 2017;58(4):1555–1559.

52. Albernaz VS, Castillo M, Mukherji SK, et al. Congenital arhinia. *AJNR Am J Neuroradiol.* 1996;17:1312–1314.

53. Tewfik TL, Der Kaloustian VM. *Congenital Anomalies of the Ear, Nose, and Throat.* New York, NY: Oxford University Press; 1997.

54. U.S. National Library of Medicine. Frontonasal dysplasia. Genetics Home Reference [Internet]. October 15, 2019; Cystic fibrosis [reviewed April 2014; cited October 18, 2019]. Bethesda, MD: U.S. National Library of Medicine. https://ghr.nlm.nih.gov/condition/frontonasal-dysplasia.

55. Cash C, Set P, Coleman N. The accuracy of antenatal ultrasound in the detection of facial clefts in a low-risk screening population. *Ultrasound Obstet Gynecol.* 2001;18:432–436.

56. Wantia N, Rettinger G. The current understanding of cleft lip malformations. *Facial Plast Surg.* 2002;18:147–153.

57. Nagase Y, Natsume N, Kato T, et al. Epidemiological analysis of cleft lip and/or palate by cleft pattern. *J Maxillofac Oral Surg.* 2010;9:389–395.

58. Yuzuriha S, Mulliken JB. Minor-form, microform, and mini-microform cleft lip: anatomical features, operative techniques, and revisions. *Plast Reconstr Surg.* 2008;122:1485–1493.

59. Yuzuriha S, Oh AK, Mulliken JB. Asymmetrical bilateral cleft lip: complete or incomplete and contralateral lesser defect (minor-form, microform, or mini-microform). *Plast Reconstr Surg.* 2008;122:1494–1504.

60. Demircioglu M, Kangesu L, Ismail A, et al. Increasing accuracy of antenatal ultrasound diagnosis of cleft lip with or without cleft palate, in cases referred to the North Thames London Region. *Ultrasound Obstet Gynecol.* 2008;31:647–651.

61. Maarse W, Bergé SJ, Pistorius L, et al. Diagnostic accuracy of transabdominal ultrasound in detecting prenatal cleft lip and palate: a systematic review. *Ultrasound Obstet Gynecol.* 2010;35:495–502.

62. Abramson ZR, Peacock ZS, Cohen HL, et al. Radiology of cleft lip and palate: imaging for the prenatal period and throughout life. *Radiographics.* 2015;35(7):2053–2063.

63. Dochez V, Corre P, Riteau AS, et al. Correlation between antenatal ultrasound and postnatal diagnosis in cleft lip or palate: a retrospective study of 44 cases. *Gynecol Obstet Fertil.* 2015;43(12):767–772.

64. Hanny KH, de Vries IA, Haverkamp SJ, et al. Late detection of cleft palate. *Eur J Pediatr.* 2016;175(1):71–80.

65. James JN, Schlieder DW. Prenatal counseling, ultrasound diagnosis, and the role of maternal-fetal medicine of the cleft lip and palate patient. *Oral Maxillofac Surg Clin North Am.* 2016;28(2):145–151.

66. Johnson MM. Prenatal imaging for cleft lip and palate. *Radiol Technol.* 2019;90(6):581–596.

67. Mak ASL, Leung KY. Prenatal ultrasonography of craniofacial abnormalities. *Ultrasonography.* 2019;38(1):13–24.

68. Ozturk S, Karagoz H, Zor F, et al. Fetal cleft lip/palate surgery: end of a dream? *Fetal Pediatr Pathol.* 2016;35(4):277–281.

69. Wirtz N, Sidman J, Block W. Clefting of the alveolus: emphasizing the distinction from cleft palate. *Am J Perinatol.* 2016;33(6):531–534.

70. Leung KY, Ngai CS, Tang MH. Facial cleft or shadowing artifact? *Ultrasound Obstet Gynecol.* 2006;27:231–232.

71. Timor-Tritsch IE, Platt LD. Three-dimensional ultrasound experience in obstetrics. *Curr Opin Obstet Gynecol.* 2002;14:569–575.

72. Zajicek M, Achiron R, Weisz B, et al. Sonographic assessment of fetal secondary palate between 12 and 16 weeks of gestation using three-dimensional ultrasound. *Prenat Diagn.* 2013;33:1256–1259.

73. Baumler M, Faure JM, Bigorre M, et al. Accuracy of prenatal three-dimensional ultrasound in the diagnosis of cleft hard palate when cleft lip is present. *Ultrasound Obstet Gynecol.* 2011;38:440–444.

74. Campbell S. Prenatal ultrasound examination of the secondary palate. *Ultrasound Obstet Gynecol.* 2007;29:124–127.

75. Chmait R, Pretorius D, Jones M, et al. Prenatal evaluation of facial clefts with two-dimensional and adjunctive three-dimensional ultrasonography: a prospective trial. *Am J Obstet Gynecol.* 2002;187:946–949.

76. Faure JM, Baumler M, Boulot P, et al. Prenatal assessment of the normal fetal soft palate by three-dimensional ultrasound examination: is there an objective technique? *Ultrasound Obstet Gynecol.* 2008;31:652–656.

77. Faure JM, Captier G, Baumler M, et al. Sonographic assessment of normal fetal palate using three-dimensional imaging: a new technique. *Ultrasound Obstet Gynecol.* 2007;29:159–165.

78. McGahan MC, Ramos GA, Landry C, et al. Multislice display of the fetal face using 3-dimensional ultrasonography. *J Ultrasound Med.* 2008;27:1573–1581.

79. Wong HS, Tait J, Pringle KC. Viewing of the soft and the hard palate on routine 3-D ultrasound sweep of the fetal face—a feasibility study. *Fetal Diagn Ther.* 2008;24:146–154.

80. Hata T, Yonehara T, Aoki S, et al. Three-dimensional sonographic visualization of the fetal face. *AJR Am J Roentgenol.* 1998;170:481–483.

81. Ramos GA, Romine LE, Gindes L, et al. Evaluation of the fetal secondary palate by 3-dimensional ultrasonography. *J Ultrasound Med.* 2010;29:357–364.

82. Offerdal K, Jebens N, Syvertsen T, et al. Prenatal ultrasound detection of facial clefts: a prospective study of 49,314 deliveries in a non-selected population in Norway. *Ultrasound Obstet Gynecol.* 2008;31:639–646.

83. Stroustrup Smith A, Estroff JA, Barnewolt CE, et al. Prenatal diagnosis of cleft lip and cleft palate using MRI. *AJR Am J Roentgenol.* 2004;183:229–235.

84. Salomon LJ, Sonigo P, Ou P, et al. Real-time fetal magnetic resonance imaging for the dynamic visualization of the pouch in esophageal atresia. *Ultrasound Obstet Gynecol.* 2009;34:471–474.

85. Kazan-Tannus JF, Levine D, McKenzie C, et al. Real-time magnetic resonance imaging aids prenatal diagnosis of isolated cleft palate. *J Ultrasound Med.* 2005;24:1533–1540.

86. Shen SH, Guo WY, Hung JH. Two-dimensional fast imaging employing steady-state acquisition (FIESTA) cine acquisition of fetal non-central nervous system abnormalities. *J Magn Reson Imaging.* 2007;26:672–677.

87. Descamps MJ, Golding SJ, Sibley J, et al. MRI for definitive in utero diagnosis of cleft palate: a useful adjunct to antenatal care? *Cleft Palate Craniofac J.* 2010;47:578–585.

88. Tonni G, Panteghini M, Pattacini P, et al. Integrating 3D sonography with targeted MRI in the prenatal diagnosis of posterior cleft palate plus cleft lip. *J Diagn Med Sonogr.* 2006;22:367–372.

89. Mailath-Pokorny M, Worda C, Krampl-Bettelheim E, et al. What does magnetic resonance imaging add to the prenatal ultrasound diagnosis of facial clefts? *Ultrasound Obstet Gynecol.* 2010;36:445–451.

90. Manganaro L, Tomei A, Fierro F, et al. Fetal MRI as a complement to US in the evaluation of cleft lip and palate. *La Radiologia Medica.* 2011;116:1134–1148.

91. Moreira NC, Ribeiro V, Teixeira J, et al. Visualization of the fetal lip and palate: is brain-targeted MRI reliable? *Cleft Palate Craniofac J.* 2013;50:513–519.

92. Wang G, Shan R, Zhao L, et al. Fetal cleft lip with and without cleft palate: comparison between MR imaging and US for prenatal diagnosis. *Eur J Radiol.* 2011;79:437–442.

93. Bekiesinska-Figatowska M, Brągoszewska H, Romaniuk-Doroszewska A, et al. The role of magnetic resonance imaging in the prenatal diagnosis of cleft lip and palate. *Dev Period Med.* 2014;18(1):27–32.

94. Dabadie A, Quarello E, Degardin N, et al. Added value of MRI for the prenatal diagnosis of isolated orofacial clefts and comparison with ultrasound. *Diagn Interv Imaging.* 2016;97(9):915–921.

95. Laifer-Narin S, Schlechtweg K, Lee J, et al. A comparison of early versus late prenatal magnetic resonance imaging in the diagnosis of cleft palate. *Ann Plast Surg.* 2019;82(4S suppl 3):S242–S246.

96. Tian M, Xiao L, Jian N, et al. Accurate diagnosis of fetal cleft lip/palate by typical signs of magnetic resonance imaging. *Prenat Diagn.* 2019;39(10):883–889.

97. Zheng W, Li B, Zou Y, et al. The prenatal diagnosis and classification of cleft palate: the role and value of magnetic resonance imaging. *Eur Radiol.* 2019;29(10):5600–5606.

98. Paterson P, Sher H, Wylie F, et al. Cleft lip/palate: incidence of prenatal diagnosis in Glasgow, Scotland, and comparison with other centers in the United Kingdom. *Cleft Palate Craniofac J.* 2011;48:608–613.

99. McDonnell R, Owens M, Delany C, et al. Epidemiology of orofacial clefts in the east of Ireland in the 25-year period 1984–2008. *Cleft Palate Craniofac J.* 2014;51(4):e63–e69.

100. Johnson CY, Honein MA, Hobbs CA, et al. Prenatal diagnosis of orofacial clefts, National Birth Defects Prevention Study, 1998–2004. *Prenat Diagn.* 2009;29:833–839.

101. Gorlin RJ, Cohen MM, Levin LS. *Syndromes of the Head and Neck.* New York, NY: Oxford University Press; 1990.

102. Wang BC, Hakimi M, Martin MC. Use of two cleft lip and palate classification systems by nonsubspecialized health care providers. *Cleft Palate Craniofac J.* 2014;51(5):540–543.

103. Mooney M. Classification of orofacial clefting. In: Losee JE, Kirschner RE, eds. *Comprehensive Cleft Care.* New York, NY: McGraw-Hill Professional; 2008:21–23.

104. Veau V. *Division Palatine.* Paris: Masson; 1931.

105. Kernahan DA. The striped Y—a symbolic classification for cleft lip and palate. *Plast Reconstr Surg.* 1971;47:469–470.

106. Kriens O. *What Is a Cleft Lip and Palate?: A Multidisciplinary Update.* Stuttgart, Germany: Thieme; 1989.

107. Tessier P. Anatomical classification of facial, cranio-facial and latero-facial clefts. *J Maxillofac Surg.* 1976;4:69–92.

108. Tewfik TL, Karsan N. Congenital malformations, mouth and pharynx. Medscape. 2008. http://emedicine.medscape.com/article/837347-print. Accessed January 13, 2009.

109. Achiron R, Ben Arie A, Gabbay U, et al. Development of the fetal tongue between 14 and 26 weeks of gestation: in utero ultrasonographic measurements. *Ultrasound Obstet Gynecol.* 1997;9:39–41.

110. Bianchi D, Crombleholme T, D'Alton M, et al. Macroglossia. In: Bianchi D, Crombleholme T, D' Alton M, et al, eds. *Fetology: Diagnosis and Management of the Fetal Patient.* New York, NY: McGraw-Hill Professional; 2010:207–213.

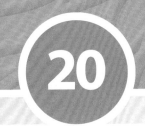

20 Mandible Emphasizing Micrognathia

Rupa Radhakrishnan • Robert J. Hopkin

MICROGNATHIA

Micrognathia is a facial malformation characterized by a small mandible. Retrognathia, which indicates a posteriorly placed chin, is invariably present with micrognathia. Micrognathia is commonly associated with multiple syndromes and associations, but may occasionally be idiopathic. The prenatal diagnosis of micrognathia is obvious in severe cases, where the chin is much posterior to the plane of the upper lip or forehead. Depending on severity, the tongue may fall backward (glossoptosis) and block the airway. In subtle micrognathia, published normal facial indices and mandibular measurements can help in diagnosis.[1,2] Agnathia or otocephaly is the most severe form of mandibular hypoplasia or aplasia.

Incidence: The incidence of micrognathia is approximately 1 in 1,600 infants.

Pathogenesis/Etiology: The mandible develops from the Meckel cartilages, which develop within the first branchial arch during the 7th and 8th weeks of gestation. Membranous ossification of the mandibular body occurs lateral to the mandibular cartilage around the 8th to 12th weeks of gestation. By the 14th to 16th week of gestation, the mandibular condyle and temporomandibular joints develop. Growth of the mandible depends on intrinsic factors, as well as interaction with the surrounding structures such as the oral cavity, muscles of mastication, tongue, maxilla and palate, developing teeth, and the inferior alveolar nerve and branches.[3] This normal development of the mandible may be disrupted by several genetic and environmental factors.[3]

Micrognathia is often associated with chromosomal anomalies and syndromes (Fig. 20.1), varying from 38% to 66% in several series.[4–6] In addition, micrognathia can be a component of various embryopathies occurring with drug and toxin exposure, including cyclophosphamide and methotrexate,[7,8] or congenital infections such as cytomegalovirus.[9] Rarely, micrognathia may be isolated and idiopathic.

Imaging: Fetal micrognathia is frequently associated with polyhydramnios due to relative obstruction to swallowing. On prenatal ultrasound (US), the fetal mandible can be identified from as early as 10 weeks' gestation, and depending on head position, the mandibular body, alveolar ridge, and rami can be evaluated.[3] On coronal plane prenatal US, the anterior echogenic tip of the mandible should be in the same plane as the lips. The diagnosis of fetal micrognathia is often made subjectively, though several authors have published nomograms for mandibular size and growth (Table 24 Appendix A1).[1,10–12]

On prenatal US or magnetic resonance imaging (MRI), the common measurements used to diagnose micrognathia and retrognathia are the inferior facial angle and jaw index. The inferior facial angle is measured on the midsagittal view of the fetal profile. The angle between a line drawn orthogonal to the vertical part of the forehead at the nasal bone synostosis and another other line drawn along the connection between the more prominent lip and the mentum has a normal value of approximately 65°.[13] An inferior facial angle of less than 49.2° is diagnostic of retrognathia (Fig. 20.2).[13]

The jaw index can be assessed sonographically or by MRI on an axial view of the fetal mandible at the base of the cranium just caudad to the lower dental arch, where the whole horseshoe mandible is imaged (Fig. 20.3). The laterolateral diameter is measured by a line connecting the bases of the two rami, and the anteroposterior diameter is measured by drawing a second line from the mentum to the midpoint of the laterolateral diameter. The jaw index is the ratio of the anteroposterior mandibular diameter to the biparietal diameter. A jaw index of less than 23 indicates micrognathia, with a sensitivity and specificity of 100% and 98.1%, respectively.[11]

In addition, multiple other measures have been described to screen for micrognathia, including the facial maxillary angle and frontal nasal–mental angle.[14] A ratio of mandible width to maxilla width of less than 0.785 indicates micrognathia on early prenatal US at 20 to 25 weeks' gestation. The absence of the mandibular gap in the retronasal triangle view is also described as a potential marker of micrognathia on first-trimester US.[15]

Three-dimensional (3D) US and fetal MRI aid greatly in assuring assessment is made on a midline sagittal view. Additional facial abnormalities involving the maxilla, orbits, and ears and commonly associated cleft lip and palate can be sometimes be seen on 2D fetal sonography and more reliably with 3D and 4D US techniques and fetal MRI.[16,17]

Associated Malformations/Conditions: Prenatal identification of micrognathia has been described with several genetic and syndromic causes. Disorders associated with micrognathia

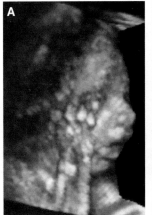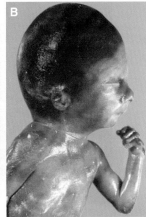

FIGURE 20.1: Micrognathia with trisomy 18. **A:** 3D sonogram showing micrognathia. **B:** Pathological photograph of another case of trisomy 18 showing micrognathia and clenched hand.

585

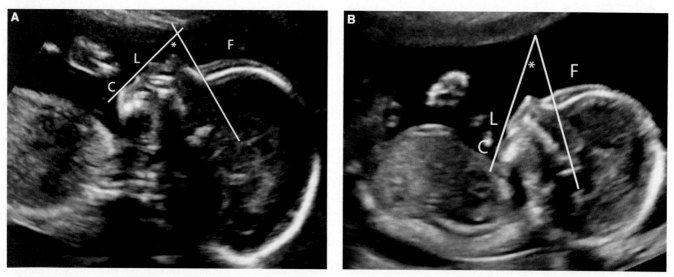

FIGURE 20.2: Inferior facial angle used to diagnose retro-micrognathia. **A:** Normal profile of a 22-week-gestational age fetus in which the angle (*asterisk*) between two lines (one line along the chin–lip anterior surface and the other line orthogonal to the forehead) should be greater than 50°. **B:** A different fetus at 19 weeks has an abnormally low inferior facial angle, signifying an abnormally posteriorly positioned mandible. *F*, forehead; *L*, lip; *C*, chin.

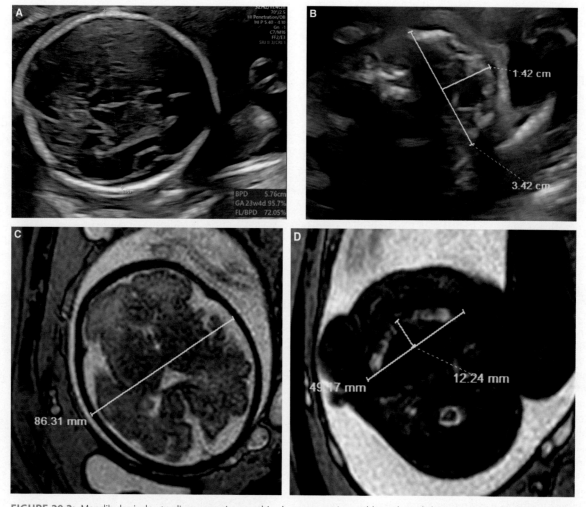

FIGURE 20.3: Mandibular index to diagnose micrognathia. Anteroposterior and laterolateral diameters are measured, and the jaw index is then calculated as follows: anteroposterior mandibular diameter/biparietal diameter (BPD). A jaw index less than 23 indicates micrognathia. **A/B:** Measurement of the mandible by US at 22 weeks. Image **A** is standard BPD measuring 5.76 cm. On second image **B**, 3.42 cm indicate laterolateral diameters and 1.42 cm anterior-to-posterior dimension of the mandible. Jaw index is borderline at 24%. **C/D:** Jaw index on MRI on the same fetus at 32 weeks Image **C** demonstrates BPD of 86.31mm. Image **D** shows anterior to posterior mandibular dimension of 12.24. Jaw index is 14.

include Goldenhar syndrome; Treacher Collins syndrome; Nager acrofacial dysostosis[18]; trisomies 3, 8, 9, 13, and 18; triploidy; tetrasomy 18p[19]; Pena–Shokeir/fetal akinesia syndrome[20]; Marshall and Stickler syndromes; diastrophic and camptomelic dysplasias; Nemaline myopathy; Smith–Lemli–Opitz syndrome[21]; Cornelia de Lange syndrome[22]; Saethre–Chotzen syndrome; multiple contractures or arthrogryposis[23]; cerebro-costo-mandibular syndrome[24]; Fryns syndrome[25]; Wolf–Hirschhorn syndrome[26]; femoral facial syndrome[27]; Meier–Gorlin syndrome; and Seckel syndrome.[28] Exposure to teratogens and medications, including epirubicin, 5-fluorouracil, cyclofphosphamid,[29] methotrexate,[8] and isotretinoin, can be associated with micrognathia. Multiple isolated genetic abnormalities are also shown to present with micrognathia, including MED12 missense mutation.[30]

Prognosis and Management: Fetuses with mandible anomalies are at risk of acute neonatal respiratory distress due to mechanical airway obstruction by the tongue in the presence of an abnormally formed mandible or due to an associated defect of the central nervous system (CNS).[5] Depending on the severity of airway obstruction, these fetuses with potential airway obstruction may need to be referred to fetal care centers to completely evaluate and manage delivery of those with severe airway obstruction. Fetuses with severe micrognathia, combined with the presence of polyhydramnios and absent stomach visualization, may require airway intubation through ex utero intrapartum treatment (EXIT) during delivery.[31,32]

Recurrence Risk: Recurrence risk is variable and depends on the etiology.

DISORDERS ASSOCIATED WITH MICROGNATHIA/AGNATHIA

Robin Sequence

Formerly called Robin or Pierre Robin syndrome, anomalad or complex, it is now called the Robin sequence because most specialists consider the abnormality to be caused by a series of developmental events causing the triad of micrognathia, glossoptosis, and cleft palate. It should be noted that there is still lack of consensus on the exact definition of the Robin sequence, with some pediatric centers considering micrognathia, glossoptosis, and airway obstruction to be diagnostic of the condition.[33]

Incidence: The incidence of Robin sequence is 1 in 8,500 to 1 in 14,000 births.[34]

Pathogenesis: The etiology of Robin sequence is uncertain. Most authors postulate that a small embryonic mandible causes the tongue to be displaced posteriorly and superiorly, thereby preventing closure of the secondary palate.

Imaging: The Robin sequence is a clinical diagnosis when there is micrognathia, cleft secondary palate, and glossoptosis, when the tongue falls posteriorly and obstructs the oral and nasal airway (Fig. 20.4). Robin sequence may be suspected on prenatal US or fetal MRI when there is severe micrognathia and a palatal cleft.[35,36]

Glossoptosis can be seen in some fetuses on sonography and more often on fetal MRI. On fetal MRI in Robin sequence, the tongue may touch the posterior pharyngeal wall in up to one-fifth of the fetuses, a finding not seen in isolated micrognathia or fetuses without craniofacial anomalies.[37] On fetal MRI, a tongue shape index (tongue height divided by tongue length) of more than 80% (Fig. 20.4), a Veau class I or II cleft palate, and an inferior facial angle of less than 48° may be independent predictors of the Robin sequence.[38] Frequently, the oropharyngeal space is also small on fetal MRI in Robin sequence.[39] Cleft of the uvula as a marker for the secondary palate can sometimes be seen on 2D fetal sonography and more reliably on fetal MRI.[16,40] Secondary cleft palate is not usually detected sonographically, although it is readily detectable on fetal MRI.

Differential Diagnosis: Agnathia, in which the mandible is absent and the mouth is small (Fig. 20.5), may resemble Robin sequence.

Prognosis and Management: Robin sequence can present as a medical emergency during delivery, as the retropositioned tongue can obstruct the airway leading to respiratory compromise.[40] When the anomaly is known prenatally, ideally, delivery should take place at a specialized center with neonatal, plastic surgical, and otolaryngology specialists in attendance to manage the airway. A surgical tongue tie may be necessary to prevent airway obstruction. EXIT to airway and/or tracheostomy may also

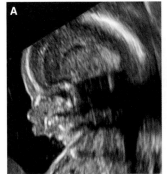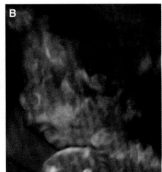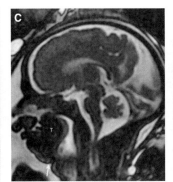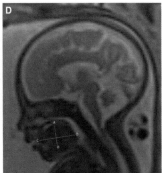

FIGURE 20.4: Robin sequence. **A:** Sagittal 2D US at 21 weeks demonstrating foreshortened mandible that is confirmed on 3D US. **B, C:** Sagittal SSFP MRI at 33 weeks demonstrating micrognathia (*arrow*) and tongue (*T*) obstructing the airway with abnormal tongue shape index (TSI) given the increased tongue height but decreased tongue length. There is absence of the secondary palate. **D:** Sagittal T2 MRI at 34 weeks in a healthy fetus showing normal measurement of the TSI, which is obtained by dividing tongue height AB, by tongue length CD.

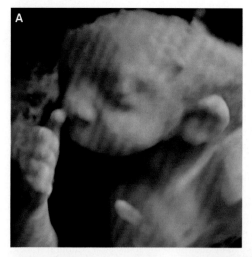
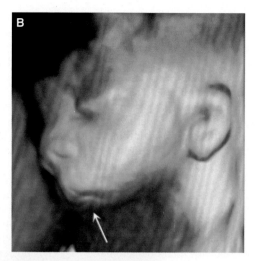
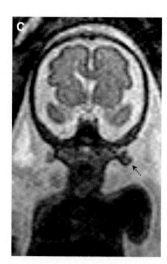
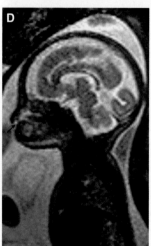
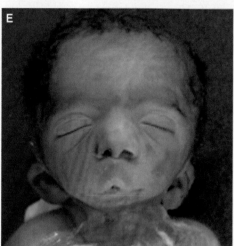

FIGURE 20.5: Otocephaly. A 25-week gestation three-dimensional fetal sonograms **(A, B)**, and coronal and sagittal MRI **(C, D)** showing small mouth (microstomia) (*solid arrow*), severe micrognathia/absent mandible, and low-set ears (*dotted arrow*). **E:** Postmortem photograph at 29 weeks after unsuccessful intubation.

be necessary. Prone or lateral positioning of the infant may keep the airway open for many affected infants. In milder cases, a nasopharyngeal tube may be used to keep the airway open.

If the airway can be managed in the neonatal period, there is often catch-up growth of the small mandible, which allows improvement in respiratory status. This catch up in growth often occurs during infancy and childhood, once the tongue has been pexed anteriorly. Children with Robin sequence have difficulty breathing and eating, and some have temporary or permanent tracheostomies. Palatal repair can be performed once the mandibular size has increased, but airway compromise remains a risk. Surgical mandibular distraction osteogenesis may also be used to accelerate mandibular growth. Approximately 60% to 90% of infants with Robin sequence have other anomalies, most frequently cardiac and renal.[41] Infants may need to be gavage fed to save energy and to gain weight.[42]

Recurrence Risk: Robin sequence recurrence is unknown but infrequent, though there are some data to suggest that there may be a genetic component involved.

Otocephaly

Otocephaly is a rare and typically a lethal malformation involving a defect in the ventral portion of the first branchial arch.

Affected fetuses have microstomia (small mouth), aglossia (absent tongue), agnathia (absent mandible), and melotia/synotia (medially positioned, low and malformed ears).

Synonyms for otocephaly are agnathia–microstomia–synotia syndrome and synotia.

Incidence: Otocephaly is rare and sporadic, occurring in less than 1 in 70,000 births.[43]

Pathogenesis/Etiology: In otocephaly, there is failure of development of the first branchial arch, with lack of ascent of the developing auricles, resulting in low set to markedly displaced ears positioned along the anterior lower neck. It is always associated with agnathia (Fig. 20.5) or severe micrognathia.[43] Both familial cases and de novo mutations in the *PRRX1* and *OTX2* genes have been described in otocephaly.[44-46]

Diagnosis: On imaging, the mandible and lower jaw cannot be seen, and the ears are extremely low (Fig. 20.5). The mouth is often small.

Associated Anomalies: Otocephaly can be associated with other facial abnormalities in the setting of agnathia–otocephaly complex or agnathia–microstomia–synotia syndrome, where there is associated small mouth (microstoma) and aglossia or macroglossia[47]; brain anomalies, such as holoprosencephaly (most commonly associated anomaly) and cephalocele; anophthalmia or microphthalmia; choanal atresia and tracheoesophageal fistula; cardiac, renal, and vertebral anomalies; and a two-vessel umbilical cord.[48–51]

Prognosis/Management: This is almost always a lethal malformation, although rare cases of survival to adulthood are described with staged facial and mandibular reconstructive surgeries.[52]

Recurrence Risk: Recurrence risk is not known, although familial cases have been described.

COMMON SYNDROMES CHARACTERIZED BY MICROGNATHIA

Goldenhar Syndrome

Goldenhar syndrome is one of the craniofacial microsomia syndromes associated with micrognathia, caused by malformations involving the first and second branchial apparatus derivatives. Goldenhar syndrome, also known as oculoauriculovertebral syndrome/spectrum/dysplasia, OAVS, and expanded-spectrum hemifacial microsomia, consists of hemifacial microsomia with characteristic aural, eye and vertebral anomalies. Facial features include lip and palate clefting, temporomandibular joint ankylosis, asymmetric mandibular hypoplasia, asymmetric palpebral fissures, and midface hypoplasia.[53] Eye findings include eyelid coloboma, microphthalmia, or anophthalmia, in addition to the presence of the characteristic epibulbar dermoid.[54] Ear findings include microtia, preauricular tragi, and hearing loss.[53] Vertebral abnormalities include malformed vertebrae, block vertebrae, or vertebral segmentation abnormalities. Other associated features include pulmonary agenesis, absent thyroid gland, multiple cranial nerve palsies, renal anomalies, radial ray anomalies, cardiac anomalies (usually atrioventricular septal defect) and intracranial anomalies such as hydrocephalus, cerebellar or cerebellar vermian hypoplasia, and lipoma of the corpus callosum.[55–57] There have been reports of bilateral hemifacial macrosomia as well.

Incidence: The prevalence of Goldenhar syndrome is approximately 1 to 9 in 100,000. The incidence of hemifacial microsomia ranges from 1 in 3,000 to 1 in 45,000 live births.[58]

Pathogenesis/Etiology: Although most cases of Goldenhar syndrome are sporadic, there may rarely be a family history of this condition, suggesting an autosomal dominant inheritance. No genetic locus is currently associated with Goldenhar syndrome. Etiology of Goldenhar syndrome is not known, although a mesodermal dysplasia complex leading to disruption in development of the first and second branchial arches, especially due to interruption of the stapedial artery or other vascular cause such as interrupted inferior vena cava with azygos continuation and persistent left superior vena cava,[55] has been suggested. However, this does not explain the associated multisystem anomalies in Goldenhar syndrome.

Diagnosis: No genetic testing is available. Amniocentesis has been noted to show inconsistent chromosomal abnormalities; however, in many cases, karyotype is normal in Goldenhar syndrome. Diagnosis is made clinically, but debate on the specific diagnostic criteria continues.[58]

Imaging: Although Goldenhar syndrome has been described as being suspected on prenatal US as early as 15 weeks' gestational age, with observations of cleft palate and unilateral severe microphthalmia, (Fig. 20.6A)[59] asymmetric facial appearance may rarely be visible on 2D US and may be better assessed on 3D US.[60] Associated anomalies, particularly vertebral, are more frequently seen on US, prompting further imaging with fetal MRI,[60,61] which can improve detection of the asymmetry and raise concern for a hemifacial microsomia syndrome (Fig. 20.6D).[62] Several primary features and additional associated anomalies in this condition are detected on fetal MRI, including microtia, ocular hypoplasia, renal anomalies, and facial asymmetry.[62] Most often, characteristic facial features are obvious after delivery, leading to diagnosis.[53] Other abnormalities such as absent nasal bones and micrognathia can also be seen on prenatal US.[61] Subtle abnormalities such as preauricular skin tags and colobomas can be recognized on late trimester imaging.[63] Additional anomalies such as pulmonary agenesis may be suggested by displacement of the fetal heart on US (Fig. 20.6B), but better imaged on fetal MRI.

Differential Diagnosis: The differential diagnosis includes other craniofacial conditions, associations, or syndromes with spine anomalies, such as Emanuel syndrome (due to an unbalanced 11/22 translocation that results in partial trisomy 11q and partial trisomy 22q); Treacher Collins Syndrome; Townes–Brocks, in which there may be asymmetry of the ear size and cupping of one ear; CHARGE syndrome (coloboma, heart defects, atresia choanae, growth retardation, genital abnormalities, ear anomalies); branchio-oto-renal; or chromosomal deletions/duplications.

Prognosis: Postnatal mortality primarily depends on the severity of congenital cardiac disease or airway malformations. If severe defects are not present, the long-term prognosis is good.[55]

Management: Infants suspected of having a craniofacial microsomia syndrome should have neonatology support at the time of delivery. Full physical examination should be performed to exclude other congenital anomalies. Ophthalmology and audiology evaluations, screening echocardiography, and renal US should be obtained.[64] Echocardiography is especially important because of the possibility of severe conotruncal defects that result in high postnatal mortality. Postnatal spine radiographs are also recommended to evaluate for vertebral malformations.[53] Most affected individuals (>90%) have normal intelligence. Long-term management should focus on hearing abnormalities and possible facial nerve weakness.[65] Reconstructive surgery to address the facial asymmetry is often helpful.

Recurrence Risk: Most cases are de novo. Recurrence risk is 2% to 3% in absence of familial transmission.[65]

Treacher Collins Syndrome

Treacher Collins Syndrome (TCS), also referred to as Treacher Collins–Franceschetti syndrome and mandibulofacial dysostosis, consists of hypoplastic zygomatic bones and mandible, ear anomalies, eyelid coloboma, absent lower eyelashes, and displaced hair growth onto cheeks.[66]

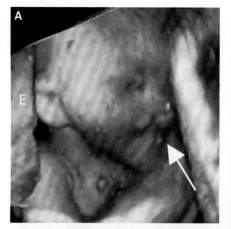

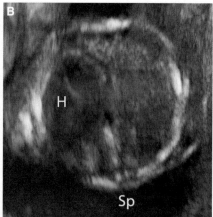

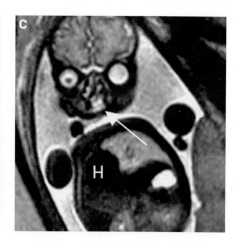

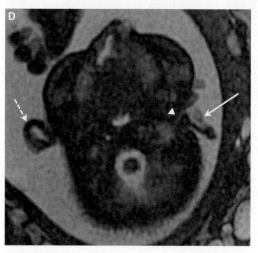

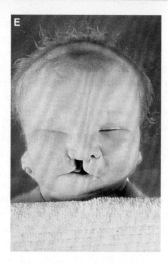

FIGURE 20.6: Goldenhar syndrome diagnosed prenatally in a 34-week-gestational age fetus. **A:** Three-dimensional US of the fetal face showing a low-set ear (*E*) and a cleft palate (*arrow*). **B:** Axial US through the chest demonstrating agenesis of one lung, with lateral displacement the fetal heart (*H*, heart; *Sp*, spine). **C:** Subsequent evaluation with fetal MRI of the same fetus readily showing aplasia of the right lung with normal left lung and cleft palate (*arrow*) on coronal SSFSE T2 image. **D:** Axial SSFP sequence through the temporal bones showing asymmetry of earlobes with the left (*solid arrow*) normal and the right malformed (*dotted arrow*). Normal external auditory canal is present on the left (*arrowhead*) but absent on the right. **E:** A postmortem photograph of a different patient with Goldenhar syndrome showing similar facial features.

Incidence: The incidence of TCS ranges from 1 in 10,000 to 1 in 50,000.[67]

Pathogenesis/Etiology: In over 95% of cases, TCS is inherited as autosomal dominant with de novo mutations in the *TCOF1* or *POLR1D* pathogenic variant. Rarely, inheritance may be autosomal recessive due to genetic mutations in the *POLR1C* or *POLR1D* pathogenic variant.[67] Mutations in the *TCOF1* gene are the most common, accounting for 71% to 93% of cases.[68]

Diagnosis: If genetic testing is performed, the *TCOF1* gene is typically evaluated first. If no mutation is found, the *POLR1D* and *POLR1C* genes are evaluated.

Imaging: The reliability of prenatal US in diagnosing TCS will depend on the severity of the findings. The principal findings in TCS are polyhydramnios, micrognathia, low-set ears, slanting palpebral fissures, and cleft palate (Fig. 20.7A). Typical facial features are better illustrated with 3D US (Fig. 20.7B) than with standard 2D imaging.[69] MRI may be helpful to evaluate airway and temporal bone anatomy (Fig. 20.7C, D).[69]

Differential Diagnosis: The differential diagnosis may include Goldenhar syndrome, though abnormalities in Goldenhar syndrome are almost always unilateral and involve notching of the upper rather than the lower lid, as well as epibulbar dermoids. Fetuses with Goldenhar may also have vertebral anomalies and cardiac defects. Nager syndrome typically has preaxial reduction

defects of the upper extremities, ranging from hypoplasia to aplasia of the thumb with or without involvement of the radius. Miller syndrome, also known as postaxial acrofacial dysostosis (POADS), may have similar findings, but is characterized by micrognathia, cleft palate, postaxial reduction defects, and vertebral anomalies.[70] Robin sequence or nonsyndromic mandibular hypoplasia is characterized by early mandibular hypoplasia alone. It should be emphasized that limb anomalies are not a feature of TCS, and if present, Miller and Nager syndromes should be considered.

Prognosis: The prognosis depends on the severity of the phenotype expressed.

Management: Craniofacial abnormalities seen in this syndrome can lead to respiratory distress, requiring special positioning or tracheostomy,[71] and an EXIT procedure may be discussed for delivery planning if micrognathia is severe and airway access is questionable.[72] In this instance, the child will remain on placental support until the airway is secured.

Management should involve a multidisciplinary craniofacial team. Surgical management is often needed for craniofacial reconstruction and cleft repair.[73] Diagnostic imaging with postnatal computed tomography (CT) of the head and face to delineate abnormalities of the zygomatic arch, malar bones, and mandible is often pursued. An ophthalmology examination is important to evaluate for vision loss, amblyopia, refractive errors, and strabismus.[74] Auricular malformations of ossicles and the tympanic

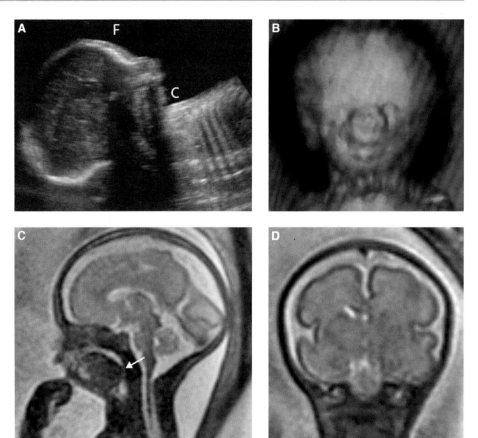

FIGURE 20.7: Treacher Collins syndrome diagnosed prenatally in a 29-week fetus. **A:** Two-dimensional sagittal US of the face showing retrognathia. *F,* forehead; *C,* chin. **B:** Three-dimensional view of the fetal face demonstrating abnormal flattening of the fetal nose and lack of visualization of the pinna bilaterally. **C:** Further evaluation with fetal MRI in sagittal plane with T2 imaging depicting the small mandible and the flattened nose. The tongue partly occludes the oropharyngeal airway (*arrow*). **D:** Coronal MRI showing the absence of the bilateral external ears.

cavity can lead to conductive hearing loss in 40% to 50% of cases.[68] Speech therapy evaluations to assess for swallowing and feeding difficulty may determine the need for gastrostomy tube.[69] Rarely, palatal clefting and abnormalities of choanae can be seen.[75] Dental anomalies are present in 60% of TCS cases and can include dental agenesis, enamel abnormalities, and ectopic molars.[76]

Recurrence Risk: The inheritance of TCS is autosomal dominant, and most mutations are de novo.[67] Intrafamilial variability is marked. It is not uncommon for a parent to be mildly affected and undetected, so parental testing should be considered to guide recurrence risk counseling.

Nager Syndrome

Nager type of acrofacial dysostosis (AFD1) is one of a group of syndromes associated with craniofacial and skeletal malformations. Of the AFDs, Nager can be distinguished by characteristic facial features, including downslanting palpebral fissures, external ear malformations, midface/malar hypoplasia, and micrognathia.[77] Cleft lip and palate are also seen.[78] Limb malformations involve the radial distribution and include small or absent thumbs, triphalangeal thumbs, radial hypoplasia/aplasia, and radioulnar synostosis. Reports of patients with typical features of Nager syndrome and other congenital anomalies, including Hirschsprung disease, CNS anomalies, congenital heart defects, and cardiac conduction abnormalities, have been described.[79]

Incidence: Nager syndrome is rare, with fewer than 100 reported cases.[80]

Pathogenesis/Etiology: Most of the cases of Nager syndrome are caused by the heterozygous mutation in the *SF3B4* gene on chromosome 1q21.2.[18,77] Frequently, these are point mutations causing haploinsufficiency, but may also be whole gene deletions.[18,81] High-resolution chromosomal microarray may be helpful to confirm Nager syndrome due to *SF3B4* mutation in early pregnancy.[18] The genetic mutation may be heritable or de novo.[81–83]

Diagnosis: *AFD1* gene testing could be offered if Nager syndrome is suspected. Postnatal assessment of clinical features is more definitive than genetic testing.

Imaging: Suspicion for Nager syndrome may be raised on prenatal US, although craniofacial and extremity findings can be subtle and are often not well delineated. As with Goldenhar syndrome and TCS, prenatal diagnosis depends on the severity of the disorder. The vast majority of these rare cases have been described in the pediatric literature, and very few fetuses with Nager have been described prenatally.[84] Prenatal diagnosis may be suspected as early as 22 weeks' gestational age based on US.[85] The most readily recognized features by prenatal 2D US are micrognathia and radial hypoplasia (Fig. 20.8A, B). Adding 3D technique will enable further detail of the external ears, which are typically small, low set, and posteriorly rotated. Sometimes, it is possible to identify downsloping palpebral fissures. Unilateral limb involvement has also been described in a prenatally diagnosed case without any family history of AFD.[86] MRI is helpful in the presence of severe micrognathia to evaluate the severity of airway obstruction (Fig. 20.8C, D).

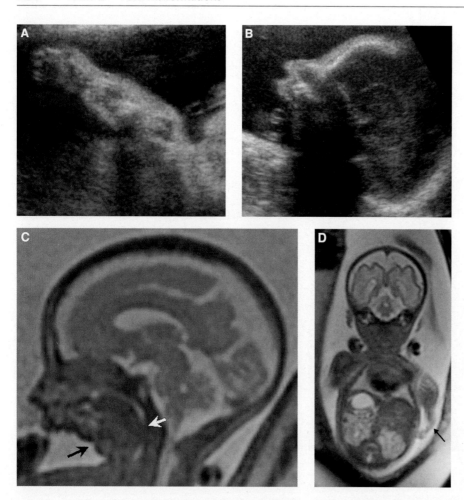

FIGURE 20.8: A 28-week fetus with confirmed Nager syndrome. **A:** US of the arm demonstrating lack of visualization of bones of the forearm. **B:** Severe micrognathia was present on US. **C:** Sagittal T2 MRI of the same fetus showing severe micrognathia (*black arrow*) with obstruction of the oropharyngeal airway (*white arrow*). **D:** Coronal T2 MRI depicting significant shortening of the arm (*arrow*). The lower extremities were normal.

Differential Diagnosis: The differential diagnosis depends on the severity of associated anomalies. Other facial dysostoses in the differential would include Treacher Collins, which is distinguished by lack of limb anomalies. Orofacial digital syndromes typically have polydactyly or bifid hallux, whereas reduction defects are noted in Nager syndrome. Other syndromes associated with radial ray anomalies include Fanconi anemia and trisomy 18. Lower extremity malformations are rarely seen in Nager syndrome. This finding may help distinguish Nager from Miller syndrome, which is another disorder within the AFDs group and is characterized by postaxial reduction defects, vertebral anomalies, and cardiac defects.[86]

Prognosis: Prognosis depends on the severity and medical management of the conductive hearing loss and upper airway obstruction that is responsible for early feeding and respiratory difficulties. Intelligence is expected to be normal, unless impacted by delayed diagnosis of these anomalies.[84]

Management: Infants born with suspected Nager syndrome often have respiratory issues related to micrognathia. In the presence of severe micrognathia, an EXIT procedure to airway may be necessary. Tracheostomy is sometimes required.[87] Feeding issues are common. Orthopedic management of extremity anomalies may be necessary, and a radiographic survey of the infant will be important to define skeletal malformations. Nearly all affected fetuses have some degree of hearing loss, and postnatal imaging with CT or MR of the temporal bones may be indicated. Because of the associated

incidence of congenital heart disease and conduction abnormalities, echocardiography should be performed to screen for structural heart disease.[87]

Recurrence Risk: Recurrence risk varies according to inheritance pattern. Both autosomal dominant and recessive inheritance have been reported. In sporadic cases, recurrence risk is cited at 3% to 5%.[87]

Mandibulofacial Dysostosis with Microcephaly

Mandibulofacial dysostosis with microcephaly (MFDM) includes a phenotype of microcephaly, choanal atresia, cleft palate, maxillary and mandibular hypoplasia, microtia, and developmental delay.[88,89] The most distinguishing finding associated with MFDM is small head circumference, which can be variable from mild to severe and even progressive.[88] The other principle facial features are similar to TCS or Nager syndrome, with malar and mandibular hypoplasia, microtia, or other ear malformations also being very common. However, microtia in most MFDM patients presents as severe symmetric hypoplasia of the upper portion of the ear with normal lobes.[88] Choanal atresia may also overlap with the CHARGE syndrome. There is often associated facial asymmetry. Epibulbar dermoids and zygomatic arch clefting can also be present.[88] Congenital heart disease (40%), esophageal atresia/tracheoesophageal fistula (40%), and thumb abnormalities (25%) are additionally common.[89] This overlap has led some patients to be misdiagnosed with either Goldenhar syndrome or VACTERL association.

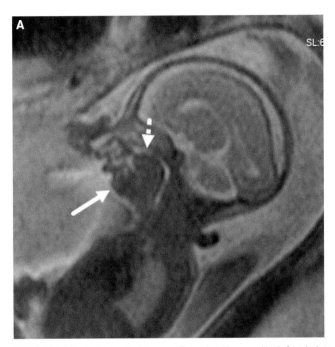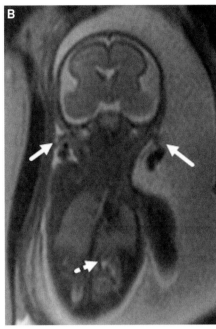

FIGURE 20.9: A 24-week fetus confirmed with mandibulofacial dysostosis with microcephaly and tracheoesophageal fistula. Brain biometrics was small for age, and polyhydramnios was present. **A:** Sagittal MRI demonstrating micrognathia (*solid arrow*) and secondary palate defect (*dotted arrow*) with tongue displaced in the posterior oropharynx obstructing airway. **B:** Coronal MRI demonstrating low-set ears (*solid arrows*) and lack of visualization of the stomach (*dotted arrow*). A tracheoesophageal fistula was noted postnatal.

Incidence: The syndrome is rare with only case reports in the literature, though the diagnosis may be underestimated.[88,89]

Pathogenesis/Etiology: MFDM is an autosomal dominant condition caused by loss-of-function mutations in the *EFTUD2* gene.[88,89] The gene is likely involved in abnormal development of derivatives of the first and second branchial arches.[88]

Diagnosis: Confirmation can be made with sequencing and deletion/duplication analysis of the *EFTUD2* gene.

Imaging: The diagnosis should be suspected in a fetus with mandibular hypoplasia and microcephaly. Measurements of the fetal brain are therefore important for diagnosis. Ear anomalies may also be detected prenatally. Dilated, obstructed nasal passages may support choanal atresia. If tracheoesophageal fistula is present, polyhydramnios, small stomach, and/or dilated esophageal pouch may be detected (Fig. 20-9).

Differential Diagnosis: Given the similar ear and mandibular anomalies, differential would include CHARGE, TCS, Miller, and Nager syndrome. However, none of these syndromes are associated with microcephaly. Severe limb anomalies are also not as common as in Nager and Miller syndromes. In CHARGE, choanal atresia is seen; however, typically ear abnormalities affect the lower portion. VACTERL and Goldenhar syndrome may be considered but are usually asymmetrical.

Prognosis: MFDM is strongly associated with intellectual disability, feeding problems in the newborn, and severe speech delays.

Management: In the presence of severe airway compromise, delivery may require EXIT or planned delivery at an institution which can perform emergent intubation or tracheostomy. Craniofacial

manifestations should be managed by a multidisciplinary team. Cardiac disorders should be managed by cardiology and esophageal atresia by surgery. Occupation, physical, and speech therapy is typically required to optimize developmental outcome.[89] It is important to distinguish MFDM from the other mandibulofacial syndromes as these children have cognitive impairment.

Recurrence: Most affected individuals have de novo mutation of the *ERTUD2* gene; however, familial recurrence can result from either germline mosaicism or inheritance from a parent with mild phenotype, resulting in 50% chance of transmission.[88,89]

Orofacial Digital Syndrome

Orofacial digital (OFD) syndrome is a heterogeneous group of disorders characterized by abnormalities in the mouth, face, and digits and with variable additional anomalies in the eyes, brain, heart, kidney, and genitalia.[90,91] At least 13 subtypes of OFD syndrome have been described so far; however, there is frequent variation in phenotypic expression within one subtype and phenotypic overlap between subtypes.[92] OFD syndrome type 1 is the only one with an established genetic defect and is described in this chapter.

Incidence: The incidence of type 1 OFD syndrome is 1 in 50,000 to 1 in 250,000 live births.[93,94]

Pathogenesis/Etiology: OFD type 1 is a ciliopathy with X-linked inheritance, and the *OFD1* gene is located on Xp22.2.[95,96] This gene has an important role in primary ciliary function and defects overlap with other ciliopathies such as X-linked Joubert syndrome and polycystic kidney disease.[97] On clinical testing of *OFD1*, a mutation is found in approximately 80% of patients with the syndrome.[98] The genetic disorder is almost always lethal in male fetuses, with intrauterine demise usually in the first or second trimester.[97] However, rare cases of males with *OFD1*, some surviving to adulthood, have recently been described and may be related to mutation type.[95]

Diagnosis: Molecular testing for *OFD1* includes single-gene testing, usually followed by the use of a multigene panel and more comprehensive genomic testing if single-gene testing is negative.[99] Molecular testing should be offered but is not required for diagnosis, as characteristic anomalies are frequently present at birth. The *OFD1* gene demonstrates X-linked inheritance in familial cases, but the mutation is frequently de novo.[99]

Imaging: Features of OFD type 1 are usually readily apparent on clinical and postnatal imaging, but some features may be identified prenatally to suggest diagnosis, especially when there is a family history of this condition. Clinical features include oral findings of lobed tongue, hamartomas or lipomas of the tongue, ankyloglossia, cleft of the hard or soft palate, alveolar clefts and accessory gingival frenula, and hypodontia or other dental abnormalities;[99] facial features such as micrognathia hypertelorism, telecanthus, hypoplastic alae nasi, clefts of upper lip (Fig. 20.10A); and digital anomalies such as brachydactyly, syndactyly, clinodactyly, duplicated digits, or polydactyly (Fig. 20.10B).[99] Renal cysts may be seen in approximately 50% of individuals with OFD1.[99] Rarely, renal cysts may be the only manifestation.[100] Brain malformations are relatively common, noted in 65% of cases, and include intracerebral cysts, agenesis of corpus callosum, cerebellar agenesis, and Dandy–Walker malformation.[99] Prenatal diagnosis of OFD syndrome has been described for types I, II, IV, and VI.[101] OFD1 is almost always diagnosed in female fetuses.

Prenatal US and fetal MRI can detect cleft lip, cleft palate, hypertelorism, micrognathia, facial asymmetry, ear anomalies, brain malformations, echogenic or cystic kidneys, and anomalies of the extremities. In pregnancies in which there is a family history of OFD1, prenatal imaging may be especially helpful in identifying fetal phenotype. Even in nonfamilial cases, the presence of intracranial and digital abnormalities may suggest prenatal diagnosis of OFD type 1.[102] In the mildest cases, diagnosis may not be made until polycystic kidney disease develops later in life.[103] In OFD type VI, hypothalamic hamartoma is a specific, but not sensitive feature, which can be identified on fetal MRI and help in making the diagnosis.[104,105]

Differential Diagnosis: The differential diagnosis for OFD type 1 would include other subtypes of OFD due to variable phenotypic expression in each subtype and overlap between subtypes. In addition, other syndromes that affect the face and extremities may also need to be considered. Smith-Lemli-Opitz syndrome is associated with facial, digital, and renal anomalies. Other syndromes not discussed in this chapter but that overlap with OFD findings include Carpenter syndrome, which features a bifid hallux and hydrolethalus syndrome, which has both CNS abnormalities and preaxial polydactyly.[106] Majewski syndrome is a skeletal dysplasia featuring a midline facial cleft, polydactyly, and short limbs. OFD type 1 also has similar features with other ciliopathies, such as primary ciliary dyskinesia, which can present with hydrocephalus, but does not have the craniofacial defect seen with OFD type 1.[107] Jeune asphyxiating thoracic dystrophy, polycystic kidney disease, Bardet–Biedl syndrome, Meckel syndrome, Ellis–Van Creveld syndrome, and nephronophthisis also have some features in common with OFD type 1 such as polydactyly, cystic kidneys, skeletal dysplasia, and CNS defects, but lack the characteristic craniofacial abnormalities.[107]

Prognosis: The prognosis of any individual with OFD syndrome depends on the phenotypic severity.

Management: Orofacial issues typically cause feeding difficulty at birth. Management includes surgery for defects, such as cleft lip/palate, tongue nodules, and accessory frenula. Nutrition consultation and speech therapy are typically necessary.[93] Postnatal brain imaging should be performed to evaluate for structural brain abnormalities.[94] Although polycystic kidney disease is common, seen in up to 50% of cases, it typically does not develop until adulthood. A screening renal US could be performed but would be expected to be negative and does not exclude the potential to develop cystic disease later in life.[103] Long-term issues include orthodontia for malocclusion, surgical management of syndactyly, and special education for developmental delay.[93] Developmental delay depends on the severity of intracranial abnormality and is seen in up to 50% of patients.[94]

Recurrence Risk: In cases of de novo mutation, the recurrence risk for subsequent pregnancies is very low. In familial cases, one-third of live-born infants are at risk of OFD type 1.[93]

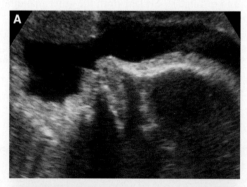

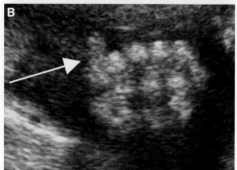

FIGURE 20.10: Imaging findings seen in orofacial digital syndrome. **A:** US of the midline face in sagittal projection showing micrognathia in a 23-week fetus. No cleft palate was found. **B:** Evaluation of the hand shows polydactyly (*arrow* indicates supernumerary digit). Abnormality was bilateral.

REFERENCES

1. Chitty LS, Campbell S, Altman DG. Measurement of the fetal mandible—feasibility and construction of a centile chart. *Prenat Diagn.* 1993;13(8):749–756.
2. Neuschulz J, Wilhelm L, Christ H, et al. Prenatal indices for mandibular retrognathia/micrognathia. *J Orofac Orthop.* 2015;76(1):30–40.
3. Paladini D. Fetal micrognathia: almost always an ominous finding. *Ultrasound Obstet Gynecol.* 2010;35(4):377–384.
4. Bromley B, Benacerraf BR. Fetal micrognathia: associated anomalies and outcome. *J Ultrasound Med.* 1994;13(7):529–533.

5. Nicolaides KH, Salvesen DR, Snijders RJ, et al. Fetal facial defects: associated malformations and chromosomal abnormalities. *Fetal Diagn Ther.* 1993;8(1):1–9.
6. Turner GM, Twining P. The facial profile in the diagnosis of fetal abnormalities. *Clin Radiol.* 1993;47(6):389–395.
7. Rengasamy P. Congenital malformations attributed to prenatal exposure to cyclophosphamide. *Anticancer Agents Med Chem.* 2017;17(9):1211–1227.
8. Kozma C, Ramasethu J. Methotrexate and misoprostol teratogenicity: further expansion of the clinical manifestations. *Am J Med Genet A.* 2011;155A(7):1723–1728.
9. Weichert A, Vogt M, Dudenhausen JW, et al. Evidence in a human fetus of micrognathia and cleft lip as potential effects of early cytomegalovirus infection. *Fetal Diagn Ther.* 2010;28(4):225–228.
10. Otto C, Platt LD. The fetal mandible measurement—an objective determination of fetal jaw size. *Ultrasound Obst Gyn.* 1991;1(1):12–17.
11. Paladini D, Morra T, Teodoro A, et al. Objective diagnosis of micrognathia in the fetus: the jaw index. *Obstet Gynecol.* 1999;93(3):382–386.
12. Nemec U, Nemec SF, Brugger PC, et al. Normal mandibular growth and diagnosis of micrognathia at prenatal MRI. *Prenat Diagn.* 2015;35(2):108–116.
13. Rotten D, Levaillant JM, Martinez H, et al. The fetal mandible: a 2D and 3D sonographic approach to the diagnosis of retrognathia and micrognathia. *Ultrasound Obstet Gynecol.* 2002;19(2):122–130.
14. Lu J, Sahota DS, Poon LC, et al. Objective assessment of the fetal facial profile at second and third trimester of pregnancy. *Prenat Diagn.* 2019;39(2):107–115.
15. Sepulveda W, Wong AE, Viñals F, et al. Absent mandibular gap in the retronasal triangle view: a clue to the diagnosis of micrognathia in the first trimester. *Ultrasound Obstet Gynecol.* 2012;39(2):152–156.
16. Wilhelm L, Borgers H. The "equals sign": a novel marker in the diagnosis of fetal isolated cleft palate. *Ultrasound Obstet Gynecol.* 2010;36(4):439–444.
17. Tonni G, Grisolia G, Santana EF, et al. Assessment of fetus during second trimester ultrasonography using HDlive software: what is its real application in the obstetrics clinical practice? *World J Radiol.* 2016;8(12):922–927.
18. Lund IC, Vestergaard EM, Christensen R, et al. Prenatal diagnosis of Nager syndrome in a 12-week-old fetus with a whole gene deletion of SF3B4 by chromosomal microarray. *Eur J Med Genet.* 2016;59(1):48–51.
19. Inan C, Sayin NC, Atli E, et al. Tetrasomy 18p in a twin pregnancy with diverse expression in both fetuses. *Fetal Pediatr Pathol.* 2016;35(5):339–343.
20. Nayak SS, Kadavigere R, Mathew M, et al. Fetal akinesia deformation sequence: expanding the phenotypic spectrum. *Am J Med Genet A.* 2014;164A(10):2643–2648.
21. Szpera-Gozdziewicz A, Ropacka-Lesiak M, Rzymski P, et al. Smith-Lemli-Opitz Syndrome—a challenging prenatal diagnosis. *Ginekol Pol.* 2016;87(1):76–78.
22. Akahori Y, Masuyama H, Masumoto Y, et al. Three-dimensional ultrasound findings in Cornelia de Lange syndrome: a case report. *Case Rep Obstet Gynecol.* 2012;2012:568351.
23. Hall JG. Arthrogryposis (multiple congenital contractures): diagnostic approach to etiology, classification, genetics, and general principles. *Eur J Med Genet.* 2014;57(8):464–472.
24. Ramaswamy P, Negus S, Homfray T, et al. Severe micrognathia with rib dysplasia: cerebro-costo-mandibular syndrome. *Arch Dis Child Fetal Neonatal Ed.* 2016;101(1):F85.
25. Slavotinek A. Fryns syndrome. In: Adam MP, Ardinger HH, Pagon RA, et al., eds. *GeneReviews®.* Seattle, WA: University of Washington; 1993.
26. Paradowska-Stolarz AM. Wolf-Hirschhorn syndrome (WHS)—literature review on the features of the syndrome. *Adv Clin Exp Med.* 2014;23(3):485–489.
27. Castro S, Peraza E, Zapata M. Prenatal diagnosis of femoral-facial syndrome: case report. *J Clin Ultrasound.* 2014;42(1):49–52.
28. Ogi T, Walker S, Stiff T, et al. Identification of the first ATRIP-deficient patient and novel mutations in ATR define a clinical spectrum for ATR-ATRIP Seckel Syndrome. *PLoS Genet.* 2012;8(11):e1002945.
29. Leyder M, Laubach M, Breugelmans M, et al. Specific congenital malformations after exposure to cyclophosphamide, epirubicin and 5-fluorouracil during the first trimester of pregnancy. *Gynecol Obstet Invest.* 2011;71(2):141–144.
30. Prescott TE, Kulseth MA, Heimdal KR, et al. Two male sibs with severe micrognathia and a missense variant in MED12. *Eur J Med Genet.* 2016;59(8):367–372.
31. Suenaga M, Hidaka N, Kido S, et al. Successful ex utero intrapartum treatment procedure for prenatally diagnosed severe micrognathia: a case report. *J Obstet Gynaecol Res.* 2014;40(8):2005–2009.
32. DaValle B, Nagel E, Gonzalez S, et al. Ex utero intrapartum treatment of fetal micrognathia. *Mil Med.* 2014;179(6):e705–e711.
33. Breugem CC, Courtemanche DJ. Robin sequence: clearing nosologic confusion. *Cleft Palate Craniofac J.* 2010;47(2):197–200.
34. Vettraino IM, Lee W, Bronsteen RA, et al. Clinical outcome of fetuses with sonographic diagnosis of isolated micrognathia. *Obstet Gynecol.* 2003;102(4):801–805.
35. Rogers-Vizena CR, Mulliken JB, Daniels KM, et al. Prenatal features predictive of robin sequence identified by fetal magnetic resonance imaging. *Plast Reconstr Surg.* 2016;137(6):999e–1006e.
36. Lind K, Aubry MC, Belarbi N, et al. Prenatal diagnosis of Pierre Robin Sequence: accuracy and ability to predict phenotype and functional severity. *Prenat Diagn.* 2015;35(9):853–858.
37. Resnick CM, Kooiman TD, Calabrese CE, et al. In utero glossoptosis in fetuses with robin sequence: measurements from prenatal MRI. *Cleft Palate Craniofac J.* 2018;55(4):562–567.
38. Resnick CM, Kooiman TD, Calabrese CE, et al. An algorithm for predicting Robin sequence from fetal MRI. *Prenat Diagn.* 2018;38(5):357–364.

39. Kooiman TD, Calabrese CE, Didier R, et al. Micrognathia and oropharyngeal space in patients with robin sequence: prenatal MRI measurements. *J Oral Maxillofac Surg.* 2018;76(2):408–415.
40. Kaufman MG, Cassady CI, Hyman CH, et al. Prenatal identification of pierre robin sequence: a review of the literature and look towards the future. *Fetal Diagn Ther.* 2016;39(2):81–89.
41. Hoffman W. Cleft palate. In: Rodriguez E, Losee J, Neligan P, eds. *Craniofacial, Head and Neck Surgery and Pediatric Plastic Surgery.* Vol 3. Philadelphia, PA: Saunders; 2012.
42. Gangopadhyay N, Mendonca DA, Woo AS. Pierre robin sequence. *Semin Plast Surg.* 2012;26(2):76–82.
43. Agarwal S, Sen J, Jain S, et al. Otocephaly: prenatal and postnatal imaging findings. *J Pediatr Neurosci.* 2011;6(1):94–95.
44. Sergouniotis PI, Urquhart JE, Williams SG, et al. Agnathia-otocephaly complex and asymmetric velopharyngeal insufficiency due to an in-frame duplication in OTX2. *J Hum Genet.* 2015;60(4):199–202.
45. Chassaing N, Sorrentino S, Davis EE, et al. OTX2 mutations contribute to the otocephaly-dysgnathia complex. *J Med Genet.* 2012;49(6):373–379.
46. Dasouki M, Andrews B, Parimi P, et al. Recurrent agnathia-otocephaly caused by DNA replication slippage in PRRX1. *Am J Med Genet A.* 2013;161A(4):803–808.
47. Wai LT, Chandran S. Cyclopia: isolated and with agnathia-otocephaly complex. *BMJ Case Rep.* 2017;2017.
48. Hersh JH, McChane RH, Rosenberg EM, et al. Otocephaly-midline malformation association. *Am J Med Genet.* 1989;34(2):246–249.
49. Persutte WH, Lenke RR, DeRosa RT. Prenatal ultrasonographic appearance of the agnathia malformation complex. *J Ultrasound Med.* 1990;9(12):725–728.
50. Cayea PD, Bieber FR, Ross MJ, et al. Sonographic findings in otocephaly (synotia). *J Ultrasound Med.* 1985;4(7):377–379.
51. Rahmani R, Dixon M, Chitayat D, et al. Otocephaly: prenatal sonographic diagnosis. *J Ultrasound Med.* 1998;17(9):595–598.
52. Golinko MS, Shetye P, Flores RL, et al. Severe agnathia-otocephaly complex: surgical management and longitudinal follow-up from birth through adulthood. *J Craniofac Surg.* 2015;26(8):2387–2392.
53. Cohen MM Jr, Rollnick BR, Kaye CI. Oculoauriculovertebral spectrum: an updated critique. *Cleft Palate J.* 1989;26(4):276–286.
54. Harris J, Kallen B, Robert E. The epidemiology of anotia and microtia. *J Med Genet.* 1996;33(10):809–813.
55. Volpe P, Gentile M. Three-dimensional diagnosis of Goldenhar syndrome. *Ultrasound Obstet Gynecol.* 2004;24(7):798–800.
56. Castori M, Brancati F, Rinaldi R, et al. Antenatal presentation of the oculo-auriculo-vertebral spectrum (OAVS). *Am J Med Genet A.* 2006;140(14):1573–1579.
57. Martinelli P, Maruotti GM, Agangi A, et al. Prenatal diagnosis of hemifacial microsomia and ipsilateral cerebellar hypoplasia in a fetus with oculoauriculovertebral spectrum. *Ultrasound Obstet Gynecol.* 2004;24(2):199–201.
58. Gougoutas AJ, Singh DJ, Low DW, et al. Hemifacial microsomia: clinical features and pictographic representations of the OMENS classification system. *Plast Reconstr Surg.* 2007;120(7):112e–120e.
59. De Catte L, Laubach M, Legein J, et al. Early prenatal diagnosis of oculoauriculovertebral dysplasia or the Goldenhar syndrome. *Ultrasound Obstet Gynecol.* 1996;8(6):422–424.
60. Guzelmansur I, Ceylaner G, Ceylaner S, et al. Prenatal diagnosis of Goldenhar syndrome with unusual features by 3D ultrasonography. *Genet Couns.* 2013;24(3):319–325.
61. Ribeiro B, Igreja J, Goncalves-Rocha M, et al. Goldenhar syndrome: a rare diagnosis with possible prenatal findings. *BMJ Case Rep.* 2016;2016.
62. Hattori Y, Tanaka M, Matsumoto T, et al. Prenatal diagnosis of hemifacial microsomia by magnetic resonance imaging. *J Perinat Med.* 2005;33(1):69–71.
63. Ghi T, Contro E, Carletti A, et al. Prenatal sonographic imaging of Goldenhar syndrome associated with cystic eye. *Prenat Diagn.* 2008;28(4):362–363.
64. Gorlin RJ, Cohen MM, Hennekam RCM, ed. *Syndromes of the Head and Neck.* Oxford, England: Oxford University Press; 2001.
65. Ala-Mello S, Siggberg L, Knuutila S, et al. Further evidence for a relationship between the 5p15 chromosome region and the oculoauriculovertebral anomaly. *Am J Med Genet A.* 2008;146A(19):2490–2494.
66. Dixon M. Treacher Collins syndrome. *Hum Mol Genet.* 1996;5:1391–1396.
67. Trainor PA, Dixon J, Dixon MJ. Treacher Collins syndrome: etiology, pathogenesis and prevention. *Eur J Hum Genet.* 2009;17(3):275–283.
68. Teber OA, Gillessen-Kaesbach G, Fischer S, et al. Genotyping in 46 patients with tentative diagnosis of Treacher Collins syndrome revealed unexpected phenotypic variation. *Eur J Hum Genet.* 2004;12(11):879–890.
69. Tanaka Y, Kanenishi K, Tanaka H, et al. Antenatal three-dimensional sonographic features of Treacher Collins syndrome. *Ultrasound Obstet Gynecol.* 2002;19(4):414–415.
70. Miller M, Fineman R, Smith DW. Postaxial acrofacial dysostosis syndrome. *J Pediatr.* 1979;95(6):970–975.
71. Moessinger AC. Fetal akinesia deformation sequence: an animal model. *Pediatrics.* 1983;72(6):857–863.
72. Duek I, Gil Z, Solt I. Modified ex utero intrapartum treatment procedure in a bicornuate uterus breech presentation Pierre Robin fetus with severe micrognathia and cleft palate. *Clin Case Rep.* 2018;6(11):2040–2044.
73. Thompson JT, Anderson PJ, David DJ. Treacher Collins syndrome: protocol management from birth to maturity. *J Craniofac Surg.* 2009;20(6):2028–2035.

74. Posnick JC. Treacher Collins syndrome: perspectives in evaluation and treatment. *J Oral Maxillofac Surg*. 1997;55(10):1120–1133.

75. Hayashi T, Sasaki S, Oyama A, et al. New grading system for patients with Treacher Collins syndrome. *J Craniofac Surg*. 2007;18(1):113–119.

76. da Silva Dalben G, Costa B, Gomide MR. Prevalence of dental anomalies, ectopic eruption and associated oral malformations in subjects with Treacher Collins syndrome. *Oral Surg Oral Med Oral Pathol Oral Radiol Endod*. 2006;101(5):588–592.

77. Bernier FP, Caluseriu O, Ng S, et al. Haploinsufficiency of SF3B4, a component of the pre-mRNA spliceosomal complex, causes Nager syndrome. *Am J Hum Genet*. 2012;90(5):925–933.

78. Richieri-Costa A, Gollop TR, Colletto GM. Brief clinical report: syndrome of acrofacial dysostosis, cleft lip/palate, and triphalangeal thumb in a Brazilian family. *Am J Med Genet*. 1983;14(2):225–229.

79. Aylsworth AS, Lin AE, Friedman PA. Nager acrofacial dysostosis: male-to-male transmission in 2 families. *Am J Med Genet*. 1991;41(1):83–88.

80. Schlieve T, Almusa M, Miloro M, et al. Temporomandibular joint replacement for ankylosis correction in Nager syndrome: case report and review of the literature. *J Oral Maxillofac Surg*. 2012;70(3):616–625.

81. Petit F, Escande F, Jourdain AS, et al. Nager syndrome: confirmation of SF3B4 haploinsufficiency as the major cause. *Clin Genet*. 2014;86(3):246–251.

82. McDonald MT, Gorski JL. Nager acrofacial dysostosis. *J Med Genet*. 1993;30(9):779–782.

83. Czeschik JC, Voigt C, Alanay Y, et al. Clinical and mutation data in 12 patients with the clinical diagnosis of Nager syndrome. *Hum Genet*. 2013;132(8):885–898.

84. Paladini D, Tartaglione A, Lamberti A, et al. Prenatal ultrasound diagnosis of Nager syndrome. *Ultrasound Obstet Gynecol*. 2003;21(2):195–197.

85. Ansart-Franquet H, Houfflin-Debarge V, Ghoumid J, et al. Prenatal diagnosis of Nager syndrome in a monochorionic-diamniotic twin pregnancy. *Prenat Diagn*. 2009;29(2):187–189.

86. Couyoumjian CA, Treadwell MC, Barr M. Prenatal sonographic diagnosis of Nager acrofacial dysostosis with unilateral upper limb involvement. *Prenat Diagn*. 2008;28(10):964–966.

87. Palomeque A, Pastor X, Ballesta F. Nager anomaly with severe facial involvement, microcephaly, and mental retardation. *Am J Med Genet*. 1990;36(3):356–357.

88. Luquetti DV, Hing AV, Rieder MJ, et al. Mandibulofacial dysostosis with microcephaly caused by EFTUD2 mutations: Expanding the phenotype. *Am J Med Genet Part A*. 2012;161A:108–113.

89. Lines M, Hartley T, Boycott KM. Mandibulofacial dysostosis with microcephaly. In: Adam MP, Ardinger HH, Pagon RA, et al., eds. *GeneReviews*®. Seattle, WA: University of Washington; 2014.

90. Fenton OM, Watt-Smith SR. The spectrum of the oro-facial digital syndrome. *Br J Plast Surg*. 1985;38(4):532–539.

91. Toriello HV. Oral-facial-digital syndromes, 1992. *Clin Dysmorphol*. 1993;2(2):95–105.

92. Toriello HV. Are the oral-facial-digital syndromes ciliopathies? *Am J Med Genet A*. 2009;149A(5):1089–1095.

93. Gurrieri F, Franco B, Toriello H, et al. Oral-facial-digital syndromes: review and diagnostic guidelines. *Am J Med Genet A*. 2007;143A(24):3314–3323.

94. Thauvin-Robinet C, Cossee M, Cormier-Daire V, et al. Clinical, molecular, and genotype-phenotype correlation studies from 25 cases of oral-facial-digital syndrome type 1: a French and Belgian collaborative study. *J Med Genet*. 2006;43(1):54–61.

95. Sakakibara N, Morisada N, Nozu K, et al. Clinical spectrum of male patients with OFD1 mutations. *J Hum Genet*. 2019;64(1):3–9.

96. Macca M, Franco B. The molecular basis of oral-facial-digital syndrome, type 1. *Am J Med Genet C Semin Med Genet*. 2009;151C(4):318–325.

97. Field M, Scheffer IE, Gill D, et al. Expanding the molecular basis and phenotypic spectrum of X-linked Joubert syndrome associated with OFD1 mutations. *Eur J Hum Genet*. 2012;20(7):806–809.

98. Ferrante MI, Giorgio G, Feather SA, et al. Identification of the gene for oral-facial-digital type I syndrome. *Am J Hum Genet*. 2001;68(3):569–576.

99. Toriello HV, Franco B, Bruel AL, et al. Oral-facial-digital syndrome type I. In: Adam MP, Ardinger HH, Pagon RA, et al., eds. *GeneReviews*®. Seattle, WA: University of Washington; 1993.

100. McLaughlin K, Neilly JB, Fox JG, et al. The hypertensive young lady with renal cysts—it is not always polycystic kidney disease. *Nephrol Dial Transplant*. 2000;15(8):1245–1247.

101. Shipp TD, Chu GC, Benacerraf B. Prenatal diagnosis of oral-facial-digital syndrome, type I. *J Ultrasound Med*. 2000;19(7):491–494.

102. Alby C, Boutaud L, Bonniere M, et al. In utero ultrasound diagnosis of corpus callosum agenesis leading to the identification of orofaciodigital type 1 syndrome in female fetuses. *Birth Defects Res*. 2018;110(4):382–389.

103. Coll E, Torra R, Pascual J, et al. Sporadic orofaciodigital syndrome type I presenting as end-stage renal disease. *Nephrol Dial Transplant*. 1997;12(5):1040–1042.

104. Poretti A, Brehmer U, Scheer I, et al. Prenatal and neonatal MR imaging findings in oral-facial-digital syndrome type VI. *AJNR Am J Neuroradiol*. 2008;29(6):1090–1091.

105. Stephan MJ, Brooks KL, Moore DC, et al. Hypothalamic hamartoma in oral-facial-digital syndrome type VI (Varadi syndrome). *Am J Med Genet*. 1994;51(2):131–136.

106. Muenke M, Ruchelli ED, Rorke LB, et al. On lumping and splitting: a fetus with clinical findings of the oral-facial-digital syndrome type VI, the hydrolethalus syndrome, and the Pallister-Hall syndrome. *Am J Med Genet*. 1991;41(4):548–556.

107. Lee JE, Gleeson JG. A systems-biology approach to understanding the ciliopathy disorders. *Genome Med*. 2011;3(9):59.

The ear develops as three distinct connected components: the external ear (formed by the auricle and the external auditory canal), the middle ear, and the inner ear. The focus of this chapter is on the most visible component of the external ear, the auricle (aka pinna or ear). Although auricle abnormalities can be an isolated event, they are frequently seen in association with other ear anomalies, facial malformations (including branchial arch syndromes), syndromic conditions, and chromosomal defects. In other cases, underlying environmental factors such as retinoid acid, alcohol, thalidomide, and maternal diabetes are at fault. Neural crest cells are essential for the formation of the face and neck, including the auricles, and also for the development of aortic and pulmonary arteries. For this reason, otofacial malformations can be seen in association with conotruncal defects, such as in the context of 22q11.2 deletion (DiGeorge syndrome), hemifacial macrosomia/oculo-auriculo-vertebral, and CHARGE syndromes as well as with exposures to retinoic acid and thalidomide.[1]

Ultrasound (US) and three-dimensional (3D) US are useful in the evaluation of size, position, orientation, and structure of the fetal auricle, unless the amniotic fluid is low or the fetal position is unfavorable. Fetal magnetic resonance imaging (MRI) can also provide further assessment of the external auditory canal, middle, and inner ear structures (Fig. 21.1).[2]

EMBRYOLOGY

The external ear starts developing between 40th and 45th day from mesenchymal hillocks 1 through 6, derived from the first and second branchial arches and first pharyngeal cleft. By 12 weeks, the hillocks have fused, and by 16 weeks, the auricle development is complete (Fig. 21.2). The position of the external ear will change during this process. It is initially located in the ventral lower neck region with horizontal long axis but, in its final stage, by 20 weeks, will lie on the side of the head at the level of the eyes in a vertical long axis. This change in position and rotation is due to differential growth between facial structures and the development of the mandible. Mild residual posterior angulation of the auricles (between 10° and 20°) represents a normal variation.[3]

The external auditory canal forms from the dorsal aspect of the first branchial cleft. By the 12th week, a solid epithelial proliferation, the meatal plug, forms at the end of this meatus and, by the 7th month, dissolves, with subsequent development of the eardrum. At the time of birth, the tympanic membrane is nearly horizontal in orientation, and the external auditory canal is short. The tympanic membrane reaches its definitive, more vertical position during the third year of life. The external auditory canal continues to elongate and attains its adult size by 9 to 10 years.

The tympanic cavity is derived from the first branchial pouch and the ossicles from cartilage of the first (malleus and incus) and second (stapes) branchial arches. The ossicles are fully formed by the 15th week, although, until the 28th week, the surrounding mesenchyma is not completely reabsorbed. At birth, some mesenchymal tissue can remain in the tympanic space, although it is soon completely replaced by air.

The development of the inner ear starts at 21 to 24 days of gestation with the development of the otic placode, which soon invaginates to form the otocyst (aka otic vesicle). At 5 to 6 weeks, diverticulum buds from the otocyst form the endolymphatic sac and, subsequently, the cochlea and the vestibule. At 7 to 8 weeks, the semicircular canals also start developing. The superior canal develops first, followed by the posterior and then by the lateral semicircular canal. The adult configuration of the cochlea is completed at 11 weeks. The otocyst also induces the surrounding mesenchyma to form cartilage around the membranous labyrinth (cochlea, vestibule, semicircular canals, and endolymphatic duct and sac) and eventually forms the bony otic capsule, which fully develops to its adult size by 21 weeks. Other structures such as the vestibular aqueduct and internal auditory canal continue to grow after birth, and by 3 years of age, the vestibular aqueduct will reach its adult size.[4]

AURICLE ANOMALIES

Auricle anomalies are not uncommon and can be detected in utero through a meticulous analysis of the face. Malformations of the auricle can, among others, affect **size** (normally formed auricle but small or large), **shape/underdevelopment** (microtia–anotia spectrum), and **position** (low-set and/or posteriorly rotated auricles). Anterior to the auricle, ear tags and ear pits can develop and may be found more frequently after birth. Ear tags are auricle appendages are more frequently present in isolation, although they may be associated with other ear malformations or an underlying syndrome. Preauricular pits are frequently associated with preauricular tags as isolated defects or in the context of a syndrome.[5]

Normal Auricle with Abnormal Size

Auricle length is determined by measuring the length from the superior helix to the tip of the lobule and can be compared with normal standards based on gestational age (Table 21.1).[6] A number of papers have addressed the fetal auricle length.[6–11] When the auricle is morphologically normal but the length is at two standard deviations or more below the mean, it is considered small. Small but structurally normal auricles have been described in the context of trisomy 21 and other chromosomal defects, although this is not specific enough to be used as a single identifying parameter.[12] More recently, Ginsberg et al. reported the use of 3D US rendering mode to further help in identifying fetuses at high risk for autosomal trisomies, assessing not only the length but also the auricle morphology, level of insertion, and auricle angle.[13] Macrotia denotes an increased length of the auricle above the 97th percentile on standard curves and is frequently seen in association with increased protrusion. Most cases are isolated and symmetric, but macrotia has also been reported in Marfan, cerebro-oculo-facio-skeletal, and Fragile X syndromes and chromosomal defects.[14]

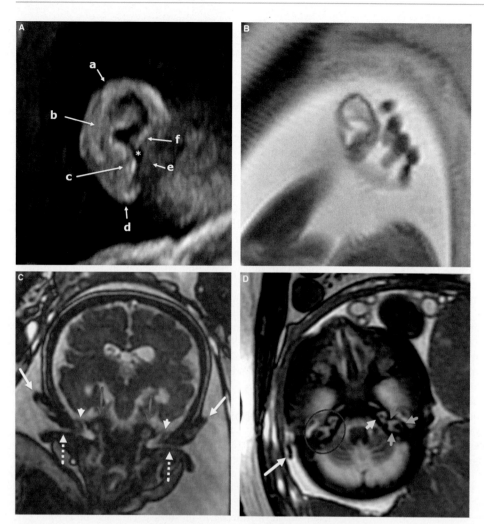

FIGURE 21.1: Normal fetal ear anatomy. US **(A)** and SSFP fetal MRI **(B)** parasagittal view of a normal auricle at 28 weeks' gestation. Helix (a), antihelix (b), antitragus (c), lobule (d), tragus (e), crus (f), and external acoustic meatus (*asterisk*). Additional coronal **(C)** and axial **(D)** SSFP fetal MRI views at 31 weeks' gestation. Auricle (*arrow*), external auditory canal (*dashed arrow*), middle ear (*arrowhead*) and inner ear structures (*red arrow and red circle*), cochlea (*yellow arrow*), vestibule (*blue arrow*), and semicircular canals (*green arrows*).

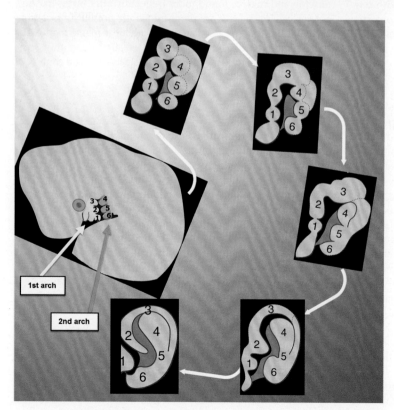

FIGURE 21.2: Diagrammatic representation of the normal auricle development.

TABLE 21.1	Ultrasound Percentile Reference Values for Ear Length						
	EAR LENGTH (mm)				EAR LENGTH (mm)		
	PERCENTILES				PERCENTILES		
GESTATIONAL AGE (wk)	5TH	50TH	95TH	GESTATIONAL AGE (wk)	5TH	50TH	95TH
15	7	9	11	28	18	24	28
16	8	10	12	29	19	25	29
17	9	11	13	30	20	26	30
18	10	12	14	31	21	27	31
19	11	13	16	32	22	28	32
20	11	15	17	33	22	28	33
21	12	16	18	34	23	29	34
22	13	17	19	35	24	30	35
23	14	18	21	36	25	30	36
24	15	19	22	37	25	31	37
25	16	20	24	38	26	31	37
26	17	22	26	39	27	32	38
27	18	23	27	40	27	32	38

Ratio biparietal diameter/ear length is 3.03 (standard deviation, 0.29), independent of gestational age.

Reprinted from Chitkara U, Lee L, El-Sayed YY, et al. Ultrasonographic ear length measurement in normal second- and third-trimester fetuses. *Am J Obstet Gynecol.* 2000;183(1):230–234. Copyright © 2000 Elsevier. With permission.
Reproduced with permission from Shimizu T, Salvador L, Allanson J, et al. Ultrasonographic measurements of fetal ear. *Obstet Gynecol.* 1992;80(3, pt 1):381–384.

Microtia/Anotia

The spectrum of auricle hypoplasia is graded from its mildest form, microtia type I, to microtia type IV, which reflects complete absence of the auricle or anotia (Fig. 21.3).[15] The defect may be unilateral or bilateral. Microtias type I to III can occasionally have associated preauricular tags, and type II or higher are frequently associated with external auditory canal atresia (aka aural or meatal atresia). The degree of hearing loss will depend on the presence of aural atresia and other middle or inner ear associated defects.[16]

Incidence: Incidence varies between ethnic groups, and males are affected twice more often than females. In general, the estimated average incidence of microtia is 1 to 2 in 10,000 in the Western world. However, it has been reported to be as low as 1 in 500 to 3,000 in South America.[17]

Pathogenesis/Etiology: It is believed that alteration in the neural crest cell migration from the hindbrain to the first and second branchial arches is responsible for a large number of craniofacial malformations that involve the ear and the face.[18] The etiology

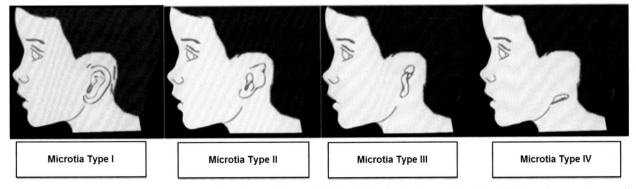

| Microtia Type I | Microtia Type II | Microtia Type III | Microtia Type IV |

FIGURE 21.3: Microtia grading. Type I: mild hypoplasia of the auricle. Type II: longitudinal mass of cartilage. "S" shaped or question-mark appearance. Type III: small rudimentary "peanut"-shaped soft tissue and no external ear canal. Type IV: absent auricle or anotia and no external ear canal.

of microtia is heterogeneous. Most cases of microtia/anotia are isolated, with a positive family history found less than 10% of the time. Forty percent of patients with microtia have associated anomalies or an identifiable syndrome, including branchial arch syndromes. Microtia type I is frequent in trisomy 21 and types II through IV in trisomies 18 and 13. Other chromosomal defects reported in association with microtia include trisomy 22 as well as mosaicism of trisomies 13 and 18, and aneusomies, as in deletion of 4p, 5p, 18p, 18q, and 22q11.2.[19,20] In other cases, a teratogen exposure such as retinoic acid, thalidomide, alcohol, or maternal diabetes is considered at fault.[16]

Diagnosis: The auricle presents different degrees of hypoplasia or is completely absent. Aural atresia as well as other craniofacial defects may also be present.[21]

Differential Diagnosis: Epidermolysis bullosa and Harlequin ichthyosis, when affecting the skin around the auricles, could mimic microtia. The presence of layering particles within the amniotic fluid, from sloughed skin, has been described in both conditions. The detection of focal areas of skin thinning and gastric outlet obstruction (pyloric atresia) in the same fetus would be useful clues to suggest epidermolysis bullosa.[22,23] The most constant imaging findings in Harlequin ichthyosis include large gaping mouth, dysplastic or swollen hands and feet, absent nose, and bulging eyes.[24] Genetic testing can further assist in the prenatal diagnosis of these skin conditions.[25,26]

Prognosis/Management: Microtia/anotia is problematic not only in the social setting but also because of common hearing loss. When it is not isolated, the prognosis and management will be guided by the type of underlying condition and extension of the defects.

Associated Anomalies: Further evaluation of the face and the rest of the fetal anatomy should be obtained in order to assess for a possible chromosomal or syndromic condition, including branchial arch syndromes (also referred to as otomandibular dysplasias).[27] The most frequent branchial arch syndrome with

unilateral or asymmetric distribution is hemifacial macrosomia/oculo-auriculo-vertebral spectrum. When the defects are bilateral, Treacher Collins syndrome (TCS), among others, should be entertained. A more detailed discussion of these two syndromes and main differential considerations are presented below.

Hemifacial Microsomia/Oculo-auriculo-vertebral Spectrum

Hemifacial microsomia is a condition in which there are unilateral auricle anomalies (microtia/anotia) and unilateral underdevelopment of the craniofacial bony structures. In 30% of cases, findings are bilateral but typically asymmetric. The term *oculo-auriculo-vertebral spectrum* (aka Goldenhar syndrome or Goldenhar–Gorlin syndrome) is used when ocular (epibulbar dermoid, upper eyelid coloboma, microphthalmia/anophthalmia) and vertebral anomalies (segmentation or dysraphic defects) are also present. Other associated malformations include cleft lip or palate (up to 15%), cardiac defects (tetralogy of Fallot, double-outlet right ventricle, ventricular septal defects, total anomalous pulmonary venous return, and even heterotaxy), renal/gastrointestinal anomalies, and lung hypoplasia/agenesis.[28,29]

Incidence/Etiology: It is the second most common facial defect after cleft lip and palate and affects males almost twice as often as females. The prevalence of oculo-auriculo-vertebral spectrum is 1 in 3,500 to 6,000 live births. Most cases are sporadic, but some familial cases exhibit autosomal dominant or autosomal recessive inheritance (1% to 2%). Nongenetic factors have been also linked to this defect, including maternal diabetes and exposure to vasoactive medications.[29,30]

Imaging Diagnosis: There will be some combination of facial asymmetry and ipsilateral microtia/anotia. Additional facial anomalies involving the eyes, such as microphthalmia/anophthalmia, and facial cleft can be present. Polyhydramnios may be present due to ineffective fetal swallowing or associated gastrointestinal anomalies such as esophageal atresia. Segmentation anomalies should be suspected if there is a persistent associated spinal curvature (Fig. 21.4).[31]

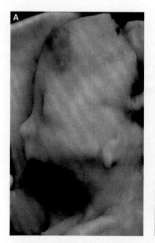 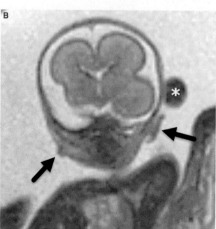 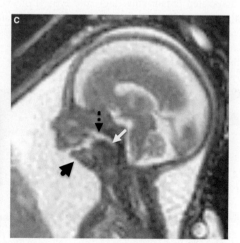

FIGURE 21.4: A 23-week fetus with Goldenhar syndrome. **A:** 3D US surface rendering image showing severe microtia with a small low-set dysmorphic auricle as well as micrognathia. **B, C:** Coronal and sagittal SSFP MRI. There are asymmetric auricles (*black arrows*), small and low-set on the right, micrognathia (*black arrowhead*), cleft palate (*black dashed arrow*), and glossoptosis (*white arrow*). The left upper extremity (*asterisk*) is incidentally noted. Right eye corneal lipodermoid was detected on ophthalmological examination after birth. No other systemic associations were present.

Differential Diagnosis: Branchio-oto-renal syndrome could present with similar facial features plus presence of a branchial cleft cyst or sinus in the neck.[32]

Prognosis/Management: The prognosis will depend on the presence of associated anomalies as well as the impact of the primary anomalies on the airway, auditory, and feeding functions. These children will require longitudinal interdisciplinary team care. Spine radiographs, renal US, and echocardiogram should be obtained after birth.[33]

Recurrence Risk: The risk is not known, but it would be increased in families of affected individuals who have a karyotype anomaly. Different chromosomal alterations have been reported with higher involvement of chromosomal regions 22q and 5p, mosaic trisomies of chromosomes 9 and 22, chromosome X aneuploidy, and, more recently, chromosomal imbalances in chromosomes 4 and 22.[30,34–40] If there is a negative family history, the recurrence risk is low (2% to 3%).[28]

Treacher Collins Syndrome

Treacher Collins Syndrome (TCS), also referred to as Treacher Collins–Franceschetti syndrome and mandibulofacial dysostosis, is characterized by symmetric distribution of facial defects, including microtia/anotia, deformity or absence of the external auditory canal, hypoplastic facial bones (zygomatic, maxillary, and mandibular bones), downslanting palpebral fissures, lower eyelid colobomas, and frequently cleft palate. The nose may be broad or protruding. Limb anomalies do not occur in TCS.[28,41]

Incidence/Etiology: TCS occurs in 1 in 50,000 live births. It is inherited in an autosomal dominant manner, with variable penetrance and phenotypic variable expression. Sixty percent of the cases represent new mutations. Mutations in the *TCOF1* gene, mapped to 5q32–q33.1, are found in most cases. Two additional genes, *POLR1D* and *POLR1C*, have been also identified. These three genes are typically evaluated if genetic testing is performed.[42,43] A very small proportion of cases (1%) are inherited in a recessive manner due to mutations in *POLR1C*.[43]

Imaging Diagnosis: US, especially 3D rendering mode, and fetal MRI can detect TCS. There is bilateral microtia or anotia and frequently aural atresia. The amniotic fluid is increased, as

expected in the context of micrognathia. There is midface hypoplasia, and cleft palate is frequently present (Fig. 21.5).[2,44–49]

Differential Diagnosis: Facial features resembling TCS can be present in fetuses with acrofacial dysostosis, although auricle anomalies are not typically as severe, and limb malformations, absent in TCS, will be expected in these syndromes. In Nager syndrome, there are preaxial digital anomalies such as hypoplastic or absent thumbs, and different degrees of radial ray deficiency.[50,51] Postaxial defects, such as the absence of the fifth digit/toe, and ulnar deficiency are described in Miller syndrome.[52]

Prognosis/Management: The prognosis depends on the severity of the phenotype expressed. When the degree of mandibular hypoplasia is severe, an ex utero intrapartum treatment (EXIT) procedure to tracheostomy at the time of delivery may be required to secure an airway.[53] The array of craniofacial defects in TCS can affect the form or function of the eyes, ears, nose, facial bones, and airway, and their management will be optimized through a multidisciplinary team approach.[54]

Recurrence Risk: TCS has a well-defined mode of inheritance, with up to 60% of the cases reflecting de novo mutations. The penetrance of the underlying mutations is high but with marked inter- and intrafamilial phenotypic variability. For this reason, parental molecular testing will help to define the recurrence risk for future pregnancies.[55]

Malposition of the Auricle

Low-set ears are auricles located low on the lateral face and, most of the time, also posteriorly rotated. In normal conditions, a perpendicular line to the lateral aspect of the orbit (outer canthi of the eye) should cross near the superior attachment of the auricle once the face and auricle have been completely formed (Fig. 21.6). Low-set ears can be seen as a common feature of many syndromes and trisomies, secondary to the effects of oligohydramnios/anhydramnios, and as a developmental arrest in association with different degrees of mandibular hypoplasia such as in 22q11.2 deletion (DiGeorge syndrome), Pierre Robin sequence, and skeletal dysplasias. In Townes–Brocks syndrome, both auricles are small with overfolded superior helix (lop/cup ear) and low set in combination with hand anomaly (triphalangeal or bifid thumb or preaxial

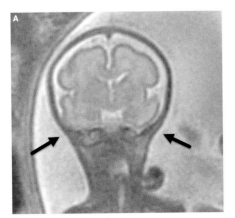
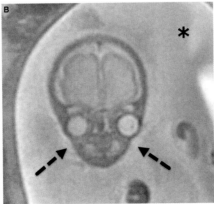
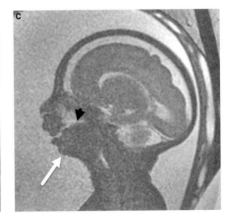

FIGURE 21.5: Treacher Collins syndrome in a 29-week fetus. Fetal MRI SSFSE T2 **(A, B)** and sagittal SSFP **(C)** images showing the absence of the auricles and external auditory canals (*black arrows*), midface (*dashed arrows*) and mandibular hypoplasia (*white arrow*), cleft palate (*arrowhead*), and polyhydramnios (*asterisk*).

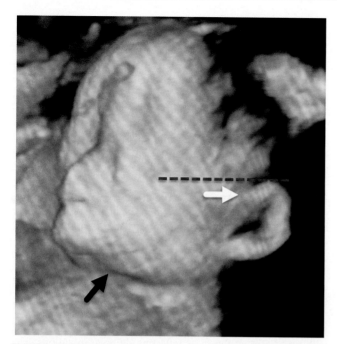

FIGURE 21.6: 3D US surface rendering image showing low-set ear in a 25-week fetus. The superior attachment of the auricle (*white arrow*) is caudal to a line traced from the outer cantus of the eye. There is associated micrognathia (*black arrow*).

polydactyly) and anorectal malformations.[56] Low-set and/or posteriorly rotated auricle is the most consistent external ear finding in CHARGE syndrome, and sometimes, a small lop/cup or "folded" ear with absent lobe or triangular concha may be seen.[5,57]

Otocephaly

Otocephaly represents the most extreme form of auricle malposition. This malformation consists of marked underdevelopment or almost complete absence of the mandible and malformed auricles in an anterior, caudal, and more horizontal position, near the midline. A very small or even absent oral opening is a consistent feature with potential additional levels of upper airway obstruction, such as persistence of the buccopharyngeal membrane and choanal atresia as well as absent or hypoplastic tongue. In the most severe form, little more than the abnormal auricles are apparent on the face. *Agnathia–otocephaly complex* or *agnathia–microstomia-synotia complex* are other terms used to describe this condition. Otocephaly may occur alone or in association with other malformations, including holoprosencephaly and heterotaxy.[58]

Incidence: It affects nearly equally both genders, with an incidence of less than 1 in 70,000 births.[59]

Pathogenesis/Etiology: Otocephaly is a first branchial arch defect believed to result from alteration in neural crest cell migration. Multiple etiologies can contribute to this pathogenesis. Several medications such as theophylline, corticosteroids, rufochromomycin, bruneomycin, and trypan blue may increase the risk among pregnancies.[60,61] Genetic etiologies include the absence or abnormal expression of the *PRRX1* gene (chromosome 1q23) and diminished expression of bone morphogenetic

protein 4 and transforming growth factor-beta. The transcriptional factor *OTX2* (chromosome 14q23) is also thought to be implicated.[59,62–65]

Imaging Diagnosis: This malformation can be associated with polyhydramnios due to impaired swallowing and airway obstruction but not always.[66] Prenatal detection with US, 3D US, and fetal MRI has been reported and will require a careful assessment of the face. The mandible is severely hypoplastic or absent, with abnormal auricles in the usual position of the mandible (melotia) or even auricular fusion (synotia) (Fig. 21.7). There is microstomia (small mouth) and other facial malformations affecting the eyes (hypotelorism, cyclopia, unilateral/bilateral microphthalmia/anophthalmia, short and laterally downward-sloping palpebral fissures) and nose (proboscis, large nose) as well as facial clefts possible. Prenatal detection is typically reported during the second and third trimesters, although it may be possible in the first trimester.[67–70]

Differential Diagnosis: Less extreme forms of mandibular hypoplasia could impair the fetal swallowing and be associated with polyhydramnios. The auricles tend to be low set but not horizontally rotated in the ventral neck as in otocephaly. Fetuses with *hypomandibular faciocranial dysostosis* may resemble otocephaly, but the auricles are only low set, and there are additional features such as craniosynostosis, midface hypoplasia, and prominent eyes.[71]

Associated Anomalies: The most frequent association is holoprosencephaly, but skeletal, genitourinary, and cardiovascular defects, including heterotaxy, may be present.[58]

Prognosis/Management: Although classically described as a lethal condition due to upper airway obstruction, several new reports describe survival past the first year and even long term.[72–76]

Prenatal detection of otocephaly will allow improved parental counseling of management options and better preparation for the delivery, including the consideration for EXIT. Planning for a premature birth and perinatal tracheostomy and gastrostomy tube would be essential for survival. The postnatal care by a specialized multidisciplinary craniofacial team from birth to adulthood would also be recommended. Facial reconstruction surgeries could possibly improve aesthetics and have a positive psychosocial impact for the patients and their families but will not, with the current therapies available, be able to restore masticatory, swallowing, or articulation functions. Cognition, unless associated with holoprosencephaly, would not be affected.[74]

Recurrent Risk: Otocephaly is sporadic in the majority of reported cases, with no known underlying molecular etiology or known recurrence risk. A balanced translocation involving 6p and 18p was found in the father of two affected siblings, and another report described a case of transmission from an affected mother to her daughter.[77–79]

CHARGE Syndrome

CHARGE syndrome is a variable nonrandom association of anomalies that includes ocular coloboma (C), heart defect (H), choanal atresia (A), retarded growth (R), genitourinary defects and/or hypogonadism (G), and ear anomalies (E), among other defects.[80]

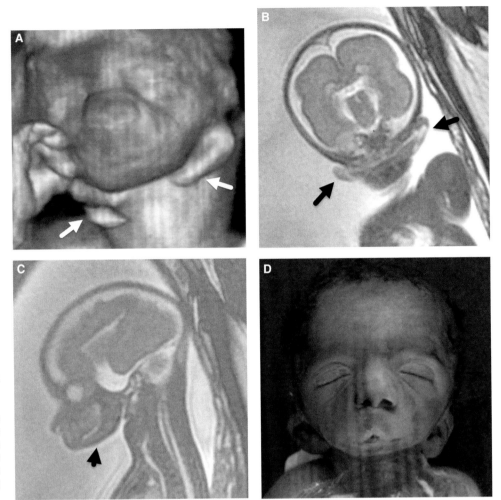

FIGURE 21.7: Otocephaly. 27-week fetus 3-D US coronal surface rendering image **(A)** and Fetal MRI coronal and sagittal SSFP images **(B-C)**. The auricles are horizontally rotated in the ventral neck (*arrows*) and the mandible is severely hypoplastic (*arrowhead*). **E:** Postmortem photograph at 29 weeks (different patient with same features) after unsuccessful intubation.

Incidence: The incidence of CHARGE syndrome has been estimated to range from 1 in 8,500 to 1 in 17,000 live births.[80–82]

Pathogenesis/Etiology: The majority of CHARGE cases occur as a new autosomal dominant condition, with no family history. The chromodomain helicase DNA-binding protein 7 (*CDH7*) has been identified as the major gene involved.[83] Loss-of-function pathogenetic variants of this gene can be seen in 70% to 90% of patients but is not necessary for establishing the diagnosis.[84,85] Most cases in prenatal series have truncated mutations. Missense mutations incidence (resulting in a single-nucleotide change rendering its encoding protein nonfunctional) is higher in postnatal series as they seem to be related to a less severe, less specific phenotype.[86,87] *CHD7* can form complexes with different proteins, including the PBAF (polybromo- and BRG1-associated factor containing complex) that are essential for neural crest gene expression and cell migration, accounting for errors in blastogenesis and neurulation when the *CHD7* protein is affected.[88,89]

Diagnosis: An amniocentesis with gene testing for *CHD7* can be offered and has been described in confirming a prenatally suspected case of CHARGE syndrome. High-resolution chromosomal microarray and exome sequencing using child–parent trios

can detect *CHD7* pathogenic variants.[90] The diagnosis can be also established with clinical criteria (Table 21.2), which is useful in the 10% to 30% of cases that lack mutations in this gene.[80,87,91–93]

Imaging: Postnatal diagnosis is based on clinical findings, temporal bone imaging, and genetic testing. Prenatal suspicion for CHARGE syndrome may be raised by abnormal prenatal US and MRI findings. Legendre et al. described a series of 40 fetuses affected by a *CDH7* gene mutation at autopsy. The most commonly seen findings included bilateral and asymmetric external ear abnormalities manifesting as small low set, posteriorly rotated and triangular- or square-shaped auricles, semicircular canal hypoplasia or agenesis, and arhinencephaly.[87] 2D and 3D US can readily evaluate the auricle; however, sonographic evaluation of the temporal bone is more challenging. Identification of the fetal cochlea caudal to the temporal lobes via US can be obtained in approximately 50% of cases in the second trimester using the fetal anterior fontanelle and coronal plane insonation.[94] The semicircular canals may be identified by second-trimester US as well, although with limited resolution. Fetal MRI has shown to distinguish the cochlea from the semicircular canals, and it also permits the identification of the middle ear after 25 weeks' gestational age and external auditory

TABLE 21.2	Fetal and Postnatal Diagnostic Criteria for CHARGE Syndrome		
	MAJOR CRITERIA	**MINOR CRITERIA**	**INCLUSION RULE**
After birth	• Coloboma • Choanal atresia and/or cleft lip or palate • Abnormal external, middle, or inner ear including semicircular canals dysplasia/aplasia • Arhinencephaly and/or anosmia • Pathogenetic CHD7 mutation	• Cranial nerve dysfunction (VII to XII). This includes hearing loss, dysphagia/feeding difficulties • Hypothalamo-hypophyseal dysfunction (gonadotropin or growth hormone deficiency)/genital anomalies • Heart defects, esophageal anomalies • Developmental delay/intellectual disabilities/autism • Structural brain anomalies • Renal anomalies • Skeletal/limb anomalies	Typical: • 3 major • 2 major + 2 minor Partial: • 2 major + 1 minor Atypical: • 2 major + 0 minor • 1 major + 3 minor Proposed by Hale et al.[91] • 2 major + any number of minor
At fetal or neonatal autopsy (unknown CDH7 mutation status)	• Same criteria as after birth (coloboma, choanal atresia, abnormal external, middle or inner ear, and arrhinencephaly) but also to include heart defects	• Brain, esophageal, renal, skeletal/limb, and genital anomalies (each considered as a criterion like postnatally) • In addition, thymic hypoplasia/agenesis and polyhydramnios are each considered prenatally	Proposed by Legendre: • 4 major • 3 major + 2 minor and absence of intrauterine growth restriction

Among the criteria, semicircular canals hypoplasia/aplasia was introduced by Verloes[93] in 2005, cleft lip/palate by Blake and Prasad[80] in 2006, arrhinencephaly/anosmia by Sanlaville et al.[92] More recently, Hale et al.[91] proposed broadening of the CHARGE clinical diagnosis and include pathogenetic CHD7 variant status as a major criterion. Legendre et al.[87] proposed the clinical criteria at fetal or neonatal autopsy. Interestingly, although postnatal growth retardation is a feature of this syndrome as a consequence of early feeding difficulties, intrauterine growth retardation is not observed.

canals after 28 weeks, with improved resolution as gestational age advances (Fig. 21.1).[2,95] Fetal MRI, performed after 29 weeks, will also depict the olfactory lobes in normal conditions.[96] Assessment of these structures is very important as absence of the olfactory lobes (arhinencephaly) or semicircular canal hypoplasia/agenesis is highly suggestive of CHARGE syndrome (Fig. 21.8).

Prenatal imaging can also define potential presence of coloboma, microphthalmia, choanal atresia, and facial clefts, although 22% of cases reported by Legendre et al. had neither choanal atresia nor facial cleft.[87,97] Brain evaluation may provide more clues to the diagnosis. In addition to arhinencephaly, which is seen in up to 90%, posterior fossa anomalies (predominantly vermian hypoplasia) and ventriculomegaly have been noted in up to 72% in Legendre series.[87] Congenital heart defects have been described in up to 85% of fetal cases with CHARGE syndrome, and these are usually complex and often involving the conotruncal region in combination with septal defects. Polyhydramnios is frequently seen in the context of esophageal defect with tracheoesophageal fistula, with a reported incidence of 10%. Inner and/or external genital anomalies can be seen in both genders (48% in males vs 36% in females), most of them being genital hypoplasia and cryptorchidism. The urinary system can be also affected in up to 28%. In addition, skeletal findings frequently involve the fifth digit of the hands, although the spectrum of limb anomalies is large.[87] Major and minor diagnostic criteria and diagnostic inclusion rules are summarized in Table 21.2.

Differential Diagnosis: Some conditions can mimic CHARGE syndrome, such as 22q11.2 deletion syndrome, VACTERL association, *SOX2* mutations, mandibulofacial dysostosis, Kabuki

syndrome, Joubert syndrome, disorders caused by teratogens (maternal diabetes, Accutane), and Kallmann syndrome.[84,98]

Prognosis: Survival depends on the severity of an individual's phenotype. Cyanotic heart disease, tracheoesophageal fistula, and bilateral choanal atresia have the lowest survival. It is highly recommended that affected infants be delivered at a tertiary care center. Although birth weight and length are normal at birth, the majority of infants experience poor growth during late infancy. Cognitive ability is often impaired.[99]

Management: An infant born with suspected CHARGE syndrome should have a full physical examination. In the newborn period, associated medical conditions can be life-threatening. Airway management typically requires tracheostomy and surgical correction of choanal atresia. Feeding difficulties are common, and evaluation by a speech pathologist should be performed. Need for gastrostomy or jejunostomy is not uncommon. Cardiology consultation, echocardiography, renal US, and hearing screening should be obtained shortly after birth. Long-term needs include hearing and vision evaluations, early and appropriate developmental interventions, assessment for hypogonadism as puberty onset can be delayed, and consideration of airway anomalies if anesthesia is required.[99]

Recurrence Risk: If parents are *unaffected*, recurrence risk is approximately 1% to 2% due to germline mosaicism.[100] If the disease-causing *CDH7* mutation is found in mosaic or nonmosaic form in one of the parents, recurrence risk is increased (up to 50%).[98] The severity of the phenotype in the offspring, however, cannot be predicted because of large intrafamilial variability.[84]

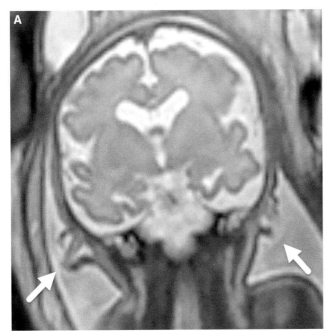

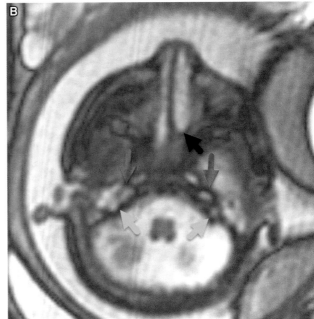

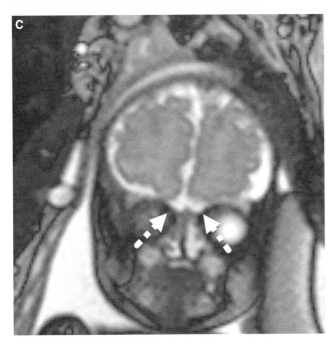

FIGURE 21.8: CHARGE syndrome. A 34-week fetus. **A:** Fetal MRI coronal SSFSE T2 image showing small, low-set auricles (*white arrows*) and mild lateral ventriculomegaly. **B:** Axial SSFP fetal MRI. There is left choanal atresia (*black arrow*) with dilated fluid-filled and blind-ending left nasal cavity. The inner ears are also abnormal with portions of the cochlea (*red arrow*) and vestibule (*green arrows*) seen but absent semicircular canals. **C:** Coronal SSFP fetal MRI along the anterior frontal lobes demonstrating absence of the olfactory bulbs (*white dashed arrows*). This fetus also presented with cardiac defect (double-outlet right ventricle), bilateral hydronephrosis, and undescended testicles (not shown here).

REFERENCES

1. Cox TC, Camci ED, Vora S, et al. The genetics of auricular development and malformation: new findings in model systems driving future directions for microtia research. *Eur J Med Genet.* 2014;57:394–401.
2. Katorza E, Nahama-Allouche C, Castaigne V, et al. Prenatal evaluation of the middle ear and diagnosis of middle ear hypoplasia using MRI. *Pediatr Radiol.* 2011;41:652–657.
3. Kagurasho M, Yamada S, Uwabe C, et al. Movement of the external ear in human embryo. *Head Face Med.* 2012;8:2.
4. Peck JE. Development of hearing. Part II. Embryology. *J Am Acad Audiol.* 1994;5:359–365.
5. Bartel-Friedrich S. Congenital auricular malformations: description of anomalies and syndromes. *Facial Plast Surg.* 2015;31:567–580.
6. Chitkara U, Lee L, El-Sayed YY, et al. Ultrasonographic ear length measurement in normal second- and third-trimester fetuses. *Am J Obstet Gynecol.* 2000;183:230–234.
7. Birnholz JC, Farrell EE. Fetal ear length. *Pediatrics.* 1988;81:555–558.
8. Lettieri L, Rodis JF, Vintzileos AM, et al. Ear length in second-trimester aneuploid fetuses. *Obstet Gynecol.* 1993;81:57–60.
9. Awwad JT, Azar GB, Karam KS, et al. Ear length: a potential sonographic marker for Down syndrome. *Int J Gynaecol Obstet.* 1994;44:233–238.
10. Chitkara U, Lee L, Oehlert JW, et al. Fetal ear length measurement: a useful predictor of aneuploidy? *Ultrasound Obstet Gynecol.* 2002;19:131–135.
11. Joshi KS, Chawla CD, Karki S, et al. Sonographic measurement of fetal pinna length in normal pregnancies. *Kathmandu Univ Med J (KUMJ).* 2011;9:49–53.
12. Chang CH, Chang FM, Yu CH, et al. Fetal ear assessment and prenatal detection of aneuploidy by the quantitative three-dimensional ultrasonography. *Ultrasound Med Biol.* 2000;26:743–749.
13. Ginsberg NA, Cohen L, Dungan JS, et al. 3-D ultrasound of the fetal ear and fetal autosomal trisomies: a pilot study of a new screening protocol. *Prenat Diagn.* 2011;31:311–314.
14. Nagarajan M, Sharbidre KG, Bhabad SH, et al. MR imaging of the fetal face: comprehensive review. *Radiographics.* 2018;38:962–980.
15. Alasti F, Van Camp G. Genetics of microtia and associated syndromes. *J Med Genet.* 2009;46:361–369.
16. Luquetti DV, Heike CL, Hing AV, et al. Microtia: epidemiology and genetics. *Am J Med Genet A.* 2012;158A:124–139.
17. Castilla EE, Orioli IM. Prevalence rates of microtia in South America. *Int J Epidemiol.* 1986;15:364–368.
18. Johnston MC, Bronsky PT. Prenatal craniofacial development: new insights on normal and abnormal mechanisms. *Crit Rev Oral Biol Med.* 1995;6:368–422.
19. Giannatou E, Leze H, Katana A, et al. Unilateral microtia in an infant with trisomy 18 mosaicism. *Genet Couns.* 2009;20:181–187.

20. Griffith CB, Vance GH, Weaver DD. Phenotypic variability in trisomy 13 mosaicism: two new patients and literature review. *Am J Med Genet A.* 2009;149A:1346–1358.
21. Milic A, Blaser S, Robinson A, et al. Prenatal detection of microtia by MRI in a fetus with trisomy 22. *Pediatr Radiol.* 2006;36:706–710.
22. Lepinard C, Descamps P, Meneguzzi G, et al. Prenatal diagnosis of pyloric atresia-junctional epidermolysis bullosa syndrome in a fetus not known to be at risk. *Prenat Diagn.* 2000;20:70–75.
23. Merrow AC, Frischer JS, Lucky AW. Pyloric atresia with epidermolysis bullosa: fetal MRI diagnosis with postnatal correlation. *Pediatr Radiol.* 2013;43:1656–1661.
24. Berg C, Geipel A, Kohl M, et al. Prenatal sonographic features of Harlequin ichthyosis. *Arch Gynecol Obstet.* 2003;268:48–51.
25. Kelsell DP, Norgett EE, Unsworth H, et al. Mutations in ABCA12 underlie the severe congenital skin disease harlequin ichthyosis. *Am J Hum Genet.* 2005;76:794–803.
26. Fassihi H, Eady RA, Mellerio JE, et al. Prenatal diagnosis for severe inherited skin disorders: 25 years' experience. *Br J Dermatol.* 2006;154:106–113.
27. Stoll C, Alembik Y, Dott B, et al. Associated anomalies in cases with anotia and microtia. *Eur J Med Genet.* 2016;59:607–614.
28. Passos-Bueno MR, Ornelas CC, Fanganiello RD. Syndromes of the first and second pharyngeal arches: a review. *Am J Med Genet A.* 2009;149A:1853–1859.
29. Barisic I, Odak L, Loane M, et al. Prevalence, prenatal diagnosis and clinical features of oculo-auriculo-vertebral spectrum: a registry-based study in Europe. *Eur J Hum Genet.* 2014;22:1026–1033.
30. Bragagnolo S, Colovati MES, Souza MZ, et al. Clinical and cytogenomic findings in OAV spectrum. *Am J Med Genet A.* 2018;176:638–648.
31. Haratz K, Vinkler C, Lev D, et al. Hemifacial microsomia with spinal and rib anomalies: prenatal diagnosis and postmortem confirmation using 3-D computed tomography reconstruction. *Fetal Diagn Ther.* 2011;30:309–313.
32. Kochhar A, Fischer SM, Kimberling WJ, et al. Branchio-oto-renal syndrome. *Am J Med Genet A.* 2007;143A:1671–1678.
33. Heike CL, Hing AV, Aspinall CA, et al. Clinical care in craniofacial microsomia: a review of current management recommendations and opportunities to advance research. *Am J Med Genet C Semin Med Genet.* 2013;163C:271–282.
34. Ladekarl S. Combination of Goldenhar's syndrome with the Cri-Du-Chat syndrome. *Acta Ophthalmol (Copenh).* 1968;46:605–610.
35. Wilson GN, Barr M Jr. Trisomy 9 mosaicism: another etiology for the manifestations of Goldenhar syndrome. *J Craniofac Genet Dev Biol.* 1983;3:313–316.
36. Garavelli L, Virdis R, Donadio A, et al. Oculo-auriculo-vertebral spectrum in Klinefelter syndrome. *Genet Couns.* 1999;10:321–324.
37. de Ravel TJ, Legius E, Brems H, et al. Hemifacial microsomia in two patients further supporting chromosomal mosaicism as a causative factor. *Clin Dysmorphol.* 2001;10:263–267.
38. Descartes M. Oculoauriculovertebral spectrum with 5p15.33-pter deletion. *Clin Dysmorphol.* 2006;15:153–154.
39. Digilio MC, McDonald-McGinn DM, Heike C, et al. Three patients with oculo-auriculo-vertebral spectrum and microdeletion 22q11.2. *Am J Med Genet A.* 2009;149A:2860–2864.
40. Ala-Mello S, Siggberg L, Knuutila S, et al. Further evidence for a relationship between the 5p15 chromosome region and the oculoauriculovertebral anomaly. *Am J Med Genet A.* 2008;146A:2490–2494.
41. Johnson JM, Moonis G, Green GE, et al. Syndromes of the first and second branchial arches, part 1: embryology and characteristic defects. *AJNR Am J Neuroradiol.* 2011;32:14–19.
42. Dauwerse JG, Dixon J, Seland S, et al. Mutations in genes encoding subunits of RNA polymerases I and III cause Treacher Collins syndrome. *Nat Genet.* 2011;43:20–22.
43. Kadakia S, Helman SN, Badhey AK, et al. Treacher Collins Syndrome: the genetics of a craniofacial disease. *Int J Pediatr Otorhinolaryngol.* 2014;78:893–898.
44. Cohen J, Ghezzi F, Goncalves L, et al. Prenatal sonographic diagnosis of Treacher Collins syndrome: a case and review of the literature. *Am J Perinatol.* 1995;12:416–419.
45. Crane JP, Beaver HA. Midtrimester sonographic diagnosis of mandibulofacial dysostosis. *Am J Med Genet.* 1986;25:251–255.
46. Meizner I, Carmi R, Katz M. Prenatal ultrasonic diagnosis of mandibulofacial dysostosis (Treacher Collins syndrome). *J Clin Ultrasound.* 1991;19:124–127.
47. Milligan DA, Harlass FE, Duff P, et al. Recurrence of Treacher Collins' syndrome with sonographic findings. *Mil Med.* 1994;159:250–252.
48. Ochi H, Matsubara K, Ito M, et al. Prenatal sonographic diagnosis of Treacher Collins syndrome. *Obstet Gynecol.* 1998;91:862.
49. Tanaka Y, Kanenishi K, Tanaka H, et al. Antenatal three-dimensional sonographic features of Treacher Collins syndrome. *Ultrasound Obstet Gynecol.* 2002;19:414–415.
50. Paladini D, Tartaglione A, Lamberti A, et al. Prenatal ultrasound diagnosis of Nager syndrome. *Ultrasound Obstet Gynecol.* 2003;21:195–197.
51. Ansart-Franquet H, Houfflin-Debarge V, Ghoumid J, et al. Prenatal diagnosis of Nager syndrome in a monochorionic-diamniotic twin pregnancy. *Prenat Diagn.* 2009;29:187–189.
52. Verrotti C, Benassi G, Piantelli G, et al. Acrofacial dysostosis syndromes: a relevant prenatal dilemma. A case report and brief literature review. *J Matern Fetal Neonatal Med.* 2007;20:487–490.
53. Trainor PA, Andrews BT. Facial dysostoses: etiology, pathogenesis and management. *Am J Med Genet C Semin Med Genet.* 2013;163C:283–294.
54. Thompson JT, Anderson PJ, David DJ. Treacher Collins syndrome: protocol management from birth to maturity. *J Craniofac Surg.* 2009;20:2028–2035.
55. Dixon J, Trainor P, Dixon MJ. Treacher Collins syndrome. *Orthod Craniofac Res.* 2007;10:88–95.
56. Powell CM, Michaelis RC. Townes-Brocks syndrome. *J Med Genet.* 1999;36:89–93.
57. Edwards BM, Van Riper LA, Kileny PR. Clinical manifestations of CHARGE Association. *Int J Pediatr Otorhinolaryngol.* 1995;33:23–42.
58. Faye-Petersen O, David E, Rangwala N, et al. Otocephaly: report of five new cases and a literature review. *Fetal Pediatr Pathol.* 2006;25:277–296.
59. Gekas J, Li B, Kamnasaran D. Current perspectives on the etiology of agnathia-otocephaly. *Eur J Med Genet.* 2010;53:358–366.
60. Ibba RM, Zoppi MA, Floris M, et al. Otocephaly: prenatal diagnosis of a new case and etiopathogenetic considerations. *Am J Med Genet.* 2000;90:427–429.
61. Pauli RM, Graham JM Jr, Barr M Jr. Agnathia, situs inversus, and associated malformations. *Teratology.* 1981;23:85–93.
62. Sergi C, Kamnasaran D. PRRX1 is mutated in a fetus with agnathia-otocephaly. *Clin Genet.* 2011;79:293–295.
63. Celik T, Simsek PO, Sozen T, et al. PRRX1 is mutated in an otocephalic newborn infant conceived by consanguineous parents. *Clin Genet.* 2012;81:294–297.
64. Herman S, Delio M, Morrow B, et al. Agnathia-otocephaly complex: a case report and examination of the OTX2 and PRRX1 genes. *Gene.* 2012;494:124–129.
65. Schmotzer CL, Shehata BM. Two cases of agnathia (otocephaly): with review of the role of fibroblast growth factor (FGF8) and bone morphogenetic protein (BMP4) in patterning of the first branchial arch. *Pediatr Dev Pathol.* 2008;11:321–324.
66. Diep J, Kam D, Munir F, et al. Otocephaly complex: case report, literature review, and ethical considerations. *A Case Rep.* 2016;7:44–48.
67. Umekawa T, Sugiyama T, Yokochi A, et al. A case of agnathia-otocephaly complex assessed prenatally for ex utero intrapartum treatment (EXIT) by three-dimensional ultrasonography. *Prenat Diagn.* 2007;27:679–681.
68. Kamnasaran D, Morin F, Gekas J. Prenatal diagnosis and molecular genetic studies on a new case of agnathia-otocephaly. *Fetal Pediatr Pathol.* 2010;29:207–211.
69. Hisaba WJ, Milani HJ, Araujo Junior E, et al. Agnathia-otocephaly: prenatal diagnosis by two- and three-dimensional ultrasound and magnetic resonance imaging. Case report. *Med Ultrason.* 2014;16:377–379.
70. Rodriguez N, Casasbuenas A, Andreeva E, et al. First-trimester diagnosis of agnathia-otocephaly complex: a series of 4 cases and review of the literature. *J Ultrasound Med.* 2019;38:805–809.
71. Thauvin-Robinet C, Rousseau T, Laurent N, et al. Hypomandibular faciocranial dysostosis in consanguineous parents revealed by ultrasound prenatal diagnosis. *Prenat Diagn.* 2002;22:710–714.
72. Brecht K, Johnson CM 3rd. Complete mandibular agenesis. Report of a case. *Arch Otolaryngol.* 1985;111:132–134.
73. Kamiji T, Takagi T, Akizuki T, et al. A long surviving case of holoprosencephaly agnathia series. *Br J Plast Surg.* 1991;44:386–389.
74. Golinko MS, Shetye P, Flores RL, et al. Severe agnathia-otocephaly complex: surgical management and longitudinal follow-up from birth through adulthood. *J Craniofac Surg.* 2015;26:2387–2392.
75. Walker PJ, Edwards MJ, Petroff V, et al. Agnathia (severe micrognathia), aglossia and choanal atresia in an infant. *J Paediatr Child Health.* 1995;31:358–361.
76. Shermak MA, Dufresne CR. Nonlethal case of otocephaly and its implications for treatment. *J Craniofac Surg.* 1996;7:372–375.
77. Pauli RM, Pettersen JC, Arya S, et al. Familial agnathia-holoprosencephaly. *Am J Med Genet.* 1983;14:677–698.
78. Krassikoff N, Sekhon GS. Familial agnathia-holoprosencephaly caused by an inherited unbalanced translocation and not autosomal recessive inheritance. *Am J Med Genet.* 1989;34:255–257.
79. Erlich MS, Cunningham ML, Hudgins L. Transmission of the dysgnathia complex from mother to daughter. *Am J Med Genet.* 2000;95:269–274.
80. Blake KD, Prasad C. CHARGE syndrome. *Orphanet J Rare Dis.* 2006;1:34.
81. Issekutz KA, Graham JM Jr, Prasad C, et al. An epidemiological analysis of CHARGE syndrome: preliminary results from a Canadian study. *Am J Med Genet A.* 2005;133A:309–317.
82. Janssen N, Bergman JE, Swertz MA, et al. Mutation update on the CHD7 gene involved in CHARGE syndrome. *Hum Mutat.* 2012;33:1149–1160.
83. Vissers LE, van Ravenswaaij CM, Admiraal R, et al. Mutations in a new member of the chromodomain gene family cause CHARGE syndrome. *Nat Genet.* 2004;36:955–957.
84. Bergman JE, Janssen N, Hoefsloot LH, et al. CHD7 mutations and CHARGE syndrome: the clinical implications of an expanding phenotype. *J Med Genet.* 2011;48:334–342.
85. Legendre M, Abadie V, Attie-Bitach T, et al. Phenotype and genotype analysis of a French cohort of 119 patients with CHARGE syndrome. *Am J Med Genet C Semin Med Genet.* 2017;175:417–430.

86. Pampal A. CHARGE: an association or a syndrome? *Int J Pediatr Otorhinolaryngol.* 2010;74:719–722.

87. Legendre M, Gonzales M, Goudefroye G, et al. Antenatal spectrum of CHARGE syndrome in 40 fetuses with CHD7 mutations. *J Med Genet.* 2012;49:698–707.

88. Bajpai R, Chen DA, Rada-Iglesias A, et al. CHD7 cooperates with PBAF to control multipotent neural crest formation. *Nature.* 2010;463:958–962.

89. Pauli S, Bajpai R, Borchers A. CHARGEd with neural crest defects. *Am J Med Genet C Semin Med Genet.* 2017;175:478–486.

90. van Ravenswaaij-Arts C, Martin DM. New insights and advances in CHARGE syndrome: diagnosis, etiologies, treatments, and research discoveries. *Am J Med Genet C Semin Med Genet.* 2017;175:397–406.

91. Hale CL, Niederriter AN, Green GE, et al. Atypical phenotypes associated with pathogenic CHD7 variants and a proposal for broadening CHARGE syndrome clinical diagnostic criteria. *Am J Med Genet A.* 2016;170A:344–354.

92. Sanlaville D, Etchevers HC, Gonzales M, et al. Phenotypic spectrum of CHARGE syndrome in fetuses with CHD7 truncating mutations correlates with expression during human development. *J Med Genet.* 2006;43:211–217.

93. Verloes A. Updated diagnostic criteria for CHARGE syndrome: a proposal. *Am J Med Genet A.* 2005;133A:306–308.

94. Leibovitz Z, Egenburg S, Arad A, et al. Sonography of the fetal cochlea in the early second trimester of pregnancy. *J Ultrasound Med.* 2013;32:53–59.

95. Moreira NC, Teixeira J, Raininko R, et al. The ear in fetal MRI: what can we really see? *Neuroradiology.* 2011;53:1001–1008.

96. Azoulay R, Fallet-Bianco C, Garel C, et al. MRI of the olfactory bulbs and sulci in human fetuses. *Pediatr Radiol.* 2006;36:97–107.

97. Tilea B, Garel C, Menez F, et al. Contribution of fetal MRI to the diagnosis of inner ear abnormalities: report of two cases. *Pediatr Radiol.* 2006;36:149–154.

98. van Ravenswaaij-Arts CM, Blake K, Hoefsloot L, et al. Clinical utility gene card for: CHARGE syndrome—update 2015. *Eur J Hum Genet.* 2015;23(11).

99. Hsu P, Ma A, Wilson M, et al. CHARGE syndrome: a review. *J Paediatr Child Health.* 2014;50:504–511.

100. Jongmans MC, Admiraal RJ, van der Donk KP, et al. CHARGE syndrome: the phenotypic spectrum of mutations in the CHD7 gene. *J Med Genet.* 2006;43:306–314.

EMBRYOLOGY

The basic tissues of the head and neck become organized in the branchial apparatus and, therefore, the origin of many fetal neck lesions reside in this embryological structure. The branchial apparatus contains five pairs of mesenchymal condensations, which develop on both sides of the pharyngeal foregut on day 22, equivalent to branchial arches 1, 2, 3, 4, and 6. The fifth arch is very small and essentially regresses. The mesodermal arches are separated externally by ectodermal grooves notated as clefts and internally by endoderm-lined pouches (Figs. 22.1 and 22.2). The core of each arch contains its own arterial element and crest cells that contribute to skeletal structures. The mesodermal component will give rise to musculature of the face and neck and carry their own nerve and cranial nerve component.

There are four ectoderm-lined clefts along the arches. In the fifth to sixth week, the second arch grows and elongates inferiorly to meet the enlarging fifth arch or developing epipericardial ridge (Fig. 22.1A). As a result, an ectoderm-lined cavity encloses the second, third, and fourth branchial clefts. This temporary cavity, known as the "Sinus of His," usually obliterates secondary to fusion of its walls. Failure of complete wall fusion can result in a branchial cleft cyst, sinus, or fistula and, depending on the level, is classified into types 1, 2, 3, or 4 (Fig. 22.1B). The first branchial cleft is the only one that will become a definitive structure, eventually giving rise to the epithelium of the external auditory canal.

There are five pharyngeal or branchial pouches lined by endoderm. The fifth develops late and is usually considered part of the fourth. The first pouch gives rise to the pharyngotympanic tube, which develops into the middle ear cavity and tympanic membrane (Fig. 22.2). The second becomes the palatine tonsil. The third and fourth branchial pouches become the thymus, parathyroid glands, and ultimobranchial body—the latter gives rise to the calcitonin-secreting parafollicular cells of the thyroid gland. Maldevelopment of the branchial pouches results in complete lack of or erroneous formation of structures to which each pouch contributes. For example, incomplete obliteration of the thymopharyngeal duct may result in a thymopharyngeal duct cyst or an ectopic thymus, persisting along the tract of the migrating tissue (Fig. 22.3).

Table 22.1 summarizes the different structures arising from the branchial arches, clefts, and pouches. First arch syndromes include anomalies secondary to abnormal development or absence of various components of the first pharyngeal arch. Examples include Treacher Collins syndrome and Pierre Robin sequence.[1]

The thyroid gland arises during the fourth week as a small mass of proliferating endoderm at the apex of the foramen cecum of the developing tongue. It descends in the neck attached to the thyroglossal duct anterior to the hyoid and laryngeal cartilage. The thyroid reaches its final location within the lower neck, anterior to the trachea, by the seventh week. At this time, the thyroglossal duct involutes. Failure of involution may result

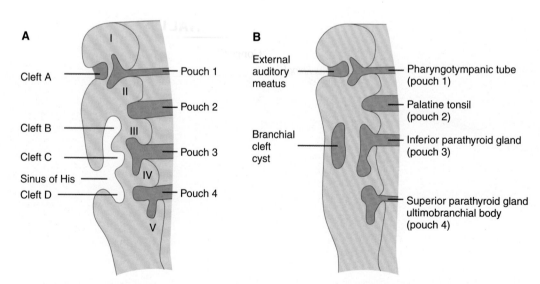

FIGURE 22.1: A: Differentiation of the pharyngeal clefts and pouches. There is elongation and growth of the second and fifth arches forming the sinus of His. **B:** Further maturation of the epithelium in the walls of the pharyngeal pouches. (Reprinted with permission from Langman J. *Medical Embryology*. 3rd ed. Baltimore, MD: Williams & Wilkins; 1975:234–236.)

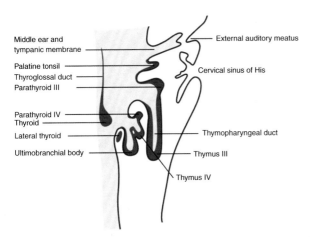

FIGURE 22.2: The structures that develop from the branchial clefts and pouches, particularly origin of the thymus, parathyroids, and ultimobranchial body. (Reprinted with permission from Zarbo RJ, Areen RG, McClatchey KD, et al. Thymopharyngeal duct cyst: a form of cervical thymus. *Ann Otol Rhinol Laryngol.* 1983;92(3, pt 1):284–289. Copyright © 1983 SAGE Publications.)

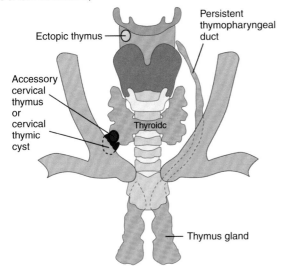

FIGURE 22.3: The course of the thymopharyngeal duct and possible locations for ectopic thymic tissue and/or thymic cyst. (Reprinted with permission from Zarbo RJ, Areen RG, McClatchey KD, Baker SB. Thymopharyngeal duct cyst: a form of cervical thymus. *Ann Otol Rhinol Laryngol.* 1983;92(3 Pt 1):284–289. Copyright © 1983 SAGE Publications.)

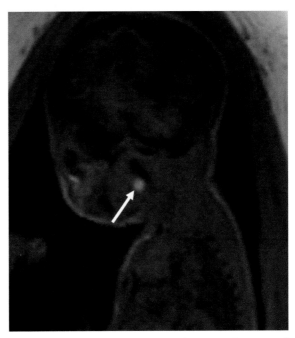

FIGURE 22.4: Ectopic thyroid tissue in a late second trimester fetus. Sagittal oblique T1 MRI shows a rounded hyperintense lesion (*white arrow*) along the base of the tongue.

in a thyroglossal cyst or sinus. Rarely, ectopic thyroid tissue may be found along the path of descent (Fig. 22.4).

The lymphatic sacs begin to develop by the end of the fifth week of gestation, approximately 2 weeks after the cardiovascular system. There are six primary lymphatic sacs: paired jugular lymphatic sacs, cisterna chyli, retroperitoneal (mesenteric), and paired iliac. They eventually evolve into groups of lymph nodes (Fig. 22.5). Lymphatic sacs develop alongside vessels and later make connections with the venous system. Lymphatic malformations (LMs) may develop secondary to incomplete or inadequate venous connections with stasis of lymphatic fluid resulting in dilated lymphatic channels.

CONGENITAL LESIONS OF THE NECK

Congenital neck lesions detected during the fetal period are very rare, with unknown incidence. A list of congenital lesions of the neck is shown in Table 22.2.

TABLE 22.1	Derivatives of the Branchial Apparatus		
LEVEL	DERIVATIVE OF BRANCHIAL POUCH (ENDODERM)	DERIVATIVE OF BRANCHIAL ARCH (MESODERM)	DERIVATIVE OF BRANCHIAL CLEFT (ECTODERM)
1	Eustachian tube, tympanum, mastoid air cells	Mandible, muscles of mastication, ear ossicles, CN V	External ear canal
2	Palatine tonsils	Muscles of facial expression, lesser horn of the hyoid bone, CN VII and VIII	Sinus of His
3	Inferior parathyroid, thymus and pyriform fossa	Superior constrictor muscle, ICA, greater horn of the hyoid bone, CN IX	Sinus of His
4	Superior parathyroid gland, apex of pyriform sinus	Most pharyngeal constrictors, laryngeal muscles, thyroid, aortic arch, right subclavian artery, CN X	None
5 and 6	Parafollicular C cells of thyroid	Laryngeal and pharyngeal muscles, CN XI	None

CN, cranial nerve; ICA, internal carotid artery.

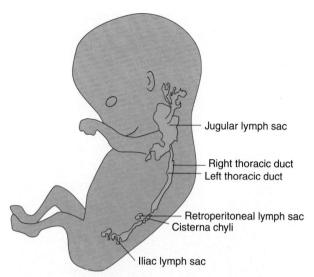

FIGURE 22.5: Seven-week embryo shows lymphatic sacs before the venous connections are formed.

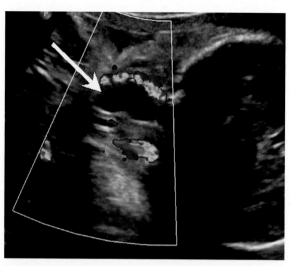

FIGURE 22.6: Branchial cyst. Coronal Doppler US shows an anechoic avascular cervical lesion (*arrow*) with acoustic enhancement in the lateral neck diagnosed as branchial cyst postnatal.

TABLE 22.2	Fetal Cervical Lesions	
CYSTIC	**SOLID**	**MIXED CYSTIC AND SOLID**
Branchial cleft cyst	Ectopic thymus	Neuroblastoma
Cervical meningocele	Ectopic thyroid	Teratoma
Cervical thymic cyst	Goiter	
Esophageal atresia	Hemangioma	
Esophageal duplication cyst	Neuroblastoma	
Laryngocele	Rhabdomyosarcoma	
Lymphatic malformations	Sarcoma	
Neuroenteric cyst	Teratoma	
Thyroglossal duct cyst	Metastasis (rare)	
Thyroid cyst		

Branchial Anomalies

Incidence: Prenatal diagnosis of branchial apparatus anomalies is very rare, with few cases described in the literature.[2–5]

Pathogenesis/Etiology: Defects of branchial apparatus embryogenesis result in branchial, parathyroid, and thymic anomalies, which may manifest as sinuses, fistulas, or cysts. These anomalies can be further classified according to their branchial pouch or cleft of origin. Histological evaluation of the epithelium lining the sinuses, fistulas, or cysts can define pouch versus cleft derivation.

The etiology of these lesions is poorly understood. The most accepted theory suggests that branchial anomalies are vestigial remnants from incomplete obliteration of the branchial apparatus or buried epithelial cell rests.[6] The most common lesion is a branchial cleft cyst type 2, which arises from a persistent cervical sinus of His. The majority are located within the anterolateral neck, most often on the left, lying anterior to the sternocleidomastoid muscle, posterior to the submandibular gland, and lateral to the carotid sheath.[2]

Diagnosis: By ultrasound (US), branchial cysts are round or ovoid, anechoic or hypoechoic, thin-walled cysts (Fig. 22.6). Real-time imaging may demonstrate movement of internal echoes, differentiating it from a solid lesion. On magnetic resonance imaging (MRI), the cysts are hypointense on T1 imaging and hyperintense on T2 imaging (Fig. 22.7).

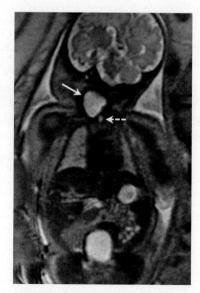

FIGURE 22.7: Branchial cyst. Same fetus as in Figure 22.6. Coronal SSFSE T2 MRI shows hyperintense lesion (*solid arrow*) in the lateral fetal neck. The airway (*dotted arrow*) is partially visualized on this image.

Associated Anomalies: Branchial cleft cysts are usually isolated lesions; however, they are associated with branchio-oto-renal syndrome.[7]

Differential Diagnosis: Differential diagnosis for branchial cleft cyst includes thymic cyst, LM, and thyroglossal duct cyst—when paramedian in location.

Prognosis/Management: Rarely, branchial cleft cyst can cause airway or esophageal obstruction and necessitate an *ex utero intrapartum treatment* (EXIT).[2] Given the risk of hemorrhage, infection, and questionable predisposition to cancer, surgical resection and marsupialization of the tract is the treatment of choice. The prognosis is excellent following excision.

Cervical Thymic Cyst

Incidence: Thymic cysts are very rare and infrequently diagnosed *in utero*.

Pathogenesis/Etiology: The thymus is derived from the ventral division of the paired third and fourth pharyngeal pouches at around 6 weeks of gestation. Thymic buds migrate inferiorly on each side of the neck forming the thymopharyngeal ducts, which extend from the angle of the mandible to the superior mediastinum along the carotid sheaths. During the seventh to ninth weeks, there is obliteration of the proximal ducts that then separate from the pharynx. Epithelial proliferation within the distal ducts gives rise to bilateral thymic tissue that fuses in the anterior mediastinum. Thymic cysts may be encountered in the neck, thoracic inlet, or mediastinum because of persistence of the thymopharyngeal duct(s). Similarly, rests of ectopic thymic tissue can also be found along the path of descent.[8,9]

Diagnosis: Cervical thymic cysts are often multilocular, but may be unilocular, and vary in size from 1.4 to 8 cm. They are intimately associated with the carotid space, splaying the carotid artery and jugular vein.[9] Thymic cysts are more common on the left, and up to 50% have a mediastinal connection. By US, they are anechoic but may have internal debris (Fig. 22.8). On MRI, the

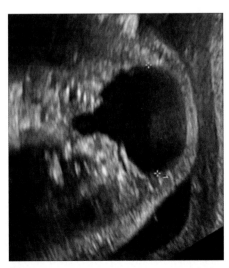

FIGURE 22.8: Thymic cyst. Axial US demonstrates lobulated anechoic lesion designated by calipers centered in the lateral neck diagnosed as thymic cyst postnatal.

lesions are hypointense on T1 imaging and hyperintense on T2 imaging (Fig. 22.9). If complicated by hemorrhage, the internal signal will be heterogeneous.[10]

Differential Diagnosis: The differential diagnosis includes LM, thyroid cyst, thyroglossal duct cyst, and branchial cleft cyst.

Prognosis/Management: Thymic cysts are usually asymptomatic, although respiratory distress, dysphagia, and vocal cord paralysis have been described.[11] Treatment consists of surgical excision of the cyst and residual tract. Spontaneous resolution has been reported.[11]

Ranula

Incidence: The incidence of congenital ranula is estimated to be 0.7%. Prenatal diagnosis is very rare.[12]

Pathogenesis/Etiology: A ranula is a sublingual or minor salivary gland retention cyst located at the floor of the mouth. They are classified by location into simple (intraoral) or plunging (oral/cervical) types. Congenital ranulas are thought to arise secondary to atresia of the salivary gland ducts or ostial adhesion.[12] Salivary duct epithelium lines the walls of the cyst, distinguishing it from a LM.

Diagnosis: By US, a ranula is a well-defined anechoic or hypoechoic cyst along the floor of the mouth that may extend into the submandibular region (Fig. 22.10). No color Doppler is usually observed. Well-delineated borders are seen on MRI with hypointense signal on T1 imaging and hyperintense signal on T2 imaging (Fig. 22.11).

Differential Diagnosis: Differential diagnosis includes LM, thyroglossal duct cyst, and dermoid cyst because of its midline/paramidline positioning.

Prognosis/Management: Congenital ranula presents as a cystic structure in the oral cavity. They elevate the floor of the mouth and displace the tongue superiorly and anteriorly. Rarely, they can grow to fill the oral cavity.[13] Infrequently, giant congenital ranula may result in airway obstruction, necessitating the EXIT procedure at birth to secure the airway.[12,13] Treatments of congenital ranula include marsupialization, aspiration of the ranula, and resection of the sublingual salivary gland, all of which showed no recurrence except for marsupialization with 61% recurrence.[14] Spontaneous resolution in the neonatal period has also been described.[12]

Thyroglossal Duct Cyst

Incidence: Prenatal diagnosis of a thyroglossal duct cyst is rare,[15] despite it being the most common midline cervical anomaly, representing 70% of all congenital neck masses.[16] The exact incidence is unknown, but 7% of the population has been shown to have a thyroglossal duct remnant.[16]

Pathogenesis/Etiology: The thyroglossal duct is an embryological structure that originates at the foramen cecum of the tongue and extends inferiorly within the midline neck, anterior to the hyoid, and terminates at the pyramidal lobe of the thyroid. Persistence of the duct results in cyst or sinus formation at any

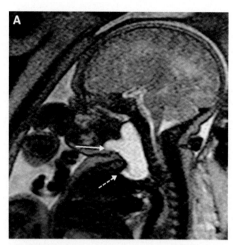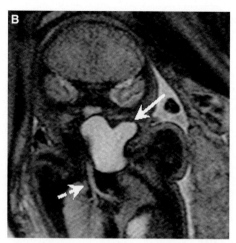

FIGURE 22.9: Thymic cyst. **A:** Sagittal T2 SSFSE MRI of same fetus in Figure 22.8. Lobular lesion is T2 hyperintense (*solid arrow*) and extends the length of neck but is also present in the mediastinum (*dotted arrow*), contiguous with thymic tissue. **B:** Coronal T2 SSFSE image in the same fetus demonstrates lesion (*solid arrow*) and patency of the airway (*dotted arrow*).

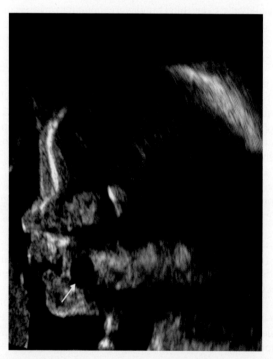

FIGURE 22.10: Ranula. Sagittal US demonstrates a round anechoic lesion (*arrow*) in the floor of the mouth, noted to represent ranula postnatal.

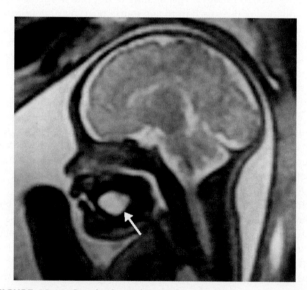

FIGURE 22.11: Ranula. Sagittal T2 SSFSE MRI shows a hyperintense cystic lesion (*arrow*) in the floor of the mouth, below the tongue.

point along its path. The majority of duct remnants are midline or parasagittal in location, adjacent to the hyoid bone.[17] Thyroglossal duct cysts may be seen in Cowden syndrome.

Diagnosis: On US, the classic appearance of a thyroglossal duct cyst is a thin-walled, anechoic, unilocular lesion. On occasion, they may be hypoechoic or heterogeneous in echotexture owing to increased protein content. Rarely, they may appear pseudosolid, mimicking ectopic tissue.[18] Posterior acoustic enhancement is present in the majority of lesions, as is absence of color Doppler flow. Demonstration of a normal thyroid gland is important in excluding the diagnosis of

ectopic tissue. On MRI, the signal depends on the protein content of the cyst, the majority of which are hyperintense on T1 and T2 sequences.[19]

Differential Diagnosis: Other cystic lesions in the midline/paramidline location include dermoid cyst, esophageal duplication cyst, and ranula. Branchial and thymic cysts tend to be located within the lateral neck. LMs and teratomas are typically complex cystic and solid masses.

Prognosis/Management: Up to one-third of patients with thyroglossal duct cyst will develop superimposed infection.[18] There is a 1% risk of cancer, primarily of the papillary type.[20] Rarely, when located within the tongue or floor of the mouth, the cyst may be large enough to cause airway obstruction and an EXIT procedure may be necessary.[15] Postnatal therapy entails surgical excision of the cyst, remnant tract, and a portion of the hyoid bone—known as the Sistrunk procedure.[20]

Dermoid/Epidermoid

Incidence: Prenatal diagnosis of dermoid/epidermoids is rare. Overall, they represent 7% of head and neck lesions and 25% of midline cervical anomalies.[20]

Pathogenesis/Etiology: Dermoid/epidermoids reflect abnormal inclusion of ectodermal tissue during the fusion of the branchial arches. Dermoid cysts contain two germ layers, ectoderm and mesoderm, whereas epidermoid cysts consist of only one germ layer, the ectoderm.[21] Although the majority of these lesions are found around the orbit or adjacent to the nose, approximately 11% of these cysts will present midline/paramidline within the oral cavity.[20] These lesions can be associated with Gardner syndrome.[19]

Diagnosis: US of dermoid/epidermoids will demonstrate a well-circumscribed, thin-walled, unilocular mass with internal echoes and little posterior acoustic enhancement. On MRI, these lesions may be isointense to hyperintense on T1 imaging, and typically hyperintense on T2 imaging. In the context of dermoid cysts, a fat–fluid level may be present. Classically, epidermoid cysts demonstrate reduced diffusivity on diffusion-weighted imaging, which may aid in the diagnosis, although this finding is variable and can sometimes be seen in dermoid cysts as well.[19]

Prognosis/Management: Rarely, the lesions at the floor of the mouth may cause airway obstruction, and EXIT may be considered. Surgical resection is the treatment of choice since these anomalies are at risk for rupture or infection. Five percent will undergo malignant degeneration to squamous cell neoplasm.[20]

INFLAMMATORY LESIONS

Thyroid Goiter

Thyroid goiter represents diffuse enlargement of the thyroid gland, often associated with decreased or increased function.

Incidence: Fetal goiter is very rare. Hypothyroidism associated with goiter is more common than hyperthyroidism, with an incidence of 1 in 3,000 to 4,000 births worldwide.[22]

Pathogenesis/Etiology: Fetal goiter associated with hypothyroidism is most often due to transplacental passage of maternal antithyroid medications (propylthiouracil, methimazole) or maternal antithyroid antibodies, or, rarely, maternal iodine deficiency. Maternal thyroid function may be normal despite fetal goiter and should not deter monitoring and treatment of fetal thyroid dysfunction. In the absence of maternal thyroid disease, fetal goiter is likely due to congenital dyshormonogenesis. If untreated in the first 3 months of life, congenital hypothyroidism can cause severe irreversible mental retardation with impairment of speech and hearing.

Fetal goiter associated with hyperthyroidism is usually secondary to transplacental passage of maternal thyroid-stimulating immunoglobulin IgG antibody, often in women with Graves disease. It is not detected in the fetus before 20 to 24 weeks' gestational age as the fetal thyroid is not mature enough to respond to antibody stimulation.

Fetal thyroid function begins in the late first trimester, around week 12.[23] The fetal thyroid slowly increases in size until week 32, after which a rapid growth pattern ensues. Reference tables correlating normal thyroid gland size to gestational age and/or biparietal diameter are available to aid in the diagnosis of thyroid gland enlargement[24–26] (see Table 26 in Appendix A1).

Diagnosis: Maternal thyroid function tests, including antithyroid antibody titers, should be obtained. That said, maternal thyroid status does not reflect fetal thyroid state and, therefore, fetal blood sampling may be required. The definitive diagnosis of fetal thyroid dysfunction is made by cordocentesis, with a risk for fetal loss of 0.5% to 1.4%.[27] Historically, amniotic fluid analysis of fetal thyroid function is considered unreliable as there is poor correlation between amniotic fluid thyroid hormone levels and fetal serum levels.[28] Fetal blood will show elevated thyroid-stimulating hormone (TSH) and low thyroxine in cases of hypothyroidism and low TSH in cases of hyperthyroidism.

Ultrasound: Fetal goiter is diagnosed by US at an average gestational age of 26 weeks.[29] The thyroid is symmetrically enlarged with bilobed configuration and varying echogenicity, either homogeneous or heterogeneous, with multiple cysts. Enlargement of the thyroid often results in neck hyperextension seen via two-dimensional US (2DUS) and three-dimensional US (3DUS). The airway and esophagus may be compressed by the gland; polyhydramnios ensues if swallowing is impaired. Color Doppler shows increased vascular flow (Fig. 22.12). The pattern of increased central flow has been associated with hyperthyroid goiter, and peripherally increased flow with hypothyroid goiter.[30] In fetuses with hyperthyroid goiter with high-output cardiac failure, Doppler may show increased velocities in the common carotid artery and descending aorta (~200 cm/s) and dilatation of the superior vena cava. Cardiomegaly and pleural effusions have been reported.

In fetuses with hyperthyroid goiter, additional US findings include tachycardia, advanced bone age, hydrops, intrauterine growth restriction, and hepatosplenomegaly. In those with hypothyroid goiter, US may reveal cardiac dysfunction and delayed bone age.

MRI: On MRI, the normal thyroid gland is hyperintense on T1 imaging and isointense on T2 imaging, relative to muscle. With

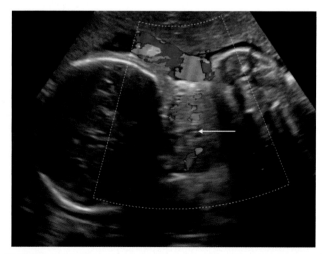

FIGURE 22.12: Thyroid goiter. Coronal Doppler US shows increased vascular flow and enlargement of the thyroid. There is questionable mass effect on the airway (*arrow*).

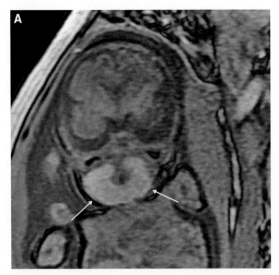 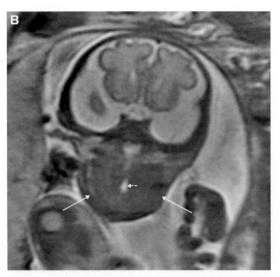

FIGURE 22.13: Thyroid goiter. **A:** Coronal T1 MRI demonstrates enlargement and hyperintensity of the thyroid gland (*arrows*). **B:** Coronal T2 SSFSE MRI shows isointense signal (with regard to muscle) of the enlarged thyroid (*solid arrows*), which encircles narrowed but patent airway (*dotted short arrow*).

fetal goiter, there is symmetric thyroid enlargement with increased signal on T1 imaging and intermediate signal on T2 imaging[31] (Fig. 22.13). Thyroid enlargement with signal on T2 imaging greater than muscle suggests thyroid dysfunction, either hypo- or hyperthyroid state. Intrinsic thyroid hyperintensity on T1 imaging persists despite hypo- or hyperthyroid state.[32] MRI is useful in the evaluation of tracheal and esophageal compression as well as in the degree of neck hyperextension. MRI is particularly helpful in delivery planning as the most severe cases may require cesarean section or EXIT procedure to secure the airway at the time of delivery. In this instance, MRI performed closer to delivery will best depict the airway.

Differential Diagnosis: The differential diagnosis for fetal thyroid enlargement includes other fetal neck masses (cystic or solid), notably LM, hemangioma, and cervical teratoma. Cervical teratomas are usually midline, mixed cystic and solid, show rapid growth, and cause greater degree of mass effect upon the airway and esophagus and secondary polyhydramnios when compared with goiter. LMs are usually lateral rather than medial and are predominantly cystic. Hemangiomas characteristically have high vessel density and flow. Thyroglossal duct cyst, thyroid cyst, branchial cleft cyst, cervical neuroblastoma, cervical rhabdomyosarcoma, and ectopic thymus are much less common.

Associated Anomalies: Rarely, fetal goiter with hypothyroidism has been associated with other congenital anomalies, such as Prader–Willi syndrome.[33]

Prognosis: Fetal goiter is usually self-limited and has good prognosis. In many cases, the thyroid decreases in size prenatally or soon after birth once treatment has been established. In fetuses born to mothers with Graves disease, the hyperthyroid goiter will resolve as circulating maternal thyroid-stimulating antibodies abate. The prognosis for newborns with congenital hypothyroidism depends on timely levothyroxine treatment.

Management: Treatment of fetal goiter depends on maternal thyroid state and medications, as well as on fetal thyroid

function. In fetal hypothyroid goiter, single or multiple intra-amniotic and fetal intramuscular injections of levothyroxine have been successful in treating hypothyroidism.[27,34–37] If cordocentesis reveals elevated thyroid-stimulating autoantibody titers, administration of antithyroid drugs, such as propylthiouracil or methimazole, to the mother is recommended. Repeat cordocentesis will demonstrate normalization of fetal thyroid function. US can aid in monitoring the fetal thyroid state by assessing the thyroid size, degree of neck hyperextension, polyhydramnios, and pleural effusions. Doppler US will show decreased vascular flow within the goiter.

Independent of fetal thyroid function, goiter may cause mass effect upon the airway and esophagus, leading to polyhydramnios, which could prompt preterm labor. Neck hyperextension may necessitate cesarean section owing to risk of dystocia. Rarely, if the goiter causes severe airway compression, EXIT procedure may be necessary to rapidly secure the fetal airway upon delivery.

Recurrence: The recurrence risk of fetal goiter in subsequent pregnancies is a concern in women with thyroid dysfunction. Of the estimated 1% of pregnant women with Graves disease,[38] the incidence of fetal hypo- or hyperthyroidism is 2% to 12%.[34,38] In mothers with hyperthyroidism taking propylthiouracil, 1% of their fetuses will have hypothyroidism.[28] Thyroid dyshormonogenesis, although rare, is transmitted as an autosomal recessive trait; therefore, the recurrence risk is 25%.

VASCULAR MALFORMATIONS

Vascular anomaly is an all-encompassing term that includes both vascular malformations and vascular tumors. Vascular malformations are classified according to hemodynamics into high-flow and low-flow malformations and are further classified according to the type of vessels present (arteries, veins, or lymphatics). Low-flow vascular malformations include pure or combined malformations of capillary, lymphatic, and venous channels. High-flow vascular malformations include both arteriovenous malformations and fistulas. Vascular tumors include hemangiomas, which are classified into congenital or infantile types.

Lymphatic Malformations

LMs contain dysplastic but mature lymphatic channels. The fetal literature frequently refers to macrocystic lesions as cystic hygroma (if in the neck) or microcystic lesions as lymphangioma. This nomenclature has largely been replaced since 1982 by Mulliken and Glowacki in that all these lesions are now referred to as LMs.[39] Therefore, for the purposes of this chapter, we refer to these as nuchal and nonnuchal LMs, respectively.

Incidence: A recent meta-analysis of 306 fetuses by Tonni et al. showed that the most common prenatally diagnosed head and neck masses are LMs/venolymphatic malformations comprising more than 50% of all lesions.[40] Seventy-five percent of LMs occurs in the neck, and the majority originate in the posterior triangle (nuchal), left side greater than right, or oral cavity.[41] The incidence of nuchal LMs, between 10 and 14 weeks of gestation, is approximately 0.35%.[42] Less is known about the incidence of nonnuchal LMs (lymphangiomas); however, they are one-fifth as common as nuchal LMs.[43] When large, LMs are often diagnosed prenatally, but the majority present by age 2 years.

Pathogenesis: The communication between jugular lymphatic sacs and jugular veins is formed by 40 days' conceptional age.[44] A failure in this communication results in dilated jugular lymphatic sacs. Nonnuchal LMs may result from noncommunication at any portion of the lymphatic or lymphovenous system. LMs are well-defined, multicystic lesions with numerous internal septa and may be infiltrative, crossing fascial planes. They are classified into microcystic, macrocystic, and combined lesions. LMs often coexist with venous malformations, termed venolymphatic malformations. Pathological biomarkers for LMs include the VEGFR-3 and PROX1 antibodies[45] and D2-40 monoclonal antibody.[46]

Etiology: Nuchal LMs diagnosed during the first trimester arc highly associated with chromosomal abnormalities (51%), the most common being trisomy 21. Other aneuploidies include Turner syndrome, trisomies 13 and 18, and deletions such as 13q and 18p.[42] In addition, cardiac and skeletal malformations are seen in 34% of cases.[42]

Nonnuchal LMs are usually isolated, yet can be associated with syndromes such as Gorham–Stout disease, Klippel–Trenaunay syndrome, and generalized lymphatic anomaly syndrome.[47]

Diagnosis

Ultrasound: LMs are multilocular cystic masses with posterior acoustic enhancement and vascular flow limited to the internal septations (Fig. 22.14). Vascular flow is not seen in pure LMs; however, venous flow will be present in a combined (venolymphatic) malformation. Macrocystic LMs are anechoic centrally when simple, although they may appear complex because of internal hemorrhage or protein. Fluid–fluid levels are not uncommon. Microcystic LMs appear hyperechoic as a result of innumerable interfaces created by multiple small cysts, often too small to resolve.

Magnetic Resonance Imaging: Classic MRI appearance is that of a multilocular, transspatial cystic mass. The cystic component is typically isointense to muscle on T1 imaging and hyperintense on T2 imaging, unless there is elevated protein content or presence of hemorrhage, in which case there may be fluid–fluid levels (Fig. 22.15). The literature shows that only 3% to 10% of

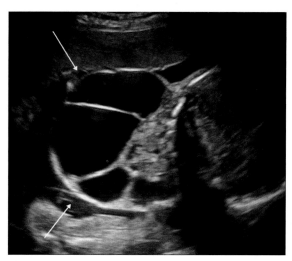

FIGURE 22.14: Lymphatic malformation. First-trimester axial US showing a septated fluid-filled lesion (*arrows*) in the anterolateral neck.

nonnuchal LMs may cause airway compromise, and, if so, they may exhibit partial effacement rather than complete collapse of the airway as may be seen in cases of cervical teratoma.[48,49] Ng and colleagues studied the predictor MRI findings of significant morbidity in cases of head and neck masses and found that the maximum vertical pocket of amniotic fluid (measured similarly to US) and mass effect on the trachea were the most contributory parameters that predicted neonatal morbidity and the need for EXIT procedures.[48] Therefore, evaluation of the fluid-filled larynx and trachea is of paramount importance by fetal MRI. The deep component of the malformation is often not well delineated by US, particularly if microcystic. Fetal MRI should be considered to evaluate deep extent and airway involvement in order to

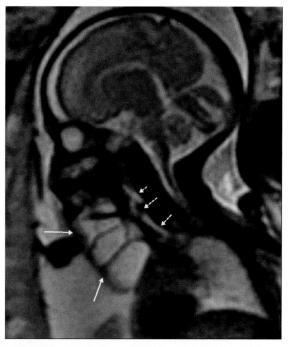

FIGURE 22.15: Lymphatic malformation. Sagittal T2 SSFSE MRI of the same fetus as in Figure 22.17 with multiseptated predominately T2 hyperintense lesion (*solid arrows*). Note the patent hypopharynx, glottis, and hypoglottic region (*dotted arrows*).

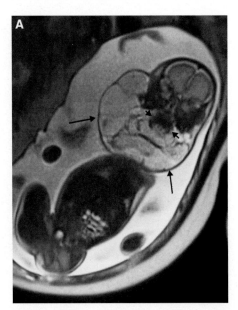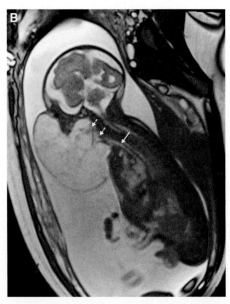

FIGURE 22.16: Lymphatic malformation with airway compromise. **A:** Coronal T2 SSFSE MRI of a fetus with a large multiseptated cystic lesion in the anterolateral neck (*long black arrows*) with suspicion for airway compromise as the lesion invades oral cavity/tongue (*short arrows*). **B:** Sagittal T2 SSFSE MRI in the same fetus showing poor delineation of the hypopharynx and proximal trachea (*dotted arrows*). Note the patent thoracic trachea (*solid arrow*).

guide perinatal management, in particular the decision for EXIT procedure (Fig. 22.16).[47,50]

Differential Diagnosis: The primary differential diagnosis for nuchal LM is increased nuchal translucency. Presence of multiple septations and posterolateral involvement of the neck aids in the diagnosis of LM. Neural tube defect, encephalocele, and cystic teratoma can sometimes have a similar appearance. For non-nuchal LM, the differential diagnosis includes cystic teratoma, hemangioma, venous malformation, arteriovenous malformation, and soft-tissue sarcoma.

Prognosis: Nearly 50% of fetuses with an US diagnosis of nuchal LM in the first trimester will have a chromosomal abnormality and, therefore, poor prognosis. The risk of fetal or perinatal death is as high as 25%. Only 17% will result in a healthy newborn. However, if the fetus has no aneuploidy, no cardiac anomalies, and has a normal anatomic sonographic evaluation at 16 to 20 weeks' gestation, there is a 95% chance of normal pediatric outcome.[42] Spontaneous regression of nuchal LM has been reported *in utero*, usually between 2 and 7 months of age.[45]

The outcome for isolated nonnuchal LM is favorable, depending on the extent and treatment response of the lesion. Approximately 3% to 10% of infants with LMs have respiratory compromise because of airway obstruction or mediastinal extension.[41]

Management: Prenatal aspiration of lymphatic fluid in macrocystic lesions is rarely performed but considered when there is rapid expansion, infection, and/or intralesional hemorrhage.[51] A few cases have been described in the literature where aspiration of macrocystic lesions immediately prior to delivery has allowed normal vaginal delivery.[52] In the presence of airway obstruction,

delivery via the EXIT procedure may be imperative. Surgical resection is the treatment of choice, but can be difficult in the presence of neural, vascular, or muscular encasement/invasion. Macrocystic LMs are often successfully treated postnatal with sclerotherapy. Other treatment strategies include radiofrequency and laser ablation.

Small, focal LMs have excellent prognoses, both with percutaneous sclerosis and with surgical resection. Large, infiltrating lesions can be difficult to treat fully. Large lesions can lead to permanent facial/neck disfiguration and often require multiple treatments with sclerotherapy. A study by Sheikh et al. evaluating the disfigurement and outcome of fetal neck lesions including LM and non-LM lesions reported that surviving patients with LMs had the highest incidence of moderate to severe disfigurement (18% to 36%), higher rate of persistent/recurrent disease (100%), and cranial nerve dysfunction (50%).[53] Overall, recurrence is seen in up to 17% of complete excisions and 40% of incomplete excisions.[54]

Venous Malformations

Incidence: Venous malformations occur in about 1% of the population. Of these, approximately 40% occur in the head and neck.[55]

Pathogenesis/Etiology: Venous malformations contain dysplastic but mature venous channels. They may be purely venous, venolymphatic (most common), or arteriovenous. Venous malformations may occur at any time during angiogenesis. Similar to LMs, these lesions are often infiltrative and cross fascial planes, usually subcutaneous tissue and muscle. Venous malformations can be associated with blue rubber bleb nevus syndrome, Maffucci syndrome, Klippel–Trenaunay syndrome, and Parkes Weber syndrome.[55]

Diagnosis: With US, Doppler is helpful in differentiating venous malformations from other vascular malformations. Pulsed Doppler shows slow velocity with monophasic to biphasic waveforms. On occasion, flow within the vessels is so slow; no color flow can be seen. Acoustic shadowing related to phleboliths may be present. On MRI, these malformations are typically isointense to muscle on T1 imaging and hyperintense on T2 imaging, but appear heterogeneous if thrombus is present. T2* gradient recalled echo (GRE) images are useful to demonstrate blooming artifact from phleboliths.

Differential Diagnosis: Differential diagnosis includes LM, arteriovenous malformation, hemangioma, and soft-tissue sarcoma.

Prognosis: Many, if not all, venous malformations are present at birth; however, most are small and often go unrecognized on prenatal imaging. After birth, they tend to grow proportional to the growth of the child. Some lesions may enlarge suddenly because of hemorrhage, infection, thrombosis, or hormonal changes.

Treatment: Most venous malformations are treated conservatively, either with elastic compression, sclerotherapy, or surgical excision.[56]

Arterial Venous Fistula or Malformation

Incidence: Arterial malformations are most common in the head and neck, yet the true incidence is unknown.

Pathogenesis/Etiology: An arterial venous malformation is a tangle of abnormally thin-walled vessels connecting dilated high-flow feeding arteries to a prominent draining vein. Arteriovenous fistulas are similar; however, these lesions lack the tangle of dysplastic vessels that are present in the malformations and are more often acquired than congenital. It is believed that arteriovenous malformations arise in the fetus from failure of regression of arteriovenous channels in the primitive retiform plexus.[57]

They can be associated with phosphatase and tensin (*PTEN*) homolog gene mutations, such as Cowden and Bannayan–Riley–Ruvalcaba syndrome, RASA (angiogenic) gene mutations (which includes some forms of Parkes Weber syndrome), and hereditary hemorrhagic telangiectasia.[55]

Diagnosis: On US, multiple hypoechoic channels with or without soft-tissue mass are noted (Fig. 22.17A). Doppler demonstrates high systolic and high diastolic flow in the arteries. Arterialized waveforms with spectral broadening are present within the veins (Fig. 22.17B). MRI may show multiple tubular

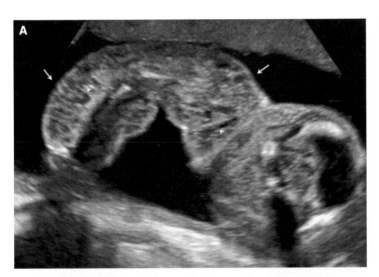

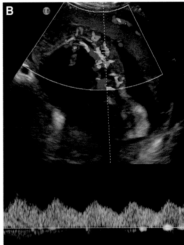

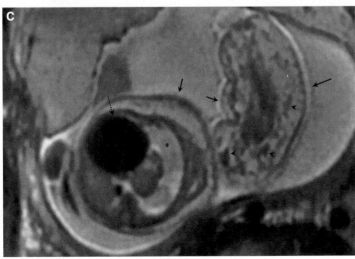

FIGURE 22.17: High-flow combined vascular malformation. Fetus at 21 weeks with diagnosis of Parkes Weber syndrome. **A:** Axial US demonstrates heterogeneous mass along upper extremity (*arrows*) containing multiple tubular hypoechoic enlarged vessels (*arrowheads*). **B:** With color Doppler, there are large arterial feeders demonstrating spectral broadening and low-impedance arterial waveform. **C:** Axial T2 SSFSE MRI demonstrates heterogeneous lesion along the upper extremity and chest (*solid arrows*) containing multiple flow voids (*arrowheads*). There is mild cardiomegaly (*dotted arrow*) and pleural effusion (*asterisk*).

structures with flow-related signal void and heterogeneous signal on T2 imaging (Fig. 22.17C). Single or multiple large vessels may be seen coursing through the mass. Cardiac failure and hydrops may develop in the presence of high arteriovenous shunting.

Management: These lesions are treated with trans-arterial embolization or surgery.

NEOPLASMS

Cervical Hemangioma

Incidence: Hemangioma is the most common vascular tumor of infancy, affecting approximately 10% of infants. Greater than 50% of hemangiomas involve the head and neck region.[58] They commonly appear in the neonatal period, although some may be present at birth and are known as congenital hemangiomas (CHs). There is a high female predilection.

Pathogenesis/Etiology: Hemangiomas arise from abnormal cellular proliferation of vascular endothelial cells. Boon et al. introduced a new classification for hemangiomas and showed a clear histological distinction between infantile hemangiomas and CHs by demonstrating that CHs are glut-1 (glucose-1 transporter 1) negative and infantile hemangiomas are glut-1 positive. CHs are further divided into rapidly involuting congenital hemangiomas

(RICHs) and noninvoluting congenital hemangiomas (NICHs) on the basis of their natural history.[59] Most CHs are solitary, as opposed to infantile hemangiomas in which 20% are multiple. CHs demonstrate steady growth *in utero* until the third trimester, at which point they stabilize in size.

Diagnosis: CHs have been diagnosed as early as 12 weeks' gestation and usually involve the posterolateral neck.[60] There is no apparent imaging distinction between RICHs and NICHs. They share location, size, and similar imaging features. On US, CHs are heterogeneous, solid, and vascular masses with high vessel density and high flow velocity. They demonstrate low-resistance index and broadening of spectrum on Doppler US (Fig. 22.18A, B). MRI will show a well-defined, solid mass in the posterolateral head and neck region with intermediate signal intensity on T1 imaging and increased signal intensity on T2 imaging (Fig. 22.18C). High signal intensity on T2 imaging is likely secondary to slow flow through small vascular spaces of the hemangioma. Flow-related signal void can be seen in high-flow vessels within the mass. Additional imaging findings including polyhydramnios, neck hyperextension, or lateral head tilting will depend on the location and size of the hemangioma and the amount of airway and esophageal compression. Congestive heart failure secondary to arteriovenous shunting can be seen. Unlike infantile hemangiomas, CHs may contain vascular aneurysms, intravascular thrombi, and arteriovenous shunting.[61]

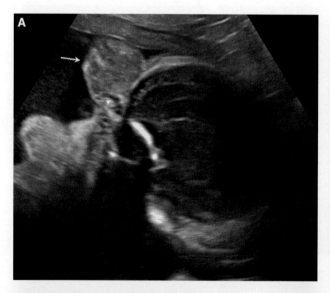

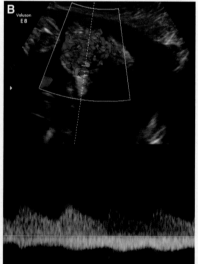

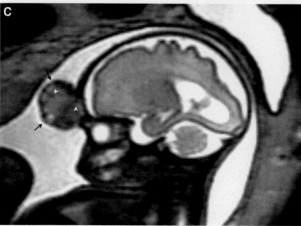

FIGURE 22.18: Congenital hemangioma. Fetus at 31 weeks. **A:** Sagittal US demonstrates echogenic mass (*arrows*) arising from the subcutaneous tissues of the forehead with prominent feeding vessel (*arrowhead*). **B:** Doppler of lesion demonstrates arterial waveform with high diastolic flow and pulsatile vein. **C:** Sagittal T2 SSFSE MRI demonstrates heterogeneous hyperintense subcutaneous lesion (*black arrows*) above the orbit containing prominent flow voids (*white arrowheads*). There is no intracranial extension.

Associated Anomalies: Several studies have reported an association of brain cortical malformations with arterial anomalies; therefore, careful scrutiny of the brain is warranted.[60,62] Hemangiomas can also be seen as part of PHACES syndrome (*p*osterior *f*ossa malformations, *h*emangiomas, *a*rterial anomalies, *c*ardiac defects, *e*ye abnormalities, and *s*ternal cleft).

Differential Diagnosis: The imaging features of hemangiomas may be difficult to distinguish from congenital fibrosarcoma. A well-defined mass with flow-related signal voids, and increased flow will be seen on US and MRI[59,60] in both entities. When located in the posterior neck, hemangiomas may mimic an occipital cephalocele on prenatal US.[63] Fetal MRI is a valuable tool to evaluate for associated intracranial anomalies and help distinguish hemangiomas from other entities.

Prognosis/Management: RICHs usually regress postnatal by 14 months of age and may leave behind atrophic skin or large veins. NICHs usually require surgical treatment. Unfortunately, there are no distinguishing imaging characteristics to predict postnatal course. Maternal administration of steroids may accelerate involution of the hemangioma. If there is compression upon the airway, delivery by cesarean section or EXIT procedure to secure the airway should be performed.

Cervical Teratoma

Teratomas are germ cell tumors that contain tissue from each of the three embryonic layers, the ectoderm, mesoderm, and endoderm.

Incidence: Cervical teratomas occur in approximately 1 in 20,000 to 40,000 live births.[64] They represent 3% to 5% of all teratomas, and approximately 300 cases have been described in the literature.[64,65] Compared with other teratomas, cervical teratomas do not have a female predominance.[65]

Pathogenesis/Etiology: Cervical teratomas arise from totipotential germ cells or as an end result of a defective twin pregnancy with fetus *in fetu*.[28,66] These masses, when occurring within the neck, are typically within the anterior midline. They

likely originate in the thyroid gland, on the basis of the presence of a thin pseudocapsule in continuity between the mass and the thyroid.[67]

Cervical teratomas are mixed cystic and solid lesions. They are composed of a combination of skin, skin appendages, cartilage, muscle, and respiratory and gastrointestinal epithelium. Teratomas can be further classified into mature and immature subtypes. The immature subtype contains embryonic cells, usually neural, and occur more commonly in the cervical region (>50%)[68] compared with other extragonadal teratomas. Importantly, most immature teratomas are not malignant; however, the presence of yolk sac tumor cells carries a higher association with malignancy and recurrence.[69]

Diagnosis: Amniotic fluid alpha-fetoprotein (AFP) has been suggested to help in the diagnosis of cervical teratomas. Unfortunately, only 30% of fetal cervical teratomas produce AFP and both maternal and fetal AFP levels may be normal.[28] However, postnatal, AFP levels are often useful to evaluate for recurrence after resection.

Ultrasound: US can detect cervical teratomas as early as 15 to 17 weeks' gestational age, although the majority are diagnosed in the late second to third trimester. They differ from LMs and branchial cleft cysts in location as these lesions predominantly occur in the posterolateral neck, whereas cervical teratomas occur anteriorly. They are usually large tumors varying in size from 4 to 12 cm in diameter. US shows a complex mass with multiloculated cystic and solid components. Hyperechoic adipose tissue and calcification with posterior acoustic shadowing may be seen. The presence of calcification is fairly specific for the diagnosis of teratoma (Fig. 22.19). Teratomas are less pliable tumors compared with LMs and may cause compression of the neck vasculature and hypopharynx. If vasculature compression is severe, high-output cardiac failure and potentially nonimmune hydrops may result, with possible intrauterine fetal demise. Polyhydramnios can occur if swallowing is impaired.

Magnetic Resonance Imaging: MRI is valuable in confirming the diagnosis of a cervical teratoma as well as aiding in perinatal planning. It can demonstrate the full extent of the mass as well as the

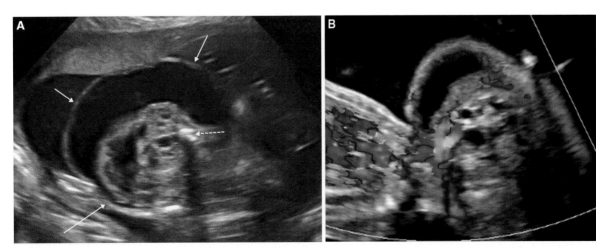

FIGURE 22.19: Cervical teratoma. **A:** Axial US of the fetal neck shows a complex solid and cystic mass (*solid arrows*) with foci of calcification (*dotted arrow*) verified by posterior acoustic shadowing. **B:** Coronal Color Doppler US of the same fetus shows increased vascular supply to the mass.

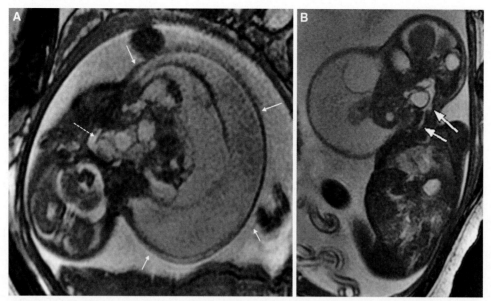

FIGURE 22.20: Cervical teratoma in a 23 week gestation fetus. **A:** Axial T2 SSFP MRI shows a large complex mass (*solid arrows*) arising from the neck and extending into the oropharynx (*dotted arrow*). **B:** Coronal T2 SSFP MRI shows a patent left piriform sinus and infraglottic airway (*white arrows*).

degree of compression of the airway and esophagus. Imaging shows a complex mass with multiloculated cystic and solid components (Fig. 22.20). Intratumoral hemorrhage can be seen as dark signal on gradient echo images and bright signal on T1 images. In large cervical teratomas, polyhydramnios and a small stomach may be present due to impaired swallowing from esophageal compression. MRI may be utilized to diagnose pulmonary hypoplasia, a severe complication in large cervical teratomas secondary to distortion of the airway by the mass. In these cases, the carina is retracted superiorly, resulting in compression of the lungs in the upper thorax with poor lung development (Fig. 22.21).[70] Three-plane T2 imaging (single-shot fast spin echo or steady-state free precession) of the neck is helpful in delineating the fluid-filled airway from the nasopharynx to the carina and should be carefully evaluated for airway deviation, effacement, or complete collapse. A recent study by Ng et al. showed that the maximum vertical pocket of amniotic fluid (measured similarly to US) and mass effect on the trachea were the most contributory MRI parameters that predicted neonatal morbidity, mortality, and the need for EXIT procedures.[48]

Associated Anomalies: Anomalies associated with cervical teratoma include agenesis of the corpus callosum, imperforate anus, hypoplastic left heart, trisomy 13, and mandibular hypoplasia.[28]

Differential Diagnosis: Vascular anomalies including LM, venous malformation, and mixed venolymphatic malformation, as well as hemangioma are the primary differential diagnoses for cervical teratoma. Macrocystic LM may mimic teratomas because of their multiloculated cystic appearance and hemorrhagic potential. However, LMs are usually located in the posterolateral neck and cause less mass effect upon the airway, esophagus, and neck vessels. Venous malformations have internal flow on color Doppler and may contain calcified phleboliths. Hemangiomas are highly vascular, and color Doppler will demonstrate increased intralesional flow.

Prognosis/Management/Recurrence: In the presence of airway obstruction, cervical teratomas have a poor prognosis and near 100% mortality, as it can be difficult to secure an airway at the time of delivery. Accurate prenatal diagnosis and perinatal planning is essential. A delay in securing an airway can lead to hypoxic ischemic brain injury. The EXIT procedure has been successful in preventing this and may be combined with surgical resection of the teratoma while on placental support (operation on placental support [OOPS]). Postnatal morbidity depends on the degree of pulmonary hypoplasia and other associated anomalies.

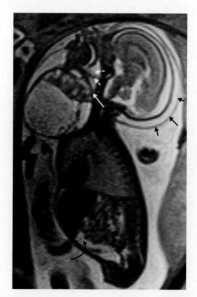

FIGURE 22.21: Cervical teratoma. Sagittal T2 SSFSE MRI shows cervical mass causing hyperextension of the neck known as "flying fetus" position. There is obstruction of the oropharynx (*solid long arrow*) with fluid distention of the proximal airway (*dotted arrows*). Hydrops with scalp edema (*black arrows*) and intra-abdominal ascites (*curved black arrow*) is noted.

Fetuses with large cervical teratomas are at increased risk for preterm labor because of polyhydramnios and premature rupture of membranes. Hyperextension of the neck can lead to dystocia, requiring cesarean section. Hypothyroidism and hypoparathyroidism may result as the thyroid may be hypoplastic and the parathyroid glands may not be easily discernible during tumor resection and thus removed. In these cases, calcium and vitamin D supplementation with or without thyroid hormone replacement may be needed.

While the majority of cervical teratomas are histologically benign, they may grow quickly and recur. Most recurrences occur within 7 months of resection. The presence of yolk sac tumor cells appears to be the only valid predictor of increased risk of malignancy and recurrence rather than the histological immaturity of the tumor. A 4% risk of death at 2 to 6 years has been reported secondary to the development of a yolk sac tumor. Close follow-up of serum AFP following resection can aid in early detection of recurrences or malignant transformation.[28,68] Malignant cervical teratomas with fetal metastatic lesions have been reported, although rarely.[71,72]

Epignathus

Incidence: The incidence of epignathus is reported as 1 in 35,000 to 200,000 live births, representing 2% to 9% of all teratomas.[73,74] They are more common in females with a 3:1 ratio.[75]

Pathogenesis/Etiology: Epignathus (also known as oral teratomas or oropharyngeal teratomas) are rare oral tumors with components of all three germ layers with similarities to teratomas arising in the neck. Oral teratomas arise from the soft or hard palate and are believed to derive from pluripotential cells in Rathke pouch that grow in a disorganized manner.[74] Approximately 6% of patients with oral teratomas have associated anomalies, including cleft palate, branchial cleft cyst, duplicated pituitary gland, agenesis of the corpus callosum, and congenital heart disease.[75,76] They usually present during the second trimester as unidirectional or bidirectional masses, involving the oral cavity and protruding forward. They may extend intracranially.

Diagnosis: On US and MRI, epignathus has similar characteristics as those described for cervical teratomas (Fig. 22.22). These tumors can vary in size: from a few centimeters to as large

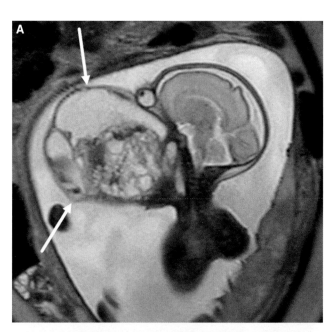

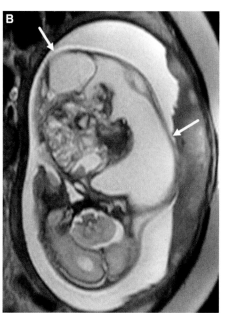

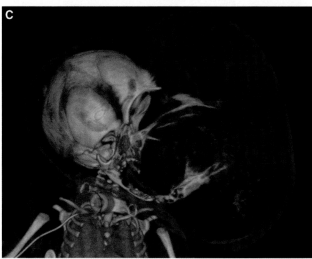

FIGURE 22.22: Epignathus. **A, B:** Sagittal and axial T2 SSFSE MRI of the fetal face and neck demonstrates a large solid and cystic mass arising from the oral cavity (*white arrows*). **C:** Coronal 3D bone computed tomography reconstruction of the same child postnatally, illustrates marked deformity of the face by the mass.

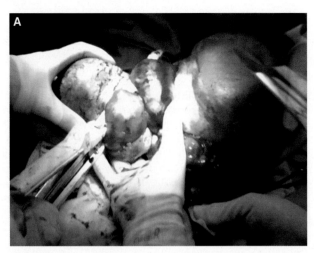
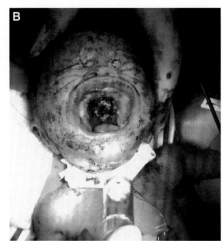

FIGURE 22.23: Epignathus. **A:** Intraoperative image during an *ex utero* intrapartum treatment procedure of a fetus with epignathus. Note the size of the oral teratoma (*right*) compared with the size of the baby's head (*left*). **B:** Same patient after resection of the epignathus showing the origin of the mass from the hard palate.

as the fetal head or body. Epignathus can rapidly grow and cause swallowing dysfunction leading to polyhydramnios or airway obstruction.

Prognosis/Management: Because of the high degree of airway obstruction, OOPS or EXIT procedures are required to secure the airway (Fig. 22.23). The prognosis is very poor in the presence of intracranial extension with rare surviving cases.[73]

Epulis

Incidence: Congenital epulis is rare, occurring almost exclusively in females.[73]

Pathogenesis/Etiology: Congenital epulis (also known as congenital gingival granular cell tumor) is a benign tumor arising from the gingival mucosa of the alveolar ridge of the maxilla and less commonly of the mandible. It is usually solitary, although a few cases of synchronous epulides have been described.[77,78] Its etiology is unknown and controversial. The term epulis and congenital gingival granular cell tumor have been used synonymously in the literature, but their histology and epidemiology are different. Epulides are gingival tumors of infancy, while granular cell tumors occur in adulthood.[77,79]

Diagnosis: Congenital epulis is a well-defined pedunculated mass protruding through the fetal mouth. On US, an epulis is a solid mass with internal blood flow via a vascular pedicle from the mouth (Fig. 22.24). Fetal swallowing is often not affected, although if the lesion becomes large it may impair fetal swallowing and ultimately lead to polyhydramnios and/or airway obstruction.[77] By MRI, epulides are hypointense on T2 imaging, and the origin from the maxilla or mandibular alveolar ridge can infrequently be seen (Fig. 22.25).

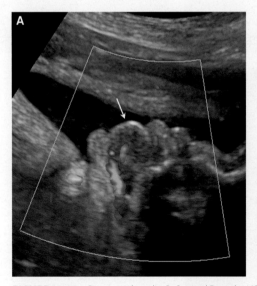
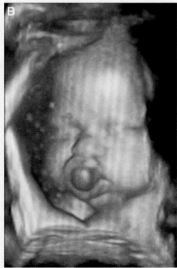

FIGURE 22.24: Congenital epulis. **A:** Sagittal Doppler US shows a rounded solid mass (*arrow*) with a vascular pedicle protruding through the fetal mouth. **B:** Three-dimensional volume rendering image of the same fetus shows the fetal profile and mass protruding through the mouth.

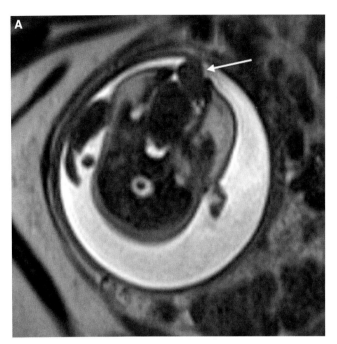
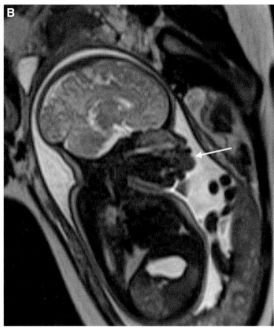

FIGURE 22.25: Congenital epulis. **(A)** Axial and **(B)** sagittal T2 SSFSE MRI demonstrates a rounded, hypointense lesion (*white arrows*) protruding through the mouth and in continuity with the maxilla.

Differential Diagnosis: Differential diagnoses include epignathus, oropharyngeal rhabdomyosarcoma, and hemangioma.

Prognosis/Management: Surgical excision is curative, with no reported recurrence in the literature.[80] Small lesions may regress spontaneously.[77]

Neuroblastoma

Incidence: Congenital cervical neuroblastoma is rarely encountered, accounting for 4.4% of congenital neuroblastomas (most common location is the adrenal gland).[81]

Diagnosis: Prenatal US findings include a solid or mixed solid and cystic mass in the lateral aspect of the neck with or without calcification. Fetal MRI shows a mass with low signal intensity on T1 imaging and high signal intensity on T2 imaging. Extension to the brain and/or metastasis is extremely rare but such cases have been reported.[82]

Prognosis/Management: As with other neck masses, neuroblastomas may cause compression of the airway and esophagus and neck hyperextension. Maternal elevation of catecholamine metabolites is present in >90% of cases and can lead to maternal hypertension. Furthermore, fetal urinary catecholamine metabolites (vanillylmandelic acid [VMA] and homovanillic acid [HVA]) may also be elevated. Congenital neuroblastoma, especially purely cystic, has a better prognosis than do those occurring during childhood.[81] Disappearance of the tumor before birth has been reported.[83]

Rhabdomyosarcoma

Incidence: Congenital rhabdomyosarcoma is extremely rare, with little information published regarding prenatal diagnosis.

Pathogenesis/Etiology: Congenital rhabdomyosarcoma is often associated with chromosomal translocations; therefore, amniocentesis for fetal karyotype should be performed. Association with Robert syndrome, Beckwith–Wiedemann syndrome, and neurofibromatosis has been reported.[84] Prenatal metastases to the sacral region have been described.[85]

REFERENCES

1. Sadler TW. *Langman's Medical Embryology*. Philadelphia, PA: Wolters Kluwer Health; 2011.
2. Lind RC, Hulscher JB, van der Wal JE, Dikkers FG, Langen ZJ. A very rare case of a giant third branchial pouch remnant discovered in utero. *Eur J Pediatr Surg*. 2010;20(5):349–351. doi:10.1055/s-0029-1246194.
3. Robichaud J, Papsin BC, Forte V. Third branchial cleft anomaly detected in utero. *J Otolaryngol*. 2000;29(3):185–187.
4. Suchet IB. Ultrasonography of the fetal neck in the second and third trimesters. Part 3. Anomalies of the anterior and anterolateral nuchal region. *Can Assoc Radiol J*. 1995;46(6):426–433.
5. Tsai PY, Chang CH, Chang FM. Prenatal imaging of the fetal branchial cleft cyst by three-dimensional ultrasound. *Prenat Diagn*. 2003;23(7):605–606. doi:10.1002/pd.639.
6. Benson MT, Dalen K, Mancuso AA, Kerr HH, Cacciarelli AA, Mafee MF. Congenital anomalies of the branchial apparatus: embryology and pathologic anatomy. *Radiographics*. 1992;12(5):943–960.
7. Smith RJH. Branchiootorenal spectrum disorders. In: Pagon RA, Adam MP, Bird TD, Dolan CR, Fong CT, Stephens K, eds. *GeneReviews*. Seattle, WA: University of Washington; 1993.
8. Nguyen Q, deTar M, Wells W, Crockett D. Cervical thymic cyst: case reports and review of the literature. *Laryngoscope*. 1996;106(3 pt 1):247–252.
9. Cigliano B, Baltogiannis N, De Marco M, et al. Cervical thymic cysts. *Pediatr Surg Int*. 2007;23(12):1219–1225. doi:10.1007/s00383-006-1822-5.
10. de Miguel Campos E, Casanova A, Urbano J, Delgado Carrasco J. Congenital thymic cyst: prenatal sonographic and postnatal magnetic resonance findings. *J Ultrasound Med*. 1997;16(5):365–367.
11. McEwing R, Chaoui R. Fetal thymic cyst: prenatal diagnosis. *J Ultrasound Med*. 2005;24(1):127–130.
12. Gul A, Gungorduk K, Yildirim G, Gedikbasi A, Ceylan Y. Prenatal diagnosis and management of a ranula. *J Obstet Gynaecol Res*. 2008;34(2):262–265. doi:10.1111/j.1447-0756.2008.00767.x.
13. Chan DF, Lee CH, Fung TY, Chan DL, Abdullah V, Ng PC. Ex utero intrapartum treatment (EXIT) for congenital giant ranula. *Acta Paediatr*. 2006;95(10):1303–1305. doi:10.1080/08035250600580545.

14. Crysdale WS, Mendelsohn JD, Conley S. Ranulas—mucoceles of the oral cavity: experience in 26 children. *Laryngoscope*. 1988;98(3):296–298.

15. Lindstrom DR, Conley SF, Arvedson JC, Beecher RB, Carr MH. Anterior lingual thyroglossal cyst: antenatal diagnosis, management, and long-term outcome. *Int J Pediatr Otorhinolaryngol*. 2003;67(9):1031–1034.

16. Keizer AL, Deurloo KL, van Vugt JM, Haak MC. A prenatal diagnosis of a thyroglossal duct cyst in the fetal anterior neck. *Prenat Diagn*. 2011;31(13):1311–1312. doi:10.1002/pd.2872.

17. Hsieh YY, Hsueh S, Hsueh C, et al. Pathological analysis of congenital cervical cysts in children: 20 years of experience at Chang Gung Memorial Hospital. *Chang Gung Med J*. 2003;26(2):107–113.

18. Kutuya N, Kurosaki Y. Sonographic assessment of thyroglossal duct cysts in children. *J Ultrasound Med*. 2008;27(8):1211–1219.

19. Mossa-Basha M, Yousem DM. Congenital cystic lesions of the neck. *Appl Radiol*. 2013;42(1):8–22.

20. Masters F, Given CA. Cystic neck masses: a pictorial review of unusual presentations and complicating features. *Appl Radiol*. 2008;37(9):26–32.

21. Lev S, Lev MH. Imaging of cystic lesions. *Radiol Clin North Am*. 2000;38(5):1013–1027.

22. Koyuncu FM, Tamay AG, Bugday S. Intrauterine diagnosis and management of fetal goiter: a case report. *J Clin Ultrasound*. 2010;38(9):503–505. doi:10.1002/jcu.20717.

23. Bromley B, Frigoletto FD, Cramer D, Osathanondh R, Benacerraf BR. The fetal thyroid: normal and abnormal sonographic measurements. *J Ultrasound Med*. 1992;11(1):25–28.

24. Ho SS, Metreweli C. Normal fetal thyroid volume. *Ultrasound Obstet Gynecol*. 1998;11(2):118–122. doi:10.1046/j.1469-0705.1998.11020118.x.

25. Ranzini AC, Ananth CV, Smulian JC, Kung M, Limbachia A, Vintzileos AM. Ultrasonography of the fetal thyroid: nomograms based on biparietal diameter and gestational age. *J Ultrasound Med*. 2001;20(6):613–617.

26. Gietka-Czernel M, Debska M, Kretowicz P, Debski R, Zgliczynski W. Fetal thyroid in two-dimensional ultrasonography: nomograms according to gestational age and biparietal diameter. *Eur J Obstet Gynecol Reprod Biol*. 2012;162(2):131–138. doi:10.1016/j.ejogrb.2012.02.013.

27. Francois A, Hindryckx A, Vandecruys H, et al. Fetal treatment for early dyshormonogenetic goiter. *Prenat Diagn*. 2009;29(5):543–545. doi:10.1002/pd.2237.

28. Bianchi DW, Crombleholme TM, D'Alton ME, Malone FD. *Fetology. Diagnosis and Management of the Fetal Patient*. 2nd ed. New York, NY: McGraw-Hill; 2010.

29. Agrawal P, Ogilvy-Stuart A, Lees C. Intrauterine diagnosis and management of congenital goitrous hypothyroidism. *Ultrasound Obstet Gynecol*. 2002;19(5):501–505. doi:10.1046/j.1469-0705.2002.00717.x.

30. Huel C, Guibourdenche J, Vuillard E, et al. Use of ultrasound to distinguish between fetal hyperthyroidism and hypothyroidism on discovery of a goiter. *Ultrasound Obstet Gynecol*. 2009;33(4):412–420. doi:10.1002/uog.6315.

31. Karabulut N, Martin DR, Yang M, Boyd BK. MR imaging findings in fetal goiter caused by maternal Graves disease. *J Comput Assist Tomogr*. 2002;26(4):538–540.

32. Kondoh M, Miyazaki O, Imanishi Y, Hayakawa M, Aikyou M, Doi H. Neonatal goiter with congenital thyroid dysfunction in two infants diagnosed by MRI. *Pediatr Radiol*. 2004;34(7):570–573. doi:10.1007/s00247-004-1145-4.

33. Insoft RM, Hurvitz J, Estrella E, Krishnamoorthy KS. Prader-Willi syndrome associated with fetal goiter: a case report. *Am J Perinatol*. 1999;16(1):29–31. doi:10.1055/s-2007-993832.

34. Friedland DR, Rothschild MA. Rapid resolution of fetal goiter associated with maternal Grave's disease: a case report. *Int J Pediatr Otorhinolaryngol*. 2000;54(1):59–62.

35. Hanono A, Shah B, David R, et al. Antenatal treatment of fetal goiter: a therapeutic challenge. *J Matern Fetal Neonatal Med*. 2009;22(1):76–80. doi:10.1080/14767050802448299.

36. Ribault V, Castanet M, Bertrand AM, et al., French Fetal Goiter Study Group. Experience with intraamniotic thyroxine treatment in nonimmune fetal goitrous hypothyroidism in 12 cases. *J Clin Endocrinol Metab*. 2009;94(10):3731–3739. doi:10.1210/jc.2008-2681.

37. Corral E, Reascos M, Preiss Y, Rompel SM, Sepulveda W. Treatment of fetal goitrous hypothyroidism: value of direct intramuscular L-thyroxine therapy. *Prenat Diagn*. 2010;30(9):899–901. doi:10.1002/pd.2560.

38. Hatjis CG. Diagnosis and successful treatment of fetal goitrous hyperthyroidism caused by maternal Graves disease. *Obstet Gynecol*. 1993;81(5 (pt 2)):837–839.

39. Donnelly LF, Adams DM, Bisset GS. Vascular malformations and hemangiomas: a practical approach in a multidisciplinary clinic. *AJR Am J Roentgenol*. 2000;174(3):597–608. doi:10.2214/ajr.174.3.1740597.

40. Tonni G, Granese R, Martins Santana EF, et al. Prenatally diagnosed fetal tumors of the head and neck: a systematic review with antenatal and postnatal outcomes over the past 20 years. *J Perinat Med*. 2017;45(2):149–165. doi:10.1515/jpm-2016-0074.

41. Fordham LA, Chung CJ, Donnelly LF. Imaging of congenital vascular and lymphatic anomalies of the head and neck. *Neuroimaging Clin N Am*. 2000;10(1):117–136, viii.

42. Malone FD, Ball RH, Nyberg DA, et al., FASTER Trial Research Consortium. First-trimester septated cystic hygroma: prevalence, natural history, and pediatric outcome. *Obstet Gynecol*. 2005;106(2):288–294. doi:10.1097/01.AOG.0000173318.54978.1f.

43. Woodward PJ, Kennedy A, Sohaey R. *Diagnostic Imaging Obstetrics*. 2nd ed. Manitoba, Canada: Amirsys; 2011.

44. Chervenak FA, Isaacson G, Blakemore KJ, et al. Fetal cystic hygroma. Cause and natural history. *N Engl J Med*. 1983;309(14):822–825. doi:10.1056/NEJM198310063091403.

45. Perkins JA, Manning SC, Tempero RM, et al. Lymphatic malformations: review of current treatment. *Otolaryngol Head Neck Surg*. 2010;142(6):795.e1–803.e1. doi:10.1016/j.otohns.2010.02.026.

46. Sherer DM, Perenyi AR, Glick SA, et al. Prenatal sonographic findings of extensive low-flow mixed lymphatic and venous malformations. *J Ultrasound Med*. 2006;25(11):1469–1473.

47. Kathary N, Bulas DI, Newman KD, Schonberg RL. MRI imaging of fetal neck masses with airway compromise: utility in delivery planning. *Pediatr Radiol*. 2001;31(10):727–731.

48. Ng TW, Xi Y, Schindel D, et al. Fetal head and neck masses: MRI prediction of significant morbidity. *AJR Am J Roentgenol*. 2019;212(1):215–221. doi:10.2214/ajr.18.19753.

49. Schindel DT, Twickler D, Frost N, Walsh D, Santiago-Munoz P, Johnson R. Prognostic significance of an antenatal magnetic resonance imaging staging system on airway outcomes of fetal craniofacial venolymphatic malformations. *J Surg Res*. 2017;217:187–190. doi:10.1016/j.jss.2017.05.024.

50. Gaffuri M, Torretta S, Iofrida E, et al. Multidisciplinary management of congenital giant head and neck masses: our experience and review of the literature. *J Pediatr Surg*. 2019;54(4):733–739. doi:10.1016/j.jpedsurg.2018.09.018.

51. Oosthuizen JC, Burns P, Russell JD. Lymphatic malformations: a proposed management algorithm. *Int J Pediatr Otorhinolaryngol*. 2010;74(4):398–403. doi:10.1016/j.ijporl.2010.01.013.

52. Kaufman GE, D'Alton ME, Crombleholme TM. Decompression of fetal axillary lymphangioma to prevent dystocia. *Fetal Diagn Ther*. 1996;11(3):218–220.

53. Sheikh F, Akinkuotu A, Olutoye OO, et al. Prenatally diagnosed neck masses: long-term outcomes and quality of life. *J Pediatr Surg*. 2015;50(7):1210–1213. doi:10.1016/j.jpedsurg.2015.02.035.

54. Alqahtani A, Nguyen LT, Flageole H, Shaw K, Laberge JM. 25 Years' experience with lymphangiomas in children. *J Pediatr Surg*. 1999;34(7):1164–1168.

55. Donnelly LF, Jones B, O'Hara S, et al. Diagnostic imaging: pediatrics. *Radiol Med*. 2006;111:1168–1169.

56. Dubois J, Alison M. Vascular anomalies: what a radiologist needs to know. *Pediatr Radiol*. 2010;40(6):895–905. doi:10.1007/s00247-010-1621-y.

57. Kohout MP, Hansen M, Pribaz JJ, Mulliken JB. Arteriovenous malformations of the head and neck: natural history and management. *Plast Reconstr Surg*. 1998;102(3):643–654.

58. Tseng JJ, Chou MM, Chen WH. Prenatal 3- and 4-dimensional ultrasonographic findings of giant fetal nuchal hemangioma. *J Chin Med Assoc*. 2007;70:460–463.

59. Boon LM, Fishman SJ, Lund DP, Mulliken JB. Congenital fibrosarcoma masquerading as congenital hemangioma: report of two cases. *J Pediatr Surg*. 1995;30:1378–1381.

60. Robson CD, Barnewolt CE. MR imaging of fetal head and neck anomalies. *Neuroimaging Clin N Am*. 2004;14:273–291, viii.

61. Alamo L, Beck-Popovic M, Gudinchet F, Meuli R. Congenital tumors: imaging when life just begins. *Insights Imaging*. 2011;2:297–308.

62. O'Connor SC, Rooks VJ, Smith AB. Magnetic resonance imaging of the fetal central nervous system, head, neck, and chest. *Semin Ultrasound CT MR*. 2012;33(1):86–101. doi:10.1053/j.sult.2011.10.005.

63. Miyakoshi K, Tanaka M, Matsumoto T, et al. Occipital scalp hemangioma: prenatal sonographic and magnetic resonance images. *J Obstet Gynaecol Res*. 2008;34:666–669.

64. Tonni G, De Felice C, Centini G, Ginanneschi C. Cervical and oral teratoma in the fetus: a systematic review of etiology, pathology, diagnosis, treatment and prognosis. *Arch Gynecol Obstet*. 2010;282(4):355–361. doi:10.1007/s00404-010-1500-7.

65. Garmel SH, Crombleholme TM, Semple JP, Bhan I. Prenatal diagnosis and management of fetal tumors. *Semin Perinatol*. 1994;18(4):350–365.

66. Hitchcock A, Sears RT, O'Neill T. Immature cervical teratoma arising in one fetus of a twin pregnancy. Case report and review of the literature. *Acta Obstet Gynecol Scand*. 1987;66(4):377–379.

67. Riedlinger WF, Lack EE, Robson CD, Rahbar R, Nose V. Primary thyroid teratomas in children: a report of 11 cases with a proposal of criteria for their diagnosis. *Am J Surg Pathol*. 2005;29:700–706.

68. Bianchi B, Ferri A, Silini EM, Magnani C, Sesenna E. Congenital cervical teratoma: a case report. *J Oral Maxillofac Surg*. 2010;68:667–670.

69. Isaacs H Jr. Perinatal (fetal and neonatal) germ cell tumors. *J Pediatr Surg*. 2004;39:1003–1013.

70. Liechty KW, Hedrick HL, Hubbard AM, et al. Severe pulmonary hypoplasia associated with giant cervical teratomas. *J Pediatr Surg*. 2006;41(1):230–233. doi:10.1016/j.jpedsurg.2005.10.081.

71. Baumann FR, Nerlich A. Metastasizing cervical teratoma of the fetus. *Pediatr Pathol*. 1993;13(1):21–27.

72. Shoenfeld A, Ovadia J, Edelstein T, Liban E. Malignant cervical teratoma of the fetus. *Acta Obstet Gynecol Scand*. 1982;61(1):7–12.

73. Clement K, Chamberlain P, Boyd P, Molyneux A. Prenatal diagnosis of an epignathus: a case report and review of the literature. *Ultrasound Obstet Gynecol*. 2001;18(2):178–181. doi:10.1046/j.1469-0705.2001.00456.x.

74. Sumiyoshi S, Machida J, Yamamoto T, et al. Massive immature teratoma in a neonate. *Int J Oral Maxillofac Surg.* 2010;39(10):1020–1023. doi:10.1016/j.ijom.2010.04.008.

75. Kaido Y, Kikuchi A, Oyama R, Kanasugi T, Fukushima A, Sugiyama T. Prenatal ultrasound and magnetic resonance imaging findings of a hypovascular epignathus with a favorable prognosis. *J Med Ultrason.* 2013;40(1):61–64.

76. Vazquez E, Castellote A, Mayolas N, Carreras E, Peiro JL, Enriquez G. Congenital tumours involving the head, neck and central nervous system. *Pediatr Radiol.* 2009;39(11):1158–1172. doi:10.1007/s00247-009-1369-4.

77. Koch BL, Myer C III, Egelhoff JC. Congenital epulis. *AJNR Am J Neuroradiol.* 1997;18(4):739–741.

78. Roy S, Sinsky A, Williams B, Desilets V, Patenaude YG. Congenital epulis: prenatal imaging with MRI and ultrasound. *Pediatr Radiol.* 2003;33(11):800–803. doi:10.1007/s00247-003-1024-4.

79. Lopez de Lacalle JM, Aguirre I, Irizabal JC, Nogues A. Congenital epulis: prenatal diagnosis by ultrasound. *Pediatr Radiol.* 2001;31(6):453–454.

80. Jiang L, Hu B, Guo Q. Prenatal sonographic diagnosis of congenital epulis. *J Clin Ultrasound.* 2011;39(4):217–220. doi:10.1002/jcu.20765.

81. Isaacs H Jr. Fetal and neonatal neuroblastoma: retrospective review of 271 cases. *Fetal Pediatr Pathol.* 2007;26:177–184.

82. Guzelmansur I, Aksoy HT, Hakverdi S, Seven M, Dilmen U, Dilmen G. Fetal cervical neuroblastoma: prenatal diagnosis. *Case Rep Med.* 2011;2011:529749. doi:10.1155/2011/529749.

83. Moore SW, Satge D, Sasco AJ, Zimmermann A, Plaschkes J. The epidemiology of neonatal tumours. Report of an international working group. *Pediatr Surg Int.* 2003;19(7):509–519. doi:10.1007/s00383-003-1048-8.

84. Onderoglu LS, Yucel A, Yuce K. Prenatal sonographic features of embryonal rhabdomyosarcoma. *Ultrasound Obstet Gynecol.* 1999;13(3):210–212. doi:10.1046/j.1469-0705.1999.13030210.x.

85. Yoshino K, Takeuchi M, Nakayama M, Suehara N. Congenital cervical rhabdomyosarcoma arising in one fetus of a twin pregnancy. *Fetal Diagn Ther.* 2005;20(4):291–295. doi:10.1159/000085088.

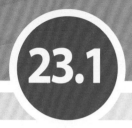

23.1 Neural Tube Defects—Cranium

Beth M. Kline-Fath • David Perry • Dorothy I. Bulas

Neural tube defects (NTDs) encompass a heterogeneous group of congenital brain and spine anomalies that result from the defective closure of the neural tube early in gestation. Acrania-exencephaly-anencephaly and spinal dysraphism are equal in prevalence, accounting for 95% of cases, whereas encephaloceles account for the remaining 5%.[1] After a review of epidemiology and embryology, this chapter discusses common cranial NTDs. The following chapter 23.2 provides a review of spinal NTDs.

EPIDEMIOLOGY

NTDs are one of the most common fetal malformations, second only to cardiac anomalies, with a worldwide prevalence of 1.86 per 1,000 live births.[2] The etiology of an NTD is not fully understood, but it is likely multifactorial encompassing chromosomal or genetic abnormalities, environmental, teratogen, and maternal predisposing factors. Despite increasing knowledge of these risk factors, most children with an NTD are born without a known cause.

Less than 10% of NTDs are due to chromosomal anomalies, such as trisomy 13 and 18.[3] Although over 400 genetic alterations have been associated with deficient neural tube closure in animals, no conclusive evidence has been found in humans. However, genetics likely has an effect as the incidence varies with family history, gender, race, and geography. For example, if one child is affected, the risk for subsequent siblings is around 3%, with two affected siblings 10%, and with three affected siblings 20%.[4,5] Female preponderance is known in pregnancies with anencephaly.[3] Prevalence differs by geography—in the United States 1 in 1,200, in Europe 1 in 1,000, and in China 3 to 5 per 1,000.[3,5] Also, ethnic difference in NTD risk persists even after migration to different geographical areas.

Environmental exposures, including air pollution, are risk factors.[3] Twin gestations, especially monochorionic, have higher association with NTD. Maternal exposures to pregestational diabetes, substance abuse, and chronic illness significantly increase the risk for NTD in the fetus.[6] Maternal obesity, hyperthermia, drug exposure, especially valproate, and poor nutrition have also been implicated.[3]

Folic acid deficiency is a well-known risk factor; therefore, women are advised to consume food high in folate or take folate supplements at least 3 months prior to pregnancy.[7] In the past few decades, the number of births with NTDs worldwide has declined because of folic acid supplementation, with countries with mandatory food fortification policies reaching a NTD prevalence of 0.6 per 1,000 total births.[8] However, it is known that some NTDs are not prevented by folic acid fortification. Inositol, a molecular vitamin which can normalize neural tube closure, has shown promise to further reduce NTD frequency.[9] Overall, there has been a significant decrease in number of children born with NTDs, partly due to supplementation strategies but also given early ultrasound (US) diagnosis followed by elective pregnancy termination.[2]

EMBRYOLOGY

Dysraphism is the result of defective closure of the neural tube and is reserved for defects of primary and secondary neurulation, which involves tubulation of the neural plate and tail bud and disjunction of the superficial ectoderm from the neural ectoderm.

Primary neurulation is the process in which formation of the brain and spinal cord arises from development of the neural tube (Fig. 23.1-1).[10] The neural plate originates from the dorsal surface ectoderm. The thickened neural plate will become paired longitudinal neural folds over the median neural groove, which will fuse to create the neural tube. Primary neurulation is initiated at day 22 at the boundary between the future hindbrain and cervical spine and extends bidirectionally to the forebrain and down the spine. Fusion of the neural folds occurs anteriorly to the lamina terminalis, also known as the anterior neuropore (cranial) on day 24. The zippering in the spine progresses caudal to the posterior neuropore in the upper sacral area at day 26.

Secondary neurulation occurs differently to form the spinal cord in the lower sacral and caudal levels. In this area, multipotential cells in the tail bud or caudal eminence, through a process known as canalization, organize into a neuroepithelium with central cavity

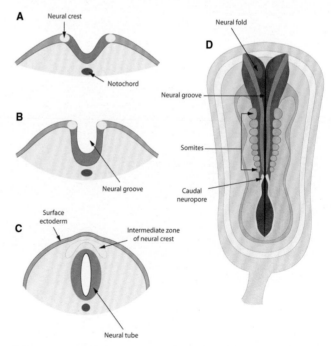

FIGURE 23.1-1: Embryology of primary neurulation in which neural plate develops **(A)** and then infolds to become a groove **(B)** and with closure a neural tube **(C)**. **D:** Diagram of the dorsal aspect of the developing craniospinal area in the embryo.

which then becomes continuous with the primary neural tube.[11] Through apoptosis, the caudal most neural tube will degenerate.

The neural tube separates from the ectoderm, and the mesoderm proliferates laterally to form the axial skeleton and dura (Fig. 23.1-1). In the tail bud, multipotential cells will give rise to sacral and coccygeal vertebrae. If the process of primary neurulation is interrupted, a defect in the neural tube will result, cranial or spinal. Disruption in secondary neurulation results in a closed spinal dysraphism.

ACRANIA-EXENCEPHALY-ANENCEPHALY (AEA) SEQUENCE

Description: *Acrania* is a defect that occurs due to complete or partial absence in the development of the cranial vault above the orbits, with absence of parietal, squamosal, occipital, temporal, and frontal bones above the supraciliary ridge.[12] *Exencephaly* is acrania with protrusion of substantial brain into the amniotic cavity.[13] *Anencephaly* or *holoanencephaly* represents absence of forebrain, midbrain, and skull. The cerebral hemispheres are replaced with residual covering of hemorrhagic, fibrotic, degenerated neurons and glia with little definable structure (Fig. 23.1-2).[3] *Craniorachischisis* is a rare malformation in which the closure defect affects both the brain and spinal neural tube.[3] *Meroanencephaly* is also an infrequent defect in which there are malformed cranial bones with an open median cranial defect that allows protrusion of exposed brain.[14]

Incidence: The incidence of anencephaly is difficult to assess, but the malformation accounts for approximately 40% of NTDs, and in the United States, frequency is estimated at up to 1 in 1,000 pregnancies or live births.[2,15] A progressive decline is suspected with periconceptional folate fortification and termination.[16] Anencephaly has a higher rate in countries such as Egypt, Lebanon, Ireland, Scotland, and New Zealand. In the United States, fetuses of Caucasian and Hispanic ethnicity are more frequently affected than those of African descent.[17] Twin gestations also have a higher risk for anencephaly. There is a female preponderance of 3:1.[16,17] Ninety-five percent of infants born with anencephaly are in families with no prior history of an NTD.[16]

Pathogenesis: The major insult in acrania, exencephaly, and anencephaly is failed closure of the rostral neural tube resulting in an open cranial defect. The unprotected cerebral tissue is progressively destroyed through exposure to amniotic fluid and mechanical trauma and disappears from 14 weeks onward.[18–20] Prior animal and US reports have demonstrated that there typically is

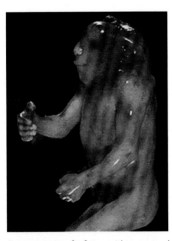

FIGURE 23.1-2: Postmortem of a fetus with anencephaly.

progression of acrania-exencephaly to anencephaly.[7,18,21] In some cases with a less severe bony defect such as meroanencephaly, residual disorganized brain may persist late in gestation or even postnatally.

Exencephaly pathologically demonstrates a highly vascular layer of epithelium with two relatively equivalent disorganized, dysplastic cerebral hemispheres.[12,13,18] With progression to anencephaly, the cerebral hemispheres are replaced by a mass of connective and vascular tissue with scattered islands of brain tissue, so-called angiomatous stroma or area cerebrovasculosa.[18,22]

In acrania, although the cerebral hemispheres are present and covered by a thin membrane, the brain tissue is similarly disorganized. Acrania, also characterized by partial or complete absence of the cranium, is hypothesized to occur at the beginning of the fourth week at the same time the anterior neuropore closes but is due to failure of the mesenchyme to migrate under the ectoderm and superficial to the cerebral hemispheres.[12]

Etiology: AEA appears to be multifactorial in origin, being from both genetic and environmental causes.[1] Associated chromosomal syndromes have been reported in 5% to 10% of these cases and include trisomy, triploidy, mosaic trisomy 11 and 20, and a number of deletions and duplications or single-gene disorders.[7] Hyperthermia, deficiency in zinc and copper, and occupation solvent exposure have been associated with a higher risk of anencephaly.[20] Most relevant is inadequate dietary consumption of folates prior to conception.[7,12]

Diagnosis: Preliminary screening for high maternal serum alpha-fetoprotein (AFP) at 10 to 15 weeks may disclose evidence of leakage from the fetal neural tube in 90% of cases.[23] The combination of elevated AFP and low estriol levels is highly predictive for anencephaly.[23,24] However, screening can be falsely positive and requires confirmation with US.

Ultrasound: Sonography can identify almost 100% of anencephalic fetuses.[1,21,25] First-trimester diagnosis benefits from transvaginal imaging where it can potentially be diagnosed shortly before 10 weeks by the presence of a widened cranial pole, altered brain echotexture, variable asymmetric or lobulated disorganized tissue, and decreased head-to-trunk ratio.[25–27] Confirmation is usually obtained after 11 to 12 weeks when hyperechogenic calvarial ossification relative to the underlying soft tissues is noted to be absent.[25,26] Echogenic amniotic fluid is a useful clue in approximately 89% of cases, believed to represent particles of degenerated brain.[20,27] Brain content is variable in appearance and may be cystic, elongated craniocaudally, overhanging anteriorly, or foreshortened.[27] From 10 to 14 weeks, the "Mickey Mouse" sign may be seen on coronal images, as cerebral lobes floating in amniotic fluid above the orbits (Fig. 23.1-3).[27,28] 3D imaging can be helpful in confirming diagnosis, excluding other anomalies that mimic AEA.[27]

Detection can improve after 14 weeks when the brain has completely formed, although a significant amount of disorganized cranial tissue may be still present as it has not yet been destroyed by amniotic fluid.[19] AEA may result in a reduced crown rump length or chin length-to-crown rump length ratio, but in some cases the measurement is normal and can lead to a false-negative study below 14 weeks.[19,29,30]

In the mid to late second trimester, the diagnosis is easier as less brain tissue is present. The typical "frog eyes" sign on coronal plane is due to prominent orbits in conjunction with the symmetric absence of a normally formed calvarium and brain (Fig. 23.1-4).[22] Exposed residual neural tissue may be echogenic,

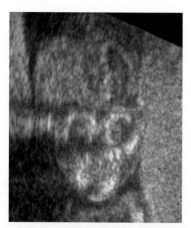

FIGURE 23.1-3: Coronal US of acrania/exencephaly with absent calvarium and protruding brain above orbits giving rise to Mickey Mouse appearance.

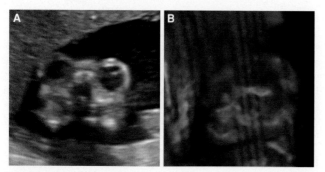

FIGURE 23.1-4: Anencephaly. **A:** Coronal 2D US shows prominent "frog eye" appearance. **B:** 3D US demonstrating lack of skull above the orbits.

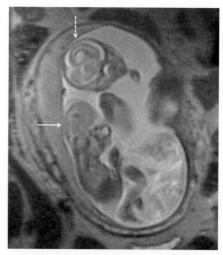

FIGURE 23.1-5: T2 fetal MRI showing lack of calvarium and dysmorphic brain in acrania/exencephaly (*solid arrow*) and normal brain and calvarium in co-twin (*dashed arrow*).

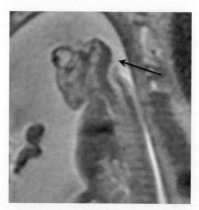

FIGURE 23.1-6: T2 sagittal MRI of fetus with anencephaly demonstrating cervical spine defect and absent brainstem and cervical cord (*arrow*).

cystic, or normally formed with pseudosulcations.[13,22] The cerebellar hemispheres may be absent, and spinal segmentation anomalies are common, especially in the cervical area. In the second or third trimester, as many as 30% to 50% of cases have associated polyhydramnios from impaired fetal swallowing, excess cerebrospinal fluid (CSF) across the meninges, or increased fetal urine output due to absent antidiuretic hormone.[22]

Magnetic Resonance Imaging: Fetal magnetic resonance imaging (MRI) is usually not required to confirm the diagnosis of anencephaly. MRI may be utilized when there is limitation in US imaging or in the case of medical, legal, or ethical issues.[31] It can be helpful to exclude other pathologies mimicking AEA, provide information in the presence of smaller defects, and is useful in multiple gestations when it is necessary to confirm normal development of the co-twin.

In AEA, the calvarium and scalp are absent above the orbits in the presence of normal development of facial structure. In exencephaly, there are disorganized cerebral hemispheres with loss of normal landmarks and associated deformity of the cerebellum and brainstem.[32] In acrania, similar or less severe deformity is noted (Fig. 23.1-5). With anencephaly, the orbits are prominent, no brain tissue is seen, and a cervical spine defect with absence of brainstem and spinal cord can be identified (Fig. 23.1-6). In meroanencephaly, there is a median bone defect, best depicted on US, with disorganized brain tissue that extends through a superior midline open calvarial defect (Fig. 23.1-7).

Associated Anomalies: Approximately 80% of fetuses with anencephaly have associated malformations.[33] Spinal lesions are the

most common, being found in up to 50% of cases. Other common anomalies include cleft lip/palate, clubbed feet and hands, genital, gastrointestinal, and cardiac anomalies.[1,33]

Differential Diagnosis: Differential includes large cephaloceles, osteogenesis imperfecta (OI), and hypophosphatasia. In both OI and hypophosphatasia, the bones are present but poorly mineralized, and other fractures, bone shortening, and/or bowing are typically present.

This disorder should be distinguished from amniotic band syndrome, in which there is an asymmetric brain defect, multiple limb or digit amputations, asymmetric ventral wall defects, and unusual craniofacial or spinal defects. The amniotic band is often associated with oligohydramnios, which is rare in anencephaly.[22]

Prognosis: Approximately 55% to 60% of pregnancies with anencephaly die *in utero* or during labor.[2,34] Affected live born fetuses have a rudimentary brainstem which may support breathing and responses to sound and touch, but long-term survival is not possible with neonatal death typically within hours to days.[2]

Management: Elective termination is often considered. In the United States, prenatal diagnosis and pregnancy termination have

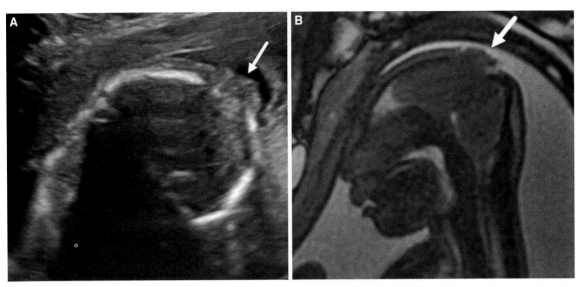

FIGURE 23.1-7: Meroanencephaly in 24-week fetus. **A:** Sagittal US demonstrating median calvarial defect with protruding brain (*arrow*). Notice the head is small. **B:** Sagittal T2 SSFP MRI in same fetus demonstrating disorganized brain protruding through midline calvarial defect (*arrow*) without covering membrane. Notice small brain without normal landmarks.

decreased the prevalence of anencephaly at birth by 60% to 70%.[35] In Europe, America, and Asia, the overall frequency for termination of anencephaly pregnancy has been reported to be 83%, ranging from 59% to 100%.[36] A worldwide review from 2015, however, noted a 33% elective termination in the presence of anencephaly.[2]

Maternal obstetric risks are not increased; however, there is a tendency toward delivery via repeated caesarean section.[32] For the 40% to 45% that are born alive, supportive care is typically provided for minutes to days.[37] The potential for neonatal organ donation has raised both legal and ethical issues.

Recurrence Risk: There is a 2% to 5% recurrence risk.[1,16] Increased risk also exists for those with relatives affected by anencephaly or those with genetic predisposition.

CEPHALOCELES

Description: A cephalocele is a closed NTD characterized by extracalvarial herniation of intracranial structures through a congenital cranial defect, typically covered with skin. These NTDs are classified according to the location and contents of the herniation. *Meningoceles* are herniations of meninges and CSF only. *Meningoencephaloceles,* the most common form, are herniations of meninges, brain, and CSF. A meningoencephalocele which includes part of a ventricle is termed *meningoencephalocystocele.* An *atretic cephalocele* is typically parietal or occipital in location and consists of a narrow meningofibrous tract extending from the posterior fossa to the scalp.[38,39]

Incidence: Cephaloceles account for 10% of all craniospinal dysraphisms. Estimated incidence is 0.8 to 5.63 per 10,000 births.[40] The actual incidence may be higher as many of these malformations result in termination, *in utero* demise, and stillbirth. There is a difference in cephalocele anatomical defect site geographically and by gender. In the West, occipital encephaloceles are most common (80%), while midline frontal and parietal are evenly divided between the remaining 20%.[41] In Southeast Asia and Russia, frontal cephaloceles are prevalent.[41] Females are affected twice as commonly as are males in the occipital location.[38]

Pathogenesis: The pathogenesis is not completely understood and multiple theories have been described. All encephaloceles have a midline defect which corresponds to abnormal neural tube closure, but, in addition, most are covered by skin or an epithelial layer, supporting a disturbance in separation of the neural tube from surface ectoderm (postneurulation disorder).[42] Disturbance of neural tube closure in multiple sites is likely the reason for different anatomical defects. For example, final closure of the rostral neuropore is between the nasal field and likely results in a frontonasal encephalocele. It is hypothesized that disturbance in this site of closure would result in persistent connections between the neuroectoderm and surface ectoderm, such that mesodermal tissue necessary for skull formation would not occur. Some hypothesize that the persistent connections may be due to lack of apoptosis.[42] Given the embryonic stage of insult, it is likely that encephaloceles occur early in embryogenesis, at between 24 and 60 days.[43]

Etiology: Cephaloceles have been associated with both genetic and environmental teratogens. A recent study found that these defects are significantly more common in Hispanic women and in pregnancies where maternal age was less than 29 years.[40] These NTDs are associated with exposure to trypan blue, irradiation, excess vitamin A, folic acid antagonists, triamcinolone, warfarin exposure, hyperthermia, and malnutrition.[39,44] Cephaloceles are also seen at a higher rate with maternal diabetes mellitus, rubella, and consanguineous marriages.[44] Increase in folic acid consumption is not likely to affect prevalence.[45] Some cephaloceles are part of recognized genetic and nongenetic syndromes (Table 23.1-1).[43,46] However, approximately 80% of cases are not associated with identifiable genetic, chromosomal, or teratogenic disorders.[45]

Diagnosis: As many cephaloceles are covered with normal or dysplastic skin, there is no elevation in AFP.[44,47] An elevated antenatal AFP, however, can sometimes be present if the lesion is incompletely covered. Because of inconsistency, prenatal diagnosis is typically dependent on US.

Most cephalocele defects are found midline or paramidline and named for their location. The most common types are occipital, frontoethmoidal, parietal, and basal. Lateral meningoceles

TABLE 23.1-1   Syndromes/Association in Cephaloceles

SYNDROME/ASSOCIATION	GENETIC TRANSMISSION
Occipital	
Meckel–Gruber	Autosomal recessive
Knobloch (eye malformations)	Autosomal recessive
Walker–Warburg (Chemke, HARD ± E)	Autosomal recessive
Cryptophthalmos	Autosomal recessive
Dyssegmental dwarfism	Autosomal recessive
Von Voss–Cherstvoy (radial ray defects and urogenital)	Autosomal recessive
Joubert	Primary autosomal recessive
Klippel–Feil	Variable
Craniostenosis	Variable syndrome
Hemifacial microsomia (oculoauriculovertebral)	Sporadic
Ectrodactyly-ectodermal dysplasia	Sporadic and familial
Warfarin embryopathy	
Dandy Walker	
Arnold Chiari, especially type III	
Iniencephaly	
Myelomeningocele	
Parietal	
Absent corpus callosum	
Atretic form	
Corpus callosum anomalies	
Midline fusion anomalies	
Schizencephaly	
Intracranial cysts	
Absent septum pellucidum	
Chiari II–III	
Frontal	
Roberts-SC phocomelia	Autosomal recessive
Frontonasal dysplasia	Autosomal recessive
Cleft lip/palate	
Absent corpus callosum	
Basal/Transsphenoidal	
Sakoda complex (with agenesis corpus callosum and midline cleft palate/lip)	
Morning glory syndrome (congenital dysplasia of optic disc)	
Cleft palate/lip	
Hypothalamic pituitary dysfunction	
Absent corpus callosum	

can very rarely occur, although the most common etiology entertained should be amniotic bands.[39]

- *Occipital:* The defect is between the lambda and the foramen magnum, can include the infratentorial and supratentorial brain, and may demonstrate anomalous venous sinus extension.[38,48]

- Chiari III is characterized by a high cervical and low occipital encephalocele in association with anatomical characteristics of a Chiari II malformation, including hindbrain herniation, medullary abnormalities, hydrocephalus (88%), and small posterior fossa (Fig. 23.1-8).[49]
- Atretic encephaloceles (see later)

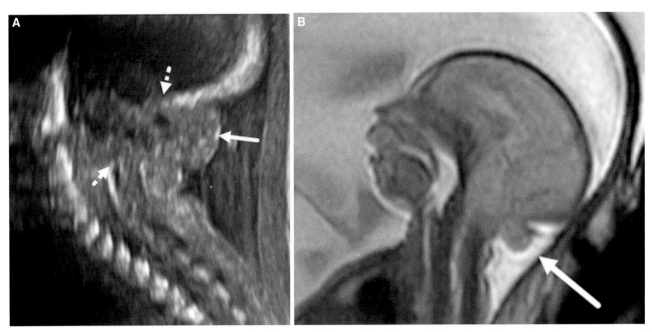

FIGURE 23.1-8: Chiari III in fetus at 25 weeks **A:** Sagittal US showing defect in the inferior occipital and cervical posterior elements (*demarcated by dotted arrows*). There is herniation of brain tissue through the defect (*solid arrow*). **B:** Sagittal T2 MRI showing encephalocele (*solid arrow*). Notice small posterior fossa and hindbrain herniation.

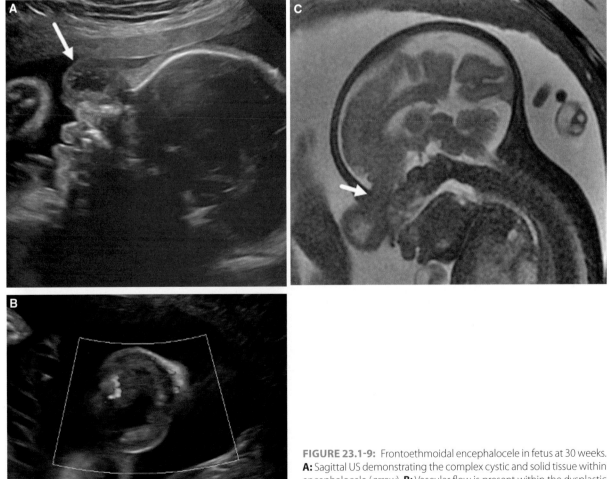

FIGURE 23.1-9: Frontoethmoidal encephalocele in fetus at 30 weeks. **A:** Sagittal US demonstrating the complex cystic and solid tissue within encephalocele (*arrow*). **B:** Vascular flow is present within the dysplastic tissue on axial color Doppler US. **C:** Sagittal SSFP MRI demonstrating continuity of the defect with intracranial contents (*arrow*).

- *Frontoethmoidal/Sincipital:* The defect is at the foramen cecum, anterior to the crista galli where the frontal and ethmoidal bones meet (Fig. 23.1-9). Hypertelorism is a common association. Smaller meningoceles may be undetectable on antenatal imaging but can present with ascending infection in childhood.[50] Failure of involution can also lead to a nasal dermal sinus or nasal glioma.[48,50–52]
  - A nasal dermal sinus occurs when there is incomplete separation of the dura from the skin, resulting in dermal inclusion cysts anywhere along the tract, including intracranial.
  - Nasal gliomas are heterotopic glial tissue without intracranial connection that can be found in the nose or, more commonly, above the nose (glabella). The tissue in the defect is typically hypoechoic and vascular on US and follows gray matter signal on fetal MRI[52] (Fig. 23.1-10).
- *Parietal:* The defect is between the intersection of coronal sutures and the lambda.
  - Atretic cephaloceles account for most of the cephaloceles in the parietal area and overall 25% to 56% of all cephaloceles.[53] The atretic lesion is typically identified in the presence of a CSF-filled, cigar-shaped tract extending posterosuperiorly from the posterior fossa, within the interhemispheric fissure, accompanied by an aberrant straight sinus (falcine sinus). The tissue in the stalk extending extracranial through the calvarial defect may contain meningeal and/or fibrous tissue, blood vessels, and/or neural or glial elements[53,54] (Fig. 23.1-11).
- *Basal:* These rare defects in the skull base occur at the junction of the sphenoid and ethmoid, and may present as a mass in the mouth or posterior pharynx, potentially obstructing the airway (Fig. 23.1-12).[51] Herniation of tissue may result in endocrine dysfunction or disruption of optic pathway. Morning glory syndrome (enlarged funnel-shaped optic disc resembling a morning glory flower) is described in 67% of basal encephaloceles.[51]

Ultrasound: Although the literature reports prenatal US detection rates of 80% to 100%, lesions such as atretic cephaloceles, small frontoethmoidal meningoceles, and basal defects may be difficult to detect.[55,56] The diagnosis of larger lesions can be confidently made during the first and second trimester.[39,55] Especially helpful in the first trimester is transvaginal imaging, which can improve diagnosis and identify sac contents, even small lesions containing less than 10% of intracranial contents (Fig. 23.1-13).[57] The utilization of 3D US can improve detection of small lesions and also provide assistance in the first-trimester imaging.[55,57]

To confidently diagnose a cephalocele, a defect in the cranial vault and continuity between the defect contents and the intracranial structures must be demonstrated[55] (Fig. 23.1-14). However, care must be taken to ensure that the calvarial defect is not an artifact related to angle dropout or the normal posterior fontanel.[56] If the skull defect is small (up to 20% of cases), diagnosis can be difficult.[41] Low amniotic fluid, maternal obesity, or fetal head positioning may also impede detection.

Cephaloceles are variable in size, shape, and echotexture, appearing solid, cystic, or mixed[41] (Fig. 23.1-15). Detection of fetal brain with a gyral pattern within the sac is helpful, although the US appearance may change throughout gestation with solid tissue becoming more cystic and the size changing over time.[55,58,59] Therefore, it can sometimes be difficult to discriminate a cranial

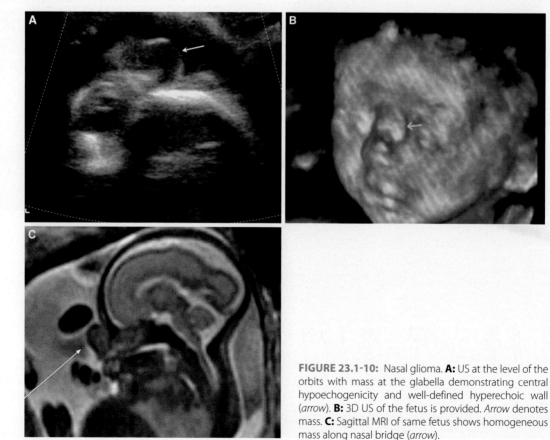

FIGURE 23.1-10: Nasal glioma. **A:** US at the level of the orbits with mass at the glabella demonstrating central hypoechogenicity and well-defined hyperechoic wall (*arrow*). **B:** 3D US of the fetus is provided. *Arrow* denotes mass. **C:** Sagittal MRI of same fetus shows homogeneous mass along nasal bridge (*arrow*).

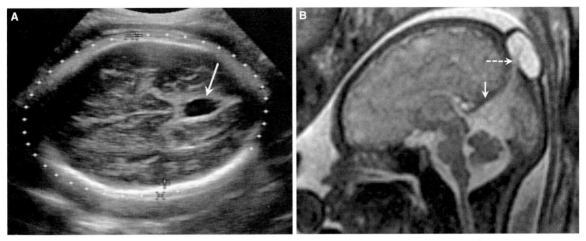

FIGURE 23.1-11: Atretic parietal cephalocele. **A:** Axial US shows cigar-shaped interhemispheric cerebrospinal fluid (CSF) collection (*arrow*) in a fetus in the third trimester. **B:** On sagittal MRI, the same fetus shows vertical persistent falcine sinus (*solid arrow*), small parietal calvarial defect (*dotted arrow*), and CSF extracranial skin covered sac containing linear tissue.

meningocele from an encephalocele. A cephalocele can be differentiated from an extracranial lesion by the acute angle with the surface of the fetal head.[44,55] Vascular flow into and around the lesion can indicate venous sinus extension and may be helpful in securing diagnosis of a cephalocele (Fig. 23.1-14B). Factors on US that can help to predict a good outcome include a sac containing only CSF or a nubbin of neural tissue, no associated anomalies, normal-sized brain, and absence of ventriculomegaly.[60] If more than 50% of the intracranial contents are exteriorized, survival and outcome are poor.[55]

Associated anomalies commonly identified on US include ventriculomegaly, microcephaly, loss of normal cerebral landmarks, lemon skull, features of Chiari II (termed Chiari III when combined with occipital cephalocele or high cervical meningoceles),

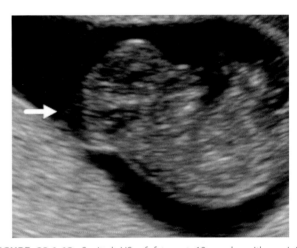

FIGURE 23.1-13: Sagittal US of fetus at 12 weeks with occipital cephalocele (*arrow*) detected via transvaginal imaging.

obliteration of cisterna magna, and flattened basiocciput.[55] Evaluation of extracranial structures should be performed with special attention to the kidneys and spine.[61] The presence of oligohydramnios, polycystic kidneys, and occipital cephalocele should raise suspicion for Meckel–Gruber syndrome.[55]

Magnetic Resonance Imaging: Fetal MRI can overcome many of the limitations of US cranial imaging and therefore improve on an already high detection rate.[31] In the presence of an NTD, MRI has been shown to detect new findings that change US diagnosis in 15% of cases and discern new findings that were not defined on US in 42% of cases. MRI has the ability to influence management decisions such as continuation of pregnancy or mode of delivery in 21%.[31]

Multiplanar imaging allows sharp delineation of the calvarial defect and can define the varying amounts of brain tissue, venous sinus extension, and CSF in the cephalocele sac, thus providing important information with regard to prognosis.[31,62] Steady-state free precession (SSFP) imaging demonstrates good contrast between water and soft tissue and can be helpful at defining borders of the defect. Echo planar imaging (EPI) can assist in definition of the venous anatomies, and diffusion imaging may improve

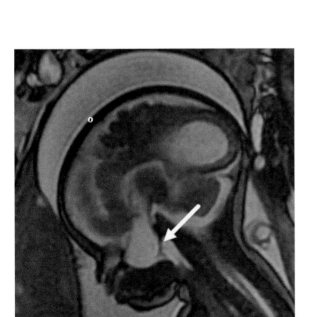

FIGURE 23.1-12: Sagittal SSFP MRI of a basal cephalocele (*arrow*) in fetus at 32 weeks referred for multiple anomalies including median cleft lip and ventriculomegaly. Notice the defect obstructs the oropharynx. The cephalocele was not well delineated on US.

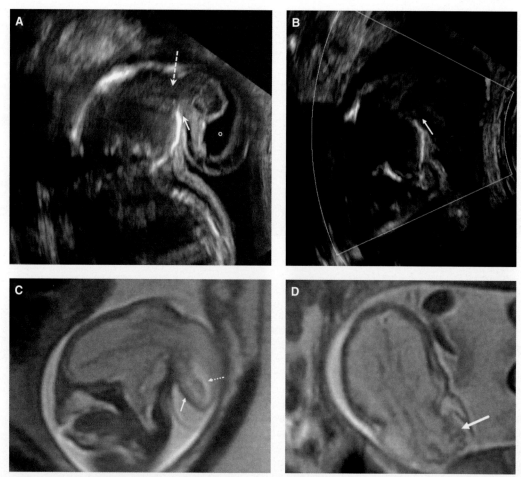

FIGURE 23.1-14: Fetus at 27 weeks with occipital meningoencephalocystocele. **A:** Sagittal US demonstrates a defect in the calvarium (*solid arrow*) and continuity of intracranial brain extending into sac (*dotted arrow*). Cystic dilatation in extracranial tissue represents dilated ventricle (*circle*). **B:** Sagittal US with color demonstrating venous extension into the defect (*arrow*). **C:** Sagittal MRI showing solid tissue (*solid arrow*) with central cerebrospinal fluid representing herniated ventricle (*dotted arrow*). The supratentorial brain demonstrates lack of normal sulcation. **D:** Axial MRI showing lobular contour (*arrow*) of the herniated brain parenchyma consistent with polymicrogyria.

detection of displaced brain, exclude ischemia, or define other lesions including a dermoid, which will show restricted diffusion. Diffusion tensor imaging (DTI) can demonstrate white matter and brainstem tracts.[63]

Fetal MRI is also extremely useful in identifying additional associated CNS anomalies, such as hindbrain malformations, corpus callosum dysgenesis, and cerebral parenchymal abnormalities[31] (Fig. 23.1-16). The externalized brain may show degenerative changes including polymicrogyria, calcification, and hemorrhage (Fig. 23.1-14D).[63] Brainstem anomalies include herniation into the encephalocele, kinked configuration between midbrain and diencephalon and medulla and cervical cord, molar tooth malformations, and Chiari malformations.[63] Excluding syndromes such as Meckel–Gruber, Walker–Warburg, and Joubert, which are seen in conjunction with occipital encephaloceles, is important for counseling and future pregnancies given the recurrence risk.

Associated Anomalies: Both intracranial and extracranial anomalies have been cited in up to 50% of children with cephaloceles.[47] Associated extracranial anomalies include facial, cardiovascular, gastrointestinal, genitourinary, limb, heterotaxy, and other NTDs.[47,64]

Intracranial associations are varied but include ventriculomegaly, microcephaly, brainstem anomalies, callosal dysgenesis, cortical malformations, and vascular abnormalities. Ventriculomegaly or hydrocephalus is the most common association, present in approximately 50% of cases.[47]

Differential Diagnosis: Demonstration of a calvarial bone defect confirms the diagnosis of cephalocele. However, if the fetus has an asymmetric cephalocele and constriction or amputation deformities, findings are more consistent with amniotic band syndrome. In the presence of a small skull defect, extracranial lesions can mimic cephaloceles. The differential diagnosis of a mass adjacent to the fetal skull includes teratoma, vascular or lymphatic malformation, congenital hemangioma, branchial cleft cyst, and scalp edema.[65] A lesion arising from the skin surface should have an obtuse angle with the skull on US.[55] Rarely, fetal hair mimicking a thin membrane on US may be misinterpreted as a defect.[65] A frontal encephalocele should be differentiated from a dermoid cyst and dacrocystocele.[66] Basal encephaloceles must be differentiated from epignathus and congenital granular epulis tumors.[67]

Prognosis: Predictors of poor outcome include associated intracranial abnormalities, development of hydrocephalus, seizure

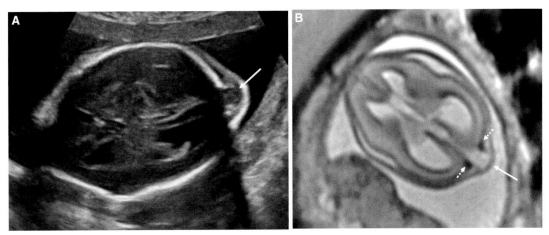

FIGURE 23.1-15: Occipital cephalocele in fetus at 23 weeks. **A:** Axial US shows small defect in calvarium is association with cystic appearance of sac (*arrow*). **B:** Axial MRI showing cystic appearance of sac (*solid arrow*) with venous sinuses along the margin of the skull defect (*dotted arrows*).

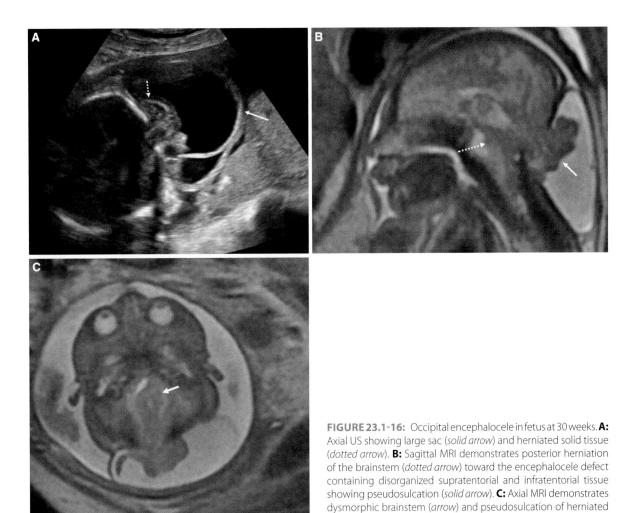

FIGURE 23.1-16: Occipital encephalocele in fetus at 30 weeks. **A:** Axial US showing large sac (*solid arrow*) and herniated solid tissue (*dotted arrow*). **B:** Sagittal MRI demonstrates posterior herniation of the brainstem (*dotted arrow*) toward the encephalocele defect containing disorganized supratentorial and infratentorial tissue showing pseudosulcation (*solid arrow*). **C:** Axial MRI demonstrates dysmorphic brainstem (*arrow*) and pseudosulcation of herniated brain tissue.

disorder, microcephaly, and presence of large brain tissue in the malformation.[68,69] The more rostral the lesion, the better the prognosis.[69,70] In the presence of hydrocephalus, other intracranial abnormalities, or genetic syndrome, the prognosis is poor.[69]

Worldwide, approximately 20% to 25% of pregnancies affected by encephaloceles result in termination and 10% to 15%

in stillbirth.[2] Of the 65% that survive, 80% die under the age of 5 years, although this number decreases to 30% in North America, likely due to better medical support.[2] Occipital lesions with large extracranial brain parenchyma, microcephaly and hydrocephalus are likely to have significant developmental delay.[69] Frontal, small parietal, or atretic cephaloceles generally have a favorable prognosis. In a North American cohort, 48% of patients with encephalocele had normal development, 11% mild delay, 16% moderate delay, and 25% severe delay.[68]

Management: In the presence of a cephalocele, genetic testing should be considered to exclude genetic or chromosomal abnormality. If the encephalocele is large, with severe microcephaly and/or association with other anomalies, termination of the pregnancy may be considered. A caesarean section is recommended to minimize trauma to the brain if the defect is large.[56] If the cephalocele is small, vaginal delivery may be considered. Most cephaloceles are treated with surgery because of risk of injury to displaced brain, leakage of CSF, infection, obstruction of the airway, or facial maldevelopment.[44,68] As the lesion is covered with skin, timing of surgery is typically elective. A staged procedure may be indicated in complex cases. Postoperatively, children with cephaloceles are at risk for hydrocephalus, CSF leak, infection, and lesion recurrence.

Recurrence: The sporadic cases do not have an increased risk of recurrence.[48] In the presence of a genetic syndrome, recurrence can be increased.

AMNIOTIC BAND SYNDROME

Synonyms: Adhesions, amniotic disruption complex, amniotic bands, constricting bands.

Description: Amniotic band syndrome is a collection of malformations thought to be secondary to fetal entanglement in membranes/bands resulting in asymmetric defects that can involve the spine or the cranium.[71]

Incidence: 1 in 1,200 to 15,000 live births.[72]

Pathogenesis: Etiology is unclear. The exogenous theory suggests early amnion rupture leading to fibrous bands, which entrap and can result in asymmetric amputation of fetal parts.[71] If it occurs early, cranial or spinal defects may develop. The endogenous theory suggests lesions are secondary to vascular compromise. Neither mechanism explains all anomalies seen in this syndrome.

Diagnosis: Whenever unusual asymmetric clefts are noted by US or MRI, such as off midline spine, cranial or facial defects particularly when in association with extremity amputation, the diagnosis should be considered. Defects within more than one region are also suggestive of the diagnosis.[72] Diagnosis has been made in the first trimester where membranes are more likely to be directly visualised.[73] On US, the bands are seen in association with a fetal deformity in a random distribution. On MRI, the bands appear as dark T2 signal linear structures in association with an affected body part (Fig. 23.1-17).[74]

Differential Diagnosis: Open NTD, anencephaly, encephalocele, limb body wall complex, and body stalk anomaly should be considered in the presence of a spine or cranial defect.

Associated Anomalies: Variable anomalies have been associated including major cranial, facial, thorax, abdomen, or spine anomalies. Limb constriction, clubfeet, scoliosis, and reduction defects of digits are often present.

Prognosis: Outcome depends on location, size and number of defects.[75–78] Termination is considered if severe craniofacial and visceral abnormalities are present.

Recurrence: Most cases are sporadic.

INIENCEPHALY

Description: Iniencephaly is a severe malformation of the craniovertebral junction and upper thoracic spine with fixed extension of the head, frequently associated with occipital encephalocele and/or myelomeningocele.[79] Inion is Greek for the nape of the neck. Iniencephaly apertus is associated with a hypoplastic occipital bone and encephalocele, while iniencephaly clausus is skin covered with no encephalocele.[80–82]

Incidence: It is 0.1 to 10 in 10,000.

Etiology: Etiology is likely similar to other open NTDs. Folic acid supplements may decrease the risk of iniencephaly. Antiepileptic

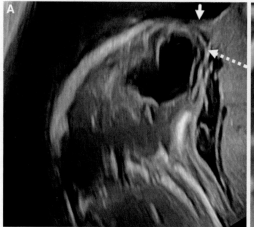
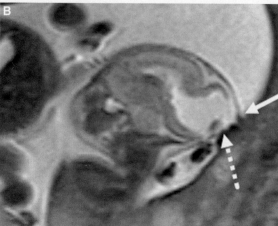

FIGURE 23.1-17: Occipital left-sided encephalocele in a fetus at 23 weeks due to amniotic band. **A:** Sagittal US showing band (*solid arrow*) and disorganized encephalocele (*dotted arrow*). **B:** Sagittal MRI in same fetus demonstrating linear dark T2 signal band (*solid arrow*) and encephalocele defect (*dotted arrow*). The fetus was also lacking the left globe and ear.

drugs, diuretics, and sulfa drugs have all been associated with increased risk.[82,83]

Pathogenesis: Onset is likely a few days later than development of anencephaly. Features include deficit of the occipital bone with enlarged foramen magnum and partial or total absence of cervical and thoracic vertebra with lack of segmentation and irregular vertebral arch fusion. There may be cervicothoracic spine duplication.[79] Shortening of the spinal column with hyperextension of the cervical thoracic spine is present. The face is upturned, with the mandibular skin continuous with the chest because of the short neck.

Diagnosis: AFP is typically elevated.[84]

Ultrasound: Fixed dorsal flexion of the head "star gazing," short cervical and thoracic spine, and irregular vertebrae can be noted by US. A common cavity between the spinal cord and the brain is present owing to the neural arch defects. The skin of the chest directly connects to the face, while the scalp is directly connected to the back.[85–87] Cephaloceles are present in the open form. Polyhydramnios is often noted. Associated anomalies such as arthrogryposis can be identified. Three-dimensional sonography has been used to further assess this complex anomaly.[88]

Magnetic Resonance Imaging: MRI can be a useful adjunct in confirming the diagnosis and is superior in the delineation of the complex brain and spinal cord anomalies[81,83] (Fig. 23.1-18).

Associated Anomalies: Associated anomalies include cleft palate, anencephaly, cephaloceles, omphalocele, gastroschisis, congenital diaphragmatic hernia, cardiac malformations, renal anomalies, arthrogryposis, and clubfoot. Polymicrogyria, heterotopias, holoprosencephaly, and vermian agenesis have been reported.[81,85]

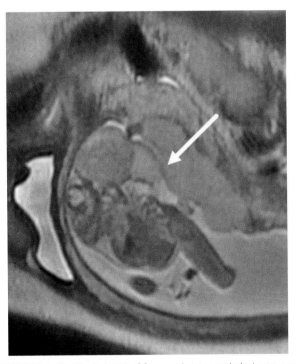

FIGURE 23.1-18: Sagittal MRI of fetus with iniencephaly. Large neural tube defect is present occipital and upper cervical spine (*solid arrow*).

Differential Diagnosis: Differential diagnosis includes Klippel–Feil syndrome, which also has a short neck due to cervical vertebrae fusion anomalies. However, retroflexion of the head is typically not as severe, and AFP is normal. Anencephaly, cervical myelomeningocele, and encephaloceles should also be considered in the differential.

Prognosis: Both types of iniencephaly are typically lethal. Cases of stillbirth or death within hours of delivery have been described.[86,89] Long-term survivors are extremely rare.[79]

Management: Decisions regarding termination of pregnancy or providing supportive care at delivery should be discussed. Dystocia has been reported, and thus avoidance of a caesarean section may require early induction.[89]

Recurrence Risk: The risk of recurrence increases to 1% to 5%.[83]

REFERENCES

1. Nicolaides KH, Campbell S. Diagnosis and management of fetal malformations. *Bailliere's Clin Obstet Gynaecol.* 1987;1:591–622.
2. Blencow H, Kancherla V, Moorthis S, et al. Estimates of global and regional prevalence of neural tube defects for 2015: a systemic analysis. *Ann N Y Acad Sci.* 2018;1414:31–46.
3. Avagliano L, Massa V, George TM, et al. Overview on neural tube defects: from development to physical characteristics. *Birth Defects Res.* 2018. doi:10.1002/bdr2.1380.
4. Frey L, Hauser WA. Epidemiology of neural tube defects. *Epilepsia.* 2003;44(suppl 3):4–13.
5. Seller MJ. Risks in spina bifida. *Dev Med Child Neurol.* 1994;36:1021–1025.
6. Liu S, Evans J, MacFarlane AJ, et al. Association of maternal risk factors with the recent rise of neural tube defects in Canada. *Paediatr Perinat Epidemiol.* 2019;33:145–153.
7. Cameron M, Moran P. Prenatal screening and diagnosis of neural tube defects. *Prenat Diagn.* 2009;29:402–411.
8. Kancheria V, Black RE. Historical perspective on folic acid and challenges in estimating global prevalence of neural tube defects. *Ann N Y Acad Sci.* 2018:1414:20–30.
9. Greene ND, Leung KY, Gay V, et al. Inositol for the prevention of neural tube defects: a pilot randomised controlled trial. *Br J Nutr.* 2016:115;974–983.
10. Copp AJ, Adzick NS, Chitty LS, et al. Spina bifida. *Nat Rev Dis Primers.* 2015;1:15007.
11. Nikolopoulou E, Galea GL, Rolo A, et al. Neural tube closure: cellular, molecular and biomechanical mechanisms. *Development.* 2017;144(4):552–566.
12. Weissman A, Diukman R, Auslender R. Fetal acrania: five new cases and review of the literature. *J Clin Ultrasound.* 1997;25:511–514.
13. Hendricks SK, Cyr DR, Nyberg DA, et al. Exencephaly—clinical and ultrasonic correlation to anencephaly. *Obstet Gynecol.* 1988;72:898–900.
14. Isada NB, Qureshi F, Jacques SM, et al. Meroanencephaly: pathology and prenatal diagnosis. *Fetal diagn Ther.* 1993;8:423–428.
15. Cook RJ, Erdman JN, Hevia M, et al. Prenatal management of anencephaly. *Int J Gynaecol Obstet.* 2008;102:304–308.
16. Stumpf DA, Cranford RE, Elias S, et al. The infant with anencephaly. *N Engl J Med.* 1990;322:669–674.
17. Mitchell LE. Epidemiology of neural tube defects. *Am J Med Genet.* 2005;135:88–94.
18. Wilkins-Haug L, Freedman W. Progression of exencephaly to anencephaly in the human fetus: an ultrasound perspective. *Prenat Diagn.* 1991;11:227–233.
19. Goldstein RB, Filly RA, Callen PW. Sonography of anencephaly: pitfalls in early diagnosis. *J Clin Ultrasound.* 1989;17:397–402.
20. Cafici D, Sepulveda W. First-trimester echogenic amniotic fluid in the acrania-anencephaly sequence. *J Ultrasound Med.* 2003;22:1075–1079.
21. Souka AP, Nicolaides KH. Diagnosis of fetal abnormalities at the 10–14 week scan. *Ultrasound Obstet Gynecol.* 1997;10:429–442.
22. Goldstein RB, Filly RA. Prenatal diagnosis of anencephaly: spectrum of sonographic appearances and distinction from the amniotic band syndrome. *AJR Am J Roentgenol.* 1988;151:547–550.
23. Gorgal R, Ramalho C, Brandao O, et al. Revisiting acrania: same phenotype, different aetiologies. *Fetal Diagn Ther.* 2011;29:164–168.
24. Yaron Y, Hamby DD, O'Brien JE, et al. Combination of elevated maternal serum alpha-fetoprotein (MSAFP) and low estriol is highly predictive of anencephaly. *Am J Med Genet.* 1998;75:297–299.
25. Campbell S, Holt EM, Johnstone FD, et al. Anencephaly: early ultrasonic diagnosis and active management. *Lancet.* 1972;9:1226–1227.
26. Machado RA, Brizot ML, Carvalho MH, et al. Sonographic markers of exencephaly below 10 weeks' gestation. *Prenat Diagn.* 2005;25:31–33.

27. Martins Santana EF, Junior AE, Tonni G, et al. Acrania-exencephaly anencephaly sequence phonotypic characterization using two and three dimensional ultrasound between 11 and 13 week and 6 days gestation. *J Ultrason*. 2018;18(74);240–246.

28. Chatzipapas IK, Whitlow BJ, Economides DL. The Mickey Mouse sign and the diagnosis of anencephaly in early pregnancy. *Ultrasound Obstet Gynecol*. 1999;13:196–199.

29. Johnson SP, Sebire NJ, Snijders RJM, et al. Ultrasound screening for anencephaly at 10–14 weeks of gestation. *Ultrasound Obstet Gynecol*. 1997;9:14–16.

30. Sepulveda W, Sebire NJ, Fung TY, et al. Crown-chin length in normal and anencephalic fetuses at 10–14 weeks' gestation. *Am J Obstet Gynecol*. 1997;176:852–855.

31. Saleem SN, Said AH, Abdel-Raouf M, et al. Fetal MRI in the evaluation of fetuses referred for sonographically suspected neural tube defects (NTDs): impact on diagnosis and management decision. *Neuroradiology*. 2009;51:761–772.

32. Sharif A, Zhou Y. Fetal MRI characteristics of exencephaly: a case report and literature review. *Case Rep Radiol*. 2016;2016:9801267.

33. Gole RA, Meshram PM, Hattangdi SS. Anencephaly and its associated malformations. *J Clin Diagn Res*. 2014;8(9);AC07–AC09.

34. Al-Obaidly S, Thomas J, Abu Jubara M, et al. Anencephaly and obstetric outcome beyond the age of viability. *J Perinat Med*. 2018;46(8):885–888.

35. Cragan JD, Roberts HE, Edmonds LD, et al. Surveillance for anencephaly and spina bifida and the impact of prenatal diagnosis: United States, 1985–1994. *MMWR CDC Surveill Summ*. 1995;44:1–13.

36. Johnson CY, Honein MA, Flanders WD, et al. Pregnancy termination following prenatal diagnosis of anencephaly or spina bifida: a systematic review of the literature. *Birth Defects Res A Clin Mol Teratol*. 2012;94:857–863.

37. Obeidi N, Russell N, Higgins JR, et al. The natural history of anencephaly. *Prenat Diagn*. 2010;30:357–360.

38. David DJ, Proudman TW. Cephaloceles: classification, pathology and management. *World J Surg*. 1989;13:349–357.

39. Naidich TP, Altman NR, Braffman BH, et al. Cephaloceles and related malformations. *AJNR Am J Neuroradiol*. 1992;13:655–690.

40. Wen S, Ethen M, Langloi PH, et al. Prevalence of encephalocele in Texas, 1999–2002. *Am J Med Genet A*. 2007;143A:2150–2155.

41. Goldstein RB, LaPidus AS, Filly RA. Fetal cephaloceles: diagnosis with US. *Radiology*. 1991;180:803–808.

42. Hoving EW. Nasal encephaloceles. *Childs Nerv Syst*. 2000;16;702–706.

43. Rapport RL, Dunn RC Jr., Alhady F. Anterior encephalocele. *J Neurosurg*. 1981;54:213–219.

44. Martinez-Lage JF, Poza M, Sola J, et al. The child with a cephalocele: etiology, neuroimaging and outcome. *Childs Nerv Syst*. 1996;12:540–550.

45. Siffel C, Wong LC, Olney RS, et al. Survival of infants diagnosed with encephalocele in Atlanta, 1979-98. *Paediatr Perinat Epidemiol*. 2003;17;40–48.

46. Cohen MM, Lemire RL. Syndromes with cephaloceles. *Teratology*. 1992;25:161–172.

47. Simpson DA, David D, White J. Cephaloceles: treatment, outcome and antenatal diagnosis. *Neurosurgery*. 1984;15:14–21.

48. Diebler C, Dulac O. Cephaloceles: clinical and neuroradiological appearances. *Neuroradiology*. 1983;25:199–216.

49. Ivashchuk G, Loukas M, Blount JP, et al. Chiari III malformation: a comprehensive review of this enigmatic anomaly. *Childs Nerv Syst*. 2015;31;2035–2040.

50. Tirumandas M, Sharma A, Gbenimache I, et al. Nasal encephaloceles: a review of etiology, pathophysiology, clinical presentations, diagnosis, treatment, and complications. *Childs Nerv Syst*. 2013;29:739–744.

51. Hedlund G. Congenital frontonasal masses: developmental anatomy, malformations, and MR imaging. *Pediatr Radiol*. 2006;36:647–662.

52. Grzegorczyk V, Brasseur-Daudruy M, Labadie G, et al. Prenatal diagnosis of a nasal glioma. *Pediatr Radiol*. 2010;40:1706–1709.

53. Demir MK, Colak A, Eksi MS, et al. Atretic cephaloceles: a comprehensive analysis of historical cohort. *Childs Nerv Syst*. 2016;32;2327–2337.

54. Patterson RJ, Egehoff JC, Crone KR, et al. Atretric parietal cephaloceles revisited: an enlarging clinical and imaging spectrum? *AJNR Am J Neuroradiol*. 1998;19:791–795.

55. Budorick NE, Pretorius DH, McGahan JP, et al. Cephalocele detection in utero: sonographic and clinical features. *Ultrasound Obstet Gynecol*. 1995;5:77–85.

56. Liao SL, Tsai PY, Chen YC, et al. Prenatal diagnosis of fetal encephalocele using three dimensional ultrasound. *J Ultrasound Med*. 2012;20:150–154.

57. Sepulveda W, Wong AE, Andreeva E, et al. Sonographic spectrum of first-trimester fetal cephalocele: review of 35 cases. *Ultrasound Obstet Gynecol*. 2015;46:29–33.

58. Bromshtein M, Zimmer EZ. Transvaginal sonographic follow up on the formation of fetal cephalocele at 13–19 weeks' gestation. *Obstet Gynecol*. 1991;78:528.

59. Tsai PY, Chang CH, Chang FM. Prenatal diagnosis of fetal frontal encephalocele by three-dimensional ultrasound. *Prenat Diagn*. 2006;26:373–394.

60. Bannister CM, Russell SA, Rimmer S, et al. Can prognostic indicators be identified in a fetus with an encephalocele? *Eur J Pediatr Surg*. 2000;10:20–23.

61. Graham D, Johnson RB Jr., Winn K, et al. The role of sonography in prenatal diagnosis and management of encephalocele. *J Ultrasound Med*. 1982;1:111–115.

62. Kojima K, Suzuki Y, Miyajima S, et al. Antenatal evaluation of an encephalocele in a dizygotic twin pregnancy using fast magnetic resonance imaging. *Fetal Diagn Ther*. 2003;18:338–341.

63. Kasprian GJ, Paldino MJ, Mehollin-Ray AR, et al. Prenatal imaging of occipital encephaloceles. *Fetal Diagn Ther*. 2014;37;241–248.

64. Wininger SJ, Donnenfeld AE. Syndromes identified in fetuses with prenatally diagnosed cephaloceles. *Prenat Diagn*. 1994;14:839–843.

65. Noriega CA, Fleming AD, Bonebrake RG. A false-positive diagnosis of a prenatal encephalocele on transvaginal ultrasonography. *J Ultrasound Med*. 2001;20:925–927.

66. Shahabi S, Busine A. Prenatal diagnosis of an epidermal scalp cyst simulating an encephalocele. *Prenat Diagn*. 1998;18:373–377

67. Carlan SJ, Angel JL, Leo J, et al. Cephalocele involving the oral cavity. *Obstet Gynecol*. 1990;75:494–495.

68. Lo BW, Kulkarni AV, Rutka JT, et al. Clinical predictors of developmental outcome in patients with cephaloceles. *J Neurosurg Pediatr*. 2008;2:254–257.

69. Thompson DNP. Postnatal management and outcome for neural tube defects including spina bifida and encephaloceles. *Prenat Diagn*. 2009;29;412–419.

70. Bui CJ, Tubbs RS, Shannon CN, et al. Institutional experience with cranial vault encephaloceles. *J Neurosurg*. 2007;107(suppl 1);22–25.

71. Sentilhes L, Verspyck E, Patrier S, et al. Amniotic band syndrome: pathogenesis, prenatal diagnosis and neonatal management. *J Gynecol Obstet Biol Reprod*. 2003;32;693–704.

72. Burton KJ, Jilly RA. Sonographic diagnosis of the amniotic band syndrome. *AJR Am J Roentgenol*. 1991;156:555.

73. Higuchi T, Tanaka M, Kuroda K, et al. Abnormal first-trimester fetal nuchal translucency and amniotic band syndrome. *J Med Ultrason*. 2012;39(3):177–180.

74. Neuman J, Calvo-Garcia MA, Kline-Fath BM, et al. Prenatal imaging of amniotic band sequence: utility and role of fetal MRI as an adjunct to prenatal ultrasound. *Pediatr Radiol*. 2012;42(5);544–551.

75. Moran SL, Jensen M, Bravo C. Amniotic band syndrome of the upper extremity: diagnosis and management. *J Am Acad Orthop Surg*. 2007;15(7):397–407.

76. Hudgins RJ, Edwards MS, Ousterhout DK, et al. Pediatric neurosurgical implications of the amniotic band disruption complex: case reports and review of the literature. *Pediatr Neurosci*. 1985–1986;12(4–5):232–239.

77. Richter J, Wergeland H, DeKoninck P, et al. Fetoscopic release of an amniotic band with risk of amputation: case report and review of the literature. *Fetal Diagn Ther*. 2012;31(2):134–137.

78. Hüsler MR, Wilson RD, Horii SC, et al. When is fetoscopic release of amniotic bands indicated? Review of outcome of cases treated in utero and selection criteria for fetal surgery. *Prenat Diagn*. 2009;29(5):457–463.

79. Holmes LB, Toufaily MH, Westgate MN. Iniencephaly. *Birth Defects Res*. 2018;110(2):128–133.

80. Aleksic S, Budzilovich G, Greco MA, et al. Iniencephaly a neuropathologic study. *Clin Neuropathol*. 1983;2:55–61.

81. Gadodia A, Gupta P, Sharma R, et al. Antenatal sonography and MRI of iniencephaly apertus and clausus. *Fetal Diagn Ther*. 2010;27(3):178–180.

82. Kulkarni PR, Rao RV, Alur MB, et al. Iniencephaly clausus: a case report with review of literature. *J Pediatr Neurosci*. 2011;6(2):121–123.

83. Pungavkar SA, Sainani NI, Karnik AS, et al Antenatal diagnosis of iniencephaly: sonographic and MR correlation: a case report. *Korean J Radiol*. 2007;8(4):351–355.

84. Mórocz I, Szeifert GT, Molnár P, et al. Prenatal diagnosis and pathoanatomy of iniencephaly. *Clin Genet*. 1986;30(2):81–86.

85. Tugrul S, Uludoğan M, Pekin O, et al. Iniencephaly: prenatal diagnosis with postmortem findings. *J Obstet Gynaecol Res*. 2007;33(4):566–569.

86. Balci S, Aypar E, Altinok G, et al. Prenatal diagnosis in three cases of iniencephaly with unusual postmortem findings. *Prenat Diagn*. 2001;21(7):558–562.

87. Sahid S, Sepulveda W, Dezerega V, et al. Iniencephaly: prenatal diagnosis and management. *Prenat Diagn*. 2000;20;202–205.

88. Sepulveda W. Three-dimensional sonography of fetal iniencephaly. *J Ultrasound Med*. 2012;31(8):1296–1298.

89. Katz VL, Aylsworth AS, Albright SG. Iniencephaly is not uniformly fatal. *Prenat Diagn*. 1989;9(8):595–599.

SPINAL DYSRAPHISM EMBRYOLOGY AND CLASSIFICATION

Neural tube defects involving the spine and spinal cord form a wide spectrum of abnormalities that can be collectively referred to as *spinal dysraphisms*, and one of the most widely cited classification systems in the pediatric neuroradiology literature is the cliniconeuroradiological classification described by Tortori-Donati et al.[1–3] This classification system divides spinal dysraphisms into two main categories: *open* versus *closed*, the distinction of which is made by the absence (open) or presence (closed) of a skin covering. Open spinal dysraphisms, mainly myelomeningoceles and myeloceles, have absence of a skin covering and are associated with a constellation of intracranial abnormalities known as Chiari II malformation.[2] These are almost always detected prenatally.[4] Closed spinal dysraphisms, of which there is a wide spectrum of abnormalities, are skin covered and, depending on the severity, are not always possible to detect by fetal imaging.[5]

Though a detailed description of spinal embryology is beyond the scope of this text, in short, spinal cord development can be divided into three stages: stage 1 is *gastrulation* (2 to 3 weeks' gestational age), during which the embryological disk converts from a bilaminar to a trilaminar disk comprising ectoderm, mesoderm, and endoderm. During gastrulation, the notochord is formed from the mesoderm. Stage 2 is *primary neurulation* (third to fourth weeks) during which the notochord interacts with the overlying ectoderm to form the neural plate, which then folds inward to form the neural tube. Stage 3 is *secondary neurulation and retrogressive differentiation* (fifth to sixth weeks), during which the secondary neural tube (which becomes the conus and filum terminale) forms by the caudal cell mass (pluripotent cells that form from fusion of the caudal neural epithelium with the notochord) followed by retrogressive differentiation (selective apoptosis).

These stages of embryology can be used to explain and categorize many of the described congenital spine abnormalities, though there is much overlap between the embryological and cliniconeuroradiological classification schemes. From a fetal imaging perspective, it may be more practical to divide the closed spinal dysraphisms into those with a sac and those without a sac, and further divide the closed spinal dysraphisms without a sac into complex and simple, with complex spinal dysraphisms being more likely to have abnormalities outside the spinal cord identifiable on prenatal imaging and simple being very challenging to confidently diagnose or detect on fetal imaging. One must also keep in mind that not all spinal dysraphisms will fit perfectly into one particular category and that more than one type of spinal dysraphism may coexist in a single fetus (Fig. 23.2-1). In this section, we discuss the embryology, fetal imaging findings, and clinical implications of some of the most common spinal dysraphisms detected prenatally.

OPEN SPINAL DYSRAPHISM

Synonyms: Open neural tube defect, spina bifida aperta, myelomeningocele myelocele, myeloschisis.

Description: What makes a spinal dysraphism "open" is a lack of skin covering at birth. The two open spinal dysraphisms that are described are myelomeningoceles and myeloceles.[2] Myelomeningoceles have a sac with the neural placode protruding posterior to the skin surface, while in myeloceles, also known as myeloschisis, the neural placode is flush with the skin surface.[3] While this distinction is important in fetal imaging for planning of fetal surgery, open spinal dysraphisms are rarely imaged postnatally prior to repair since these are typically repaired within the first 48 hours of life in order to decrease the risk of infection from the exposed neural elements.[6] Open spinal dysraphisms are associated with intracranial findings of Chiari II malformation.[7]

Epidemiology: Open spinal dysraphisms comprise one of the most common congenital abnormalities of the central nervous system. The worldwide prevalence is highly variable, and in the United States, it has been reported to occur in 5.3 per 10,000 births from 1999 to 2007.[8] Folate deficiency during pregnancy is one of the primary described risk factors of open spinal dysraphisms, and folic acid supplementation is believed to be the leading cause of decreased incidence of the disease.[9] However, the etiology is likely multifactorial as genetic factors have been implicated in the pathogenesis, and open spinal dysraphisms can be seen in many described syndromes.[10,11]

Embryology/Pathogenesis: *Disjunction* occurs during primary neurulation immediately after neural tube closure, during which the cutaneous ectoderm separates from the neural ectoderm. Large areas of nondisjunction are believed to result in open spinal dysraphisms, either myelomeningocele or myelocele.

Open spinal dysraphism is classically associated with intracranial findings of Chiari II malformation.[1,2,12,13] One of the most widely accepted theories for this is the unified theory of McLone and Knepper, which describes how defective occlusion caused by an open neural tube defect precludes cerebrospinal fluid (CSF) accumulation and pressure within the developing cerebral ventricles, causing the findings of Chiari II malformation.[14] These include a small posterior cranial fossa with hindbrain herniation (Fig. 23.2-2).

Diagnosis: Maternal serum screening for open neural tube defects (which includes open spinal dysraphisms and anencephaly) by measuring maternal serum alpha-fetoprotein (AFP) can be performed between 15 and 18 weeks' gestational age, with 16 to 18 weeks being optimal. Elevated AFP can detect up to 90% of open spinal dysraphisms and more than 95% of anencephaly

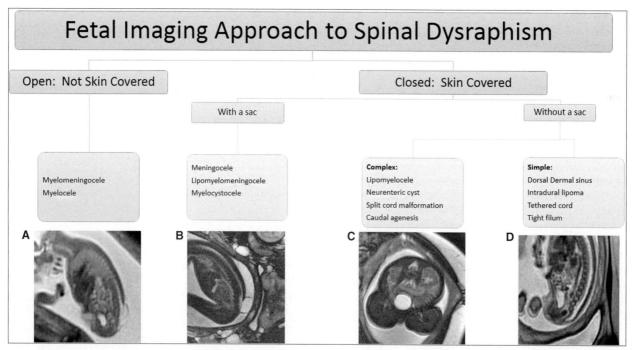

Fetal Imaging Approach to Spinal Dysraphism

Open: Not Skin Covered

Closed: Skin Covered

With a sac

Without a sac

Myelomeningocele
Myelocele

Meningocele
Lipomyelomeningocele
Myelocystocele

Complex:
Lipomyelocele
Neurenteric cyst
Split cord malformation
Caudal agenesis

Simple:
Dorsal Dermal sinus
Intradural lipoma
Tethered cord
Tight filum

A **B** **C** **D**

FIGURE 23.2-1: Fetal imaging approach to classifying spinal dysraphism: **A:** Open spinal dysraphism: fetal MRI of myelomeningocele with no skin covering and neural placode outside the spinal canal. **B:** Closed spinal dysraphism with a sac: fetal MRI of skin-covered sac without neural elements consistent with a meningocele. **C:** Complex closed spinal dysraphism without a sac: axial fetal MRI of a split cord malformation. **D:** Simple closed spinal dysraphism without a sac: fetal MRI of low conus.

prenatally.[15] However, given that second-trimester fetal ultrasound (US) has been shown to detect more open neural tube defects than AFP alone, some believe this screening test is no longer useful.[16] Elevated AFP and a substance called acetylcholinesterase (AChE) can be evaluated in the patient's amniotic fluid as an additional screening tool, as patients who are interested in pursuing fetal surgery will require an amniocentesis in order to confirm a normal fetal karyotype.[17] Though the roles of these amniotic fluid screening studies have been called into question given the high accuracy of US, this tool may be of value for diagnosis in select patients where it is not clear if there is an open or closed spinal dysraphism prenatally.[18,19]

Ultrasound: There are multiple characteristic brain and spine sonographic findings seen in open spinal dysraphisms (Table 23.2-1). Chiari II malformation is the constellation of brain abnormalities associated with an open spinal dysraphism. On fetal US, two of the most sensitive imaging findings of Chiari II malformation include the "lemon sign" and the "banana sign."[20] The "lemon sign" is the description given to the bifrontal concavity of the calvarium in these patients, which can be seen in 98% of cases before 24 weeks and has been described as early as 13 weeks' gestation.[20,21] The "lemon sign" is present in up to 1% to 2% of normal fetuses and typically resolves by the third trimester of fetuses with open spinal dysraphism (present in

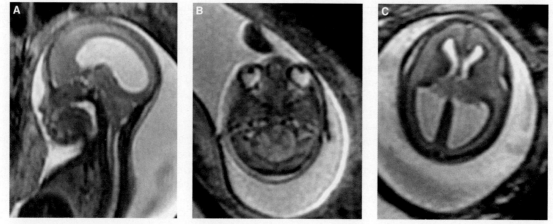

FIGURE 23.2-2: Chiari II malformation. **A:** Sagittal MRI at 21 weeks gestation demonstrating hindbrain herniation below the foramen magnum with complete effacement of the fourth ventricle and near-complete effacement of the cisterna magna. **B:** Axial T2 image of the posterior fossa demonstrating cerebellum wrapping around the brainstem. **C:** Axial T2 image through the supratentorial compartment demonstrating posterior predominant ventriculomegaly with near-complete effacement of the extra-axial cerebrospinal fluid spaces.

TABLE 23.2-1	Sonographic Features of Open Spinal Dysraphism

Small BPD and HC

Bi-frontal concavity (lemon sign)

Small/absent cisternal magna

Rounded small cerebellum (banana sign)

Lateral ventriculomegaly

Dorsal vertebral arches separated or absent

No skin covering

Overlying sac with thin membrane

BPD, biparietal diameter; HC, head circumference.

only 13% of affected fetuses after 24 weeks). Biparietal diameter (BPD) and head circumference (HC) measurements can be below the fifth percentile in the early second trimester, which typically normalize by the third trimester. Microcephaly has been described in up to 69% of cases between 16 and 24 weeks.[22,23]

Dolichocephaly can also be seen marked by decreased cephalic index.[7] The "banana sign" is the description of the cerebellum wrapping around the brainstem, with associated effacement of the fourth ventricle. The cisterna magna is also often effaced (Fig. 23.2-3). Ventriculomegaly is a common associated finding, and reporting ventricular size may be important since it has been suggested that patients with severe ventriculomegaly are less likely to benefit from fetal surgery.[24] Also, macrocephaly can be seen in the presence of ventriculomegaly from obstructive hydrocephalus, though this is more likely to be seen postnatally after the spinal defect has been closed.

Ossification of vertebral bodies progresses through the second trimester with the L5 arch ossified by 16 weeks' gestation, S1 by 19 weeks' gestation, and S2 by 22 weeks' gestation[25] (Fig. 23.2-4). One can count the vertebral body level using the lowest rib as T12 or identifying the lowest horizontal disk space at the lumbosacral junction. The associated open spinal dysraphism, usually located in the lumbosacral region, can be identified by US by identifying the absence of the posterior elements, both skin and bone, overlying the dorsal spinal canal with associated widening or "splaying" of the lamina. Evaluation of the spine in all three planes is necessary to provide the most accurate information about the defect. In a myelomeningocele, a sac can be seen at the defect level, while

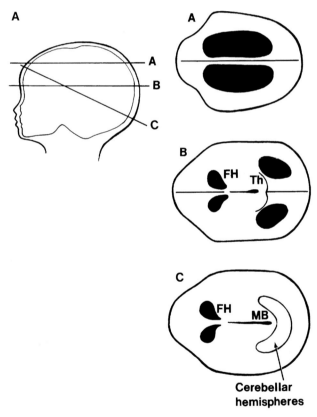

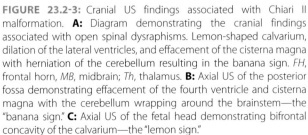

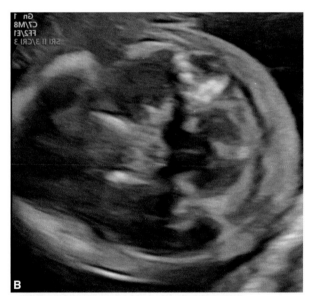

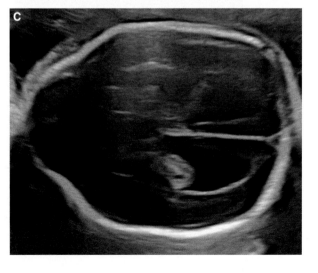

FIGURE 23.2-3: Cranial US findings associated with Chiari II malformation. **A:** Diagram demonstrating the cranial findings associated with open spinal dysraphisms. Lemon-shaped calvarium, dilation of the lateral ventricles, and effacement of the cisterna magna with herniation of the cerebellum resulting in the banana sign. *FH*, frontal horn, *MB*, midbrain; *Th*, thalamus. **B:** Axial US of the posterior fossa demonstrating effacement of the fourth ventricle and cisterna magna with the cerebellum wrapping around the brainstem—the "banana sign." **C:** Axial US of the fetal head demonstrating bifrontal concavity of the calvarium—the "lemon sign."

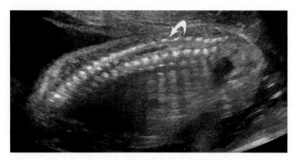

FIGURE 23.2-4: Oblique US of a normal spine at 22 weeks' gestation. Note conus at L3 (*arrow*).

in myeloceles, no measurable myelomeningocele sac is present[26,27] (Figs. 23.2-5 and 23.2-6). The myelomeningocele sac wall when present should be very thin rather than thick in a closed or skin-covered spinal dysraphism. Three-dimensional (3D) US can be of benefit over 2D US in identifying the exact level of the osseous spinal dysraphic defect, allowing for a single volume acquisition to be viewed in the axial, sagittal, and coronal planes simultaneously.[28]

Sonographic evaluation of the lower extremities is important from an anatomic and functional perspective. Equinovarus or clubfoot deformity is the most common foot deformity identified prenatally in patients with open spinal dysraphism and seen in roughly one-third of affected patients.[29] Some advocate for

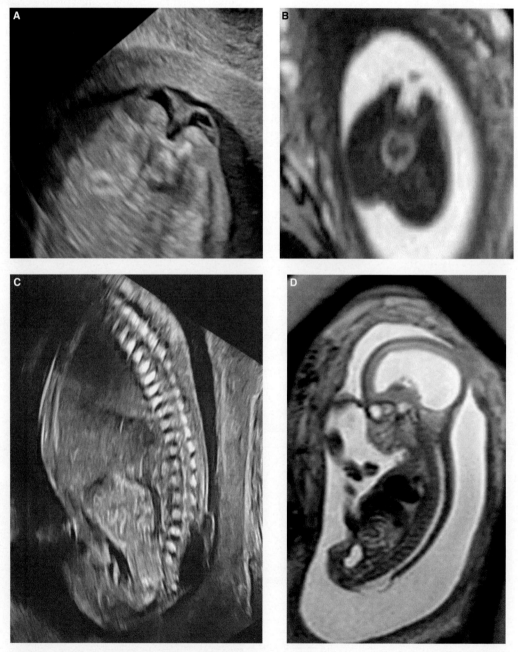

FIGURE 23.2-5: Myelomeningocele at 20 weeks' gestational age. **A:** Axial US of the myelomeningocele sac demonstrating the neural placode outside the spinal canal. **B:** Axial SSFP image of the myelomeningocele sac demonstrating the nearly imperceptible sac wall characteristic of open spinal dysraphisms with the neural placode outside the spinal canal. **C:** Sagittal US of the fetal spine demonstrating open spinal dysraphism of the lumbosacral spine with a myelomeningocele sac. **D:** Sagittal T2 image from fetal MRI of the same patient demonstrating the lumbosacral myelomeningocele with hindbrain herniation.

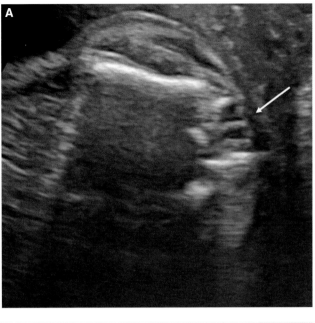

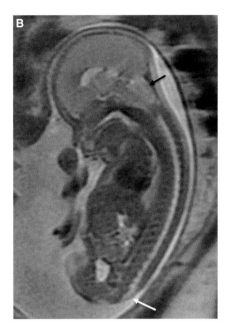

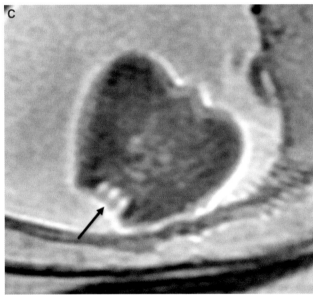

FIGURE 23.2-6: Myelocele (aka myeloschisis). **A:** Axial US of the fetal spine at 21 weeks' gestational age demonstrating an open sacral spinal dysraphism without a measurable sac (*arrow*). **B:** Sagittal T2 MRI demonstrating the sacral myelocele (*white arrow*) with posterior fossa findings consistent with Chiari II malformation (*black arrow*). **C:** Axial T2 MRI showing the open spinal dysraphism with the neural placode flush with the level of the skin surface (*arrows*). There is question of coexisting split cord malformation in this patient.

prenatal sonographic evaluation of lower extremity movement in order to predict the functional level of the spinal deficit. Early research has suggested that the functional level of the lower extremity can be evaluated prenatally by US and correlates with the postnatal segmental level of the neurological lesion, which is the best predictor of future ability to walk. Examination for the absence or presence of ankle plantar flexion (S1), ankle dorsal flexion (L5), knee flexion (L4), knee extension (L3), hip adduction (L2), and hip flexion (L1) can allow for prenatal assignment of a functional level in addition to the vertebral anatomic level.[30] Though evaluation for all of these movements may seem labor intensive, by simply identifying the lowest functional level of movement in a given fetus, an assignment can be made.

Magnetic Resonance Imaging: Fetal magnetic resonance imaging (MRI) has become an important tool in further evaluation of fetuses with open spinal dysraphisms aiding in prenatal counseling and perinatal management. It has become an essential tool in selecting candidates for fetal surgery. The degree of hindbrain herniation is described on fetal MRI by examining the posterior fossa for patency of the fourth ventricle and cisterna magna. We grade these 1 to 3, with grade 1 having a patent fourth ventricle and cisterna magna, grade 2 having an effaced fourth ventricle and a patent cisterna magna, and grade 3 having effacement of both the cisterna magna and fourth ventricle[7] (Fig. 23.2-7). Patients with grade 3 Chiari II malformation are the best candidates for fetal surgery.[31] Subependymal gray matter heterotopias, while common in patients with Chiari II, cannot be reliably diagnosed on fetal MRI and are of unclear clinical significance in this patient population.[32] Fetal MRI, in addition to US, can be used to identify the level of the spinal dysraphic defect and also has a high specificity for detecting associated spinal cord syrinx, particularly in the third trimester. The size of the dysraphic defect can be accurately measured for surgical planning as well. Differentiation

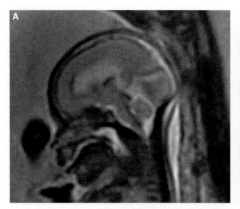
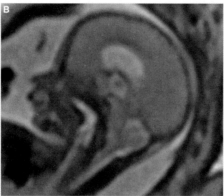
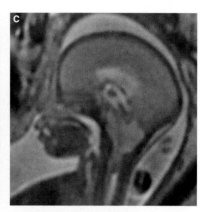

FIGURE 23.2-7: Chiari II malformation grading system. **A:** Grade 1: patent cisterna magna and fourth ventricle without significant hindbrain herniation below the foramen magnum. **B:** Grade 2: effaced fourth ventricle and patent cisterna magna with hindbrain herniation below the foramen magnum. **C:** Grade 3: effacement of the fourth ventricle and cisterna magna with hindbrain herniation.

between myelomeningocele and myelocele is of importance for surgical planning since the absence of a sac is technically more challenging from a neurosurgical perspective as graft closure is often necessary.[33]

When creating an imaging protocol, small field-of-view images at 2- to 4-mm slice thickness in three orthogonal planes of the brain and spine are necessary. T2 single-shot fast spin echo and balanced steady-state free precession (SSFP), also known as TrueFISP (Siemens Medical Solutions) and FIESTA (GE Healthcare), provide a combination of soft-tissue contrast and spatial resolution to help best define the spinal defect and intracranial abnormalities.[34] Additional axial diffusion-weighted images (DWI), echo-planar imaging (EPI), and fast T1 gradient echo images of the brain can aid in identification of cerebral injury. T1 and EPI sequences can also be helpful in the spine for evaluation of fat and osseous structures, respectively.[35] With postprocessing, MR sequences can be used to create models either virtual or using various materials such as paper for surgical planning[36] (Figs. 23.2-8 and 23.2-9).

Associated Anomalies: In addition to the intracranial findings of Chiari II malformation, open spinal dysraphisms are associated with equinovarus or clubfoot deformity, which can be seen on both fetal MRI and US.[37] Decreased rectal meconium signal is commonly seen on fetal MRI in patients with open spinal dysraphism. The presence of coexisting anorectal malformation is rare, though has been described in the setting of caudal agenesis.[38] Coexisting split cord malformation has also been reported in these patients, though fetal MRI is limited in its ability to detect this abnormality in these patients.[39–41]

Differential Diagnosis: Closed spinal dysraphisms such as lipomyelomeningocele or terminal myelocystocele may potentially be difficult to differentiate from open spinal dysraphisms prenatally. However, closed spinal dysraphisms tend to have fewer posterior fossa anomalies, decreased frequency of ventriculomegaly, and high association with the OEIS (omphalocele–exstrophy–imperforate anus–spinal defects) complex when compared with open spinal dysraphisms.[19] A primarily cystic sacrococcygeal teratoma may potentially be in the differential, particularly in a patient without intracranial findings of Chiari II malformation. Identification of solid components in the mass, calcifications, fat, and/or intra-abdominal extension

on both fetal MRI and US can usually allow for accurate distinction of this entity.[42]

Management: Prenatal imaging is very important in counseling, management of the pregnancy, labor and delivery planning, and selecting candidates for fetal surgery. Amniocentesis is recommended in patients with open spinal dysraphism for chromosomal microarray, particularly if additional fetal anomalies are identified. Also, a normal fetal karyotype is required for selection of candidates for fetal surgery. AFP and AChE can also be analyzed at the same time to confirm the diagnosis of open spinal dysraphism. A cesarean section is recommended to minimize trauma to the spine before the onset of labor.[43] Postnatally, the spinal defect is typically closed surgically within the first 48 hours of life in order to stabilize neurological deficits and prevent infection.

Since the Management of Myelomeningocele (MOMS) trial was published in 2013, fetal surgery has become an acceptable method of treatment for open spinal dysraphism.[6,44] In the MOMS trial, prenatal surgery reduced the need for shunting and improved motor outcomes in some patients; however, it was associated with maternal and fetal risks. Inclusion criteria seen on imaging for prenatal repair include patients with a spinal dysraphic defect at the S1 level or higher and the presence of hindbrain herniation, which is best delineated on fetal MRI. Exclusion criteria by imaging include fetal kyphosis ≥30° and identification of fetal anomalies unrelated to the known open spinal dysraphism.[17] A follow-up to the MOMS trial described decreased benefit of fetal surgery in fetuses with lateral ventriculomegaly of 15 mm or larger, making the reporting of ventricle size important in counseling when selecting candidates for fetal surgery.[24]

Prognosis: Open spinal dysraphisms are associated with significant lifelong morbidity, including cognitive impairment, orthopedic disabilities, and bowel and bladder dysfunction. Lifelong multidisciplinary care from neurosurgery, neurology, orthopedics, urology, and physical and occupational therapy are often required.

Outcomes are highly variable around the world and are in part affected by medical resources. Intrauterine demise is seen in fewer than 5%, with the majority of fetuses (≈80%) being born at term. Nearly 90% of patients require ventriculoperitoneal shunt placement, which carries risks of shunt failure or infection.[45,46] Approximately 80% of those born are expected to survive past

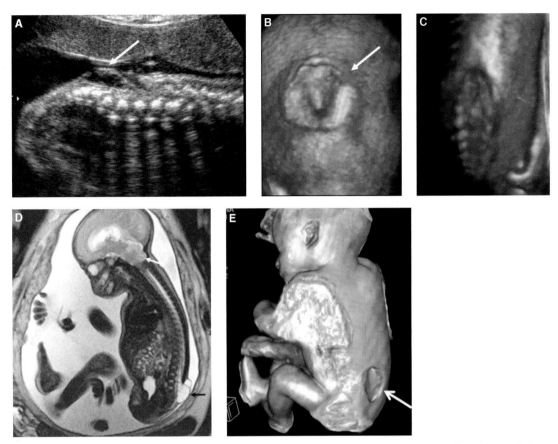

FIGURE 23.2-8: Myelomeningocele at 26 weeks' gestation. **A:** Sagittal US demonstrating overlying thin-walled sac (*arrow*) with cord tethering. 3D US of the sac in surface mode **(B)** and spinal dysraphism in skeletal mode **(C)**. **D:** Sagittal MRI demonstrating the Chiari malformation (*white arrow*) and MMC sac containing neural elements (*black arrow*). **E:** 3D MR surface model demonstrating skin defect (*arrow*). (Courtesy of Heron Werner.)

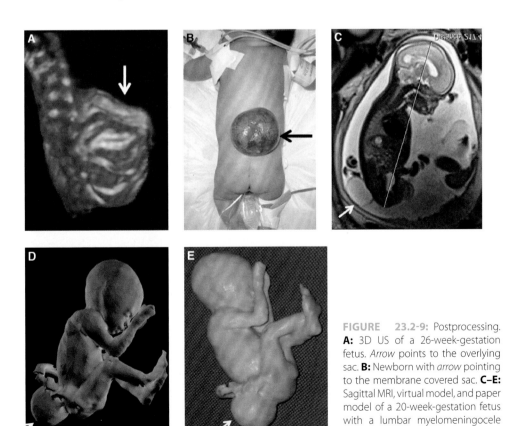

FIGURE 23.2-9: Postprocessing. **A:** 3D US of a 26-week-gestation fetus. *Arrow* points to the overlying sac. **B:** Newborn with *arrow* pointing to the membrane covered sac. **C–E:** Sagittal MRI, virtual model, and paper model of a 20-week-gestation fetus with a lumbar myelomeningocele (*arrows*). (Courtesy of Heron Werner.)

5 years of age, with approximately 75% of patients reaching adulthood.[47] Long-term outcomes are highly variable, adults range from near-normal to severe mental and physical disability. Approximately two-thirds of adult survivors will have normal IQ scores, and up to one-third can ambulate independently. However, up to one-third of adult survivors require daily care.[48]

Despite the wide variability of outcomes, efforts to accurately predict outcomes based on imaging findings have been of limited success, though a few small series have been published. Higher degrees of cerebellar herniation have been described in association with increased childhood seizure activity, bladder dysfunction, and decreased independent ambulation.[49] When examining the spine, larger and higher spinal dysraphic defects have been described in association with full-time wheelchair use.[50] Gray matter heterotopias, which are associated with epilepsy and disorders of cognition in other patient populations, are of unclear clinical significance in patients with open spinal dysraphism.[51] The clinical implications of a myelomeningocele versus a myelocele are still unclear. While myeloceles are shown to be associated with higher degrees of hindbrain herniation, along with increased scoliosis and bladder dysfunction, a 30-month follow-up study to the MOMS trial described the absence of a sac on fetal MRI positively correlated with independent ambulation in patients who underwent prenatal repair.[50,52,53] More studies in this area will be valuable to aid in counseling and management.

CLOSED SPINAL DYSRAPHISM

Synonyms: Spina bifida occulta, skin-covered neural tube defects, closed neural tube defects.

Description: Congenital abnormalities of the spine that are covered by skin can be collectively referred to as closed spinal dysraphisms, under which a variety of spinal abnormalities can be categorized. Though the often-cited cliniconeuroradiological classification proposed by Tortori-Donati et al. subdivides closed spinal dysraphisms into those with and without a subcutaneous mass, from a fetal imaging perspective, it may make more sense to subdivide these into those with a sac (meningocele, lipomyelomeningocele, myelocystocele), which may be readily detected on screening US, and those without a sac.[3] Closed spinal dysraphisms without a sac may be further categorized into those that are "complex" and will have abnormalities outside the spinal cord that may be detected on fetal MRI (lipomyelocele, neurenteric cyst, split cord malformation, caudal agenesis) and those that are "simple" and will unlikely be diagnosed prenatally in isolation, though they may have a low conus on fetal MRI (dorsal dermal sinus, intradural lipoma, tight filum, and tethered cord) (Fig. 27.2-1).

Meningocele

Description: Congenital spinal meningoceles are closed spinal dysraphisms characterized by a skin-covered CSF-filled sac lined by dura and arachnoid mater protruding outside the spinal canal. This sac classically does not contain neural elements, though nerve roots can occasionally be displaced into a meningocele sac. The spinal cord itself is completely within the spinal canal, though it is often tethered to the neck of the meningocele sac.[3] These are most commonly seen at the thoracic level, though they can be present in the cervical and lumbosacral regions as well[54] (Fig. 23.2-10).

Incidence: Up to 10% of patients with spinal dysraphism have a meningocele.[55] Anterior or anterolateral meningoceles are less common, though can be seen. An anterior sacral meningocele with an associated anorectal malformation has been described in the setting of Currarino triad.[56–58]

Embryology/Pathogenesis: Though the exact embryology of dorsal congenital meningoceles is unknown, anterior sacral meningoceles in association with Currarino triad may be related to a complex of abnormal endoectodermal adhesions and notochordal defects beginning during gastrulation in the second to third weeks of gestation.[3,59,60]

Diagnosis: AFP levels are typically normal, as the defects are skin covered.

Ultrasound: Typically, there is no association with hindbrain herniation, as is seen with Chiari II malformation. With no cranial findings to suggest a spinal dysraphism, US may miss an isolated small meningocele if the spine lies adjacent to the uterine wall or is not carefully searched for. The spine should be evaluated in both sagittal and axial planes. The overlying fluid-filled sac is typically thick walled as it is covered by skin. There should typically be the absence of visible neural elements in the meningocele sac.[5]

Magnetic Resonance Imaging: MRI can be a useful adjunct in evaluating the sac wall, contents of the sac, and conus level. The absence of hindbrain herniation and presence of a continuous sac-wall sign can be particularly helpful[19,61,62] (Fig. 23.2-11).

Differential Diagnosis: Differential includes myelomeningocele, sacrococcygeal teratoma, myelocystocele, and lipomyelomeningocele.

Prognosis and Management: Meningoceles are skin covered and typically not associated with hindbrain herniation; hence, they are not the candidates for fetal surgery. As the neuroglial tissue is covered by the thick layer of skin, the neurological examination is often normal or near-normal after delivery. Tethered cord syndrome may result in impaired bowl and bladder control as well as spasticity.[63,64]

Given the heterogeneity of terminology in the literature in regard to spinal dysraphisms, the true incidence of Chari malformation in the setting of a meningocele is unknown but is likely rare. When hindbrain herniation is present however, these patients may require shunting, as in the setting of Chiari II malformation with an open spinal dysraphism.[65]

Mode of delivery is dependent on the size of the sac. Large sacs may require cesarean section to prevent rupture at delivery. Following delivery, early repair may be needed to prevent sac injury, CSF leak, and infection.

Lipomyelomeningocele and Lipomyelocele

Synonym: Lipoma with dorsal defect, lipomyeloschisis.

Description: This is a closed spinal dysraphism (skin-covered) with the neural placode attached to lipomatous tissue in continuity with the subcutaneous fat through a dorsal spinal dysraphic defect. When the placode–lipoma interface is located within the spinal canal, it is referred to as a lipomyelocele, and when located outside the spinal canal, it is referred to as

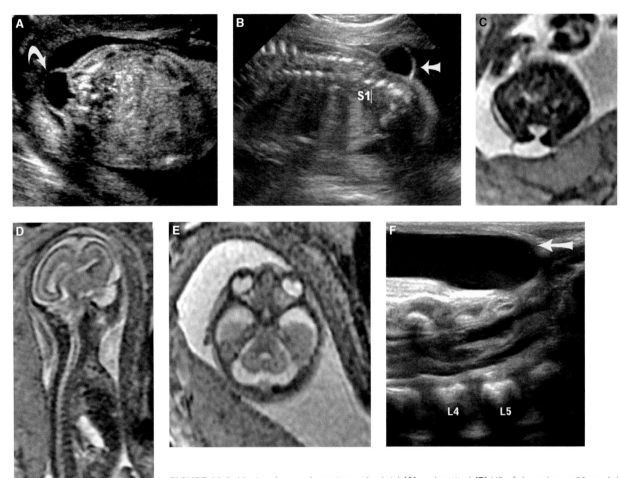

FIGURE 23.2-10: Lumbosacral meningocele. Axial **(A)** and sagittal **(B)** US of the spine at 20 weeks' gestation demonstrating a thick-walled sac containing fluid and no neural elements (*arrow*). Axial **(C)** and sagittal **(D)** T2 MRI at 20 weeks' confirming the lack of appreciable neural elements in the thick-walled sac. Notice subcutaneous fat along margins of sac are continuous or wrap around sac wall. **E:** Axial MRI of the posterior fossa demonstrating normal cerebellum and cisterna magna with no hindbrain herniation. **F:** Postnatal US demonstrating low conus with skin-covered fluid-filled sac (*arrow*).

as a lipomyelomeningocele, though these two entities do fall along a spectrum and can be difficult to distinguish from each other.[2,3]

Incidence: Incidence is 0.3 to 0.6 per 10,000 live births and accounts for 14% to 20% of closed spinal dysraphisms.[66–68] Lipomyelomeningocele has higher reported rates in infants born to mothers in younger and older age groups. Compared with non-Hispanic whites, Hispanics have a higher prevalence of lipomyelomeningoceles and related subtypes than myelomeningoceles and related subtypes.[69,70] Familial forms of lipomyelomeningocele are rare. There is no reduction in rates of lipomyelomeningocele following folic acid supplementation.[71,72]

Embryology/Pathogenesis: Disjunction is the process by which the cutaneous ectoderm separates from the neural ectoderm during primary neurulation immediately after neural tube closure. Lipomyelomeningoceles and lipomyeloceles are thought to be the result of premature disjunction, which allows mesenchyme to enter the closing neural tube, thus focally preventing neurulation to proceed.[3] As a result, the spinal cord is elongated with a

low-lying neural placode attached to lipomatous tissue, resulting in a tethered cord.[73]

Diagnosis: These skin-covered defects have normal AFP and AChE levels.

Ultrasound: Since this category of spinal dysraphisms is not typically associated with Chiari malformation, the diagnosis is heavily dependent on the US findings.[74] The diagnosis can be difficult to make by US if the spine lies adjacent to the uterine wall with limited visualization of the subcutaneous mass. Axial images of the spine can be helpful to identify absent or deficient posterior osseous elements. The brain is typically normal (Fig. 23.2-12).

Magnetic Resonance Imaging: MRI can be key in diagnosing lipomyelomeningoceles by identifying a low-lying distal spinal cord; however, the presence or absence of an intraspinal lipomatous tissue may be challenging. MRI can help to look at the associated sac in a lipomyelomeningocele, which typically has a thick wall from the skin covering (Fig. 23.2-12). Though fat within the defect on T1 images has been described on fetal MRI, the absence of fat within the defect does not exclude the diagnosis and can be a false negative.[19,61] This is particularly true at

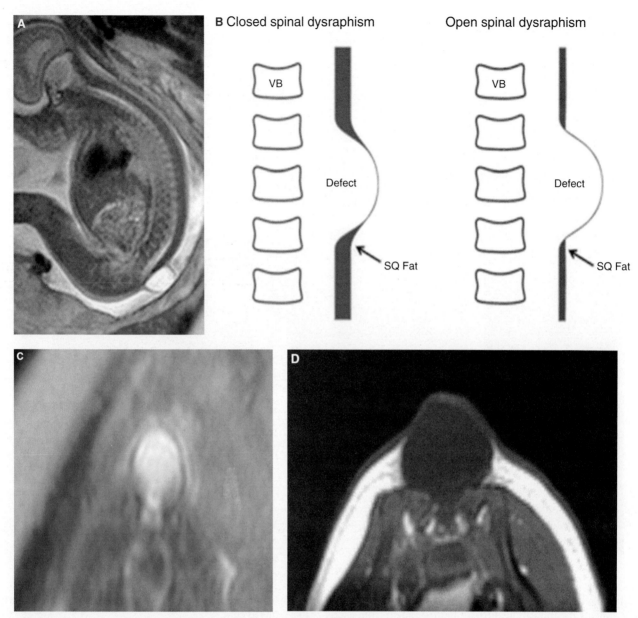

FIGURE 23.2-11: Meningocele. **A:** Sagittal T2 image in a 25-week-gestation fetus with sacral meningocele. Though the wall of the sac appears relatively thin, the sac margins appear continuous with the adjacent subcutaneous tissues (continuous sac-wall sign). **B:** Drawings depicting continuous sac-wall sign. In closed spinal dysraphisms, subcutaneous (SQ) fat and epidermal soft tissues have gradual smooth tapering transition with sac wall of spinal dysraphic defect (*arrow, left*). This is in contrast to open spinal dysraphisms in which transition is more abrupt (*arrow, right*). VB, vertebral body. **C:** Axial T2 image demonstrating the focal osseous spinal dysraphic defect with no neural elements extending into the meningocele sac. **D:** Postnatal axial T1 spine MRI confirming a skin-covered meningocele.

earlier gestational ages (<29 weeks) due to relative underdevelopment of fetal fat.[75]

Associations: Associated anomalies include caudal agenesis (group 2), segmentation anomalies, anal atresia, genitourinary anomalies, split cord malformation, and scoliosis.[76] On fetal imaging, there is also an association with the OEIS complex, for which fetal MRI can be helpful in delineating the coexisting abnormalities.[19] Despite being a closed spinal dysraphism, there is an increased incidence of Chiari malformation or hindbrain herniation compared with the general population.[77] Associated cutaneous stigmata include subcutaneous lipoma, vestigial tail (which can sometimes be detected on prenatal imaging), hairy patch, and dysplastic skin.[78,79]

Management: Because the sac is skin covered, cesarean section can be reserved for those masses that are particularly large. Most will require prophylactic surgery in the postnatal period to prevent tethered cord syndrome.[73]

Prognosis: The placode–lipoma interface in a lipomyelomeningocele is often deformed and frequently rotates away from the protruded meninges, resulting in asymmetric lengths of the associated nerve roots. This makes repair difficult as the distorted nerve roots require careful repositioning at surgery.[67,80–82] Compared with open spinal dysraphisms, patients with lipomyelomeningoceles and lipomyeloceles tend to have milder neurological deficits, including preserved bowel and bladder continence, despite significant dysplasia of

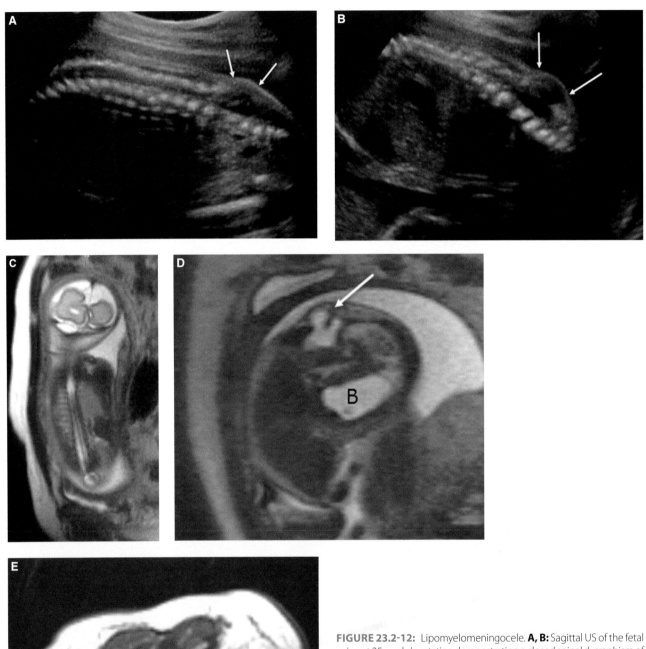

FIGURE 23.2-12: Lipomyelomeningocele. **A, B:** Sagittal US of the fetal spine at 25 weeks' gestation demonstrating a closed spinal dysraphism of the lumbosacral spine. There is continuity of the overlying skin with the thick sac wall **(A)**, and there is a clear protruding sac containing neural elements **(B)**. **C:** Coronal T2 MRI at 27 weeks' gestation demonstrating elongation of the spinal cord with low-lying neural placode inserting onto the back of a skin-covered sac. **D:** Axial SSFP MRI demonstrating the neural placode attached to the overlying subcutaneous fat (*arrow*). **E:** Axial T1 image from postnatal spine MRI confirming the diagnosis of a lumbosacral lipomyelomeningocele.

the caudal spinal cord.[83,84] Incidence of retethering, however, is 10% to 30%.[73,82,84]

Myelocystocele

Description: This is a relatively rare form of closed spinal dysraphism characterized by a skin-covered spinal dysraphic defect containing herniated spinal cord with syringohydromyelia or

cystic dilatation of the central canal. They can be divided into terminal and nonterminal subtypes.[85]

Embryology/Pathogenesis: Terminal myelocystocele is believed to be the result of a disruption in embryogenesis during the later phases of secondary neurulation, during which time the secondary neural tube forms; however, an arrest of normal apoptosis during retrogressive differentiation results in a persistent attachment of the secondary neural tube to the cutaneous ectoderm, which invariably dilates.[86] Nonterminal myelocystoceles, which occur at locations other than the end of the spinal cord, are believed to have a unique embryological etiology and are the result of partial failure of late primary neurulation with focal incomplete fusion of the apposed neural folds after most of primary neurulation has been completed.[54] Two forms of nonterminal myelocystoceles have been described. First is the abortive form or "myelocystocele manqué" in which what appears to be a skin-covered meningocele is crossed by a fibroneurovascular stalk that extends from the dorsal aspect of the spinal cord to attach to the dome of the meningocele sac. Second is the complete form in which a hydromyelic cavity is continuous with the ependymal canal of the spinal cord[85] (Fig. 23.2-13).

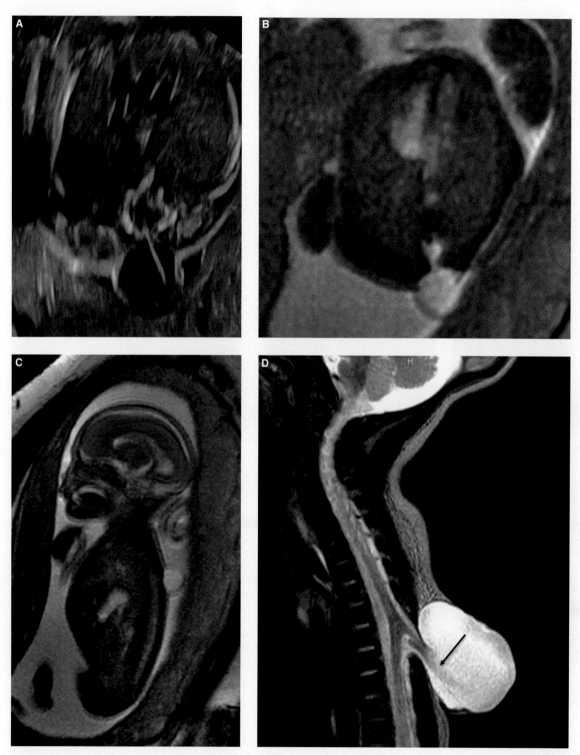

FIGURE 23.2-13: Abortive nonterminal myelocystocele (aka myelocystocele manqué). **A:** Axial US of 22 weeks' gestation fetus demonstrating closed spinal dysraphism of the thoracic spine with a sac containing linear neural elements. Axial **(B)** and sagittal **(C)** SSFP MRI demonstrating a skin-covered closed spinal dysraphism with a sac, though the neural elements in the sac are difficult to appreciate. **D:** Postnatal spine MRI confirming focal tethering of the thoracic spinal cord toward the sac with a neurovascular stalk (*arrow*) within the sac, consistent with an abortive nonterminal myelocystocele.

While closed spinal dysraphisms are usually not associated with Chiari malformation or hindbrain herniation, myelocystoceles differ in that they have a significant association with Chiari malformation and have been described to have an incidence as high as 40%.[87,88] This can make these difficult to differentiate from open spinal dysraphisms prenatally.[89]

Diagnosis: AFP should be normal.

Ultrasound: Findings suggestive of a myelocystocele by US include the presence of a thick-walled protruding sac (due to skin coverage) with the absence of Chiari II malformation (particularly in the second trimester). In the early second trimester, the spine should be carefully examined to identify the thick skin-covered sac overlying the lower spine with neural elements present within the sac. The diagnosis may be missed if the spine is lying against the adjacent uterine wall.[90] In the third trimester, hindbrain herniation may develop. Thus, this anomaly can be particularly difficult to distinguish from a myelomeningocele[91] (Fig. 23.2-14A, B).

Magnetic Resonance Imaging: MRI can help assess the contents within the herniated sac with associated dilated central canal.[92] Much like on postnatal MRI, in terminal myelocystoceles, the neural placode will appear to split within the skin-covered sac with a "trumpet" morphology.[93] Fetal MRI is particularly useful in evaluating for the presence or absence of hindbrain herniation in the late second and early third trimesters. It can also help delineate associated anomalies, such as caudal agenesis and cloacal malformations[19] (Fig. 23.2-14C, D).

Differential Diagnosis: Differentiating a myelocystocele from a myelomeningocele can be challenging, particularly in the presence of hindbrain herniation. In a retrospective series of 16 prenatally diagnosed closed spinal dysraphisms, we found that myelocystoceles tend to have a sac wall in continuity with the epidermal and subcutaneous tissues ("continuous sac-wall" sign), a thicker sac wall, and a high association with the OEIS complex.[19] Evaluation for skin coverage, sac contents, and severity of hindbrain herniation all must be carefully assessed in these cases on both US and MRI.

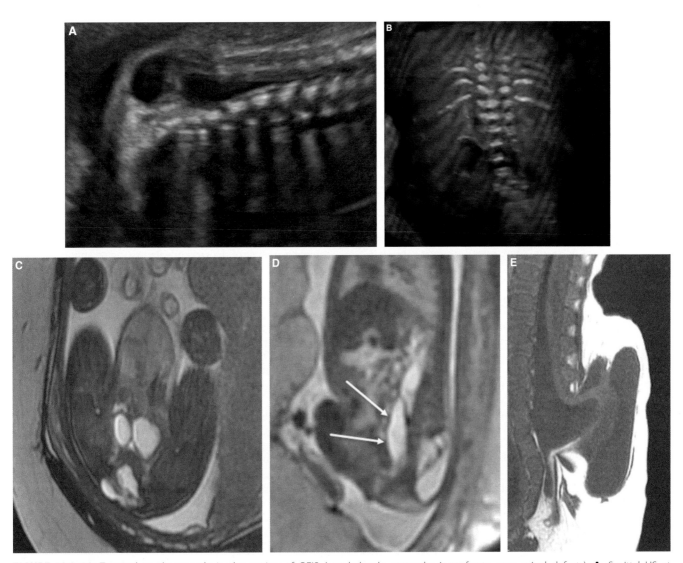

FIGURE 23.2-14: Terminal myelocystocele in the setting of OEIS (omphalocele–exstrophy–imperforate anus–spinal defects). **A:** Sagittal US at 27 weeks gestation demonstrating a closed lumbosacral spinal dysraphism with spitting of the neural placode within a protruding sac. **B:** Coronal 3D US demonstrating sacral hypoplasia and angulation, consistent with coexisting caudal agenesis. Axial SSFP **(C)** and sagittal T2 image **(D)** of the fetal pelvis in the same patient demonstrating anterior abdominal wall protuberance consistent with omphalocele. There is a bilobed cystic structure in the pelvis (arrows) and absence of a normal urinary bladder compatible with coexisting cloacal malformation. **E:** Sagittal T1 image from postnatal MRI in the same patient clearly delineating the splitting of the neural placode in a "trumpet" shape consistent with a terminal myelocystocele.

Associated Anomalies: Terminal myelocystocele is often associated with maldevelopment of the lower spine, pelvis, genitalia, bowel, bladder, kidney, and the abdominal wall, including cloacal extrophy.[94] OEIS complex is known to be associated with terminal myelocystoceles.[19]

Management/Prognosis: Outcome is dependent on the severity of anorectal and other visceral anomalies. Neurologically, patients may be intact but can progressively lose neurological function.[88,94]

Neurenteric Cyst: See chapter 25.3

Split Cord Malformation

Synonyms: Diastematomyelia, diplomyelia.

Description: Though sometimes referred to as diastematomyelia and diplomyelia, these terms have fallen out of favor in the neurosurgical literature, given that they are difficult to differentiate on imaging and in the operating room. Split cord malformation is the sagittal division of the spinal cord into two hemicords.[95]

Incidence: Existing literature on incidence of prenatal diagnosis of split cord malformation is limited; however, it has been reported.[96,97] It is overall rare representing a small percentage of all spinal anomalies.

Pathogenesis/Embryology: Split cord malformation is believed to be the result of an abnormal adhesion between the ectoderm and the endoderm during gastrulation in the second to third weeks of gestation, which splits the notochord and neural plate. There are two types described in the neurosurgical literature, which can have implications for treatment.[98] Type I split cord malformation consists of two separate dural tubes, usually in association with a bony or cartilaginous cleft. Type II split cord malformation is contained within a single dural sac, usually with a thin separating fibrous band.[99] The hemicords can have variable symmetry and sometimes unite below the cleft.[100]

Diagnosis
Ultrasound: Split cord malformation is often associated with vertebral segmentation anomalies. With type I, an intraspinal echogenic focus marking the osseous septum may potentially be seen.[101–104] However, a fibrous septum or cord duplication may not be identified by US.[97]

Magnetic Resonance Imaging: Two- to three-millimeter high-resolution axial MRI of the spine can be helpful to demonstrate a split cord malformation with two hemicords (Fig. 23.2-15). In open spinal dysraphisms, one may be able to see coexisting split cord malformation involving the neural placode; however, this cannot be reliably diagnosed by fetal MRI.[41]

Associated Anomalies: Split cord malformation is usually associated with other spinal anomalies, including coexisting open spinal dysraphisms (hemimyelomeningocele or hemimyelocele).[105] Associated spinal anomalies include segmentation anomalies, scoliosis, and kyphosis. Equinovarus foot deformity is common. Dorsal midline cutaneous lesions can be present, including telangiectasias, hemangiomas, lipomas, and cutaneous nevi.

Prognosis/Management: When isolated, prognosis may be favorable depending on neurological and orthopedic surgical outcome.[106] Prophylactic surgical treatment for type I split cord malformations is recommended to resect the spur, lyse-associated fibrous adhesions, and cord detethering.[107] The timing for intervention for type II split cord malformations, however, is less clear in the neurosurgical literature.[98,99,108]

Caudal Agenesis

Synonyms: Caudal regression syndrome, sacral agenesis, caudal dysplasia, and caudal dysgenesis.

Description: Caudal agenesis is characterized by congenital absence of a portion of the caudal spine usually in association with spinal cord, anorectal, and/or genitourinary anomalies. There is a wide spectrum of presentations ranging from isolated coccygeal aplasia to sirenomelia.[109] There are two groups described based on morphology. Group 1 patients have a high (L1 or higher) blunted conus and tend to be associated with more severe osseous anomalies and anorectal and genitourinary malformations. Group 2 patients have a low-lying tethered cord and may have an additional closed spinal dysraphism, such as an intradural lipoma or lipomyelomeningocele.[110,111]

Incidence: Incidence is 0.1 to 0.25 per 10,000 in normal pregnancies and 200 times higher in diabetic pregnancies. Though usually occurs sporadically, up to 16% of cases are associated with infants of diabetic mothers.[112]

Pathogenesis/Embryology: Caudal agenesis is likely the result of abnormalities of secondary neurulation and retrogressive differentiation during the fifth to sixth gestational weeks; however, it is believed that group 1 caudal agenesis is also the result of an abnormality of primary neurulation in addition to secondary neurulation.[109]

Diagnosis
Ultrasound: Sonographic findings are variable. There may be complete absence of the sacrum with associated abnormalities of the lumbar spine and lower extremities, including club feet and knee and hip contractions. Absence of several vertebrae, fused iliac wings, and medialization of the femoral heads can be noted. Axial views of the abdomen may fail to show the normal spine. Decreased motion of the lower extremities may be present. Polyhydramnios has also been described.[113,114] However, in cases of mild caudal agenesis when only a few distal sacral elements are missing or in coccygeal aplasia, the diagnosis can be missed prenatally by both US and MRI (Fig. 23.2-16A).

Magnetic Resonance Imaging: MRI can potentially confirm the diagnosis of caudal agenesis and identify a blunted conus in group 1 patients. Both sagittal and axial images are helpful in assessing the number of sacral elements. When oligohydramnios is present due to coexisting renal anomalies, MRI is superior to US in the assessment of associated fetal anomalies (Fig. 23.2-16B, C).

Associated Anomalies: Caudal agenesis can be seen in the setting of OEIS, VACTERL (vertebral, anal, cardiac, tracheoesophageal fistula, renal and limb anomalies), and Currarino triad. Coexisting spinal anomalies include segmentation anomalies and other closed spinal dysraphisms. Genitourinary abnormalities are more common in group 1 than group 2 caudal agenesis and can range from renal agenesis/ectopia, hydronephrosis, Müllerian duct malformations, and urinary bladder

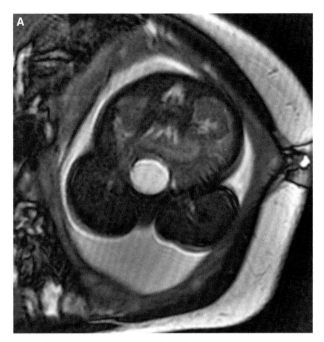

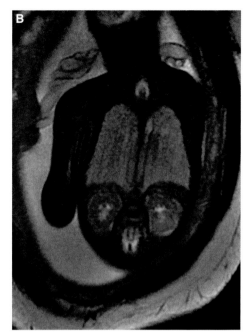

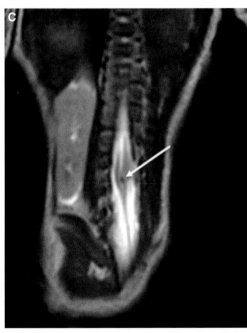

FIGURE 23.2-15: Split cord malformation: **A:** Axial SSFP of the spine in a 31-week-gestation fetus demonstrating splitting of the spinal cord into two hemicords consistent with split cord malformation. **B:** Coronal SSFP image demonstrating the appearance of a bony spur at the lower level of the split, suggestive of a type I split cord malformation. **C:** Coronal T2 image from postnatal spine MRI in the same patient confirming the split cord with osseous spur (arrow). Note that the cord joins to form a single filum terminale caudal to the spur.

malformations. Anorectal malformations, particularly anal atresia, are more common the more severe the degree of lumbosacral agenesis. Patients can also suffer orthopedic abnormalities, including hip dysplasia, and even varying degrees of the absence of the lower extremities.[110,115,116]

Prognosis and Management: Prognosis depends on the severity of the defect and associated anomalies. Often, urological and orthopedic long-term care is required.

Recurrence Risk: Recurrence risk is thought to be small, though higher in diabetic mothers.

Sirenomelia

Synonym: Mermaid syndrome.

Description: Lethal anomaly in the caudal agenesis spectrum with fusion or near-complete fusion of the lower extremities.

Incidence: Incidence is 1 in 60,000 live births, with a male-to-female ratio of 2.7:1.[117] Maternal diabetes is associated with a higher incidence. There is a 100-fold increased incidence in monozygotic twins. Cocaine and high doses of vitamins A and E have been associated with this anomaly.

Embryology/Pathogenesis: The cause is thought to be a localized insult to the caudal end of the developing embryo between days 13 and 22 gestation. A persistent vitelline artery has been noted with a dorsal hypoplastic distal aorta.[118,119] Shunting of nutrients away from the caudal structure may result in malrotation, merging, and dysgenesis of the lower extremities.[120] Chromosomes are typically normal. With a high association with

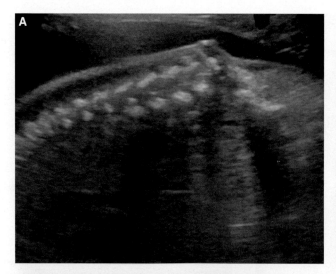

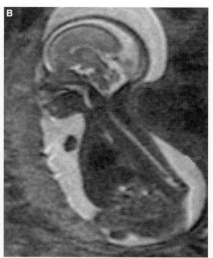

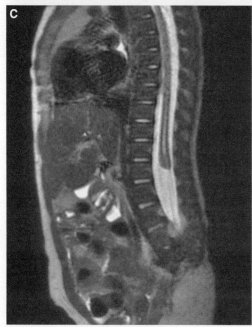

FIGURE 23.2-16: Caudal agenesis. **A:** Sagittal US image in a 22 week gestation demonstrating focal kyphotic angulation of the lumbar spine with absence of the sacrum. Iliac bones are present. **B:** Sagittal T2 MRI demonstrating blunted high-ending conus consistent with group 1 caudal agenesis. Sacrum is absent. **C:** Postnatal sagittal T2 MRI of the spine in a different patient with group 1 caudal agenesis demonstrating complete sacral agenesis and blunted conus with characteristic "double-bundle" nerve roots of the cauda equina.

monozygotic twinning, a vascular steal phenomenon could explain the high incidence in this group.

In 1987, Stocker and Heifetz classified sirenomelia into seven types: type I (thigh and leg bones present), type II (single fibula), type III (no fibula), type IV (femurs partially fused and fibula completely fused), type V (femurs partially fused), type VI (single femur and single tibia), and type VII (single femur and absent tibia).[121]

Associated Anomalies: Associated anomalies include sacral agenesis, anorectal atresia, renal agenesis, bladder agenesis, urethral agenesis, single umbilical artery, and ambiguous genitalia. Oligohydramnios is common.[117]

Diagnosis
Ultrasound: In the first trimester, fused lower limbs may be seen with an increased nuchal translucency present.[122–127] A single umbilical artery is common. In the second trimester, a single large intra-abdominal vessel, the vitelline artery, may be seen coursing to the umbilical cord. Oligohydramnios, renal agenesis, and

intrauterine growth restriction are typically present with a single lower extremity.[128] When two femurs are present, the diagnosis can be difficult.[128] Color Doppler can be useful to search for the presence of renal arteries and the single vitelline artery.[129,130]

3D US can delineate the extremity anomalies if amniotic fluid is present.[127] However, with renal anomalies common, oligohydramnios often limits the resolution of US, particularly 3D.

Magnetic Resonance Imaging: When oligohydramnios is present, MRI is a useful adjunct to confirm the diagnosis of renal agenesis and fused lower extremities[113,131,132] (Fig. 23.2-17).

Differential Diagnosis: Bilateral renal agenesis. Milder cases of caudal agenesis typically have a normal amount of amniotic fluid.

Prognosis: Typically lethal.

Recurrence Risk: Families at risk of increased incidence of monozygotic twins may have an increased risk of sirenomelia.

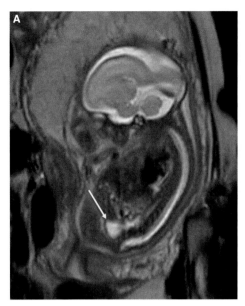
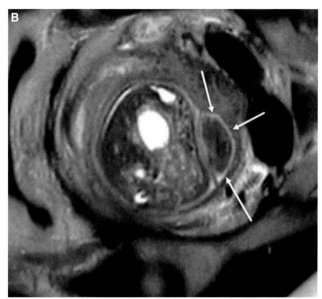

FIGURE 23.2-17: Severe caudal agenesis/sirenomelia: **A:** Sagittal T2 MRI at 25 weeks gestation demonstrating abnormal angulation of the lumbar spine and absence of the normal sacrum. No normal renal tissue was identified with associated anhydramnios, and there is a fluid-filled rectum (*arrow*) suspicious for coexisting cloacal malformation. **B:** Axial T2 MRI demonstrating a single-thickened lower extremity (*arrows*) consistent with sirenomelia.

"Simple" Closed Spinal Dysraphism

Synonym: Tethered cord syndrome and spina bifida aperta.

Description: There are a group of spinal dysraphisms listed under the cliniconeuroradiological classification system that are termed "simple dysraphic states without a subcutaneous mass." These include, but are not limited to, entities such as intradural lipomas, tight filum terminale, and low-lying conus. A dorsal dermal sinus tract is also a closed spinal dysraphism without a subcutaneous mass; however, it is considered a "complex dysraphic state."[3] These closed spinal dysraphisms are extremely challenging to identify prenatally and may be missed, though they can result in tethered cord syndrome.[5,133] This group of spinal dysraphisms is embryologically heterogeneous and includes abnormalities of both primary and secondary neurulation. True incidence is difficult to determine, particularly when many are clinically occult and controversial descriptions of occult tethered cord syndrome exist.[134] The reason to mention is to keep in mind that simple closed spinal dysraphisms are difficult to entirely exclude on fetal imaging.[5]

Diagnosis
Ultrasound: Though imaging of the spine is performed routinely on second-trimester screening USs, identification of the conus medullaris is not a part of the American Institute of Ultrasound in Medicine (AIUM) practice guidelines for obstetric US examinations.[135] While evaluation of the conus medullaris may be feasible in most cases, it is frequently limited by maternal obesity, advanced gestational age, and fetal positioning.[136,137] Since a low-lying conus medullaris may be one of the only prenatal imaging clues for simple closed spinal dysraphism and potentially tethered cord syndrome, when identified, its location should be noted.[138]

Magnetic Resonance Imaging: A low-lying conus medullaris can be detected on fetal MRI and should be routinely examined. Postmortem MR studies have demonstrated that the conus ends between the L2 and L5 levels in fetuses less than 35 weeks' gestational age and ends between L1 and L3 after 35 weeks.[139] Since vertebral bodies can be challenging to reliably count on fetal MRI particularly in the second trimester, the kidneys can be used as a landmark since they are usually located between T12 and L4 in both the second and third trimesters.[140] In general, the conus should not end below the lower margin of the kidneys, assuming the kidneys are normally positioned. A low conus on fetal MRI can be further evaluated by postnatal spinal US.

Segmentation Anomalies

Description: Congenital abnormalities of formation and/or segmentation of the vertebral bodies include a wide range of abnormalities, including vertebral body asomia (agenesis), hypoplastic vertebra, hemivertebra, coronal clefting, butterfly vertebra (sagittal clefting), and block vertebra (vertebral body fusion).[141]

Incidence: Estimated incidence is 0.5 to 1.0 in 1,000 births; however, it remains unclear, since it can be incidental and involve just a single vertebral body or the entire spinal column.[142]

Pathogenesis: These are the result of aberrant vertebral column formation during the 9th to 12th gestational weeks. They can be isolated or syndromal. Genetics may play a role. Homeobox, or *Hox*, genes regulate the differentiation process of the axial and appendicular skeleton, and mutations of these genes may result in congenital abnormalities of the cervical spine.[143] Deranged *PAX1* gene expression, resulting in abnormal notochord signaling in developing vertebral column, has also been implicated.[144] There are numerous genetic and nongenetic syndromes that include segmentation anomalies as descriptors.

Diagnosis
Ultrasound: US findings include irregular shape of the spine, best demonstrated on sagittal and coronal views. A triangular vertebral body structure smaller than the adjacent vertebra may be

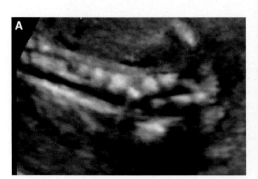
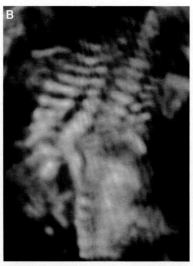
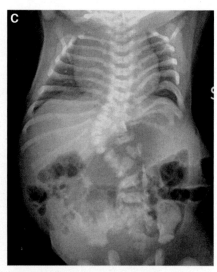

FIGURE 23.2-18: Hemivertebra. **A:** Coronal US demonstrating hemivertebra with acute angulation. **B:** 3D US skeletal mode rendering of the spine and ribs confirming the lower thoracic scoliosis. **C:** Postnatal radiograph revealing multiple lower left thoracic rib anomalies in addition to thoracolumbar hemivertebra and butterfly vertebra in this patient with spondylocostal dysplasia.

seen at the site of angulation. Though scoliosis is commonly seen in association when multiple levels are affected, the alignment may be balanced with no significant resultant scoliosis.[145–148] 3D US is particularly useful for assessing scoliosis and associated vertebral and rib anomalies[149] (Fig. 23.2-18).

Magnetic Resonance Imaging: Though fetal MRI may be limited in the assessment of an isolated hemivertebra particularly in the early second trimester, echo-planar or susceptibility weighted sequences (aka "black bone") may increase its utility in further delineating segmentation anomalies.[150,151] Fetal MRI can also be extremely useful in evaluating associated anomalies such as associated spinal dysraphisms, cloacal anomalies, and VACTERL association[5] (Fig. 23.2-19).

Computed Tomography: The use of intrauterine 3D CT for the assessment of fetal skeletal anomalies has been described (for technique description, see Chapter 29).[152,153] Spinal anomalies delineated by this technique include platyspondyly, hemivertebrae, decreased intervertebral distance, and vertebral agenesis.

Using a multislice scanner with relatively low mAs (40 to 80) and kVp (80 to 120), the mean CT-dose index has been reported to be approximately 3 mGy per study. The acquisitions are performed during breath-hold with the mother supine. Postprocessing 3D reconstruction of the fetal skeleton involves using maximum intensity projection and segmentation with removal of the overlying maternal pelvic bones. Centers using this technique typically perform the examination in the third trimester. Decreased skeletal ossification, increased fetal movement, smaller size of the fetus, and increased radiation sensitivity may limit the use of this technique earlier in pregnancy (Fig. 23.2-20).

Differential Diagnosis: Anomalies associated with scoliosis include open spinal dysraphisms, closed spinal dysraphisms, OEIS, limb body wall complex, and Currarino triad. However, segmentation anomalies can coexist many other conditions and genetic disorders.

Associated Anomalies: Segmentation anomalies are seen in up to 30% of cases of congenital scoliosis.[154] Segmentation anomalies

are commonly seen in association with other musculoskeletal anomalies, including spine, ribs, and limbs. Multiple syndromes including Jarcho–Levin, Klippel–Feil, VATER, VACTERL, spondylocostal dysostosis, Alagille syndrome, and Goldenhar syndrome are seen with segmentation anomalies.[142,155] Chromosomal anomalies are uncommon, though should also be considered.[156]

Prognosis: Prognosis is related to the presence of associated anomalies. Spinal fusion is the treatment of choice with congenital scoliosis that is progressive, which can result in a markedly short spine and low lung volumes.[154,157]

Management: Close evaluation for other anomalies is critical. Vaginal delivery may be appropriate if the anomaly is isolated. Orthopedic follow-up is important.

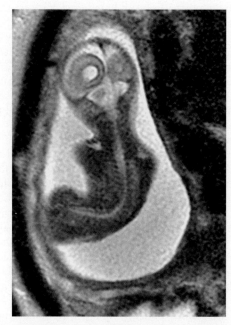

FIGURE 23.2-19: Coronal T2 MRI demonstrating severe lower thoracic scoliosis.

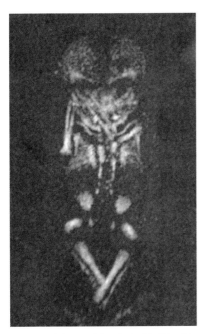

FIGURE 23.2-20: Spondylocostal dysplasia. 3D CT at 21 weeks' gestation demonstrates abnormal ribs and vertebra. (Courtesy of Teresa Victoria.)

Recurrence Risk: Congenital scoliosis has reported 4% increased risk of spinal dysraphism in siblings.[158]

Sacrococcygeal Teratoma

Description: Germ cell tumor composed of cells from all three germ cell layers (ectoderm, mesoderm, and endoderm) in the sacrococcygeal region.

TABLE 23.2-2 The American Academy of Pediatric Surgery Staging Classification of Sacrococcygeal Teratomas

TYPE	DESCRIPTION
I	External with minimal presacral component
II	External with intrapelvic component
III	External and primarily internal component with abdominal extension
IV	Entirely internal with no external component

Incidence: Incidence is 1 per 35,000 to 40,000 births. Sacrococcygeal teratomas (SCTs) represent 25% to 35% of all neonatal tumors and are the most common fetal tumor. Teratomas can be seen anywhere from the head to the pelvis; however, they are most commonly seen in the sacrococcygeal region in the fetus.[159]

Pathogenesis: These tumors arise from totipotent cells of the caudal cell mass. Approximately two-thirds are mature teratomas and the other one-third are split almost equally between immature teratomas and anaplastic carcinomas.

Diagnosis: SCT has been classified by the amount of presacral and external components of the mass by the American Academy of Pediatric Surgery Section.[160] There are four types (Table 23.2-2, Fig. 23.2-21):

- Type I: Nearly entirely external mass and is usually identified prenatally. This is the easiest to resect and has the lowest malignancy potential.

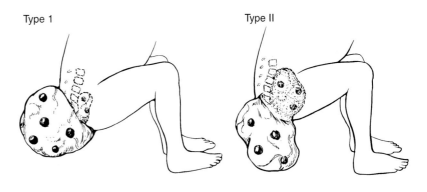
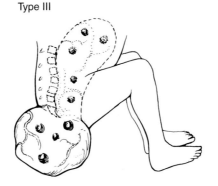
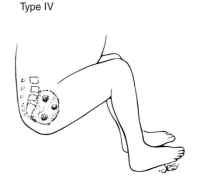

FIGURE 23.2-21: Types of sacrococcygeal teratomas. SCT may be almost entirely external or combined internal and external, or, as in type IV, mainly internal. Those that are mainly external are less commonly malignant, whereas those that are mainly internal usually have a delayed diagnosis and are often malignant. (Adapted from Altman RP, Randolph JG, Lilly JR. Sacrococcygeal teratoma: American Academy of Pediatrics Surgical Section Survey. *J Pediatr Surg.* 1974;9:389–398. Copyright © 1974 Elsevier. With permission.)

- Type II: Tumor is mostly external; however, there is a significant intrapelvic component.
- Type III: External tumor with intrapelvic and intra-abdominal component, with tumor extending above the pelvic inlet.
- Type IV: Completely internal mass without visible external component. This is difficult to diagnose prenatally. Malignant transformation is most common with type IV tumors.

Ultrasound: On screening fetal US, SCT is usually identified as an external mass from the sacrococcygeal region. These masses are usually cystic and solid in appearance on US, though tumors of mostly solid or cystic tissue can be seen[161] (Figs. 23.2-22A and 23.2-23A, B). The presence of shadowing calcifications within the mass is highly suggestive of the diagnosis, an advantage that US has over fetal MRI (Fig. 23.2-24). The intrapelvic and/or intra-abdominal component of the mass can be difficult to evaluate on

US; however, the presence of mass effect on the urinary bladder can be helpful. Findings of fetal hydrops secondary to high-output cardiac failure is a poor prognostic sign, making evaluation for the presence of pericardial effusion, pleural effusion, fetal ascites, and skin thickening important.[162]

In the evaluation of candidates for fetal intervention, additional sonographic markers are helpful in selecting the best candidates, including combined cardiac output (mean ± standard deviation [SD]: normal 553 ± 153 mL/kg/min, cardiac-to-thoracic ratio (normal <0.33), descending aortic blood flow (mean ± SD: normal 184 ± 20 mL/kg/min), inferior vena cava diameter (normal 2.9 to 4.1 mm from 21 to 28 weeks' gestational age), placental thickness, umbilical artery Doppler systolic-to-diastolic (S/D) ratio (<3 at 30 weeks' gestation), and amniotic fluid index.[163] Reporting peak systolic velocities in the descending aorta at the thoracic, upper abdominal, and lower abdominal levels as well as the peak systolic velocity in the middle cerebral artery can

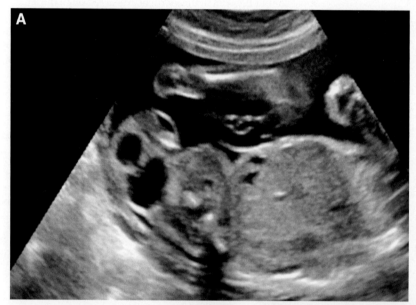

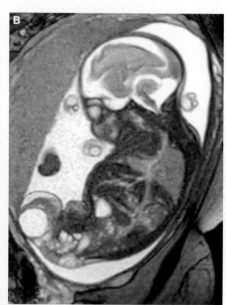

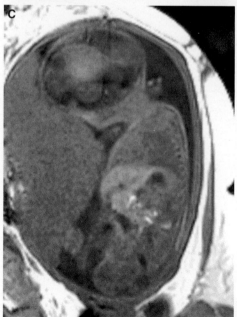

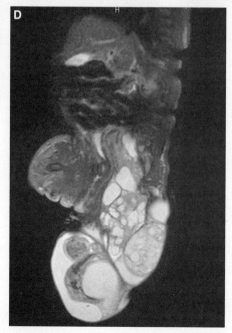

FIGURE 23.2-22: SSFP Types II and III SCT. **A:** Oblique sagittal/coronal US at 24 weeks' gestation demonstrating large cystic and solid mass consistent with SCT, though intrapelvic extent not well visualized. **B:** Oblique sagittal SSFP MRI at 26 weeks' gestation demonstrating the intrapelvic and intra-abdominal extension of the tumor with mass effect on the urinary bladder. **C:** Sagittal T1 image in the same fetus demonstrating the absence of normal rectal meconium signal, a common finding in SCT. **D:** Postnatal sagittal T2 image in the same patient showing the same findings, though a patent rectum can be more clearly delineated (confirmed on physical examination).

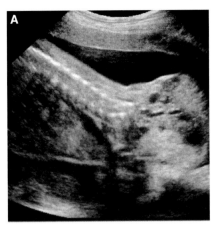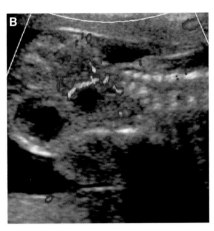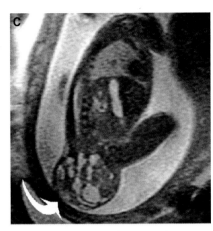

FIGURE 23.2-23: Type I cystic and solid SCT at 24-week gestation. **A:** Sagittal US demonstrating a mixed external mass adjacent to the coccyx. **B:** Doppler US demonstrating moderate vascularity. **C:** Sagittal T2 image demonstrating the solid and cystic mass at the base of the buttocks with no internal component (*arrow*).

also be helpful in the assessment of the degree of vascular steal by the tumor.[164]

Magnetic Resonance Imaging: Fetal MRI can be an important tool in further workup of these patients and can help better delineate the degree of intra-abdominal and intrapelvic extension, as well as determine its relationship to the fetal spine, rectum, and urinary bladder for preoperative planning (Figs. 23.2-22B, C and 23.2-23C). Rectal meconium signal on T1 images is often absent, with the presence of SCT secondary to mass effect; however, anorectal malformation can present in the setting of SCT and cannot entirely be excluded prenatally in many cases.[165] Fetal MRI findings of associated urinary tract obstruction and gastrointestinal obstruction have been associated with worsening postnatal functional outcomes.[166]

Associated Anomalies: Up to 18% of SCTs are associated with other anomalies. If a sacral malformation is associated with SCT, it suggests a rare familial form of tumor with an autosomal dominant inheritance. Anorectal stenosis, vesicoureteral reflux, and cutaneous stigmata are frequently present in children with the familial form. The sporadic and familial forms are indistinguishable on imaging. SCT can also be associated with anorectal malformations and caudal agenesis in Currarino triad.[60]

Differential Diagnosis: When a sacral mass is identified, the primary differential considerations include a myelomeningocele or a closed spinal dysraphism with an associated subcutaneous mass, such as a terminal myelocystocele, meningocele, or lipomyelomeningocele. These entities can usually be differentiated from SCT on US by lack of shadowing calcifications or vascularity on color Doppler. AFP may be elevated in both myelomeningoceles and SCT; however, myelomeningoceles should not have large solid components and are associated with intracranial findings of Chiari II malformation. Rare mimics of SCT include neuroblastoma or congenital hemangioma.[167]

Prognosis: Prenatally diagnosed SCT has a higher mortality rate than postnatally diagnosed SCT. Prognosis is related to the development of fetal hydrops, histology, and size of mass.[168] Larger tumors, particularly with high solid component, have a worse prognosis with increased risk of hydrops and greater surgical risk as well as hemorrhage at delivery. Tumor volume-to-fetal weight ratio (TFR) greater than 0.12 prior to 24 weeks' gestational age has been described as a poor prognostic indicator.[169] Good outcomes are associated with small tumors, along with external primarily cystic masses that are avascular. Long-term sequela includes radicular pain, constipation, or urinary frequency and incontinence. Best prognosis is seen with complete surgical excision.[170]

Management: Given that these tumors have the potential for rapid growth, close monitoring for prenatally diagnosed SCT is generally advised to evaluate for poor prognostic signs, such as cardiomegaly or fetal hydrops.[171] Though exact criteria for what constitutes a high-risk SCT are evolving, large highly vascular tumors may require early elective delivery after 28 weeks' gestational age.[172] Before 28 weeks' gestational age, fetal interventions including amnioreduction, cyst aspiration, and surgical debulking have been described as successful in selected cases.[163] Small SCTs without other complications can be delivered vaginally, while elective

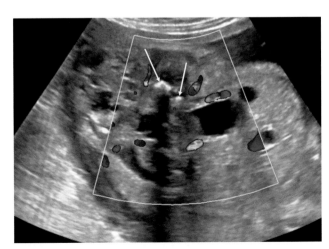

FIGURE 23.2-24: Selected US of sacrococcygeal teratoma at 26 weeks' gestation with color Doppler demonstrating internal vascularity in the tumor. Also note the shadowing calcifications (*arrows*) within the tumor, consistent with the diagnosis.

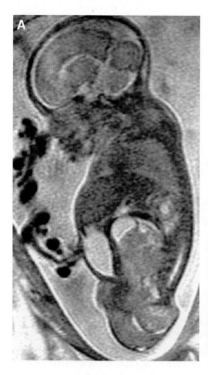

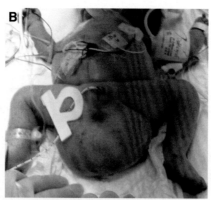

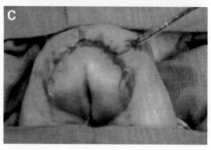

FIGURE 23.2-25: Type III sacrococcygeal teratoma. **A:** Sagittal T2 MRI demonstrating a mixed solid and cystic mass with internal and external components. The bladder is deviated anteriorly by the internal mass. **B:** Newborn with large skin-covered SCT. **C:** The infant was taken to surgery without additional imaging. Postoperative image of the buttock following successful resection.

cesarean delivery is recommended for SCTs measuring greater than 5 cm in diameter due to risk of traumatic vascular injury and tumor hemorrhage. After a period of stabilization and preoperative workup, elective removal of the tumor is usually performed within the first few days of life[173] (Fig. 23.2-25).

Recurrence Risk: While typically sporadic, some cases appear to be familial with an autosomal dominant inheritance, particularly type IV.[174] Familial cases are associated with anorectal malformations and Currarino triad (presacral mass, anorectal malformation, and sacral anomaly). Chromosomal abnormalities are rare but have been described with trisomy 1q.[175]

REFERENCES

1. Barkovich A, Raybaud C. *Pediatric Neuroimaging.* 5th ed. Philadelphia, PA: Lippincott Williams & Wilkins; 2012.
2. Rufener SL, Ibrahim M, Raybaud CA, et al. Congenital spine and spinal cord malformations—pictorial review. *Am J Roentgenol.* 2010;194(3 suppl):26–37.
3. Tortori-Donati P, Rossi A, Cama A. Spinal dysraphism: a review of neuroradiological features with embryological correlations and proposal for a new classification. *Neuroradiology.* 2000;42(7):471–491.
4. Blumenfeld Z, Siegler E, Bronshtein M. The early diagnosis of neural tube defects. *Prenat Diagn.* 1993;13(9):851–861.
5. Bulas D. Fetal evaluation of spine dysraphism. *Pediatr Radiol.* 2010;40(6):1029–1037.
6. Adzick NS, Thom EA, Spong CY, et al. A randomized trial of prenatal versus postnatal repair of myelomeningocele. *N Engl J Med.* 2013;364(11):993–1004.
7. Nagaraj UD, Bierbrauer KS, Zhang B, et al. Hindbrain herniation in Chiari II malformation on fetal and postnatal MRI. *Am J Neuroradiol.* 2017;38(May):1031–1036.
8. Zaganjor I, Sekkarie A, Tsang BL, et al. Describing the prevalence of neural tube defects worldwide: a systematic literature review. *PLoS One.* 2016;11(4):1–31.
9. De Wals P, Tairou F, Van Allen MI, et al. Reduction in neural-tube defects after folic acid fortification in Canada. *N Engl J Med.* 2007;357(2):135–142.
10. Ross ME, Mason CE, Finnell RH. Genomic approaches to the assessment of human spina bifida risk. *Birth Defects Res.* 2017;109(2):120–128.
11. Chen C-P. Syndromes, disorders and maternal risk factors associated with neural tube defects. *Taiwan J Obstet Gynecol.* 2008;47(3):259–266.
12. Wolpert S, Anderson M, Scott RM, et al. Chiari II malformation: MR imaging evaluation. *AJR.* 1987;149(5):1033–1042.
13. el Gammal T, Mark EK, Brooks BS. MR imaging of Chiari II malformation. *AJR.* 1988;150(1):163–170.
14. McLone DG, Knepper P. The cause of Chiari II malformation: a unified theory. *Pediatr Neurosci.* 1989;15(1):1–12.
15. Driscoll DA, Gross SJ. Screening for fetal aneuploidy and neural tube defects. *Genet Med.* 2009;11(11):818–821.
16. Roman AS, Gupta S, Fox NS, et al. Is MSAFP still a useful test for detecting open neural tube defects and ventral wall defects in the era of first-trimester and early second-trimester fetal anatomical ultrasounds? *Fetal Diagn Ther.* 2015;37(3):206–210.
17. Adzick NS. Fetal surgery for myelomeningocele: trials and tribulations. Isabella Forshall Lecture. *J Pediatr Surg.* 2012;47(2):273–281.
18. Flick A, Krakow D, Martirosian A, et al. Routine measurement of amniotic fluid alpha-fetoprotein and acetylcholinesterase: the need for a reevaluation. *Am J Obstet Gynecol.* 2014;211(2):139.e1–139.e6.
19. Nagaraj UD, Bierbrauer KS, Peiro JL, et al. Differentiating closed versus open spinal dysraphisms on fetal MRI. *Am J Roentgenol.* 2016;207(6).
20. Van den Hof MC, Nicolaides KH, Campbell J, et al. Evaluation of the lemon and banana signs in one hundred thirty fetuses with open spina bifida. *Am J Obstet Gynecol.* 1990;162(2):322–327.
21. Blaas H, Eik-Nes S. Sonoembryology and early prenatal diagnosis of neural anomalies. *Prenat Diagn.* 2009;29:312–325.
22. Campbell J, Gilbert W, Nicolaides K, et al. Ultrasound screening for spina bifida: cranial and cerebellar signs in a high-risk population. *Obstet Gynecol.* 1987;70(2):247–250.
23. Thiagarajah S, Henke J, Hogge W, et al. Early diagnosis of spina bifida: the value of cranial ultrasound markers. *Obstet Gynecol.* 1990;76(1):54–57.
24. Tulipan N, Wellons J, Thom EA, et al. Prenatal surgery for myelomeningocele and the need for cerebrospinal fluid shunt placement. *Neurosurg Pediatr.* 2015;16(6):613–620.
25. Tutschek B, Pilu G. Virtual reality ultrasound imaging of the normal and abnormal fetal central nervous system. *Ultrasound Obstet Gynecol.* 2009;34(3):259–267.
26. Coleman BG, Langer JE, Horii SC. The diagnostic features of spina bifida: the role of ultrasound. *Fetal Diagn Ther.* 2015;37(3):179–196.
27. McEwing RL, Pretorius DH, James HE, et al. Prenatal assignation of lesion levels in neural tube defects by using ultrasonography. Case report and review of the literature. *J Neurosurg.* 2005;102(2 suppl):248–251.
28. Leung KY, Ngai CSW, Chan BC, et al. Three-dimensional extended imaging: a new display modality for three-dimensional ultrasound examination. *Ultrasound Obstet Gynecol.* 2005;26(3):244–251.
29. Westcott MA, Dynes MC, Remer EM, et al. Congenital and acquired orthopedic abnormalities in patients with myelomeningocele. *RadioGraphics.* 1992;12(6):1155–1173.
30. Carreras E, Maroto A, Illescas T, et al. Prenatal ultrasound evaluation of segmental level of neurological lesion in fetuses with myelomeningocele: development of a new technique. *Ultrasound Obstet Gynecol.* 2016;47(2):162–167.
31. Sutton LN, Adzick NS, Bilaniuk LT, et al. Improvement in hindbrain herniation demonstrated by serial fetal magnetic resonance imaging following fetal surgery for myelomeningocele. *J Am Med Assoc.* 1999;282(19):1826–1831.

32. Nagaraj UD, Peiro JL, Bierbrauer KS, et al. Evaluation of subependymal gray matter heterotopias on fetal MRI. *Am J Neuroradiol.* 2016;37(4).
33. Heuer GG, Adzick NS, Sutton LN. Fetal myelomeningocele closure: technical considerations. *Fetal Diagn Ther.* 2015;37(3):166–171.
34. Abele TA, Lee SL, Twickler DM. MR imaging quantitative analysis of fetal Chiari II malformations and associated open neural tube defects: balanced SSFP versus half-Fourier RARE and interobserver reliability. *J Magn Reson Imaging.* 2013;38(4):786–793.
35. Nemec U, Nemec SF, Krakow D, et al. The skeleton and musculature on foetal MRI. *Insights Imaging.* 2011;2(3):309–318.
36. Werner H, Lopes Dos Santos JR, Fontes R, et al. Virtual bronchoscopy for evaluating cervical tumors of the fetus. *Ultrasound Obstet Gynecol.* 2013;41(1):90–94.
37. Servaes S, Hernandez A, Gonzalez L, et al. Fetal MRI of clubfoot associated with myelomeningocele. *Pediatr Radiol.* 2010;40(12):1874–1879.
38. Nagaraj UD, Calvo-Garcia MA, Merrow AC, et al. Decreased rectal meconium signal on MRI in fetuses with open spinal dysraphism. *Prenat Diagn.* 2018;38(11):870–875.
39. Higashida T, Sasano M, Sato H, et al. Myelomeningocele associated with split cord malformation type I -three case reports-. *Neurol Med Chir (Tokyo).* 2010;50(5):426–430.
40. Ansari S, Nejat F, Yazdani S, et al. Split cord malformation associated with myelomeningocele. *J Neurosurg.* 2007;107(4 suppl):281–285.
41. Nagaraj UD, Bierbrauer KS, Stevenson CB, et al. Spinal imaging findings of open spinal dysraphisms on fetal and postnatal MRI. *Am J Neuroradiol.* 2018;39(10):1947–1952.
42. Danzer E, Hubbard AM, Hedrick HL, et al. Diagnosis and characterization of fetal sacrococcygeal teratoma with prenatal MRI. *AJR Am J Roentgenol.* 2006;187(4):350–356.
43. Luthy D, Wardinsky T, Shurtleff D, et al. Cesarean section before the onset of labor and subsequent motor function in infants with meningomyelocele diagnosed antenatally. *N Engl J Med.* 1991;324(10):662–666.
44. Committee on Obstetric Practice Society for Maternal-Fetal Medicine. Maternal-fetal surgery for myelomeningocele. 2017;130(720):164–167.
45. Kellogg R, Lee P, Deibert CP, et al. Twenty years' experience with myelomeningocele management at a single institution: lessons learned. *J Neurosurg Pediatr.* 2018:1–5.
46. Januschek E, Röhrig A, Kunze S, et al. Myelomeningocele—a single institute analysis of the years 2007 to 2015. *Child's Nerv Syst.* 2016;32(7):1281–1287.
47. Shaer CM, Chescheir N, Schulkin J. Myelomeningocele: a review of the epidemiology, genetics, risk factors for conception, prenatal diagnosis, and prognosis for affected individuals. *Obstet Gynecol Surv.* 2007;62(7):471–479.
48. Oakeshott P, Hunt GM. Long-term outcome in open spina bifida. *Br J Gen Pract.* 2003;53(493):632–636.
49. Chao TT, Dashe JS, Adams RC, et al. Central nervous system findings on fetal magnetic resonance imaging and outcomes in children with spina bifida. *Obstet Gynecol.* 2010;116(2):323–329.
50. Chao TT, Dashe JS, Adams RC, et al. Fetal spine findings on MRI and associated outcomes in children with open neural tube defects. *Am J Roentgenol.* 2011;197(5):956–961.
51. Barkovich AJ, Kuzniecky RI. Gray matter heterotopia. *Neurology.* 2000;55(11):1603–1608.
52. Nagaraj UD, Bierbrauer K, Stevenson CB, et al. Myelomeningocele versus myelocele on fetal MR images: are there differences in brain findings? *AJR Am J Roentgenol.* 2018;211(December):1376–1380.
53. Farmer DL, Thom EA, Brock JW, et al. The management of myelomeningocele study: full cohort 30 month pediatric outcomes. *Am J Obstet Gynecol.* 2017;218(2):256.e1–256.e13.
54. Steinbok P, Cochrane D. Cervical meningoceles and myelocystoceles: a unifying hypothesis. *Pediatr Neurosurg.* 1995;23(6):317–322.
55. Marks J, Khoshnood B. Epidemiology of common neurosurgical diseases in the neonate. *Neurosurg Clin N Am.* 1998;9(1):63–72.
56. Feltes CH, Fountas KN, Dimopoulos VG, et al. Cervical meningocele in association with spinal abnormalities. *Child's Nerv Syst.* 2004;20(5):357–361.
57. Göçer AI, Tuna M, Gezercan Y, et al. Multiple anterolateral cervical meningoceles associated with neurofibromatosis. *Neurosurg Rev.* 1999;22(2–3):124–126.
58. Salomao J. Cervical meningocele in association with spinal abnormalities. *Child's Nerv Syst.* 2005;20(21):4–5.
59. Schwartz ES, Barkovich A. Congenital anomalies of the spine. In: Barkovich AJ, Raybaud C, eds. *Pediatric Neuroimaging.* 5th ed. Philadelphia, PA: Lippincott Williams & Wilkins; 2012:857–922.
60. Currarino G, Coln D, Votteler T. Triad of anorectal, sacral, and presacral anomalies. *Am J Roentgenol.* 1981;137:395–398.
61. Simon EM, Pollock AN. Prenatal and postnatal imaging of spinal dysraphism. *Semin Roentgenol.* 2004;39(2):182–196. doi:10.1053/j.ro.2003.12.004.
62. Duczkowska A, Bekiesinska-Figatowska M, Herman-Sucharska I, et al. Magnetic resonance imaging in the evaluation of the fetal spinal canal contents. *Brain Dev.* 2011;33(1):10–20.
63. Pang D, Dias M. Cervical myelomeningoceles. *Neurosurgery.* 1993;33(3):363–372.
64. Cornette L, Verpoorten C, Lagae L, et al. Closed spinal dysraphism: a review on diagnosis and treatment in infancy. *Eur J Paediatr Neurol.* 1998;2(4):179–185.
65. Singh S, Mehrotra A, Pandey S, et al. Cystic cervical dysraphism: experience of 12 cases. *J Pediatr Neursci.* 2018;13(1):39–45.
66. Northrup H, Volcik KA. Spina bifida and other neural tube defects. *Curr Probl Pediatr.* 2000;30(10):317–332.
67. Pierre-Kahn A, Zerah M, Renier D, et al. Congenital lumbosacral lipomas. *Child's Nerv Syst.* 1997;13(6):298–335.
68. Forrester MB, Merz RD. Descriptive epidemiology of lipomyelomeningocele, Hawaii, 1986-2001. *Birth Defects Res A Clin Mol Teratol.* 2004;70(12):953–956.
69. Agopian AJ, Canfield MA, Olney RS, et al. Spina bifida subtypes and sub-phenotypes by maternal race/ethnicity in the National Birth Defects Prevention Study. *Am J Med Genet Part A.* 2012;158A(1):109–115.
70. Canfield MA, Marengo L, Ramadhani TA, et al. The prevalence and predictors of anencephaly and spina bifida in Texas. *Paediatr Perinat Epidemiol.* 2009;23(1):41–50.
71. De Wals P, Van Allen MI, Lowry RB, et al. Impact of folic acid food fortification on the birth prevalence of lipomyelomeningocele in Canada. *Birth Defects Res A Clin Mol Teratol.* 2008;82(2):106–109.
72. McNeely DP, Howes W. Ineffectiveness of dietary folic acid supplementation on the incidence of lipomyelomeningocele. *J Neurosurg Pediatr.* 2004;100(Pediatrics 2):98–100.
73. Sutton L. Lipomyelomeningocele. *Neurosurg Clin N Am.* 1995;6(2):325–338.
74. Kim SY, Mcgahan JP, Boggan JE, et al. Prenatal diagnosis of lipomyelomeningocele. *J Ultrasound Med.* 2000;19(11):801–805.
75. Berger-Kulemann V, Brugger P, Reisegger M, et al. Quantification of the subcutaneous fat layer with MRI in fetuses of healthy mothers with no underlying metabolic disease vs. fetuses of diabetic and obese mothers. *J Perinat Med.* 2011;40(2):179–184.
76. Pang D. Sacral agenesis and caudal spinal cord malformations. *Neurosurgery.* 1993;32(5):755–778.
77. Tubbs R, Bui C, Rice W, et al. Critical analysis of the Chiari malformation Type I found in children with lipomyelomeningocele. *J Neurosurg Pediatr.* 2007;106:196–200.
78. O'Neill BR, Gallegos D, Herron A, et al. Use of magnetic resonance imaging to detect occult spinal dysraphism in infants. *J Neurosurg Pediatr.* 2017;19(2):217–226.
79. Abbott JF, Davis GH, Endicott B, et al. Prenatal diagnosis of vestigial tail. *J Ultrasound Med.* 1992;11(1):53–55.
80. Huang SL, Shi W, Zhang LG. Surgical treatment for lipomyelomeningocele in children. *World J Pediatr.* 2010;6(4):361–365.
81. Cochrane DD. Cord untethering for lipomyelomeningocele: expectation after surgery. *Neurosurg Focus.* 2007;23(2):e9.
82. Arai H, Sato K, Okuda O, et al. Surgical experience of 120 patients with lumbosacral lipomas. *Acta Neurochir (Wien).* 2001;143(9):857–864.
83. Atala A, Bauer S, Dyro F, et al. Bladder functional changes resulting from lipomyelomeningocele repair. *J Urol.* 1992;148(2 pt 2):592–594.
84. Colak A, Pollack I, Albright A. Recurrent tethering: a common long-term problem after lipomyelomeningocele repair. *Pediatr Neurosurg.* 1998;29(4):184–190.
85. Muthukumar N. Terminal and nonterminal myelocystoceles. *J Neurosurg Pediatr.* 2007;107(2):87–97.
86. Pang D, Zovickian J, Lee JY, et al. Terminal myelocystocele: surgical observations and theory of embryogenesis. *Neurosurgery.* 2012;70(6):1383–1404.
87. Byrd SE, Harvey C, Mclone DG, et al. Imaging of terminal myelocystoceles. *Radiology.* 1996;88(8):510–516.
88. Tandon V, Garg K, Mahapatra AK. Terminal myelocystocele: a series of 30 cases and review of the literature. *Pediatr Neurosurg.* 2013;48(4):229–235.
89. Midrio P, Silberstein H, Bilaniuk L, et al. Prenatal diagnosis of a terminal myelocystocele in the fetal surgery era: case report. *Neurosurgery.* 2002;50(5):1152–1154.
90. Bhargava R, Hammond D, Benzie R, et al. Prenatal demonstration of a cervical myelocystocele. *Prenat Diagn.* 1992;12(8):653–659.
91. Husler M, Danzer E, Johnson M, et al. Prenatal diagnosis and postnatal outcome of fetal spinal defects without Arnold-Chiari II malformation. *Prenat Diagn.* 2006;26(10):980–984.
92. Kolble N, Huisman TA, Stallmach T, et al. Prenatal diagnosis of a fetus with lumbar myelocystocele. *Ultrasound Obstet Gynecol.* 2001;18(5):536–539.
93. Hung BH, Chiang CL, Wang PC, et al. Teaching neuroimages: terminal myelocystocele. *Neurology.* 2011;76(14):75–76.
94. Choi SH, McComb JG. Long-term outcome of terminal myelocystocele patients. *Pediatr Neurosurg.* 2000;32(2):86–91.
95. Erşahin Y, Mutluer S, Kocaman S, et al. Split spinal cord malformations in children. *J Neurosurg.* 1998;88(1):57–65.
96. Sonigo-Cohen P, Schmit P, Zerah M, et al. Prenatal diagnosis of diastematomyelia. *Child's Nerv Syst.* 2003;19(7–8):555–560.
97. Kutuk MS, Ozgun MT, Tas M, et al. Prenatal diagnosis of split cord malformation by ultrasound and fetal magnetic resonance imaging: case report and review of the literature. *Child's Nerv Syst.* 2012;28(12):2169–2172.
98. Ayvaz M, Akalan N, Yazici M, et al. Is it necessary to operate all split cord malformations before corrective surgery for patients with congenital spinal deformities? *Spine (Phila Pa 1976).* 2009;34(22):2413–2418.
99. Erşahin Y. Split cord malformation types I and II: a personal series of 131 patients. *Child's Nerv Syst.* 2013;29(9):1515–1526.
100. Pang D, Dias M, Ahab-Barmada M. Split cord malformation: part I: a unified theory of embryogenesis for double spinal cord malformations. *Neurosurgery.* 1992;31(3):451–480.
101. Allen LM, Silverman RK. Prenatal ultrasound evaluation of fetal diastematomyelia: two cases of type I split cord malformation. *Ultrasound Obstet Gynecol.* 2000;15(1):78–82.

102. Sepulveda W, Kyle P, Hassan J, et al. Prenatal diagnosis of diastematomyelia: case reports and review of the literature. *Prenat Diagn.* 1997;17(2):161–165.

103. Has R, Yuksel A, Buyukkurt S, et al. Prenatal diagnosis of diastematomyelia: presentation of eight cases and review of the literature. *Ultrasound Obstet Gynecol.* 2007;30(6):845–849.

104. Anderson NG, Jordan S, MacFarlane MR, et al. Diastematomyelia: diagnosis by prenatal sonography. *Am J Roentgenol.* 1994;163(4):911–914.

105. Kaffenberger DA, Heinz ER, Oakes JW, et al. Meningocele manqué: radiologic findings with clinical correlation. *AJNR Am J Neuroradiol.* 1992;13(4):1083–1088.

106. Proctor MR, Bauer SB, Scott RM. The effect of surgery for split spinal cord malformation on neurologic and urologic function. *Pediatr Neurosurg.* 2000; 32(1):13–19.

107. Liu W, Zheng D, Cui S, et al. Characteristics of osseous septum of split cord malformation in patients presenting with scoliosis: a retrospective study of 48 cases. *Pediatr Neurosurg.* 2009;45(5):350–353.

108. Mahapatra A. Split cord malformation—a study of 300 cases at AIIMS 1990-2006. *J Pediatr Neursci.* 2011;6(suppl 1):S41–S45.

109. Nievelstein RA, Valk J, Smit LM, et al. MR of the caudal regression syndrome: embryologic implications. *Am J Neuroradiol.* 1994;15(6):1021–1029.

110. Balioglu MB, Akman YE, Ucpunar H, et al. Sacral agenesis: evaluation of accompanying pathologies in 38 cases, with analysis of long-term outcomes. *Child's Nerv Syst.* 2016;32(9):1693–1702.

111. Jeelani Y, Mosich GM, McComb JG. Closed neural tube defects in children with caudal regression. *Child's Nerv Syst.* 2013;29(9):1451–1457.

112. Dunn V, Nixon G, Jaffe R, et al. Infants radiographic of diabetic mothers: radiographic manifestations. *AJR Am J Roentgenol.* 1981;137(1):123–128.

113. Twickler D, Budorick N, Pretorius D, et al. Caudal regression versus sirenomelia: sonographic clues. *J Ultrasound Med.* 1993;12(6):323–330.

114. Sonek JD, Gabbe SG, Landon MB, et al. Antenatal diagnosis of sacral agenesis syndrome in a pregnancy complicated by diabetes mellitus. *Am J Obstet Gynecol.* 1990;162(3):806–808.

115. Torre M, Buffa P, Jasonni V, et al. Long-term urologic outcome in patients with caudal regression syndrome, compared with meningomyelocele and spinal cord lipoma. *J Pediatr Surg.* 2008;43(3):530–533.

116. Nievelstein RA, Vos A, Valk J, et al. Magnetic resonance imaging in children with anorectal malformations: embryologic implications. *J Pediatr Surg.* 2002;37(8):1138–1145.

117. Valenzano M, Paoletti R, Rossi A, et al. Sirenomelia. Pathological features, antenatal ultrasonographic clues, and a review of current embryogenic theories. *Hum Reprod Update.* 1999;5(1):82–86.

118. Stevenson RE, Jones KL, Phelan MC, et al. Vascular steal: the pathogenetic mechanism producing sirenomelia and associated defects of the viscera and soft tissues. *Pediatrics.* 1986;78(3):451–457.

119. Talamo T, Macpherson T, Dominquez R. Sirenomelia. Angiographic demonstration of vascular anomalies. *Arch Pathol Lab Med.* 1982;106(7):347–348.

120. Kapur R, Mahony B, Nyberg D, et al. Sirenomelia associated with a "vanishing twin." *Teratology.* 1991;43(2):103–108.

121. Stocker J, Heifetz S. Sirenomelia. A morphological study of 33 cases and review of the literature. *Perspect Pediatr Pathol.* 1987;10:7–10.

122. Schiesser M, Holzgreve W, Lapaire O, et al. Sirenomelia, the mermaid syndrome—detection in the first trimester. *Prenat Diagn.* 2003;23(6):493–495.

123. Akbayir O, Gungorduk K, Sudolmus S, et al. First trimester diagnosis of sirenomelia: a case report and review of the literature. *Arch Gynecol Obstet.* 2008;278(6):589–592.

124. Blaicher W, Lee A, Deutinger J, et al. Sirenomelia: early prenatal diagnosis with combined two- and three-dimensional sonography. *Ultrasound Obstet Gynecol.* 2001;17(6):542–543.

125. Keirsbilck J, Cannie M, Robrechts C, et al. First trimester diagnosis of sirenomelia. *Prenat Diagn.* 2006;26:684–688.

126. Contu R, Zoppi MA, Axiana C, et al. First trimester diagnosis of sirenomelia by 2D and 3D ultrasound. *Fetal Diagn Ther.* 2009;26(1):41–44.

127. Monteagudo A, Mayberry P, Rebarber A, et al. Sirenomelia sequence: first-trimester diagnosis with both two- and three-dimensional sonography. *J Ultrasound Med.* 2002;21(8):915–920.

128. Chenoweth C, Kellogg S, Abu-Yousef M. Antenatal sonographic diagnosis of sirenomelia. *J Clin Ultrasound.* 1991;19(3):167–171.

129. Sepulveda W, Corral E, Sanchez J, et al. Sirenomelia sequence versus renal agenesis: prenatal differentiation with power Doppler ultrasound. *Ultrasound Obstet Gynecol.* 1998;11(6):445–449.

130. Patel S, Suchet I. The role of color and power Doppler ultrasound in the prenatal diagnosis of sirenomelia. *Ultrasound Obstet Gynecol.* 2004;24(6):684–691.

131. Bravo C, De León-Luis J, Gámez F, et al. Fetal MRI as a complementary technique after prenatal diagnosis of persistent vitelline artery in an otherwise normal fetus. *J Magn Reson Imaging.* 2013;38(4):951–954.

132. Fitzmorris-Glass R, Mattrey R, Cantrell C. Magnetic resonance imaging as an adjunct to ultrasound in oligohydramnios. Detection of sirenomelia. *J Ultrasound Med.* 1989;8(3):159–162.

133. Agarwalla PK, Dunn IF, Scott RM, et al. Tethered cord syndrome. *Neurosurg Clin N Am.* 2007;18(3):531–547.

134. Tu A, Steinbok P. Occult tethered cord syndrome: a review. *Child's Nerv Syst.* 2013;29(9):1635–1640.

135. American Institute of Ultrasound in Medicine. AIUM practice guideline for the performance of obstetric ultrasound examinations. *J Ultrasound Med.* 2013;32(6):1038–1101.

136. Mottet N, Saada J, Jani J, et al. Sonographic evaluation of fetal conus medullaris and filum terminale. *Fetal Diagn Ther.* 2016;40(3):224–230.

137. Rodriguez M, Prats P, Rodriguez I, et al. Prenatal evaluation of the fetal conus medullaris on a routine scan. *Fetal Diagn Ther.* 2016;39(2):113–116.

138. Melikhov IV, Makogon YF, Gorbatchevskii AY, et al. Prenatal ultrasound evaluation of the position of conus medullaris for the diagnosis of tethered cord syndrome. *Ultrasound Q.* 2016;32(4):356–360.

139. Widjaja E, Whitby EH, Paley MN, et al. Normal fetal lumbar spine on postmortem MR imaging. *Am J Neuroradiol.* 2006;27(3):553–559.

140. Sulak O, Özgüner G, Malas MA. Size and location of the kidneys during the fetal period. *Surg Radiol Anat.* 2011;33(5):381–388.

141. Kumar R, Guinto FC, Madewell JE, et al. The vertebral body: radiographic configurations in various congenital and acquired disorders. *RadioGraphics.* 1988;8(3):455–485.

142. Eckalbar WL, Fisher RE, Rawls A, et al. Scoliosis and segmentation defects of the vertebrae. *Wiley Interdisc Rev Dev Biol.* 2012;1(3):401–423.

143. Thawait GK, Chhabra A, Carrino JA. Spine segmentation and enumeration and normal variants. *Radiol Clin North Am.* 2012;50(4):587–598.

144. Barnes GL, Hsu CW, Mariani BD, et al. Chicken Pax-1 gene: structure and expression during embryonic somite development. *Differentiation.* 1996;61(1):13–23.

145. Abrams SL, Filly RA. Curvature of the fetal femur: a normal sonographic finding. *Radiology.* 1985;156(2):490.

146. Benacerraf BR, Greene MF, Barss VA. Prenatal sonographic diagnosis of congenital hemivertebra. *J Ultrasound Med.* 1986;5(5):257–259.

147. Goldstein I, Makhoul IR, Weissman A, et al. Hemivertebra: prenatal diagnosis, incidence and characteristics. *Fetal Diagn Ther.* 2005;20(2):121–126.

148. Harrison LA, Pretorius DH, Budorick NE. Abnormal spinal curvature in the fetus. *J Ultrasound Med.* 1992;11(9):473–479.

149. Ruano R, Molho M, Roume J, et al. Prenatal diagnosis of fetal skeletal dysplasias by combining two-dimensional and three-dimensional ultrasound and intrauterine three-dimensional helical computer tomography. *Ultrasound Obstet Gynecol.* 2004;24(2):134–140.

150. Nemec U, Nemec SF, Weber M, et al. Human long bone development in vivo: analysis of the distal femoral epimetaphysis on MR images of fetuses. *Radiology.* 2013;267(2):570–580.

151. Robinson AJ, Blaser S, Vladimirov A, et al. Foetal "black bone" MRI: utility in assessment of the foetal spine. *Br J Radiol.* 2015;88(1046):1–6.

152. Cassart M, Massez A, Cos T, et al. Contribution of three-dimensional computed tomography in the assessment of fetal skeletal dysplasia. *Ultrasound Obstet Gynecol.* 2007;29(5):537–543.

153. Victoria T, Epelman M, Bebbington M, et al. Low-dose fetal CT for evaluation of severe congenital skeletal anomalies: preliminary experience. *Pediatr Radiol.* 2012;42(suppl 1):142–149.

154. Jaskwhich D, Ali R, Patel T, et al. Congenital scoliosis. *Curr Opin Pediatr.* 2000;12(1):61–66.

155. Lawson M, Share J, Benacerraf B, et al. Jarcho-Levin syndrome: prenatal diagnosis, perinatal care, and follow-up of siblings. *J Perinatol.* 1997;17(5):407–409.

156. Zelop C, Pretorius D, Benacerraf B. Fetal hemivertebrae: associated anomalies, significance, and outcome. *Obstet Gynecol.* 1993;81(3):412–416.

157. McMaster M, Ohtsuka K. The natural history of congenital scoliosis: a study of two hundred and fifty-one patients. *J Bone Joint Surg.* 1982;64(8):1128–1147.

158. Connor J, Conner A, Connor R, et al. Genetic aspects of early childhood scoliosis. *Am J Med Genet.* 1987;27(2):419–424.

159. Kocaoglu M, Frush DP. Pediatric presacral masses. *Radiographics.* 2006; 26:833–857.

160. Altman R, Randolph J, Lilly J. Sacrococcygeal teratoma: American Academy of Pediatrics Surgical Section Survey 1973. *J Pediatr Surg.* 1974;9(3):389–398.

161. Sheth S, Nussbaum A, Sanders R, et al. Prenatal diagnosis of sacrococcygeal teratoma: sonographic-pathologic correlation. *Radiology.* 1988;169(1):131–134.

162. Gucciardo L, Uyttebroek A, De Wever I, et al. Prenatal assessment and management of sacrococcygeal teratoma. *Prenat Diagn.* 2011;31(7):678–688.

163. Hedrick HL, Flake AW, Crombleholme TM, et al. Sacrococcygeal teratoma: prenatal assessment, fetal intervention, and outcome. *J Pediatr Surg.* 2004; 39(3):430–438.

164. Van Mieghem T, Al-Ibrahim A, Deprest J, et al. Minimally invasive therapy for fetal sacrococcygeal teratoma: case series and systematic review of the literature. *Ultrasound Obstet Gynecol.* 2014;43(6):611–619.

165. Moazam F, Talbert JL. Congenital anorectal malformations. Harbingers of sacrococcygeal teratomas. *Arch Surg.* 1985 Jul;120(7):856–859.

166. Partridge EA, Canning D, Long C, et al. Urologic and anorectal complications of sacrococcygeal teratomas: prenatal and postnatal predictors. *J Pediatr Surg.* 2014;49(1):139–143.

167. Tanaka K, Kanai M, Yosizawa J, et al. A case of neonatal neuroblastoma mimicking Altman type III sacrococcygeal teratoma. *J Pediatr Surg.* 2005; 40(3):578–580.

168. Langer JC, Harrison MR, Schmidt KG, et al. Fetal hydrops and death from sacrococcygeal teratoma: rationale for fetal surgery. *Am J Obstet Gynecol.* 1989;160(5 pt 1):1145–1150.

169. Akinkuotu AC, Coleman A, Shue E, et al. Predictors of poor prognosis in prenatally diagnosed sacrococcygeal teratoma: a multiinstitutional review. *J Pediatr Surg.* 2015;50(5):771–774.

170. Marina NM, Cushing B, Giller R, et al. Complete surgical excision is effective treatment for children with immature teratomas with or without malignant elements: a Pediatric Oncology Group/Children's Cancer Group Intergroup Study. *J Clin Oncol.* 1999;17(7):2137–2143.

171. Wilson RD, Hedrick H, Flake AW, et al. Sacrococcygeal teratomas: prenatal surveillance, growth and pregnancy outcome. *Fetal Diagn Ther.* 2009;25(1):15–20.

172. Roybal JL, Moldenhauer JS, Khalek N, et al. Early delivery as an alternative management strategy for selected high-risk fetal sacrococcygeal teratomas. *J Pediatr Surg.* 2011;46(7):1325–1332.

173. Peiró JL, Sbragia L, Scorletti F, et al. Management of fetal teratomas. *Pediatr Surg Int.* 2016;32(7):635–647.

174. Gopal M, Turnpenny PD, Spicer R. Hereditary sacrococcygeal teratoma—not the same as its sporadic counterpart! *Eur J Pediatr Surg.* 2007;17(3):214–216.

175. Wax JR, Benn P, Steinfeld JD, et al. Prenatally diagnosed sacrococcygeal teratoma: a unique expression of trisomy 1q. *Cancer Genet Cytogenet.* 2000;117(1):84–86.

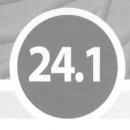

24.1   Cardiac Anomalies

Sarah B. Clauss • Neeta Jain Sethi • Mary T. Donofrio

Approximately 1% of all children are born with a congenital heart defect (CHD), making cardiac disease the most common congenital malformation. Ventricular septal defects (VSDs) are the most common, comprising 26% of all congenital cardiac lesions followed by tetralogy of Fallot (TOF), atrioventricular (AV) septal defects, atrial septal defects (ASDs), pulmonary stenosis, coarctation of the aorta, hypoplastic left heart syndrome, and transposition of the great arteries, all of which occur with a frequency of approximately 5% to 10% (Table 24.1-1). The percentage of fetuses with heart defects is up to five-fold higher, many of which are lethal. Cardiac defects account for more than 20% of perinatal deaths from congenital abnormalities. Fetal echocardiography is widely available, and current technology allows for definitive diagnosis or exclusion of congenital heart disease in most patients. This chapter reviews diagnostic utility and impact on management of fetal echocardiography.

TIMING AND INDICATIONS

Fetal echocardiography has been in use since the late 1980s, and current technology allows for diagnostic testing as early as the first trimester with transvaginal imaging.[1,2] Ideal imaging usually occurs between 20 and 28 weeks' gestation, but it can be performed up to delivery. Third-trimester imaging may be limited by a lack of amniotic fluid and limited variability in fetal position. Indications for fetal echocardiography can be related to maternal and/or fetal risk factors (see Chapter 5).[3] The most common reasons for referral are family history of congenital heart disease, fetal dysrhythmia, maternal diabetes, and noncardiac fetal defect (i.e., increased nuchal fold). Indications that are most predictive of cardiac disease are an abnormal four-chamber view on routine ultrasound (30% to 50%), fetal dysrhythmia (30%), hydrops (30%), and polyhydramnios (25%). See Chapter 5 for detailed discussion of indications.

CLASSIFICATION OF DEFECTS

Septal Defects

Atrial Septal Defects

Definition: An ASD is a defect within the atrial septum that leads to a communication between the right and left atrium.

Incidence: In total, ASDs comprise 8% of CHD in live births, although prenatal diagnosis can be challenging due to the expected opening of the foramen ovale in normal fetal hearts.[4] Both prenatally and within the initial postnatal period, a normal patent foramen ovale (PFO) can be difficult to distinguish from a small secundum ASD.

Pathology and Hemodynamics: ASDs are classified by location within the atrial septum. The most common ASD is a secundum ASD, followed by primum, sinus venosus, and coronary sinus defects. A PFO is an opening in the atrial septum and is a normal structure in the fetus (allowing right to left shunting of oxygenated blood from the umbilical vein to the left side of the heart) (Fig. 24.1-1). An aneurysm of the atrial septum is common, giving the septum a "wind sock" appearance. It is difficult to use fetal echocardiography to predict persistence of the foramen ovale or a small secundum ASD after birth. Secundum ASDs represent a defect within the septum primum, often adjacent to the foramen ovale. A primum ASD represents a defect in the endocardial cushion, adjacent to the AV valves, and is the second most common type of ASD. If a primum ASD is suspected, the presence of an AV septal defect must be considered and the ventricular septum and mitral valve should be closely evaluated. Sinus venosus defects are located posteriorly and adjacent to the superior vena cava or inferior vena cava (IVC). In case of a sinus venosus ASD, the pulmonary veins should be carefully imaged, as superior sinus venosus defects are often associated with anomalous drainage of the right pulmonary veins. The least common ASD is the coronary sinus ASD, which is located at the coronary sinus ostium within the left atrium. If a coronary sinus defect is suspected, the possibility of a left superior vena cava should be considered.

Associated Anomalies: Most major types of CHD can be associated with an ASD, including endocardial cushion defect,

TABLE 24.1-1	The Baltimore–Washington Infant Study	
DIAGNOSIS	**CHILDREN WITH CHD (%)**
Ventricular septal defect	26
Tetralogy of Fallot	9
Atrioventricular septal defect	9
Atrial septal defect	8
Pulmonary valve stenosis	7
Coarctation of the aorta	7
Hypoplastic left heart syndrome	6
D-Transposition of the great arteries	5
Other	23

CHD, congenital heart defect.
From Ferencz C, Rubin JD, McCarter RJ, et al. Congenital heart disease: prevalence at livebirth. The Baltimore-Washington infant study. *Am J Epidemiol.* 1985;121(1):31–36. Copyright © 1985 by The Johns Hopkins University School of Hygiene and Public Health. Reproduced by permission of Oxford University Press.

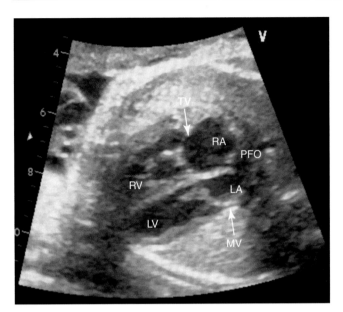

FIGURE 24.1-1: Four-chamber view obtained by cross-sectional imaging of the chest. The four chambers are readily visualized, right atrium (*RA*), left atrium (*LA*), right ventricle (*RV*), left ventricle (*LV*). In addition, the two atrioventricular valves are seen, tricuspid valve (*TV*), and mitral valve (*MV*). The heart is perpendicular to the plan of imaging and the ventricular septum is well visualized and appears intact. The patent foramen ovale (*PFO*) is also visualized.

anomalous pulmonary venous return, TOF, double-outlet right ventricle (DORV) and hypoplastic left heart syndrome. These anomalies are discussed later in the chapter. Specific genetic defects are also associated with an atrial level shunt. Holt–Oram syndrome consists of a secundum ASD, hypoplasia of the thumbs and radius, triphalangeal thumbs, abrachia, and phocomelia. Other congenital syndromes in which a secundum ASD may occur include Noonan syndrome, Treacher Collins syndrome, and the thrombocytopenia–absent radii (TAR) syndrome.

Treatment/Outcome: Postnatally, small secundum ASDs can be followed clinically as these defects often spontaneously close. Secundum ASDs that do require intervention are often amenable to percutaneous device closure in the cardiac catheterization laboratory, although some require surgical intervention depending on size and location. All other types of ASDs require surgical closure, although timing is dependent on exact diagnosis, clinical situation, and associated cardiac abnormalities.

Ventricular Septal Defects
Definition: A VSD is a defect in the ventricular septum that causes a communication between the two ventricles.

Incidence: VSDs are the most commonly diagnosed CHD, involving 25% of live births with CHD.[4]

Pathology and Hemodynamics: Like ASDs, VSDs are classified by their location within the ventricular septum, although various classification systems exist. VSDs can be classified as muscular, AV, conoventricular (including membranous/perimembranous, and malalignment-type defects), and conoseptal. Muscular VSDs are defects within the muscular septum and are entirely surrounded by muscle. These defects can be further classified by location within the muscular septum, such as apical (below the

moderator band), mid-muscular, posterior, and anterior. Atrioventricular ([AV] or inlet) defects are defects in the posterior ventricular septum abutting the AV valves. These defects may or may not be associated with an atrioventricular canal (AVC) defect. Membranous defects involve the membranous septum with the defect bordering the tricuspid valve. Perimembranous defects are around the membranous septum. Conoventricular VSDs encompass those defects that involve the conal or outlet septum. The malalignment-type VSD is a type of conoventricular VSD. Defects of conal septal position result in malalignment, yielding the potential for outflow tract obstruction. The conal septum can be anteriorly displaced (as in TOF) or posteriorly displaced (often associated with interrupted aortic arch). Defects of the conal septum resulting in conal hypoplasia are closely associated with the semilunar valves. These defects can lead to aortic insufficiency due to lack of support of the aortic valve and distortion of the right coronary cusp if the valve gets pulled into the defect.

Associated Anomalies: Most VSDs are isolated, but they can be found with almost all other CHDs. Therefore, when a VSD is identified, all other cardiac structures must be thoroughly evaluated (i.e., to exclude more extensive anomalies, such as TOF and coarctation of the aorta). VSDs are also seen in fetuses with chromosomal abnormalities, including trisomies 21, 18, and 13.

Imaging: VSDs often are best seen when the ultrasound beam is perpendicular to the septum, as "false dropout" occurs when the beam is parallel to the septum (Fig. 24.1-2). However, in some cases, the VSD may not be seen when the beam is perpendicular to the septum and other views are needed. Large defects will be easily visible; however, small defects are often missed. Color Doppler demonstrates bidirectional shunting. Perimembranous defects will be wedged under the tricuspid valve; these types of defects are best seen from the short- and long-axis views of the heart. Conal septal defects occur in outlet septum in the muscle that supports the aortic valve adjacent to the pulmonary valve. These defects

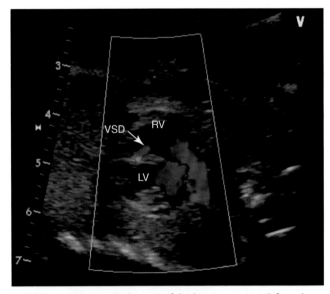

FIGURE 24.1-2: A sagittal image of the heart, sweeping leftward, one can see the anterior right ventricle (*RV*) and the posterior left ventricle (*LV*). The *red* flow represents a muscular ventricular septal defect (*VSD*). The *blue* color flow demonstrates the laminar flow in the right ventricular outflow tract.

are best seen in short-axis imaging. Anterior malalignment of the conal septum is typically seen in conjunction with aortic override, making the diagnosis of TOF. The conal septum may also be posteriorly malaligned, which may be associated with subaortic narrowing, aortic valve stenosis, and coarctation of the aorta or interrupted aortic arch. AVC-type VSDs or inlet defects are well seen in the four-chamber view under the AV valves.

Treatment/Outcome: Postnatally, small VSDs can be followed up clinically as perimembranous and muscular defects often close spontaneously (more likely when the defects are smaller than 3 mm in a term infant). Moderate to large defects often require surgical closure in the setting of congestive heart failure that cannot be managed medically. In older patients, muscular VSDs are sometimes amenable to percutaneous device closure in the cardiac catheterization laboratory, although most VSDs that require closure necessitate surgical intervention. Malalignment and AVC-type defects will not close spontaneously and therefore need surgical closure. Typically, conal septal hypoplasia defects do not close, but the decision to operate depends on the amount of left to right shunting and the effect the defect has on the aortic valve.

Endocardial Cushion Defects

Definition: Endocardial cushion defects include the spectrum of diseases involving the endocardial cushion and include complete atrioventricular canal (CAVC), transitional AVC defects, and isolated primum ASD with cleft mitral valve. These defects can be classified by size/presence of the VSD, the balance of the AV valve over the ventricles, and the anatomy of the common valve.

Incidence: Endocardial cushion defects account for 5% to 7% of all live births with CHD.[4]

Pathology and Hemodynamics: A CAVC defect includes defects of the atrial septum (primum ASD) and ventricular septum (AV VSD) with a common AV valve. A partial AVC is comprised

of a primum ASD and a cleft mitral valve. A transitional AVC is similar to a complete CAVC, except there is a small restrictive VSD. CAVCs can be further classified by the anatomy of the anterior bridging leaflet of the common AV valve. Using the classification system of Rastelli,[5] in type A defects, the anterior bridging leaflet is divided and has attachments to the crest of the ventricular septum. In type B defects, the anterior bridging leaflet is partially divided, but with no attachments to the ventricular septum. In type C defects, the anterior bridging leaflet is both undivided and unattached to the ventricular septal crest (Fig. 24.1-3). The Rastelli classification is best determined by short-axis imaging of the ventricles, noting the valve *en face*.

Further classification of endocardial cushion defects must include a description of the absolute and relative size of the ventricles. In a balanced CAVC, both ventricles are approximately equal in size and the common valve is positioned symmetrically over both ventricles. In an unbalanced CAVC, the AVC sits predominantly over either the right ventricle (RV) or left ventricle (LV); flow is toward that ventricle and the contralateral ventricle is usually small.

Associated Anomalies: Defects associated with endocardial cushion defects include TOF, DORV, coarctation of the aorta, subaortic stenosis, pulmonary valve stenosis, and single ventricle. In the case of multiple defects (i.e., CAVC with DORV and/or with complete heart block [CHB]), heterotaxy syndrome should be considered. When CAVC exists as an isolated lesion, trisomy 21 is present in 60% of the cases.[6] Endocardial cushion defects may also occur with trisomies 13, 18, and 21.

Imaging: Endocardial cushion defects are easily seen in the four-chamber view, with the components of the ASD, VSD, and common valve easily visible (Figs. 24.1-4 to 24.1-6). The details of the common AV valve (*en face* view) are best seen in short-axis imaging of the ventricle (Fig. 24.1-7). The cleft of the anterior leaflet refers to the division of the leaflet with the attachment to

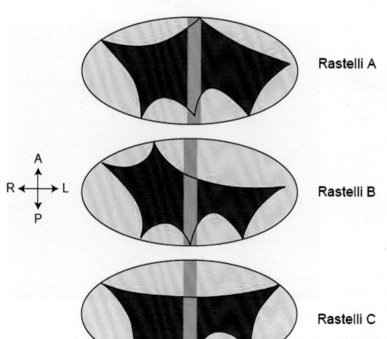

Rastelli A

Rastelli B

Rastelli C

FIGURE 24.1-3: Illustration of Rastelli classification of complete atrioventricular canal. In type A (*top*) the superior bridging leaflet is divided at the level of the ventricular septum. In type B (*center*) division of the superior bridging leaflet occurs to a right ventricular papillary muscle. In type C (*bottom*) the superior bridging leaflet is undivided or "free floating." (From Lai W. *Echocardiography in Pediatric and Congenital Heart Disease.* Chicester, UK: Wiley-Blackwell; 2009. Copyright © 2009 by John Wiley & Sons, Inc. Reprinted by permission of John Wiley & Sons, Inc.)

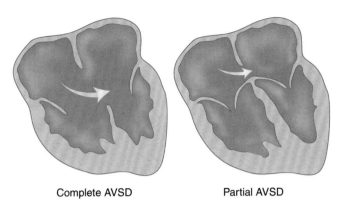

Complete AVSD   Partial AVSD

FIGURE 24.1-4: Illustration of partial and complete atrioventricular canal. AVSD, atrioventricular septal defect. (Reprinted with permission from Rice MJ, McDonald RW, Pilu G, et al. Cardiac malformations. In: Nyberg DA, McGahan JP, Pretorius DH, et al., eds. *Diagnostic Imaging of Fetal Anomalies*. Philadelphia, PA: Lippincott Williams & Wilkins; 2003:459.)

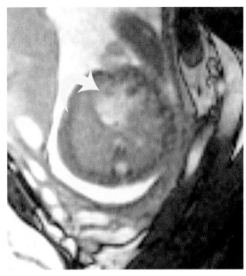

FIGURE 24.1-6: Atrioventricular canal. Axial SSFP MRI of the fetal heart demonstrates a single common valve (*curved arrow*). A large primum atrial septal defect and ventricular septal defect are also present.

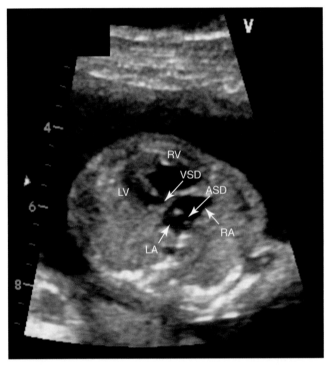

FIGURE 24.1-5: Four-chamber view of a complete atrioventricular canal. The crux of the heart is absent in this view, demonstrating both the inlet ventricular septal defect (*VSD*) and the primum atrial septal defect (*ASD*). The patent foramen ovale is also present in this image. In this systolic view, the single or common valve is also appreciated. *LA*, left atrium; *LV*, left ventricle; *RA*, right atrium; *RV*, right ventricle.

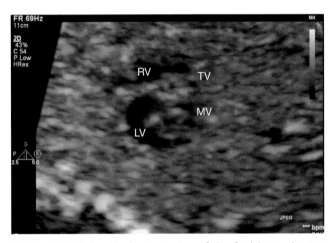

FIGURE 24.1-7: In this short-axis view of the fetal heart, the two components of the right and left side of the atrioventricular valves are well seen. This image will aid in determining Rastelli classification and balance of the valves over the ventricles. Here, the right-sided atrioventricular valve is labeled as the tricuspid valve (*TV*), and the left-sided atrioventricular valve is labeled as the mitral valve (*MV*). *LV*, left ventricle; *RV*, Right ventricle.

repair of CAVCs can vary widely, and be comprised of a single patch, two-patch, or modified patch technique. Short- and long-term outcomes are greatly dependent on associated cardiac defects, residual AV valve regurgitation, outflow tract obstruction, and chromosomal anomalies.

Inflow Defects

Diseases of the Tricuspid Valve

Ebstein Anomaly of the Tricuspid Valve Definition
Ebstein anomaly of the tricuspid valve is defined by specific anatomical features including apical displacement of the septal and posterior leaflets of the tricuspid valve within the RV (Fig. 24.1-8). This creates a displaced tricuspid valve orifice into the body of the ventricle with the proximal RV becoming functionally part of the right atrium.

the left ventricular septal surface. Loss of the normal offsetting between the septal insertions of the mitral and tricuspid valves can be a clue that a CAVC is present. Color Doppler ultrasound should be performed to evaluate for AV valve regurgitation in the four-chamber view.

Treatment/Outcome: CAVC defects always require surgical correction, although the type of repair can be dependent on other anatomical factors (e.g., a significantly unbalanced CAVC may require single-ventricle palliation). The technique of the surgical

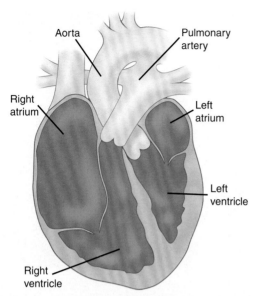

FIGURE 24.1-8: Illustration of Ebstein anomaly of the tricuspid valve. The tricuspid valve is displaced into the right ventricle. (Reprinted with permission from Rice MJ, McDonald RW, Pilu G, et al. Cardiac malformations. In: Nyberg DA, McGahan JP, Pretorius DH, et al., eds. *Diagnostic Imaging of Fetal Anomalies*. Philadelphia, PA: Lippincott Williams & Wilkins; 2003:461.)

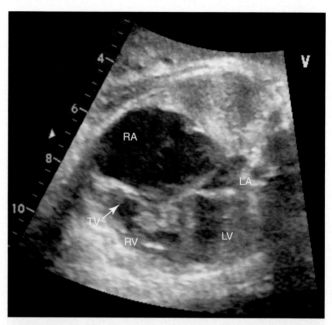

FIGURE 24.1-9: Four-chamber view of Ebstein anomaly of the tricuspid valve in systole. Note the severely enlarged right atrium (*RA*) and the abnormal tricuspid valve (*TV*). *LA*, left atrium; *LV*, left ventricle; *RV*, right ventricle.

Incidence: Ebstein anomaly accounts for 0.5% of live births with CHD, although it occurs in approximately 3% to 8% of fetal CHD, with a 44% rate of fetal demise.[4]

Pathology and Hemodynamics: There is a wide spectrum of disease related to Ebstein anomaly, ranging from minimal displacement of the tricuspid valve, to severe apical displacement wherein nearly the entire RV is "atrialized" and there is little to no functional RV. Severe tricuspid regurgitation can be associated with secondary hydrops fetalis and *in utero* fetal demise. In some cases, there is associated pulmonary stenosis or atresia.

Associated Anomalies: Ebstein anomaly may be associated with other CHDs, such as severe pulmonary stenosis or pulmonary atresia, ASDs, Wolf–Parkinson–White syndrome and congenitally corrected transposition of the great arteries.[7] In addition, severe cardiomegaly may contribute to lung hypoplasia, increasing the risk of death.

Imaging: Ebstein anomaly is well seen in the four-chamber view (Fig. 24.1-9). The displacement of the hinge point of the septal leaflet of the tricuspid valve is quantified by measuring the distance between the crux of the heart (from the mitral valve hinge point) to the hinge point of the septal leaflet of the tricuspid valve; this distance should be less than 5 mm at birth. Cardiomegaly secondary to atrial or ventricular dilation may be present. Color Doppler should be used to evaluate the degree of tricuspid regurgitation (Fig. 24.1-10). Tricuspid regurgitation may progress during fetal life. When severe tricuspid regurgitation exists, the RV may not be able to generate sufficient pressure to open the pulmonary valve even though it may be patent; this is termed functional pulmonary atresia. The "sail-like" anterior leaflet of the tricuspid valve may also contribute to right ventricular outflow tract obstruction. The branch pulmonary arteries can be best seen in short-axis imaging; these may be normal in size or hypoplastic. The ductus arteriosus flow may be normal or reversed. If flow is

reversed, associated "functional" or anatomical pulmonary atresia is likely present. Finally, the right heart may be dilated, causing the left heart to be compressed and appear hypoplastic.

Prognosis: A neonate with significant Ebstein anomaly associated with pulmonary stenosis or atresia will present with cyanosis in the immediate newborn period. The presence of severe pulmonary regurgitation in neonates with severe tricuspid insufficiency and a patent ductus arteriosus may cause a circulatory shunt and severe cardiogenic shock. Postnatally when the pulmonary vascular resistance falls, antegrade pulmonary blood flow may improve if the valve is not atretic. If there is pulmonary atresia or a delayed decrease in pulmonary vascular resistance, prostaglandin is often used to maintain ductal patency and pulmonary blood flow. These neonates may need a surgical systemic to pulmonary artery shunt to ensure adequate pulmonary blood flow. Additional surgeries such as right ventricular outflow patch reconstruction or single-ventricle palliation may need to be performed depending on the degree of right ventricular outflow tract obstruction, right ventricular hypoplasia, or tricuspid valve competency. Alternatively, if the tricuspid valve displacement is minimal and the tricuspid valve regurgitation is mild, patients may not be diagnosed until adulthood (often due to associated atrial arrhythmias).

Tricuspid Valve Dysplasia
Tricuspid valve dysplasia is a nonspecific term that can include various abnormalities of tricuspid valve anatomy. Unlike Ebstein anomaly, in tricuspid valve dysplasia, the tricuspid valve leaflet attachments are at the level of the valve annulus. The leaflets are often thickened, with poor coaptation, and have abnormal papillary muscle and chordae. Various amounts of tricuspid valve regurgitation will often be present and the degree of the regurgitation will determine severity and outcome of the disease. Tricuspid valve dysplasia is associated with varying degrees of right ventricular hypoplasia, pulmonary stenosis, or pulmonary atresia.

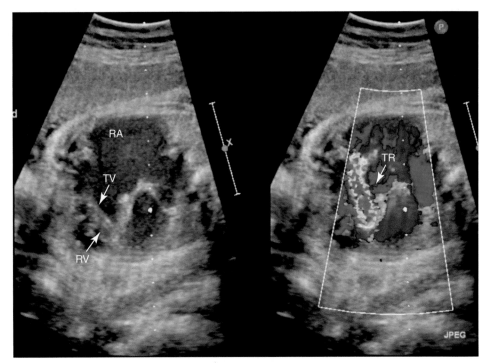

FIGURE 24.1-10: Four-chamber color compare view of Ebstein anomaly of the tricuspid valve in diastole. The apical displacement of the tricuspid valve leaflets (*TV*) into the right ventricle is readily visualized. There is moderate to severe tricuspid insufficiency (*TR*) with severe right atrial (*RA*) enlargement. *RV*, right ventricle.

Isolated Tricuspid Valve Regurgitation

Tricuspid valve regurgitation can vary in severity and clinical significance. An attempt to quantify the regurgitation can be made by evaluating the duration of the insufficiency during systole, the peak velocity of the regurgitant jet, the diameter of the regurgitant jet, and how far back within the right atrium the jet reaches.[8] Trivial tricuspid valve regurgitation may be found in up to 5% of fetuses with structurally normal hearts and resolution is usually expected.[9] More significant amounts of tricuspid valve regurgitation can be associated with structural heart defects, volume overload states (such as fetal anemia or vein of Galen aneurysms), poor fetal cardiac function, or in fetuses of SSA antibody–positive women.[10]

Cor Triatriatum Dexter

Cor triatriatum dexter is an extremely rare condition whereby there is a persistence of a right venous valve that results in septation of the smooth and trabeculated portions of the right atrium. Normal venous valves exist to help direct oxygenated blood flow from the placenta across the foramen ovale. Complete persistence of the right venous valve or prominent chiari network may result in cor triatriatum dexter. The physiology and presentation is dependent on the degree of septation of the right atrium. Cor triatriatum dexter can occur in isolation or with other right-sided defects, such as pulmonary stenosis or atresia, tricuspid valve anomalies, ASD, or Ebstein anomaly.

Tricuspid Stenosis and Tricuspid Atresia

Tricuspid stenosis and tricuspid atresia are typically associated with varying degrees of right ventricular hypoplasia. Either of these lesions may be associated with a VSD. It is important to evaluate the size of the RV and the source of pulmonary blood flow (antegrade via a pulmonary artery or retrograde via a ductus arteriosus). These lesions are typically classified in the single-ventricle lesion and are discussed further in the section "Single-Ventricle Anomalies."

Diseases of the Mitral Valve

Dysplastic Mitral Valve

A dysplastic mitral valve with primary mitral regurgitation is rare. Mitral regurgitation is more often associated with severe aortic stenosis and left ventricular injury, endocardial cushion defects, or primary left ventricular heart failure. Mitral regurgitation is also seen in fetuses of SSA antibody–positive mothers or in those with myocarditis. Often, the LV is dilated and the endocardium and papillary muscles are echo bright.

Mitral Stenosis

Congenital mitral stenosis is a rare condition. Congenital mitral stenosis can occur with other left-sided obstructive lesions. Shone syndrome is a term used for patients with multiple left-sided obstructions. Severe mitral stenosis may lead to progressive aortic and left ventricular hypoplasia *in utero*. In congenital mitral stenosis, the annulus, leaflets, chordae, and/or the papillary muscles may be abnormal.[11] The chordae may be absent or extremely short so that the valve apparatus attaches directly to the papillary muscles; this is named a mitral valve arcade. The chordae may attach to a single papillary muscle; this is termed a parachute mitral valve. Imaging of the heart in the short axis will demonstrate the papillary muscles. Imaging from the apical four-chamber view will demonstrate the mitral valve annulus diameter and chords. Color and pulsed-wave Doppler should be used to identify the degree of stenosis or regurgitation. Ventricular size and function should be assessed, as should the direction of foramen ovale flow. Reversed foramen ovale flow suggests severe disease. Some patients may be candidates for mitral valvuloplasty postnatally. However, patients are generally managed conservatively and surgical intervention is delayed as long as possible; valve replacement may be needed.

Cor Triatriatum Sinister

Cor triatriatum sinister describes a membrane within the body of the left atrium, proximal to the left atrial appendage, which causes a varying degree of obstruction to pulmonary venous return to the left side of the heart. Developmentally, this is thought to be due to incomplete incorporation of the pulmonary veins into the left atrium. There is usually a communication between the superior and inferior chambers of the left atrium of variable size. There may be an ASD or PFO with the right atrium connecting to the distal chamber, and there may be anomalous pulmonary venous drainage. The physiology of this lesion depends on the degree of restriction between the superior and inferior chambers caused by the cor triatriatum membrane. If the opening is large, the neonate will be asymptomatic. If the opening is small, there will be venous obstruction with subsequent pulmonary edema, pulmonary hypertension, and decreased cardiac output. The echocardiographic evaluation should include the size of the foramen ovale, the communication between the superior and inferior chambers, and pulmonary venous return. Color and pulsed-wave Doppler should be performed to evaluate restriction of the communication. The treatment includes resection of the left atrial membrane if it is restrictive or in patients who are symptomatic or have pulmonary artery hypertension.

Supravalvar Mitral Ring

A supravalvar mitral ring consists of a ring of tissue that adheres to the atrial surface of the mitral valve leaflets. This tissue is distal to the left atrial appendage (thus differentiating it from a cor triatriatum membrane). This may be associated with other left-sided defects such as subaortic stenosis, coarctation of the aorta, and VSD. There will be varying degrees of mitral regurgitation and mitral stenosis. The membrane will be best seen in the long axis or posteriorly tipped in four-chamber views adherent to the mitral valve annulus. Surgical resection is the treatment of choice.

Outflow Defects

Pulmonary Valve Stenosis

Definition: Pulmonary valve stenosis is an abnormality in the pulmonary valve leading to varying degrees of obstruction to the right ventricular outflow tract, often due to fusion of the valve commissures.

Incidence: Isolated pulmonary valve stenosis accounts for approximately 7% of live births.[1]

Pathology and Hemodynamics: Pulmonary valve stenosis, like stenosis at any valve, can progress during gestation. Interval imaging should be performed as the disease can evolve. Serial fetal echocardiograms will allow for postnatal planning to assess for disease progression. Severe pulmonary stenosis may cause inadequate pulmonary blood flow and require postnatal initiation of prostaglandin to maintain patency of the ductus arteriosus.

Associated Anomalies: Complete fetal echocardiogram should include evaluation for commonly associated cardiac anomalies, such as an ASD, TOF, Ebstein anomaly, and DORV. Associated genetic anomalies and syndromes should be considered, such as Noonan syndrome and Beckwith–Wiedemann syndrome. Rubella is a known teratogen causing both pulmonary stenosis and peripheral pulmonic stenosis.

Imaging: The pulmonary valve can be visualized from several different views and should be assessed for thickening, doming, and poor excursion of the valve leaflets. The amount and velocity of antegrade blood flow can be assessed with color and pulsed-wave

Doppler. Pulsed-wave Doppler can be used to calculate the gradient across the valve using the modified Bernoulli equation, where the pressure gradient across a discrete stenosis is equal to $4 \times$ (velocity).[5,6] Right ventricular hypertrophy and/or hypoplasia and tricuspid valve regurgitation may be seen in the four-chamber view. Right ventricular hypertension may develop and right ventricular pressures can be estimated by measuring the velocity of the tricuspid regurgitation and calculating right ventricular pressure by the simplified Bernoulli's equation where the pressure gradient is proportional to 4v squared.[5,6] Poststenotic dilatation of the main pulmonary artery may be associated with pulmonary stenosis. In some cases, mild pulmonary stenosis may not be visualized, and the only indicator of valve disease is poststenotic dilation of the main pulmonary artery. In severe or critical pulmonary stenosis, there will be reversed flow in the ductus arteriosus.

Treatment/Outcome: The prognosis for pulmonary valve stenosis is dependent on the severity of the outflow tract obstruction and associated defects. Mild or moderate pulmonary stenosis has an excellent prognosis and often requires no immediate postnatal intervention, although percutaneous balloon valvuloplasty may be required in infancy or early childhood. More severe forms of pulmonary stenosis or functional pulmonary atresia may require urgent neonatal intervention. Reversal of flow in the ductus arteriosus prenatally can be indicative of ductal-dependent pulmonary blood flow and need for early initiation of prostaglandin to maintain ductal patency until balloon valvuloplasty or surgical intervention in the immediate neonatal period can be undertaken.

Pulmonary Atresia

Definition: In pulmonary atresia, no antegrade flow is present across the pulmonary valve leaflets and the leaflets are often fused (Fig. 24.1-11). The diagnosis of pulmonary atresia with intact ventricular septum is used to distinguish this disease from TOF with pulmonary atresia.

Incidence: Pulmonary atresia with intact ventricular septum occurs in 1% to 2% of all live births with CHD.

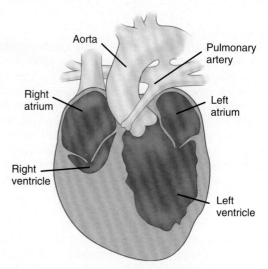

FIGURE 24.1-11: Illustration of pulmonary atresia with intact ventricular septum. (Reprinted with permission from Rice MJ, McDonald RW, Pilu G, et al. Cardiac malformations. In: Nyberg DA, McGahan JP, Pretorius DH, et al, eds. *Diagnostic Imaging of Fetal Anomalies.* Philadelphia, PA: Lippincott Williams & Wilkins; 2003:464.)

Pathophysiology and Hemodynamics: The pulmonary valve is atretic in pulmonary atresia/intact ventricular septum. There are usually varying degrees of tricuspid valve and right ventricular hypoplasia. The pulmonary valve leaflets are often present but fused, and the branch pulmonary arteries are typically small but not severely hypoplastic. Coronary artery fistulous connections to the RV may be present and are related to right ventricular pressure elevation. In severe forms, there may be right ventricular–dependent coronary artery circulation with severe proximal

stenosis or atresia of at least one major coronary artery, and myocardial perfusion is dependent on distal coronary fistulous connections from the RV.

Imaging: In the four-chamber view, the tricuspid valve will be patent but is usually small. The RV may be hypoplastic and echogenic (Fig. 24.1-12). There may be tricuspid insufficiency as there is no other egress from the RV (Fig. 24.1-13). Use of pulsed-wave Doppler of the tricuspid insufficiency will allow

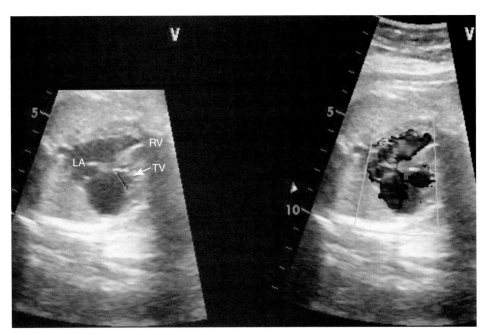

FIGURE 24.1-12: Color compare view of pulmonary atresia with intact ventricular septum demonstrating a hypoplastic tricuspid valve (*TV*) annulus. Note that in the color image the foramen ovale is widely patent, allowing unrestrictive right to left atrial flow. *LA*, left atrium; *RV*, right ventricle.

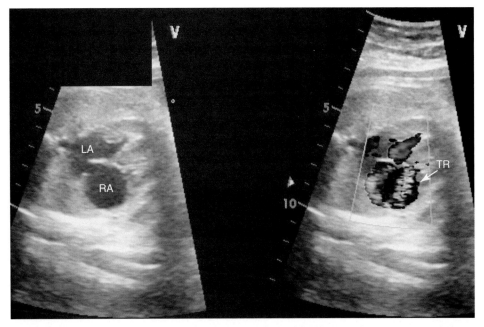

FIGURE 24.1-13: Color compare view of four-chamber view of fetal heart with pulmonary atresia intact ventricular septum. The *blue* color Doppler demonstrates severe tricuspid regurgitation (*TR*). *LA*, left atrium; *RA*, right atrium.

an estimation of right ventricular pressure, which may be supra-systemic (Fig. 24.1-14). Imaging from the short axis and ductal views will demonstrate no antegrade flow across the pulmonary valve and reversed flow in the ductus arteriosus. A main pulmonary artery will be present and give rise to continuous, although small, pulmonary arteries. Finally, coronary fistulae may be present and are best visualized in either the four-chamber view or short axis of the ventricles with color Doppler (Fig. 24.1-15). Typically, there is a stretched PFO or secundum ASD.

Treatment/Outcome: By definition, newborns with pulmonary atresia are ductal dependent and therefore prostaglandin should be initiated immediately after delivery. In addition to echocardiography, cardiac catheterization is performed to evaluate coronary artery anatomy. Right ventricular–dependent coronary arteries are a significant risk factor for death. A small percentage of patients will have an adequate size tricuspid valve (> -2 to -3 z-score), a well-developed RV, and normal coronary arteries with flow not dependent on the RV. These patients may

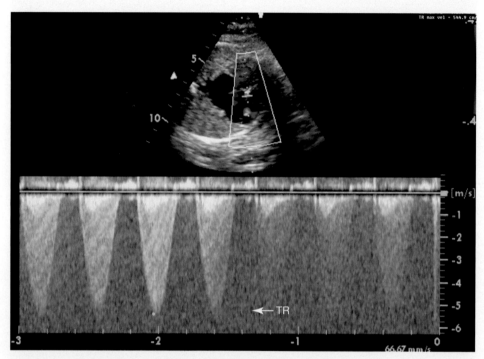

FIGURE 24.1-14: Pulsed-wave Doppler imaging of the tricuspid regurgitation (*TR*) demonstrates a high velocity, 5.3 m/s, predicting a right ventricular pressure of 112 mm Hg.

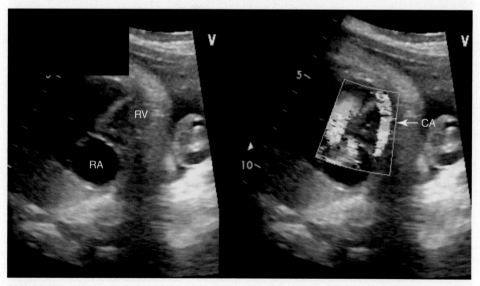

FIGURE 24.1-15: Color compare four-chamber view of pulmonary atresia intact ventricular septum with a fistula from the right ventricle (*RV*) to the coronary artery (*CA*). Color Doppler is necessary to show this diagnosis. *RA*, right atrium.

be candidates for radiofrequency ablation to open up the right ventricular outflow tract. The remainder of patients will need a systemic to pulmonary artery shunt. Patients are followed up over the first year of life, and if the tricuspid valve z-score is greater than -2 and the RV is adequate, a two-ventricular repair may be undertaken later. If the RV is small but has some output, a "one-and-a-half ventricular repair" may be performed. This repair includes a Glenn shunt (superior vena cava anastomosis to the pulmonary artery) with the IVC flow returning to the RV to be pumped to the lungs. Finally, some patients must follow a single-ventricle approach to repair. One indication for single-ventricle palliation is right ventricular–dependent coronary circulation. In these patients, "decompressing" the RV with pulmonary balloon valvuloplasty is contraindicated in that it can result in myocardial infarction. Primary cardiac transplantation may be considered as well in these patients. Other indications for single-ventricle palliation is an extremely small tricuspid valve (z-score < -4) or severely hypoplastic RV. In these patients, a systemic to pulmonary artery shunt will be placed in the newborn period. These patients will then ultimately undergo Glenn shunt and Fontan procedure (see section "Hypoplastic Left Heart Syndrome" for further discussion of these surgeries).

A small subset of fetuses with pulmonary atresia/intact ventricular septum may be considered for fetal intervention; however, there is debate if intervention should be offered.[12-14] The goal of intervention is to promote right ventricular growth and avoid single-ventricle palliation or as a lifesaving measure if severe tricuspid regurgitation and hydrops exist and there is impending fetal demise.[15] The technique for intervention is difficult given the right ventricular cavity is small, hypertrophied, and located behind the sternum.[16]

Long-term prognosis for children with pulmonary atresia intact ventricular septum depends on the degree of tricuspid, degree of right ventricular hypoplasia, and the presence of coronary abnormalities. The outcome is good for those who undergo pulmonary valve dilation or right ventricular outflow plasty with a two-ventricular repair. In patients who undergo single-ventricle palliation, early deaths have been reported secondary to coronary ischemia, but long-term survival is reported to be 83% at 5 years.[17]

Aortic Stenosis

Definition: Aortic stenosis is an abnormality in the aortic valve leading to left-sided outflow tract obstruction at the level of the aortic valve. The valve may be bicuspid, unicuspid, or thickened with fused commissures.

Incidence: Aortic stenosis accounts for 5% to 7% of children with cardiac disease. A bicuspid nonstenotic aortic valve may be as common as 3% of the population, but it does not always present as heart disease in childhood.

Pathology and Hemodynamics: The abnormal aortic valve itself may have three leaflets; more commonly, there may be fusion of the leaflets resulting in unicuspid or bicuspid valve. Aortic stenosis, like stenosis at any valve, can progress during gestation. Interval imaging should be performed as the disease can evolve. Serial fetal echocardiograms will allow for postnatal planning to assess for disease progression. Severe aortic stenosis may cause inadequate systemic blood flow and require postnatal initiation of prostaglandin to maintain patency of the ductus arteriosus.

Associated Anomalies: Aortic stenosis is often familial. Bicuspid aortic valve and coarctation of the aorta can be seen in association with Turner syndrome. Supravalvar aortic stenosis can be associated with Williams syndrome. Subvalvar aortic stenosis does not typically present in the fetus. Associated abnormalities include hypoplasia of the LV, mitral valve, or aortic arch (see section "Hypoplastic Left Heart Syndrome").

Imaging: Ultrasound findings vary depending on the severity of disease. The aortic leaflets will be best visualized in a short-axis view and they may appear thickened and fused. Color and pulse Doppler should be performed to accurately determine degree of stenosis (Fig. 24.1-16). Aortic flow gradient can be calculated by the Bernoulli equation (aortic gradient $4 \times$ velocity^2). In the presence of severe left ventricular dysfunction, the gradient may be minimal. Dilation of the ascending aorta is a subtle clue of mild aortic stenosis and is best seen in the long-axis evaluation of the left ventricular outflow tract. Significant mitral regurgitation may be present and is best visualized in the four-chamber view. Severe aortic stenosis may cause left ventricular dysfunction, resulting in retrograde aortic arch and foramen flow; this may be a precursor to hypoplastic left heart syndrome.

Treatment/Outcome: Postnatal management of aortic stenosis is dependent on severity of the disease. With critical aortic stenosis, there is little to no antegrade blood flow, and prostaglandin is necessary to supply sufficient cardiac output. Balloon aortic valvuloplasty is performed if there is aortic stenosis with ventricular dysfunction, or the peak gradient is greater than 70 to 80 mm Hg. Balloon angioplasty is typically successful, although most patients will need further procedures and ultimate aortic valve replacement. Morbidity and mortality will be dependent on the degree of stenosis or left ventricular dysfunction.

Conotruncal Defects

Conotruncal defects encompass a wide spectrum of CHD with abnormalities of the connection between the ventricles and great vessels including TOF, transposition of the great arteries, truncus arteriosus, and DORV. Conotruncal anomalies account for 20% to 30% of all live births with structural CHD.

Tetralogy of Fallot

Definition: The anatomical features of TOF include infundibular and valvar pulmonary stenosis, a malalignment-type VSD, overriding aorta, and right ventricular hypertrophy (a late sequelae of the outflow tract obstruction and not observed *in utero*) (Fig. 24.1-17). The aortic valve is in continuity with the RV.

Incidence: TOF is the most common type of cyanotic congenital heart disease, accounting for approximately 9% of CHD live births.[4]

Pathophysiology and Hemodynamics: If not diagnosed prenatally, timing of presentation can vary significantly depending on the severity of the right ventricular outflow tract obstruction. Postnatally, patients with TOF become cyanotic because of right to left shunting across the VSD in the presence of severe right ventricular outflow tract obstruction. The degree of shunting and cyanosis is secondary to the right ventricular outflow tract obstruction. Newborns with little right to left shunting will be "pink" and will have clinical symptoms of a large VSD.

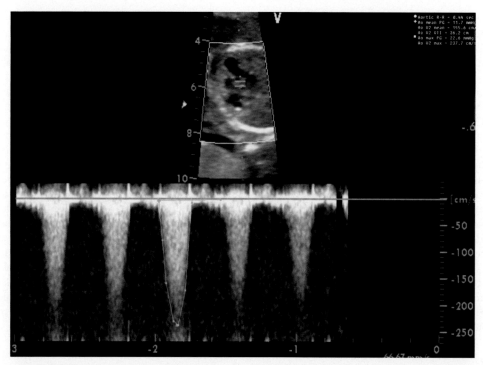

FIGURE 24.1-16: In the upper panel, the heart is imaged in a four-chamber view angled cranially. The aortic valve and left ventricle appear echo bright. Pulsed-wave Doppler demonstrates increased velocity across the aortic valve of 4.1 m/s or a peak gradient of 67 mm Hg.

The right ventricular outflow tract obstruction may progress and therefore warrants close observation. During a "tet spell," there is dynamic muscular obstruction of the right ventricular outflow tract causing severe cyanosis. "Tet spells" may be precipitated by crying, illness, or decreased systemic vascular resistance. Treatment includes oxygen, intravenous (IV) fluids, morphine, knee to chest position, and often emergency surgery.

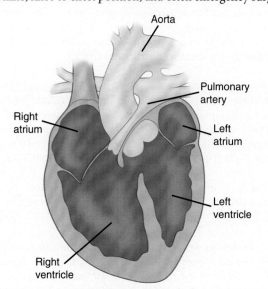

FIGURE 24.1-17: Illustration of tetralogy of Fallot. A large aorta overrides a ventricular septal defect, and the pulmonary outflow tract is hypoplastic. (Reprinted with permission from Rice MJ, McDonald RW, Pilu G, et al. Cardiac malformations. In: Nyberg DA, McGahan JP, Pretorius DH, et al., eds. *Diagnostic Imaging of Fetal Anomalies.* Philadelphia, PA: Lippincott Williams & Wilkins; 2003:475.)

Associated Anomalies: TOF is often associated with genetic and extracardiac anomalies such as DiGeorge syndrome, VACTERL (verterbral anomalies, anal atresia, cardiac anomalies, tracheosophageal fistula, renal anomalies, and limb anomalies) association, and Goldenhar syndrome, among many others. A right aortic arch suggests a deletion on chromosome 22q11. TOF can also be found in association with endocardial cushion defects, most commonly in those fetuses diagnosed with trisomy 21. A variation of TOF with significant hypoplasia of the conal septum is more commonly found in Asian and Native American populations. In some cases, the distinction between TOF and DORV can be difficult. DORV can be classified with TOF-like physiology if the aorta overrides the ventricular septum more than 50% toward the RV with a lack of fibrous continuity between the aortic and mitral valves.

Imaging: The anterior malalignment-type VSD is best viewed in the long axis of the heart where the overriding aorta can be easily appreciated (Fig. 24.1-18). The VSD will not be seen in the four-chamber view as it is located in the outlet conal septum. The short-axis views will demonstrate the VSD and the anterior deviation of the conal septum and allow for assessment of right ventricular outflow obstruction. The degree of pulmonary stenosis may progress *in utero*, and, therefore, serial imaging should be performed. The pulmonary valve, main pulmonary artery, and branch pulmonary arteries should be carefully measured as they may be hypoplastic (Fig. 24.1-19). The direction of ductus arteriosus flow is important because with severe obstruction there will be reversed flow, and these babies will have significant right to left ventricular-level shunting and will be ductal dependent at birth. There can be varying degrees of abnormalities of the pulmonary valve (see sections "Tetralogy

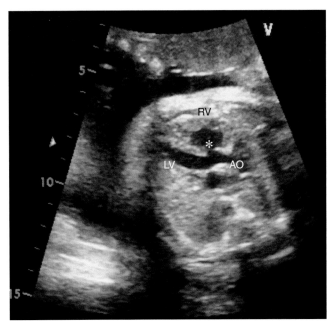

FIGURE 24.1-18: Long-axis view of tetralogy of Fallot with an overriding aorta (*AO*). The *asterisk* denotes the ventricular septal defect. *LV*, left ventricle; *RV*, right ventricle.

of Fallot with Pulmonary Atresia" and "Tetralogy of Fallot with Absent Pulmonary Valve").

Treatment/Outcome: Surgical repair is necessary in TOF and usually occurs between 2 to 6 months of age or earlier if cyanosis is present. Surgical repair includes closure of the VSD and relief of the right ventricular outflow tract obstruction. If the

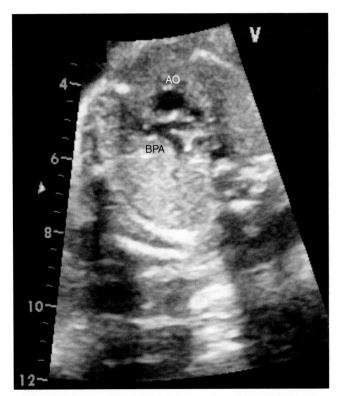

FIGURE 24.1-19: Three-vessel view in tetralogy of Fallot demonstrating hypoplastic branch pulmonary arteries (*BPA*) relative to the aorta (*AO*).

pulmonary valve annulus is small, a patch may be placed across the right ventricular outflow tract to relieve valvar obstruction ("transannular patch repair"). If the valve size is within normal limits (> -2 standard deviation [SD]), then an infundibular patch may be considered. Finally, stenosis or discontinuity of the branch pulmonary arteries, if present, is usually also corrected. Outcomes are good, although some patients may need catheter intervention for residual right ventricular outflow tract or branch pulmonary artery stenosis.

Tetralogy of Fallot with Pulmonary Atresia
Tetralogy of Fallot with pulmonary atresia (TOF/PA) is a severe form of TOF in which the pulmonary valve is atretic and there is no antegrade pulmonary blood flow. TOF/PA is typically associated with good-sized branch pulmonary arteries if there is a large patent ductus arteriosus. However, it may be associated with hypoplastic branch pulmonary arteries and major aortopulmonary collateral arteries (MAPCAs) arising from the aorta if the ductus is absent. A diagnostic cardiac catheterization is often indicated to delineate the size and distribution of the true pulmonary arteries and MAPCAs. The type and timing of surgical repair of TOF/PA is dependent on the nature of the pulmonary blood supply. Outcome is typically not as good, especially in the presence of hypoplastic pulmonary arteries.

Tetralogy of Fallot with Absent Pulmonary Valve
Tetralogy of Fallot with absent pulmonary valve (TOF/APV) is a rare variant of TOF. The pulmonary valve is not truly absent, but it is primitive with underdeveloped leaflets that do not function effectively. This abnormality leads to severe or "wide open" pulmonary insufficiency with severe dilatation of the main pulmonary arteries, branch pulmonary arteries, and the RV (Figs. 24.1-20 to 24.1-22). There may be airway compression from the massive dilation of the pulmonary arteries and the lungs can be hypoplastic[18] (Fig. 24.1-23). There may also be significant tracheobronchial anomalies including significant malacia. Typically, there is no patent ductus arteriosus. There is a high risk for hydrops and *in utero* fetal demise, as well as postnatal demise due to respiratory complications.

Transposition of the Great Arteries
D-Transposition
Definition: In D-transposition of the great arteries (D-TGA), there is normal AV relationship with ventricular-arterial discordance; the aorta is connected to the RV and the pulmonary artery is connected to the LV (Fig. 24.1-24).

Incidence: D-TGA is the second most common (5% to 7% live births) form of cyanotic heart disease and the most common cyanotic lesion presenting in the newborn period.

Pathology and Hemodynamics: Embryologically, D-TGA results from abnormal neural crest cell migration and failure of normal twisting during truncal septation.[19] Postnatally, the abnormal connection of the aorta and pulmonary artery results in two parallel circulations: with deoxygenated blood circulating to the body and oxygenated blood recirculating to the lungs. Patency of the foramen ovale and ductus arteriosus allows for mixing until surgical repair is performed. Prostaglandin is utilized to ensure the patency of the ductus arteriosus. In most newborns, cyanosis is present and the foramen ovale needs to be enlarged to promote effective pulmonary blood flow. To enlarge the ASD, a balloon

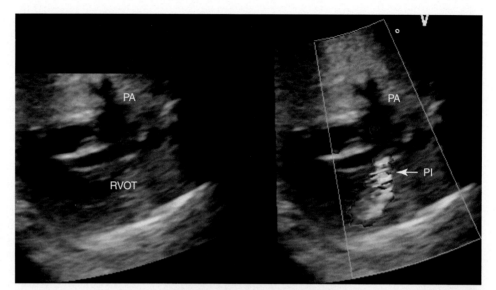

FIGURE 24.1-20: Color compare view of the short-axis view of the heart showing significantly dilated pulmonary artery (*PA*). Color Doppler demonstrates severe pulmonary insufficiency (*PI*). *RVOT*, right ventricular outflow tract.

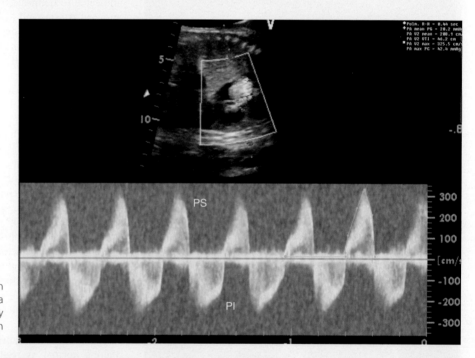

FIGURE 24.1-21: Pulsed-wave Doppler in the right ventricular outflow tract shows a to-and-fro pattern with systolic pulmonary stenosis (*PS*) with a peak gradient of 32 mm Hg and diastolic pulmonary insufficiency (*PI*).

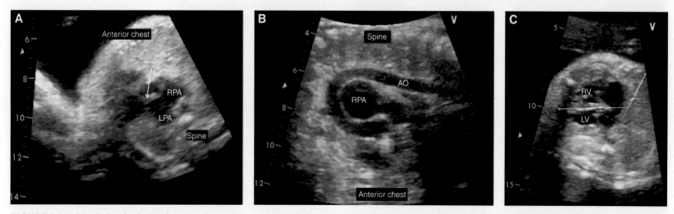

FIGURE 24.1-22: A: Fetal echocardiogram demonstrating severely dilated main and branch pulmonary arteries. *Arrow* indicates rudimentary pulmonary valve leaflets. **B:** Sagittal image showing a dilated right pulmonary artery in cross section. **C:** Transverse image of the fetal chest demonstrating marked left shift of the heart with right lung overexpansion and left lung hypoplasia versus compression. *AO*, aorta; *LPA*, left pulmonary artery; *LV*, left ventricle; *RPA*, right pulmonary artery; *RV*, right ventricle.

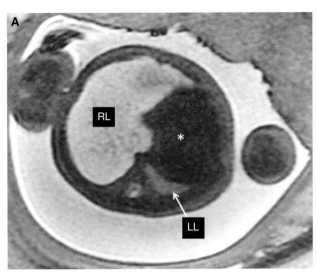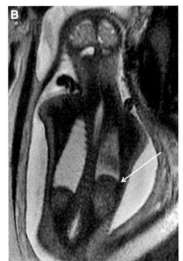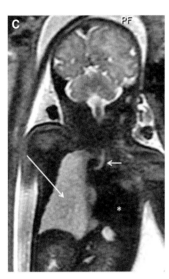

FIGURE 24.1-23: A: Axial SSFSE MRI shows a hyperinflated right lung and severe left shift of the cardiac silhouette. *LL*, left lung, *RL*, right lung, *asterisk*, heart. **B:** Coronal SSFSE MRI demonstrating hyperinflated T2-bright right lung and decreased signal and volume of the left lung volume. *Arrow* points to elevated left hemidiaphragm. **C:** Additional coronal image demonstrates high-signal hyperinflated right lung (*long arrow*), severe leftward cardiac shift (*asterisk*), and compressed trachea (*short arrow*).

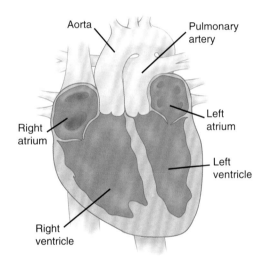

FIGURE 24.1-24: Illustration of complete transposition of the great arteries (D-TGA). (Reprinted with permission from Rice MJ, McDonald RW, Pilu G, et al. Cardiac malformations. In: Nyberg DA, McGahan JP, Pretorius DH, et al., eds. *Diagnostic Imaging of Fetal Anomalies*. Philadelphia, PA: Lippincott Williams & Wilkins; 2003:481.)

atrial septostomy is performed by introducing an umbilical or venous balloon-tipped catheter into the femoral vein. The balloon is inflated in the left atrium and then pulled across the septum, creating an ASD. This allows mixing between the two parallel circuits. Adequate shunting at the atrial level is the only way to improve arterial oxygenation and maintain hemodynamic stability prior to surgery. If there is associated coarctation of the aorta or persistent pulmonary hypertension with ductal patency, there will be reversed differential cyanosis.

Imaging: D-TGA can be very difficult to identify on routine prenatal ultrasound because the four-chamber view will be normal. In D-TGA with cranial angulation from the four-chamber view, the first great vessel that is visualized will be the pulmonary artery originating from the LV. The second great vessel originating from

the RV will be the aorta. In addition, the great vessels rise in a parallel manner more superiorly instead of the normal crossing orientation (Figs. 24.1-25 and 24.1-26). The foramen ovale should be evaluated in the bicaval view or a short-axis view. Deviation of the atrial septum into the right atrium suggests restriction of

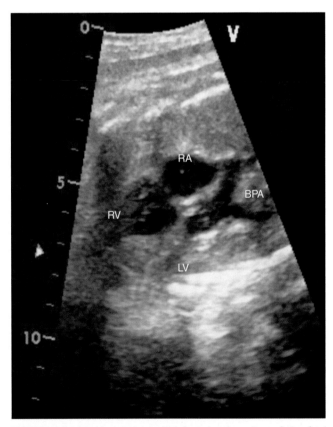

FIGURE 24.1-25: Anteriorly angled four-chamber view of the fetal heart. The first great vessel that is visualized is the pulmonary artery with the branch pulmonary arteries (*BPA*). *LV*, left ventricle; *RA*, right atrium; *RV*, right ventricle.

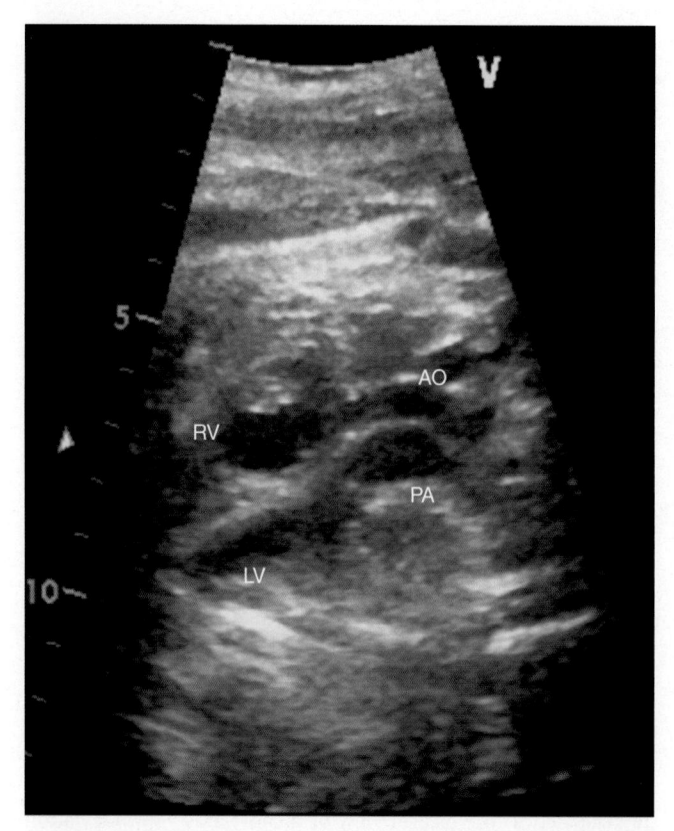

FIGURE 24.1-26: Anteriorly angled four-chamber view of the fetal heart demonstrating parallel great arteries; *AO*, aorta; *LV*, left ventricle; *PA*, pulmonary artery; *RV*, right ventricle.

the foramen ovale. The presence of significant flow reversal on Doppler interrogation of the pulmonary veins is also suggestive of atrial restriction, but predicting the need for urgent septostomy after delivery can be challenging. It is important to evaluate semilunar valvar size and presence of pulmonary or aortic valve stenosis as these may impact surgical repair.

Associated Anomalies: D-TGA is more common in males (3:1 ratio). Babies usually have normal chromosomes, and D-TGA is more common in infants of diabetic mothers. D-TGA may be associated with pulmonary stenosis, ASD, VSD (30% to 50%), and left ventricular outflow tract obstruction. If the aorta is hypoplastic, there may be hypoplasia of the arch (with coarctation of the aorta and interrupted aortic arch) or the pulmonary valve may be hypoplastic with associated main pulmonary artery/branch pulmonary artery hypoplasia.

Treatment/Outcome: D-TGA is often difficult to diagnose prenatally. Reports suggest that in the United Kingdom, there is only a 25% prenatal detection rate without a VSD, and a 40% detection rate with a VSD. In the United States, there is only a 19% prenatal detection rate.[20,21] Prenatal diagnosis is important for D-TGA because newborns rely on patency of the foramen ovale for mixing of the oxygenated and deoxygenated blood, and with foramen ovale closure, newborns become extremely compromised in the delivery room.[22] Optimally, delivery should be at a tertiary care center with cardiology available if an urgent balloon septostomy is needed. The arterial switch is the operation of choice for D-TGA. The great vessels are transected and connected to the appropriate ventricle and the coronary arteries

are translocated to the neoaorta. The operative mortality is low and long-term outcome is good, but pulmonary artery reintervention may be required secondary to "stretching" from the LeCompte maneuver.

L-Transposition

Congenitally corrected transposition of the great arteries or L-TGA results from abnormal heart tube looping (L loop) resulting in ventricular inversion and AV discordance in which the right atrium is connected to the LV to the pulmonary artery and the left atrium to the RV to the aorta (Fig. 24.1-27). AV discordance is associated with transposition of the great arteries and, therefore, the blue blood goes to the lungs and the red blood to the body. Usually, these babies are not cyanotic unless there are associated defects. Inversion of the ventricles is recognized by identifying a right-sided mitral valve and a left-sided tricuspid valve. In addition, the left-sided ventricle will be coarsely trabeculated and have a moderator band. L-TGA is commonly associated with a VSD or pulmonary stenosis. Heart block may be associated with L-TGA. The outcome of patients with L-TGA is dependent on the associated anomalies, including VSD, pulmonary stenosis, and heart block. Given that patients with L-TGA have an RV as their systemic pump, over their lifetime, significant tricuspid regurgitation and heart failure may develop.[23]

Truncus Arteriosus

Definition: In truncus arteriosus, a single outflow tract originates from the heart, with a conoventricular-type VSD. The single outflow tract gives rise to the systemic, pulmonary and coronary circulation.

Incidence: Truncus arteriosus occurs in 1% to 1.5% of all live births with CHD.[4]

Pathology and Hemodynamics: Truncus arteriosus is classified into four subtypes.[24] Type I has a main pulmonary artery segment that gives rise to confluent branch pulmonary arteries with no patent ductus arteriosus; type II has no main pulmonary artery

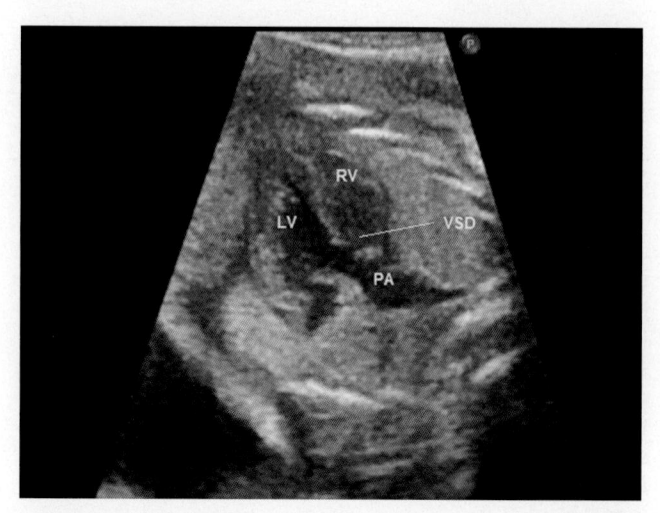

FIGURE 24.1-27: Illustration of corrected transposition of the great arteries (L-TGA). *LV*, left ventricle; *RV*, right ventricle; *PA*, pulmonary artery; *VSD*, ventricular septal defect. (From Rice MJ, McDonald RW, Pilu G, et al. Cardiac malformations. In: Nyberg DA, McGahan JP, Pretorius DH, et al., eds. *Diagnostic Imaging of Fetal Anomalies*. Philadelphia, PA: Lippincott Williams & Wilkins; 2003:483.)

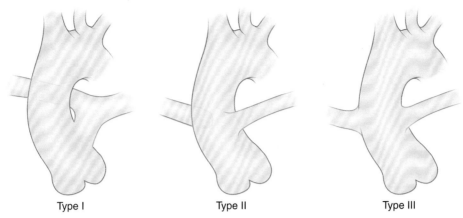

Type I   Type II   Type III

FIGURE 24.1-28: Illustration of the types of truncus arteriosus. (Reprinted with permission from Rice MJ, McDonald RW, Pilu G, et al. Cardiac malformations. In: Nyberg DA, McGahan JP, Pretorius DH, et al., eds. *Diagnostic Imaging of Fetal Anomalies*. Philadelphia, PA: Lippincott Williams & Wilkins; 2003:483.)

segment and the branch pulmonary arteries arise from the back of the truncus in close proximity to one another with no PDA; type III the branch pulmonary arteries arise separately and one may originate from the ductus arteriosus; and type IV is associated with coarctation of the aorta and interrupted aortic arch (Fig. 24.1-28). Types I and II do not require prostaglandin after birth. If not diagnosed prenatally, newborns will often present early with congestive heart failure secondary to pulmonary overcirculation with continuous systolic and diastolic blood flow into the pulmonary vascular bed. Concomitant truncal valve insufficiency may compromise coronary artery perfusion with low diastolic blood pressures.

Associated Anomalies: One-third of babies with truncus arteriosus will have 22q11 deletion.

Imaging: The four-chamber view will show four normal chambers; however, with cranial angulation, the VSD and single-outflow tract will be appreciated (Fig. 24.1-29). The VSD is large and also seen in short- and long-axis images. Delineation of the pulmonary arteries is important as they can have variable origins. The truncal valve is best seen in the short axis. Most of the time the truncal valve is tricuspid; however, it can be unicuspid or quadricuspid. The truncal valve may be both stenotic and insufficient and, therefore, color and pulsed-wave Doppler interrogation should be performed (Fig. 24.1-30).

Treatment/Outcome: Neonatal repair is typically performed. The repair usually includes closing the VSD to the aortic trunk and placement of a valved homograft from the RV to the pulmonary arteries; often, they are transected from the main trunk. Additional surgeries are needed to replace the RV to pulmonary artery conduit, and possibly repair or replace the truncal valve.

Double-Outlet Right Ventricle

Definition: In DORV, both the aorta and the pulmonary artery arise from the RV (Fig. 24.1-31). The ventricles can be normal in size and position, or there can be right or left ventricular hypoplasia.

Incidence: DORV constitutes 1% to 1.5% of all live births with CHD.[4]

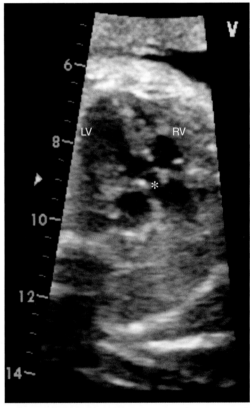

FIGURE 24.1-29: Anteriorly angled four-chamber image of truncus arteriosus with a single large vessel, the common trunk (*asterisk*), overriding a large ventricular septal defect. *LV*, left ventricle; *RV*, right ventricle.

Pathology and Hemodynamics: DORV can be classified into subtypes by VSD location and postnatal cardiac physiology. The VSD can be described as subaortic (50%), subpulmonary (30%), doubly committed, or remote. DORV with a subaortic VSD will have physiology similar to that of a large VSD, although some may be cyanotic ("tetralogy-like") if there is associated pulmonary stenosis. DORV with a subpulmonary-type VSD will have pathophysiology similar to that of D-TGA with large VSD. A Taussig-Bing-type of DORV consists of a subpulmonary VSD, no pulmonary stenosis, side-by-side great vessels, and bilateral

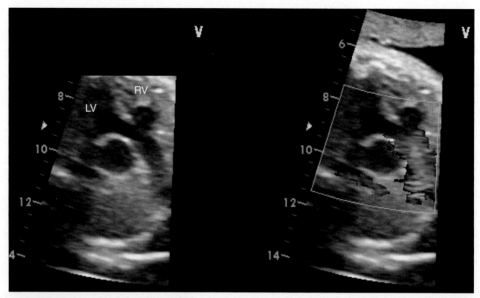

FIGURE 24.1-30: Color compare view of the truncal valve. Color Doppler should be performed to evaluate for truncal stenosis or insufficiency. The origins of the branch pulmonary arteries should be identified. *LV*, left ventricle; *RV*, right ventricle.

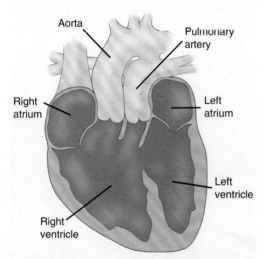

FIGURE 24.1-31: Illustration of double-outlet right ventricle. (Reprinted with permission from Rice MJ, McDonald RW, Pilu G, et al. Cardiac malformations. In: Nyberg DA, McGahan JP, Pretorius DH, et al., eds. *Diagnostic Imaging of Fetal Anomalies.* Philadelphia, PA: Lippincott Williams & Wilkins; 2003:478.)

conus. A doubly committed VSD sits below both arterial valves. A remote VSD is typically inlet or muscular and remote from both the aorta and the pulmonary valves. The relationship of the VSD to the great vessels and the presence of outflow tract obstruction determine postnatal hemodynamics and symptoms that may include congestive heart failure or cyanosis.

Associated Anomalies: Chromosomal anomalies may be seen including trisomies 13 and 18, 22q11, and heterotaxy syndrome. There may be varying anomalies of the AV valves with straddling, atresia, or overriding. Heterotaxy syndrome should be considered especially if there is an associated AVC defect or if there are anomalies of abdominal and atrial situs and/or pulmonary and systemic venous return.

Imaging: Definitive diagnosis is demonstrated by visualizing both great vessels arising from the RV. There may be valvar or subvalvar obstruction of either outflow tract. The four-chamber view may be normal or show hypoplasia of either ventricle. Careful sweeps cranially of the outflow tracts will demonstrate the VSD and that the RV gives rise to both the great vessels. If there is aortic stenosis, there may be coarctation of the aorta or interrupted aortic arch. Similarly, with valvar or subvalvar pulmonary obstruction, there may be hypoplasia of the branch pulmonary arteries.

Treatment/Outcome: These patients most often undergo surgery in the neonatal period, with the ultimate goal of establishing unobstructed flow to both outflow tracts and closure of the VSD. In some cases, associated defects prohibit a two-ventricle repair and single-ventricle palliation is warranted.

Single-Ventricle Anomalies

Hypoplastic Left Heart Syndrome

Definition: Hypoplastic left heart syndrome (HLHS) is a spectrum of disease in which the left side of the heart cannot support the systemic circulation. HLHS may be secondary to mitral atresia or stenosis, aortic atresia or stenosis, DORV with mitral atresia or stenosis, unbalanced AVC to the right with left ventricular hypoplasia, or critical aortic stenosis with evolving HLHS (Fig. 24.1-32).

Incidence: HLHS accounts for 1.2% to 1.5% of all CHD live births.

Associated Anomalies: HLHS may be associated with Turner syndrome (XO), Jacobsen syndrome (deletion of distal 11q), and trisomies 13 and 18.[25,26] However, most children with HLHS do not have a syndrome or significant extracardiac anomalies. HLHS is more common in males than in females.

Pathology and Hemodynamics: The most common form of HLHS is due to aortic atresia. Many of these children will

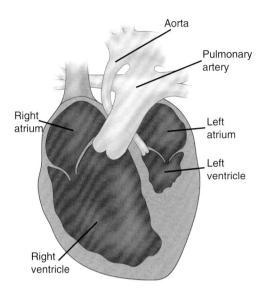

FIGURE 24.1-32: Illustration of hypoplastic left heart syndrome. (Reprinted with permission from Rice MJ, McDonald RW, Pilu G, et al. Cardiac malformations. In: Nyberg DA, McGahan JP, Pretorius DH, et al., eds. *Diagnostic Imaging of Fetal Anomalies*. Philadelphia, PA: Lippincott Williams & Wilkins; 2003:472.)

also have mitral valve abnormalities (mitral valve hypoplasia, stenosis, or atresia). The ascending aorta will be diminutive with retrograde flow. Survival after birth with aortic valve atresia is dependent on patency of the ductus arteriosus. The RV supplies both pulmonary and systemic blood flow with the ductus arteriosus open. Blood flow to the coronary arteries and head and neck vessels are supplied in a retrograde manner. This is noted as reversed flow in the isthmus and transverse aortic arch. The size and restriction of the foramen ovale will impact both systemic and pulmonary blood flow at delivery.

HLHS with an intact or nearly intact atrial septum is associated with significant morbidity and mortality. This may be in part due to "arterialization" of the lung parenchyma *in utero* from elevated pulmonary venous pressures. Pulmonary lymphangiectasia may develop, resulting in echogenic pulmonary parenchyma and effusions by ultrasound and "nutmeg" appearance by fetal magnetic resonance imaging (MRI) (see Chapter 11).[27] If HLHS with a restrictive/intact atrial septum is not diagnosed prenatally, these newborns become severely ill in the delivery room, given that blood is unable to exit the left atrium. This results in hypoxemia, acidosis, and pulmonary edema. Even when identified prenatally and an urgent balloon septostomy is performed, outcomes are poor. Fetal intervention to open the atrial septum with either septoplasty or stent placement to minimize damage to the pulmonary bed has been reported.[27-31]

An important subtype of HLHS is severe aortic stenosis with evolving HLHS.[32-34] HLHS secondary to aortic stenosis is believed to have had a normally formed LV early in gestation.[35,36] As the aortic stenosis becomes more severe, the LV becomes injured with left ventricular dilation, scarring, and reversal of flow at the foramen ovale and transverse arch. With scarring, seen as bright endocardium (endocardial fibroelastosis) on imaging, blood is diverted away from the left ventricular cavity, which ultimately becomes hypoplastic. Some centers perform fetal intervention to prevent the development of HLHS in this disease.[32] In one large experience, of 70 fetuses that had *in utero* aortic balloon valvuloplasty, the procedure was technically successful in 74%, and greater than 30% of babies went on to have a biventricular repair,

and another 8% were converted to a biventricular repair after initial univentricular palliation.[32]

In utero, the presence of HLHS is well tolerated as the RV can support the fetal circulation. After delivery, the systemic and the coronary circulation is dependent on the patency of the ductus arteriosus. As the patent ductus arteriosus closes, infants not prenatally diagnosed may present with lethargy, pallor, difficulty breathing, low cardiac output, and acidosis. Of note, there is usually no heart murmur. Prostaglandin is indicated immediately after delivery to maintain ductal patency. Even this circulation is tenuous as there is a delicate balance between pulmonary and systemic circulation; and, therefore, these infants should be cared for by centers with significant experience in pediatric cardiology.

Imaging: Left ventricular hypoplasia is recognizable in the four-chamber view, although early in pregnancy if there are patent mitral and aortic valves, left ventricular hypoplasia may be subtle. The LV may appear hyperechoic from endocardial fibroelastosis (Figs. 24.1-33 and 24.1-34). The mitral and aortic annuli usually measure small with decreased leaflet motion. Retrograde flow in the transverse arch suggests that there is inadequate left ventricular outflow (Fig. 24.1-35). Another important finding is abnormal reversed color Doppler flow across the foramen ovale. Foramen ovale flow and pulmonary venous Doppler should be evaluated to assess degree of foramen ovale obstruction given that an associated restrictive or intact atrial septum is associated with poor outcomes. Pulmonary venous Doppler with reversed flow (f/r < 3) suggests severe restriction and has been shown to be associated with need for intervention (Fig. 24.1-36).[37-39] The use of color Doppler is also important in the four-chamber view to evaluate for tricuspid insufficiency. Finally, right ventricular function should be assessed. Decreased right ventricular function and significant tricuspid insufficiency may be associated with hydrops and poor outcomes.

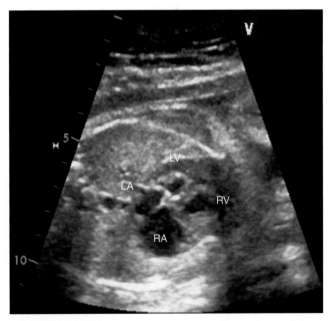

FIGURE 24.1-33: Apical four-chamber view of hypoplastic left heart syndrome. A hypoplastic, echogenic left ventricle (*LV*) is easily visualized. The left atrium (*LA*) appears hypoplastic and the mitral valve appears bright and abnormal as well. *RA*, right atrium; *RV*, right ventricle.

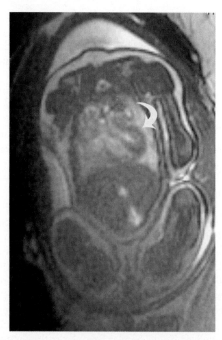

FIGURE 24.1-34: Coronal steady-state free precession sequence magnetic resonance demonstrates a hypoplastic left ventricle with thick walls (*arrow*).

Treatment/Outcome: Surgical repair for HLHS consists of a three-staged palliation. The Norwood operation, introduced in the 1980s, includes reconstruction of the aortic arch using the pulmonary valve and main pulmonary artery and establishment of pulmonary blood flow via a Blalock–Taussig shunt (aortic to pulmonary artery shunt). More recently, the Blalock–Taussig shunt has been replaced by the Sano shunt (RV to PA conduit) in many centers. The second stage is the bidirectional Glenn or hemi-Fontan, which entails connecting the superior vena cava to the pulmonary artery with take down of the Blalock–Taussig or Sano shunt at 4 to 6 months. In some instances, an initial hybrid approach to palliation is considered with stenting of the ductus arteriosus and bilateral pulmonary artery banding, followed by a comprehensive stage II procedure with Norwood arch reconstruction and placement of a bidirectional Glenn as the second surgery. The third surgery is the Fontan, which baffles the IVC and hepatic veins to the branch pulmonary arteries at 2 to 4 years of age. Overall surgical survival is ~80%. HLHS with an intact atrial septum has a worse prognosis with early survival at only 33% due to damage to lung parenchyma and vasculature from left atrial hypertension.[40]

Tricuspid Atresia

Definition: In tricuspid atresia, the tricuspid valve is absent with usually some degree of associated right ventricular hypoplasia.

Incidence: Tricuspid atresia occurs in 1% to 3% of all live births with CHD.[4]

Pathology and Hemodynamics: Tricuspid atresia is divided into two types, type I with normally related great vessels (70%) and type II with transposition of the great arteries (30%). There may be an associated VSD or ASD and there is usually some degree of right ventricular hypoplasia (Fig. 24.1-37). Postnatal presentation depends on the size of VSD if present, the degree of right outflow tract obstruction, and the position of the great vessels.

Imaging: Atresia of the tricuspid valve and hypoplasia of the RV is readily apparent in the four-chamber view. The foramen ovale must be patent with right to left flow to allow egress from the right atrium. A large VSD will apparent in the four-chamber view. The great vessels should carefully be inspected as they may be normally related or transposed. There will usually be some degree of pulmonary stenosis if the great vessels are normally related; therefore, careful color and pulsed Doppler should be performed. Alternatively, there may be aortic stenosis, coarctation of the aorta, or interrupted aortic arch if there is transposition of the great arteries. Reversal of ductal flow suggests ductal-dependent pulmonary circulation. Tricuspid atresia may be associated with ventricular inversion.

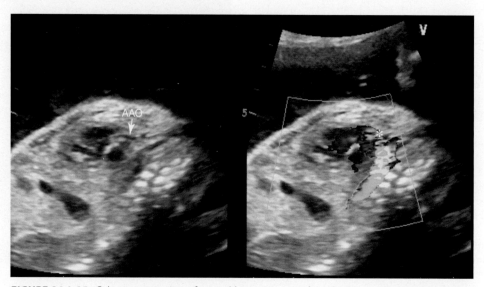

FIGURE 24.1-35: Color compare view of sagittal long-axis view of the fetal heart. The ascending aorta (*AAO*) is labeled and may be overlooked given its diminutive size. Color Doppler demonstrates retrograde flow, denoted by the *red* flow and *asterisk*.

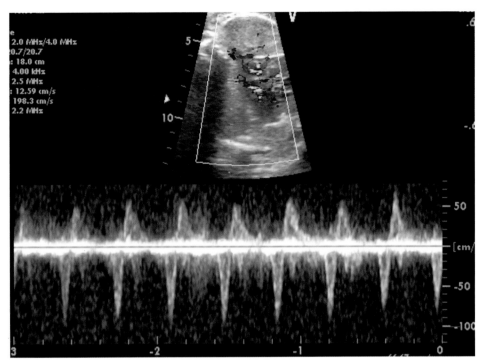

FIGURE 24.1-36: Pulsed Doppler in the pulmonary vein shows no diastolic flow and a biphasic pattern with an f/r <3 suggesting significant obstruction.

Treatment/Outcome: Palliation for tricuspid atresia is dependent on additional defects present. Depending on the degree of pulmonary blood flow, infants may have no operation at birth, pulmonary artery banding, or a Blalock–Taussig shunt. If transposition is present, the aortic arch may need repair. Infants will ultimately undergo staged single-ventricle repair with a bidirectional Glenn and then Fontan. Outcomes for patients with a Fontan palliation for tricuspid atresia are similar to that for HLHS, with approximately 80% survival at 10 years. Long-term complications include heart failure, arrhythmias, and the need for reoperation.

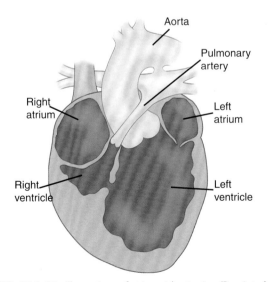

FIGURE 24.1-37: Illustration of tricuspid atresia. (Reprinted with permission from Rice MJ, McDonald RW, Pilu G, et al. Cardiac malformations. In: Nyberg DA, McGahan JP, Pretorius DH, et al, eds. *Diagnostic Imaging of Fetal Anomalies*. Philadelphia, PA: Lippincott Williams & Wilkins; 2003:484.)

Double-Inlet Left Ventricle

Definition: Double-inlet left ventricle (DILV) is diagnosed when both AV valves empty into a single dominant LV with a right ventricular outlet chamber giving rise to one or both great arteries originating. The LV is connected to the RV via a VSD or "bulboventricular foramen."

Incidence: DILV is an uncommon lesion occurring in 0.01% of CHD live births. It is usually associated with ventricular inversion, although it can occur with AV concordance.

Diagnosis: From a four-chamber view, the single LV is seen with two AV valves emptying into it. The AV valves may be normal, or one may be stenotic or atretic. Typically, the pulmonary artery arises from the LV and the aorta from an outlet chamber (transposed great vessels). Color and pulsed-wave Doppler should be performed to determine if there is associated aorta or pulmonary obstruction. Color Doppler should also be performed to evaluate for AV valve regurgitation. Significant valve regurgitation may be associated with the development of hydrops. CHB may be present, especially if there is ventricular inversion.

Treatment/Outcome: Surgical management and outcome depends on the associated defects. Ultimately, single-ventricle palliation with Fontan is performed.

Arterial Abnormalities

Coarctation of the Aorta

Definition: Coarctation of the aorta is a narrowing of the aorta typically just distal to the origin of the left subclavian artery (juxtaductal).

Incidence: Coarctation of the aorta represents 3% to 4% of all live births with CHD.

Pathophysiology and Hemodynamics: Coarctation of the aorta typically presents in the first days of life as the ductus arteriosus closes. Ductal tissue is present around the posterior aspect of the aorta; and as the ductus constricts, the arch narrows. Postnatally, coarctation should be considered if the lower extremity pulses are decreased and there is greater than a 20 mm Hg gradient between the upper and lower extremity blood pressures. At birth, decreased saturations in the lower extremities indicate right to left shunting at the level of the ductus arteriosus in severe coarctation. Prostaglandin infusion is needed to maintain ductal flow to ensure adequate perfusion to the lower extremities.

Associated Anomalies: Coarctation of the aorta may be associated with many other types of heart disease, most often other left-sided defects. Fifty percent of the cases with coarctation will have a bicuspid aortic valve.[41] Approximately one-third of infants with Turner syndrome will have coarctation. Coarctation of the aorta may also be seen in conjunction with ASDs, VSDs, DORV, or HLHS.

Imaging: Coarctation is difficult to diagnose in the fetus. Signs that suggest a coarctation include right ventricular dilation, hypertrophy, or dysfunction, or tricuspid insufficiency. Imaging of the aortic arch may reveal aortic isthmus hypoplasia, aliasing color Doppler, or increased pulsed-wave Doppler velocity (Fig. 24.1-38). In addition, in the three-vessel view, a size discrepancy between the transverse aorta and the ductus or abnormal color flow may be noted. If coarctation is suspected, other left-sided structures should be closely examined, as there is an increased incidence of aortic and mitral valve anomalies. Color Doppler should also be performed to evaluate for VSDs.

Treatment/Outcome: Definitive diagnosis of coarctation of the aorta cannot be made until after delivery. If a significant coarctation is diagnosed at less than 2 years of age, then surgical repair is indicated. Older patients may be eligible for catheter-based intervention with stent angioplasty. Patients with coarctation of the aorta need lifelong monitoring. Patients have increased rates of hypertension, atherosclerotic heart disease, and may have residual or recurrent obstruction. For those patients with recurrent obstruction, catheter-based intervention with angioplasty/stent placement is generally recommended.

Interrupted Aortic Arch

Interrupted aortic arch is a severe type of coarctation in which the ascending and descending aorta are discontinuous, with the descending aorta supplied by the ductus arteriosus. There are three types of arch interruption. In type A, the interruption occurs distal to the left subclavian artery. In type B, interruption occurs between the left carotid and left subclavian arteries. Type C interruption occurs after the innominate artery and is very rare (Fig. 24.1-39). Interrupted aortic arch may be overlooked on fetal

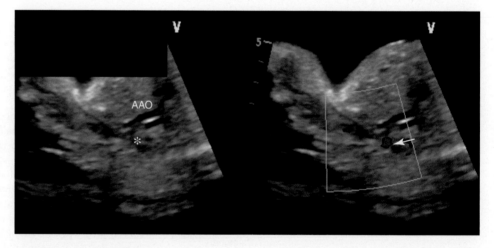

FIGURE 24.1-38: Sagittal long-axis imaging of the fetal aortic arch with color compare demonstrates a very hypoplastic aortic isthmus (*asterisk*) in comparison with the ascending aorta (*AAO*). Color compare denotes continuous diastolic flow as indicated by the *blue* color and *arrow*.

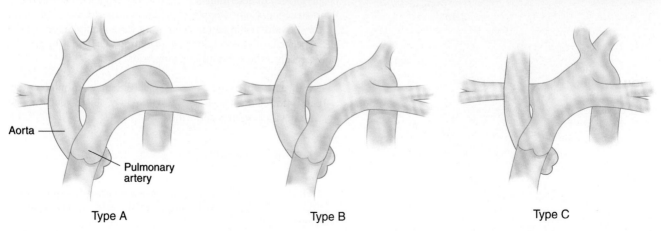

Aorta

Pulmonary artery

Type A   Type B   Type C

FIGURE 24.1-39: Illustration of the types of interrupted aortic arch. (Reprinted with permission from Rice MJ, McDonald RW, Pilu G, et al. Cardiac malformations. In: Nyberg DA, McGahan JP, Pretorius DH, et al., eds. *Diagnostic Imaging of Fetal Anomalies*. Philadelphia, PA: Lippincott Williams & Wilkins; 2003:470.)

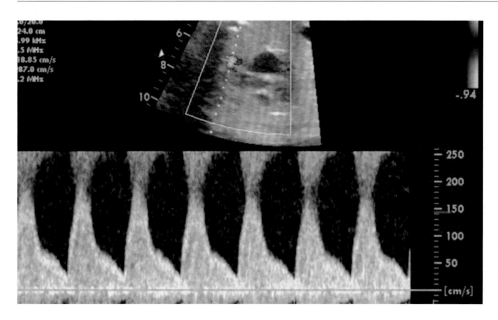

FIGURE 24.1-40: Pulsed-wave Doppler in a fetus with ductal restriction showing continuous diastolic flow and increased systolic velocity.

imaging because there will be a normal four-chamber image, normal crossing outflow tracts, and good heart function. However, there may be right ventricular dilation in the four-chamber view. In the aortic arch views, there will be an inability to connect the ascending and descending aorta. A malalignment-type VSD is usually present with a type B interruption and present in about in half of type A cases. Interrupted aortic arch may be associated with 22q11 deletion. All neonates with interrupted aortic arch will need prostaglandin infusion to maintain ductal patency. Surgical repair is performed in the newborn period.

Restriction or Closure of the Ductus Arteriosus

A patent ductus arteriosus is a normal fetal structure, and premature closure can lead to right-sided heart failure *in utero*. Treatment with indomethacin or other nonsteroidal anti-inflammatory drugs for tocolysis may result in premature restriction or closure of the ductus. Fetal echocardiographic features of restrictive or closure of the ductus include right ventricular dilation with right ventricular dysfunction, tricuspid insufficiency, and ductal narrowing with aliasing color Doppler and increased pulsed-wave Doppler in the ductal arch (Fig. 24.1-40). Typically, if the causative drug is discontinued, ductal patency is restored and the heart normalizes. However, in some cases, premature closure of the ductus *in utero* is associated with postnatal right ventricular dysfunction and pulmonary artery hypertension.[42]

Venous Anomalies

Anomalies of Systemic Venous Connections

A common anomaly of the systemic veins is bilateral superior vena cavae with drainage of the left superior vena cava into the coronary sinus. This defect is usually suspected when an enlarged coronary sinus is noted in the four-chamber view (Fig. 24.1-41). This anatomy exists in 3% of the normal population; however, it is much more prevalent in patients with CHD.

Interrupted Inferior Vena Cava

Interruption of the hepatic portion of the IVC is the most common anomaly of the IVC. Venous blood from the lower half of the body reaches the heart via the azygous vein that drains into

the superior vena cava. This finding may occur in isolation or can be associated with heterotaxy syndrome. An interrupted IVC is diagnosed when the hepatic portion of the inferior cava is absent; usually, the azygous vein is visualized as a venous vessel posterior to the aorta. The presence of two large vessels posterior to the four-chamber view is a clue that there is an interrupted IVC with an extra vessel (right azygous vein or left hemiazygous vein) adjacent to the descending aorta. Color Doppler interrogation will demonstrate opposite color flow compared to the aorta (Fig. 24.1-42). If an interrupted IVC is documented, the heart should be examined to evaluate for complex congenital heart disease.

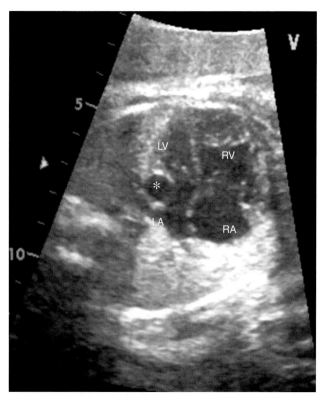

FIGURE 24.1-41: Apical four-chamber view showing a significantly dilated coronary sinus (*asterisk*) indicating a left-sided superior vena cava. *LA*, left atrium; *LV*, left ventricle; *RA*, right atrium; *RV*, right ventricle.

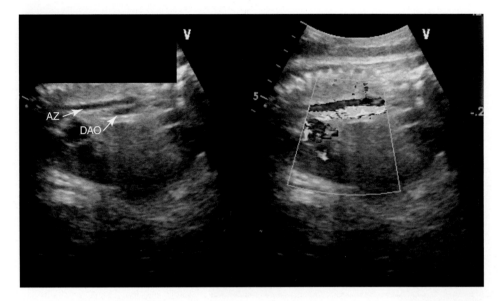

FIGURE 24.1-42: Color compare view of the azygous vein (*AZ*) located more posteriorly to the descending aorta (*DAO*). Color Doppler demonstrates *blue*, superiorly directed blood, in the azygous vein compared to descending aortic flow directly inferiorly in *red*.

Absent Ductus Venosus

The ductus venosus connects the portal and umbilical veins with the IVC. The ductus venosus acts as a sphincter to placental flow to protect the fetus from placental overcirculation. An absent ductus venosus results in umbilical venous flow directly to the IVC, another venous structure, or the right atrium. An absent ductus venosus may cause congestive heart failure or hydrops fetalis. In addition, with absent ductus venosus, there is an increased rate of chromosomal anomalies and congenital malformations.[43] If an absent ductus venosus is identified, a full cardiac evaluation should be performed (Fig. 24.1-43).

Anomalies of Pulmonary Venous Connections

Some or all of the pulmonary veins can drain into the systemic circulation, entering above the heart (usually through a vertical vein into the innominate vein), into the heart (directly into the right atrium or into the coronary sinus), or below the heart (through the liver). If the pulmonary venous drainage becomes obstructed postnatally, infants will be critically ill and require lifesaving surgery in the newborn period. This most often occurs if the drainage is below the diaphragm. Abnormal drainage of all pulmonary veins, total anomalous pulmonary venous return, is suspected on fetal echocardiography when a small left atrium is seen in combination with a large right atrium and RV and the pulmonary venous flow cannot be confirmed entering into the left atrium. In addition, in most fetuses, an abnormal venous structure can be identified coursing behind the heart. Anomalous pulmonary venous drainage may be difficult to diagnose in the fetus because of the limited amount of the fetal cardiac output that enters the pulmonary circulation. Surgical repair is the only therapy for this condition. The prognosis is typically good if there is no venous obstruction; however, long-term follow-up is needed.

Fetal Cardiac Tumors

The prevalence of cardiac tumors is approximately 0.14% in pregnancies referred for fetal echocardiography.[44] Rhabdomyomas are the most common, followed by fibromas and hemangiomas. Associated findings include hydrops fetalis, pericardial effusion, or a family history of tuberous sclerosis.[44-47]

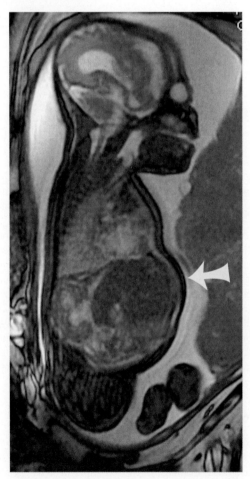

FIGURE 24.1-43: Sagittal steady-state free precession sequence image demonstrates absence of the ductus venosus (*arrow*).

Rhabdomyomas tend to increase in size prenatally and then regress after birth.[48-52] The association of rhabdomyomas with tuberous sclerosis is well documented.[51-54] Tuberous sclerosis has been found in 100% of cases of fetuses with multiple rhabdomyomas, and approximately 50% of fetuses with single tumors and no family history. Arrhythmias may be seen with

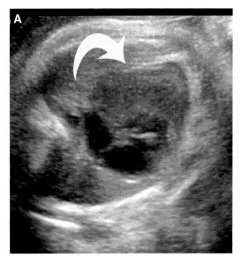
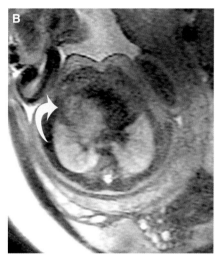
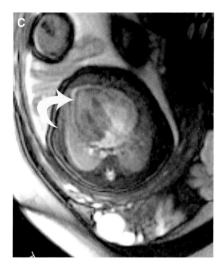

FIGURE 24.1-44: Rhabdomyoma. At 35 weeks' gestation. **A:** Axial ultrasound demonstrates a large echogenic homogeneous mass filling the left ventricle (*arrows*). Axial steady-state free precession **(B)** and axial SSFSE **(C)** MRI confirm the presence of the intraventricular mass, intermediate in signal.

rhabdomyomas.[51] Rhabdomyomas are homogeneous and more echogenic than in the surrounding myocardium. They may be found in the ventricular septum or free wall and may extend into the cardiac chambers (Fig. 24.1-44).

Fibromas represent 5% to 7% of all fetal cardiac tumors.[44,55] Fibromas are more likely to be associated with pericardial effusion, hydrops, heart failure, and fetal demise.[55] Fibromas often are single and appear homogeneous.[44] Hemangiomas are uncommon in fetuses and children. They typically have mixed echogenicity due to cysts and calcifications.[44] Hemangiomas may also invade the AV node, and varying degrees of heart block may be seen.[51] Ultimately, hemangiomas may regress after birth.[55] Teratomas are rare as well and are typically extracardiac, intrapericardial, and attached to the aortic root or pulmonary artery.[56] These also have mixed echogenicity secondary to cysts and calcifications.[44] Fibromas and teratomas will not regress and may require surgery.

Fetal cardiac tumors can be visualized using the four-chamber view and outflow. Imaging can identify size, location, and hemodynamic significance of the tumor. It is important to image with color Doppler to evaluate for AV valve regurgitation. Other important measures include assessment of heart function, presence of pericardial or pleural effusion, and heart rate (HR) and rhythm.

Echogenic foci are usually found in the LV within a papillary muscle. In one study, 20% of second- and third-trimester fetuses had echogenic foci.[57] These foci may be distinguished from true tumors in that they are usually smaller and intensely echogenic (Fig. 24.1-45). Autopsies done on fetuses with abnormal chromosomes (most frequently trisomies 13 and 21) have demonstrated papillary calcification.[58-60] Echogenic foci do not increase in size and do not become clinically significant.[60-62] In a large prospective study of greater than 10,000 fetuses, isolated echogenic foci were benign and did not increase the risk for fetal aneuploidy. Advanced maternal age (>35 years), abnormal biochemical markers, and/or other ultrasound markers were present in all fetuses found to have aneuploidy.[63]

Cardiomyopathy

Definition: Primary hypertrophic cardiomyopathy is defined as hypertrophy of the ventricles, not in response to a pressure or volume overload. There is often normal systemic function but

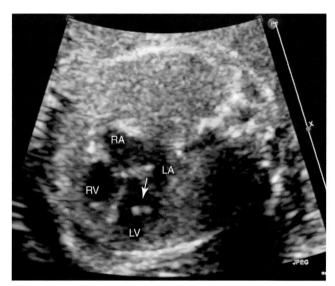

FIGURE 24.1-45: Four-chamber view demonstrates the hyperechoic echogenic foci (*arrow*). *LA*, left atrium; *LV*, left ventricle; *RA*, right atrium; *RV*, right ventricle.

abnormal diastolic function. Dilated cardiomyopathy refers to primary dilation of the ventricles due to muscle dysfunction.

Incidence: Fetal cardiomyopathies are infrequent. Hypertrophic cardiomyopathy can be associated with genetic disorders (i.e., Noonan syndrome, mitochondrial disorders) or familial idiopathic hypertrophic cardiomyopathy. Dilated cardiomyopathies are rarer and are typically due to a myocarditis. The most common cause of myocarditis are coxsackievirus, cytomegalovirus, parvovirus, adenovirus, and herpes.[64,65]

Imaging: Imaging of a fetus with hypertrophic cardiomyopathy will demonstrate increased thickness of the septum and free wall. The systolic function will be normal. When hypertrophy is identified, evaluation for outflow tract obstruction should be performed with color and pulsed-wave Doppler to rule out primary valve disease. Fetuses with hypertrophic cardiomyopathies are at increased risk for arrhythmias. In dilated cardiomyopathy, the

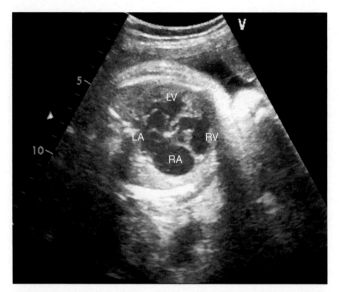

FIGURE 24.1-46: Apical four-chamber view demonstrating a severely dilated right atrium (*RA*) and right ventricle (*RV*). The left-sided chambers are also dilated. *LA*, left atrium; *LV*, left ventricle.

ventricles are enlarged, there is decreased function, and the septum and free wall are thin (Fig. 24.1-46). In both hypertrophic and dilated cardiomyopathies, AV valve regurgitation may be present and may be a precursor to heart failure and *in utero* fetal demise.

Prognosis: Hypertrophy secondary to maternal diabetes has a good outcome, with spontaneous resolution of the cardiomyopathy by 3 to 6 months of age. After delivery, infants with significant ventricular hypertrophy should have adequate preload, as dehydration can result in dynamic outflow tract obstruction. In addition, inotropes should be avoided. Infants can be observed for symptoms and supportive measures should be utilized, if needed. Outcomes of the dilated cardiomyopathies are generally associated with a poor outcome, especially in the presence of hydrops or significant AV valve regurgitation.

Fetal Arrhythmias

Definition: The normal fetal HR usually ranges from 120 to 160 bpm. Tachycardia is defined as greater than 180 bpm and bradycardia below 120 bpm.[66]

Incidence: Fetal arrhythmia is a common indication for referral for fetal echocardiogram. Premature atrial contractions (PACs) account for 70% to 80% of fetal arrhythmia, tachycardia for 10% to 15%, and bradycardia 8% to 12%.[67]

Imaging: The mechanism of fetal arrhythmia can be determined using several modalities. Simultaneous M-mode echocardiography of the atrial and ventricular wall or semilunar valve can be used to assess the atrial and ventricular contraction and atrial-ventricular synchrony (Fig. 24.1-47). Alternatively, pulsed Doppler can be performed within the LV sampling mitral inflow (EA wave = atrial contraction) and aortic outflow (V = ventricular contraction) (Fig. 24.1-48). Simultaneous superior vena cava flow and aortic outflow can also be used (Fig. 24.1-49).

Often, analysis of the initiation and termination of the tachycardia or bradycardia is helpful in determining the mechanism of arrhythmia. A complete evaluation of the fetal heart structures should be performed to evaluate for structural heart disease. There may be ventricular dysfunction or AV valve insufficiency secondary to persistent arrhythmia. All fetuses with persistent arrhythmias (excluding occasional PACs) should be followed up for development of hydrops or other signs of fetal distress.

Premature Atrial Contractions

PACs are very common and most often are benign (Fig. 24.1-50). Frequent PACs in a bigeminy pattern with block will result in a fetal HR between 75 and 90 bpm when conduction is a 2:1 pattern.[68] No treatment is required unless supraventricular tachycardia (SVT) occurs. A baseline fetal echocardiogram to assess cardiac structure and auscultation of the fetal HR by the obstetrician or maternal fetal medicine specialist is recommended. Close follow-up is recommended to monitor for sustained SVT, which

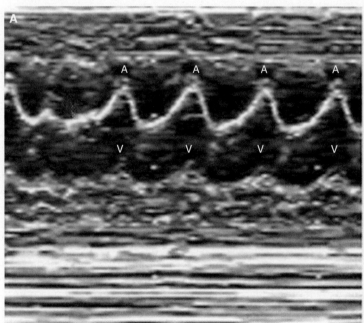
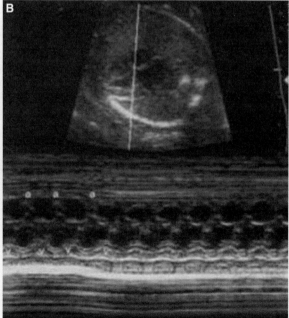

FIGURE 24.1-47: A, B: M-mode image of normal sinus rhythm. Atrial contraction is noted by an *A* and ventricular contraction by a *V*.

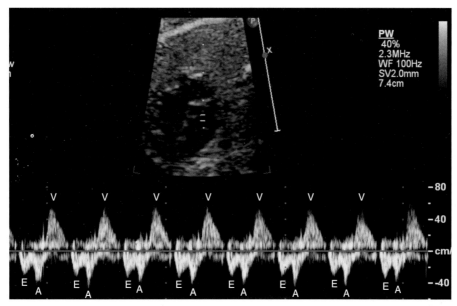

FIGURE 24.1-48: Pulse Doppler obtaining mitral inflow (*E, A*) and aortic outflow (*V*) demonstrating normal sinus rhythm.

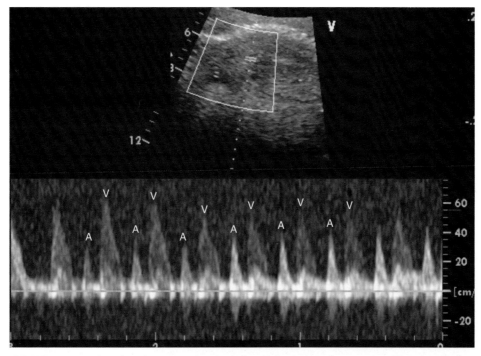

FIGURE 24.1-49: Doppler of superior vena cava flow indicating atrial contraction (*A*) and aortic flow indicating ventricular (*V*) contraction. This image demonstrates normal sinus rhythm.

occurs in approximately 10% of fetuses with frequent premature atrial contractions.

Supraventricular Tachycardia

SVT is typically due to an accessory conduction pathway between the atrium and ventricle. The rate is usually 220 to 280 bpm (Fig. 24.1-51). There is 1:1 conduction between the atrium and the ventricle. Maternal administration of digoxin is often successful as a first-line drug in fetuses with SVT. Second-line drugs include sotalol, flecainide, and amiodarone. Drug initiation requires hospitalization for close monitoring of the mother and fetus.

Atrial Flutter

Atrial flutter accounts for about 30% of fetal tachyarrhythmias and can be seen with myocarditis, CHD, or SSA/SSB isoimmunization.[69] Atrial flutter is due to a reentry circuit within the atrium. Typically, the atrial rate is greater than 300 bpm. There may be varying levels of block at the AV node (2:1 or 3:1 AV conduction) (Fig. 24.1-52). Sotalol is generally recommended as the first-line agent, although digoxin and amiodarone may be used.[70,71] After delivery, transesophageal pacing or synchronized cardioversion will convert the neonate to normal sinus rhythm. Typically, once converted to normal sinus rhythm, postnatal atrial flutter does not recur.

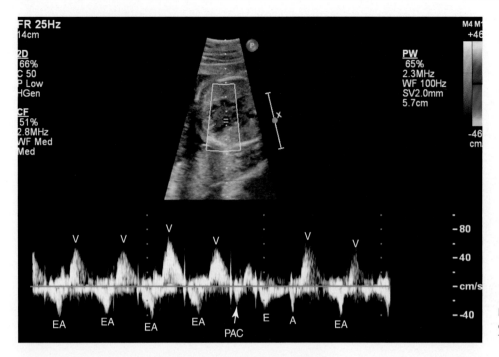

FIGURE 24.1-50: Pulse Doppler pattern of a premature atrial contraction (*PAC*). The normal *EA* wave pattern is disrupted.

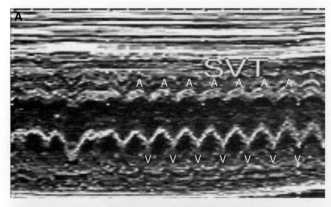

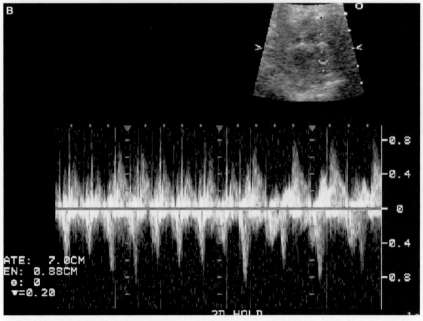

FIGURE 24.1-51: A: M-mode Doppler of supraventricular tachycardia; the heart rate is about 230 bpm. Note that the atrial (*A*) and ventricular (*V*) waves occur in a 1 to 1 pattern. **B:** Left-sided inflow and outflow Doppler demonstrating supraventricular tachycardia (*SVT*).

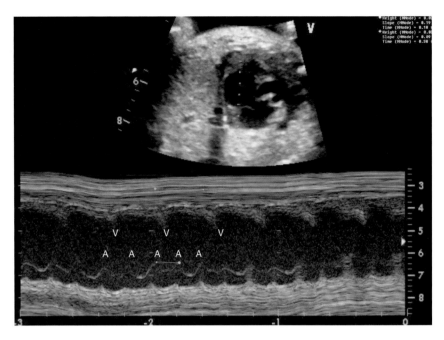

FIGURE 24.1-52: M-mode Doppler of atrial flutter. Note that the atrial rate (A) is twice that of the ventricular (V) rate.

Chaotic or Multifocal Atrial Tachycardia

Chaotic or multifocal atrial tachycardia is rare and is usually seen in the last trimester of pregnancy. The HR will be 180 to 220 bpm. Treatment is indicated if there is cardiac dysfunction or if the average HR is above 200 bpm. These arrhythmias are difficult to treat; however, digoxin, flecainide, or sotalol can be used.

Ventricular Tachycardia

Ventricular tachycardia is rare in the fetus and the HRs are usually 150 to 250 bpm; and there is dissociation between ventricular and atrial contraction. Ventricular tachycardia secondary to long QT syndrome (LQTS) is usually associated with both tachy- and bradyarrhythmias. Ventricular tachycardia may also be a complication of AV block, cardiac tumors, or myocarditis. Treatment is dependent on the etiology of the ventricular tachycardia, and may include dexamethasone, intravenous immunoglobulin (IVIG), magnesium, IV lidocaine, oral propranolol, or mexiletine.[71-75]

Bradycardia

Long QT Syndrome

LQTS may present with persistent sinus bradycardia.[66,76-78] Management of the fetus with suspected LQTS includes close observation and postnatal evaluation. Fetal treatment is not recommended for bradycardia; however, torsade de pointes and ventricular tachycardia require treatment if they occur. Maternal electrolyte abnormalities (hypomagnesemia and hypocalcemia) should be avoided as well as drugs/anesthetics that prolong the QT interval.

Atrioventricular Heart Block

Definition: First-degree heart block is defined as a PR interval greater than 150 ms. Second-degree heart block defined as intermittent AV dissociation can be subdivided into type I or type II. Type I is also known as Wenckebach and is characterized by progressive PR prolongation until there is a blocked atrial beat. Type II is an abrupt failure of AV conduction without prior PR prolongation. Type II second-degree heart block may progress to CHB. During second-degree AV block, there may be a repetitive conduction drop between the atrium and ventricle, whereby there is a regular conduction ratio between atrial and ventricular beats (2:1 block, 3:1 block, etc.).

Incidence: CHB occurs when there is complete dissociation between the atria and the ventricle. The electrical impulses from the atrium do not signal the ventricle and the ventricle beats independently. CHB may be due to congenitally malformed conduction system secondary to complex congenital heart disease (50% to 55%), to maternal autoantibodies (SSA/SSB) (40%), or to an undetermined etiology. In mothers with SSA antibodies, there is a 1% to 5% risk of CHB in the fetus if there is no prior affected pregnancy. The recurrence risk is 11% to 19% for woman who have had a previously affected pregnancy.[79,80]

Imaging: CHB can be diagnosed by M-mode or Doppler echocardiography. Serial Doppler assessment of the time between atrial and ventricular contraction is used for surveillance in maternal SSA-positive patients to measure the PR interval to detect primary heart block (Fig. 24.1-53).[81] Serial assessment at 1- to 2-week intervals starting at 16 weeks and continuing through 28 weeks' gestation is suggested. For previously affected pregnancies, weekly evaluation is recommended.

Treatment: Treatment of the CHB depends on etiology, ventricular rate, and presence and degree of heart failure. HRs below 55 to 60 bpm increase fetal risk. Maternal steroid, beta agonist, and IVIG treatment have been used with variable success in these patients, although timing of dosing and efficacy is still controversial.[82-84]

The majority of fetal arrhythmias can be controlled *in utero*. The prognosis is poor with hydrops. Most tachycardias, with the exception of atrial flutter, will need postnatal medical therapy. Fetuses with CHB will often ultimately need a pacemaker and fetuses with LQTS will need continued medical therapy and monitoring.

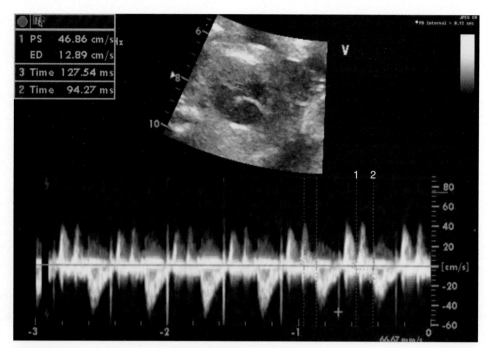

FIGURE 24.1-53: Assessment of the PR interval by mitral valve inflow Doppler and aortic outflow. The PR interval is measured by the time between the occurrence of the A wave (*1*) and ventricular systole (*2*).

DELIVERY PLANNING

Delivery brings a transition from fetal to postnatal circulation. In fetal life, the right and left circulations are functionally connected in parallel; however, with delivery, the low-resistance placental circulation is eliminated and the pulmonary vascular bed and lungs expand. The pulmonary vascular resistance falls, causing increased pulmonary blood flow that results in a rise in left atrial pressure, which closes the foramen ovale. In addition, smooth muscle cells begin to close the ductus. Postnatally, after foramen ovale and ductus arteriosus closure, the circulation functions in series, with the right heart ejecting to the lungs and the left heart to the body. The parallel circulation *in utero* allows major cardiac malformations with obstructed outflow to be well tolerated. However, after delivery, the change in the circulation may result in inadequate pulmonary or systemic blood flow. Infants may present with cyanosis, hypotension, acidosis, heart failure, and shock.

TABLE 24.1-2   Definition of Congenital Heart Disease Level of Care Assignment and Coordinating Action Plan

LOC	EXPECTED PHYSIOLOGY	EXAMPLE CHD	DELIVERY RECOMMENDATIONS	CARDIAC DR RECOMMENDATIONS
1	No instability expected in first weeks of life	ASD, VSD, AVSD, mild valve disease	Delivery at local hospital	Arrange outpatient follow up
2	Stability in DR expected although requiring postnatal catheter/surgery	Ductal-dependent lesions including HLHS, PA/IVS, severe TOF	Planned vaginal induction at ~39 wk at local hospital; transport to CNMC	Neonatalogist in DR; PGE if indicated
3	Instability requiring immediate specialty care in DR prior to catheter/surgery	HLHS or TGA with RFO, CHD or arrhythmia with decreased heart function	Planned vaginal induction at WHC at ~38–39 wk with "bailout" to C/S if necessary	CNMC specialists in DR; medications predetermined by care plan
4	Instability requiring immediate catheter/surgery in DR	HLHS or TGA with severe RFO or IAS, CHD or arrhythmia with hydrops	Planned C/S at CNMC usually at 38 wk; for EXIT, maternal general anesthesia	Multidisciplinary specialized care team in DR; medications/equipment predetermined by care plan including ECMO if indicated

ASD, atrial septal defect; AVSD, atrioventricular septal defect; CHD, congenital heart defect; CNMC, Children's National Medical Center; C/S, cesarean section; DR, delivery room; ECMO, extracorporeal membrane oxygenation; EXIT, *ex utero* intrapartum treatment; HLHS, hypoplastic left heart syndrome; LOC, level of care; PA/IVS, pulmonary atresia/intact ventricular septum; RFO, restrictive foramen ovale; TGA, transposition of the great arteries; TOF, tetralogy of Fallot; VSD, ventricular septal defect.
Reprinted from Donofrio MT, Levy RJ, Schuette JJ, et al. Specialized delivery room planning for fetuses with critical congenital heart disease. *Am J Cardiol.* 2013;111(5):737–747. Copyright © 2013 Elsevier. With permission.

Most fetuses with CHD will not have ductal- or systemic-dependent pulmonary blood flow. These babies can be delivered and cared for in local community hospitals. Some babies with significant heart disease can be born at an outlying hospital and stabilized by a neonatologist and then transferred to a tertiary care center for further care. A small subset will need pediatric cardiology care and intervention immediately after delivery. Babies with defects at risk for compromise in the delivery room include hypoplastic left heart syndrome with restrictive foramen ovale or intact atrial septum, D-TGA, uncontrolled tachycardia, heart block with low ventricular rate, severe Ebstein anomaly, TOF/PA, and others with cardiac dysfunction and heart failure. A risk stratification system developed at the Children's National Medical Center to help guide postnatal delivery and management is summarized in Table 24.1-2.[85] Most infants with CHD are assigned level of care (LOC) 1 and can be delivered at an outlying hospital with elective cardiology consultations. Newborns with ductal-dependent pulmonary or systemic circulation are assigned LOC 2. These babies will require initiation of prostaglandin to maintain ductal patency by a neonatologist prior to transfer to the tertiary care center. Babies that need urgent intervention after delivery by a pediatric cardiologist, such as balloon atrial septostomy, are assigned LOC 3 or 4 depending on disease severity. Delivery in these complex cases is planned with a neonatology and cardiology team available to assess and care for the infant immediately after birth. For all CHD, regulation of systemic and pulmonary blood flow is critical to ensure adequate oxygenation and optimal organ perfusion.

Accurate prenatal diagnosis and understanding of the physiology of specific heart defects allow for a safe delivery at a local hospital when possible, or adequate planning for a multidisciplinary delivery at the tertiary hospital if indicated. Success is ultimately dependent on essential collaborations between the prenatal diagnostic team and the postnatal care team.

REFERENCES

1. Rasiah SV, Publicover M, Ewer AK, et al. A systematic review of the accuracy of first-trimester ultrasound examination for detecting major congenital heart disease. *Ultrasound Obstet Gynecol.* 2006;28:110–116.
2. Sinkovskaya ES, Chaoui R, Karl K,et al. Fetal cardiac axis and congenital heart defects in early gestation. *Obstet Gynecol.* 2015;125(2):453–460. doi:10.1097/AOG.0000000000000608.
3. Donofrio MT, Moon-Grady AJ, Hornberger LK, et al. Diagnosis and treatment of fetal cardiac disease: a scientific statement from the American Heart Association. *Circulation.* 2014;129(21):2183–2242. doi:10.1161/01.cir.0000437597.44550.5d.
4. Fyler DC. Report of the New England Regional Infant Cardiac Program. *Pediatrics.* 1980;65:375–461.
5. Rastelli GC, Kirklin JW, Titus JL. Anatomic observations on complete form of persistent common atrioventricular canal with special reference to atrioventricular valves. *Mayo Clin Proc.* 1966;41:296–308.
6. Ferencz C, Rubin JD, McCarter RJ, et al. Congenital heart disease: prevalence at livebirth. The Baltimore-Washington infant study. *Am J Epidemiol.* 1985;121:31–36.
7. Sharland GK, Chita SK, Allan LD. Tricuspid valve dysplasia or displacement in intrauterine life. *J Am Coll Cardiol.* 1991;17:944–949.
8. Hornberger LK, Sahn DJ, Kleinman CS, et al. Tricuspid valve disease with significant tricuspid insufficiency in the fetus: diagnosis and outcome. *J Am Coll Cardiol.* 1991;17:167–173.
9. Respondek ML, Kammermeier M, Ludomirsky A, et al. The prevalence and clinical significance of fetal tricuspid valve regurgitation with normal heart anatomy. *Am J Obstet Gynecol.* 1994;171:1265–1270.
10. Krishnan AN, Sable CA, Donofrio MT. Spectrum of fetal echocardiographic findings in fetuses of women with clinical or serologic evidence of systemic lupus erythematosus. *J Matern Fetal Neonatal Med.* 2008;21:776–782.
11. Nakano H, Ueda K, Saito A. Acute hemodynamic effects of nitroprusside in children with isolated mitral regurgitation. *Am J Cardiol.* 1985;56:351–355.
12. Roman KS, Fouron JC, Nii M, et al. Determinants of outcome in fetal pulmonary valve stenosis or atresia with intact ventricular septum. *Am J Cardiol.* 2007;99:699–703.
13. Salvin JW, McElhinney DB, Colan SD, et al. Fetal tricuspid valve size and growth as predictors of outcome in pulmonary atresia with intact ventricular septum. *Pediatrics.* 2006;118:e415–e420.
14. Gardiner HM, Belmar C, Tulzer G, et al. Morphologic and functional predictors of eventual circulation in the fetus with pulmonary atresia or critical pulmonary stenosis with intact septum. *J Am Coll Cardiol.* 2008;51:1299–1308.
15. Tulzer G, Arzt W, Franklin RC, et al. Fetal pulmonary valvuloplasty for critical pulmonary stenosis or atresia with intact septum. *Lancet.* 2002;360:1567–1568.
16. Tworetzky W, McElhinney DB, Marx GR, et al. In utero valvuloplasty for pulmonary atresia with hypoplastic right ventricle: techniques and outcomes. *Pediatrics.* 2009;124:e510–e518.
17. Jahangiri M, Zurakowski D, Bichell D, et al. Improved results with selective management in pulmonary atresia with intact ventricular septum. *J Thorac Cardiovasc Surg.* 1999;118:1046–1055.
18. Chelliah A, Berger JT, Blask A, Donofrio MT. Clinical utility of fetal magnetic resonance imaging in tetralogy of Fallot with absent pulmonary valve. *Circulation.* 2013;127(6):757–759.
19. Bockman DE, Kirby ML. Dependence of thymus development on derivatives of the neural crest. *Science.* 1984;223:498–500.
20. Blyth M, Howe D, Gnanapragasam J, Wellesley D. The hidden mortality of transposition of the great arteries and survival advantage provided by prenatal diagnosis. *BJOG.* 2008;115:1096–1100.
21. Friedberg MK, Silverman NH, Moon-Grady AJ, et al. Prenatal detection of congenital heart disease. *J Pediatr.* 2009;155:26–31.
22. Bonnet D, Coltri A, Butera G, et al. Detection of transposition of the great arteries in fetuses reduces neonatal morbidity and mortality. *Circulation.* 1999;99:916–918.
23. Graham TP Jr, Bernard YD, Mellen BG, et al. Long-term outcome in congenitally corrected transposition of the great arteries: a multi-institutional study. *J Am Coll Cardiol.* 2000;36:255–261.
24. Van Praagh R, Van Praagh S. The anatomy of common aorticopulmonary trunk (truncus arteriosus communis) and its embryologic implications: a study of 57 necropsy cases. *Am J Cardiol.* 1965;16(3):406–425.
25. Allan LD, Sharland GK, Milburn A, et al. Prospective diagnosis of 1,006 consecutive cases of congenital heart disease in the fetus. *J Am Coll Cardiol.* 1994;23:1452–1458.
26. Raymond FL, Simpson JM, Sharland GK, et al. Fetal echocardiography as a predictor of chromosomal abnormality. *Lancet.* 1997;350:930.
27. Victoria T, Andonikou S. The fetal MR appearance of "nutmeg lung": findings in 8 cases lined to pulmonary lymphangiectasia. *Pediatr Radiol.* 2014:444:1237–1242.
28. Marshall AC, Levine J, Morash D, et al. Results of in utero atrial septoplasty in fetuses with hypoplastic left heart syndrome. *Prenat Diagn.* 2008;28:1023–1028.
29. Selamet Tierney ES, Wald RM, McElhinney DB, et al. Changes in left heart hemodynamics after technically successful in-utero aortic valvuloplasty. *Ultrasound Obstet Gynecol.* 2007;30:715–720.
30. Marshall AC, van der Velde ME, Tworetzky W, et al. Creation of an atrial septal defect in utero for fetuses with hypoplastic left heart syndrome and intact or highly restrictive atrial septum. *Circulation.* 2004;110:253–258.
31. Xu Z, Owens G, Gordon D, et al. Noninvasive creation of an atrial septal defect by histotripsy in a canine model. *Circulation.* 2010;121:742–749.
32. McElhinney DB, Marshall AC, Wilkins-Haug LE, et al. Predictors of technical success and postnatal biventricular outcome after in utero aortic valvuloplasty for aortic stenosis with evolving hypoplastic left heart syndrome. *Circulation.* 2009;120:1482–1490.
33. Maxwell D, Allan L, Tynan MJ. Balloon dilatation of the aortic valve in the fetus: a report of two cases. *Br Heart J.* 1991;65:256–258.
34. Mizrahi-Arnaud A, Tworetzky W, Bulich LA, et al. Pathophysiology, management, and outcomes of fetal hemodynamic instability during prenatal cardiac intervention. *Pediatr Res.* 2007;62:325–330.
35. Hornberger LK, Sanders SP, Rein AJ, et al. Left heart obstructive lesions and left ventricular growth in the midtrimester fetus. A longitudinal study. *Circulation.* 1995;92:1531–1538.
36. Hornberger LK, Need L, Benacerraf BR. Development of significant left and right ventricular hypoplasia in the second- and third-trimester fetus. *J Ultrasound Med.* 1996;15:655–659.
37. Divanovic A, Hor K, Cnota J, et al. Prediction and perinatal management of severely restrictive atrial septum in fetuses with critical left heart obstruction: clinical experience using pulmonary venous doppler analysis. *J Thorac Cardiovasc Surg.* 2011;141:988–994.
38. Chintala K, Tian Z, Du W, et al. Fetal pulmonary venous doppler patterns in hypoplastic left heart syndrome: relationship to atrial septal restriction. *Heart.* 2008;94:1446–1449.
39. Michelfelder E, Gomez C, Border W, et al. Predictive value of fetal pulmonary venous flow patterns in identifying the need for atrial septoplasty in the newborn with hypoplastic left ventricle. *Circulation.* 2005;112:2974–2979.
40. Rychik J, Rome JJ, Collins MH, et al. The hypoplastic left heart syndrome with intact atrial septum: atrial morphology, pulmonary vascular histopathology and outcome. *J Am Coll Cardiol.* 1999;34:554–560.
41. Becker AE, Becker MJ, Edwards JE. Anomalies associated with coarctation of aorta: particular reference to infancy. *Circulation.* 1970;41:1067–1075.
42. Huhta JC, Cohen AW, Wood DC. Premature constriction of the ductus arteriosus. *J Am Soc Echocardiogr.* 1990;3:30–34.
43. Berg C, Kamil D, Geipel A, et al. Absence of ductus venosus-importance of umbilical venous drainage site. *Ultrasound Obstet Gynecol.* 2006;28:275–281.

44. Holley DG, Martin GR, Brenner JI, et al. Diagnosis and management of fetal cardiac tumors: a multicenter experience and review of published reports. *J Am Coll Cardiol.* 1995;26:516–520.

45. Gresser CD, Shime J, Rakowski H, et al. Fetal cardiac tumor: a prenatal echo-cardiographic marker for tuberous sclerosis. *Am J Obstet Gynecol.* 1987; 156:689–690.

46. Harding CO, Pagon RA. Incidence of tuberous sclerosis in patients with cardiac rhabdomyoma. *Am J Med Genet.* 1990;37:443–446.

47. Wu CT, Chen MR, Hou SH. Neonatal tuberous sclerosis with cardiac rhabdomyomas presenting as fetal supraventricular tachycardia. *Jpn Heart J.* 1997;38:133–137.

48. Groves AM, Fagg NL, Cook AC, et al. Cardiac tumours in intrauterine life. *Arch Dis Child.* 1992;67:1189–1192.

49. Smythe JF, Dyck JD, Smallhorn JF, et al. Natural history of cardiac rhabdomyoma in infancy and childhood. *Am J Cardiol.* 1990;66:1247–1249.

50. Fesslova V, Villa L, Rizzuti T, et al. Natural history and long-term outcome of cardiac rhabdomyomas detected prenatally. *Prenat Diagn.* 2004;24:241–248.

51. Boxer RA, Seidman S, Singh S, et al. Congenital intracardiac rhabdomyoma: prenatal detection by echocardiography, perinatal management, and surgical treatment. *Am J Perinatol.* 1986;3:303–305.

52. Goh RH, Lappalainen RE, Mohide PT, et al. Multiple cardiac masses diagnosed with prenatal ultrasonography in the fetus of a woman with tuberous sclerosis. *Can Assoc Radiol J.* 1995;46:461–464.

53. Bader RS, Chitayat D, Kelly E, et al. Fetal rhabdomyoma: prenatal diagnosis, clinical outcome, and incidence of associated tuberous sclerosis complex. *J Pediatr.* 2003;143:620–624.

54. Lethor JP, de Moor M. Multiple cardiac tumors in the fetus. *Circulation.* 2001;103:E55.

55. Isaacs H Jr. Fetal and neonatal cardiac tumors. *Pediatr Cardiol.* 2004;25:252–273.

56. De Geeter B, Kretz JG, Nisand I, et al. Intrapericardial teratoma in a newborn infant: use of fetal echocardiography. *Ann Thorac Surg.* 1983;35:664–666.

57. Levy DW, Mintz MC. The left ventricular echogenic focus: a normal finding. *AJR Am J Roentgenol.* 1988;150:85–86.

58. Roberts DJ, Genest D. Cardiac histologic pathology characteristic of trisomies 13 and 21. *Hum Pathol.* 1992;23:1130–1140.

59. Veldtman GR, Blackburn ME, Wharton GA, et al. Dystrophic calcification of the fetal myocardium. *Heart.* 1999;81:92–93.

60. Brown DL, Roberts DJ, Miller WA. Left ventricular echogenic focus in the fetal heart: pathologic correlation. *J Ultrasound Med.* 1994;13:613–616.

61. Petrikovsky B, Klein V, Herrera M. Prenatal diagnosis of intra-atrial cardiac echogenic foci. *Prenat Diagn.* 1998;18:968–970.

62. Petrikovsky B, Challenger M, Gross B. Unusual appearances of echogenic foci within the fetal heart: are they benign? *Ultrasound Obstet Gynecol.* 1996;8:229–231.

63. Bradley KE, Santulli TS, Gregory KD, et al. An isolated intracardiac echogenic focus as a marker for aneuploidy. *Am J Obstet Gynecol.* 2005;192:2021–2026.

64. Bennet P, Nicolini U. Fetal infections. In: Fisk MN, Moise KJ, eds. *Fetal Therapy: Invasive and Transplacental.* Cambridge, MA: Cambridge University Press; 1997:92–116.

65. Wagner HR. Cardiac disease in congenital infections. *Clin Perinatol.* 1981;8:481–497.

66. Serra V, Bellver J, Moulden M, et al. Computerized analysis of normal fetal heart rate pattern throughout gestation. *Ultrasound Obstet Gynecol.* 2009;34:74–79.

67. Southhall DP, Richards J, Hardwick RA, et al. Prospective study of fetal heart rate and rhythm patterns. *Arch Dis Child.* 1980;55:506–511.

68. Eliasson H, Wahren-Herlenius M, Sonesson SE. Mechanisms in fetal bradyarrhythmia: 65 cases in a single center analyzed by doppler flow echocardiographic techniques. *Ultrasound Obstet Gynecol.* 2011;37:172–178.

69. Strasburger JF, Wakai RT. Fetal cardiac arrhythmia detection and in utero therapy. *Nat Rev Cardiol.* 2010;7:277–290.

70. Shah A, Moon-Grady A, Bhogal N, et al. Effectiveness of sotalol as first-line therapy for fetal supraventricular tachyarrhythmias. *Am J Cardiol.* 2012;109:1614–1618.

71. Strasburger JF, Cuneo BF, Michon MM, et al. Amiodarone therapy for drug-refractory fetal tachycardia. *Circulation.* 2004;109:375–379.

72. Cuneo BF, Strasburger JF, Niksch A, et al. An expanded phenotype of maternal SSA/SSB antibody-associated fetal cardiac disease. *J Matern Fetal Neonatal Med.* 2009;22:233–238.

73. Zhao H, Cuneo BF, Strasburger JF, et al. Electrophysiological characteristics of fetal atrioventricular block. *J Am Coll Cardiol.* 2008;51:77–84.

74. Cuneo BF, Ovadia M, Strasburger JF, et al. Prenatal diagnosis and in utero treatment of torsades de pointes associated with congenital long QT syndrome. *Am J Cardiol.* 2003;91:1395–1398.

75. Horigome H, Nagashima M, Sumitomo N, et al. Clinical characteristics and genetic background of congenital long-QT syndrome diagnosed in fetal, neonatal, and infantile life: a nationwide questionnaire survey in japan. *Circ Arrhythm Electrophysiol.* 2010;3:10–17.

76. Simpson JM, Maxwell D, Rosenthal E, et al. Fetal ventricular tachycardia secondary to long QT syndrome treated with maternal intravenous magnesium: case report and review of the literature. *Ultrasound Obstet Gynecol.* 2009;34:475–480

77. Roberts JFE. *Pregnancy Related Hypertension.* Philadelphia, PA: WB Saunders; 2009.

78. Mitchell JL, Cuneo BF, Etheridge SP, et al. Fetal heart rate predictors of long QT syndrome. *Circulation.* 2012;126:2688–2695.

79. Brucato A, Frassi M, Franceschini F, et al. Risk of congenital complete heart block in newborns of mothers with anti-Ro/SSA antibodies detected by counterimmunoelectrophoresis: a prospective study of 100 women. *Arthritis Rheum.* 2001;44:1832–1835.

80. Buyon JP, Hiebert R, Copel J, et al. Autoimmune-associated congenital heart block: demographics, mortality, morbidity and recurrence rates obtained from a national neonatal lupus registry. *J Am Coll Cardiol.* 1998;31:1658–1666.

81. Nii M, Hamilton RM, Fenwick L, et al. Assessment of fetal atrioventricular time intervals by tissue doppler and pulse doppler echocardiography: normal values and correlation with fetal electrocardiography. *Heart.* 2006;92:1831–1837.

82. Cuneo BF, Lee M, Roberson D, et al. A management strategy for fetal immune-mediated atrioventricular block. *J Maternal-Fetal Neonatal Med.* 2010;23:1400–1405.

83. Eliasson H, Sonesson SE, Sharland G, et al. Isolated atrioventricular block in the fetus: a retrospective, multinational, multicenter study of 175 patients. *Circulation.* 2011;124:1919–1926.

84. Skog A, Wahren-Herlenius M, Sundstrom B, et al. Outcome and growth of infants fetally exposed to heart block-associated maternal anti-Ro52/SSA autoantibodies. *Pediatrics.* 2008;121:e803–e809.

85. Donofrio MT, Levy RJ, Schuette JJ, et al. Specialized delivery room planning for fetuses with critical congenital heart disease. *Am J Cardiol.* 2013;111:737–747.

Maria A Calvo-Garcia • David N. Schidlow

Heterotaxy

Synonyms: Heterotaxy, cardiosplenic syndrome, right and left isomerism, and situs ambiguous.

Definition: Heterotaxy syndrome is a disorder leading to abnormal arrangement of the abdominal viscera, thoracic organs, and cardiac atria across the left–right axis. In this disease, some organs are in the correct side, while others will be found on the opposite of expected side, and the cardiac axis can be variable. Cardiac defects are usually present.

Incidence: The incidence of heterotaxy syndrome is 1 per 10,000 live births with a male-to-female ratio of about 2:1. It accounts for approximately 3% of congenital heart defects.[1]

Embryology/Genetics: Left to right axis formation or impairment starts during the third week of embryonic development and depends on the establishment of the primitive node, at the cranial end of the primitive streak. The motile cilia contained in the primitive node will determine a clockwise movement and leftward flow of the extraembryonic fluid. The node cilia function is critical to the development of proper organ laterality and several linked processes mediate an ordered cascade of patterning. Disruption of the right to left axis determination would lead to the clinical phenotype of heterotaxy. There are at least 20 genes known to be involved in the early left to right pattering, including *ZIC3, NODAL, CFC1, LEFTYA, CRYPTIC, ACVR2B, NKX2.5,* and *CRELD1.*

Nongenetic, environmental factors are also thought to be able to alter this process, especially maternal diabetes. Monozygotic twin gestation and maternal cocaine use are also known risk factors.[2,3]

Clinical Presentations: There are two recognized subtypes of heterotaxy syndrome; *heterotaxy syndrome with asplenia* (characterized by isomerism of right atrial appendages) and *heterotaxy syndrome with polysplenia* (associated with isomerism of the left atrial appendages) (Fig. 24.2-1). However, not all patients show all the expected combinations for each category, and in other cases, the spleen is normal in number and position.[4] A detailed description of the cardiac and extracardiac findings should be provided for each individual case.

Associated Anomalies: In addition to right to left axis displacement, organs that typically are asymmetric, such as the lungs and atrial appendages, will develop in a symmetrical or mirror-image way. It is usual to find associated complex congenital heart malformations, and in some forms there are rhythm disturbances, such as complete heart block. There are also noncardiac abnormalities. The splenic function may be normal, marginal (if polysplenia), or absent (if asplenia), leading to potential immune deficiency. There might be gastrointestinal complications from increased incidence of malrotation, biliary atresia, microgastria, duodenal or jejunal atresia, and anorectal malformations. Other systems can also be affected and craniofacial, renal, central nervous system (CNS) and musculoskeletal abnormalities as well as abdominal wall defects

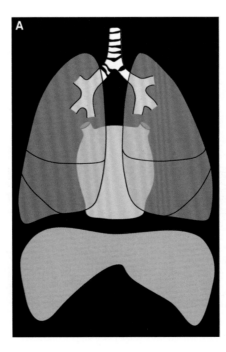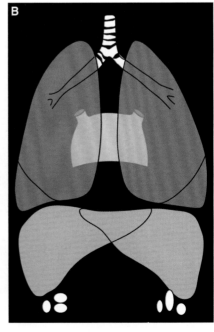

FIGURE 24.2-1: Diagrams of classic features in heterotaxy syndrome. **A:** Heterotaxy syndrome with asplenia, characterized by symmetric development of typical right-sided structures. There are trilobed lungs with bilateral minor fissures, eparterial bronchi (main bronchi superior to the ipsilateral pulmonary artery), bilateral systemic atria, midline liver, absent spleen, and variable position of the stomach. **B:** Heterotaxy syndrome with polysplenia, characterized by symmetric development of typical left-sided structures. There are bilateral bilobed lungs with hyparterial bronchi (main bronchi caudal to ipsilateral pulmonary arteries), bilateral pulmonary atria, midline/right or left-sided liver, variable position of the stomach, and multiple spleens along the greater curvature of the stomach.

have been observed in association with heterotaxy syndrome.[5] In addition, heterotaxy can be seen in up to 6.3% of patients with primary ciliary dyskinesia.[6] Most patients with heterotaxy syndrome have a normal karyotype. However, fetal karyotyping might be considered as there are several reports describing cases with microdeletion of chromosome 22q11, trisomy 18, and trisomy 13.[7]

Imaging

Ultrasound and Fetal Magnetic Resonance Imaging (MRI)

Prenatal ultrasound and fetal MRI detection of heterotaxy syndrome requires a systematic approach that will start by describing the fetal right and left side. This will be determined by the fetal orientation within the uterus and fetal lie and should be performed at the beginning of any examination.[8] Then, the position of the organs will be defined and the abdominal situs will be determined by the position of the stomach, liver, and spleen. The thoracic situs is determined by the atrial morphology, which is defined during fetal echocardiographic evaluation of the atrial appendages and/or the venoatrial concordance. The thoracic situs is also supported by the bronchial anatomy and fetal MRI could help in this process (Fig. 24.2-2). Under normal conditions (*situs solitus*), the right main bronchus is shorter, with early branching of the right upper lobe bronchus (called *eparterial bronchus*). The right main pulmonary artery will be in front or slightly below the right main bronchus. On the left, the main pulmonary artery crosses above the left main bronchus (called *hyparterial bronchus*). In left isomerism, there are bilateral hyparterial bronchi with the main pulmonary arteries on top. In right isomerism, the main right and left pulmonary arteries lie in front or slightly below the main bronchi.

Fetal imaging can provide clues for defining the subtype of heterotaxy based on the systemic vascular anatomy and noncardiac anomalies. Evaluation of the aorta and inferior vena cava is valuable in particular. In a transverse view of the upper abdomen of a fetus with situs solitus, the descending aorta is to the left and close to the spine, while the inferior vena cava is more anterior and to the right. Any variation from this standard arrangement can raise concern for heterotaxy syndrome, particularly if both vessels are on the same side. Another frequent variation of the venous system seen in heterotaxy syndrome is azygous continuation of the interrupted inferior vena cava. In this specific situation, the azygous vein is dilated, with similar size and is parallel to the adjacent thoracic aorta (Fig. 24.2-3).

Careful assessment of the fetal anatomy will be able to define potential associated noncardiac anomalies. In *heterotaxy syndrome with asplenia*, the spleen is most frequently absent, and microgastria, hiatal hernia, and imperforate anus can be present. In *heterotaxy syndrome with polysplenia*, multiple, small, poorly functioning spleens are noted and biliary atresia (typically represented by a persistently absent gallbladder) is present in up to 10% of cases. It is noted that *in utero*, it might not be possible to detect more than one spleen, given the small size of the splenules. However, this assessment should be attempted by looking for splenic tissue posterior to the stomach. Color Doppler evaluation of the splenic artery and vein can be useful as well (Fig. 24.2-4). The liver may be midline. In both subtypes, intestinal malrotation may be present in up to 70% of cases. This may be detected by reviewing the meconium and small bowel distribution in the third trimester by MRI (Figs. 24.2-4 and 24.2-5).[9] Fetal cardiac MRI has been used for the characterization of cardiovascular morphology and function as well.[10-12]

Fetal Echocardiography

A detailed echocardiographic evaluation is essential as part of the assessment of a fetus with suspected heterotaxy syndrome.

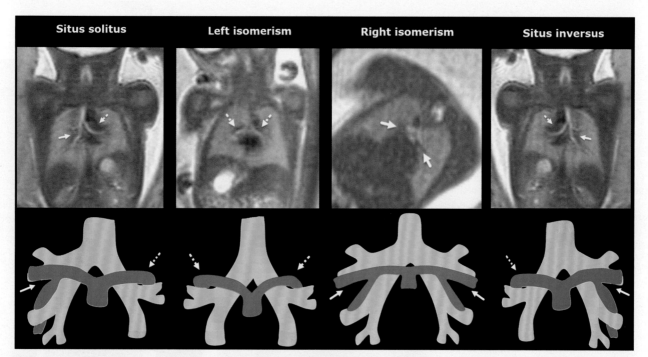

FIGURE 24.2-2: Determination of thoracic situs supported by bronchial anatomy and relation of bronchi to pulmonary arteries. Right pulmonary artery morphology (*arrows*). Left pulmonary artery morphology (*dashed arrows*).

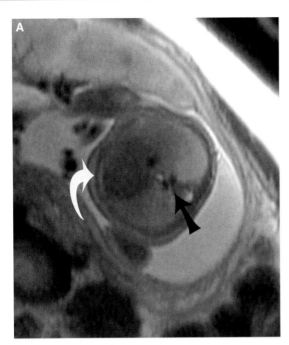
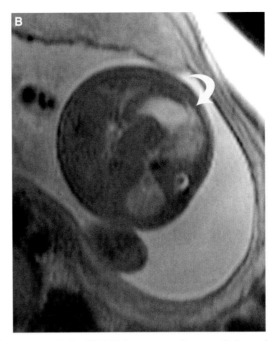

FIGURE 24.2-3: Heterotaxy syndrome with asplenia—26 weeks' gestation. **A:** Axial T2 MRI demonstrate dextrocardia (*curved arrow*) and asplenia (*curved arrow*) **(B)** as well as interrupted inferior vena cava with azygous continuation (*black arrow*).

The spectrum of congenital cardiovascular abnormalities in heterotaxy syndrome is extraordinarily broad. It ranges from benign variants of virtually no clinical consequence to complex single-ventricle malformations, and some fetuses have substantial risk of *in utero* or perinatal demise.[13] In addition, cardiac arrhythmias are often associated with heterotaxy syndrome due to perturbations in the cardiac conduction system. Complete heart block is encountered in polysplenia, and pathological tachyarrhythmias are relatively frequent in asplenia due to the presence of accessory conduction pathways and, in some cases, dual sinoatrial and/or atrioventricular nodes.[14,15]

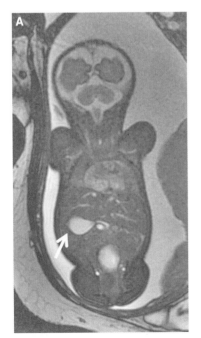
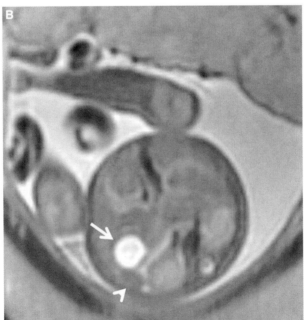
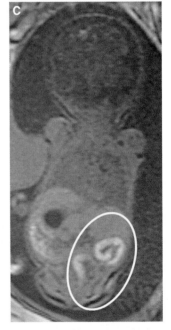

FIGURE 24.2-4: Heterotaxy syndrome with polysplenia—28 weeks' gestation. **A:** T2 coronal 2D steady-state free process, axial half Fourier single-shot echo T2 **(B)** as well as T1 coronal fast spoiled gradient echo magnetic resonance images **(C)**. There is a discordant abdominal situs with a right-sided stomach (*arrow*). The liver is symmetric. Splenic tissue was noted adjacent and posterior to the greater curvature of the stomach (*arrowhead*). T1 image shows meconium-filled colon located only in the left abdomen (*ellipse*), supporting the presence of intestinal malrotation.

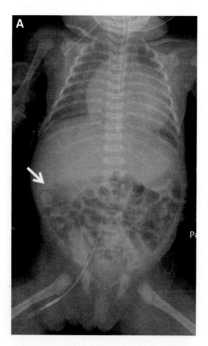

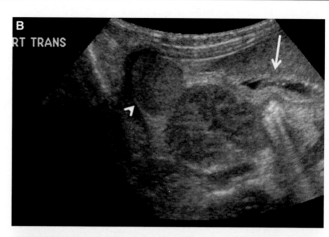

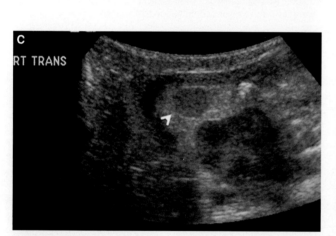

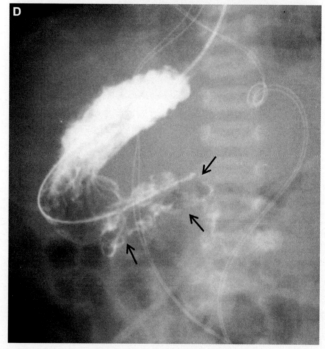

FIGURE 24.2-5: Heterotaxy syndrome with polysplenia. Postnatal assessment of the same patient as in Figure 24-4. Chest-abdomen X-ray on first day of life **(A)** and axial ultrasound images **(B, C)**. Two spleens (*arrowhead*) are noted adjacent to the right-sided stomach (*white arrow*). The most caudal spleen was not detectable *in utero*. **D:** Frontal view during upper gastrointestinal series with contrast in the duodenum (*black arrows*), which never crossed the midline, in concordance with the prenatal concern for malrotation.

Certain patterns of cardiac malformations are more likely in polysplenia versus asplenia (Table 24.2-1). In the setting of *heterotaxy syndrome with asplenia*, typical findings include intact inferior vena cava on the same side of the aorta (aka juxtaposition of the aorta and inferior vena cava), bilateral superior vena cavae (70%), total anomalous pulmonary venous return (TAPVR) to a systemic vein (58%), complete common atrioventricular canal (CAVC) (69%), double-outlet right ventricle (DORV) (82%), pulmonary atresia and stenosis (80%), single ventricle (50%), and dextrocardia (36%).

Typical features of *heterotaxy syndrome with polysplenia* include interrupted inferior vena cava with azygous continuation (80%), bilateral superior vena cavae (50%), partial anomalous pulmonary venous return (40%), left ventricular outflow tract obstruction (40%), CAVC (33%), DORV (37%), and complete heart block (40%).

In up to 20% of cases in both subtypes, there is absence of the right superior vena cava with an isolated left superior vena cava.[7,16,17] Bearing these associations in mind during fetal cardiac assessment is valuable, but it must be noted that there is substantial overlap among the two categories.[18] In all cases, detailed fetal echocardiography in experienced hands is required to accurately define the anatomy and its associated physiology. The components of the fetal echocardiogram are beyond the scope of this chapter and are readily available from multiple sources.[19] Briefly, a detailed anatomical assessment using the segmental approach should be undertaken. Thoracoabdominal situs, cardiac position, atrial anatomy, ventricular looping and morphology, atrioventricular connections and alignments, ventriculoarterial alignments, venous drainage, arterial exit, and any abnormalities in septation should be identified. Assessment of valvar function, ventricular function, and cardiac rhythm must be performed. Of note, assessment of atrial appendage morphology has utility in categorizing a specific fetus into the polyspenia or asplenia subtype (Fig. 24.2-6), but it is of limited practical utility without additional details of the cardiac anatomy.[20]

TABLE 24.2-1 Cardiovascular Abnormalities Commonly Associated with Asplenia and Polysplenia Syndromes

	ASPLENIA	POLYSPENIA
Systemic veins	Normal IVC	Interrupted IVC Bilateral SVCs
Pulmonary veins	TAPVR	Normal Ipsilateral
Atria	Bilateral RAA Primum ASD	Bilateral LAA Primum ASD
Atrioventricular valves	Single	Normal Single
Ventricles	Single ventricle CAVC defect	Two ventricles CAVC defect
Great arteries	DORV TGA Pulmonary stenosis/atresia	DORV TGA Pulmonary stenosis/atresia
Electrophysiology	Bilateral SA nodes Bilateral AV nodes	Superior P axis Heart block

ASD, atrial septal defect; AV, atrioventricular; CAVC, complete common atrioventricular canal defect; DORV, double-outlet right ventricle; IVC, inferior vena cava; LAA, left atrial appendage; NRGA, normally related great arteries; RA, right atrium; RAA, right atrial appendage; SA sinoatrial; SVC, superior vena cava; TAPVR, total anomalous pulmonary venous connection; TGA, transposition of the great arteries.

With currently available ultrasound equipment, the complete cardiac diagnosis can be made with a reasonable degree of confidence.[16] Nevertheless, it is prudent to be somewhat circumspect due to the many nuances associated with heterotaxy syndrome, especially with regard to the variations in systemic and pulmonary venous anatomy. Clinicians should be especially cautious when making predictions regarding postnatal surgical interventions, as the complex cardiac anatomy makes many cardiac surgical interventions challenging or even prohibitive.

Despite multisystem involvement in many cases of heterotaxy syndrome, cardiac abnormalities are, in many cases, the largest driver of early outcomes. Therefore, two of the primary benefits of prenatal characterization of the cardiac anatomy and physiology are (1) to appropriately counsel families such that they are provided reasonable expectations regarding pregnancy and postnatal outcomes and (2) to plan for the perinatal care of the infant.

Differential Diagnosis: Situs inversus totalis (situs inversus with dextrocardia or mirror-image reversal of situs solitus) is a form of visceral malposition but, by definition, it was excluded from heterotaxy as there is no association with asplenia/polysplenia or intestinal malrotation.[18] Nonetheless, these cases will require a complete assessment as there is a higher incidence of congenital heart defects than in situs solitus, a positive association with primary ciliary dyskinesia (up to 20%), and cases reported with similar genetic mutations also seen in heterotaxy.[21]

Thoracic and abdominal organs could be displaced in the presence of thoracic masses, unilateral lung agenesis, diaphragmatic hernia, and skeletal chest wall anomalies. In these cases, a careful analysis will clarify the correct diagnosis.

Prognosis/Management: The prognosis and management is dependent on the presence and type of congenital heart defect and associated malformations. Intracardiac malformations may be absent in up to 13% of patients with left isomerism.[22] The majority of heterotaxy cases, however, are associated with complex heart diseases and therefore have significant morbidity

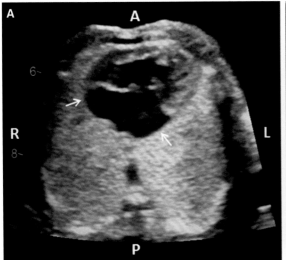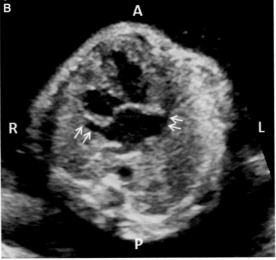

FIGURE 24.2-6: Heterotaxy with asplenia **(A)** and polysplenia **(B)**. The fetus with asplenia has right atrial appendage (denoted by *single arrows*) isomerism. The right atrial appendages have their typical broad pyramidal shape and wide atrial junction. Also present is a common atrium and right-dominant complete common atrioventricular canal defect. This functionally represents single-ventricle congenital heart disease. The fetus with polysplenia **(B)** has left atrial appendage (denoted by *double arrows*) isomerism. The left atrial appendages have their typical fingerlike shape and narrow atrial junction. Also present is dextrocardia, ventricular inversion, a common atrium, and a complete common atrioventricular canal defect. Two normally sized ventricles are present. *A*, anterior; *P*, posterior; *R*, right; *L*, left.

and mortality. Fetal mortality is increased in left isomerism in the presence of heart block and hydrops. Another risk factor for poor outcome is the presence of extracardiac TAPVR, which is almost always seen in right isomerism.[16] After birth, patients with right isomerism face higher morbidity and mortality due to more complex cardiac malformations and more frequent need for neonatal cardiac surgery and single-ventricle palliation.[1,13]

From a clinical management perspective, a well-defined system of care graduated to meet the needs of increasingly complex disease is useful in delivery preparation and marshaling appropriate resources for optimal outcomes.[23,24] An intravenous prostaglandin infusion is typically necessary in disease with ductus-dependent systemic or pulmonary blood flow, although most such infants are perfectly stable after delivery. In cases where complete heart block is present, immediate access to chronotropic medications and/or cardiac pacing modalities may be beneficial. In extreme cases, such as when obstructed total anomalous pulmonary venous connection is present, a well-coordinated multidisciplinary team including cardiac intensivists, extracorporeal membrane oxygenation specialists, and cardiothoracic surgeons may be required to offer the maximum likelihood of survival. In some instances where medical and surgical interventions are unlikely to be of benefit, it may be reasonable to consider palliative care. After stabilization in the neonatal period, attention can be turned to surgical or catheter-based strategies to treat the cardiac disease. In the most benign cases, no intervention is necessary. In some cases, complete physiological biventricular repair of the heart disease is possible.[25,26] Alternatively, single-ventricle palliation culminating in total cavopulmonary anastomosis (Fontan circulation) is frequently required; this is often the case even when two normally sized ventricles are present due to the associated lesions. In all cases of heterotaxy, the surgical risk is greater than that for comparatively similar disease without heterotaxy.[25] Furthermore, the complexity of care for these patients is increased because of comorbid diagnosis such as immune deficiency, malrotation, biliary atresia, or other anomalies. Specifically, the combination of complex cardiac disease and biliary atresia has a very poor outcome. Depending on the degree of splenic dysfunction, antibiotic prophylaxis and vaccination against pneumococcus may be required.[27] Especial consideration should be also given to the evaluation for possible associated ciliary dysfunction and primary ciliary dyskinesia in the neonatal period. This assessment could optimize respiratory management and improve surgical outcomes.[28]

Recurrence Risk: There is evidence for multiple modes of inheritance that include autosomal dominant, autosomal recessive, X-linked, and single-gene mutation. Approximately 10% of infants with heterotaxy have a family history of a close relative with congenital heart defects. Most cases, however, are single occurrences.[29] Without an identified cause, the recurrence risk for a pregnancy to have a form of heterotaxy is estimated between 5% and 10%.[2,30]

REFERENCES

1. Lin AE, Ticho BS, Houde K, et al. Heterotaxy: associated conditions and hospital-based prevalence in newborns. *Genet Med.* 2000;2:157–172.
2. Belmont JW, Mohapatra B, Towbin JA, et al. Molecular genetics of heterotaxy syndromes. *Curr Opin Cardiol.* 2004;19:216–220.
3. Kuehl KS, Loffredo C. Risk factors for heart disease associated with abnormal sidedness. *Teratology.* 2002;66:242–248.
4. Ware SM, Peng J, Zhu L, et al. Identification and functional analysis of ZIC3 mutations in heterotaxy and related congenital heart defects. *Am J Hum Genet.* 2004;74:93–105.
5. Cohen MS, Anderson RH, Cohen MI, et al. Controversies, genetics, diagnostic assessment, and outcomes relating to the heterotaxy syndrome. *Cardiol Young.* 2007;17(suppl 2):29–43.
6. Kennedy MP, Omran H, Leigh MW, et al. Congenital heart disease and other heterotaxic defects in a large cohort of patients with primary ciliary dyskinesia. *Circulation.* 2007;115:2814–2821.
7. Berg C, Geipel A, Kamil D, et al. The syndrome of left isomerism: sonographic findings and outcome in prenatally diagnosed cases. *J Ultrasound Med.* 2005;24:921–931.
8. Barboza JM, Dajani NK, Glenn LG, et al. Prenatal diagnosis of congenital cardiac anomalies: a practical approach using two basic views. *Radiographics.* 2002;22:1125–1137; discussion 1137–1138.
9. Nemec SF, Brugger PC, Nemec U, et al. Situs anomalies on prenatal MRI. *Eur J Radiol.* 2012;81:e495–e501.
10. Saleem SN. Feasibility of MRI of the fetal heart with balanced steady-state free precession sequence along fetal body and cardiac planes. *AJR Am J Roentgenol.* 2008;191:1208–1215.
11. Yamamura J, Kopp I, Frisch M, et al. Cardiac MRI of the fetal heart using a novel triggering method: initial results in an animal model. *J Magn Reson Imaging.* 2012;35:1071–1076.
12. Dong SZ, Zhu M, Li F. Preliminary experience with cardiovascular magnetic resonance in evaluation of fetal cardiovascular anomalies. *J Cardiovasc Magn Reson.* 2013;15:40.
13. Escobar-Diaz MC, Friedman K, Salem Y, et al. Perinatal and infant outcomes of prenatal diagnosis of heterotaxy syndrome (asplenia and polysplenia). *Am J Cardiol.* 2014;114:612–617.
14. Escobar-Diaz MC, Tworetzky W, Friedman K, et al. Perinatal outcome in fetuses with heterotaxy syndrome and atrioventricular block or bradycardia. *Pediatr Cardiol.* 2014;35:906–913.
15. Niu MC, Dickerson HA, Moore JA, et al. Heterotaxy syndrome and associated arrhythmias in pediatric patients. *Heart Rhythm.* 2018;15:548–554.
16. Cohen MS, Schultz AH, Tian ZY, et al. Heterotaxy syndrome with functional single ventricle: does prenatal diagnosis improve survival? *Ann Thorac Surg.* 2006;82:1629–1636.
17. Lapierre C, Dery J, Guerin R, et al. Segmental approach to imaging of congenital heart disease. *Radiographics.* 2010;30:397–411.
18. Jacobs JP, Anderson RH, Weinberg PM, et al. The nomenclature, definition and classification of cardiac structures in the setting of heterotaxy. *Cardiol Young.* 2007;17(suppl 2):1–28.
19. Donofrio MT, Moon-Grady AJ, Hornberger LK, et al. Diagnosis and treatment of fetal cardiac disease: a scientific statement from the American Heart Association. *Circulation.* 2014;129:2183–2242.
20. Berg C, Geipel A, Kohl T, et al. Fetal echocardiographic evaluation of atrial morphology and the prediction of laterality in cases of heterotaxy syndromes. *Ultrasound Obstet Gynecol.* 2005;26:538–545.
21. Evans WN, Acherman RJ, Restrepo H. Heterotaxy in southern Nevada: prenatal detection and epidemiology. *Pediatr Cardiol.* 2015;36:930–934.
22. Gilljam T, McCrindle BW, Smallhorn JF, et al. Outcomes of left atrial isomerism over a 28-year period at a single institution. *J Am Coll Cardiol.* 2000; 36:908–916.
23. Donofrio MT, Levy RJ, Schuette JJ, et al. Specialized delivery room planning for fetuses with critical congenital heart disease. *Am J Cardiol.* 2013;111: 737–747.
24. Schidlow DN, Donofrio MT. Prenatal maternal hyperoxygenation testing and implications for critical care delivery planning among fetuses with congenital heart disease: early experience. *Am J Perinatol.* 2018;35:16–23.
25. Anagnostopoulos PV, Pearl JM, Octave C, et al. Improved current era outcomes in patients with heterotaxy syndromes. *Eur J Cardiothorac Surg.* 2009;35:871–877; discussion 877–878.
26. Lim HG, Bacha EA, Marx GR, et al. Biventricular repair in patients with heterotaxy syndrome. *J Thorac Cardiovasc Surg.* 2009;137:371–379.e373.
27. Gottschalk I, Stressig R, Ritgen J, et al. Extracardiac anomalies in prenatally diagnosed heterotaxy syndrome. *Ultrasound Obstet Gynecol.* 2016;47:443–449.
28. Nakhleh N, Francis R, Giese RA, et al. High prevalence of respiratory ciliary dysfunction in congenital heart disease patients with heterotaxy. *Circulation.* 2012;125:2232–2242.
29. Sutherland MJ, Ware SM. Disorders of left-right asymmetry: heterotaxy and situs inversus. *Am J Med Genet C Semin Med Genet.* 2009;151C:307–317.
30. Ware SM, Harutyunyan KG, Belmont JW. Heart defects in X-linked heterotaxy: evidence for a genetic interaction of Zic3 with the nodal signaling pathway. *Dev Dyn.* 2006;235:1631–1637.

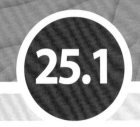

25.1

Pulmonary Hypoplasia and Chest Wall Abnormalities

Jennifer H. Johnston

Fetal anomalies of the chest include a heterogeneous group of abnormalities with diverse etiologies, presentations, natural histories, and prognoses. Sonography is a key tool not only for screening and diagnosis of fetal chest disorders but also for detection of potential prognostic indicators and identification of unstable fetuses requiring urgent therapy. Magnetic resonance imaging (MRI) can be valuable as an adjunct to ultrasound (US) as it has excellent soft-tissue contrast and can provide detailed information about the contents and structure of the fetal chest.

The clinical relevance and prognosis of chest lesions is generally related to the degree of mass effect on the adjacent structures, including the heart, great vessels, lungs, trachea, and esophagus. While some lesions may be self-resolving, others can result in serious *in utero* distress with subsequent hydrops and fetal demise. Moreover, fetuses with chest abnormalities that survive may bear the postnatal consequences of lung disease.

FETAL LUNG DEVELOPMENT

Embryological Considerations

The salient features required for a functioning pulmonary system include a branching conducting airway, adequate gas-exchange surface area with a thin air–blood barrier, surfactant, and vasculature to supply deoxygenated blood and carry away oxygenated blood.

The development of the lung is divided into five stages: embryological (26 days to 6 weeks), pseudoglandular (6 to 16 weeks), canalicular (16 to 28 weeks), saccular (28 to 36 weeks), and alveolar (36 weeks to childhood).[1–3] There is significant overlap between these stages due to differing speeds of maturation between the central and peripheral lung regions, as well as cephalad and caudal segments.[4]

Lung development begins at 26 days when the respiratory diverticulum arises as an outpouching from the ventral surface of the embryological foregut.[5] The lung bud initially communicates with the foregut but is eventually separated by two longitudinal ridges (the tracheoesophageal ridges), leaving behind the dorsal portion of the foregut, which is the precursor of the esophagus (Fig. 25.1-1A, B).

The respiratory diverticulum elongates to form the trachea and two lung buds, each of which enlarges to form the main bronchi at the fifth week of gestation. Branching morphogenesis is driven by signals received in the epithelium of the lung bud from the surrounding mesenchyme. The lung buds divide successively in a dichotomous manner, resulting in 10 right segmental bronchi and 8 left by the end of six weeks' gestation, the precursors of the bronchopulmonary segments in the adult lung (Fig. 25.1-1C–E). By 16 weeks, after additional rounds of

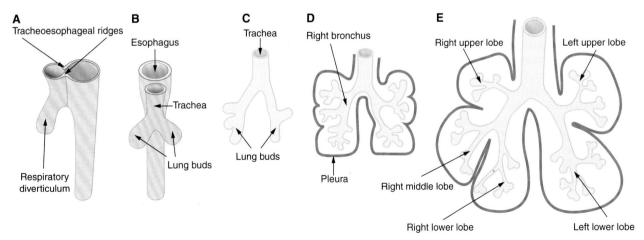

FIGURE 25.1-1: Embryological development of the respiratory diverticulum, lung buds, trachea, and bronchi. **A:** Formation of the respiratory diverticulum from the ventral surface of the embryological foregut, from which it is eventually separated by two tracheoesophageal ridges. **B:** Elongation of the respiratory diverticulum with subsequent formation of the lung buds. **C–E:** Development of the trachea and lungs at 5 weeks **(C)**, 6 weeks **(D)**, and 8 weeks **(E)**. (Adapted from Sadler TW. *Langman's Medical Embryology*. 12th ed. Philadelphia, PA: Lippincott Williams & Wilkins; 2012.)

branching, the basic conducting architecture of the lung has been established.

The development of the pulmonary vasculature closely mirrors that of the bronchial tree. After their appearance at approximately five weeks' gestation, the sixth branchial arches develop into the main pulmonary artery and its right and left branches.[1] The pre-acinar pulmonary arteries and veins form by vasculogenesis using the budding airways as a scaffold through the 17th week of gestation. Post-acinar pulmonary vessels subsequently form by angiogenesis in a network closely associated with the growing alveoli.[6] The bronchial arteries develop later than do the pulmonary arteries, arising during the eighth week of gestation from the dorsal aorta and entering the lungs alongside the main bronchi.

The peripheral airways enlarge during the canalicular period, and the capillaries in the surrounding mesenchyme undergo massive proliferation and become closely apposed to the airway epithelium.[6] Type II epithelial cells are derived from the cuboidal epithelium of the bronchial tree and begin to produce surfactant at approximately 22 to 24 weeks. The acinar epithelium also differentiates into type I epithelial cells, which contribute to formation of the first functional gas-exchange surfaces.[5] During the subsequent saccular phase, an increase in the number of terminal sacs (primitive alveoli) results in a rapid expansion of the gas-exchanging surface area. By 26 to 28 weeks' gestation, there is sufficient vascularization of the lungs, surfactant, and terminal sacs to potentially allow survival of a prematurely born infant who receives intensive neonatal care.

Alveolarization commences at 36 weeks' gestation; however, the vast majority of alveoli develop after birth.[2] This process continues until late childhood, approximately 8 years of age.[1] Postnatal growth of lung is due primarily to an increase in the number of respiratory bronchioles and alveoli as opposed to an increase in alveolar size.

Factors Affecting Lung Growth

The most important factors needed for normal lung development and growth include amniotic and lung fluid and adequate thoracic space. The formation and clearance of fetal lung fluid is a dynamic process. Lung liquid is formed by active transport across the pulmonary epithelium into the bronchial system, establishing positive transpulmonary pressure. Clearance of this fluid is achieved by fetal breathing movements[7] and by peristaltic airway contractions.[8] Approximately 50% of lung fluid is swallowed by the fetus, the principal mechanism of amniotic fluid resorption, with the other 50% effluxed through the trachea into the amniotic space, comprising 30% of the amniotic fluid.[9] The efflux of lung liquid and intratracheal pressures are carefully regulated by the larynx.

Inadequate amniotic fluid is well documented to be associated with pulmonary hypoplasia, although the exact mechanism remains unclear. Proposed mechanisms include physical compression of the thorax by the uterine wall, inhibition of fetal breathing movements, and increased efflux of lung liquid into the amniotic space.[1] Limited intrathoracic space also has a detrimental effect on lung growth and can result in pulmonary hypoplasia, as seen in the case of congenital diaphragmatic hernia (CDH), pulmonary masses, and skeletal malformations. Fetal breathing movements,

which appear as early as 11 weeks' gestation, produce changes in intrathoracic pressure, and there is experimental evidence that these movements also contribute to normal lung development.[10,11]

A balance between lung volume and pressure is required for appropriate growth as adequate transpulmonary pressure maintains lung expansion. Lung liquid both distends the developing airways and stimulates proliferation of alveolar cells. Disruption of this balance in either direction has significant consequences on lung development, as seen in the opposing examples of pulmonary hypoplasia and congenital high airway obstruction syndrome (CHAOS).

Increased knowledge of fetal lung fluid dynamics has resulted in the development of fetoscopic tracheal occlusion for treatment of CDH and the use of amnioinfusion for pulmonary hypoplasia related to oligohydramnios.

PULMONARY HYPOPLASIA

Pulmonary underdevelopment has been categorized into three groups[12]:

1. Pulmonary agenesis: complete absence of lung and bronchus
2. Pulmonary aplasia: incomplete development of lung parenchyma with a rudimentary bronchus
3. Pulmonary hypoplasia: underdevelopment of the pulmonary parenchyma

The formal histological diagnosis of pulmonary hypoplasia is determined by postmortem measurements including lung weight to body weight ratio, radial alveolar count, and DNA estimation,[13] and therefore limited for clinical use. US and MRI, however, are noninvasive tools that can aid in the antenatal prediction of and differentiation between lethal and nonlethal forms of pulmonary hypoplasia.

Pulmonary hypoplasia can be included under the category of alveolar growth disorders, which are histologically characterized by enlarged and simplified alveolar spaces (alveolar simplification). Common secondary changes seen with alveolar simplification are (1) interstitial thickening related to pulmonary interstitial glycogenesis (PIG) and (2) hypertensive vascular changes, likely due to increased vascular resistance related to reduced vascularization.[14]

Incidence: Pulmonary hypoplasia occurs with a reported incidence of 9 to 11 per 10,000 live births and 14 per 10,000 of all births.[15,16] The prevalence of this condition in autopsies ranges between 4.9% and 22%.[15,17,18]

Pathogenesis/Etiology: Bilateral pulmonary hypoplasia may be the result of various congenital abnormalities or complications of pregnancy that inhibit lung development (Table 25.1-1). Pulmonary hypoplasia most commonly occurs in the setting of oligohydramnios due to preterm premature rupture of membranes (PPROM) or fetal renal abnormalities, reportedly occurring with oligohydramnios for as short as 6 days.[13] CDH and intrathoracic masses such as congenital pulmonary airway malformations (CPAMs) may also cause pulmonary hypoplasia. Other potential etiologies include skeletal malformations deforming the thoracic cavity, pleural effusions, neuromuscular

TABLE 25.1-1	Anomalies Associated with Pulmonary Hypoplasia
Oligohydramnios, renal or urinary	Renal agenesis/dysplasia or multicystic dysplastic kidneys
	Bladder outlet obstruction
	Autosomal recessive (infantile) polycystic kidney disease
	Meckel–Gruber syndrome
	Renal dysplasia-limb defects syndrome
Oligohydramnios, nonrenal	Prolonged preterm rupture of membranes
	Idiopathic
Intrathoracic masses	Congenital diaphragmatic hernia
	Pulmonary masses (congenital pulmonary airway malformation, bronchopulmonary sequestration, bronchogenic cyst)
	Pleural effusions or chylothoraces
	Thoracic neuroblastoma (rare)
	Chest wall hamartoma (rare)
Skeletal malformations	Thanatophoric dwarfism
	Osteogenesis imperfecta
	Asphyxiating thoracic dystrophy (Jeune syndrome)
	Atelosteogenesis, type II
	Tetra-amelia
	Other skeletal dysplasias
Neuromuscular and central nervous system anomalies	Fetal akinesia deformation sequence
	Cerebrooculofacioskeletal syndrome
	Intrauterine anoxic or ischemic damage
	Anencephaly
	Phrenic nerve abnormalities
Cardiac lesions	Hypoplastic left or right heart, pulmonary stenosis, and so forth
	Cardiomyopathy
	Ebstein anomaly
Abdominal wall defects	Omphalocele
	Gastroschisis
Syndromes associated with pulmonary hypoplasia	Trisomy 13
	Trisomy 18
	Trisomy 21
	Roberts syndrome
	Matthew-Wood syndrome
	Familial pulmonary hypoplasia
	Larson-like syndrome, lethal type
	Aphalangy with hemivertebrae
	Fryns syndrome
	Goldenhar syndrome

Adapted from Goldstein RB. The thorax. In: Nyberg DA, McGahan JP, Pretorius DH, Pilu G, eds. *Diagnostic Imaging of Fetal Anomalies*. Philadelphia, PA: Lippincott Williams & Wilkins; 2002:381–420.

anomalies, abdominal wall defects, and cardiac lesions. The etiology of pulmonary agenesis is unknown but may be due to failure of the development of bronchial buds or an *in utero* vascular accident.

Numerous syndromes are associated with primary abnormalities in lung development, including trisomies 13, 18, and 21. Other syndromes associated with pulmonary hypoplasia include fetal akinesia deformation sequence (FADS), cerebrooculofacioskeletal (COFS) syndrome due to hypotonia and decreased fetal breathing, and various skeletal dysplasias that cause restriction of thoracic volume. Primary isolated pulmonary hypoplasia in the absence of an underlying disorder is extremely uncommon, usually sporadic, but may have rare familial occurrence.[19]

Unilateral pulmonary hypoplasia is typically secondary to conditions that limit the thoracic space available for lung growth and is rarely due to a primary embryological defect.[20] Less common etiologies for congenital unilateral pulmonary hypoplasia include main pulmonary artery atresia or thrombus, lobar agenesis–aplasia complex (including pulmonary venolobar or scimitar syndrome), and accessory diaphragm.[20–22]

Abnormalities associated with alveolar growth disorders in general include congenital heart disease and chromosomal anomalies such as trisomy 21 and X-linked filamin-A mutation.[23] Alveolar growth disorders have more recently been described in infants with TTF-1 (thyroid transcription factor-1, also known as NKX2.1) deficiency.[24]

Diagnosis US/MRI: In the setting of pulmonary hypoplasia, a reduction in pulmonary lung volumes will be observed on both US and MRI. A bell-shaped chest is common. Decreased T2 parenchymal signal intensity for gestational age is typically seen on MRI.[25,26] Both US and MRI may show ancillary findings that can explain the presence of pulmonary hypoplasia (Fig. 25.1-2). In unilateral pulmonary agenesis or hypoplasia, the affected lung and pulmonary artery are absent or small, and there is shift of mediastinal structures toward that side (Fig. 25.1-3). The contralateral lung may be normal in size but is often overdistended. MRI may be helpful to exclude an underlying lung mass. Diminished lung volumes may also be seen in alveolar growth deficiencies (Fig. 25.1-4).

Prognosticators: *Gray-scale US* can assess fetal lung size by *2D sonographic parameters*, including thoracic circumference (TC) (See Appendix Table 27), lung area, thoracic area, and lung length. The TC is measured in the axial plane at the level of the four chambers of the heart and the atrioventricular valves during fetal diastole (Fig. 25.1-5). Ratios utilizing these

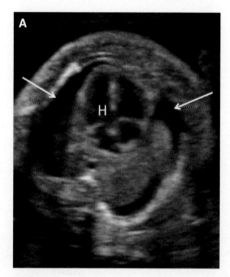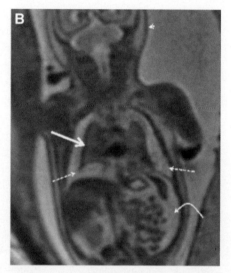

FIGURE 25.1-2: Pulmonary hypoplasia and hydrops in a fetus at 27 weeks' gestational age. **A:** Axial US image of small lungs and bilateral pleural effusions (*arrows*). H, heart. **B:** Coronal T2 MRI of the chest demonstrates marked pulmonary hypoplasia. The lungs are small and dark T2 signal (*solid straight arrow*) and are surrounded by hyperintense pleural fluid (*dashed arrows*). Ascites (*curved arrow*) and skin thickening are also present.

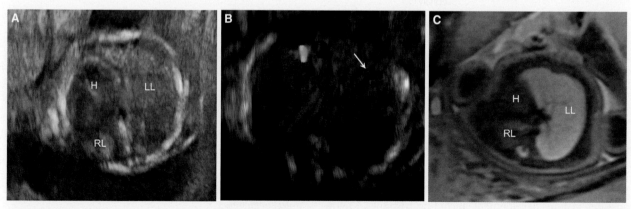

FIGURE 25.1-3: Unilateral pulmonary hypoplasia in a fetus at 25 weeks' gestational age. Gray-scale US **(A)** and color Doppler **(B)** axial images through the chest demonstrate markedly small right lung with rightward mediastinal shift and overexpansion of the left lung. Arrow in **(B)** shows normal-sized left pulmonary vessels but lack of visualization of the right. **C:** Axial T2 MRI demonstrates diminished signal intensity in the affected right lung. *H*, heart; *LL*, left lung; *RL*, right lung.

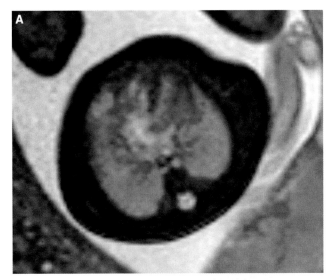

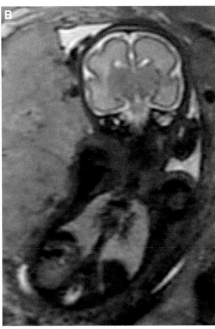

FIGURE 25.1-4: Congenital alveolar growth dysplasia in a fetus at 29 weeks' gestational age. T2 MRI with axial SSFP **(A)** and coronal SSFSE **(B)** planes through the chest demonstrate bell-shaped chest with small lungs that are decreased in T2 signal intensity for age; microcephaly was also present. The fetus demised at birth due to pulmonary hypoplasia. *H*, heart.

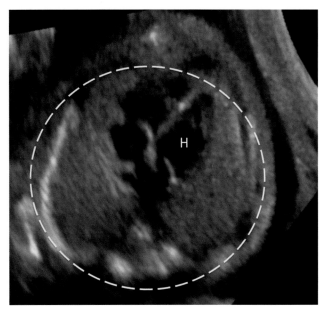

FIGURE 25.1-5: Normal thoracic circumference. Axial view through the chest at the level of the atrioventricular valves shows normal thoracic circumference measurement. *H*, heart.

parameters may be calculated to adjust for gestational age or fetal size, most commonly TC/abdominal circumference (AC) ratio,[27,28] which is normally 0.89 to 1.0. Other ratios include TC/ gestational age or femur length,[29] thoracic area/heart area,[30] and (thoracic area − heart area) × 100/thoracic area.[30] 2D sonographic parameters, with the exception of lung area-to-head circumference ratio (LHR) in fetuses with congenital diaphragmatic hernia (discussed in Chapter 25.2), have been shown to be less sensitive than is preferred for clinical practice.[31]

3D US, which accounts better for contour irregularities, has been shown to produce reliable lung volume measures[32–34] (Fig. 25.1-6; Tables 28-30 in Appendix A1). There

are two main approaches to obtaining lung volume measurements by 3D US. The multiplanar approach involves scrolling through the lungs in one reference plane while simultaneously displaying three orthogonal planes. Alternatively, VOCAL (virtual organ computer-aided analysis) allows volume calculation around a fixed axis in a sequential number of steps.[35] 3D lung volume measurements appears to be more robust in predicting pulmonary hypoplasia when compared to 2D techniques, particularly if estimated fetal weight is taken into consideration.[36]

Fetal MRI may also be used in the assessment for pulmonary hypoplasia, particularly in fetuses with CDH in which lung and liver parenchyma may be difficult to differentiate sonographically. While 3D US has the advantage of lower cost and quicker volume acquisition, benefits of MRI include increased spatial resolution and greater contrast between the lungs and adjacent structures. Lung volumes can be calculated by planimetric analysis in which the area of the lungs, excluding the mediastinum and hilar vessels, is measured on a series of images through the fetal chest that have little motion and multiplied by section thickness to obtain the section volume. The sum of the section volumes is then taken as the total lung volume. Lung volumes are also commonly performed on 3D reconstruction software (Fig. 25.1-7). Although some studies suggest that measurements obtained in the axial plane yield more accurate volumes than those in the coronal or sagittal planes,[25,37] more recent studies have reported no significant difference in lung volumes with regard to imaging planes.[38–40]

Nomograms of MRI-determined fetal lung volume in relation to gestational age have been constructed and may be useful in evaluation for pulmonary hypoplasia (Tables 31 and 32 Appendix A1). Rypens et al. measured lung volumes in 215 fetuses between 21 and 38 weeks' gestation and has been widely used for determination of normal fetal lung volumes.[41] More recently, lung volumes have also been reported by Meyers et al. in 665 fetuses between 18 and 38 weeks.[40] There is overall good correlation between these two nomograms, with the caveat that

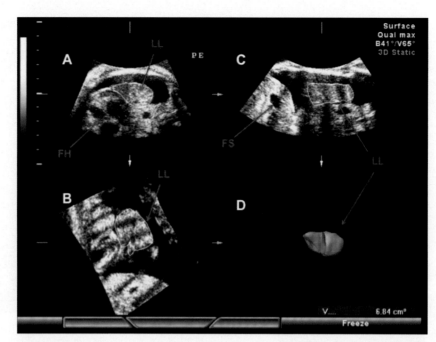

FIGURE 25.1-6: Three-dimensional multiplanar imaging of left lung (LL) volume in a fetus with pleural effusion at 31 gestational weeks. **A:** Transverse plane. **B:** Sagittal plane. **C:** Frontal plate. **D:** 3D rendering of the LL volume. *FH,* fetal heart; *FS,* fetal stomach; *RL,* right lung. (Reproduced with permission from Ruano R, Ramalho AS, de Freitas RC, et al. Three-dimensional ultrasonographic assessment of fetal lung volume as a prognostic factor in primary pleural effusion. *J Ultrasound Med.* 2012;31:1731–1739.)

Meyers et al. is likely more robust at 19 to 22 weeks due to the small number of fetuses at these gestational ages included in Rypens et al. In general, however, there remains variability in calculated fetal lung volumes that is likely due to heterogeneity in methodologies.[42] Improved standardization of MR image acquisition and measurement of lung volumes will be helpful for further investigations into the role of MRI-based evaluation of pulmonary hypoplasia.

Assessment of fetal lung maturity using MRI is another approach that has been studied in fetuses at risk for pulmonary hypoplasia. Lung-to-liver signal-intensity ratio (LLSIR), derived from signal intensities of regions of interest drawn on the lung and liver on single-shot fast spin-echo sequences, normally increases as gestational age progresses.[43] LLSIR has been shown to be lower than expected for gestational age in fetuses with autopsy-proven pulmonary hypoplasia,[44] and persistent low LLSIR during gestation may be a marker for poor prognosis postnatally in patients with CDH.[45]

Doppler velocimetry of fetal pulmonary circulation has been studied as another method to predict pulmonary hypoplasia since maldevelopment of the pulmonary vasculature parallels development of the pulmonary airways. Decreased peak

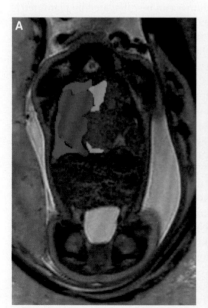

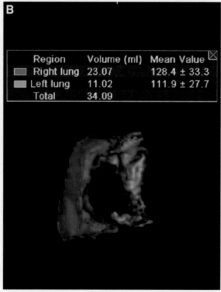

FIGURE 25.1-7: Determination of fetal lung volumes by MRI in a fetus at 34 weeks with left-sided congenital diaphragmatic hernia. The boundaries of the lungs, excluding the mediastinum and hilar vessels, are drawn on consecutive coronal images through the chest, and the subsequent area of these regions of interest is multiplied by the section thickness to obtain the lung volume. **A:** Right lung, blue; left lung, aquamarine; mediastinum, red. **B:** 3D rendering of the right and left lung volumes.

systolic velocity (PSV) and increased pulsatility index in the main pulmonary arteries, likely due to high peripheral vascular resistance, and decreased acceleration to ejection time have been reported to be associated with pulmonary hypoplasia[27,46,47] but have shown mixed results with regard to their clinical reliability.[36]

It may be that the most accurate prediction of lethal pulmonary hypoplasia requires an approach integrating clinical data with imaging parameters. In cases of mid-trimester PPROM, gestational age at time of rupture, degree of oligohydramnios, and latency time between rupture and delivery have been studied extensively with regard to pulmonary hypoplasia. A meta-analysis of 28 studies found that gestational age at PPROM performed significantly better than did the two other parameters.[48] An approach combining clinical (degree and duration of oligohydramnios, and gestational age at PROM), biometric (TC/AC), and Doppler (PSV in the proximal pulmonary arterial branch) parameters yielded positive predictive value of 100%, accuracy of 93%, and sensitivity of 71%.[27]

Differential Diagnosis: A small chest circumference may be related to various skeletal dysplasias. When the lungs appear relatively small in comparison to the heart, fetal cardiomegaly should be excluded by careful examination.

Prognosis: The perinatal mortality rate related to pulmonary hypoplasia is approximately 70% in most investigative series.[13] Although most cases of pulmonary hypoplasia are lethal, a spectrum of manifestations exists, ranging from neonatal death due to respiratory failure to mild respiratory disease. Mortality is increased in infants with associated anomalies, particularly renal agenesis and CDH.

Management: The management of pulmonary hypoplasia depends mainly on the underlying etiology. Large pleural effusions may be treated with thoracentesis or thoracoabdominal shunting to increase thoracic space available for lung development. Removal of an intrathoracic mass is usually performed soon after birth to permit reexpansion of the lung. In the setting of PPROM, the use of amnioinfusion to normalize amniotic fluid volume and potentially prevent pulmonary hypoplasia has shown promise, but more data is needed to assess its utility in routine clinical practice.[49] While fetoscopic tracheal occlusion can improve survival in fetuses with CDH, this procedure would be significantly more technically challenging in cases of oligohydramnios related to PPROM due to limited access and maneuverability.[50]

Recurrence Risk: The recurrence risk of pulmonary hypoplasia depends primarily on the underlying etiology. The reported recurrence of PPROM ranges between 16% and 32%.[51]

CHEST WALL

Chest wall abnormalities encompass deformities related to anomalies in growth and masses.

Chest Wall Deformities

Congenital chest wall deformities include pectus excavatum, pectus carinatum, and sternal defects, including ectopic cordis and pentalogy of Cantrell. Pectus excavatum (funnel chest) is characterized by depression of the sternum and the adjacent costal cartilages. Pectus carinatum refers to outward protrusion of the sternal body and adjacent ribs and may be isolated or may occur in combination with pectus excavatum.

The chest wall shape may also be deformed in fetuses with skeletal dysplasias such as thanatophoric dysplasia, achondrogenesis, asphyxiating thoracic dysplasia (Jeune syndrome), Ellis Van-Creveld syndrome, and rib polydactyly syndromes. In osteogenesis imperfecta, multiple rib fractures may be present.

Incidence: Pectus excavatum is the most common congenital chest wall deformity and occurs in 0.1 to 0.8 per 100 persons.[52] Pectus carinatum is second most common with an incidence of approximately 1 in 2,500 live births.[53] Both pectus excavatum and carinatum affect boys more commonly than girls.

Pathogenesis: The thoracic cavity is formed after the establishment of the intraembryonic cavity at approximately the fourth week of gestation. A group of mesenchymal cells pass ventrolaterally from the developing vertebrae to form the ribs and costal cartilages at the beginning of the fifth gestational week; the ribs fuse with the developing sternum one week later.[52] The sternum arises from paired parallel mesenchymal bands that migrate from the lateral plates and fuse by the 10th gestational week, from cranial to caudal.[53,54]

The pathogenesis of pectus excavatum and carinatum are unclear, but chief hypotheses focus on defective metabolism of the sternocostal cartilage leading to biomechanical weakness and overgrowth.[52]

Etiology: Pectus excavatum is often an isolated abnormality but can be associated with connective tissue disorders such as Marfan syndrome, Ehlers–Danlos syndrome, Sprengle deformity, and scoliosis.[54] Among numerous other syndromes associated with pectus excavatum and/or pectus carinatum are Noonan syndrome, cardiofaciocutaneous syndrome, Holt–Oram syndrome, Turner syndrome, and osteogenesis imperfecta.[55] Cases of familial nonsyndromic pectus excavatum and carinatum have been reported but may represent multifactorial inheritance.[54]

Diagnosis US/MRI: The contour of the fetal chest wall can be evaluated both by US and MRI. Pectus excavatum will be evident by an abnormal fetal contour related to a ventral depression in the thoracic wall (Fig. 25.1-8). In pectus carinatum, the sternum and adjacent ribs protrude anteriorly. In the setting of skeletal dysplasia, a chest wall deformity will be accompanied by other skeletal abnormalities.

Differential Diagnosis: Pectus excavatum should be differentiated from depressions in the ventral thoracic wall caused by oligohydramnios, which may deform the fetal contour by uterine wall compression, or umbilical cord loops that may simulate indentations.

Prognosis: Depending on the degree of sternal depression and resultant displacement of the heart and diminished pulmonary volume, pectus excavatum may result in measurable pulmonary and cardiac dysfunction. Mitral valve prolapse, mitral valve regurgitation, and ventricle compression may occur.[52] Most patients with pectus carinatum are asymptomatic, although some patients with severe deformity may complain of pain.

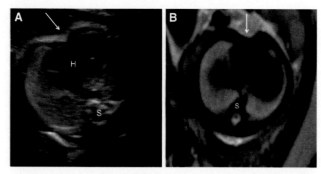

FIGURE 25.1-8: Pectus excavatum. Axial images through the lower chest in two different fetuses at gestational age of 33 weeks demonstrate depression of the sternum (*arrow*) on ultrasound **(A)** and T2 MRI **(B)**. *H*, heart; *S*, spine.

Management: Pectus excavatum may be surgically repaired postnatally depending on the severity. Nonoperative management with a brace for patients with pectus carinatum may achieve progressive remodeling; surgical correction is often reserved for when conservative management fails.[53]

Recurrence Risk: Pectus excavatum may be sporadic; however, a genetic predisposition is likely as positive family history is noted in up to 43% of cases.[52] Recurrence of pectus excavatum or pectus carinatum related to genetic syndromes or chromosomal aberrations depends on the specific genetic abnormality.

Chest Wall Masses

Soft-tissue masses that occur elsewhere in the body may potentially arise in the chest wall, including fibromatosis, myofibromatosis, fibrous hamartoma, and infantile fibrosarcoma. A handful of soft-tissue masses, however, are found typically or characteristically in the chest. Mesenchymal hamartomas of the chest wall are relatively rare but occur as benign lesions that always arise from the ribs. Previous names for this entity in the literature include mesenchymoma, infantile osteochondroma, and infantile cartilaginous hamartoma.[56] Vascular lesions, including hemangiomas, lymphatic malformations (LMs), and arteriovenous malformations, may also occur within the chest wall.

Incidence: Chest wall mesenchymal hamartomas are extremely rare, representing approximately 1 in 3,000 of primary bone tumors, or less than 1 in 1 million of the general population.[57] LMs of the chest wall are uncommon as 75% to 80% of LMs occur in the nuchal region.[58]

Pathogenesis/Etiology: Mesenchymal hamartomas are composed of benign proliferations of skeletal tissue with a prominent cartilaginous component and dilated hemorrhagic spaces. Mesenchymal hamartomas are predominantly nonfamilial, with all but one reported case in the literature having a familial association.[57] LMs are believed to be related to abnormal development during embryonic lymphangiogenesis. Although classic posterior cervical LMs carry a high risk of chromosomal abnormalities, LMs found elsewhere in the body, including the chest wall, may generally represent a separate entity with a relatively low rate of structural and genetic abnormalities.[58] LMs in the chest wall and axilla, however, can also be seen in syndromes such as Klippel–Trenaunay, Gorham–Stout disease, and CLOVES syndrome (Congenital Lipomatous Overgrowth, Vascular malformations, Epidermal nevi and Spinal abnormalities).[59]

Diagnosis US/MR: Mesenchymal hamartomas of the chest wall typically appear as large expansile extrapleural lesions arising from the center of one or more ribs away from the costochondral and costovertebral junctions. These masses characteristically demonstrate prominent secondary aneurysmal bone cystic components. On US, they appear as well-circumscribed, heterogeneous, and usually intrathoracic masses (Fig. 25.1-9). MRI shows heterogeneous masses with mixed T1 and T2 signal intensity. Hemorrhage in the mass as evidenced by focally increased T1 signal intensity is common, and fluid-fluid levels may be seen on both prenatal and postnatal imaging.[60] Calcification within the mass and rib involvement aid in differentiating mesenchymal hamartomas from pulmonary masses such as CPAMs.[61] In general, these lesions demonstrate rapid growth initially, subsequently showing slower growth, plateauing, or regressing.[61] Depending on the size of the lesion, mediastinal displacement or scoliosis may be present.

Chest wall LMs may be unilocular or multilocular and are similar in appearance to LMs elsewhere in the body (Fig. 25.1-10).[58]

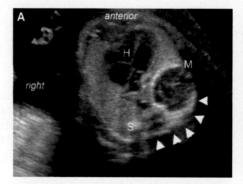
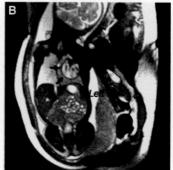

FIGURE 25.1-9: Mesenchymal hamartoma. **A:** Axial US of the chest in a fetus at 32 weeks' gestational age demonstrates a heterogeneous mass with echogenic capsule that appears to be related to the posterior rib (*arrowheads*). **B:** Steady-state free precession fetal magnetic resonance imaging in the coronal plane demonstrates a well-circumscribed mass (*arrows*) associated with the lateral chest wall. *H*, heart; *M*, mass; *S*, spine. (Reproduced with permission from Chu L, Seed M, Howse E, et al. Mesenchymal hamartoma: prenatal diagnosis by MRI. *Pediatr Radiol.* 2011;41:781–784.)

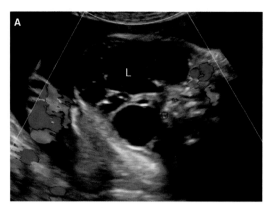
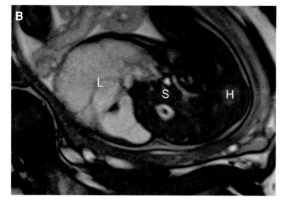

FIGURE 25.1-10: Chest wall lymphatic malformation. **A:** Color Doppler US image in the axial plane through a fetus at 26 weeks' gestational age demonstrates a predominantly cystic structure in the right upper chest wall containing numerous septations without detectable hypervascularity. **B:** Steady-state free precession magnetic resonance image in the axial plane shows an infiltrating multiloculated cystic lesion at the superior right chest wall. *H*, humeral head; *L*, lymphatic malformation; *S*, spine.

Differential Diagnosis: Differential considerations for mesenchymal hamartomas of the chest wall include congenital fibrosarcoma, neuroblastoma, or chondrosarcoma, although the latter is exceedingly uncommon in children.[56] A chest wall mass must also be differentiated from other masses occurring within the chest cavity, including a mass of pulmonary origin, such as CPAM or, rarely, pleuropulmonary blastoma, mediastinal or pericardial tumors, and CDH.

Prognosis: Mesenchymal hamartomas of the chest wall have a benign histology and self-limiting natural history. Many of these pregnancies are complicated, however, with fetal pleural effusions in 50% and polyhydramnios in 50% of cases.[61] If not diagnosed *in utero*, these masses come to light postnatally due to chest wall deformity or respiratory symptoms, or incidentally on chest imaging. Scoliosis can occur due to deformity of adjacent skeletal structures. In the case of chest wall and axillary LMs, the major risks are dystocia during labor and, in the long term, infiltration and organ involvement with potential infection and hemorrhage.[58]

Management: Mesenchymal hamartomas associated with large pleural effusions may require *in utero* treatment with thoracoamniotic shunting. Postnatal treatment for symptomatic patients typically consists of wide *en bloc* resection. Scoliosis is a postsurgical concern and related to the number of resected ribs.[56] Radiofrequency thermoablation is a minimally invasive technique that may have utility in treatment of mesenchymal hamartomas.[62] In the absence of symptoms, conservative management with observation can be considered as spontaneous regression has been reported.[57,61] Possible treatments for LMs include sclerotherapy, medical therapy, surgical resection, and laser therapy.

Recurrence Risk: Recurrence of mesenchymal hamartomas has been reported in cases with incomplete resection.[56] Following surgical excision of chest wall LMs, the recurrence risk is 10% to 15%.[58]

REFERENCES

1. Laudy JA, Wladimiroff JW. The fetal lung. 1: developmental aspects. *Ultrasound Obstet Gynecol.* 2000;16:284–290.
2. Burri PH. Structural aspects of postnatal lung development—alveolar formation and growth. *Biol Neonate.* 2006;89:313–322.
3. Pringle KC. Human fetal lung development and related animal models. *Clin Obstet Gynecol.* 1986;29:502–513.
4. Langston C, Kida K, Reed M, et al. Human lung growth in late gestation and in the neonate. *Am Rev Respir Dis.* 1984;129:607–613.
5. Schittny JC. Development of the lung. *Cell Tissue Res.* 2017;367:427–444.
6. Hislop A. Developmental biology of the pulmonary circulation. *Paediatr Respir Rev.* 2005;6:35–43.
7. Harding R, Hooper SB. Regulation of lung expansion and lung growth before birth. *J Appl Physiol.* 1996;81:209–224.
8. Schittny JC, G. Miserocchi, and Sparrow MP. Spontaneous peristaltic airway contractions propel lung liquid through the bronchial tree of intact and fetal lung explants. *Am J Respir Cell Mol Biol.* 2000;23:11–18.
9. Brace RA, Wlodek ME, Cock ML, et al. Swallowing of lung liquid and amniotic fluid by the ovine fetus under normoxic and hypoxic conditions. *Am J Obstet Gynecol.* 1994;171:764–770.
10. Adzick NS, Harrison MR, Glick PL, et al. Experimental pulmonary hypoplasia and oligohydramnios: relative contributions of lung fluid and fetal breathing movements. *J Pediatr Surg.* 1984;19:658–665.
11. Wigglesworth JS, Desai R. Effect on lung growth of cervical cord section in the rabbit fetus. *Early Hum Dev.* 1979;3:51–65.
12. Schneider P, Schwalbe E. Die morphologic der missbildungen des menschen und der thiere. *Jena: Fischer.* 1912;3:812–822.
13. Laudy JA, Wladimiroff JW. The fetal lung. 2: pulmonary hypoplasia. *Ultrasound Obstet Gynecol.* 2000;16:482–494.
14. Armes JE, Mifsud W, Ashworth M. Diffuse lung disease of infancy: a pattern-based, algorithmic approach to histological diagnosis. *J Clin Pathol.* 2015;68:100–110.
15. Knox WF, Barson AJ. Pulmonary hypoplasia in a regional perinatal unit. *Early Hum Dev.* 1986;14:33–42.
16. Moessinger AC, Santiago A, Paneth NS, et al. Time-trends in necropsy prevalence and birth prevalence of lung hypoplasia. *Paediatr Perinat Epidemiol.* 1989;3:421–431.
17. Gupta K, Das A, Menon P, et al. Revisiting the histopathologic spectrum of congenital pulmonary developmental disorders. *Fetal Pediatr Pathol.* 2012;31:74–86.
18. Husain AN, Hessel RG. Neonatal pulmonary hypoplasia: an autopsy study of 25 cases. *Pediatr Pathol.* 1993;13:475–484.
19. Frey B, Fleischhauer A, Gersbach M. Familial isolated pulmonary hypoplasia: a case report, suggesting autosomal recessive inheritance. *Eur J Pediatr.* 1994;153:460–463.
20. Abrams ME, Ackerman VL, Engle WA. Primary unilateral pulmonary hypoplasia: neonate through early childhood—case report, radiographic diagnosis and review of the literature. *J Perinatol.* 2004;24:667–670.
21. van Schendel MP, Visser DH, Rammeloo LA, et al. Left pulmonary artery thrombosis in a neonate with left lung hypoplasia. *Case Rep Pediatr.* 2012;2012:314256.
22. Currarino G, Williams B. Causes of congenital unilateral pulmonary hypoplasia: a study of 33 cases. *Pediatr Radiol.* 1985;15:15–24.
23. Liszewski MC, Lee EY. Neonatal lung disorders: pattern recognition approach to diagnosis. *Am J Roentgenol.* 2018;210:964–975.
24. Galambos C, Levy H, Cannon CL, et al. Pulmonary pathology in thyroid transcription factor-1 deficiency syndrome. *Am J Respir Crit Care Med.* 2010;182:549–554.
25. Kasprian G, Balassy C, Brugger PC, et al. MRI of normal and pathological fetal lung development. *Eur J Radiol.* 2006;57:261–270.
26. Kuwashima S, Nishimura G, Iimura F, et al. Low-intensity fetal lungs on MRI may suggest the diagnosis of pulmonary hypoplasia. *Pediatr Radiol.* 2001;31:669–672.
27. Laudy JA, Tibboel D, Robben SG, et al. Prenatal prediction of pulmonary hypoplasia: clinical, biometric, and Doppler velocity correlates. *Pediatrics.* 2002;109:250–258.

28. Yoshimura S, Masuzaki H, Gotoh H, et al. Ultrasonographic prediction of lethal pulmonary hypoplasia: comparison of eight different ultrasonographic parameters. *Am J Obstet Gynecol*. 1996;175:477–483.

29. Fong K, Ohlsson A, Zalev A. Fetal thoracic circumference: a prospective cross-sectional study with real-time ultrasound. *Am J Obstet Gynecol*. 1988;158:1154–1160.

30. Vintzileos AM, Campbell WA, Rodis JF, et al. Comparison of six different ultrasonographic methods for predicting lethal fetal pulmonary hypoplasia. *Am J Obstet Gynecol*. 1989;161:606–612.

31. Vergani P. Prenatal diagnosis of pulmonary hypoplasia. *Curr Opin Obstet Gynecol*. 2012;24:89–94.

32. Peralta CF, Cavoretto P, Csapo B, et al. Lung and heart volumes by three-dimensional ultrasound in normal fetuses at 12-32 weeks' gestation. *Ultrasound Obstet Gynecol*. 2006;27:128–133.

33. Vergani P, Andreani M, Greco M, et al. Two- or three-dimensional ultrasonography: which is the best predictor of pulmonary hypoplasia? *Prenat Diagn*;30:834–838.

34. Gerards FA, Twisk JW, Fetter WP, et al. Predicting pulmonary hypoplasia with 2- or 3-dimensional ultrasonography in complicated pregnancies. *Am J Obstet Gynecol*. 2008;198:140 e1–e6.

35. Kalache KD, Espinoza J, Chaiworapongsa T, et al. Three-dimensional ultrasound fetal lung volume measurement: a systematic study comparing the multiplanar method with the rotational (VOCAL) technique. *Ultrasound Obstet Gynecol*. 2003;21:111–118.

36. Triebwasser JE, Treadwell MC. Prenatal prediction of pulmonary hypoplasia. *Semin Fetal Neonatal Med*. 2017;22:245–249.

37. Jani J, Breysem L, Maes F, et al. Accuracy of magnetic resonance imaging for measuring fetal sheep lungs and other organs. *Ultrasound Obstet Gynecol*. 2005;25:270–276.

38. Busing KA, Kilian AK, Schaible T, et al. Reliability and validity of MR image lung volume measurement in fetuses with congenital diaphragmatic hernia and in vitro lung models. *Radiology*. 2008;246:553–561.

39. Ward VL, Nishino M, Hatabu H, et al. Fetal lung volume measurements: determination with MR imaging—effect of various factors. *Radiology*. 2006;240:187–193.

40. Meyers ML, Garcia JR, Blough KL, et al. Fetal lung volumes by MRI: normal weekly values from 18 through 38 weeks' gestation. *Am J Roentgenol*. 2018;211:432–438.

41. Rypens F, Metens T, Rocourt N, et al. Fetal lung volume: estimation at MR imaging-initial results. *Radiology*. 2001;219:236–241.

42. Deshmukh S, Rubesova E, Barth R. MR assessment of normal fetal lung volumes: a literature review. *AJR Am J Roentgenol*. 2010;194:W212–W217.

43. Moshiri M, Mannelli L, Richardson ML, et al. Fetal lung maturity assessment with MRI fetal lung-to-liver signal-intensity ratio. *Am J Roentgenol*. 2013;201:1386–1390.

44. Brewerton LJ, Chari RS, Liang Y, et al. Fetal lung-to-liver signal intensity ratio at MR imaging: development of a normal scale and possible role in predicting pulmonary hypoplasia in utero. *Radiology*. 2005;235:1005–1010.

45. Yamoto M, Iwazaki T, Takeuchi K, et al., The fetal lung-to-liver signal intensity ratio on magnetic resonance imaging as a predictor of outcomes from isolated congenital diaphragmatic hernia. *Pediatr Surg Int*. 2018;34:161–168.

46. Fuke S, Kanzaki T, Mu J, et al. Antenatal prediction of pulmonary hypoplasia by acceleration time/ejection time ratio of fetal pulmonary arteries by Doppler blood flow velocimetry. *Am J Obstet Gynecol*. 2003;188:228–233.

47. Chaoui R, Kalache K, Tennstedt C, et al. Pulmonary arterial Doppler velocimetry in fetuses with lung hypoplasia. *Eur J Obstet Gynecol Reprod Biol*. 1999;84:179–185.

48. van Teeffelen AS, van der Ham DP, Oei SG, et al. The accuracy of clinical parameters in the prediction of perinatal pulmonary hypoplasia secondary to midtrimester prelabour rupture of fetal membranes: a meta-analysis. *Eur J Obstet Gynecol Reprod Biol*. 2010;148:3–12.

49. Hofmeyr GJ, Eke AC, Lawrie TA. Amnioinfusion for third trimester preterm premature rupture of membranes. *Cochrane Database Syst Rev*. 2014:CD000942.

50. Williams O, Hutchings G, Hubinont C, et al. Pulmonary effects of prolonged oligohydramnios following mid-trimester rupture of the membranes—antenatal and postnatal management. *Neonatology*. 2012;101:83–90.

51. Lee T, Carpenter MW, Heber WW, et al. Preterm premature rupture of membranes: risks of recurrent complications in the next pregnancy among a population-based sample of gravid women. *Am J Obstet Gynecol*. 2003;188:209–213.

52. Brochhausen C, Turial S, Müller FK, et al. Pectus excavatum: history, hypotheses and treatment options. *Interact Cardiovasc Thorac Surg*. 2012;14:801–806.

53. Blanco FC, Elliott ST, Sandler AD. Management of congenital chest wall deformities. *Semin Plast Surg*. 2011;25:107–116.

54. Cobben JM, Oostra RJ, van Dijk FS. Pectus excavatum and carinatum. *Eur J Med Genet*. 2014;57:414–417.

55. Kotzot D, Schwabegger AH. Etiology of chest wall deformities—a genetic review for the treating physician. *J Pediatr Surg*. 2009;44:2004–2011.

56. Groom KR, Murphey MD, Howard LM, et al. Mesenchymal hamartoma of the chest wall: radiologic manifestations with emphasis on cross-sectional imaging and histopathologic comparison. *Radiology*. 2002;222:205–211.

57. Braatz B, Evans R, Kelman A, et al. Perinatal evolution of mesenchymal hamartoma of the chest wall. *J Pediatr Surg*. 2012;45:e37–e40.

58. Goldstein I, Leibovitz Z, Noi-Nizri M. Prenatal diagnosis of fetal chest lymphangioma. *J Ultrasound Med*. 2006;25:1437–1440.

59. Blei F. Congenital lymphatic malformations. *Ann N Y Acad Sci*. 2008;1131:185–194.

60. Chu L, Seed M, Howse E, et al. Mesenchymal hamartoma: prenatal diagnosis by MRI. *Pediatr Radiol*. 2011;41:781–784.

61. Jozaghi Y, Emil S, Albuquerque P, et al. Prenatal and postnatal features of mesenchymal hamartoma of the chest wall: case report and literature review. *Pediatr Surg Int*. 2013;29:735–740.

62. Falappa P, Natali GL, Bertocchini A, et al. Minimal invasive technique in mesenchymal hamartoma of the chest wall: use of radiofrequency thermoablation. *J Pediatr Surg*. 2010;45:1072–1073; author reply 1074.

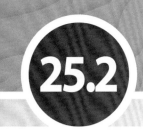

Congenital Diaphragmatic Hernia

Amy R. Mehollin-Ray • Beth M. Kline-Fath

Congenital diaphragmatic hernia (CDH) occurs when there is a defect in the fetal diaphragm allowing herniation of intra-abdominal structures into the thoracic cavity. The most common type of CDH is *intrapleural*, accounting for 90% to 95% of CDH cases.[1] The less common type is *mediastinal*, which can be either ventral as in *pentalogy of Cantrell* or dorsal as in *hiatal* hernia, through the esophageal hiatus. The *Morgagni* hernia is a subtype of ventral mediastinal hernia that occurs through the potential space between the sternal and costal heads of the diaphragm muscle. *Eventrations* are extreme elevations of all or part of the diaphragm that occur because of thinning or atrophy of the muscle.

Incidence: CDH occurs at an incidence of 1 in 2,500 with inclusion of stillborn pregnancies.[2] In the neonatal population, the incidence is 1 in 5,000 live born infants.[2] About 85% to 90% of CDH are left sided, 10% to 15% right sided, and 1% to 2% bilateral. A hernia sac can develop when the diaphragm muscle is absent and the remaining parietal layers of pleura and peritoneum fuse to form a covering membrane, present in approximately 15% of cases.[3] CDH occurs in isolation, in the absence of additional congenital malformations, in about 60% of cases.

Pathogenesis: The diaphragm develops between the 4th and 12th weeks of gestation. The current understanding is that the diaphragm forms first as a nonmuscular primitive anlage termed the pleuroperitoneal fold.[4] From the 4th to 10th weeks of gestation, this mesenchymal substrate originates from the lateral cervical wall to fuse with the esophageal mesentery and ventral septum transversum. Sequentially, cervical neural and myogenic cells then migrate across the fold to form the diaphragm. When there is a "hole" in the primitive mesenchymal anlage, a CDH develops.[3,4] If there is thinning or undermuscularization of the diaphragm, an eventration may result.[3] Left-sided CDH being more common than right is thought to be due to the muscularization being completed later on the left side.[5] True agenesis of the hemidiaphragm may also rarely occur.[6] In the presence of CDH, a spectrum of complicating diseases that occur secondary to the defect is often present (Table 25.2-1).[1]

The severity of pulmonary hypoplasia in patients with CDH is dependent on the timing of the insult and the duration of the herniation, as well as on the amount of viscera displaced into the thorax. The pathophysiology is believed to result from a "dual hit hypothesis", in which the lungs develop abnormally and are then further compressed by the herniated abdominal viscera, resulting in injury to both the ipsilateral and contralateral lungs.[5] First, early in gestation (5 to 16 weeks), there is a direct insult to the developing lung that results in decreased bronchial branching and reduction in alveoli. Second, with diminished fetal breathing movements and increasing compression of the growing lungs, there is a decrease in airway size, reduced alveoli, increased interstitial tissue, abnormal sacculoalveolar maturation, and diminished alveolar air space

TABLE 25.2-1 Complicating Diseases in Congenital Diaphragmatic Hernia
Pulmonary hypoplasia
Malrotation or incomplete rotation of bowel
Patent ductus arteriosus
Patent foramen ovale
Heart hypoplasia and/or dextroposition
Tricuspid/mitral valve regurgitation
Undescended testes
Accessory spleen

and gas-exchange surface area. At the same time that the lung parenchyma is affected, pulmonary vascular changes, which include reduction in the number of vessels and abnormal extension of the muscular layer into the small intra-acinar arterioles, are also occurring. The result of these parenchymal and vascular alterations becomes evident postnatally as pulmonary hypoplasia and pulmonary arterial hypertension (PAH). It is the severity of these changes that has the most impact on postnatal survival.

Etiology and Detection: The causes of CDH are incompletely understood. It is believed that the majority of CDH cases develop secondary to a complex inheritance pattern in which chromosomal aberrations and environmental factors cause a defect in the genes that guide normal diaphragm growth.[3] Familial CDH is rare, comprising 2% of cases.[7] Toxins, such as maternal anti-epileptic medication and thalidomide, have been implicated as causative of CDH, but the most important environmental factor known to cause CDH is disturbance in the retinol pathways.[1,8] Vitamin A (retinol) and its derivatives (retinoids) play a central role in embryonic morphogenesis and are important in the development of the diaphragm and lung.[1,9] In humans with CDH, vitamin A deficiency and genetic mutations tightly related to retinoid signaling have been noted.[1,9]

Chromosomal anomalies have been described in 10% of affected individuals.[10,11] The most common aneuploidies associated with CDH include trisomy 13, trisomy 18, trisomy 21, 45 X, and tetrasomy 12p (Pallister–Killian syndrome).[1] The most frequently diagnosed syndrome in association with CDH is Fryns syndrome, which also includes coarse facial features, cleft lip and palate, cardiac and cerebral malformations, and hypoplastic fingernails and toenails.[1] Many syndromes are linked with CDH at higher rates than in the general population (Table 25.2-2).[1]

Diagnosis: Because of known genetic associations, amniocentesis with karyotype is imperative in patients with CDH. As routine amniocentesis can miss cryptic deletions and duplications, obtaining higher resolution cytogenetic testing such as

TABLE 25.2-2 Syndromes Associated with Congenital Diaphragmatic Hernia

SYNDROME	INHERITANCE
Cornelia de Lange	Autosomal dominant
Craniofrontonasal	X-linked dominant
Denys–Drash	Autosomal dominant
Donnai–Barrow	Autosomal recessive
Fryns	Autosomal recessive
Matthew–Wood	Autosomal recessive
Pallister–Killian	Random, mosaic tetrasomy 12p
Pentalogy of Cantrell	Sporadic
Simpson–Golabi–Behmel	X-linked recessive
Thoracoabdominal	X-linked dominant
Wolf–Hirschhorn	Random, deletion 4p16

chromosomal microarray is also regularly recommended.[1] Prenatal diagnosis is typically via ultrasound (US). Additional imaging with fetal magnetic resonance imaging (MRI) and echocardiography is helpful to exclude associated anomalies, assist in predicting prognosis, and guide prenatal counseling. Although fetal MRI may occasionally detect additional anatomic abnormalities not seen on US, its greatest benefit is its ability to provide prognostic data.

Ultrasound: US evaluation of the fetal chest should be performed in all three anatomical planes, but the most important view is the axial. Diagnosis of CDH via US requires detecting direct signs of an intrathoracic mass containing stomach, bowel, and/or liver or indirect evidence such as abnormal cardiac axis and mediastinal shift. Identification of the diaphragm as a thin hypoechoic line on a sagittal or coronal image is helpful but not always sufficient to exclude a hernia, as only a portion of the diaphragm may be absent.[12] When diagnosing a CDH, it is important to identify associated anomalies that may support the presence of an underlying syndrome.

Left CDH, representing 85% to 90% of CDH cases, is usually first suspected when the stomach is not observed in the normal left upper abdominal quadrant location. In a true transverse plane through the fetal chest, the two cardinal findings of left CDH are (1) identification of a fluid-filled stomach at the level of the heart and (2) displacement of the heart to the right of midline (Fig. 25.2-1). It must be remembered, however, that the stomach is herniated in only 90% of left CDH, with the remaining 10% being intra-abdominal.[13] In these situations, other secondary findings must be utilized to diagnose CDH.

Early in gestation, bowel loops are usually decompressed and echogenic, making it difficult to separate the bowel from the lung and liver (Fig. 25.2-2A). However, later in gestation, the small bowel is better discriminated as it is filled with fluid, and the presence of intrathoracic bowel peristalsis is confirmative of CDH (Fig. 25.2-2B). Indirect signs of left CDH, in addition to displacement of the heart and mediastinum, include a scaphoid abdomen and small abdominal circumference due to absence of expected intra-abdominal structures (Fig. 25.2-3). Polyhydramnios may occur because of impaired fetal swallowing and/or partial gastric outlet obstruction due to kinking of the gastroduodenal junction.[14] Hydrothorax occurs in 5% of left CDH cases, but hydrops rarely develops despite significant heart and vascular compression.[15]

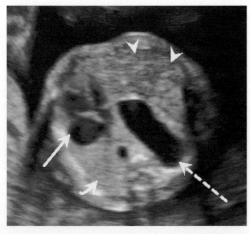

FIGURE 25.2-1: Left congenital diaphragmatic hernia with liver up. Axial US of the chest showing fluid-filled stomach (*dashed arrow*) in left thorax and heart (*straight arrow*) displaced into the right chest. Notice tissue anterior to the stomach, consistent with herniated liver (*arrowheads*), which is of lower echogenicity than normal lung (*curved arrow*).

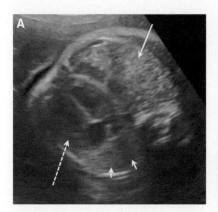

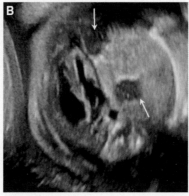

FIGURE 25.2-2: Left congenital diaphragmatic hernia and intrathoracic bowel. **A:** Axial US of chest in a 24-week fetus with left CDH without stomach herniation. In the left chest, the bowel has heterogeneous increased echogenicity (*long arrow*). The heart is shifted into the right chest (*dashed arrow*) and normal homogeneous right lung is noted posterior to the heart (*short arrows*). **B:** Axial US of the chest in same fetus as in **(A)** at 32 weeks. Note fluid-dilated bowel in left thorax (*arrows*).

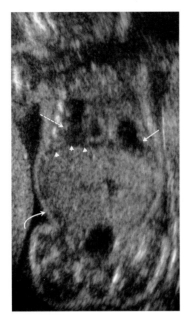

FIGURE 25.2-3: Left congenital diaphragmatic hernia. Coronal US demonstrates stomach (*straight arrow*) in the left thorax with displacement of the heart into the right chest (*dashed arrow*). The hypoechoic diaphragm (*arrowheads*) is seen on the right but absent on the left. The abdomen is scaphoid (*curved arrow*).

Identification of herniated liver can be difficult because of similar echogenicity to fetal lung and collapsed bowel. When the liver herniates into the left chest in a CDH, the left lobe lies perpendicular to the normal liver axis and immediately adjacent to the heart, in the anterior aspect of the left hemithorax. The position of the stomach can be helpful in supporting the presence of liver herniation (LH): If the herniated stomach occupies the anterior left hemithorax adjacent to the heart, the likelihood of LH is low (Fig. 25.2-4A). If the stomach is displaced posteriorly away from the left anterior chest and heart, LH is responsible (Fig. 25.2-4B). When the left lobe of the liver is herniated, the gallbladder, identified separate from the stomach, is often pulled over into the left upper quadrant or into the thorax. However, the most accurate way to validate liver positioning is via color Doppler, as

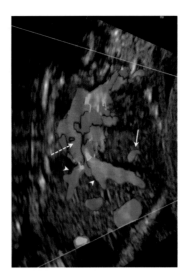

FIGURE 25.2-5: Left congenital diaphragmatic hernia with liver up. Coronal color Doppler US demonstrates the heart displaced into the right thorax (*dashed arrow*). The right and middle hepatic veins (*arrowheads*) are intra-abdominal, but the left hepatic vein (*solid arrow*) projects at the same level as the heart in the herniated liver.

intrathoracic extension of the portal or hepatic venous structures will confirm herniated liver (Fig. 25.2-5).[16,17]

Right CDH represents 10% to 15% of CDH cases. The right lobe of the liver is displaced with or without the gastrointestinal tract, resulting in a shift of the heart and mediastinum to the left. The fetal stomach almost always remains intra-abdominal. Given that right CDH primarily contains a solid, herniated liver, the defect can sometimes be confused with a lung lesion. On grayscale US, the easiest structure to identify is the gallbladder, which is often displaced high in the right abdomen or into the right hemithorax (Fig. 25.2-6). Confirmation is best achieved with color Doppler by demonstrating kinking of the sinus venosus, bowing of the umbilical segment of the portal vein, and/or coursing portal and venous structures extending into the right thoracic cavity (Fig. 25.2-7).[16] Right-sided hernias are not uncommonly—approximately 30%—associated with intrathoracic and intra-abdominal fluid,

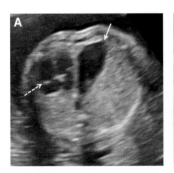 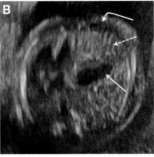

FIGURE 25.2-4: Left congenital diaphragmatic hernia without and with liver up. **A:** Axial thoracic US of left CDH with liver down. The stomach (*arrow*) is along the anterior thoracic wall. Note the heart at the same level as the stomach, shifted into the anterior right chest (*dashed arrow*). **B:** Axial thoracic US of fetus with left CDH with liver up. The stomach (*solid arrow*) is displaced from the anterior thoracic wall (*curved arrow*) because of liver herniated anteriorly (*dotted arrow*). The heart is shifted into the anterior right chest.

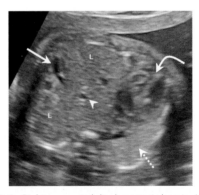

FIGURE 25.2-6: Right congenital diaphragmatic hernia. Axial US shows that the heart (*curved arrow*) is displaced into the left chest. Tubular anechoic structure consistent with gallbladder (*long arrow*) is within the right thorax, providing a clue to liver herniation (*L*). The liver is slightly less echogenic when compared with the normal left lung (*dashed arrow*) posterior to the heart. Also note portal triads in the herniated liver (*arrowhead*).

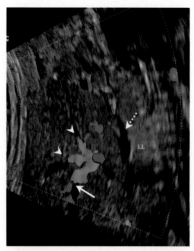

FIGURE 25.2-7: Right congenital diaphragmatic hernia. Coronal color Doppler US demonstrates kinking of the ductus venosus (*arrow*) and extension of right and middle hepatic veins (*arrowheads*) into the chest. Descending aorta (*dotted arrow*) and left lung (*LL*) are delineated.

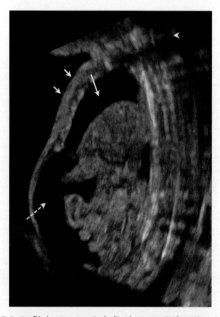

FIGURE 25.2-8: Right congenital diaphragmatic hernia with hydrops. Sagittal US of fetus with liver within the thorax. There is a large pleural effusion (*long arrow*), ascites (*dotted arrow*), chest wall edema (*short arrows*), and nuchal edema (*arrowhead*) consistent with hydrops. Despite thoracoamniotic shunting, neonatal demise occurred.

which may indicate that a hernia sac is present (Fig. 25.2-8).[15] Occasionally, hydrops may incur, thought to be related to cardiac tamponade.[16]

Bilateral CDH is rare, occurring in 1% to 2% of CDH cases. Complete absence of the diaphragm is even more uncommon but can be considered the most extreme form of bilateral CDH. Diagnosis of bilateral CDH is a challenge as the heart is typically midline, which gives the false impression of a lack of mass effect. Diagnosis relies on visualization of the stomach and bowel in the left thorax and liver in the right or in both thoraces.[18,19] The herniated stomach is often identified posterior or lateral to the heart, which may be shifted anteriorly and

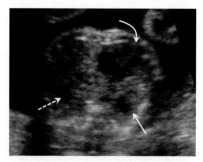

FIGURE 25.2-9: Bilateral congenital diaphragmatic hernia. Axial US of chest in a fetus with bilateral CDH. The heart (*curved arrow*) is not significantly deviated. There is a fluid-filled stomach (*arrow*) posterior to the heart in the left chest, and the gallbladder (*dotted arrow*) is present in the right posterior thorax.

superiorly but still midline (Fig. 25.2-9).[15,18] Herniation of the liver is demonstrated by verifying intrathoracic hepatic vessels with color Doppler.[18] Bilateral CDH has a higher incidence of associated anomalies and chromosomal aberrations and is present in 10% of familial cases.[20,21]

Unless a systematic approach is utilized when imaging the fetal chest, diagnosis of CDH can be missed. Although Guibaud et al. found that the prenatal sonography detection rate was 93% at a mean gestational age (GA) of 19 weeks, in the European literature, sonographic screening for CDH resulted in only an overall detection rate of 54% to 59% at an average GA of 24 weeks, improving later in gestation and in the presence of associated anomalies.[10,13,22] Prenatal detection rate has also been reported to be different depending on CDH type: 31% for right, 52% for left, and 63% in bilateral.[22] Although much less common than is left CDH, right CDH is missed disproportionately, thought to be due to the greater challenge of recognizing a herniated solid liver on the right compared to a herniated fluid-filled stomach on the left. For a similar reason, left-sided CDH is more likely to be missed when the stomach is not herniated. In a study that reviewed missed CDH diagnosis by prenatal US, the authors found that the most significant factors were quality of the imaging, lack of standard views in 55%, and missed findings in 30%.[23]

Magnetic Resonance Imaging: In many institutions, fetal MRI is performed at age of diagnosis and again at late gestation (32 to 36 weeks). Prenatal MRI easily discriminates between lung, herniated liver, other herniated intra-abdominal organs, and mediastinal structures. The early imaging confirms the presence of CDH, identifying herniated tissue, lung distribution, and associated malformations, and may also be used to identify candidacy for fetal intervention.[24] Late gestation MRI is primarily obtained for lung volume analysis.

In left CDH, the stomach is typically intrathoracic and may be distended due to impaired gastric emptying. If the liver is not herniated, the stomach will occupy the anterior left hemithorax adjacent to the heart. In the presence of a herniated liver, the stomach will be displaced posteriorly in the lower left chest, and may even be anterior to the spine or herniated into the right lower thorax.[24] Malrotation of the stomach both organoaxial and mesenteroaxial is almost always present when the stomach is herniated (Fig. 25.2-10). Typically, all of the small bowel and most of the large bowel,

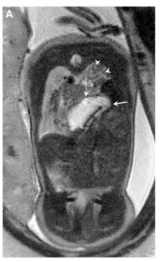

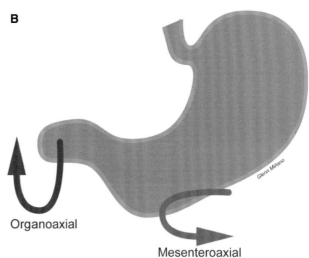

FIGURE 25.2-10: Left congenital diaphragmatic hernia with stomach up. **A:** Coronal MRI in a fetus at 22 weeks. *Dotted arrow* points to the greater curvature of the stomach, now oriented superiorly, consistent organoaxial rotation. *Solid arrow* demonstrates the antrum directed to the left consistent with mesenteroaxial rotation. *Arrowheads* show collapsed dark tubular bowel. **B:** Diagram of the stomach demonstrating organoaxial and mesenteroaxial rotation.

except the left colon, is intrathoracic. Depending on GA, the small bowel will appear as tubular dark structures earlier in pregnancy or as fluid-filled loops later (Fig. 25.2-11), and the large bowel will have variable meconium T1 hyperintensity and T2 hypointensity (Fig. 25.2-12). In most cases, the bowel is abnormally rotated. If the stomach is herniated, the spleen is typically also intrathoracic and tends to lie adjacent to the stomach, likely because of intact gastrosplenic ligaments (Fig. 25.2-13). The liver is herniated in approximately 50% of cases, and the left lobe, contiguous with the intra-abdominal liver, will extend for variable degrees into the anterior left thorax and, in the presence of severe herniation, into the right thorax. T1 imaging helps verify liver positioning (Fig. 25.2-14). Fetal MRI may also identify displacement of

the left adrenal and/or kidney into the lower posterior thorax (Fig. 25.2-15).

In Right CDH, the right lobe of the liver is always herniated into the right chest. The gallbladder may be displaced into the right upper abdomen or into the right lower thorax. LH in a right CDH can result in liver lock, in which the herniated liver is constricted by the diaphragm remnants.[24,25] In this instance, hepatic venous obstruction and liver edema develop in the herniated liver. On fetal MRI, this is manifested as an increased T2 signal in the herniated liver when compared with the intra-abdominal portion. This phenomenon of liver lock and resulting hepatic congestion may explain the development of ipsilateral pleural effusion and ascites in right CDH (Fig. 25.2-16).[16]

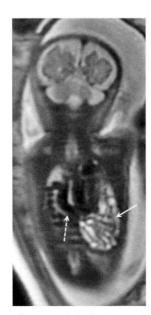

FIGURE 25.2-11: Left congenital diaphragmatic hernia with fluid-filled bowel. Coronal T2 MRI of fetus at gestational age of 33 weeks with fluid-filled small bowel (*solid arrow*). Notice dark T2 signal meconium in herniated colon (*dotted arrow*).

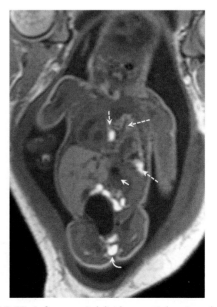

FIGURE 25.2-12: Left congenital diaphragmatic hernia and meconium. Coronal T1 MRI of fetus at 32 weeks with stomach down (*short arrow*). Meconium can be seen in multiple bowel loops in the left chest (*dashed arrows*) and in the rectum (*curved arrow*).

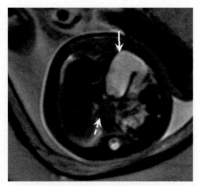

FIGURE 25.2-13: Left congenital diaphragmatic hernia and herniated spleen. Axial MRI shows herniated stomach (*solid arrow*). Near the stomach in the prespinal area is a wedge-shaped T2 hypointense tissue consistent with herniated spleen (*dashed arrow*).

Bilateral CDH is well delineated on fetal MRI as the liver is easily discriminated from the lung despite the absence of cardio-mediastinal shift (Fig. 25.2-17).[25]

Sac-type hernias, which generally have a better prognosis, can be suggested by the presence of a well-defined rounded border of the hernia capped superiorly by normal lung.[26,27] A sac may also be supported by pleural or peritoneal fluid lining the membrane of the hernia (Fig. 25.2-18).[26,28] Sensitivity and specificity for a single finding suggestive of hernia sac is 48% and 97%, respectively.[27]

On fetal MRI, lung signal in the presence of a CDH is typically not as T2 hyperintense as is expected for GA because of hypoplasia and compression.[29] If there is a dilated proximal esophageal segment with polyhydramnios, esophageal atresia and tracheoesophageal fistula may be present. MRI is also helpful in defining associated anomalies, including lung lesions that can be seen in conjunction with CDH (Fig. 25.2-19).[30,31]

Differential Diagnosis: Differential diagnosis for a fetal intrathoracic mass includes congenital lung malformation, primary lung tumor, and mediastinal mass such as teratoma or lymphatic malformation. Pulmonary agenesis/hypoplasia can present with displacement of the heart into one hemithorax

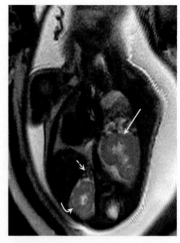

FIGURE 25.2-15: Left congenital diaphragmatic hernia with kidney up. Coronal MRI of a fetus at 32 weeks' gestation with left kidney (*solid arrow*) partly herniated. Right adrenal (*dashed arrow*) and right kidney (*curved arrow*) are within the abdomen.

with the absent/small lung and may mimic CDH. Diaphragmatic eventrations, especially when large, may be difficult to distinguish from CDH.

Associated Anomalies: Associated anomalies occur commonly in CDH, in as many as 40% of cases. In those cases associated with stillbirth or intrauterine demise, this figure rises to 95%.[32] Anomalies identified commonly include, in descending order of frequency: cardiac, renal, central nervous system, and gastrointestinal.[33] Sequestrations of the lung have been associated in less than 5% of CDH cases.[26] Cardiac anomalies have been noted in 15% of CDH patients.[34]

Prognosis: In a large multicenter retrospective study, the overall survival of CDH was 71%. Patients with CDH diagnosed prenatally had lower survival at 65% in comparison to those whose CDH was only diagnosed postnatally (83% survival).[35] This difference is felt

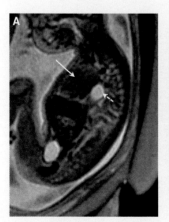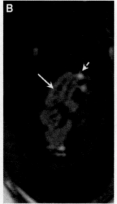

FIGURE 25.2-14: Left congenital diaphragmatic hernia with liver up. **A:** Sagittal T2 MRI. Notice liver (*solid arrow*) herniated in the anterior chest. The stomach (*dashed arrow*) is posterior to the liver. **B:** Sagittal T1 MRI in same fetus as in **(A)**. *Solid arrow* indicates herniated liver, mildly hyperintense on the T1 imaging. *Dashed arrow* indicates higher T1 signal meconium-filled bowel within the thorax.

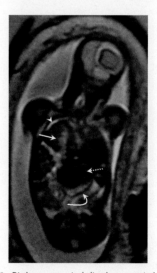

FIGURE 25.2-16: Right congenital diaphragmatic hernia with liver lock. Coronal T2 MRI in a 28-week fetus. *Solid arrow* points to an edematous portal triad within the herniated liver. Notice that the herniated liver demonstrates higher T2 signal than intra-abdominal liver (*dotted arrow*). *Arrowhead* shows small pleural effusion likely related to hepatic venous obstruction. *Curved arrow* identifies the stomach within the abdomen.

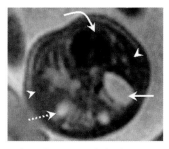

FIGURE 25.2-17: Bilateral congenital diaphragmatic hernia. Axial MRI of same fetus as in Figure 25.2-9. *Curved arrow* shows a relatively normally positioned heart. In the left thorax, the *solid arrow* identifies stomach. In the right thorax, *dotted arrow* indicates gallbladder. *Arrowheads* demarcate herniated liver in both thoracic cavities.

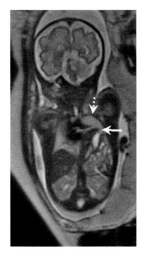

FIGURE 25.2-18: Sac-type left congenital diaphragmatic hernia. Coronal MRI demonstrates that the superior border of the hernia is rounded and well defined (*solid arrow*), and there is a "cap" of left lung tissue (*dotted arrow*) consistent with sac-type hernia.

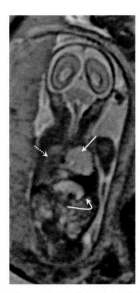

FIGURE 25.2-19: Left congenital diaphragmatic hernia with lung lesion. Coronal MRI of fetus at 23 weeks with left CDH containing stomach and liver (*curved arrow*). There is a T2 hyperintense lung lesion (*solid arrow*) in the left upper chest that demonstrates higher signal than normal right lung (*dotted arrow*).

to reflect higher prenatal detection rates for more severe hernias compared to those that are less severe; for example, a relatively minor CDH without liver and stomach herniation might be missed on prenatal imaging and not detected until postnatal life when the infant develops respiratory symptoms. Differences in outcome may also reflect cases in which the fetus was stillborn or did not make it to transfer to an appropriate referral center. It is therefore important to determine which fetuses are likely to have a poor prognosis and will need immediate support (Table 25.2-3).

The identification of *additional anomalies* is imperative as these fetuses have an overall poor prognosis, with survival

TABLE 25.2-3	Markers of Poor Prognosis

US/MRI Anatomic Markers

Additional anomalies
Stomach up in L CDH
Liver up
Bilateral CDH

Pulmonary Hypoplasia

US Tools

Lung
  LHR < 1
  o/e LHR < 25%
  3D o/e TFLV < 35%
Pulmonary artery
  Low o/e PA ratios

MRI Tools

Lung
  o/e TFLV < 25%
  PPLV < 15%
  Late gestation TLV < 20 mL
Liver
  LiTR ≥ 20%
  %LH > 20%

Pulmonary Hypertension

US Tools

Doppler waveform
  PI > 1
  PEDRF > 3.5
Maternal hyperoxygenation
  HPVR ≤ 20% PI
Power Doppler
  <3 divisions PA branching
  3D o/e perfusion indices <25%
  Lower FMBV

MRI Tools

Modified McGoon
  MMG < 1
Diffusion (?)

3D, three-dimensional; CDH, congenital diaphragmatic hernia; FMBV, fractional moving blood volume; HPVR, hyperoxygenation test for pulmonary vascular reactivity; L, left; LHR, lung head ratio; LiTR, liver to thoracic volume ratio; MMG, modified McGoon ratio; MRI, magnetic resonance imaging; o/e, observed-to-expected ratio; PA, pulmonary artery; PEDRF, peak end diastolic reversed flow; PI, pulsatility index; PPLV, percent predicted lung volume; TFLV, total fetal lung volume; TLV, total lung volume; US, ultrasound.

ranging between 50% for genetic syndromes and 30% for fetuses with CDH in conjunction with major cardiac anomalies.[36] In the presence of *diaphragmatic agenesis*, a worse outcome has been cited.[37] *Bilateral hernias* have a guarded prognosis with survival at highest 30% to 35%.[19,20,38] Right-sided hernias have been previously suggested to have less,[39] no different,[22] and increased morbidity with regard to left hernias.[40] A sac-type hernia has improved outcome.[25,27]

The position of the liver is one of the most important prognostic factors, as the liver up is associated with survival rates of 45% and liver down with 74%.[41,42] The existence of the *stomach in the chest* in a left CDH patient has a worse outcome, versus a survival rate of 90% to 100% when the stomach is intra-abdominal.[42–45] Hydrothorax and ascites have not shown to affect outcome, but may be a source for worsening pulmonary hypoplasia if large, and in the presence of cardiac/venous compression, can be lethal.[15,16,33] Several US markers remain controversial, including diagnosis prior to 25 weeks' gestation, polyhydramnios, and left ventricular hypoplasia/disproportion.[42,43,46] Ultimately, prognosis is related to multiple factors, some of which are likely more important than others, and this is the subject of ongoing research.

US Prognostic Tools: *Pulmonary hypoplasia* is an important factor in the survival of a patient with CDH. The *LHR* or *lung-to-head ratio* is an US tool that was devised to predict the severity of pulmonary hypoplasia and fetal outcome. The measurement is obtained by quantifying the area of the lung contralateral to the hernia at the level of the four-chamber view of the heart and then, to standardize for body size, dividing the product (in square millimeters) by head circumference in millimeters. In 1996, Metkus et al.[43] described the technique and showed that a fetus with CDH and LHR less than 0.6 did not survive despite postnatal therapy. In 2003, Laudy et al.[47] demonstrated that fetuses with CDH and LHR less than 1 had 100% mortality, whereas those with LHR greater than 1.4 had 100% survival. Recent studies have suggested that the LHR is most reliable at predicting outcome when performed between 24 and 34 weeks.[48]

Three LHR techniques have been described. Using the original University of California San Francisco method, the largest transverse dimension of the contralateral lung is drawn parallel to the sternum at the level of the four-chambered heart.

The largest anterior to posterior (AP) measurement is then obtained by drawing a line perpendicular to the transverse (Fig. 25.2-20A). The second technique quantifies the longest measurement, regardless of plane, and then multiplies by longest orthogonal dimension (Fig. 25.2-20B). The third method is a tracing technique in which the outline of the contralateral lung is performed at the level of the four-chambered heart (Fig. 25.2-20C). When comparing the three techniques, the lung tracing method has been shown be the most reproducible and accurate in predicting survival.[40,49]

Since lung growth increases between 12 and 32 weeks at a rate of four times the head circumference, it has been suggested that the LHR should be expressed as a ratio divided by the mean LHR of the same lung in a normal fetus for a given GA.[49,50] The expected lung-to-head ratio (eLHR) is obtained by an equation devised for GA, and the observed-to-expected (o/e) LHR ratio is then multiplied by 100 to obtain a percentage (Table 25.2-4).[51] In other words, an LHR of 1.3 at 24 weeks' gestation and an LHR of 1.3 at 34 weeks' gestation are not equivalent, so translating those numbers into percentages of expected (o/e) LHR allows for more realistic representation of the severity of mass effect and pulmonary hypoplasia. Using this technique, it has been demonstrated that fetuses with left intrapleural CDH and o/e LHR less than 15% have *extreme* pulmonary hypoplasia with virtually no survivors, those between 15% and 25% have *severe* pulmonary hypoplasia with survival of 20%, those between 26% and 35% or 36% and 45% with liver up are *moderate* with expected survival of 30% to 60%, and those with ratios 36% to 45% with liver down or greater than 45% have *mild* hypoplasia and a survival of greater than 75%.[52] For simplification, most utilize an o/e LHR of less than 25% as at risk for severe pulmonary hypoplasia (see Table 25.2-3).[51,53]

The primary measurement for LHR is dependent on obtaining a true transverse plane of the fetal chest at the level of the four-chambered heart. Many have questioned the accuracy, stating that there can be difficulty in reproducibility.[54,55] In addition, LHR underestimates the actual total lung volume and leaves a significant group of fetuses between the two extremes in the "gray" area. For this reason, some centers do not routinely perform LHR. Most that do note that there is a learning curve and that education of the technique is best taught in experienced referral centers.[56,57]

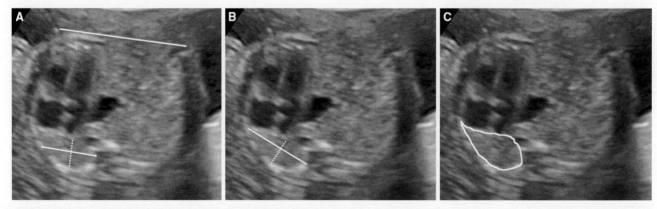

FIGURE 25.2-20: Lung-to-head ratio techniques. **A:** San Francisco method: axial US at level of four-chamber heart in a fetus with left congenital diaphragmatic hernia. The *long solid line* represents line drawn parallel to sternum. Transverse right lung dimension demarcated by the *shorter solid line* is parallel to the sternal line. Perpendicular anteroposterior (AP) measurement is shown with *dotted line*. **B:** Longest-axis method: maximum transverse dimension (*solid line*) with AP drawn perpendicular (*dotted line*). **C:** Tracing method: the circumference of the right lung is traced.

TABLE 25.2-4   Important Prognosticator Equations

Ultrasound

LHR[49]

Right eLHR $= -2.2481 + (0.2712 \times GA) - (0.0033 \times GA^2)$

Left eLHR $= -1.4815 + (0.1824 \times GA) - (0.0023 \times GA^2)$

3D US TFLV[61]

eTFLV (mL) $= \exp(4.72/(1 + \exp(20.32 - GA)/6.05))$

Pulmonary arteries[65]

MPA (mm) $= -2.77 + (0.30 \times GA)$

RPA (mm) $= -1.71 + (0.18 \times GA)$

LPA (mm) $= -1.95 + (0.19 \times GA)$

Doppler waveform

PI: P50th: $Y = 0.537 + (0.246 \times GA) - (0.005 \times GA^2)$

SD: 0.57

PEDRF (cm/s): P50th: $Y = -7.465 + (1.049 \times GA) - (0.015 \times GA^2)$

SD: $Y = -7.128 + (0.56 \times GA) - (0.008 \times GA^2)$

MRI

TLV or TFLV[76,79]

By GA eFLV (mL) $= 0.0033 \times (GA)^{2.86}$

By GA eFLV (mL) $= 0.000865 \times (GA)^{3.254}$

By FBV eFLV (mL) $= (0.04 \times FBV) + 3.82$

3D US, three-dimensional ultrasound; FBV, fetal body volume; GA, gestational age in weeks; LHR, lung to head circumference ratio; LPA, left pulmonary artery; MRI, magnetic resonance imaging; MPA, main pulmonary artery; PI, pulsatility index; RPA, right pulmonary artery; SD, standard deviation; TLV or TFLV, total (fetal) lung volume.

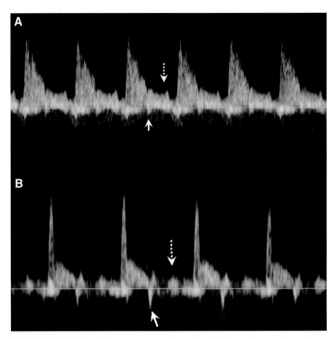

FIGURE 25.2-21: Pulmonary artery Doppler. **A:** Doppler waveform from a normal fetus. There is small peak early diastolic reversed flow (PEDRF; *solid arrow*) and antegrade diastolic flow (*dotted arrow*). **B:** Doppler waveform from a fetus with left congenital diaphragmatic hernia and liver up. The PEDRF is increased (*solid arrow*). There is intermittent loss of diastolic flow (*dotted arrow*).

Three-dimensional ultrasound (3D US) has been utilized in fetuses with CDH. Using nomograms of normal 3D US lung volume (Table 28 in Appendix A1), a fetus with CDH and 3D US o/e total fetal lung volume (TFLV) less than 35% has been shown to predict survival, even more accurately than does contralateral 3D US lung volume or LHR (see Tables 25.2-3 and 25.2-4).[58–60] However, comparative studies have demonstrated that the 3D US technique is suboptimal to LHR and MR lung volumes, as in up to 45% of cases, it is difficult to measure ipsilateral lung on US, and measurements are consistently 25% lower than those obtained from MRI.[61]

Prenatal pulmonary artery (PA) measurements have been performed at the hila at the level of the four-chamber view of the heart. Although intuitively it was thought to reflect pulmonary hypertension, it has been documented that these measurements more likely reflect lung mass.[62] Measuring the main, right, and left PAs and comparing with normal fetuses via the o/e ratio showed a significant reduction in the measurements in those fetuses with CDH and pulmonary hypoplasia (see Tables 25.2-3 and 25.2-4).[63,64]

Although predicting pulmonary hypoplasia is important, it is well known that despite adequate lung volumes some infants die of pumonary arterial hypertension (PAH). *Doppler waveform analysis* has proved helpful to further stratify infants, defining the most severe CDH cases at risk for lung hypoplasia and PAH. Increased PA pulsatility index (PI) and especially peak early diastolic reversed flow (PEDRF) in the right and left PA branches have been found not only to correlate with lung growth in fetuses but also reflect high resistance in the pulmonary vascular bed and preferential flow through the ductus arteriosus

(Fig. 25.2-21).[65] In the presence of o/e LHR less than 26%, PI and PEDRF transformed to Z-score (Z-score = [measured fetus − mean$_{GA}$]/SD$_{GA}$) documented limited survival after fetoscopic tracheal occlusion (FETO) when the PI is greater than 1 and PEDRF is greater than 3.5.[61,65]

Maternal hyperoxygenation, with oxygen provided at 60%, can normally lower fetal pulmonary arterial resistance in the third trimester. The hyperoxygenation test for pulmonary vascular reactivity (HPVR) performed in fetuses with CDH at 31 to 36 weeks and after fetoscopic occlusion therapy demonstrated a good outcome when a reactive test, greater than or equal to 20% reductions in PA pretest PI, was noted.[66,67]

Power Doppler may also provide important information about changes in lung tissue perfusion. When the contralateral lung is evaluated at the level of the four-chamber view of the heart, PAH has been predicted if there is visualization of less than three divisions of vascular branching on 2D US or when 3D volume-rendered perfusion indices compared with normal were less than 25%.[68,69] However, these methods are qualitative or limited by lack of correction for attenuation and depth or variation in power Doppler setting.[67] *Fractional moving blood volume (FMBV)* is a quantitative technique that depicts the percentage of moving blood in a specific region of interest (ROI).[70] Decreased FMBV has been shown to correlate with decreased lung growth and increased intrapulmonary artery impedance in CDH and has proved helpful in evaluating the potential of survival after tracheal occlusion, with delayed imaging documenting a ≥30% of FMBV, ≥50% LHR change, and 100% survival.[71,72]

MRI Prognostic Tools: MRI imaging has become a well-documented technique when evaluating for *pulmonary hypoplasia*. The least validated method is the use of *lung signal intensity*, as a compressed and hypoplastic lung demonstrates decreased signal when compared with a normal lung for GA. Fetal lung-to-liver signal intensity ratio (LLSIR) has been shown to increase with GA; however, recent literature has shown that the ratio is not useful when predicting CDH outcome.[69,73]

Volumetric analysis of the lung with MRI has become the method of choice to obtain *total fetal lung volume (TLV or TFLV)*. MRI-derived TFLV is utilized to predict severity of hypoplasia in CDH and response to fetoscopic occlusion therapy. Several researchers have developed GA-based nomograms of lung volumes with 3D processing (Tables 31 and 32 in Appendix A1).[74-80]

When describing fetal lung volume in CDH, the amount of lung present in the fetus with CDH is often related to expected lung volumes from normal fetuses, most commonly those that reflect normal volumes for GA or fetal body volume.[77] Multiple researchers have noted a strong correlation with outcome when utilizing these ratios, known as *relative fetal lung volume (rFLV)* or *observed to expected total fetal lung volume (o/e TFLV)*. Paek et al.[78] found that an rFLV less than 40% suggested poor outcome, whereas Datin-Dorriere et al.[42] noted an rFLV cutoff at 30%. Gorincour et al.[80] and Jani et al.[81] noted poor survival in those fetuses in which the o/e TFLV was less than 25%.

Regression analyses of GA-based data have led to the creation of formulae to predict expected lung volumes at various GAs. The use of nomograms or formulae to obtain expected lung volume varies by institution, and the method used should be decided with input from the entire fetal care team, including pediatric surgeons and maternal fetal medicine specialists. The more recent publication from Meyers et al. was powered by a larger number of early second-trimester fetuses, resulting in lower expected FLV in fetuses between 18 and 22 weeks' GA than predicted by earlier studies, so that data is preferred for calculating rFLV or o/e TFLV in the early second trimester.[76,79]

An innovative technique to standardize lung volume includes the *percent predicted lung volume (PPLV)*, a calculation that utilizes the mediastinal volume subtracted from the total thoracic volume to estimate expected lung volume (Fig. 25.2-22). The PPLV is obtained by dividing the actual lung volume in the CDH fetus by this estimated lung volume.[82] Barnewolt et al.[82] found that fetuses with PPLV of less than 15% had 40% survival, whereas fetuses with PPLV of greater than 20% had 100% survival.

The rFLV or o/e TFLV ratios have also been compared with TFLV, with studies demonstrating that both techniques are equally predictable of survival and morbidity in CDH.[83,84] Because lung growth is accelerated later in gestation, some hypothesized that MRI fetal lung volumes later in gestation, at 34 to 35 weeks, may be a better gauge of outcome and need for postnatal support. Lee et al.[85] noted that a late gestation TLV of less than 20 mL was associated with 35% survival and 86% extracorporeal membrane oxygenation (ECMO) utilization, whereas those above 40 mL had a survival of 90%, with only 10% needing ECMO.

Despite different methodologies and GA at time of assessment, there remain questions regarding the validity of volumetric analysis. Assessment of normal fetal lung volume literature demonstrates that there is no standardization of the technique, including pulse sequence parameters, plane of imaging to assess volume, and ROI with inclusion or exclusion of pulmonary hila.[86] In defense, studies directed at obtaining MR lung volumetry in CDH cases demonstrated good interobserver reliability, independent of sequence or imaging plane.[79,87]

Since MRI easily discriminates liver from lung, the technique is extremely helpful in confirming liver up or down morphology. *Volumetric analysis of the liver* with fetal MRI has been performed and compared as a ratio or percentage with total thoracic volume. This liver-to-thoracic ratio (LiTR) was predictive of postnatal survival in CDH, with neonatal death more likely when greater than or equal to 20% of fetal thoracic volume was occupied by the liver.[88,89] Another method of quantifying LH involves reporting intrathoracic liver volume as a ratio to total liver volume, or percent liver herniation (%LH). This ratio was also shown to predict mortality, pulmonary morbidity, and need for ECMO when %LH was greater than 20%.[90,91]

Fetal MRI may be helpful in the prediction of *PAH*. The modified McGoon (MMG) index, previously described as a US technique, has also been performed on late gestation fetal MRI. On an axial T2 image, maximum diameters are obtained of the right and left PA and aorta at the level of the diaphragm (Fig. 25.2-23). Vuletin et al.[92] found that an index greater than 1 correlated with severe postnatal pulmonary hypertension at 3 weeks of age.

Diffusion imaging may also hold promise in providing functional information with regard to lung development, since the apparent diffusion coefficient (ADC) measurement reveals capillary perfusion and water diffusion in the extravascular space. In the presence of CDH, however, a difference in the ADC values compared with normal fetuses did not predict survival and did not correlate with fetal lung volume.[93] These findings may reflect the limitations of the technique, which include high sensitivity to fetal motion, lower signal, and longer scan times.

Management: Prenatal surgical intervention for CDH has been evaluated for years with first attempts at open repair failing because of kinking of the umbilical vein during liver reduction and preterm labor from uterine irritability. Utilizing fetal sheep with CDH, it was proved that tracheal obstruction accelerated lung growth and pushed viscera back into the abdomen, resulting in significant improvement in outcome (Fig. 25.2-24).[94] Because of these experiments, tracheal occlusion in the human fetus was first attempted as an open fetal procedure with placement of a clip across the trachea and then via fetoscopic placement of a

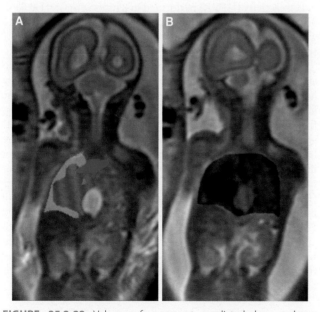

FIGURE 25.2-22: Volumes for percent predicted lung volume. **A:** Coronal MRI with superimposed 3D rendered lung volume of the right lung (*orange*), left lung (*blue*), and mediastinal volume (*pink*) in a fetus with left congenital diaphragmatic hernia. **B:** Coronal MRI with superimposed 3D total thoracic volume.

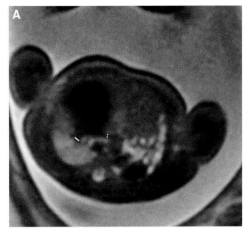
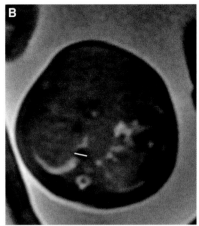

FIGURE 25.2-23: Modified McGoon index. **A:** The right (*solid line*) and left (*dotted line*) pulmonary artery transverse dimensions obtained on an axial MRI in a fetus with left congenital diaphragmatic hernia. **B:** The transverse dimension of the descending aorta (*line*) at the level of the diaphragm.

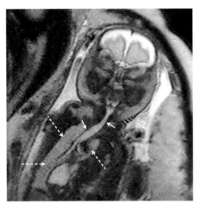

FIGURE 25.2-24: Tracheal balloon occlusion in congenital diaphragmatic hernia. Coronal T2 MRI shows dilatation of the airway (*solid arrow*) and hyperintense lungs (*dashed arrows*) because of balloon tracheal occlusion. (Image courtesy of Chris Cassady, MD.)

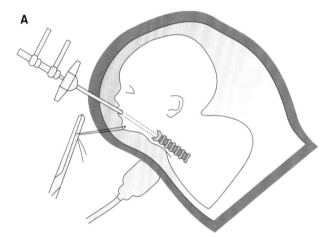
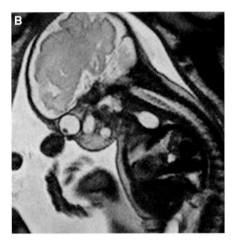

FIGURE 25.2-25: Fetoscopic endotracheal balloon occlusion. **A:** The diagram demonstrates placement of the balloon into the trachea under ultrasound guidance. **B:** Corresponding sagittal T2 MRI shows the balloon (*arrow*) positioned in the trachea. (Image courtesy of Chris Cassady, MD.)

detachable endoluminal balloon.[95] This early randomized trial, however, was terminated when it was found that the standard care group had the same 90-day survival (77%) as the tracheal occlusion group (73%).

Fetoscopic endotracheal occlusion (FETO) has reemerged and is currently performed via balloon occlusion (Fig. 25.2-25).[96] The surgery is offered to those CDH fetuses with extreme or severe hypoplasia represented by an LHR less than 1 and/or o/e LHR less than 25% with LH. The balloon is inserted at 26 to 28 weeks and then removed at 34 weeks. As with all fetal interventions, there is an increased risk of premature rupture of membranes. If preterm labor and delivery ensues, ex *utero intrapartum treatment* (EXIT) to balloon retrieval would be required. However, FETO has shown improved survival in severe left CDH from 24% with conventional therapy to 49% with FETO, and in severe right CDH from 0% to 35%, respectively.[97] Another similar study cited 52% survival in the severe CDH group treated with FETO compared to 5% with conservative therapy.[98] FETO has also been shown to improve PAH in survivors.[99] Major predictors for survival in FETO include GA at delivery and lung measurements (o/e TFLV and o/e LHR) pre-FETO.[52,53] An increase in lung volume after FETO was an independent variant for survival, while pulmonary vascular reactivity was a predictor for both survival and PAH.[53] Improvements in lung volume and growth after FETO for severe CDH may outweigh potential negative effects related to premature

delivery, as shown by similar survival in infants not eligible for FETO.[100] Future work is focused on prospective trials of FETO for both severe and moderate CDH, with a large international multicenter study under way (TOTAL, or Tracheal Occlusion To Accelerate Lung growth).

If the pregnancy is continued without prenatal intervention, US is recommended once a month prior to 32 weeks and at least weekly as term approaches. Close observation late in gestation is necessary to manage developing polyhydramnios and evaluate fetal well-being. Arrangements should be made for planned delivery at a tertiary care center with availability of neonatal intensive and surgical care at 39 weeks.

Prior to the 1990s, neonatal management of CDH included emergent repair followed by aggressive ventilation. Evidence now suggests that better outcome may be achieved by delivering at an experienced center and delaying surgery until acceptable hemodynamic and respiratory stability has been attained with nonaggressive mechanical ventilation.[101] Nonaggressive ventilation, also known as gentle ventilation or "gentilation," is aimed at reducing barotrauma and pneumothorax by limiting inflation pressure and preventing hyperventilation. Nitrous oxide is utilized to treat pulmonary hypertension, and prostaglandins are commonly administered to keep the ductus arteriosus patent, especially with severe right ventricular dysfunction.[2] ECMO is utilized in 15% to 54% of neonates with CDH and may be a rescue therapy after birth in those infants with significant pulmonary hypertension, hypoplasia, or ventilator lung injury.[102] In the presence of poor prognosticators, some centers have delivered the infant EXIT to ECMO; however, recent studies have shown no outcome benefit.[103,104] The decision to utilize ECMO has shifted to early use after delivery to achieve lung preservation when medical therapy has failed.

When appropriate respiratory and hemodynamic stability is achieved, surgical repair is currently favored to be done thoracoscopically rather than via thoracotomy.[105] In neonates with a large defect, a patch of synthetic or bioprosthetic material may be necessary to close the defect. Some centers will attempt repair of the defect while the infant remains on ECMO, a practice which has recently been shown to improve survival although not to shorten ECMO duration.[106]

The long-term outcome for these children remains complicated. Approximately 50% of these children have chronic respiratory disease.[52,105] Gastroesophageal reflux is frequent, and as many as 30% will have failure to thrive between 6 months and 2 years of life.[105] Neurodevelopmental deficits are possible, particularly when ECMO is required, but is also seen in 23% to 46% of children not requiring ECMO.[107] Sensorineural hearing loss is common.[52] Vertebral anomalies may originate because of abnormal fetal development, and chest asymmetry may persist into childhood and adolescence.[108]

Recurrence: Most cases are sporadic with recurrence risk at 2%, increasing to 10% in a family with two affected siblings.[3,7] Familial CDH inheritance is either multifactorial or autosomal recessive, but in the presence of diaphragmatic agenesis or bilateral CDH, autosomal recessive inheritance is likely.[7,52,108]

REFERENCES

1. Holder AM, Klaassens M, Tibboel D, et al. Genetic factors in congenital diaphragmatic hernia. *Am J Hum Genet.* 2007;80:825–845.
2. Deprest JA, Gratacos E, Nicolaides K, et al. Changing perspectives on the perinatal management of isolated congenital diaphragmatic hernia in Europe. *Clin Perinatol.* 2009;36:329–347.
3. Pober BR. Genetic aspects of human congenital diaphragmatic hernia. *Clin Genet.* 2008;74:1–15.
4. Babiuk RP, Greer JP. Diaphragm defects occur in a CDH hernia model independently of myogenesis and lung formation. *Am J Physiol Lung Cell Mol Physiol.* 2002;283:L1310–L1314.
5. Ackerman KG, Pober BR. Congenital diaphragmatic hernia and pulmonary hypoplasia: new insights from developmental biology and genetics. *Am J Med Genet C Semin Med Genet.* 2007;145C:105–108.
6. Tovar JA. Congenital diaphragmatic hernia. *Orphanet J Rare Dis.* 2012;7:1–15.
7. Nagase H, Ishikawa H, Kurosawa K, et al. Familial severe congenital diaphragmatic hernia: left herniation in one sibling and bilateral herniation in another. *Congenit Anom.* 2013;53:54–57.
8. Waag KL, Loff S, Zahn K, et al. Congenital diaphragmatic hernia: a modern day approach. *Semin Pediatr Surg.* 2008;17:244–254.
9. Goumy C, Gousas L, Marceau G, et al. Retinoid pathway and congenital diaphragmatic hernia: hypothesis from the analysis of chromosomal abnormalities. *Fetal Diagn Ther.* 2010;28:129–139.
10. Garne E, Haeusler M, Barisic I, et al. Congenital diaphragmatic hernia: evaluation of prenatal diagnosis in 20 European regions. *Ultrasound Obstet Gynecol.* 2002;19:329–333.
11. Howe DT, Kilby MD, Sirry H, et al. Structural chromosome anomalies in congenital diaphragmatic hernia. *Prenat Diagn.* 1996;16:P1003–P1009.
12. Claus F, Sandaite I, Dekoninck P, et al. Prenatal anatomical imaging in fetuses with congenital diaphragmatic hernia. *Fetal Diagn Ther.* 2011;29:88–100.
13. Guibaud L, Filiatrault D, Garel L, et al. Fetal congenital diaphragmatic hernia: accuracy of sonography in the diagnosis and prediction of the outcome after birth. *AJR Am J Roentgenol.* 1996;166:1195–1202.
14. Bianchi DW, Crombleholme TM, D'Alton ME, et al. *Fetology: Diagnosis and Management of the Fetal Patient.* 2nd ed. New York, NY: McGraw Hill Medical; 2010.
15. Mieghem TV, Cruz-Martinez R, Allegaerts K, et al. Outcome of fetuses with congenital diaphragmatic hernia and associated intrafetal fluid effusions managed in the era of fetal surgery. *Ultrasound Obstet Gynecol.* 2012;39:50–55.
16. Salmanian B, Shamshirsaz AA, Cass DL, et al. Fetal cardiac tamponade in a case of right-sided congenital diaphragmatic hernia. *Obstet Gynecol.* 2014;123:447–450.
17. Bootstaylor BS, Filly RA, Harrison MR. Prenatal sonographic predictors of liver herniation in congenital diaphragmatic hernia. *J Ultrasound Med.* 1995;14:515–520.
18. Song MS, Yoo SJ, Smallhorn JF, et al. Bilateral congenital diaphragmatic hernia: diagnostic clues at fetal sonography. *Ultrasound Obstet Gynecol.* 2001;17:255–258.
19. Kamata S, Sawai T, Usui N, et al. Bilateral diaphragmatic hernia followed by fetal ultrasonography. A report of two cases. *Fetal Diagn Ther.* 2001;16(4):248–250.
20. Eroglu D, Yanik F, Sakallioglu AE, et al. Prenatal diagnosis of bilateral diaphragmatic hernia by fetal sonography. *J Obstet Gynaecol Res.* 2006;32:90–93.
21. Neville HL, Jaksic T, Wilson JM, et al. Bilateral congenital diaphragmatic hernia. *J Pediatr Surg.* 2003;38:522–524.
22. Gallot D, Boda C, Ughetto S, et al. Prenatal detection and outcome of congenital diaphragramtic hernia: a French registry-based study. *Ultrasound Obstet Gynecol.* 2007;29:276–283.
23. Lewis DA, Reickert C, Bowerman R, et al. Prenatal ultrasonography frequently fails to diagnose congenital diaphragmatic hernia. *J Pediatr Surg.* 1997;32:352–356.
24. Leung JW, Coakley FV, Hricak H, et al. Prenatal MR imaging of congenital diaphragmatic hernia. *AJR Am J Roentgenol.* 2000;174:1607–1612.
25. Mehollin-Ray AR, Cassady CI, Cass DL, et al. Fetal MR imaging of congenital diaphragmatic hernia. *Radiographics.* 2012;32:1067–1084.
26. Zamora IJ, Mehollin-Ray AR, Sheikh F, et al. Predictive value of MRI findings for the identification of a hernia sac in fetuses with congenital diaphragmatic hernia. *AJR Am J Roentgenol.* 2015;205(5):1121–1125.
27. Oliver ER, DeBari SE, Adams SE, et al. Congenital diaphragmatic hernia sacs: prenatal imaging and associated postnatal outcomes. *Pediatr Radiol.* 2019;49:593–599.
28. Zamora IJ, Cass DL, Lee TC, et al. The presence of a hernia sac in congenital diaphragmatic hernia is associated with better fetal lung growth and outcomes. *J Pediatr Surg.* 2013;48(6):1165–1171.
29. Barth RA, Rubesova E. Fetal magnetic resonance imaging: anomalies of the neck, chest and abdomen. *Neoreviews.* 2007;8:e313–e335.
30. Hubbard AM, Crombleholme TM, Adzick NS, et al. Prenatal MRI evaluation of congenital diaphragmatic hernia. *Am J Perinatol.* 1999;16:407–413.
31. Hubbard AM, Adzick NS, Crombleholme TM, et al. Congenital chest lesions: diagnosis and characterization with prenatal MR imaging. *Radiology.* 1999;212:43–48.
32. Puri P, Gorman F. Lethal nonpulmonary anomalies associated with congenital diaphragmatic hernia: implications for early intrauterine surgery. *J Pediatr Surg.* 1984;19:29–32.
33. Graham G, Devine PC. Antenatal diagnosis of congenital diaphragmatic hernia. *Semin Perinatol.* 2005;29:69–76.
34. Ruano R, Javadian P, Kailin JA, et al. Congenital heart anomaly in newborns with congenital diaphragmatic hernia: a single-center experience. *Ultrasound Obstet Gynecol.* 2015;45(6):683–688.
35. Burgos CM, Frenckner B, Luco M, et al. Prenatally versus postnatally diagnosed congenital diaphragmatic hernia—side, stage, and outcome. *J Pediatr Surg.* 2019;54:651–655.
36. Akinkuotu AC, Cruz SM, Cass DL, et al. An evaluation of the role of concomitant anomalies on the outcomes of fetuses with congenital diaphragmatic hernia. *J Pediatr Surg.* 2016;51:714–717.
37. Gibbs DL, Rice HE, Farrell JA, et al. Familial diaphragmatic agenesis: an autosomal-recessive syndrome with a poor prognosis. *J Pediatr Surg.* 1997;32:366–368.
38. Hiasa KI, Fujita Y, Fukushima K, et al. Ultrasound and MR images of prenatally diagnosed bilateral congenital diaphragmatic hernia, a rare variation of CDH. *Clin Imaging.* 2012;36:639–642.

39. Hedrick HL, Crombleholme TM, Flake AW, et al. Right congenital diaphragmatic hernia. *J Pediatr Surg.* 2004;39:319–323.
40. Fisher JC, Jefferson RA, Arkovitz MS, et al. Redefining outcomes in right congenital diaphragmatic hernia. *J Pediatr Surg.* 2008;43:373–379.
41. Mullassery D, Ba'ath ME, Jesudason EC, et al. Value of liver herniation in prediction of outcome in fetal congenital diaphragmatic hernia: a systematic review of meta-analysis. *Ultrasound Obstet Gynecol.* 2010;35:609–614.
42. Datin-Dorriere V, Rouzies S, Taupin P, et al. Prenatal prognosis in isolated congenital diaphragmatic hernia. *Am J Obstet Gynecol.* 2008;198:80.e1–80.e5.
43. Metkus AP, Filly RA, Stringer MD, et al. Sonographic predictors of survival in fetal diaphragmatic hernia. *J Pediatr Surg.* 1996;31:148–152.
44. Hatch EI Jr, Kendall J, Blumhagen J. Stomach position as an in utero predictor of neonatal outcome in left-sided diaphragmatic hernia. *J Pediatr Surg.* 1992;27:776–779.
45. Hedrick HL, Danzer E, Merchant A. Liver position and lung-to-head ratio for prediction of extracorporeal membrane oxygenation and survival in isolated left congenital diaphragmatic hernia. *Am J Obstet Gynecol.* 2007;197:422.e1–422.e4.
46. Thebaud B, Azancot A, de Lagausie P. Congenital diaphragmatic hernia: antenatal prognostic factors: does cardiac ventricular disproportion in utero predict outcome and pulmonary hypoplasia? *Intensive Care Med.* 1997;23:1062–1069.
47. Laudy JA, Van Gucht M, Dooren MF, et al. Congenital diaphragmatic hernia: an evaluation of the prognostic value of the lung-to-head ratio and other prenatal parameters. *Prenat Diagn.* 2003;23:634–639.
48. Yang SH, Nobuhara KK, Keller RL, et al. Reliability of the lung-to-head ratio as a predictor of outcome in fetuses with isolated left congenital diaphragmatic hernia at gestation outside 24–26 weeks. *Am J Obstet Gynecol.* 2007;197:30.e1–30.e7.
49. Peralta CF, Cavoretto P, Csapo B, et al. Assessment of lung area in normal fetuses at 12–32 weeks. *Ultrasound Obstet Gynecol.* 2005;26:718–724.
50. Jani JC, Peralta CF, Ruano R, et al. Comparison of fetal lung area to head circumference ratio with lung volume in the prediction of postnatal outcome in diaphragmatic hernia. *Ultrasound Obstet Gynecol.* 2007;30:850–854.
51. Jani J, Nicolaides KH, Keller RL, et al. Observed to expected lung area to head circumference ratio in the prediction of survival in fetuses with isolated diaphragmatic hernia. *Ultrasound Obstet Gynecol.* 2007;30:67–71.
52. Deprest JA, Flemmer AW, Gratacos E, et al. Antenatal prediction of lung volume and in-utero treatment by fetal endoscopic tracheal occlusion in severe isolated congenital diaphragmatic hernia. *Semin Fetal Neonatal Med.* 2009;14:8–13.
53. Jani JC, Nicolaides KH, Gratacos E, et al. Fetal lung-to-head ratio in the prediction of survival in severe left-sided diaphragmatic hernia treated by fetal endoscopic tracheal occlusion (FETO). *Am J Obstet Gynecol.* 2006;195:1646–1650.
54. Arkovitz MS, Russo M, Devine P. Fetal lung-head ratio is not related to outcome for antenatal diagnosed congenital diaphragmatic hernia. *J Pediatr Surg.* 2007;42:107–111.
55. Ba'ath ME, Jesudason EC, Losty PD. How useful is the lung-to-head ratio in predicting outcome in the fetus with congenital diaphragmatic hernia? A systematic review and meta-analysis. *Ultrasound Obstet Gynecol.* 2007;30:897–906.
56. Britto IS, Sananes N, Olutoye O, et al. Standardization of sonographic lung-to-head ratio measurements in isolated congenital diaphragmatic hernia: impact on the reproducibility and efficacy to predict outcomes. *J Ultrasound Med.* 2015;34:1721–1727.
57. Cruz-Martinez R, Figueras F, Moreno-Alvarez O. Learning curve for lung area to head circumference ratio measurement in fetuses with congenital diaphragmatic hernia. *Ultrasound Obstet Gynecol.* 2010;36:32–36.
58. Ruano R, Takashi E, Da Silva MM, et al. Prediction and probability of neonatal outcome in isolated congenital diaphragmatic hernia using multiple ultrasound parameters. *Ultrasound Obstet Gynecol.* 2012;39:42–49.
59. Ruano R, Benachi A, Joubin L, et al. Three-dimensional ultrasonographic assessment of fetal lung volume as a prognostic factor in isolated congenital diaphragmatic hernia. *BJOG.* 2004;111:423–429.
60. Ruano R, Aubry MC, Barthe B, et al. Three-dimensional sonographic measurement of contralateral lung volume in fetuses with isolated congenital diaphragmatic hernia. *J Clin Ultrasound.* 2008;36:273–278.
61. Jani JC, Cannie M, Peralta CFA, et al. Lung volumes in fetuses with congenital diaphragmatic hernia: comparison of 3D US and MR imaging assessments. *Radiology.* 2007;244:575–582.
62. Sokol J, Bohn D, Lacro RV, et al. Fetal pulmonary artery diameters and their association with lung hypoplasia and postnatal outcome in congenital diaphragmatic hernia. *Am J Obstet Gynecol.* 2002;186:1085–1090.
63. Ruano R, de Fatima M, Maeda Y, et al. Pulmonary artery diameters in healthy fetuses from 19 to 40 weeks' gestation. *J Ultrasound Med.* 2007;26:309–316.
64. Ruano R, Aubry MC, Barthe B, et al. Predicting perinatal outcome in isolated congenital diaphragmatic hernia using fetal pulmonary artery diameters. *J Pediatr Surg.* 2008;43:606–611.
65. Moreno-Alvarez O, Hernandez-Andrade E, Oros D, et al. Association between intrapulmonary arterial Doppler parameters and degree of lung growth as measured by lung-to-head ratio in fetuses with congenital diaphragmatic hernia. *Ultrasound Obstet Gynecol.* 2008;31:164–170.
66. Broth RE, Wood DC, Rasanen J, et al. Prenatal prediction of lethal pulmonary hypoplasia: the hyperoxygenation test for pulmonary artery reactivity. *Am J Obstet Gynecol.* 2002;187:940–945.
67. Cruz-Martinez R, Hernandez-Andrade E, Moreno-Alvarez O, et al. Prognostic value of pulmonary Doppler to predict response to tracheal occlusion in fetuses with congenital diaphragmatic hernia. *Fetal Diagn Ther.* 2011;29:18–24.
68. Ruano R, Aubry MC, Barthe B, et al. Quantitative analysis of fetal pulmonary vasculature by 3-dimensional power Doppler ultrasonography in isolated congenital diaphragmatic hernia. *Am J Obstet Gynecol.* 2006;195:1720–1728.
69. Mahieu-Caputo D, Aubry MC, El Sayed M, et al. Evaluation of fetal pulmonary vasculature by power Doppler imaging in congenital diaphragmatic hernia. *J Ultrasound Med.* 2004;23:1011–1017.
70. Hernandez-Andrade E, Thuring-Jonsson A, Jasson T, et al. Fractional moving blood volume estimation in the fetal lung using power Doppler ultrasound: a reproducibility study. *Ultrasound Obstet Gynecol.* 2004;23:369–373.
71. Moreno-Alvarez O, Cruz-Martinez R, Hernandez-Andrade E, et al. Lung tissue perfusion in congenital diaphragmatic hernia and association with the lung-to-head ratio and intrapulmonary artery pulsed Doppler. *Ultrasound Obstet Gynecol.* 2010;35:578–582.
72. Cruz-Martinez R, Moreno-Alvarez O, Hernandez-Andrade E, et al. Changes in lung tissue perfusion in the prediction of survival in fetuses with congenital diaphragmatic hernia treated with fetal endoscopic tracheal occlusion. *Fetal Diagn Ther.* 2011;29:101–107.
73. Brewerton LJ, Chair RS, Liang Y, et al. Fetal lung-to-liver signal intensity ratio at MR imaging: development of a normal scale and possible role in predicting pulmonary hypoplasia in utero. *Radiology.* 2005;235:1005–1010.
74. Balass C, Kasprian G, Brugger PC, et al. Assessment of lung development in isolated congenital diaphragmatic hernia using signal intensity ratios on fetal imaging. *Eur Radiol.* 2010;20:829–837.
75. Coakley FV, Lopoo JB, Lu Y, et al. Normal and hypoplastic fetal lungs: volumetric assessment with prenatal signal-shot rapid acquisition with relaxation enhancement MR imaging. *Radiology.* 2000;216:107–111.
76. Rypens F, Metens T, Rocourt N, et al. Fetal lung volume: estimation at MR imaging—initial results. *Radiology.* 2001;219:236–241.
77. Cannie M, Jani JC, DeKeyzer F, et al. Fetal body volume: use at MR imaging to quantify relative lung volume in fetuses suspected of having pulmonary hypoplasia. *Radiology.* 2006;241:847–853.
78. Paek BW, Coakley FV, Lu Y, et al. Congenital diaphragmatic hernia: prenatal evaluation with MR lung volumetry: preliminary experience. *Radiology.* 2001;220:63–67.
79. Meyers ML, Garcia JR, Blough KL, et al. Fetal lung volumes by MRI: normal weekly values from 18 through 38 weeks' gestation. *AJR Am J Roentgenol.* 2018;211:432–438.
80. Gorincour G, Bouvenot J, Mourot MG, et al. Prenatal prognosis of congenital diaphragmatic hernia using magnetic resonance imaging measurement of fetal lung volume. *Ultrasound Obstet Gynecol.* 2005;26:738–744.
81. Jani J, Cannie M, Sonigo P, et al. Value of prenatal magnetic resonance imaging in the prediction of postnatal outcome in fetuses with diaphragmatic hernia. *Ultrasound Obstet Gynecol.* 2008;32:791–799.
82. Barnewolt CE, Kunisaki SM, Fauza DO, et al. Percent predicted lung volumes as measured on fetal magnetic resonance imaging: a useful biometric parameter for risk stratification in congenital diaphragmatic hernia. *J Pediatr Surg.* 2007;42:193–197.
83. Busing KA, Killian AK, Schaible T, et al. MR relative fetal lung volume in congenital diaphragmatic hernia: survival and need for extracorporeal membrane oxygenation. *Radiology.* 2008;248:240–246.
84. Killian AK, Schaible T, Hofmann V, et al. Congenital diaphragmatic hernia: predictive value of MRI relative lung-to-head ratio compared with MRI fetal lung volume and sonographic lung-to-head ratio. *AJR Am J Roentgenol.* 2009;192:153–158.
85. Lee TC, Lim FY, Keswani SG, et al. Late gestation fetal magnetic resonance imaging-derived total lung volume predicts postnatal survival and need for extracorporeal membrane oxygenation support in isolated congenital diaphragmatic hernia. *J Pediatr Surg.* 2011;46:1165–1171.
86. Deshmukh S, Rubesova E, Barth R. MR assessment of normal fetal lung volumes: a literature review. *AJR Am J Roentgenol.* 2010;194:W212–W217.
87. Busing KA, Killian AK, Schaible T, et al. Reliability and validity of MR image lung volume measurement in fetuses with congenital diaphragmatic hernia and in vitro lung models. *Radiology.* 2008;246:533–561.
88. Cannie M, Jani J, Chaffiotte C, et al. Quantification of intrathoracic liver herniation by magnetic resonance imaging and prediction of postnatal survival in fetuses with congenital diaphragmatic hernia. *Ultrasound Obstet Gynecol.* 2008;32:627–632.
89. Worley KC, Dashe JS, Barber RG, et al. Fetal magnetic resonance imaging in isolated diaphragmatic hernia: volume of herniated liver and neonatal outcome. *Am J Obstet Gynecol.* 2009;200:318.e1–318.e6.
90. Ruano R, Lazar DA, Cass DL, et al. Fetal lung volume and quantification of liver herniation by magnetic resonance imaging in isolated congenital diaphragmatic hernia. *Ultrasound Obstet Gynecol.* 2014;43:662–669.
91. Zamora IJ, Olutoye OO, Cass DL, et al. Prenatal MRI fetal lung volumes and percent liver herniation predict pulmonary morbidity in congenital diaphragmatic hernia (CDH). *J Pediatr Surg.* 2014;49:688–693.
92. Vuletin JF, Lim FY, Cnota J, et al. Prenatal pulmonary hypertension index: novel prenatal predictor of severe postnatal pulmonary artery hypertension in antenatally diagnosed congenital diaphragmatic hernia. *J Pediatr Surg.* 2010;45:703–708.
93. Cannie M, Janis J, De Keyyzer F, et al. Diffusion-weighted MRI in lungs of normal fetuses and those with congenital diaphragmatic hernia. *Ultrasound Obstet Gynecol.* 2009;34:678–686.
94. Hedrick MH, Estes JM, Sullivan KM, et al. Plug the lung until grows (PLUG): a new method to treat congenital diaphragmatic hernia in utero. *J Pediatr Surg.* 1994;29:612–617.

95. Harrison MR, Keller RL, Hawgood SB, et al. A randomized trial of fetal endoscopic tracheal occlusion for severe fetal congenital diaphragmatic hernia. *N Engl J Med.* 2003;349:1916–1924.

96. Deprest JA, Hyett JA, Flake AW, et al. Current controversies in prenatal diagnosis 4: should fetal surgery be done in all cases of severe diaphragmatic hernia? *Prenat Diagn.* 2009;29:15–19.

97. Jani JC, Nicolaides KH, Gratacos E, et al. Severe diaphragmatic hernia treated by fetal endoscopic tracheal occlusion. *Ultrasound Obstet Gynecol.* 2009;34:304–310.

98. Ruano R, Yoshisaki CT, Da Silva MM, et al. A randomized controlled trial of fetal endoscopic tracheal occlusion versus postnatal management of severe isolated congenital diaphragmatic hernia. *Ultrasound Obstet Gynecol.* 2012;39:20–27.

99. Style CC, Olutoye OO, Belfort MA, et al. Fetal endoscopic tracheal occlusion reduces pulmonary hypertension in severe congenital diaphragmatic hernia. *Ultrasound Obstet Gynecol.* 2019. doi:10.1002/uog.20216.

100. Ali K, Bendapudi P, Polubothu S, et al. Congenital diaphragmatic hernia: influence of feta tracheal occlusion on outcomes and predictors of survival. *Eur J Pediatr.* 2016;175(8):1071–1076.

101. Downard CD, Jaksic T, Garza JJ, et al. Analysis of an improved survival rate for congenital diaphragmatic hernia. *J Pediatr Surg.* 2003;38:729–732.

102. Kays DW. Congenital diaphragmatic hernia: real improvements in survival. *Neoreviews.* 2006;7:e428–e439.

103. Rollins MD. Recent advances in the management of congenital diaphragmatic hernia. *Curr Opin Pediatr.* 2012;24:379–385.

104. Hedrick HL. Management of prenatally diagnosed congenital diaphragmatic hernia. *Semin Pediatr Surg.* 2013;22:37–43.

105. Haroon J, Chamberlain RS. An evidence-based review of the current treatment of congenital diaphragmatic hernia. *Clin Pediatr.* 2012;52:115–124.

106. Glenn IC, Abdulhai S, Lally PA, et al. Early CDH repair on ECMO: improved survival but no decrease in ECMO duration (A CDH Study Group Investigation). *J Pediatr Surg.* 2019. doi:10.1016/j.jpedsurg.2019.01.063.

107. Frisk V, Jakobson LS, Unger S, et al. Long-term neurodevelopmental outcomes of congenital diaphragmatic hernia survivors not treated with extracorporeal membrane oxygenation. *J Pediatr Surg.* 2011;46:1309–1318.

108. Hitch DC, Carson JA, Smith EI, et al. Familial congenital diaphragmatic hernia is an autosomal recessive variant. *J Pediatr Surg.* 1989;24:860–864.

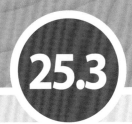
AIRWAY ANOMALIES

Congenital High Airway Obstruction Syndrome

Congenital high airway obstruction syndrome (CHAOS) is a rare fetal anomaly resulting from airway obstruction secondary to laryngeal atresia, or, less commonly, a laryngeal cyst, laryngeal web, laryngeal stenosis, or tracheal atresia.[1,2] CHAOS is typically bilateral; however, sporadically it can be unilateral secondary to central bronchial atresia.

Incidence: The incidence of CHAOS is unknown as only a few cases have been reported in the literature.[3,4]

Pathogenesis/Associated Anomalies: The pathogenesis relates to a complete airway obstruction resulting in trapping and accumulation of fluid within the fetal airways and lungs. Pathological findings include severe distension of the fetal trachea, bronchi, and hyperplastic lungs. The markedly enlarged fetal lungs compress the heart and inferior vena cava, decreasing venous return to the heart, which often results in fetal ascites, cardiac compression resulting in dysfunction, placentomegaly, and hydrops fetalis.[1] Isolated CHAOS is a sporadic fetal malformation with a low risk of associated anomalies or chromosomal abnormalities. Less commonly, CHAOS can be associated with Fraser syndrome, which is an autosomal recessive disorder characterized by laryngeal atresia secondary to underlying fusion of the false vocal cords. Other associations with Fraser syndrome include renal agenesis, microphthalmia, cryptophthalmos, polydactyly, syndactyly, cleft lip/palate, ear anomalies, ambiguous genitalia, congenital heart disease, and severe oligohydramnios secondary to bilateral renal agenesis.[5,6]

Diagnosis: *US:* The characteristic findings of CHAOS include hyperechogenic and hyperexpanded lungs, resulting in flattening or inversion of the diaphragms (Fig. 25.3-1A, B).[3,6] A dilated fluid-filled trachea and bronchi are often identified below the level of the airway obstruction, which most commonly occurs at the level of the larynx. Color Doppler will allow separation of the dilated airway from adjacent vasculature. Fetal ascites is a common feature of CHAOS resulting from obstructed venous return to the heart.

MRI: T2 sequences show similar findings including hyperinflated high-signal lungs, inverting diaphragms, and severely dilated bronchi distal to the more proximal airway obstruction (see Fig. 25.3-1C, D). Fetal ascites is also frequently seen. MRI may complement US by demonstrating the precise level of airway obstruction in preparation for the mandatory tracheostomy required as a lifesaving intervention during the delivery process (see Fig. 25.3-1E).

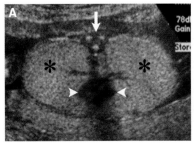
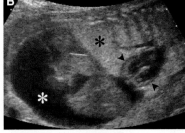
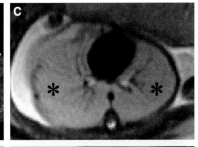
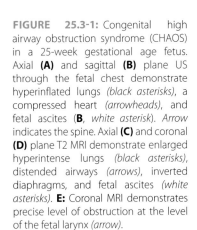
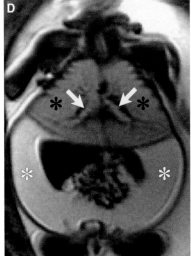
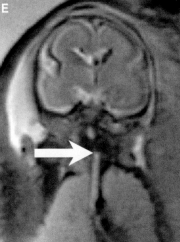

FIGURE 25.3-1: Congenital high airway obstruction syndrome (CHAOS) in a 25-week gestational age fetus. Axial **(A)** and sagittal **(B)** plane US through the fetal chest demonstrate hyperinflated lungs *(black asterisks)*, a compressed heart *(arrowheads)*, and fetal ascites *(B, white asterisk)*. *Arrow* indicates the spine. Axial **(C)** and coronal **(D)** plane T2 MRI demonstrate enlarged hyperintense lungs *(black asterisks)*, distended airways *(arrows)*, inverted diaphragms, and fetal ascites *(white asterisks)*. **E:** Coronal MRI demonstrates precise level of obstruction at the level of the fetal larynx *(arrow)*.

Differential Diagnosis: Congenital pulmonary airway malformation (CPAM) is the primary differential diagnosis. In distinction to CHAOS, the majority of CPAMs are unilateral lesions; however, the rare case of bilateral type 3 microcystic CPAM or the even rarer variant of type 0 CPAM composed of acinar dysplasia affecting all lobes may appear similar to CHAOS.[7,8] In a single case report of confirmed alveolar capillary dysplasia, fetal MRI demonstrated bilateral small lungs with decreased single intensity on T2 imaging.[9]

Prognosis: CHAOS is usually a lethal anomaly with mortality in approximately 80% to 100% of cases.[1] This is especially true when CHAOS is associated with Fraser syndrome. In the absence of additional congenital malformations, prognosis depends on lung size and presence of hydrops. In the absence of hydrops, some cases may be salvageable with proper perinatal management. Rarely, a spontaneous *in utero* fistula between the obstructed airway and esophagus may develop, improving survival postnatal.

Management: In most cases, the natural history of CHAOS includes a progressive enlargement of both lungs with secondary hydrops and a high association with perinatal demise. Termination of pregnancy is a reasonable option to be discussed with the parents. The perinatal outcome of CHAOS is 100% mortality without intervention to secure an airway. Fetuses with CHAOS may benefit from *in utero* fetal therapy via a fetoscopic tracheostomy to ameliorate the intrapulmonary hyperexpansion, and to provide mediastinal decompression, thereby improving venous return to the heart.[10] The only viable perinatal management option to improve survival is delivery via the *ex utero* intrapartum treatment (EXIT) procedure.[11,12] Even with tracheostomy and delivery via the EXIT procedure, only a few survivors have been reported.[1,12,13]

Recurrence: Isolated CHAOS is a sporadic event with no known recurrence risk.

Overinflation/Congenital Lobar Overinflation/Emphysema

Congenital lobar overinflation (CLO; aka congenital lobar emphysema [CLE]) is an overinflation of a lung lobe, characterized on microscopic analysis by air space enlargement without maldevelopment.[14] Congenital lung overinflation is likely a better descriptor than CLO as the abnormality often involves only a lung segment or subsegment. The designation of overinflation is preferred to that of emphysema since the lung is hyperinflated, with intact alveolar walls.

Incidence: Overinflation accounts for approximately 20% of all prenatally diagnosed fetal lung malformations (Table 25.3-1).[15]

Pathogenesis: Pathologically, CLO is composed of two subgroups. The first group is associated with an overinflated lung lobe caused by an intrinsic cartilage abnormality of the airway, absent bronchial cartilage, or extrinsic compression of the airway by an enlarged pulmonary artery or bronchogenic cyst.[16] The collapsed airway acts as a one-way valve resulting in air trapping, and, historically, the majority of cases presented with respiratory distress in the newborn or infant. This form of CLO, previously known as CLE, occurs most frequently in the left upper lobe followed by the right middle and right upper lobes, with the lower lobes involved in less than 1% of cases.[17] A second subgroup of patients with overinflation has emerged largely via prenatal diagnosis. This group is characterized by lobar, segmental, or subsegmental overinflation and a high association with bronchial atresia. This subgroup has a predisposition to the lower lobes and lower symptomatology.[18,19]

Diagnosis: *US:* CLO appears as a primarily homogeneous hyperechogenic mass compared with normal lung tissue (Fig. 25.3-2A). A central dilated bronchus distal to an atretic bronchus helps confirm the diagnosis of associated bronchial atresia/anomaly.[17–19] In addition, mass effect with mediastinal shift may be identified. On color Doppler, CLO demonstrates blood supply from the pulmonary artery and drainage via the pulmonary vein.[20]

MRI: CLO typically appears as a homogeneous high-signal lung mass compared with normal lung tissue on T2 sequences (see Fig. 25.3-2B, C). On MRI, it is often possible to identify the central dilated mucoid-impacted bronchus distal to an atretic or abnormal bronchus (see Fig. 25.3-2D).[19]

Differential Diagnosis: The microcystic form of CPAM is the primary differential diagnosis for CLO. Microcystic CPAM appears similar on US and MRI, and is often an incorrect default prenatal diagnosis when an echogenic mass is detected on US. Pacharn et al.[21] reported high accuracy of prenatal MRI for the diagnosis of the specific type of bronchopulmonary malformation (BPM) with postnatal confirmation of the correct diagnosis on pathology or postnatal imaging in 98% of the cases utilizing a designated algorithm (Fig. 25.3-3). On MRI, CPAMs may have a more heterogeneous appearance with architectual distortion associated with small cystic areas. Identification of a central dilated bronchus and homogenous lesion without architectual distortion suggests bronchial atresia and favors the diagnosis of CLO. Bronchopulmonary sequestrations (BPSs) may also appear similar to CLO on US and MRI; however, identification of a systemic arterial feeder in a sequestration should allow for accurate diagnosis.

Prognosis: Prenatal complications and postnatal sequelae of prenatally diagnosed CLO are rare. The majority of prenatally

TABLE 25.3-1 Distribution of Pathologically Proven Fetal Lung Lesions (108 Cases)	
CPAM	47%
Hybrid (CPAM and sequestration)	25%
Overinflation/bronchial atresia	20%
Sequestration	8%

CPAM, congenital pulmonary airway malformation.
Adapted from Epelman M, Kreiger PA, Servaes S, et al. Current imaging of prenatally diagnosed congenital lung lesions. *Semin Ultrasound CT MR.* 2010;31(2):141–157. Copyright © 2010 Elsevier. With permission

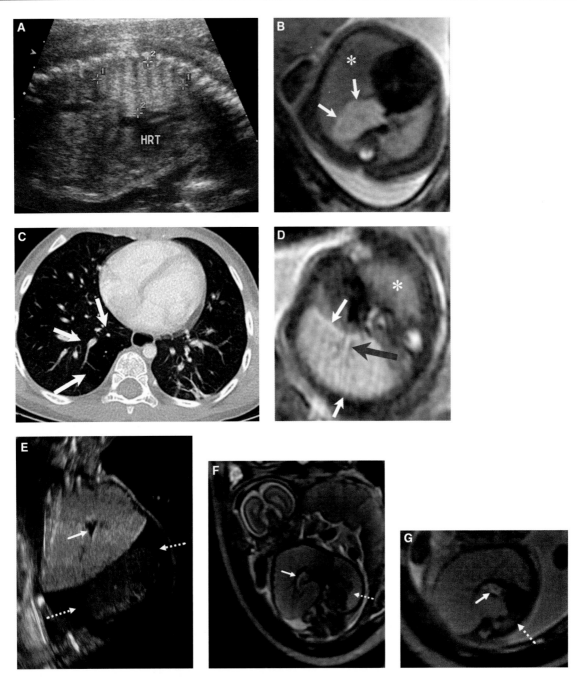

FIGURE 25.3-2: Congenital lobar overinflation (CLO) in multiple fetuses. **A:** Sagittal plane US through the fetal chest in a fetus at 22 weeks demonstrates a homogeneous hyperechogenic mass in the right lower lobe *(calipers)*. *HRT*, heart. **B:** Axial plane T2 MRI in same fetus as image A demonstrates a homogeneous high-signal-intensity mass *(arrows)* in the right lower lung *(asterisk)*. **C:** Computed tomography in the same patient as a newborn demonstrates a hyperlucent segment in the right lower lobe *(arrows)* with otherwise normal architecture. **D:** Axial T2 MRI in a different fetus with confirmed right lower lobe CLO *(white arrows)* and bronchial atresia. Dilated mucoid impacted bronchus *(red arrow)*. *Asterisk* indicates normal lung. Images **E–G** are of a fetus at 19 weeks with central right main bronchus obstruction and CHAOS pathology. Fetus demised intrauterine. **E:** Coronal US demonstrating a homogeneous echogenic mass with central branching hypoechogenicity which lacked color flow consistent with dilated bronchus *(solid arrow)*. Notice everted diaphragms and large intraabdominal ascites *(dotted arrow)*. **F:** Coronal T2 MRI again demonstrates homogeneous mass with central tubular cystic area consistent with dilated bronchus *(solid arrow)*. Notice ascites (dotted arrow) **G:** Axial MRI of the lung mass with dilated bronchus (solid arrow). Notice compressed normal left lung *(dotted arrow)*.

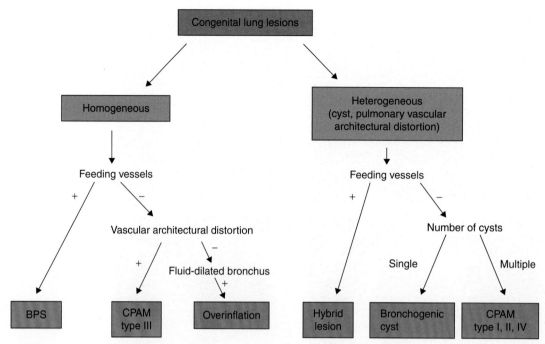

FIGURE 25.3-3: Algorithm for diagnosing lung lesions on fetal MRI. *BPS,* bronchopulmonary sequestration; *CPAM,* congenital pulmonary airway malformation. (Adapted from Pacharn P, Kline-Fath B, Calvo-Garcia M, et al. Congenital lung lesions: comparison between prenatal magnetic resonance imaging (MRI) and postnatal findings. In: *Radiological Society of North America 95th Scientific Assembly & Annual Meeting*; November 29–December 4, 2009; Chicago, IL.)

diagnosed CLO cases are asymptomatic at birth.[18,19] However, in the presence of a main bronchial obstruction and unilateral CHAOS pathology, the prognosis is poor (Fig. 25.3-2 E-G). [19]

Management: Prenatal management of CLO consists of serial USs to assess for the infrequent case associated with a large degree of mass effect, which is more likely to be associated with respiratory distress at birth. Fetal intervention is rarely indicated for CLO. Accurate diagnosis of CLO is important since the incidence of fetal and postnatal complications are uncommon compared with CPAM, and the postnatal management of asymptomatic CLO may be conservative without surgical intervention.

Recurrence: There is no known recurrence risk for isolated CLO.

Esophageal Atresia/Tracheoesophageal Fistula

Esophageal atresia (EA) is characterized by interruption of the esophagus, resulting in a blind-ending pouch. Often, there is an associated fistula between the trachea and the esophagus.

Incidence: The incidence of EA is approximately 1:4,000 live births.[22,23] More than 90% have an associated tracheoesophageal fistula.[24,25]

Pathogenesis/Associated Anomalies: EA results when the tracheoesophageal septum of the foregut fails to complete division of the foregut into the ventral respiratory and dorsal digestive portions. EA can be subclassified into five major types (Fig. 25.3-4). Type A is the most common anatomical configuration, representing proximal EA with a tracheoesophageal fistula to the distal esophageal segment. The other types

of EA in decreasing order of frequency are type B: EA without tracheoesophageal fistula; type C: tracheoesophageal fistula with no EA; type D: EA with tracheoesophageal fistula to both the proximal and the distal esophageal segments; and type E: EA with tracheoesophageal fistula to the proximal esophageal segment.

Other associated malformations are seen in up to 70% of fetuses with EA, with the incidence for the most frequent abnormalities as follows: cardiovascular (35%) (most commonly patent ductus arteriosus [PDA] and ventricular septal defect [VSD]), gastrointestinal (24%) (most commonly anal atresia and duodenal atresia), genitourinary (20%) (most commonly unilateral renal agenesis or renal dysplasia), skeletal (13%) (most commonly vertebral, rib, or radial ray), and neurological (10%) (most commonly hydrocephalus).[22,24–27] EA may also occur in association with other gastrointestinal tract atresias.[28,29] The association of EA and duodenal atresia in the absence of a tracheoesophageal fistula results in a closed-loop bowel obstruction involving the distal esophagus, stomach, and duodenum.[30] Approximately 10% of cases of EA are part of the VACTERL association (*v*ertebral anomalies, *a*nal atresia, *c*ardiac anomalies, *t*racheoesophageal fistula, *r*enal anomalies, and *l*imb anomalies).[31,32] Careful search for these associated anomalies should be performed on prenatal US and MRI when EA is suspected.

Aneuploidy, most commonly trisomies 18 and 21, is relatively common in EA ranging from 5% to 10% in different series.[31,33] The risk of trisomy 21 is 30 times higher than expected in the general population.[34,35]

Diagnosis: *US:* Prenatal US detection of EA is challenging; however, the constellation of a small or absent stomach,

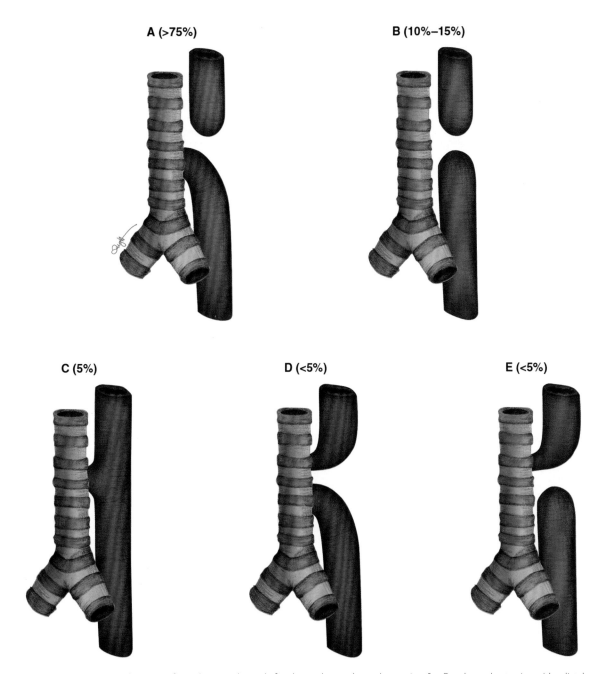

FIGURE 25.3-4: Five subtypes of tracheoesophageal fistula and esophageal atresia. **A:** Esophageal atresia with distal tracheoesophageal fistula. **B:** Esophageal atresia with no tracheoesophageal fistula. **C:** H-type tracheoesophageal fistula with no esophageal atresia. **D:** Esophageal atresia with both proximal and distal tracheoesophageal fistulas. **E:** Esophageal atresia with proximal tracheoesophageal fistula.

polyhydramnios, and a pouch sign is highly suggestive of EA (Fig. 25.3-5A).[36,37] The pouch sign represents the proximal fluid-containing esophageal blind pouch located in the neck or the superior mediastinum. The detection of the proximal esophageal pouch is not straightforward because it fills and empties periodically, likely related to fetal swallowing. Furthermore, depending on the nature of the anomaly, the pouch may be located in the cervical region or superior mediastinum. The sensitivity to and accuracy of identifying the proximal esophageal pouch has not been carefully examined. Diagnosis of EA with an absent stomach and polyhydramnios

is rare prior to 22 weeks' gestation. In fact, a normal appearing stomach and a normal amount of amniotic fluid may be seen earlier in gestation. Overall sensitivity for detecting EA associated with tracheoesophageal fistula is low, cited at 30% prenatal detection rate.[38,39] Limited detection may be explained by the fact that in the presence of EA with tracheoesophageal fistula, the stomach may fill with fluid via the fistula. It is possible that in many cases of EA, the tracheoesophageal fistula maintains flow into the stomach early in pregnancy, but that the fistula progressively narrows as pregnancy continues, resulting in a small or nonvisualized stomach.

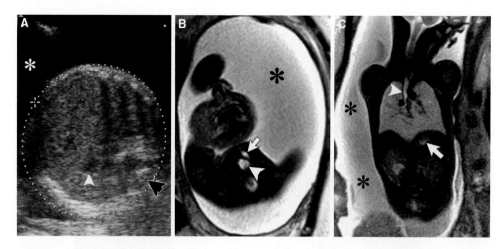

FIGURE 25.3-5: Esophageal atresia with tracheoesophageal fistula in a 30-week gestational age fetus. **A:** Axial US through the upper abdomen demonstrates a very small fetal stomach *(white arrowhead)* and polyhydramnios *(asterisk)*. The spine is indicated by a *black arrowhead*. T2 MRI axial scan through the neck **(B)** and coronal view of the chest **(C)** demonstrate the proximal esophageal pouch *(arrowheads)*, posterior to the trachea *(arrow in B)*, and polyhydramnios *(asterisks)*. The *arrow in* **(C)** indicates the small stomach.

Stringer et al.[38] reported a predictive value for EA ranging from 39% with identification of a small stomach and polyhydramnios to 56% for polyhydramnios in the absence of an identifiable fetal stomach. When EA without a tracheoesophageal fistula is associated with duodenal atresia, US will typically reveal significant polyhydramnios in association with a severely distended stomach because of the closed-loop obstruction.[30,40]

MRI: Diagnostic accuracy is increased with the use of MRI.[41–43] MRI may demonstrate a small stomach, distended hypopharynx, and/or proximal fluid-filled blind-ending esophageal pouch on T2 sequences (see Fig. 25.3-5B, C).[42,43] In a recent study, these findings were detected on US in 36% but visualized in 78% when utilizing MRI.[43] Both distended hypopharynx (high sensitivity) and visualization of the esophageal pouch (high specificity) are strong predictors in the diagnosis of EA.[42,43] MRI may also rarely identify the tracheoesophageal fistula. MRI may also be useful to identify associated anomalies not definitively diagnosed on US, including anal atresia and vertebral anomalies.

Differential Diagnosis: Nonvisualization of the fetal stomach has been reported in approximately 0.07% to 0.4% of pregnancies with abnormal outcome in 48% to 100% of the cases.[44,45] In addition to EA, lack of visualization of the fluid-filled stomach may be seen in conditions associated with abnormal swallowing and passage of amniotic fluid into the esophagus and stomach, including severe fetal central nervous system disorders, neck masses (particularly anterior neck teratomas or fetal goiter), anatomical disorders of swallowing (such as severe cleft palate), diaphragmatic hernia with an intrathoracic stomach, and any cause of oligohydramnios, which limits the available fluid for swallowing.

A small stomach may also be seen with congenital microgastria, which is an extremely rare anomaly believed to result from impairment of normal foregut development. On sonography,

these cases demonstrate a very small stomach on serial scans. Of note, in congenital microgastria, the amniotic fluid may be normal, whereas in EA, polyhydramnios is usually present late in gestation.[46–48]

Prognosis: The outcome of fetuses and infants with EA has been reported as unfavorable with perinatal mortality of 21%, primarily as a result of associated congenital malformations and prematurity.[22,49–51]

Morbidity in survivors depends mostly on the timing of diagnosis and the presence of associated anomalies. Prenatal diagnosis does not change the morbidity and mortality, but can improve prenatal care leading to an average of 2-week later gestation at birth and planned delivery at a site which can provide appropriate neonatal and surgical intervention.[52] Postoperative mortality in infants surviving to undergo primary surgery has been reported at 9%.[22] The prognosis for EA without associated anomalies or genetic disorder is good.[52,53] However, in the first year of life, 59% have gastroesophageal reflux, with 33% requiring fundoplication.[53] In addition, greater than 65% develop anastomotic strictures requiring therapy and enteral nutrition via nasogastric tube.[53]

Management: All patients suspected to have EA should undergo genetic counseling and are referred for karyotype evaluation given the increased risk for trisomies 18 and 21. In addition, a fetal cardiac echo is important to assess for associated cardiac anomalies. EA is usually well managed after birth with surgical correction, and therefore fetal intervention is not indicated.[49]

Recurrence: EA can occur as an isolated finding, as part of a genetic syndrome, or as part of a nonisolated (but not syndromic) set of findings. Most individuals with EA are the only affected member of the family, and when EA is the only abnormality without a clear etiology, the recurrence risk for siblings is approximately 1%.[54] When EA is associated with an inherited chromosomal abnormality or specific syndrome, genetic counseling for recurrence risk is indicated.[54]

LUNG LESIONS

Congenital Pulmonary Airway Malformations (aka Congenital Cystic Adenomatoid Malformation)

Congenital Pulmonary Airway Malformations (CPAMs) are part of the BPM spectrum, which includes BPS, hybrid lesions (CPAM and sequestration), and CLO/bronchial atresia.

Incidence: CPAMs are the most common lung anomaly diagnosed in the fetus, accounting for approximately half of all lesions (see Table 25.3-1).[15] The estimated incidence for prenatal diagnosis is 1:4,000 to 1:6,000 pregnancies.[55,56]

Pathogenesis: The definite etiology is unknown, but several mechanisms have been referenced. A gene interaction (Hox B-5; FGF-7; PDGFB Gene) has been a suggested cause of CPAMs.[57,58] Homeobox genes control axial identity and organ-specific patterning during embryogenesis.[59] Abnormal Hox B-5 expression during human lung branching morphogenesis has been implicated in the development of CPAMs.[57,58] Airway obstruction in the developing fetus has also been cited as the etiology of most BPMs, with the type of malformation depending on the severity and timing of airway obstruction during lung development.[12,60,61] Supporting this conclusion is the associated pathological diagnosis of bronchial atresia in 70% of CPAMs.[60]

CPAMs represent a benign hamartomatous or dysplastic tumor, which are composed of a mass of abnormal solid or cystic pulmonary tissue in which there is proliferation of bronchial structures at the expense of alveolar development. These lesions are thought to result from abnormal endodermal and mesodermal differentiation between the fifth to seventh weeks of gestation.

These lesions typically involve one pulmonary lobe and usually communicate with the tracheobronchial tree, although the communication is abnormal. CPAMs receive blood supply from the pulmonary artery and drain via the pulmonary veins with the exception of hybrid lesions (CPAM and sequestration), which have a systemic arterial blood supply. CPAMs may be predominately cystic, solid, or mixed pathologically.

Stocker et al.[56] has pathologically classified CPAMs into three types according to cyst size and histological resemblance to the segments of the developing bronchial tree and airspaces (Fig. 25.3-6). Type 1 macrocystic CPAM lesions are characterized by single or multiple cysts greater than 2 cm in diameter lined by ciliated pseudostratified columnar epithelium.[62] These account for approximately half of all CPAM lesions in postnatal series.[62] Type 2 lesions are characterized by macroscopic cysts ranging from 0.5 to 2.0 cm in diameter and lined with mixed ciliary, columnar, and cuboidal epithelium.[62] Type 3 lesions are predominantly solid with microcystic components and are histologically composed of alveolus-like structures lined by ciliated cuboidal epithelium.[62] Type 3 CPAM comprises approximately 10% of all CPAMs. Type 1 lesions represent an anomaly of the more

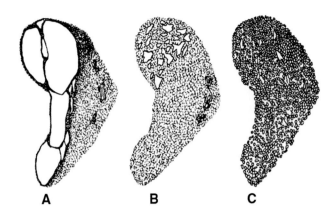

FIGURE 25.3-6: The three original types of congenital pulmonary airway malformation of the fetus as described by Stocker et al.[56] **A:** Type I lesions have large cysts of variable sizes. **B:** Type II lesions have smaller cysts. **C:** Type III lesions are microcystic and appear solid on US owing to reflections from numerous microscopically dilated bronchioles. (Reprinted from Stocker JT, Madewell JE, Drake RM. Congenital cystic adenomatoid malformation of the lung: classification and morphologic spectrum. *Hum Pathol.* 1977;8(2):155–171. Copyright © 1977 Elsevier. With permission.)

proximal bronchial tree affecting primarily the bronchioles, whereas type 3 lesions affect the more distal portion of the bronchial tree at the level of the alveoli.[63] Recently, two additional subtypes of CPAM have been added to the classification (types 0 and 4).[62] Type 0 is characterized by acinar dysplasia or agenesis and is very rare, involving all of the lung lobes, and is incompatible with postnatal survival.[62] Type 4 lesions, which cannot be differentiated from type 1 and 2 lesions by imaging, are characterized by large peripheral cysts of the distal acinus lined predominately by alveolar-type cells. With this new classification, Stocker[62] proposed that the prior designation of congenital cystic adenomatoid malformation (CCAM) be changed to CPAM as the lesions are cystic in only three of the five pathological classifications and adenomatoid in one type.

Diagnosis: *US:* Most CPAMs are detected as an incidental finding. CPAMs may appear as a predominately macrocystic mass, microcystic or a homogeneous hyperechogenic solid mass, or a complex mass with both cystic and echogenic components (Fig. 25.3-7). Solid masses are typically hyperechogenic compared with normal fetal lung in the second trimester, and often become isoechoic with the normal fetal lung and invisible on sonography in the third trimester (Fig. 25.3-8). The decreasing conspicuity relates to both the increasing echogenicity of the normal fetal lungs as pregnancy progresses and the propensity of solid masses to decrease in size as pregnancy progresses. When solid masses are isoechoic to normal lung, the sonographic diagnosis is more challenging and relies on mass effect, including mediastinal shift, altered cardiac position or axis, or an inverted diaphragm to confirm the diagnosis (Fig. 25.3-9A). Color Doppler US is useful in demonstrating pulmonary artery blood supply to the mass and drainage via the pulmonary vein (see Fig. 25.3-9B). Identification of an associated systematic arterial blood supply confirms the diagnosis of a

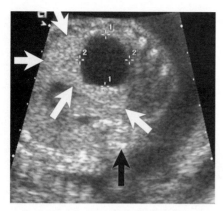

FIGURE 25.3.3-7: Complex cystic lung malformation detected as incidental finding on US at 22 weeks' gestational age. Axial sonogram through the fetal chest shows a complex mass composed of macrocystic (*calipers*) and solid (*white arrows*) components. Fetal spine is indicated by a *black arrow*.

hybrid BPM composed of both CPAM and sequestration components (Fig. 25.3-10).

Adzick[64] suggested a sonographic characterization based on a predominately macrocystic or microcystic appearance of CPAMs as a more clinically useful classification. The macrocystic lesions are composed of single or multiple cysts larger than 5 mm in diameter on US, and microcystic lesions appear as a solid hyperechogenic mass because of the numerous acoustic interfaces created by small cysts measuring less than 5 mm in diameter (Fig. 25.3-11).[64] The presence or absence of macroscopic cysts may be important as these can predispose to rapid growth and complications, and also in determining therapy for

cases complicated by fetal hydrops. CPAMs are usually unilateral and unilobar with a slight predisposition to the lower lobes. Approximately 40% of CPAMs increase in size during pregnancy, with the most rapid growth occurring between 20 and 26 weeks' gestational age, after which growth peaks and plateaus.[65,66]

MRI: Utilizing MRI, diagnosis and further characterization of CPAMs may be useful. MRI is reported to provide alternative or additional diagnoses compared with US in 38% to 50% of fetuses with chest anomalies.[41,67] In the second trimester, CPAMs usually appear as a hyperintense mass compared with normal lung tissue on T2 MRI sequences (Fig. 25.3-12A). However, in the third trimester, CPAMs may appear high signal, isointense, or lower signal compared with lung tissue. The identification of a high-signal mass alone on MRI is not specific for the type of BPM; however, identification of a macrocystic component and/or distortion of the vascular architecture is highly suggestive for CPAM (see Fig. 25.3-12B).[41,68]

Rarely, a CPAM may be T2 hypointense and hypoechoic on US and have a rosette pattern.[69] These CPAMs have more immature parenchymal development with increased mesenchymal tissue and usually are large with polyhydramnios that may result in preterm delivery.[69] These masses can have similar imaging characteristics to congenital myofibroblastic tumors.[69]

MRI may be useful during the third trimester of pregnancy in evaluating for pulmonary hypoplasia via lung volume measurements and confirming the presence and size of a CPAM when solid masses may not be visualized on US.[70] In our experience, the latter is helpful in planning delivery location (see Fig. 25.3-8B). In addition, measurements of the lesion volume divided by head circumference can provide a lung mass volume ratio, which, if greater than 2, increases the risk of hydrops and worse perinatal outcome.[70] When the mass is ascertained to be small on MRI,

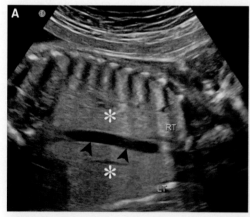

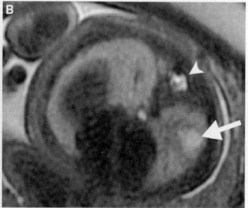

FIGURE 25.3-8: Disappearing fetal lung mass in the third trimester. **A:** Coronal plane US through the fetal chest shows no evidence of a fetal lung mass. Normal lungs are indicated by *asterisks* and the aorta by *arrowheads*. **B:** Axial plane fetal MRI confirms a small high-signal bronchopulmonary malformation (*arrow*). The *arrowhead* indicates the spine.

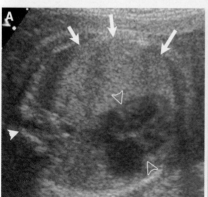

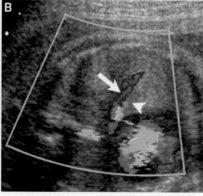

FIGURE 25.3-9: Isoechoic lung mass. **A:** Axial US through the fetal chest demonstrates dextroposition of the heart (*open arrowheads*) secondary to an isoechoic lung mass (*arrows*). The spine is indicated by a *closed arrowhead*. **B:** Axial plane Doppler US demonstrates pulmonary artery blood supply to the mass (*arrow*) and drainage via the pulmonary vein (*arrowhead*). Postnatal surgical resection confirmed congenital pulmonary airway malformation.

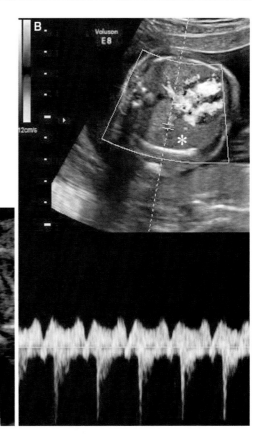

FIGURE 25.3-10: Hybrid bronchopulmonary malformation at 22 weeks' gestational age. Coronal **(A)** and axial **(B)** plane US through the fetal chest demonstrates a systemic artery *(arrowhead)* arising from the lower thoracic aorta and the pulmonary artery *(spectral tracing)* supplying the hybrid bronchopulmonary malformation *(asterisks)*. Spectral tracing demonstrates both pulmonary arterial supply and pulmonary venous drainage.

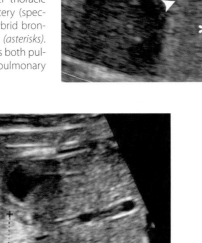

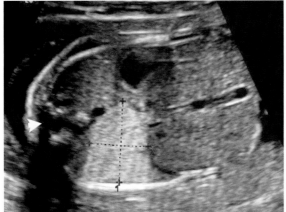

FIGURE 25.3-11: Microcystic CPAM at 22 weeks' gestational age. Axial US through the fetal chest demonstrates a hyperechogenic mass *(calipers)* representing a microcystic CPAM. Spine *(arrowhead)*.

patients can safely deliver in their local community and undergo elective evaluation of the mass after birth.

Differential Diagnosis: Differential diagnosis for a CPAM includes multiple entities including congenital lung lesions, congenital diaphragmatic hernia (CDH), lymphatic malformation, primary lung tumor, or pulmonary agenesis/hypoplasia.

Differential diagnosis for a solid microcystic CPAM includes hybrid BPMs (CPAM and BPS), congenital lobar or segmental overinflation, CDH, and congenital myofibroblastic tumor, especially if the lesion is T2 hypointense. Solid hybrid lesions may be differentiated by identification of both pulmonary artery and systemic arterial blood supply to the mass on US or MRI. Lobar or segmental overinflation may appear similar to a CPAM on prenatal imaging but lacks architectural distortion. Identification of a dilated central bronchus with mucoid impaction also suggests CLO. CDH can usually be differentiated from CPAM by identification of the fetal stomach in the thorax and observation of peristalsis of herniated intestinal loops in the chest. A right-sided

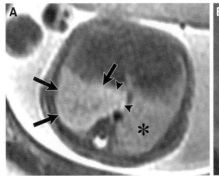

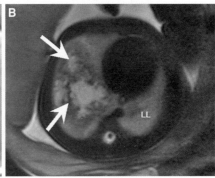

FIGURE 25.3-12: MRI of congenital pulmonary airway malformation. **A:** Axial T2 MRI of fetus at a gestational age of 22 weeks demonstrates a high-signal-intensity CPAM *(arrows)* with small peripheral cysts *(arrowheads)* in the right lower lobe. Normal lung is indicated by *asterisk*. **B:** Axial T2 MRI of fetus at 21 weeks with confirmed CPAM showing complex lesion of mixed signal containing multiple cysts *(arrows)*. *LL*, normal left lung.

CDH associated with liver herniation may appear similar to a microcystic CPAM presenting as a solid intrathoracic mass. In contrast to CPAMs, the herniated liver does not appear as hyperechogenic on US. Color Doppler US should correctly diagnose the herniated liver by identifying the intrahepatic portal veins and the inferior vena cava within the mass.

An intrapulmonary bronchogenic cyst is the main differential diagnosis for a macrocystic CPAM. Bronchogenic cysts are usually unilocular cystic lesions, which can occur in the pulmonary parenchyma and are unassociated with a solid component. A dilated stomach in a left congenital diaphragmatic may also be considered. A primary lung mass, which should include pleuropulmonary blastoma (PPB), may present with both large and small cysts with or without solid tissue. In the presence of a primary lung mass, the lesion will typically continue to grow beyond 26 weeks, past the time a typical CPAM will plateau.

Pulmonary lymphatic malformations (PLMs) may also mimic a macrocystic CPAM. PLMs can be a primary lung developmental abnormality due to failure of the normal regression processes of the lymphatic channels in the fetal lungs or secondary, usually associated with congenital hypoplastic left heart with pulmonary venous obstruction. On US, PLMs can manifest as bilateral small intrapulmonary cysts. Fetal MRI has been reported to demonstrate a typical heterogeneous "nutmeg" appearance of the lungs on T2 images in fetuses with hypoplastic left heart and pulmonary venous obstruction.[71–73]

Pulmonary hypoplasia or agenesis may also present with ipsilateral mediastinal shift, thereby mimicking an isoechoic mass such as a CPAM on US.[74] MRI can confirm the correct diagnosis by excluding an underlying lung mass as the cause of the mediastinal shift, thereby confirming the presence of a hypoplastic right lung.

Associated Anomalies: Isolated CPAMs are not associated with increased risk for chromosomal abnormalities[75,76]; however, prenatal series have reported associated anomalies in 8% to 12% of CPAMs. Associated anomalies include renal abnormalities, CDH, tracheoesophageal fistula, and congenital heart defects.[75,77,78] Genetic counseling for fetal karyotyping should be offered when associated anomalies are identified.[79,80]

Prognosis: Imaging plays a key role in predicting the clinical outcome for a fetus diagnosed with a CPAM. Prognosis depends on the size of the mass and the presence or absence of hydrops fetalis. Small isolated fetal lung malformations with no mass effect have excellent outcomes and usually are asymptomatic at birth. A subset of fetuses with large CPAMs have mass effect, resulting in mediastinal shift and can develop life-threatening complications including hydrops fetalis or, less commonly, severe pulmonary hypoplasia. Earlier literature reported that 30% to 50% of fetuses with CPAMs developed hydrops fetalis with an associated mortality approaching 100% without intervention.[81] More recent literature suggests that hydrops is less frequent and occurs in 9% to 21% of cases.[82,83]

The pathophysiology for hydrops fetalis is felt to be secondary to compression of the heart and inferior vena cava, obstructing venous return to the heart. Large masses may also be associated with isolated polyhydramnios secondary to compression of the esophagus, obstructing normal passage of amniotic fluid into the gastrointestinal tract. In a prospective series, Crombleholme et al.[65] reported that sonographic measurement of the CPAM volume ratio (CVR) predicted the risk of hydrops in fetuses with CPAM (aka CCAM). CVR is the measured CPAM volume divided by the head circumference (Fig. 25.3-13). The CPAM volume is a calculated measurement utilizing the formula for a prolate ellipse (mass length × height × width × 0.52). In the Crombleholme series, a CVR greater than 1.6 predicted an increased risk of hydrops fetalis occurring in 75% of cases.[65] A CVR less than or equal to 1.6 in the absence of a dominant cyst was associated with a less than 3% risk of hydrops fetalis. Crombleholme et al. noted that in addition to the absolute size of the mass, the rate of lesion growth, particularly when associated with a macroscopic cyst, is a risk factor for developing hydrops fetalis. Prenatal US and MRI measurements of fetal lung mass volumes can predict neonatal respiratory distress, even when obtained before 24 weeks' gestational age.[84]

Management: The vast majority of CPAMs are managed conservatively with sonographic surveillance every 1 to 2 weeks to assess for the complication of hydrops fetalis. After 30 weeks' gestational age, the risk of developing hydrops fetalis is unlikely, and the frequency of surveillance can be decreased.

In the presence of large lesions with high CVR, maternal administration of betamethasone may have a beneficial effect on microcystic CPAMs in preventing or reversing hydrops fetalis.[85–87] The exact mechanism is unknown, but it is postulated that

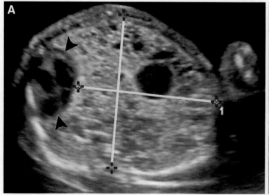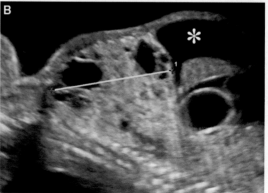

FIGURE 25.3-13: CPAM volume ratio (CVR): Large congenital pulmonary airway malformation of mixed increased echogenicity and cystic components complicated by early hydrops in a 24-week gestational age pregnancy. CVR = 2.6. CVR is calculated as the CPAM volume divided by head circumference. CVR = $L \times H \times W \times 0.52$/head circumference. Axial **(A)** and sagittal **(B)** US demonstrate measurement of the CPAM volume (calipers). Displaced heart is indicated by arrowheads and ascites by asterisk.

TABLE 25.3-2	Prenatal Steroids for Microcystic CPAM (Data from Three Centers)				
	PATIENTS	CVR	HYDROPS	HYDROPS RESOLVED	SURVIVAL
UCSF	13	2.7	9 (69%)	7 (78%)	11 (85%)
CHOP	10	2.2	5 (50%)	4 (80%)	10 (100%)
Cincinnati	8	2.5	6 (75%)	5 (83%)	6 (75%)
Total	**31**	**2.5**	**20/31(65%)**	**16/20(80%)**	**27/31(87%)**

CPAM, congenital pulmonary airway malformation; CHOP, Children's Hospital of Philadelphia; CVR, CPAM volume ratio; UCSF, University California San Francisco.
Adapted from Curran PF, Jelin EB, Rand L, et al. Prenatal steroids for microcystic congenital cystic adenomatoid malformations. *J Pediatr Surg.* 2010;45(1):145–150. Copyright © 2010 Elsevier. With permission.

steroids may accelerate lung maturation or mass involution. Reports from three centers have shown resolution of hydrops fetalis in approximately 80% of CPAMs treated with maternal steroids (Table 25.3-2).[87] In addition, Curran et al.[87] reported survival to discharge ranging from 75% to 100% for large microcystic CPAMs managed with maternal betamethasone. Macrocystic CPAMs do not seem to respond as well to treatment with betamethasone.[85] Loh et al. reported a series comparing steroid treatment to surgical treatment for CPAMs associated with fetal hydrops in the second trimester. Improved survival, particularly for microcystic CPAMs, was noted in the steroid-treated group compared with the open surgery group (Table 25.3-3).[88]

The current consensus in many centers is to administer maternal steroids as the first line of treatment prior to surgical intervention in fetuses at high risk for fetal hydrops. Multiple courses of betamethasone may result in favorable outcomes in high-risk CPAMs.[89] In fetuses with large CPAMs complicated by hydrops fetalis, who are unresponsive to maternal steroid administration, a spectrum of interventional procedures, including cyst aspiration, placement of a thoracoamniotic shunt, percutaneous laser ablation, or surgical resection, may be considered prior to 32 weeks' gestational age.[90–93] Open surgery with mass resection has been reported to be approximately 50% successful in managing CPAMs; however, it is controversial because of complications related to the procedure, which include increased risk for premature rupture of the membranes, preterm delivery, and fetal demise.[94] Percutaneous laser ablation of microcystic lesions may be an alternative

TABLE 25.3-3	Steroid Rx vs. Fetal Surgery in 24 Fetuses with CPAM and Fetal Hydrops	
	STEROID RX	SURGICAL RX
Mean GA age	23 wk	24 wk
CVR	2.68 ± 0.29	2.95 ± 0.31
Survival to delivery	12/13 (92%)	9/11 (82%)
Survival to discharge	10/12 (83%)	5/9 (56%)

CPAM, congenital pulmonary airway malformation; CVR, CPAM volume ratio; GA, gestational age.
Adapted from Loh KC, Jelin E, Hirose S, et al. Microcystic congenital pulmonary airway malformation with hydrops fetalis: steroids vs open fetal resection. *J Pediatr Surg.* 2012;47(1):36–39. Copyright © 2012 Elsevier. With permission.

treatment to surgical resection for microcystic lesions, but additional studies are necessary to consider this as a valid therapeutic option.[95] Fetal percutaneous sclerotherapy has also been reported as a minimally invasive and effective palliative strategy to ameliorate hydrops fetalis associated with predominately solid types of CPAMs, and may represent an alternative to surgical resection.[96]

Postnatal management of symptomatic lesions is surgical resection. However, treatment for asymptomatic CPAMs remains controversial. In a recent survey of surgeons, 75% operate on asymptomatic patients typically between 6 and 12 months of age due to risk of infection and cancer, of which 17% noted they have seen at least one patient with lung cancer in a CPAM.[97] However, some believe conservative management is a reasonable option given that in their review of CPAMs the risk of recurrent infection is less than 10% and no malignancy was confirmed.[98]

Recurrence: There is no known recurrence risk for isolated CPAM.

Bronchopulmonary Sequestration

Bronchopulmonary sequestrations (BPSs) represent a cystic developmental lung malformation composed of nonfunctioning pulmonary tissue, which lacks communication to the tracheobronchial tree and is supplied by a systemic artery.

Incidence: BPS is the second most common cause of a congenital lung mass, occurring in approximately 1.1% to 1.8% of all pulmonary resections.[99] In the fetus, BPS occurs primarily as an isolated lesion, but it can have associated anomalies in approximately 8% of cases and is associated with a CPAM in 25% of cases (see Table 25.3-1).[15]

Pathogenesis/Associated Anomalies: BPS is thought to originate from a supernumerary caudally positioned lung bud and has a preferential location for the left lower thorax in 65% to 90% of cases.[99,100] BPSs are characterized as intralobar sequestration (ILS) or extralobar sequestration (ELS).[101] ELS is completely separated from the adjacent normal lung tissue and invested in its own pleural covering. Late development of the lung bud after formation of the pleura leads to formation of a separate pleural covering surrounding the ELS. ILS shares common pleura with the normal lung tissue. On occasion, ELS and ILS forms of BPS can coexist.[102] ELS accounts for the majority of BPSs diagnosed prenatally and approximately 25% to 50% of cases of BPS diagnosed postnatally.[101] Bronchial atresia affecting the lobar, segmental, or subsegmental bronchi has been reported in 100% of ELS and 82% of ILS cases.[60] Approximately 10% to 15% of ELSs are found within or below the diaphragm.[100,103] All BPSs receive blood supply from an anomalous systemic feeding artery usually arising from the lower thoracic aorta, upper abdominal aorta, or the celiac artery. Multiple systematic artery feeders may be identified on imaging and at pathology. Venous drainage is via the pulmonary veins in ILS.[104] The venous drainage of ELS is usually systemic through the azygous vein, hemi azygous vein, or the superior vena cava.[99,105] ELS may be associated with other fetal anomalies, most commonly CDH and foregut abnormalities.[100,106]

Diagnosis: *US:* BPS appears as a homogeneous hyperechogenic mass compared with the normal lung in the vast majority of cases (Fig. 25.3-14).[101] Less commonly, there may be a cystic component, with a high percentage attributed to hybrid lesions. Large masses may result in mass effect with mediastinal shift or compression of the diaphragm. BPSs are usually detected in the second trimester as an incidental finding and are most commonly localized in the left lower hemithorax or below the diaphragm in approximately 10% of cases.[100,103] Hybrid lesions composed of both CPAM and ELS components are described in approximately 50% of cases (see Fig. 25.3-10).[107,108] A systematic feeding artery or multiple arteries arising from the lower thoracic or abdominal upper aorta can be identified on color Doppler US in the majority of cases, thereby confirming the diagnosis.[108] US has been shown to be more accurate than is MRI in identification of the systemic vessel, and can define ILS versus ELS based on draining veins.[109] On rare occasions, ELS may be complicated by a large ipsilateral hydrothorax, which is thought to occur secondary to torsion of the sequestration, resulting in obstruction of the efferent venous and lymphatic drainage.[110] ELS may be associated with other congenital anomalies, including CDH, cardiac abnormalities, or foregut duplications.[111]

MRI: BPSs usually appear as a high-signal mass compared with normal fetal lung on T2-fluid-sensitive sequences (see Fig. 25.3-14C). The lesions are typically homogeneous, of high-signal intensity, and only slightly less intense than that of amniotic fluid. The presence of an associated cyst suggests a hybrid lesion with a CPAM component. Systematic feeding vessels may be identified, usually arising from the lower thoracic or upper abdominal aorta.

Differential Diagnosis: Differential diagnosis for an intrathoracic BPS includes other causes of a solid intrathoracic mass—CPAM, CLO or segmental overinflation, and CDH. The identification of a systematic arterial feeder to the BPS should allow for a specific diagnosis. Differential diagnosis for a subdiaphragmatic suprarenal BPS includes adrenal neuroblastoma and adrenal hemorrhage, and, again, a systemic feeder to a hyperechogenic mass in a subdiaphragmatic location should allow for accurate diagnosis of BPS. On MRI, congenital neuroblastoma can appear as a predominately cystic or solid mass in a fetus. Solid neuroblastomas tend to be heterogeneous with intermediate signal intensity on T2 sequences in contrast to BPS, which are usually high-signal-intensity lesions on fluid-sensitive T2 MRI sequences. Adrenal hemorrhage is usually diagnosed in the subacute phase and appears as intermediate to high signal on both T2 and T1 sequences.

Prognosis: Most BPSs decrease in size after 26 to 28 weeks' gestation and rarely require fetal intervention.[112] Approximately 68% of BPS lesions regress dramatically before birth, and most are generally associated with an outstanding prognosis.[64] Hydrops fetalis is a rare complication of BPS and much less frequent than in CPAM. BPS may be complicated by a large ipsilateral pleural effusion secondary to torsion, which may then progress to hydrops, particularly when it is of the extralobar type.[14,112]

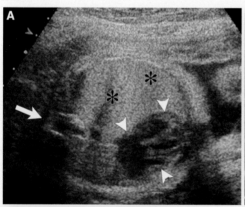
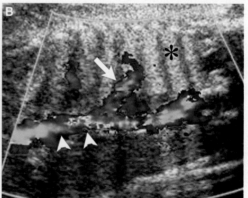
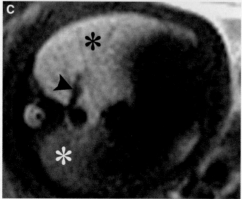

FIGURE 25.3-14: Bronchopulmonary sequestration at 22 weeks' gestational age. **A:** Axial US through the fetal chest shows a homogeneous hyperechoic left-sided solid chest mass *(asterisks)* displacing the heart *(arrowheads)* to the right. Fetal spine is indicated by *arrow.* **B:** Coronal color Doppler through the fetal chest and abdomen shows a systemic arterial feeder *(arrow)* arising from the lower thoracic aorta *(arrowheads)* supplying the fetal chest mass *(asterisk).* **C:** Axial plane T2 MRI demonstrates a homogeneous high-signal mass *(black asterisk)* compared with normal lung *(white asterisk)*; systemic arterial feeder *(arrowhead)* is seen arising from the lower thoracic aorta.

Management: Prenatal management consists of surveillance via US. No intervention is required in the vast majority of cases. Early delivery may be contemplated after 32 weeks' gestation in the rare case complicated by hydrops fetalis. Maternal betamethasone and thoracoamniotic shunt may be considered for treatment of the infrequent case complicated by a large ipsilateral pleural effusion as the associated mortality is very high in the absence of intervention.[90,91] Open fetal surgical resection is considered controversial because of the maternal risks associated with surgery.

Recurrence: There is no known recurrence risk for isolated BPS.

MASSES

Pleuropulmonary Blastoma

Pleuropulmonary Blastoma (PPB) is also known as pulmonary sarcoma and pulmonary rhabdomyosarcoma.

Incidence: PPB is a rare tumor but represents the most common cause of a primary lung malignancy in childhood.[113] The incidence of PPB in the fetus is unknown.

Pathogenesis: Although rare, PPB occurs predictably in certain clinical and familial circumstances. Approximately 20% of children with PPB have a family history of pediatric neoplasia, most commonly cystic nephroma of the kidney and rhabdomyosarcoma.[114] Families with PPB may harbor heterozygous germline mutations in the *DICER1* gene, which have been shown to predispose to PPB.[114] PPB is a dysembryonic malignancy, which is believed to arise from pleuropulmonary germ cells and is composed of both epithelial and mesenchymal components.[113] Mesenchymal cells susceptible to malignant transformation reside within cyst walls and may evolve into sarcomas. Priest et al.[115] subclassified PPB as type 1 (purely cystic), type 2 (cystic and solid), or type 3 (purely solid) lesions. The type 1 (predominately cystic) lesion represents the early form of the disease and is the type most commonly reported in the fetus or young infant.[115,116] The cystic nature of the mass renders it difficult to distinguish from CPAM as it is pathologically deceptive because of its resemblance to developmental lung cysts.[117] PPB may be unilateral or bilateral.

Diagnosis: On imaging with prenatal US or MRI, PPB appears as a primarily cystic or a complex mass with cystic and solid components, which are usually indistinguishable from the findings in CPAM (Fig. 25.3-15). Findings which may help differentiate a PPB from a CPAM include a positive family history, multifocal disease, associated pleural effusion, or continued growth late in gestation past the typical plateau of CPAM growth.[113,118]

Differential Diagnosis: CPAM, or hybrid lesion, is the primary differential diagnosis and may appear identical to PPB on prenatal imaging, although the presence of a systemic vessel should exclude PPB.[119] A positive family history, continued interval growth beyond 28 weeks, bilateral or multisegmental parenchymal involvement, and the presence of pleural effusion should raise consideration for a PPB. Timing of lesion detection should differentiate PPB from bronchopulmonary malformations. The vast majority of bronchopulmonary malformations are detected in the mid-second trimester and PPB has not been reported in the second trimester.

Prognosis: Complete surgical resection of PPB may be curative, particularly for type 1 (cystic) disease, with 91% 5-year overall survival.[120] Type 2 and especially type 3 diseases are often progressive and carry a much worse prognosis.[120]

Management: PPB is a very rare lesion in the fetus, and most are presumed to represent a CPAM and, therefore, undergo US surveillance to assess for the complication of hydrops fetalis. In the majority of cases, the diagnosis is not confirmed until after birth, when the lesion is surgically resected. No fetal intervention has been reported in PPB. PPB survival statistics suggest that it is vital to diagnose and treat children at an early age, at which time the lesion is more curable.[117]

Recurrence: The recurrence risk for PPB is increased in patients with a familial predisposition associated with the *DICER1* gene mutation.[114]

Congenital Peribronchial Myofibroblastic Tumor

Congenial peribronchial myofibroblastic tumor (CPMT) is also known as bronchopulmonary leiomyosarcoma, bronchopulmonary fibrosarcoma, congenital fibroleiomyosarcoma, hamartoma, and congenital mesenchymal/adenomatoid malformation.

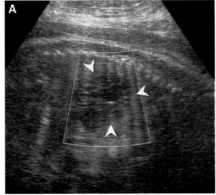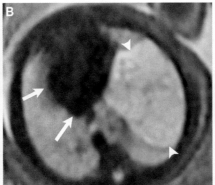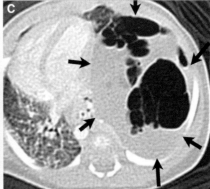

FIGURE 25.3-15: Cystic pleuropulmonary blastoma. **A:** Sagittal plane US through the fetal chest demonstrates complex cystic and solid lung mass *(arrowheads)*. **B:** Axial T2 MRI demonstrates high-signal mass *(arrowheads)* within the left chest displacing the heart *(arrows)* to the right. **C:** Axial computed tomography scan after birth demonstrates a solid and air-containing cystic mass *(arrows)*, confirmed on surgical pathology to represent a cystic pleuropulmonary blastoma. Images courtesy of Beth Kline-Fath, MD.

Incidence: CPMT is a rare benign primary lung tumor, which is usually detected by prenatal imaging or diagnosed in the neonate presenting with respiratory distress.[121,122] The incidence in the fetus is unknown.

Pathogenesis: CPMT is a benign lung tumor which usually is detected in the fetus as a large solid lung mass associated with hydrops fetalis or presents with respiratory distress at birth. The tumor histology shows proliferation of myofibroblasts around a bronchus with invasion into the surrounding lung parenchyma.[122] CPMT is thought to arise from pluripotent peribronchial mesenchymal cells and may share pathogenesis similar to other mesenchymal lesions such as pleuropulmonary blastoma or fetal lung interstitial tumor. There is no destruction or invasion of the airway.[121] Mitotic figures can be seen, but there is no significant cytologic atypia or atypical mitoses. There is no predilection for gender, lobe, or laterality.

Diagnosis: On imaging with prenatal US or MRI, CPMT manifests as a large primary lung mass. The mass does not demonstrate the typical imaging patterns described for bronchopulmonary malformations. On US, the mass is hypoechoic and heterogeneous compared with normal lung in the third trimester (Fig. 25.3-16A).[122] On MRI, CPMT appears hypointense compared with normal lung on fluid-sensitive images. No cystic components are identified. It is the only congenital lung tumor that has been reported as early as the second trimester.[122] Imaging findings are not entirely specific but support a solid fibrous tumor.

Differential diagnosis: Differential diagnosis includes PPB, congenital fibrosarcoma, and fetal lung interstitial tumor (FLIT). PPB would be expected to be cystic in the fetus. Congenital fibrosarcoma may present as a solid mass; however, it is typically found in the soft tissues and rarely in the lung.[123] FLIT is a congenital pulmonary tumor with a solid or mixed cystic appearance and has been reported as T2 hyperintense on MRI in a single case report.[122,124]

Prognosis: Surgical resection is felt to be curative with no recurrence risk. CPMT complicated by nonimmune hydrops fetalis may be associated with intrauterine fetal demise.[121]

Management: Treatment is complete surgical resection postnatal. Lobectomy or pneumectomy is often required. Chemotherapy or radiation treatment is not indicted for this benign tumor. Fetal surgical resection or EXIT to extracorporeal membrane oxygenation (ECMO) delivery may be considered for cases complicated by hydrops or for large masses likely to be associated with respiratory distress.

Recurrence risk: Recurrences have not been reported after surgical resection.[121]

MEDIASTINUM

Thymus

The thymus is a normal lymphoid organ which is important for immune function during both intrauterine and extrauterine life.[125,126]

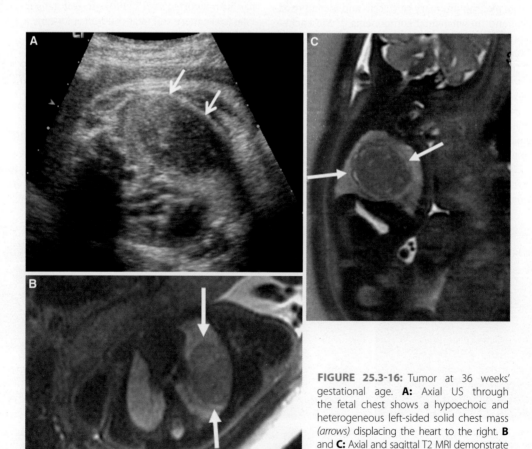

FIGURE 25.3-16: Tumor at 36 weeks' gestational age. **A:** Axial US through the fetal chest shows a hypoechoic and heterogeneous left-sided solid chest mass *(arrows)* displacing the heart to the right. **B** and **C:** Axial and sagittal T2 MRI demonstrate a homogeneous low-signal mass *(arrows)* compared with normal lung.

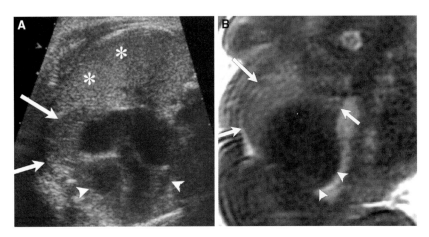

FIGURE 25.3-17: Normal thymus gland in a third-trimester fetus. **A:** Axial US through the chest demonstrates a normal thymus gland *(arrows)*, which is hypoechoic relative to the normal lung *(asterisks)*. *Arrowheads* indicate the heart. **B:** Coronal T2 MRI through the fetal chest demonstrates the thymus gland as an intermediate signal bilobed structure *(arrows)*. Note normal asymmetry of lobes. Heart is indicated by *arrowheads.*

Embryology: The thymus is derived embryologically from the third pharyngeal pouch and the third pharyngeal cleft, which gives rise respectively to the endodermal (cortical) and ectodermal (medullary) components of the thymus. The pouch is anterior to the aorta in the anterior mediastinum.

Diagnosis: *US:* The normal thymus gland can be identified in the majority of fetuses in the second and third trimesters. The thymus gland appears as a bilobed structure in the anterior superior mediastinum ventral to the pericardium and great vessels of the heart. The thymus echogenicity is similar or slightly more echogenic than that of the fetal lungs early in the second trimester and less echogenic than normal fetal lung tissue in the later part of pregnancy (Fig. 25.3-17A).[127] Occasionally, nonshadowing linear or punctate echogenic foci may be seen in the thymus gland, likely corresponding to normal connective tissue septa and blood vessels. Nomograms for normal fetal thymic size have been reported with no substantial size difference between male and female fetuses.[127–130]

MRI: The thymus gland should be identified in all normal fetuses in the second and third trimesters with the gland appearing bilobed and intermediate signal intensity on T2 sequences (see Fig. 25.3-17B). The thymus gland is higher in signal than is the adjacent muscle in the chest wall but of lesser signal intensity than that of adjacent lung tissue in the late second and third trimesters. The two lobes of the thymus gland may substantially differ in size. The normal thymus gland is very pliable, and even when appearing large on US or MRI, does not exhibit compression or displacement of adjacent mediastinal structures.

Differential Diagnosis: Solid masses in the thymus gland are extremely rare, and the primary consideration for a solid mass in the anterior/superior mediastinum is a teratoma. Teratomas are usually complex masses with cystic and solid components. Ectopic thyroid or fetal goiter may also mimic a thymic region mass. MRI should accurately characterize the tissue as thyroid gland by identifying the typical bilobed appearance and homogeneous bright signal on T1 sequences. Differential diagnosis for an apparently absent thymus gland includes ectopic thymus. Early in development, the thymus may fail to normally descend from the neck into the mediastinum as part of normal embryogenesis, in which case the thymus gland can be partially or completely ectopic in the cervical region. The latter is important to recognize as a potential explanation for nonvisualization of the thymus gland in its expected normal location in the superior mediastinum.[131]

Associated Anomalies: Prenatal diagnosis of a thymic mass is a rare occurrence. There have been case reports of prenatally diagnosed thymic cysts. Absence of the thymus gland is indicative of thymic aplasia, and a small gland is associated with thymic hypoplasia (Fig. 25.3-18). These findings are of high concern because of the association in various diseases, including DiGeorge syndrome, Ellis–Van Creveld syndrome, and severe combined immunodeficiency.[132–134] Other associations with an underdeveloped or absent thymus include human immunodeficiency virus, infection, intrauterine growth restriction, acute illnesses, and chorioamnioitis.[135–137] Others have reported that an absent or hypoplastic thymus on US is a marker for deletion 22q11.1 associated with fetal cardiac defects.[138,139] Focused imaging of the thymus gland on US or MRI may be indicated in fetuses at risk for a hypoplastic or absent thymus gland.[128]

Bronchogenic Cyst

A bronchogenic cyst is a cystic duplication of the tracheobronchial tree.

Incidence: Bronchogenic cysts are relatively rare but represent the most common cystic lesion of the mediastinum and account for approximately 20% of surgically resected cystic lung lesions.[140]

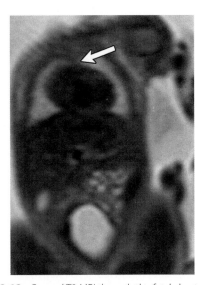

FIGURE 25.3-18: Coronal T2 MRI through the fetal chest demonstrates absence of the thymus gland in the superior mediastinum.

Prevalence may be underestimated because of cases not coming to clinical recognition.[101]

Pathogenesis: Bronchogenic cysts result from abnormal budding of the ventral diverticulum of the foregut, which leads to a focal cystic duplication of the tracheobronchial tree.[101] The cyst walls are lined with ciliated columnar epithelium and often contain fibrous tissue and small amounts of cartilage. Cyst contents may vary from a thin watery fluid collection to thicker mucoid material.[101] The majority of bronchogenic cysts (approximately 85%) are located in the mediastinum most commonly adjacent to the distal trachea or proximal main stem bronchi. The remainder of bronchogenic cysts occurs within the lung parenchyma. If the budding abnormality occurs early in bronchial development, the cyst is mediastinal in location, and when abnormal budding occurs later in development, the result is usually an intrapulmonary bronchogenic cyst.[141]

Diagnosis: *US:* Bronchogenic cysts usually appear as a well-defined unilocular hypoechoic mass within the fetal mediastinum near the carina of the trachea or, less commonly, within the lung parenchyma (Fig. 25.3-19A). The cysts are typically solitary or, less commonly, manifest as multiple lesions.[141] Large mediastinal bronchogenic cysts may compress the tracheobronchial tree and esophagus, and result in lung overinflation and polyhydramnios.[142]

MRI: A bronchogenic cyst appears as a high-signal-intensity fluid-containing structure on T2 sequences (Figs. 25.3-19B and 25.3-20).[143,144] MRI may complement US by ascertaining the precise location of the cyst and assessing for any associated lung parenchyma abnormalities.

Differential Diagnosis: The differential diagnosis for a mediastinal bronchogenic cyst includes an enteric duplication cyst involving the esophagus. Enteric duplication cysts are rare congenital anomalies that may arise anywhere in the gastrointestinal tract. Approximately one-third of cases involve the foregut, which includes the esophagus, stomach, and proximal duodenum. A large neurenteric cyst may also mimic a

bronchogenic cyst; however, accurate localization of the cyst between the esophagus and the trachea should confirm the correct diagnosis of a bronchogenic cyst. The differential diagnosis for an intrapulmonary bronchogenic cyst includes a unilocular CPAM with a single dominant cyst or the very rare case of a cystic PPB.

Prognosis: Limited data are available for the prognosis of prenatally diagnosed bronchogenic cysts. Most lesions are small and unassociated with mass effect, and fare well with no significant complications. Some lesions that compress the bronchial tree may cause overinflation of the adjacent lung parenchyma.

Management: Most cysts require no fetal intervention and are managed with serial US to assure stability in size. A very large bronchogenic cyst associated with mediastinal shift may have improved outcome with percutaneous drainage, but the experience is very limited.[142,145]

Most are removed postnatally to prevent superimposed infection, hemorrhage, or growth that could impinge on adjacent structures.

Recurrence: There is no known recurrence risk.

Neurenteric Cyst

Neurenteric cysts represent enteric remnants, which result from incomplete separation of the notochord from the foregut during early embyrogenesis.[146–148]

Incidence: Neurenteric cysts are rare lesions, and the incidence in the fetus is not known.

Pathogenesis: Neurenteric cysts are felt to occur due to incomplete notochord separation in the presence of a persistent communication between the ectoderm of the spinal cord and the endoderm of the foregut before closure of the neural tube. Neurenteric cysts are characterized by an intraspinal cystic component

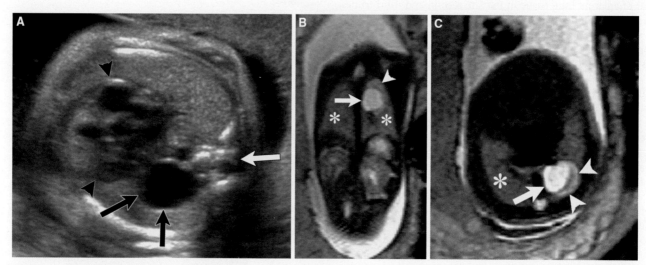

FIGURE 25.3-19: Intrapulmonary bronchogenic cyst in a 25-week gestational age fetus. **A:** Axial US through the fetal chest demonstrates an intrapulmonary unilocular hypoechoic lesion with through transmission *(black arrows)*. The heart is indicated by *arrowheads* and the spine by a *white arrow*. Coronal **(B)** and axial **(C)** T2 MRI demonstrate a left-sided high-signal mass *(arrow)* confirmed to be a bronchogenic cyst. High-signal-intensity lung *(arrowheads)* surrounding the cyst corresponded to fluid trapped in the lung distal to the bronchogenic cyst. Normal lungs are indicated by *asterisks*.

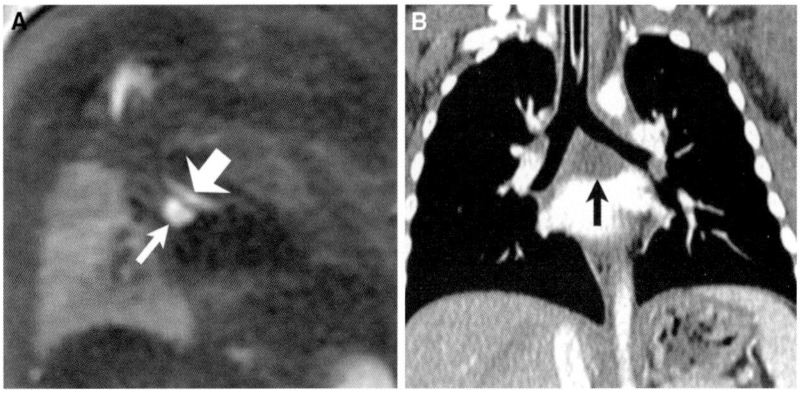

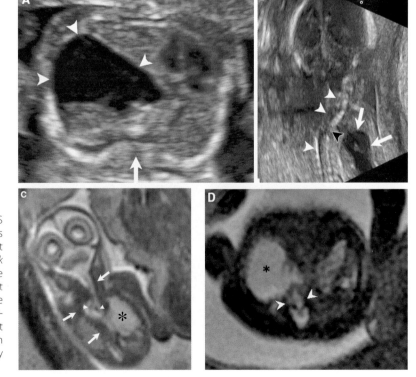

FIGURE 25.3-20: Mediastinal bronchogenic cyst causing lung hyperinflation in a 23-week gestational age fetus. **A:** Coronal T2 fetal MRI demonstrates a subcarinal bronchogenic cyst *(thin arrow)*. Left main stem bronchus is indicated by *thick arrow*. **B:** Newborn coronal computed tomography confirms subcarinal bronchogenic cyst *(arrow)*.

that is connected to a mediastinal or thoracic cyst.[149] Approximately 90% of all neurenteric cysts are localized to the posterior mediastinal compartment superior to the carina; however, the cysts may occur at any location throughout the spinal column. The most common locations are in the lower cervical and upper thoracic regions. Most are associated with an intradural extamedullary cystic component within the spinal canal. Connections with the gastrointestinal tract may also be identified.[150] Approximately 50% are associated with vertebral body segmentation anomalies and scoliosis.[146,148,151] Serpentine syndrome, likely sporadic, is described in the presence of brachioesophagus, thoracic stomach, and congenital vertebral anomalies including failure of fusion, segmentation, and/or formation resulting in rachischisis.[152]

Neurenteric cysts are usually unilocular and appear as a round or tubular mediastinal cystic mass with connection to the spinal canal. Large mediastinal neurenteric cysts may result in mass effect on the adjacent lung, airways, heart, and vessels, and when coexisting with intraspinal lesions may result in signs and symptoms of central nervous system abnormalities after birth.

Diagnosis: *US:* Neurenteric cysts appear as a posterior mediastinal unilocular or septated cyst with a thin wall, most commonly superior to the carina (Fig. 25.3-21A, B). Large cysts with mass effect may result in cardiac malposition or hydrops fetalis. Associated spinal findings include vertebral segmentation anomalies (hemivertebra or butterfly vertebra) and scoliosis.[146,148,151]

MRI: T2 fluid-sensitive sequences demonstrate a high-signal-intensity, well-marginated cyst in the posterior mediastinum (see Fig. 25.3-21B, C). MRI may also show the extent of the lesion into the spinal canal. Neurenteric cysts may be associated with the rare split notochord syndrome characterized by a cleft of the vertebral column. Gastrointestinal and other central nervous system anomalies have been described.[153–155]

Differential Diagnosis: Differential diagnosis for a neurenteric cyst includes BPMs, including a macrocystic CPAM. Other considerations include a bronchogenic cyst, pericardial cyst, CDH with herniated stomach, and cystic pleural pulmonary blastoma. The presence of associated spinal anomalies should confirm the correct diagnosis of neurenteric cyst.

FIGURE 25.3-21: Neurenteric cyst. **A:** Axial US shows a large mediastinal cyst *(arrowheads)*. Spine is indicated by an *arrow*. **B:** Coronal US demonstrates cyst *(arrows)* communicating with the spinal canal *(black arrowhead)*. Scoliotic spine with abnormal curvature *(white arrowheads)*. **C:** Coronal T2 MRI demonstrates split spinal cord *(arrowheads)* and abnormal curvature to the spine *(arrows)*. Neurenteric cyst *(asterisk)*. **D:** Axial steady-state free precession MRI demonstrates neurenteric cyst *(asterisk)* and open communication of spinal canal with posterior mediastinal cyst *(arrowheads)*. Images courtesy of Beth Kline-Fath.

Prognosis: The outcome of a neurenteric cyst depends largely on the extent of the mass, mass effect on adjacent organs, and the presence of associated central nervous system abnormalities. Large cysts may compress the developing lung and result in pulmonary hypoplasia or hydrops fetalis. Pulmonary hypoplasia secondary to a neurenteric cyst can be associated with respiratory distress after birth.[76,151]

Management: There is minimal literature regarding the role of surgical intervention in fetuses diagnosed with a neurenteric cyst.[149] Prenatal intervention is rarely indicated, although there have been case reports of treatment by aspiration or placement of a shunt if the cystic mass is large enough to raise concern for pulmonary hypoplasia.[149] Postnatal surgical correction is indicated.

Recurrence: The lesion is sporadic with no known recurrence risk.

Teratoma

Teratomas are a type of germ cell tumor that histologically contains tissue elements of ectodermal, mesodermal, and endodermal origin.

Incidence: Prenatal diagnosis of a mediastinal teratoma is a rare occurrence, and pericardial lesions are extremely rare with fewer than 100 cases reported.[156,157] Teratomas are the most common congenital neoplasm in children, and the vast majority of prenatally diagnosed teratomas are sacrococcygeal, accounting for approximately 80% of all teratomas.[156] Approximately 10% of teratomas are localized in the mediastinum, most commonly in the anterior superior compartment, and when large may result in severe compression of adjacent mediastinal structures and the developing lung.[157]

Pathogenesis: Teratomas are neoplasms composed of all three germ layers or multiple foreign tissues without organ specificity. Etiology is yet unknown, but hypothesized to result from aberrant twinning, totipotent cells from Hensen node or from reproductive gland analog. The majority of teratomas in children are benign.

Diagnosis: *US:* Mediastinal teratomas are localized to the anterior/superior mediastinum and appear as a cystic, solid, or a complex mass with heterogeneous echogenicity (Fig. 25.3-22A). Hyperechogenic foci associated with acoustic shadowing are indicative of internal calcifications and are helpful to confirm diagnosis. Pericardial teratomas may be differentiated from mediastinal teratoma by the association with pericardial effusion in the majority of cases.[158]

MRI: On T2 sequences, mediastinal and pericardial teratomas appear as cystic, solid, or complex masses in the superior

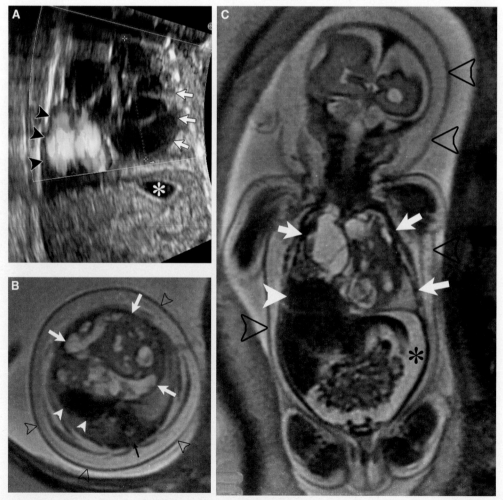

FIGURE 25.3-22: Mediastinal teratoma. **A:** Coronal US demonstrates a large complex cystic mediastinal mass *(arrows)* displacing the heart *(arrowheads)*. *Asterisk* indicates the stomach. Axial **(B)** and coronal **(C)** T2 MRI demonstrate a large complex mediastinal teratoma *(white arrows)* displacing the heart *(white arrowheads)* inferiorly into the right chest and associated fetal hydrops. Skin thickening *(black arrowheads)* and fetal ascites *(black asterisk)*. *Black arrow* indicates the spine. Images courtesy of Beth Kline-Fath, MD.

anterior mediastinum (see Fig. 25.3-22B, C). High-signal foci on T1 sequences are indicative of internal fat, calcification, or hemorrhage into the cystic components. The lesion usually displaces the heart inferiorly.

Differential Diagnosis: Differential diagnosis for a mediastinal or pericardial teratoma includes mediastinal bronchogenic cyst or enteric duplication cyst. Bronchogenic cysts or enteric duplication cysts tend to be in the middle or posterior mediastinum respectively and are not associated with solid components. When large, the lesion may mimic a CPAM, but can be differentiated by inferior more than right or leftward displacement of the heart. The anterior mediastinal location of teratomas and the frequent presence of solid components or calcifications should also allow for accurate diagnosis.

Prognosis: Complications of teratomas in the fetus are uncommon, and prognosis is expected to be good for small lesions. Large mediastinal or pericardial teratomas may cause significant mass effect on airway, heart, lungs, and esophagus, resulting in airway obstruction, diminished cardiac output, pulmonary hypoplasia, and polyhydramnios.[157,159] In the presence of polyhydramnios, the fetus is at risk for preterm labor. Hydrops fetalis likely results when a large mass inhibits venous return to the heart and is associated with high morbidity and mortality.[156]

Management: Management is surveillance with serial USs to assess for the rare complication of airway obstruction, hydrops fetalis, or diminished cardiac output. If hydrops occurs late in gestation greater than 30 weeks, the fetus may be delivered preterm or EXIT to airway if airway compression is noted.[159] If the fetus is less than 30 weeks with large pericardial effusion or dominant lesion cyst, pericardiocentesis and/or cyst aspiration may be considered.[160] In the absence of drainable fluid in a severely less than 30-week hydropic fetus, *in utero* resection may be attempted. In the presence of compression of intrathoracic structures, EXIT procedure may rarely be considered.[161] Postnatal resection is mandated because of risk of malignancy.

Recurrence: Most cases are sporadic with no recurrence risk; however, there is a small group that is inherited as a familial genetic disturbance.

Fetal Pleural Effusion (Hydrothorax)

Incidence: Fetal pleural effusions are relatively uncommon, manifesting in approximately 1:10,000 to 15,000 pregnancies.[162]

Pathogenesis: Fetal pleural effusion may occur as a primary abnormality, usually associated with chylothorax, or as part of hydrops fetalis.[162–166] Most commonly, a pleural effusion in the fetus is associated with hydrops fetalis, which may be caused by numerous conditions, including cardiovascular disease, underlying BPMs, chromosomal abnormalities (most commonly trisomy 21 and Turner syndrome), CDH, cystic hygroma, or infection.[163–165] Cardiac, pulmonary, or chromosomal abnormalities are associated in approximately 80% of cases.[163,166]

Maternal parvovirus infection has been associated with transient isolated pleural effusions, which often resolve spontaneously before term and are thought to result from direct pleural inflammation.[167]

Chylothorax is the most common cause of a primary congenital pleural effusion in a fetus and is a diagnosis to be considered

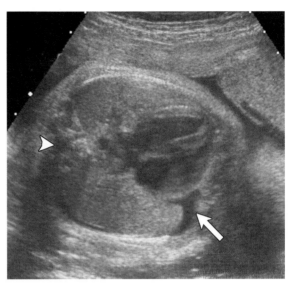

FIGURE 25.3-23: Pleural effusion. Axial US demonstrates a right pleural effusion *(arrow)* secondary to maternal parvovirus infection, which resolved spontaneously without postnatal sequelae. *Arrowhead* indicates spine.

after excluding other causes.[168] Chylothorax is commonly due to a primary defect in the lymphatic system, caused either via inflammation or genetic origin or, less likely, as a secondary finding in the presence of an underlying lymphatic malformation. When a primary pleural effusion is large, it may result in mediastinal compression and lead to hydrops fetalis, thereby making it difficult to distinguish between primary and secondary effusions.[168–170]

Diagnosis: *US:* Fetal pleural effusion is usually detected as an incidental finding by identifying an intrathoracic fluid collection surrounding the fetal lung, most often on the right side but may be bilateral (Fig. 25.3-23). It is often the first sign of fetal hydrops; therefore, identification of pleural effusion should trigger an investigation to exclude the more common causes of fetal hydrops prior to assuming the diagnosis of a chylothorax. A search for additional anomalies, including lymphatic malformation or sequestration, should be performed. When pleural effusions are large, the underlying lung will appear to float freely in the pleural cavity.

MRI: Pleural effusions can also be readily identified on MRI, which by itself does not add significant information to that provided by US. The potential value of MRI in the setting of a hydrothorax is to identify an associated underlying mass as the etiology of the effusion. For example, torsion of an ELS may present with a large ipsilateral pleural effusion (Fig. 25.3-24).

Differential Diagnosis: Diagnosis of pleural effusion is usually straightforward. Occasionally, a massive pericardial effusion may mimic a pleural effusion; however, the appearance of the fluid surrounding the heart should allow for distinction. The main challenge in diagnosis of pleural effusion is to distinguish a primary from a secondary effusion. Careful scrutiny to exclude an underlying mass or other anomalies is important for patient counseling and pregnancy management.

Prognosis: The prognosis for pleural effusion in the fetus is variable. Some cases resolve or remain stable throughout pregnancy, whereas others evolve to severe hydrothorax, which can result in hydrops fetalis. Approximately 10% of isolated hydrothoraces

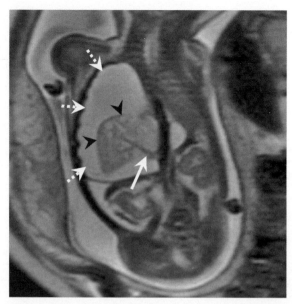

FIGURE 25.3-24: A 31-week gestation fetus with large pleural effusion. Coronal T2 MRI identified a heterogeneous lung lesion *(arrowheads)* supplied by a feeding vessel from aorta *(white arrow)* in association with large pleural effusion *(dotted arrows)*. Postnatal confirmed hybrid lesion. Images courtesy of Beth Kline-Fath, MD.

resolve spontaneously with good postnatal outcome. Mild-to-moderate pleural effusions which remain stable throughout pregnancy are associated with good postnatal outcome.[166,168,171] Cases associated with hydrops fetalis have a high mortality rate, reported as greater than 50%.[172] Large bilateral pleural effusions with significant mediastinal compression associated with hydrops fetalis constitute poor prognostic signs with a high likelihood for fatal outcome, reported as greater than 90% in the absence of intervention.[165,169,170,172-177] Large pleural effusions may also compress the underlying lung and result in pulmonary hypoplasia or compress the esophagus, causing polyhydramnios. Karyotyping to exclude trisomy 21 or Turner syndrome is indicated.

Management: Small-to-moderate isolated pleural effusions, which remain stable, can undergo surveillance with serial USs without intervention. Given the high mortality in the presence of large effusions and propensity to develop hydrops, prenatal intervention is typically considered. If the karyotype is normal, maternal diet modification by supplementation with medium-chain triglycerides may decrease or resolve the effusion.[178] If titers are negative for infection and effusion persists, thoracentesis may aid in confirming chylothorax by documenting lymphocyte predominance (>95%). Thoracoamniotic shunting is the gold standard therapy in the presence of large effusion or hydrops. Shunting may reduce the risk of lung hypoplasia and hydrops and has been reported to improve the outcome.[170,174,175,179,180] With thoracoamniotic shunting, mortality rates are reduced; however, they still remain high at 10% to 30% for non hydropic cases and 50% to 60% for hydropic cases.[168,170,180] Some centers will consider a thoracentesis prior to placing a thoracoamniotic shunt since decompression of fluid may enhance sonographic examination of the fetal heart and the underlying lungs. However, in the majority of cases, the fluid will reaccumulate within 24 hours, and a shunt will need to be placed if prolonged decompression is desired.[168,169,171,181]

Recurrence: Risk of recurrence is dependent on the etiology of the effusion. Chylothorax is usually sporadic with low recurrence, although familial cases have been cited.[182]

REFERENCES

1. Lim FY, Crombleholme TM, Hedrick HL, et al. Congenital high airway obstruction syndrome: natural history and management. *J Pediatr Surg.* 2003;38:940–945.
2. Barth RA. Imaging of fetal chest masses. *Pediatr Radiol.* 2012;42(suppl 1):S62–S73.
3. Gilboa Y, Achiron R, Katorza E, et al. Early sonographic diagnosis of congenital high-airway obstruction syndrome. *Ultrasound Obstet Gynecol.* 2009;33:731–733.
4. Vidaeff AC, Szmuk P, Mastrobattista JM, et al. More or less CHAOS: case report and literature review suggesting the existence of a distinct subtype of congenital high airway obstruction syndrome. *Ultrasound Obstet Gynecol.* 2007;30:114–117.
5. Kassanos D, Christodoulou CN, Agapitos E, et al. Prenatal ultrasonographic detection of the tracheal atresia sequence. *Ultrasound Obstet Gynecol.* 1997;10:133–136.
6. Berg C, Geipel A, Germer U, et al. Prenatal detection of Fraser syndrome without cryptophthalmos: case report and review of the literature. *Ultrasound Obstet Gynecol.* 2001;18:76–80.
7. Mong A, Johnson AM, Kramer SS, et al. Congenital high airway obstruction syndrome: MR/US findings, effect on management, and outcome. *Pediatr Radiol.* 2008;38:1171–1179.
8. Guimaraes CV, Linam LE, Kline-Fath BM, et al. Prenatal MRI findings of fetuses with congenital high airway obstruction sequence. *Korean J Radiol.* 2009;10:129–134.
9. Girsen AI, Hintz SR, Sammour R, et al. Prediction of neonatal respiratory distress in pregnancies complicated by fetal lung masses. *Prenat Diagn.* 2017;37(3):266–272.
10. Kohl T, Van de Vondel P, Stressig R, et al. Percutaneous fetoscopic laser decompression of congenital high airway obstruction syndrome (CHAOS) from laryngeal atresia via a single trocar—current technical constraints and potential solutions for future interventions. *Fetal Diagn Ther.* 2009;25:67–71.
11. DeCou JM, Jones DC, Jacobs HD, et al. Successful ex utero intrapartum treatment (EXIT) procedure for congenital high airway obstruction syndrome (CHAOS) owing to laryngeal atresia. *J Pediatr Surg.* 1998;33:1563–1565.
12. Bui TH, Grunewald C, Frenckner B, et al. Successful EXIT (ex utero intrapartum treatment) procedure in a fetus diagnosed prenatally with congenital high-airway obstruction syndrome due to laryngeal atresia. *Eur J Pediatr Surg.* 2000;10:328–333.
13. Nolan HR, Gurria J, Peiro JL, et al. Congenital high airway obstruction syndrome (CHAOS): natural history, prenatal management strategies, and outcomes at a single comprehensive fetal center. *J Pediatr Surg* 2019, 54(6):1153–1158.
14. Langston C. New concepts in the pathology of congenital lung malformations. *Semin Pediatr Surg.* 2003;12:17–37.
15. Epelman M, Kreiger PA, Servaes S, et al. Current imaging of prenatally diagnosed congenital lung lesions. *Semin Ultrasound CT MR.* 2010;31:141–157.
16. Biyyam DR, Chapman T, Ferguson MR, et al. Congenital lung abnormalities: embryologic features, prenatal diagnosis, and postnatal radiologic-pathologic correlation. *Radiographics.* 2010;30:1721–1738.
17. Stigers KB, Woodring JH, Kanga JF. The clinical and imaging spectrum of findings in patients with congenital lobar emphysema. *Pediatr Pulmonol.* 1992;14:160–170.
18. Barth RA, Newman B, Rubesova E, et al. Congenital lobar overinflation (CLO)/congenital lobar emphsysema (CLE)—not an uncommon cause for a fetal chest mass (Paper # PA9). *Pediatr Radiol.* 2009;39(suppl 2):S252–S255.
19. Johnston J, Kline-Fath BM, Bitters C, et al. Congenital overinflation: prenatal MRI and US findings and outcomes. *Prenat Diagn.* 2016;36:568–575.
20. Olutoye OO, Coleman BG, Hubbard AM, et al. Prenatal diagnosis and management of congenital lobar emphysema. *J Pediatr Surg.* 2000;35:792–795.
21. Pacharn P, Kline-Fath B, Calvo-Garcia M, et al. Congenital lung lesions: prenatal MRI and postnatal findings. *Pediatr Radiol.* 2013;43(9):1136–1143.
22. Sparey C, Jawaheer G, Barrett AM, et al. Esophageal atresia in the Northern Region Congenital Anomaly Survey, 1985–1997: prenatal diagnosis and outcome. *Am J Obstet Gynecol.* 2000;182:427–431.
23. Depaepe A, Dolk H, Lechat MF. The epidemiology of tracheo-oesophageal fistula and oesophageal atresia in Europe: EUROCAT Working Group. *Arch Dis Child.* 1993;68:743–748.
24. Torfs CP, Curry CJ, Bateson TF. Population-based study of tracheoesophageal fistula and esophageal atresia. *Teratology.* 1995;52:220–232.
25. Forrester MB, Merz RD. Epidemiology of oesophageal atresia and tracheo-oesophageal fistula in Hawaii, 1986–2000. *Public Health.* 2005;119:483–488.
26. Pringle KC. Human fetal lung development and related animal models. *Clin Obstet Gynecol.* 1986;29:502–513.
27. Slovis TL. *Caffey's Pediatric Diagnostic Imaging.* 11th ed. Philadelphia, PA: Mosby Elsevier; 2008.
28. Pameijer CR, Hubbard AM, Coleman B, et al. Combined pure esophageal atresia, duodenal atresia, biliary atresia, and pancreatic ductal atresia: prenatal diagnostic features and review of the literature. *J Pediatr Surg.* 2000;35:745–747.
29. Marquette GP, Skoll MA, Yong SL, et al. First-trimester imaging of combined esophageal and duodenal atresia without a tracheoesophageal fistula. *J Ultrasound Med.* 2004;23:1232.

30. Estroff JA, Parad RB, Share JC, et al. Second trimester prenatal findings in duodenal and esophageal atresia without tracheoesophageal fistula. *J Ultrasound Med.* 1994;13:375–379.
31. Genevieve D, de Pontual L, Amiel J, et al. An overview of isolated and syndromic oesophageal atresia. *Clin Genet.* 2007;71:392–399.
32. Holder TM, Cloud DT, Lewis JE Jr, et al. Esophageal atresia and tracheoesophageal fistula: a survey of its members by the surgical section of the American Academy of Pediatrics. *Pediatrics.* 1964;34:542–549.
33. Bundy AL, Saltzman DH, Emerson D, et al. Sonographic features associated with cleft palate. *J Clin Ultrasound.* 1986;14:486–489.
34. Kallen B, Mastroiacovo P, Robert E. Major congenital malformations in Down syndrome. *Am J Med Genet.* 1996;65:160–166.
35. Matsuoka S, Takeuchi K, Yamanaka Y, et al. Comparison of magnetic resonance imaging and ultrasonography in the prenatal diagnosis of congenital thoracic abnormalities. *Fetal Diagn Ther.* 2003;18:447–453.
36. Satoh S, Takashima T, Takeuchi H, et al. Antenatal sonographic detection of the proximal esophageal segment: specific evidence for congenital esophageal atresia. *J Clin Ultrasound.* 1995;23:419–423.
37. Centini G, Rosignoli L, Kenanidis A, et al. Prenatal diagnosis of esophageal atresia with the pouch sign. *Ultrasound Obstet Gynecol.* 2003;21:494–497.
38. Stringer MD, McKenna KM, Goldstein RB, et al. Prenatal diagnosis of esophageal atresia. *J Pediatr Surg.* 1995;30:1258–1263.
39. Langer JC, Hussain H, Khan A, et al. Prenatal diagnosis of esophageal atresia using sonography and magnetic resonance imaging. *J Pediatr Surg.* 2001;36:804–807.
40. Mitani Y, Hasegawa T, Kubota A, et al. Prenatal findings of concomitant duodenal and esophageal atresia without tracheoesophageal fistula (Gross type A). *J Clin Ultrasound.* 2009;37:403–405.
41. Levine D, Barnewolt CE, Mehta TS, et al. Fetal thoracic abnormalities: MR imaging. *Radiology.* 2003;228:379–388.
42. Ethun CG, Fallon SC, Cassady CI, et al. Fetal MRI improves diagnostic accuracy in patients referred to a fetal center for suspected esophageal atresia. *J Pediatr Surg.* 2014;49(5):712–715.
43. Tracy S, Buchmiller TL, Ben-Ishay O, et al. The distended fetal hypopharynx: a sensitive and novel sign for the prenatal diagnosis of esophageal atresia. *J Pediatr Surg.* 2018;53(6):1137–1141.
44. McKenna KM, Goldstein RB, Stringer MD. Small or absent fetal stomach: prognostic significance. *Radiology.* 1995;197:729–733.
45. Brumfield CG, Davis RO, Owen J, et al. Pregnancy outcomes following sonographic nonvisualization of the fetal stomach. *Obstet Gynecol.* 1998;91:905–908.
46. Hill LM. Congenital microgastria: absence of the fetal stomach and normal third trimester amniotic fluid volume. *J Ultrasound Med.* 1994;3:894–896.
47. Kroes EJ, Festen C. Congenital microgastria: a case report and review of literature. *Pediatr Surg Int.* 1998;13:416–418.
48. Menon P, Rao KL, Cutinha HP, et al. Gastric augmentation in isolated congenital microgastria. *J Pediatr Surg.* 2003;38:E4–E6.
49. Spitz L. Oesophageal atresia. *Orphanet J Rare Dis.* 2007;2:24.
50. Lopez PJ, Keys C, Pierro A, et al. Oesophageal atresia: improved outcome in high-risk groups? *J Pediatr Surg.* 2006;41:331–334.
51. Sinha CK, Haider N, Marri RR, et al. Modified prognostic criteria for oesophageal atresia and tracheo-oesophageal fistula. *Eur J Pediatr Surg.* 2007;17:153–157.
52. Garabedian C, Bonnard A, Rousseau V, et al. Management and outcome of neonates with a prenatal diagnosis of esophageal atresia type A: a population-based study. *Prenat Diagn.* 2018;38(7):517–522. doi:10.1002/pd.5273.
53. Hölscher AC, Laschat M, Choinitzki V, et al. Quality of life after surgical treatment for esophageal atresia: long-term outcome of 154 patients. *Eur J Pediatr Surg.* 2017;27(5):443–448. doi:10.1055/s-0036-1597956.
54. Scott DA. Esophageal atresia/tracheoesophageal fistula overview. In: *GeneReviews [Internet].* Seattle, WA: University of Washington; 2009.
55. Burge D, Wheeler R. Increasing incidence of detection of congenital lung lesions. *Pediatr Pulmonol.* 2010;45:103; author reply 104.
56. Stocker JT, Madewell JE, Drake RM. Congenital cystic adenomatoid malformation of the lung: classification and morphologic spectrum. *Hum Pathol.* 1977;8:155–171.
57. Simonet WS, DeRose ML, Bucay N, et al. Pulmonary malformation in transgenic mice expressing human keratinocyte growth factor in the lung. *Proc Natl Acad Sci U S A.* 1995;92:12461–12465.
58. Volpe MV, Pham L, Lessin M, et al. Expression of Hoxb-5 during human lung development and in congenital lung malformations. *Birth Defects Res A Clin Mol Teratol.* 2003;67:550–556.
59. Volpe MV, Archavachotikul K, Bhan I, et al. Association of bronchopulmonary sequestration with expression of the homeobox protein Hoxb-5. *J Pediatr Surg.* 2000;35:1817–1819.
60. Riedlinger WF, Vargas SO, Jennings RW, et al. Bronchial atresia is common to extralobar sequestration, intralobar sequestration, congenital cystic adenomatoid malformation, and lobar emphysema. *Pediatr Dev Pathol.* 2006;9:361–373.
61. Kunisaki SM, Fauza DO, Nemes LP, et al. Bronchial atresia: the hidden pathology within a spectrum of prenatally diagnosed lung masses. *J Pediatr Surg.* 2006;41:61–65.
62. Stocker JT. Congenital pulmonary airway malformation: a new name for and an expanded classification of congenital cystic adenomatous malformation of the lung. *Histopathology.* 2002;41:424–431.
63. Stocker JT. The respiratory tract. In: Stocker JT, Dehner LP, eds. *Pediatric Pathology.* Philadelphia, PA: Lippincott Williams & Wilkins; 2001:445.
64. Adzick NS. Management of fetal lung lesions. *Clin Perinatol.* 2003;30:481–492.
65. Crombleholme TM, Coleman B, Hedrick H, et al. Cystic adenomatoid malformation volume ratio predicts outcome in prenatally diagnosed cystic adenomatoid malformation of the lung. *J Pediatr Surg.* 2002;37:331–338.
66. Azizkhan RG, Crombleholme TM. Congenital cystic lung disease: contemporary antenatal and postnatal management. *Pediatr Surg Int.* 2008;24:643–657.
67. Hubbard AM, Adzick NS, Crombleholme TM, et al. Congenital chest lesions: diagnosis and characterization with prenatal MR imaging. *Radiology.* 1999;212:43–48.
68. Hubbard AM. Prenatal magnetic resonance imaging for fetal abnormalities. In: Milunsky A, ed. *Genetic Disorders and the Fetus: Diagnosis, Prevention, and Treatment.* Baltimore, MD and London: Johns Hopkins University Press; 2004:944.
69. Victoria T, Srinivasan AS, Pogoriler J, et al. The rare solid fetal lung lesion with T2-hypointense components: prenatal imaging findings with postnatal pathological correlation. *Pediatr Radiol.* 2018;48(11):1556–1566. doi:10.1007/s00247-018-4174-0.
70. Zamora IF, Sheikh F, Cassady CI, et al. Fetal MRI lung volumes are predictive of perinatal outcomes in fetuses with congenital lung masses. *J Pediatr Surg.* 2014;49(6):853–858.
71. Toru HS, Sanhal CY, Yilmaz GT, et al. Rare congenital pulmonary malformation with diagnostic challenging: congenital pulmonary lymphangiectasia, report of four autopsy cases and review of literature. *J Matern Fetal Neonatal Med.* 2015;28(12):1457–1460.
72. Seed M, Bradley T, Bourgeois J, et al. Antenatal MR imaging of pulmonary lymphangiectasia secondary to hypoplastic left heart syndrome. *Pediatr Radiol.* 2009;39(7):747–749.
73. Saul D, Degenhardt K, Iyoob SD, et al. Hypoplastic left heart syndrome and the nutmeg lung pattern in utero: a cause and effect relationship or prognostic indicator? *Pediatr Radiol.* 2016;46(4):483–489.
74. Abdullah MM, Lacro RV, Smallhorn J, et al. Fetal cardiac dextroposition in the absence of an intrathoracic mass: sign of significant right lung hypoplasia. *J Ultrasound Med.* 2000;19:669–676.
75. Cavoretto P, Molina F, Poggi S, et al. Prenatal diagnosis and outcome of echogenic fetal lung lesions. *Ultrasound Obstet Gynecol.* 2008;32:769–783.
76. Adzick NS, Harrison MR, Crombleholme TM, et al. Fetal lung lesions: management and outcome. *Am J Obstet Gynecol.* 1998;179:884–889.
77. Wilson RD, Hedrick HL, Liechty KW, et al. Cystic adenomatoid malformation of the lung: review of genetics, prenatal diagnosis, and in utero treatment. *Am J Med Genet A.* 2006;140:151–155.
78. Husler MR, Wilson RD, Rychik J, et al. Prenatally diagnosed fetal lung lesions with associated conotruncal heart defects: is there a genetic association? *Prenat Diagn.* 2007;27:1123–1128.
79. Bromley B, Parad R, Estroff JA, et al. Fetal lung masses: prenatal course and outcome. *J Ultrasound Med.* 1995;14:927–936; quiz p1378.
80. Thorpe-Beeston JG, Nicolaides KH. Cystic adenomatoid malformation of the lung: prenatal diagnosis and outcome. *Prenat Diagn.* 1994;14:677–688.
81. Miller JA, Corteville JE, Langer JC. Congenital cystic adenomatoid malformation in the fetus: natural history and predictors of outcome. *J Pediatr Surg.* 1996;31:805–808.
82. Duncombe GJ, Dickinson JE, Kikiros CS. Prenatal diagnosis and management of congenital cystic adenomatoid malformation of the lung. *Am J Obstet Gynecol.* 2002;187:950–954.
83. Illanes S, Hunter A, Evans M, et al. Prenatal diagnosis of echogenic lung: evolution and outcome. *Ultrasound Obstet Gynecol.* 2005;26:145–149.
84. Zirpoli S, Munari AM, Rustico M, et al. Fetal-MRI prenatal diagnosis of severe bilateral lung hypoplasia: alveolar capillary dysplasia case report. *J Prenat Med.* 2016;10(3–4):15–19.
85. Morris LM, Lim FY, Livingston JC, et al. High-risk fetal congenital pulmonary airway malformations have a variable response to steroids. *J Pediatr Surg.* 2009;44:60–65.
86. Peranteau WH, Wilson RD, Liechty KW, et al. Effect of maternal betamethasone administration on prenatal congenital cystic adenomatoid malformation growth and fetal survival. *Fetal Diagn Ther.* 2007;22:365–371.
87. Curran PF, Jelin EB, Rand L, et al. Prenatal steroids for microcystic congenital cystic adenomatoid malformations. *J Pediatr Surg.* 2010;45:145–150.
88. Loh KC, Jelin E, Hirose S, et al. Microcystic congenital pulmonary airway malformation with hydrops fetalis: steroids vs open fetal resection. *J Pediatr Surg.* 2012;47:36–39.
89. Derderian SC, Coleman AM, Jeanty C, et al. Favorable outcomes in high-risk congenital pulmonary airway malformations treated with multiple courses of maternal betamethasone. *J Pediatr Surg.* 2015;50:515–528.
90. Brown MF, Lewis D, Brouillette RM, et al. Successful prenatal management of hydrops, caused by congenital cystic adenomatoid malformation, using serial aspirations. *J Pediatr Surg.* 1995;30:1098–1099.
91. Ryo E, Okai T, Namba S, et al. Successful thoracoamniotic shunting using a double-flower catheter in a case of fetal cystic adenomatoid malformation associated with hydrops and polyhydramnios. *Ultrasound Obstet Gynecol.* 1997;10:293–296.
92. Wilson RD, Baxter JK, Johnson MP, et al. Thoracoamniotic shunts: fetal treatment of pleural effusions and congenital cystic adenomatoid malformations. *Fetal Diagn Ther.* 2004;19:413–420.
93. Yokoyama T, Yamashita K, Nishiyama T, et al. A case of thoraco-amniotic shunt for congenital cystic adenomatoid malformation [in Japanese]. *Masui.* 2005;54:283–290.

94. Harrison MR, Adzick NS, Jennings RW, et al. Antenatal intervention for congenital cystic adenomatoid malformation. *Lancet.* 1990;336:965–967.
95. Bruner JP, Jarnagin BK, Reinisch L. Percutaneous laser ablation of fetal congenital cystic adenomatoid malformation: too little, too late? *Fetal Diagn Ther.* 2000;15:359–363.
96. Lee FL, Said N, Grikscheit TC, et al. Treatment of congenital pulmonary airway malformation induced hydrops fetalis via percutaneous sclerotherapy. *Fetal Diagn Ther.* 2012;31:264–268.
97. Morini F, Zani A, Conforti A, et al. Current management of congenital pulmonary airway malformations: a "European Pediatric Surgeon Association" Survey. *Eur J Pediatr Surg.* 2018;28(1):1–5.
98. Cook J, Chitty LS, De Coppi P, et al. The natural history of prenatally diagnosed congenital cystic lung lesions: long-term follow-up of 119 cases. *Arch Dis Child.* 2017;102(9):798–803.
99. Rosado-de-Christenson ML, Frazier AA, Stocker JT, et al. From the archives of the AFIP. Extralobar sequestration: radiologic-pathologic correlation. *Radiographics.* 1993;13:425–441.
100. Stocker JT. Sequestrations of the lung. *Semin Diagn Pathol.* 1986;3:106–121.
101. Winters WD, Effmann EL. Congenital masses of the lung: prenatal and postnatal imaging evaluation. *J Thorac Imaging.* 2001;16:196–206.
102. Wesley JR, Heidelberger KP, DiPietro MA, et al. Diagnosis and management of congenital cystic disease of the lung in children. *J Pediatr Surg.* 1986;21:202–207.
103. Lager DJ, Kuper KA, Haake GK. Subdiaphragmatic extralobar pulmonary sequestration. *Arch Pathol Lab Med.* 1991;115:536–538.
104. Johnson AM, Hubbard AM. Congenital anomalies of the fetal/neonatal chest. *Semin Roentgenol.* 2004;39:197–214.
105. Frazier AA, Rosado de Christenson ML, Stocker JT, et al. Intralobar sequestration: radiologic-pathologic correlation. *Radiographics.* 1997;17:725–745.
106. Gerle RD, Jaretzki A III, Ashley CA, et al. Congenital bronchopulmonary-foregut malformation: pulmonary sequestration communicating with the gastrointestinal tract. *N Engl J Med.* 1968;278:1413–1419.
107. Conran RM, Stocker JT. Extralobar sequestration with frequently associated congenital cystic adenomatoid malformation, type 2: report of 50 cases. *Pediatr Dev Pathol.* 1999;2:454–463.
108. Cass DL, Crombleholme TM, Howell LJ, et al. Cystic lung lesions with systemic arterial blood supply: a hybrid of congenital cystic adenomatoid malformation and bronchopulmonary sequestration. *J Pediatr Surg.* 1997;32:986–990.
109. Oliver ER, DeBari SE, Giannone MM, et al. Going with the flow: an aid in detecting and differentiating bronchopulmonary sequestrations and hybrid lesions. *J Ultrasound Med.* 2018;37(2):371–383.
110. Hernanz-Schulman M, Stein SM, Neblett WW, et al. Pulmonary sequestration: diagnosis with color Doppler sonography and a new theory of associated hydrothorax. *Radiology.* 1991;180:817–821.
111. Newman B. Congenital bronchopulmonary foregut malformations: concepts and controversies. *Pediatr Radiol.* 2006;36:773–791.
112. Riley JS, Urwin JW, Oliver ER, et al. Prenatal growth characteristics and pre/postnatal management of bronchopulmonary sequestrations. *J Pediatr Surg.* 2018;53(2):265–269.
113. Priest JR, Williams GM, Hill DA, et al. Pulmonary cysts in early childhood and the risk of malignancy. *Pediatr Pulmonol.* 2009;44:14–30.
114. Hill DA, Ivanovich J, Priest JR, et al. DICER1 mutations in familial pleuropulmonary blastoma. *Science.* 2009;325:965.
115. Priest JR, McDermott MB, Bhatia S, et al. Pleuropulmonary blastoma: a clinicopathologic study of 50 cases. *Cancer.* 1997;80:147–161.
116. Miniati DN, Chintagumpala M, Langston C, et al. Prenatal presentation and outcome of children with pleuropulmonary blastoma. *J Pediatr Surg.* 2006;41:66–71.
117. Hill DA, Jarzembowski JA, Priest JR, et al. Type I pleuropulmonary blastoma: pathology and biology study of 51 cases from the international pleuropulmonary blastoma registry. *Am J Surg Pathol.* 2008;32:282–295.
118. Naffaa LN, Donnelly LF. Imaging findings in pleuropulmonary blastoma. *Pediatr Radiol.* 2005;35:387–391.
119. Feinberg A, Hall NJ, Williams GM, et al. Can congenital pulmonary airway malformation be distinguished from Type I pleuropulmonary blastoma based on clinical and radiological features? *J Pediatr Surg.* 2016;51(1):33–37.
120. Messinger YH, Stewart DR, Priest JR, et al. Pleuropulmonary blastoma: a report on 350 central pathology-confirmed pleuropulmonary blastoma cases by the International Pleuropulmonary Blastoma Registry. *Cancer.* 2015;121(2):276–285.
121. Brock KE, Wall J, Esquivel M, et al. Congenital peribronchial myofibroblastic tumor: case report of an asymptomatic infant with a rapidly enlarging pulmonary mass and review of the literature. *Ann Clin Lab Sci.* 2015;45(1):83–89.
122. Calvo-Garcia MA, Lim FY, Stanek J, et al. Congenital peribronchial myofibroblastic tumor: prenatal imaging clues to differentiate from other fetal chest lesions. *Pediatr Radiol.* 2014;44(4):479–483.
123. Dishop MK, Kuruvilla S. Primary and metastatic lung tumors in the pediatric population: a review and 25-year experience at a large children's hospital. *Arch Pathol Lab Med.* 2008;132(7):1079–1103.
124. Lazar DA, Cass DL, Dishop MK, et al. Fetal lung interstitial tumor: a cause of late gestation fetal hydrops. *J Pediatr Surg.* 2011;46(6):1263–1266.
125. Haynes BF, Hale LP. The human thymus: a chimeric organ comprised of central and peripheral lymphoid components. *Immunol Res.* 1998;18:175–192.
126. Schwartz RH. Acquisition of immunologic self-tolerance. *Cell.* 1989;57:1073–1081.
127. Cho JY, Min JY, Lee YH, et al. Diameter of the normal fetal thymus on ultrasound. *Ultrasound Obstet Gynecol.* 2007;29:634–638.
128. De Leon-Luis J, Gamez F, Pintado P, et al. Sonographic measurements of the thymus in male and female fetuses. *J Ultrasound Med.* 2009;28:43–48.
129. Felker RE, Cartier MS, Emerson DS, et al. Ultrasound of the fetal thymus. *J Ultrasound Med.* 1989;8:669–673.
130. Li L, Bahtiyar MO, Buhimschi CS, et al. Assessment of the fetal thymus by two- and three-dimensional ultrasound during normal human gestation and in fetuses with congenital heart defects. *Ultrasound Obstet Gynecol.* 2011;37:404–409.
131. Han BK, Yoon HK, Suh YL. Thymic ultrasound, II: diagnosis of aberrant cervical thymus. *Pediatr Radiol.* 2001;31:480–487.
132. Dodson WE, Alexander D, Al-Aish M, et al. The DiGeorge syndrome. *Lancet.* 1969;1:574–575.
133. Ichijima K, Yamabe H, Kobashi Y, et al. An unusual case of metaphyseal chondrodysplasia with an abnormal perilacunar matrix associated with agranulocytosis and hypoplasia of the thymus. *Virchows Arch.* 1981;391:275–289.
134. Martin JP, Aguilar FT. Thymic hypoplasia with severe combined immunodeficiency. *Ann Allergy.* 1977;39:196–200.
135. Hartge R, Jenkins DM, Kohler HG. Low thymic weight in small-for-dates babies. *Eur J Obstet Gynecol Reprod Biol.* 1978;8:153–155.
136. Zalel Y, Gamzu R, Mashiach S, et al. The development of the fetal thymus: an in utero sonographic evaluation. *Prenat Diagn.* 2002;22:114–117.
137. Toti P, De Felice C, Stumpo M, et al. Acute thymic involution in fetuses and neonates with chorioamnionitis. *Hum Pathol.* 2000;31:1121–1128.
138. Chaoui R, Kalache KD, Heling KS, et al. Absent or hypoplastic thymus on ultrasound: a marker for deletion 22q11.2 in fetal cardiac defects. *Ultrasound Obstet Gynecol.* 2002;20:546–552.
139. Barrea C, Yoo SJ, Chitayat D, et al. Assessment of the thymus at echocardiography in fetuses at risk for 22q11.2 deletion. *Prenat Diagn.* 2003;23:9–15.
140. Shanti CM, Klein MD. Cystic lung disease. *Semin Pediatr Surg.* 2008;17:2–8.
141. Young G, L'Heureux PR, Krueckeberg ST, et al. Mediastinal bronchogenic cyst: prenatal sonographic diagnosis. *AJR.* 1989;152:125–127.
142. Barbut J, Fernandez C, Blanc F, et al. Pulmonary sequestration of the left upper lobe associated with a bronchogenic cyst: case report of an exceptional association. *Pediatr Pulmonol.* 2011;46:509–511.
143. Levine D, Jennings R, Barnewolt C, et al. Progressive fetal bronchial obstruction caused by a bronchogenic cyst diagnosed using prenatal MR imaging. *AJR.* 2001;176:49–52.
144. Ward VL. MR imaging in the prenatal diagnosis of fetal chest masses: effects on diagnostic accuracy, clinical decision making, parental understanding, and prediction of neonatal respiratory health outcomes. *Acad Radiol.* 2002;9:1064–1069.
145. Bayar UO, Numanoglu V, Bektas S, et al. Management of fetal bronchogenic lung cysts: a case report and short review of literature. *Case Rep Med.* 2010;2010:751423.
146. Uludag S, Madazli R, Erdogan E, et al. A case of prenatally diagnosed fetal neurenteric cyst. *Ultrasound Obstet Gynecol.* 2001;18:277–279.
147. Reed JC, Sobonya RE. Morphologic analysis of foregut cysts in the thorax. *AJR.* 1974;120:851–860.
148. Strollo DC, Rosado-de-Christenson ML, Jett JR. Primary mediastinal tumors, part II: tumors of the middle and posterior mediastinum. *Chest.* 1997;112:1344–1357.
149. Aydin AL, Sasani M, Ucar B, et al. Prenatal diagnosis of a large, cervical, intraspinal, neurenteric cyst and postnatal outcome. *J Pediatr Surg.* 2009;44:1835–1838.
150. Fernandes ET, Custer MD, Burton EM, et al. Neurenteric cyst: surgery and diagnostic imaging. *J Pediatr Surg.* 1991;26:108–110.
151. Ryckman FC, Rosenkrantz JG. Thoracic surgical problems in infancy and childhood. *Surg Clin North Am.* 1985;65:1423–1454.
152. Beleza-Meireles A, Steenhaut P, Hocq C, et al. "Serpentine-like syndrome": a very rare multiple malformation syndrome characterised by brachioesophagus and vertebral anomalies. *Eur J Med Genet.* 2017;60(2):100–104.
153. Perera GB, Milne M. Neurenteric cyst: antenatal diagnosis by ultrasound. *Australas Radiol.* 1997;41:300–302.
154. Almog B, Leibovitch L, Achiron R. Split notochord syndrome—prenatal ultrasonographic diagnosis. *Prenat Diagn.* 2001;21:1159–1162.
155. Agangi A, Paladini D, Bagolan P, et al. Split notochord syndrome variant: prenatal findings and neonatal management. *Prenat Diagn.* 2005;25:23–27.
156. Schild RL, Plath H, Hofstaetter C, et al. Prenatal diagnosis of a fetal mediastinal teratoma. *Ultrasound Obstet Gynecol.* 1998;12:369–370.
157. Liang RI, Wang P, Chang FM, et al. Prenatal sonographic characteristics and Doppler blood flow study in a case of a large fetal mediastinal teratoma. *Ultrasound Obstet Gynecol.* 1998;11:214–218.
158. Tollens M, Grab D, Lang D, et al. Pericardial teratoma: prenatal diagnosis and course. *Fetal Diagn Ther.* 2003;18:432–436.
159. Merchant A, Hedrick H, Johnson M, et al. Management of fetal mediastinal teratoma. *J Pediatr Surg.* 2005;40:228–231.
160. Takayasu H, Yoshihiro K, Kuroda T, et al. Successful management of a large fetal mediastinal teratoma complicated by hydrops fetalis. *J Pediatr Surg.* 2010;45:621–624.
161. Agarwal A, Rosenkranz E, Yasin S, et al. EXIT procedure for fetal mediastinal teratoma with large pericardial effusion: a case report with review of literature. *J Matern Fetal Neonatal Med.* 2018;31(8):1099–1103.
162. Yinon Y, Grisaru-Granovsky S, Chaddha V, et al. Perinatal outcome following fetal chest shunt insertion for pleural effusion. *Ultrasound Obstet Gynecol.* 2010;36:58–64.

163. Ruano R, Ramalho AS, Cardoso AK, et al. Prenatal diagnosis and natural history of fetuses presenting with pleural effusion. *Prenat Diagn*. 2011;31:496–499.

164. Yinon Y, Kelly E, Ryan G. Fetal pleural effusions. *Best Pract Res Clin Obstet Gynaecol*. 2008;22:77–96.

165. Gratacos E. *Medicina Fetal*. Barcelona: Ed Medica Panamericana (ME); 2007.

166. Aubard Y, Derouineau I, Aubard V, et al. Primary fetal hydrothorax: a literature review and proposed antenatal clinical strategy. *Fetal Diagn Ther*. 1998;13:325–333.

167. Parilla BV, Tamura RK, Ginsberg NA. Association of parvovirus infection with isolated fetal effusions. *Am J Perinatol*. 1997;14:357–358.

168. Deurloo KL, Devlieger R, Lopriore E, et al. Isolated fetal hydrothorax with hydrops: a systematic review of prenatal treatment options. *Prenat Diagn*. 2007;27:893–899.

169. Hayashi S, Sago H, Kitano Y, et al. Fetal pleuroamniotic shunting for bronchopulmonary sequestration with hydrops. *Ultrasound Obstet Gynecol*. 2006;28:963–967.

170. Alkazaleh F, Saleem M, Badran E. Intrathoracic displacement of pleuroamniotic shunt after successful in utero treatment of fetal hydrops secondary to hydrothorax: case report and review of the literature. *Fetal Diagn Ther*. 2009;25:40–43.

171. National Institute for Health and Clinical Excellence. *Insertion of Pleuro-Amniotic Shunt for Fetal Pleural Effusion*. London: National Institute for Health and Clinical Excellence; 2006.

172. Longaker MT, Laberge JM, Dansereau J, et al. Primary fetal hydrothorax: natural history and management. *J Pediatr Surg*. 1989;24:573–576.

173. Paladini D, Volpe P. *Ultrasound of Congenital Fetal Anomalies: Differential Diagnosis and Prognostic Indicators*. London: Informa Health Care, Informa UK Ltd; 2007.

174. Blott M, Nicolaides KH, Greenough A. Pleuroamniotic shunting for decompression of fetal pleural effusions. *Obstet Gynecol*. 1988;71:798–800.

175. Rodeck CH, Fisk NM, Fraser DI, et al. Long-term in utero drainage of fetal hydrothorax. *N Engl J Med*. 1988;319:1135–1138.

176. Pumberger W, Hörmann M, Deutinger J, et al. Longitudinal observation of antenatally detected congenital lung malformations (CLM): natural history, clinical outcome and long-term follow-up. *Eur J Cardiothorac Surg*. 2003;24:703–711.

177. Knox EM, Kilby MD, Martin WL, et al. In-utero pulmonary drainage in the management of primary hydrothorax and congenital cystic lung lesion: a systematic review. *Ultrasound Obstet Gynecol*. 2006;28:726–734.

178. Yang Y, Ma G, Shih J, et al. Experimental treatment of bilateral fetal chylothorax using in-utero pleurodesis. *Ultrasound Obstet Gynecol*. 2012;39:56–62.

179. Witlox RS, Lopriore E, Walther FJ, et al. Single-needle laser treatment with drainage of hydrothorax in fetal bronchopulmonary sequestration with hydrops. *Ultrasound Obstet Gynecol*. 2009;34:355–357.

180. Bianchi S, Lista G, Castoldi F, et al. Congenital primary hydrothorax: effect of thoracoamniotic shunting on neonatal clinical outcome. *J Matern Fetal Neonatal Med*. 2010;23:1225–1229.

181. Picone O, Benachi A, Mandelbrot L, et al. Thoracoamniotic shunting for fetal pleural effusions with hydrops. *Am J Obstet Gynecol*. 2004;191:2047–2050.

182. Battin M, Yan J, Aftimos S, et al. Congenital chylothorax in siblings. *Br J Obstet Gynaecol*. 2000;107:1516–1518.

26.1 Bowel Abnormalities

Dorothy I. Bulas • Eva Ilse Rubio

Prenatal detection of a wide variety of anomalies and masses of the gastrointestinal tract is possible with ultrasonography and, in selected cases, with magnetic resonance imaging (MRI). Familiarity with the underlying disease process, associated malformation, and outcomes is important for determining the best obstetric management, mode of delivery, and postnatal care.

EMBRYOLOGY

The primitive gut forms at 20 days postfertilization, with the dorsal yolk sac invaginating into the growing embryonic disc. The foregut, midgut, and hindgut are supplied by the celiac artery, superior mesenteric artery, and inferior mesenteric artery, respectively. The foregut gives rise to the pharynx, respiratory tract, esophagus, stomach, duodenum, liver, and pancreas. The small bowel and proximal colon arise from the midgut. The distal colon and rectum as well as portions of the vagina and urinary bladder are derived from the hindgut (Fig. 26.1-1).

The fetal gastrointestinal tract forms and undergoes its rotational process in the first trimester, returning into the abdomen by 11 weeks' gestation. In the first trimester, meconium is produced from secretions of the liver and intestinal glands. Desquamated intestinal epithelium and amniotic fluid mix with meconium and migrate from the small bowel to the rectum with increasing gestational age.

Fetal swallowing begins at 14 weeks' gestation with the advent of bowel peristalsis. The fetus swallows 2 to 7 mL/day by 16 weeks' gestation, 16 mL/day by 20 weeks, and 450 mL/day by term.[1]

THE NORMAL ABDOMEN

Ultrasound

Physiological midgut herniation into the umbilical cord can be visualized as early as 8 weeks' gestation with transvaginal scanning (see Fig. 26.2-5).[2–4]

Because of the greater supply of oxygenated blood to the left lobe of the liver, the left lobe is larger than the right in utero. The spleen may be visualized posterior to the stomach on the left. Normal measurements of the fetal liver, spleen, pancreas, stomach, gallbladder, and intestine are available (see Appendix Tables 40–44).

Normally, the collapsed esophagus is not visualized by prenatal ultrasound (US).[5] Fluid may be observed within the lumen of the small bowel by 13 weeks' gestation.[6,7] Meconium accumulates in the small bowel and colon throughout the second and

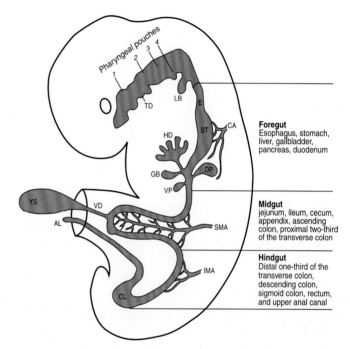

FIGURE 26.1-1: Development of gastrointestinal tract showing the foregut, midgut, and hindgut along with the adult derivatives. The entire length of the endodermal gut tube is shown from the mouth to the anus. *1–4*, pharyngeal pouches; *AL*, allantois; *CA*, celiac artery; *CL*, cloaca; *DP*, dorsal pancreas; *E*, esophagus; *GB*, gallbladder; *HD*, hepatic ducts; *IMA*, inferior mesenteric artery; *LB*, lung bud; *SMA*, superior mesenteric artery; *ST*, stomach; *TD*, thyroid diverticulum; *VD*, vitelline duct; *VP*, ventral pancreas; *YS*, yolk sac. (Reprinted with permission from Dudek RW, ed. *High-Yield Systems: Gastrointestinal Tract.* Philadelphia, PA: Wolters Kluwer Health/Lippincott Williams & Wilkins; 2010.)

third trimesters.[8,9] Bowel normally is collapsed and can be variably echogenic, at times similar in echogenicity to adjacent liver, spleen, and kidneys. Higher resolution linear transducers can be helpful in differentiating these organs. However, linear transducers can make normal bowel look unusually echogenic. This must be carefully differentiated from truly echogenic bowel that can be associated with infections, intrauterine growth restriction (IUGR), and cystic fibrosis (CF) (see section "Meconium Ileus") (Fig. 26.1-2).

Swallowing occurs by 14 weeks' gestation, so a fluid-filled stomach should always be detectable by the second trimester.[10,11] Echogenic debris can sometimes be seen layering in the stomach

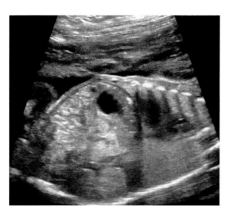

FIGURE 26.1-2: Echogenic bowel at 25 weeks' gestation. Coronal US demonstrates abnormally echogenic bowel in a fetus with cystic fibrosis.

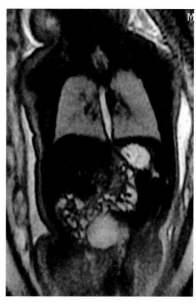

FIGURE 26.1-3: Normal esophagus. Coronal T2 MRI of a fluid-filled esophagus at 33 weeks' gestation.

and can represent vernix, protein, or intra-amniotic hemorrhage.[12] It is important to confirm situs (see Chapter 24.2). An absent or small stomach on serial fetal US examinations can suggest a mechanical obstruction secondary to esophageal atresia or neck mass, central nervous system (CNS) anomalies or syndromes in which fetal swallowing is depressed, or oligohydramnios.

Fluid-filled bowel lumen is not seen in the first trimester, but is generally noted by US by 20 weeks' gestation. Peristalsis may be observed by 18 weeks' gestation. Small bowel should not exceed 5 mm in diameter. The presence of dilated loops (>15 mm in length and 7 mm in diameter) suggests fetal bowel obstruction.[13]

Colon is best seen after 24 weeks' gestation as hypoechoic regions along the periphery of the abdomen.[8] The colon fills with meconium, progressively distending throughout the third trimester measuring 3 to 5 mm at 20 weeks and by term measuring up to 28 mm in diameter.[14] While variable, lumen diameter tables are available for gestational ages.[4,14] At times, normal colon can be mistaken for dilated small bowel or masses.[13]

The prenatal US diagnosis of bowel atresia can be difficult and is dependent on the site of obstruction, presence of associated anomalies, and timing of the study. The prenatal detection rate for obstruction is highest with duodenal obstruction and lowest for esophageal (24%) and anal atresia (6% to 8%).[15–17] There is poor sensitivity in the prenatal US diagnosis of colonic lesions, and misdiagnosis between small and large bowel obstruction is common.[18] Overall prenatal detection rate of gastrointestinal obstruction by US has varied from 24% to 34%.[16,17] With confounding variables such as maternal obesity, overlying gas and bone, transient normal variant, and late presentation, prenatal diagnosis and assessment of potential prognosis of fetuses with gastrointestinal abnormalities can be difficult by US.

Magnetic Resonance Imaging

Fetal bowel is well visualized by MRI and can be easily differentiated from adjacent liver, spleen, kidneys, bladder, and gallbladder.[19–24]

Fluid-filled small bowel loops are high signal on T2 imaging and low signal on T1, while meconium is low signal on T2 sequences and high signal on T1. Thus, MRI can be a useful tool to help characterize bowel anomalies.[19,20,23,24]

The gastrointestinal tract is progressively filled by swallowed amniotic fluid that is T2 hyperintense and T1 hypointense.

The esophagus may be transiently seen with fluid (Fig. 26.1-3). The stomach and duodenum should always be filled with T2 hyperintense fluid.

The jejunum is typically of high T2 and low T1 signal after 33 weeks' gestation. The distal small bowel has a more variable appearance, dependent on gestational age. Before 32 weeks, 50% of distal small bowel remains high signal on T1 imaging owing to slow protein-rich meconium progression.[19,25] T1 high signal may remain in proximal dilated loops because of lack of progression of meconium if bowel atresia is present or there is delayed peristalsis.[23–25]

By 20 weeks' gestation, the rectum normally is of high T1 and low T2 signal owing to the protein and mineral content of the meconium accumulating near the functionally closed anus. The rectum should be posterior to the bladder and 5 to 10 mm below the bladder base, depending on gestational age. The rectal anteroposterior diameter increases with gestational age, measuring 4 to 8 mm at 24 weeks and 9 to 15 mm by 35 weeks.[19] Colonic luminal volume increases exponentially with gestational age. Colonic luminal volumes at 20 to 37 weeks' gestational age range between 1.1 and 65 mL, with greater variations in the later gestation.[23]

With advancing gestation, the accumulating meconium not only distends the colon but also begins to progressively fill the entire colon in a retrograde manner. The descending colon is filled with meconium by 24 weeks' gestation (Fig. 26.1-4). However, there is greater variability proximally, with only half of normal cases having meconium-filled ascending colon by 31 weeks' gestation.[19]

BOWEL DISORDERS

The most common bowel abnormalities involve a mechanical or functional obstruction that results in proximal bowel dilatation. Common causes of dilated bowel are listed in Table 26.1-1. At times, associated anomalies are present (Table 26.1-2). Associated anomalies are more common with esophageal atresia, duodenal atresia, and anal atresia, while jejunal and ileal atresia are more

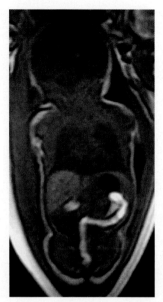

FIGURE 26.1-4: Meconium. Coronal T1 MRI demonstrates high signal within the descending colon and rectosigmoid at 33 weeks' gestation.

TABLE 26.1-2	Abnormalities Associated with Atresias	
ABNORMALITY	**PRENATAL FINDINGS**	**ASSOCIATED ABNORMALITIES**
Esophageal atresia/ TEF	Absent or small stomach Polyhydramnios	VACTERL
Duodenal atresia	Double bubble	Trisomy 21
Jejunal atresia	Dilated small bowel	Isolated
Meconium ileus	Hyperechoic bowel	Cystic fibrosis
Anal atresia	Rarely dilated colon	VACTERL Trisomy 21 OEIS Caudal regression

OEIS, omphalocele-exstrophy-imperforate anus-spinal defects; *TEF*, tracheo-esophageal fistula; *VACTERL*, vertebral defects, anal atresia, cardiac defects, tracheo-esophageal fistula, renal anomalies, and limb abnormalities.

TABLE 26.1-1	Etiology of Dilated Bowel

Esophagus
  Esophageal atresia
Small bowel
  Jejunal atresia
  Ileal atresia
  Meconium ileus
  Enteric duplication
  Congenital diarrhea
  Hirschsprung disease
Large bowel
  Hirschsprung disease
  Anorectal atresia
Pitfalls
  Hydroureter
  Normal bowel/meconium

likely isolated (with the exclusion of CF). Dilated bowel loops may contain fluid or meconium. It is important to consider normal bowel in the differential when dilated bowel is questioned. Other intra-abdominal cystic masses should also be considered when a dilated loop of bowel is thought to be present. Differentiating dilated ureter from bowel may be difficult as well.

It can take time for bowel dilatation to become apparent. Distal atresias, such as anal atresia, may never develop dilated bowel because of the absorption of fluid by the multiple proximal bowel loops. Jejunal and ileal atresias secondary to vascular ischemia may not develop until the second trimester, with bowel dilatation progressing only later in gestation. Conversely, proximal obstructions from duodenal atresia may be easily identified in the early second trimester.

Polyhydramnios can develop with bowel obstruction, but its presence is variable and its absence should not exclude the diagnosis. Esophageal atresia may present with early polyhydramnios, but if a tracheoesophageal fistula (TEF) accompanies the atresia, the presence of a fluid-filled stomach and normal amniotic fluid can result in a missed diagnosis prenatally. In cases of duodenal obstructions, polyhydramnios may only develop in 50% of cases owing to the absorption of fluid within the dilated stomach and duodenum. It is common for more distal small bowel and colonic obstructions to have normal amniotic fluid volumes.[26]

The following sections discuss the major bowel disorders that can be identified by US. MRI has become a useful adjunct in helping assess meconium location and further defining pathology. Accurate diagnosis allows for improved counseling, appropriate delivery planning, and postnatal care.[27–30]

Proximal Gastrointestinal Disorders

Esophageal Atresia

Incidence: Esophageal atresia with or without TEF occurs in 1 in 2,500 to 1 in 4,000 live births. Males are slightly more affected than females.[31]

Embryology and Pathology: Tracheoesophageal anomalies are the result of incomplete division of the foregut into the ventral respiratory portion and dorsal digestive portion by the tracheoesophageal septum. At the fourth week of gestation, the growth of the ectodermal ridge is interrupted, resulting in a TEF.

There are five types of tracheoesophageal anomalies (see Fig. 25.3-4):

Type A: Esophageal atresia with a TEF to the distal esophageal segment (>75%)
Type B: Esophageal atresia without TEF (10% to 15%)
Type C: H-type TEF with no esophageal atresia (5%)

Type D: Esophageal atresia with TEF to both the proximal and the distal esophageal segments (<5%)

Type E: Esophageal atresia with a TEF to the proximal esophageal segment (<5%)

Diagnosis

Ultrasound: Esophageal atresia, with or without a distal fistula, can be difficult to diagnose prenatally, with sonographic detection rate for esophageal obstruction ranging from 24% to 30%.[15,32–36] When a TEF is present, the sensitivity of US in prospectively making the diagnosis drops to 12%. Diagnosis often relies on indirect sonographic findings including polyhydramnios and a persistently small or absent stomach, though a false-positive rate can be as high as 27%[34] (Fig. 26.1-5).

Associated anomalies suggesting VACTERL association (vertebral, renal, radial ray, cardiac, two-vessel cord) may help in suspecting this diagnosis prenatally.[35]

Type A isolated esophageal atresias are the most likely to be diagnosed prenatally by US. If there is failure to visualize the fetal stomach over several hours, the diagnosis of esophageal atresia should be considered, particularly in the presence of polyhydramnios. At times, a dilated proximal esophageal pouch may be noted in the neck or upper mediastinum.[36–45]

The high false-negative rate of identifying a TEF is due to the fact that the amniotic fluid from the proximal pouch can pass into the stomach through the TEF with a resultant fluid-filled stomach present. Polyhydramnios develops in only one-third of these cases. The proximal pouch is often missed because of intermittent filling and emptying.[37,39]

If the stomach is small, TEF should be considered, particularly if polyhydramnios is also present. If there is marked polyhydramnios with a visualized stomach, and no additional findings, the diagnosis of TEF should still be considered in the differential.

The presence of vertebral, cardiac, renal, or limb anomalies or a two-vessel cord is suggestive of VACTERL. Up to 60% of individuals with VACTERL association have either esophageal atresia or TEF.[43] Thus, in cases with one or two of the previous findings, careful evaluation for TEF should be performed. The presence of polyhydramnios and small stomach in addition to a two-vessel cord is highly suggestive of a TEF and should be counseled appropriately.[35]

Magnetic Resonance Imaging: MRI can be a useful adjunct in the prenatal diagnosis of esophageal atresia. Dilated proximal esophageal pouches have been identified by MRI.[19,21,46] However, this finding may be transient by both US and MR, and the esophagus can be collapsed throughout either study.

MRI is also useful in the identification of associated VACTERL anomalies, such as pulmonary atresia, vertebral anomalies, and, at times, anal atresia (see later).

Differential Diagnosis: The absence of a fluid-filled stomach by US or MRI can be due to multiple etiologies. A repeat scan should be performed to confirm that the stomach has not simply emptied during the study.

If no normal stomach is identified, differential includes displacement of the stomach into the chest, or heterotaxy. Oligohydramnios is the most common cause of an empty stomach, and microgastria is the least common.

Oral and neck masses occluding the pharynx may result in a small or empty stomach. Sonographic observation of swallowing and muscular activity may help exclude a neuromuscular etiology.

Associated Findings: Up to 50% of patients with esophageal atresia have other anomalies. Cardiac malformations are the most common (25%) and result in the highest morbidity and mortality.[47] Additional anomalies include gastrointestinal (28%), genitourinary (13%), musculoskeletal (11%), CNS (7%), and facial anomalies (6%).[48]

Gastrointestinal anomalies include malrotation, anorectal atresia, duodenal atresia, and annular pancreas.[48] In Down syndrome, the combination of esophageal and duodenal atresia has been reported.[49–53]

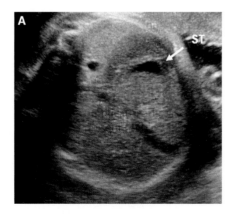
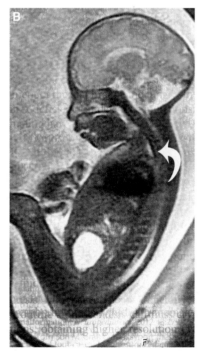

FIGURE 26.1-5: Tracheoesophageal fistula in a 32-week-gestation fetus with two-vessel cord. **A:** Axial US demonstrates a small stomach (*arrow*). Polyhydramnios was present. **B:** Sagittal T2 MRI demonstrates small fluid in the proximal esophageal pouch (*arrow*). Following delivery, an esophageal atresia with distal TEF was diagnosed.

The VACTERL association typically presents with several anomalies, including TEF (see section on VACTERL in Chapter 30).[54]

The risk of aneuploidy includes trisomies 18 and 21. Prenatal series report a wide incidence of aneuploidy ranging from 6% to 44%.[32,35,41] In a large postnatal series, however, chromosomal abnormalities were reported in 5% of cases.[51]

Management: If the diagnosis of TEF is suspected, serial USs may be needed to confirm the diagnosis. Careful assessment for potential associated anomalies should include echocardiography. Karyotype should be performed because of the risk of chromosomal abnormalities, including trisomies 21 and 18.[35]

Polyhydramnios develops in up to 60% of cases of esophageal atresia/TEF, typically in the third trimester.[32] Thus, follow-up studies to assess amniotic fluid volume are important because of the added risk of preterm labor with polyhydramnios. Bed rest, tocolytic agents, and reduction amniocenteses may be required. Betamethasone can be administered to promote fetal lung maturity if preterm labor develops.

Delivery should be planned at a center that has appropriate neonatal support. Cesarean section should be reserved for obstetric indications. If esophageal atresia is confirmed postnatally, the infant should be transferred to a tertiary care center. Intravenous fluid should be administered. A sump tube should be placed in the proximal esophageal pouch to prevent aspiration.

Abdominal radiographs will demonstrate absent air in the bowel with esophageal atresia without fistula. If there is a TEF, air typically will course into the stomach with normal-appearing distal bowel. Chest and abdominal films are helpful to exclude associated spine anomalies.

Surgery is performed depending on the gestational age, birth weight, and presence of other anomalies. A decision is made as to whether a primary repair or a staged repair is to be executed. If the gap between the proximal and the distal pouch is long, a gastrostomy tube is placed for a staged repair. Growth of the two pouches typically occurs over several weeks and often results in successful reconstruction.

Prognosis: It is unclear whether the prenatal diagnosis of esophageal atresia/TEF actually improves the prognosis. Early diagnosis allows for appropriate counseling, screening for associated anomalies, and planned delivery at an appropriate center. Immediate supportive management may decrease the risk of aspiration.

Increased perinatal loss rates have been noted in several series because of the high incidence (60%) of associated anomalies.[41,49,51]

The overall prognosis depends on associated anomalies, gestational age, and respiratory complications. When there are no severe cardiac anomalies or chromosomal anomalies, survival is reported to be greater than 95% in infants weighing over 2.5 kg.[54] Infants may require mechanical ventilation and prolonged hospital stays due to gastrointestinal issues. Short- and long-term follow-up is required after tracheoesophageal repair is performed to monitor for possible complications such as leakage at the anastomosis or the development of esophageal strictures and gastrointestinal reflux.

Hiatal Hernia
Incidence: Rare in the prenatal and newborn period.

Pathology/Embryology: The gastroesophageal junction slides above the diaphragm through the esophageal hiatus.

Diagnosis: A dilated esophagus may be seen in the chest prenatally by both US and MRI.[55–59] The stomach may be small[60,61] (Fig. 26.1-6).

Differential Diagnosis: Esophageal atresia may present with a dilated proximal esophageal pouch and small stomach mimicking a hiatal hernia. Esophageal duplication cyst could be considered in the differential. Hiatal hernia may be mistaken for a congenital diaphragmatic hernia.[62]

Associated Anomalies: Hiatal hernias have been associated with heterotaxy and Marfan syndrome.

Prognosis and Management: Isolated hiatal hernias typically have a good prognosis following surgical repair. There is a report of two giant hiatal hernias with associated anomalies having poor outcomes following delivery.[63]

Recurrence Risk: Familial cases have been reported rarely.[64]

Duodenal Atresia/Obstruction
Incidence: Duodenal atresia or stenosis is the most common type of intestinal atresia detected in the fetus, occurring in 1 in 10,000 live births.[27] Atresia is more common than stenosis, occurring in up to 75% of cases.[65] Approximately 30% of infants with duodenal atresia have trisomy 21.

Embryology/Pathology: The most common type of obstruction detected in the fetus is duodenal atresia or stenosis, thought to result from a failure of recanalization of the bowel at 8 to 10 weeks' gestation. The blockage may be associated with an annular pancreas.

There are three types of duodenal atresia:

Type 1—Membranous mucosal atresia with an intact muscular wall (most common 69%)
Type 2—Short fibrous cord connecting the two ends of the atretic duodenum
Type 3—Complete separation of the two ends associated with biliary tract anomalies[65,66]

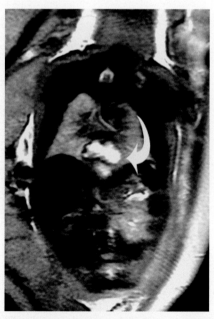

FIGURE 26.1-6: Hiatal hernia. Coronal T2 MRI demonstrates a fluid-filled structure above the diaphragm (curved arrow) with a small infradiaphragmatic stomach consistent with a hiatal hernia.

Duodenal obstruction can be associated with annular pancreas either by extrinsic compression or more commonly complete intrinsic atresia. The remaining 25% of cases are stenosis.

More than half of fetuses with duodenal atresia have associated anomalies. Trisomy 21 is the most frequent, occurring in up to 30% of cases. Increased incidence of duodenal atresia has been reported with gestational and preexisting diabetes, VACTERL association, and malrotation.[67,68]

Diagnosis

Ultrasound: Sonographic findings of duodenal atresia include a dilated fluid-filled stomach and proximal duodenum (fetal "double bubble"). The two structures should be contiguous to confirm the diagnosis (Fig. 26.1-7).[69–71] A dilated duodenum that persists is abnormal. Prior to 24 weeks, the duodenum may not be sufficiently dilated to make the diagnosis.[72–74] There are reports of the diagnosis being made in the first trimester.[75] The diagnosis can be noted in the early second trimester but is more likely confirmed in the third trimester when the duodenum becomes more dilated.[73,74] Polyhydramnios may develop in up to 50% of cases.[69]

In cases of incompletely obstructing duodenal stenosis or associated esophageal atresia, the diagnosis can be missed prenatally if the duodenum does not become sufficiently dilated.[76] At times, the stomach becomes extremely dilated, and the duodenal bulb may be difficult to visualize, resulting in a missed diagnosis.[77]

As 30% of fetuses with duodenal atresia have trisomy 21, other sonographic features of Down syndrome should be sought.[72,78,79] Anomalies associated with trisomy 21 include small or absent nasal bone, nuchal fold thickening, hypoplastic middle phalanx of the fifth digit, short humeri and femura, echogenic bowel, mild cerebral ventriculomegaly, mild pyelectasis, and cardiac anomalies such as atrioventricular (AV) canal and ventriculoseptal defects (see section "Trisomy 21" in Chapter 30).

Duodenal atresia and stenosis can be part of the VACTERL association. In these cases, hemivertebra, radial ray, and renal anomalies may be identified.[79] When a TEF and duodenal atresia are present together, a markedly dilated stomach may develop. If esophageal atresia without fistula and duodenal atresia are present together, the stomach may be small with a collapsed duodenum, making the diagnosis difficult to detect prenatally.[49,50,53,79]

Magnetic Resonance Imaging: MRI can be used as an adjunct in the diagnosis of duodenal atresias. On T2, the fluid-filled dilated stomach and duodenum will be of high signal with decompressed bowel loops distally (see Fig. 26.1-7B). The normal caliber fluid-filled small bowel loops and normal meconium-filled colon and rectum should be easily visualized. The dilated duodenum is easily differentiated from adjacent gallbladder, and duplication cysts by MRI.[18]

Associated anomalies in the brain, spine, limbs, lung, and anal atresia may be confirmed and further evaluated by MRI.[80]

Differential Diagnosis: The differential diagnosis includes annular pancreas, malrotation with Ladd's bands, duplication cysts, preduodenal portal vein, and choledochal cyst.[76] Documenting that the fluid-filled structure is contiguous with the stomach can help differentiate duodenal atresia/stenosis from a duplication or choledochal cyst.[81,82]

Associated Anomalies: Duodenal atresia is an isolated finding in one-third to one-half of cases. However, it is often associated with other malformations, including cardiac, gastrointestinal (biliary atresia, agenesis of the gallbladder), renal, and vertebral anomalies.[72,78,79]

Thirty percent of newborns with duodenal atresia or stenosis have Down syndrome. Conversely, approximately 2.5% of patients with Down syndrome have duodenal atresia or stenosis.[72]

Prenatal Management: If the diagnosis of duodenal atresia or stenosis is suspected, serial USs may be needed to confirm the diagnosis. As 30% of fetuses with duodenal atresia have trisomy 21 and 20% to 30% have congenital heart disease, fetal karyotype analysis and detailed fetal survey, including fetal echocardiography, are indicated.[83]

Amniotic fluid digestion enzyme assays, including gamma-glutamyl transpeptidase (GGTP), aminopeptidase (AMP), total alkaline phosphatase (ALP), and intestinal form (iALP) and total

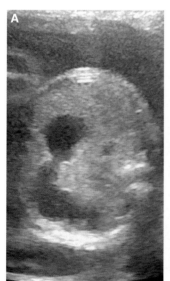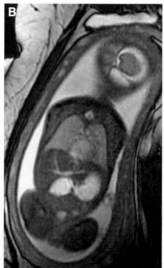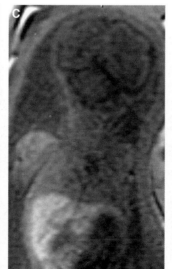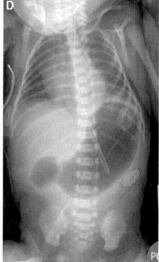

FIGURE 26.1-7: Duodenal atresia. **A:** Axial US demonstrates a fluid-filled double bubble at 28 weeks' gestation. **B, C:** T2 and T1 MRI, respectively, confirm the presence of a fluid-filled double bubble. **D:** Postnatal radiograph demonstrates the presence of an air-filled double bubble.

protein have been evaluated. Muller et al. correlated elevations of GGTP and iALP with duodenal and small bowel atresias. For duodenal atresia, sensitivity was reported to be 71% with a 100% specificity, while distal bowel sensitivity was 69% with 83% specificity.[20,84] Normal values in amniotic fluid do not exclude the diagnosis of obstructions.

As duodenal atresia can be complicated by polyhydramnios in up to 50% of cases,[69,83] follow-up sonograms are useful to monitor amniotic fluid volume. Polyhydramnios can result in preterm labor, so close monitoring is useful. Prenatal pediatric surgical consultation with parents can be helpful in alleviating anxiety and planning postnatal care.

The fetus will usually not need delivery at a high-risk center and can be safely transported after birth to a pediatric center after enteric tube decompression of the intestinal tract to prevent aspiration of gastric contents. Intravenous fluid should be administered to replace volume with attention to electrolyte imbalance.

Abdominal radiographs will demonstrate the typical air-filled "double bubble" with absent gas distally (see Fig. 26.1-7D). If there is a stenosis or the biliary tree bridges the atresia, air may be seen in the small bowel. Radiographs should be interpreted with caution as a postnatal double-bubble appearance may also be seen in the setting of malrotation of the midgut with or without associated volvulus.

Surgery is typically performed in the early postnatal period after assessment of other associated anomalies, volume resuscitation, and correction of electrolyte imbalances.

Prognosis/Outcome: Several series suggest that prenatal diagnosis does reduce morbidity and shortens hospitalization.[85–87] Survival has improved over the past two decades, with a 95% survival reported.[76,78,88,89] Outcome now is more related to associated anomalies, particularly cardiac defects.[83] Potential late complications include dysmotility of the proximal duodenum, resulting in gastroesophageal reflux, gastritis, pancreatitis, and/or cholecystitis.[89]

Jejunal and Ileal Atresia

Incidence: The incidence of small bowel atresia is 1 per 1,500 to 5,000 births.[29,90] Atresias can occur anywhere in the small bowel but is most commonly present in the proximal jejunum (30%) or distal ileum (35%) with multiple atresias in up to 6% of cases.[28,91]

Embryology/Pathology: Jejunal and ileal atresia are a complete obstruction of the bowel lumen and are more common than small bowel stenosis. Small bowel atresias are thought to be caused by vascular ischemia in the second trimester with the ischemic necrosis leading to resorption of the segment or fibrous scarring.[92–94]

Type 1—32%; lumen is obstructed by an intact diaphragm or membrane made of mucosa and submucosa. The muscularis and serosa are intact with continuity of the proximal and distal segments. If the membrane stretches, it takes the shape of a windsock.

Type 2—25%; fibrotic cord connecting two blind-ending bowel segments

Type 3

3a—15%; complete separation of blind-ending loops

3b—11%; mesenteric defect with large gap in small bowel mesentery. The distal small bowel is short and coiled like an apple peel. Terminal ileum is perfused from a single ileocolic artery (can be familial).

Type 4—6%; multiple atresias[95,96]

Lesions can range from a focal atresia to extensive atresia of the entire bowel possibly related to constriction/volvulus.[97] Placental vascular abnormalities have also been associated with small bowel atresias.[93] Atresias have been reproduced in experimental animals by ligation of mesenteric blood vessels.[98] Maternal use of vasoconstrictive medications may contribute to interruption of mesenteric blood flow.[99] Inherited thrombophilia leading to spontaneous thrombosis may play a role in some cases.[100]

Gastroschisis has been associated with bowel atresia because of ischemic injury from bowel kinking.[101–104] In rare cases, the entire extruded bowel mass of gastroschisis volvulizes, resulting in necrotic bowel that involutes and is resorbed with spontaneous closure of the abdominal wall defect, a phenomenon known as "vanishing gastroschisis." The prognosis is poor due to extensive loss of small bowel.

The incidence of small bowel atresia secondary to meconium ileus is reported to be 10% of cases. The incidence of associated aneuploidy and extraintestinal anomalies is low.

Diagnosis

Ultrasound: Obstruction of the fetal bowel may be sonographically diagnosed when dilated bowel loops are detected proximal to a point of obstruction. Hyperperistalsis of the proximal bowel may be observed. The diagnosis of obstruction before 18 weeks' gestation is rare and may even be difficult to diagnose before 24 weeks' gestation. Bowel loops become progressively more dilated with vigorous peristalsis in the third trimester.

The presence of dilated loops (>15 mm in length and 7 mm in diameter) and/or mural thickness of greater than 3 mm is most suggestive of fetal bowel obstruction.[4,105,106] The abdomen can be distended with disproportionate increase in the abdominal circumference. A proximal or jejunal atresia may show a sonographic fetal "triple bubble," representing the dilated stomach, duodenum, and proximal jejunum (Figs. 26.1-8A and 26.1-9A). The jejunum's capacity to dilate is greater than that of the ileum and is, therefore, less likely to be associated with the complications of perforation, such as meconium peritonitis and meconium pseudocyst. The presence of multiple dilated loops of bowel is more suggestive of a distal obstruction such as an ileal atresia. If meconium ileus is present, increased bowel echogenicity may be noted.

Bowel distal to the most proximal level of obstruction is difficult to assess by US. Thus, differentiating an isolated atresia from multiple atresias is difficult sonographically.[16,107] The presence of multiple atresias is often only confirmed at surgery postnatally.

While proximal gastrointestinal obstruction can lead to polyhydramnios, increased amniotic fluid is seen in fewer than 50% of cases with jejunal obstruction and rarely with more distal obstructions.[108–112] Iacobelli et al.[26] suggested that polyhydramnios and dilated bowel loops are markers of more severe obstruction with a longer predicted length of stay when present.

Other clues to sonographic diagnosis include ascites and echogenic bowel.[18] In cases of more proximal small bowel obstruction, the dilated loops are generally filled with hypoechoic or anechoic fluid. With the increasingly distal location of small bowel obstruction, the luminal contents tend to become progressively echogenic and complex as there is more accumulated meconium within the loops.[113]

A perforation at the site of ischemia may result in leakage of fluid and meconium. This can result in ascites and meconium peritonitis. Loculated collections of fluid and debris may develop, which

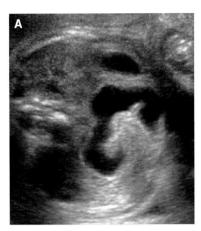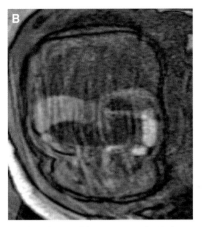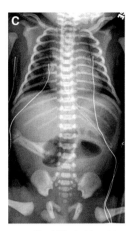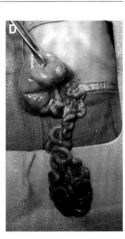

FIGURE 26.1-8: Jejunal atresia with fluid-filled dilated jejunal loops. **A:** Axial US demonstrates a fluid-filled dilated loop of bowel. **B:** Coronal T1 MRI demonstrates a dilated fluid-filled loop of bowel containing no high-signal meconium. **C:** Postnatal radiograph demonstrates air in the stomach and proximal jejunum. **D:** Surgical image of jejunal atresia.

calcify, developing into meconium pseudocysts (Fig. 26.1-10). Scattered peritoneal calcifications with posterior acoustical shadowing may be noted[111,113] (Fig. 26.1-11).

US has limitations in the assessment of bowel anomalies. Maternal obesity, overlying gas, and maternal pelvic bones may obscure imaging of the fetus. Expertise of the sonographer is important in the assessment of more complex anomalies. At times, it may be difficult to differentiate dilated small bowel loops from colon or megaureters sonographically. US lacks the specificity to identify the number and location of obstructions and is limited in assessing the viability of unobstructed distal bowel.

A multicenter retrospective sonographic study from Europe in an unselected study showed an overall detection rate of bowel atresia of 34%, with 40% of those detected at less than 24 weeks' gestation.[15,16,107]

Magnetic Resonance Imaging: MRI has been used as an adjunct in the characterization of bowel obstruction, including the level of obstruction.[9,19,20,22,23,112–117] In a series by Veyrac et al.,[18] MRI provided more accurate findings than US in the assessment of small bowel atresias.

Bowel loops proximal to the obstruction are dilated (13 to 30 mm). The signal characteristics are variable, depending on the gestational age and level of obstruction.

Dilated bowel loops in more proximal jejunal atresias are typically filled with simple fluid that is high signal on T2 and low signal on T1 sequences, while distal jejunal and proximal ileal bowel obstruction may present with bowel loops containing fluid of intermediate signal. With distal small bowel obstruction and in particular with meconium ileus, the intraluminal contents of the dilated small bowel contain increasing amounts of meconium and are commonly lower signal on T2 and higher signal on T1 sequences, a reverse appearance of more proximal obstructions. The signal may approach that of colonic meconium (see Figs. 26.1-8 and 26.1-9).

Distally, the colon and rectum may contain overall less meconium and thus be decreased in size (2 to 7 mm).[18,23] However, with isolated atresias, the distal rectal meconium descent is still expected to lie below the level of the urinary bladder base, with an exception to this possible in fetuses with CF and meconium ileus, presumably because the tenacious nature of the meconium in these cases results in poor or incomplete migration.[113]

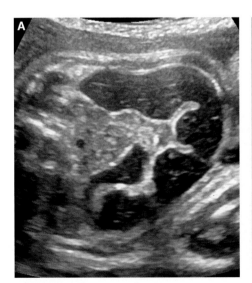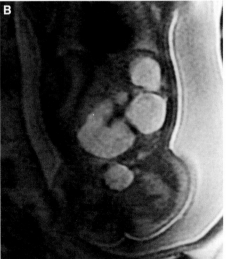

FIGURE 26.1-9: Jejunal atresia with meconium-filled dilated jejunal loops. **A:** Axial US demonstrates a dilated loop of bowel filled with echogenic material. **B:** Coronal T1 MRI demonstrates dilated high-signal meconium-filled loops of small bowel. At surgery, jejunal atresia was confirmed.

The absence of loops distal to the level of obstruction may suggest multiple atresias.[18] Shinmoto and Kuribayashi[115] described dilated loops with two different signals in a case with two levels of atresia. Other factors such as the presence of volvulus or bowel hemorrhage may confound the earlier described imaging findings and specific diagnosis (see Fig. 26.1-9). In a series by Colombani et al.,[24] of the 11 patients between 23 and 35 weeks' gestation with T1 high signal in dilated bowel, nine had proximal jejunal atresia (five with short bowel syndrome), and two had meconium ileus at delivery.

Differential Diagnosis: The differential for dilated tubular loops within the abdomen includes jejunal or ileal atresia, total colonic aganglionosis, malrotation with volvulus, meconium ileus, and meconium peritonitis. Rarer entities to consider include megacystis-microcolon-intestinal hypoperistalsis syndrome and fetal diarrhea. At times, hydronephrosis, duplication cysts, ovarian cysts, and abdominal mesenteric cysts can mimic dilated bowel loops.

Associated Anomalies: Other gastrointestinal anomalies can be present in up to 45%. These include malrotation (23%), microcolon (3%), duplication cysts (3%), esophageal atresia (3%), and meconium peritonitis (8%).[118] In rare cases, the fetus may have associated chromosomal anomalies, or an underlying syndrome coexisting with multiple other anomalies. However, in most instances, jejunal and ileal atresia are isolated, in contrast to esophageal, duodenal, or anal atresia.

Management: Once the diagnosis of small bowel atresia is made, a complete anatomic survey should be performed. If echogenic bowel is present, amniocentesis for fetal karyotype and CF DNA mutation analysis should be performed. As congenital infections have also been associated with echogenic bowel, a close evaluation for additional anomalies as well as TORCH titers may be useful.

Severe polyhydramnios rarely develops with small bowel atresias, though mild polyhydramnios can occur. Follow-up sonograms, once the diagnosis is confirmed, can be spread apart. Amniotic fluid digestion enzymes assays, including GGTP, AMP, ALP, and iALP, and total protein have been evaluated, though sensitivity of 69% and specificity of 83% limit its utility in distal obstructions.[20,84]

Prenatal pediatric surgical consultation with parents is helpful in alleviating anxiety and planning delivery and postnatal care. Fetuses with more proximal bowel obstructions can deliver early, particularly in the presence of polyhydramnios. If meconium peritonitis is present without bowel obstruction, the outcome is typically favorable and may not require surgery. Large meconium pseudocysts with or without associated bowel atresias, however, require surgery.[17,27,110,119,120]

Delivery of fetuses with bowel obstruction can be at term and vaginal. Delivery should be planned at a center with appropriate neonatal support. Postnatal management of small bowel atresias includes gastric decompression and intravenous fluid to correct fluid and electrolyte imbalances.

Postnatal radiographs will document dilated small bowel loops. A water-soluble contrast enema is useful in the assessment of colonic caliber and to exclude concomitant colonic atresia. If the colon and rectum are normal in caliber, a more proximal atresia is likely present. If diffuse microcolon is present with poor rectal distension, a diagnosis of ileal atresia or meconium ileus or rarely total aganglionic Hirschsprungs should be considered.[113] If the obstruction is secondary to meconium ileus, sequential enemas may help relieve the obstruction by breaking up the inspissated meconium.

Prognosis/Outcome: Surgery is performed after associated anomalies are excluded and the infant is adequately resuscitated. The proximal dilated bowel may be resected to prevent functional obstruction at the anastomosis.[121] A disproportionately dilated loop may have poor motility and can develop blind loop syndrome. Short bowel syndrome can result in cases of multiple atresias or with the apple-peel deformity.

In proximal atresias, enteral feedings can begin quickly. More distal atresias may require longer periods of rest until normal gut activity returns.

Long-term outcome is typically excellent with survival of 95%. Most of the mortality occurs in infants with medical conditions such as prematurity, respiratory distress syndrome, associated anomalies, CF, or short gut syndrome. Late complications include recurrent obstruction from strictures, adhesions, and liver abnormalities from prolonged total parenteral nutrition (TPN).[122]

Recurrence Risk: Most small bowel atresias are sporadic. However, with type 3b atresias, apple-peel deformity, short bowel, and retrograde perfusion of the distal ileum, there is an 18% recurrence risk, suggesting a genetic component.[123] Type 4 also has been described as recurring in families. Hereditary multiple atresias have be noted.[124]

Meconium Ileus/Cystic Fibrosis

Meconium ileus should always be included in the differential when small bowel obstruction is identified. In these cases, obstruction of the small bowel occurs from impacted thick meconium. Perforation with secondary ileal atresia and meconium peritonitis may develop. An additional known complication is volvulus, intrauterine or postnatal, resulting from the dense meconium accumulation acting as a lead point.

Incidence: CF is one of the most common autosomal recessive disorders in the United States, present in 1 per 3,000 newborns. Up to 15% of fetuses with CF present with meconium ileus.[125,126] Up to 50% of these cases will be complicated with an atresia, volvulus, perforation, and/or meconium pseudocysts.

CF is rare in African American and Asian populations.

Embryology and Pathology: The fetus with CF may present prenatally with a distal small bowel obstruction due to meconium ileus. The obstruction of the terminal ileum is from the thick viscous meconium that can develop in the fetus and neonate with CF. A microcolon can be present due to the lack of passage of the meconium into the colon and rectum.

Diagnosis

Ultrasound: CF is diagnosed in approximately 3% to 9.9% of fetuses with echogenic bowel.[127–129] Echogenic bowel associated with bowel dilatation is suspicious for meconium ileus (Fig. 26.1-12). In these cases, there is a high incidence of complications (up to 50%), including small bowel atresia and volvulus. A mixed picture of dilated fluid-filled loops and echogenic collapsed loops should prompt consideration of CF.

Perforation in cases of meconium ileus or small bowel atresia can result in leakage of meconium and fluid, with ascites, meconium peritonitis, and, occasionally, a meconium pseudocyst formation (see Fig. 18.1-11).[130–132] Sonogram may demonstrate scattered calcifications in the fetal abdomen and along the liver margin.

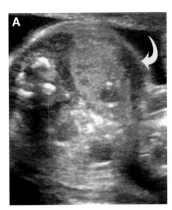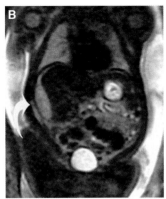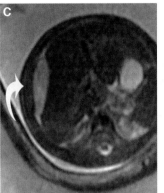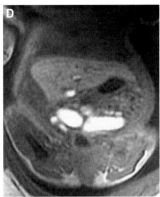

FIGURE 26.1-10: Ileal atresia with meconium peritonitis. **A:** Axial US demonstrates dilated bowel loops, echogenic bowel, and fluid adjacent to the liver (*arrow*) at 32 weeks' gestation. **B, C:** Coronal and axial T2 MRI, respectively, demonstrate a perihepatic collection of fluid consistent with a loculated meconium pseudocyst (*arrow*). Dilated low-signal bowel loops are present as well. **D:** Coronal T1 MRI demonstrates high-signal meconium-filled dilated small bowel.

Lack of visualization of the fetal gallbladder may be another clue to the diagnosis.[125,133]

Magnetic Resonance Imaging: MRI may be useful as an adjunct in the demonstration of meconium distribution. In a series by Carcopino et al.,[116] two cases of meconium ileus were noted to have unusual hyperintense T1 and intermediate T2 signal within dilated bowel loops.

Meconium peritonitis can be diagnosed by the demonstration of extraluminal fluid collections scattered through the abdomen. MR can distinguish meconium cysts from adjacent bowel because of different signal characteristics as well as improved soft-tissue detail and large field of view of the abdominal contents (see Fig. 26.1-10). Peritoneal calcifications, however, are more reliably characterized by US.[18,130–132]

Differential Diagnosis: Prenatal differentiation between distal ileal atresia and meconium ileus may be challenging, because both have a meconium-filled dilated distal ileum and a microcolon.[9] However, patients with CF may have a striking near-absent distal colorectal meconium due to the abnormal meconium tenacity, a finding not noted in fetuses with isolated jejunal or ileal atresia.

Echogenic bowel is nonspecific and may also be seen with bleeding in the amniotic cavity, aneuploidy, fetal growth restriction, infection, gastrointestinal obstruction, and biliary atresia.[134–140] Although associated with a higher rate of fetal loss, the majority of neonates with echogenic bowel are normal at delivery. Echogenic bowel is diagnosed in 0.2% to 1.4% of second-trimester studies.[141] The diagnosis of fetal echogenic bowel can be made by comparing the echogenicity with adjacent bone or liver (Fig. 26.1-13). Bowel that is as echogenic as adjacent bone has been proposed as an objective marker to decrease the subjectivity of assessing echogenic bowel, particularly when using higher frequency linear transducers.[135,141]

A rare cause of dilated bowel includes megacystis-microcolon-intestinal hypoperistalsis syndrome.[142]

Associated Anomalies: Fetuses with confirmed meconium ileus have CF. Long-term complications include pulmonary, pancreatic, and bowel sequelae.

Prognosis and Management: If CF is suspected, a sweat chloride test or CF DNA mutation analysis should be performed after delivery if not prenatally.[125,129,137,139]

Severe polyhydramnios rarely develops with small bowel atresias, so follow-up sonograms, once the diagnosis is confirmed, can be timed according to obstetrical indications. Prenatal pediatric surgical consultation with parents is helpful in alleviating anxiety and planning delivery and postnatal care.

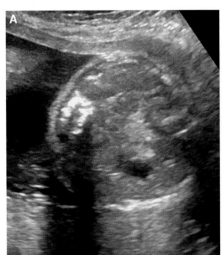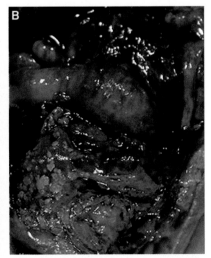

FIGURE 26.1-11: Meconium peritonitis. **A:** Axial US at 26 weeks' gestation demonstrates echogenic foci with posterior acoustical shadowing in the anterior abdomen. **B:** Surgical image of a different patient with meconium scattered within the peritoneum.

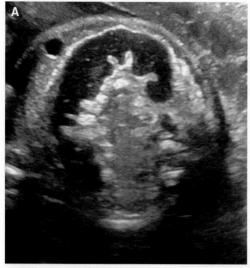
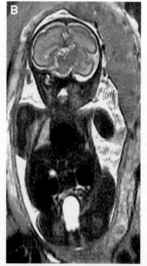
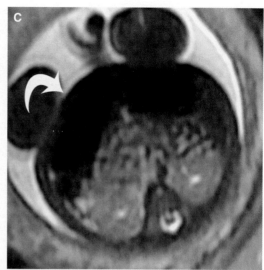
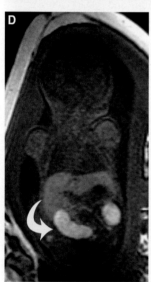
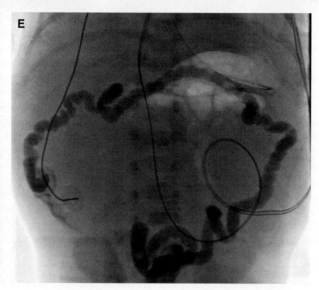

FIGURE   26.1-12: Meconium ileus with jejunal volvulus. **A:** Axial US at 28 weeks' gestation demonstrates a dilated loop anteriorly containing particulate matter and more distal echogenic bowel collapsed. **B, C:** Coronal and axial T2 MRI, respectively, demonstrate that the dilated loop contains low-signal meconium (*arrow*). **D:** T1 coronal MRI confirms the dilated bowel loop contains meconium (*arrow*), with no meconium in the rectosigmoid. **E:** Enema following delivery demonstrates microcolon. Infant was diagnosed with cystic fibrosis following delivery.

Delivery of fetuses with meconium ileus can be at term and vaginal. Delivery should be planned at a center with appropriate neonatal support. Postnatal management of small bowel atresias includes gastric decompression and intravenous fluid to correct fluid and electrolyte imbalances. Radiographs will document dilated small bowel loops. A water-soluble contrast enema is performed in an attempt to dissolve the inspissated meconium. Sequential enemas may be required to relieve the obstruction. If unsuccessful, the infant may require surgery to relieve the obstruction, which may be the result of a stenosis/atresia or meconium.[143]

Recurrence Risk: CF is autosomal recessive with a 25% risk of recurrence.

Preimplantation genetic diagnosis and DNA prenatal diagnosis are available for future pregnancies if CF is indeed confirmed.[128,143]

Congenital Diarrhea
Incidence: Rare case reports in the literature.[144–147]

Pathology: Congenital diarrhea is a rare disorder in which the infant has watery diarrhea for which no infectious agent is identified in at least three stool samples, lasting 2 weeks in an infant under 3 months of age. Chloride diarrhea is a rare form caused by an

autosomal recessive gene, with a few hundred cases reported primarily in Saudi Arabia, Finland, and Poland. The chloride bicarbonate channels are abnormal with resultant hypochloremia and hypokalemia. Sodium diarrhea is also recessive and causes metabolic disturbances because of sodium loss. Over 30 genetic mutations have been identified, including *SCL26A3* on chromosome 7.[144]

Diagnosis: Assessment of amniotic fluid reveals normal cytogenetic and microbiological results. Chloride or sodium levels can be elevated.

Ultrasound: Moderately generalized bowel dilatation and polyhydramnios between 24 and 32 weeks' gestation are typically noted.[144–147]

Magnetic Resonance Imaging: MRI can play an important role in the diagnosis of this prenatally. In a series of four cases, all four were correctly diagnosed prospectively with MRI.[145] T2 high-signal intraluminal fluid is seen throughout the small bowel and colon. In addition, there is an absence of T1 meconium in the colon and rectum.

Management: Close prenatal follow-up is required owing to the potential development of polyhydramnios and risk of premature

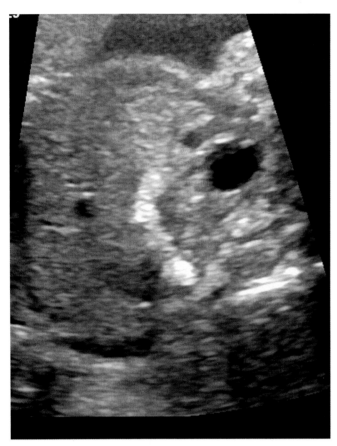

FIGURE 26.1-13: Echogenic bowel. Coronal US demonstrates echogenic bowel at 25 weeks' gestation. The fetus died a few days later.

delivery. Following delivery, aggressive fluid replacement is required. Colostomy may be indicated.

Outcome: Significant fluid loss and electrolyte disorders can be lethal if not properly managed.

The prognosis for sodium diarrhea appears worse than that for chloride diarrhea with a higher death rate.

Recurrence Risk: Autosomal recessive disorders with frequency higher in some countries than others.

Abnormalities of the Colon, Rectum, and Anus

Colonic obstruction includes colonic atresias, anorectal malformations, and Hirschsprung disease. The presence of anal and colorectal obstruction is often missed prenatally. This is due to the fact that fluid is often resorbed in the small bowel and colonic loops. Thus, the small bowel and colon typically remain normal in caliber despite a distal obstruction. Each diagnosis has its own etiology and outcome, with diagnosis usually confirmed following delivery.

Imperforate Anus

Incidence: Anorectal malformations affect 1 in 5,000 live births and range from isolated imperforate anus to persistent cloaca (female) or anorectal malformation (males).

Embryology/Pathology: Abnormalities of the rectum and anus are thought to be due to an arrest of the caudal descent of the urorectal septum to the cloacal membrane.[148] By 6 weeks' gestation, the cloacal membrane divides into the anterior urogenital sinus and posterior anorectum by the urorectal septum. Fusion of the hindgut mesoderm with the ectoderm occurs at the dentate line. Failure of Rathke folds to develop results in the arrest of the inferior urorectal septum, causing a high termination of the rectum and rectourethral fistula in males and cloaca in females. Isolated imperforate anus without fistula occurs from failure of the anal pit to form.

Bourdelat studied sphincter development in the fetus by US and noted slow growth from 14 to 19 weeks. There was rapid growth from 19 to 30 weeks. After 30 weeks, contractions were noted, with no further growth.[14]

Diagnosis

Ultrasound: Anorectal malformations are often missed by prenatal US because fluid is resorbed in the small bowel and colonic loops typically remain normal in caliber.[149–151] Polyhydramnios is rare and, when present, suggest a more proximal concomitant obstruction. Perforation with ascites and meconium peritonitis are rare as well. In females with a cloaca, the urinary system may be obstructed, resulting in oligohydramnios.

Transient bowel dilatation and a dilated distal colon are potential prenatal findings.[150,152,153] Colonic dilatation has been described in fetuses greater than 26 weeks' gestation and may have a V- or U-shaped configuration.[150,154] Transiently dilated rectum supportive of the diagnosis has been described at 12 to 13 weeks with a transvaginal scan and at 16 weeks with transabdominal images.[3,152,153,155]

Vesicorectal fistulas are associated with anorectal malformations. In these cases, urine mixes with meconium and intraluminal calcifications (enterolithiasis) develop. The presence of enterolithiasis can be seen by US as punctate foci of echogenicity in the rectum mixed with fluid.[156–159] The entire colon may become fluid filled and can be mistaken for a dilated small bowel loop[8] (Fig. 26.1-14).

Prenatal US diagnosis of anorectal disorders may improve with careful analysis of the fetal anus with high-resolution sonographic scanning. The rectum can be seen in the normal fetus posterior to the bladder as a hypoechoic target-like structure with lack of visualization highly suggestive of anal atresia[160–163] (Fig. 26.1-15). Reference values for the in utero development of the fetal anal sphincter are available.[161] Three-dimensional US can further aid in the evaluation of the fetal anal canal.[162,163] The fetal perianal muscular complex (PAMC), which includes the internal and external anal sphincter and puborectalis muscle,[163,164] appears as a hypoechogenic ring in the axial plane (target sign) and two hypoechogenic parallel stripes in the coronal and sagittal plane just posterocephalad to the external genitalia. In a series by Ochoa et al.,[164] the absence of the PAMC had a high sensitivity and specificity for the diagnosis of anorectal atresia.

An anorectal malformation or cloaca should be suspected when associated abnormalities, such as sacral agenesis, hemivertebrae, caudal regression syndrome, and VACTERL sequence, are detected. The presence of these anomalies should prompt a closer inspection of the anus to determine whether indeed a target sign is absent or the colon appears dilated.

Magnetic Resonance Imaging: MRI is useful as an adjunct in the assessment of distal colonic obstruction.[18] Abnormally high termination of the rectum has been described by MRI in cases of anal atresia (see Fig. 26.1-15). The detection of abnormal fluid in the rectum has been noted in cases with vesicorectal fistulas (see Fig. 26.1-14B).[165] Assessment of the rectal cul-de-sac by MRI has allowed for differentiation between a high anorectal malformation and cloaca.[18]

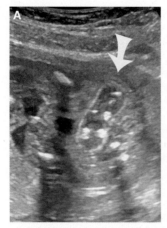
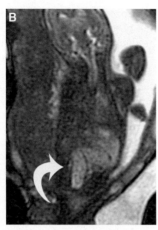

FIGURE 26.1-14: Anal atresia with vesicourethral fistula. **A:** Coronal US at 20 weeks' gestation demonstrates dilated rectosigmoid filled with fluid and calcifications—enteroliths (*arrow*). Two-vessel cord was present. **B:** Coronal T2 MRI confirms fluid-filled rectosigmoid (*arrow*), enteroliths not as well visualized. Infant was found to have a vesicorectal fistula at delivery and diagnosed with VACTERL sequence.

MRI is useful in further assessment of complex associated anomalies, including omphalocele-exstrophy-imperforate anus-spinal defects (OEIS) complex, cloaca, and VACTERL.[166–170]

Differential Diagnosis: The differential for distal obstruction includes colonic atresia, meconium ileus, persistent cloaca, meconium plug syndrome, and megacystis-microcolon-hypoperistalsis syndrome. Urachal cysts, ovarian cysts, and hydrometrocolpos should also be considered.

When calcifications are noted, it is important to determine whether they are intraluminal or extraluminal. Intraluminal calcifications suggest a rectovesicle fistula, while extraluminal calcifications may be secondary to meconium peritonitis.

Associated Anomalies: Anorectal malformations are associated with additional anomalies in up to 50% to 70% of cases. These malformations are separated into "high" supralevator lesions that end above the levator sling and are typically associated with fistulas. "Low" infralevator lesions end below the levator sling and are not associated with fistulas to the urinary tract, although there may be a fistula to the perineum.

Anal atresia is most commonly associated with the VACTERL association. Cloaca, OEIS complex, and caudal regression syndrome[148,150,152] are also associated with anal atresia. Anorectal malformations are also seen in association with trisomy 21.[171–176]

Management: If an anorectal abnormality is suspected, careful sonographic evaluation for associated anomalies of the spine, skeleton, kidneys, and umbilical cord should be performed. Because of the increased risk of cardiac disease, a fetal echocardiogram should be performed. Karyotype should be reserved for cases with associated anomalies that are linked with chromosome abnormalities, such as trisomy 21 and long-segment aganglionosis.

Prenatal pediatric surgical consultation with the parents can be helpful in alleviating anxiety. The diagnosis of a distal colorectal obstruction is not typically associated with prematurity or polyhydramnios. If isolated, the diagnosis has no implications for timing or route of delivery. Delivery should be planned at a center with appropriate high-risk obstetric and neonatal support.

Following delivery, the infant will develop abdominal distension and fail to pass meconium. A nasogastric tube should be placed to relieve abdominal distension. An intravenous line should be placed for fluid resuscitation.

If an imperforate anus is present, the diagnosis needs to be further defined into low, intermediate, or high lesions. Low lesions, typically with a perineal fistula, have a perineal anoplasty performed soon after birth. Intermediate and high lesions require a diverting colostomy in the first few days of life.[177] Anorectal reconstruction is then carried out at a later age following MR of the spine and pelvis to assess for associated tethered cord.[178] Pressure colostogram can be performed preoperatively to define the course of the rectourethral fistula and demonstrate the level of rectal termination.

Outcome: Mortality rate of anorectal abnormalities is usually related to associated cardiac or renal anomalies.[177–180] Voiding

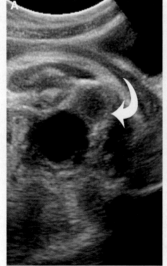
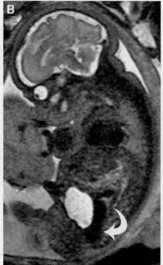
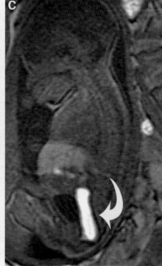

FIGURE 26.1-15: Anal atresia in a 31-week-gestation fetus with a two-vessel cord. **A:** Axial US demonstrates distended rectum (*arrow*) measuring 13 mm (*arrow*) posterior to the bladder at 31 weeks' gestation. **B:** Sagittal T2 MRI confirms the presence of distended rectosigmoid (*arrow*). At delivery, anal atresia was noted in this infant with VACTERL sequence. **C:** Note prominent rectum (*arrow*) in a different 31-week-gestation fetus. This infant was normal at delivery with no anal atresia.

dysfunction, stenosis, and chronic constipation can occur. Fecal continence is a major issue in these cases. While 90% of children with low imperforate anus achieve fecal continence, those with high or intermediate imperforate anus have a much higher risk of long-term incontinence.[179,180]

Recurrence Risk: Recurrence depends on whether the atresia is isolated or syndromic. Isolated cases are thought to be sporadic with rare familial cases reported.[173]

Cloaca
See Chapter 27.2.

Hirschsprung Disease
Incidence: Hirschsprung disease is one of the most common causes of intestinal obstruction in the newborn. The incidence is 1 in 5,000.[181] Males are more affected than females, 4:1. Up to 25% have concurrent anomalies with a strong association with trisomy 21.

Embryology/Pathology: Aganglionosis of the distal colon results in a functionally obstructed distal segment with a dilated proximal segment that tapers at a transition zone. As fetuses do not stool, it takes time after delivery for a transition zone with a dilated proximal segment to become apparent. Thus, prenatal diagnosis is rare, with obstructive symptoms and constipation typically developing only after birth.[182,183]

Diagnosis: Echogenic bowel has been described with fetal Hirschsprung disease,[184] but is not specific to this diagnosis. Enterolithiasis owing to functional obstruction and precipitation of urates within the lumen may be seen.

Cases of total aganglionosis have been diagnosed in the third trimester with polyhydramnios and small bowel dilatation.[184-186] Total colonic aganglionosis is rare, accounting for only 3% to 12% of cases and can mimic ileal atresia or meconium ileus prenatally and postnatally.[187]

Differential Diagnosis: Differential for distal bowel dilatation with polyhydramnios includes colonic atresia, ileal atresia, meconium ileus, meconium plug, small left colon, and imperforate anus.[188-190]

Associated Anomalies: Up to 25% of patients with Hirschsprung disease have associated anomalies, including heart disease, renal anomalies, imperforate anus, colonic atresia, and hypospadias.[188] About 2% of patients with Hirschsprung disease have trisomy 21. Genetic conditions including Bardet–Biedl, cartilage hair hypoplasia, Riley–Day, and Smith–Lemli–Opitz syndromes have been associated with Hirschsprung disease.[191]

Prognosis and Management: If an anus is patent but distal obstruction is suspected, an abdominal radiograph can help document the level of the distal obstruction by demonstrating multiple loops of dilated bowel with air fluid levels. A water-soluble contrast enema may demonstrate the level of obstruction. However, the colon is often normal in caliber as a transition zone has not yet developed. An abnormal sigmoid rectal ratio may provide the diagnosis. If the entire colon is small, total aganglionosis, distal ileal atresia, or meconium ileus should be considered in the differential.[192,193] Total aganglionosis of the colon may also appear as a diffusely stiff, pipe-like colon with broad splenic and hepatic flexures, without conspicuous narrowing. With a persistently abnormal stooling pattern, a biopsy is indicated.

If Hirschsprung disease is confirmed with biopsy, a pull-through procedure is typically performed. Hirschsprung disease often results in good long-term function.[193,194] However, complications including enterocolitis (23%), fecal incontinence (3% to 10%), and chronic constipation (6% to 34%) can occur. Deaths can be secondary to associated anomalies or a delay in diagnosis.[193,195-197]

Recurrence Risk: Typically sporadic. Four percent to 8% of cases are familial with an increased risk of recurrence in siblings.[198] The association with trisomy 21 and other chromosomal abnormalities suggests a genetic component.[191,199,200]

Colonic Atresia
Incidence: Colonic atresias are a rare cause of intestinal obstruction and account for up to 10% of all bowel atresias.[201] Incidence has been reported to be around 1 in 20,000.[202]

Embryology/Pathology: Colonic atresias are thought to be secondary to a vascular or mechanical event (such as intestinal volvulus) similar to jejunal and ileal atresia.[203-207] The majority of colonic atresias occur proximal to the splenic flexure with resultant distal microcolon. In two-thirds of cases, colonic atresia occurs as an isolated defect without associated abnormalities. Colonic atresia may occur in combination with Hirschsprung disease.[208,209]

Diagnosis: The US appearance is indistinguishable from other distal obstructions and difficult to make prenatally. Bowel dilatations and polyhydramnios may rarely develop and suggest a more proximal obstruction. Perforation has been reported with the development of ascites and meconium peritonitis.[210]

A paucity of meconium in the rectum by MRI may help suggest the diagnosis, although if the vascular accident occurred later in gestation, the distal colon and rectum may have already filled with meconium by the time the obstruction occurred.

Associated Anomalies: Anomalies associated with colonic atresia include gastroschisis, omphalocele, Hirschsprung disease, and ocular and skeletal anomalies.[204,209,211] Cardiac anomalies and genetic defects have rarely been described.

Management: Primary repair is often technically feasible in colonic atresia. A suction rectal biopsy prior to the primary repair, to rule out Hirschsprung disease, is recommended.

At times, a colostomy is performed so that the infant can be discharged earlier from the hospital than with a primary repair.[212]

Prognosis/Outcome: Colonic atresia typically has an excellent prognosis with survival greater than 90%.

Recurrence Risk: Recurrence is rare. Cases of colonic atresia because of genetic or familial occurrence have been reported.[206,207,213]

REFERENCES

1. Pritchard JA. Fetal swallowing and amniotic fluid volume. *Obstet Gynecol.* 1966;28:606–610.
2. Cyr DR, Mack LA, Schoenecker SA, et al. Bowel migration in the normal fetus: US detection. *Radiology.* 1986;161:119.
3. Lam YH, Shek T, Tang MH. Sonographic features of anal atresia at 12 weeks. *Ultrasound Obstet Gynecol.* 2002;19:523–524.
4. Nyberg DA, Mack LA, Patten RM, et al. Fetal bowel: normal sonographic findings. *J Ultrasound Med.* 1987;6:3–6.
5. Hertzberg BS. The fetal gastrointestinal tract. *Semin Roentgenol.* 1998;33:360–368.
6. Hertzberg BS. Sonography of the fetal gastrointestinal tract: anatomic variants, diagnostic pitfalls, and abnormalities. *AJR Am J Roentgenol.* 1994;162:1175–1182.

7. Parulekar SG. Sonography of normal fetal bowel. *J Ultrasound Med.* 1991;10:211–220.
8. Zalel Y, Perlitz Y, Gamzu R, et al. In-utero development of the fetal colon and rectum: sonographic evaluation. *Ultrasound Obstet Gynecol.* 2003;21:161–164.
9. Rubesova E. Fetal bowel anomalies—US and MR assessment. *Pediatr Radiol.* 2012;42(suppl 1):S101–S106.
10. Sase M, Asada M, Okuda M, et al. Fetal gastric size in normal and abnormal pregnancies. *Ultrasound Obstet Gynecol.* 2002;19:467–470.
11. Goldstein I, Reece EA, Yarkoni S, et al. Growth of the fetal stomach in normal pregnancies. *Obstet Gynecol.* 1987;70:641.
12. Fakry J, Shapiro LR, Schechter A, et al. Fetal gastric pseudomasses. *J Ultrasound Med.* 1987;6:177–180.
13. Karnik TJ, Rubenstein JB, Swayne LC. The fetal presacral pseudomass: a normal sonographic variant. *J Ultrasound Med.* 1991;10:579–581.
14. Bourdelat D, Muller F, Droullé P, et al. Anatomical and sonographical studies of the development of fecal continence and sphincter development in human fetuses. *Eur J Pediatr Surg.* 2001;11:124–130.
15. Haeusler MC, Berghold A, Stoll C, et al; EUROSCAN Study Group. Prenatal ultrasonographic detection of gastrointestinal obstruction: results from 18 European congenital anomaly registries. *Prenat Diagn.* 2002;22(7):616–623.
16. Stoll C, Alembik Y, Dott B, et al. Evaluation of prenatal diagnosis of congenital gastrointestinal atresias. *Eur J Epidemiol.* 1996;12:611–616.
17. Corteville JE, Gray DL, Langer JC. Bowel abnormalities in the fetus—correlation of prenatal ultrasonographic findings with outcome. *Am J Obstet Gynecol.* 1996;175:724–729.
18. Veyrac C, Couture A, Saguintaah M, et al. MRI of fetal GI tract abnormalities. *Abdom Imaging.* 2004;29:411–420.
19. Huisman T, Kellenberger C. MR imaging characteristics of the normal fetal gastrointestinal tract and abdomen. *Eur J Radiol.* 2008;65:170–181.
20. Garel C, Dreux S, Philippe-Chomette P, et al. Contribution of fetal magnetic resonance imaging and amniotic fluid digestive enzyme assays to the evaluations of gastrointestinal tract abnormalities. *Ultrasound Obstet Gynecol.* 2006;28:282–291.
21. Barnewolt CE. Congenital abnormalities of the gastrointestinal tract. *Semin Roentgenol.* 2004;39(2):263–281.
22. Saguintaah M, Couture A, Veyrac C, et al. MRI of the fetal gastrointestinal tract. *Pediatr Radiol.* 2002;32:395–404.
23. Rubesova E, Vance CJ, Ringertz HG, et al. Three-dimensional MRI volumetric measurements of the normal fetal colon. *AJR Am J Roentgenol.* 2009;192(3):761–765.
24. Colombani M, Ferry M, Garel C, et al. Fetal gastrointestinal MRI: all that glitters in T1 is not necessarily colon. *Pediatr Radiol.* 2010;40:1215–1221.
25. Farhatazia N, Engels JE, Ramus RM, et al. Fetal MRI of urine and meconium by gestational age for the diagnosis of genitourinary and gastrointestinal abnormalities. *AJR Am J Roentgenol.* 2005;184(6):1891–1897.
26. Iacobelli BD, Zaccara A, Spirydakis I, et al. Prenatal counseling of small bowel atresia: watch the fluid! *Prenat Diagn.* 2006;26:214–217.
27. Forrester MB, Merz RD. Population-based study of small intestinal atresia and stenosis, Hawaii, 1986–2000. *Public Health.* 2004;118:434–438.
28. Robertson FM, Crombleholme TM, Paidas M, et al. Prenatal diagnosis and management of gastrointestinal anomalies. *Semin Perinatol.* 1994;18:182–195.
29. Rowe MI, O'Neill JA Jr, Grosfeld JL, et al. Intestinal atresia and stenosis. In: Rowe MI, O'Neill JA Jr, Grosfeld JL, et al., eds. *Essentials of Pediatric Surgery.* St Louis, MO: Mosby; 1995:508–514.
30. Aite L, Trucchi A, Nahom A, et al. Antenatal diagnosis of surgically correctable anomalies: effects of repeated consultations on parental anxiety. *J Perinatol.* 2003;23:652–654.
31. Depaepe A, Dolk H, Lechat MF. The epidemiology of TEF and esophageal atresia in Europe EURO-CAT Working Group. *Arch Dis Child.* 1993;68:743–748.
32. Pretorius DH, Drose JA, Dennis MA, et al. Tracheoesophageal fistula in utero: twenty-two cases. *J Ultrasound Med.* 1987;6(9):509–513.
33. Sparey C, Robson SC. Oesophageal atresia. *Prenat Diagn.* 2000;20(3):251–253.
34. Borsellino A, Zaccara A, Nahom A, et al. False-positive rate in prenatal diagnosis of surgical anomalies. *J Pediatr Surg.* 2006;41(4):826–829.
35. Shaw-Smith C. Oesophageal atresia, tracheo-oesophageal fistula, and the VACTERL association: review of genetics and epidemiology. *J Med Genet.* 2006;43:545.
36. Solt I, Rotmensch S, Bronshtein M. The esophageal "pouch sign": a benign transient finding. *Prenat Diagn.* 2010;30(9):845–848.
37. Estroff JA, Parad RB, Share JC, et al. Second trimester prenatal findings in duodenal and esophageal atresia without tracheoesophageal fistula. *J Ultrasound Med.* 1994;13:375.
38. Shulman A, Mazkereth R, Zalel Y, et al. Prenatal identification of esophageal atresia: the role of ultrasonography for evaluation of functional anatomy. *Prenat Diagn.* 2002;22:669–674.
39. Kalache KD, Wauer R, Mau H, et al. Prognostic significance of the pouch sign in fetuses with prenatally diagnosed esophageal atresia. *Am J Obstet Gynecol.* 2000;182:978–981.
40. Mourali M, Essoussi-Chikhaoui J, Fatnassi A, et al. Prenatal diagnosis of esophageal atresia. *Tunis Med.* 2011;89(2):213–214.
41. Stringer MD, McKenna KM, Goldstein RB, et al. Prenatal diagnosis of esophageal atresia. *J Pediatr Surg.* 1995;30:1258–1263.
42. Develay-Morice E, Rathat G, Duyme M, et al. Ultrasonography of fetal esophagus: healthy appearance and prenatal diagnosis of a case of esophagus atresia with esotracheal fistula. *Gynecol Obstet Fertil.* 2007;35:249–257.
43. Botto LD, Khoury MJ, Mastroiacovo P, et al. The spectrum of congenital anomalies of the VATER association: an international study. *Am J Med Genet.* 1997;71(1):8–15.
44. Eyheremendy E, Pfister M. Antenatal real-time diagnosis of esophageal atresias. *J Clin Ultrasound.* 1983;11(7):395–397.
45. Has R, Günay S, Topuz S. Pouch sign in prenatal diagnosis of esophageal atresia. *Ultrasound Obstet Gynecol.* 2004;23(5):523–524.
46. Langer JC, Hussain H, Khan A, et al. Prenatal diagnosis of esophageal atresia using MRI. *J Pediatr Surg.* 2001;36:804–807.
47. Olgun H, Karacan M, Caner I, et al. Congenital cardiac malformations in neonates with apparently isolated gastrointestinal malformations. *Pediatr Int.* 2009;51(2):260–262.
48. Holder TM, Cloud DT, Lewis JE Jr, et al. Esophageal atresia and TEF: a survey of its members by the Surgical Section of the American Academy of Pediatrics. *Pediatrics.* 1964;34:542.
49. Mitani Y, Hasegawa T, Kubota A, et al. Prenatal findings of concomitant duodenal and esophageal atresia without tracheoesophageal fistula (Gross type A). *J Clin Ultrasound.* 2009;37(7):403–405.
50. Dave S, Shi E. The management of combined oesophageal and duodenal atresia. *Pediatr Surg Int.* 2004;20:689–691.
51. Beasley SW, Allen M, Myers N. The effects of Down syndrome and other chromosomal abnormalities on survival and management in esophageal atresia. *Pediatr Surg.* 1997;12:550–551.
52. Pameijer CR, Hubard AM, Coleman B, et al. Combined pure esophageal atresia, duodenal atresia, biliary atresia, and pancreatic ductal atresia: prenatal diagnostic features and review of the literature. *J Pediatr Surg.* 2000;35:745–747.
53. Chitty LS, Goodman J, Seller MF. Esophageal and duodenal atresia in a fetus with Down's syndrome: prenatal sonographic features. *Ultrasound Obstet Gynecol.* 1996;7:450–452.
54. Spitz L. Esophageal atresia: past, present, and future. *J Pediatr Surg.* 1996;31:19.
55. Bahado-Singh RO, Romero R, Vecchio M, et al. Prenatal diagnosis of congenital hiatal hernia. *J Ultrasound Med.* 1992;11:297–300.
56. Ogunyemi D. Serial sonographic findings in a fetus with congenital hiatal hernia. *Ultrasound Obstet Gynecol.* 2001;17:350–353.
57. Chacko J, Ford WD, Furness ME. Antenatal detection of hiatus hernia. *Pediatr Surg Int.* 1998;13:163–164.
58. Ruano R, Benachi A, Aubry MC, et al. Prenatal sonographic diagnosis of congenital hiatal hernia. *Prenat Diagn.* 2004;24(1):26–30.
59. Yamamoto N, Hidaka N, Anami A, et al. Prenatal sonographic diagnosis of a hiatal hernia in a fetus with asplenia syndrome. *J Ultrasound Med.* 2007;26(9):1257–1261.
60. Al-Assiri A, Wiseman N, Bunge M. Prenatal diagnosis of intrathoracic stomach (gastric herniation). *J Pediatr Surg.* 2005;40(2):E15–E17.
61. Parida SK, Driss VM, Hall BD. Hiatus/paraesophageal hernias in neonatal Marfan syndrome. *Am J Med Genet.* 1995;72:156–158.
62. Yadav K, Myers NA. Paraesophageal hernia in the neonatal period another differential diagnosis of esophageal atresia. *Pediatr Surg Int.* 1997;12:420–421.
63. Al-Arfaj AL, Khwaja MS, Upadhyaya P. Massive hiatal hernia in children. *Eur J Surg.* 1991;157:465–468.
64. Baglaj SM, Noblett HR. Paraoesophageal hernia in children: familial occurrence and review of the literature. *Pediatr Surg Int.* 1999;15:85–87.
65. Skandalakis JE, Gray SW. The small intestines. In: Skandalakis JE, Gray SW, eds. *Embryology for Surgeons.* Baltimore, MD: Williams & Wilkins; 1994:184.
66. Boyden EA, Cope JG, Bill AH. Anatomy and embryology of congenital intrinsic obstruction of the duodenum. *Am J Surg.* 1967;114:190–195.
67. Schaefer-Graf UM, Buchanan TA, Xiang A, et al. Patterns of congenital anomalies and relationship to initial maternal fasting glucose levels in pregnancies complicated by type 2 and gestational diabetes. *Am J Obstet Gynecol.* 2000;182(2):313–320.
68. Ben Ahmed Y, Ghorbel S, Chouikh T, et al. Combination of partial situs inversus, polysplenia and annular pancreas with duodenal obstruction and intestinal malrotation. *JBR-BTR.* 2012;95(4):257–260.
69. Farrant P, Dewbury KC, Meire HB. Antenatal diagnosis of duodenal atresia. *Br J Radiol.* 1981;54(643):633–635.
70. Zimmer EZ, Bronshtein M. Early diagnosis of duodenal atresia and possible sonographic pitfalls. *Prenat Diagn.* 1996;16:564–566.
71. Lawrence M, Ford A, Furness M, et al. Congenital duodenal obstruction: early antenatal ultrasound diagnosis. *Pediatr Surg Int.* 2000;16:342–345.
72. Balcar I, Grant DC, Miller WA, et al. Antenatal detection of Down syndrome by sonography. *AJR Am J Roentgenol.* 1984;143(1):29–30.
73. Nelson LH, Clark CE, Fishburn JI, et al. Value of serial sonography in the in utero detection of duodenal atresia. *Obstet Gynecol.* 1982;59:657–661.
74. Bovicelli L, Rizzo N, Orsini LF, et al. Prenatal diagnosis and management of fetal gastrointestinal abnormalities. *Semin Perinatol.* 1983;7(2):109–117.
75. Petrikovsky BM. First trimester diagnosis of duodenal atresia. *Am J Obstet Gynecol.* 1994;171:569–570.
76. Stauffer UG, Schwoebel M. Duodenal atresia and stenosis annular pancreas. In: O'Neill JA, Rowe MI, Grosfeld JL, et al., eds. *Pediatric Surgery.* 5th ed. St Louis, MO: Mosby-Year Book; 1998:1133–1143.
77. Pariente G, Landau D, Aviram M, et al. Prenatal diagnosis of a rare sonographic appearance of duodenal atresia: report of 2 cases and literature review. *J Ultrasound Med.* 2012;31(11):1829–1833.

78. Choudhry MS, Rahman N, Boyd P, et al. Duodenal atresia: associated anomalies, prenatal diagnosis and outcome. *Pediatr Surg Int.* 2009;25(8):727–730.

79. Fujishiro E, Suziki Y, Sato T, et al. Characteristics findings for diagnosis of baby complicated with both VACTERL association and duodenal atresia. *Fetal Diagn Ther.* 2004;19:134–137.

80. Obata-Yasuoka M, Hamada H, Ohara R, et al. Alveolar capillary dysplasia associated with duodenal atresia: ultrasonographic findings of enlarged, highly echogenic lungs and gastric dilatation in a third-trimester fetus. *J Obstet Gynaecol Res.* 2011;37(7):937–939.

81. Gilbertson-Dahdal DL, Dutta S, Varich LJ, et al. Neonatal malrotation with midgut volvulus mimicking duodenal atresia. *AJR Am J Roentgenol.* 2009;192(5):1269–1271.

82. Malone F, Crombleholme TM, Nores J, et al. Pitfalls of the "double bubble" sign: a case of congenital duodenal duplication. *Fetal Diagn Ther.* 1997;12:298–300.

83. Hancock BJ, Wiseman NE. Congenital duodenal obstruction: the impact of an antenatal diagnosis. *J Pediatr Surg.* 1989;24:1027–1031.

84. Muller F, Dommergues M, Ville Y, et al. Amniotic fluid digestive enzymes: diagnostic value in fetal gastrointestinal obstructions. *Prenat Diagn.* 1994;14(10):973–979.

85. Murshed R, Nicholls G, Spitz L. Intrinsic duodenal obstruction: trends in management and outcome over 45 years (1951–1995) with relevance to prenatal counseling. *Br J Obstet Gynaecol.* 1999;106:1197–1199.

86. Bittencourt DG, Barini R, Marba S, et al. Congenital duodenal obstruction does prenatal diagnosis improve the outcome? *Pediatr Surg Int.* 2004;20:582–585.

87. Cohen-Overbeek T, Grijseels E, Niemeijer N, et al. Isolated or nonisolated duodenal obstruction: perinatal outcome following prenatal or postnatal diagnosis. *Ultrasound Obstet Gynecol.* 2008;32:784–792.

88. Grosfeld JL, Rescorla FJ. Duodenal atresia and stenosis: reassessment of treatment and outcome based on antenatal diagnosis, pathologic variances, and long-term follow-up. *World J Surg.* 1993;17:301–309.

89. Escobar MA, Ladd AP, Grosfeld JL, et al. Duodenal atresia and stenosis: long-term follow-up over 30 years. *J Pediatr Surg.* 2004;39(6):867–871.

90. Touloukian RJ. Diagnosis and treatment of jejunoileal atresia. *World J Surg.* 1993;17:310–319.

91. Baglaj M, Carachi R, Lawther S. Multiple atresia of the small intestine: a 20 year review. *Eur J Pediatr Surg.* 2008;18:13–18.

92. Foucade L, Shima H, Miyazaki E, et al. Multiple gastrointestinal atresias result from disturbed morphogenesis. *Pediatr Surg Int.* 2001;17:361–364.

93. Kumuro H, Amagai T, Hori T, et al. Placental vascular compromise in jejunoileal atresia. *J Pediatr Surg.* 2004;39:1701–1705.

94. Sweeney B, Surana R, Puri P. Jejunoileal atresia and associated malformations: correlation with the timing of in utero insult. *J Pediatr Surg.* 2001;35:774–776.

95. Martin LW, Zerella JT. Jejuno-ileal atresia: a proposed classification. *J Pediatr Surg.* 1976;11:399–403.

96. Ahlgren LS. Apple peel jejunal atresia. *J Pediatr Surg.* 1987;22:451–453.

97. Komuro H, Hori T, Amagai T, et al. The etiologic role of intrauterine volvulus and intussusception in jejunoileal atresia. *J Pediatr Surg.* 2004;39:1812–1814.

98. Patricolo M, Noia G, Rossi L. An experimental animal model of intestinal obstruction to simulate in utero therapy for jejunoileal atresia. *Fetal Diagn Ther.* 1998;13(5):298–301.

99. Graham JM Jr, Marin-Padilla M, Hoefnagel D. Jejunal atresia associated with Cafergot ingestion during pregnancy. *Clin Pediatr (Phila).* 1983;22(3):226–228.

100. Lubinsky M. Hypothesis: estrogen related thrombosis explains the pathogenesis and epidemiology of gastroschisis. *Am J Med Genet A.* 2012;158A(4):808–811.

101. Basaran UN, Inan M, Gucer F, et al. Prenatally closed gastroschisis with midgut atresia. *Pediatr Surg Int.* 2002;18:550–552.

102. Ghionzoli M, James CP, David AL, et al. Gastroschisis with intestinal atresia—predictive value of antenatal diagnosis and outcome of postnatal treatment. *J Pediatr Surg.* 2012;47(2):322–328.

103. Kumar T, Vaughan R, Polak M. A proposed classification for the spectrum of vanishing gastroschisis. *Eur J Pediatr Surg.* 2013;23(1):72–75.

104. Ogunyemi D. Gastroschisis complicated by midgut atresia, absorption of bowel, and closure of the abdominal wall defect. *Fetal Diagn Ther.* 2001;16(4):227–230.

105. Langer JC, Adzick NS, Filly RA, et al. Gastrointestinal tract obstruction in the fetus. *Arch Surg.* 1989;124(10):1183–1186.

106. Langer JC, Khanna J, Caco C, et al. Prenatal diagnosis of gastroschisis: development of objective sonographic criteria for predicting outcome. *Obstet Gynecol.* 1993;81(1):53–56.

107. Wax J, Hamilton T, Cartin A, et al. Congenital jejunal and ileal atresia. *J Ultrasound Med.* 2006;25:337–342.

108. Damato N, Filly RA, Goldstein RB, et al. Frequency of fetal anomalies in sonographically detected polyhydramnios. *J Ultrasound Med.* 1993;12:11–15.

109. Touloukian RJ. Composition of amniotic fluid with experimental jejuno-ileal atresia. *J Pediatr Surg.* 1977;12:397–401.

110. Estroff J, Bromley B, Benacerraf B. Fetal meconium peritonitis without sequelae. *Pediatr Radiol.* 1992;22:277–278.

111. Dirkes K, Crombleholme TM, Craigo SD, et al. The natural history of meconium peritonitis diagnosed in utero. *J Pediatr Surg.* 1995;30:979–982.

112. Benachi A, Sonig P, Jouannic JM, et al. Determination of the anatomical location of an antenatal intestinal occlusion by magnetic resonance imaging. *Ultrasound Obstet Gynecol.* 2001;18:163–165.

113. Rubio EI, Blask AR, Badillo AT, et al. Prenatal magnetic resonance and ultrasonographic findings in small-bowel obstruction: imaging clues and postnatal outcomes. *Pediatr Radiol.* 2017;47(4):411–421.

114. Brugger PC, Prayer D. Fetal abdominal magnetic resonance imaging. *Eur J Radiol.* 2006;57:278–293.

115. Shinmoto H, Kuribayashi S. MRI of fetal abdominal abnormalities. *Abdom Imaging.* 2003;28:877–886.

116. Carcopino X, Chaumoitre K, Shojai R, et al. Use of fetal magnetic resonance imaging in differentiating ileal atresia from meconium ileus. *Ultrasound Obstet Gynecol.* 2006;28(7):976–977.

117. Whitby EH, Paley MN, Sprigg A, et al. Comparison of ultrasound and magnetic resonance imaging in 100 singleton pregnancies with suspected brain abnormalities. *BJOG.* 2004;111:784–792.

118. Nixon HH. Small intestinal atresia. *Proc R Soc Med.* 1971;64(4):372–374.

119. Shawis R, Antao B. Prenatal bowel dilatation and the subsequent postnatal management. *Early Hum Dev.* 2006;82(5):297–303.

120. Basu R, Burge DM. The effect of antenatal diagnosis on the management of small bowel atresia. *Pediatr Surg Int.* 2004;20:177–179.

121. Ozguner IF, Savas C, Ozguner M, et al. Intestinal atresia with segmental musculature and neural defect. *J Pediatr Surg.* 2005;40(8):1232–1237.

122. DallaVecchia LK, Grosfeld JL, West KW, et al. Intestinal atresia and stenosis: a 25 year experience with 277 cases. *Arch Surg.* 1998;133:490–496.

123. Arnal-Monreal F, Pombo F, Capdevila-Puerta A. Multiple hereditary gastrointestinal atresias: study of a family. *Acta Paediatr Scand.* 1983;72:773–777.

124. Shorter NA, Georges A, Perenyi A, et al. A proposed classification system for familial intestinal atresia and its relevance to the understanding of the etiology of jejunoileal atresia. *J Pediatr Surg.* 2006;41(11):1822–1825.

Meconium Ileus

125. Muller F, Frot JC, Aubry MC, et al. Meconium ileus in cystic fibrosis fetuses. *Lancet.* 1984;1:223.

126. Caspi B, Elchalal U, Lancet M, et al. Prenatal diagnosis of cystic fibrosis: ultrasonographic appearance of meconium ileus in the fetus. *Prenat Diagn.* 1988;8:379–382.

127. Barki Y, Bar-Ziv J. Meconium ileus: ultrasonic diagnosis of intraluminal inspissated meconium. *J Clin Ultrasound.* 1985;13(7):509–512.

128. Bulas D. Prenatal diagnosis of gastrointestinal atresia and obstruction. In: Basow DS, ed. UpToDate. Waltham, MA: Wolters Kluwer Health; 2012.

129. Scotet V, De Braekeleer M, Audrezet MP, et al. Prenatal detection of cystic fibrosis by ultrasonography: a retrospective study of more than 346,000 pregnancies. *J Med Genet.* 2002;39:443–448.

130. Degnan AJ, Bulas DI, Sze RW. Ileal atresia with meconium peritonitis: fetal MRI evaluation. *J Radiol Case Rep.* 2010;4:15–18.

131. Wong A, Toh CH, Lien R, et al. Prenatal MR imaging of a meconium pseudocyst extending to the right subphrenic space with right lung compression. *Pediatr Radiol.* 2006;36:1208–1211.

132. Simonovsky V, Lisy J. Meconium pseudocyst secondary to ileal atresia complicated by volvulus: antenatal MR demonstration. *Pediatr Radiol.* 2007;37:305–309.

133. Blazer S, Zimmer EZ, Bronshtein M. Nonvisualization of the fetal gallbladder in early pregnancy: comparison with clinical outcome. *Radiology.* 2002;224(2):379–382.

134. Carcopino X, Chaumoitre K, Shojai R, et al. Foetal magnetic resonance imaging and echogenic bowel. *Prenat Diagn.* 2007;27:272–278.

135. Al-Kouatly HB, Chasen ST, Streltzoff J, et al. The clinical significance of fetal echogenic bowel. *Am J Obstet Gynecol.* 2001;185:1035–1038.

136. Kesrouani AK, Guibourdenche J, Mullr F, et al. Etiology and outcome of fetal echogenic bowel: ten years of experience. *Fetal Diagn Ther.* 2003;18:240–246.

137. Scotet V, Dugueperoux I, Audrezet MP, et al. Focus on cystic fibrosis and other disorders evidenced in fetuses with sonographic finding of echogenic bowel: 16-year report from Brittany, France. *Am J Obstet Gynecol.* 2010;203:592.e1–e6.

138. Sepulveda W, Leung KY, Roberson ME, et al. Prevalence of cystic fibrosis mutations in pregnancies with fetal echogenic bowel. *Obstet Gynecol.* 1996;87:103–106.

139. Chasen ST. Fetal echogenic bowel. In: Wilkins-Haug L, ed. UpToDate. Waltham, MA: Wolters Kluwer Health; 2012.

140. Jackson CR, Orford J, Minutillo C, et al. Dilated and echogenic fetal bowel and postnatal outcomes: a surgical perspective. Case series and literature review. *Eur J Pediatr Surg.* 2010;20(3):191–193.

141. Bashiri A, Burstein E, Hershkowitz R, et al. Fetal echogenic bowel by ultrasound: what is the clinical significance? *Harefuah.* 2007;146(12):964–969, 996–997.

142. Oka Y, Asabe K, Shirakusa T, et al. An antenatal appearance of megacystis-microcolon-intestinal hypoperistalsis syndrome. *Turk J Pediatr.* 2008;50(3):269–274.

143. Gaillard D, Bouvier R, Scheiner C, et al. Meconium ileus and intestinal atresia in fetuses and neonates. *Pediatr Pathol Lab Med.* 1996;16:25–40.

144. Kirkinen P, Jouppila P. Prenatal ultrasonic findings in congenital chloride diarrhea. *Pernat Diagn.* 1984;4:457.

145. Colombani M, Ferry M, Toga CV, et al. Magnetic resonance imaging in the prenatal diagnosis of congenital diarrhea. *Ultrasound Obstet Gynecol.* 2010;35:560–565.

146. Usui N, Kamiyama M, Tani G, et al. Prenatal differential diagnosis of congenital chloride diarrhea: the importance of a dilated fluid-filled rectum. *Eur J Pediatr Surg.* 2011;21(3):193–194.

147. Langer JC, Winthrop AL, Burrows RF. False diagnosis of intestinal obstruction in a fetus with congenital chloride diarrhea. *Pediatr Surg.* 1991;26(11):1282–1284.

148. Hohlschneider AM, Hutson JM. *Anorectal Malformations in Children: Embryology, Diagnosis, Surgical Treatment, Follow-up.* Berlin, Germany: Springer-Verlag; 2006.

149. Bean WJ, Calonje MA, Aprill CN, et al. Anal atresia: a prenatal ultrasound diagnosis. *J Clin Ultrasound.* 1978;6:111–114.

150. Harris RD, Nyberg DA, Mack LA, et al. Anorectal atresia: prenatal sonographic diagnosis. *AJR Am J Roentgenol.* 1987;149:395–400.

151. Brantberg A, Blass HGK, Haugen SE, et al. Imperforate anus: a relatively common anomaly rarely diagnosed prenatally. *Ultrasound Obstet Gynecol.* 2006;28:904–910.

152. Gilbert CE, Hamil J, Metcalfe RF, et al. Changing antenatal sonographic appearance of anorectal atresia from first to third trimesters. *J Ultrasound Med.* 2006;25:781–784.

153. Kaponis A, Paschopoulos M, Parakevaidis E, et al. Fetal anal atresia presenting as transient bowel dilatation at 16 weeks of gestation. *Fetal Diagn Ther.* 2006;21:383–385.

154. Taipale P, Rovamo L, Hiilesmaa V. First-trimester diagnosis of imperforate anus. *Ultrasound Obstet Gynecol.* 2005;25:187–188.

155. Chen M, Meagher S, Simpson I, et al. Sonographic features of anorectal atresia at 12 weeks. *J Matern Fetal Neonatal Med.* 2009;22:931–933.

156. Mandell J, Lillehei C, Greene M, et al. The prenatal diagnosis of imperforate anus with rectourinary fistula: dilated fetal colon with enterolitiasis. *J Pediatr Surg.* 1992;27(1):82–84.

157. Grant T, Newman M, Gould R, et al. Intraluminal colonic calcifications associated with anorectal atresia: prenatal sonographic detection. *J Ultrasound Med.* 1990;9:411–413.

158. Sepulveda W, Romero R, Qureshi F, et al. Prenatal diagnosis of enterolithiasis: a sign of fetal large bowel obstruction. *J Ultrasound Med.* 1994;13:581–585.

159. Bergholz R, Wenke K. Enterolithiasis: a case report and review. *J Pediatr Surg.* 2008;44:828–830.

Anus

160. Vijayaraghavan SB, Prema AS, Suganyadevi P. Sonographic depiction of the fetal anus and its utility in the diagnosis of anorectal malformations. *J Ultrasound Med.* 2011;30:37–45.

161. Moon MH, Cho JY, Kim JH, et al. In utero development of the fetal anal sphincter. *Ultrasound Obstet Gynecol.* 2010;35:556–559.

162. Elchalal U, Yanai N, Valsky DV, et al. Application of 3-dimensional ultrasonography to imaging the fetal anal canal. *J Ultrasound Med.* 2010;29:1195–1201.

163. Gindes L, Weissmann-Brenner A, Achiron R, et al. 3-Dimensional demonstration of fetal anal canal and sphincter. *Ultraschall Med.* 2012;33(7):E25–E30.

164. Ochoa JH, Chiesa M, Vildoza RP, et al. Evaluation of the perianal muscular complex in the prenatal diagnosis of anorectal atresia in a high-risk population. *Ultrasound Obstet Gynecol.* 2012;39(5):521–527.

165. Lubusky M, Prochazka M, Dhaifalah I, et al. Fetal enterolithiasis: prenatal sonographic and MRI diagnosis in two cases of urorectal septum malformation (URSM) sequence. *Prenat Diagn.* 2006;26(4):345–349.

166. Chen CP, Chang TY, Liu YP, et al. Prenatal 3-dimensional sonographic and MRI findings in omphalocele-exstrophy-imperforate anus-spinal defects complex. *J Clin Ultrasound.* 2008;36(5):308–311.

167. Warne S, Chitty LS, Wilcox DT. Prenatal diagnosis of cloacal anomalies. *BJU Int.* 2002;89:78–81.

168. Witters I, Meylaerts L, Peeters H, et al. Fetal hydrometrocolpos, uterus didelphys with low vaginal and anal atresia: difficulties in differentiation from a complex cloacal malformation: a case report. *Genet Couns.* 2012;23(4):513–517.

169. Goto S, Suzumori N, Obayashi S, et al. Prenatal findings of omphalocele-exstrophy of the bladder-imperforate anus-spinal defects (OEIS) complex. *Congenit Anom (Kyoto).* 2012;52(3):179–181.

170. Vasudevan PC, Cohen MC, Whitby EH, et al. The OEIS complex: two case reports that illustrate the spectrum of abnormalities and a review of the literature. *Prenat Diagn.* 2006;26(3):267.

171. Nour S, Kumor D, Dickson JAS. Anorectal malformations with sacral bony abnormalities. *Arch Dis Child.* 1989;64:1618–1624.

172. Jaramillo D, Lebowitz RL, Hendren WH. The cloacal malformation: radiologic findings and imaging recommendations. *Radiology.* 1990;177:441–448.

173. Boocock GR, Donnai D. Anorectal malformation: familial aspects and associated anomalies. *Arch Dis Child.* 1987;62:576–579.

174. Cuschieri A. EROCAT Working Group: anorectal anomalies associated with or as part of other anomalies. *Am J Med Genet.* 2002;110:122–130.

175. Cho S, Moore SP, Fangman T. One hundred three consecutive patients with anorectal malformations and their associated anomalies. *Arch Pediatr Adolesc Med.* 2001;155:587–591.

176. Stoll C, Alembik Y, Dott B, et al. Associated malformations in patients with anorectal anomalies. *Eur J Med Genet.* 2007;50:281–290.

177. Livingston J, Elicevik M, Crombleholme T, et al. US findings in neonates with anorectal malformations: a review of 95 cases. *Am J Obstet Gynecol.* 2006; 195:S63.

178. Peña A, Devries P. Posterior sagittal anorectoplasty: important technical considerations and new applications. *J Pediatr Surg.* 1982;17:796–802.

179. Kazizoke H. Preexisitng neurogenic voiding dysfunction in children with imperforate anus: problems in management. *J Urol.* 1994;151:1041–1045.

180. Rintala R, Lindahl H, Louchimo I. Anorectal malformations—results of treatment and long-term follow-up in 208 patients. *Pediatr Surg Int.* 1991;6:36–42.

181. Parisi MA, Kapur RP. Genetics of Hirschsprung's disease. *Curr Opin Pediatr.* 2000;12:610–617.

182. Bickler SW. Long-segment Hirschsprung disease. *Oral Surg.* 1992;127:1047–1051.

183. Puri P. Hirschsprung's disease: clinical and experimental observations. *World J Surg.* 1993;17:374–384.

184. Wrobleski D, Wesselhoeft C. US diagnosis of prenatal intestinal obstruction. *J Pediatr Surg.* 1979;14:598–600.

185. Vermesh M, Mayden KL, Confino E, et al. Prenatal sonographic diagnosis of Hirschsprung's disease. *J Ultrasound Med.* 1986;5:37–39.

186. Eliyahu S, Yanai N, Blondheim O, et al. Sonographic presentation of Hirschsprung's disease: a case of an entirely aganglionic colon and ileum. *Prenat Diagn.* 1994;14:1170–1172.

187. Wildhaber BE, Teitelbaum DH, Coran AG. Total colonic Hirschsprung's disease: a 28-year experience. *J Pediatr Surg.* 2005;40:203–207.

188. Cowles RA, Berdon WE, Holt PD, et al. Neonatal intestinal obstruction simulating meconium ileus in infants with long-segment intestinal aganglionosis: radiographic findings that prompt the need for rectal biopsy. *Pediatr Radiol.* 2006;36:133–137.

189. Johnson JF, Dean BL. Hirschsprung's disease co-existing with colonic atresia. *Pediatr Radiol.* 1981;11:97–98.

190. Arbell D, Gross E, Orkin B, et al. Imperforate anus, malrotation, and Hischsprung's disease: a rare and important association. *J Pediatr Surg.* 2006;41:1335–1337.

191. Kusafuha T, Puri P. Genetic aspects of Hirschsprung's disease. *Semin Pediatr Surg.* 1998;7:148–155.

Management

192. Bodian M, Carter CO, Ward BCH. Hirschsprung disease (with radiological observations). *Lancet.* 1951;1:302–309.

193. Swenson O, Sherman JO, Fisher JH, et al. The treatment and post-operative complications of congenital megacolon: a twenty-five year follow-up. *Ann Surg.* 1985;182:266–273.

194. Teitelbaum DH, Coran AG, Primary pull-through in the newborn. *Semin Pediatr Surg.* 1998;7:103–107.

195. Craigie RJ, Conway SJ, Cooper L, et al. Primary pull-through for Hirschsprung's disease: comparison of open and laparoscopic assisted procedures. *J Laparoendosc Adv Surg Tech A.* 2007;17:809–812.

196. Rescorla F, Morrison A, Engles D, et al. Hirschsprung's disease: evaluation of mortality and long-term outcome in 260 cases. *Arch Surg.* 1992;127:934–941.

197. Suita S, Taguchi T, Ieiri S, et al. Hirschsprung's disease in Japan: analysis of 3852 patients based on a national wide survey in 30 years. *J Pediatr Surg.* 2005;40:197–202.

198. Raffensperger JG, ed. *Swenso's Pediatric Surgery.* 5th ed. Norwalk, CT: Appleton and Lange; 1990.

199. Martucciello G, Bicocchi MP, Dodero P, et al. Total colonic aganglionosis associated with interstitial deletion of the long arm of chromosome 10. *Pediatr Surg Int.* 1992;7:300–310.

200. Edery P, Pelet A, Mulligan LM, et al. Long segment and short segment familial Hirschsprung's disease variable clinical expression of the RET locus. *J Med Genet.* 1994;31:602–606.

201. Touloukian RI. Diagnosis and treatment of jejunoileal atresia. *World J Surg.* 1993;17:310–317.

202. Philippart AI. Atresia stenosis and other obstructions of the colon. In: Welch KI, Randolph IT, eds. *Pediatric Surgery.* Chicago, IL: Year Book Medical Publishers; 1986:984–985.

203. Boweles ET, Vassy LE, Ralston M. Atresia of the colon. *J Pediatr Surg.* 1976; 11:69–75.

204. Etensel B, Temir G, Karkiner A, et al. Atresia of the colon. *J Pediatr Surg.* 2005; 40:1258–1268.

205. Sturim HA, Ternberg JL. Congenital atresia of the colon. *Surgery.* 1966; 59:458–464.

206. Guttman FM, Braun P, Garanace PH, et al. Multiple atresias involving the GI tract form the stomach to rectum. *J Pediatr Surg.* 1973;8:633–640.

207. Puri P, Fujimoto T. New observation on the pathogenesis of multiple intestinal atresia. *J Pediatr Surg.* 1988;23:221.

208. Currie ABM, Hemalatha AH, Doraiswomy NV, et al. Colonic atresia in association with Hirschsprung's disease. *J R Coll Surg Edinb.* 1983;28:31–34.

209. Draus JM, Maxfield CM, Bond SJ. Hirschsprung's disease in an infant with colonic atresia and normal fixation of the distal colon. *J Pediatr Surg.* 2007;42:E5–E8.

210. Agrawala G, Predanic M, Perni SC, et al. Isolated fetal ascites caused by bowel perforation due to colonic atresia. *J Matern Fetal Neonatal Med.* 2005;17:291–294.

211. Saxonhouse MA, Kays DW, Burchfield DJ, et al. Gastroschisis with jejunal and colonic atresia, and isolated colonic atresia in dichorionic, diamniotic twins. *Pediatr Surg Int.* 2009;25(5):437–439.

212. Davenport M, Bianchi A, Doig CM, et al. Colonic atresia: current results of treatment. *J R Coll Surg Edinb.* 1990;35:25–28.

213. Benawra R, Puppla BL, Mangurten HH, et al. Familial occurrence of congenital colonic atresia. *J Pediatr.* 1981;99:435–436.

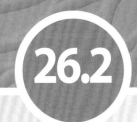

26.2 Ventral Wall Defects

Leann E. Linam

Ventral wall defects are commonly occurring malformations, seen in approximately 1 in 2,000 live births. This group of defects includes complex lethal anomalies that develop early in gestation, such as limb–body wall complex (LBWC), as well as pentalogy of Cantrell, ectopia cordis, bladder exstrophy, omphalocele, cloacal exstrophy, and the later occurring gastroschisis. Urachal anomalies can also be included in this classification. With appropriate prenatal evaluation, including maternal serum alpha-fetoprotein (AFP) screening and ultrasound, many of these anomalies are successfully detected prenatally.

When evaluating a fetus sonographically, it is important to obtain views of the anterior abdominal wall and abdominal umbilical cord (UC) insertion (Fig. 26.2-1) and critical to avoid missing small defects during screening examinations.[1] Once identified, the malformation should be further categorized and associated anomalies described (Table 26.2-1). Fetal magnetic resonance imaging (MRI) can be useful in confirming the diagnosis and identifying additional abnormalities. Accurate diagnosis is important for parental counseling, pregnancy management, delivery planning, and prognosis.

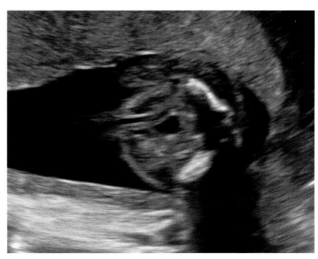

FIGURE 26.2-1: Normal cord insertion at 20 weeks' gestation. Transverse sonogram of the abdomen shows a normal insertion of the umbilical cord (UC) into the anterior abdominal wall.

TABLE 26.2-1	Typical Features of Ventral Wall Defects and Associated Conditions		
TYPE OF DEFECT	**DESCRIPTION**	**SONOGRAPHIC FEATURES**	**ASSOCIATED ANOMALIES**
Gastroschisis	Paraumbilical defect	Typically, only bowel is eviscerated; occasionally other organs, rarely liver No membrane Defect to the right of cord insertion	Associated anomalies uncommon; low risk of aneuploidy; high rate of bowel-related complications
Omphalocele	Midline defect, contained by membrane	Large—extracorporeal liver Small—intracorporeal liver Membrane covered Central cord insertion	High risk of anomalies/aneuploidy; isolated extracorporeal liver—low risk of aneuploidy/high rate of cardiac anomalies; intracorporeal liver—>50% risk of aneuploidy
Beckwith–Wiedemann syndrome	Syndromic	Macroglossia, omphalocele typically intracorporeal liver type, visceromegaly	Wilms tumor Hepatoblastoma
Pentalogy of Cantrell	(1) Omphalocele, (2) anterior diaphragmatic hernia, (3) distal partial sternal defect, (4) pericardial defect, (5) cardiac defect	High omphalocele; pleural effusion suggestive of diaphragmatic hernia	Cardiac defects
Ectopia cordis	Thoracic defect of sternum and skin	Ectopic heart not covered by skin	Cardiac defects; high omphalocele
Limb–body wall complex	Multiple anomalies	Complex ventral wall defect, close attachment to placenta, short umbilical cord scoliosis	Limb, spine, short umbilical cord, lethal

EMBRYOLOGY

In the third gestational week (menstrual week 5), the embryo is an elongated disc consisting of two cell layers (Fig. 26.2-2A).[2,3] Late in this week, gastrulation converts the two layers into the three germ cell layers (Fig. 26.2-3A): dorsally, the ectoderm will become the central nervous system, skin, and sensory organs; the mesoderm (middle layer) will become the skeletal system, heart and blood vessels, and urogenital system; ventrally, the endoderm becomes abdominal organs, including the gastrointestinal (GI) tract.[2] The process of gastrulation begins in the cranial portion of the embryo and proceeds caudally. As a region develops, the mesoderm layer divides into three types: paraxial, intermediate, and lateral plate mesoderm. The lateral plate mesoderm splits into two layers. The parietal mesoderm adheres to the ectoderm and becomes the body wall; the visceral mesoderm covers the gut tube and becomes the smooth muscle, and the visceral and parietal membranes that cover the surfaces of organs (Fig. 26.2-3).[2,3]

The parietal mesoderm, together with the ectoderm, makes up the lateral body folds. These folds grow ventrally (Figs. 26.2-3D and 26.2-4A), eventually fusing to become the ventral body wall.[2] This movement narrows the connection between the yolk sac and the ventral portion of the embryo to form the midgut (Fig. 26.2-4). The body stalk and the yolk stalk come together at 5 to 6 fetal weeks (7 to 8 menstrual weeks) to form the UC.

Development of the midgut is followed by rapid elongation of the gut and its mesentery, forming a primary intestinal loop. This primary intestinal loop elongates so much that there is no room in the abdominal cavity for the contents, and the intestinal loop herniates into the base of the UC (Fig. 26.2-5).[4] Within the UC, the midgut loop rotates 90° counterclockwise around the axis of the superior mesenteric artery. During the 10th fetal week (12th menstrual week), the bowel begins to return to the abdomen, undergoing another 180° rotation during this return. During this time of physiologic gut herniation, it is possible to mistake this normal process for a ventral wall defect.

GASTROSCHISIS

Gastroschisis is a full-thickness defect in the umbilical wall that occurs lateral to the normally inserted UC (Fig. 26.2-6). This defect is nearly always to the right of the abdominal cord insertion, but left-sided defects have been reported, but are likely a different entity.[5] The small intestine is typically herniated outside the abdominal cavity, and occasionally stomach, colon, and gonads are herniated as well. There is no covering membrane.[6]

Incidence: The incidence of gastroschisis is approximately 1 in 2,200 births.[7] Variability of prevalence is seen with maternal age, with the highest incidence being in younger women (1 in ~1,100 births for women younger than 20 years of age).[8] The incidence of gastroschisis has steadily increased worldwide since the first case was described in 1963,[7,9–13] suggesting a new environmental teratogen combining with behaviors of young mothers to produce the defect.[6]

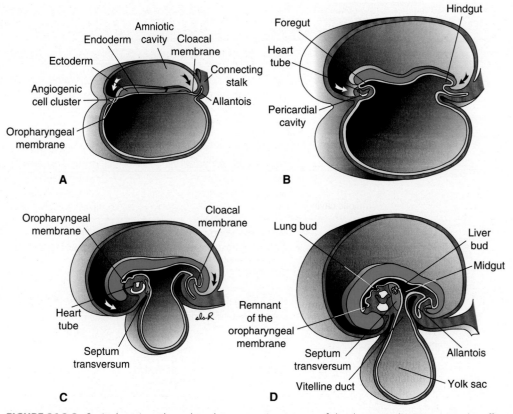

FIGURE 26.2-2: Sagittal sections through embryos at various stages of development demonstrating the effect of cephalocaudal and lateral folding on the position of the endoderm-lined cavity. Note formation of the foregut, midgut, and hindgut. **A:** Presomite embryo. **B:** Embryo with seven somites. **C:** Embryo with 14 somites. **D:** At the end of the first month. (Reprinted with permission from Sadler TW. *Langman's Medical Embryology*. 12th ed. Philadelphia, PA: Wolters Kluwer Health/Lippincott Williams & Wilkins; 2012:87.)

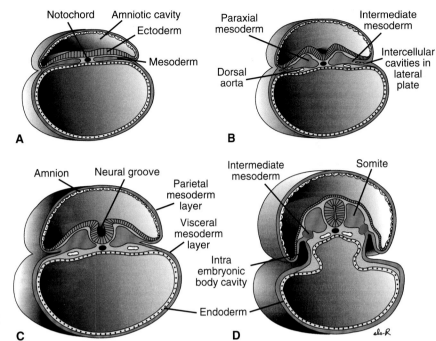

FIGURE 26.2-3: Transverse sections showing development of the mesodermal germ layer. **A:** Day 17. **B:** Day 19. **C:** Day 20. **D:** Day 21. The thin mesodermal sheet gives rise to paraxial mesoderm (future somites), intermediate mesoderm (future excretory units), and lateral plate, which is split into parietal and visceral mesoderm layers lining the intraembryonic cavity. (Reprinted with permission from Sadler TW. *Langman's Medical Embryology.* 12th ed. Philadelphia, PA: Wolters Kluwer Health/ Lippincott Williams & Wilkins; 2012:71.)

Embryology and Pathology: There are many theories regarding the embryologic origin of gastroschisis. Recent research by Bargy and Beaudoin suggests that the physiologic umbilical hernia is located to the right side of the cord, because after 6 weeks of development the left umbilical vein is predominant. The normal UC is divided into the pars vasculosa and pars flaccida. The midgut extends into the pars flaccida, which is very thin and more likely to rupture since the pars flaccida contains no vessels. A rupture of the cord in this place would allow the bowel to extend extracorporally without a covering.[14]

Another current hypothesis is that one or more of the folds responsible for closure of the abdominal wall fails. This prevents the yolk stalk from merging with the connecting stalk; part of the primary intestinal loop then herniates through this defect.[15] Other theories include the following:

- Gastroschisis is the result of abnormal involution of the right umbilical vein.[16]
- Disruption of the omphalomesenteric artery results in infarction of a portion of the abdominal wall.[17]
- Embryonic mesenchyme fails to differentiate as the result of teratogenic exposure during the 4th week after conception.[18]

Most cases of gastroschisis are sporadic, but rare cases of familial gastroschisis have been reported.[6] The cause of gastroschisis is unknown. Young maternal age is a risk factor in nearly every epidemiologic study conducted on gastroschisis. Behaviors typically found in younger mothers are also associated, such as primigravida and short cohabitation time with the father and change in paternity.[6] Non-Hispanic and white race has an increased risk of gastroschisis.[13] Other risk factors include low socioeconomic

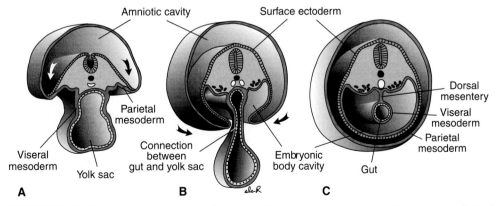

FIGURE 26.2-4: Cross sections through embryos at various stages of development to show the effect of lateral folding on the embryonic cavity. **A:** Folding is initiated. **B:** Transverse section through the midgut to show the connection between the gut and the yolk sac. **C:** Section just below the midgut to show the closed ventral abdominal wall and gut suspended from the dorsal abdominal wall by its mesentery. *Arrows,* lateral folds. (Reprinted with permission from Sadler TW. *Langman's Medical Embryology.* 12th ed. Philadelphia, PA: Wolters Kluwer Health/Lippincott Williams & Wilkins; 2012:79.)

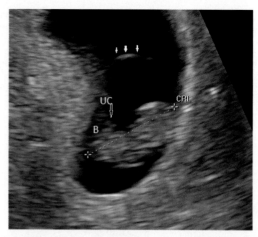

FIGURE 26.2-5: Normal gut migration. Longitudinal sonogram shows echogenic bowel *(B)* herniated into the base of the umbilical cord *(UC)*. The *small arrows* indicate amnion. Crown rump length *(CRL)* consistent with a 9-week gestation.

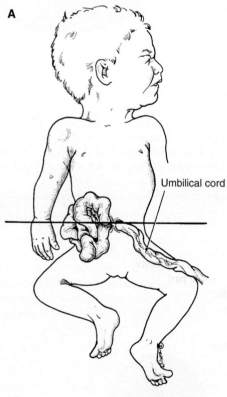

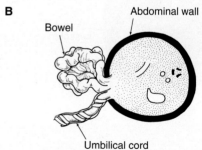

FIGURE 26.2-6: Typical features of gastroschisis shown on external examination **(A)** and on cross-sectional view **(B)**. (Reprinted with permission from Hertzberg BS, Nyberg DA, Neilson IA. Ventral wall defects. In: Nyberg DA, McGahan JP, Pretorius DH, et al., eds. *Diagnostic Imaging of Fetal Anomalies*. Philadelphia, PA: Lippincott Williams & Wilkins; 2003:519–520.)

status, low income, and poor nutrition. Maternal obesity is thought to be protective.

Because of the theory that gastroschisis is the result of vascular disruption, vasoactive drugs have been investigated as potential teratogens. However, acetaminophen and pseudoephedrine are the only two legal drugs implicated in the literature.[6] Illicit drugs, on the other hand, have been found to be significant risk factors for the development of gastroschisis, including cocaine, methamphetamines, and marijuana. Maternal smoking and alcohol consumption have been implicated in some studies, but not others.

Diagnosis: Although prenatal diagnosis of gastroschisis has not been shown to improve postnatal outcome,[19] accurate prenatal diagnosis allows for physicians to counsel families, adequately monitor the pregnancy, and prepare for transferring the infant to a pediatric specialty center for immediate treatment. Elevated AFP in the second trimester is a diagnostic clue, which should lead the clinicians to perform a detailed ultrasound looking for specific structural anomalies. However, maternal serum AFP is now only measured in women who do not undergo first-trimester screening.[11] Thus, routine first- and second-trimester screening sonography has led to the detection of the majority of cases of gastroschisis.[20]

Ultrasound: The classic sonographic appearance of gastroschisis is multiple loops of free-floating bowel herniating through a defect to the right of the UC insertion (Fig. 26.2-7). There is no surrounding membrane. The small bowel is uniformly involved; variable amounts of colon, the stomach, and the urinary bladder may also herniate into the amniotic fluid. The presence of eviscerated solid organs suggests a ruptured omphalocele or diagnosis other than gastroschisis.[21] Gastroschisis tends to be isolated, although a search for additional anomalies should always be performed.

Serial sonographic evaluation with amniotic fluid assessment is important in pregnancies with gastroschisis. These fetuses are at risk for intrauterine growth restriction (IUGR), although this can be difficult to measure because of the herniated abdominal contents, resulting in a small abdominal circumference. Abdominal circumference less than 5th percentile is associated with

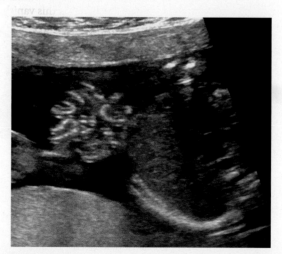

FIGURE 26.2-7: Gastroschisis at 19 weeks' gestational age. Transverse sonogram demonstrates bowel floating outside the abdomen with no covering membrane.

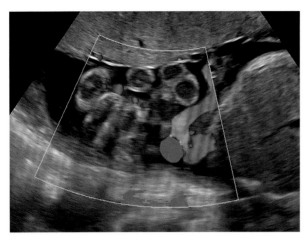

FIGURE 26.2-8: Gastroschisis at 32 weeks. Transverse Doppler sonogram shows the cord in color. The bowel is dilated with a thickened wall.

morbidity.[22] Injury to the exposed bowel can occur. A fibrous peel may develop owing to a sterile inflammatory reaction to amniotic fluid. This causes the bowel to appear echogenic and thick-walled on ultrasound.[20] Sudden increase in echogenicity of the bowel or loss of peristaltic activity should be concerning for bowel ischemia.[23] Polyhydramnios may indicate the development of a bowel atresia.

Mild bowel dilatation is commonly seen in gastroschisis and may be related to a difference in transmural pressure when it is outside the abdomen[23] (Fig. 26.2-8). It has been suggested that more severe bowel dilatation is an indicator of poor postnatal outcome, and multiple studies have undertaken to evaluate this further. Recent studies suggest that both intra- and extra-abdominal bowel dilation are indicators of complex gastroschisis, causing a prolonged neonatal intensive care unit (NICU) stay, but that intra-abdominal bowel dilation is associated with a worse prognosis, that is, higher risk of atresia or short bowel syndrome.[22,24] However, progressive dilation of the bowel with decreased peristalsis is considered a more reliable indicator of poor prognosis than is bowel dilation alone.[25]

Occasionally, in severe cases, the extruded bowel can vanish completely. In these cases, the ventral wall defect may spontaneously close *in utero* ("vanishing gastroschisis" or "vanishing gut"). Often, the remaining bowel within the abdomen is dilated and thickened with atretic portions.[26] It is thought that this vanishing gut and atresia is because of ischemia from a tight defect. These fetuses have an extremely poor prognosis.

Magnetic Resonance Imaging: Because gastroschisis tends to be an isolated GI anomaly and well delineated by sonogram, MRI is not routinely recommended. Prenatal MRI does allow for improved soft-tissue contrast and assessment of meconium. In addition, MRI has a larger field of view, allowing more detailed evaluation of complex anomalies. Single-shot rapid acquisition sequence with multiple 180° refocusing echoes should be obtained in the axial and sagittal planes. T1 images can assess for liver and meconium position. MRI shows free-floating bowel loops herniating through an abdominal wall defect to the right of an intact UC insertion[21] (Fig. 26.2-9). The abdominal wall defect can be visualized and bowel mucosa assessed.[27]

Differential Diagnosis: The major differential diagnosis of gastroschisis is a bowel-containing omphalocele. Other ventral wall defects such as LBWC, cloacal exstrophy, and pentalogy of Cantrell should be excluded. In omphalocele, the bowel has a peritoneal covering and the UC inserts at the base of the defect. LBWC often has herniated liver, characteristic cranial and limb defects, scoliosis, and a short UC. Cloacal exstrophy is an infra-umbilical defect, with absent bladder.

Prognosis: Long-term prognosis for gastroschisis is generally excellent. Mortality rate has continually decreased, and survival now exceeds 90%.[11,20,28] Improved perinatal care, fetal monitoring, surgical management, and neonatal intensive care all contribute to the improved survival. The major causes of neonatal death in gastroschisis are bowel ischemia, necrotizing enterocolitis, sepsis, and liver failure.[28]

Fetal distress is common in fetuses with gastroschisis, and these pregnancies have a higher rate of third-trimester intrauterine fetal demise.[20] Fetal distress is hypothesized to arise from cord compression by extruded bowel,[29] but may also be related to oligohydramnios. IUGR has been reported to affect 30% to 70% of fetuses.[11] Bowel dilatation may indicate a poor prognosis, but this is controversial and does not warrant early delivery at this time.

About 10% to 20% of newborns with gastroschisis have associated anomalies, predominantly involving the GI tract.[6] Bowel complications include intestinal atresia, stenosis, necrosis, and perforation. In the past, atresia has been the major determining prognostic factor, but patients with atresias can now do very well as long as the bowel is not irreversibly damaged.[30] Necrosis is usually related to a small abdominal wall defect that cuts off blood supply to the extruded bowel, and often results in short bowel syndrome.[30] Perforation can often be managed by resection and primary anastomosis.[30]

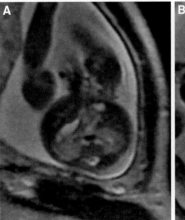
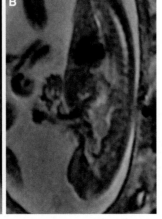

FIGURE 26.2-9: Gastroschisis at 26-week fetus. **A:** Axial MRI shows defect lateral to cord insertion. **B:** Sagittal MRI shows bowel outside the abdominal cavity with no covering membrane.

About 60% of infants are preterm (mean 35.7 weeks) and low birth weight (mean 2,492 g).[31] Gestational age at delivery is the most important prognostic indicator,[32] with an association between early gestational age and increased length of stay and prolonged time to enteral feeds.[33] In general, most children with gastroschisis will have no long-term physical complications, and normal physical growth after 5 years of age.[31] Earlier studies suggested that infants with gastroschisis are at risk for developmental or neurologic abnormalities. A recent study showed that children with gastroschisis performed along test norms for cognitive, language, and motor skills at both 2 and 5 years of age.[34] However, school age children with gastroschisis have been shown to have decreased verbal intelligence, abnormal response inhibition, and visual and auditory attention.[35]

Management: The majority of fetuses with gastroschisis are detected in early second trimester with maternal serum AFP and sonogram. Once diagnosis is established, counseling should be performed by a multidisciplinary team that includes perinatologists, neonatologists, and pediatric surgeons. Assuming the pregnancy is continued, a targeted ultrasound including an echocardiogram should be performed, followed by serial sonograms and evaluation by a perinatologist. At each visit, fetal growth, amniotic fluid volume, bowel dilatation, bowel wall thickness, and peristalsis should be assessed.[25]

Animal research suggests that amnioinfusion with warm saline may reduce bowel inflammation.[36] The potential benefit of amnioinfusion is thought to be related to dilution of GI waste products that cause bowel wall damage. However, studies performed in humans have shown no benefit.[37,38]

The mode and timing of delivery for fetuses with gastroschisis was a past source of debate. It was earlier thought that much of the bowel injury occurs because of exposure to amniotic fluid in late pregnancy, suggesting that early delivery is beneficial. However, a randomized controlled trial comparing elective delivery at 36 weeks to spontaneous delivery at term showed no significant difference in neonatal outcomes,[39] and later retrospective studies support this finding.[40,41] In addition, preterm infants with gastroschisis are more likely to develop sepsis and have longer hospital courses than do full-term infants with gastroschisis.[42] Most centers recommend spontaneous or planned vaginal delivery at 36 to 37 weeks. Cesarean section was originally thought to be the optimal mode of delivery of fetuses with gastroschisis, because it was thought that the bowel would undergo further trauma during vaginal delivery. Data have failed to show a difference in outcomes between vaginal delivery and cesarean section. A large proportion (up to 39% in two studies) is delivered via cesarean section because of fetal distress.[11] Immediately following delivery, appropriate fluid resuscitation should be initiated; high water losses can occur from evaporation through the exposed bowel (Fig. 26.2-10). The herniated bowel should be placed in a sterile covering, and the bowel should be placed in the midline of the abdomen to prevent kinking of the mesentery. Once the baby has been assessed and initial resuscitation performed, the abdominal wall defect should be assessed and treatment determined.

Primary closure of the abdominal wall defect has long been the standard of care. In this method, the bowel is reduced into the abdominal cavity, and a primary suture repair of the fascia is performed. When primary repair is performed, intra-abdominal or bladder pressure must be monitored during the procedure, as abdominal compartment syndrome can occur, causing intestinal and renal ischemia, as well as respiratory distress.

With the development of a preformed, spring-loaded silo, staged reduction with delayed primary suture closure has largely supplanted immediate primary closure in the management of gastroschisis.[43] In this method, a prefabricated silo with a circular spring is placed into the abdominal defect at the patient's bedside (Fig. 26.2-10). The bowel is reduced daily into the abdominal cavity, and the silo is sequentially shortened.[30] Multiple studies, predominantly retrospective, have undertaken to determine the most beneficial method of closure; the best level of evidence shows no survival difference between immediate closure and silo placement with delayed closure.[44] In addition, a CAPSnet study showed no difference in ventilation time, length of stay, or length of total parenteral nutrition (TPN).[44] One recent retrospective study showed that while preformed silo placement may be associated with decreased ventilation days and shorter time to full enteral feeds, this treatment method has a longer hospital stay.[43]

In 2004, a nonoperative technique was introduced, termed *sutureless closure*. This closure method involves placement of a preformed silo, with sequential reduction of the intestines. Once the intestines are reduced, the defect is covered with the UC, and an occlusive plastic dressing is used. Two retrospective studies evaluating this closure technique[45,46] showed no

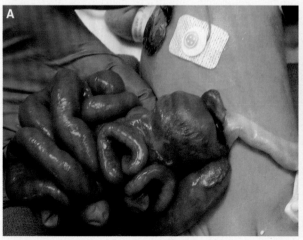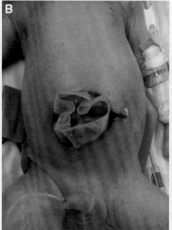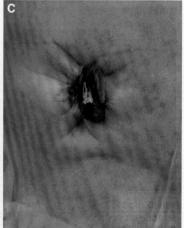

FIGURE 26.2-10: Newborn with gastroschisis. **A:** Immediately after birth. **B:** Bowel is completely reduced into the abdomen and suture closure has been performed. **C:** After closure with neoumbilicus formation.

statistically significant differences between sutureless closure closure and suture closure with regard to length of stay, ventilation days, or time to feeding.

Following closure, infants with gastroschisis have abnormal intestinal motility and nutrient absorption, generally requiring these infants to remain on TPN until bowel function returns. Infants with simple gastroschisis can usually begin enteral feeds approximately 14 days postclosure.[47] Infants with gastroschisis experience a dysmotility syndrome causing intermittent feeding intolerance. Studies have not shown benefit with erythromycin for dysmotility,[30] but cisapride has shown some benefits. Because of the high risk of cardiovascular side effects, cisapride is only recommended with infants with severe dysmotility who have not responded to other treatments and have been cleared by cardiovascular evaluation.[30] The median time of parenteral nutrition is in the range of 22 to 36 days, time to full oral feeding is 25 to 44 days, and median hospitalization time is 1 to 2 months.[20,39,43,48] However, patients with gastroschisis complicated by intestinal atresia or perforation may take significantly longer to achieve full feeds.

Recurrence Risk: Gastroschisis is typically sporadic, although occasional familial cases have been reported. A recent study summarizing all population-based studies of familial recurrence of gastroschisis (412 cases) suggests a 2.4% recurrence risk.[49]

OMPHALOCELE

Omphalocele is a midline abdominal wall defect containing variable amounts of viscera that is covered by a membrane made up of peritoneum and amnion, and Wharton jelly between the two layers. The UC inserts directly onto the membrane (Fig. 26.2-11).

Incidence: Omphalocele occurs in approximately 1 in 5,000 live births. This incidence increases to 1 in 1,100 if the incidence is based on 14 to 18 week fetuses.[50,51] These defects have a high rate of termination and still birth. The incidence of omphalocele increases with increasing maternal age.[52] There is a lower incidence in non-Hispanic black mothers, and a higher incidence in infants of Hispanic mothers.[7]

Embryology and Pathology: As with gastroschisis, there is no consensus for the embryology of omphalocele. There have been a number of theories described, but many are based on clinical observation. The current accepted cause is a combination of two theories[53]:

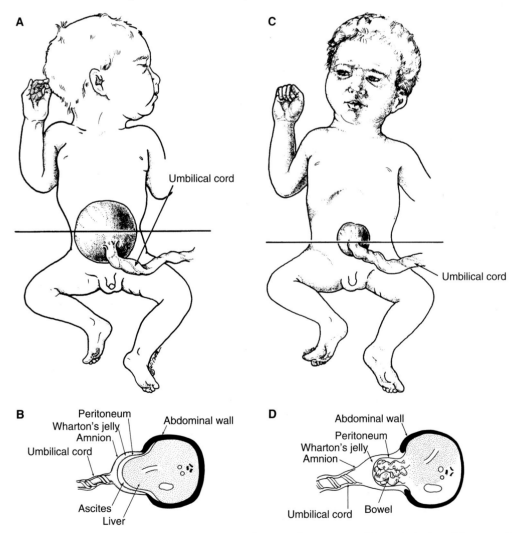

FIGURE 26.2-11: **A, B:** Omphalocele with typical features of extracorporeal liver. **C, D:** Typical features of omphalocele with intracorporeal liver. (Reprinted with permission from Hertzberg BS, Nyberg DA, Neilson IA. Ventral wall defects. In: Nyberg DA, McGahan JP, Pretorius DH, et al., eds. *Diagnostic Imaging of Fetal Anomalies.* Philadelphia, PA: Lippincott Williams & Wilkins; 2003:519–520.)

1. The embryonic dysplasia theory suggests that early defects in the germinal disc lead to malformations later in development.[53]
2. Malfunction of the ectodermal placodes in early development leads to a disruption of the folding process.[53]

A specific etiology for omphalocele has not been identified. Most cases are sporadic, but familial cases of omphalocele have been reported.[54] Risk factors for omphalocele include advanced maternal age, African American race, and maternal obesity.[53] Teratogens have not been implicated in the etiology of omphalocele.

Omphalocele is frequently associated with chromosomal anomalies, predominantly trisomies 13, 18, and 21. These chromosomal anomalies are also associated with advanced maternal age. Other genetic variations identified include mutations in the PITX2 protein, which is thought to be responsible for Axenfeld–Rieger syndrome (congenital malformations of the face, teeth, and skeletal system). A mutation in the *CDKN1C* gene, which encodes a kinase inhibitor, has also been associated with omphalocele; this mutation is often diagnosed in Beckwith–Wiedemann syndrome (macroglossia, macrosomia, midline abdominal wall defects, ear creases or ear pits, and neonatal hypoglycemia). Autosomal dominant and x-linked forms of omphalocele have also been reported.[6]

Diagnosis

Ultrasound: Current sensitivity of prenatal ultrasound in the diagnosis of omphalocele is 97%.[55] The ultrasound appearance of omphalocele is variable. Size can range from a small umbilical hernia to a giant omphalocele greater than 5 cm. Eviscerated organs can vary; ascites may be present, and there is a range of associated anomalies. Therefore, it is important to keep in mind those features that reliably diagnose omphalocele and differentiate omphalocele from gastroschisis.

Omphalocele is a central abdominal wall defect, located at the base of the UC. The cord typically inserts on the apex of the defect.[56] This can be demonstrated in transverse images, but sagittal imaging may also be helpful in demonstrating the cord insertion (Fig. 26.2-12). Observing the intrahepatic umbilical vein coursing through the defect can also be helpful in confirming the central location of the defect.

A surrounding membrane is another characteristic unique to omphalocele. However, the membrane may be difficult to visualize or may rupture *in utero*. If the membrane is present, but unapparent, its presence can be inferred by the eviscerated organs appearing contained rather than freely floating. The presence of ascites is also a helpful indicator of omphalocele[57] (Fig. 26.2-13). The membrane covering the omphalocele allows fluid to accumulate within the peritoneal cavity; this fluid can also help delineate

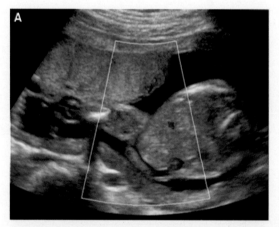
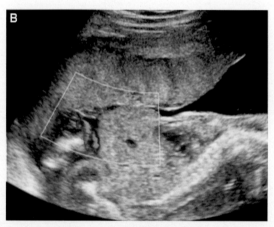

FIGURE 26.2-12: Omphalocele. **(A)** Transverse and **(B)** sagittal color Doppler US of 23-week fetus with omphalocele demonstrating cord insertion at the base of the defect (*color*).

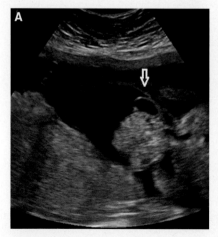
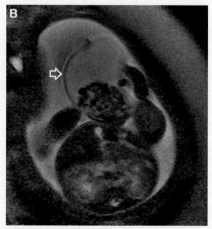

FIGURE 26.2-13: Omphalocele with ascites. Transverse US **(A)** and axial T2 MRI **(B)** of omphalocele with ascites. The membrane (*arrow*) is delineated by the fluid on both sides.

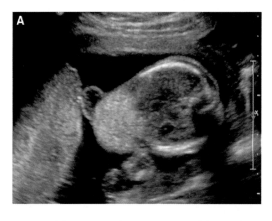
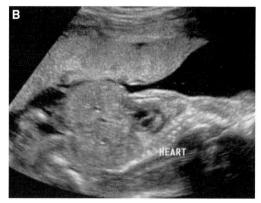
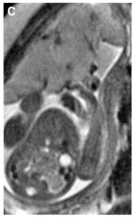
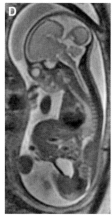

FIGURE 26.2-14: Omphalocele. Transverse **(A)** and sagittal **(B)** US and axial **(C)** and sagittal **(D)** T2 MRI show an omphalocele containing only liver.

the covering membrane on ultrasound. However, a large amount of ascites may be confused for amniotic fluid and misdiagnosis of gastroschisis can be made; in distinction to gastroschisis, the bowel within an omphalocele will not be thickened or dilated.

Approximately 80% of prenatally diagnosed omphaloceles contain liver[51] (Fig. 26.2-14). Liver is never seen outside the abdominal cavity during normal development, so omphalocele with extracorporeal liver can be diagnosed at any gestational age. Liver has a homogeneous sonographic appearance, and hepatic vessels can be demonstrated within it. The amount of extruded liver and size of the defect are variable, but an omphalocele is generally termed "giant" when the majority of the liver is extra-abdominal.[51] There is no strict definition for giant omphaloceles.

Polyhydramnios has been associated with omphalocele in approximately 10% of cases.[58] Although the etiology is unclear, it is associated with a more complicated postnatal course.[57]

Magnetic Resonance Imaging: Omphalocele is frequently associated with other anomalies; recent studies have shown detection rate of these associated anomalies to range from 30% to 70%.[55,58] Therefore, MRI is useful for improved delineation of associated anomalies. On MRI, an omphalocele appears as a central abdominal wall defect. The viscera can be seen herniating into a membrane-covered sac.[21] Liver is easily distinguished from bowel on MRI as opposed to ultrasound (Fig. 26.2-15).

MRI is useful in evaluating the size of the abdominal wall defect. In addition, MRI shows promise as a predictor of

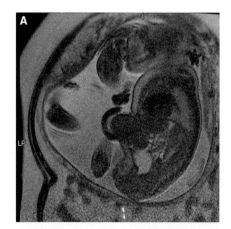
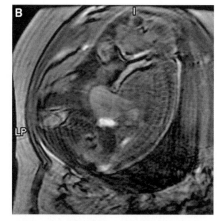

FIGURE 26.2-15: Omphalocele. Sagittal T2 **(A)** and T1 **(B)** MRI of a fetus with omphalocele containing liver. The cord inserts onto the base of the defect.

pulmonary hypoplasia.[59] A study by Danzer et al. measured total lung volume in fetuses with omphalocele and compared this as a ratio to the expected lung volume based on age-matched nomograms, and found that fetuses with giant omphalocele had significantly lower than expected lung volumes compared with age-matched nomograms. In addition, they found that a ratio less than 50% predicted a more complicated postnatal/postrepair course.[59]

Differential Diagnosis: Because the ultrasound appearance of omphalocele is variable, they can be difficult to distinguish from other types of ventral wall defects. When the liver is within the defect, the main differential is LBWC. At least two of the typical findings of LBWC must be present to make the diagnosis. These include anterior body wall defect, limb defect, exencephaly, and/or encephalocele. Additional findings of LBWC that may be seen are kyphoscoliosis, short- or single-artery UC, neural tube defects, genitourinary (GU) malformations, chest wall, lung, and/or diaphragm abnormalities.[61]

If the liver is not extracorporeal and only the bowel is eviscerated, then the differential considerations include gastroschisis and umbilical hernia. The gastroschisis defect is located to the right of the umbilicus, does not have a covering membrane, and ascites is not present.[30] A small omphalocele may be more difficult to distinguish from an umbilical hernia since both defects are located in the midline at the abdominal cord insertion site. An umbilical hernia is a defect only in the abdominal wall muscles; therefore, the intestine protrudes only into the base of the UC, and the defect is covered by skin as well as a membrane.[62] An omphalocele defect is covered only by a membrane.

Simple omphalocele should be differentiated from other complex syndromes, which may include omphalocele. Pentalogy of Cantrell, a defect in the cephalic fold, includes not only omphalocele but also diaphragmatic defect, sternal cleft, pericardial defect, and cardiovascular malformations (see section on pentalogy of Cantrell later in this chapter). Cloacal exstrophy is a defect of the caudal fold; this includes a low ventral wall defect associated with bladder or cloacal exstrophy.

Occasionally, a false-positive diagnosis of omphalocele, or pseudo-omphalocele, may occur. Two clinical settings may cause this appearance. The first is in the setting of oligohydramnios; the uterine wall causes the fetal abdominal wall to elongate anterior–posterior and narrow transverse, giving the appearance of herniated abdominal contents. The second setting is when the fetal abdomen is wedged in the uterus, in direct contact with the myometrium or placenta. The angle between the abdominal wall and the defect in these two settings should be an obtuse angle, as opposed to an acute angle in a true omphalocele.[63]

Prognosis: Prognosis of omphalocele depends on, primarily, the presence and severity of associated anomalies. Approximately 70% of fetuses with omphalocele have additional malformations.[8] Musculoskeletal malformations are seen in 23%, including clubfoot, polydactyly, limb deficiency, and vertebral anomalies. Urinary anomalies comprise approximately 17% of associated malformations and include renal agenesis, polycystic kidney, hydronephrosis, ureteral anomalies, and vesicoureteral reflux. Approximately 15% of patients with omphalocele have associated heart defects, including ventricular septal defect, tetralogy of Fallot, and dextrocardia. Anomalies of the bowel are less common than is gastroschisis, but are seen in approximately 10% of cases. Central nervous system anomalies can also be present. Other less common anomalies include diaphragmatic hernias, facial anomalies, and genital and pulmonary abnormalities.[8]

Chromosomal abnormalities are present in up to 30% of omphalocele cases.[8] The most common chromosomal abnormalities are trisomy 18 (68%) and trisomy 13 (20%). The risk of chromosomal abnormalities is increased when the liver is not within the omphalocele sac.[64]

Beckwith–Wiedemann syndrome, a complicated genetic condition that can involve 11p15 deletion or mutations in the *CDKN1C* gene, is also associated with omphalocele.[64] This is defined as a large-for-gestational-age fetus with omphalocele and macroglossia.[64] These infants also have early hypoglycemia, and increased risk of Wilms tumor, hepatoblastoma, and neuroblastoma in childhood.

Many studies have been performed to evaluate the size of omphalocele and contents of omphalocele sac in relation to prognosis. Small omphaloceles generally have intracorporeal liver, and have been found to have a higher association with chromosomal anomalies.[64] However, extracorporeal liver and larger defects are associated with a poorer prognosis.[64-67]

Giant omphalocele is generally defined as a defect larger than 5 cm, or containing greater than 50% of the liver in the omphalocele sac,[68] but there is no universal consensus on this definition (Fig. 26.2-16). In addition, the size can change as the fetus grows in gestation. In a study in 2011, Montero et al.[69] suggested a standard that is based on a ratio of the omphalocele size to the head circumference (O/HC ratio). In this study, they found that an O/HC ratio greater than 0.21 predicts inability to achieve primary closure of the defect. In addition, they found that this ratio was a better predictor of prognosis than was the measurement of

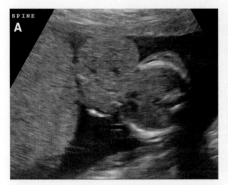
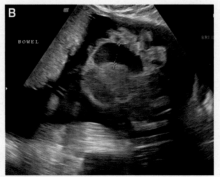
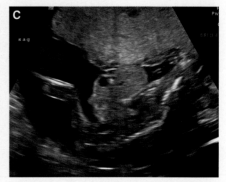

FIGURE 26.2-16: Giant omphalocele. Transverse **(A, B)** and sagittal **(C)** US of a fetus show a giant omphalocele that contains liver, stomach, and bowel. The bowel is dilated **(B)**. Some of the bowel appears free-floating, suggesting rupture of the membrane.

the defect alone.[69] Giant omphalocele is associated with a poorer prognosis, with 75% developing respiratory insufficiency in the first 24 hours of life and 57% developing pulmonary hypertension[70]; these children have narrow chest width and smaller lung areas and can have long-term pulmonary issues such as asthma.[66] Pregnancies with giant omphalocele can be complicated by polyhydramnios, indicating a more complicated postnatal course.[66]

Management: When a diagnosis of omphalocele is made prenatally, further evaluation is required. A detailed ultrasound evaluation should be performed to evaluate other structural abnormalities; MRI should also be offered to identify structural anomalies that may not be seen with ultrasound. Given the frequency of major cardiac defects, a fetal echocardiogram should also be performed. The patient should be offered chromosomal analysis.[71] Serial ultrasounds are recommended, as these fetuses can be at increased risk for IUGR and polyhydramnios.[5,30,60]

Delivery at a tertiary care center at or near term is recommended. Mode of delivery is controversial, and neither vaginal delivery nor cesarean section has been shown to be superior.[30,51,71] However, caesarian section is usually performed for large omphaloceles to prevent rupture or dystocia of the omphalocele sac or trauma to the visceral contents of the sac.[71]

Following delivery, cardiopulmonary status should be carefully assessed; these infants may have unsuspected pulmonary hypoplasia or a cardiac defect requiring immediate intubation and ventilation.[30,71] The UC should be cut generously, as abdominal contents may protrude further into the cord than appreciated.[71] The omphalocele should be covered with saline gauze or other nonadherent dressing until the infant is stabilized and further assessment is possible (Fig. 26.2-17).

The method of closure of omphalocele is dependent on the size of the defect. If the defect is small, primary closure can be performed. However, in large defects, primary closure can cause increased abdominal pressure because of the small size of the peritoneal cavity[30]; this increased pressure, if not relieved, can lead to abdominal compartment syndrome, with bowel necrosis, respiratory compromise, and loss of blood flow to kidneys and liver.[30] When the defect is too large to accomplish primary closure, either a staged or delayed closure can be performed. There are multiple reported staged techniques: reduction using a pressure dressing, prosthetic silo placement with gradual reduction, as in gastroschisis, vacuum-assisted closure,[72] tissue expanders,[73] and other types of mesh to close the defect.

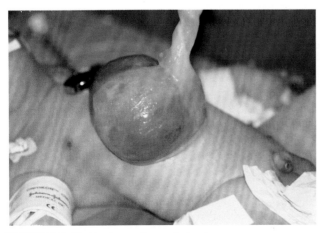

FIGURE 26.2-17: Newborn with omphalocele.

Nonsurgical delayed closure is often employed when the defect is large and the infant is not stable enough to undergo surgical repair of the defect.[71] This technique is referred to as "paint and wait." Several different substances have been employed in this technique: mercurochrome, povidone–iodine, silver sulfadiazine, and neomycin–bacitracin ointments. Silver sulfadiazine is currently the most widely used agent. It is inexpensive and requires only daily application, and associated with very little toxicity.[74] In addition, it has antibacterial and antifungal properties, allowing prevention of infection.[74] One study showed that patients managed with delayed closer had length of mechanical ventilation and hospital stay.[68] Delayed closure allows time for thoracic and abdominal growth and enables a more successful definitive repair.[68]

Recurrence Risk: Omphalocele is typically sporadic, although occasional familial cases have been reported. Syndromic forms of omphalocele are typically associated with chromosomal abnormalities, including trisomies 13, 18, and 21. Beckwith–Wiedemann syndrome has a mutation in the *CDKN1C* gene. Isolated omphalocele should be considered to have a low recurrence risk; syndromic omphalocele recurrence is that of the chromosomal abnormality.

CLEFT STERNUM, ECTOPIA CORDIS, PENTALOGY OF CANTRELL

Cleft sternum, ectopia cordis, and pentalogy of Cantrell share a defect of the sternum. Cleft sternum has partial or absent sternum without ectopia. In true ectopia cordis, only the heart is displaced outside of the thoracic cavity and lacks pericardial coverage.[75] Pentalogy of Cantrell includes a midline, supraumbilical abdominal wall defect; defect of the lower sternum; deficiency of the anterior diaphragm; defect in the diaphragmatic pericardium; and congenital intracardiac defects.[76]

Incidence: All are rare. Ectopia cordis occurs in approximately 5.5 to 7.9 per million live births.[77] Pentalogy of Cantrell occurs in fewer than five per million live births.[78]

Embryology and Pathology: The embryological defect is poorly understood; the most common theory is that a defect in the maturation of midline mesodermal components causes failure of fusion of the cephalic lateral body folds. These abnormal midline mesodermal components include failure of the transverse septum to develop, causing a diaphragmatic hernia, and abnormal development of myocardium, resulting in heart defects.

Ectopia cordis can also result from amniotic band syndrome.[79] The normal descent of the heart is interrupted by mechanical compression from tissue bands in thoracic ectopia cordis; tethering of the heart to paraumbilical structures is thought to be a cause of thoracoabdominal ectopia cordis.[79]

There is a weak association with trisomy 18, and x-linked recessive cases have been reported.[80] Pentalogy of Cantrell has also been seen in trisomy 21 and Turner syndrome.[81] Teratogenesis can occur with amniotic bands.

Diagnosis
Ultrasound
Pentalogy of Cantrell: Early prenatal diagnosis of pentalogy of Cantrell is possible. The primary finding on ultrasound is a supraumbilical omphalocele.[82] A pericardial effusion is an indicator

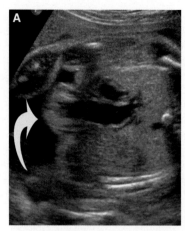 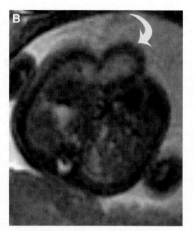 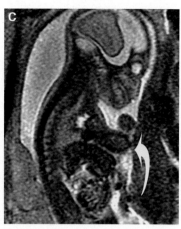

FIGURE 26.2-18: Pentalogy of Cantrell. **A:** US shows left ventricle protruding through a defect in the sternum *(arrow)*. Axial SSFP **(B)** and sagittal T2 **(C)** MRI demonstrates heart protruding outside the chest *(arrow)*.

of diaphragmatic pericardial defects, and pleural effusion may signal an associated anterior diaphragmatic hernia.[82,83] The pericardial effusion may be transient. Other anomalies associated with pentalogy of Cantrell include cleft lip/palate, encephalocele, hydrocephalus, limb defects, gall bladder agenesis, and polysplenia[83] (Fig. 26.2-18). Echocardiograms are important to assess the complexity of cardiac anomalies.

Ectopia Cordis: The heart is identified by ultrasound as either completely or partially displaced outside the thoracic cavity with lack of skin covering. Classification is based on the location of the heart and is divided into cervical, cervicothoracic, thoracic, and thoracoabdominal. Displacement may be only partial or may be transient[82] (Fig. 26.2-19). Cardiac anomalies can be complex.

Cleft Sternum: The anterior chest wall is dynamic when the sternum is absent. The heart may appear to protrude through the chest, yet the chest wall is intact.

Magnetic Resonance Imaging: MRI provides soft-tissue differentiation and can delineate the extent of the thoracoabdominal defect.[84] The diaphragmatic defects should be searched for, but may be difficult to detect if small. Lung volumes can be calculated (Figs. 26.2-20 and 26.2-21).

Differential Diagnosis: The major differential consideration for ectopia cordis and pentalogy of Cantrell is amniotic band syndrome. This syndrome is heterogeneous in presentation and can cause a broad range of abnormalities.[85] The characteristic finding in amniotic band syndrome is echogenic bands that attach to the fetus.[85] Other differentials include LBWC and omphalocele.

Prognosis: Cervical and cervicothoracic forms of ectopia cordis are considered fatal.[77] Thoracic or true ectopia cordis is associated with a poor prognosis. Survivors tend to have limited intracardiac defects.[75,77] Abdominal ectopia cordis, or displacement of the heart into the abdomen, has a better prognosis, and often does not require surgery to survive.[77]

Thoracoabdominal ectopia cordis is the classification associated with pentalogy of Cantrell, and it is the most common form of cardiac displacement. Overall survival rate is approximately 50%,[75,77] and is dependent on the severity of the cardiac and associated malformations. Cardiac defects include ventricular septal defect (100%), atrial septal defect (53%), tetralogy of Fallot (20%), and left ventricular diverticulum (20%).[75,77] There have been reports of hypoplastic left heart syndrome[86] and tricuspid atresia.[87] A review in 2008 by van Hoorn et al.[83] found that prognosis is worse in complete pentalogy, isolated ectopia cordis, and patients with non–cardiac-associated anomalies. This review did not find cardiac defects to affect prognosis.

Management: Following prenatal diagnosis, a detailed ultrasound and echocardiogram should be performed to evaluate for associated anomalies and cardiac defects. Delivery should be performed by cesarean section to avoid compression of the exposed heart during labor.[77] Routine resuscitation of the neonate should be performed, beginning with airway management. These neonates are more likely to have pulmonary hypoplasia because of the chest wall defect and possible diaphragmatic hernia.[77]

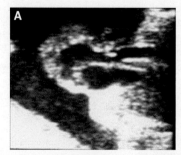 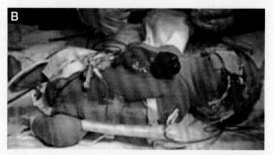

FIGURE 26.2-19: Ectopia cordis. **A:** Transverse US through the chest demonstrates the heart protruding through a thoracic wall defect. There was no associated omphalocele. **B:** Postnatal image of the infant demonstrating the ectopic heart.

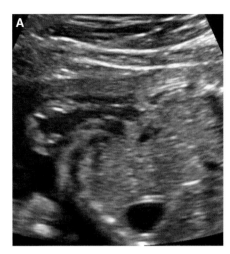
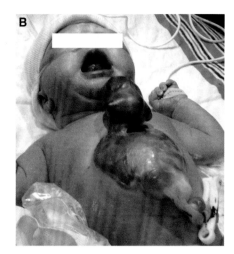

FIGURE 26.2-20: Thoracoabdominal ectopia cordis. **A:** Transverse US at 25 weeks' gestation demonstrates the heart protruding into the amniotic fluid. **B:** Postnatal image of thoracoabdominal ectopia cordis. (Courtesy of Renee Bornemeier.)

Milder cases can be repaired in a single stage, but two- or three-stage repair is common.[75,77] In general, symptomatic cardiac anomalies should be corrected first. The exception is in cases of complete thoracoabdominal ectopia, because of the lack of skin coverage of the heart.[75] In this case, the first stage provides soft-tissue coverage of the heart and hemodynamic palliation, and the second stage repairs the intracardiac defects and reduces the heart into the thoracic cavity.[74,75,77]

Recurrence Risk: Sporadic, there is no known genetic origin, making the recurrence risk low.[77]

LIMB–BODY WALL COMPLEX, BODY STALK ANOMALY

Limb body wall complex (LBWC) is a complex congenital defect that includes at least two of the following three abnormalities: neural tube defect (exencephaly, encephalocele, myelomeningocele); thoraco- and/or abdominoschisis; and limb anomalies. Body stalk anomaly includes a large abdominal defect, absent or abnormal UC, and severe kyphoscoliosis. These two anomalies overlap and can be considered two points on a spectrum.

Incidence: The incidence of LBWC is estimated at 1 in 14,000 to 1 in 31,000 live births.[88] However, in a study of 106,727 cases of 10- to 14-week pregnancies, the prevalence was approximately 1 in 7,500 pregnancies, suggesting a high spontaneous abortion and planned termination rate.

Embryology and Pathology: There is no known genetic anomaly. Embryology is poorly understood. Three hypotheses have been proposed, but none of these has been supported in animal studies. These hypotheses include the following:

1. The amniotic band theory: In this theory, it is postulated that the amnion ruptures before the obliteration of the celomic cavity. The lower half of the fetal body then passes into the celomic cavity through the defect in the amniotic sac, causing the abdominal and spinal defects.[89–91] However, this theory does not explain the coexistent internal defects seen in the majority of cases.[91]
2. The theory of vascular disruption: A vascular disturbance causes a general disruption of blood supply during embryogenesis. This causes failure of closure of the ventral abdominal wall and persistence of celomic cavity.[89,91]

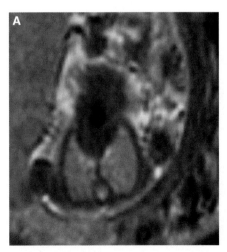
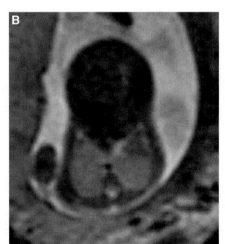
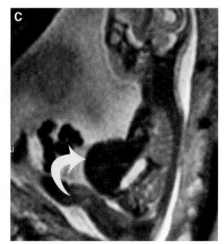

FIGURE 26.2-21: Pentalogy of Cantrell. **A:** Axial T2 MRI of the thorax shows thoracic defect with ectopic heart. **B:** Axial MRI at the level of the chest shows the defect with ectopic heart. **C:** Sagittal MRI shows heart and liver protruding through thoracoabdominal defect (arrow).

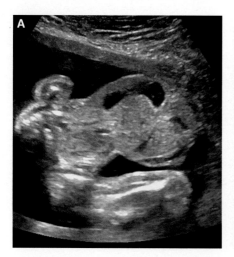
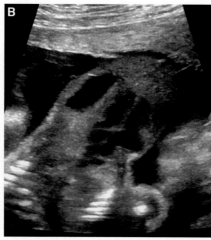

FIGURE 26.2-22: Limb–body wall complex. **A:** Axial US at 23 weeks' gestational age show large membrane-covered anterior midline thoracoabdominal wall defect containing liver and stomach. **B:** A majority of the heart is external as well. The defect is in close approximation to the placenta.

3. The theory of abnormal embryonic folding: In this theory, LBWC is the result of faulty folding in the cephalic, lateral, and caudal axes.[89]

There have been two cases reported in which the mother abused cocaine.[92] One case has been reported after *in vitro* fertilization and embryo transfer.[93] A single case has been reported with antiepileptic use during pregnancy.[94]

Diagnosis

Ultrasound: Prenatal ultrasound findings include abdominal wall defect, scoliosis, attachment of the head or body to the placenta, limb reduction anomalies, and short- or two-vessel (or both) UC.[95] The body wall defect is eccentric and typically large; left-sided defects are much more common.[56] Three-dimensional (3D) ultrasound can be helpful in differentiating the abdominal wall defect from other forms of ventral wall defects by showing adjacent structures in relation to the defect[96] (Fig. 26.2-22).

Magnetic Resonance Imaging: MRI can be helpful in further delineating the associated anomalies and providing a large field of view. MRI will show an abnormally located placenta often directly adjacent to the fetus.[20] The herniated abdominal organs are well delineated (Fig. 26.2-23). Amniotic bands may be seen.[20]

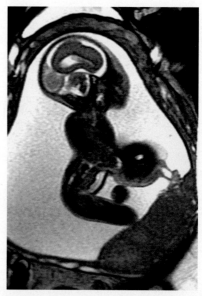

FIGURE 26.2-23: Limb–body wall complex at 23 weeks' gestation. Sagittal T2 MRI demonstrates a large membrane-covered anterior midline thoracoabdominal wall defect containing liver and bowel. There is kyphoscoliosis. The umbilical cord is short.

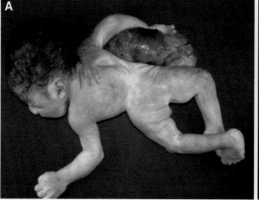
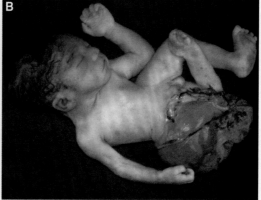

FIGURE 26.2-24: **A, B:** Postmortem images of an infant with limb–body wall complex. The ventral wall is plastered to the placenta. Note the limb anomalies and kyphosis.

Differential Diagnosis: The major differential consideration is amniotic band syndrome. This syndrome is heterogeneous in presentation and can cause a broad range of abnormalities.[85] The characteristic finding in amniotic band syndrome is echogenic bands that attach to the fetus.[85]

Pentalogy of Cantrell and OEIS (omphaloceles-exstrophy of the bladder-imperforate anus-spinal defects) should be included in the differential. Bladder exstrophy should be suspected if there is nonvisualization of the fetal urinary bladder, and the expected T1 hyperintensity of meconium late in gestation will be absent if a cloacal anomaly allows for mixing of urine and meconium.

Prognosis and Management: LBWC is lethal (Fig. 26.2-24). Many pregnancies spontaneously terminate.[89] Many patients choose to terminate electively. Prenatal management should emphasize maternal safety. Management is supportive following delivery.

Recurrence Risk: The majority of cases of LBWC are sporadic. The development of this disorder has been associated with the use of the cigarette smoking, alcohol use, and illicit drug use.[94,97]

REFERENCES

1. American Institute of Ultrasound Medicine. AIUM—ACR-ACOG-SMFM—SRU practice parameter for the performance of standard diagnostic obstetric ultrasound examinations. *J Ultrasound Med.* 2018;9999:1–12.
2. Sadler TW. The embryologic origin of ventral body wall defects. *Semin Pediatr Surg.* 2010;19(3):209–214.
3. Sadler TW, Feldkamp ML. The embryology of body wall closure: relevance to gastroschisis and other ventral body wall defects. *Am J Med Genet C Semin Med Genet.* 2008;148C(3):180–185.
4. Sadler TW. *Langman's Medical Embryology.* 12th ed. Baltimore, MD: Lippincott Williams & Wilkins; 2012.
5. Beaudoin S. Insights into the etiology and embryology of gastroschisis. *Semin Pediatr Surg.* 2018;27:283–288.
6. Frolov P, Alali J, Klein MD. Clinical risk factors for gastroschisis and omphalocele in humans: a review of the literature. *Pediatr Surg Int.* 2010;26(12):1135–1148.
7. Kirby RS. The prevalence of selected major birth defects in the United States. *Semin Perinatol.* 2017;41:338–344.
8. Stoll C, Alembik Y, Dott B, et al. Omphalocele and gastroschisis and associated malformations. *Am J Med Genet A.* 2008;146A(10):1280–1285.
9. Collins SR, Griffin MR, Arbogast PG, et al. The rising prevalence of gastroschisis and omphalocele in Tennessee. *J Pediatr Surg.* 2007;42(7):1221–1224.
10. Fillingham A, Rankin J. Prevalence, prenatal diagnosis and survival of gastroschisis. *Prenat Diagn.* 2008;28(13):1232–1237.
11. Holland AJ, Walker K, Badawi N. Gastroschisis: an update. *Pediatr Surg Int.* 2010;26(9):871–878.
12. Mastroiacovo P, Lisi A, Castilla EE, et al. Gastroschisis and associated defects: an international study. *Am J Med Genet A.* 2007;143(7):660–671.
13. Kirby RS, Marshall J, Tanner JP, et al. Prevalence and correlates of gastroschisis in 15 states, 1995 to 2005. *Obstet Gynecol.* 2013;12(2):275–281.
14. Bargy F, Beaudoin S. Comprehensive developmental mechanisms in gastroschisis. *Fetal Diagn Ther.* 2914;36:223–230.
15. Feldkamp ML, Carey JC, Sadler TW. Development of gastroschisis: review of hypotheses, a novel hypothesis, and implications for research. *Am J Med Genet A.* 2007;143(7):639–652.
16. deVries PA. The pathogenesis of gastroschisis and omphalocele. *J Pediatr Surg.* 1980;15(3):245–251.
17. Hoyme HE, Higginbottom MC, Jones KL. The vascular pathogenesis of gastroschisis: intrauterine interruption of the omphalomesenteric artery. *J Pediatr.* 1981;98(2):228–231.
18. Duhamel B. Embryology of exomphalos and allied malformations. *Arch Dis Child.* 1963;38(198):142–147.
19. Murphy FL, Mazlan TA, Tarheen F, et al. Gastroschisis and exomphalos in Ireland 1998–2004: does antenatal diagnosis impact on outcome? *Pediatr Surg Int.* 2007;23(11):1059–1063.
20. David AL, Tan A, Curry J. Gastroschisis: sonographic diagnosis, associations, management and outcome. *Prenat Diagn.* 2008;28(7):633–644.
21. Daltro P, Fricke BL, Kline-Fath BM, et al. Prenatal MRI of congenital abdominal and chest wall defects. *AJR Am J Roentgenol.* 2005;184(3):1010–1016.
22. Andrade WS, Brizot ML, Rodrigues AS, et al. Sonographic markers in the prediction of fetal complex gastroschisis. *Fetal Daign Ther.* 2018;43:45–52.
23. Badillo AT, Hedrick HL, Wilson RD, et al. Prenatal ultrasonographic gastrointestinal abnormalities in fetuses with gastroschisis do not correlate with postnatal outcomes. *J Pediatr Surg.* 2008;43(4):647–653.
24. Goetzinger KR, Tuul MG, Longman RE, et al. Sonographic predictors of postnatal bowel atresia in fetal gastroschisis. *Ultrasound Obstet Gynecol.* 2014;43:420–425.
25. Vegunta RK, Wallace LJ, Leonardi MR, et al. Perinatal management of gastroschisis: analysis of a newly established clinical pathway. *J Pediatr Surg.* 2005;40(3):528–534.
26. Tawil A, Comstock CH, Chang CH. Prenatal closure of abdominal defect in gastroschisis: case report and review of the literature. *Pediatr Dev Pathol.* 2001;4(6):580–584.
27. Tonni G, Pattaccini P, Ventura A, et al. The role of ultrasound and antenatal single-shot fast spin-echo MRI in the evaluation of herniated bowel in case of first trimester ultrasound diagnosis of fetal gastroschisis. *Arch Gynecol Obstet.* 2011;283(4):903–908.
28. Bradnock TJ, Marven S, Owen A, et al. Gastroschisis: one year outcomes from national cohort study. *BMJ.* 2011;343:d6749.
29. Kalache KD, Bierlich A, Hammer H, et al. Is unexplained third trimester intrauterine death of fetuses with gastroschisis caused by umbilical cord compression due to acute extra-abdominal bowel dilatation? *Prenat Diagn.* 2002;22(8):715–717.
30. Christison-Lagay ER, Kelleher CM, Langer JC. Neonatal abdominal wall defects. *Semin Fetal Neonatal Med.* 2011;16(3):164–172.
31. Gorra AS, Needelman H, Azarow KS, et al. Long-term neurodevelopmental outcomes in children born with gastroschisis: the tiebreaker. *J Pediatr Surg.* 2012;47(1):125–129.
32. Meyer MR, Shaffer BL, Doss AE, et al. Prospective risk of fetal death with gastroschisis. *J Matern Fetal Neonatal Med.* 2015;28(17):2126–2129.
33. Carnaghan H, Baud D, Lapidus-Krol E, et al. Effect of gestational age at birth on neonatal outcomes in gastroschisis. *J Pediatr Surg.* 2016;51:734–738.
34. Burnett AC, Gunn JK, Hutchinson EA, et al. Cognition and behavior in children with congenital abdominal wall defects. *Early Hum Dev.* 2018;116:47–52.
35. Lap CC, Bolhuis SW, Van Braeckel KN. Functional outcome at school age of children born with gastroschisis. *Early Hum Dev.* 2017;106–107:47–52.
36. Luton D, de Lagausie P, Guibourdenche J, et al. Influence of amnioinfusion in a model of in utero created gastroschisis in the pregnant ewe. *Fetal Diagn Ther.* 2000;15(4):224–228.
37. Midrio P, Stefanutti G, Mussap M, et al. Amnioexchange for fetuses with gastroschisis: is it effective? *J Pediatr Surg.* 2007;42(5):777–782.
38. Luton D, Mitanchez D, Winer N, et al. A randomized control trial of amnioexchange for fetal gastroschisis. *BJOG.* 2019. doi:10.1111/1471-0528.15804.
39. Logghe HL, Mason GC, Thornton JG, et al. A randomized controlled trial of elective preterm delivery of fetuses with gastroschisis. *J Pediatr Surg.* 2005;40(11):1726–1731.
40. Ergün O, Barksdale E, Ergün FS, et al. The timing of delivery of infants with gastroschisis influences outcome. *J Pediatr Surg.* 2005;40(2):424–428.
41. Henrich K, Huemmer HP, Reingruber B, et al. Gastroschisis and omphalocele: treatments and long-term outcomes. *Pediatr Surg Int.* 2008;24(2):167–173.
42. Wilson MS, Carroll MA, Braun SA, et al. Is preterm delivery indicated in fetuses with gastroschisis and antenatally detected bowel dilation? *Fetal Diagn Ther.* 2012;32:262–266.
43. Weil BR, Leys CM, Rescorla FJ. The jury is still out: changes in gastroschisis management over the last decade are associated with both benefits and shortcomings. *J Pediatr Surg.* 2012;47(1):119–124.
44. Mortellaro VE, St Peter SD, Fike FB, et al. Review of the evidence on the closure of abdominal wall defects. *Pediatr Surg Int.* 2011;27(4):391–397.
45. Bonnard A, Zamakhshary M, de Silva N, et al. Non-operative management of gastroschisis: a case-matched study. *Pediatr Surg Int.* 2008;24(7):767–771.
46. Orion KC, Krein M, Liao J, et al. Outcomes of plastic closure in gastroschisis. *Surgery.* 2011;150(2):177–185.
47. Skarsgard ED. Management of gastroschisis. *Curr Opin Pediatr.* 2016;28:363–369.
48. Bucher BT, Mazotas IG, Warner BW, et al. Effect of time to surgical evaluation on the outcomes of infants with gastroschisis. *J Pediatr Surg.* 2012;47(6):1105–1110.
49. Kohl M, Wiesel A, Schier F. Familial recurrence of gastroschisis: literature review and data from the population-based birth registry "Mainz Model." *J Pediatr Surg.* 2010;45(9):1907–1912.
50. Islam S. Advances in surgery for abdominal wall defects: gastroschisis and omphalocele. *Clin Perinatol.* 2012;39(2):375–386.
51. Wilson RD, Johnson MP. Congenital abdominal wall defects: an update. *Fetal Diagn Ther.* 2004;19(5):385–398.
52. Bird TM, Robbins JM, Druschel C, et al. Demographic and environmental risk factors for gastroschisis and omphalocele in the National Birth Defects Prevention Study. *J Pediatr Surg.* 2009;44(8):1546–1551.
53. Khan FA, Hashmi A, Islam S. Insights into embryology and development of omphalocele. *Semin Pediatr Surg.* 2019;28:80–83.
54. Port-Lis M, Leroy C, Manouvrier S, et al. A familial syndromal form of omphalocele. *Eur J Med Genet.* 2011;54(3):337–340.
55. Faugstad EM, Brantberg A, Blaas HK, Vogt C. Prenatal examination and postmortem findings in fetuses with gastroschisis and omphalocele. *Prenat Diagn.* 2014;34:570–576.
56. Emanuel PG, Garcia GI, Angtuaco TL. Prenatal detection of anterior abdominal wall defects with US. *Radiographics.* 1995;15(3):517–530.
57. Bair JH, Russ PD, Pretorius DH, et al. Fetal omphalocele and gastroschisis: a review of 24 cases. *AJR Am J Roentgenol.* 1986;147(5):1047–1051.
58. Conner P, Vejde JH, Burgos CM. Accuracy and impact of prenatal diagnosis in infants with omphalocele. *Pediatr Surg Int.* 2018;34:629–633.

59. Juhasz-Boss I, Goelz R, Solomayer EF, et al. Fetal and neonatal outcome in patients with anterior abdominal wall defects (gastroschisis and omphalocele). *J Perinat Med.* 2011;40(1):85–90.
60. Danzer E, Victoria T, Bebbington MW, et al. Fetal MRI-calculated total lung volumes in the prediction of short-term outcome in giant omphalocele: preliminary findings. *Fetal Diagn Ther.* 2012;31(4):248–253.
61. Hacivelioglu S, Tarim E. Limb body wall defect: three different presentations with abdominal wall defects. *J Obstet Gynaecol.* 2010;30(7):737–738.
62. Haas J, Achiron R, Barzilay E, et al. Umbilical cord hernias: prenatal diagnosis and natural history. *J Ultrasound Med.* 2011;30(12):1629–1632.
63. Salzman L, Kuligowska E, Semine A. Pseudoomphalocele: pitfall in fetal sonography. *AJR Am J Roentgenol.* 1986;146(6):1283–1285.
64. Hidaka N, Tsukimori K, Hojo S, et al. Correlation between the presence of liver herniation and perinatal outcome in prenatally diagnosed fetal omphalocele. *J Perinat Med.* 2009;37(1):66–71.
65. Kominiarek MA, Zork N, Pierce SM, et al. Perinatal outcome in the live-born infant with prenatally diagnosed omphalocele. *Am J Perinatol.* 2011;28(8):627–634.
66. Biard JM, Wilson RD, Johnson MP, et al. Prenatally diagnosed giant omphaloceles: short- and long-term outcomes. *Prenat Diagn.* 2004;24(6):434–439.
67. Cohen-Overbeek TE, Tong WH, Hatzmann TR, et al. Omphalocele: comparison of outcome following prenatal or postnatal diagnosis. *Ultrasound Obstet Gynecol.* 2010;36(6):687–692.
68. Akinkuotu AC, Sheikh F, Olutoye OO, et al. Giant omphaloceles: surgical management and perinatal outcomes. *J Surg Res.* 2015;198(2):388–392.
69. Montero FJ, Simpson LL, Brady PC, et al. Fetal omphalocele ratios predict outcomes in prenatally diagnosed omphalocele. *Am J Obstet Gynecol.* 2011;205(3):284.e1–284.e7.
70. Hutson S, Baerg J, Deming D, et al. High prevalence of pulmonary hypertension complicates the care of infants with omphalocele. *Neonatology.* 2017;112:281–286.
71. Mann S, Blinman TA, Douglas Wilson R. Prenatal and postnatal management of omphalocele. *Prenat Diagn.* 2008;28(7):626–632.
72. Kilbride KE, Cooney DR, Custer MD. Vacuum-assisted closure: a new method for treating patients with giant omphalocele. *J Pediatr Surg.* 2006;41(1):212–215.
73. Martin AE, Khan A, Kim DS, et al. The use of intraabdominal tissue expanders as a primary strategy for closure of giant omphaloceles. *J Pediatr Surg.* 2009;44(1):178–182.
74. Ein SH, Langer JC. Delayed management of giant omphalocele using silver sulfadiazine cream: an 18-year experience. *J Pediatr Surg.* 2012;47(3):494–500.
75. Morales JM, Patel SG, Duff JA, et al. Ectopia cordis and other midline defects. *Ann Thorac Surg.* 2000;70(1):111–114.
76. Cantrell JR, Haller JA, Ravitch MM. A syndrome of congenital defects involving the abdominal wall, sternum, diaphragm, pericardium, and heart. *Surg Gynecol Obstet.* 1958;107(5):602–614.
77. Lampert JA, Harmaty M, Thompson EC, et al. Chest wall reconstruction in thoracoabdominal ectopia cordis: using the pedicled osteomuscular latissimus dorsi composite flap. *Ann Plast Surg.* 2010;65(5):485–489.
78. Carmi R, Boughman JA. Pentalogy of Cantrell and associated midline anomalies: a possible ventral midline developmental field. *Am J Med Genet.* 1992;42(1):90–95.
79. Engum SA. Embryology, sternal clefts, ectopia cordis, and Cantrell's pentalogy. *Semin Pediatr Surg.* 2008;17(3):154–160.
80. Martin RA, Cunniff C, Erickson L, et al. Pentalogy of Cantrell and ectopia cordis, a familial developmental field complex. *Am J Med Genet.* 1992;42(6):839–841.
81. Williams AP, Marayati R, Beierle EA. Pentalogy of Cantrell. *Semin Pediatr Surg.* 2019;28:106–110.
82. Desselle C, Herve P, Toutain A, et al. Pentalogy of Cantrell: sonographic assessment. *J Clin Ultrasound.* 2007;35(4):216–220.
83. van Hoorn JH, Moonen RM, Huysentruyt CJ, et al. Pentalogy of Cantrell: two patients and a review to determine prognostic factors for optimal approach. *Eur J Pediatr.* 2008;167(1):29–35.
84. Peixoto-Filho FM, do Cima LC, Nakamura-Pereira M. Prenatal diagnosis of Pentalogy of Cantrell in the first trimester: is 3-dimensional sonography needed? *J Clin Ultrasound.* 2008;37(2):112–114.
85. Stein W, Haller F, Hawighorst T, et al. Pentalogy of Cantrell vs. limb body wall complex: differential diagnosis of a severe malformation in early pregnancy. *Ultraschall Med.* 2009;30(6):598–601.
86. Wheeler DS, St Louis JD. Pentalogy of Cantrell associated with hypoplastic left heart syndrome. *Pediatr Cardiol.* 2007;28(4):311–313.
87. Yuan SM, Shinfeld A, Mishaly D. An incomplete pentalogy of Cantrell. *Chang Gung Med J.* 2008;31(3):309–313.
88. Murphy A, Platt LD. First-trimester diagnosis of body stalk anomaly using 2- and 3-dimensional sonography. *J Ultrasound Med.* 2011;30(12):1739–1743.
89. Daskalakis G, Sebire NJ, Jurkovic D, et al. Body stalk anomaly at 10–14 weeks of gestation. *Ultrasound Obstet Gynecol.* 1997;10(6):416–418.
90. Hunter AG, Seaver LH, Stevenson RE. Limb-body wall defect. Is there a defensible hypothesis and can it explain all the associated anomalies? *Am J Med Genet A.* 2011;155A(9):2045–2059.
91. Pumberger W, Schaller A, Bernaschek G. Limb-body wall complex: a compound anomaly pattern in body-wall defects. *Pediatr Surg Int.* 2001;17(5–6):486–490.
92. Viscarello RR, Ferguson DD, Nores J, et al. Limb-body wall complex associated with cocaine abuse: further evidence of cocaine's teratogenicity. *Obstet Gynecol.* 1992;80(3, pt 2):523–526.
93. Litwin A, Fisch B, Tadir Y, et al. Limb-body wall complex with complete absence of external genitalia after in vitro fertilization. *Fertil Steril.* 1991;55(3):634–636.
94. Negishi H, Yaegashi M, Kato EH, et al. Prenatal diagnosis of limb-body wall complex. *J Reprod Med.* 1998;43(8):659–664.
95. Chen CP, Lin CJ, Chang TY, et al. Second-trimester diagnosis of limb-body wall complex with literature review of pathogenesis. *Genet Couns.* 2007;18(1):105–112.
96. Liu IF, Yu CH, Chang CH, et al. Prenatal diagnosis of limb-body wall complex in early pregnancy using three-dimensional ultrasound. *Prenat Diagn.* 2003;23(6):513–514.
97. Luehr B, Lipsett J, Quinlivan JA. Limb-body wall complex: a case series. *J Matern Fetal Neonatal Med.* 2002;12:132–137.

CYSTIC MASSES

Cystic abdominal masses in the fetus are common. The etiology of fetal intra-abdominal cysts can be prenatally diagnosed in 70% to 75% of cases.[1,2] Since the diagnosis rarely affects prenatal intervention or delivery, it is important to recognize the abnormality, provide a differential diagnosis, and obtain postnatal follow-up to document resolution or make a definitive diagnosis for possible postnatal therapy.

Ovarian Cyst

Incidence: The presence of small (<1 cm) cysts in the perinatal period is normal. The incidence of clinically significant fetal ovarian cysts is estimated at 1 in 2,500 pregnancies.[3]

Embryology and Pathology: Fetal ovarian follicles are thought to undergo maturation and enlargement when the ovary is exposed to fetal pituitary gonadotropins (FSH), placental human chorionic gonadotropins (HCG), and maternal estrogens, particularly when hormone levels are high in the third trimester. There may be increased incidence of fetal ovarian cysts in cases of maternal diabetes, rhesus sensitization, and preeclampsia, all of which are associated with increased serum chorionic gonadotropins, but this has not been confirmed in large studies.[3]

After birth, HCG and estrogen drop, while FSH and luteinizing hormone (LH) increase until 3 months and then fall as the hypothalamic-pituitary axis matures. Cysts typically regress with time, likely due to hormonal changes.

Diagnosis

Ultrasound: Fetal ovarian cysts are most often seen by imaging in the third trimester after 28 weeks, although they are also reported in the second trimester. They are typically unilateral but may be bilateral.[3]

Ovarian cysts may be simple (Fig. 26.3-1) or complicated (Fig. 26.3-2). Simple cysts are anechoic and smooth, with thin or imperceptible walls on ultrasound (US). Complicated cysts demonstrate hemorrhage as a fluid-debris level, retracting clot, multiple internal septations, or a solid mass on US. The wall may be thick and echogenic from dystrophic calcification.[4] A "daughter cyst sign," with a small round cyst within a cyst, is pathognomonic for ovarian origin.[3]

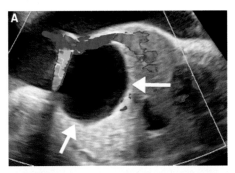

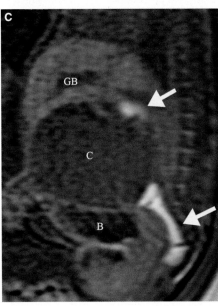

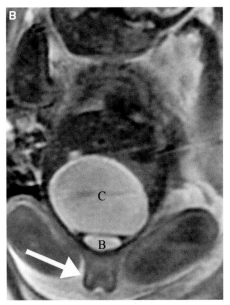

FIGURE 26.3-1: Simple ovarian cyst at 32 weeks' gestation. **A:** Axial color Doppler US demonstrates a large simple anechoic cyst *(arrows)* filling the pelvis and lower abdomen. **B:** Coronal fetal MRI demonstrates a large simple pelvic cyst *(C)* filling the pelvis and lower abdomen with hyperintense T2 signal. This cyst displaces the bladder *(B)* inferiorly. Gender is female *(arrow)*. **C:** Sagittal T1 fetal MRI demonstrates hypointense T1 fluid signal in this simple cyst *(C)* separate from the bladder *(B)* and gallbladder *(GB)*. Hyperintense signal posteriorly is from meconium in the rectum and colon *(arrows)*.

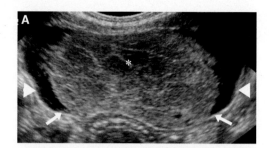

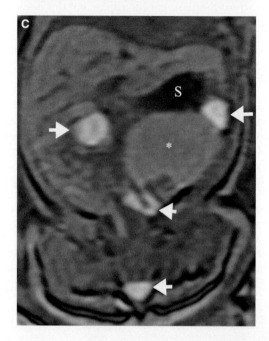

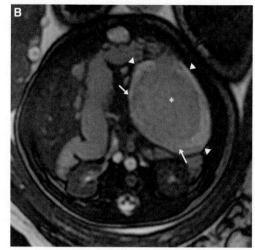

FIGURE 26.3-2: Complicated ovarian cyst secondary to ovarian torsion at 30 weeks' gestation. **A:** Axial US demonstrates peripheral anechoic fluid *(arrowheads)* and central lacelike echogenic mass *(asterisk)* representing retracting clot with acute margins *(arrows)* between the mass and the cyst wall. **B:** Axial fetal MRI demonstrates a complicated pelvic cyst with peripheral hyperintense T2 signal corresponding with fluid *(arrowheads)* and central intermediate signal *(asterisk)* with acute margins *(arrows)*, corresponding to retracting clot. **C:** Coronal MRI demonstrates mildly hyperintense T1 signal in this complicated cyst corresponding with clot *(asterisk)*. It is a higher signal than the fluid-filled stomach *(S)*, but less intense than the bright meconium in the adjacent colon *(arrows)*.

MRI: Simple cysts are hyperintense on T2 imaging and hypointense on T1 imaging, following fluid signal. On T2 imaging, the blood products in complicated cysts are lower signal than in fluid. Marked hypointensity on gradient echo or echoplanar imaging indicates hemosiderin deposition. Hemorrhage causes hyperintense T1 signal on magnetic resonance imaging (MRI). Nemac et al.[5] describe restricted diffusion and hyperintense fluid-attenuated inversion recovery (FLAIR) signal with intracystic hemorrhage. MRI can be useful to evaluate soft-tissue components, but for the vast majority of cases, US diagnosis and follow-up is the imaging standard.[5]

Suggested criteria for the diagnosis of enlarged fetal ovarian cysts include (1) female gender, (2) unilateral or bilateral pelvic or lower abdominal location, and (3) normal kidneys, bladder, and intestines. Cysts may be located anywhere in the abdomen or pelvis due to ligamentous laxity and a relatively long mesosalpynx, or due to torsion with autoamputation.[4,6] Cysts are considered pathological if they measure 2 cm or greater. When very large, a cyst may fill the abdomen and pelvis, displacing normal structures and making it difficult or impossible to determine the source.[3]

Cyst hemorrhage, with or without torsion, is the most common complication and is suspected when the cyst appears complicated. Ovarian cyst hemorrhage is highly associated with torsion. Ascites may occur with cyst rupture or torsion.[6] Anemia has been reported. Other complications can be due to mass effect. Polyhydramnios occurs in up to 18% of cases[3] and is likely secondary to extrinsic bowel obstruction by large cysts.[6] Severe mass effect may rarely result in elevation of the diaphragm and pulmonary hypoplasia.[6]

Differential Diagnosis: The differential diagnosis for a cyst in the fetal abdomen or pelvis includes lymphangioma, gastrointestinal (GI) duplication cyst, cystic teratoma, hydrocolpos, urachal cysts, and persistent cloaca. Identifying a normal urinary system excludes bladder outlet obstruction, megacystis microcolon intestinal hypoperistalsis syndrome, prune belly syndrome, and hydroureteronephrosis.

When a cyst is very large, it may not be possible to determine if it arises from the abdomen or pelvis, and abdominal cysts should also be considered (Tables 26.3-1 and 26.3-2). Extremely rare fetal ovarian tumors such as benign cystic teratomas, mucinous and serous cystadenomas, and a single case of carcinoma have been reported.[6]

Prognosis: In a meta-analysis including 954 fetuses with ovarian cysts from 2000 to 2016, 53.8% of all ovarian cysts undergo regression either prenatally or postnatally; 70% of simple cysts and 85% of cysts less than 4 cm resolve. Complicated cysts and cysts measuring 4 cm or larger are less likely to regress. The overall incidence of ovarian torsion in this meta-analysis was 21.8%, with 6% occurring in simple cysts and 44.9% in complicated cysts. More than 20% of simple cysts change appearance and become complex during pregnancy or at birth. This occurs more often in cysts measuring greater than 4 cm (odds ratio [OR] 3.16), and there is a higher rate of ovarian loss

TABLE 26.3-1 Differential Diagnosis of Fetal Abdominal Cysts Based on Location

Right upper quadrant
  Choledochal
  Hepatic cyst or cystic tumor
  Duodenal duplication
  Duodenal atresia
  Pancreatic (head)
Left upper quadrant
  Splenic
  Gastric duplication
  Pancreatic
Mid-abdomen
  Lymphatic (mesenteric, omental)
  Meconium pseudocyst
  Umbilical vein varix
Retroperitoneal
  Common
    Urinary tract dilation
    Renal cystic disease
  Uncommon
    Urinoma
    Adrenal cyst
    Cystic neuroblastoma
    Lymphatic (retroperitoneal)
Lower abdomen and pelvis
  Common
    Hydrometrocolpos
    Ovarian
    Ureterocele
    Urachal
    Megacystis
  Uncommon
    Persistent cloaca
    Anterior sacral meningocele
    Sacrococcygeal teratoma
Any location
  Alimentary duplication
  Dilated bowel (obstruction, atresia)
  Cystic teratoma

by autoamputation or surgery in those patients. Whether simple or complex, cysts measuring 4 cm or larger are more likely to be associated with torsion (OR 59.1).[7]

Management: Most authors recommended serial US follow-up for cysts less than 4 cm to document size and monitor for increasing complexity associated with hemorrhage/torsion. *In utero* needle aspiration appears to be safe and effective but is used rarely. In a meta-analysis, about half of aspirated cysts resolve, 38% recur, and 7% increase in size.[7] In a small prospective randomized trial of 61 participants with anechoic cysts, 31 *in utero* aspirations were uneventful and resulted in greater *in utero* resolution of the cyst (47.1% vs. 18.5%) and reduced rate of oophorectomy (3% vs. 22%) versus expectant management.[8] Since torsion often occurs *in utero*, postnatal surgery is primarily for the purpose of preventing complications such as hemorrhage, rupture with peritonitis,

and intestinal obstruction from adhesions, rather than for ovarian salvage.

Recurrence Risk: Since the hormonal stimulation is removed in the neonatal period, they are not expected to recur after they spontaneously resolve or are surgically treated.

Hepatic Cysts

Incidence: Low but not precisely known.[9] There is a female predominance.

Embryology and Pathology: Simple hepatic cysts are presumed secondary to interruption of the intrahepatic biliary system with growth arrest and dilation, representing cysts of biliary origin.

Most antenatally diagnosed hepatic cysts are simple cysts.[9] They most commonly have a cuboidal epithelial lining with positive CK-7 staining and a fibrous wall with occasional smooth muscle fibers, suggesting bile origin and supporting a biliary growth arrest etiology.[10] However, no epithelial lining[11] and simple squamous lining has also been reported.[9] Avni et al.[11] hypothesize that some hepatic cysts may represent areas of necrosis from an ischemic event, particularly those without an epithelial lining.

Diagnosis
Ultrasound: A hepatic cyst is most commonly seen in the second trimester (median gestational age 22 weeks), but has been reported in the third and first trimesters as well.[9,10] Hepatic cysts may be unilocular or multilocular. They may be clearly intrahepatic or subhepatic and attached to the liver capsule. Cysts as large as 20 cm have been reported.[12] Antenatally detected liver cysts are more often present in the left lobe.[9,12] On US, hepatic cysts are round, well-defined, anechoic structures with posterior acoustical enhancement.

A large cyst may compress the umbilical vein, resulting in hydrops and fetal demise, may elevate the diaphragm and cause pulmonary hypoplasia, or may compress the bowel and cause polyhydramnios.[9,12]

MRI: Hepatic cysts follow fluid signal on MRI with hyperintense T2 signal and hypointense T1 signal surrounded by higher signal liver parenchyma (Fig. 26.3-3).

Differential Diagnosis: Simple hepatic cysts, intrahepatic choledochal cysts (Caroli disease), and mesenchymal hamartomas (MHs) may look identical on prenatal imaging,[9] although simple hepatic cysts are statistically more common.[9,10] Consider rare entities like cystic hepatoblastoma, cystic teratoma, and hemangioma, particularly if there is question of a solid component or multilocularity. If the cyst is large and/or subhepatic it may be difficult to differentiate from extrahepatic fetal abdominal cysts (Tables 26.3-1 and 26.3-2).

Prognosis: Most simple hepatic cysts are asymptomatic and remain unchanged or regress over time.[9] Complications are rare and secondary to large size and mass effect. Infection, hemorrhage, and torsion of the cyst are theoretical complications. In a meta-analysis including 49 fetuses with hepatic cysts, 59.3% resolved or regressed prenatally or postnatally and 8.7% increased in size. Clinical symptoms were present in 14.8% and none had abnormal liver function tests at birth.[13]

TABLE 26.3-2 Comparison of Fetal Abdominal Cysts

CYST	LOCULARITY	TRIMESTER	GENDER	LOCATION
Ovarian	U > M	3rd >> 2nd	F	Pelvis ± abdomen
Hepatic	U >> M	2nd > 3rd > 1st	F >> M	RUQ
Choledochal	U	2nd > 3rd	F >> M	RUQ
Gallbladder duplication	U	2nd or 3rd	—	RUQ
Enteric	U >> M	2nd or 3rd	M > F	Any
Lymphatic	M or U	2nd > 3rd	M ≥ F	Any
Splenic	U	3rd	—	LUQ
Pancreatic-isolated	M or U	3rd > 2nd	F > M	Upper abdomen
Pancreatic-with anomalies	M or U	2nd > 3rd	F ≥ M	Upper abdomen

F, female; LUQ, left upper quadrant; M, male; M, multilocular; RUQ, right upper quadrant; trimester, trimester at diagnosis; U, unilocular.

Management: Hepatic cysts are typically managed with serial prenatal US examinations to document size and mass effect on adjacent structures. A very large cyst resulting in mass effect on the chest, umbilical cord, or bowel may require *in utero* aspiration to allow normal fetal development.[14]

Postnatally, cholangiography, and/or hepatobiliary scan may differentiate a choledochal cyst from a simple hepatic cyst, which is managed differently. Postnatal surgery for simple cysts, including aspiration, fenestration, cystectomy, or hepatic lobectomy, is typically reserved for patients with symptoms due to cyst size or uncertainty about the diagnosis.[9,10]

Postnatally, 18.3% of prenatally diagnosed hepatic cysts undergo surgery, with no reported complications.[13]

Recurrence Risk: Surgically resected cysts have not demonstrated recurrence.[9,10]

Choledochal Malformation/Cyst

Incidence: The incidence is unknown, but choledochal cysts are more prevalent in Asian populations and there is a 4:1 overall female predominance.[15]

Embryology and Pathology: The bile duct elongates and begins to recanalize at the end of the fifth week. By the 12th week, bile is secreted from the liver and transported to the duodenum by the extrahepatic biliary system.[16] The pancreas secretes enzymes in the fifth month of gestation.

Pathogenesis/Etiology: The etiology is not proved. The most widely cited theory states that pancreaticobiliary reflux secondary to an abnormal pancreaticobiliary duct junction (APBDJ) results in increased pressure, inflammation, and weakening resulting in cystic dilation. While a long common channel has been described (1 to 4.5 cm range in the literature), it is probably more accurate to describe the abnormal junction as one occurring outside the duodenal wall, allowing pancreatobiliary reflux and mixing. This does not explain cysts seen before pancreatic enzyme production. Alternatively, choledochal cysts may be due to distal obstruction by a web, stricture, biliary atresia, or sphincter of Oddi dysfunction. There may be varying pathogenesis related to the location and shape of the malformation. The theory of the APBDJ best explains type 1 and 4 cysts. There is also a theory that type 2 diverticula and type 3 choledochoceles may represent a biliary duplication cyst.

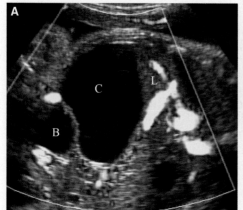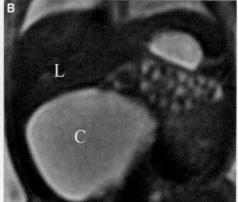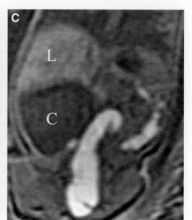

FIGURE 26.3-3: Hepatic cyst at 27 weeks' gestation. **A:** Coronal color Doppler US demonstrates a large anechoic cyst *(C)* along the inferior margin of the right lobe of the liver *(L)*, separate from the bladder *(B)*. There is no internal Doppler flow. **B:** Coronal MRI demonstrates hyperintense T2 fluid signal in the cyst *(C)* at the inferior margin of the right hepatic lobe *(L)*. **C:** Coronal T1 MRI demonstrates hypointense fluid signal of the cyst *(C)* at the inferior margin of the right hepatic lobe *(L)*.

Intrahepatic dilation, Caroli disease, is postulated to arise from a ductal plate malformation. Round cysts tend to have fewer neurons and ganglion cells, leading to a hypothesis that they are due to functional obstruction from aganglionosis (analogous to Hirschsprung disease).[17]

Choledochal cysts are most commonly classified by the Todani modified Alonso-Lej classification (Fig. 26.3-4).[18,19] Some authors have challenged this and advocate a descriptive nomenclature, since the classification may group together disease entities with different pathogenesis, clinical courses, surgical approaches, and outcomes.[15,17]

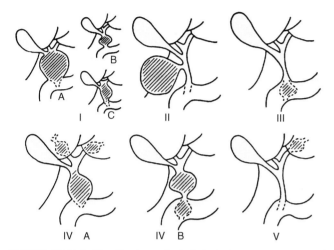

FIGURE 26.3-4: Classification of choledochal cysts as proposed by Alonso-Lej et al.[18] and modified by Todani et al.[19] Type IA, cystic extrahepatic biliary dilation; type IB, segmental extrahepatic biliary dilation; type IC, diffuse extrahepatic biliary dilation; type II, saccular diverticulum of extrahepatic bile duct; type III, choledochocele; IVA, multiple cysts of the intrahepatic and extrahepatic biliary tree; type IVB, multiple cysts of the extrahepatic biliary tree only; type V, intrahepatic cysts only (Caroli disease). (Reprinted with permission from Novak DA, Suchy FJ, Balistreri WF. Disorders of the liver and biliary system. In: McMillan JA, Feigin RD, DeAngelis C, et al., eds. *Oski's Solution*. Philadelphia, PA: Lippincott Williams & Wilkins; 2006:2035.)

There is evidence that 22% of U.S. patients with choledochal cysts have associated congenital cardiac anomalies including atrial septal defect (ASD), ventricular septal defect (VSD), patent ductus arteriosus (PDA), congenital anomaly not otherwise specified (NOS) and persistent fetal circulation.[20] Other associations include colon atresia, duodenal atresia, imperforate anus, pancreatic divisum, pancreatic aplasia, multiseptate gallbladder, aortic hypoplasia, congenitally absent portal vein, heterotopic pancreatic tissue, OMENS-plus syndrome, and familial adenomatous polyposis.[17]

Choledochal cysts may also be associated with concurrent biliary atresia or be confused with cystic biliary atresia, another type of choledochal malformation.[15,17,21]

Diagnosis

Ultrasound: A choledochal cyst is a cystic mass at the liver hilum, subhepatic, or in the liver parenchyma (type V), that is separate from the gallbladder. Choledochal cysts have been detected during second- or third-trimester US. It can be differentiated from other cystic masses if one can demonstrate continuity with the biliary system. Choledochal cysts tend to taper inferomedially to terminate in the midline epigastrium.[22] On US, it is typically anechoic with posterior enhancement, separate from the stomach, duodenum, and gallbladder, and without peristalsis (Fig. 26.3-5). Choledochal cysts with internal echoes have been reported.[23] Doppler US demonstrates lack of internal flow and intimate relationship with the portal vein and hepatic artery at the hilum.

MRI: Choledochal cysts follow fluid signal on MRI with hypointense T1 signal and hyperintense T2 signal. In some cases, MRI may be more useful than US in demonstrating the relationship to the biliary tree (Fig. 26.3-5).

Differential Diagnosis: If a cyst is in the porta hepatis and demonstrates intimate association with the portal vein and hepatic artery, the differential diagnosis includes choledochal cyst, cystic biliary atresia, duodenal duplication cyst, and pancreatic head cyst (Fig. 26.3-6). Biliary atresia with cystic dilation is uncommon but may be indistinguishable from

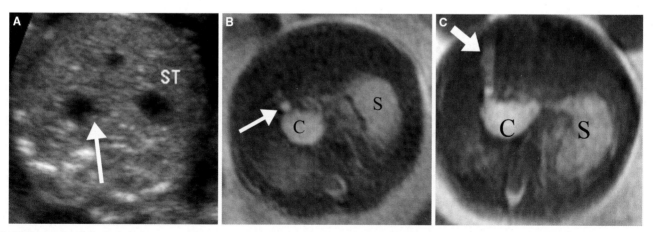

FIGURE 26.3-5: Choledochal cyst at 20 weeks' gestation. **A:** Transverse US through the fetal abdomen demonstrates a cyst in the liver hilum that tapers medially *(arrow)*. *ST*, stomach. **B:** Axial MRI demonstrates T2 hyperintense fluid signal of the cyst *(C)* at the hepatic hilum, separate from the stomach *(S)* and communicating with the bile duct *(arrow)* at the liver hilum. **C:** The next slice demonstrates the proximity of the cyst *(C)* to the gallbladder *(arrow)*, but separate from it. *S*, stomach.

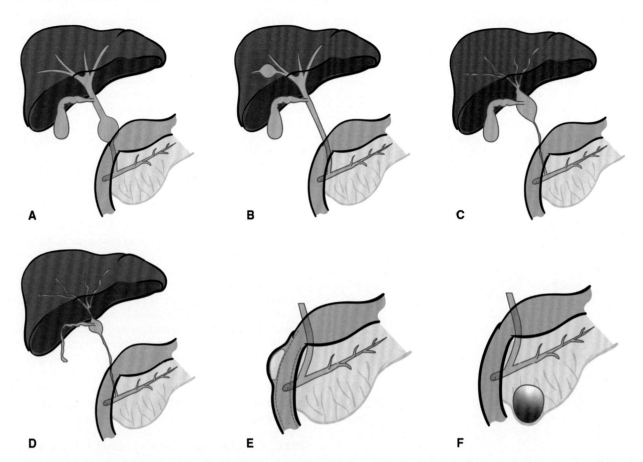

FIGURE 26.3-6: Schematic diagram of cystic lesions identified prenatally at the porta hepatis in intimate association with the portal vein and hepatic artery. **A:** Type I-c choledochal cyst. **B:** Type V choledochal cyst. **C:** Type 1 biliary atresia. **D:** Type 3 biliary atresia with segmental cyst. **E:** Duodenal duplication cyst *(yellow)*. **F:** Pancreatic head cyst *(red)*. (Illustration courtesy of Mr. Bryan Moss.)

a choledochal cyst on imaging. Amniotic fluid analysis for digestive enzymes may help differentiate them *in utero*; biliary atresia demonstrates decreased gamma-glutamyl transferase.[24] Redkar et al.[25] evaluated infants with postnatal biliary disease and abnormal prenatal US; postnatal diagnoses include choledochal cysts, type 1 biliary atresia (atresia of the common bile duct with mild proximal dilation) and type 3 biliary atresia with segmental cyst (cyst along the course of the atretic common bile duct).[25] Some authors suggest that (1) choledochal cysts increase in size over time, whereas cystic biliary atresia does not; (2) cysts of biliary atresia tend to be less than 2.5 cm, whereas choledochal cysts tend to be greater than 4 cm or have intrahepatic biliary dilation; or (3) anechoic cysts correspond to atresia, whereas large, echoic, or enlarging cysts correspond with choledochal cysts. However, the number of cases is small and exceptions are reported, so these criteria should not be used for definitive prenatal diagnosis.[24,25]

Other abdominal or pelvic cysts, including hepatic cysts, MHs, ovarian cysts, renal cysts, and adrenal cysts, should be considered in the differential diagnosis for a right upper quadrant cyst.

Prognosis: Untreated choledochal cysts may be complicated by rupture with peritonitis, biliary obstruction, recurrent cholangitis, pancreatitis, cirrhosis, portal hypertension, liver failure, and malignant degeneration. With modern early surgical treatment, symptoms resolve and the prognosis is good, with increasing morbidity and mortality with delayed surgery.[25,26] Choledochal cysts left *in situ* carry a risk of malignancy as high as 50%[27] with the youngest diagnosis at 3 years of age.[15]

There is evidence that choledochal cysts are associated with congenital cardiac anomalies in U.S. pediatric patients, so echocardiographic screening may be warranted before surgery.[20]

Management: Postnatal US and hepatobiliary scan confirm hepatobiliary origin and further differentiate a choledochal cyst from the rare cystic biliary atresia. Tanaka el al.[21] found a statistically significant increase in choledochal cyst size and significant decrease in biliary atresia cyst size between birth and surgery in a small group of patients. Small or absent gallbladder supports a diagnosis of biliary atresia,[21] while dilated intrahepatic ducts support a diagnosis of choledochal cyst.[28] Intraoperative cholangiography and/or pathology may be necessary to definitively exclude biliary atresia.[21]

Complete surgical excision of type 1 and 4 choledochal cysts with bilioenteric reconstruction, typically Roux-en-Y hepaticojejunostomy, is the preferred treatment. This has historically been performed as an open surgery, but laparoscopic and robot-assisted surgery are emerging. Type 2 and 3 cysts are very low risk for malignancy, so complete excision is not necessary. Simple excision of type 2 cysts and sphincterotomy of type 3 cysts may be adequate. Intrahepatic disease in type

4a and 5 disease is more complex and may involve some combination of wide excision, hepatic lobectomy, cyst unroofing, hepaticoenterostomy, or liver transplant.[27]

Early surgery in the first month of life may be warranted since even asymptomatic (not jaundiced) patients tend to develop liver fibrosis immediately after birth.[26]

Recurrence Risk: Postsurgical follow-up of antenatally diagnosed, postnatally resected choledochal cysts has not demonstrated cyst recurrence. There is risk of recurrent cholangitis in unresected cysts. Many authors advocate lifelong surveillance with US and liver enzymes for postexcisional malignancy (0.7% to 6%) potentially due to remnant tissue.[27]

Gallbladder Duplication

Incidence: One in 3,800 is based on literature from Boyden's 1926 work citing only 5 cases out of 19,000 autopsy and patient cases.[29] Bronshtein et al.[30] found two gallbladders described as septated, bilobed, or duplicated in 10,016 prenatal USs, for an estimated incidence of 1 in 5,008 screening USs.

Embryology and Pathology: The gallbladder arises from the caudal aspect of the hepatic diverticulum of the foregut in the 4th week and canalizes by the 12th week.[30]

In true duplication there are two gallbladders, each with its own cystic duct.[31] It may result from continued growth, rather than the expected regression of diverticula that arise from the cystic or common bile duct in the fifth and sixth weeks.[29] Alternatively, two cystic primordia may arise separately from the common bile duct resulting in an accessory gallbladder.[31]

A disturbance of cell division of the cystic primordium in the fifth or sixth week may result in splitting with two gallbladders in a septate, V-shaped, or Y-shaped duplication, but only one cystic duct entering the common duct.[31]

Diagnosis

Ultrasound: A duplicated gallbladder appears as parallel elongated cysts in the gallbladder fossa. Duplicated gallbladder has been reported on prenatal imaging between 20 and 32 weeks' gestation.[32–34] On US, fluid in the gallbladder is typically anechoic.

MRI: The duplicated gallbladder follows fluid signal with hyperintense T2 signal (Fig. 26.3-7) and hypointense T1 signal. In the third trimester, gallbladder content signal is more variable.

Differential Diagnosis: The primary differential consideration is a gallbladder fold, but this is oriented along the short axis of the gallbladder. Other considerations include choledochal, hepatic, enteric duplication, or lymphatic cysts. Its parallel configuration in the gallbladder fossa is characteristic.[33]

Prognosis: Duplicated gallbladder is an incidental finding with a good prognosis. The greatest importance lies in knowledge of the anatomy prior to cholecystectomy for symptomatic disease later in life, and for differentiating it from prenatal cysts that require postnatal surgery.

Management: If the diagnosis is uncertain prenatally, postnatal US or MRI may be useful for diagnosis. No intervention is required.

Recurrence Risk: None.

Enteric Duplication Cyst

Incidence: Prenatal detection is reported to be 1 in 18,333 live births, compared to 1 in 4,500 detected by autopsy, suggesting that prenatal US detects approximately 25% of duplication cysts.[35]

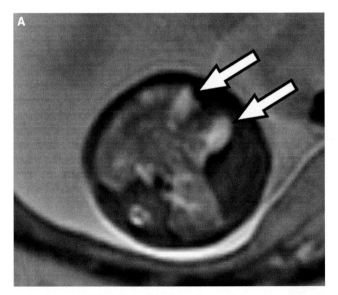 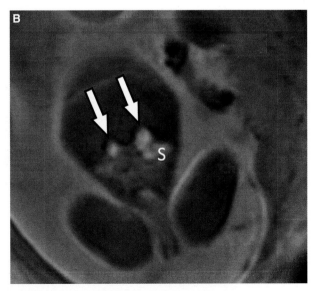

FIGURE 26.3-7: Gallbladder duplication on prenatal magnetic resonance. **A:** Axial T2 image demonstrates two parallel, elongated, hyperintense fluid-filled structures *(arrows)* in the gallbladder fossa. **B:** Coronal T2 image demonstrates the two gallbladders in the gallbladder fossa, separate from the stomach *(S)*.

Embryology and Pathology: Between the sixth and eighth weeks of gestation, the solid GI tract canalizes via coalescence of multiple vacuoles. Duplications of the esophagus and intestines may be related to an error of canalization according to the "aberrant recanalization theory." The split notochord theory states that an adhesion between the endoderm and ectoderm during the fifth gestational week causes the notochord to split, resulting in vertebral abnormality and an intraspinal or extraspinal neurenteric cyst, mostly applying to foregut duplications. Other theories include incomplete twinning, persistent embryological diverticula, and intrauterine vascular accident theories.[36]

Duplication cysts are spherical (80%) or tubular (20%), typically unilocular structures. They are typically single but may be multiple in up to 7%. Duplication cysts occur anywhere along the alimentary tract from the mouth/tongue to the rectum, but most commonly involve the ileum. The spherical type usually does not communicate with the lumen, whereas the tubular type frequently communicates. Intestinal duplications typically occur along the mesenteric border and gastric duplications typically occur along the greater curvature. Rarely, a duplication cyst may have its own separate mesentery. They should be associated with the GI tract, but there are reports of cysts separate from the GI tract with the same histology as duplication cysts, called isolated or atypical duplication cysts.[37]

Diagnosis

Ultrasound: On US, duplication cysts are typically anechoic. Intracystic hemorrhage results in internal echoes. Rarely, duplication cysts communicate with the bowel lumen and enteric content/meconium is present in the cyst, causing internal echoes.[38] Enteric duplication cysts may demonstrate peristalsis and gut signature with echogenic mucosal and echolucent muscular layers. However, gut signature is easier to see on postnatal imaging and may not be detectable on prenatal US (Fig. 26.3-8). Polyhydramnios may be present if the cyst results in GI obstruction or if there is concurrent bowel atresia, but this is uncommon. There is an association of bowel atresia with ileojejunal duplications in about 11%.[39] Half of foregut duplication cysts are associated with skeletal malformations and one-third of midgut and hindgut duplications are associated with GI or genitourinary (GU) anomalies.[40]

MRI: On MRI, duplication cysts follow fluid signal, unless hemorrhage or meconium is present resulting in hyperintense T1 and hypointense T2 signal (Fig. 26.3-8). The larger field of view provided by MRI compared to US may help identify the cyst origin and identify additional cysts. Associated GI or GU anomalies may be further assessed by MRI.

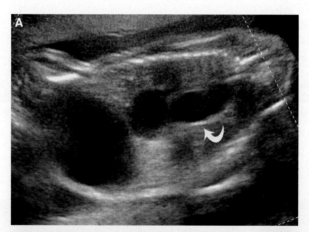

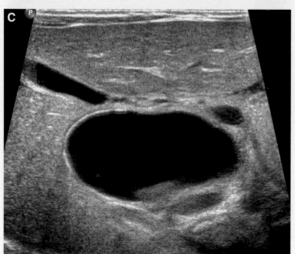

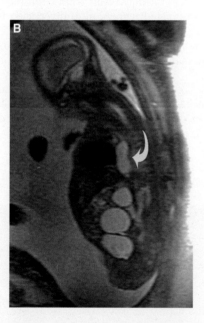

FIGURE 26.3-8: Multiple duplication cysts. **A:** Coronal prenatal US at 25 weeks demonstrates three cystic lesions in the chest and abdomen (*arrow* points to esophageal cyst). **B:** Sagittal MRI demonstrates hyperintense T2 fluid signal in multiple cysts (*arrow* points to esophageal cyst). **C:** Postnatal US documents gut signature sign with internal debris. Infant presented with vomiting at 2 weeks of age requiring surgery.

Differential Diagnosis: The differential diagnosis depends on location (Tables 26.3-1 and 26.3-2). Features that make a duplication cyst more likely include a thick wall with gut signature and peristalsis. Identification in the second trimester favors duplication cyst over ovarian cyst or bowel obstruction. Lymphatic cyst may be indistinguishable unless there is peristalsis.

Prognosis: Prognosis is good with surgical resection. Duplication cysts may be complicated by ulceration and hemorrhage if acid secreting gastric mucosa is present. Ectopic pancreatic tissue is most commonly found in gastric duplications and may cause pancreatitis. Duplications may result in mass effect on adjacent structures and intestinal obstruction. They may undergo torsion, become a lead point for intussusception or intestinal volvulus, or become infected or inflamed and perforate. Foley et al.[35] found that of 4 of 12 prenatally detected duplications required surgery in the first 2 months for symptoms of bowel obstruction. Of the asymptomatic patients, five out of eight duplications demonstrated ulcerated acid secreting mucosa.[35] A systematic review indicates that 41% of all prenatally diagnosed enteric duplication cysts become symptomatic early and are resected at a median age of 2 days.[41]

Management: Since most enteric duplications become symptomatic in the first 2 years of life, they are typically completely excised, with or without segmental bowel resection. A systematic review indicates that asymptomatic prenatally diagnosed cysts tend to be prophylactically resected at a median of 90 days.[41] In a recent study, 37% of the resected duplication cysts were prenatally diagnosed, and were laparoscopically resected at a median of 4.3 months of age without complication.[42] The risk of anesthesia in infants has not been objectively weighed against the risk of an enteric cyst complication in the literature to determine the best timing for surgery.[41]

Recurrence Risk: They do not recur after resection.

Lymphatic Malformations (Mesenteric, Omental, Retroperitoneal Cysts, and Abdominal Lymphangioma)

Lymphatic cysts include mesenteric, omental, and retroperitoneal cysts. Lymphangioma is a term historically used to describe a lymphatic malformation that is infiltrative. These terms are often used interchangeably in the literature, although some authors separate them on the basis of histology and clinical course. For this discussion of prenatal imaging, all the lymphatic malformations will be grouped together with an emphasis on imaging follow up to assess behavior.

Incidence: Lymphatic malformation of any location is common, occurring in 1 in 6,000 pregnancies, but most of these involve the neck and axilla (95%).[43] Abdominal lymphatic malformations account for less than 5%.[44] Localized lymphatic cysts are often asymptomatic, and the incidence is not known.

Embryology and Pathology: Abdominal lymphatic cysts are hypothesized to arise from abnormal development of the lymphatic system in the sixth week of gestation, with lack of lymphatic drainage resulting in cystic collections.[45]

Obstructed lymphatic drainage results in a benign cystic mass of lymphatic channels; in the abdomen, this most commonly occurs in the small bowel mesentery, but may occur in the large bowel mesentery, omentum, or retroperitoneum.[46] Some authors describe them as obstructed lymphatics and others as hamartomatous lymphatic tumors.

Diagnosis
Ultrasound: Review of case reports indicates that lymphatic cysts are discovered on prenatal imaging in the second and early third trimesters (19 to 31 weeks), they increase in size over time, are more often left sided, and they may change from unilocular to multilocular over time. Small localized cysts are most often centrally located in the abdomen but may be anywhere in the abdomen or pelvis and may change position because of attachment to the mobile mesentery or omentum. Infiltrating lymphatic malformations (lymphangiomas) may be isolated to the abdomen or may infiltrate surrounding structures and may extend to the abdominal wall, chest, or legs.[45,47–49]

On US, lymphatic cysts are typically thin-walled anechoic unilocular or multilocular structures. Hemorrhage or chylous fluid may cause internal echoes. There may be associated skin edema, polyhydramnios, and hydrops.

MRI: MRI is useful for large field of view assessment. Lymphatic malformations follow fluid signal with hypointense T1 signal and hyperintense T2 signal. If there is hemorrhage, T1 signal is hyperintense, T2 signal is more hypointense, and there may be marked hypointense signal on gradient echo imaging with hemosiderin deposition (Fig. 26.3-9).

Differential Diagnosis: Enteric duplication cysts and ovarian cysts may look identical to unilocular lymphatic cysts. Other cystic differential considerations depend on location (Tables 26.3-1 and 26.3-2). Pedunculated MH and cystic teratoma are also considerations.

Prognosis: The prognosis depends on the location, rate of growth, extent, and effect on adjacent structures. The prognosis is good for small mesenteric cysts localized to the abdomen, where there is often complete postnatal resection without recurrence. Poor prognosis is associated with early diagnosis, rapid growth, large size, hydrops/polyhydramnios, and extra-abdominal extension. Postnatally, localized cysts result in abdominal pain and/or distension from mass effect, torsion, hemorrhage, rupture, intussusception, or volvulus.[43]

Management: Serial prenatal US is recommended to monitor growth. Fetal karyotype is suggested because lymphatic malformations of the neck are associated with chromosomal abnormalities, but thus far the few reported cases of abdominal lymphatic malformations have not demonstrated abnormal karyotype or other congenital abnormalities.[43]

The few cysts detected by prenatal imaging have either been postnatally resected,[50–52] monitored clinically,[48] or pregnancy was terminated because of the extent and fast growth of the lesion.[44,45,47,49]

Postnatally diagnosed symptomatic cysts have been treated surgically, preferably with complete enucleation. Bowel resection may be necessary. Marsupialization is the least preferable choice since incomplete resection may result in recurrence.[46]

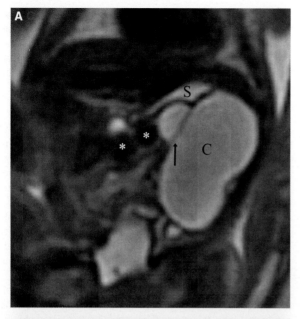

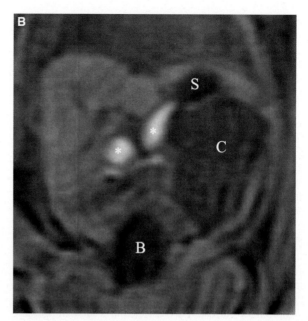

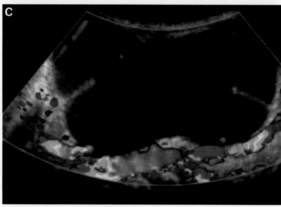

FIGURE 26.3-9: Mesenteric cyst. **A:** Coronal prenatal MRI at 30 weeks' gestation demonstrates a septated cyst (*C, arrow*) with hyperintense T2 signal, slightly less bright than fluid in the stomach (*S*), suggesting hemorrhage or debris. Adjacent hypointense meconium *(asterisks)* in the colon. **B:** Coronal T1 MRI demonstrates subtle hyperintense signal in the cyst *(C)* when compared with the stomach *(S)* and bladder *(B)*, representing hemorrhage or debris. There is hyperintense meconium *(asterisks)* in the adjacent colon. **C:** Postnatal color Doppler US demonstrates a large avascular, anechoic cyst containing septations.

Recurrence Risk: In children younger than 10 years of age, there is a 2% recurrence rate after resection. Recurrence is more likely for retroperitoneal cysts than for mesenteric cysts.[46]

Splenic Cyst

Incidence: Not precisely known; but splenic cysts are rare, with currently 55 cases reported in the literature. Dankovcik et al. found 3 fetal splenic cysts in 7,897 (0.04%) screening USs performed from 1997 to 2007.[53] Sauvageot et al. found 14 of 5,450 (0.3%) fetuses with splenic cysts at a tertiary referral center from 2007 to 2017.[54] There is likely a difference due to the evolution of better imaging equipment, although population bias and gestational age at the time of imaging may have an effect as well. Fetal splenic cysts are more common in males.[54]

Embryology and Pathology: The spleen begins development in the sixth to seventh week.

Splenic cysts are classified as true cysts (with an epithelial lining) or pseudocysts (no epithelial lining, secondary to trauma or infection). True cysts are divided into parasitic and nonparasitic classifications. Prenatally diagnosed splenic cysts are most commonly congenital, nonparasitic true cysts, which include epidermoid, polycystic, or mesothelial (simple) cysts.[55] The pathogenesis is not proved, and theories include (1)

pluripotent cell invasion of the spleen with subsequent metaplasia, (2) inclusion of coelomic mesothelial cells with squamous metaplasia, (3) invagination of peritoneal endothelial cells, and (4) lymphatic dilation.[53]

Diagnosis
Ultrasound: A splenic cyst is unilocular with a thin or imperceptible smooth wall most often diagnosed in the third trimester at a median of 30 weeks' gestation (range 17 to 37 weeks). On US, it is an anechoic round unilocular left upper quadrant mass, separate from organs other than the spleen. Rarely, a septation has been noted. Cysts are typically single; rarely, there are two to three cysts present in one fetus.[54] Splenic cysts commonly measure 1 to 2 cm or less, with the largest reported case measuring 4.5 cm prenatally.[55] With modern imaging equipment, splenic location can usually be diagnosed with US.

MRI: Splenic cysts follow fluid signal with hyperintense T2 signal and hypointense T1 signal. MRI is useful in the rare cases in which splenic location is not confirmed with US and other differential diagnoses need to be excluded.

Differential Diagnosis: Differential considerations include pancreatic cyst, hepatic cyst, lymphatic cyst, duplication cyst, renal cyst, urinoma, urinary collecting system dilation, and adrenal cyst.

Prognosis: Prenatally detected splenic cysts tend to be small and more than half decrease in size or resolve *in utero* or in the first 2 years of life. Some remain unchanged, and rarely do cysts enlarge.[53–56] They are almost always asymptomatic. There is one reported case of resection for symptoms; this was an epidermoid cyst that measured 4.5 cm antenatally and grew to 7 cm postnatally with compression of adjacent structures. Splenic cyst complications of torsion, hemorrhage, rupture, and infection described in children and adults have not been described in the perinatal period.[55]

Fetal splenic cyst is typically an isolated finding. Of the 55 reported cases, 3 fetuses had other abnormalities (megaureter, cleft lip/palate, talipes) which may have been unrelated to the splenic cyst.[55]

Management: US monitoring *in utero* and postnatally is recommended to document cyst regression or stability and exclude growth, subsequent complications, or alternative diagnoses.

Recurrence Risk: Case reports of antenatally diagnosed splenic cysts indicate stability or regression. They are rarely resected, so the recurrence rate is unknown.

Pancreatic Cyst

Incidence: Fetal pancreatic cysts are rare, with case reports of isolated congenital cysts[57–59] and rare cases associated with other congenital anomalies.[59–61]

Embryology and Pathogenesis: True pancreatic cysts are epithelium-lined cysts hypothesized to result from anomalous development of the pancreatic ducts.

It is suggested that anomalous development of the pancreatic ductal system sequesters secretory cells, giving rise to cysts.[62] There is a predilection for female gender and body/tail location for isolated cysts. Prenatal pancreatic cysts have been prenatally associated with Beckwith–Wiedemann syndrome, asphyxiating thoracic dysplasia, renal-hepatic-pancreatic dysplasia, and narrow thorax with short limb dwarfism.[59,61] Small cysts have been reported with short rib polydactyly syndrome type 1.[60] Postnatally, there is an association with polycystic renal disease, anorectal malformation, and von Hippel Lindau disease.[62]

Diagnosis

Ultrasound: Reported cases without congenital anomalies have been diagnosed between 21 and 38 weeks' gestation with cyst size of 21 to 58 mm. They may stay the same or increase in size.[57–59] Those with other congenital anomalies have been diagnosed between 15 and 32 weeks with varied size, number, and appearance of cysts.[59–61]

Pancreatic cysts may be unilocular, multilocular, or transition from a unilocular to septated cyst. They may be single or multiple. They are anechoic on US.

MRI: Pancreatic cysts follow fluid signal on MRI with hyperintense T2 signal and hypointense T1 signal.

Differential Diagnosis: Consider renal, liver, biliary, adrenal, or alimentary duplication cyst.

Prognosis: The prognosis is good for fetal pancreatic cysts without other congenital abnormalities, where postnatal resection is successful; however, no long-term follow-up has been

documented. Potential serious postnatal complications of pancreatic cysts include infection, cholangitis, pancreatitis, cyst rupture, and peritonitis if not resected.

Prognosis is worse with concurrent congenital anomalies.

Management: Pancreatic cysts located in the body and tail are treated with surgical excision. Cysts in the pancreatic head are treated with internal drainage procedures.[59]

Recurrence Risk: There is a paucity of data to determine recurrence risk. There is one case report of recurrence in an incompletely resected antenatally diagnosed pancreatic cyst.[63]

LIVER/SPLEEN

Hepatosplenomegaly

Fetal hepatosplenomegaly (HSM) may be secondary to immune or nonimmune hydrops, congenital infection, cardiac failure, hemolytic anemia, metabolic disease, overgrowth disorders, myeloproliferative disorders, or tumors (Table 26.3-3).[64–70] Detection of hepatic and/or splenic enlargement should prompt careful evaluation of the entire anatomy for other anomalies and clinical screening for congenital infection.

A myeloproliferative disorder may result in hepatomegaly or HSM, with or without hydrops. It may either represent transient abnormal myelopoiesis or acute leukemia; definitive

TABLE 26.3-3   Causes of Fetal Hepatosplenomegaly

Immune hydrops
Nonimmune hydrops
Cardiac failure
Congenital infection
  Toxoplasmosis
  CMV
  Syphilis
  Rubella
  Tuberculosis
Metabolic
  Hyperthyroidism
  Storage disease (Hunter, Gaucher, Niemann Pick, Wolman, and Glycogen storage disease type IV have been described with prenatal hepatosplenomegaly)
  Congenital disorders of glycosylation
  Mitochondrial hepatopathy
  Smith–Lemli–Opitz syndrome (defect in cholesterol synthesis)
  Enzyme deficiencies resulting in hemolytic anemia
    Congenital erythropoietic porphyria
    Pyruvate kinase deficiency
    Glucose-phosphate isomerase deficiency
    Transaldolase deficiency
Overgrowth disorders (Beckwith–Wiedemann syndrome)
Zellweger syndrome
Hemophagocytic lymphohistiocytosis
Myeloproliferative disorder/leukemia (usually associated with trisomy 21)
Primary tumor
Metastases

diagnosis requires cordocentesis and analysis of blast forms. The liver is often hypoechoic. Myeloproliferative disorders have mostly been described in infants with trisomy 21 but also have been noted in those with normal karyotype. Patients require intensive care after birth, so prenatal assessment of severity may be helpful. Ogawa et al. suggest that the degree of HSM may correlate with severity of postnatal disease, but there are no large studies to prove this.[71,72]

Studies have demonstrated that splenic circumference is an excellent predictor of severe fetal anemia secondary to Rh alloimmunization in nonhydropic fetuses not treated with transfusion, and is more useful late in pregnancy (after 30 weeks).[73] It was less sensitive and specific, but still useful, in the second-trimester evaluation of hemoglobin Bart (homozygous alpha thalassemia 1).[66]

SOLID MASSES

Solid hepatic masses of the fetus and neonate are rare and account for approximately 5% of total neoplasms in this age group. Primary hepatic tumors include congenital vascular masses, MH, and hepatoblastoma. Liver metastases may be secondary to neuroblastoma, leukemia, or renal tumors. Less common liver metastases may be secondary to yolk sac tumor, rhabdomyosarcoma, or rhabdoid tumor.[74] Rare cases of fetal focal nodular hyperplasia, and hepatic adenomas have been reported.[75,76]

Hepatic Vascular Lesions

Incidence: Hepatic vascular tumors account for 60% of perinatal liver tumors.[74] A large study from southern China found an incidence of 0.64/10,000 diagnosed on prenatal screening.[77]

Embryology and Pathology: North's placental theory suggests that placental mesodermal progenitor cells or placental angioblasts are responsible for the "vasculogenesis" of vascular tumors, as evidenced by the striking similarity of glucose transporter protein (GLUT)-1 positive infantile hemangioma tissue to placental tissue and supported by increased incidence after chorionic villous sampling.[78] This suggests hemangiomas may represent embolized placental implants. GLUT 1 negative congenital hemangiomas are more difficult to explain; cases of combined congenital and infantile histology suggest transformation may be possible.[79] Alternatively, a vascular precursor cell may undergo somatic mutation or may be influenced by local inductive influences to proliferate.[78] Presence of cutaneous hemangiomas along embryological fusion lines raises the question of neuroectoderm origin.[79]

Hemangioendothelioma is a term historically applied to a benign vascular lesion of the liver. In the literature, several terms have been used, sometimes considered synonymous and sometimes discussed as separate entities (Table 26.3-4). Vascular liver lesions were later grouped into solitary, multiple, and diffuse lesions in a liver hemangioma registry to study the natural history and response to treatment.[80,81] More recently, the International Society for the Study of Vascular Anomalies (ISSVA) updated its classification of vascular lesions; benign vascular neoplasms of the liver are subdivided into infantile and congenital hemangiomas.[82] Congenital hemangiomas are further subdivided into rapidly involuting congenital

hemangiomas (RICH), noninvoluting congenital hemangiomas (NICH), and partially involuting hemangiomas (PICH). Congenital hemangiomas are associated with an activating mutation in GNAQ or GNA11.[82]

Benign vascular liver neoplasms are classified as congenital or infantile depending on the timing of diagnosis, pattern of growth or regression, and GLUT 1 reactivity (Table 26.3-4).

Congenital hemangiomas are GLUT 1 (−) and typically present prenatally—either fully grown or already involuting at birth. There is no sex predilection. RICH regress by 1 to 2 years, whereas NICH do not regress and may grow with the child. PICH begin to involute like RICH and then stop before resolving, like NICH, suggesting these entities are part of a spectrum.[82,83] Congenital hemangiomas are more likely to be seen on prenatal imaging and are more commonly a solitary mass.[75,84]

Infantile hemangiomas are GLUT 1 (+) and typically present between 2 weeks and 2 months of postnatal life. They are more common in premature low-birth-weight white female infants. They rapidly proliferate in the first year and then regress over 1 to 8 years. They are unlikely to be seen on prenatal imaging. They may be solitary but are more commonly multiple or diffuse.[75,79,84] Maternal risk factors include advanced age, preeclampsia, and placental abnormalities.[85]

Multifocal and diffuse *infantile hemangiomas* express type 3 iodothyronine deiodinase, which degrades thyroid hormone and causes hypothyroidism. It is theorized that multifocal lesions may coalesce and become diffuse.[81]

Diagnosis

Ultrasound: On US, the GLUT-1 (−) congenital hemangiomas are typically large, well-circumscribed, solitary lesions with heterogeneous echogenicity from central necrosis and hemorrhage, and may have echogenic shadowing dystrophic calcification. They sometimes demonstrate high-flow arteriovenous or portovenous shunts with large tubular anechoic vessels at the periphery and may show intravascular thrombus (Fig. 26.3-10).[84,86]

On US, the GLUT-1 (+) infantile hemangioma may be a solitary mass similar to the congenital hemangioma, although calcification and vascular thrombosis are more rare. More often, infantile hemangiomas of the liver present as multiple small round masses that are of variable echogenicity.[84,86] When diffuse tumors are present, it may be difficult to discern on prenatal US because of near complete replacement of the liver parenchyma with hepatomegaly and heterogeneous echotexture.[80]

Doppler may demonstrate hypervascularity with high-velocity arterial waveforms and arterialized venous waveforms. Decreased aortic caliber below the celiac axis with hepatic artery, hepatic vein, and cardiac dilation suggest shunting.[86]

MRI: All types are predominantly T2 hyperintense and T1 hypointense, but large solitary tumors may be heterogeneous secondary to central necrosis, hemorrhage, thrombus, fibrosis, and calcification (Fig. 26.3-10). Dilated vessels are tubular flow voids on T2 MRI. Shunting is suspected when there are large flow voids with aortic caliber change. Small nodules of multifocal or diffuse subtypes may be more apparent on MRI than on US because of the soft-tissue contrast and they tend to be homogeneous in signal.[80]

TABLE 26.3-4	Comparison of Hepatic Hemangioma Subtypes[79-82]	
SUBTYPE	**CONGENITAL**	**INFANTILE**
Synonyms	Hemangioendothelioma, cavernous hemangioma, arteriovenous malformation, solitary hemangioma, RICH, NICH, hepatic vascular malformation with associated capillary proliferation	Hemangioendothelioma, capillary hemangioma, cellular hemangioma, infantile hepatic hemangioma, hemangiomatosis
GLUT 1 reactivity	GLUT 1 negative (−)	GLUT 1 positive (+)
Time of clinical presentation	Prenatal imaging or first few weeks of life	First weeks–months of life
Natural history	Fully grown at birth RICH: involute in infancy NICH: stabilize or grow PICH: partially involute then stabilize	Proliferate in infancy, then involute over 1–8 y
Sex predilection	None	Female
Prenatal appearance	Usually solitary Large, spherical, often heterogeneous with central necrosis/fibrosis, calcification	Multiple or diffuse > solitary Multiple: spherical homogeneous mass(es), hepatomegaly Solitary: similar to congenital
Postnatal enhancement	Peripheral rim enhancement with no central enhancement of necrotic areas on delay	Multiple: centripetal enhancement with delayed homogeneous enhancement Solitary: similar to congenital
Cutaneous	15.3%	77% multifocal, 53% diffuse
Complications	High-flow shunts → CHF RICH: transient mild/moderate thrombocytopenia ± consumptive coagulopathy and elevated D-dimer	Occasional high-flow shunts → CHF, anemia, thrombocytopenia, impaired venous flow from liver enlargement
Hypothyroidism	No association	21% multifocal, 100% diffuse
Treatment	Asymptomatic: monitor regression Symptomatic RICH: treat symptoms, consider antiangiogenic drugs Rarely: embolize shunts in refractory disease NICH: surgical resection	Asymptomatic: monitor regression Symptomatic: treat symptoms, begin antiangiogenic drugs Rarely: embolization, liver transplant in refractory disease
Response to medical therapy	Steroids used in symptomatic CHF, no strong evidence to support propranolol, vincristine	Favorable, especially multifocal

CHF, congestive heart failure; NICH, noninvoluting congenital hemangiomas; PICH, partially involuting hemangiomas; RICH, rapidly involuting congenital hemangiomas.

There is an association with cutaneous hemangiomas (Table 26.3-4). When hemangiomas are diffuse, there may be extrahepatic involvement of many organs.[74] Liver hemangioma is rarely associated with other congenital anomalies.

Differential Diagnosis: Other hepatic tumors including MH, hepatoblastoma, and metastases are the primary differential considerations. Solid versus cystic nature discriminates hemangioma from MH. Urine catecholamines and imaging exclusion of a primary tumor help differentiate neuroblastoma metastases in the case of diffuse or multifocal disease. Alpha fetoprotein (AFP) does not definitely differentiate it from hepatoblastoma since AFP may be elevated in hemangioma,[87] is elevated in the immediate newborn period, and is not elevated in some congenital hepatoblastomas. Following up on serial quantitative AFP over time in the perinatal period may be useful.

Prognosis: Asymptomatic patients have an excellent prognosis. Prognosis is poorer for patients with the diffuse form, hydrops, cardiac failure, jaundice, or thrombocytopenia.[81,88] Disseminated intravascular coagulation (DIC) rarely occurs.

Management: Most fetuses are managed prenatally with serial US to monitor for complications of anemia and hydrops. Prenatal fetal blood sampling to diagnose DIC with subsequent *in utero* platelet transfusion,[89] prenatal treatment with maternal oral steroids,[90] and intrauterine steroids via the umbilical vein and amniotic fluid[91] have been described. Rarely, tumor rupture during delivery may result in massive hemorrhage, so cesarean section should be considered.[74]

Postnatally, asymptomatic patients are monitored with serial imaging. Symptomatic patients are treated medically with antiangiogenic drugs. Corticosteroids are first-line treatment to hasten involution and close shunts. Propranolol,

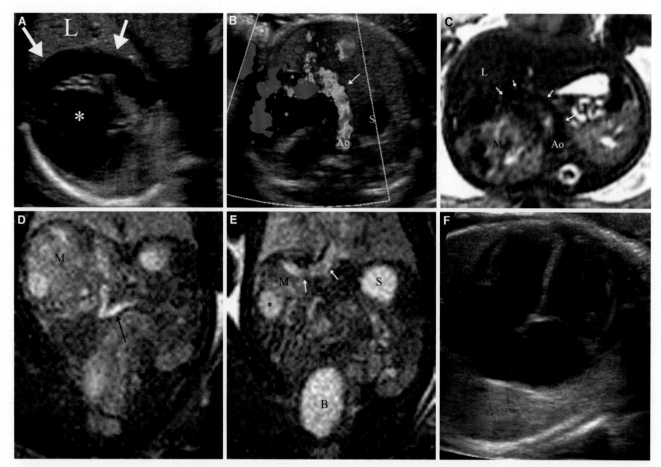

FIGURE 26.3-10: Hepatic hemangioma. **A:** Axial US of the right lobe of the liver *(L)* demonstrates a heterogeneous, predominantly hypoechoic mass with a large round anechoic area centrally *(asterisk)* and a tubular anechoic structure anteriorly *(arrows)*. **B:** Doppler confirms that the tubular structure is a large celiac and hepatic artery *(arrow)* arising from the aorta *(Ao)*. There is no Doppler flow in anechoic cystic areas *(asterisks)* of degeneration. *S,* stomach. **C:** Axial T2 MRI demonstrates the heterogeneous, predominantly hyperintense mass *(M)*. The tubular hypointense flow void of the large artery *(arrows)* is displaced by the mass. Coronal steady-state free process images demonstrates **(D)** the large feeding artery *(arrow)* supplying the heterogeneous hepatic mass *(M)* and **(E)** large hepatic vein drains into the IVC *(arrows)*. *S,* stomach; *B,* bladder; *asterisk,* cystic degeneration. **F:** Four-chamber heart view demonstrates cardiomegaly secondary to high-flow shunt. (Courtesy of Chris Cassady, MD.)

vincristine, or interferon may be used in addition to steroids or separately. Medical therapy is often effective for GLUT-1 (+) infantile tumors, but effectiveness is unknown for GLUT-1 (−) congenital tumors.[81] Approximately one-third of patients with shunts fail pharmacological therapy and require embolization. If medical management is ineffective, surgical options include hepatic artery ligation or embolization of shunts, rarely resection, and as a last resort, liver transplant. Symptomatic patients with diffuse disease should be quickly referred for transplant consideration while attempting medical therapy since their course is often short with high mortality. Thyroid function screening is recommended, since consumptive hypothyroidism associated with the multifocal and diffuse forms requires high-dose supplementation.[80] Hypothyroidism, thrombocytopenia, anemia, and heart failure are more common with multiple tumors.

Recurrence Risk: There are reports of hepatic infantile hemangiomas regressing, and then recurring between 2½ and 5 years of age with malignant histology, and often metastatic disease, considered synonymous with angiosarcoma.[92]

Mesenchymal Hamartoma

Incidence: MHs account for 23% of liver tumors diagnosed in the perinatal period.[74]

Embryology and Pathology: Several chromosomal translocations have been described, favoring the hypothesis that MH may actually represent a neoplasia. There are four hypotheses: (1) developmental, arising from a ductal plate malformation, (2) the result of a local vascular insult/ischemia, (3) a response to a toxic insult, or (4) a neoplasia rather than a hamartoma. MH is associated with placental mesenchymal stem villous hyperplasia (vascular malformation) and is not typically associated with other congenital anomalies.[93]

Diagnosis

Ultrasound: MH is more common in the right lobe. Twenty percent are pedunculated and may not appear intrahepatic.[93] It has been diagnosed as early as 19 weeks. On US, MH is a multilocular cystic structure with a variable soft-tissue component (Fig. 26.3-11). There are typically multiple thin mobile septations and hyperechoic intracystic nodules. Rare appearances include

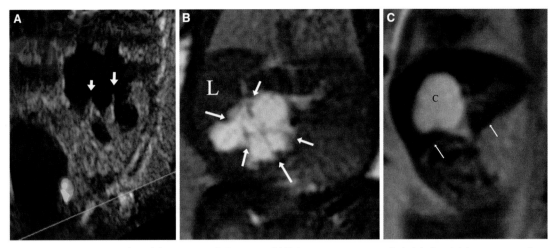

FIGURE 26.3-11: Mesenchymal hamartoma. **A:** Parasagittal US demonstrates an anechoic lobulated right upper quadrant abdominal mass with septations *(arrows)* and lack of internal Doppler signal. **B:** Coronal SSFP image demonstrates hyperintense signal in the lobulated mass in the liver *(L)* with several thin hypointense septations *(arrows)*. **C:** A sagittal T2 image best depicts its location within the liver (inferior margin of the liver is denoted by *arrows*). C, cyst.

intracystic hemorrhage or debris, hypervascular angiomatous component or mixed MH-hemangioma, cysts so small that the mass appears solid on imaging, or echogenic calcifications.

Look for complications related to mass effect such as polyhydramnios, hydrops, and diaphragm elevation with pulmonary hypoplasia.

MRI: Large field of view is useful in assessing the origin of these masses by MRI. MH is T1 hypointense, but variable signal intensity in T2 imaging (Fig. 26.3-11).[93] Lung hypoplasia can be assessed on MRI in the case of large space-occupying lesions.

Differential Diagnosis: The differential diagnosis for lesions in the liver includes hepatic cyst, hemangioma, and cystic hepatoblastoma. Pedunculated tumors may mimic intra-abdominal cysts, particularly lymphatic cysts or cystic teratoma because of the septations.[93]

Prognosis: The prognosis is poorer for those diagnosed *in utero* than in childhood, with 29% mortality, predominantly due to mass effect.[94] There are reports of partial spontaneous regression, particularly in cases with a prominent angiomatous component. There are also rare reports of undifferentiated embryonal cell carcinoma of the liver arising within mesenchymal hamartoma or after incomplete resection.[93]

Management: Prenatal follow-up with US is important to monitor cyst size. They often enlarge quickly and can cause significant mass effect. Prenatal cyst decompression may alleviate mass effect and allow more normal fetal development, but fluid typically reaccumulates quickly. If the cyst is large, cesarean section may be performed for potential dystocia. Postnatally, symptomatic cysts are usually treated with surgical resection. Imaging and clinical follow-up is recommended for 5 years.[93]

Recurrence Risk: Recurrence rate is not documented, but recurrence of MH is reported after incomplete resection, and there are also cases of recurrence from small unrecognized satellite lesions.[93]

Hepatoblastoma

Incidence: The incidence of hepatoblastoma in U.S. children younger than age 1 is 10.5/1,000,000, and has been increasing.[95] Less than 10% of all hepatoblastomas occur in the perinatal period. It accounts for 17% of liver tumors diagnosed in the perinatal period.[74]

Embryology and Pathology: Multiple cytogenetic abnormalities have been described in association with childhood hepatoblastoma, including gain of chromosome 20, 2, or 8. There is also an association with trisomy 18.[95] An association with familial adenomatous polyposis has led to the discovery of adenomatous polyposis coli (APC)/beta-catenin gene mutations found even in some sporadic hepatoblastoma cases. Changes in expression of *H19* and *IGF2* have been described, and are also commonly seen in Beckwith–Wiedemann syndrome, with which hepatoblastoma is associated.[95,96]

Pathogenesis/Etiology: It is hypothesized that oxygen free radicals may impede hepatocyte differentiation. There is also a high incidence of hepatoblastoma in very low-birth-weight infants, but whether the tumor is initiated or promoted by environmental factors of the neonatal intensive care unit (NICU) or due to a common etiology is controversial and not proved.[95]

Hepatoblastoma is derived from undifferentiated embryonal tissue and may be classified as epithelial (subclassified as fetal, embryonal, or small cell undifferentiated) or mixed epithelial/mesenchymal subtypes. Congenital hepatoblastomas are more often the pure fetal histology. In childhood, metastases occur in the lung. In prenatal cases, the lungs are spared, presumably due to fetal circulation, and metastases occur in the brain, bone, and placenta.[97]

Diagnosis
Ultrasound: Review of the antenatally diagnosed case reports indicates that fetal hepatoblastomas are typically diagnosed by US late in the third trimester as a large mass measuring 6 to 10 cm, although it has been seen as early as 30 weeks, and as small as 2.5 cm.[98] They are typically single, but may be multiple,

and are more common in the right lobe.[74] On US, it is usually hyperechoic but may be heterogeneous with areas of degeneration demonstrating necrosis, hemorrhage, and calcification. It is a vascular, predominantly solid tumor. It may appear polylobular with a "spoke-wheel appearance."[98]

Mass effect may result in compression of vessels (umbilical vein, portal vein, and inferior vena cava [IVC]), hydrops, and compression of the lungs resulting in respiratory distress.

MRI: Hepatoblastoma is typically T2 hyperintense, and T1 hypointense, but there may be heterogeneity in large tumors if there is associated degeneration (Fig. 26.3-12). MRI is useful for lung volume calculation and metastasis detection.

Differential Diagnosis: The differential diagnosis includes hemangioma, metastases, and mesenchymal hamartoma. The serum AFP is not a reliable discriminator. It is only elevated in half of congenital cases, and may rarely be elevated in hemangioma and mesenchymal hamartoma.[74]

Prognosis: Prenatally, mass effect may result in compression of vessels, hydrops and stillbirth. Diaphragmatic elevation may compress the lungs resulting in respiratory distress. Tumor hemorrhage, spontaneous or related to vaginal delivery, may result in anemia or death. Rarely, metastases contribute to mortality.[99]

Previous data (1970 to 2005) implied a worse prognosis for congenital hepatoblastoma[74] with a 40% survival rate for treated disease. A recent review of databases of multicenter group studies (1993 to 2013) shows that congenital hepatoblastoma has a 3-year survival of 86%, which is comparable to cohorts unselected for age.[100] Modern treatment for hepatoblastoma seems to have improved mortality for those diagnosed in the perinatal period as well.

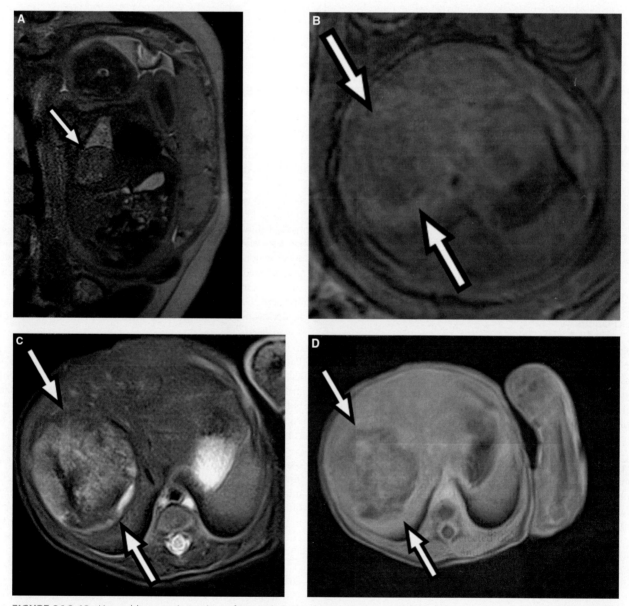

FIGURE 26.3-12: Hepatoblastoma *(arrows)* in a fetus with Beckwith–Wiedemann syndrome. **A:** Coronal T2 MRI at 37 weeks' gestation demonstrates a heterogeneous mass that is mildly hyperintense relative to the liver. **B:** On T1 prenatal MRI the mass is hypointense. **C:** T2 MRI 1 week after birth by induction demonstrates a heterogeneous, hyperintense mass that has rapidly grown from an average diameter of 3 to 5 cm. **D:** Postnatal contrast enhanced MRI demonstrates heterogeneous enhancement of the mass. (Courtesy of Rachelle Goldfisher, MD.)

Management: Prenatally, hepatic masses are followed up with imaging to assess growth, mass effect on adjacent structures, and to monitor for hydrops. Cesarean section should be considered since these tumors are known to bleed and rupture during delivery and are typically large and may cause dystocia.[74] Postnatally, they are treated with surgical resection. Chemotherapy may be used preoperatively to shrink the tumor, and/or postnatally to control microscopic disease.

Recurrence Risk: Hepatoblastoma diagnosed in childhood recurs at a rate of 12% after complete remission.[101] A review of 27 cases of congenital hepatoblastoma found one recurrence (3.7%), which was successfully treated.[100]

Other Masses

Teratoma and fetus in fetu both demonstrate heterogeneous appearance on US and MR, often with soft tissue, bone, and fat elements, and with varying degree of organization. *Fetus in fetu* is a rare diagnosis in which a monochorionic, monozygotic twin is incorporated into the host twin. Some authors believe that presence of four limbs appropriately arranged relative to a vertebral column differentiates it from a teratoma, and others believe that a vertebral column is not required for the diagnosis.[102,103] Both *fetus in fetu* and teratoma are completely surgically excised with their surrounding membranes to reduce the risk of recurrence.[103]

Gastric pseudomass is a rounded echogenic area in the lumen of the stomach, possibly as a result of swallowed cells or hemorrhage in the amniotic fluid, which aggregates due to poor peristalsis in the second trimester. They resolve on follow-up imaging.[104]

Meconium pseudocyst is a well-defined hypoechoic mass with a hyperechoic calcified wall and indicates bowel perforation.[104]

Extralobar pulmonary sequestration occurs more commonly on the left (4:1) as an echogenic subdiaphragmatic mass, and the diagnosis is supported by identifying a thoracic aortic feeding vessel with Doppler. On MRI, it is homogeneously T2 hyperintense and a feeding artery may be seen as a hypointense tubular flow void on T2 imaging. They are typically seen in the second trimester and more often on the left, as opposed to neuroblastomas that are more hypoechoic and seen more often seen in the third trimester on the right.[104]

The Gallbladder

The gallbladder is first visible by US at 13 to 14 weeks' gestation as a fluid-filled, anechoic structure in the right upper quadrant, subhepatic or intrahepatic in location, and to the right of the umbilical vein. Size increases linearly with gestational age and plateaus at 32 to 35 weeks. It has a sinusoidal contractility pattern over a 3-hour interval that is independent of maternal meals. While the percent contractility increases through the third trimester, the minimum volume is relatively constant, so the gallbladder should be visible on imaging throughout the cycle.[105] The MRI signal of the gallbladder contents is variable and is age dependent. Before 27 weeks, gallbladder contents are T1 hypointense and T2 hyperintense. After 30 weeks, T1 and T2 signals are variable. This is likely due to sludge or accumulation of paramagnetic substances in the gallbladder secretions.[106]

Nonvisualization of the Fetal Gallbladder

This is defined as not seeing the gallbladder on two USs within 7 to 15 days. With modern equipment and transvaginal technique at 14 to 16 weeks, the gallbladder is absent in only 0.1% of pregnancies.[107] Blazer found that absent gallbladder was isolated in 59% (incidence 1 in 6,000 pregnancies) with normal outcome. Associated structural malformations were present in 41% and 36% of those also had abnormal karyotype. The gallbladder was detected later in pregnancy or postnatally in 4 out of 5 structurally abnormal babies that were not terminated, and in 13 out of 20 normal babies.[107] Nonvisualization of the gallbladder is associated with cystic fibrosis, biliary atresia, and aneuploidy, so amniocentesis with karyotype and evaluation of amniotic digestive enzymes may be useful.

Cholecystomegaly

This is defined as gallbladder area more than 2 standard deviations above the mean for gestational age. Despite small retrospective studies suggesting an association with aneuploidy or biliary abnormalities, a large prospective study found cholecystomegaly in 43 of 775 (5.5%) fetuses and no such association.[108]

Gallbladder Stones and Sludge

Echoes in the gallbladder with posterior acoustic shadowing suggest stones, and without shadowing suggest sludge. There are few reported cases with an estimated incidence of 1% after 28 weeks' gestation.[109] They often resolve *in utero* or in the first year of life without symptoms. Management includes follow-up US and possibly postnatal ursodeoxycholic acid.[110]

REFERENCES

1. Ozyuncu O, Canpolat FE, Ciftci AO, et al. Perinatal outcomes of fetal abdominal cysts and comparison of prenatal and postnatal diagnoses. *Fetal Diagn Ther.* 2010;28:153–159.
2. Catania VD, Briganti V, DiGiacomo V, et al. Fetal intra-abdominal cysts: accuracy and predictive value of prenatal ultrasound. *J Matern Fetal Neonatal Med.* 2016;29(10):1691–1699.
3. Trinh TW, Kennedy AM. Fetal ovarian cysts: review of imaging spectrum, differential diagnosis, management and outcome. *Radiographics.* 2015;35:621–635.
4. Ozcan HN, Balci S, Ekinci S, et al. Imaging findings of fetal-neonatal ovarian cysts complicated with ovarian torsion and autoamputation. *AJR Am J Roentgenol.* 2015;205:185–189.
5. Nemac U, Nemac SF, Bettelheim D, et al. Ovarian Cysts on Prenatal MRI. *Eur J Radiol.* 2012;81:1937–1944.
6. Dimitraki M, Koutlaki N, Nikas I, et al. Fetal ovarian cysts. Our clinical experience over 16 cases and review of the literature. *J Matern Fetal Neonatal Med.* 2012;25(3):222–225.
7. Bascietto F, Liberati M, Marrone L, et al. Outcome of fetal ovarian cysts diagnosed on prenatal ultrasound examination: systematic review and meta-analysis. *Ultrasound Obstet Gynecol.* 2017;50:20–31.
8. Diguisto C, Winer N, Benoist G, et al. In-utero aspiration vs expectant management of anechoic fetal ovarian cysts: open randomized controlled trial. *Ultrasound Obstet Gynecol.* 2018;52:159–164.
9. Charlesworth P, Ade-Ajayi N, Davenport M. Natural history and long-term follow-up of antenatally detected liver cysts. *J Pediatr Surg.* 2007;42(3):494–499.
10. Rogers T, Woodley H, Ramsden W, et al. Solitary liver cysts in children: not always so simple. *J Pediatr Surg.* 2007;42(2):333–339.
11. Avni EF, Rypens F, Donner C, et al. Hepatic cysts and hyperechogenicities: perinatal assessment and unifying theory on their origin. *Pediatr Radiol.* 1994;24(8):569–572.
12. Hackmon-Ram R, Wiznitzer A, Gohar J, et al. Prenatal diagnosis of a fetal abdominal cyst. *Eur J Obstet Gynecol Reprod Biol.* 2000;91(1):79–82.
13. Leombroni M, Buca D, Celentano C, et al. Outcomes associated with fetal hepatobiliary cysts: systematic review and meta-analysis. *Ultrasound Obstet Gynecol.* 2017;50:167–174.
14. Ito M, Yoshimura K, Toyoda N, et al. Aspiration of giant hepatic cyst in the fetus in utero. *Fetal Diagn Ther.* 1997;12(4):221–225.
15. Friedmacher F, Ford KE, Davenport M. Choledochal malformations: global research, scientific advances and key controversies. *Pediatr Surg Int.* 2019;35:273–282.
16. Ando H. Embryology of the biliary tract. *Dig Surg.* 2010;27:87–89.
17. Singham J, Yoshida EM, Scudamore CH. Choledochal cysts. Part 1 of 3: classification and pathogenesis. *Can J Surg.* 2009;52(5):434–440.
18. Alonso-Lej F, Rever WB Jr, Pessagno DJ. Congenital choledochal cyst, with a report of 2, and an analysis of 94, cases. *Int Abstr Surg.* 1959;108(1):1–30.

19. Todani T, Watanabe Y, Narusue M, et al. Congenital bile duct cysts: classification, operative procedures, and review of thirty-seven cases including cancer arising from choledochal cyst. *Am J Surg.* 1977;134(2):263–269.

20. Murphy A, Axt J, Lovvorn H. Associations between pediatric choledochal cysts, biliary atresia, and congenital cardiac anomalies. *J Surg Res.* 2012; 177(2):59–63.

21. Tanaka H, Sasaki H, Wada M, et al. Postnatal management of prenatally diagnosed biliary cystic malformation. *J Pediatr Surg.* 2015;50:507–510.

22. Cong X, Sun X, Liu S. Evaluation and screening ultrasonic signs in the diagnosis of fetal biliary cystic malformation. *J Matern Fetal Neonatal Med.* 2015;28(17):2100–2105.

23. Casaccia G, Bilancioni E, Nahom A, et al. Cystic anomalies of biliary tree in the fetus: is it possible to make a more specific prenatal diagnosis? *J Pediatr Surg.* 2002;37(8):1191–1194.

24. Mackenzie TC, Howell LJ, Flake AW, et al. The management of prenatally diagnosed choledochal cysts. *J Pediatr Surg.* 2001;36(8):1241–1243.

25. Redkar R, Davenport M, Howard ER. Antenatal diagnosis of congenital anomalies of the biliary tract. *J Pediatr Surg.* 1998;33(5):700–704.

26. Diao M, Li L, Cheng W. Timing of surgery for prenatally diagnosed asymptomatic choledochal cysts: a prospective randomized study. *J Pediatr Surg.* 2012;47(3):506–512.

27. Singham J, Yoshida EM, Scudamore CH. Choledochal cysts. Part 3 of 3: management. *Can J Surg.* 2009;53(1):51–56.

28. Morel B, Kolanska K, Dhombres F, et al. Prenatal ultrasound diagnosis of cystic biliary atresia. *Clin Case Rep.* 2015;3(12):1050–1051.

29. Boyden EA. The accessory gall-bladder: an embryological and comparative study of aberrant biliary vesicles occurring in man and the domestic mammals. *Am J Anat.* 1926;38:177–231.

30. Bronshtein M, Weiner Z, Abramovici H, et al. Prenatal diagnosis of gall bladder anomalies—report of 17 cases. *Prenat Diagn.* 1993;13(9):851–861.

31. Harlaftis N, Gray SW, Skandalakis JE. Multiple gallbladders. *Surg Gynecol Obstet.* 1977;145(6):928–934.

32. Gerscovich E, Towner D, Sanchez T, et al. Fetal gallbladder duplication. *J Ultrasound Med.* 2011;30(9):1310–1312.

33. Kinoshita L, Callen P, Filly R, et al. Sonographic detection of gallbladder duplication: two cases discovered in utero. *J Ultrasound Med.* 2002;21(12):1417–1421.

34. Sifakis S, Mantas N, Koumantakis G, et al. Prenatal diagnosis of gallbladder duplication. *Ultrasound Obstet Gynecol.* 2007;30(3):362–363.

35. Foley P, Sithasanan N, McEwing R, et al. Enteric duplications presenting as antenatally detected abdominal cysts: is delayed resection appropriate? *J Pediatr Surg.* 2003;38(12):1810–1813.

36. Macpherson RI. Gastrointestinal tract duplications: clinical, pathologic, etiologic, and radiologic considerations. *Radiographics.* 1993;13(5):1063–1080.

37. Nebot CS, Salvador RL, Palacios, et al. Enteric duplication cysts in children: varied presentations, varied imaging findings. *Insights Imaging.* 2018;9(6):1097–1106.

38. Tseng JJ, Chou MM, Ho ES. In utero sonographic diagnosis of a communicating enteric duplication cyst in a giant omphalocele. *Prenat Diagn.* 2001;21(7):540–542.

39. Holcomb GW III, Gheissari A, O'Neill JA, et al. Surgical management of alimentary tract duplications. *Ann Surg.* 1989;209(2):167–174.

40. Ildstad ST, Tollerud DJ, Weiss RG, et al. Duplications of the alimentary tract. Clinical characteristics, preferred treatment, and associated malformations. *Ann Surg.* 1988;208(2):184–189.

41. Fahy A, Pierro A. A systematic review of prenatally diagnosed intra-abdominal enteric duplication cysts. *Eur J Pediatr Surg.* 2019;29:68–74.

42. Sujka JA, Sobrino J, Benedict LA, et al. Enteric duplication in children. *Pediatr Surg Int.* 2018;34:1329–1332.

43. Arisoy R, Erdogdu E, Kumru P, et al. Prenatal diagnosis and outcome of lymphangiomas and its relationship with fetal chromosomal abnormalities. *J Matern Fetal Neonatal Med.* 2016;29(3):466–472.

44. Giacalone PL, Boulot P, Deschamps F, et al. Prenatal diagnosis of a multifocal lymphangioma. *Prenat Diagn.* 1993;13(12):1133–1137.

45. Deshpande P, Twining P, O'Neill D. Prenatal diagnosis of fetal abdominal lymphangioma by ultrasonography. *Ultrasound Obstet Gynecol.* 2001;17(5):445–448.

46. Kurtz RJ, Heimann TM, Holt J, et al. Mesenteric and retroperitoneal cysts. *Ann Surg.* 1986;203(1):109–112.

47. Kozlowski KJ, Frazier CN, Quirk JG. Prenatal diagnosis of abdominal cystic hygroma. *Prenat Diagn.* 1988;8(6):405–409.

48. Katz VL, Watson WJ, Thorp JM, et al. Prenatal sonographic findings of massive lower extremity lymphangioma. *Am J Perinatol.* 1992;9(2):127–129.

49. Kaminopetros P, Jauniaux E, Kane P, et al. Prenatal diagnosis of an extensive fetal lymphangioma using ultrasonography, magnetic resonance imaging and cytology. *Br J Radiol.* 1997;70(835):750–753.

50. Santo S, Marques J, Veca P, et al. Prenatal ultrasonographic diagnosis of abdominal cystic lymphangioma: a case report. *J Matern Fetal Neonatal Med.* 2008;21(8):565–566.

51. Devesa R, Muñoz A, Torrents M, et al. Prenatal ultrasonographic findings of intra-abdominal cystic lymphangioma: a case report. *J Clin Ultrasound.* 1997;25(6):330–332.

52. Salvador A, Rosenberg HK, Horrow MM, et al. Abdominal lymphangioma in a preterm infant. *J Perinatol.* 1996;16(4):305–308.

53. Dankovcik R, Urdzik P, Lazar I, et al. Conservative management in three cases of prenatally recognized splenic cyst using 2D, 3D, multi-slice and Doppler ultrasonography. *Fetal Diagn Ther.* 2009;26(3):177–180.

54. Sauvageot C, Faure JM, Mousty E, et al. Prenatal and postnatal evolution of isolated fetal splenic cysts. *Prenat Diagn.* 2018;38:390–394.

55. Sepulveda W, Ochoa JH, Cafici D, et al. Splenic cyst as a rare cause of fetal abdominal cystic mass: a multicenter series of nine cases and review of the literature. *Ultrasound.* 2018;26(1):22–31.

56. Garel C, Hassan M. Foetal and neonatal splenic cyst-like lesions. US follow-up of seven cases. *Pediatr Radiol.* 1995;25(5):360–362.

57. Gerscovich EO, Fiels NT, Sanchez T, et al. Fetal true pancreatic cysts. *J Ultrasound Med.* 2012;31:811–813.

58. Choi SJ, Kang MC, Kim YH, et al. Prenatal detection of a congenital pancreatic cyst by ultrasound. *J Korean Med Sci.* 2007;22(1):156–158.

59. Liao Y, Chen H, Chou C, et al. Antenatal detection of a congenital pancreatic cyst. *J Formos Med Assoc.* 2003;102(4):273–276.

60. Balci S, Altinok G, Tekşen F, et al. A 34-week-old male fetus with short rib polydactyly syndrome (SRPS) type I (Saldino-Noonan) with pancreatic cysts. *Turk J Pediatr.* 2003;45(2):174–178.

61. Boopathy Vijayaraghavan S, Kamalam M, Raman ML. Prenatal sonographic appearance of congenital bile duct dilatation associated with renal-hepatic-pancreatic dysplasia. *Ultrasound Obstet Gynecol.* 2004;23(6):609–611.

62. Auringer ST, Ulmer JL, Sumner TE, et al. Congenital cyst of the pancreas. *J Pediatr Surg.* 1993;28(12):1570–1571.

63. Ishimaru T, Uchida H, Yotsumoto K, et al. Recurrence of a congenital pancreatic cyst mimicking omental cyst after laparoscopic cyst resection. *Eur J Pediatr Surg.* 2009;19(1):53–54.

64. Clayton P. Diagnosis of inherited disorders of liver metabolism. *J Inherit Metab Dis.* 2003;26(2–3):135–146.

65. Chen C, Lin S, Tzen C, et al. Prenatal diagnosis and genetic counseling of mucopolysaccharidosis type II (Hunter syndrome). *Genet Couns.* 2007;18(1):49–56.

66. Srisupundit K, Tongprasert F, Luewan S, et al. Splenic circumference at midpregnancy as a predictor of hemoglobin Bart's Disease among fetuses at risk. *Gynecol Obstet Invest.* 2011;72:63–67.

67. Mignot C, Gelot A, Bessières B, et al. Perinatal-lethal Gaucher disease. *Am J Med Genet A.* 2003;120A(3):338–344.

68. Mochel F, Grébille AG, Benachi A, et al. Contribution of fetal MR imaging in the prenatal diagnosis of Zellweger syndrome. *AJNR Am J Neuroradiol.* 2006;27(2):333–336.

69. Patel S, DeSantis E. Treatment of congenital tuberculosis. *Am J Health Syst Pharm.* 2008;65(21):2027–2031.

70. Williams D, Gauthier D, Maizels M. Prenatal diagnosis of Beckwith-Wiedemann syndrome. *Prenat Diagn.* 2005;25(10):879–884.

71. Ogawa H, Hosoya N, Sato A, et al. Is the degree of fetal hepatosplenomegaly with transient abnormal myelopoiesis closely related to the postnatal severity of hematological abnormalities in Down syndrome? *Ultrasound Obstet Gynecol.* 2004;24(1):83–85.

72. Kikuchi A, Tamura N, Ishii K, et al. Four cases of fetal hypoechoic hepatomegaly associated with trisomy 21 and transient abnormal myelopoiesis. *Prenat Diagn.* 2007;27:665–669.

73. Bahado-Singh R, Oz U, Mari G, et al. Fetal splenic size in anemia due to Rh-alloimmunization. *Obstet Gynecol.* 1998;92(5):828–832.

74. Isaacs H. Fetal and neonatal hepatic tumors. *J Pediatr Surg.* 2007;42(11):1797–1803.

75. Applegate KE, Ghei M, Perez-Atayde AR. Prenatal detection of a solitary liver adenoma. *Pediatr Radiol.* 1999;29(2):92–94.

76. Petrikovsky BM, Cohen HL, Scimeca P, et al. Prenatal diagnosis of focal nodular hyperplasia of the liver. *Prenat Diagn.* 1994;14(5):406–409.

77. Jiao-ling L, Xiu-ping G, Kun-shan C, et al. Huge fetal hepatic hemangioma: prenatal diagnosis on ultrasound and prognosis. *BMC Pregnancy Childbirth.* 2018;18(1):2.

78. North P, Waner M, Brodsky M. Are infantile hemangioma of placental origin? *Ophthalmology.* 2002;109(2):223–224.

79. Kollipara R, Dinneen L, Rentas KE, et al. Current classification and terminology of pediatric vascular anomalies. *AJR Am J Roentgenol.* 2013;201:1124–1135.

80. Christison-Lagay ER, Burrows PE, Alomari A, et al. Hepatic hemangiomas: subtype classification and development of a clinical practice algorithm and registry. *J Pediatr Surg.* 2007;42(1):62–67; discussion 67–68.

81. Kulungowski A, Alomari A, Chawla A, et al. Lessons from a liver hemangioma registry: subtype classification. *J Pediatr Surg.* 2012;47(1):165–170.

82. International Society for the Study of Vascular Anomalies. Classification. http://issva.org/classification. Published April 2014. Revised May 2018. Accessed January 22, 2019.

83. Nasseri E, Piram M, McCuaig CC, et al. Partially involuting congenital hemangiomas: a report of 8 cases and review of the literature. *J Am Acad Dermatol.* 2014;70:75–79.

84. Mo JQ, Dimashkieh HH, Bove K. GLUT 1 endothelial reactivity distinguishes hepatic infantile hemangioma from congenital hepatic vascular malformation with associated capillary proliferation. *Hum Pathol.* 2004;35(2):200–209.

85. Lowe LH, Marchant TC, Rivard DC, et al. Vascular malformations: classification and terminology the radiologist needs to know. *Semin Roentgenol.* 2012;47(2):106–117.

86. Johnson CM, Navarro OM. Clinical and sonographic features of pediatric soft-tissue vascular anomalies part 1: classification, sonographic approach and vascular tumors. *Pediatr Radiol.* 2017;47:1184–1195.
87. Lehrnbecher T, Frauendienst-Egger G, Schrod L, et al. Haemangioendothelioma in a preterm infant associated with highly elevated alpha-fetoprotein. *Eur J Pediatr.* 1996;155(5):423–424.
88. Kuroda T, Kumagai M, Nosaka S, et al. Critical infantile hepatic hemangioma: results of a nationwide survey by the Japanese Infantile Hepatic Hemangioma study group. *J Pediatr Surg.* 2011;46(12):2239–2243.
89. Gembruch U, Baschat AA, Gloeckner-Hoffmann K, et al. Prenatal diagnosis and management of fetuses with liver hemangiomata. *Ultrasound Obstet Gynecol.* 2002;19(5):454–460.
90. Morris J, Abbott J, Burrows P, et al. Antenatal diagnosis of fetal hepatic hemangioma treated with maternal corticosteroids. *Obstet Gynecol.* 1999;94(5, pt 2):813–815.
91. Mejides AA, Adra AM, O'Sullivan MJ, et al. Prenatal diagnosis and therapy for a fetal hepatic vascular malformation. *Obstet Gynecol.* 1995;85(5, pt 2):850–853.
92. Ackermann O, Fabre M, Franchi S, et al. Widening spectrum of liver angiosarcoma in children. *J Pediatr Gastroenterol Nutr.* 2011;53(6):615–619.
93. Stringer M, Alizai N. Mesenchymal hamartoma of the liver: a systematic review. *J Pediatr Surg.* 2005;40(11):1681–1690.
94. Cornette J, Festen S, van den Hoonaard T, et al. Mesenchymal hamartoma of the liver: a benign tumor with deceptive prognosis in the perinatal period. *Fetal Diagn Ther.* 2009;25(2):196–202.
95. Spector L, Birch J. The epidemiology of hepatoblastoma. *Pediatr Blood Cancer.* 2012;59(5):776–779.
96. Herzog CE, Andrassy RJ, Eftekhari F. Childhood cancers: hepatoblastoma. *Oncologist.* 2000;5(6):445–453.
97. Makin E, Davenport M. Fetal and neonatal liver tumours. *Early Hum Dev.* 2010;86(10):637–642.
98. Catanzarite V, Hilfiker M, Daneshmand S, et al. Prenatal diagnosis of fetal hepatoblastoma: case report and review of the literature. *J Ultrasound Med.* 2008;27(7):1095–1098.
99. Ammann RA, Plaschkes J, Leibundgut K. Congenital hepatoblastoma: a distinct entity? *Med Pediatr Oncol.* 1999;32(6):466–468.
100. Trobaugh-Lotrario AD, Chaiyachati BH, Meyers RL, et al. Outcomes for patients with congenital hepatoblastoma. *Pediatr Blood Cancer.* 2013;60:1817–1825.
101. Semeraro M, Branchereau S, Maibach R, et al. Relapses in hepatoblastoma patients: clinical characteristics and outcome-experience of the international childhood liver tumour strategy group (SIOPEL). *Eur J Cancer.* 2013;49:915–922.
102. Escobar M, Rossman J, Caty M. Fetus-in-fetu: report of a case and a review of the literature. *J Pediatr Surg.* 2008;43(5):943–946.
103. Basu A, Jagdish S, Iyengar K, et al. Fetus in fetu or differentiated teratomas? *Indian J Pathol Microbiol.* 2006;49(4):563–565.
104. McNamara A, Levine D. Intraabdominal fetal echogenic masses: a practical guide to diagnosis and management. *Radiographics.* 2005;25(3):633–645.
105. Tanaka Y, Senoh D, Hata T. Is there a human fetal gallbladder contractility during pregnancy? *Hum Reprod.* 2000;15(6):1400–1402.
106. Brugger P, Weber M, Prayer D. Magnetic resonance imaging of the fetal gallbladder and bile. *Eur Radiol.* 2010;20(12):2862–2869.
107. Blazer S, Zimmer EZ, Bronshtein M. Nonvisualization of the fetal gallbladder in early pregnancy: comparison with clinical outcome. *Radiology.* 2002;224(2)379–382.
108. Hertzberg BS, Kliewer MA, Bowie JD, et al. Enlarged fetal gallbladder: prognostic importance for aneuploidy or biliary abnormality at antenatal US. *Radiology.* 1998;208(3):795–798.
109. Kiserud T, Gjelland K, Bognø H, et al. Echogenic material in the fetal gallbladder and fetal disease. *Ultrasound Obstet Gynecol.* 1997;10(2):103–106.
110. Iroh Tam P, Angelides A. Perinatal detection of gallstones in siblings. *Am J Perinatol.* 2010;27(10):771–774.

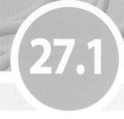

27.1 Renal and Adrenal Abnormalities

Fred E. Avni

INTRODUCTION

Congenital malformations of the urinary tract are among the most commonly identified abnormalities at antenatal ultrasound (US) with an incidence between 1 in 250 and 1 in 1,000 pregnancies. Abnormalities range from benign and simple conditions such as unilateral renal pelvic dilatation up to complex malformations or even life-threatening conditions, such as bilateral multicystic dysplasia. Kidney malformation can be an isolated finding or part of a polymalformative syndrome.[1-3]

US plays a central role in assessing the normal and abnormal fetal urinary tract. Fetal magnetic resonance imaging (MRI) has become a complementary examination in cases of complex malformations or when US is limited because of fetal or maternal limiting factors (e.g., oligohydramnios, fetal lie, maternal obesity). The findings of both techniques must be interpreted conjointly in order to provide the most accurate information to determine prognosis and appropriate management for delivery and postnatal care.[4-7]

Integrating imaging data along with familial, biological, and genetic data are of utmost importance as they can provide additional information for a proper diagnosis. Familial diseases clearly influence the course of the fetal development, as do maternofetal diseases. Advances in genetic research in isolated or polymalformative kidney diseases are obvious and increasing day after day; this has led to two important concepts: congenital anomalies of the kidney and urinary tract (CAKUT) (Table 27.1-1) and ciliopathies (Table 27.1-2). CAKUT account for the largest group of pediatric patients with end-stage renal diseases encompassing a broad phenotype spectrum. There is wide variability in genotype–phenotype correlation, indicating

TABLE 27.1-1 Principal Congenital Anomalies of the Kidney and Urinary Tract

Duplex kidneys
Horseshoe kidneys
Multicystic dysplastic kidney
Polycystic kidneys
Posterior urethral valves
Renal agenesis
Renal dysplasia
Renal hypoplasia
Vesicoureteric reflux

Modified from Toka HR, Toka O, Hariri A, et al. Congenital anomalies of the urinary tract. *Semin Nephrol.* 2010;30:374–386; Song R, Yosypiv IV. Genetics of congenital anomalies of the kidney and urinary tract. *Pediatr Nephrol.* 2011;26:353–364.

TABLE 27.1-2 Principal Ciliary Disorders Associated with Congenital Hepatorenal Fibrocystic Diseases (Including Major Gene Mutations)

Autosomal dominant polycystic kidney disease (PKD1-PKD2)
Autosomal recessive polycystic kidney disease (PKHD-1)
Bardet–Biedl syndrome (BBSI → BBS10, MSK1)
Ellis–van Creveld syndrome (EVC1-EVC2)
Glomerulocystic kidney disease (HNF-1Beta)
Jeune chondrodysplasia (IFT80)
Joubert syndrome (NHPH1)
Meckel–Gruber syndrome (MSK1, MSK3)
Nephronophthisis (NPH1, NPH3, NPH4, NPH8)
Orofaciodigital syndrome (OFD1)
Renal hepatic pancreatic dysplasia (NPHP3) (Zellweger syndrome)

Modified from Woolf AS. A molecular and genetic view of human renal and urinary tract malformations. *Kidney Int.* 2000;58:500–512; Rizk D, Chapman AB. Cystic and inherited kidney diseases. *Am J Kidney Dis.* 2003;42:1305–1307; Gunay-Aygun M. Liver and kidney disease in ciliopathies. *Am J Med Genet.* 2009;151C:269–306.

a complex process depending on many factors. Ciliopathies have brought a unifying concept in relation to hepatorenal fibrocystic diseases. In selected patients with urinary tract abnormalities, chromosomal analysis needs to be performed and will provide information as well.[8-12]

EMBRYOLOGY

The development of the human kidney starts when the primitive nephritic duct is formed on the embryonic day 22 from the intermediate mesoderm. The human urinary tract results from the progressive development and subsequent degeneration of three overlapping systems: the pronephros, the mesonephros, and the metanephros (Fig. 27.1-1). The *pronephros* forms a vestigial excretory unit that disappears by the end of the fourth week. The *mesonephros* development starts during the fourth week and results in primitive excretory tubules that eventually form primitive glomeruli at their medial extremity. These excretory tubules and primitive glomeruli form the renal corpuscle. These early structures degenerate rapidly, although some mesonephritic tubules remain and participate in the formation of the male reproductive system. The third system, the *metanephros* or permanent kidney, appears during the fifth week. On day 28, the definitive excretory units start to develop from

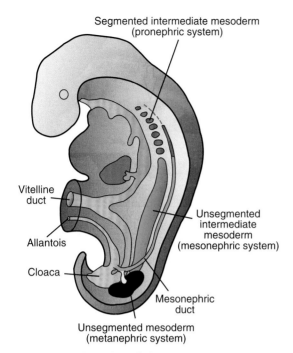

FIGURE 27.1-1: Relationship of the intermediate mesoderm of the pronephric, mesonephric, and metanephric systems. (Reprinted with permission from Sadler TW. The urogenital system. In: Sadler TW, ed. *Langman's Medical Embryology.* 9th ed. Philadelphia, PA: Lippincott Williams & Wilkins; 2004:321–362.)

the metanephric mesoderm; the definitive collecting ducts of the permanent kidney develop from the ureteric bud, an outgrowth of the vestigial mesonephritic duct. The ureteral bud invades the adjacent metanephric mesenchyme. Further development of the metanephros occurs via reciprocal inductive interactions between the ureteral bud and the mesenchyme. The ureteral bud end dilates progressively, forming the renal pelvis and subsequently, it splits into the future calyces. Each calyx forms new buds while penetrating the metanephritic tissue. At the periphery of the ureteral bud, initial generations of the ureteral bud are remodeled into the ureter, renal pelvis, and calyces; subsequent generations develop into collecting tubules (Fig. 27.1-2). The capillaries grow parallel to the collecting tubules and differentiate into the final glomeruli. The association of glomeruli and tubules represents a nephronic unit (Fig 27.1-3). Nephrons are formed until the 36th week.

The embryo–fetal differentiation of the kidney involves epithelial/mesenchymal interactions under the regulation of many genes, the so-called renal developmental genes (RDGs) that include transcription/growth factors and intracellular signaling molecules (e.g., RET, PAX2, HNF1Beta, UMOD, WT1); malfunction or mutation of these genes would induce urinary tract malformation.

The kidneys develop originally within the pelvis and ascend progressively to the lumbar areas (Fig. 27.1-4). The ureteral orifices move cranially into the bladder trigone, whereas the ejaculatory ducts, remains of the mesonephritic ducts, move closer to the midline and enter the prostatic urethra where they open.

The bladder and urethra originate from the cloacal partition by the urorectal septum between the seventh and the eighth weeks. This partition separates the cloaca into the primitive urogenital sinus anteriorly and the anal canal posteriorly (Fig. 27.1-4). Subsequently, the urogenital sinus develops into three parts: *first,* the urinary bladder; *second,* the pelvic part of the urogenital sinus, which gives rise to the urethra (prostatic and membranous in the male, entire urethra in the female), and, *third,* the phallic part that will correspond to the genital tubercle. The anterior urethra in the male develops as an ingrowth of the phallic ectoderm and closure of the urethral folds. Finally, the urogenital membrane breaks during the seventh week, establishing continuity between the developing urinary tract and the amniotic cavity. Chwalla membrane at the ureterovesical junction (UVJ) disappears during the eighth week. Intrinsic narrowings persist and can be discerned at the ureteropelvic and UVJ up to the 18th week.

If development is normal, urine production starts at the ninth week.[8–11,13,14]

IMAGING OF THE NORMAL URINARY TRACT

Ultrasound Imaging

The normal development of the urinary tract is well depicted by US. The bladder and kidney are clearly visible during the first trimester (Fig. 27.1-5). The fetal bladder is the first structure of the urinary tract to be visualized on US, appearing as an anechoic cystic structure within the fetal pelvis around 9 to 10 weeks' gestation. The kidneys themselves are visualized slightly later, appearing as two hyperechoic oval nodules, one at each side of the lumbar spine. During the first trimester, the kidneys appear globally hyperechoic, without corticomedullary differentiation (CMD). Throughout the rest of the pregnancy, the kidneys

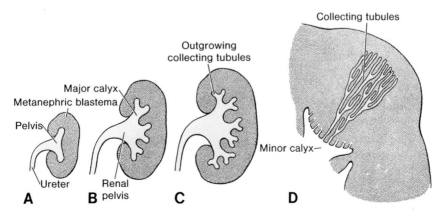

FIGURE 27.1-2: Development of the renal pelvis calyces and collecting tubules of the metanephros at 6 weeks **(A)**, at the end of 6 weeks **(B)**, at 7 weeks **(C)**, and in the newborn **(D)**. (Reprinted with permission from Sadler TW. The urogenital system. In: Sadler TW, ed. *Langman's Medical Embryology.* 9th ed. Philadelphia, PA: Lippincott Williams & Wilkins; 2004:321–362.)

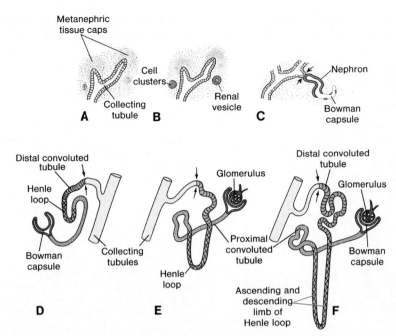

FIGURE 27.1-3: Stages in the development of a metanephric excretory unit (nephron). **A:** Metanephric cap stage. **B:** Renal vesicle stage. **C:** S-shape tubule stage. **D:** Bowman capsule stage. **E:** Glomerulus and proximal tubule stage. **F:** Distal convoluted tubule stage. The *arrows* point to the place where the excretory unit establishes an open communication that allows a flow of urine from the glomerulus into the collecting system. (Reprinted with permission from Sadler TW. The urogenital system. In: Sadler TW, ed. *Langman's Medical Embryology*. 9th ed. Philadelphia, PA: Lippincott Williams & Wilkins; 2004:321–362.)

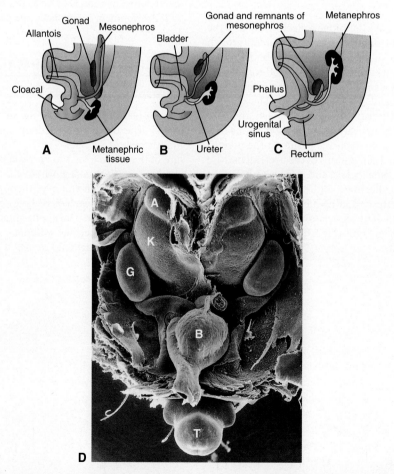

FIGURE 27.1-4: A–C: Cloacal partition into urogenital sinus and bladder anteriorly and rectum posteriorly. The ascent of the kidney is illustrated as well. **D:** Scanning electron micrograph of a mouse embryo showing the kidneys in the pelvis. *A*, adrenal gland; *B*, bladder; *G*, gonad; *K*, kidney; *T*, tail. (Reprinted with permission from Sadler TW, ed. *Langman's Medical Embryology*. 9th ed. Philadelphia, PA: Lippincott Williams & Wilkins; 2004:321–362.)

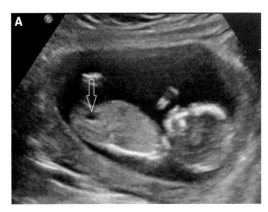
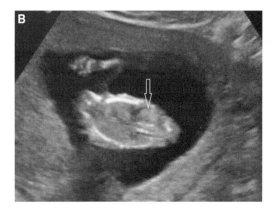

FIGURE 27.1-5: Fetal urinary tract at 13 weeks' gestation. **A:** The *arrow* points to the fluid-filled bladder. **B:** Coronal view. The *arrow* points to a hyperechoic normal kidney. Note the hypoechoic adrenal lying above the kidney.

will grow and their echogenicity will evolve. The renal growth can be assessed by the measurement of the sagittal length compared with established nomograms (Table 33 in Appendix A1). Renal length can be evaluated through the formula "renal length in cm = number of gestation weeks $\times$ 1.1." This growth can also be assessed by the evaluation of renal parenchymal area or even volume calculation, although these types of measurements are not performed routinely. With evolving gestational age, the echogenicity of the renal cortex decreases with respect to the liver, and should be less echogenic than the liver by the third trimester.

CMD should be progressively demonstrated—hypoechoic medulla compared to relatively hyperechoic cortex—starting at the fourth month of gestation (Figs. 27.1-6A and 27.1-7A). The renal vessels can easily be demonstrated with color or power Doppler (see Fig. 27.1-6B).[15-20]

The fetal bladder becomes larger, containing more urine (see Figs. 27.1-6C and 27.1-7B), and cycles of filling and emptying will be observed. These cycles slow at the end of the pregnancy especially in female fetuses. Even almost empty, it should be possible to identify the bladder using the umbilical arteries as

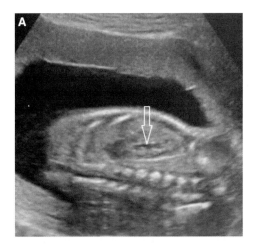
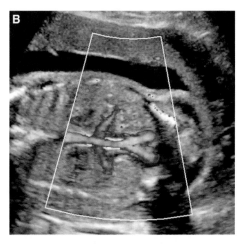
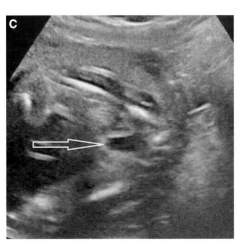
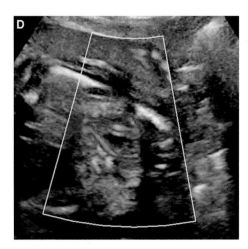

FIGURE 27.1-6: Fetal urinary tract. **A:** Sagittal US of a normal kidney in the second trimester. The renal cortical echogenicity has reduced as compared with Figure 27.1-5B. Some urine (*arrow*) distends the renal pelvis. A corticomedullary differentiation is beginning to appear (hyperechoic cortex/hypoechoic medulla). **B:** Coronal view of the fetal trunk with power Doppler displaying the aorta and renal vessels. **C:** Axial view of the lower pelvis and bladder (*arrow*). **D:** Color Doppler demonstrates the two umbilical arteries along each side of the bladder.

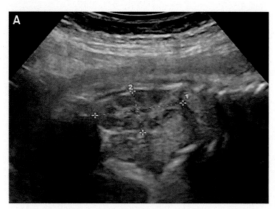 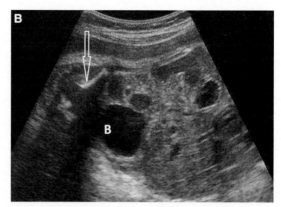

FIGURE 27.1-7: Fetal urinary tract. **A:** Sagittal view through the left kidney (limited by the *crosses*) in the third trimester. A corticomedullary differentiation is now obvious (hypoechoic medulla). The kidney measures 36 mm at 32 weeks, appropriate for the calculated length (number of weeks × 1.1 cm). **B:** Oblique view of the fetal abdomen; a round urine-filled bladder (*B*) is visible. The *arrow* points to the iliac wing.

landmarks (see Fig. 27.1-6D). Filling of the bladder is influenced by maternal hydration. Normally, the fetal ureters are not visualized.[21]

Amniotic fluid volume should always be assessed. The kidney contributes by two-third to the amniotic fluid volume at the beginning of the fourth month of gestation.[22]

Information regarding the normal urinary tract can be obtained at each trimester of the pregnancy using US. In the first trimester, a fluid-filled bladder and hyperechoic kidneys should be identified. In the second and third trimesters, a systematic approach to evaluate the urinary tract includes identifying two kidneys, assessing size and echogenicity, including CMD, identifying the bladder, including size and contour, and evaluating the amniotic fluid volume. If an anomaly is identified, it should be determined whether it is isolated or part of a polymalformative syndrome. MRI should be considered if assessment is incomplete.

Magnetic Resonance Imaging

The advantages of MRI in the fetus with renal anomalies include a large field of view and multiplanar approach that can help assess complex and large urinary tract abnormalities and also associated malformations. In cases with oligohydramnios, MRI can provide better resolution of anomalies and lung volumes for assessment of pulmonary hypoplasia. T2 sequences are well adapted for the visualization of the kidneys, renal pelvis, and bladder. The fetal

kidneys display a homogeneous intermediate hypersignal signal as compared with the liver. Urine in the renal pelvis and bladder is high in signal (Fig. 27.1-8). The use of T1 sequences is useful when a urodigestive fistula is suspected.[7,23–28] Diffusion-weighted sequences can be helpful in locating renal parenchyma in cases of possible pelvic kidneys.

URINARY TRACT ABNORMALITIES

Bilateral Renal Agenesis

Definition: Congenital absence of both kidneys.

Incidence: Bilateral renal agenesis occurs in 1:4,000 births. The condition is three-fold more common in male fetuses, with increased incidence in the offspring of diabetic mothers. It can be isolated or associated with other system malformations and part of syndromes (Table 27.1-3). Bilateral renal agenesis determines the so-called Potter syndrome or sequence (see later).[1,9,29–31]

Embryology and Pathogenesis: Renal agenesis can be explained from either failure of the ureteric bud to develop or from absent interaction between the ureteral bud and the metanephritic mesenchyma. Whatever the embryological "explanation," it is obvious that mutations of the different genes that are involved in the normal renal development (RET, PAX2, WT1, HNFB1) are

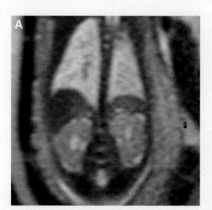 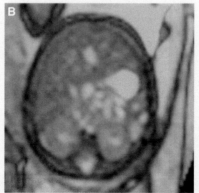 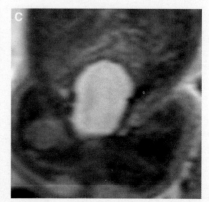

FIGURE 27.1-8: T2 MRI of the normal urinary tract. **A:** Coronal view through both kidneys, intermediate signal compared with the liver and spleen. **B:** Axial scan through the kidneys (and liver). **C:** Coronal view through the bladder.

TABLE 27.1-3 Syndromes Including Unilateral or Bilateral Renal Agenesis

Autosomal Dominant

Acro-renal-ocular syndrome
Branchio-oto-renal syndrome
Ectrodactyly–ectodermal dysplasia—cleft palate (EEC) syndrome
Pallister–Hall syndrome
Renal coloboma syndrome
Townes–Brocks syndrome
HNF1Beta (also sporadic)

Autosomal Recessive

Acro-renal-mandibular syndrome
Antley–Bixler syndrome
Fraser syndrome
Fryns syndrome
Rokitansky sequence
Smith–Lemli–Opitz syndrome

X-linked

Goltz–Gorlin syndrome
Kallmen syndrome
Lenz microphthalmia syndrome

Sporadic

Caudal regression syndrome
Goldenhar syndrome
Mullerian duct aplasia – renal agenesis – cervicothoracic somite dysplasia (MURCS) association
Kabuki syndrome
VATER syndrome
HNF1Beta

Chromosomal

Miller–Dieker syndrome
XXX
Deletion 22q

Modified from Desphande C, Hennekam RC. Genetic syndromes and prenatally detected renal anomalies. *Semin Fetal Neonatal Med.* 2008;13:171–180.

responsible for a wide range of anomalies that include uni- or bilateral renal agenesis, (multicystic) dysplasia, or hypoplasia. This explains the recurrence of the disease, sometimes under another phenotype; furthermore, these various genes are also involved in the development of the genital tract, and this explains why genital tract anomalies are associated in the case of their mutations.[2,9–11,14,32]

Diagnosis

Ultrasound: The sonographic diagnosis of bilateral renal agenesis can be difficult during the first trimester since at this stage, the amniotic fluid volume is normal as it is mainly produced by the placenta; the diagnosis is easier during the second and third trimesters, when it can be based on direct and indirect signs (Fig. 27.1-9). The main direct sign is the lack of visualization of kidneys in the lumbar fossae. Indirect signs include nonvisualization of the bladder (Fig. 27.1-9B), absent renal arteries on color Doppler, oligohydramnios, small chest, and club feet. In most cases, the urine-filled bladder is absent (still, a bladderlike structure can be filled backward through a patent urachus). The combination of renal agenesis, small chest, oligohydramnios, club feet, low-set ears, and facial deformation constitutes the so-called Potter syndrome or sequence. Other causes for bilateral nonfunctioning kidneys—for example, bilateral multicystic dysplastic kidneys (MCDKs)—are able to display the same sequence. With bilateral renal agenesis, the adrenals are present and appear elongated (Fig. 27.1-10).[33–35]

MRI: MRI is useful to confirm the absence of renal parenchyma and bladder on T2 sequences. Diffusion-weighted sequences may help identify residual renal parenchyma. Associated malformations may be better assessed by MRI in the presence of oligohydramnios and lung volumes can be better measured to document pulmonary hypoplasia.[7,36]

Differential Diagnosis: The differential diagnosis of bilateral renal agenesis includes cases with poorly or nonfunctioning kidneys such as bilateral renal dysplasia or bilateral MCDK (Fig. 27.1-11). Other diagnoses to consider include bilateral pelvic kidneys or a solitary pelvic kidney (Fig. 27.1-12) (see later). Other causes of oligohydramnios such as intrauterine growth retardation or premature rupture of the membranes should also be considered.

Prognosis: Bilateral renal agenesis has been lethal.[2,36] There have been a few case reports using serial amnioinfusion with resultant improved pulmonary function at delivery. Dialysis and transplantation remain a significant issue long term.[37]

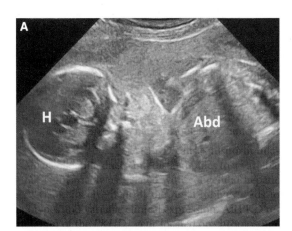
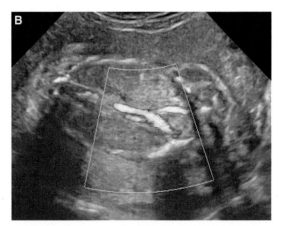

FIGURE 27.1-9: Bilateral renal agenesis. **A:** US through the fetal head (*H*) and abdomen (*Abd*). There is a striking anamnios; no renal structure could be demonstrated. **B:** Color Doppler US enhancing the umbilical vessels. No urine-filled bladder is visible. (Courtesy of B. Broussin, MD.)

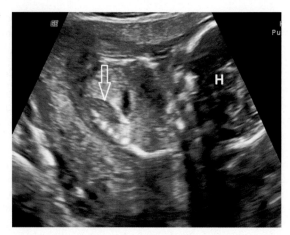

FIGURE 27.1-10: Bilateral renal agenesis. Sagittal US of the fetal body. A hypertrophied globular adrenal appears as a hypoechoic ovoid mass (*arrow*). *H*, fetal head. (Courtesy of R. De Maubeuge, MD.)

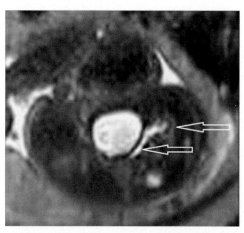

FIGURE 27.1-12: Hypoplastic solitary pelvic kidney. Axial T2 MRI through the fetal pelvis and bladder demonstrates a dilated ureter connected to a hypoplastic kidney (*arrows*) that was not visualized on simultaneous ultrasound.

Management: Genetic counseling is important to evaluate the risk of recurrence.

Chromosomal analysis prenatally may be difficult because of the lack of amniotic fluid.

Recurrence Risk: The recurrence risk ranges between 3% and 6%. There are cases of autosomal dominant and recessive conditions with higher recurrence risks.[1-3]

Unilateral Renal Agenesis

Definition: Congenital absence of one kidney.

Incidence: Unilateral renal agenesis occurs in about 1:500 to 1:1,000 births. There is a male predominance, and the left kidney is more often the one missing. The condition can be isolated or part of polymalformative syndromes (Table 27.1-3). The solitary kidney itself can display anomalies such as ureteropelvic junction (UPJ) or UVJ obstruction as well as vesicoureteric reflux (VUR). Associated genital tract anomalies are commonly encountered.[1,9,38]

Embryology and Pathogenesis: Renal agenesis can be explained from either failure of the ureteric bud to develop or from absent interaction between the ureteral bud and the metanephritic mesenchyma. Mutations of the different genes that are involved in the normal renal development (RET, PAX2, WT1, HNFB1) are responsible for a wide range of anomalies that include renal agenesis, multicystic dysplasia, and hypoplasia. This explains the recurrence of the disease, sometimes under another phenotype; furthermore, these mutations also explain why genital tract anomalies are associated as some of these genes are also involved in its development.

A pseudorenal agenesis can be the result of a complete involution of an MCDK (see later).[2,9-11,14,32]

Diagnosis
Ultrasound: The sonographic diagnosis of a unilateral renal agenesis is based on the inability to visualize the kidney in one of the renal fossae. The corresponding renal artery tends to be absent on color Doppler (Fig. 27.1-13). The corresponding adrenal fills the empty space, as does the colon with left renal agenesis. Colonic loops should not be misinterpreted as a dilated

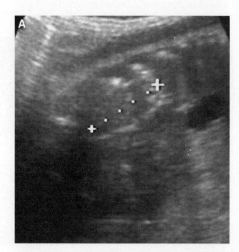
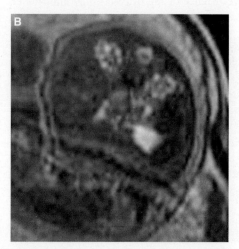

FIGURE 27.1-11: Bilateral multicystic dysplastic kidneys. **A:** Sagittal US through one kidney (between *crosses*), which appears small (20 mm at 30 weeks) and homogeneous, without corticomedullary differentiation. Oligohydramnios is striking. **B:** T2 MRI. The kidneys have multiple tiny cysts.

2">2

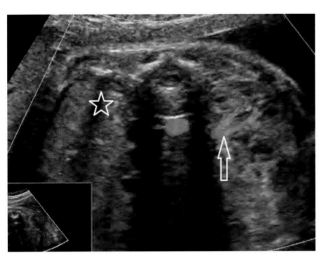

FIGURE 27.1-13: Unilateral renal agenesis. On US with color Doppler in the second trimester, neither renal parenchyma nor renal vessels can be visualized in the right renal fossa (*star*), whereas both are visible present on the left side (*arrow*). (Courtesy of R. De Maubeuge, MD.)

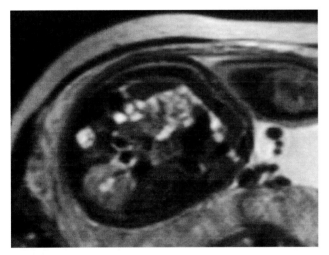

FIGURE 27.1-14: Unilateral renal agenesis. On this T2 MRI, only one kidney is visualized.

ureter. Renal abnormalities such as UPJ, UVJ obstruction, or VUR can be associated findings within the solitary kidney. Often, the solitary kidney undergoes compensatory hypertrophy *in utero*.[33–35,38,39]

Whenever a renal fossa appears empty, one should look for an ectopic location. Renal agenesis can be the result of a complete involution of an MCDK.[32,37,40]

MRI: MRI is rarely performed for a diagnosis of solitary kidney. T2 and diffusion-weighted images can help search for a potential ectopic kidney. Assessment of other anomalies is useful in polymalformative syndromes (Fig. 27.1-14).[5,8,9]

Differential Diagnosis: Unilateral renal hypoplasia, crossed fused ectopia (CFE), involuting MCDK, pelvic kidney.[40]

Prognosis: Excellent if isolated. Poor if the remaining kidney is dysplastic or obstructed and poorly functioning or the anomaly is part of a severe polymalformative syndrome. Solitary kidneys are at higher risk for developing cardiovascular diseases and renal failure.[41,42]

Management: Assessment of the remaining kidney is important to exclude UPJ, UVJ, and VUR.

Recurrence Risk: About 12%, possibly under other phenotypes.

Renal Ectopia

Definition: Abnormal location of one or both kidneys. There are different types of ectopia: simple pelvic ectopia corresponds to a kidney that has not migrated from the pelvis, whereas complex ectopia with fusion that includes horseshoe kidneys (HSKs) and CFE. HSK corresponds to kidneys that fuse through an isthmus that connects (most usually) their lower poles. They are usually located lower than are the normal kidneys. In CFE, both kidneys are fused on the same side. The ureters open within the bladder trigone in the normal location.[43–45]

Incidence: The incidence of pelvic kidneys is estimated at 1:2,500, HSK about 1:400 births and CFE around 1:7,500 births. All forms of renal ectopia are associated with a wide range of other renal anomalies, the commonest being UPJ and VUR. There is also a high prevalence of associated other system malformations, most commonly skeletal and genital (~25%).[43,44]

Embryology and Pathogenesis: Ectopia results from an abnormal ascent of the kidney(s) during embryology. HSK may result from coalescence of the kidney poles during ascent, possibly in relation to abnormal caudal tilting. An abnormal tilting to a higher extent may explain the occurrence of CFE. Vascular and genetic factors are probably involved as well.[43,44]

Diagnosis: The discovery of an empty renal fossa (or bilateral fossae) may lead to the diagnosis of renal ectopia versus renal agenesis. An ectopic pelvic kidney tends to be small and malrotated. CMD in the renal parenchyma should be searched for (Fig. 27.1-15). The ectopic kidney may have a dilated collecting system, or it could be dysplastic or be multicystic dysplastic (Fig. 27.1-16A).

HSKs may be more difficult to diagnose prenatally since the isthmus can be thin. The axis of the fused kidneys may be a hint for the diagnosis as the lower poles are more oblique toward the midline than normal. The demonstration of CMD within

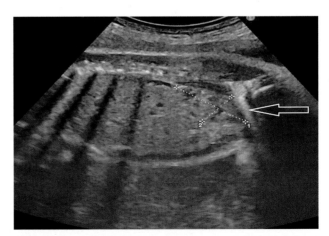

FIGURE 27.1-15: Pelvic kidney. Parasagittal US of the fetal abdomen shows the pelvic kidney is delineated by the *crosses*. The *arrow* points to the right iliac wing. No renal parenchyma could be demonstrated in the left lumbar fossa.

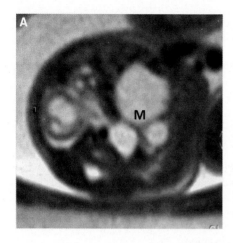 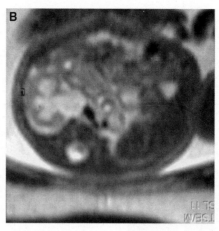

FIGURE 27.1-16: Pelvic MCDK and contralateral ureteropelvic junction (UPJ) obstruction. **A:** Axial MRI through the fetal pelvis displays the multicystic dysplastic kidney (*M*). **B:** Axial MRI through the left kidney shows UPJ obstruction. *MCDK*, multicystic dysplastic kidneys.

the renal parenchyma, especially the isthmus, is confirmatory (Fig. 27.1-17). Each kidney can be affected by UPJ obstruction or MCDK.

CFE is even more difficult to diagnose prenatally. It may be confused with a solitary kidney and/or unilateral renal duplication. The

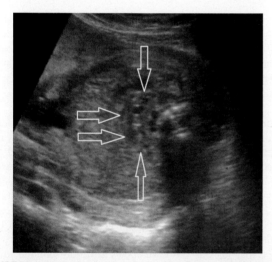

FIGURE 27.1-17: Horseshoe kidney. On axial US through fetal abdomen in the third trimester, the horseshoe kidney (*arrows*) can be identified by demonstration of the corticomedullary differentiation.

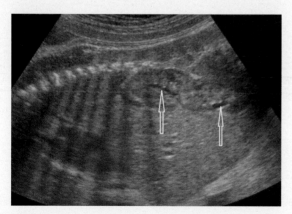

FIGURE 27.1-18: Crossed fused ectopia. On left parasagittal US in the third trimester, the kidney appears elongated owing to the fusion of both kidneys. Two renal pelves (*arrows*) are visualized. (Courtesy of C. Garel, MD.)

clue to the diagnosis is the axes of both kidneys that can be either parallel to each other or at right angles (L-ectopia). The CFE kidney is typically lower than is the normally located one (Fig. 27.1-18).[46,47]

MRI may be useful in evaluating complicated ectopic kidneys, especially those presenting with a multicystic portion or with dilatation.[7]

Differential Diagnosis: A pelvic kidney may be confused with a nonrenal pelvic mass, such as a pelvic teratoma. CFE can be confused with renal duplication or with solitary kidney.

Prognosis: Ectopic kidneys have a good prognosis unless associated with a significant renal malformation or part of a severe polymalformative syndrome.

Management: There is no specific *in utero* management. Chromosomal analysis should be considered in the case of polymalformative syndrome.

Recurrence Risk: Around 10% potentially under another phenotype.[44]

Simple Renal Cyst

Definition: Unilateral, solitary, nongenetically transmitted cystic lesion within the renal parenchyma.[48]

Incidence: Rare, most resolving by 24 weeks' gestation.

Embryology and Pathogenesis: The origin of simple renal cysts is unclear; it may correspond to a sequel of localized ischemia.

Diagnosis
Ultrasound: A simple renal cyst appears as a single cystic structure without septa or calcifications; its size varies from a few millimeters to several centimeters (Fig. 27.1-19). It is localized within the renal cortex. Color Doppler is helpful in order to confirm the intrarenal location of the cyst (Fig. 27.1-19B).

MRI: At MRI, on T2, a renal cyst will appear as a cystic high-signal structure within the kidney.

Differential Diagnosis: The differential diagnosis includes a calyceal diverticulum, a hydrocalyx, and a cystic tumor. In the case of calyceal diverticulum and hydrocalyx, the diagnosis

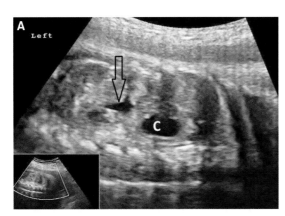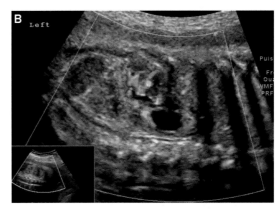

FIGURE 27.1-19: Simple renal cyst. **A:** On parasagittal US through the left kidney in the third trimester, a cystic structure (*C*) is visible within the upper pole of the kidney, and some urine distends the renal pelvis (*arrow*). **B:** Color Doppler US, same view as in (**A**), confirms the intrarenal location of the cyst. (Courtesy of R. De Maubeuge, MD.)

would be confirmed by the demonstration of a connection with the pyelocalyceal system. A tumor will usually appear as a cystic multiseptated mass. A hereditary renal cystic disease may start with a unilateral cyst; follow-up and familial history would help reassess the diagnosis. Cysts in the upper pole of a kidney should be differentiated from a dilated upper pole moiety of a duplex kidney.

Prognosis: Excellent if isolated with no specific management *in utero.*

Cystic Renal Diseases

Definition: Uni- or bilateral presence of multiple cystic lesions within the renal cortex or medulla or both. The cystic lesions may have a genetic (bilateral diseases) or nongenetic transmission (uni- or bilateral diseases). Obstructive cystic dysplasia and MCDK are the commonest diseases without genetic transmission. Autosomal recessive polycystic kidney disease (ARPKD) and autosomal dominant polycystic kidney disease (ADPKD) are the commonest ones with genetic transmission. Cystic renal diseases can present as isolated renal anomalies or as part of a syndrome.[12,48–54]

Embryology and Pathogenesis: The Potter classification of renal cystic diseases has been replaced by a classification based on the genetic or nongenetic origin of the renal cystic diseases. Genetic renal cystic diseases include ARPKD and ADPKD as well as glomerulocystic kidney disease (GCKD), medullary cystic dysplasia associated with syndromes and nephronophthisis (NPHP)/medullary cystic dysplasia complex.[49–53] Among the nongenetic cystic diseases, obstructive cystic dysplasia and MCDK are the most common. Obstructive dysplasia is associated with urinary tract dilatation and various congenital uropathies. Of note, some cases of MCDK are genetically transmitted.

A further step in the characterization and understanding of genetically transmitted cystic renal diseases has been achieved through their recognition as part of the group of *ciliopathies* (Table 27.1-2). Primary cilia are microtubules, antenna-like cellular organelles that extend outward from the surface of many cells of the renal tubule epithelium. These organelles are rich in receptors, ion channels, and signaling proteins activated by mechanical or chemical stimuli. Cilia regulate cell proliferation and differentiation in the developing and mature kidneys. Any defect

in the structures or function of primary cilium may lead to various cystic phenotypes. Cilia are encountered in various sites and organs of the human body (i.e., liver, lungs), and this explains the potential association of cystic renal changes and other malformations encountered in various syndromes.[10–12,48–50] The cilia concept has induced a more global approach in renal cystic diseases combining renal and hepatic diseases. Hepatorenal fibrocystic diseases are characterized by developmental abnormalities of the portociliary hepatic system in association with cystic degeneration of the kidney. They encompass various inherited diseases. The hepatic lesions are usually demonstrated by histology only and to a lesser extent by imaging. One or several genetic defects have been demonstrated (Table 27.1-2). As some genetic loci mutations can be located close one to another, not surprisingly, different diseases may have similar sonographic appearances (i.e., tuberous sclerosis and ADPKD → the so-called contiguous genes syndrome).[50–54]

Diagnosis
Ultrasound: Imaging plays an essential role in detecting and characterizing renal cystic diseases as well as follow-up.[53–56]

Standard high-resolution sonographic images are essential. The knowledge of histological changes that occur in cystic diseases helps one to understand their sonographic appearance (Table 27.1-4).[52] The examination includes measuring renal size, defining echogenicity of the cortex compared with liver and medulla (hypoechoic, absent, or hyperechoic), assessment of the CMD (present, absent, or reversed) and presence of cysts (number, size, and location), or calcifications as well as evaluation of the pelvicalyceal system.[53–57]

Two main sonographic features lead to the suspicion of renal cystic diseases: the presence of renal cysts and the detection of hyperechoic kidneys (Figs. 27.1-20 and 27.1-21).[53–57] The "cysts" that are visualized on US result either from renal tubular dilatation, glomerular cysts, or from real cysts. They develop anywhere in the kidney and can be uni- or bilateral. Renal hyperechogenicity may involve the entire kidney, only the cortex, or only the medulla. The discovery of hyperechoic kidneys can be challenging as there are no objective US criteria defined up to 32 weeks' gestation; after 32 weeks, the hyperechogenicity is less subjective and should be considered abnormal whenever the renal cortex appears more echoic than the liver or spleen.[20] Once a suspicion of a renal cystic disease has arisen, the evaluation of the US findings should be standardized in a decision tree–type approach (Fig. 27.1-22).[51]

TABLE 27.1-4	Main Histological Changes in Renal Cystic Diseases
DISEASE	**HISTOLOGICAL CHANGES**
Autosomal dominant polycystic kidney disease	Rounded cysts (from a few millimeters to several centimeters) developing in the medulla and cortex anywhere on the renal tubules or collecting tubules. Glomerular cysts can be present
Autosomal recessive polycystic kidney disease	Fusiform dilatation (1–2 mm in diameter) of the collecting ducts, mainly into the medulla but extending toward the cortex with normal glomeruli
Bardet–Biedl syndrome	Medullary cystic dysplasia with preservation of superficial cortex. Progressive tubulointerstitial nephropathy
Glomerulo-cystic kidney disease	Glomerular cysts without tubular dilatation anywhere in the renal cortex; most visible in the subcapsular areas
Nephro-nophthisis	Tubular distension. Cysts at the corticomedullary junction with nonspecific tubulointerstitial nephritis and varying degrees of glomerulosclerosis
Medullary cystic dysplasia	Extensive dilatation of the medullary tubules extending toward the cortex, which is compressed and thinned
Obstructive dysplasia	Cystic dilatation of primitive ducts. Nodules of metaplastic cartilage and renal dysplasia may be present
Multicystic dysplastic kidney disease	Ductal dilatations, most marked peripherally. Paucity of nephrons. Diffuse renal dysplasia with occasional metaplastic cartilage

Modified from Bisaglia M, Galliani CA, Senger C, et al. Renal cystic diseases: a review. *Adv Anat Pathol.* 2006;13:26–56.

TABLE 27.1-5	Differential Diagnosis of Fetal Hyperechoic and Cystic Kidneys

Hyperechoic Kidneys with Normal or Moderately Enlarged Kidneys

Renal cystic diseases
TCF2-gene mutation
Autosomal recessive polycystic kidney disease
Autosomal dominant polycystic kidney disease

Maternally induced diseases
Diabetes
Neutral endopeptidase autoimmune glomerulopathy
Cytomegalovirus infection
Antagonists
Angiotensin II

Metabolic diseases
Nephrotic syndromes, Finnish type
Obstructive dysplasia
"Transient"

Bilateral Multiple Cysts

Autosomal recessive polycystic kidney disease
Autosomal dominant polycystic kidney disease
Bilateral multicystic dysplastic kidney disease (only in fetus)
Bilateral obstructive dysplasia
Syndromes (e.g., Bardet–Biedl, Zellweger)

Fetal Macrocysts (>2 cm)

Tuberous sclerosis
Simpson–Golabi–Behmel syndrome
TCF2-gene mutation
Joubert syndrome

Color Doppler assessment is useful in selected cases.[9] Associated malformations should be searched for with particular assessment of the liver and genital tract. Family history is important, and whenever cystic kidneys are suspected, it is useful to perform a sonographic examination to the parents to check for "unknown" familial disease.[58]

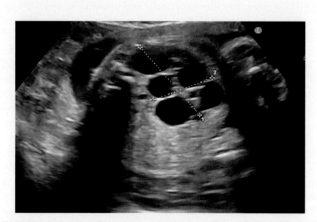

FIGURE 27.1-20: Left multicystic dysplastic kidney. US in the second trimester shows typical multicystic patter, and no renal parenchyma or renal pelvis can be visualized.

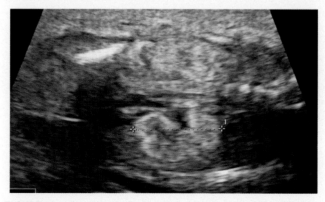

FIGURE 27.1-21: Glomerulocystic disease. Coronal US of both kidneys, which appear hyperechoic but normal sized. Family history was positive. (Reproduced from Avni FE, Garel C, Cassart M, et al. Imaging and classification of congenital cystic renal diseases. *AJR Am J Roentgenol.* 2012;198:1004–1013. Copyright © 2012 American Roentgen Ray Society.)

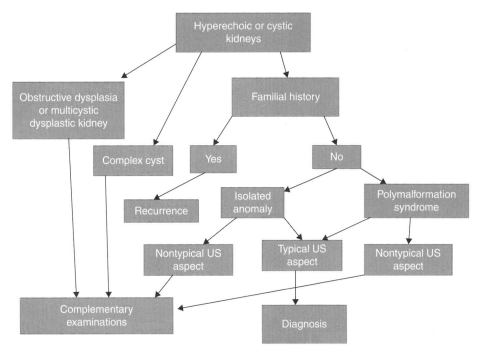

FIGURE 27.1-22: Decision tree approach to renal cystic diseases. US, ultrasound.

MRI: In some patients, MRI provides additional information by demonstrating the renal cysts or associated brain malformation.[7,58]

Management: When bilateral renal cystic disease is identified, the evaluation of the US findings can be standardized in a decision tree–type approach (Fig. 27.1-22). The first step is to rule out dysplasia associated with an obstructive uropathy (with dilatation of the collecting system). Obstructive dysplasia is the commonest cause for a hyperechoic cortex with or without cysts. MCDK is the second diagnosis to consider. If these diagnoses are unlikely, inherited renal cystic diseases should be considered.

Knowledge of any familial history is essential. If *positive*, the finding of abnormal kidneys suggests recurrence (Fig. 27.1-21).

TABLE 27.1-6   Syndromes that Include Cystic Kidneys

Bardet–Biedl syndrome
COACH syndrome
Ellis–van Creveld syndrome
Fryns syndrome
Glutaric acid II
Jeune syndrome
Marden–Walker syndrome
Joubert syndrome
Meckel–Gruber syndrome
Orofaciodigital syndrome
Roberts syndrome
Smith–Lemli–Opitz syndrome
Zellweger syndrome
Tuberous sclerosis
Trisomy 13
Deletion 22q

From Desphande C, Hennekam RC. Genetic syndromes and prenatally detected renal anomalies. *Semin Fetal Neonatal Med.* 2008;13:171–180.

If no familial history is present, cases can be further separated in patients where the renal findings are isolated and limited to the kidney and those where the renal anomalies are associated with malformations of other organs.

There are typical US patterns suggestive of specific diagnoses and nontypical US patterns. A "typical" pattern means typical pattern of all sonographic features that lead to a specific diagnosis (isolated or in association with other malformations). Nonspecific (or nontypical) means that there are no significant features that can lead to a specific diagnosis. For the latter, the diagnosis can be approached using tables of differential diagnosis and syndromes that include renal cysts (Tables 27.1-5 and 27.1-6; Fig. 27.1-23). In undetermined cases, supplementary examinations may help, such as genetic studies or MRI to reach the most accurate diagnosis.

For example, in the fetus, bilateral, very large (>4 standard deviation [SD]) hyperechoic kidneys with hyperechoic medulla (reversed CMD) is a typical pattern for fetal ARPKD (Fig. 27.1-24). The association of "renal cystic changes + malformations" can be characteristic of a specific syndrome (Table 27.1-6). For example, GCKD plus molar tooth sign in the CNS establishes the diagnosis of Joubert syndrome (Fig. 27.1-25).[53,54,57]

Cystic Obstructive Dysplasia

See section on "Urinary Tract Dilatation."

Multicystic Dysplastic Kidney Disease

Definition: Multiple cysts of varying size that do not connect to a central pelvis. No functioning renal parenchyma.[39,40,59–64]

Incidence: Unilateral MCDK occurs in 1:2,500 births, bilateral MCDK occurs in 1:12,000 births.

Embryology and Pathogenesis: MCDK is classically considered to result from aberrant interactions between the ureteral bud and

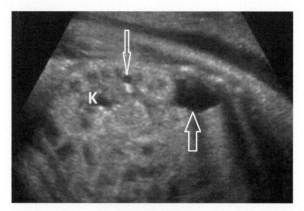

FIGURE 27.1-23: Simpson–Golabi–Behmel syndrome with renal cysts. Sagittal US shows a kidney (K) that appears hyperechoic and contains one large and one tiny (arrows) cyst. Small cysts were visualized in the other kidney as well. Anomalies included signs of an overgrowth syndrome.

the metanephritic blastema. Most cases are sporadic, yet a genetic origin has been established in some cases. Mutations of PAX2, TCF2 (HNF1Beta), and uroplakin have been identified.

On histology, the kidney is highly dysplastic, displaying cysts, primitive abnormal tubules, a few abnormal nephrons,

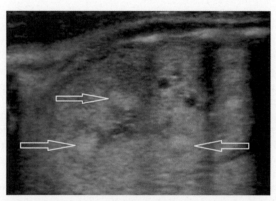

FIGURE 27.1-24: Autosomal recessive polycystic kidney disease with hyperechoic medulla. Sagittal US of one kidney (both displayed the same pattern) shows areas of mottled hyperechogenicities within the renal pyramids (arrows). (Courtesy of C. Garel, MD.)

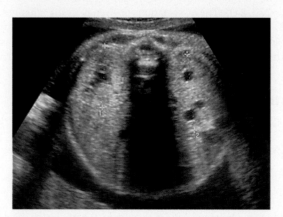

FIGURE 27.1-25: Joubert syndrome. Axial US shows both kidneys to be hyperechoic without corticomedullary differentiation. There are scattered cysts within the parenchyma around the corticomedullary junction. The fetus displayed a molar tooth sign on fetal MRI (not shown). (Courtesy of M. Molho, MD.)

and foci of cartilage. In rare instances, a few functioning normal nephrons are present and the kidney would display some function. It can be uni- or bilateral (lethal form). It can develop in ectopic or duplex kidneys. Unilateral MCDK is associated with contralateral renal anomalies such as UPJ or VUR in 30% to 40% of cases. It can be associated with malformations of several other systems, especially of the genital tract.

Ultrasound: MCDK is usually detected during the second-trimester US examination. Its diagnosis is straightforward in typical cases: multiple cysts of varying sizes without normal renal parenchyma and without recognized renal pelvis (Fig. 27.1-20). The cysts may be tiny (microcystic form) (Fig. 27.1-26) or very large (giant form) (Fig. 27.1-27). The homolateral ureter may be enlarged. Furthermore, an MCDK may affect an ectopic kidney (Fig. 27.1-16A) or any moiety of a duplex one (Fig. 27.1-28). Once an MCDK has been detected, associated anomalies should be searched for at the level of the contralateral kidney (Fig. 27.1-16B), the genital tract, or other systems. The contralateral kidney may undergo compensatory hypertrophy already *in utero*, which can be assessed through measurement of the contralateral kidney (Fig. 27.1-26).[39] Furthermore, MCDK

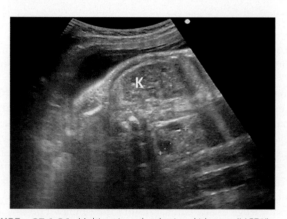

FIGURE 27.1-26: Multicystic dysplastic kidney (MCDK) with contralateral hypertrophy. Oblique US in the third trimester shows the small MCDK (limited by the crosses), which is displaying small cysts. The contralateral kidney (K) measures 42 mm in length at 30 weeks, which confirms hypertrophy.

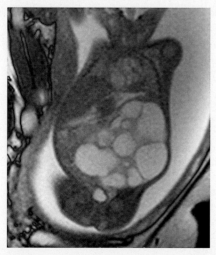

FIGURE 27.1-27: Multicystic dysplastic kidney (MCDK). T2 coronal MRI shows a large MCDK occupying a large part of the fetal abdomen. (Courtesy of K. Chaumoitre, MD.)

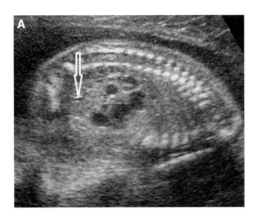
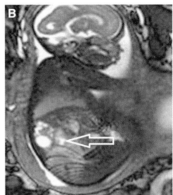

FIGURE 27.1-28: Multicystic dysplastic kidney developing within the upper poles of a duplex kidney bilaterally. **A:** Parasagittal US of one kidney demonstrates multicystic appearance of the upper moiety. The lower pole pelvis is slightly dilated (*arrow*). **B:** Parasagittal MRI confirms the lower moiety is displaced anteriorly and slightly distended (*arrow*).

may undergo regression *in utero* or after birth, resulting eventually in a pseudorenal agenesis.[40,64]

MRI: MRI may be helpful to characterize very large or ectopic MCDK and unusual complications of the anomaly as well as complications of the contralateral kidney (see Fig. 27.1-16). In the case of bilateral MCDK, cysts are present in both kidneys, and oligohydramnios is the rule as both kidneys are nonfunctioning. MRI is helpful to differentiate bilateral hypoplasia from bilateral MCDK by showing the cystic lesions (Fig. 27.1-11).[7]

Differential Diagnosis: The differential diagnosis of unilateral MCDK includes unusual UPJ obstruction, obstructive cystic dysplasia, cystic mesoblastic nephroma, and segmental dysplasia. The differential diagnosis of bilateral MCDK includes bilateral hypodysplasia, cystic dysplasia, and other inherited cystic renal diseases (see later).

Prognosis: The prognosis of unilateral MCDK is excellent as isolated anomaly. Bilateral MCDK is lethal, however.

Management: With unilateral MCDK, the other kidney, if abnormal on postnatal US, should be evaluated for possible UPJ, UVJ, and VUR.

Recurrence Rate: About 12% in the case of genetic transmission.

Autosomal Recessive Polycystic Kidney Disease

Definition: ARPKD is an autosomal recessively transmitted disease that causes fusiform dilatation of the renal collecting ducts and distal tubules, resulting in large echogenic kidneys.[12,49,65–69]

Incidence: Estimated at 1:20,000 births.[66–69]

Embryology and Pathogenesis: ARPKD causes fusiform dilatation of the renal collecting ducts and distal tubules to a variable extent, and that is invariably associated with congenital hepatic fibrosis. The variable involvement of the renal tubules leads to variable phenotypes and variable clinical expression. ARPKD results from mutation of the *PKHD1* gene located on chromosome 6p12. Truncating mutations are associated with a higher perinatal mortality, whereas missense mutations are associated with milder

forms of the diseases. The disease has a variable expressivity even in the same family.[66–69]

Diagnosis

Ultrasound: The diagnosis of ARPKD is usually achieved in the second and third trimesters, although there have been reports of cases detected in the first trimester.

Because of the histological variability, ARPKD displays a variety of US patterns; still, "markedly enlarged hyperechoic kidneys (4 to 8 SD above the mean) without CMD" is the most frequent pattern encountered on obstetrical US examination performed during the second and third trimesters (Fig. 27.1-29). Other possible appearances include hyperechoic very large kidneys with reversed CMD (very specific pattern; see Fig. 27.1-24), moderately enlarged hyperechoic kidneys, or even normal kidneys (at least at the start of the disease). Renal cysts may be observed already *in utero*; they tend to be located within the medulla (Fig. 27.1-30). The US patterns may evolve during pregnancy.

In cases with recurring disease, the US appearance may vary from one pregnancy to another.

Severely affected fetuses display a "Potter"-like phenotype as oligohydramnios and pulmonary hypoplasia are associated findings.

At the level of the liver, small hilar cysts can rarely be visualized. The hepatic fibrosis will not be detected *in utero*.

MRI: MRI may potentially display tiny cysts not visualized on US and help characterize the diseases.[7,58]

Differential Diagnosis: The differential diagnosis of ARPKD includes the other causes of enlarged hyperechoic kidneys, including Bardet–Biedl syndrome (BBS), HNF1Beta mutation, other disorders with glomerulocystic kidneys, and rarely ADPKD.[50–55,57]

Prognosis: Of those affected, 50% will die in the perinatal period because of pulmonary hypoplasia and renal failure.

Survivors will display features of renal failure leading to renal transplantation in childhood. Some patients with a mild form of the disease will be detected only later in childhood.[12,49,65–68]

Genetic counseling and evaluation of the postnatal prognosis in the light of US, genetic results, and degree of renal failure.

Recurrence Risk: ARPKD is transmitted as an autosomal recessive trait.

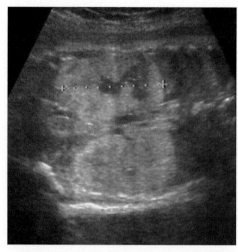

FIGURE 27.1-29: Autosomal recessive polycystic kidney disease. Coronal US through both kidneys demonstrates enlarged (8 cm), diffusely hyperechoic kidneys without corticomedullary differentiation. (Reproduced from Avni FE, Garel C, Cassart M, et al. Imaging and classification of congenital cystic renal diseases. *AJR Am J Roentgenol.* 2012;198:1004–1013. Copyright © 2012 American Roentgen Ray Society.)

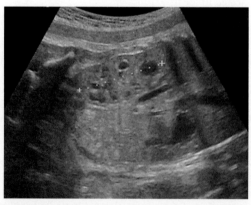

FIGURE 27.1-30: Autosomal recessive polycystic kidney disease with intramedullary cysts. Sagittal US through the enlarged right kidney shows cysts within several pyramids.

Autosomal Dominant Polycystic Kidney Disease

Definition: ADPKD is the most common genetically transmitted renal cystic disease in humans and is characterized by the presence of multiple large cysts developing at any level of the nephron. The disease affects not only the kidneys but also the liver and the pancreas. There is also an increased risk of associated intracranial aneurisms and subarachnoid cysts.[12,41,53,70,71]

Incidence: One or 2 per 1,000 births.

Embryology, Genetics, and Pathogenesis: ADPKD includes at least three phenotypically similar but genetically different entities. Mutations of the gene *PKD1*, located on chromosome 6, and gene *PKD2*, located on chromosome 4, have been described. A 3D gene mutation PKD3 is suspected but not demonstrated. Ten percent *de novo* mutations occur as well. About 15% of cases may present asynchronously with the involvement of only one kidney first.[53,55]

Diagnosis: A typical pattern suggesting fetal ADPKD includes normal-sized kidneys with a hyperechoic cortex leading to an increased CMD (Fig. 27.1-31). Some cortical renal cysts may be observed already *in utero*. In the case of US suspicion, US of the parents may reveal cystic disease as well. Normally appearing renal US in the fetus or in the parents does not exclude the disease. Associated urinary tract malformation such as duplex kidney or UPJ obstruction can be observed.

In rare cases, hyperechoic large kidneys with subcortical and/or diffuse parenchymal cysts associated with oligohydramnios may lead to a diagnosis of glomerulocystic type of ADPKD (see later) (Fig. 27.1-32).[55,71,72]

Differential Diagnosis: Hyperechoic kidneys with increased CMD can result from various anomalies, including consequences of infectious or vascular insults to the kidneys or fetuses affected by congenital nephrotic syndromes. It can also correspond to a normal variant.[52-56]

Prognosis: The disease becomes clinically obvious in the fourth and fifth decades of life, but because of US screening, fetal and

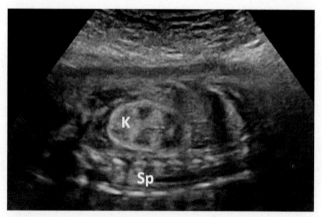

FIGURE 27.1-31: Autosomal dominant polycystic kidney disease. Sagittal US shows an enlarged kidney (*K*) with an echogenic cortex. The corticomedullary differentiation is increased. *Sp*, fetal spine.

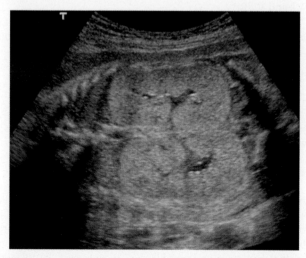

FIGURE 27.1-32: Autosomal dominant polycystic kidney disease, glomerulocystic type (GLMC). Coronal US in the third trimester shows both kidneys are markedly enlarged and hyperechoic and lack corticomedullary differentiation. (Courtesy of C. Garel, MD.)

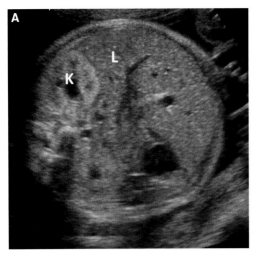
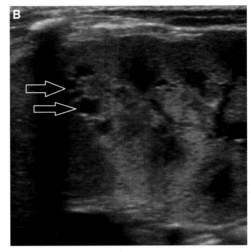

FIGURE 27.1-33: TCF2/HNF1Beta mutation. **A:** Transverse US in the third trimester demonstrates hyperechoic parenchyma compared with the liver (*L*). Its corticomedullary differentiation is preserved; the renal size is normal. *K*, kidney. **B:** Postnatal image of the right kidney. Tiny subcapsular cysts are visible (*arrows*). These are typical for glomerulocystic pattern of the disease.

neonatal cases are increasingly detected. Patients with the GLMK type of ADPKD may develop neonatal hypertension and renal failure.

Management: Familial enquiry is mandatory and renal US should be performed on both parents (and if possible on grandparents). One should keep in mind that absence of cysts in young parents does not exclude the disease as cysts may start to appear as late as 36 years of age.

Recurrence: ADPKDs are transmitted as an autosomal dominant trait.

Anomalies of the gene TCF2 (or HNF1Beta mutations)

Definition: Anomalies of the gene TCF2 encompass a spectrum of diseases of the kidney that includes renal cystic disease, various renal malformations (uni- or bilateral agenesis, hypoplasia, dysplasia, MCDK) as well as pancreatic (diabetes-type MODY V) and genital malformations. Histologically, the main feature is the demonstration of glomerular cysts—in over 5% of the surface of the renal parenchyma—without dilated tubules.[51,73–77]

Incidence: The incidence is unknown, but the condition is increasingly being detected.

Embryology, Genetics, and Pathogenesis: Transcription gene factor 2 (TCF2) is localized on chromosome 17 and encodes the protein hepatocyte nuclear factor-1Beta (HNF1Beta). It is one of the principal genes involved in the development of the kidney, pancreas, and genital tract. HNF1Beta is also expressed in the neural tube, the biliary tract, the esophagus, and the lungs. HNF1Beta regulates various genes involved (in the mouse) in cilium formations (UMOD, PKHD1, PKD2). The genetic transmission is autosomal dominant but cases of sporadic occurrence are very common.[73–77]

Histologically, the main feature is the demonstration of glomerular cysts—in over 5% of the surface of the renal parenchyma—without dilated tubules.[73–77]

Diagnosis: The TCF2 mutation has become the most frequently recognized cause of hyperechoic kidneys in the fetus (usually normal-sized kidneys) (Fig. 27.1-33). Cysts may be either tiny and subcapsular or very large, resembling postnatal ADPKD. The amniotic fluid volume is typically normal.

MRI may display the very characteristic subcapsular cysts (Fig. 27.1-34).[76,77]

Differential Diagnosis: Hyperechoic kidneys with increased CMD can result from various anomalies, including infectious or vascular insults to the kidneys, congenital nephrotic syndromes. It can also correspond to a normal variant[51–53,55] (Table 27.1-5).

Prognosis: *In utero*, the prognosis is good and depends on the presence of associated malformation. Postnatally, the prognosis will depend upon the progression of renal disease and diabetes.

Recurrence: HNF1Beta is transmitted through a dominant trait, but a large number of sporadic mutations do occur.

Other Renal Genetically Transmitted Renal Cystic Diseases

Renal cystic diseases can present as an isolated renal disease or can be a symptom of syndromes associating the renal cysts and other system anomalies. The kidney patterns can point to the diagnosis. See Figure 27.1-22 decision tree approach to renal cystic disease.

- BBS: BBS associates hyperechoic large kidneys resembling ARPKD because of medullary cystic dysplasia. Associated postaxial polydactyly is the clue to the diagnosis (Fig. 27.1-35).[78]
- Meckel–Gruber syndrome (MGS): MGS includes cystic kidneys, CNS anomalies, and polydactyly. Because of massive medullary cystic dysplasia, the renal pyramids will appear cystic and hypoechoic as early as in the first trimester (Fig. 27.1-36).[79]
- Nephronophtisis (NPHPH): NPHPH consists of a group of tubule–interstitial disorders that can be isolated or

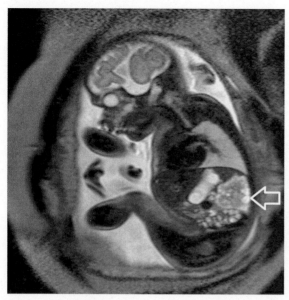

FIGURE 27.1-34: TCF2 mutation. Sagittal T2 MRI of the left kidney shows typical subcapsular cysts (*arrow*). (Courtesy of L. Rausin, MD.)

associated with other organs anomalies (e.g., Joubert or Jeune syndrome). The renal cysts develop mainly in the corticomedullary junction (Fig. 27.1-25). Associated anomalies are the clue to the diagnosis.[80-83]

- Glomerulocystic kidney diseases (GMCK): GMCK can be observed in ADPKD and HNF1Beta mutation as well as in Zellweger syndrome, trisomies, and with urinary tract dilatation (Fig. 27.1-37; see Figs. 27.1-21 and 27.1-33)[84]

Urinary Tract Dilatation

Definition: Dilatation of the renal pelvis, calyces, and/or ureters. The urinary bladder may be dilated as well. Dilatation may result from obstruction, VUR, both, or any.

Incidence: Prenatal renal pelvis dilatation is observed in 1% to 5% of pregnancies; the male-to-female ratio is 2:1. Some 40% to 80% of cases will regress spontaneously.

Embryology and Pathogenesis: Ureteral kinks, delays in openings of the Chwalla membrane, or of the permeation of the urethra can explain the occurrence of some of the dilatation. VUR has been identified in 50% of parents and siblings of affected individuals consistent with a genetic transmission.

Diagnosis: Various criteria are used to standardize urinary tract dilatation. The criterion usually used is the measurement of the anteroposterior (AP) diameter of the renal pelvis on a transverse scan of the fetal abdomen. Many authors agree that the upper limit of the normal pelvic diameter should be 4 mm during the second and 7 mm during the third trimester of the pregnancy. These limits are set in order to detect not only patients who will need corrective surgery (in the case of obstructive dilatation) but also fetuses and neonates with VUR who can be at risk for infections that can cause renal scarring.[4,6,85-90] There is a relation between higher degrees of dilatation and postnatal decreased renal function and need for corrective surgery; therefore, dilatation has been separated into groups of mild (7 to 9 mm), moderate (10 to 15 mm), and severe (>15 mm in the third trimester) dilatation (Fig. 27.1-38). Pyelectasis (Fig. 27.1-39) refers to a visible renal pelvis below the significant threshold. During the second trimester, this can be considered a minor sign of chromosomal anomaly.

Other sonographic evidence includes dilatation of the ureters or calyces (Fig. 27.1-40) or the demonstration of an enlarged bladder (over 12 mm long on a sagittal scan during the first, 3 cm during the second, and 5 cm during the third trimester; Fig. 27.1-41).

Once a dilatation has been detected *in utero*, usually through US, the subsequent evaluation should answer three questions: the origin of the dilatation, the coexistence of associated anomalies, and, finally, the prognosis of the malformation. The most common cause for urinary tract dilatation is UPJ obstruction (around 30%; Fig. 27.1-42). Other causes include nonobstructive and nonrefluxing dilatation (around 20%), UVJ obstruction (around 15%), VUR (around 25%), complicated duplex kidneys, and posterior urethral valves (PUVs).

In selected cases, fetal MRI can be useful, particularly when oligohydramnios is present. Assessment of ureteral dilatation and insertion may be better demonstrated by MRI. MRI provides additional information regarding associated malformations. T2 sequences are useful for assessing the dilated collecting system.

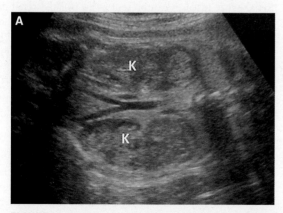
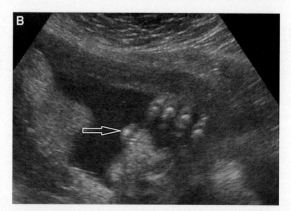

FIGURE 27.1-35: Bardet–Biedl syndrome. **A:** Coronal US in the third trimester shows kidneys (*K*) that are enlarged, hyperechoic, and without corticomedullary differentiation . **B:** Postaxial polydactyly was present (the *arrow* points to a supernumerary digit). Both hands and feet were involved. (Courtesy of C. Garel, MD.)

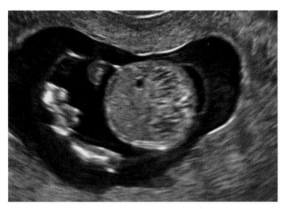

FIGURE 27.1-36: Meckel–Gruber syndrome. Transverse US in the first trimester shows cystic changes at the level of the renal pyramids. There was an associated central nervous system malformation. (Reproduced from Avni FE, Garel C, Cassart M, et al. Imaging and classification of congenital cystic renal diseases. *AJR Am J Roentgenol.* 2012;198:1004–1013. Copyright © 2012 American Roentgen Ray Society.)

T1 sequence can demonstrate the relationship of the bladder to the rectum. Diffusion-weighted images can assess location of renal tissue.[7]

Prognosis and Prenatal Management: Whenever renal dilatation is detected, a complete survey of the fetal anatomy should be performed to detect associated malformations that would indicate the need for chromosomal analysis or the possibility of polymalformative syndromes. Bilateral renal dilatation and bladder outlet obstruction (BOO) have an increased risk of associated chromosomal anomalies.

In the case of dilatation, the prognosis will depend upon the type and extent of anomalies; features of severity include early diagnosis, bilateral marked dilatation, obstructive dysplasia, persistently obstructed bladder, oligohydramnios, and secondary lung hypoplasia. The finding of associated echogenic and/or cystic renal parenchyma is frequently, but only partially, informative about renal function. Conversely, normal cortical echogenicity does not exclude dysplasia.

Still, for most uropathies, the prognosis is good, and the prenatal diagnosis will allow proper management after birth in order to apply best treatment and to prevent any further renal damage.[89,90]

Postnatal Management: After birth, any information relevant to the proper postnatal management should be transmitted to the postnatal team in charge of the newly born and, when necessary, delivery should occur in a tertiary care center. Some conditions require an immediate confirmation and treatment. For example, severe PUVs or prolapsed ectopic ureterocele into the urethra leading to oligoanuria necessitate immediate treatment. Giant UPJ or MCDK—crossing the midline—may interfere with normal digestion with gastric compression, requiring close follow-up as well. Fetuses with oligohydramnios/renal failure may have pulmonary hypoplasia with pneumothoraxes requiring immediate support. In these cases, US and voiding cystourethrography may need to be performed immediately after birth in order to confirm the anomaly. In all other cases, the workup can be planned on an outpatient basis following a decision tree based on postnatal US findings (Fig. 27.1-43). US should be performed after a few days of age to decrease false-negative studies that may occur in the first days of life due to the dehydrated status of the newborn. Only patients with persistent ureteral dilatation should undergo a voiding cystourethrogram (VCUG) and possible renal Lasix scans.[4,6,91–95]

UPJ Obstruction

Definition: Obstruction at the level of the UPJ.

Incidence: The commonest cause for renal dilatation; approximately 1:2,000 births.

Embryology and Pathogenesis: The origin of the obstruction is unclear (ureteral kinking and/or vascular crossing). In most cases, the junction is patent, and the problem is likely functional.

Diagnosis
Ultrasound: The classic appearance is dilation of the renal pelvis and calyces without hydroureter (Figs. 27.1-38 and 27.1-42). UPJ obstruction is most commonly diagnosed in the second

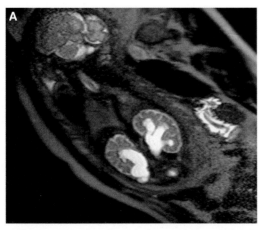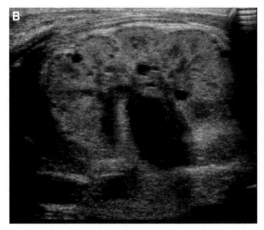

FIGURE 27.1-37: Glomerulocystic disease. **A:** Coronal T2 MRI of the fetal kidney shows bilateral urinary tract dilatation with multiple tiny cysts all around the kidney surfaces on both sides. **B:** Postnatal US of one kidney confirms the dilatation of the renal pelvis and the microscopic subcapsular tiny cysts. (Courtesy of L. Rausin, MD.)

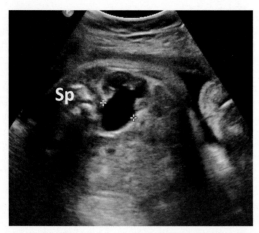

FIGURE 27.1-38: Ureteropelvic junction obstruction with significant dilatation. Transverse US in the second trimester shows the diameter of the dilatation (between the crosses) to be 21 mm. *Sp*, fetal spine.

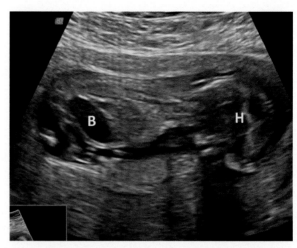

FIGURE 27.1-41: Megacystis (first trimester), prune belly sequence. Sagittal US demonstrates a distended bladder (*B*). *H*, fetal head.

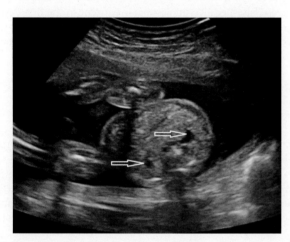

FIGURE 27.1-39: Bilateral mild pyelectasis (second trimester). Transverse US of the fetal abdomen reveals that some urine distends both renal pelves (*arrows*).

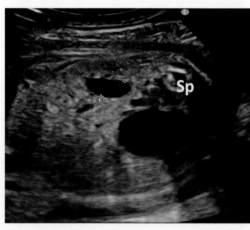

FIGURE 27.1-42: Bilateral ureteropelvic junction obstruction (third trimester). Transverse US of the fetal abdomen shows bilateral asymmetrical dilatation. *Sp*, fetal spine.

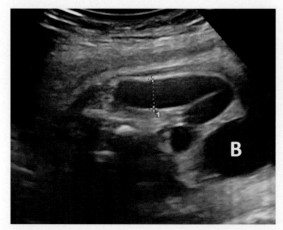

FIGURE 27.1-40: Primary megaureter (third trimester). Oblique US demonstrates a tortuous and dilated ureter (12 mm between *crosses*) above the bladder (*B*).

and/or third trimester. There might be an involution or a progression of the dilatation during pregnancy.[5,88–90]

With marked obstruction, the calyces may enlarge, and echogenic precipitates may be observed at the level of the precalyceal area. Obstruction may lead to rupture of renal calyces, and urinary extravasation collected as a perirenal urinoma (Fig. 27.1-44) or ascitis. In some instances, leakage may protect the renal parenchyma, while in others, renal growth is impaired.

MRI: MRI may be helpful in order to characterize the amount of leakage, as well as underlying renal parenchyma (Fig. 27.1-44B).

Differential Diagnosis: The main differential diagnosis includes nonobstructive, nonrefluxing dilatation that accounts for a large proportion of urinary tract dilatation (~20%) as well as MCDK, VUR, and UVJ obstruction.

Associated Anomalies: Renal anomalies in the contralateral kidney are commonly present in up to 25% of cases. This includes renal agenesis, MCDK, and vesicoureteral reflux. Extrarenal anomalies are noted in up to 12% of affected fetuses.

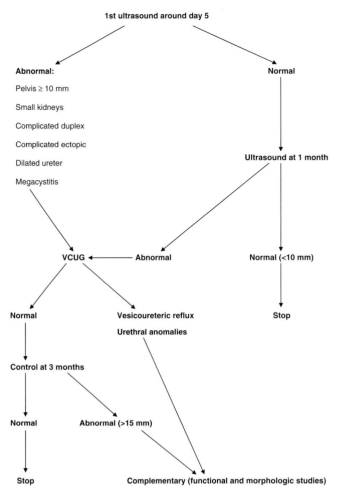

FIGURE 27.1-43: Postnatal workup of antenatally diagnosed urinary tract dilatation.

Prognosis: Outcome is usually good. There is poor correlation between prenatal pelvic dilatation and postnatal function. Thinned, echogenic cortex containing cortical cysts corresponds most likely to obstructive cystic dysplasia with potentially postnatal impaired renal function.

Management: Follow-up US in the third trimester is useful to assess progression and amniotic fluid volume.

Following delivery, in severe cases, evaluation includes ultrasound, VCUG, and renal Lasix scans to assess severity of obstruction. Most cases are managed conservatively unless there is poor differential renal function and/or progressive obstruction. Pyeloplasty is performed in these cases to prevent further deterioration of renal function.

UVJ Obstruction

Definition: Obstruction at the level of the UVJ.

Incidence: 1:6,500. Bilateral in up to 25% of cases. More common in males 2:1.

Embryology and Pathogenesis: Obstruction may be due to a localized region of dysfunction or secondary to an ectopic insertion, or ureterocele.

Diagnosis

Ultrasound: The diagnosis of UVJ obstruction is suspected whenever the fetal ureter is visible and dilated (see Fig. 27.1-40). This can be differentiated from bowel as the urine is clear and then can be followed to the pelvis and/or bladder. The renal pelvic and calyces may be dilated as well. The dilatation may increase *in utero* but usually decreases progressively after birth.

MRI: MRI is helpful in the evaluation of ureteral insertion.

Differential Diagnosis: It can be difficult to differentiate UVJ obstruction from dilatation secondary to high-grade VUR.[96,97] Differential diagnosis includes nonobstructive, nonrefluxing dilatation as well as UPJ obstruction and PUVs.

Prognosis and Management: Follow-up scans are required to follow amniotic fluid stability. Prophylactic antibiotics is started until diagnosis is confirmed. Postnatal assessment includes US, VCUG, and renal Lasix scans. Reimplantation is performed on those with poor or deteriorating renal function. Patients with good renal function can be managed conservatively. Prognosis is generally good even when bilateral.

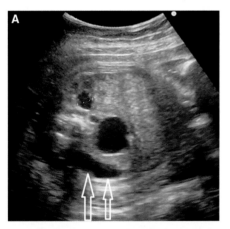

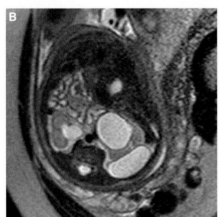

FIGURE 27.1-44: Urinoma associated with ureteropelvic junction obstruction (third trimester). **A:** Transverse US displays asymmetrical dilatation in the right kidney, with perirenal fluid collection (*arrows*) corresponding to the urinoma. **B:** Axial T2 MRI of the fetal abdomen. The urinoma is well demarcated. The renal parenchyma has a homogeneous "normal" signal.

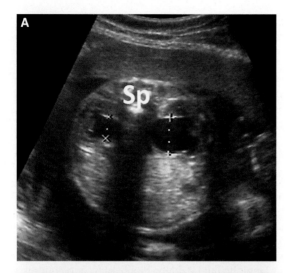

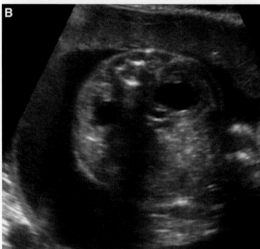

FIGURE 27.1-45: Vesicoureteric reflux (third trimester). **A:** Transverse US of the fetal abdomen through the kidneys. Bilateral dilatation 10 mm to the right and 16 mm to the left. *Sp*, fetal spine. **B:** Transverse scan at same level as in **(A)**, a few seconds later. The dilatation has modified.

Vesicoureteric Reflux

Definition: Retrograde flow of urine from the bladder into the ureter and pelvicalyceal system.

Incidence: Reflux is estimated to occur in up to 1% of all children. Up to 10% of neonates with antenatal diagnosis of dilatation likely have reflux.

Embryology and Pathogenesis: There are two types of reflux: low-grade VUR more commonly diagnosed in girls after a urinary tract infection, and high-grade VUR associated with dilated collecting systems, dysplastic kidneys that occur mainly in boys. The latter is more commonly detected *in utero* with damage occurring *in utero* prior to postnatal infections.

Diagnosis: The diagnosis can be suggested in patients where the dilatation varies at different moments of the same examination (Fig. 27.1-45) or in cases where renal dilatation is associated with impaired renal growth (Fig. 27.1-46).

Differential Diagnosis: Direct diagnosis of VUR *in utero* is difficult. Differential includes UPJ, UVJ obstruction, and PUVs. VUR should be included in the list of differential diagnosis of fetal megacystis, especially in female fetuses—in relation to the pseudo—megacystis–megaureters syndrome (Fig. 27.1-47).[98]

Associated Anomalies: Associated with contralateral renal anomalies, including UPJ obstruction, MCKD, duplex kidney, and renal agenesis.

Prognosis: The majority of VURs resolve by age 2 years. In the rare cases of severe reflux nephropathy, the outcome can be poor in terms of renal function.

Renal Duplication

Definition: Presence of two distinct renal moieties with two separated collecting systems.

Incidence: Occurs in 1:500 births.

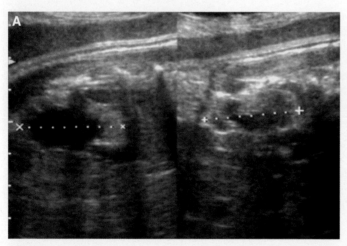
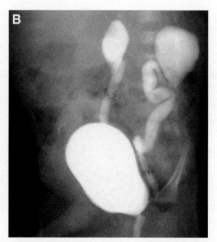

FIGURE 27.1-46: Vesicoureteric reflux associated with hypodysplastic kidneys (third trimester). **A:** Sagittal US through both kidneys (limited by *crosses*) shows that both are dilated and small, measuring 25 and 22 mm in length at 31 weeks. **B:** Postnatal voiding cystography shows bilateral grade IV VUR.

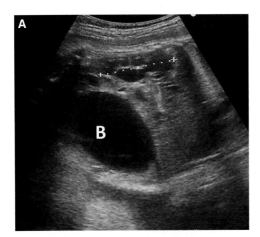

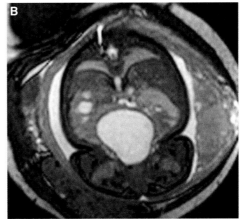

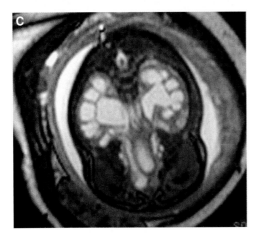

FIGURE 27.1-47: Megacystis associated with massive bilateral vesicoureteric reflux. **A:** Sagittal US through one kidney (delineated by the *crosses*) and the enlarged bladder (*B*). Amniotic fluid volume was normal. **B:** Coronal T2 MRI shows the enlarged bladder. **C:** Coronal T2 MRI through the dilated kidneys and ureters. T1 images demonstrated a normal colon, excluding megacystis, microcolon, and hypoperistalsis syndrome (not shown).

Embryology and Pathology: It results from a supernumerary ureteral bud budding from the primitive nephritic duct.

Diagnosis

Ultrasound: Shows two collecting systems separated by a cortical band that can be visualized (Fig. 27.1-48) unless an associated urinary tract malformation is observed, it should be considered to be a normal variant. If dilatation is demonstrated in either upper or lower moiety, the condition should be considered abnormal and requires a complete workup postnatally (Figs. 27.1-49 and 27.1-50).

Obstruction (Fig. 27.1-49), MCDK or reflux, may develop in either moiety of the duplication (see Fig. 27.1-28). The upper pole may be completely dysplastic and small (Fig. 27.1-50A) or very large. The upper pole may be associated with extravesical insertion of a ureter (Fig. 27.1-49C). An ectopic ureterocele is seen as a septum within the bladder (Fig. 27.1-50B). The ureterocele may collapse because of bladder filling or protrude into the bladder neck, inducing BOO. "Disappearance" of a ureterocele has been described as urine production of the dysplastic upper pole may reduce. The renal parenchyma related to an obstructive moiety may display evidence for obstructive (cystic) dysplasia (Fig. 19-50A). Dysplastic parenchyma may also be associated with high-grade reflux.[99–101]

MRI: MRI may better demonstrate an extravesical insertion of a ureter (see Fig. 27.1-49B, C).

Differential Diagnosis: VUR, UVJ obstruction, upper pole renal cysts, and adrenal anomalies could be considered in the differential.

Outcome/Management: Prognosis is generally good. The function of the kidney depends on the degree of dysplasia affecting the upper pole moiety. The lower pole moiety may have severe VUR that may be associated with marked dysplasia. Large ureteroceles or bilateral ureteroceles can obstruct both kidneys, resulting in oligohydramnios; therefore, follow-up sonograms are recommended.

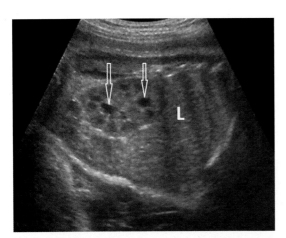

FIGURE 27.1-48: Uncomplicated duplex kidney (third trimester). Sagittal US through the kidney shows two separated collecting systems (*arrows*). *L*, fetal liver.

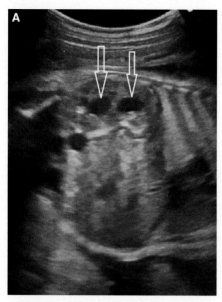
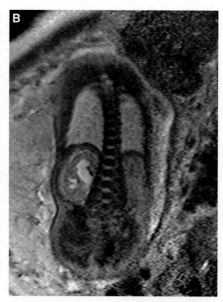
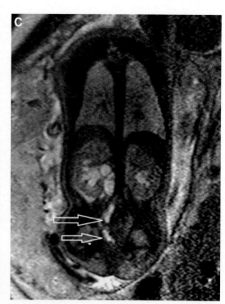

FIGURE 27.1-49: Duplex system with ectopic insertion of the upper pole ureter (third trimester). **A:** Sagittal US of the right kidney shows that the upper and lower moieties are dilated (*arrows*). **B:** Coronal T2 MRI of the fetal urinary tract shows a dilated upper pole. **C:** Coronal T2 MRI demonstrates the dilated lower pole as well as the distended upper pole ectopic ureter (*arrows*) that inserts below the bladder neck. (Courtesy of M. Cassart, MD.)

Following delivery, infants are placed on prophylactic antibiotics. US, VCUG, and renal Lasix scans are performed postnatally at 2 to 3 weeks of age. In case of large ureterocele, US should be performed during the first days of life as the ureterocele may protrude in the urethra and induce BOO. Cystoscopy with puncture of the ureterocele may be performed to preserve function in the upper pole and prevent obstruction; yet rupture of the ureterocele predisposes to VUR. If the upper pole is nonfunctioning, heminephrectomy may be considered.

Posterior Urethral Valves

Definition: BOO at the level of the posterior urethra.

Incidence: Occurs in 1:5,000 males. The commonest cause of BOO in male fetuses.

Embryology and Pathology: Incomplete regression of a urogenital membrane that develops during early embryological development.

Diagnosis
Ultrasound: The degree of obstruction and the timing of diagnosis vary greatly. Some cases are detected early during the first or early second trimester because of megacystis (see Figs. 27.1-41 and 27.1-51) and/or oligohydramnios, while others will be detected during the third trimester or only after birth.

An enlarged bladder with thickened wall (above 3 mm) and a dilated posterior urethra are common findings (Fig. 27.1-51).[102–105] Associated upper urinary tract dilatation is frequent but variable. Renal dilatation can be uni- or bilateral, related to obstruction and/or to VUR (Fig. 27.1-52). The degree of associated renal dysplasia is variable as well. There seems to be a correlation between cortical echogenicity, cystic changes, and the degree of obstructive dysplasia (Fig. 27.1-52). Unusual presentations include bladder rupture with ascitis and perirenal urinoma.

MRI: MRI may provide additional information, particularly when oligohydramnios is present.[7,106]

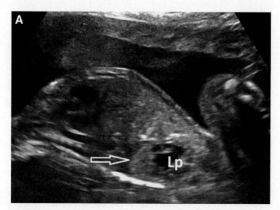
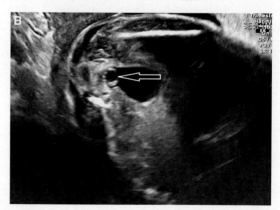

FIGURE 27.1-50: Duplex system. **A:** Sagittal US shows echogenic dysplastic upper pole (*arrow*) and dilated lower pole (*Lp*). **B:** Endovaginal US demonstrates a ureterocele within the bladder (*arrow*). (Courtesy of M. van Rysselberghe.)

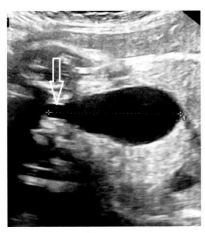

FIGURE 27.1-51: Posterior urethral valve (third trimester). Sagittal US shows a fetal megacystis (6 cm in length). The posterior urethra is dilated (*arrow*). (Courtesy of B. Broussin.)

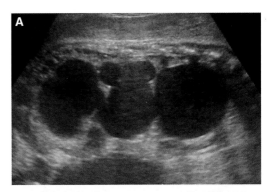

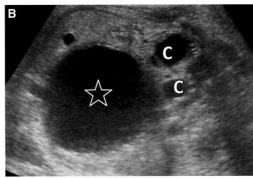

FIGURE 27.1-52: Obstructive cystic dysplasia in a case of posterior urethral valve (third trimester). **A:** Sagittal US of one kidney shows a marked dilatation with cortical thinning and cortical cysts. **B:** Close-up of the dilated renal pelvis (*star*). There are numerous cysts (*C*) within the renal cortex, consistent with obstructive cystic dysplasia. (Courtesy of C. Garel, MD.)

Differential Diagnosis: In the second and third trimesters, the differential diagnosis of enlarged bladder includes severe VUR (pseudomegacystis megaureter syndrome), megacystis–micro-colon–hypoperistalsis syndrome, and prune belly syndrome (Fig. 27.1-53). Medication-induced megabladder (e.g., cocaine) and a pseudoenlarged bladder in the female fetus should be considered. Anterior valves can very rarely be demonstrated *in utero*. A megalourethra (Fig. 27.1-54) is a particular abnormality of the urethra wherein the corpus spongiosa are lacking and where the urethra is dilated. Differential diagnosis includes megameatus and meatal stenosis.[104,107–111]

Bladder enlargement due to obstruction secondary to PUV must be differentiated from other causes of BOO (Table 27.1-7). During the first and early second trimesters, BOO could result from urethral atresia (Fig. 27.1-41). The kidneys will appear hyperechoic because of obstructive dysplasia. The prognosis is poor. Megabladder of the first trimester may be transitory or also associated with trisomies.

Outcome: The outcome is variable and depends on the severity of the obstruction. Postnatal mortality is around 8%, although prenatal mortality rates are higher—23% to 54%.

Management: The role of measuring urinary electrolytes in the fetal urine obtained through transabdominal puncture is controversial. Fetuses with renal damage show increased urinary concentration, especially of Na and Ca, without clear convincing confirmation. Measurements of B2-immunoglobulin on C cystatin in the fetal urine allow a better accuracy. Karyotyping can bring additional important information as chromosomal anomalies can be detected.

The role of vesicoamniotic shunting is controversial. Although technically easy, the long-term results of shunting have not been validated.[112–117]

In the poor prognosis group with severe oligohydramnios, bilateral hydroureteronephrosis, and echogenic dysplastic kidneys, termination may be offered because of the poor outcome in the neonatal period from pulmonary hypoplasia. Close follow-up with determination of optimal delivery coincides with the gestation age and timing of oligohydramnios. Before 32 weeks'

gestation if oligohydramnios is developing, shunting may be useful. After 32 weeks' gestation if oligohydramnios develops, early delivery should be considered.

Postnatally, the patient should be placed on antibiotics, and emergency VCUG performed. If PUV is confirmed, urethral valve ablation or vesicostomy may be performed, depending on the size of the infant.

Prune Belly Syndrome

Definition: Also known as Eagle Barret or triad syndrome, prune belly syndrome includes poor abdominal wall muscle development, undescended testicles, and urinary tract abnormalities.

TABLE 27.1-7 Differential Diagnosis of Fetal Megabladder

Posterior urethral valves
Prune belly sequence
Megacystis–megaureter syndrome (massive vesicoureteric reflux)
Megacystis–microcolon–hypoperistalsis syndrome
Maternal sedative medication
Physiological (female, late third trimester)

Incidence: Occurring in 1 in 40,000 live births, with 3% to 4% occurring in females. Four percent are associated with twinning.[117,118]

Embryology and Pathology: Several theories have been suggested. One theory focuses on functional obstruction due to prostatic hypoplasia. The obstruction may be transient and result in reflux as well as an overdistended bladder that results in abnormal development of the abdominal wall musculature and prevents descent of testis. The mesodermal arrest theory is supported by histological findings in the abdominal wall and urinary tract, where sparsely placed smooth muscle suggests a mesodermal differentiation problem rather than an obstruction problem.[118–120]

Diagnosis: Typically, megacystis is noted with a large protruberant abdomen. Obstruction can occur as high as the UPJ to as low as the prostatic membranous urethra, with megalourethra observed at times. Dilated tortuous ureters are often present. Patent urachus is often associated with prune belly syndrome.

MRI can be useful in assessment of the ureters, bladder, and urachus, particularly if oligohydramnios develops.

Differential Diagnosis: PUVs, severe VUR, and megacystis–microcolon–hypoperistalsis syndrome should be considered

(Figs. 27.1-46 and 27.1-53). Isolated megalourethra (Fig. 27.1-54) with absent corpus spongiosa is rare but should be included in the differential.[107–111,118–121]

Associated Anomalies: Patent urachus is commonly present. Anterior urethral abnormalities from atresia to megalourethra have been described.

Orthopedic anomalies, including scoliosis and hip dislocation, can affect up to 50% of patients. Cardiac anomalies are noted in 10% of cases. Gastrointestinal abnormalities, including malrotation, atresia, and volvulus, affect up to one-third of patients.[118]

Outcome: Prognosis is variable. The spectrum extends from still birth due to severe pulmonary hypoplasia to undescended testis with minimal abdominal wall weakness. Long-term medial issues include renal failure, bladder incontinence, and infertility.[117–122]

Management: Vesicoamniotic shunting has had little effect in reducing the incidence of renal failure and need for transplantation.

In severe cases, immediate care is required because of pulmonary hypoplasia.

Prophylactic antibiotics should be initiated. US, VCUG, and renal Lasix scans should be performed to assess renal status. Urethral stenosis must be treated immediately. If there is

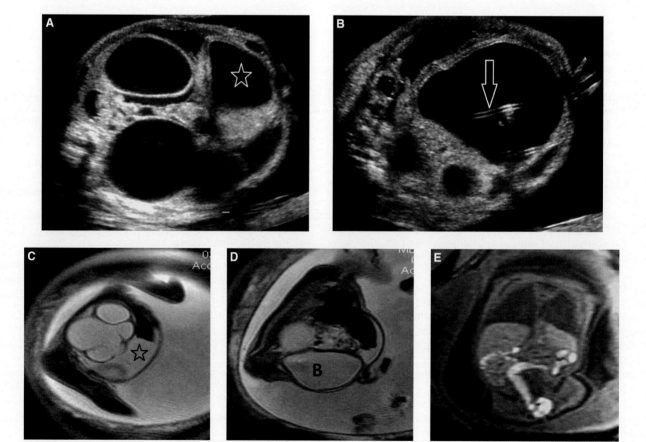

FIGURE 27.1-53: Megacystis–microcolon–hypoperistalsis syndrome (third trimester). **A:** Transverse US of the fetal abdomen at the level of the markedly dilated kidneys. Ascitis is also visible (*star*). **B:** Transverse US through the fetal megacystis. A catheter had been inserted within the bladder (*arrow*). **C:** Sagittal T2 MRI through one of the dilated kidneys. *Star*, ascites. **D:** Sagittal T2 MRI through the distended bladder (*B*) surrounded by ascitis. **E:** T1 MRI displays a short colon in the left upper quadrant. (Courtesy of L. Guibaud, MD.)

no obstruction or reflux, management can be conservative. Abdominal wall reconstruction, vesicostomies, ureteral reimplantations, nephrostomies, and/or pyeloplasties may be required to help preserve renal function. Some individuals eventually require renal transplantation.[117–122]

Mesoblastic Nephroma

Incidence: The most common congenital renal neoplasm, representing 2% to 5% of all pediatric renal tumors.[122,123]

Pathology: There are two main subtypes, a classical (resembling fibromatosis) and a cellular type (resembling fibrosarcoma).

Diagnosis: In the fetus, it appears as a solid tumor that is sometimes difficult to delineate from the adjacent renal normal parenchyma (Fig. 27.1-55). The tumor can display a partially cystic and septated pattern. *In utero*, polyhydramnios is typically present. MRI can provide better anatomical delineation of the mass from surrounding structures (Fig. 27.1-56).

Differential Diagnosis: Rare cases of fetal renal Wilms tumor have been reported. Some syndromes, especially those associated with a mutation of *WT1* gene, are at risk for developing Wilms tumor (e.g., Beckwith–Wiedemann, Wilms-Aniridia, or Drash syndrome). Bilateral involvement suggests bilateral Wilms or nephroblastomatosis (Fig. 27.1-57). The main differential diagnoses of cystic renal tumors include MCDK, cystic dysplasia, intrarenal lymphangiectasia, segmental dysplasia, and renal cysts.[122–127]

Prognosis and Management: The prognosis is usually good.[122–127] Hypertension may develop after birth but resolves after nephrectomy. Survival rate is 95% after resection; a worse prognosis is reported with advanced stages of the cellular type and whenever excision is incomplete.

Renal Hypodysplasia/Tubular Dysgenesis-Oligomeganephronia

Definition: A congenital small kidney is defined by a sagittal length below 2 SD compared to normal gestational age (Table 38 in Appendix A1). The exact definitions of hypoplasia, dysplasia, tubular dysgenesis, or oligomeganephronia are histological ones.

Embryology, Genetics, and Pathogenesis: The origin of a congenital small kidney is multifactorial; it may be related to genetic mutations (e.g., HNF1Beta mutation, renin angiotensin system mutation), associated with VUR or other uropathies, or acquired. Medications such as angiotensin-converting enzyme inhibitors and cocaine can cause hypodysplastic kidney. The condition can also be associated with chromosomal abnormalities.[128–131]

Diagnosis: Standard measures by gestation age are available (Tables 33 and 34 renal measures in Appendix A1). Associated urinary tract dilatation should suggest VUR and renal dysplasia (Fig. 27.1-45A).

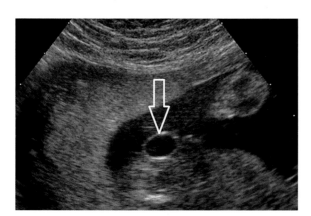

FIGURE 27.1-54: Megalourethra (second trimester). US shows distension of the intrapenile urethra (*arrow*).

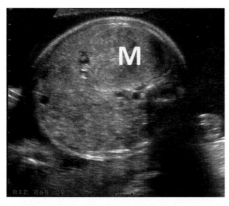

FIGURE 27.1-55: Mesoblastic nephroma (third trimester). Transverse US of the fetal abdomen shows a large solid-type mass (*M*) occupying the right renal fossa.

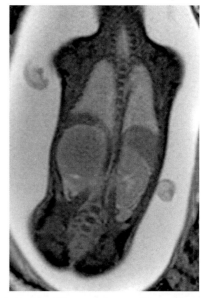

FIGURE 27.1-56: Mesoblastic nephroma (third trimester). Coronal T2 MRI of the kidneys shows a large mass, hyposignal compared with the rest of the kidney, occupying the upper pole of the right kidney. (Courtesy of K. Chaumoitre.)

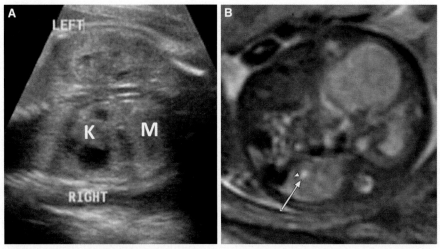

FIGURE 27.1-57: Bilateral Wilms tumor (third trimester). **A:** Coronal US of both kidneys shows solid-type mass (*M*) and the lower pole of the right kidney (*K*). **B:** Axial T2 MRI demonstrates a large mass at the lower pole of the kidney. The *arrow* points to a contralateral Wilms tumor. (Courtesy of Beth Kline-Fath, MD.)

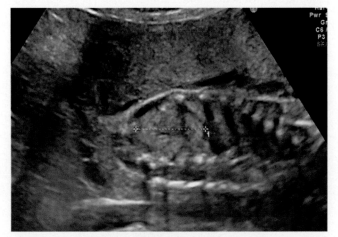

FIGURE 27.1-58: Tubular dysgenesis (third trimester). Sagittal US shows one kidney (limited by the *crosses*) that appears hyperechoic and small (the other kidney had similar findings). Oligohydramnios was present. The baby died at birth from pulmonary hypoplasia.

Hyperechoic small kidneys with oligohydramnios is suggestive of tubular dysgenesis. The CMD is potentially preserved in these cases (Fig. 27.1-58).[131]

Prognosis: The prognosis depends on the degree of renal failure and oligohydramnios.

Recurrence: Recurrence depends on the etiology. Cases that have genetic origin have a higher risk.

Acquired Renal Pathologies

Renal anomalies can develop during pregnancy because of vascular impairment, maternal preexisting disease, maternofetal acquired disease, or toxic medications.[128–131] Fetal renal vein thrombosis (RVT) may develop with maternal diabetes at any stage of the pregnancy. Sonographically, during the acute stage of the thrombosis, the kidney enlarges markedly and its echogenicity becomes heterogeneous (Fig. 27.1-59A). Doppler analysis may in some cases confirm the thrombosis. A thrombus within the

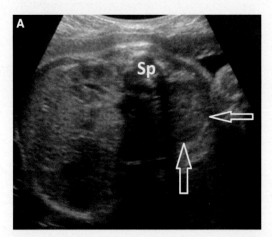

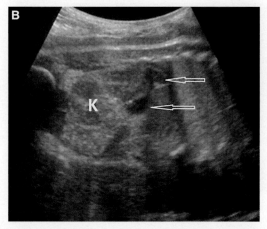

FIGURE 27.1-59: Renal vein thrombosis, acute phase. **A:** On transverse US of the kidneys on each side of the spine (*Sp*), the left kidney (*arrows*) appears globular and lacks corticomedullary differentiation. **B:** On sagittal US, the kidney (*K*) displays a heterogeneous pattern, and there is an associated acute adrenal hemorrhage (*arrows*).

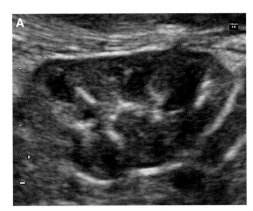
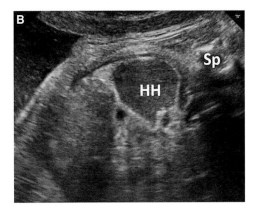

FIGURE 27.1-60: Renal vein thrombosis follow-up. **A:** Sagittal US in the third trimester reveals hyperechoic streaks in the interlobar areas, corresponding to calcifications. **B:** Transverse US of the corresponding adrenal gland shows an adrenal hemorrhage (*HH*). *Sp*, fetal spine.

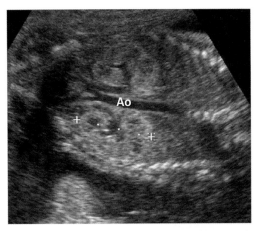

FIGURE 27.1-61 Ischemic kidney, twin–twin transfusion syndrome. On coronal US in the third trimester, both kidneys appear hyperechoic but normal in size. *Ao*, aorta. Cursor length left kidney.

inferior vena cava and adrenal hemorrhage may be associated findings (Fig. 27.1-59B). Rapidly, collateral vessels develop and the renal revascularization may resume. Vascular calcifications in the interlobar areas may remain as sequelae (Fig. 27.1-60).[132–135] Kidney growth will be impaired in more severe cases with poorer prognosis.

Twin–twin transfusion syndrome, the death of one twin, may render the surviving one more vulnerable to ischemia. The ischemic kidneys might appear hyperechoic (Fig. 27.1-61).

Maternal deficit in neuropeptidase may induce an acute transient glomerulonephritis in the fetus, which will determine increased renal volume and cortical echogenicity. Transient renal failure may develop at birth. The renal appearance will return to normal progressively.[136–137]

Furthermore, maternofetal infection may involve the kidneys and determine increased echogenicity, as demonstrated in some cases with cytomegalovirus (CMV).[136]

As mentioned earlier, some medications may result in impaired renal growth, neonatal renal failure, and intractable pneumothoraces.[132–135]

Congenital Nephrotic Syndromes

Congenital nephrotic syndrome may start in fetal life. The kidneys appear diffusely hyperechoic (Fig. 27.1-62). The placenta

is thick and polyhydramnios is present. Affected fetuses are growth retarded, and birth is usually premature. The proteinuria can be detected in the amniotic fluid. A particular association is the Drash syndrome that includes disorders of sexual differentiation and a particular nephrotic syndrome (mesangial sclerosis). Patients affected by the syndrome carry an increased risk for Wilms tumor.[138]

FETAL ADRENALS

Embryology

The adrenal develops from two components: mesothelial cells and neural crest cells. During the fifth week of development, mesothelial cells close to the urogenital ridge proliferate and penetrate the underlying mesenchyme, where they differentiate into large acidophilic organs that will constitute the primitive fetal cortex. Thereafter, a second wave of cells surround the first ones and form the definitive cortex. Only the outermost layer will remain after birth. Simultaneously, neural crest cells invade the sympathetic system, where they are arranged in cords; they will form the adrenal medulla. These cells will migrate and penetrate the fetal cortex and coalesce within it. Both components, cortex and medulla, will remain separated in the definitive adrenal (Fig. 27.1-63).[139]

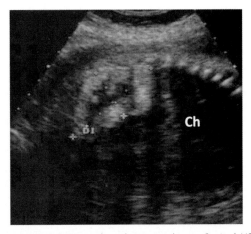

FIGURE 27.1-62: Congenital nephrotic syndrome. Sagittal US in the third trimester shows one kidney (limited by *crosses*) that is hyperechoic and heterogeneous. It corresponded to a mesangial sclerosis. *Ch*, fetal chest; *D1*, length of the kidney – 3.5 cm.

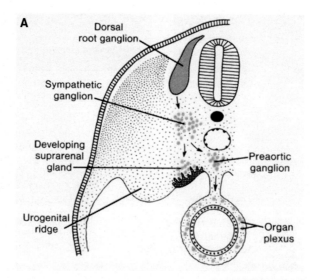

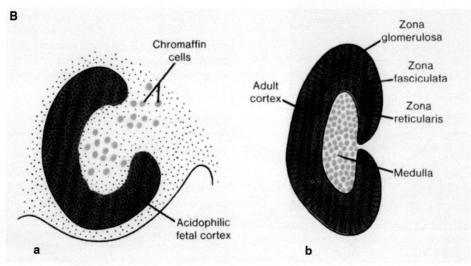

FIGURE 27.1-63: Embryology of the human adrenals. **A:** Formation of the sympathetic ganglia. A portion of neuroblasts migrates toward the mesothelium (*shaded area*) to form the medulla of the adrenal. **B:** The neuroblasts became the chromaffin cells; they penetrate the fetal cortex but remain separated from it in the definitive gland. (Reprinted with permission from Sadler TW. The urogenital system. In: Sadler TW, ed. *Langman's Medical Embryology*. 9th ed. Philadelphia, PA: Lippincott Williams & Wilkins; 2004:321–362.)

Normal Ultrasound Appearance

The fetal adrenals are easily visualized and measured during obstetrical ultrasound as early as 13 to 14 weeks. They appear as hypoechoic, triangular-shaped structures above the kidneys (Fig. 27.1-5B). During this period, the fetal adrenals are globular and large (their height is half of the kidney height). Progressively, during the second and third trimesters a CMD will become obvious (Fig. 27.1-64A, B). The cortex appears hypoechoic, while the medulla is hyperechoic. The gland will display a Y or reverted V shape. The adrenal height should be one-third of that of the kidneys.[140,141]

Normal MRI Appearance

MRI can be a useful adjunct for the evaluation of the fetal adrenal. In the second trimester, the adrenal glands are low in signal intensity on T2 and are surrounded by hyperintense perirenal fat. In the third trimester, the glands become less conspicuous with increasing T2 signal and decreasing perirenal fat. The glands are of moderate high signal on T1 throughout pregnancy.[142]

Tumors and Pseudotumors of the Adrenal Glands

Differential Diagnosis: The differential diagnosis of enlargement of the fetal adrenals includes tumoral and pseudotumoral enlargement. They must be differentiated from extra-adrenal tumors (Table 27.1-8).

Tumoral enlargement includes cysts and solid-type tumors. Simple adrenal cysts are detected during routine examinations. Their evolution is benign, and they may resolve spontaneously. Some syndromes (e.g., Beckwith–Wiedemann syndrome) include dysplastic, usually bilateral dysplastic cortical cysts. These cysts may become large and bleed (Fig. 27.1-65). Adrenal hemorrhage may develop *in utero*, associated or not with RVT (Fig. 27.1-59B).

Neuroblastoma is the main tumor affecting the fetal adrenals. Neuroblastomas represent 30% to 40% of fetal tumors and are the most common congenital malignancy (1:10,000 live births).

TABLE 27.1-8	Differential Diagnosis of Adrenal Masses

Adrenal cortical cyst
Adrenal dysplastic cortical cyst
Adrenal hemorrhage
Neuroblastoma
Cortical adenoma
Congenital adrenal hyperplasia
Inflammatory hypertrophy
Upper pole of a duplex kidney
Intra-abdominal pulmonary sequestration
Hepatic and splenic cyst
Duplication cyst

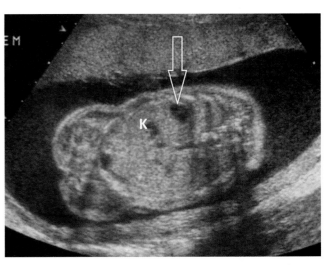

FIGURE 27.1-65: Adrenal dysplastic cyst, Beckwith–Wiedemann syndrome. Coronal US in the second trimester shows a hypoechoic mass (*arrow*) above the kidney (*K*).

The tumor is usually detected during the second trimester. The classic US appearance includes a suprarenal well-defined echogenic mass (Fig. 27.1-66A). Cystic changes may develop within the mass, and the tumor will become hypoechoic; at this stage, it becomes difficult to differentiate it from adrenal hemorrhage. The latter may develop isolated or in association with RVT. Color Doppler may demonstrate vascularization within the tumor helping the differentiation. Liver metastasis may develop already *in utero* in the case of neuroblastoma (pepper syndrome). MRI may help delineate the tumor or the metastasis (Figs. 27.1-66

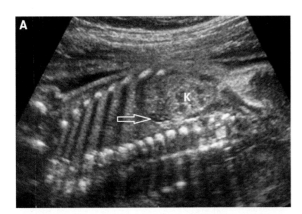

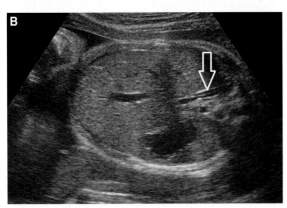

FIGURE 27.1-64: Normal adrenals. **A:** On parasagittal US in the second trimester, the adrenal (*arrow*) appears linear with an outer hypoechoic and central hyperechoic layer above the kidney (*K*). **B:** On transverse US, the two-layered adrenal is visible (*arrow*).

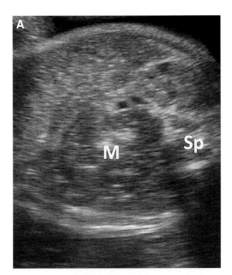

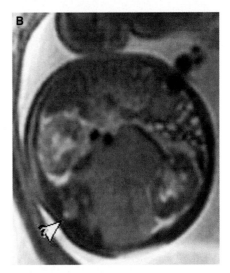

FIGURE 27.1-66: Neuroblastoma. **A:** US in the third trimester demonstrates a heterogeneous solid-type mass (*M*) anterior to the fetal spine (*Sp*). **B:** Axial MRI shows the mass displacing the left kidney anteriorly. Fetal spine (*arrowhead*).

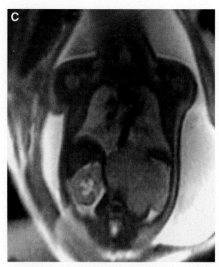

FIGURE 27.1-66: (*continued*) **C:** On coronal MRI, the neuroblastoma crosses the midline.

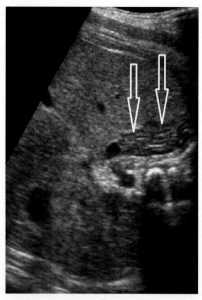

FIGURE 27.1-68: Congenital adrenal hyperplasia. On transverse US in the third trimester, the right adrenal appears multilayered (*arrows*) as compared with a normal adrenal as seen in Figure 27.1-64B.

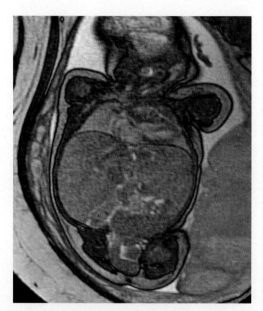

FIGURE 27.1-67: Neuroblastoma, Pepper syndrome. On coronal MRI, the liver is enlarged and has a heterogeneous pattern, related to the neuroblastoma metastasis. (Courtesy of O. Prodhomme, MD.)

and 27.1-67). Despite the malignant nature of neuroblastoma, the overall prognosis is excellent, even though metastasis has developed. Furthermore, cases of spontaneous regression have been described.[132–135,143–147]

Congenital Adrenal Hyperplasia

Congenital adrenal hyperplasia (CAH) is the main cause of pseudotumoral enlargement. The clue to the prenatal diagnosis of CAH is usually the detection of a disorder of the sexual differentiation (DSD) (ambiguous genitalia) (see Chapter 27.3). Such a finding should prompt a detailed analysis of the fetal adrenals. In the case of CAH, the glands are

markedly enlarged because of cortical hypertrophy; in typical cases, they would display the specific cerebriform pattern (Fig. 27.1-68). In the case of CAH, whenever a corticoid treatment is initiated *in utero*, sonography is helpful while demonstrating the progressive reduction in adrenal size. Enlargement of fetal adrenals due to CAH must be differentiated from the other causes of pseudotumoral enlargement.[148–151]

REFERENCES

1. Wiesel A, Queisser-Luft A, Clementi M, et al. Prenatal detection of congenital renal malformations by fetal ultrasonographic examination: an analysis of 709,030 births in 12 Europeans countries. *Eur J Med Genet.* 2005;48:131–144.
2. Carpenter MW, Corrado F, Sung J. Lethal fetal renal anomalies and obstetrics outcome. *Eur J Obstet Gynecol Reprod Biol.* 2000;89:149–153.
3. Desphande C, Hennekam RC. Genetic syndromes and prenatally detected renal anomalies. *Semin Fetal Neonatal Med.* 2008;13:171–180.
4. Nguyen HT, Herndon CD, Cooper C, et al. The Society for Fetal Urology consensus statement on the evaluation and management of antenatal hydronephrosis. *J Pediatr Urol.* 2010;6:212–231.
5. Riccabona M, Avni FE, Blickman JG, et al. Imaging recommendations in paediatric uroradiology: minutes of the ESPR workgroup session on urinary tract infection, fetal hydronephrosis, urinary tract US and voiding cystourethrography. *Pediatr Radiol.* 2008;38:138–145.
6. Hubert KC, Palmer JS. Current diagnosis and management of fetal genitourinary abnormalities. *Urol Clin North Am.* 2007;34:89–101.
7. Cassart M, Massez A, Metens T, et al. Complementary role of MRI after sonography in assessing bilateral urinary tract anomalies in the fetus. *AJR Am J Roentgenol.* 2004;182:689–695.
8. Wynyard P, Chitty LS. Dysplastic kidneys. *Semin Fetal Neonatal Med.* 2008;13:142–151.
9. Toka HR, Toka O, Hariri A, et al. Congenital anomalies of the urinary tract. *Semin Nephrol.* 2010;30:374–386.
10. Song R, Yosypiv IV. Genetics of congenital anomalies of the kidney and urinary tract. *Pediatr Nephrol.* 2011;26:353–364.
11. Woolf AS. A molecular and genetic view of human renal and urinary tract malformations. *Kidney Int.* 2000;58:500–512.
12. Deltas C, Papagregoriou G. Cystic diseases of the kidney. *Arch Pathol Lab Med.* 2010;134:569–582.
13. Sadler TW. The urogenital system. In: Sadler TW, ed. *Langman's Medical Embryology.* 9th ed. Baltimore, MD: Lippincott Williams & Wilkins; 2004:321–362.
14. Cuckow PM, Nyirady P, Winyard PJ. Normal and abnormal development of the urogenital tract. *Prenat Diagn.* 2001;21:908–916.

15. Zalel Y, Lotan D, Achiron R, et al. The early development of the fetal kidney—an in utero sonographic evaluation between 13 and 22 weeks' gestation. *Prenat Diagn.* 2002;22:962–965.
16. Brohnstein M, Kushnir O, Ben Zalel Z, et al. Transvaginal sonographic measurement of fetal kidneys in the first trimester of pregnancy. *J Clin Ultrasound.* 1990;18:299–301.
17. Chitty LS, Altman DG. Charts of fetal size: kidney and renal pelvis measurements. *Prenat Diagn.* 2003;23:891–897.
18. Kennedy WA II, Chitkara U, Abidari JM, et al. Fetal renal growth as assessed through renal parenchymal area derived from prenatal and perinatal US. *J Urol.* 2003;169:298–302.
19. Yu C, Chang C, Chang F, et al. Fetal renal volume in normal gestation: a three dimensional US study. *Ultrasound Med Biol.* 2000;26:1253–1256.
20. Devriendt A, Cassart M, Massez A, Donner C, Avni EF. Fetal kidneys: additional sonographic criteria of normal development. *Prenat Diagn.* 2013;33:1248–1252.
21. Oosterhof H, Haak MC, Aarnouche JG. Acute maternal rehydration increases the urine production rate in the near-term human fetus. *Am J Obstet Gynecol.* 2000;183:226–229.
22. Ross MG, Brace RA. Amniotic fluid biology: basic and clinical aspects. *J Matern Fetal Med.* 2001;10:2.
23. Hubbard AM. Ultrafast fetal MRI and prenatal diagnosis. *Semin Pediatr Surg.* 2003;12:143–153.
24. Farhataziz N, Engels JE, Ramus RM, et al. Fetal MRI of urine and meconium by gestational age for the diagnosis of genitourinary and gastrointestinal abnormalities. *AJR Am J Roentgenol.* 2005;184:1891–1897.
25. Abdelazim IA, Abdelrazak KM, Ramy RM, et al. Complementary roles of prenatal US and MR imaging in diagnosis of fetal renal anomalies. *Aust N Z J Obstet Gynaecol.* 2010;50:237–241.
26. Savelli S, Di Maurizio M, Perrone A, et al. MRI with diffusion weighted imaging (DWI) and apparent diffusion coefficient (ADC) assessment in the evaluation of normal and abnormal fetal kidneys: preliminary experience. *Prenat Diagn.* 2007;27:1104–1111.
27. Chaumoitre K, Colavolpe N, Shojah R, et al. DW MRI with ADC determination in normal and pathological fetal kidneys. *Ultrasound Med Gynecol.* 2007;29:22–31.
28. Lubusky M, Prochazka M, Dhaifalah I, et al. Fetal enterolithiasis: prenatal sonographic and MRI diagnosis in two cases of urorectal septum malformation (URSM) sequence. *Prenat Diagn.* 2006;26:345–349.
29. Schwarderer AL, Bates CM, McHugh KM. Renal anomalies in family members of infants with bilateral renal agenesis/adysplasia. *Pediatr Nephrol.* 2007;22:52–56.
30. Harewood L, Liu M, Keeling J, et al. Bilateral renal agenesis/hypoplasia/dysplasia (BRAHD): postmortem analysis of 45 cases with breakpoint mapping of two de novo translocations. *PLoS One.* 2010;5:e12375.
31. Nielsen BL, Norgard B, Puho E, et al. Risk of specific congenital anomalies in offspring of women with diabetes. *Diabet Med.* 2005;22:693–696.
32. Skinner MA, Safford SD, Reeves JG. Renal aplasia in humans is associated with RET mutations. *Am J Hum Genet.* 2008;82:344–351.
33. Hoffman CK, Filly RA, Callen PW. The lying down adrenal sign: a sonographic indicator of renal agenesis or ectopia in fetuses and neonates. *J Ultrasound Med.* 1992;11:533–536.
34. DeVore GR. The value of color Doppler US in the diagnosis of renal agenesis. *J Ultrasound Med.* 1995;14:443–449.
35. Bronshtein M, Amit A, Achiron R. The early prenatal US diagnosis of renal agenesis: technique and possible pitfalls. *Prenat Diagn.* 1994;14:291–297.
36. Hawkin JS, Dashe JS, Twickler DM. MRI diagnosis of severe fetal renal anomalies. *Am J Obstet Gynecol.* 2008;198:328.
37. Thomas AN, McCullough LB, Chervenak FA, et al. Evidence-based ethically justified counseling for bilateral renal agenesis. *J Perinat Med.* 2017;45:585–594.
38. Ciasco S, Paran S, Puri P. Associated urological anomalies in children with unilateral renal agenesis. *Pediatr Nephrol.* 1992;6:412–416.
39. Cho JY, Moons MH, Lee YH, et al. Measurement of compensatory hyperplasia of the contralateral kidney: usefulness for differential diagnosis of fetal unilateral empty renal fossa. *Ultrasound Obstet Gynecol.* 2009;34:515–520.
40. Mesrobian HG, Rushton HG, Bulas D. Unilateral renal agenesis may result from in utero regression of multicystic renal dysplasia. *J Urol.* 1993;150:793–794.
41. Westland R, Schreuer MF, Ket JC, et al. Unilateral renal agenesis: a systematic review on associated anomalies and renal injury. *Nephrol Dial Transplant.* 2013;28:1844–1855.
42. Sanna-Cherchi S, Ravani P, Corbani V, et al. Renal outcome in patients with congenital anomalies of the kidney and urinary tract. *Kidney Int.* 2009;76:528–533.
43. Glodny B, Peterson J, Hofmann KJ, et al. Kidney fusion anomalies revisited: clinical and radiological analysis of 209 cases of crossed fused ectopia and horseshoe kidney. *BJU Int.* 2009;103:224–235.
44. Decter RM. Renal duplication and fusion anomalies. *Pediatr Clin North Am.* 1997;44:1323–1341.
45. Guarino N, Tadini B, Camardi P, et al. The incidence of associated urological abnormalities in children with renal ectopia. *J Urol.* 2004;172:1757–1759.
46. Hill LM, Grysbeck P, Mills A. Antenatal diagnosis of fetal pelvic kidneys. *Obstet Gynecol.* 1994;83:333–336.
47. Zajicek M, Perlman S, Dekel B, et al. Crossed ectopic kidneys: prenatal diagnosis and postnatal follow-up. *Prenat Diagn.* 2017;37:1–4.
48. Blazer S, Zimmer EZ, Blumenfeld Z, et al. Natural history of fetal renal cysts detected in early pregnancy. *J Urol.* 1999;162:812–814.
49. Rizk D, Chapman AB. Cystic and inherited kidney diseases. *Am J Kidney Dis.* 2003;42:1305–1307.
50. Gunay-Aygun M. Liver and kidney disease in ciliopathies. *Am J Med Genet.* 2009;151C:269–306.
51. Hildebrandt F, Benzing T, Katsanis N. Ciliopathies. *N Engl J Med.* 2011;364:1533–1543.
52. Bisaglia M, Galliani CA, Senger C, et al. Renal cystic diseases: a review. *Adv Anat Pathol.* 2006;13:26–56.
53. Gimpel C, Avni FE, Bergmann C, et al. Perinatal diagnosis, management and follow-up of cystic renal diseases: a clinical practice recommendation with systematic literature reviews. *JAMA Pediatr.* 2018;172:74–86.
54. Avni FE, Hall M. Renal cystic diseases in children: new concepts. *Pediatr Radiol.* 2010;40:939–946.
55. Avni FE, Garel C, Cassart M, et al. Imaging and classification of congenital cystic renal diseases. *AJR Am J Roentgenol.* 2012;198:1004–1013.
56. De Bruyn R, Gordon I. Imaging in cystic renal disease. *Arch Dis Child.* 2000;83:401–407.
57. Chaumoitre K, Brun M, Cassart M, et al. Differential diagnosis of fetal hyperechogenic cystic kidneys unrelated to renal tract anomalies: a multicenter study. *Ultrasound Obstet Gynecol.* 2006;28:911–917.
58. Breysem L, Bosmans H, Dymarkowski S, et al. The value of fast MR imaging as an adjunct to ultrasound in prenatal diagnosis. *Eur Radiol.* 2003;13:1538–1548.
59. Aubertin G, Cripps S, Coleman G, et al. Prenatal diagnosis of apparently isolated unilateral multicystic kidney: implications for counseling and management. *Prenat Diagn.* 2002;22:388–394.
60. Schreuder MF, Wesland R, van Wijk JA. Unilateral MDK: a meta-analysis of observational studies on the incidence, associated urinary tract malformations and the contralateral kidney. *Nephrol Dial Transplant.* 2009;24:1810–1818.
61. Hains DS, Bates CM, Ingraham S, et al. Management and etiology of unilateral MDK: a review. *Pediatr Nephrol.* 2009;24:233–241.
62. Dahmen-Elias HA, Stoutenbeek PH, Visser GH, et al. Concomitant anomalies in 100 children with unilateral multicystic kidney. *Ultrasound Obstet Gynecol.* 2005;25:384–388.
63. Aslam M, Watson AR. Unilateral MDK: long term outcome. *Arch Dis Child.* 2006;91:820–823.
64. Siqueira Rabelo EA, Oliveira EA, Silva JM, et al. US progression of prenatally detected MDK. *Urology.* 2006;68:1098–1102.
65. Bergman C, Senderek J, Windelen E, et al. Clinical consequences of PKHD1 mutations in 164 patients with ARPKD. *Kidney Int.* 2005;65:829–848.
66. Denamur E, Delezoide A, Alberti C, et al. Genotype-phenotype correlations in fetuses and neonates with ARPKD. *Kidney Int.* 2010;77:350–358.
67. Guay-Woodford LM, Desmond RA. Autosomal recessive polycystic kidney disease: the clinical experience in North America. *Pediatrics.* 2003;111:1072–1080.
68. Okumura M, Bunduki V, Shiang C, et al. Unusual sonographic features of ARPKD. *Prenat Diagn.* 2006;26:330–332.
69. Turkbey B, Ocak I, Daryanani K, et al. ARPKD and congenital hepatic fibrosis. *Pediatr Radiol.* 2009;39:100–111.
70. Wilson PO. Polycystic kidney disease. *N Engl J Med.* 2004;350:151–164.
71. Brun M, Maugey-Laulom B, Eurin D, et al. Prenatal sonographic patterns in autosomal dominant polycystic kidney disease: a multicenter study. *Ultrasound Obstet Gynecol.* 2004;24:55–61.
72. Mashiach R, Davidovits M, Einsenstein B, et al. Fetal hyperechogenic kidney with normal amniotic fluid volume: a diagnostic dilemma. *Prenat Diagn.* 2005;25:553–558.
73. Nakayama M, Nozu K, Goto Y, et al. HNF1B alterations with congenital anomalies of the kidney and urinary tract. *Pediatr Nephrol.* 2010;25:1073–1079.
74. Edghill EL, Bingham C, Ellard S, et al. Mutations in hepatocyte nuclear factor-1beta and their related phenotypes. *J Med Genet.* 2006;43:84–90.
75. Ulinski T, Lescure S, Beaufils S, et al. Renal phenotypes related to hepatocyte nuclear factor-1beta (TCF2) mutations in a pediatric cohort. *J Am Soc Nephrol.* 2006;17:497–503.
76. Decramer S, Parant O, Beaufils S, et al. Anomalies of the TCF2 gene are the main cause of fetal bilateral hyperechogenic kidneys. *J Am Soc Nephrol.* 2007;18:923–933.
77. Faguer S, Bouissou F, Dumazer P, et al. Massively enlarged polycystic kidneys in monozygotic twins with TCF2/HNF-1ß heterozygous whole gene deletion. *Am J Kidney Dis.* 2007;50:1023–1027.
78. Cassart M, Eurin D, Didier F, et al. Antenatal renal sonographic anomalies and postnatal follow-up of renal involvement in Bardet-Biedl syndrome. *Ultrasound Obstet Gynecol.* 2004;24:51–54.
79. Ickowicz V, Eurin D, Maugey-Laulom B, et al. Meckel-Grüber syndrome: sonography and pathology. *Ultrasound Obstet Gynecol.* 2006;27:296–300.
80. Hildebrandt F, Zhou W. Nephronophthisis-associated ciliopathies. *J Am Soc Nephrol.* 2007;18:1855–1871.
81. Salomon R, Saunier S, Niaudet P. Nephronophthisis. *Pediatr Nephrol.* 2009;24:2333–2344.
82. Blowey DL, Querfeld U, Geary D, et al. Ultrasound findings in juvenile nephronophthisis. *Pediatr Nephrol.* 1996;10:22–24.
83. Valente EM, Marsh SE, Castori M, et al. Distinguishing the four genetic causes of Jouberts syndrome-related disorders. *Ann Neurol.* 2005;57:513–519.
84. Lennerz JK, Spence DC, Iskandar SS, et al. Glomerulocystic kidney: one-hundred-year perspective. *Arch Pathol Lab Med.* 2010;134:583–605.

85. Pates JA, Dashe JS. Prenatal diagnosis and management of hydronephrosis. *Early Hum Dev*. 2006;82:3–8.

86. Ismaili K, Hall M, Piepz A, et al. Insight into the pathogenesis and natural history of foetuses with renal pelvis dilatation. *Eur Urol*. 2005;48:207–214.

87. Thorup J, Jokela R, Cortes D, et al. The results of 15-years of consistent strategy in treating antenatally suspected PUJ obstruction. *BJU Int*. 2003;91:850–852.

88. Ismaili K, Hall M, Donner C, et al. Results of systematic screening for minor degrees of fetal renal pelvis dilatation in an unselected population. *Am J Obstet Gynecol*. 2003;188:242–246.

89. John U, Kahler C, Schulz S, et al. The impact of fetal renal pelvic diameter on postnatal outcome. *Prenat Diagn*. 2004;24:591–595.

90. Lee RS, Kinnamon DD, Nguyen HT. Antenatal hydronephrosis as a predictor of postnatal outcome: a meta-analysis. *Pediatrics*. 2006;118:586–593.

91. Carr MC. Prenatal management of urogenital disorders. *Urol Clin North Am*. 2004;31:389–397.

92. Thomas DF. Prenatal diagnosis: what do we know of long-term outcomes? *J Pediatr Urol*. 2010;6:204–211.

93. Valentin L, Marsal K. Does the prenatal diagnosis of fetal urinary tract anomalies affect perinatal outcome. *Ann N Y Acad Sci*. 1998;847:59–73.

94. Nakai H, Asanuma H, Shishido S, et al. Changing concepts in urological management of the congenital anomalies of kidney and urinary tract (CAKUT). *Pediatr Int*. 2003;45:634–641.

95. Riccabona M, Avni FE, Blickman JG, et al. Imaging recommendations in pediatric uroradiology: childhood obstructive uropathy, high grade fetal hydronephrosis, childhood haematuria, and urolithiasis in childhood. *Pediatr Radiol*. 2009;39:891–898.

96. Shukla AR, Cooper J, Paytel RK, et al. Prenatally detected primary megaureter: a role for extended follow-up. *J Urol*. 2005;173(4):1353–1356.

97. Van Eerde AM, Meutgeert MH, de Jong TP, et al. VUR in children with prenatally detected hydronephrosis: a systematic review. *Ultrasound Obstet Gynecol*. 2007;29:463–469.

98. Ismaili K, Hall M, Piepz A, et al. Primary VUR detected in neonates with a history of fetal pelvis dilatation: a prospective clinical and imaging study. *J Pediatr*. 2006;148:222–227.

99. Whitten SM, Wilcox DT. Duplex systems. *Prenat Diagn*. 2001;21:952–957.

100. Uphadhyay J, Bolduc S, Braga L, et al. Impact of prenatal diagnosis on the morbidity associated with ureterocele management. *J Urol*. 2002;167:2560–2565.

101. Austin PF, Cain MP, Casale AJ, et al. Prenatal bladder outlet obstruction secondary to ureterocele. *Urology*. 1998;52:1132–1135.

102. Harvie S, McLeod L, Acott P, et al. Abnormal antenatal sonogram: an indicator of disease severity in children with PUV. *Can Assoc Radiol J*. 2009;60:185–189.

103. Kousidis G, Thomas DF, Morgan H, et al. The long term follow-up of prenatally detected PUV: a 10 to 23 year follow-up study. *BJU Int*. 2008;102:1020–1024.

104. Anumba DO, Scott JE, Plant ND, et al. Diagnosis and outcome of fetal lower urinary tract obstruction in the northern region of England. *Prenat Diagn*. 2005;25:7–13.

105. Morris RK, Malin GL, Khan KS, et al. Antenatal US to predict post natal renal function in congenital lower urinary tract obstruction: systematic review of test accuracy. *BJOG*. 2009;116:1290–1299.

106. Miller OF, Lashley DB, McAleer IM, et al. Diagnosis of urethral obstruction with prenatal MRI. *J Urol*. 2002;168:1158–1159.

107. Carlsson SA, Hokegard KH, Mattson LA. Megacystis-microcolon-hypoperistalsis syndrome: antenatal appearance in two cases. *Acta Obstet Gynecol Scand*. 1992;71:645–648.

108. McHugo J, Witthle M. Enlarged fetal bladders: aetiology, management and outcome. *Prenat Diagn*. 2001;21:958–963.

109. Osborne NG, Bonilla-Musoles F, Machado LE, et al. Fetal megacystis: differential diagnosis. *J Ultrasound Med*. 2011;30:833–841.

110. Gonzalez R, De Filippo R, Jednak R, et al. Urethral atresia: long term outcome in 6 children who survived the neonatal period. *J Urol*. 2001;165:2241–2244.

111. Stephens FD, Fortune DW. Pathogenesis of megalourethra. *J Urol*. 1993;149:1512–1516.

112. Klaassen I, Neuhaus TJ, Mueller-Wiefel DE, et al. Antenatal oligohydramnios of renal origin: long term outcome. *Nephrol Dial Transplant*. 2007;22:432–439.

113. Muller F, Dreux S, Audibert F, et al. Fetal serum B2-microglobulin and cystatin C in the prediction of post-natal renal function in bilateral hypoplasia and hyperechogenic enlarged kidneys. *Prenat Diagn*. 2004;24:327–332.

114. Morris RK, Quinlan-Jones E, Kilby MD, et al. Systematic review of accuracy of fetal urine analysis to predict poor postnatal renal function in cases of congenital urinary tract obstruction. *Prenat Diagn*. 2007;27:900–911.

115. Morris RK, Khan KS, Kilby MD. Vesico-amniotic shunting for lower urinary tract obstruction: an overview. *Arch Dis Child*. 2007;92:F166–F168.

116. Makino Y, Kobayashi H, Kyono K, et al. Clinical results of fetal obstructive uropathy treated by vesico-amniotic shunting. *Urology*. 2000;55:118–122.

117. Biard JM, Johnson MP, Carr MC, et al. Long-term outcomes in children treated by prenatal vesicoamniotic shunting for lower urinary tract obstruction. *Obstet Gynecol*. 2005;106(3):503–508.

118. Terada S, Suzuki N, Uchide K, et al. Etiology of prune belly syndrome: evidence of megalocystic origin in an early fetus. *Obstet Gynecol*. 1994;83:865–868.

119. Tonni G, Ida V, Alessandro V, et al. Prune-belly syndrome: case series and review of the literature regarding early prenatal diagnosis, epidemiology, genetic factors, treatment, and prognosis. *Fetal Pediatr Pathol*. 2013;31(1):13–24.

120. Woods AG, Brandon DH. Prune belly syndrome: a focused physical assessment. *Adv Neonatal Care*. 2007;7:132–143.

121. Duckett J, Knutrud O, Hohenfellner R. Prune belly syndrome. *J Urol*. 1980;3:9.

122. Chan KL, Tang MH, Tse HY, et al. Factors affecting outcomes of prenatally-diagnosed tumors. *Prenat Diagn*. 2002;22:437–444.

123. Woodward PJ, Sohaey R, Kennedy A, et al. A comprehensive review of fetal tumors with pathologic correlation. *Radiographics*. 2005;25:215–242.

124. Sebire NJ, Jauniaux E. Fetal and placental malignancies: prenatal diagnosis and management. *Ultrasound Obstet Gynecol*. 2009;33:235–244.

125. Avni FE, Massez A, Cassart M. Tumors of the fetal body: a review. *Pediatr Radiol*. 2009;39:1147–1157.

126. Linam LE, Yu X, Clvo-Garcia MA, et al. Contribution of MR imaging to prenatal differential diagnosis of renal tumors: report of two cases and review of the literature. *Fetal Diagn Ther*. 2010;28:100–108.

127. Ferguson MR, Chapman T, Dighe M. Fetal tumors: imaging features. *Pediatr Radiol*. 2010;40:1263–1273.

128. Celsi G, Kistner A, Aizman R, et al. Prenatal dexamethasone causes oligonephronia, sodium retention, and higher blood pressure in the offspring. *Pediatr Res*. 1998;44:317–322.

129. Peruzzi L, Gianoglio B, Porcellini MG, et al. Neonatal end-stage renal failure associated with maternal ingestion of COX-1 selective inhibitor nimesulide as tocolytic. *Lancet*. 1999;354:1615.

130. Saji H, Yamanaka M, Hagiwara A, et al. Losartan and fetal toxic effects. *Lancet*. 2001;357:363.

131. Lambot MA, Vermeylen D, Noel JC. Angiotensin II receptor inhibitors in pregnancy. *Lancet*. 2001;357:1619–1620.

132. Winyard PJ, Bharucha T, De Bruyn R, et al. Perinatal renal venous thrombosis: presenting renal length predicts outcome. *Arch Dis Child*. 2006;91:F273–F278.

133. Kraft JK, Brandao LR, Navarro OM. Sonography of renal venous thrombosis in neonates and infants: can we predict outcome? *Pediatr Radiol*. 2011;41:299–307.

134. Lau KK, Fernandez y Garcia E, Kwan WY, et al. Bilateral renal venous thrombosis and adrenal hemorrhage: sequential prenatal US with postnatal recovery. *Pediatr Radiol*. 2007;37:912–915.

135. Sohdi KS, Khandelwal S, Ray M, et al. Calcified neonatal renal vein and caval thrombosis. *Pediatr Radiol*. 2006;36:437–439.

136. Nortier JL, Debiec H, Tourney Y, et al. Neonatal disease in neutral endopeptidase alloimmunization: lessons for immunological monitoring. *Pediatr Nephrol*. 2006;10:1399–1405.

137. Chan M, Hecht JL, Boyd T, et al. Congenital CMV: a cause for renal dysplasia? *Pediatr Dev Pathol*. 2007;10:300–304.

138. Hofstaetter C, Neumann I, Lennert T, et al. Prenatal diagnosis of diffuse mesangial sclerosis by US: a longitudinal study of a case in an affected family. *Fetal Diagn Ther*. 1996;11:126–131.

139. Sadler TW. Central nervous system: sympathetic nervous system. In: Sadler TW, ed. *Langman's Medical Embryology*. 9th ed. Philadelphia, PA: Lippincott Williams & Wilkins; 2004:474–477.

140. Van Vuuren SH, Dahmen-Elias HA, Stigter RH, et al. Size and volume of the fetal kidney, renal pelvis and adrenal gland. *Ultrasound Obstet Gynecol*. 2012;40(6):659–664.

141. Turan OM, Turan S, Funai EF, et al. US measurements of fetal adrenal gland enlargement on accurate predictor of preterm birth. *Am J Obstet Gynecol*. 2011;204:e1–e10.

142. Smiththimedhin A, Rubio E, Blask A, et al. Normal size of the fetal adrenal gland on prenatal MR imaging. Abstract presented at the Society for Pediatric Radiology; 2018.

143. Lin J, Lin G, Hung I, et al. Prenatally detected tumor mass in the adrenal gland. *J Pediatr Surg*. 1999;34:1620–1623.

144. Rubenstein SC, Benaceraff BR, Retik AB, et al. Fetal suprarenal masses: US appearance and differential diagnosis. *Ultrasound Obstet Gynecol*. 1995;5:164–167.

145. Sherer DM, Dalloul M, Wagreich A, et al. Prenatal sonographic findings of congenital adrenal cortical adenoma. *J Ultrasound Med*. 2008;27(7):1091–1093.

146. McCauley RG, Beckwith JB, Elias ER, et al. Benign hemorrhagic adrenocortical macrocysts in Beckwith-Wiedemann syndrome. *AJR Am J Roentgenol*. 1991;157:549–552.

147. Niemec SF, Horcher E, Kasprian G, et al. Tumor disease and associated congenital abnormalities on prenatal MRI. *Eur J Radiol*. 2012;81:e15–e22.

148. Chambrier ED, Heinrichs C, Avni EF. US appearance of congenital adrenal hyperplasia in utero. *J Ultrasound Med*. 2002;21:97–100.

149. Saada J, Grebille A, Aubry MC, et al. Sonography in prenatal diagnosis of congenital adrenal hyperplasia. *Prenat Diagn*. 2004;24:627–630.

150. Cassart M, Massez A, Donner C, et al. Sonographic diagnosis of fetal adrenal hyperplasia: utility for prenatal corticotherapy. *Prenat Diagn*. 2005;25:1060–1061.

151. Buhimschi CS, Turan OM, Funai EF, et al. Fetal adrenal gland volume and cortisol/DHEA sulfate ratio in inflammation-associated preterm birth. *Obstet Gynecol*. 2008;111:715–722.

Anorectal and Complex Urogenital Malformations

Maria A. Calvo-Garcia

FETAL ANORECTAL MALFORMATIONS

Anorectal malformations (ARMs) are complex anomalies that can affect both genders and involve the distal anus and rectum. In most cases, the anus is not perforated and the distal bowel ends blindly or through a fistula. If a fistula is present, it could connect with the urinary system, the genital tract, or the perineum (Table 27.2-1).[1–3] More than half of these patients have associated findings. Genitourinary malformations are the most frequently noted (up to 60%), followed by cardiovascular (30% to 35%), spinal (25% to 30%), gastrointestinal (5% to 10%) defects, and VACTERL association (vertebral, anorectal, cardiac, tracheo-esophageal fistula, renal, limb; 4% to 9%).[4,5]

Incidence: The most frequent ARM, imperforate anus, has an incidence of 1 in 5,000 live births, whereas in cloaca the incidence is 1 in 20,000 to 50,000 and in cloacal exstrophy 1 in 200,000 to 400,000 live births.[5]

Embryology: ARMs are thought to result from abnormal development of the primitive cloaca and urorectal septum (Fig. 27.2-1). Several animal models have been studied allowing for a better understanding of the embryologic process involved. The studies in SD mutant mice, by Dietrich Kluth, demonstrated that in all abnormal SD mouse embryo, the dorsal cloacal membrane and the dorsal cloaca were not formed, accounting for an absent or misplaced anal opening and ventral urogenital communications.[6]

Etiology: Environmental and genetic factors, including homeobox and sonic hedgehog signaling pathways, are thought to be implicated. The genetic basis for the VACTERL association is still unknown, but mutations in the SALL1-zinc-finger protein and the homeobox HLXB9 gene have been linked with Townes–Brock syndrome and Currarino triad, respectively. Another specific association with ARM is seen in caudal regression syndrome, in which 15% to 25% of cases are seen in the context of maternal diabetes.[7,8]

Diagnosis: Analysis of the perineum and anal sphincter can provide the most important clue in the prenatal diagnosis of ARM. In normal conditions, on a tangential sonographic view, the anal sphincter will be seen as a hypoechoic ring with an echogenic center from 20 weeks onward and more confidently identified during the third trimester (Fig. 27.2-2). Absent visualization of the anal sphincter, especially in high-risk fetuses, would support the presence of an underlying ARM.[9–11]

However, evaluation of the anal sphincter is not part of the routine fetal anatomic sonogram and, more frequently, this assessment will be triggered by the presence of suspicious features such as megacystis with oligohydramnios, urinary tract dilatation and renal/external genitalia anomalies, fetal ascites, abdominopelvic cystic masses, and dilated distal bowel.[12,13] Depending on the type of defect and degree of patency of potential fistulas, imaging findings could be more specific. Detection of urine or meconium in the wrong anatomic compartment would support those connections, and when meconium is mixed with urine,

TABLE 27.2-1   Main Types of Anorectal Malformations Adopting the International Krickenbeck Nomenclature

TYPE OF DEFECT	GENDER AFFECTED	SURGICAL MANAGEMENT AT BIRTH	FORMER TERMINOLOGY (WINGSPREAD CLASSIFICATION)
Imperforate anus with rectoperineal fistula	(♂ / ♀)	No need for colostomy	Low type
Imperforate anus with rectovestibular fistula	♀		
Imperforate anus without fistula	(♂ / ♀)	Colostomy Delayed repair	Intermediate type
Imperforate anus with rectourethral bulbar fistula	♂		
Imperforate anus with rectourethral prostatic fistula	♂		High type
Imperforate anus with rectovesical fistula	♂		
Rectal atresia or stenosis (with patent anus)	(♂ / ♀)		
Cloaca	♀		Cloaca
Rare malformations	(♂ / ♀)		Rare malformations

Note: Rare malformations were not alluded to in either the Krickenbeck or the Wingspread classifications. Cloacal dysgenesis (aka urorectal septum malformation), cloacal exstrophy, and covered cloacal exstrophy, among others, would be included in that last group.

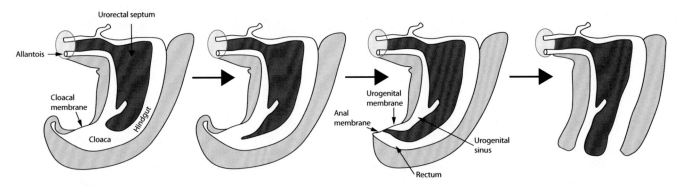

FIG. 27.2-1: Normal development of the urorectal septum. The urorectal septum grows in a caudal direction to separate the cloaca into the dorsal rectum and the ventral urogenital sinus. The urorectal septum also divides the cloacal membrane into the urogenital and anal membranes. These structures will grow caudal, so they will be no longer part of the ventral wall. Both membranes will subsequently rupture.

focal intraluminal calcifications, known as enteroliths, could be formed. Ultrasound (US) and fetal magnetic resonance imaging (MRI) will potentially detect rectal fluid content, sometimes with dilatation and enteroliths and layering meconium or enteroliths within the genitourinary system (Fig. 27.2-3).[14,15]

A meticulous systematic approach, ideally combining US and fetal MRI and review of any prior imaging, will help increase the detection of fetal ARMs.

The evaluation of prior examinations or reports could provide important clues as well. Cloaca and urogenital sinus should be strongly suspected if there is description of transient ascites, followed by subsequent development of progressive hydrocolpos and worsening hydronephrosis and oligohydramnios. Another clinical scenario that should alert about possible exstrophies (cloacal exstrophy or bladder exstrophy) would be persistent absent visualization of the bladder in the presence of normal amniotic fluid volume.

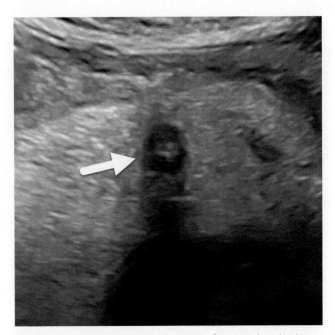

FIG. 27.2-2: Tangential sonographic view of a normal anal sphincter at 33 weeks' gestation. Note the circular hypoechoic sphincter muscle *(arrow)* around the echogenic central anal mucosa.

Differential Diagnosis: The presence of combined genitourinary and rectal findings will increase the level of suspicion and will allow differentiation from rare processes such as congenital diarrhea, where the rectum and the rest of the bowel contain fluid, or multiple intestinal atresias, where enteroliths could be also present.[16] The distal rectal pouch could be further evaluated with fetal MRI and could be seen in normal position, high and dilated within the pelvis, or even undetectable, depending on the type of defect.[17–19] A short rectum is not always linked to an underlying ARM, especially if it is not dilated and is seen in the presence of another potential anatomic or functional condition that could account for a delayed or interrupted transfer of meconium to the rectum. Conditions that could impair swallowing, other types of bowel obstruction, and open neural tube defects could account for this appearance.[20,21]

Prognosis: The prognosis will be dictated by the specific type of defect, the degree of genitourinary compromise altering amniotic fluid volume and lung development, and potential associated malformations.

Management: The more detailed the prenatal diagnosis, the better the multidisciplinary counseling and planning for the neonatal management. Perineal and vestibular fistulas will be eligible for a primary repair or sequential dilatation and will not need decompression surgery in the neonatal period. Otherwise, a colostomy will be performed after the first 24 to 48 hours of life (Table 27.2-1). These more complex cases with delayed repair will benefit from management in specialized centers. Surgical decisions, in these cases, will be made during the initial operation in the hands of a multidisciplinary expert team to optimize the functional outcome of subsequent reconstructive surgeries.[22]

Recurrence Risk: There is increased risk for siblings of patients affected with specific forms of ARM. A 3% chance of another family member being affected has been reported with perineal and vestibular fistulas. However, there is less family transmission in the context of cloaca or prostatic fistulas.[23]

PERSISTENT CLOACA

Persistent cloaca (aka cloaca, classic cloaca, or cloacal malformation) is a type of ARM in which the urinary tract, the vagina,

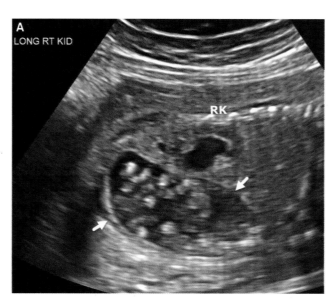
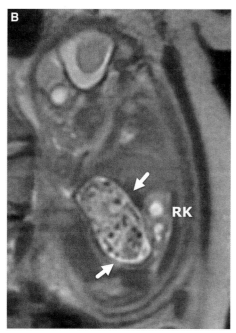

FIG. 27.2-3: Imperforate anus with rectourinary fistula in a 27-week-gestation male fetus. Sagittal US **(A)** and T2 MRI **(B)**. The rectum is markedly dilated *(arrows)* and contains fluid and enteroliths. There is associated anhydramnios and hydronephrosis. RK, right kidney.

and the rectum converge above the level of the perineum, creating a single channel and perineal opening, the cloaca (Latin for "sewer") (Fig. 27.2-4). Virilization of the external genitalia, with clitoral enlargement, sometimes is present but generally normalizes spontaneously after birth.[24] Because of prognostic and therapeutic implications, cloacas can be subdivided depending on the length of the common channel. Cloacal malformations with a short common channel (<3 cm) have a lower incidence of associated defects and less difficult repair. Cloacas with a long common channel (>3 cm) have a high incidence of associated defects, complex anatomy, more difficult repair, and inferior functional results.[25]

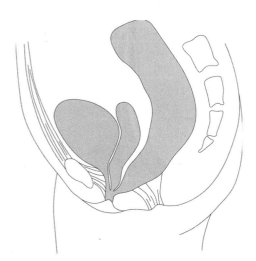

FIG. 27.2-4: Diagram of a cloaca. Sagittal view of the pelvis. The rectum, vagina, and urethra are fused together forming a single common channel opening to the perineum.

Incidence: The condition is typically seen in females with an approximate incidence of 1 in 40,000 to 50,000 births, although it could be estimated as frequent as 1 in 20,000 births accounting for cases misdiagnosed as rectovaginal fistulas in the past.[5]

Embryology: The most widely accepted theory is that cloacal malformations are related to failure in development of the urorectal septum. This is a structure that normally fuses with the cloacal membrane by the 6th week of gestation and subdivides the primitive cloaca into the urogenital sinus in front and the rectum posteriorly (Fig. 27.2-1). A normal dorsal cloaca and cloacal membrane is required for this process to take place.[6] Development of these structures may be altered at any stage, leading to a wide spectrum of defects (Fig. 27.2-5). Recently, this arrested urorectal septum has been linked with defects in embryonic cloacal epithelial differentiation and altered sonic hedgehog and bone morphogenetic protein signaling.[26]

The aberrant drainage of urine through the common channel can lead to bladder obstruction. The fetal urine could then exit through the vagina and uterus causing hydrocolpos and transient urinary ascites. Colonic dilatation can also be present. It is also thought that abnormalities in cloacal septation and urogenital sinus formation could interfere with normal mesonephric and paramesonephric duct development, explaining the high incidence of genital tract duplication or agenesis and increase anomalies of number and position of the kidneys in these patients. Associated anomalies of the lower spinal cord, lumbosacral spine, lower limbs, and bladder as well as ambiguous genitalia also suggest multiple disturbances during the embryonic development of the caudal pole.[27]

Etiology: The etiology is unknown but genetic factors, including homeobox and sonic hedgehog signaling pathways, are thought to be implicated. Defects in early embryonic cloacal epithelial differentiation and abnormal development of the dorsal

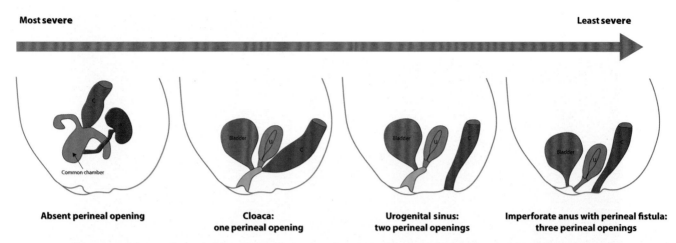

Most severe   **Least severe**

| Absent perineal opening | Cloaca: one perineal opening | Urogenital sinus: two perineal openings | Imperforate anus with perineal fistula: three perineal openings |

FIG. 27.2-5: Spectrum of abnormalities related to the urorectal septum. Variations of these forms may also occur. The most severe form, with absent perineal opening, is referred as urorectal septum malformation (URSM) sequence or cloacal dysgenesis. Partial URSM is synonymous with cloaca. C, colon; K, kidney; U, uterus.

cloaca and dorsal cloacal membrane have been identified using animal models.[6,26]

Diagnosis: US diagnosis of cloacal malformations is challenging and usually considered when a pelvic cyst is seen in a female fetus (Fig. 27.2-6). In this situation, a differential diagnosis should include hydrocolpos or megacystis in the setting of cloaca, isolated hydrocolpos, urogenital sinus, obstructive uropathy, and other pelvic cystic lesions such as ovarian cyst, enteric duplication cyst, bowel atresia, cystic type IV sacrococcygeal teratoma, and anterior meningocele. In addition, the sequence of findings on serial sonograms of transient ascites (from escape of urine via the fallopian tubes), progressive hydrocolpos, hydronephrosis, oligohydramnios, with or without development of peritoneal calcifications, has been described as suggestive of this malformation.[28–31] More specific sonographic signs supporting this diagnosis and the communication between the urinary system and the distal bowel in a female fetus are fluid-filled dilated rectum with intraluminal

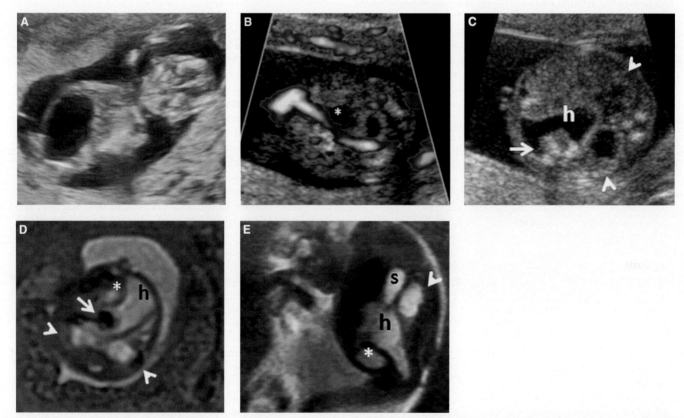

FIG. 27.2-6: Cloacal malformation with hydrocolpos. **A:** Coronal US at 13 weeks' gestational age (GA) shows a large abdominopelvic cyst. Axial US **(B)**, axial 2D SSFP, and sagittal fetography **(C)** fetal MRI on same fetus at 17 weeks' GA. There is bilateral hydronephrosis, large hydrocolpos (h) containing intraluminal echogenic foci with posterior shadowing (*arrow* in **C**), or dark T2 material as expected for meconium (*arrow* in **D**). The bladder is anterior to the hydrocolpos *(asterisk)* and the stomach (S) anterior to the left kidney (*arrowhead* in **E**).

calcifications (enteroliths) and the detection of calcified or echogenic meconium in the genitourinary system.[14,32] Unfortunately, these signs are not always present or easily detected on US. Assessment for the presence or absence of the anal sphincter complex would be helpful in cases where several fetal malformations are detected, especially if the genitourinary and skeletal systems are involved. In those fetuses, the concern for an underlying ARM should be raised and the sonographic absence of the anal dimple would further help support it.[11]

Fetal MRI can assess the pelvic organs, including the rectum. Starting around 20 to 21 weeks of gestation, meconium is expected to fill the rectum, and by 26 weeks, the entire colon is visualized with its characteristic bright T1 and dark T2 signal. The rectum is close to the bladder and its cul-de-sac at least 10 mm below the bladder neck.[33] In cloacas, the rectal content could be normal or alternatively increased in fluid signal depending on the degree of patency of the existing fistulous connections. In a series of long common channel cloacas, the rectum was dilated and high, not extending below the bladder. In addition, abnormal content signal could be also detected layering within the bladder, or in a hydrocolpos due to the presence of meconium.[18]

Differential Diagnosis: The differential diagnosis includes other etiologies presenting with megacystis and/or hydrocolpos. Megacystis can be seen in the setting of mechanical obstruction such as urethral atresia, or in the setting of megacystis-microcolon intestinal hypoperistalsis syndrome and prune belly syndrome. Urethral atresia is typically associated with early development of oligo/anhydramnios, typically with normal rectal anatomy. Megacystis-microcolon intestinal hypoperistalsis syndrome, a process more frequently affecting females, is typically associated with polyhydramnios during the third trimester, and fetal MRI will be extremely helpful in defining the presence of microcolon. Megacystis is also seen in prune belly syndrome, characterized by deficient abdominal musculature, urinary tract abnormalities, and cryptorchidism in males or major genital tract malformations in females including cloacal malformation.[13,18]

Hydrocolpos due to underlying isolated genital tract obstruction or urogenital sinus has a normal rectum, and fetal MRI is helpful in differentiating this process from cloacas.[18,34] Further analysis of the hydrocolpos and bladder content signal will help differentiate isolated hydrocolpos from urogenital sinus.[35,36]

Transient ascites and meconium peritonitis can be seen with cloacal malformation in the absence of bowel perforation (from urine and meconium escape through the fallopian tubes). Fetal MRI will help define the appearance of the bowel and the pelvic structures to support one of the two possibilities.[17]

Prognosis: The prognosis will be dictated by the presence of oligohydramnios and renal dysplasia, the type of cloaca, and the presence of other associated malformations. Postnatal management of associated anomalies and efficient meticulous and coordinated surgical repair by an experienced surgical team can provide the best chance for a good anatomic outcome. Functional results will depend as well on the degree of sacral development/hypoplasia, nerve supply, and spinal cord anomalies. In cases with incontinence despite excellent anatomic repair, effective bowel and bladder management programs have been devised to improve the patient's quality of life.[22]

Management: Once the diagnosis is suspected with US, fetal MRI will help better characterize the defect, assess renal parenchyma, and help identify potential associated malformations.

Fetal echocardiogram is recommended to rule out congenital heart defect. This approach provides more accurate information. The comprehensive multidisciplinary counseling session with the parents will be possible in the presence of pediatric and colorectal surgeons, pediatric urologist, neonatologist, pediatric nephrologist, and pediatric neurosurgeons.[37]

Attempts to restore the amniotic fluid volume with amnioports have been described in cases of bladder outlet obstruction to avoid lung hypoplasia.[38]

Delivery is recommended at a tertiary center, and these infants will need urgent clinical and radiologic evaluation by experienced pediatric surgeons and radiologists with crucial management decisions taking place during the first 24 hours.[39]

Recurrence Risk: The condition is sporadic, with low recurrence risk.[23]

UROGENITAL SINUS

Urogenital sinus is the persistence of an embryonic state in which there is a single-exit chamber for the bladder and the vagina in the presence of a normal rectum and anus. On physical examination, there are two perineal openings, one anterior for the urogenital sinus and the other for the anus (Fig. 27.2-5).[40]

Incidence: The condition affects females and is rare.[40] Its exact incidence is not well defined in the literature.

Embryology: The anomaly is the result of abnormal development of the lower vagina and failure of urethrovaginal septation. In this situation, urine flow can be impaired, leading to potential development of cystic dilatation of the vagina, also known as hydrocolpos (or hydrometrocolpos if the uterus is also involved). The hydrocolpos can compress the bladder forward, and can result in obstructive uropathy. Rarely, urine can reach the peritoneum through the fallopian tubes and present as urinary ascites.

Etiology: The most common etiology for persistent urogenital sinus is adrenogenital syndrome (congenital adrenal hyperplasia) or other in utero exposure to androgenic stimuli, with expected clitoral enlargement/ambiguous genitalia. It may also occur as pure urogenital sinus with normal external genitalia, or associated with gonadal dysgenesis and disorders of sexual development.[40]

Diagnosis: Prenatal cystic dilatation of the vagina will compress and displace the bladder anteriorly. A pelvic cystic mass with fluid-debris levels, representing mixing of urine and thick, mucoid cervical or vaginal secretions, should be highly concerning for hydrocolpos in the context of urogenital sinus.[41] Associated findings could include hydroureteronephrosis, urinary ascites, and, in severe cases, renal dysplasia and oligohydramnios (Fig. 27.2-7).[42] Enlarged adrenal glands with a cerebriform pattern, typically seen in neonates with congenital adrenal hyperplasia, might not be detected in utero until the late third trimester.[43] Babies with urogenital sinus can present with normal or ambiguous genitalia.

Fetal MRI could detect the cervical imprint on the vagina confirming the diagnosis of hydrocolpos and will define the presence or absence of meconium in the rectum or potential abnormal content. With normal meconium in the rectum, normal sonographic appearance of the anal sphincter and a hydrocolpos, urogenital sinus or vaginal obstruction should be suspected. If there is absence of meconium in the rectum or the rectum is

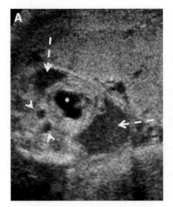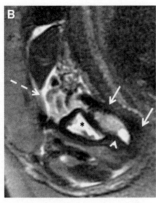

FIG. 27.2-7: At 26 weeks' gestation with urogenital sinus and severe oligohydramnios. **A:** Axial US. **B:** Sagittal heavily T2 hydrography MRI. There is a septated hydrocolpos *(arrowheads)* posterior to a thick-walled bladder *(asterisk)*. There is ascites *(dashed arrow)* and normal meconium-filled (dark T2 signal) rectum *(arrow)* posterior to the hydrocolpos.

identified but high, with fluid content or enteroliths, or there is sonographic absence of the anal dimple, the underlying malformation is a cloaca.[10,18,34] Additional clues to differentiate hydrocolpos in the context of urogenital sinus versus isolated genital tract obstruction were suggested in a small series comparing the T2 signal content between the bladder and the hydrocolpos. In four cases of urogenital sinus, both structures had a similar signal. On the other hand, in three cases of isolated genital tract obstruction pathology, the hydrocolpos showed a lower T2 signal.[35] These observations have been corroborated in another small series subsequently.[36]

Differential Diagnosis: One difficulty in diagnosing pelvic cystic masses in female fetuses is the potential confusion of the bladder with the hydrocolpos and an initial consideration of megacystis. However, the fetal bladder is outlined by the umbilical arteries, has an anterior midline position, and its volume is expected to change, allowing its correct identification.[13] In the setting of hydrocolpos, the possibility of cloaca, urogenital sinus, or obstructive vagina should be entertained. Other pelvic cystic lesions would be considered in the differential such as ovarian cyst, anterior meningocele, type IV sacrococcygeal teratoma, enteric duplication cyst, lymphatic malformations, and ectopic multicystic dysplastic kidney.[42]

Prognosis: The prognosis will be dictated by the degree of obstructive uropathy, and potential associated malformations. In survivors, the long-term outlook is reasonably good after reconstructive surgery. In the neonatal period, a correct prenatal diagnosis, absence of renal dysplasia, and coordinated work between the involved teams (obstetricians, neonatologists, radiologist, pediatric urologists, and pediatric surgeons) will significantly impact the clinical outcome.[42]

Management: Multidisciplinary counseling and delivery in a tertiary center is indicated. In the neonatal period, vaginal drainage will alleviate the abdominal distension and potential cardiorespiratory compromise and will improve any obstructive uropathy associated. Metabolic assessment and treatment in cases of congenital adrenal hyperplasia and chromosomal studies will be indicated in cases of ambiguous genitalia.[40,44]

In families with known history of congenital adrenal hyperplasia, early medical treatment can start *in utero* with maternal glucocorticoid administration before the development of the urogenital sinus (6th to 7th week of gestation) and be maintained after confirmation of gene mutation and female karyotype (usually by the 13th week of gestation).[43]

Recurrence Risk: Persistent urogenital sinus, in the absence of congenital adrenal hyperplasia, is usually a sporadic condition with low recurrence risk. On the other hand, congenital adrenal hyperplasia is a genetic disorder with an autosomal recessive transmission.[43]

HYDROCOLPOS

Hydrocolpos is the cystic dilatation of the vagina. Hydrometrocolpos is distension of the uterus and vagina. The term hydrocolpos is used here to refer to both conditions.

Incidence: The condition is rare. The prevalence of congenital hydrocolpos is less than 1 per 30,000 births and represents 15% of the abdominal masses in female fetuses.[34]

Embryology: There are two types of hydrocolpos. The **urinary type** is related to a urogenital sinus or cloacal malformation. The **secretory type** is related to vaginal obstruction due to abnormal development of the lower vagina presenting as imperforate hymen, vaginal agenesis or hypoplasia, and transverse septum.[44]

Etiology: Most cases of hydrocolpos are sporadic, but the **secretory type** can also be seen with genetic conditions associated with postaxial polydactyly such as McKusick–Kaufmann, Bander–Bielt, Langer–Giedion (thrico–rhino–pharyngeal syndrome) and Pallister–Hall syndromes. Hydrocolpos can be also seen with VACTERL and Mayer–Rokitansky–Küster–Hauser syndrome/MURCS (Müllerian duct aplasia/hypoplasia, renal agenesis/ectopia, and cervicothoracic somite dysplasia such as Klippel–Feil anomaly, abnormal ribs, or Sprengel deformity) associations (Fig. 27.2-8) and in Herlyn–Werner–Wunderlich syndrome (aka OHVIRA [obstructive hemivagina and ipsilateral renal agenesis]).[44]

Diagnosis: A pelvic cystic mass posterior to the bladder, with or without fluid–fluid levels, should be highly concerning for hydrocolpos in a female fetus. When there are Müllerian duct anomalies, it may appear as a septated cyst. Hydroureteronephrosis and ascites can be associated.[42] Fetal MRI can define the appearance of the rectum after 21 weeks of gestation. With a normal rectal cul-de-sac filled with meconium, and normal sonographic appearance of the anal sphincter, cloacal malformation is excluded, and hydrocolpos could be related to urogenital sinus or vaginal obstruction.[35] If there is absence of meconium in the distal rectum or the rectum is identified but with fluid content, enteroliths, or dilatation, the underlying malformation is cloaca.[34] Additional clues to differentiate hydrocolpos in the context of urogenital sinus versus isolated genital tract obstruction were suggested in a small series comparing the T2 signal content between the bladder and the hydrocolpos. In four cases of urogenital sinus, both structures had a similar signal. On the other hand, in three cases of isolated genital tract obstruction pathology, the hydrocolpos showed lower T2 signal.[35] These observations have been corroborated in another small series subsequently.[36]

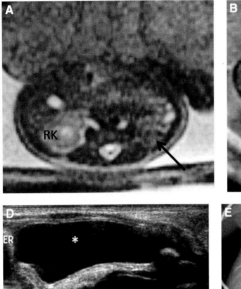
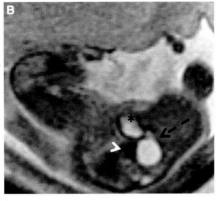
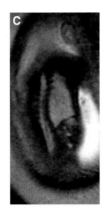
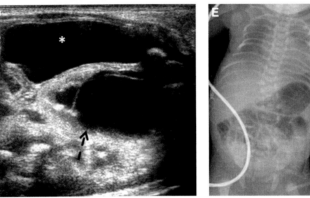

FIG. 27.2-8: Hydrocolpos in the setting of MURCS association, also known as type II Mayer–Rokytansky–Küster–Hauser syndrome. Axial (**A, B**) and coronal (**C**) T2 fetal MRI at 29 weeks' gestational age. **A:** There is left kidney renal agenesis with bowel filling the left renal fossa (arrow). A normal right kidney (RK) is present. **B:** Posterior to the bladder (asterisk), normal rectum (white arrowhead) and hydrocolpos (black dashed arrow) are noted. **C:** There is rightward thoracic scoliosis. Pelvic US (**D**) and chest-abdomen x-ray (**E**) on first day of life showing hydrocolpos (black dashed arrow) and focal segmentation vertebral anomaly at the lower thoracic spine accounting for thoracic scoliosis and short fourth ribs. There is also cardiomegaly and increased lung vascularity due to truncus arteriosus.

At birth, patients can present with a large abdominal mass with hydroureteronephrosis and possible respiratory distress from elevation of the diaphragm. If diagnosis and treatment are delayed, infection may follow, resulting in pyocolpos and sepsis.[25,44]

Differential Diagnosis: Differential diagnosis includes other cystic masses, such as ovarian cyst, enteric duplication cyst, megacystis, duplicated urinary bladder, anterior meningocele, and type IV sacrococcygeal teratoma.

In the setting of hydrocolpos, the possibility of cloaca, urogenital sinus, or obstructive vagina should be entertained. Complete assessment of the fetus will also help define the defect as potentially isolated or in the setting of a syndromic association or genetic disease.[36,42]

Prognosis: The prognosis will be dictated by the type of underlying defect (isolated vaginal obstruction versus urogenital sinus or cloacal malformation), the degree of obstructive uropathy present, and potential associated malformations or genetic syndromes. In isolated forms with preserved renal function, the outlook is excellent after final surgical reconstruction.[44]

Management: A complete assessment of the fetal anatomy is recommended to rule out other structural defects. Amniocentesis could be considered when there is concern for a major genetic anomaly. Multidisciplinary counseling and delivery in a tertiary center is indicated. In the immediate neonatal period, vaginal drainage will alleviate the abdominal distension and potential cardiorespiratory compromise and will improve urinary obstruction, if present. To rule out syndromes, high-resolution chromosome studies as well as long-term clinical follow-up could be needed.[44]

Recurrence Risk: Hydrocolpos is usually a sporadic condition with low recurrence risk. However, some syndromic forms are genetically transmitted.[41]

CLOACAL EXSTROPHY/OEIS

Cloacal exstrophy, also known as the OEIS complex (omphalocele, cloacal exstrophy, imperforate anus, spinal defects) is one of the rarest and most complex anorectal and urogenital malformations. The entity represents an anterior wall defect that includes the persistence and exstrophy of a common cloaca that receives ureters, ileum, and a rudimentary blind-ending hindgut (Fig. 27.2-9). It is commonly associated with omphalocele, spinal dysraphism, and incompletely formed external genitalia, and is always associated with an imperforate anus.[45] In females, there are usually two vaginal openings, widely separated and entering the lower aspect of each hemibladder and bilateral hemiuteri as well as two widely separated clitoral halves. In males, there is usually a rudimentary hemipenis on each side caudal to the exstrophy.[40] The terminal ileum could prolapse, giving the appearance of an elephant's trunk (Fig. 27.2-10).[46]

Incidence: The reported incidence is 1 in 200,000 to 400,000 live births, although recent epidemiologic studies provide a higher prevalence of 1 in 100,000 births when accounting for stillbirths and elective terminations.[40,47]. The condition can affect males and females, with most recent studies suggesting predilection toward female gender.[47] An increased incidence of cloacal exstrophy in monozygotic twins has also been described.[48]

Embryology: Cloacal exstrophy is a severe and rare malformation thought to be a developmental field defect affecting the mesoderm that later contributes to infraumbilical

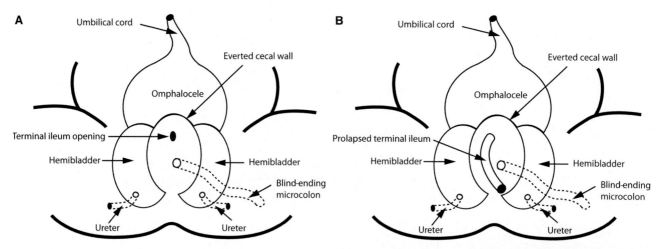

FIG. 27.2-9: Diagrams of typical anatomic appearances of cloacal exstrophy without **(A)** and with **(B)** prolapse terminal ileum. (Reproduced by permission from Springer: Calvo-Garcia MA, Kline-Fath BM, Rubio EI, et al. Fetal MRI of cloacal exstrophy. *Pediatr Radiol.* 2013;43(5):593–604. Copyright © 2012 Springer-Verlag Berlin Heidelberg.)

mesenchyme, urorectal septum, and caudal vertebrae during early embryogenesis.[48]

Before the 5th week of development, the urinary, genital, and gastrointestinal tracts empty into a common chamber, the cloaca. At the caudal end of the cloaca, the ectoderm lies directly over endoderm, forming the cloacal membrane, which at this stage forms part of the ventral wall. During the 6th week of development, the mesoderm grows toward the midline, forming the infraumbilical abdominal wall. Simultaneously, the urorectal septum extends caudally toward the cloacal membrane, and by the 8th week of

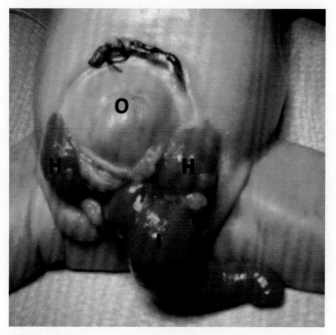

FIG. 27.2-10: Cloacal exstrophy with prolapsed terminal ileum photograph. There is a low-lying omphalocele (O). Extending from the back of the cecal plate is a prolapsed terminal ileum (I). The exstrophied hemibladders (H) are seen on each side. (Reprinted from Bischoff A, Calvo-Garcia MA, Baregamian N, et al. Prenatal counseling for cloaca and cloacal exstrophy: challenges faced by the pediatric surgeons. *Pediatr Surg Int.* 2012;28:781–788. https://creativecommons.org/licenses/by/2.0. Copyright © 2012 The Author(s).)

gestation, the cloaca is divided into an anterior chamber, the primitive urogenital sinus, and a posterior chamber, the rectum. There is also caudal retraction of the cloacal membrane, so that it is no longer part of the abdominal wall and eventually ruptures at the end of the 10th week of gestation (Fig. 27.2-1).

Different hypotheses have been elaborated along the years trying to explain the pathogenesis in cloacal exstrophy. Muecke suggested that abnormal mesodermal migration between the ectodermal and endodermal layers of the cloacal membrane or failure of the mesoderm to grow between those two layers led to its premature rupture. The stage of development when the abnormality occurs would determine the type of defect: cloacal exstrophy, bladder exstrophy, or isolated epispadias. Early damage would affect the mesenchyme that contributes to the infraumbilical mesoderm, the urorectal septum, and the lumbosacral somites. This results in failure of cloacal septation with a persistent cloaca and rudimentary hindgut with imperforate anus. A breakdown of the cloacal membrane causes exstrophy of the cloaca, failure of fusion of the genital tubercles, and diastasis of the pubic rami. Occasionally, there is also an omphalocele, and incomplete development of the lumbosacral vertebrae with, commonly, a closed neural tube defect. This constitutes what has been classically recognized as cloacal exstrophy. A later failure in migration of the infraumbilical mesoderm, after the caudal movement of the urorectal septum has been completed would result in bladder exstrophy.[49,50] However, this hypothesis has been challenged more recently by other histopathologic studies on human embryos where a very early defect in the caudal eminence instead of premature rupture of the cloacal membrane is thought to represent the triggering mechanism. Prenatally diagnosed cases of cloacal exstrophy with delayed rupture of the cloacal membrane, and rare malformation variants such as covered cloacal exstrophy would be better explained through that second hypothesis.[47]

Etiology: The underlying cause remains unknown, but genetic and environmental factors are thought to play a role.[50] Alterations in hedgehog signaling pathways and gene mutations have been detected by studying animal models, and individual cases in humans have been reported with chromosomal alterations. The most recent comprehensive clinical and risk factor analysis study identified statistically significant positive associations with prepregnancy obesity.[51]

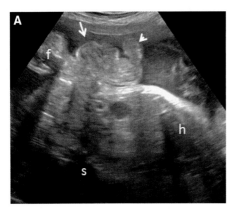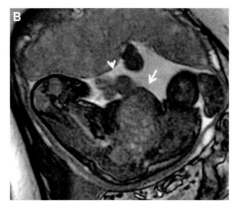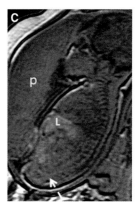

FIG. 27.2-11: Cloacal exstrophy. US and fetal MRI at 33 weeks of gestation. **A:** Sagittal oblique US shows a protruding "mass" *(arrow)* in the infraumbilical abdominal wall with a tubular extension *(arrowhead)* representing the "elephant trunk-like" image. Spine (s), femur (f), and heart (h) are labeled. **B:** Axial 2D SSFP. There is absent bladder, despite normal amniotic fluid volume, and protruding anterior pelvic contour *(arrow)* with a tubular extension *(arrowhead)*, the prolapsed terminal ileum. **C:** Sagittal midline T1 MRI shows lack of bright meconium signal in the rectum *(dashed arrow)*. Liver (L) and placenta (p) are labeled.

Diagnosis: Prenatal diagnosis with US has been suggested with the following criteria: failure to visualize the bladder in the presence of normal amniotic fluid volume, large midline infraumbilical anterior wall defect, omphalocele, cystic anterior wall structure, and/or neural tube defect.[52] In 1999, Hamada et al. reported the "elephant trunk-like" image as a new criterion for the diagnosis. This sign represents the prolapse of the terminal ileum through the exstrophy, and it is the most specific sonographic sign supporting this diagnosis (Fig. 27.2-11).[46] However, it is inconsistently found as the prolapse can be intermittent or potentially obscured by an adjacent omphalocele or umbilical cord.[53]

In the case of delayed rupture of the cloacal membrane, a protruding infraumbilical cyst will be seen outlined by the umbilical arteries. Later in the pregnancy, usually it breaks down, and by the time of delivery, a classic cloacal exstrophy is observed.[19,54]

When the elephant trunk-like sign is not seen, fetal MRI will be able to define the infraumbilical anterior wall defect with or without associated omphalocele. It will provide improved renal and spine assessment, and will help confirm a primitive hindgut with imperforate anus in the absence of meconium signal in the expected distribution of the colon and rectum.19

Differential Diagnosis: In the absence of an elephant trunk-like sign, a prenatal diagnosis with US can be challenging, and several cases have been misdiagnosed as omphalocele, gastroschisis, or sacrococcygeal teratoma.[52] In other cases, a differential diagnosis with bladder exstrophy is considered. The first clues for the correct diagnosis would be the absence of the bladder despite normal amniotic fluid and a protuberant anterior pelvic contour with or without associated omphalocele. In that situation, cloacal or bladder exstrophy should be considered, and US assessment of the anal sphincter and fetal MRI performed after 21 weeks, when meconium is expected to fill the rectum, could provide a definitive diagnosis.[19]

Prognosis: With modern surgical and medical treatment and in the absence of other severe malformations, the long-term survival rate is 83% to 100%. However, the challenge remains in how to improve the quality of life of these children, and to optimize functional results, it is paramount that a correct unified surgical management plan be instituted from birth.[37] Lifelong colostomy could be necessary, but pull-through procedures of the distal colon to the perineum might be successful together with the use of daily enemas. The majority of the patients achieve urinary continence with modern surgical reconstructive techniques, but most of them require intermittent bladder catheterization. Renal function has also a great impact on long-term outcome. Sexual function might be impaired and reproduction is unlikely.[50]

Management: Once a confident diagnosis is established, parental counseling with a multidisciplinary team, including colorectal surgeons, pediatric urologists, pediatric neurosurgeons, and neonatologists must be provided. After thorough patient education and counseling, parents can make an informed decision about available options. If parents choose postnatal treatment, referral to centers with experience in treating cloacal exstrophy is recommended.[37]

Recurrence Risk: The vast majority of cases are sporadic without a recognized associated chromosomal abnormality. There is, however, a higher reported incidence of cloacal exstrophy in monozygotic twins and in families in which one member is affected.[51,55]

BLADDER EXSTROPHY

Bladder exstrophy is characterized by a defect involving the infraumbilical abdominal wall and anterior wall of the urinary bladder. As a result, the open bladder mucosa becomes exposed and everted through the wall defect (Fig. 27.2-12). The umbilical cord is low set and the pubic symphysis is always widened. In males, there is complete epispadias with the urethral plate open to the tip of the phallus, resulting in a short, wide, anteriorly displaced penis. In females, there is an open urethral plate, a bifid clitoris, and wide separation of the labia.[50,56] In the most severe form, it may be accompanied by omphalocele, inguinal hernia, undescended testis, ventrally located anal orifice, relaxed anal sphincter, and intermittent rectal prolapse. Imperforate anus, spine defects, and spina bifida, more typical in cloacal exstrophy, have been found only in a low number of cases.[48]

Incidence: It occurs in 1 per 30,000 live births and is more common in males, with a close to 2:1 male-to-female ratio.[50,57]

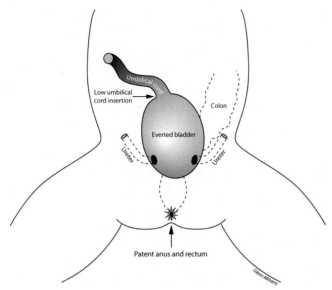

FIG. 27.2-12: Diagram of typical anatomic appearance of bladder exstrophy. The everted and opened bladder is exposed through an infraumbilical wall defect. There is a patent anus with normal rectum. (Reproduced by permission from Springer: Calvo-Garcia MA, Kline-Fath BM, Rubio EI, et al. Fetal MRI of cloacal exstrophy. *Pediatr Radiol.* 2013;43(5):593–604. Copyright © 2012 Springer-Verlag Berlin Heidelberg.)

Embryology: All authors agree that bladder exstrophy represents a slightly later abnormality in embryogenesis than in cloacal exstrophy. Several hypotheses attempt to explain the embryologic origin of the exstrophy spectrum including premature rupture of the cloacal membrane, mechanical obstruction of the mesodermal migration, and disruption of cellular function resulting in abnormal development. All those hypotheses are supported by animal studies and a final explanation possibly lies in a combination of those events but is still not resolved.[57]

Etiology: The etiology remains unclear, but it is thought to represent a multifactorial disorder in which environmental and genetic factors are likely to play a role.[57]

Diagnosis: Usual sonographic findings include persistent nonvisualization of the fetal bladder despite a normal amniotic fluid volume with a lower abdominal bulge, low umbilical insertion, small penis with anteriorly displaced scrotum, and widening of the iliac crests (Fig. 27.2-13). Color Doppler can help identify the

umbilical arteries running alongside the bulging mass, also noted in the case of cloacal exstrophy and linking the bulging mass with the exstrophic bladder.[58]

Similar findings will be noted with fetal MRI. In addition, normal appearance of the rectum and colon will allow a more definitive diagnosis, excluding cloacal exstrophy, especially in cases where omphalocele or other malformations are noted.[59]

Differential Diagnosis: The main differential diagnosis is cloacal exstrophy. The absence of associated malformations such as omphalocele or spinal defects would make cloacal exstrophy less likely. However, bladder exstrophy has been reported in a low number of cases with those same associated defects, and cases of cloacal exstrophy might not show obvious spinal defects. Fetal MRI will be able to differentiate between the two in those situations.

Other abdominal wall defects, such as omphalocele and gastroschisis, need to be considered, but they are easily differentiated and there should be a normally filled bladder.

Prognosis: The prognosis for bladder exstrophy has improved quite significantly. The overall outcome is relatively good, with expected urinary continence and normal sexual function in many patients.[60]

Management: Prenatal diagnosis will allow appropriate parental counseling, as well as optimal perinatal management and prompt postnatal surgical intervention. Early intervention, in the first 48 hours of life, minimizes damage to the exposed bladder and permits early closure and possibly avoids the need for pelvic osteotomy.[56,60]

Recurrence Risk: Most cases of bladder exstrophy are sporadic. The recurrence risk for offspring of affected individuals is 1 in 70. Among siblings, the estimated recurrence risk is been reported between 0.3% and 1%.[57]

PATENT URACHUS

The urachus is a vestigial remnant of the allantois, extending from the anterosuperior aspect of the bladder toward the umbilicus. Complete or partial persistence of its lumen gives rise to urachal disorders. The anomalies of the urachus are classified according to the persisting patent segment and include congenital

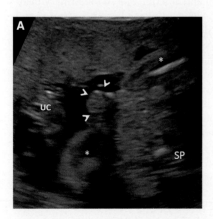

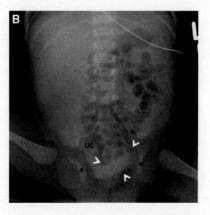

FIG. 27.2-13: Bladder exstrophy. **A:** Axial US at 24 weeks of gestation shows a protruding anterior pelvic wall "mass" (*arrowheads*) and lack of visualization of fluid-filled bladder in the presence of normal amniotic fluid volume. The spine (SP) and thighs (*white asterisks*) and umbilical cord (UC) are denoted for orientation. **B:** Postnatal frontal abdomen x-ray on the first day of life. Note also the pubic symphysis diastasis (*black asterisks*).

patent urachus, urachal cyst, umbilical-urachal sinus, and vesico-urachal diverticulum (Fig. 27.2-14).[61]

Incidence: Urachal anomalies are uncommon, with a male-to-female ratio of 2:1. Patent urachus accounts for about 50% of all cases, urachal cyst 30%, umbilical-urachal sinus about 15%, and vesico-urachal diverticulum 3% to 5%.[62]

Embryology: The urachus is the intra-abdominal remnant of the embryonic allantois (Fig. 27.2-1). The allantois appears on approximately the 16th day of gestation as a small diverticulum from the caudal wall of the yolk sac that extends into the connecting stalk. The allantois is involved with development of the dome of the urinary bladder and the umbilical vessels, and forms a hollow tube that connects the superior aspect of the urogenital sinus with the anterior abdominal wall at the umbilicus. As the bladder enlarges, the allantois becomes obliterated to form a thick tube, the urachus, also known as the median umbilical ligament, situated in the prevesical space, between the peritoneum behind and the transversalis fascia in front. Defective closure may happen and leads to congenital pathology of the urachus.[62]

Etiology: The etiology of urachal anomalies is unknown. Urachal anomalies, particularly patent urachus, have been reported, in up to one-third of these cases, in the setting of bladder outlet obstruction as a "pop-off" mechanism to protect the upper urinary tract.[61]

Diagnosis: A patent urachus results from persistent communication between the bladder lumen and the umbilicus. The bladder dome will show an elongated appearance toward the abdominal cord insertion (Fig. 27.2-15). In some cases, it could lead to the development of a true cyst at the base of the umbilical cord, which communicates with the bladder dome and will

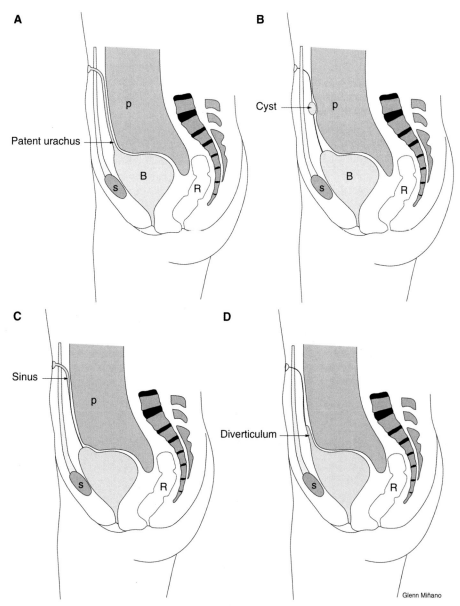

Glenn Miñano

FIG. 27.2-14: Types of congenital urachal anomalies. **A:** Patent urachus. **B:** Urachal cyst. **C:** Urachal sinus. **D:** Urachal diverticulum. B, bladder; P, peritoneal cavity; R, rectum; S, symphysis pubis.

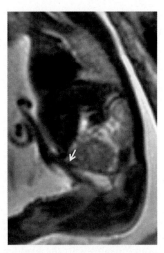

FIG. 27.2-15: A 25-week-old fetus with patent urachus. T2 sagittal MRI demonstrates elongation of the bladder dome toward the abdominal cord insertion (*white arrow*).

lead to separation of the umbilical cord vessels (Fig. 27.2-16). The cyst is known as allantoic, or vesico-allantoic cyst. US with color Doppler, 3D, 4D US, and fetal MRI can characterize these lesions. Some of these cysts can be very large and progress to diffuse cord edema.[63] Alternatively, they can rupture, leading to different degrees of bladder prolapse through the patent urachus. In most of these fetuses with subsequent bladder prolapse, the bony pelvis and the external genitalia have been described as normal.[64–66] However, there are two fetal reports with associated pubic symphysis diastasis and external genitalia abnormalities that would fit better with exstrophy variants.[67,68]

Urachal cysts are noted as anterior midline cysts, cranial to the bladder without dynamic changes in size or shape.[69]

Differential Diagnosis: Allantoic cysts in the setting of patent urachus will present as a cyst near the fetal anterior abdominal wall. Omphalomesenteric cysts are also true umbilical cord cysts and present in this same location, but they do not separate the cord vessels and do not communicate with the bladder dome. Umbilical cord pseudocysts will affect more distal segments of the cord.[63] Color Doppler US will be able to differentiate from umbilical vein varix or umbilical artery aneurysm.[62]

The differential diagnosis of an urachal cyst includes ovarian cyst, mesenteric cyst, omphalomesenteric duct remnant, and bowel atresia.

Prognosis: Allantoic cysts have no increased risk for chromosomal anomaly. One-third of these cases occur in association with bladder outlet obstruction, and its presence supports a patent urachus with urine leakage from the umbilicus noted in the neonatal period.[63]

Potential umbilical cord vessel compression, umbilical cord hematoma, or torsion leading to fetal distress and even fetal death has been described as potential rare complications in the setting of umbilical cord cysts.[70]

Associated anomalies are uncommon but include omphalocele and omphalomesenteric remnants as well as other genitourinary conditions such as hypospadias, undescended testicles, crossed renal ectopia, vesicoureteral reflux, hydronephrosis, and lower urinary tract obstruction.[63,64]

Postnatally, all urachal malformations have a high incidence of recurrent infection, stone formation, and may develop benign and malignant neoplasms.[61]

Management: In the presence of an allantoic cyst, some authors recommend close prenatal surveillance, including assessment of the size of the cyst, Doppler analysis of the umbilical circulation, and delivery as soon as fetal maturity is demonstrated.[70] Attempts to assess the pelvic ring and external genitalia as well as pediatric urology consultation would improve

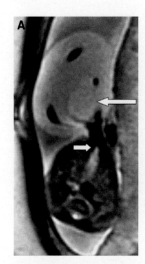
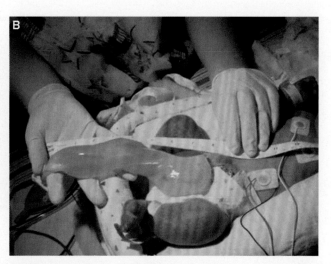

FIG. 27.2-16: Patent urachus with allantoic cyst. **A:** Fetal MRI axial T2 image shows elongation of the bladder dome toward the abdominal cord insertion (*short arrow*) with a cyst (*long arrow*) at the base of the cord. Note the splaying of the umbilical vessels (*dark structures*). **B:** First day of life photograph. There is a large edematous mass in the umbilical cord. (Reproduced by permission from Springer: Bunch PT, Kline-Fath BM, Imhoff SC, et al. Allantoic cyst: a prenatal clue to patent urachus. *Pediatr Radiol.* 2006;36(10):1090–1095. Copyright © 2006 Springer Nature.)

parental counseling. Cesarean section can be considered in cases of large allantoic cysts to better define the site of cord ligation. After delivery, surgical consult of all urachal malformations is recommended.[63]

Recurrence Risk: These conditions are sporadic with a low recurrence risk.

REFERENCES

1. Holschneider A, Hutson J, Pena A, et al. Preliminary report on the International Conference for the Development of Standards for the Treatment of Anorectal Malformations. *J Pediatr Surg.* 2005;40:1521–1526.
2. Levitt MA, Pena A. Anorectal malformations. *Orphanet J Rare Dis.* 2007;2:33.
3. Pena A. Anorectal malformations. *Semin Pediatr Surg.* 1995;4:35–47.
4. Alamo L, Meyrat BJ, Meuwly JY, et al. Anorectal malformations: finding the pathway out of the labyrinth. *Radiographics.* 2013;33:491–512.
5. Podberesky DJ, Towbin AJ, Eltomey MA, et al. Magnetic resonance imaging of anorectal malformations. *Magn Reson Imaging Clin N Am.* 2013;21:791–812.
6. Kluth D. Embryology of anorectal malformations. *Semin Pediatr Surg.* 2010;19:201–208.
7. Mo R, Kim JH, Zhang J, et al. Anorectal malformations caused by defects in sonic hedgehog signaling. *Am J Pathol.* 2001;159:765–774.
8. Jo Mauch T, Albertine KH. Urorectal septum malformation sequence: insights into pathogenesis. *Anat Rec.* 2002;268:405–410.
9. Moon MH, Cho JY, Kim JH, et al. In-utero development of the fetal anal sphincter. *Ultrasound Obstet Gynecol.* 2010;35:556–559.
10. Vijayaraghavan SB, Prema AS, Suganyadevi P. Sonographic depiction of the fetal anus and its utility in the diagnosis of anorectal malformations. *J Ultrasound Med.* 2011;30:37–45.
11. Ochoa JH, Chiesa M, Vildoza RP, et al. Evaluation of the perianal muscular complex in the prenatal diagnosis of anorectal atresia in a high-risk population. *Ultrasound Obstet Gynecol.* 2012;39:521–527.
12. Taipale P, Rovamo L, Hiilesmaa V. First-trimester diagnosis of imperforate anus. *Ultrasound Obstet Gynecol.* 2005;25:187–188.
13. Calvo-Garcia MA. Imaging evaluation of fetal megacystis: how can magnetic resonance imaging help? *Semin Ultrasound CT MR.* 2015;36:537–549.
14. Mandell J, Lillehei CW, Greene M, et al. The prenatal diagnosis of imperforate anus with rectourinary fistula: dilated fetal colon with enterolithiasis. *J Pediatr Surg.* 1992;27:82–84.
15. Lubusky M, Prochazka M, Dhaifalah I, et al. Fetal enterolithiasis: prenatal sonographic and MRI diagnosis in two cases of urorectal septum malformation (URSM) sequence. *Prenat Diagn.* 2006;26:345–349.
16. Jerdee T, Newman B, Rubesova E. Meconium in perinatal imaging: associations and clinical significance. *Semin Ultrasound CT MR.* 2015;36:161–177.
17. Veyrac C, Couture A, Saguintaah M, et al. MRI of fetal GI tract abnormalities. *Abdom Imaging.* 2004;29:411–420.
18. Calvo-Garcia MA, Kline-Fath BM, Levitt MA, et al. Fetal MRI clues to diagnose cloacal malformations. *Pediatr Radiol.* 2011;41:1117–1128.
19. Calvo-Garcia MA, Kline-Fath BM, Rubio EI, et al. Fetal MRI of cloacal exstrophy. *Pediatr Radiol.* 2013;43:593–604.
20. Nagaraj UD, Calvo-Garcia MA, Merrow AC, et al. Decreased rectal meconium signal on MRI in fetuses with open spinal dysraphism. *Prenat Diagn.* 2018;38:870–875.
21. Furey EA, Bailey AA, Twickler DM. Fetal MR imaging of gastrointestinal abnormalities. *Radiographics.* 2016;36:904–917.
22. Bischoff A, Bealer J, Pena A. Controversies in anorectal malformations. *Lancet Child Adolesc Health.* 2017;1:323–330.
23. Falcone RA Jr, Levitt MA, Pena A, et al. Increased heritability of certain types of anorectal malformations. *J Pediatr Surg.* 2007;42:124–127; discussion 127–128.
24. Chauvin NA, Epelman M, Victoria T, et al. Complex genitourinary abnormalities on fetal MRI: imaging findings and approach to diagnosis. *AJR Am J Roentgenol.* 2012;199:W222–W231.
25. Pena A, Levitt MA, Hong A, et al. Surgical management of cloacal malformations: a review of 339 patients. *J Pediatr Surg.* 2004;39:470–479; discussion 470–479.
26. Runck LA, Method A, Bischoff A, et al. Defining the molecular pathologies in cloaca malformation: similarities between mouse and human. *Dis Model Mech.* 2014;7:483–493.
27. Martinez-Frias ML, Bermejo E, Rodriguez-Pinilla E. Anal atresia, vertebral, genital, and urinary tract anomalies: a primary polytopic developmental field defect identified through an epidemiological analysis of associations. *Am J Med Genet A.* 2000;95:169–173.
28. Cilento BG Jr, Benacerraf BR, Mandell J. Prenatal diagnosis of cloacal malformation. *Urology.* 1994;43:386–388.
29. Warne S, Chitty LS, Wilcox DT. Prenatal diagnosis of cloacal anomalies. *BJU Int.* 2002;89:78–81.
30. Shono T, Taguchi T, Suita S, et al. Prenatal ultrasonographic and magnetic resonance imaging findings of congenital cloacal anomalies associated with meconium peritonitis. *J Pediatr Surg.* 2007;42:681–684.
31. Winkler NS, Kennedy AM, Woodward PJ. Cloacal malformation: embryology, anatomy, and prenatal imaging features. *J Ultrasound Med.* 2012;31:1843–1855.
32. Chaubal N, Dighe M, Shah M, et al. Calcified meconium: an important sign in the prenatal sonographic diagnosis of cloacal malformation. *J Ultrasound Med.* 2003;22:727–730.
33. Saguintaah M, Couture A, Veyrac C, et al. MRI of the fetal gastrointestinal tract. *Pediatr Radiol.* 2002;32:395–404.
34. Picone O, Laperelle J, Sonigo P, et al. Fetal magnetic resonance imaging in the antenatal diagnosis and management of hydrocolpos. *Ultrasound Obstet Gynecol.* 2007;30:105–109.
35. Capito C, Belarbi N, Paye Jaouen A, et al. Prenatal pelvic MRI: additional clues for assessment of urogenital obstructive anomalies. *J Pediatr Urol.* 2014;10:162–166.
36. Millischer AE, Grevent D, Rousseau V, et al. Fetal MRI compared with ultrasound for the diagnosis of obstructive genital malformations. *Prenat Diagn.* 2017;37:1138–1145.
37. Bischoff A, Calvo-Garcia MA, Baregamian N, et al. Prenatal counseling for cloaca and cloacal exstrophy-challenges faced by pediatric surgeons. *Pediatr Surg Int.* 2012;28:781–788.
38. Polzin WJ, Lim FY, Habli M, et al. Use of an amnioport to maintain amniotic fluid volume in fetuses with oligohydramnios secondary to lower urinary tract obstruction or fetal renal anomalies. *Fetal Diagn Ther.* 2017;41:51–57.
39. Levitt MA, Pena A. Cloacal malformations: lessons learned from 490 cases. *Semin Pediatr Surg.* 2010;19:128–138.
40. Hendren WH. Urogenital sinus and cloacal malformations. *Semin Pediatr Surg.* 1996;5:72–79.
41. Taori K, Krishnan V, Sharbidre KG, et al. Prenatal sonographic diagnosis of fetal persistent urogenital sinus with congenital hydrocolpos. *Ultrasound Obstet Gynecol.* 2010;36:641–643.
42. Pauleta J, Melo MA, Borges G, et al. Prenatal diagnosis of persistent urogenital sinus with duplicated hydrometrocolpos and ascites—a case report. *Fetal Diagn Ther.* 2010;28:229–232.
43. Chambrier ED, Heinrichs C, Avni FE. Sonographic appearance of congenital adrenal hyperplasia in utero. *J Ultrasound Med.* 2002;21:97–100.
44. Khanna K, Sharma S, Gupta DK. Hydrometrocolpos etiology and management: past beckons the present. *Pediatr Surg Int.* 2018;34:249–261.
45. Carey JC. Exstrophy of the cloaca and the OEIS complex: one and the same. *Am J Med Genet A.* 2001;99:270.
46. Hamada H, Takano K, Shiina H, et al. New ultrasonographic criterion for the prenatal diagnosis of cloacal exstrophy: elephant trunk-like image. *J Urol.* 1999;162:2123–2124.
47. Feldkamp ML, Botto LD, Amar E, et al. Cloacal exstrophy: an epidemiologic study from the International Clearinghouse for Birth Defects Surveillance and Research. *Am J Med Genet C Semin Med Genet.* 2011;157C:333–343.
48. Martinez-Frias ML, Bermejo E, Rodriguez-Pinilla E, et al. Exstrophy of the cloaca and exstrophy of the bladder: two different expressions of a primary developmental field defect. *Am J Med Genet A.* 2001;99:261–269.
49. Muecke EC. The role of the cloacal membrane in exstrophy: the first successful experimental study. *J Urol.* 1964;92:659–667.
50. Ebert AK, Reutter H, Ludwig M, et al. The exstrophy-epispadias complex. *Orphanet J Rare Dis.* 2009;4:23.
51. Keppler-Noreuil KM, Conway KM, Shen D, et al. Clinical and risk factor analysis of cloacal defects in the National Birth Defects Prevention Study. *Am J Med Genet A Part A.* 2017;173:2873–2885.
52. Austin PF, Homsy YL, Gearhart JP, et al. The prenatal diagnosis of cloacal exstrophy. *J Urol.* 1998;160:1179–1181.
53. Richards DS, Langham MR Jr, Mahaffey SM. The prenatal ultrasonographic diagnosis of cloacal exstrophy. *J Ultrasound Med.* 1992;11:507–510.
54. Langer JC, Brennan B, Lappalainen RE, et al. Cloacal exstrophy: prenatal diagnosis before rupture of the cloacal membrane. *J Pediatr Surg.* 1992;27:1352–1355.
55. Smith NM, Chambers HM, Furness ME, et al. The OEIS complex (omphalocele-exstrophy-imperforate anus-spinal defects): recurrence in sibs. *J Med Genet.* 1992;29:730–732.
56. Gearhart JP, Ben-Chaim J, Jeffs RD, et al. Criteria for the prenatal diagnosis of classic bladder exstrophy. *Obstet Gynecol.* 1995;85:961–964.
57. Siffel C, Correa A, Amar E, et al. Bladder exstrophy: an epidemiologic study from the International Clearinghouse for Birth Defects Surveillance and Research, and an overview of the literature. *Am J Med Genet C Semin Med Genet.* 2011;157C:321–332.
58. Wu JL, Fang KH, Yeh GP, et al. Using color Doppler sonography to identify the perivesical umbilical arteries: a useful method in the prenatal diagnosis of omphalocele-exstrophy-imperforate anus-spinal defects complex. *J Ultrasound Med.* 2004;23:1211–1215.
59. Hsieh K, O'Loughlin MT, Ferrer FA. Bladder exstrophy and phenotypic gender determination on fetal magnetic resonance imaging. *Urology.* 2005;65:998–999.
60. Goyal A, Fishwick J, Hurrell R, et al. Antenatal diagnosis of bladder/cloacal exstrophy: challenges and possible solutions. *J Pediatr Urol.* 2012;8:140–144.
61. Cilento BG Jr, Bauer SB, Retik AB, et al. Urachal anomalies: defining the best diagnostic modality. *Urology.* 1998;52:120–122.

62. Sepulveda W, Bower S, Dhillon HK, et al. Prenatal diagnosis of congenital patent urachus and allantoic cyst: the value of color flow imaging. *J Ultrasound Med.* 1995;14:47–51.
63. Bunch PT, Kline-Fath BM, Imhoff SC, et al. Allantoic cyst: a prenatal clue to patent urachus. *Pediatr Radiol.* 2006;36:1090–1095.
64. Matsui F, Matsumoto F, Shimada K. Prenatally diagnosed patent urachus with bladder prolapse. *J Pediatr Surg.* 2007;42:e7–e10.
65. Sepulveda W, Rompel SM, Cafici D, et al. Megacystis associated with an umbilical cord cyst: a sonographic feature of a patent urachus in the first trimester. *J Ultrasound Med.* 2010;29:295–300.
66. Riddell JV, Houle AM, Franc-Guimond J, et al. Prenatal vesico-allantoic cyst outcome—a spectrum from patent urachus to bladder exstrophy. *Prenat Diagn.* 2015;35:1342–1346.
67. Tong SY, Lee JE, Kim SR, et al. Umbilical cord cyst: a prenatal clue to bladder exstrophy. *Prenat Diagn.* 2007;27:1177–1179.
68. Choi SM, Park T, Park JK, et al. Pseudoexstrophy of the bladder diagnosed prenatally. *Prenat Diagn.* 2013;33:1002–1003.
69. Goldstein I, Shalev E, Nisman D. The dilemma of prenatal diagnosis of bladder exstrophy: a case report and a review of the literature. *Ultrasound Obstet Gynecol.* 2001;17:357–359.
70. Sepulveda W, Wong AE, Gonzalez R, et al. Fetal death due to umbilical cord hematoma: a rare complication of umbilical cord cyst. *J Matern Fetal Neonatal Med.* 2005;18:387–390.

27.3 Fetal Sex and Ambiguous Genitalia

Christopher Ian Cassady

Genetic, or chromosomal, sex is determined at conception by the absence or presence of a Y chromosome. The complex process of sexual differentiation then unfolds with the expression of a gonadal (or internal) sex, and a phenotypic (or external, anatomical) sex. When these three facets of sex expression are inconsistent, there is sexual ambiguity, or what is preferentially termed a *disorder of sex development (DSD)*.

Distinction should be made between sex differentiation and gender determination. The former is a biological term, the latter a social construct. Although often historically used interchangeably, these terms are best used specifically for clarity.

INCIDENCE

Nearly all of the time, an XY genotype results in a baby with a typical male phenotype of penis and scrotum with median raphe, testes, vas deferens, and a prostate gland; likewise, an XX genotype has labia majora and minora, a clitoris, and a uterus with fallopian tubes and ovaries. However, approximately 1/5,000 liveborn infants has a disorder of sexual development in which the genotype and classic phenotype are not consistently aligned.[1,2] This may occur for any number of complex reasons, including both in isolated instances and with other manifestations of syndromic or chromosomal anomalies (Table 27.3-1).

EMBRYOLOGY

While it is true that without the protein encoded by the sex-determining region Y (SRY) gene on the short arm of the Y chromosome there can be no male gonadal or phenotypic sexual expression, it would be incorrect to believe that the absence of SRY alone produces a normal female; genes on the X and other chromosomes, including WNT4 on chromosome 1, are necessary for ovarian development.[3] Internal differentiation begins in the fourth gestational week with the migration of primitive germ cells from the yolk sac to form genital ridges medial to both the lateral paramesonephric (Müllerian) ducts and the mesonephric (Wolffian) ducts that will end caudally in the cloaca. In week 8, gonadal differentiation is thought to begin in the fetus. The SRY protein differentiates Sertoli cells in the testes to secrete Müllerian inhibitory factor (MIF) or substance (also called anti-Müllerian hormone, AMH), inducing degeneration of paramesonephric ducts. The gonadal ridges form testes, and the mesonephric ducts form the rete testis, efferent ducts, and vas deferens under the influence of testosterone secreted by testicular Leydig cells beginning in week 9. Over weeks 9 to 20 in the female, the gonad becomes the ovary, and, under the influence of ovarian follicular estrogen, the paramesonephric ducts form the fallopian tubes, uterus, and upper vagina; the mesonephric duct regresses because of a lack of MIF and testosterone. Ovarian follicles appear after week 14.

Externally, fetuses are identical early. In week 5, cloacal folds form on either side of the cloacal membrane, and then join to make a genital tubercle and the urogenital (UG) folds on each side of the UG membrane that has been subdivided separately

TABLE 27.3-1 Conditions Associated with Nonisolated Ambiguous Genitalia

Chromosomal abnormalities and gene disorder syndromes
Abnormal sex chromosome complements
Aarskog–Scott (X-linked)
Antley–Bixler (AR)
Axenfeld–Rieger (AD)
ATRX (X-linked)
Carpenter (AR)
CAH (X-linked)
Cornelia de Lange (AD)
del(11)(q23.3)
del(13)(q33.2)
Denys–Drash (AD)
DREAM-PL
46XY t(7;16)
Fraser (AR)
Frasier (AD)
Fryns (AR)
Genitopalatocardiac (Gardner–Silengo–Wachtel)
Kallmann (AR)
MCA/MR (AR)
McKusick–Kaufman (AR)
MFRG (AD)
Noonan (AD)
Ohtahara (AR)
Opitz type I: X-linked, type II: del (22q11.2)
Persistent Müllerian duct (AR, X-linked)
Prader–Willi (15q11-q13 dysfunction)
Proud (X-linked)
Robinow (AR and AD)
Rubinstein–Taybi (AD)
Russell–Silver (AR and AD)
Smith–Lemli–Opitz (AR)
Trisomies 13 and 18
Triploidy
WAGR (AD)
Wolf–Hirschhorn (Deletion 4p)
Associations
CHARGE (AD)
EEC (epispadias, exstrophy, OEIS)
MURCS (Müllerian duct, renal, and cervicothoracic somite a/dysplasia)
VACTERL (Wernestrup)

From Chitayat D, Glanc P. Diagnostic approach in prenatally detected genital abnormalities. *Ultrasound Obstet Gynecol.* 2010;35(6):637–646. Copyright © 2010 ISUOG. Published by John Wiley & Sons, Ltd.; and Adapted by permission from Nature: Hutson JM, Grover SR, O'Connell M, et al. Malformation syndromes associated with disorders of sex development. *Nat Rev.* 2014;10(8):476–487. Copyright © 2014 Springer Nature.

from the anal orifice out of the cloacal membrane in week 7. Two additional labioscrotal folds form alongside the UG folds. After 7 (generally by 9 to 12) weeks, in a female phenotype, the genital tubercle becomes the clitoris and the UG sinus becomes the lower vagina and the urethra. The UG folds make the labia minora, and the labioscrotal folds make the labia majora. For a male phenotype, the genital tubercle becomes the penis and the UG folds the penile urethra, while the UG sinus becomes the proximal urethra and the prostate. The labioscrotal folds form the scrotum.[3-5] Initially, the phallus created by the genital tubercles is identical in length in both males and females, and it is not until 11 weeks that the external genitalia begin to become more distinct.[6]

Testicular descent begins from a gonadal position in the abdomen and continues to the inguinal canals and then to the scrotum. Between **10 and 23 weeks**, nearly 10% of testes have migrated from the abdomen and are situated in the inguinal canal. At **24 to 26 weeks**, 58% have migrated from the abdomen and descent of the testes from the inguinal canal to the scrotum begins. By **29 weeks**, less than 20% have not descended to the scrotum, and by **32 weeks**, 90% to 95% of testes are intrascrotal.[7,8]

PATHOGENESIS

When there is a disruption in the coordination among all the processes involved from genotypic sex establishment through phenotypic expression, a disorder of sex development occurs. DSDs have been categorized by the International Intersex Consensus Conference, which in 2006 published a revised nomenclature incorporating genetic assignment and description, and removing reference to gender.[9] Classification systems vary because some diagnoses overlap categories, but, in general, pathologies can be assigned to one of six groups,[10] as described here.

46, XX Disorder of Sex Development (Female Pseudohermaphroditism)

This is the most common DSD. Ovaries and Müllerian structures are normal, but external genitalia are masculinized secondary to androgen exposure. Although the exposure could be exogenous, the most common cause is congenital adrenal hyperplasia (CAH), a collection of autosomal recessive disorders from five genes that code for enzymes involved in cortisol synthesis. CAH can affect either genetic sex, but only when there is masculinization of a genetic female is it considered a cause of 46, XX DSD. Depending on the enzyme deficiency, there may be an overproduction of adrenal androgens (masculinized female genitalia, normal male genitalia) or a lack of gonadal steroid production (normal female genitalia and undermasculinized male genitalia) (Fig. 27.3-1).

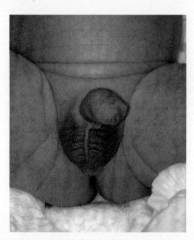

FIGURE 27.3-1: Congenital adrenal hyperplasia. Newborn with XX genotype and male phenotype.

46, XY Disorder of Sex Development (Male Pseudohermaphroditism)

Testes are at least initially present, but internal or external genitalia are not at all or incompletely masculinized. There are eight categories, and these are generally assigned after birth (Table 27.3-2).

Ovotesticular Disorder of Sex Development (True Hermaphroditism)

Both testicular and ovarian tissues are present. There are three types: lateral, with a testis on one side and ovary on the other (typically left); bilateral ovotestis; or ovotestis on one side and either testis or ovary on the other, which is most common. External genitalia are ambiguous: There may be hypospadias, cryptorchidism, and incomplete labioscrotal fold fusion. Internal genitalia generally follow the gonad per side.

Gonadal Dysgenesis

There is ambiguous development of internal genitalia, the genitourinary sinus, and external genitalia with dysgenetic gonads from lack of development or loss of primordial germ cells. Phenotypic variability occurs from mixed or partial to pure gonadal dysgenesis (GD), a term that describes conditions with normal sets of sex chromosomes (e.g., 46, XX or 46, XY) but with no gonads, including Swyer syndrome (46, XY with female external genitalia because of a lack of testicular development) and Perrault syndrome (46, XX without ovaries). Partial GD has a streak gonad on one side and a typically dysgenetic testis on the other; these patients are at risk for development of gonadal tumors, including dysgerminoma.[11] This category includes patients with Denys–Drash syndrome, WAGR (Wilms tumor, aniridia, genitourinary abnormalities, mental retardation), and Frasier syndrome, each of which can express "sex reversal," in which the phenotypic sex appears normal but is discordant with the chromosomal sex (Table 27.3-3).

Sex Chromosome Disorder of Sex Development

There is an abnormal number or complement of sex chromosomes. Examples include Klinefelter syndrome (XXY/XXXY), triple X (47XXX), or Turner syndrome (45XO or 45XO/46XX). This would also include individuals with four or more sex chromosomes. These will not be diagnosed *in utero* other than by karyotype as there is typically no genital abnormality appreciated.

TABLE 27.3-2   Etiologies of Male Pseudohermaphroditism

Leydig cell failure
Testosterone biosynthesis enzyme defects
Androgen insensitivity syndrome (testicular feminization syndrome), complete or partial
5-Alpha reductase deficiency
Persistent Müllerian duct syndrome
Congenital anorchia (vanishing testes syndrome)
Exogenous progesterone exposure
Smith–Lemli–Opitz syndrome

TABLE 27.3-3 Sex Reversal ("Chromosome–Phenotype Discordance")

Deletion 9p
Monosomy 10q25
Smith–Lemli–Opitz syndrome
Campomelic dysplasia
Gonadal dysgenesis DSD
   Swyer syndrome (XY female)
   WT1 gene alterations (chromosome 11)
   WAGR (Wilms tumor, aniridia, genitourinary abnormalities, mental retardation)
   Frasier syndrome
   Denys–Drash syndrome
Sex chromosome DSD
- Functional disomy of Xp
- Mosaicism (e.g., 45XO/46XY)
46, XX DSD
- Congenital adrenal hyperplasia
46, XY DSD
- Complete androgen insensitivity syndrome (testicular feminization syndrome)
46, XX testicular DSD
- De la Chapelle syndrome

46, XX Testicular/Ovotesticular Disorder of Sex Development

The genotype is 46, XX with male external genitalia. Nearly all (80% to 90%) are from anomalous Y-X translocation involving the SRY gene in meiosis; the greater the amount of Y DNA, the more virilized the phenotype. Therefore, there is wide variability in appearance, including what looks like "sex reversal" (de la Chapelle syndrome or XX male syndrome). Differentiation between testicular and ovotesticular varieties is made by histology. These are mostly SRY+, in comparison with 46, XX DSD (female pseudohermaphroditism), which is SRY−; note, however, that the phenotypes overlap.

IMAGING

Although parental curiosity often drives the initial imaging investigation of fetal sex, there are medical reasons for understanding sex assignment, as with fetuses at risk for x-linked and sex-specific conditions. It can be important in the determination of zygosity in multiple gestations. In addition, abnormal genitalia may be among the clues to a potentially antenatally diagnosable syndrome or chromosomal defect.[7] However, even when fetal sex is medically determined, ethical concerns around communicating this information to families remain subject to ongoing debate.[12,13]

Given the embryology, it is unsurprising that distinguishing male from female external genitalia is not reliably possible before 12 weeks. However, using the "sagittal sign" and transabdominal scanning in patients with body mass index (BMI) less than 24, many report extremely high levels of accuracy from 12 weeks onward in fetal sex assignment. Male sex is assigned if the angle of the phallus at the genital tubercle is greater than 30° from parallel to the fetal lumbosacral skin, and female if the angle is less than 10°. Angles between 10° and 30° are labeled "indeterminate,"

and this small number of fetuses (3% to 4%) is scanned again at later gestational ages (GAs)[14-16] (Figs. 27.3-2 and 27.3-3). It has been suggested that the ultrasonographer also verify a male phenotype by recognizing the "dome sign," which is the rounded scrotum and its midline echogenic median raphe, both at the penile base, as differentiated from the parallel and separate echogenic lines of the labia in a female phenotype.[17,18] Knowing that there is a normally larger anogenital distance in males starting at 12 weeks' gestation also can prove to be useful in certain cases.[19-21]

From the early second trimester on both ultrasound (US) and magnetic resonance imaging (MRI), female external genitalia in the axial plane can be seen as a series of parallel lines and three to five protuberances, with the labia majora on the periphery, and the clitoris ± the labia minora more centrally[22] (Fig. 27.3-4). Data on normal bilabial diameter are available for both US and MRI.[23,24] In males, the scrotum has a midline raphe, and the penis is tapered distally because of the foreskin; apCh, or foreskin aplasia, is exceedingly uncommon.[25] **Testicular descent** is first observed on MRI at 25 + 4 weeks. Starting at **27 weeks**, approximately 50% of testicles are bilaterally descended; at **28 weeks**, about two-thirds are intrascrotal; and from **30 weeks** less than 5% are nondescended. The testes do not necessarily descend simultaneously. Testes are hypointense on T2 imaging[26] (Fig. 27.3-5). In US studies, bilateral testicular descent has been documented in 97% of males by 32 weeks.[27]

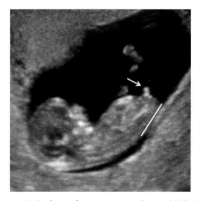

FIGURE 27.3-2: Male fetus first trimester. Sagittal US demonstrating the oblique angulation of the phallus (*arrow*) from a line parallel to the lumbosacral skin.

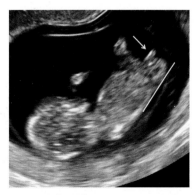

FIGURE 27.3-3: Female fetus first trimester. Sagittal US demonstrates the parallel configuration of the phallus (*arrow*) with the lumbosacral line.

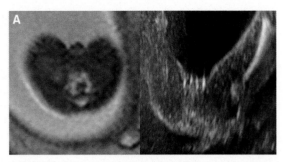 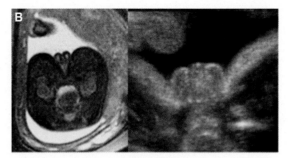

FIGURE 27.3-4: Female fetus. T2 MRI (*left*) and US in axial plane at 20 weeks, **(A)** and 32 weeks, **(B)** gestational age. Note the parallel lines on US representing the interfaces between labia and clitoris. It is neither unusual nor abnormal to see a small amount of high signal in the labia on MRI.

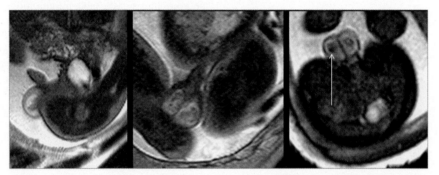

FIGURE 27.3-5: Male fetus. Sagittal, coronal, and axial T2 MRI of the male external genitalia. Testes (*arrow*) are intermediate to low signal and typically surrounded by a small volume of high-signal fluid. The median raphe is equal to or of lesser thickness than the scrotal wall. The normal penis is tapered and central.

General consensus would suggest that surface-rendered three-dimensional (3D) and virtual reality US does not provide an advantage over 2D US in the routine assignment of fetal sex, and, while occasionally useful, is potentially misleading in cases of sexual ambiguity.[1,28–33]

Because a sex assignment may need to rely on more than an assessment of the external genitalia, pelvic content evaluation can be important. Measurements of the distance between the bladder and the rectum are useful to distinguish the presence of a uterus between them. Males lie below the line determined by **distance (mm) = (0.26 × weeks' GA) − 2.17**, and 99% of females lie above.[34] A convex uterine impression on the dorsum of the bladder may also be detectable. Using 3D volume contrast imaging (VCI), approximately 85% of fetal uteri may be confirmed after 20 weeks, increasing to nearly 100% after 32 weeks' GA.[35]

Occasionally, findings other than those associated with ambiguous genitalia can affect the fetal genital system, and this pertains in particular to the scrotum. A small amount of simple fluid (hydrocele) is often seen and is normal (Fig. 27.3-5). Complex fluid, or debris, is characteristic of contamination that has flowed through the patent processus vaginalis into the scrotum from the peritoneal space, and meconium peritonitis from a gastrointestinal tract perforation, or blood product, should be considered first.[36–38] Solid-appearing masses other than the testis in the scrotum are extremely rare prenatally; inguinal hernia has been reported.[39] Also, testes can undergo *in utero* torsion and enlarge the scrotum, just as ovarian torsion can present as a fetal abdominal mass. Color or pulsed-wave Doppler is very useful in this circumstance to show a lack of internal vascularity to the mass.[40–42] The prostatic utricle can persist in the midline just caudal to the bladder as a Müllerian derivative in a male

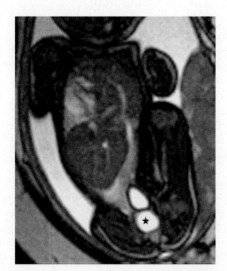

FIGURE 27.3-6: Prostatic utricle. Coronal T2 MRI in a patient with left congenital diaphragmatic hernia and an incidental cyst (*star*) in the midline caudal to the bladder.

fetus, and is typically incidental, although it may be persistent secondary to bladder outlet obstruction, as with posterior urethral valves (Fig. 27.3-6).

DIFFERENTIAL DIAGNOSIS

When the external genitalia do not appear as expected, further investigation is initiated. The anatomy should be characterized as precisely as the imaging allows:

- *Aphallia*—A failure of the fetal genital tubercle to form. The urethra opens directly onto the perineum.[43]
- *Micropenis*—A stretched penile length of less than 2 cm in a term neonate. There are penile length charts for the fetus on both US and MRI, although norms vary among investigators[44–47] (Fig. 27.3-7).
- *Hypospadias*—The penis is short and broad, and the urination stream (with color Doppler) is directed caudally and comes not from the penile tip but from the midshaft or base. Associated with a short anogenital distance for GA.
- *Chordee*—Atresia of the corpus spongiosum distal to the abnormally placed urethral meatus in hypospadias, causing an angulation to the penis (Fig. 27.3-8).
- *Penoscrotal transposition*—A ventrally bent penis between scrotal folds owing to severe hypospadias and a bifid (or shawl) scrotum. On imaging, this has been dubbed the "tulip sign"[48] (Fig. 27.3-9).
- *Epispadias*—The meatal orifice is on the dorsal side of the penis. In severe cases, the penis is split; this condition is associated with bladder or omphalocele, exstrophy of cloaca, imperforate anus, spinal Malformation (OEIS).
- *Concealed (or "buried") penis*—A syndrome consisting of a paucity of penile shaft skin and a short penile shaft, not associated typically with a DSD.[49]
- *Clitoromegaly*—A clitoris 5 mm or more beyond the labia majora. Serial US is generally indicated, as clitoromegaly may resolve over time; however, it would be prudent to examine the fetal adrenal glands for enlargement and/or a cerebriform configuration if considering CAH.[50] Should there be fused labia, the imaging can be indistinguishable from a hypospadic male. Several sonographic examinations and karyotyping may be needed to assign sex correctly.
- *Split labia and clitoris, or scrotum and penis* (in conjunction with lack of a normal bladder)—cloacal or bladder exstrophy[51] (Fig. 27.3-10).

In terms of the revised DSD classifications,[52] *46, XX DSD* is not very accurately recognized prenatally. Clitoromegaly is the sign, but as a single finding overestimates an abnormality, resulting in false positives. Vulvar or vaginal abnormalities may be more specific. *46, XY DSD* is the most reliably identified by an experienced ultrasonographer, and the imaging findings include hypospadias with chordee and scrotal anomaly ± cryptorchidism.[52] However, none of the imaging findings is diagnostic of a particular category of DSD, and each case needs a complete evaluation to arrive at an appropriate diagnosis. Even then, it will not be possible to determine many etiologies prenatally

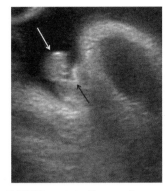
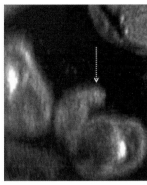

FIGURE 27.3-8: Hypospadias on axial US. On the left, the penile tip is clubbed and rounded (*white arrow*), and there is a bifid (shawl) scrotum (*black arrow*). The *dotted arrow* on the right indicates the lateral angulation of the penis that results from the chordee often associated with hypospadias.

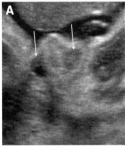
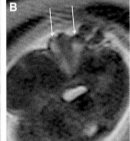

FIGURE 27.3-9: Penoscrotal hypospadias—the "tulip sign." The shortened penis is interposed between the hemiscrota (*arrows*), resembling a flower in axial US **(A)** and MRI **(B)**.

since only about half of children ultimately diagnosed with 46, XY DSD, for example, will reach a definitive clinical diagnosis.[53] A specific molecular diagnosis for chromosomal gonadal differentiation defects is identified postnatally in fewer than one-quarter of cases.[10] In addition, for ultimate differential diagnosis and treatment purposes, the identification of zero, one, or two gonads and the determination about the presence of a uterus are critical, and some of these findings are not reliably made antenatally. Finally, some disorders typically present past infancy because they are phenotypically unremarkable, and

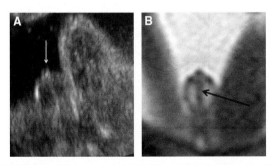

FIGURE 27.3-7: Micropenis. Axial US **(A)** and T2 MRI **(B)** in this XY fetus demonstrate both a micropenis (*white arrow*) and a thickened median raphe (*black arrow*).

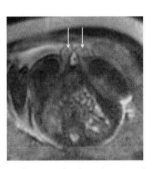

FIGURE 27.3-10: XY fetus with cloacal exstrophy. Axial T2 MRI at the expected level of the scrotum showing complete division of the hemiscrota containing the testes (*arrows*). (Courtesy of Maria Calvo-Garcia, MD, Cincinnati Children's Hospital, Cincinnati, OH.)

therefore will have a very low prenatal detection rate unless there is a specific history to prompt investigation.

A differential diagnostic algorithm for the fetus with ambiguous genitalia (Fig. 27.3-11) should include both phenotypic (external) and gonadal (internal) genitourinary tract evaluation by imaging, and chromosomal evaluation with microarray analysis if at all possible. In the absence of other fetal anomalies or intrauterine growth retardation (IUGR), a prenatal karyotype with fluorescence *in situ* hybridization (FISH) for SRY is the most useful test to work up ambiguous genitalia.[54] A maternal and family history should be taken, assessing ingestion of exogenous maternal hormones (as in assisted reproductive technology [ART]), oral contraceptives during pregnancy, neonatal deaths, urological abnormalities, precocious puberty, amenorrhea, infertility, and consanguinity; a maternal physical examination for virilization or cushingoid appearance may be appropriate. Once chromosomal, urinary tract, and syndromic etiologies are excluded, consideration should turn to steroid profiling or sequencing of the androgen receptor gene.[55]

PROGNOSIS AND MANAGEMENT

The prognosis in these cases is highly variable, depending first on whether there is a chromosomal anomaly with systemic expression of abnormalities or whether the anomalies are isolated to the genitourinary system. Isolated disorders of sexual differentiation have no impact on mode of delivery, and are not life threatening with the exception of CAH, the most common cause for the most common category of DSD at approximately 1/16,000 live births.[56] These children need to be medically managed carefully and immediately at birth.[10] If a prenatal diagnosis is made early enough (as early as 8 weeks with noninvasive cell-free techniques), steroid administered antenatally has been used to prevent virilization; however, the use of prenatal dexamethasone for CAH has been challenged on an ethical basis.[57–59] Even if there is no immediate concern for the infant's stability, most clinicians involved with caring for a child diagnosed with any DSD consider the evaluation psychosocially urgent for the family, requiring a high degree of sensitivity. In addition, some disorders, particularly those with gonadal dysgenesis, are at high risk for gonadal malignancies in childhood.

RECURRENCE RISK

Isolated DSD is not thought to have significant recurrence risk, but multiple chromosomal disorders that carry a certain risk for subsequent pregnancies have been identified, depending on the type of transmission (Table 27.3-1).

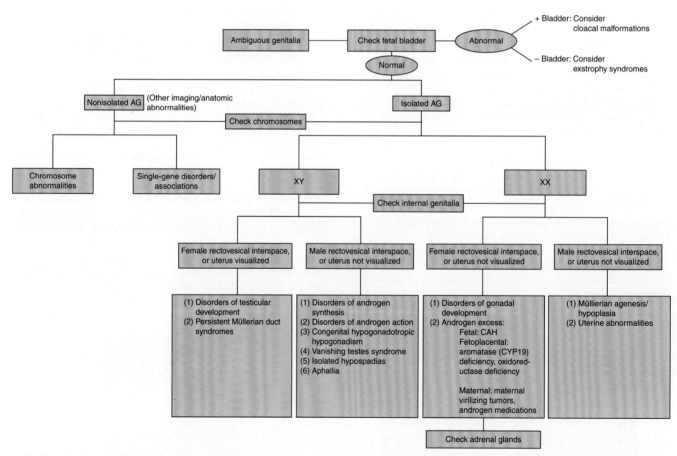

FIGURE 27.3-11: An algorithm for the workup of genital abnormalities in the fetus. AG, ambiguous genitalia; CAH, congenital adrenal hyperplasia. (From Chitayat D, Glanc P. Diagnostic approach in prenatally detected genital abnormalities. *Ultrasound Obstet Gynecol.* 2010;35(6):637–646. Copyright © 2010 ISUOG. Adapted by permission of John Wiley & Sons, Inc.)

REFERENCES

1. Naylor CS, Carlson DE, Santulli T Jr, et al. Use of three-dimensional ultrasonography for prenatal diagnosis of ambiguous genitalia. *J Ultrasound Med.* 2001;20:1365–1367.

2. Hamerton JL, Canning N, Ray M, et al. A cytogenetic survey of 14,068 newborn infants, I: incidence of chromosome abnormalities. *Clin Genet.* 1975;4:223–243.

3. Parker KL, Schimmer BP. Embryology and genetics of the mammalian gonads and ducts. In: Neill JD, ed. *Knobil and Neill's Physiology of Reproduction.* 3rd ed. St Louis, MO: Elsevier; 2006:313–336.

4. Carlson BM. *Human Embryology and Developmental Biology.* 4th ed. Philadelphia, PA: Mosby Elsevier; 2009.

5. Schoenwolf GC, Bleyl SB, Brauer PR, et al, eds. *Larsen's Human Embryology.* 4th ed. Philadelphia, PA: Churchill Livingstone Elsevier; 2009.

6. Ammini AC, Pandey J, Vijyaraghavan M, et al. Human female phenotypic development: role of fetal ovaries. *J Clin Endocrinol Metab.* 1994;79(2):604–608.

7. Smith DP, Felker RE, Noe HN, et al. Prenatal diagnosis of genital anomalies. *Urology.* 1996;47(1):114–117.

8. Sampaio FJ, Favorito LA. Analysis of testicular migration during the fetal period in humans. *J Urol.* 1998;159(2):540–542.

9. Houk CP, Hughes IA, Ahmed SF, et al. Summary of consensus statement on intersex disorders and their management. International Intersex Consensus Conference. *Pediatrics.* 2006;118:753–757.

10. Lambert SM, Vilain EJN, Kolon TF. A practical approach to ambiguous genitalia in the newborn period. *Urol Clin North Am.* 2010;37:195–205.

11. Casey AC, Bhodauria S, Shapter A, et al. Dysgerminoma: the role of conservative surgery. *Gynecol Oncol.* 1996;63:352–357.

12. Browne TK. Why parents should not be told the sex of their fetus. *J Med Ethics.* 2017;43:5–10.

13. Davis DS. A bar too high. *J Med Ethics.* 2017;43:17–18.

14. Manzanares S, Benitez A, Naveiro-Fuentes M, et al. Accuracy of fetal sex determination on ultrasound examination in the first trimester of pregnancy. *J Clin Ultrasound.* 2016;44:272–277.

15. Efrat Z, Perri T, Ramati E, et al. Fetal gender assignment by first-trimester ultrasound. *Ultrasound Obstet Gynecol.* 2006;27:619–621.

16. Emerson DS, Felker RE, Brown DL. The sagittal sign: an early second trimester sonographic indicator of fetal gender. *J Ultrasound Med.* 1989;8:293–297.

17. Odeh M, Ophir E, Bornstein J. Hypospadius mimicking female genitalia on early second trimester sonographic examination. *J Clin Ultrasound.* 2008;36(9):581–583.

18. Bronshtein M, Rottem S, Yoffe N, et al. Early determination of fetal sex using transvaginal sonography: technique and pitfalls. *J Clin Ultrasound.* 1990;18(4):302–306.

19. Natsuyama E. Sonographic determination of fetal sex from 12 weeks of gestation. *Am J Obstet Gynecol.* 1984;149:748–757.

20. Gilboa Y, Perlman S, Kivilevitch Z, et al. Prenatal anogenital distance is shorter in fetuses with hypospadius. *J Ultrasound Med.* 2017;36:175–182.

21. Gilboa Y, Kivilevitch Z, Oren M, et al. Anogenital distance in male and female fetuses at 20 to 35 weeks of gestation: centile charts and reference ranges. *Prenatal Diag.* 2014;34:946–951.

22. Martin C, Darnell A, Duran C, et al. Magnetic resonance imaging of the intrauterine fetal genitourinary tract: normal anatomy and pathology. *Abdom Imaging.* 2004;29:286–302.

23. Pinette MG, Wax JR, Blackstone J, et al. Normal growth and development of fetal external genitalia demonstrated by sonography. *J Clin Ultrasound.* 2003;31:465–472.

24. Nemec SF, Nemec U, Weber M, et al. Female external genitalia on fetal magnetic resonance imaging. *Ultrasound Obstet Gynecol.* 2011;38:695–700.

25. James T. Aplasia of the male prepuce with evidence of hereditary transmission. *J Anat.* 1951;85(4):370–372.

26. Nemec SF, Nemec U, Weber M, et al. Male sexual development *in utero*: testicular descent on prenatal magnetic resonance imaging. *Ultrasound Obstet Gynecol.* 2011;38:688–694.

27. Achiron R, Pinhas-Hamiel O, Zalel Y, et al. Development of male fetal gender: prenatal sonographic measurement of the scrotum and evaluation of testicular descent. *Ultrasound Obstet Gynecol.* 1998;11:242–245.

28. Cafici D, Iglesius A. Prenatal diagnosis of severe hypospadias with 2- and 3-dimensional sonography. *J Ultrasound Med.* 2002;21:1423–1426.

29. Hackett LK, Tarsa M, Wolfson TJ, et al. Use of multiplanar 3-dimensional ultrasonography for prenatal sex identification. *J Ultrasound Med.* 2010;29:195–202.

30. Abu-Rustum R, Chaaban M. Is 3-dimensional sonography useful in the diagnosis of ambiguous genitalia? *J Ultrasound Med.* 2009;28:95–97.

31. Wang Y, Cai A, Sun J, et al. Prenatal diagnosis of penoscrotal transposition with 2- and 3-dimensional ultrasonography. *J Ultrasound Med.* 2011;30(10):1397–1401.

32. Verwoerd-Dikkeboom CM, Koning AHJ, Groenenberg IAL, et al. Using virtual reality for evaluation of fetal ambiguous genitalia. *Ultrasound Obstet Gynecol.* 2008;32:510–514.

33. Bogers H, Rifouna M, Koning AHJ, et al. Accuracy of fetal sex determination in the first trimester of pregnancy using 3D virtual reality ultrasound. *J Clin Ultrasound.* 2018;46:241–246.

34. Glanc P, Umranikar S, Koff D, et al. Fetal sex assignment by sonographic evaluation of the pelvic organs in the second and third trimesters of pregnancy. *J Ultrasound Med.* 2007;26:563–569.

35. Jouannic J-M, Rosenblatt J, Demaria F, et al. Contribution of three-dimensional volume contrast imaging to the sonographic assessment of the fetal uterus. *Ultrasound Obstet Gynecol.* 2005;26:567–570.

36. Cesca E, Midrio P, Tregnaghi A, et al. Meconium periorchitis: a rare cause of fetal scrotal cyst—MRI and pathologic appearance. *Fetal Diagn Ther.* 2009;26:38–40.

37. Gililland A, Carlan SJ, Greenbaum LD, et al. Undescended testicle and a meconium-filled hemiscrotum: prenatal ultrasound appearance. *Ultrasound Obstet Gynecol.* 2002;20(2):200–202.

38. Regev RH, Markovich O, Arnon S, et al. Meconium periorchitis: intrauterine diagnosis and neonatal outcome: case reports and review of the literature. *J Perinatol.* 2009;29(8):585–587.

39. Frati A, Ducarme G, Vuillard E, et al. Prenatal evaluation of a scrotal mass using a high-frequency probe in the diagnosis of inguinoscrotal hernia. *Ultrasound Obstet Gynecol.* 2008;32(7):949–950.

40. Herman A, Schvimer M, Tovbin J, et al. Antenatal sonographic diagnosis of testicular torsion. *Ultrasound Obstet Gynecol.* 2002;20(5):522–524.

41. Devesa R, Muñoz A, Torrents M, et al. Prenatal diagnosis of testicular torsion. *Ultrasound Obstet Gynecol.* 1998;11(4):286–288.

42. Youssef BA, Sammak BM, Al Shahed M. Prenatally diagnosed testicular torsion ultrasonographic features. *Clin Radiol.* 2000;55(2):150–151.

43. Skoog SJ, Belman AB. Aphallia: its classification and management. *J Urol.* 1989;41(3):589–592.

44. Perlitz Y, Keselman L, Haddad S, et al. Prenatal sonographic evaluation of the penile length. *Prenat Diagn.* 2011;31(13):283–285.

45. Danon D, Ben-Shitrit G, Bardin R, et al. Reference values for fetal penile length and width from 22 to 36 gestational weeks. *Prenat Diagn.* 2012;32(9):829–832.

46. Johnson P, Maxwell D. Fetal penile length. *Ultrasound Obstet Gynecol.* 2000;15(4):308–310.

47. Nemec SF, Nemec U, Weber M, et al. Penile biometry on prenatal magnetic resonance imaging. *Ultrasound Obstet Gynecol.* 2012;39(3):330–335.

48. Meizner I, Mashiach R, Shalev J, et al. The "tulip sign": a sonographic clue for in-utero diagnosis of severe hypospadius. *Ultrasound Obstet Gynecol.* 2002;19:250–253.

49. Redman JF. Buried penis: congenital syndrome of a short penile shaft and a paucity of penile shaft skin. *J Urol.* 2005;173(5):1714–1717.

50. Chambrier ED, Heinrichs C, Avni FE. Sonographic appearance of congenital adrenal hyperplasia in utero. *J Ultrasound Med.* 2002;21(1):97–100.

51. Calvo-Garcia MA, Kline-Fath BM, Rubio EI, et al. Fetal MRI of cloacal exstrophy. *Pediatr Radiol.* 2013;43(5):593–604.

52. Cheikhelard A, Luton D, Philipp-Chomette P, et al. How accurate is the prenatal diagnosis of abnormal genitalia? *J Urol.* 2000;164:984–987.

53. Morel Y, Rey R, Teinturier C, et al. Aetiological diagnosis of male sex ambiguity: a collaborative study. *Eur J Pediatr.* 2002;161:49.

54. Adam MP, Fechner PY, Ramsdell LA, et al. Ambiguous genitalia: what prenatal genetic testing is practical? *Am J Med Genet A.* 2012;158A:1337–1343.

55. Katorza E, Pinhas-Hamiel O, Mazkereth R, et al. Sex differentiation disorders (SDD): prenatal sonographic diagnosis, genetic and hormonal work-up. *Pediatr Endocrinol Rev.* 2009;7:12–21.

56. Speiser PW, White PC. Congenital adrenal hyperplasia. *N Engl J Med.* 2003;349:776.

57. Dreger A, Feder EK, Tamar-Mattis A. Prenatal dexamethasone for congenital adrenal hyperplasia: an ethics canary in the modern medical mine. *J Bioeth Inq.* 2012;9(3):277–294.

58. Colmant C, Morin-Surroca M, Fuchs F, et al. Non-invasive prenatal testing for fetal sex determination: is ultrasound still relevant? *Eur J Obstet Gynecol Repro Biol.* 2013;171:197–204.

59. Mersy E, Faas BHW, Spiers S, et al. Cell-free RNA is a reliable fetoplacental marker in noninvasive fetal sex determination. *Clin Chem.* 2015;61:1515–1523.

28.1

Immune Fetal Hydrops

William T. Schnettler

Immune hydrops represents the visible manifestation of complex pathophysiological processes initiated by red blood cell alloimmunization (also known as hemolytic disease of the fetus and newborn, or HDFN)—the maternal immunological response to "nonself" fetal red blood cell antigens. Historians theorize that Catherine of Aragon's recurrent fetal and neonatal demises were attributable to red cell alloimmunization and ultimately led to Henry VIII's decision to divorce her without a papal annulment.[1] This led to England's split from the Roman Catholic Church and the subsequent creation of the Church of England—highlighting the morbid and historic impact of HDFN. Advances in the understanding, detection, management, and prevention of pregnancies complicated by red cell alloimmunization stand among quintessential achievements of the 20th century. However, perinatal morbidity and mortality attributable to red cell alloimmunization continue to plague the developing world at rates comparable to those of prior centuries.[2] In the absence of effective identification and preventative strategies, alloimmunization claims hundreds of thousands of fetuses and neonates every year.[2]

INCIDENCE

Fetal and neonatal effects of red cell alloimmunization range from mild hyperbilirubinemia to hydrops and death. The frequency of these effects depends upon the prevalence of specific antigens among the population and whether an effective prevention program utilizing antepartum and postpartum Rhesus immunoglobulin (RhIg) is in place. The prevalence of Rh(D) negativity varies considerably by ethnicity from less than 5% among Southeast Asian and individuals of African descent to 30% among the Basque population of Spain.[3] In the United States, 14.6% of the total population demonstrates Rh(D) negativity, with rates ranging from 1.7% among those of Asian ethnicity to 17.6% among non-Hispanic whites.[4] The rates of immune hydrops and stillbirth due to Rh-alloimmunization are highest in South Asia and Africa, where little prevention or treatment with RhIg occurs.[3] The percentage of Rh(D)-negative women who become alloimmunized after giving birth to an Rh(D)-positive baby in those countries approximates 15% compared with 1% to 2% in the industrialized world.[3] Alloimmunized pregnancies have a 14% risk for stillbirth, and up to 50% of the surviving newborns will die or experience brain injury due to severe hyperbilirubinemia.[2] In 2010, rates for stillbirth and kernicterus attributable to Rh disease are an estimated 20- to 40-fold greater in South Asia and sub-Saharan Africa than in high-income countries.[3] Data from the 2008 U.S. National Vital Statistics Report revealed that 540 out of 100,000 live births with HDFN resulted in neonatal death.[5]

Alloantibodies other than the anti-Rh(D) antibody have begun to contribute to a larger proportion of the responsibility for HDFN and immune hydrops.[6] Dutch scientists published a large prospective cohort study in 2008 that yielded a prevalence of 400 per 100,000 (0.4%) first-trimester pregnancies with a positive screen for alloantibodies capable of causing hemolytic disease.[6] Of these, 79% were antibodies other than anti-D, and the most common were anti-E, anti-c, and anti-K (Kell). Among at-risk pregnancies, the incidence of severe HDFN was 26.3% of those who screened positive for anti-K, 10.2% for anti-c, 2.1% for anti-E, and 5% for those positive for anti-Rh antibodies other than c, D, and E.[6]

GENETICS

The Rhesus blood antigen group was discovered nearly 75 years ago and includes the D, C, c, E, and e antigens.[7,8] Two linked genes on chromosome 1 encode for the red cell transmembrane proteins RhD and RhCcEe such that an individual's red blood cells display either the C or c antigen, E or e antigen, and D or no "D" antigen.[9] While all Rhesus antigens have the potential to cause immune hydrops, the D antigen is the most immunogenic and historically responsible for more than 50% of cases of maternal alloimmunization.[6,9] Common nomenclature denotes individuals lacking the D antigen as Rh negative without regard to the genotypic presence of the other antigens. Most Caucasian, Rh(D)-negative individuals lack the *RHD* gene altogether. In other populations, certain individuals possess a normal *RHD* gene, but display the Rh(D)-negative phenotype owing to an error at the level of transcription or pre-mRNA processing (known as "partial D").[9] This regional genetic heterogeneity suggests a possible "founder effect" within the Spanish population of the RHD gene deletion. Figure 28.1-1 depicts the *RHD* and *RHCE* genes with their possible phenotypic outcomes. The risk for HDFN is determined by whether the fetus is suspected or confirmed to carry the red cell antigen against which maternal alloantibodies are directed. Paternal zygosity denotes whether the risk is 50% (father is heterozygous for the gene) or 100% (father is homozygous).

PATHOGENESIS

As Levine and Stetson[7] first reported in 1939, a breach in the fetal–maternal interface may expose the mother to various fetal red cell antigens, inciting an immunological response. The antigen is presented to B lymphocytes of the maternal reticuloendothelial system (RES), activating a primary immune response characterized by large-scale immunoglobulin (Ig) M antibody production over the first several weeks. These antibodies are large and do not cross the placenta, posing no risk to the fetus. Following the initial phase, the maternal response shifts to clonal expansion of IgG-type antibodies and maturation of small resting lymphocytes into memory B lymphocytes targeted against the specific antigen. Memory B lymphocytes can persist in the mother for decades awaiting reappearance of the relevant antigen to differentiate into

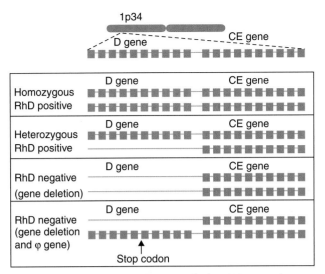

FIGURE 28.1-1: Schematic diagram of the RH gene locus on chromosome 1 with the four possible genotypes, including the "partial D" genotype phenotypically mimicking RhD negative. (Reprinted from Moise KJ Jr. Hemolytic disease of the fetus and newborn. In: Creasy RK, Resnick R, Iams JD, et al., eds. *Creasy and Resnik's Maternal-Fetal Medicine: Principles and Practice.* 6th ed. Philadelphia, PA: Saunders; 2009:479. Copyright © 2009 Elsevier. With permission.)

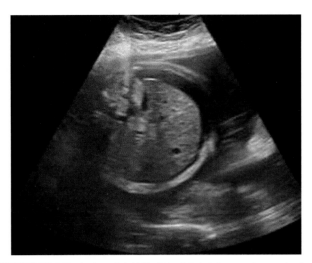

FIGURE 28.1-2: Ascites. Axial US of the fetal abdomen demonstrating ascites.

plasma cells. If the antigen is presented in a subsequent pregnancy, plasma cells can rapidly proliferate and produce large quantities of IgG antibodies that can cross the placenta and bind to fetal red cells. Factors that increase the likelihood of alloimmunization include the volume of fetal-maternal transplacental hemorrhage (0.2 mL or greater), antigen density, gestational age, and ABO compatibility. Maternal destruction of ABO-incompatible fetal red cells often occurs prior to presentation of other antigens such that the risk of Rh-alloimmunization is reduced from 16% to 2%.[10]

Once maternal alloantibodies bind fetal red cells, macrophages within the fetal circulation and spleen adhere and lyse the cells. To counter this destruction, the fetus increases plasma erythropoietin, prompting extramedullary erythropoiesis (primarily in the liver) and release of immature erythroblasts.[11] The resultant hepatosplenomegaly may alter the portal and venous architecture leading to portal hypertension and decreased hepatic albumin production. Increased umbilical venous pressure and decreased colloid oncotic pressure trigger extravasation of fluid from the fetal vasculature into the fetal and placental interstitial spaces.[12] The fetus attempts to compensate and maintain intravascular volume by increasing plasma aldosterone concentration, but this further decreases the fetal osmolality and hematocrit in a feed-forward cycle, ultimately resulting in the visible fetal and placental edema seen with immune hydrops.[13]

The mechanism underlying fetal anemia and the development of immune hydrops in fetuses affected by Kell alloimmunization differs from the processes taking place in the Rh-alloimmunized fetus. *In vitro* studies of hematopoietic progenitor cells from cord blood reveal suppressed growth of the erythroid progenitor cells in the presence of monoclonal anti-K antibodies but not anti-Rh(D) antibodies.[14] Anti-K antibodies cause fetal anemia by inhibiting erythropoiesis at the progenitor-cell level rather than by RES-mediated hemolysis, as seen in Rh-alloimmunization. This finding becomes important in differentiating the diagnostic workup of Kell-mediated alloimmunization from that caused by most of the other blood group alloantigens.

DIAGNOSIS

Imaging: Immune hydrops is generally defined by the sonographic detection of excess fluid accumulation within two separate fetal body compartments in conjunction with a positive maternal indirect Coombs test for an antibody known to cause HDFN. Excess fluid accumulation may manifest as ascites, pleural effusion, pericardial effusion, polyhydramnios, skin edema, and placental enlargement. True ascites appears as an echolucent rim of fluid encircling the entire contents of the fetal abdomen such that bowel, liver, and spleen are more easily identified (Fig. 28.1-2). Pleural effusions are often seen bilaterally compressing the lungs and mediastinum, potentially leading to pulmonary hypoplasia (Fig. 28.1-3). The diagnosis of pericardial effusion requires visualization of at least 3 mm of fluid surrounding both cardiac ventricles (Fig. 28.1-4). Skin edema must measure 5 mm or greater in thickness (Fig. 28.1-5), and placentomegaly must measure 5 cm or greater in thickness (Fig. 28.1-6). If one such finding is seen in isolation, it should simply be described in terms of its location and not as hydrops fetalis. Although fluid accumulation in two separate fetal compartments

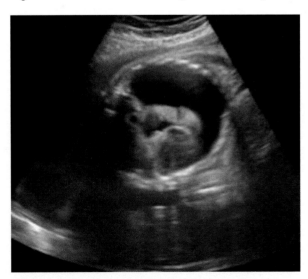

FIGURE 28.1-3: Pleural effusions. Axial US of the fetal thorax demonstrating bilateral pleural effusion with lung compression and mediastinal displacement.

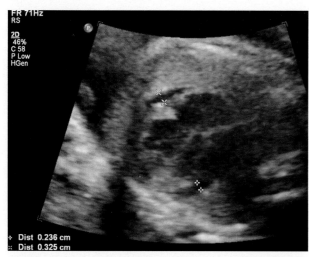

FIGURE 28.1-4: Pericardial effusion. Axial view of the fetal thorax at the level of the four-chamber cardiac view demonstrating more than 3 mm of fluid surrounding both cardiac ventricles. Markers identify measurements of the described sonographic finding.

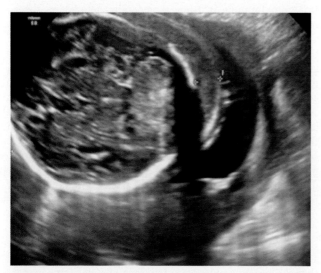

FIGURE 28.1-5: Skin edema of more than 5 mm. Markers identify measurements of the described sonographic finding.

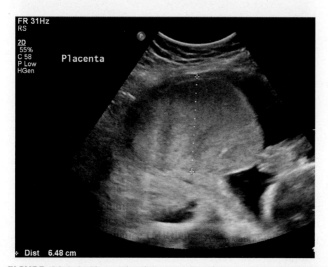

FIGURE 28.1-6: Placental edema greater than 5 cm in thickness. Markers identify measurements of the described sonographic finding.

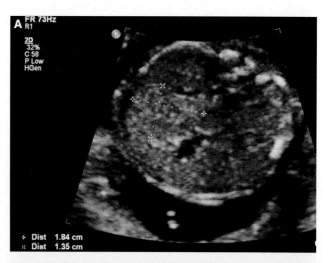

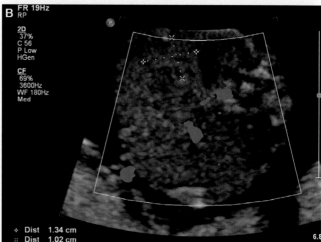

FIGURE 28.1-7: Splenic circumference. **A:** Axial view of the fetal abdomen at the standard level for abdominal circumference measurement. Splenic circumference (millimeters) = (length + width) × 1.57. **B:** Color Doppler identifying the splenic artery can aid in location of the spleen. Markers identify measurements of the described sonographic findings.

denotes hydrops, no sonographic pattern specifies the etiology or severity of anemia.[15,16]

A variety of fetal sonographic measures have been investigated in attempts at identifying methods for noninvasive quantification of fetal anemia. Measurement of the axial splenic circumference (Fig. 28.1-7) demonstrated 100% sensitivity and 94.7% specificity for severe anemia in cases without prior intrauterine transfusion (IUT) in one prospective study.[17] The pathophysiological association of splenomegaly with hemolytic anemia is easily understood, and this finding was promising. Unfortunately, enlargement of the splenic circumference was not predictive of mild anemia or the decrease in hematocrit following IUT. To achieve earlier detection and follow-up, investigators have employed Doppler assessment of the fetal blood velocity in the umbilical artery, umbilical vein, descending aorta, ductus venosus, splenic artery, and middle cerebral artery.

In 2000, Mari and coauthors[18] presented convincing evidence supporting the hypothesis that the decreased blood viscosity associated with fetal anemia manifests as an elevation in peak systolic velocity of blood flow within the middle cerebral artery. They prospectively compared cordocentesis-derived

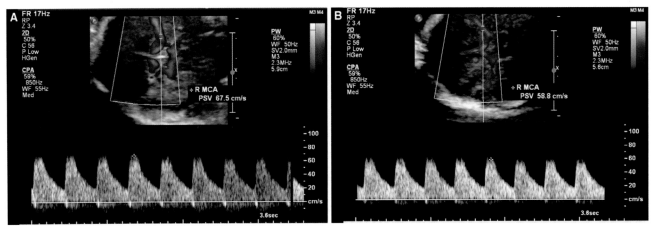

FIGURE 28.1-8: Doppler imaging of the middle cerebral artery. **A:** Transverse view of the fetal head shows Doppler sampling and peak systolic velocity measurement of the middle cerebral artery with the correct angle of insonation. **B:** Note the change in the measured value with too large an angle of insonation. MCA, middle cerebral artery; PSV, peak systolic velocity.

hemoglobin concentrations with middle cerebral artery peak systolic velocity measurements in 111 fetuses deemed as being at risk for anemia and 265 nonanemic "normal" fetuses. Their findings provided essential normative data and threshold values representing mild, moderate, and severe anemia (see Table 53 in Appendix A1). With the appropriate technique (Fig. 28.1-8), this measurement can noninvasively diagnose early anemia prior to the development of hydrops and provide surveillance following IUT to guide timing of repeat percutaneous umbilical cord blood sampling (PUBS) and transfusion. The measurements can be initiated at 18 weeks' gestation, and the fetal middle cerebral artery closest to the transducer should be evaluated with the Doppler gate placed immediately distal to the bifurcation of the carotid siphon. The angle of insonation should be as close to zero degrees (parallel) to the vessel direction as possible, and the baseline should be adjusted close to zero. Values greater than 1.50 multiples of the median (MoM) for gestational age denote moderate or severe anemia with 100% sensitivity and 88% specificity. The test's validity is preserved in the cases of Kell-mediated fetal anemia and hydrops.

Additional diagnostic tools may be employed for situations where the cause of hydrops fetalis is less clear. Fetal echocardiography may be reserved for nonimmune causes of hydrops. Magnetic resonance imaging may prove useful for investigating brain abnormalities resulting from infectious causes such as congenital parvovirus B19 infection, but its use has been limited to cases of nonimmune hydrops.[19]

Laboratory Testing: Maternal Rh typing and antibody screening are typically performed in the first trimester, but should be repeated if sonographic evidence of hydrops develops. Although a woman may demonstrate Rh(D) positivity and have a negative first-trimester antibody screen, she may acquire atypical blood group antibodies or become alloimmunized during gestation (e.g., following packed red blood cell or platelet transfusion).[20] Antibody titers may vary slightly among different laboratories, but most consider titers greater than 1:16 potentially causative of severe fetal anemia. When a maternal antibody screen is positive for non-Kell antibodies and the titer is at or below 1:16, titers are repeated monthly. Maternal Kell antibody titers are not correlative with risk for fetal anemia.[14]

To determine the likelihood of fetal expression of the suspected antigen, paternal zygosity may be accurately determined by quantitative polymerase chain reaction (PCR) for the *RHD* gene or by serology for the other blood group antigens with a nondominant allele such as the "k" of the (K1) Kell gene.[21] Paternal homozygosity essentially confers a 100% likelihood that the fetus is a carrier of the putative blood group antigen. However, paternal heterozygosity equates to a 50% risk, and determination of fetal antigen status is required. Cell-free fetal DNA testing is now available in the United States such that the exon sequences (exons 4, 5, 7) of the *RHD* gene are detected accurately with sensitivities and specificities of 97% to 99% using reverse transcriptase PCR.[22,23] This technology also has the ability to detect the Rh(D) pseudogene using specific exon primers, and the cell-free fetal DNA result will read as "indeterminant," prompting the need for amniocentesis and Rh(D) genetic testing of the amniocytes.[24] The only available assay in the United States is made by Integrated Genetics, Inc and is called "SensiGene RHD." It tests for exons 4, 5, and 7 of the Rh(D) gene, and if all three are identified the fetus is reported to be Rh(D) positive. If only 1 or 2 exons are identified, continued serial surveillance of antibody titers is indicated and consideration for amniocentesis if the anti-D titer is greater than 1:16. This technology has proved reliable for predicting fetal K, C, c, and E phenotypes as well.[25]

Invasive techniques have historically been required to confirm fetal antigen status and quantify anemia as the cause of hydrops fetalis. Amniocentesis accurately determines fetal Rh(D) status with a sensitivity of 98.7% and a specificity of 100%, and it is equally reliable for identifying dominant and nondominant alleles of the other blood group antigens.[26] Amniocentesis for spectrophotometric analysis of amniotic fluid bilirubin levels was first described by Bevis[27] and then further characterized by Liley[28] and Queenan et al.[29] The shift in optical density of amniotic fluid at a wavelength of 450 nm (ΔOD_{450}) correlates with the concentration of bilirubin and provides an indirect measure of fetal hemolysis. Liley was first to plot ΔOD_{450} values as three "zones" of anemia severity according to gestational age (weeks 27 through 42). Queenan and colleagues[29] extrapolated this concept to earlier gestational ages and additional zones in a study of 789 amniotic fluid samples with improved sensitivity and specificity (Fig. 28.1-9). Serial amniotic fluid assessments demonstrating elevation to the IUT zone on the Queenan curve or the 80th percentile of zone 2 on the Liley curve suggest severe anemia and warranted premature delivery or attempts at fetal intraperitoneal

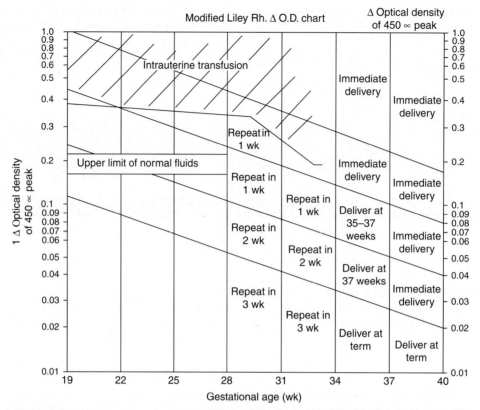

FIGURE 28.1-9: Normal Liley curves. Modification of Liley ΔOD_{450} reading zone boundaries before 24 weeks' gestation is the same as the zone boundary angle of inclination after 24 weeks' gestation. (Reprinted with permission from Ulreich S, Gruslin A, Nodell CG, et al. Fetal hydrops and ascites. In: Nyberg DA, McGahan JP, Pretorius DH, et al., eds. *Diagnostic Imaging of Fetal Anomalies*. Philadelphia, PA: Lippincott Williams & Wilkins; 2003:713–744.)

transfusion (IPT). Unfortunately, nonhemolytic anemia, as in Kell-mediated erythropoiesis inhibition, was not identifiable with this method. The 1980s witnessed the advent of fetoscopic and ultrasound-guided umbilical vein needle sampling (also called PUBS—percutaneous umbilical blood sampling, cordocentesis, or funipuncture), which allowed for direct measurement of the fetal serum bilirubin concentration and hematocrit.[30] An umbilical venous total bilirubin concentration greater than 3 mg/dL and a hematocrit less than 30% denote severe anemia, warranting potential IUT. This procedure is successful in more than 95% of cases and applicable to all causes of anemia, but is not employed on a routine basis owing to the associated 1% to 2% fetal loss rate and potential for worsened fetomaternal hemorrhage.[31]

Additional diagnostic tools may be employed for situations where the cause of hydrops fetalis is less clear. Fetal karyotype and microarray analysis are generally not required for cases of hydrops in the setting of a positive maternal indirect Coombs test unless concern exists for additional fetal abnormalities. Maternal and paternal serologies in combination with two-dimensional and Doppler sonography comprise the standard tools for diagnosis of immune hydrops.

DIFFERENTIAL DIAGNOSIS

If excess fluid is identified in only one fetal compartment, organ-specific causes of fluid accumulation such as cardiomyopathy or thoracic duct abnormalities should be considered. Aneuploidies, skeletal dysplasias, and certain fetal structural

anomalies may result in true fetal hydrops, and these should be considered even in the presence of a maternal antibody known to cause HDFN. Initial assessment should also include Doppler evaluation of the middle cerebral artery peak systolic velocity. If this velocity is found to be normal, additional anatomical abnormalities are identified, or maternal indirect Coombs testing is negative, one should consider nonimmune causes of hydrops as described later in this chapter.

PROGNOSIS

The finding of immune hydrops signifies progression of the pathophysiological processes involved in fetal alloimmune anemia toward the near-fatal stages. If left uncorrected, the prognosis is invariably fatal for the fetus or neonate. Intrauterine fetal transfusion provides an effective therapy temporarily correcting the anemia and potentially reversing the hydrops. This benefit was demonstrated in a large retrospective cohort study from the national referral center for management of fetal anemia in the Netherlands.[32] Of 210 fetuses with alloimmune anemia, 80 (36%) were hydropic and underwent intrauterine fetal transfusion with a survival rate of 78%. Logistic regression revealed that survival was decreased among cases where the first transfusion occurred prior to 20 weeks (55%), among cases in which the hydrops was not reversed (55%), and among cases of Kell alloimmunization (60%). A meta-analysis of 19 publications demonstrated a similar rate of survival (74%) among hydropic fetuses following IUT.[33]

Concern exists for the long-term neurodevelopmental outcomes of fetuses that have successfully undergone treatment for immune hydrops. Anemia may lead to hypoxemia and hyperbilirubinemia that potentially impairs critical brain development. However, a report on 18 consecutively treated hydropic fetuses revealed that physical and neurological outcomes were similar in comparison with that of their unaffected siblings for most immune hydrops survivors (13 of 16 children; 81%) at a mean age of 10 years.[34] A large national cohort study of 291 survivors of immune hydrops evaluated at a median age of 8.2 years revealed rates of cerebral palsy of 2.1%, severe developmental delay of 3.1%, bilateral deafness of 1.0%, and overall neurodevelopmental impairment of 4.8%.[35] Thus, the risk of neurodevelopmental impairment among survivors of IUT for fetal alloimmune anemia appears low.

MANAGEMENT

Management begins with prevention against alloimmunization. Although the exact mechanism is unknown, exogenous RhIg reduces the risk of alloimmunization to the Rh(D) antigen to 0.1% to 0.2% when given at 28 weeks' gestation and again within 72 hours of delivery.[36] Once bound to the RhD sites on red cells, the RhIg can bind to the IgG Fc receptors on macrophages and natural killer cells, resulting in clearance of the RhD-positive red cells from circulation prior to activation of memory B lymphocytes.[37] The standard intramuscular dose of 300 μg protects against 30 mL of fetal blood or 15 mL of packed fetal red cells, but a Kleihauer–Betke test can quantify the amount of fetal-maternal hemorrhage to further guide dosing of RhIg. Since it is derived from pooled donors' sera, the potential to transmit hepatitis C infection has been reported in a case report.[38] The cold alcohol fractionation used in isolating the antibodies appears to destroy the human immunodeficiency virus such that the possibility for transmission of HIV is considered nonexistent.

Differentiation between immune hydrops and other nonimmunological fetal conditions relies on an algorithmic approach beginning with a detailed fetal sonographic assessment and maternal blood type assessment and indirect Coombs testing (Fig. 28.1-10). Confirmed cases of immune hydrops should be assessed for maternal transport to a tertiary care center with expertise in management of this potentially critical situation. The team should include experienced perinatologists, sonographers, blood bank personnel, neonatologists, and anesthesia and nursing staff. If the gestational age lies between 24 and 34 weeks, maternal administration of an antenatal course of corticosteroids is advised. Preparations for PUBS are undertaken, including the early notification of the blood bank and collection of a maternal blood sample for typing, antibody determination, and preparation of appropriate blood for fetal transfusion. This blood should be irradiated group O negative red cells packed to a hematocrit of at least 75% and negative for Kell, cytomegalovirus (CMV), and the putative antigen. If the fetal blood type is known from a prior PUBS and there is no maternal ABO incompatibility, red cells of the same ABO status of the fetus may be used for transfusion. A detailed ultrasound should be performed to evaluate the severity of the hydrops, the estimated fetal weight, and the target for fetal intravascular sampling and transfusion.

In 1963, prior to the technological advancement of sonography, Liley[39] introduced the concept of IUT and ushered in the age of fetal therapeutics. The technique involved IPT of packed red cells to allow for lymphatic and venous absorption into the anemic fetus, and this remained the standard approach until the method of direct intravascular transfusion (IVT) under fetoscopic and sonographic guidance was introduced in the mid-1980s.[30] Direct comparison of these two techniques revealed a 13% increased survival rate for nonhydropic fetuses undergoing IVT in comparison with those undergoing IPT; the survival advantage was nearly twofold among hydropic fetuses.[40] The lymphovascular congestion and distortion of the portal and hepatic venous architecture associated with fetal hydrops likely prohibit timely absorption of transfused packed red cells from the peritoneal cavity. Thus, the intravascular approach is preferred, and the placental insertion of the umbilical vein often offers the most reliable intravascular access with minimal risk for fetal bradycardia (approximately 3%).[31] Free-floating and periumbilical portions of the cord can be more challenging to puncture (often requiring fetal paralysis), and have demonstrated higher rates of fetal bradycardia.[31] If the placental insertion site is not accessible, one may safely attempt to access the intrahepatic portion of the umbilical vein with similar low likelihood of fetal bradycardia.[41]

Once the access site has been determined, a sedative or regional neuraxial anesthesia is administered to the mother. A neuromuscular blocker may also be directly injected into the fetal circulation. An operating room is prepared for both the procedure and for possible emergent cesarean delivery of the viable fetus should severe complications arise. The appropriate blood for transfusion should be available in the operating room, and the hematology laboratory should be immediately available to quickly analyze and report results of the fetal blood samples. A broad-spectrum cephalosporin with coverage against gram-positive skin flora can be given as prophylaxis. The patient's abdomen is then prepared for surgery, and sterile technique is used while a 20- or 22-gauge spinal needle is advanced through the maternal abdomen into the fetal umbilical vein under direct ultrasound guidance (Fig. 28.1-11). Free return of blood confirms venous entry, and a 1- or 2-mL sample should be drawn into a heparinized tuberculin syringe for immediate analysis of hematocrit, hemoglobin, and mean corpuscular volume (values greater than 110 μm^3 confirm the source as fetal). Fetal blood should also be measured for platelet count, total bilirubin concentration, blood type, antibody screen, and reticulocyte count. Given that the hematocrit is less than 30% in most cases of immune hydrops, the fetal transfusion can be started while awaiting results from the laboratory.

Calculation of the total volume to transfuse relies on determination of the estimated fetal weight, the correction factor for the volume of blood in the fetoplacental circulation, the initial fetal hematocrit, the hematocrit of the transfused blood, and the target hematocrit. The following formula is commonly used for determining the total milliliters of transfusion volume (V_T):

$$V_T = \frac{V_{(fetoplacental)} \times (\text{Target fetal hematocrit} - \text{Initial fetal hematocrit})}{\text{Hematocrit of transfused blood}}$$

where $V_{(fetoplacental)}$ (mL) is calculated by multiplying the estimated fetal weight in grams by 0.14. The target fetal hematocrit should approximate the physiological fetal value (45% to 50%), but should not increase 25% above the initial fetal hematocrit, owing to concerns for fluid overload and intrauterine fetal demise.[42]

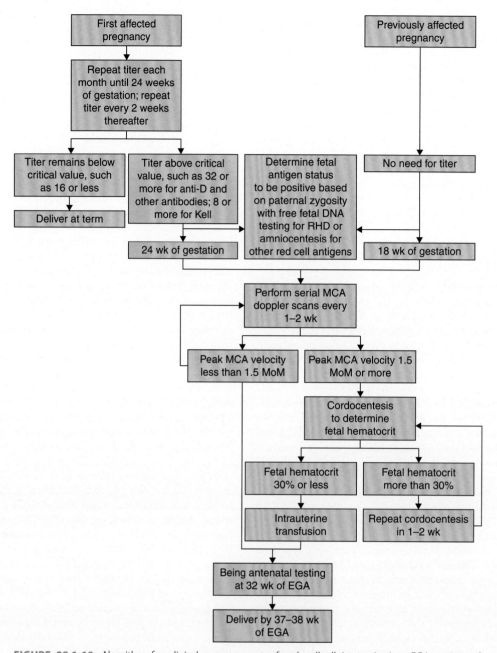

FIGURE 28.1-10: Algorithm for clinical management of red cell alloimmunization. EGA, estimated gestational age; MCA, middle cerebral artery; MoM, multiples of the median. (Reprinted with permission from Moise KJ Jr, Argoti PS. Management and prevention of red cell alloimmunization in pregnancy: a systematic review. *Obstet Gynecol.* 2012;120(5):1132–1139.)

In general, initial fetal hematocrit values less than 30% warrant IVT. Severely anemic fetuses with hematocrits below 10% should potentially undergo a two-step IVT with the initial goal of achieving a hematocrit of 25% to 30% followed by a second transfusion 48 to 72 hours later to achieve a final hematocrit of 45% to 50%. Another option for severe anemia is to perform a combined intravascular and IPT, where the IVT is performed to reach a hematocrit of 35% to 40%.[43] The needle is then inserted into the fetal peritoneal cavity, where a portion of the ascites can be aspirated and replaced with a volume (mL) of packed red cells determined by Bowman's formula, subtracting 20 from the gestational age in weeks and multiplying the result by 10.[44] This method has been shown to provide a more stable fetal hematocrit, declining only 0.01% per day rather than the 1% per day with IVT alone.[45]

Timing of subsequent transfusions depends on the final hematocrit achieved and whether a combined approach or IVT alone was performed. In addition, weekly measurement of the peak systolic velocity of the middle cerebral artery can help time subsequent transfusions. Values greater than 1.32 MoM demonstrate 100% sensitivity and 63% specificity in predicting reoccurrence of moderate anemia and warrant repeat IUT.[46] Fetal surveillance with twice-weekly biophysical profiles, including nonstress test, should be instituted until delivery. The last transfusion is typically performed around 35 weeks' gestation, with planned delivery near 37 weeks. The false-positive rate of middle cerebral artery peak systolic velocity measurement increases after 35 weeks, but its sensitivity remains excellent and may convey reassurance against moderate to severe anemia until delivery.[47]

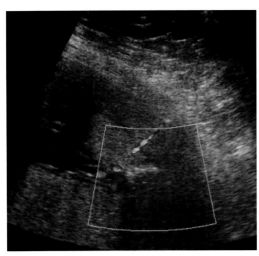

FIGURE 28.1-11: Percutaneous umbilical blood sampling. Color Doppler US demonstrating aspiration of fetal blood from the umbilical vein at the placental cord insertion site with a 20-gauge spinal needle.

RECURRENCE RISK

The recurrence risk for immune hydrops is substantial and dependent upon the gestational age and severity of the first alloimmunized pregnancy. Among women with a history of a prior perinatal loss attributable to HDFN, prior need for IUT, or delivery of an infant requiring neonatal exchange transfusion, maternal titers are not reliable in predicting HDFN in subsequent pregnancies. Paternal homozygosity for the responsible antigen confers a 100% risk for recurrence, whereas heterozygosity equates to a 50% risk. Preimplantation genetic diagnosis can accurately determine the fetal antigen status in situations of paternal heterozygosity, but this is costly and requires *in vitro* fertilization.[48] In subsequent pregnancies following Rh(D) alloimmunization with documented fetal or neonatal anemia, cell-free fetal DNA analysis can accurately determine the fetal antigen status beginning around 10 weeks of gestation, and can determine the need to initiate surveillance at 18 weeks with serial Doppler evaluation of the middle cerebral artery. While the utility of serial anti-D antibody titers in subsequent affected pregnancies is of limited value, a markedly elevated early maternal anti-D antibody titer may suggest the presence of very early severe alloimmunization. This scenario is technically challenging because the success rate and ability to perform fetal intraperitoneal blood transfusion under 18 weeks are poor. Investigators have demonstrated feasibility and success with early administration of intravenous immunoglobulin G (IVIG) and plasma exchange in the mother as a means of arresting antibody-mediated fetal red blood cell destruction.[49,50] While the gold standard of treatment remains intrauterine blood transfusion, the American Society for Apheresis guidelines state that IVIG and/or therapeutic plasma exchange are acceptable alternative therapies when the risk of fetal demise is high and signs of fetal hydrops are present prior to 20 weeks' gestation.[51]

REFERENCES

1. Moise KJ Jr. Hemolytic disease of the fetus and newborn. In: Creasy RK, Resnik R, eds. *Maternal-Fetal Medicine*. 6th ed. Philadelphia, PA: Saunders Elsevier; 2009:191–207.
2. Zipursky A, Paul VK. The global burden of Rh disease. *Arch Dis Child Fetal Neonatal Ed.* 2011;96(2):F84–F85.
3. Bhutani VK, Zipursky A, Blencowe H, et al. Neonatal hyperbilirubinemia and Rhesus disease of the newborn: incidence and impairment estimates for 2010 at regional and global levels. *Pediatr Res.* 2013;74(suppl 1):86–100.
4. Garratty G, Glynn SA, McEntire R. ABO and Rh(D) phenotype frequencies of different racial/ethnic groups in the United States. *Transfusion.* 2004;44(5):703–706.
5. Martin JA, Hamilton BE, Sutton PD, et al. Births: final data for 2008. *Natl Vital Stat Rep.* 2010;59(1):1–71.
6. Koelewijn JM, Vrijkotte TG, van der Schoot CE, et al. Effect of screening for red cell antibodies, other than anti-D, to detect hemolytic disease of the fetus and newborn: a population study in the Netherlands. *Transfusion.* 2008;48(5):941–952.
7. Levine P, Stetson RE. An unusual case of intragroup agglutination. *JAMA.* 1939;113:126–127.
8. Fisher RA, Race RR. Rh gene frequencies in Britain. *Nature.* 1946;157:48.
9. Avent ND, Reid ME. The Rh blood group system: a review. *Blood.* 2000;95(2):375–387.
10. Nevanlinna HR. ABO protection in Rh immunization. *Ann Med Exp Biol Fenn.* 1966;44(2):318–321.
11. Moya FR, Grannum PA, Widness JA, et al. Erythropoietin in human fetuses with immune hemolytic anemia and hydrops fetalis. *Obstet Gynecol.* 1993;82(3):353–358.
12. Ville Y, Sideris I, Hecher K, et al. Umbilical venous pressure in normal, growth-retarded, and anemic fetuses. *Am J Obstet Gynecol.* 1994;170(2):487–494.
13. Ville Y, Proudler A, Kuhn P, et al. Aldosterone concentration in normal, growth-retarded, anemic, and hydropic fetuses. *Obstet Gynecol.* 1994;84(4):511–514.
14. Vaughan JI, Manning M, Warwick RM, et al. Inhibition of erythroid progenitor cells by anti-Kell antibodies in fetal alloimmune anemia. *N Engl J Med.* 1998;338(12):798–803.
15. Chitkara U, Wilkins I, Lynch L, et al. The role of sonography in assessing severity of fetal anemia in Rh- and Kell-isoimmunized pregnancies. *Obstet Gynecol.* 1988;71(3 pt 1):393–398.
16. Nicolaides KH, Fontanarosa M, Gabbe SG, et al. Failure of ultrasonographic parameters to predict the severity of fetal anemia in rhesus isoimmunization. *Am J Obstet Gynecol.* 1988;158(4):920–926.
17. Bahado-Singh R, Oz U, Mari G, et al. Fetal splenic size in anemia due to Rh-alloimmunization. *Obstet Gynecol.* 1998;92(5):828–832.
18. Mari G, Deter RL, Carpenter RL, et al. Noninvasive diagnosis by Doppler ultrasonography of fetal anemia due to maternal red-cell alloimmunization. *N Engl J Med.* 2000;342(1):9–14.
19. Courtier J, Schauer GM, Parer JT, et al. Polymicrogyria in a fetus with human parvovirus B19 infection: a case with radiologic-pathologic correlation. *Ultrasound Obstet Gynecol.* 2012;40(5):604–606.
20. Yun JW, Kang ES, Ki CS, et al. Sensitization to multiple rh antigens by transfusion of random donor platelet concentrates in a -D- phenotype patient. *Ann Lab Med.* 2012;32(6):429–432.
21. Pirelli KJ, Pietz BC, Johnson ST, et al. Molecular determination of RHD zygosity: predicting risk of hemolytic disease of the fetus and newborn related to anti-D. *Prenat Diagn.* 2010;30(12–13):1207–1212.
22. Bombard AT, Akolekar R, Farkas DH, et al. Fetal RHD genotype detection from circulating cell-free fetal DNA in maternal plasma in non-sensitized RhD negative women. *Prenat Diagn.* 2011;31(8):802–808.
23. Wikman AT, Tiblad E, Karlsson A, et al. Noninvasive single-exon fetal RHD determination in a routine screening program in early pregnancy. *Obstet Gynecol.* 2012;120(2 pt 1):227.
24. Tynan JA, Angkachatchai V, Ehrich M, et al. Multiplexed analysis of circulating cell-free fetal nucleic acids for noninvasive prenatal diagnostic RHD testing. *Am J Obstet Gynecol.* 2011;204(3):251.
25. Finning K, Martin P, Summers J, et al. Fetal genotyping for the K (Kell) and Rh C, c, and E blood groups on cell-free fetal DNA in maternal plasma. *Transfusion.* 2007;47(11):2126–2133.
26. Van den Veyver IB, Moise KJ Jr. Fetal RhD typing by polymerase chain reaction in pregnancies complicated by rhesus alloimmunization. *Obstet Gynecol.* 1996;88:1061–1067.
27. Bevis DC. Blood pigments in haemolytic disease of the newborn. *J Obstet Gynaecol Br Emp.* 1956;63(1):68–75.
28. Liley AW. Liquor amnii analysis in the management of the pregnancy complicated by rhesus sensitization. *Am J Obstet Gynecol.* 1961;82:1359–1370.
29. Queenan JT, Tomai TP, Ural SH, et al. Deviation in amniotic fluid optical density at a wavelength of 450 nm in Rh immunized pregnancies from 14 to 40 weeks' gestation: a proposal for clinical management. *Am J Obstet Gynecol.* 1993;168(5):1370–1376.
30. Rodeck CH, Kemp JR, Holman CA, et al. Direct intravascular fetal blood transfusion by fetoscopy in severe rhesus isoimmunization. *Lancet.* 1981;1(8221):625–627.
31. Weiner CP, Wenstrom KD, Sipes SL, et al. Risk factors for cordocentesis and fetal intravascular transfusion. *Am J Obstet Gynecol.* 1991;165:1020–1025.
32. van Kamp IL, Klumper FJ, Meerman RH, et al. Treatment of fetal anemia due to red-cell alloimmunization with intrauterine transfusions in the Netherlands, 1988–1999. *Acta Obstet Gynecol Scand.* 2004;83(8):731–737.
33. Schumacher B, Moise KJ Jr. Fetal transfusion for red blood cell alloimmunization in pregnancy. *Obstet Gynecol.* 1996;88(1):137–150.

34. Harper DC, Swingle HM, Weiner CP, et al. Long-term neurodevelopmental outcome and brain volume after treatment for hydrops fetalis by in utero intravascular transfusion. *Am J Obstet Gynecol.* 2006;195(1):192–200.
35. Lindenburg IT, Smits-Wintjens VE, van Klink JM, et al; for the LOTUS Study Group. Long-term neurodevelopmental outcome after intrauterine transfusion for hemolytic disease of the fetus/newborn: the LOTUS study. *Am J Obstet Gynecol.* 2012;206(2):141.e1–141.e8.
36. Bowman JM. The prevention of Rh immunization. *Transfus Med Rev.* 1988;2(3):129.
37. Siberil S, de Romeuf C, Bihoreau N, et al. Selection of human anti-RhD monoclonal antibody for therapeutic use: impact of IgG glycosylation on activating and inhibitory Fc gamma R functions. *Clin Immunol.* 2006;118(2–3):170–179.
38. Power JP, Lawlor E, Davidson F, et al. Molecular epidemiology of an outbreak of infection with hepatitis C virus in recipients of anti-D immunoglobulin. *Lancet.* 1995;345(8959):1211–1213.
39. Liley AW. Intrauterine transfusion of foetus in haemolytic disease. *Br Med J.* 1963;2(5365):1107–1109.
40. Harman CR, Bowman JM, Manning FA, et al. Intrauterine transfusion—intraperitoneal versus intravascular approach: a case-control comparison. *Am J Obstet Gynecol.* 1990;162(4):1053–1059.
41. Nicolini U, Santolaya J, Ojo OE, et al. The fetal intrahepatic umbilical vein as an alternative to cord needling for prenatal diagnosis and therapy. *Prenat Diagn.* 1988;8(9):665–671.
42. Radunovic N, Lockwood CJ, Alvarez M, et al. The severely anemic and hydropic isoimmune fetus: changes in fetal hematocrit associated with intrauterine death. *Obstet Gynecol.* 1992;79(3):390–393.
43. Moise KJ Jr, Carpenter RJ Jr, Kirshon B, et al. Comparison of four types of intrauterine transfusion: effect on fetal hematocrit. *Fetal Ther.* 1989;4(2–3):126–137.
44. Bowman JM. The management of Rh-isoimmunization. *Obstet Gynecol.* 1978;52:1–16.
45. Moise KJ Jr, Argoti PS. Management and prevention of red cell alloimmunization in pregnancy: a systematic review. *Obstet Gynecol.* 2012;120(5):1132–1139.
46. Detti L, Oz U, Guney I, et al; for the Collaborative Group for Doppler Assessment of Blood Velocity in Anemic Fetuses. Doppler ultrasound velocimetry for timing the second intrauterine transfusion in fetuses with anemia from red cell alloimmunization. *Am J Obstet Gynecol.* 2001;185(5):1048–1051.
47. Zimmerman R, Carpenter RJ Jr, Durig P, et al. Longitudinal measurement of peak systolic velocity in the fetal middle cerebral artery for monitoring pregnancies complicated by red cell alloimmunisation: a prospective multicentre trial with intention-to-treat. *BJOG.* 2002;109(7):746–752.
48. Van den Veyver IB, Chong SS, Cota J, et al. Single-cell analysis of the RhD blood type for use in preimplantation diagnosis in the prevention of severe hemolytic disease of the newborn. *Am J Obstet Gynecol.* 1995;172:533–540.
49. Zwiers C, van der Bom JG, van Kamp IL, et al. Postponing early transfusion with intravenous immunoglobulin treatment; the PETIT study on severe hemolytic disease of the fetus and newborn. *Am J Obstet Gynecol.* 2018;219(3):291.
50. Nwogu LC, Moise KJ Jr, Klein KL, et al. Successful management of severe red blood cell alloimmunization in pregnancy with a combination of therapeutic plasma exchange, intravenous immune globulin, and intrauterine transfusion. *Transfusion.* 2018;58(3):677–684.
51. Schwartz J, Padmanabhan A, Aqui N, et al. Guidelines on the use of therapeutic apheresis in clinical practice-evidence-based approach from the writing committee of the American Society for Apheresis: the Seventh Special Issue. *J Clin Apher.* 2016;31(3):149–162.

Nonimmune Hydrops Fetalis and Isolated Fetal Ascites

Beth M. Kline-Fath • Eva Ilse Rubio

NONIMMUNE HYDROPS FETALIS

Hydrops fetalis is a Greek term that describes pathological fluid in fetal soft tissue or serous spaces. The term is utilized in nonimmune hydrops when there is abnormal fluid accumulation in two or more spaces in the absence of red cell alloimmunization. The distinction between nonimmune hydrops and immune hydrops was first noted in 1943 by Edith Potter.[1] At that time, in the mid-20th century, nonimmune hydrops was comparatively uncommon, representing less than a quarter of all infants born with fetal hydrops. Today, in developed countries, owing to successful prophylactic Rh immunization, nonimmune hydrops represents approximately 90% of all cases of fetal hydrops.[2,3]

Incidence: The prevalence of nonimmune hydrops remains at approximately 1 in 1,700 to 3,000 pregnancies.[3–5]

Pathogenesis: Nonimmune hydrops fetalis (NIHF) is an end-stage manifestation of any one of a growing list of maternal, fetal, and placental etiologies that result in an imbalance in the regulation of fluid movement between the fetal vascular and interstitial spaces.[5,6]

In normal physiology, fluid is released into the interstitial space by the capillary circulation and is returned to the vascular space by lymphatic vessels. The pathophysiological mechanisms leading to hydrops result in either an increase in interstitial fluid production and/or an obstruction to normal lymphatic return. The fetus is at high risk for hydrops, given that the body has higher water content (90% to 95% at 8 weeks decreasing to 70% at term) and also a highly compliant interstitial compartment, greater capillary permeability, and a lymphatic return that is strongly influenced by central venous pressure.[2] Underlying pathophysiology may be organized into the following categories. However, in reality, these mechanisms often occur together in a cascade of systemic failure (Fig. 28.2-1).[3,5,6]

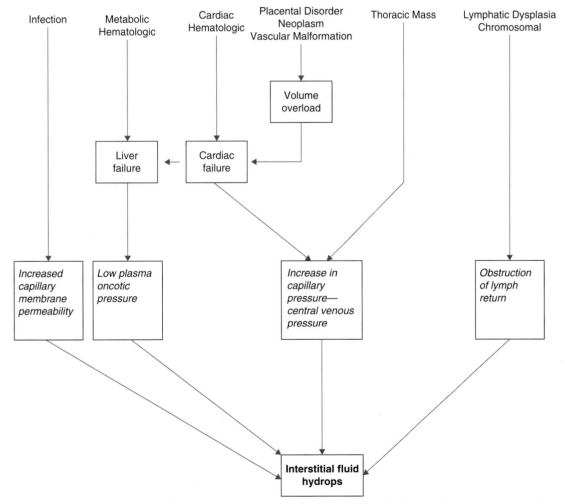

FIGURE 28.2-1: Etiologies and mechanisms for hydrops. (From Bellini C, Hennekam RC. Etiology of nonimmune hydrops fetalis: a systematic review. Am J Med Genet A. 2009;149A(5):844–851. Copyright © 2009 Wiley-Liss, Inc. Adapted by permission of John Wiley & Sons, Inc.))

Increase in Capillary/Venous Pressure is among the most common mechanisms. Pressure can rise in the capillary bed when there is increased central venous pressure, increased arterial pressure, or obstruction in venous drainage.[3] Increased fetal central venous pressure may result from cardiac failure or thoracic mass effect. Cardiac failure may be primary (arrhythmias, structural defects, and viral or autoimmune myocarditis) or secondary, resulting from high-output conditions (twin–twin transfusion syndrome [TTTS], anemia, vascular malformations, and high-flow tumors). The subsequent impedance of lymphatic flow occurring with venous hypertension also results in accumulation of fluid in the highly compliant fetal interstitial space.[6]

Increased Capillary Membrane Permeability is the result of injury to the capillary endothelium, allowing efflux of plasma proteins from the vascular space into the interstitial tissues. The fluid follows the proteins into the interstitium because of a reversal in the osmotic pressure gradient, being higher in the protein-filled interstitial space than in the vasculature. The injury may result from hypoxia, inflammatory mediators or endotoxins in the setting of infection.[3]

Diminished Plasma Oncotic Pressure occurs when large intravascular molecules, such as albumin, are decreased. In their absence in the plasma, the intravascular osmotic pressure is decreased, causing loss of fluid to the interstitial space. Most hypoproteinemic states indicate a degree of liver impairment or, less commonly, renal disease that results in loss of protein in the urine. Organ damage resulting from infection, hepatic congestion, or hypoxic injury leads to an overall reduction in plasma albumin levels.[3,6]

Impedance of Lymphatic Flow may occur via several mechanisms. Lymph vessels are made of smooth muscle with one-way valves that contract when filled. However, other important factors for lymph flow include body and limb movement, skeletal muscle contraction, arterial pulsations, and tissue compression.

The lymph flow may be impaired due to intrinsic lymphatic aberrations, decreased activity in a fetus with severe musculoskeletal or central nervous system abnormalities, or intrathoracic/cardiac abnormalities characterized by increased central venous pressure.[3]

Etiology: Identifying hydrops via ultrasound (US) is not difficult, but defining the etiology can be more challenging. The differential diagnosis of NIHF is extensive, with the most common pathologies listed in Table 28.2-1. Although in many cases the etiology of NIHF is unknown, the cause can be detected prenatally in 60% of cases and postnatally in 85% of cases, with the most common disorders resulting in NIHF being cardiovascular, chromosomal/syndromic, lymphatic dysplasia, infection, and hematological abnormalities.[5,7,8] Further discussion of causes of NIHF are provided separately later in the chapter.

Diagnosis: The primary goal of investigation in NIHF is to identify a treatable condition or diagnose genetic syndromes that may have a risk of recurrence. A thorough assessment of family history and ethnic background in conjunction with detailed maternal history, including prior pregnancies (especially those resulting in fetal or neonatal loss), medication, bleeding tendencies, exposures, and travel, should be performed. As genetic disorders account for approximately one-third of cases, knowledge of familial inherited disorders and consanguinity is extremely important.[5]

Maternal physical examination and laboratory testing should include evaluation for preeclampsia and chronic illnesses such as Sjögren, lupus, diabetes, and Graves disease. Imaging and, often, more invasive diagnostic testing will be necessary to explore all possible diagnostic entities. Stepwise evaluation of a pregnancy affected by NIHF begins with a detailed US with Doppler and fetal echocardiogram. Doppler of the middle cerebral artery (MCA) is important to assess for fetal anemia. An abnormal ductus venosus waveform

TABLE 28.2-1   Etiologies of Nonimmune Hydrops Fetalis

CAUSE	CASES (%)	MECHANISM
Cardiovascular	17–35	Increased CVP
Chromosomal	7–16	Cardiac, lymphatic, hematological
Hematological	4–12	Anemia, HOCF, hypoxia
Infectious	5–7	Anemia, anoxia, endothelial cell damage, increased capillary permeability
Thoracic	2–7	IVR
Twin–twin transfusion	3–10	Hypervolemia, increased CVP
Urinary abnormalities	0.9–3	Urinary ascites, hypoproteinemia
Gastrointestinal	0.5–4	Obstruction of venous return, protein loss, decreased colloid osmotic pressure
Lymphatic dysplasia	5–15	IVR, lymphatic
Tumors	0.7–3	Anemia, HOCF, hypoproteinemia
Skeletal dysplasia	3–4	Hypoproteinemia, IVR
Syndromic	3–12.5	Various
Inborn errors of metabolism	1–2	IVR, decreased erythropoiesis, anemia, hypoproteinemia, visceromegaly
Miscellaneous/rare	3–15	
Unknown	15–25	

Abbreviations: CVP, central venous pressure; HOCF, high-output cardiac failure; IVR, impaired venous return.
Adapted from Society for Maternal-Fetal Medicine (SMFM), Norton ME, Chauhan SP, Dashe JS. Society for Maternal-Fetal Medicine (SMFM) Clinical Guideline #7: nonimmune hydrops fetalis. *Am J Obstet Gynecol.* 2015;212(2):127–139. Copyright © 2015 Elsevier. With permission.

can help identify a fetus at risk for cardiac anomalies, which should be further evaluated via fetal echocardiogram. Utilizing these investigative tools, etiology of NIHF can be determined in 50% of cases.[9] In the presence of associated anomalies or fetal mass or in cases where the diagnosis is unknown, fetal magnetic resonance imaging (MRI) may be helpful for further definition.

If there are no fetal abnormalities detected on imaging studies, maternal blood type and Rh (D) antigen and indirect Coombs test are evaluated to exclude alloimmunization. Maternal blood tests should also include complete blood count with differential and exclusion of alpha thalassemia, particularly in mothers of Southeast Asia. Other blood test workup should consist of Kleihauer–Betke stain for fetal hemoglobin, serology for parvovirus B19, and serological testing for syphilis, cytomegalovirus (CMV), and toxoplasmosis.[5] As chromosomal abnormalities are a common cause of NIHF, cell-free DNA can be obtained to determine the presence of fetal aneuploidies.

If minimally invasive studies are negative and the fetus is normal or with findings suggesting genetic disorder, amniocentesis or fetal blood sampling should be offered for fetal karyotype and microarray genetic molecular analysis. Fetal blood sampling to determine fetal hematocrit or hemoglobin may be preferred if MCA Doppler suggests anemia, fetal bleeding is documented, or parental anemia or parvovirus B19 seroconversion is discovered. Amniotic fluid testing in a normal fetus with no other cause may include viral/bacterial cultures, polymerase chain reaction for parvovirus, CMV or toxoplasmosis, and laboratory studies for metabolic disorders such as lysosomal storage, pyruvate kinase deficiency, and glucose-6-phosphate dehydrogenase deficiency. Fetal cavity aspiration, especially pleural, should include lymphocyte count, biochemical and protein/albumin labs, as well as viral and bacterial cultures.

Imaging: Confirmation of hydrops is generally accepted as the presence of excess fluid in two or more compartments of the fetal body. On US or MRI, compartments assessed include skin thickening that should be greater than 5 mm, pericardial fluid greater than 3 mm, and presence of pleural or abdominal cavity (ascites) fluid (Fig. 28.2-2). It must be remembered that fluid accumulation in a single space such as plural or abdominal should not be interpreted

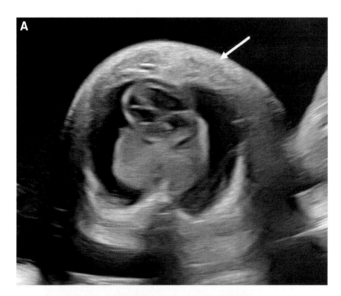

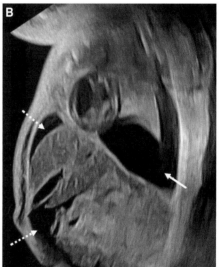

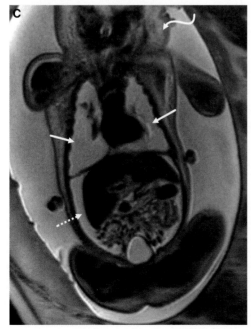

FIGURE 28.2-2: A 33-week fetus with trisomy 21 and NIHF. **A:** Axial US of the lower chest demonstrates collapsed echogenic lungs, pleural effusions, and skin edema (*solid arrow*). **B:** Sagittal US of the chest and abdomen demonstrates pleural fluid (*solid arrow*) and ascites (*dotted arrows*) anteriorly surrounding the liver and collapsed bowel. **C:** Coronal T2 MRI of same fetus demonstrating large bilateral effusions (*solid arrows*), ascites (*dotted arrow*) and skin edema (*curved arrow*).

or anticipated to evolve to hydrops. Those with isolated ascites and pleural effusion will not evolve to NIHF in 42% and 14% of cases, respectively.[7] An edematous placenta (≥4 cm in second trimester and ≥6 cm in third trimester) and polyhydramnios are often present in NIHF but not required for diagnosis.

In many cases, the pattern of the hydropic findings offers few, if any, clues to the diagnosis. A detailed and systematic approach to the fetal anatomical survey is helpful. Fluid complexity and the presence of calcifications may offer signs to a diagnosis. Anasarca is best reserved for diffuse skin thickening without septations, and often progresses in a cephalocaudal direction. It may herald impending hydrops and should be followed up closely once identified. Fetal MRI is often performed in cases where masses or anomalies are denoted and sometimes in cases where US, Doppler, and echocardiogram are normal (Fig. 28.2-3).

Doppler is essential in a fetus with NIHF. Careful interrogation of the MCA after 16 weeks' gestation for elevated peak systolic velocity greater than 1.5 multiples of the mean (MoM) may indicate fetal anemia.[5] Abnormal ductus venous or umbilical venous waveforms often suggest elevated venous pressure and/or cardiac dysfunction. Loss of diastolic flow in the umbilical artery reflects high placental resistance and/or increased cardiac afterload.

Because a significant percentage of cases of NIHF stem from a cardiac cause, a fetal echocardiogram with complete assessment of cardiac structure, contractility, and rhythm is imperative. Attention to M-mode is essential to evaluate for subtle arrhythmias.

Differential Diagnosis: Fluid in one space is not consistent with NIHF. Obliquity in the plane of imaging can create a spuriously thickened appearance of normal fetal skin. In cases of arthrogryposis and other musculoskeletal disorders, fatty replacement of the fetal musculature may create a featureless and redundant appearance of the skin and soft tissues that should be considered when diagnosing subcutaneous edema. Severe hydrops and large cystic hygromas may be mistaken for amniotic fluid (Fig. 28.2-4).

Prognosis: The prognosis in the setting of NIHF remains poor, with overall survival of 38% after excluding pregnancy terminations.[10] Reviewing several studies, intrauterine demise occurs in 15% to 60% of pregnancies with NIHF, and of those live-born, 35% to 50% will not survive the neonatal period.[3,9,11,12] However, one should bear in mind that this generalization may not apply to all cases.

The outcome is dependent on many factors including underlying etiology. Congenital heart defects have a high mortality at 51% and a fetal loss rate of 80%.[9,10] There is a worse outcome for those diagnosed at an earlier gestational age.[5,11] Fetuses presenting earlier in pregnancy are much more likely to have an underlying chromosomal disorder (80%), and carry a poor prognosis with a mortality rate of 70%.[9,11] However, many fetuses diagnosed after 24 weeks have a favorable outcome as etiology is more likely amenable to intrauterine therapy such as anemia, drainable cystic or fluid collections (chylothorax), parvovirus infection, cardiac arrhythmias, and aneurysms of the vein of Galen.[11,12] These observations are supported by postnatal studies that also describe a much higher mortality rate of 57.7% among hydropic newborns with congenital anomalies as compared with a mortality rate of 5.9% among newborns presenting with isolated, treatable abnormalities such as congenital chylothorax.[13]

Antenatal resolution of hydrops also has a favorable prognosis, seen in up to 32% of NIHF (Fig. 28.2-5).[14] In the presence of complete resolution, there is a 100% survival and with partial resolution, 76% survival prior to birth.[10] Overall, neonatal survival is noted in 76% of cases with complete or partial resolution of NIHF.[14]

Delivery statistics are also important, with outcome being less favorable with delivery at early gestational age, low birth weight, low Apgars, or needing transport after birth.[5,11] Long-term outcome data for surviving children with NIHF is limited, but it also depends on the underlying etiology. In a single-center study, approximately 39% had comorbidity.[12] Some had mild disorders such as feeding difficulty and recurrent tachyarrhythmia, but approximately 11% were found to have significant developmental delay.[12]

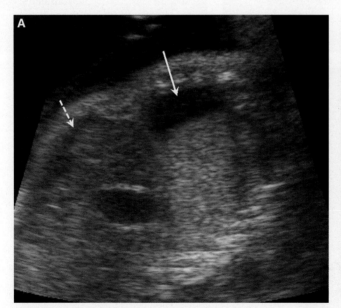
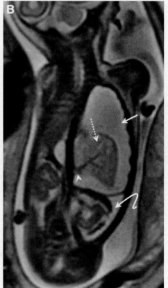

FIGURE 28.2-3: Hybrid sequestration and NIHF in a fetus at 31 weeks. **A:** Sagittal US of chest and abdomen demonstrated large pleural effusion (*solid arrow*) and small ascites (*dotted arrow*) without defined cause. The fetus also had skin edema and presented with polyhydramnios. **B:** Coronal T2 MRI of the fetal chest demonstrated a complex lung lesion (*dotted arrow*) with feeding vessel (*arrowhead*). Note large pleural effusion (*solid arrow*) and small ascites (*curved arrow*).

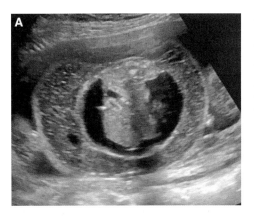

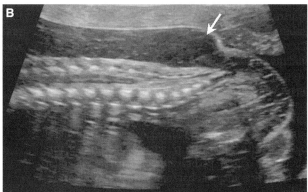

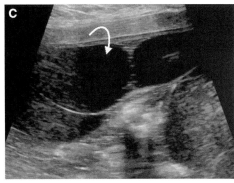

FIGURE 28.2-4: Turner syndrome, 23-week fetus. **A:** Axial US, thorax. Skin edema and large bilateral effusions. **B:** Sagittal US shows skin edema (*solid arrow*) filling the amniotic cavity. **C:** Cystic hygroma may easily be mistaken for amniotic fluid (*curved arrow*).

Management: Decisions regarding counseling and management of a pregnancy complicated by NIHF depend directly upon determination of the underlying cause. Therefore, urgent referral to a maternal fetal medicine specialist and initiation of an organized search for a diagnosis is crucial.

Some causes for NIHF are amendable to fetal therapy, which may require prompt intervention and/or referral to a specialized center. The cases where fetal intervention can be initiated are listed in Table 28.2-2. If the Doppler of the MCA is abnormal or if anemia is suspected, fetal blood sampling should be obtained with intrauterine transfusion as indicated.

Pregnancies with lethal or poor prognosis may be counseled with regard to termination or comfort care at birth. The difficult cases are those that are idiopathic, in which prognosis is uncertain. In women at risk for infection or blood dyscrasias, other directed laboratory testing may be performed. Referral to a geneticist may help guide management and therapy and direct further enzymatic testing for metabolic abnormalities.

Given that 40% of cases are associated with polyhydramnios, preterm labor is a significant risk. Maternal edema, also known as mirror syndrome, is higher in pregnancies with NIHF that may also necessitate preterm delivery. There is a three-fold increased risk of severe preeclampsia; therefore, serial evaluation of maternal blood pressure is recommended.[15]

Antenatal surveillance should be considered in those fetuses with nonlethal NIHF and/or when the pregnancy has reached a viable gestational age and imaging would assist in planning delivery.[5] There is no evidence that preterm labor will improve outcome; therefore, if NIHF worsens, delivery after 34 weeks is typically advised. In cases of absent deterioration or mirror syndrome, delivery by 37 to 38 weeks should be considered.[5] Predelivery cavity aspiration may facilitate neonatal and maternal management.

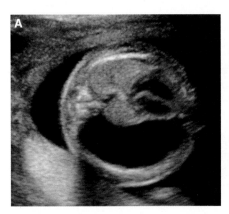

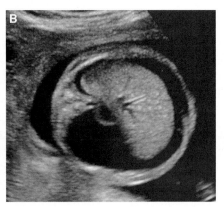

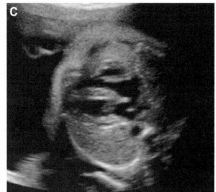

FIGURE 28.2-5: A 20-week pregnancy complicated by NIHF of unknown etiology. **A:** Axial US of the lower thorax demonstrates large effusion and compressed echogenic lungs. **B:** Axial US of the abdomen demonstrates large volume anechoic ascites. **C:** Same fetus 7 weeks later. There was spontaneous interval resolution of pleural effusions; only trace ascites (not shown) remained.

TABLE 28.2-2   Intrauterine Therapies to Treat NIHF

FETAL CONDITIONS WITH NIHF	INTRAUTERINE INTERVENTION
Anemia	Fetal intravascular blood transfusion
Cardiac arrhythmias	Maternal transplacental or direct administration antiarrhythmic, fetal ventricular pacing
Cardiac defects	Intrauterine heart surgery
Infection	Transplacental antiviral or antibiotic therapy
Obstructive uropathy	Fetal bladder decompression with vesicoamniotic shunt or open fetal surgery
Hydrothorax, chylothorax, BPS with pleural effusion	Fetal needle drainage or thoracoamniotic shunt
CPAM	Microcystic: maternal corticosteroid Macrocystic: fetal needle drainage/thoracoamniotic shunt/rare fetal surgery
Thoracic congenital anomaly	EXIT procedure/fetal surgery
Tumor/SCT	EXIT procedure/fetal surgery
TTTS or TAPS	Fetoscopic laser photocoagulation with NIHF <26 wk
TRAP	Radiofrequency ablation of acardiac twin

Abbreviations: BPS, bronchopulmonary sequestration; CPAM, congenital pulmonary airway malformation; NIHF, nonimmune hydrops fetalis; SCT, sacrococcygeal teratoma; TAPS, twin anemia polycythemia syndrome; TRAP, twin reversed arterial perfusion syndrome; TTTS, twin–twin transfusion syndrome.

Corticosteroid administration is recommended if fetal therapy is planned or preterm labor occurs between the gestational ages of 24 and 34 weeks.[5] Cesarean delivery in a center with a level III neonatal intensive care unit is suggested when intervention and resuscitation of the infant is to be instituted. If only comfort care is to be provided, vaginal delivery may be preferred.

Postnatally, infants born with hydrops are typically critically ill and require intensive therapy, including assisted ventilation and fluid resuscitation due to low intravascular volume.[6] Postnatal evaluation by a comprehensive medical team including genetics is warranted. X-ray should be considered to exclude dysmorphic syndrome or skeletal dysplasia. If demise occurs without a known cause, autopsy and placental examination is strongly suggested to exclude etiologies with recurrence risk.[16]

Recurrence: NIHF has a low recurrence risk; however, in the presence of genetic abnormalities, the risk may be as high as 25%.[5]

Conditions Associated with NIHF

Fetal Cardiac Anomalies

Cardiac abnormalities are one of the most common underlying etiologies for NIHF, especially after 22 to 24 weeks, representing approximately 10% to 20% of all cases.[16] The most common

cardiac causes are *structural abnormalities, rhythm disorders, physiological dysfunction, and tumors.*[3,16] The mechanisms by which congestive heart failure causes hydrops include one or more of the following: elevated central venous pressures or volume overload, decreased ventricular output affecting fluid balance at the capillary level, fetal capillary damage due to hypoxia, insufficient oncotic pressure due to hepatic dysfunction and protein loss, and decreased lymphatic drainage.[3] For reasons not readily apparent, fetal hydrops will manifest in some cases of cardiac anomalies, while other fetuses remain unaffected. However, the prognosis is guarded, with a live-born rate of 48% and a combined fetal and infant mortality rate in approximately 70% of cases with NIHF and an underlying cardiogenic cause.[17]

Structural defects known to be associated with nonimmune fetal hydrops tend to be anomalies of the right heart as an increase in right atrial pressure will increase venous pressure/and or volume load.[3,18] Transposition of great vessels, truncus arteriosus, double-outlet right ventricle, absent pulmonary valve, and Ebstein anomaly are known causes (Fig. 28.2-6). However, left heart defects with obstructive outflow can be transmitted to the right heart via the foramen ovale, thereby also increasing pressures. Types of lesions include hypoplastic left heart, often with restrictive foramen ovale, large atrioventricular defect, and critical aortic stenosis.[3,5] Hydrops occurring in the setting of a structural defect indicates an especially poor prognosis, with a combined fetal and infant mortality of 92% in one meta-analysis.[17] A significant percentage will also have a chromosomal anomaly.

Arrhythmias include tachycardia, bradycardia, and heart block, all of which may result in hydrops due to elevated central venous pressure, decreased cardiac output resulting in congestive heart failure, and impaired tissue perfusion.[3,18] Fetal tachyarrhythmias including supraventricular tachycardia (SVT) and atrial flutter are the most common arrhythmias causing NIHF, present in 35% to 60% of these cases.[6,18] Fetal bradycardia is a rare source, occurring primarily when fetal heart rate is persistently less than 50 per minute.[18] Fetuses with congenital heart block with heart rates of less than 90 bpm frequently have NIHF, with the most common

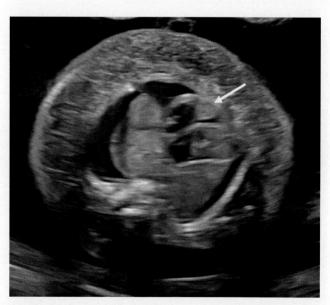

FIGURE 28.2-6: A 23-week fetus with double-outlet right ventricle and pulmonic stenosis. Axial US of the thorax. The myocardium is conspicuously thickened (*solid arrow*). Note bilateral pleural effusions and extensive skin thickening.

etiology being a maternal autoimmune disorder.[6] Fortunately, fetal dysrhythmias, with the exception of difficult to manage bradycardia, are treatable by way of maternal medications with conversion of fetal sinus rhythm typically within 3 to 14 days.[18]

Dysfunction may arise from one of many pathological entities, including infection, inflammation, infarction, or arterial calcification. The most common infectious agent is parvovirus B19, which can result in high cardiac output failure related to anemia and fetal viral myocarditis.[19,20] Other causes of inflammation includes maternal insulin-dependent diabetes and autoimmune disorders such as lupus. In a pregnancy with maternal systemic lupus erythematosus, anticardiolipin antibodies cross the placenta, causing fetal heart dysfunction. Fetal/neonatal lupus complicated by hydrops carries a significantly higher risk of demise with typical manifestations including fetal heart block, dilated cardiomyopathy, and endocardial fibroelastosis.[21]

Tumors are uncommon, but carry a risk of precipitating hydrops. Fetal intracardiac tumors include rhabdomyomas, myxomas, fibromas, and hemangiomas, although rhabdomyomas are by far the most common in this category, representing up to 80% to 90% of prenatally diagnosed cardiac tumors.[22] Pericardial tumors are rare, with the most common being teratoma. Hydrops develops in these cases by either mass effect or by obstruction of flow resulting in impedance of venous return to the heart.[3] Rhabdomyomas are commonly associated with tuberous sclerosis and only rarely lead to hydrops.[22] Pericardial teratomas have a significantly higher risk for NIHF, seen in up to 70% of cases.[18] Treatment in these cases would include thoraco/pericardial amniotic shunt, open fetal resection, or early delivery.

Fetal Chromosome Abnormalities

Chromosomal anomalies have one of the highest associations with NIHF. Although estimates vary, and a causal relationship is not always clear, approximately 25% to 75% of NIHF are caused by a chromosomal defect.[18,23] The favored pathophysiology is incomplete formation of the lymphatics and hypoalbuminemia, with less likely contributing factors being hypotonia and hematological disturbances.[6] The mortality rate with NIHF is 58% for live-born, but increases to 98% with combined fetal and infant data.[17]

The likelihood of an underlying chromosomal abnormality is increased when hydrops is discovered earlier in gestation. The most common chromosomal abnormalities associated with hydrops are Turner syndrome and trisomy 21, although other culprits include trisomies 13, 18, 16, 15, 10, triploidy or tetraploidy and various chromosomal rearrangements (Figs. 28.2-2 and 28.2-4).[3]

Lymphatic Dysplasias

Lymphatic lesions, which include *lymphatic malformations (LMs), lymphangiectasia, and chylothorax,* typically result in reduced lymphatic clearance. Mortality rate for lymphatic abnormalities in the presence of NIHF is 24% for live-born, and 66% for fetal and infant data.[17]

LMs contain dysplastic lymph channels. Terminology for these lesions in the past included cystic hygroma, lymphangioma, and venolymphatic malformation, but was replaced with LMs for standardization and to decrease confusion. LMs commonly associated with NIHF were previously known as cystic hygromas. These malformations are complex, septated, anomalous lymphatic tissue located in the posterior neck and are commonly identified earlier in pregnancy and have a high association with genetic or chromosomal abnormalities (especially Turner syndrome)[3] (Figs. 28.2-4 and 28.2-7). LMs localized in the anterolateral soft tissues of the fetal neck are usually isolated entities,

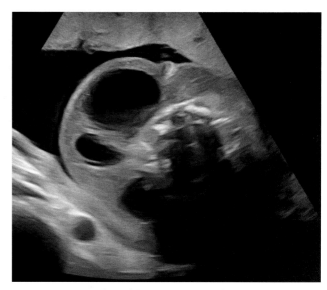

FIGURE 28.2-7: Axial US of the posterior neck of a 22-week fetus with a large, septated lymphatic malformation, in the setting of additional anomalies.

appearing somewhat later in pregnancy, and are typically not associated with chromosomal abnormalities or NIHF.

Congenital pulmonary lymphangiectasia (CPL) is a pathological dilatation of lymph vessels, and when primary or congenital is a rare severe and extensive lymphatic aberration that may only affect lung or be generalized to involve many organs. Previous autopsy studies have shown that CPL accounts for 0.5% to 1% of all fetal neonatal deaths.[23] Etiology is unclear, but some hypothesize that lack of normal regression of lymphatics at 18 to 20 weeks or mutations of genes in the vascular endothelial growth factor receptor may be the cause.[23] The onset of CPL is at an average of 21.6 weeks, presenting with NIHF and polyhydramnios with male predominance. CPL should be considered in the presence of bilateral chylothorax. Prognosis is poor, with stillbirth or neonatal death.[23] Secondary lymphangiectasia is due to obstructive cardiac disorders such as hypoplastic left heart, total anomalous pulmonary venous return, and/or thoracic duct anomalies and typically presents as pulmonary interstitial findings.

Congenital chylothorax (CC) is the most common cause for fetal hydrothorax, occurring in 1:15,000 pregnancies.[24] CC occurs more frequently on the right and has a male predominance. The etiology is often idiopathic, but pathogenesis is aplasia, hypoplasia, or obstruction of the thoracic duct. Large unilateral or bilateral effusions may lead to pulmonary hypoplasia and/or precipitate frank hydrops due to cardiomediastinal compression and impaired venous return. Loss of lymphocytes may result in malnutrition, dehydration, and increased risk for infection; and loss of albumin in the chyle of the pleural space may also aggravate interstitial fluid accumulation.[6,24] Diagnosis of chylous fluid requires greater than 1,000 white blood cells per microliter with more than 70% to 80% lymphocytes.[24] Management options include thoracentesis, thoracoamniotic shunting, maternal diet of low-fat medium-chain triglyceride diet, and/or expectant management/counseling. Timely shunting can successfully reverse fetal deterioration, decrease morbidity, and improve survival to as high as 72% (Fig. 28.2-8).[24,25] Secondary causes for chylothorax include LMs, CPL, lung lesions, congenital diaphragmatic hernia, and syndromes such as Turner, Noonan, trisomy 21, and Ehler–Danlos.[24]

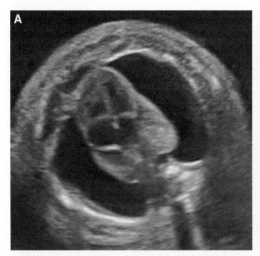
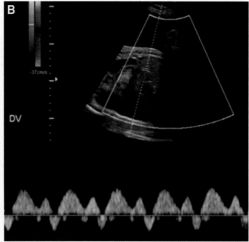
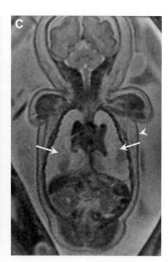

FIGURE 28.2-8: Primary chylothorax in a 31-week fetus. **A:** Axial US of the thorax demonstrates large bilateral effusions with collapsed lungs and central compression of the heart. Note skin edema. **B:** A-wave reversal of the ductus venosus. **C:** Coronal T2 MRI: large effusions (*solid arrows*) and skin edema (*arrowhead*). No mass was identified. The pleural effusions were successfully treated with thoracoamniotic shunts.

Infection

Intrauterine infection is a common cause of NIHF, present in 4% to 15% of cases.[16] Infection primarily targets the fetal bone marrow, myocardium, and vascular endothelium. Heart failure, anemia, fetal sepsis leading to anoxia, and endothelial cell damage may result in hepatic dysfunction and increased capillary permeability, which are likely mechanisms for interstitial fluid accumulation. Mortality rates are 37% in live-born and 72% in fetal and neonatal groups.[3]

Common etiologies include parvovirus B19, toxoplasma, *Treponema pallidum*, CMV, herpes simplex virus, congenital hepatitis, coxsackie virus, hepatitis B, adenovirus, human immunodeficiency virus, and *Listeria monocytogenes*.[3] Pregnancies affected by infection with subsequent hydrops have variable outcomes, and additional characteristic sonographic features may help in elucidating the diagnosis (see Chapter 31).

Parvovirus B19 is the most common organism known to cause hydrops, being the etiology of 8% to 30% of all cases of NIHF.[3,20] The pathogen is a small, single-stranded DNA virus spread primarily by respiratory secretions. The mechanisms for development of fetal hydrops in the setting of parvovirus B19 infection can be characterized as both direct and indirect and includes destruction of fetal red blood cell progenitor cells resulting in both anemia and hypoxia, fetal viral myocarditis and output failure associated with anemia, liver failure due to hepatocyte damage and hemosiderin deposits, and placentitis.[19,20] The fetus is at highest risk for adverse outcome in the first and second trimesters because of increased vulnerability and red blood cell requirements earlier in gestation, as well as changes in placental receptors over the course of the pregnancy.[20] NIHF is present in approximately 10% of pregnancies affected by parvovirus B19 infection (Fig. 28.2-9). Infected fetuses with NIHF have an increased risk for intrauterine and perinatal death as well as brain injury (10%) and sequential abnormal neurodevelopmental outcome (10%).[26,27] Early clues to diagnosis may be elevated peak systolic velocity of the MCA due to anemia. Establishment of the diagnosis of acute parvovirus B19 infection begins with maternal immunoglobulin IgM and IgG serological testing and may proceed to amniotic fluid or fetal cord blood polymerase chain reaction (PCR) testing for viral RNA or DNA.[20] In the presence of anemia, intrauterine blood transfusion or early delivery of the fetus are the most favored

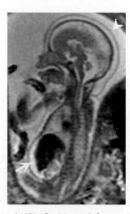

FIGURE 28.2-9: Sagittal MRI of a 20-week fetus with parvovirus B19. Note diffuse skin thickening (*arrowhead*) and ascites (*arrow*).

means of treatment.[27] When NIHF develops in the setting of parvovirus B19, fetal blood transfusion has been shown to decrease the likelihood of fetal demise by five- to seven-fold.[19,20] Although most (>80%) pregnancies affected by parvovirus have no fetal sequelae, overall fetal mortality is approximately 5% to 10% of cases.[19,20,26] The infection may affect fetuses of a twin pregnancy with asymmetric severity, and can even mimic other conditions such as TTTS and intrauterine growth restriction.

Anemia and Hematological Disorders

NIHF is the result of hematological abnormalities in approximately 10% of cases.[2] The primary pathophysiological mechanism precipitating hydrops is anemia, but other contributing factors include high-output cardiomyopathy[19,20] and liver failure with associated fetal hypoalbuminemia.[28] Differential diagnostic considerations should include alpha thalassemia, parvovirus B19, and transient abnormal myelopoiesis. The mortality rate is 57% in live-born and 88% in fetal and infant data.[17]

Alpha thalassemia is commonly found among southeastern Asian populations and Mediterranean countries. The two severe forms at risk of developing fetal hydrops include Hb Bart, characterized by total absence of hemoglobin alpha chains, and Hb H, in which three of four alpha chain genes are absent.[28] These conditions result in NIHF with anemia, hypoxemia, and marked hepatosplenomegaly, which is explained by both congestive heart failure and extramedullary hematopoiesis.[28] Hb Bart is considered essentially incompatible with survival of the fetus. Significant maternal morbidity in the form of mirror syndrome may occur and should be recognized promptly. Beta thalassemia is not associated with fetal hydrops.

Transient abnormal myelopoiesis is usually seen in fetuses with trisomy 21. Well-known postnatally, the condition affects 10% of newborns with trisomy 21.[29] It has also been documented prenatally via percutaneous umbilical cord sampling.[28,30] Imaging findings in the hydropic fetus with trisomy 21 that may raise suspicion for this entity include hepatosplenomegaly and declining cardiac function.[29,30]

Genetic and Metabolic Disorders

Genetic and metabolic disorders may cause hydrops, and identification of these entities is important, as some are inherited with a recurrence risk of 25%. Extensive genetic testing with chromosomal microarray should be considered as 19% of NIHF have been attributed to rare genetic syndromes and one third of idiopathic cases due to lysosomal storage disorders.[31] Mortality with these disorders in the presence of NIHF is high; 67% in live-born and 93% in studies with combined fetal and infant data.[17]

In genetic disorders, many mechanisms are suggested to cause NIHF, including increased venous pressure due to low thoracic volume, hypomobility, lymphatic abnormalities, and hemolytic anemias. Skeletal dysplasias and other assorted autosomal recessive and autosomal dominant single gene disorders have been cited.[3,32,33] Some skeletal dysplasias that can lead to NIHF include achondrogenesis, thoracic asphyxiating dysplasia (Jeune syndrome), osteogenesis imperfecta, and the short-rib polydactyly syndromes[32] (Fig. 28.2-10).

The percentage of cases of NIHF caused by inborn errors of metabolism was previously estimated at approximately 1%.[34] However, more recent studies indicate that inborn errors of metabolism may be more common than once assumed, accounting for up to 15% of NIHF cases.[35] Proposed mechanisms for precipitating hydrops include organomegaly causing impedance of venous return, lymph dysplasia, anemia, hypoproteinemia, and

congestive heart failure.[34] The most common metabolic etiologies of NIHF are severe forms of lysosomal storage diseases including Gaucher disease, sialidosis, I-cell disease, Niemann–Pick, GM1 gangliosidosis, infantile sialic acid storage disease, mucopolysaccharidoses, Wolman disease, and Farber disease.[34] However, multiple other metabolic disorders have been cited and include glycogenesis type IV, peroxisomal disorders, transaldolase deficiency, cholesterol metabolism inborn errors, citric cycle defects, and congenital disorders of glycosylation.[35] Most genetic and metabolic disorders are autosomal recessive in their inheritance pattern. Diagnosis can be difficult, as current testing is only directed at lysosomal storage disease with biochemical analysis of oligosaccharides, mucopolysaccharides, sialic acid, and lysosomal enzyme activities from amniotic fluid. Directed next-generation sequencing panels and biochemical testing may increase sensitivity.[35] NIHF affecting multiple pregnancies in a family, in ethnic groups with higher risk, or with consanguinity should prompt further investigation.[34]

Congenital/Thoracic Abnormalities

Intrathoracic structural abnormalities are a recognized cause of fetal nonimmune hydrops, estimated to be the underlying cause in approximately 6% of cases.[2] The mechanism for development of NIHF is generally accepted as a combination of impaired venous return, obstructed lymphatics, and direct impingement upon the cardiac chambers negatively affecting contractility.[3] Mortality is high in the setting of hydrops, 73% for fetal and 85% for combined fetal and neonatal data.[17] In-depth review with treatment options for these lesions are discussed in Chapter 25.3.

Thoracic lesions that are most likely to result in fetal hydrops are large congenital pulmonary airway malformations (CPAMs), mediastinal teratomas, and fetal chylothorax (Fig. 28.2-11). Other lesions such as congenital diaphragmatic hernias, LMs, pulmonary sequestrations, and bronchogenic cysts arc also candidates, but are less likely to be complicated by hydrops (see Fig. 28.2-3). CPAMs range in size from subcentimeter to massive lesions that occupy a majority of the fetal thorax. Although the vast majority of these lesions carry a favorable prognosis, the larger masses carry a risk of hydrops and fetal demise. A CPAM volume ratio (CVR)

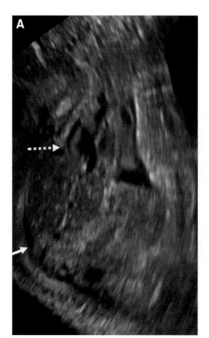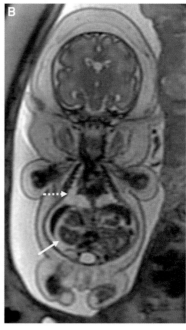

FIGURE 28.2-10: Achondrogenesis and hydrops in a 29-week fetus **A:** Coronal US demonstrates small chest with small bilateral effusions (*dotted arrow*), ascites (*solid arrow*), and soft tissue edema. **B:** Coronal T2 MRI of same fetus with small chest and limbs. Bilateral effusions (*dotted arrow*), ascites (*solid arrow*), and extensive soft-tissue edema is noted.

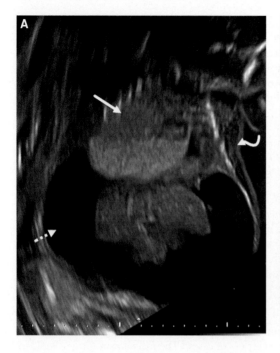

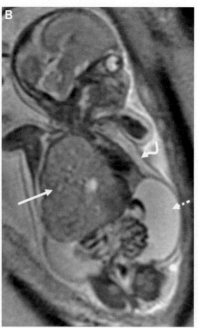

FIGURE 28.2-11: Hydrops complicating a large congenital pulmonary airway malformation in a 23 week fetus. **A:** Coronal US demonstrates an echogenic lesion (*solid arrow*) displacing heart and mediastinum. Severe ascites (*dotted arrow*) is present as well as soft-tissue edema (*curved arrow*). **B:** Coronal T2 MRI depicts heterogeneous lung mass (*solid arrow*) occupying the right thoracic cavity displacing heart into the left chest. Severe ascites (*dotted arrow*) and soft-tissue edema (*curved arrow*) again noted. Steroids were administered but intrauterine demise occurred.

is calculated by obtaining three orthogonal lesional measurements, multiplying by 0.52, and dividing this value by the head circumference. A CVR of greater than 1.6 indicates a high risk of development of hydrops. A CVR of less than 1.6 without a dominant intralesional cyst indicates a low risk of hydrops, being less than 3%.[36]

Fetal mediastinal teratomas are exceedingly rare lesions that are typically complicated by hydrops and cardiovascular compromise due to compression. The imaging appearance reflects their complex composition of fat, cysts, calcifications, and various soft tissues. Not infrequently mistaken for other diagnoses (in particular CPAMs), mediastinal teratomas often displace the heart inferiorly, a feature not demonstrated by masses arising from the lung. Mediastinal teratomas portend a grim prognosis

unless intervention is carried out in a timely manner, either during fetal life or soon after delivery (Fig. 28.2-12).

A distinct entity in which hydrops is commonly seen is congenital high airway obstruction syndrome (CHAOS). CHAOS results from upper airway (often laryngeal) atresia or occlusion and is characterized by severely hyperexpanded lungs and dilated central airways that compress central cardiomediastinal structures and evert diaphragms. Due to obstructed venous and lymphatic return in the presence of cardiomediastinal compression, anasarca and large ascites is present, often in conjunction with placentamegaly and polyhydramnios[37] (Fig. 28.2-13).

High-Flow Tumors and Vascular Malformations
Tumors and vascular anomalies are a well-known cause of fetal nonimmune hydrops, accounting for 6% to 7% of all cases.[6] Fetal neoplasms and vascular lesions can precipitate high-output cardiac failure owing to demands of increased flow volume.[38]

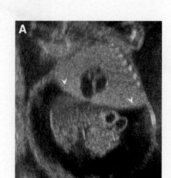

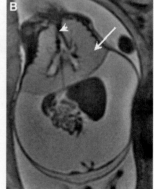

FIGURE 28.2-12: Mediastinal teratoma. Coronal SSFP MRI of a complex fetal mediastinal mass (*solid arrow*) displacing the heart (*arrowheads*) inferiorly. Note effusion (*dotted arrow*) and ascites. Mild skin thickening is also present. The fetus died shortly after the study.

FIGURE 28.2-13: A 19-week fetus with congenital high airway obstruction syndrome. **A:** Coronal US depicts echogenic, hyperexpanded lungs and ascites. Note everted diaphragms (*arrowheads*). **B:** Coronal T2 MRI demonstrates hyperexpanded increased signal lungs (*solid arrow*) and large ascites. *Arrowhead* indicates area of airway obstruction. Fluid-dilated trachea and bronchi are noted below the obstruction.

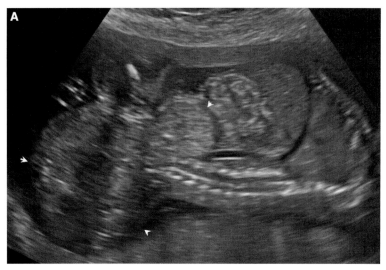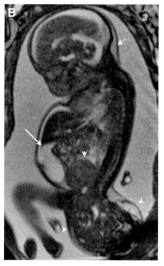

FIGURE 28.2-14: Hydrops in a fetus at 20 weeks with large sacrococcygeal teratoma. **A:** Sagittal US demonstrates large exophytic mass with extension into the pelvis and lower abdomen (*arrowheads*). There is small ascites and pleural fluid. **B:** Sagittal SSFP MRI from same fetus shows complex mass (*arrowheads*), ascites (*solid arrow*), and nuchal thickening (*dotted arrow*).

Common tumors with high flow and known association with NIHF include cervical and sacrococcygeal teratomas and liver lesions. Sacrococcygeal teratomas, in particular, may grow rapidly and/or with high solid content, placing the fetus at risk for high cardiac output hydrops (Fig. 28.2-14).[39,40] The development of hydrops indicates a high likelihood of intrauterine demise.[41] Other specific indicators of high-risk lesions include elevated aortic velocity, increased inferior vena cava (IVC) diameter, high cardiac output, and umbilical arterial diastolic flow reversal.[41] Liver tumors diagnosed in the prenatal period are an uncommon cause of hydrops. Hepatic hemangiomas or hemangioendotheliomas may precipitate hydrops via high cardiac output physiology.

Vein of Galen aneurysm is a well-known, high-flow arteriovenous anomaly in the fetus. While commonly associated with cardiomegaly, hydrops may occur when the lesion results in high-output cardiac failure. MRI can be useful to evaluate brain parenchymal injury (Fig. 28.2-15).[39]

Monozygotic Twin Pregnancies

Monozygotic pregnancies have a higher risk for fetal hydrops due to the presence of vascular anastomoses across the single placenta. In TTTS, the occurrence of hydrops in either twin is approximately 8%.[42] The donor twin is characterized by oligohydramnios, nonfilling of the urinary bladder, and smaller size. In

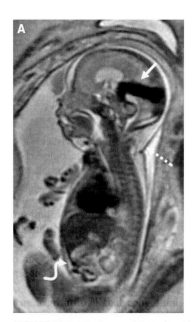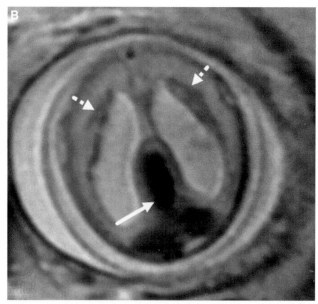

FIGURE 28.2-15: Fetus at 27 weeks with vein of Galen malformation and hydrops. **A:** Sagittal T2 MRI demonstrates large Vein of Galen aneurysm (*solid arrow*), cardiomegaly, ascites (*curved arrow*), and soft-tissue edema (*dotted arrows*). **B:** Axial T2 MRI of the brain demonstrates the large vascular malformation (*solid arrow*). The ventricles are dilated, and there is abnormal dark T2 signal in the white matter (*dotted arrows*) consistent with injury.

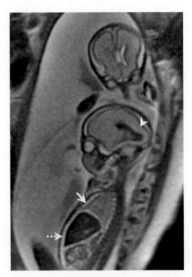

FIGURE 28.2-16: Complications of twin–twin transfusion syndrome at 21 weeks. Sagittal MRI demonstrates recipient intraventricular hemorrhage (arrowhead), small pleural effusion (solid arrow) and ascites (*dotted arrow*).

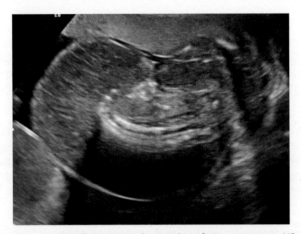

FIGURE 28.2-17: Twin reversed arterial perfusion sequence. US of dysmorphic and diffusely edematous acardiac twin.

the recipient, expected findings include polyhydramnios, urinary tract distension, and cardiomegaly.[42] The recipient twin tends to develop hydrops due to a hypertensive cardiomyopathy (Fig. 28.2-16). The donor is less likely to manifest hydrops, which, when present, is typically the consequence of severe anemia resulting in hypoxia and increased cardiac output, eventually precipitating cardiac failure.[6] Pregnancies affected by TTTS are organized according to imaging signs into stages established by Quintero, and subsequently revised by the Cincinnati staging system.[41] Development of hydrops indicates stage IV, which is uniformly fatal without therapeutic intervention.

In the infrequent scenario of acardiac twinning, also referred to as twin reversed arterial perfusion (TRAP) sequence, the acardiac twin is typically hydropic due to lymphatic abnormalities (Fig. 28.2-17).[43] However, the pump twin is at risk of developing myocardial failure, subsequent hydrops, and fetal demise. Volume calculations of the acardiac twin are assessed as a ratio to the pump twin to predict the risk of morbidity and mortality for the pump twin. The pump twin is at increased risk for demise when the acardiac twin's calculated weight is greater than 70% of the pump twin.[44]

Placental/Umbilical Cord Anomalies

Placental or umbilical cord abnormalities account for approximately 10% of cases of NIHF, with a mortality rate of 51% in live-born and 71% among combined fetal and neonatal deaths.[17] Hydrops may result from one or more of the following mechanisms: high-output failure from arteriovenous shunting[3,45]; hemolytic anemia due to intralesional trapping of fetal erythrocytes[3,45]; or fetal hypoxia with subsequent organ and tissue damage due to both abnormal shunting of unoxygenated blood and concomitant anemia.

NIHF may occur due to fetal anemia secondary to fetomaternal hemorrhage from malformation of the placenta, umbilical cord accident, or obstetric accident. Other placental abnormalities associated with NIHF include chorioangioma,[3,45] choriocarcinoma,[46] chorionic vein thrombosis, and hemorrhagic endovasculitis.[41] Chorioangioma of the placenta is a benign but vascular lesion with potential for high-flow shunting (Fig. 28.2-18). Cord abnormalities that may be associated

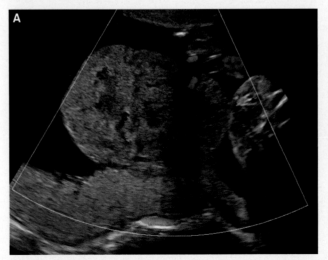
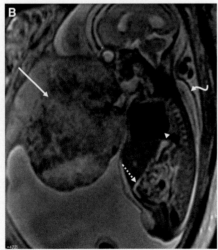

FIGURE 28.2-18: Pregnancy complicated by chorioangioma at 26 weeks. **A:** Color Doppler US shows large vascular placental mass. **B:** Sagittal T2 MRI through the fetus shows large inhomogeneous placental mass (*solid arrow*). The fetus has cardiomegaly (*arrowhead*), skin edema (*curved arrow*), and ascites (*dotted arrow*).

with fetal hydrops include umbilical vein thrombosis, umbilical cord knot, and umbilical cord tumors such as angiomyxoma.[41] Monochorionic monoamniotic twins are at particularly high risk of developing true knots of the umbilical cord(s).

Miscellaneous Conditions

In addition to the disease entities reviewed in the foregoing sections, a growing number of other disorders are reported to be associated with nonimmune fetal hydrops. These include neurological abnormalities, multiple pterygium syndrome, and arthrogryposis multiplex syndromes, which may cause hypomobility with secondary decreased respiratory movements and increased intrathoracic and venous pressure.[3,33] Urinary obstructive abnormalities may result in increase in venous pressure and lymphatic overload, while congenital nephrotic diseases, such as polycystic disease, can cause hypoalbuminemia. Gastrointestinal disorders, such as bowel perforation, bowel obstruction, or mass, may increase venous pressure, prevent normal lymphatics drainage, or injure capillaries due to infection or inflammation.[3] These are only representative samples in their respective categories. The complete lists are exhaustive and include many rare etiologies.

ISOLATED FETAL ASCITES

When fetal ascites is identified, it may be an isolated finding or the first manifestation of impending NIHF. For the purposes of this discussion, isolated ascites is defined as intra-abdominal fluid without other manifestations of hydrops such as pleural fluid, pericardial effusion, or skin thickening.

Incidence: The incidence of isolated ascites is considered rare.[47,48]

Pathogenesis: Isolated fetal ascites that does not progress to fetal hydrops is more likely to result from an intra-abdominal disturbance, and less likely to indicate an underlying systemic mechanism. Pathophysiology includes abnormal lymphatic drainage, obstruction of venous return, cardiac failure, decreased plasma oncotic pressure, hepatic insufficiency, congenital nephrosis, increased capillary permeability, urinary tract obstruction, and meconium peritonitis.[49]

Etiology: Potential etiologies of isolated fetal ascites are many, and include intestinal and genitourinary, cardiac disorders, chromosomal and genetic abnormalities, infection, LMs, liver disease, and pulmonary abnormalities.[49] Up to 15% of cases are classified as idiopathic.[50] Many cases of isolated ascites resolve spontaneously.[48,49]

Intestinal abnormalities are a common source of isolated fetal ascites, accounting for greater than 30% of cases.[50] Not uncommonly, meconium peritonitis accounts for unexplained fetal ascites, particularly in the presence of ileal or jejunal atresia. The prenatal imaging manifestations are variable and range from no detectable abnormalities to dilated bowel loops and meconium pseudocyst.[51] Additional intestinal abnormalities with isolated ascites include malrotation, intussusception, and bands.[51]

Genitourinary tract abnormalities are frequently cited as a common cause of isolated ascites, representing greater than 20% of cases, with the most frequent culprit being posterior urethral valves.[49,50] Urinary ascites may result from rupture of the bladder, pelvocalyceal system, ureters, or a perinephric urinoma. Less common genitourinary sources of ascites include cloacal anomalies, ruptured ovarian cysts, polycystic kidneys, and nephrotic syndrome.[49]

Ascites may also result from *cardiac abnormalities*, either structural or arrhythmias, noted in up to 15% of cases.[50]

Approximately 15% of isolated ascites are related to *chromosomal disorders* and 6% to 7% of cases to a *genetic disorder*, which includes *inborn errors of metabolism, especially lysosomal diseases*.[48,50]

An *infectious origin* should be considered a potential cause for isolated fetal ascites. Well-known agents include parvovirus B19, CMV, toxoplasmosis, hepatitis A, and *Escherichia coli*.[49] Varicella and congenital syphilis have also been implicated.

Isolated primary fetal chylous ascites may result from congenital lymphatic dysplasia, lymphatic vessel obstruction, or lymphatic duct leakage. Cases of isolated chyloperitoneum are commonly idiopathic in origin.[49]

The classic imaging presentation of *congenital high airway obstruction* sequence includes ascites, in addition to massively hyperexpanded lungs, laryngeal obstruction, and dilated central airways. Presumably, the ascites results from profound mass effect on the heart and inferior vena cava by the tense, fluid-filled lungs, causing obstruction of venous return.[37] CHAOS is typically complicated by development of NIHF.

Diagnosis A complete anatomical survey and search for a diagnosis is warranted in these cases, to allow for optimal counseling and therapeutic guidance. A detailed US and Doppler, fetal echocardiogram, and maternal blood testing for blood rhesus factor and type as well as antibody viral, parasitic, and bacterial titers. Fetal blood may be obtained for blood type, complete blood count, titers, and DNA analysis for chromosomal anomalies and/or cystic fibrosis.[48,50] A cause or associated anomaly can typically be identified in 80% to 90% of cases.[47,50]

Imaging: On US, fetal ascites appears as fluid around the liver or spleen, among bowel loops, or outlining the umbilical vein or falciform ligament. The smallest volume of ascites is most easily identified around the liver (Fig. 28.2-19). Specific features that deserve particular attention include location of the fluid, the presence of calcifications, the echogenicity and the sonographic appearance of the fetal bowel, kidneys, and the liver. Calcifications intraperitoneally suggest meconium peritonitis, whereas hepatic calcifications may be seen in infection or aneuploidy (Fig. 28.2-20A). Massive fluid collections that displace bowel loops posteriorly or laterally may represent meconium pseudocyst formation (Fig. 28.2-20B, C). Echogenic or cystic dysplastic kidneys suggest an underlying urinary tract obstruction. Large perinephric urinomas should not be mistaken for ascites (Fig. 28.2-21). Fetal MRI may be helpful in evaluation of anatomic abnormalities or in the absence of identified cause via US.

Differential Diagnosis: The thin hypoechoic rim of abdominal wall musculature seen on transverse views of the abdomen should not be mistaken for small free fluid. This has been described as pseudoascites. Sagittal or coronal views of the abdomen should help clarify this observation.

Prognosis: Fetuses with isolated ascites that do not go on to develop NIHF have a better prognosis, with overall survival in

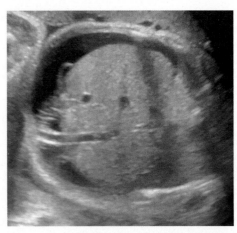

FIGURE 28.2-19: Unexplained progressive isolated ascites in a 34-week fetus being followed up for a low-risk lung lesion; note the outlines of the umbilical vein. The fetus was delivered early, and the ascites resolved spontaneously.

90% of cases.[47,49,50,52] Unfavorable outcome is noted when isolated ascites is severe or progressive and/ or presents before 24 weeks' gestation, increasing the risk of perinatal death.[47,50,53] Fetuses with abnormal karyotype or positive infection screen have a worse prognosis.[48] Greater than 85% of fetuses with ascites after 30 weeks can regress without surgical intervention, often due to complications of gastrointestinal disease such as meconium peritonitis; whereas those before 30 weeks typically require surgical intervention, many as a result of lymphatic abnormalities.[50,53] Spontaneous resolution, possible in 30% of cases, is also associated with better outcome.[50]

Management: Newly identified fetal ascites deserves repeat US evaluation in 1 to 2 weeks, to evaluate for ascites stability or progression and a biophysical profile to document fetal well-being.[48] Biochemical testing of the ascites fluid may be considered as it may improve detection of etiology.[54] Clues on biochemical analysis include low protein in cases of urinary or genitourinary abnormality, high digestive enzymes with

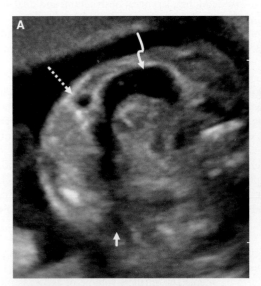

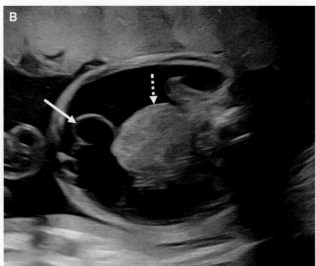

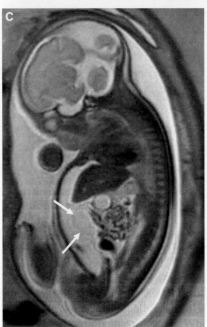

FIGURE 28.2-20: A: Fetus at 23 weeks with small ascites (*solid arrow*), peritoneal calcification (*dotted arrow*), and dilated bowel loop (*curved arrow*). Postnatal meconium peritonitis due to ileal atresia was confirmed. **B:** Fetus at 28 weeks with large intra-abdominal ascites with bowel centralized (*dotted arrow*). There is an encapsulated collection within the fluid consistent with meconium pseudocyst (*solid arrow*). **C:** Same fetus as in B. Sagittal T2 MRI, again demonstrates large ascites and encapsulated pseudocyst. (*solid arrows*).

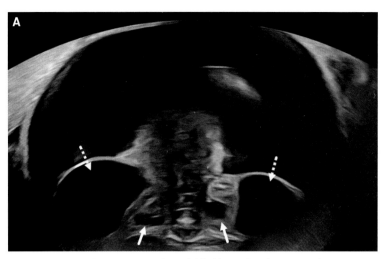
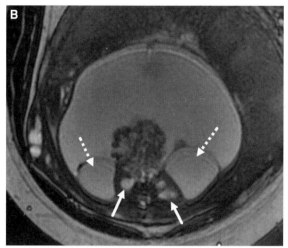

FIGURE 28.2-21: Fetus at 23 weeks with bladder outlet obstruction due to posterior urethral valves. **A:** Axial US demonstrates dilated renal collecting systems (*solid arrows*) and bilateral urinomas (*dotted arrows*) in association with severe ascites. **B:** Axial T2 MRI of the same fetus also showing bilateral urinomas (*dotted arrows*) and dilated collecting systems (*solid arrows*).

intestinal origin, high B_2-microglobulin with infectious or urinary disorder in the presence of renal failure, greater than 80% lymphocytes due to lymphatic pathology, and presence of vacuolated cells with metabolic storage diseases.[54] Intrauterine paracentesis or abdominoamniotic shunting should be considered when increasing ascites compromises normal fetal development.[50] With increasing ascites or deterioration of the biophysical profile score, depending on gestational age, early delivery may be warranted. Postnatally, approximately 50% of cases require surgery for gastrointestinal, urinary, or other malformation.[50] Greater than 60% have no long-term consequence from the initial pathology.[50]

Recurrence: There is no recurrence risk, except when the cause is a genetic syndrome with inheritable transmission.

REFERENCES

1. Potter EL. Universal edema of fetus unassociated with erythroblastosis. *Am J Obstet Gynecol.* 1943;46:130–134.
2. Bellini C, Hennekam RC. Non-immune hydrops fetalis: a short review of etiology and pathophysiology. *Am J Med Genet A.* 2012;158A(3):597–605.
3. Randenberg AL. Nonimmune hydrops fetalis, part I: etiology and pathophysiology. *Neonatal Netw.* 2010;29(5):281–295.
4. Carlson DE, Platt LD, Medearis AL, et al. Prognostic indicators of the resolution of nonimmune hydrops fetalis and survival of the fetus. *Am J Obstet Gynecol.* 1990;163(6 pt 1):1785–1787.
5. Norton ME, Chauhan SP, Dashe JS. Society for maternal-fetal medicine clinical guideline #7: nonimmune hydrops fetalis. *Am J Obstet Gynecol.* 2015;212(2):127–139.
6. Bellini C, Hennekam RC. Etiology of nonimmune hydrops fetalis: a systematic review. *Am J Med Genet A.* 2009;149A:844–851.
7. Laterrre M, Bernard P, Vikkula M, et al. Improved diagnosis of nonimmune hydrops fetalis using standardized algorithm. *Prenat Diagn.* 2018;38:337–343.
8. Bellini C, Donarini G, Paladini D, et al. Etiology of non-immune hydrops fetalis: an update. *Am J Med Genet.* 2015;152A(5);1189–1196.
9. Steurer MA, Peyvandi S, Baer RJ, et al. Epidemiology of live born infants with nonimmune hydrops fetalis- insights from a population based dataset. *J Pediatr.* 2017;187:182–188.
10. Gilgy DM, Mee JB, Farouk Kamlin CO, et al. Outcomes following antenatal identification of hydrops fetalis: a single-centre experience from 2001-2012. *Arch Dis Child fetal Neonatal Ed.* 2018. http://dx.doi.org/10.1136/archdischild-2017-313604
11. Turgal M, Ozyuncu O, Boyraz G, et al. Non-immune hydrops fetalis as a diagnostic and survival problems: what do we tell the parents? *J Perinat Med.* 2015;43(3):353–358.
12. Santo S, Mansour S, Thilaganathan B, et al. Prenatal diagnosis of non-immune hydrops fetalis: what do we tell the parents? *Prenat Diagn.* 2011;31:186–195.
13. Abrams ME, Meredith KS, Kinnard P, et al. Hydrops fetalis: a retrospective review of cases reported to a large national database and identification of risk factors associated with death. *Pediatrics.* 2007;120(1):84–89.
14. Derderian SC, Jeant C, Fleck SR, et al. The many faces of hydrops. *J Pediatr Surg.* 2015;50(1):50–54.
15. Burwick RM, Pilliod RA, Dukhovny SE, et al. Fetal hydrops and the risk of severe preeclampsia. *J Matern Fetal Neonatal Med.* 2019;32(6):961–965.
16. Desilets V, De Bie I, Audiber F. No. 363-Investigation and management of non-immune fetal hydrops. *J Obstet Gynaecol Can.* 2018;40(8):1077–1090.
17. Randenberg AL. Nonimmune hydrops fetalis, part II: does etiology influence mortality? *Neonatal Netw.* 2010;29(6):367–380.
18. Yuan, SM. Cardiac etiologies of hydrops fetalis. *Z Geburtshilfe Neonatol.* 2017;221:67–72.
19. Giorgio E, De Oronzo MA, Iozza I, et al. Parvovirus B19 during pregnancy: a review. *J Prenat Med.* 2010;4(4):63–66.
20. Lamont R, Sobel J, Vaisbuch E, et al. Parvovirus B19 in human pregnancy. *BJOG.* 2011;118:175–186.
21. Izmirly PM, Saxena A, Kim MY, et al. Maternal and fetal factors associated with mortality and morbidity in a multi-racial/ethnic registry of anti-SSA/RO-associated cardiac neonatal lupus. *Circulation.* 2011;124(18):1927–1935.
22. Pruksanusak N, Suntharasaj T, Suwanrath C, et al. Fetal cardiac rhabdomyoma with hydrops fetalis: report of 2 cases and literature review. *J Ultrasound Med.* 2012;31(11):1821–1824.
23. Yuan SM. Congenital pulmonary lymphangiectasia. *J Perinat Med.* 2017;45(9):1023–1030.
24. Attar MA, Donn SM. Congenital chylothorax. *Semin Fetal Neonatal Med.* 2017;22:234–239.
25. Chon AH, Chmait HR, Korst LM, et al. Long-term outcomes after thoracoamniotic shunt for pleural effusion with secondary hydrops. *J Surg Res.* 2019;233:304–309.
26. Xiong YQ, Tan J, Liu YM, et al. The risk of maternal parvovirus B19 infection during pregnancy on fetal and fetal hydrops: a systemic review and meta-analysis. *J Clin Virol.* 2019;114:12–20.
27. Bascietto F, Liberati M, Margano D, et al. Outcome of fetuses with congenital parvovirus B19 infection: systemic review and meta-analysis. *Ultrasound Obstet Gynecol.* 2018;52:569–576.
28. Taweevisit M, Thorner PS. The contribution of extramedullary hematopoiesis to hepatomegaly in anemic hydrops fetalis: a study in alpha-thalassemia hydrops fetalis. *Pediatr Dev Pathol.* 2012;15(3):206–212.
29. Kim GJ, Lee ES. Prenatal diagnosis of transient abnormal myelopoiesis in a Down syndrome fetus. *Korean J Radiol.* 2009;10(2):190–193.
30. Baschat AA, Wagner T, Malisius R, et al. Prenatal diagnosis of a transient myeloproliferative disorder in trisomy 21. *Prenat Diagn.* 1998;18:731–736.
31. Sparks TN, Thao K, Lianoglou R, et al. Nonimmune hydrops fetalis: identifying the underlying genetic etiology. *Genet Med.* 2019;21(6):1339–1344.
32. Van Maldergem L, Jauniaux E, Fourneau C, et al. Genetic causes of hydrops fetalis. *Pediatrics.* 1992;89(1):81–86.
33. Jauniaux E, Van Maldergem L, De Munter C, et al. Nonimmune hydrops fetalis associated with genetic abnormalities. *Obstet Gynecol.* 1990;75(3 pt 2):568–572.

34. Staretz-Chacham O, Lang TC, LaMarca ME, et al. Lysosomal storage disorders in the newborn. *Pediatrics.* 2009;123(4):1191–1207.

35. Sudrie-Arnaud B, Marguet F, Patrier S, et al. Metabolic causes of nonimmune hydrops fetalis: a next generation sequencing panel as a first line investigation. *Clin Chim Acta.* 2018;481:1–8.

36. Crombleholme TM, Coleman B, Hedrick H, et al. Cystic adenomatoid malformation volume ratio predicts outcome in prenatally diagnosed cystic adenomatoid malformation of the lung. *J Pediatr Surg.* 2002;37(3):331–338.

37. Guimaraes CVA, Linam LE, Kline-Fath BM, et al. Prenatal MRI findings of fetuses with congenital high airway obstruction sequence. *Korean J Radiol.* 2009;10(2):129–134.

38. Woodward PJ, Sohaey R, Kennedy A, et al. A comprehensive review of fetal tumors with pathologic correlation. *Radiographics.* 2005;25:215–242.

39. Cass DL, Olutoye OO, Ayres NA, et al. Defining hydrops and indications for open fetal surgery for fetuses with lung masses and vascular tumors. *J Pediatr Surg.* 2012;47:40–45.

40. Coleman A, Kline-Fath BM, Keswani S, et al. Prenatal solid tumor volume index: novel prenatal predictor of adverse outcome in sacrococcygeal teratoma. *J Surg Res.* 2013;184(1):330–336.

41. Bianchi D, Crombleholme T, D'Alton M, et al. *Fetology: Diagnosis and Management of the Fetal Patient.* 2nd ed. New York, NY: McGraw Hill; 2010.

42. Kline-Fath BM, Calvo-Garcia MA, O'Hara SM, et al. Twin-twin transfusion syndrome: cerebral ischemia is not the only fetal MR imaging finding. *Pediatr Radiol.* 2007;37:47–56.

43. Guimaraes CV, Kline-Fath BM, Linam LE, et al. MRI findings in multifetal pregnancies complicated by twin reversed arterial perfusion sequence (TRAP). *Pediatr Radiol.* 2011;41(6):694–701.

44. Moore TR, Gale S, Benirschke K. Perinatal outcome of 49 pregnancies complicated by acardiac twinning. *Am J Obstet Gynecol.* 1990;163:907–912.

45. D'Ercole C, Cravello L, Boubli L, et al. Large chorioangioma associated with hydrops fetalis: prenatal diagnosis and management. *Fetal Diagn Ther.* 1996;11(5):357–360.

46. Santamaria M, Benirschke K, Carpenter PM, et al. Transplacental hemorrhage associated with placental neoplasms. *Pediatr Pathol.* 1987;7(5–6):601–615.

47. Baccega F, Brizot ML, Krebs VLJ, et al. Nonimmune fetal ascites: identification of ultrasound findings predictive of perinatal death. *J Perinat Med.* 2016;44(2):195–200.

48. El Bishry G. The outcome of isolated fetal ascites. *Eur J Obstet Gynecol Reprod Biol.* 2008;137(1):43–46.

49. Favre R, Dreux S, Dommergues M, et al. Nonimmune fetal ascites: a series of 79 cases. *Am J Obstet Gynecol.* 2004;190(2):407–412.

50. Catania VD, Muru A, Pellegrino M, et al. Isolated fetal ascites, neonatal outcome in 51 cases observed in a tertiary referral center. *Eur J Pediatr Surg.* 2017;27:102–108.

51. Jo YS, Jang DG, Nam SY, et al. Antenatal sonographic features of ileal atresia. *J Obstet Gynaecol Res.* 2012;38(1):215–219.

52. Winn HN, Stiller R, Grannum PAT, et al. Isolated fetal ascites: prenatal diagnosis and management. *Am J Perinatol.* 1990;7(4);370-373.

53. Nose S, Usui N, Soh H, et al. The prognostic factors and the outcome of primary isolated fetal ascites. *Pediatr Surg Int.* 2011;27(8):799–804.

54. Dreux S, Saloman LJ, Rosenblatt J, et al. Biochemical analysis of ascites fluid as an aid to etiological diagnosis: a series of 100 cases of nonimmune fetal ascites. *Prenat Diagn.* 2015;35:214–220.

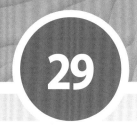

29 Skeletal Dysplasia

Teresa Victoria • Dorothy I. Bulas • Juan S. Martin-Saavedra

Skeletal dysplasias (SDs) are a heterogeneous group of disorders resulting from a generalized abnormality of the skeleton. Individually rare, collectively they occur in approximately 1/5,000 live births.[1] Clinically, these disorders may manifest as short stature, with malformation and deformation of the skeleton. Severity ranges among individuals, from minor handicaps to death in the perinatal period.

Historically, individuals with disproportionate stature were classified as belonging to short-limb or short-trunked groups. In the 1970s, the classification became more clinical and descriptive. As the complexity of information increased, a group of experts convened to discuss an approach to classify the dysplasias with a more inclusive clinical, radiographic, and molecular description of entities. Their work, which has been revised on several occasions, is presented under the umbrella name of the Nosology and Classification of Genetic Skeletal Disorders. In their 2015 revision, it included 436 conditions placed in 42 groups according to their molecular, biochemical, and/or radiographic criteria, with 364 described genes.[2] A hundred or so dysplasias have prenatal onset, while others may present during the newborn period or beyond 2 or 3 years of age.[3]

Broadly, SDs can be classified as osteochondrodysplasias, osteodystrophies, and dysostosis.[4,5] *Osteochondrodysplasias* refer to a disturbance in growth intrinsic to bone or cartilage as a result of gene expression. These usually affect multiple bones, with progressive abnormalities that may lead to changes in size and shape of limbs, trunk, and/or skull, and frequently resulting in short stature. As a result of varied gene expression through fetal and postnatal life, the phenotype of an osteochondrodysplasia may change throughout life, such that previously unaffected bones may eventually become involved. This is in contraposition with the *dysostosis*, which are malformations of individual bones or group of bones, the result of abnormal blastogenesis during the first 6 weeks of fetal life. In contrast to the osteochondrodysplasias, the phenotype in the dysostosis is static, such that the malformations do not spread to involve previously normal bones. Osteodystrophies are the result of a disturbance in nutrition or metabolism extrinsic to bone. Examples include rickets and mucopolysaccharidosis, which typically will not present in the perinatal period and so are not discussed in this chapter.

SDs are difficult entities to diagnose both pre- and postnatally. The large phenotypic variability among different patients with the same disease, or just within the same patient at different times of life, the overlapping features of some syndromes, and the lack of precise molecular diagnosis in certain entities, presents considerable diagnostic challenges. In this chapter, we review the different imaging modalities utilized prenatally to evaluate and diagnose the fetus with suspected SD and discuss the most commonly encountered dysplasias prenatally. Some of the entities discussed later, including arthrogryposis and craniosynostosis, are not strictly SDs, but are included in this chapter because they are severe osseous abnormalities that may be included in the differential diagnosis of the fetus with marked abnormalities of the skeleton.

EMBRYOLOGY

The fetal skeleton develops relatively early during gestation through two well-programmed events, *endochondral* and *intramembranous* ossification. The more common one, the *endochondral* type, responsible for the appendicular and axial skeleton, requires a cartilage template of mesenchymal cell chondrocytes (the primary cell type of cartilage) which eventually differentiate into osteocytes. These chondrocytes are selectively situated at the growth plate. Ossification of the terminal cartilage along its length and at the ends of the bones is ultimately responsible for a person's final stature. The second and less common form of ossification accounts for the calvarium and portions of the clavicle and pubis, which ossify via membranous ossification whereby mesenchymal cells differentiate directly into osteoblasts.[6]

Limb buds begin to develop during the fourth week of embryonic life as clusters of mesenchymal cells covered by a layer of ectoderm. Mesenchymal models of bone or anlages form during the fifth week of gestation. Development of the upper limb antecedes that of the lower limbs in bud appearance, differentiation, and final size. The limbs develop in a proximodistal sequence, with the humerus and femur forming first, followed by the radius and ulna, tibia and fibula, metacarpals and metatarsals, and, finally, the phalanges. Clavicles and mandibles ossify at 8 weeks of gestation; appendicular skeleton, ileum, and scapula by 12 weeks; metacarpals and metatarsals are ossified by 12 to 16 weeks.[7]

The skeleton is composed of two tissues (bone and cartilage), three cell types (osteoblasts, osteoclasts, and chondrocytes), and more than 200 skeletal elements. This intricate interplay among the different components allows for inborn errors of metabolism to occur along the path, giving rise to the SDs. These genetic "errors" may be inherited as autosomal dominant, autosomal recessive, or X-linked disorders; while other SDs are due to imprinting errors, somatic mosaicism, or teratogen exposure.[8] Within the past few decades, there has been marked progress in the field of molecular genetics, advancing the knowledge and genetic cause of many of these disorders. Yet, in order to fully evaluate the fetus with a suspected SD, highly detailed prenatal imaging is crucial, so that tailored genetic testing can be done. All prenatal dysplasias should ideally have a final diagnosis: Some SDs are prone to recurrence in subsequent pregnancies and some patients may receive the wrong treatment or incorrect preventive therapy if misdiagnosed. In addition, accurate diagnosis improves nondirected counseling and enhances determination of appropriate delivery method and perinatal care.

PRENATAL IMAGING OF SKELETAL DYSPLASIA

Ultrasound

Ultrasound (US) is the primary imaging modality in the evaluation of the affected fetus. By US, the fetal skeleton is readily visualized by 14 weeks of gestation. Suspicion of a possible fetal SD is usually first suggested when the measurement of the long bones is more than 3 standard deviations from the mean for gestational age (GA), or when focal abnormalities, such as bone bowing or fractures, are detected. The presence of an increased nuchal translucency may be the first sign of a dysplasia in the first trimester (Fig. 29.1). When evaluating a fetus for SD, a systematic and meticulous evaluation of the fetal skeleton must be undertaken, including length of the long bones (femurs, humerus, radius, ulna, tibia, fibula, and clavicle), shape of long bones (straight, curved, bilateral, or unilateral), appearance of the metaphyseal ends (spikes, irregularities), echodensity of long bones, foot size and shape, hands (number of digits, shape of phalanges), circumferences (head, abdomen, chest), size and contour of ribs (beaded if fractures), mineralization and shape of the cranium, mineralization and shape of the vertebral bodies, size and shape of scapula, presence of the secondary epiphyses (**calcaneus at 20 weeks, knee epiphyses at 28 weeks**), mandibular size and shape, fetal profile (frontal bossing, presence of nasal bone, micrognathia), abnormal posturing of the extremities (equinovarus), other congenital anomalies, evaluation of amniotic fluid volume, and presence of hydrops.[8] Detailed evaluation of additional abnormalities may provide clues to reach a more specific diagnosis. A proposed systematic approach of the fetal skeleton is discussed here.

1. *Skull.* Examination of the acoustic shadow behind the calvarium and the echogenicity of the bone itself allows evaluation for possible demineralization. Compression of the skull is suggestive of demineralization present in severe forms of osteogenesis imperfecta (OI) or hypophosphatasia. Frontal bossing, craniosynostosis, cleft palate, micrognathia, or hypertelorism are features that may help suggest a specific SD.
2. *Clavicle, scapula.* A hypoplastic scapula may be seen in campomelic dysplasia or cleidocranial dysplasia; total or partial aplasia of the clavicles may occur in cleidocranial dysplasia.
3. *Spine.* The presence of segmentation anomalies, platyspondyly, abnormal curvature of the spine, and possible nonossification of the spine must be carefully evaluated. Platyspondyly can be seen in lethal OI and thanatophoric dysplasia (TD), nonossification noted in achondrogenesis, and segmentation anomalies in VACTERL (*v*ertebral anomalies, *a*nal atresia, *c*ardiac anomalies, *t*racheoesophageal fistula, *r*enal anomalies, and *l*imb anomalies) sequence.

4. *Thorax.* Detailed examination of the thorax is crucial. Chest restriction leads to pulmonary hypoplasia, a frequent cause of death in the neonate with a lethal SD. While a chest circumference measured at the level of the four-chamber heart of less than the fifth percentile for GA can suggest pulmonary hypoplasia, additional measurements are useful for further documentation. Other parameters indicative of pulmonary hypoplasia and/or lethality include the following:
   - **Chest-circumference–abdominal circumference ratio** less than the fifth percentile
   - **Chest-trunk length ratio** less than 0.32
   - **Femur length–abdominal circumference ratio** less than 0.16.[9] Evaluation of the thorax should include a full analysis of the ribs, including number, shape, presence of fractures (beaded appearance), and overall configuration.
5. *Long bones.* Evaluation of the long bones includes analysis of the degree of mineralization, presence of fractures or abnormal curvature of the long bones, as well as absence, hypoplasia, and malformation of the bone. Comparison among segments for shortening establishes if the entity is a rhizomelic, mesomelic, or acromelic dysplasia, or if it involves all the segments of the extremities (micromelia) (Fig. 29.2). Femur length/abdominal circumference ratio of less than 0.16 suggests a lethal SD.
6. *Pelvis.* Abnormalities in the shape of the pelvis can provide clues to the diagnosis of the SD at hand. A flared iliac wing may be found in entities such as mucopolysaccharidosis or Kniest dysplasia, a small pelvis may be seen in achondrogenesis or campomelic dysplasia, delayed ossification of the pubic bones may occur in ischiopatellar dysplasia.
7. *Hands and feet.* Polydactyly (more than five digits per hand), is classified as pre- or postaxial when the extra digits are located on the radial or ulnar side of the hand respectively (Fig. 29.3). Other abnormalities, such as syndactyly (soft-tissue or bone fusion of adjacent digits), clinodactyly (deviation of the finger), postural deformities ("hitchhiker's thumb," "sandal toe deformity," clenched hands) or abnormal extremities (broad tubular phalanges) must be evaluated (Fig. 29.4). A femur/foot length ratio should approach 1 throughout pregnancy.

One the most important determinations when evaluating the fetus with presumed dysplasia by US is the assessment and prediction of postnatal lethality. Lethality is mainly determined by the risk of pulmonary hypoplasia, whereby the small lungs are unable to maintain adequate oxygen exchange postnatally. Sonographic indicators of pulmonary hypoplasia were discussed previously.[10,11]

Yet, despite being the main imaging modality in the prenatal evaluation of the fetus, US has limited sensitivity in diagnosing SD prenatally. The peak of diagnosis of a SD by US is between 15 and 29 weeks' GA. Some nonlethal forms, however, do not

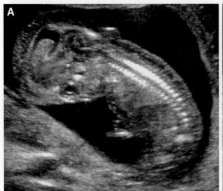
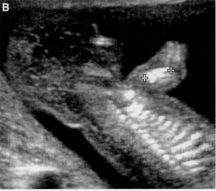

FIGURE 29.1: Cystic hygroma. Osteogenesis imperfecta type II at 14 weeks' gestation. **A:** Sagittal US demonstrates subcutaneous edema along the cranium and spine. **B:** Coronal view demonstrates markedly short-bowed humerus *(cursers)* and irregular beaded appearance of the ribs consistent with fractures.

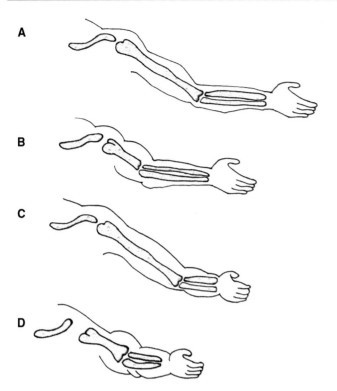

FIGURE 29.2: Nomenclature for long bone shortening. The schematic of a normal upper extremity, demonstrating relatively normal length of the proximal and mid segments of the arm, is depicted in **(A)**. **B:** shows shortening of the proximal segment, named *rhizomelia*. **C:** shows shortening of the mid segments (in this case, radius and ulna) or *mesomelia*. **D:** shows *micromelia*, where the overall extremity length is small. Not depicted is *acromelia*, where the distal segments are short in length.

become apparent until the third trimester. The diagnostic accuracy by US ranges from 35% to 68%,[12,13] opening the door to other imaging modalities.

Magnetic Resonance Imaging

The use of magnetic resonance imaging (MRI) in the assessment of the fetal skeleton has advanced as technology improves.[14,15] The development of fast echoplanar imaging (EPI) has been valuable in the evaluation of fetal cartilage and bone (Figs. 29.5 and 29.6). Nemec et al.[14] published the MRI findings of the knee joint through gestation, remarking that the unossified epiphysis displays a round contour in mid gestation, whereas in late gestation, the spherical form becomes hemispherical and interrupted by a central notch. They also showed the metaphyseal progression through gestation of the knee, flat in mid gestation and undulated toward term, while the perichondrium progressed from fairly visible to barely notable at similar GAs. Robinson et al. created a fetal black bone sequence that contrasts the fetal bones optimally against the soft-tissue background,[15] while Nogueira et al. created a 3D-modified volumetric interpolated brain examination (VIBE) sequence that constructs a complete 3D model of the fetal skeleton.[16]

Fetal MRI is particularly useful in the assessment of certain anomalies associated with SD and can help lead to a more specific diagnosis. Temporal and occipital lobe dysplasia present in some cases of thanatophoric dysplasia (TD) and achondroplasia is best demonstrated by MRI.[17–19] The evolution of craniosynostosis (Apert),[20] narrow foramen magnum (achondroplasia) and assessment of midface hypoplasia (Binder-type chondrodysplasia punctata [CDP]) may be best demonstrated by multiplanar imaging by MRI.[21] MRI can provide a second chance to evaluate hands and feet (polydactyly, vertical talus).[22]

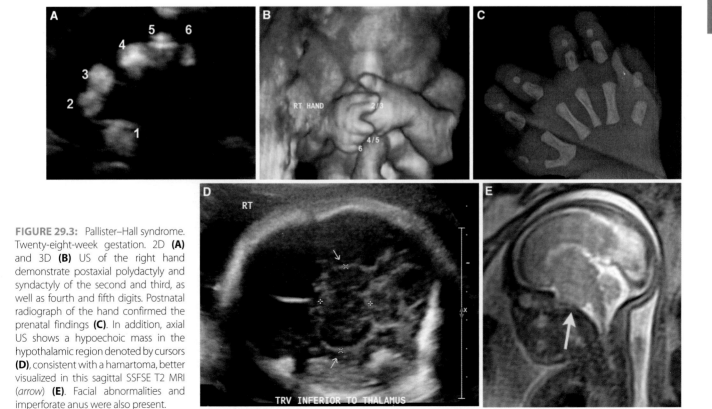

FIGURE 29.3: Pallister–Hall syndrome. Twenty-eight-week gestation. 2D **(A)** and 3D **(B)** US of the right hand demonstrate postaxial polydactyly and syndactyly of the second and third, as well as fourth and fifth digits. Postnatal radiograph of the hand confirmed the prenatal findings **(C)**. In addition, axial US shows a hypoechoic mass in the hypothalamic region denoted by cursors **(D)**, consistent with a hamartoma, better visualized in this sagittal SSFSE T2 MRI (*arrow*) **(E)**. Facial abnormalities and imperforate anus were also present.

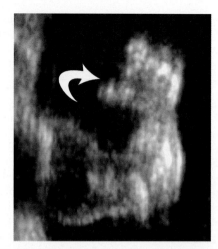

FIGURE 29.4: Diastrophic dysplasia. An 18-week fetus with short limbs. US of the hand demonstrates a classic "hitchhiker thumb" *(arrow)* with thumb abducted, helping confirm the diagnosis.

When oligohydramnios is present limiting US evaluation, MRI may be able to better define specific anomalies.

The prediction of pulmonary hypoplasia remains difficult in equivocal cases of SD. The ability to measure total lung volumes can help guide delivery management and counseling.[23,24] In a series by Weaver et al., lethality was significantly associated with a total lung volume O/E below 47.9%.[24]

Computed Tomography

In the past decades, a number of papers have been published on the use of low-dose fetal computed tomography (CT) in the evaluation of the fetal skeleton.[25–27] The main advantage of this fetal imaging modality is exquisite depiction of the fetal bones and 3D rendering of the fetal skeleton. The reconstructed skeleton can be rotated in space at the postprocessing console with partial sectioning as needed. One series noted CT can outperform US in the evaluation of SDs, in the third trimester.[28] Additional advantages include retrospective analysis of the skeleton

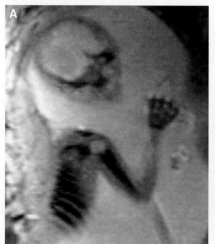
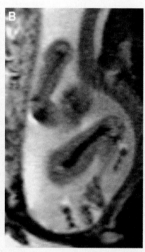
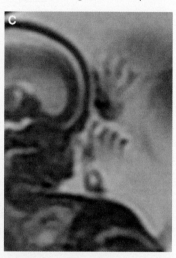

FIGURE 29.5: MRI of the fetal skeleton. Echoplanar image of a 22-week fetus demonstrates low-signal skeleton and high-signal cartilage of the humerus, ribs, and hand **(A)** and humerus, femur, and portion of the tibia **(B)**. **C:** SSFSE T2 MRI of a 17-week fetus demonstrates hands and fingers.

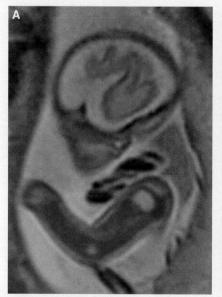
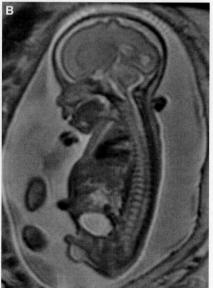

FIGURE 29.6: Kneist dysplasia. SSFSE T2 MRI demonstrates unusually prominent high-signal epiphysis **(A)** and bright discs **(B)** in this fetus with moderate micromelia and platyspondyly. This nonlethal dysplasia is caused by mutations in *COL2A1* with resultant joint contractures, scoliosis, and premature arthropathy.

if further genetic details are available about that or a subsequent pregnancy, and more intuitive visualization and understanding of the anatomical abnormalities for the parents and clinicians alike. However, given the obvious radiation dose to the fetus, this type of study is relegated exclusively to the fetus in the second and third trimester with *severe* osseous abnormalities, when the diagnosis is still in question after a detailed US and/or MRI.

When the decision is made to undergo a low-dose fetal CT, the patient is placed supine on the CT table. The top and bottom of the uterus are marked by US, providing the strict borders for CT scanning. The study is done without contrast and at such low radiation dose that only the fetal bones (and not the solid organs) are visualized. Images are reviewed in the 3D console, following sectioning of the maternal structures, rendering exquisite detail of the fetal skeleton (Fig. 29.7). By CT, the skull, clavicles, scapula, ribs, vertebral bodies, and long bones should be visualized in a normal fetus in the second and third trimester and their absence implies pathology. Because of the low radiation used, the fetal hands and feet may not be seen, particularly in the second trimester.

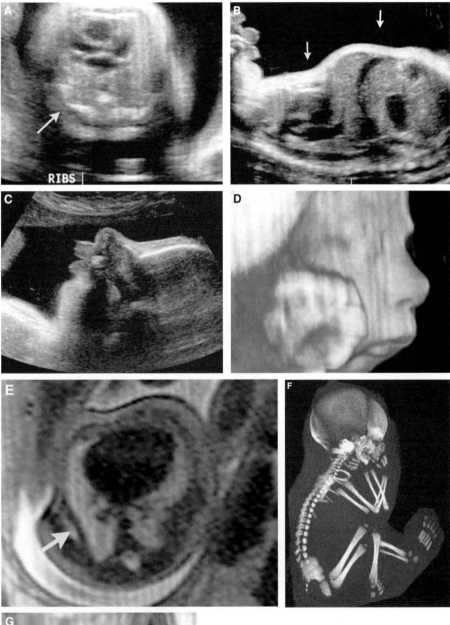

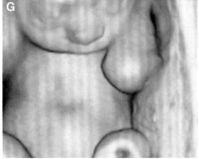

FIGURE 29.7: Cerebrocostomandibular syndrome. Thirty-four-week fetus with abnormally short ribs *(arrow)* **(A)**, protuberant abdomen *(white arrow)* and small thorax *(yellow arrow)* **(B)**. 2D **(C)** and 3D US **(D)** showed pronounced micrognathia. Single-shot fast spin-echo T2 MRI confirms short ribs *(arrow)* **(E)**. Low-dose fetal computed tomography demonstrates numerous rib defects and gaps **(F)**. The existing ribs were markedly hypoplastic. 3D US reconstruction of the chest in the coronal plane depicts a pectus excavatum deformity **(G)**.

When performing a fetal CT, the goal is to use the lowest radiation dose possible while still having a diagnostically adequate study. A study by McCollough et al. postulates that the absolute risk of fetal effects (including cancer induction) is small at a conceptus dose of 100 mSv, and negligible at a dose of less than 50 mSv.[29] Assuming a 0.07% incidence of childhood cancer and a natural incidence of malformation risk in the order of 4% in the normal population, the risk to the conceptus given a fetal dose of about 50 mSv results in a 96% probability of birthing a child with no malformation, or a 99.9% chance that the child will not develop cancer, or a 95.9% chance that the child will have no malformation nor cancer.[25–30]

The radiation dose with newer protocols can be decreased by as much as 70%, with the radiation dose now reported as low as 1.5 mSv while still giving excellent depiction of the fetal skeleton (Figs. 29.7 to 29.10). The key changes to the protocol are discussed in a recent review article[31] and summed as follows: keeping a relatively high kVp (usually 100) with modulated, relatively low mAs. A key factor in decreasing radiation dose in fetal CT is in the shape of iterative reconstruction (IR), an image post-processing method that does not decrease the radiation dose per se but does allow protocols to be changed such that lower doses can be used while maintaining diagnostic accuracy. These IR

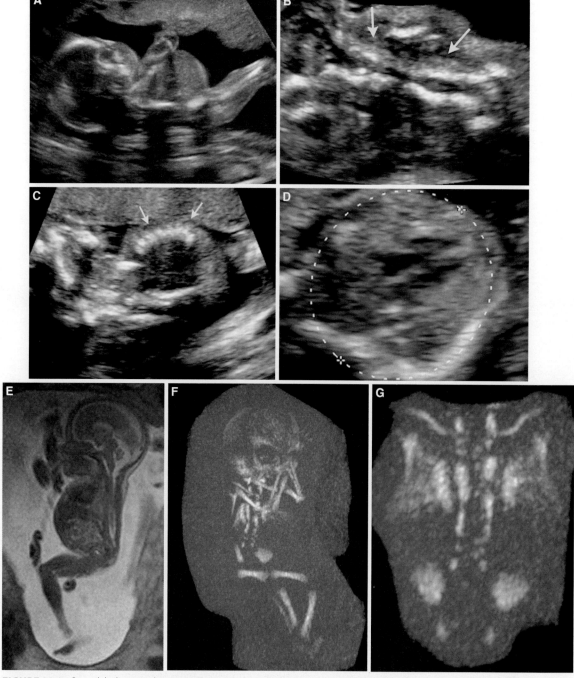

FIGURE 29.8: Spondylothoracic dysostosis. Twenty-one-week fetus with an overall short trunk and small chest/abdomen, as seen in the sagittal plane US **(A)**. The vertebral bodies are disorganized (*arrows* in **B**). The ribs (*arrows*) appeared close together **(C)**. On axial US, the ribs were short **(D)**. **(E)** Sagittal SSFSE T2 MRI confirmed short spine and provided detail about the internal organs. Low-dose fetal computed tomography showed an overall short spine with normal-size long bones and head **(F)**. The ribs were fused posteriorly and appeared to separate anteriorly, resembling a crablike configuration. Magnified view **(G)** demonstrates multiple segmentation anomalies.

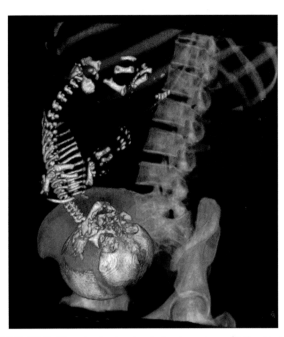

FIGURE 29.9: Thanatophoric dysplasia. Low-dose fetal computed tomography 3D rendering of a 34-week fetus with thanatophoric dysplasia (image courtesy of Monica Epelman, MD).

algorithms are vendor specific and work by decreasing the overall image noise, thus allowing use of protocols that utilize lower radiation doses while maintaining diagnostic accuracy. In essence, IR algorithms work by creating CT correction loops which continuously compare the ideal image with the reconstructed image until a final desired image is attained, thus reaching an image with decreased noise in protocols performed with a lower radiation dose. This manner of postprocessing CT reconstruction is particularly desired for fetal CT with the aim of minimizing radiation dose while still obtaining a diagnostic image.

The radiation risk to the fetus from a low-dose fetal CT is small, but real. A great deal of care must be placed in proceeding with this type of study, and taken by consensus with the family and geneticists only if the information will truly change management.

COMMONLY ENCOUNTERED PRENATAL SKELETAL DYSPLASIAS

Achondrogenesis

Description: The term "achondrogenesis" (Greek for "not producing cartilage") was coined by Marco Fraccaro, an Italian pathologist who observed a stillborn female with severe micromelia and marked histological changes of the cartilage.[32]

This is a lethal entity characterized by a relatively large head, short neck, extreme micromelia, and a defect in vertebral ossification.

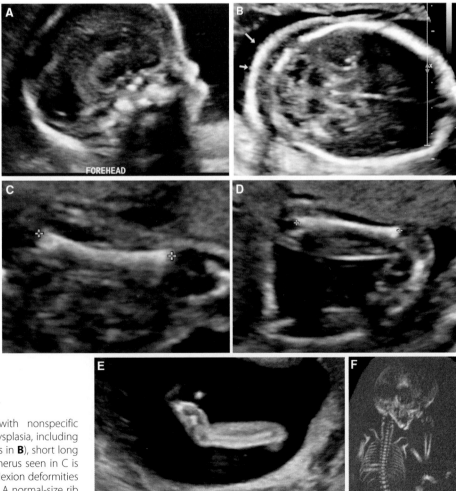

FIGURE 29.10: Twenty-two-week fetus with nonspecific findings suggestive of a nonlethal skeletal dysplasia, including frontal bossing **(A)**, nuchal thickening (arrows in **B**), short long bones without bowing or fractures (the humerus seen in C is 4 weeks behind expected gestational age), Flexion deformities at the ankle **(D)** and wrist **(E)** were present. A normal-size rib cage seen in this low-dose fetal computed tomography **(F)** Pallister–Killian syndrome was confirmed with the finding of an isochromosome at 12p.

Incidence and Molecular Pathology: Birth prevalence is about 0.2 in 10,000 live births. It is inherited as autosomal recessive **(type IA and IB)** and autosomal dominant **(type II).** The locus for type IA is not yet known; the gene for type IB is responsible for a sulfate transporter, DTDST, located on chromosome 5q,[32] also responsible for other forms of SDs including diastrophic dysplasia, atelosteogenesis type II, and multiple epiphyseal dysplasia. Type II achondrogenesis belongs to the type II collagenopathies and has a defect in the *COL2A1* gene located in chromosome 12.

Radiological Manifestations: Type I manifests with poorly mineralized skull, absent or minimal ossification of the vertebral bodies, pubis, and sacrum, as well as short and thin ribs (with fractures, in the case of the fetus with type IA), short and deformed iliac wings, and marked shortness and bowing of the tubular bones.

 Type II has variable degrees of shortness of the long bones (from near normal to very short), lack of mineralization of many vertebral bodies, nonossified sacrum and ischium, and small iliac wings with concave inferior and medial margins and shortening of the ribs. Unlike type I, the calvaria demonstrates normal mineralization in type II achondrogenesis.

Diagnosis: Achondrogenesis can be diagnosed as early as the second trimester by US (Fig. 29.11). Limbs are abnormally short with a small chest circumference. Unossified vertebra may be missed if not carefully looked for. At times, hydrops can be present Figure 29.12. Fetal CT can be helpful in demonstrating the unossified spine and short long bones.

Course and Prognosis: Achondrogenesis is lethal. Infants are either stillborn or die in the neonatal period. Polyhydramnios may be present and may accelerate delivery.

Differential Diagnosis: In **achondrogenesis IB,** there are no rib fractures and the vertebral pedicles may be ossified, whereas **type IA** may have rib fractures. In **achondrogenesis type II,** the ribs are not as thin and show no fractures. Differential includes OI and hypophosphatasia, which have absent or delayed ossification of the calvaria that can be compressible.

Achondroplasia

Description: The term "achondroplasia" was used in the past to define all short-limb dysplasias. With recognition of the heterogeneity of these disorders, this term is currently used to describe a specific disease characterized by predominantly rhizomelic shortening, lordotic spine, large head, and depressed nasal bridge.

Incidence and Molecular Pathology: Most common nonlethal SD (approximately 1 in 25,000 births) which may be transmitted as an autosomal dominant pattern or, in 80% to 90% of cases, a spontaneous mutation. It is caused by a gain-of-function mutation in the fibroblast growth receptor 3 gene (*FGFR3*), a transmembrane tyrosine kinase receptor that binds fibroblast growth factors. The gene is located in the short arm of chromosome 4 and codifies a highly conserved protein. The most common mutation, a G greater than A transition at nucleotide 1,138 (Gly380Arg), is

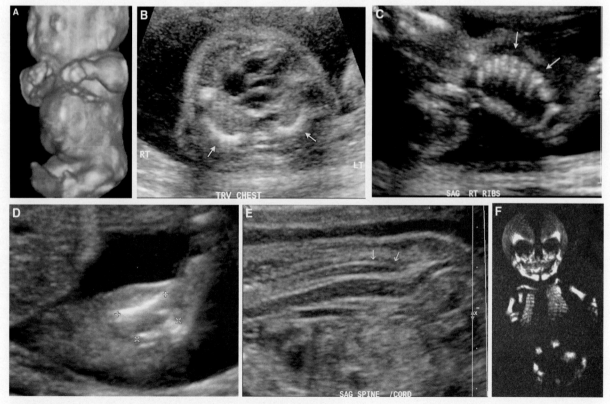

FIGURE 29.11: Achondrogenesis. 3D US rendering of this 21-week fetus demonstrates overall shortening of the upper and lower extremities and a protuberant stomach **(A)**. Axial US at the level of the heart shows short ribs *(arrows)* **(B)**, which appear stacked *(arrows)* **(C)**. The long bones are short **(D)**. The spine is nonossified *(arrows)* **(E)**. Coronal 3D CT shows nonossification of the spine **(F)**. Nonossification of the cervical spine projects as a "floating skull" appearance. The ribs are short, as are the long bones. The iliac bones are small and acetabula are flat.

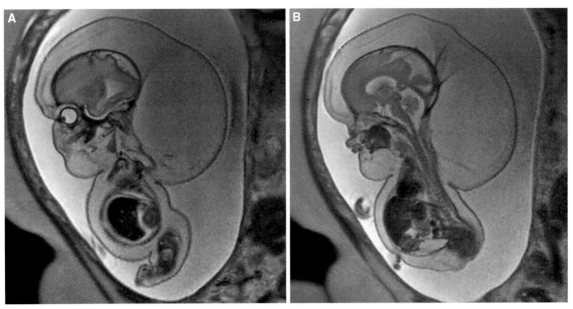

FIGURE 29.12: Achondrogenesis. **A:** SSFSE T2 MRI demonstrates severe hydrops, hygroma, and ascites. The long bones are markedly short and bowed, and the ribs short. **B:** The vertebrae are small and unossified.

observed in 95% of affected patients. The gain-of-function mutation causes ligand-independent activation of *FDFR3*, resulting in inappropriate cartilage growth plate differentiation and deficient endochondral growth and ossification.[33] The homozygous form resembles thanatophoric dysplasia (TD) and is lethal.

Radiological Manifestations: Achondroplasia is a rhizomelic micromelia with mild bowing of the long bones and a disproportionately large head. The nasal bridge is depressed, there is frontal bossing, and decreased size of the skull base and foramen magnum. Short, flat vertebral bodies which may be bullet shaped, progressive narrowing of the interpediculate distance in the lumbar spine, square iliac wings, short narrow sciatic notch, and flat acetabular roofs are findings encountered in achondroplasia. A trident hand with fingers of equal length and separation of the third and fourth fingers may be present, although this can be found in other entities such as TD.

TD, hypochondroplasia, and achondroplasia are all caused by FGFR3 (fibroblast growth factor receptor 3) mutations. Neuropathological findings of temporal lobe dysplasia are most commonly found in TD, although cases of temporal and occipital lobe abnormalities have been described in children with hypochondroplasia and achondroplasia.[19,34]

Diagnosis: Heterozygous achondroplasia is typically not diagnosed in the first and early second trimester. Femoral length crosses below the third percentile only after 18 to 26 weeks' gestation with the affected fetus having relatively normal long bone growth before then. Establishment of a femoral growth curve in the second trimester helps to distinguish between homozygous, heterozygous, and unaffected fetuses. Fetal size charts show femoral length on or below the third percentile by 25 weeks' gestation and always below the third percentile by 30 weeks.[35] The head circumference increases to above the 95th percentile in a majority of cases, with a slight increase in abdominal circumference as well. Additional US findings include frontal bossing, slightly bowed femora, short fingers, small chest, and polyhydramnios (Fig. 29.13).

Homozygous achondroplasia can be diagnosed much earlier due to the presence of severe micromelia. Femoral length will fall below the third percentile by 14 to 16.5 weeks' gestation.[36]

There have been reports of fetal MRI demonstrating temporal and occipital lobe dysplasia in achondroplasia as well as TD. When cortical dysplasia is present, it may be useful in the confirmation of the diagnosis. MRI can also document narrowing of the foramen magnum prenatally (Fig. 29.13C).

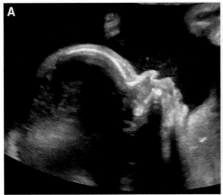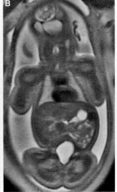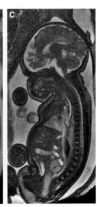

FIGURE 29.13: Achondroplasia. **A:** Sagittal US demonstrates frontal bossing at 32 weeks' gestation. **B:** Coronal SSFSE T2 MRI demonstrates short humeri but normal lung volume. **C:** Sagittal SSFP MRI confirms frontal bossing and documents narrowing of the foramen magnum.

Course and Prognosis: Intelligence and life span are usually normal. Postnatal complications are mainly neurological and are inversely related to the degree of foramen magnum narrowing and spinal cord compression.

Homozygosity for achondroplasia (when both parents are affected) is lethal, with either stillbirth or early neonatal death from respiratory failure.

Differential Diagnosis: Differential diagnosis includes asymmetric intrauterine growth restriction (IUGR) and familial short stature. Assessment for fetal health and family history is important in distinguishing between these entities. Hypochondroplasia is a relatively milder form that varies within and between families and lacks the cranial complications and has no frontal bossing.[37]

Fetuses with the severe form of homozygous achondroplasia present early in the second trimester with severe micromelia. In these cases, other lethal SDs such as thanatophoric should be included in the differential and correlated with family history.[38]

Arthrogryposis

Description: The term "arthrogryposis multiplex congenital" (AMC) is a descriptive term that refers to multiple joint contractures present at birth. This term is often misused as a specific diagnosis instead of a descriptor or clinical finding. Arthrogryposis is not a specific disorder nor a SD, but the consequence of neurological, muscular, connective tissue and skeletal abnormalities, or intrauterine crowding which may lead to limitation of fetal joint mobility and subsequent development of contractures. Potential etiologies include neuropathical abnormalities (brain, spine, or peripheral nerve), abnormalities of muscle structure or function (muscular dystrophies, mitochondrial abnormalities), abnormalities of connective tissue (diastrophic dysplasia), space limitation (multiple gestations, oligohydramnios), maternal diseases (multiple sclerosis, myasthenia gravis), and impaired intrauterine or fetal vascularity.[39] The common outcome is the decrease or lack of fetal movement leading to collagen proliferation, fibrotic replacement of the muscle, and marked thickening of the joint capsules.

Incidence and Molecular Pathology: Approximately 1% of all live births demonstrate some type of contracture involving one or more joints. The overall incidence of arthrogryposis, with multiple joint involvement, is 1 in 3,000 live births.[40] Arthrogryposis may be caused by genetic and environmental factors. Among the genetic factors, more than 35 specific genes have been associated with this condition. Since the evaluation of every single one is beyond the scope of this article, the reader is directed to a comprehensive review of the genetic etiologies.[41]

Diagnosis
Ultrasound: Decreased fetal motion as detected by US during the second or third trimester or by maternal perception may be the first clues in detecting prenatal arthrogryposis. Real-time sonographic evaluation may show contractures with decreased fetal motion or severe flexion/extension deformities, unchanged in appearance during the time of scanning.

MRI: Magnetic resonance (MR) cine sequences may be helpful in evaluating fetal movement as well. Fetal MRI may also be helpful in delineating intracranial pathology that may be directly responsible for decreased fetal movement. Subjective

evaluation of muscle mass can also be provided by US and MRI (Fig. 29.14).

CT: Fetal CT may provide 3D rendering of the fetal bones that may be easier to visually relate to for parents, obstetricians, and orthopedic surgeons (Fig. 29.14E).

Course and Prognosis: The prognosis is related to the specific etiology. In some severe cases, the underlying disease is lethal, with death occurring shortly after birth. In other cases, musculoskeletal impairment is minimal and intelligence is normal. And in between these two extremes, infants may have different degrees of handicap. It is estimated that up to 50% of children born with arthrogryposis and central nervous system (CNS) involvement will die in the neonatal period.[26] For those with contractures, treatment is directed toward achieving stable functional weight-bearing and manual dexterity.

Campomelic Dysplasia

Description: The term is derived from the Greek language meaning "bent bones," a condition characterized by bowing of the long bones, particularly lower extremities, hypoplastic scapulae, and a number of other associated abnormalities, including hydrocephalus, congenital heart disease, and hydronephrosis. Craniofacial abnormalities (macrocephaly, cleft palate, micrognathia) have been reported in 90% to 99% of cases.[34] Approximately 75% of individuals with a 46, XY karyotype have either ambiguous or normally appearing female external genitalia. The internal genitalia are variable, often with a mixture of Müllerian and Wolffian duct structures. Pretibial skin dimples may be seen in the neonate with campomelic dysplasia.

Incidence and Molecular Pathology: This is reported in 0.05 per 10,000 births. Inherited as an autosomal dominant manner as a *de novo* mutation in the *SOX9* gene mapped to chromosome 17 (17q24.3-q25.1). The *SOX9* gene is a transcription factor involved in chondrogenesis and sex determination.

Radiological Manifestations: Enlarged, elongated skull, hypoplasia and poor ossification of the cervical vertebrae, small bell-shaped thorax with 11 pairs of ribs, hypoplastic scapula, short and angulated long bones, narrow and tall iliac wings, poor or absent ossification of the pubis, angulated proximal femoral shaft with apex located anterolaterally, hypoplasia, and angulation of tibia and hypoplastic fibula

Diagnosis: US can demonstrate marked anterior bowing of the tibia and femora. Bowing may be unilateral and mimic fractures. Other findings include hypoplastic scapulae, small thorax, and vertically narrowed iliac bones

Flat face, micrognathia, hypertelorism, hydrocephalus, and ambiguous genitalia have also been described. 3D is useful in further assessment of hypoplastic scapula. As with other SDs, nuchal thickening may be noted early in gestation. Polyhydramnios, CNS, cardiac, and renal anomalies can be present (Fig. 29.15).

When campomelic dysplasia is being considered, genetic analysis of the *SOX9* gene is recommended.

Course and Prognosis: Many newborns with campomelic dysplasia die shortly after birth secondary to respiratory insufficiency. However, unlike other SDs, the cause of death is not related to thoracic cage hypoplasia, but rather to airway instability (tracheobronchomalacia) or to cervical instability.

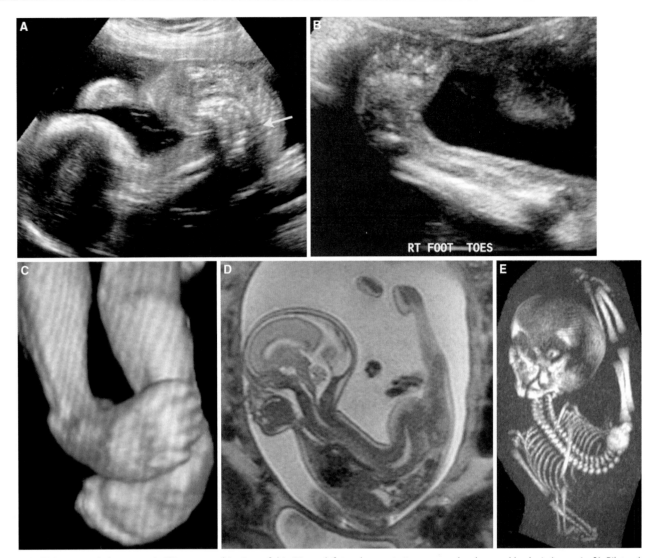

FIGURE 29.14: Arthrogryposis. 2D sonographic view of this 23-week fetus demonstrates a severe lumbosacral lordosis (*arrow* in **A**). Bilateral clubfeet are shown in this 2D image (**B**) and 3D US rendering (**C**). T2 sagittal MRI of the fetus demonstrates the scoliosis to better advantage, with marked extension contractures of the lower extremities and partial visualization of the clubfoot deformity (**D**). Low-dose fetal CT shows exquisite detail of the fetal spine, its abnormal spinal curvature, and the abnormal posturing of the extremities (**E**).

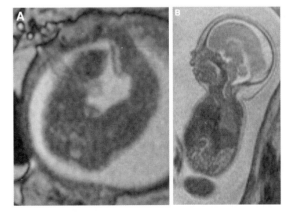

FIGURE 29.15: Campomelic dysplasia. **A:** SSFSE T2 axial MRI demonstrates short-bowed tibia and equinovarus deformity. **B:** Sagittal image demonstrates micrognathia and cystic hygroma.

Differential Diagnosis: The most common error is to confuse campomelic dysplasia with OI. Campomelic dysplasia is characterized by hypoplastic scapula and may have renal anomalies. Facial features of campomelic dysplasia are not present in OI. Irregular beaded ribs representing fractures in OI are not present in campomelic dysplasia. Bowing of long bones in the fetus with OI may be more asymmetric secondary to healing fractures. Other differentials include hypophosphatasia, TD, mesomelic dysplasia, and diastrophic dysplasia.

Craniosynostosis

Description: Abnormal development or premature closure of one or more cranial sutures resulting in abnormal head shape. It may occur in isolation or in the presence of a syndrome. The syndromic form tends to be associated with multiple sutures, whereas the isolated form tends to involve a single suture, most commonly the sagittal followed by the coronal, metopic, and lambdoid sutures. In severe cases, craniosynostosis can cause compression of cranial nerves and increased pressure on the growing brain.

Incidence and Molecular Pathology: Isolated craniosynostosis occurs in about 3.4 per 1,000 live births. When associated with a syndrome, it is a rare occurrence (<1 in 50,000 to 100,000). Most isolated cases have multifactorial or sporadic inheritance; as part of a syndrome, inheritance is usually autosomal dominant, depending on the specific syndrome. The causes of craniosynostosis are numerous and include chromosomal, metabolic, teratogenic (aminopterin, sodium valproate), and infection as possible culprits. For a more extensive list, the reader is referred to the excellent review compiled by Dr. Lachman in his well-known comprehensive book on SDs.[36]

Radiologic Manifestations: The findings seen in each fetus with craniosynostosis depend on the underlying syndrome. For example, in Crouzon syndrome, sonographic findings may include premature fusion of the coronal sutures leading to brachycephaly and, in severe cases, a cloverleaf skull. In Apert syndrome, cloverleaf deformity of the skull may also be found, along with hypertelorism, ventriculomegaly, and "mitten hands" or osseous/cutaneous syndactyly of the second, third, and fourth fingers (Fig. 29.16). In Pfeiffer syndrome, brachycephaly and acrocephaly relate to fusion of the coronal and sometimes sagittal sutures.

Diagnosis: US is usually the first imaging modality that suggests the possibility of craniosynostosis. Although the cranial sutures can be visualized by 3D sonography as early as the 13 weeks' gestation, the prenatal diagnosis of craniosynostosis is usually made on the basis of secondary features such as cranial deformation, and hyper- or hypotelorism.[42]

MRI has been shown to be a helpful imaging adjunt,[43,20] providing additional detail about the brain and possible cranial dysmorphism (Fig. 29.17).

Expected findings if there is premature fusion of a single coronal suture include ipsilateral cranial flattening or plagiocephaly

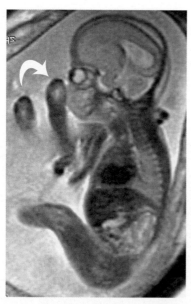

FIGURE 29.16: Apert syndrome. Sagittal SSFSE T2 MRI demonstrates mitten hands *(arrow)* as well as brachycephaly in this fetus with evolving craniosynostosis.

with elevation and posterior displacement of the ipsilateral orbit and anterior displacement of the ipsilateral ear canal. If two coronal sutures are fused, the result is brachycephaly or turribrachycephaly, with decreased anteroposterior dimension of the skull (Fig. 29.17). Premature fusion of the metopic suture leads to a triangular shape of the anterior skull (trigonocephaly), resulting in bitemporal narrowing and hypotelorism as seen in prenatal US and MRI. Synostosis of the sagittal suture results in a decreased biparietal dimension of the cranium (scaphocephaly or dolichocephaly). Premature closure of the coronal and lambdoid sutures may result in the cloverleaf deformity of the skull or Kleeblattschädel, with bitemporal and bifrontal bulging, findings that

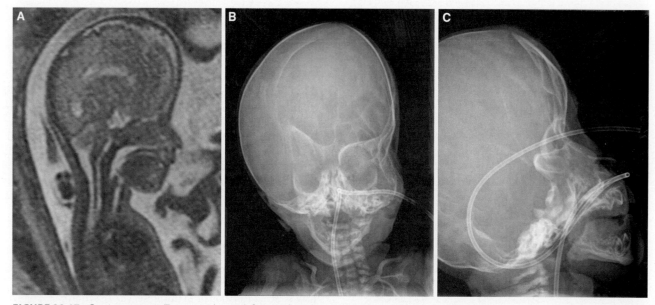

FIGURE 29.17: Craniosynostosis. Twenty-eight-week fetus with turricephaly (increased craniocaudal and decreased anteroposterior diameter of the head) and a flattened facial profile as seen in this sagittal T2 MRI **(A)**. Postnatal radiographs of the skull in the anteroposterior **(B)** and lateral **(C)** position confirm prenatal findings. The child was found to have bicoronal craniosynostosis, resulting in marked brachycephaly, and partial closure of the lambdoid suture with pronounced left plagiocephaly.

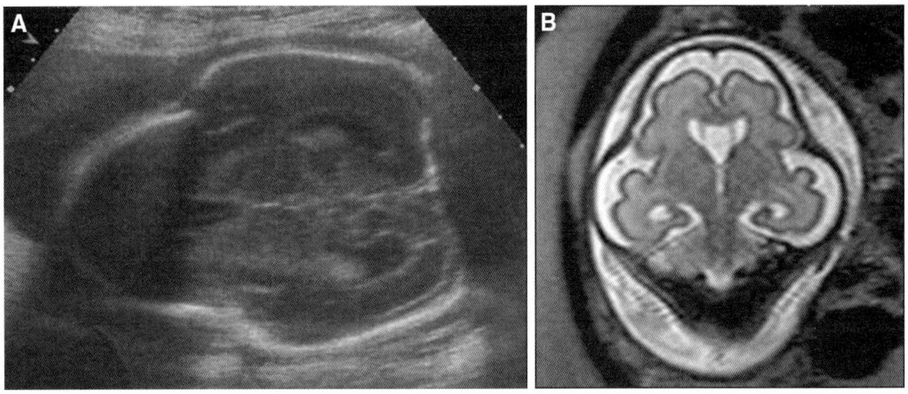

FIGURE 29.18: Craniosynostosis. US **(A)** and SSFSE T2 MRI **(B)** in this 29-week fetus with a cloverleaf deformity of the skull (*kleeblattschädel*), characterized by a trilobar skull with bossing of the forehead, temporal bulging, and a flat posterior skull.

may be seen in entities such as TD (Figs. 29.18 and 29.19). Early fusion of the lambdoid suture may produce parieto-occipital plagiocephaly.

Course and Prognosis: A prenatal diagnosis of craniosynostosis carries significant cosmetic and surgical implications. The prognosis for isolated craniosynostosis is very good with reconstructive surgery. Prognosis for individuals with a genetic syndrome with craniosynostosis ranges from very good (Crouzon, Jackson–Weiss syndrome) to developmental delay and mental retardation (Apert and Pfeiffer syndromes) or lethality (TD type II).

Chondrodysplasia Punctata

Synonyms: Conradi–Hünermann syndrome, chondrodystrophia calcificans congenita

Description: Chondrodysplasia Punctata (CDP) describes the radiographic appearance of abnormal cartilaginous stippling, the result of abnormal deposition of calcium during endochondral bone formation. Stippling may arise secondary to premature calcification of the cartilage in the epiphyseal growth plate, later resolving during the first year of life, or may also be found in cartilaginous sites not expected to calcify, like the trachea.[44,45]

These findings are caused by a diverse spectrum of etiologies including errors of metabolism, chromosomal abnormalities, syndromes, prenatal exposures, and abnormal vitamin K metabolism resulting in varied outcomes ranging from neonatal demise to a normal life span. Irving et al. proposed the following classification of disorders with cartilage stippling: (1) metabolic abnormalities, including errors of peroxisomal function, cholesterol biosynthesis, and other inborn errors of metabolism, (2) disorders resulting in disruption of vitamin K metabolism

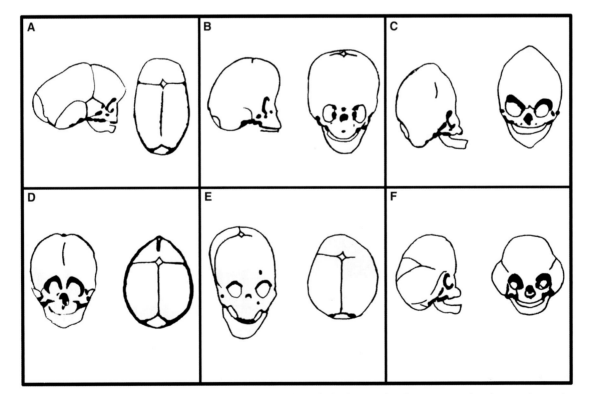

FIGURE 29.19: Common forms of craniosynostosis. **A:** *Scaphocephaly*: elongated and narrow cranial vault secondary to the premature closure of the sagittal suture. **B:** *Turricephaly* or *oxycephaly*: tall head with respect to its width and length. **C:** *Oxycephaly* with prominent bregmatic junction. **D:** *Trigonocephaly*: premature fusion of the metopic suture resulting in a triangular-shaped anterior skull. **E:** *Plagiocephaly*: asymmetric distortion and flattening of one side of the head. **F:** *Cloverleaf skull* or *kleeblattschädel*: deformity of the skull resulting in a trilobed cranium.

with deficiency of the arylsulfatase E enzyme (hyperemesis), and (3) various chromosomal abnormalities, including among others trisomies 13 and 21 as well as Turner syndrome.[44] The association with autoimmune disorders such as systemic lupus erythematosus (SLE), mixed connective tissue disorders, and scleroderma has also been reported.[21] It is important to note that CDP does not constitute a diagnosis, and that, as such, an appropriate investigation must be done in order to find the underlying diagnosis. Classifications include the rhizomelic form (potentially lethal), the brachytelephalangic type with short distal phalanges, and the Binder phenotype with severe hypoplasia of the nasal pyramid and midface and nonrhizomelic (Conradi–Hünermann syndrome, more common and generally benign).

Incidence and Molecular Pathology: The estimated incidence is approximately 0.09 per 10,000 births. CDP is seen in a number of different conditions, as noted. For a detailed list of known genetic causes, we refer the reader to a comprehensive list of disorders associated with puncta.[25,38] In general, the rhizomelic type is inherited as an autosomal recessive pattern and is lethal. The nonrhizomelic type may be inherited as an autosomal dominant or a recessive and X-linked pattern and can present with asymmetric short stature, scoliosis, cataracts, and/or flat facies with nasal hypoplasia (Binder phenotype) (Fig. 29.20).

Radiologic Manifestations: The rhizomelic type is characterized by marked limb shortening. Contractions, flexed fingers, and hypertelorism are commonly seen. There is calcific stippling of the epiphyses. Metaphyseal splaying and coronal clefts of the spine may be seen. The nonrhizomelic, or Conradi–Hünermann type, is a milder form of the disease, with mild or no limb shortening. The metaphyses are not splayed. Stippling is very fine and may be limited to the tarsal or carpal bones.[34]

Diagnosis: Prenatal findings are variable. A number of case reports have identified short limbs, unusual calcifications, and spine anomalies by US in the second or third trimester of gestation. One study describes a pregnancy with a normal first-trimester US which on follow-up US at week 19 showed profound shortening of the humeri with hypomineralization, epiphyseal fractures, and stippled hyperechoic foci in the epiphyseal cartilage.[46] All other bones were normal. A repeat US at 21 weeks demonstrated further, more profound shortening of the humeri, which also appeared bowed. Findings had propagated to the femora, with shortening below the fifth percentile, decreased echodensity of

the bones and abnormalities of the epiphyseal cartilage. Another published report describes a 23-week fetus with rhizomelic limb shortening and epiphyseal calcifications. A fetal CT was also able to demonstrate the epiphyseal calcifications, bowing of the long bones, scoliosis, and distal phalangeal hypoplasia.[47]

With milder forms, isolated midface hypoplasia may be the only finding and best seen by MRI[21] (Fig. 29.20C). MRI may be able to demonstrate the epiphyseal calcifications by EPI sequences.

Course and Prognosis: There is a wide spectrum of outcomes. The rhizomelic type of CDP is often fatal within the first year of life secondary to respiratory failure. Severe mental deficiency and psychomotor delay is present in survivors. The nonrhizomelic type, however, is compatible with life. Complications include orthopedic problems and recurrent infections.[34] The only marker in adults may be midface hypoplasia of the Binder phenotype.[44]

Differential Diagnosis: Other forms of CDP such as Warfarin embryopathy, aneuploidy, phenytoin and alcohol exposure, Smith–Lemli–Opitz syndrome, and GM1 gangliosidosis

Hypophosphatasia

Description: Congenital disease characterized by demineralization of bones and low activity of alkaline phosphatase (ALP) in the tissue and serum. ALP acts on pyrophosphate and other phosphate esters, leading to the accumulation of inorganic phosphates that are crucial for the formation of bone crystals. Bone fragility is thought to be the result of deficient generation of bone crystals. The severity of the disease is inversely related to the serum levels of ALP activity.[48–51] Hypophosphatasia has been subdivided into various forms according to the age of onset and severity: (1) perinatal severe, (2) perinatal benign, (3) infantile, (4) childhood and (5) adult, and (6) odontohypophosphatasia.

The severe perinatal form is lethal due to respiratory insufficiency and hypercalcemia. The benign perinatal form has skeletal manifestations that slowly resolve with variable infant and childhood presentations. Infantile hypophosphatasia develops rickets between birth and 6 months of age without elevated ALP activity.

Incidence and Molecular Pathology: Estimated to occur in 1 per 100,000 live births. It is inherited as autosomal recessive in the infantile/childhood type and autosomal dominant for the adult form of the disease. Loss of function of the ALP liver gene, also called tissue-nonspecific alkaline phosphatase (*TNSALP*) located

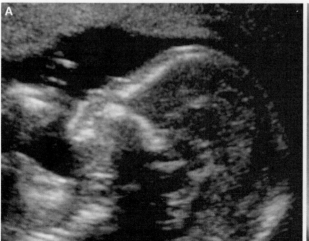
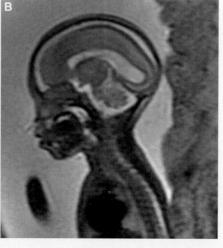

FIGURE 29.20: Chondrodysplasia punctata. Family history of chondrodysplasia punctata X-linked. In this 20-week fetus, isolated midface hypoplasia with a small nose was identified by 2D **(A)** and 3D **(B)** US consistent with Conradi–Hünermann syndrome **(C)** SSFSE T2 MRI of a 23-week gestational age also demonstrates Binder phenotype.

on chromosome 1p36.1-p34, is responsible for the genotype in hypophosphatasia. A large spectrum of mutations has been observed, resulting in different ranges of enzymatic activity, perhaps leading to the wide phenotypic variability seen in hypophosphatasia.

Radiological Manifestations: The perinatal severe form, which is the type relevant to antenatal diagnosis, is characterized by marked demineralization of the calvarium. The skull appears soft ("caput membranaceum"). Tubular bones are short and may have numerous fractures. The skeleton may be poorly and irregularly ossified.

The perinatal benign form may present with variable skeletal involvement including short-bowed long bones, asymmetric fractures that can resolve (Fig. 29.21).

Diagnosis

Severe: By US, demineralization of the skull is present when there is increased echogenicity of the falx cerebri, attributed to enhanced sound transmission in a poorly mineralized skull. Deformation of the skull from external compression with the US transducer is consistent with skull demineralization. Short limbs with multiple fractures can be noted. Amniotic fluid may be increased.

Benign: Rhizomelic shortening with bowing and rib fractures may be noted mimicking OI. The skull appears normally mineralized by US.

Course and Prognosis: The perinatal severe form is lethal and is associated with stillbirth or early neonatal birth due to intracranial hemorrhage or respiratory insufficiency secondary to the poorly developed ribs and reduced thoracic cavity volume. The benign form may have a variable outcome with self-resolution of bowing (Fig. 29.21). Treatment with Asfotase Alfa enzyme replacement can improve mineralization and bone health.

In the infantile or juvenile form, symptoms may appear shortly after birth (failure to thrive, irritability, convulsion, cyanotic episodes, angulated limbs, and other signs of hypercalcemia) or early in childhood (delayed onset of walking, myopathy, weakness).

In the adult form, bone pain, tendency to fracture, and abnormal teeth may be presenting symptoms.[51]

Differential Diagnosis: In achondrogenesis, there is lack of ossification of the spine; however, it is the vertebral bodies that are not ossified as opposed to the neural arches in hypophosphatasia. In addition, the calvarium will be ossified in achondrogenesis, as opposed to hypophosphatasia where it will be absent. Fractures and bowed and short bones may be found in OI, but the calvarium may be partially ossified in OI.

Mesomelic Dysplasia

Description: A group of disorders with disproportionate limb shortening of the middle segments of the extremities. It includes dyschondrosteosis, Nievergelt mesomelic dysplasia, Langer mesomelic dysplasia, Reinhardt mesomelic dysplasia, Robinow (fetal face syndrome) mesomelic dysplasia, and Werner mesomelic dysplasia.

Incidence and Molecular Pathology: These are rare entities, with no known incidence defined in the literature. Many, but not all, of the mesomelic dysplasias are autosomal dominant. For a detailed listing of known genes involved in these disorders, the reader is directed to Dr. Spranger's review in his book on SDs.[38]

Radiological Manifestations: Variable. *Langer mesomelic dysplasia* is characterized by a hypoplastic ulna, fibula, and mandible, with the ulna being shorter than the radius. The lower extremities are more affected than are the upper extremities. Some people consider the Langer type as the homozygous state of *dyschondrosteosis*, a mesomelic dysplasia recognized in late childhood and characterized by mesomelic shortening with Madelung deformity.

In *Nievergelt mesomelic dysplasia*, there is mesomelia and the presence of clubfoot deformity.

Robinow mesomelic dysplasia has acromelic brachymelia with short hands and feet and stubby fingers and toes. The face has been described as that of an 8-week fetus, with macrocephaly,

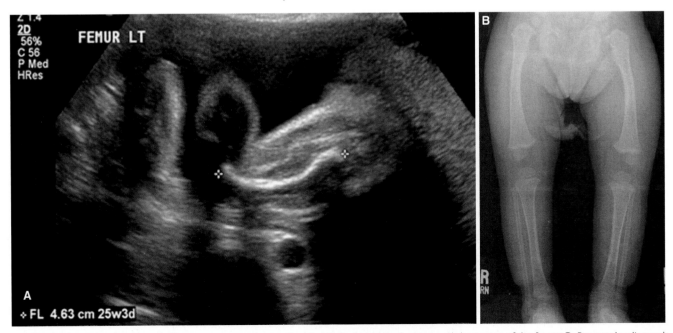

FIGURE 29.21: Hypophosphatasia. Twenty-seven-week gestation. **A:** US demonstrates bowing and shortening of the femur. **B:** Postnatal radiograph demonstrates minimal residual bowing at 1.5 months of age.

prominent forehead, hypertelorism, and hypoplastic mandible. *Werner mesomelic dysplasia* is characterized by extreme bilateral hypoplasia of the tibia, polydactyly, absence of the thumbs, and, frequently, webbing of the fingers.

Prenatal Diagnosis: Mainly, case reports have been published in the literature on the prenatal detection of mesomelic disorders.[52,53] By US, shortening of the midsegments of the limbs is identified. Ribs, scapula, and clavicles are typically normal. Increased nuchal translucency has been described in the first trimester.[52]

Course and Prognosis: These disorders are associated with normal intelligence, with the exception of the Robinow type. Orthopedic problems are expected.

Differential Diagnosis: These are other mesomelic dysplasias, VACTERL sequence, thrombocytopenia absent radius (TAR) syndrome, chondroectodermal dysplasia.

Osteogenesis Imperfecta

Description: Heritable disorder of connective tissue whose cardinal manifestation is bone fragility caused by abnormal collagen microfibril assembly. About 90% of cases are caused by mutations in genes that encode the proα1 and proα2 polypeptide chains that comprise the type I collagen molecule. Type I collagen is the most abundant type of collagen and is widely distributed in almost all connective tissues with the exception of hyaline cartilage. It is the major protein in bone, skin, tendon, ligament, sclera, cornea, and blood vessels. It comprises approximately 95% of the entire collagen content of bone and about 80% of the total protein content in bone.[54] Type I collagen is composed of two identical α1 polypeptide chains and one α2 chain, with the three strands twisted in a triple helix. Each polypeptide chain is composed of about 1,000 amino acids arranged in uninterrupted repeats of Gly-X-Y triplets. A complex pathway of postprocessing occurs with the triple helix as its final form. A mutation in one of the two genes that comprise the proα1 and proα2 polypeptide chains may induce a change either in the structure of the protein or in the number of collagen molecules made, resulting in OI. Both severe and mild forms of the disease have in common the presence of bone fractures after no or little trauma and low bone mass.

Classification: The classification of OI is disputed. In its original form, it is divided into four subtypes, as proposed by Sillence in 1979, based on clinical, genetic, and radiographic findings.[55]

- **Type I** OI is the most common and the mildest form, characterized by relatively mild bone fragility, blue sclera, and conductive hearing loss.
- **Type II** OI is the most severe form, with findings seen prenatally expressed as intrauterine fractures resulting in micromelia, and is essentially fatal.
- **Type III** is the most severe form that is compatible with survival with findings that may range between mild to severe.
- **Type IV** may present with dentinogenesis imperfecta and fractures in later life. There are other subtypes of OI that escape the Sillence classification, prompting investigators to add the additional **types V** to **VII** OI.[56] These are thought not to be associated with type I collagen mutations.

Incidence and Molecular Pathology: The precise incidence depends on the criterion used to define this entity, with reports ranging between 1 in 25,000 to 1 in 100,000.[46] The genes that encode the α1 and α2 polypeptide chains of type 1 collagen are referred to as *COL1A1* and *COL1A2*, respectively, located on chromosome17q21.31-q22 and chromosome 7q22.1. **Type I** OI, the relatively mild form, is inherited as an autosomal dominant pattern, caused by a mutation in the type I collagen gene which results in normal type I collagen, but in reduced amounts. **Type II** OI is predominantly autosomal dominant (<5% are autosomal recessive), inherited as a *de novo* mutation in the type I collagen gene. **Type III** is a predominantly autosomal dominant mutation, also called progressively deforming OI, as the incidence of fractures usually increases with age. The autosomal dominant **type IV** OI has marked intra- and interfamilial expression with clinical and radiographic manifestations that may overlap with type I in mild cases, and with type II/III in severe cases.

Radiologic Manifestations: **Types I** and **IV** demonstrate one or more fractures with normal or mildly shortened long bones which may appear angulated, with irregular contour of the bone and evidence of callus formation. Fractures may not occur until the postnatal period.

Type II is the most common type identified prenatally, demonstrated by generalized bone deossification, a crumpled and coarsened appearance of the long bones, and irregularity and beading of the ribs (Fig. 29.22).

In **type III**, fractures may be present in the second trimester, although not as severe as in type II.

Diagnosis: Types I and IV may not demonstrate prenatal deformities, and the diagnosis may be made after birth when limb deformities become apparent.

Type II presents with wrinkling of the surface of the bones due to fractures. The bones are typically less than 3% by the second trimester, and nuchal thickening can be present in the first trimester. The ribs are beaded from multiple rib fractures with the chest bell shaped. There is significant demineralization of the skull. The head may be compressible and the intracranial structures easily seen (see Fig. 29.22). Because of the degree of demineralization, both cortices of the bone may be visualized by US. Polyhydramnios may be present.

Type III may present as an isolated fracture or multiple short-bowed bones. Findings may be similar to type II, but less severe, with long bones not severely micromelic in the early second trimester unlike type II OI.

While the diagnosis can be made by US, MRI and CT have been used as an adjunct to confirm findings and help differentiate from other dysplasias. Temporal lobe dysplasias noted in TD are not present in OI (Figs. 29.22 and 29.23).

Course and Prognosis: Prognosis depends on the severity and type of the disease. Infants with type II are born with multiple fractures and most often die in the neonatal period from respiratory compromise. In the milder types, fractures may not occur until later in life.

Differential Diagnosis: Differential diagnosis includes TD, hypophosphatasia, achondrogenesis, and campomelic dysplasia. The key in differentiation includes asymmetric fractures in various stages of healing and beaded ribs.

Short-Rib Thoracic Dysplasia with/without Polydactyly

Description: Heterogeneous group of autosomal recessive ciliopathies. Characterized by short ribs with thoracic hypoplasia,

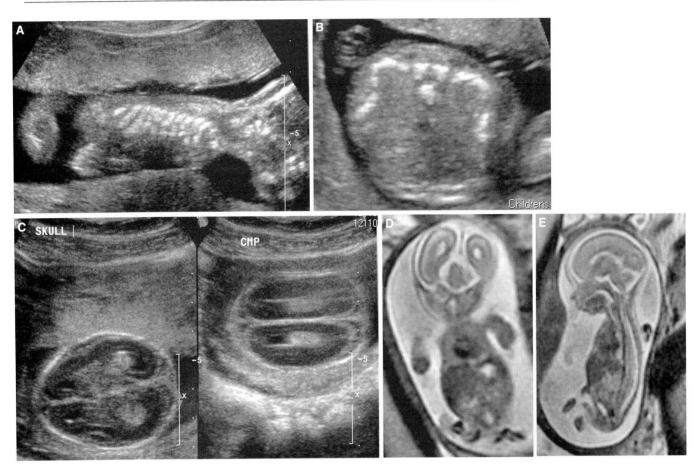

FIGURE 29.22: Osteogenesis imperfecta type II. Sagittal **(A)** and axial **(B)** US of the chest at 18 weeks' gestation demonstrate multiple irregular rib fractures. **C:** Axial image of the skull without and with compression demonstrates decreased skull echogenicity with compressibility *(right)*. SSFSE T2 coronal MRI **(D)** demonstrates unossified calvarium, small chest, and accordion appearance to the humerus. **E:** Sagittal MRI demonstrates lack of vertebral ossification.

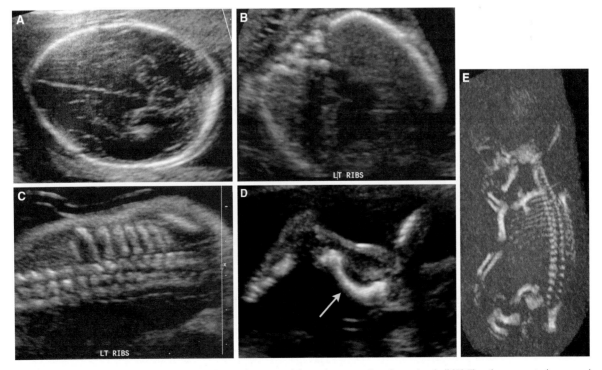

FIGURE 29.23: Osteogenesis imperfecta. 2D US in this 21-week fetus shows a pointed anterior skull **(A)**. The ribs appear to be normal in length and morphology **(B,C)**, with no definite fractures. The long bones of the lower extremity appear bowed *(arrow)* and coarse **(D)**. Low-dose fetal computed tomography shows with greater detail the degree of irregularity and coarseness of the long bones, particularly the lower extremities, findings consistent with fractures.

short tubular bones, and trident appearance of the acetabular roof.[57] Polydactyly occurs frequently but is not obligatory.

Short rib thoracic dysplasia (SRTD) encompasses Jeune syndrome (asphyxiating thoracic dystrophy), the less severe chondroectodermal dysplasia (Ellis–van Creveld syndrome), and the lethal short-rib polydactyly syndromes (SRPSs I–V).

Phenotypically, these overlap, differing by visceral malformations and metaphyseal appearance.

Asphyxiating Thoracic Dysplasia
Synonym: Jeune syndrome

Description: Autosomal recessive **SRTD** osteochondrodysplasia. Characteristic skeletal abnormalities include small and narrow thorax, short ribs, short squared iliac wings, and limb shortening. The spectrum of clinical manifestations is wide, ranging from lethal to mild forms without respiratory compromise. Renal (hypertension/failure), hepatic (polycystic liver disease and cirrhosis), pancreatic cystic disease, and retinal complications may also occur. Other pathological findings, including agenesis of the corpus callosum or Dandy Walker malformation, may be present.

Incidence and Molecular Pathology: The estimated prevalence is 0.14 per 10,000 births. Most mild and severe forms map to chromosome 15q1.[29,58] The causative gene has not yet been found.

Radiologic Manifestations: Short, horizontally directed ribs with bulbous anterior ends, narrow, bell-shaped thorax, horizontal or handlebar configuration of the clavicles, small pelvis, trident acetabulum, and normal vertebrae are some of the findings.[30,59] The extremities, including hand and feet, may be short.

Prenatal Diagnosis: May be detected by US early in the second trimester if the findings are severe.[59,60] MRI can be helpful to confirm small rib cage and low lung volumes, although the osseous findings may be difficult to delineate, particularly in the second trimester (Fig. 29.24).

Course and Prognosis: Depends on the severity of symptoms. In severe cases, thoracic narrowing is responsible for pulmonary hypoplasia, respiratory failure, and death. In the milder forms, it is the degree of renal involvement that constitutes the main prognostic indicator.

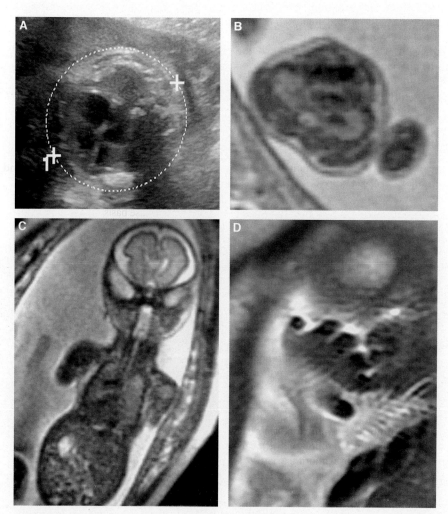

FIGURE 29.24: Asphyxiating thoracic dystrophy. **A:** Axial US demonstrates a small chest circumference (calipers). SSFSE T2 MRI axial **(B)** and coronal **(C)** images confirm the short ribs and small lung volume. **D:** Postaxial polydactyly is also present.

Differential Diagnosis: Absence of mesomelic shortness and smooth metaphyseal margins differentiate asphyxiating thoracic dysplasia from other short-rib (minus polydactyly) syndromes. The pelvic configuration is indistinguishable from chondroectodermal dysplasia (Ellis–van Creveld), but polydactyly is a constant feature in this syndrome that may not necessarily be present in asphyxiating thoracic dysplasia.

Chondroectodermal Dysplasia
Synonym: Ellis–van Creveld syndrome

Description: An autosomal recessive **SRTD** characterized by disproportionate short-limb dwarfism with centrifugal shortening, short ribs, postaxial polydactyly (generally involving the fingers, less commonly the toes), and dysplasia of ectodermal derivatives (hypoplastic or absent nails, partial anodontia, scant or fine hair). Approximately 60% of patients have congenital heart malformations, especially atrial septal defects.

Incidence and Molecular Pathology: 0.9 per 10,000 births, with a high incidence among the Amish community of Lancaster, Pennsylvania. Two EVC genes, linked to the 4p16 chromosome, are thought to be causative of the disease, although these may not be the only genes involved in this phenotype.

Radiological Manifestations: Disproportionate short-limb dwarfism with progressive distal shortening of the extremities, bony spike in the medial side of distal metaphysis of humerus in newborns, polydactyly of hands (almost 100%) and feet (about 25%), short ribs, narrow thorax, dysplasia of the pelvis with low iliac wings and hooklike protrusion of the medial and/or lateral aspect of the acetabulum (trident pelvis), often premature ossification of the capital femoral epiphysis, slanting of the proximal medial tibial metaphysis, and cone-shaped epiphysis of the middle phalanges

Diagnosis: Abnormal osseous findings may be detected during the second or third trimester of pregnancy, although distinction with other short ribs dysplasia is challenging by US. The presence of mesomelic shortened long bones, polydactyly, small chest with small ribs, and cardiac defects are clues suggestive of this entity.

Course and Prognosis: One-third of the infants die in the first month of life because of cardiopulmonary problems. Survivors may reach adulthood, usually with normal intellectual development but short stature.

Differential Diagnosis: Differentiating between chondroectodermal dysplasia and asphyxiating thoracic dysplasia (Jeune syndrome) is challenging because of the significant overlap: polydactyly, narrow thorax, and similar but less severe pelvic dysplasia occur in asphyxiating thoracic dysplasia as well. Hexadactyly of the fingers is a constant finding in chondroectodermal dysplasia but rare in asphyxiating thoracic dysplasia.

Short-Rib Polydactyly Syndromes
Synonyms: SRPS Types I-IV

Description: SRPSs are a group of lethal congenital disorders characterized by shortening of the ribs and long bones, polydactyly, and a range of extraskeletal anomalies (heart, intestine, genitalia, kidney, liver, and pancreas).[57] These short-rib dysplasias appear to share a common primary cilium function defect and form a subset of ciliopathy disease.[61]

Incidence and Molecular Pathology: Because of the rarity, its true incidence is not known. The genetic candidates for the different SRPSs are delineated in the revision of the Nosology and Classification of Genetic Skeletal Disorders from 2010.[62]

Radiologic Manifestations

SRPS Type I or Saldino–Noonan Syndrome: Findings include dolichocephaly; poor mineralization of the frontal bones, metacarpals, metatarsal, and phalanges; severe micromelia; hypoplastic tubular bones; narrow thorax; extremely short and horizontally oriented ribs; pointed femurs; and absent fibula. Cardiac, gastrointestinal, and urogenital malformations can be found. Polydactyly can be pre- or postaxial.

SRPS Type II or Majewski Syndrome: Findings include extremely short and horizontally located ribs, mesomelia with marked shortening of the tubular bones, extremely short tibia with an ovoid configuration, rounded metaphyseal ends of the long tubular bones, pre- and postaxial polysyndactyly, and distal phalangeal hypoplasia. Genitalia may be ambiguous. Hydrops and polyhydramnios have been described.

SRS Type III or Verma–Naumoff Syndrome: Similar to type I, but with milder findings, including vertebral hypoplasia, short ribs, short base of skull, shortening of all short tubular bones, and long bones with widened metaphyseal ends that contain lateral spikes.

SRPS Type IV or Beemer–Langer Syndrome: Same as SRPS type II but without polydactyly.

Diagnosis: Short long bones and ribs and polydactyly are suggestive of SRPS. By US, these findings may be detected in the early second trimester. MRI or CT may be helpful in further evaluation on a case-by-case basis.

Course and Prognosis: All four types are uniformly fatal and need to be differentiated from the potentially surviving SRTD conditions of asphyxiating thoracic dystrophy (Jeune syndrome) and chondroectodermal dysplasia (Ellis–van Creveld syndrome).

Differential Diagnosis: Included in the differential diagnoses are the different types of SRPSs, including Jeune and Ellis–van Creveld syndrome. TD, CDP, OI, and orofaciodigital syndrome type II should also be considered. Often, diagnosis can only be confirmed after birth.

Thanatophoric Dysplasia

Description: The term "thanatophoric" is derived from the Greek word thanatophorus, which means "death bringing" or "death bearing." Salient features of this phenotype include macrocephaly, narrow bell-shaped thorax, normal trunk length, and severe shortening of all the limbs (micromelia).

Incidence and Molecular Pathology: Thanatophoric dysplasia (TD) is the most common lethal SD with incidence of about 0.5 in 10,000 births. Two forms have been described: TD type I, which

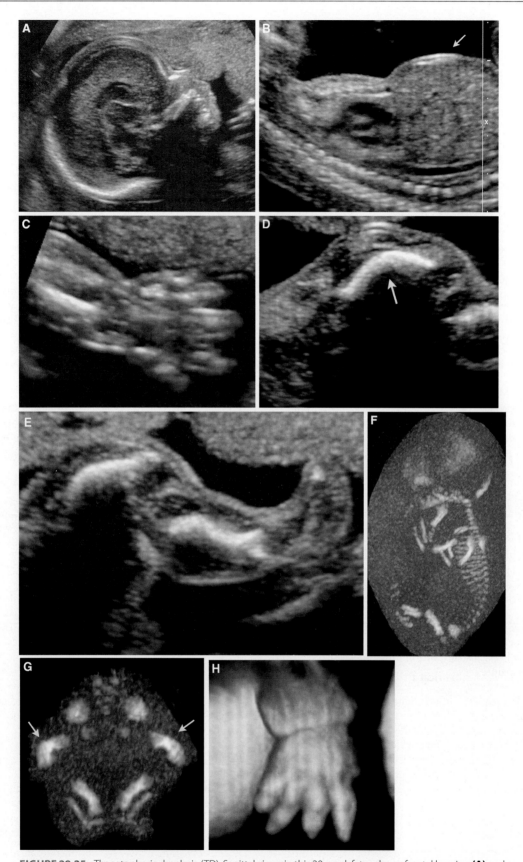

FIGURE 29.25: Thanatophoric dysplasia (TD). Sagittal views in this 20-week fetus shows frontal bossing **(A)** and a protuberant abdomen (*arrow* in **B**). The hand shows short tubular bones **(C)**. Selective views of the left lower extremity demonstrate bowing of the femur (*arrow*), which otherwise appears to have normal mineralization (observe posterior shadowing) and no fractures **(D)** and deformity of the tibia **(E)**. Low-dose fetal computed tomography reveals short ribs and extremities, subjective demineralization of the skull and platyspondyly **(F)**. Coned view of the pelvis demonstrates characteristic bowing deformity of the femora *(arrows)*, decreased vertical diameter of the ischial bones and flattened acetabula **(G)**. 3D reconstruction of the hand in another fetus with TD demonstrating brachydactyly with equal length of the digits in this 34-week fetus **(H)**.

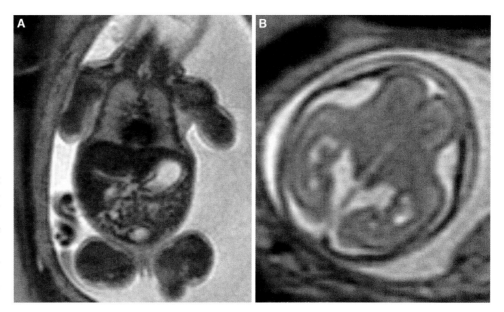

FIGURE 29.26: Thanatophoric dysplasia at 22-week gestation. **A:** SSFSE T2 MRI confirms the presence of short ribs with small lung volume. **B:** Axial image of the brain demonstrates mild changes of craniosynostosis. Deep sulci at the medial temporal lobes are present consistent with temporal lobe dysplasia.

originates from several described mutations in the *FGFR3* gene,[49] and TD type II, accounted for by a single described mutation in the same *FGFR3* gene (Lys650Glu).

Radiological Manifestations: Prenatally, the findings of TD are characteristic: A relatively large head, marked shortening of the long bones, normal trunk length, small thoracic cage with very short ribs, platyspondyly, U- or H-shaped vertebral bodies seen in AP view, small iliac bones, flat acetabular roofs, and trident hands. In TD type I, the affected fetus has bowing of the long bones and a characteristic "telephone receiver" appearance of the femora. In TD type II, the long bones are short, but straight. The morphology of the skull also differs and is typically described as cloverleaf deformity in TD type I, but normal in shape in TD type II.

Brain findings include temporal lobe dysplasia, hydrocephalus, encephaloceles, and brainstem hypoplasia.

Diagnosis: By US, the diagnosis can be made early in the second trimester with severe micromelia (long bones <3% for GA). Chest circumference is small with a bell-shaped thorax. The ribs are short but not beaded. No discreet fractures are present, although the short bones may appear bowed, which can be confused with fractures. Symmetrical findings and lack of callous formation can help differentiate these findings from OI. In addition, the skull should be normally mineralized and not compressible (see Fig. 29.25).[63,64]

MRI can confirm the diagnosis if temporal and occipital lobe dysplasias are present Figure 29.26.

CT may increase diagnostic accuracy and confidence if the sonographic findings are still in question (see Figs. 29.7, 29.8, 29.14, 29.23, and 29.25)[17–19] (Fig. 29.9).

Course and Prognosis: TD is fatal in the prenatal period. With intensive medical intervention, a few patients have survived relatively longer periods, but remained ventilator dependent and mentally deficient.

Differential Diagnosis: Type II OI is often confused with TD prenatally by US due to the severe micromelia and short ribs present in both. Key differentiating features include asymmetric beading and irregular bowing of the long bones and ribs in OI.

Homozygous achondroplasia may appear similar to TD, the final verdict ultimately in the hands of the genetic analysis of the *FGFR3* gene. It is fascinating that several SDs are caused by different mutations in one single gene, *FGFR3*. Although all *FGFR3*-related SDs manifest with shortening of the long bones, they display a graded spectrum of phenotypic severity, ranging from the relatively mild (hypochondroplasia) to the more severe form (achondroplasia), to the invariably lethal type (TD),[63–65] in all cases the result of gain-of-function mutations that deregulate the receptor gene, leading to inhibition of chondrocyte growth and proliferation.

Thrombocytopenia Absent Radius Syndrome

Description: Syndrome characterized, as its name implies, by thrombocytopenia that is generally transient (platelet count of <100,000/mm³) and bilateral absence of radii. Other anomalies of the skeleton (upper and lower limbs, ribs and vertebrae), heart, and genitourinary system (renal anomalies and agenesis of the uterus, cervix, and upper part of the vagina) may occur.

Incidence and Molecular Pathology: Thought to be autosomal recessive. Although a microdeletion at chromosome band 1q21.1 has been involved, deletion of this segment is not sufficient to cause the phenotype and suggests an additional modifier gene.[66]

Radiological Manifestations: Bilateral absent radii. The lower limbs may be short or absent. The ulna and humerus may be unilaterally or bilaterally absent. Thumbs and metacarpals are always present. Clubfoot deformity may occur.

Prenatal Diagnosis: Highly suggested when there is bilateral absence of the radii in the presence of both thumbs, findings that can be well seen by US. In the early second trimester, CT may not be useful as there is limited visualization of the hands at this relatively early GA.[15] Other manifestations in the limbs, as mentioned previously, may be also found prenatally.

Course and Prognosis: Delivery by caesarian section is recommended because these fetuses are at risk for intracranial hemorrhage. There is a high fatality rate within the first months of life, but prognosis improves considerably after the first year of life.[32] Mental retardation may be present in 8% of patients, thought to be related to intracranial bleeding. Long-term disability is related to skeletal deformity with orthopedic intervention as needed to maximize function of limbs.

Differential Diagnosis: Holt–Oram syndrome: The thumb is often absent or hypoplastic in this condition; Roberts syndrome: at times the thumb may be present, thrombocytopenia not reported; Fanconi anemia: absent thumbs, marrow failure.

CONCLUSION

The evaluation of a fetus carrying a presumed diagnosis of SD can be very challenging. Different phenotypes for a single disorder, evolving manifestations of the disease through gestation and the postnatal period, lack of specific genetic testing of certain entities, and overlapping features among syndromes make this a complex group of disorders to evaluate. US is the gold standard for initial evaluation of the fetus with abnormal bones. MRI can be a useful adjunct in the assessment of associated anomalies and may further assess bone and cartilage providing a large field of view of the limbs. Low-dose fetal CT has emerged as a method of delineating boney anomalies. Due to the low but real risk of radiation exposure to the fetus, its use is limited to a small subset of cases with severe osseous abnormalities in which accurate diagnosis will impact management.

Once all of the fetal imaging is obtained, it is usually helpful to discuss the observed findings with consultants in radiology, genetics, and in maternal fetal medicine, so that appropriate additional genetic testing, if available, can be planned for.

REFERENCES

1. Orioli IM, Castilla EE, Barbosa-Neto JG. The birth prevalence rates for the skeletal dysplasias. *J Med Genet.* 1986;23:328–332.
2. Bonafe L, Cormier-Daire V, Hall C, et al. Nosology and classification of genetic skeletal disorders: 2015 revision. *Am J Med Genet A.* 2015;167A:2869–2892.
3. Alanay Y, Lachman RS. A review of the principles of radiological assessment of skeletal dysplasias. *J Clin Res Pediatr Endocrinol.* 2011;3:163–178.
4. Hall CM. International nosology and classification of constitutional disorders of bone (2001). *Am J Med Genet.* 2002;113:65–77.
5. Offiah AC, Hall CM. Radiological diagnosis of the constitutional disorders of bone. As easy as A, B, C? *Pediatr Radiol.* 2003;33:153–161.
6. Eames BF, de la Fuente L, Helms JA. Molecular ontogeny of the skeleton. *Birth Defects Res C.* 2003;69:93–101.
7. Schoenwolf GC, Larsen WJ. *Larsen's Human Embryology.* 4th ed. Philadelphia, PA: Elsevier Churchill Livingstone; 2009.
8. Krakow D, Lachman RS, Rimoin DL. Guidelines for the prenatal diagnosis of fetal skeletal dysplasias. *Genet Med.* 2009;11:127–133.
9. Dighe M, Fligner C, Cheng E, et al. Fetal skeletal dysplasia: an approach to diagnosis with illustrative cases. *Radiographics.* 2008;28:1061–1077.
10. Milks KS, Hill LM, Hosseinzadeh K. Evaluating skeletal dysplasias on prenatal ultrasound: an emphasis on predicting lethality. *Pediatr Radiol.* 2017;47(2):134–145.
11. Schramm T, Gloning KP, Minderer S, et al. Prenatal sonographic diagnosis of skeletal dysplasias. *Ultrasound Obstet Gynecol.* 2009;34(2):160–170.
12. Doray B, Favre R, Viville B, et al. Prenatal sonographic diagnosis of skeletal dysplasias. A report of 47 cases. *Ann Genet.* 2000;43:163–169.
13. Parilla BV, Leeth EA, Kambich MP, et al. Antenatal detection of skeletal dysplasias. *J Ultrasound Med.* 2003;22:255–258; quiz 9–61.
14. Nemec U, Nemec SF, Weber M, et al. Human long bone development in vivo: analysis of the distal femoral epimetaphysis on MR images of fetuses. *Radiology.* 2013;267:570–580.
15. Robinson AJ, Blaser S, Vladimirov A, et al. Foetal "black bone" MRI: utility in assessment of the foetal spine. *Br J Radiol.* 2015;88:20140496.
16. Nogueira RDA, Werner Junior H, Daltro P, et al. The role of a novel magnetic resonance imaging sequence in the evaluation of the fetal skeleton: a pilot study. *Radiol Bras.* 2018;51:303–307.
17. Philpott C, Widjaja E, Raybaud C, et al. Temporal and occipital lobe features in children with hypochondroplasia/FGFR3 gene mutation. *Pediatr Radiol.* 2013;43(9):1190–1195.
18. Fink AM, Hingston T, Sampson A, et al. Malformation of the fetal brain in thanatophoric dysplasia: US and MRI findings. *Pediatr Radiol.* 2010;40(suppl 1): S134–S137.
19. Pugash D, Lehman AM, Langlois S. Prenatal ultrasound and MRI findings of temporal and occipital lobe dysplasia in a twin with achondroplasia. *Ultrasound Obstet Gynecol.* 2014;44(3):365–368.
20. Rubio EI, Blask A, Bulas DI. Ultrasound and MR imaging findings in prenatal diagnosis of craniosynostosis syndromes. *Pediatr Radiol.* 2016;46(5):709–718.
21. Blask AR, Rubio EI, Chapman KA, et al Severe nasomaxillary hypoplasia (Binder phenotype) on prenatal US/MRI: an important marker for the prenatal diagnosis of chondrodysplasia punctata. *Pediatr Radiol.* 2018;48(7):979–991.
22. Rubio EI, Mehta N, Blask AR, Bulas DI Prenatal congenital vertical talus (rocker bottom foot): a marker for multisystem anomalies. *Pediatr Radiol.* 2017;47(13):1793–1799.
23. Berceanu C, Gheonea IA, Vlădăreanu S, et al. Ultrasound and MRI comprehensive approach in prenatal diagnosis of fetal osteochondrodysplasias. Cases series. *Med Ultrason.* 2017;19(1):66–72.
24. Weaver KN, Johnson J, Kline-Fath B, et al. Predictive value of fetal lung volume in prenatally diagnosed skeletal dysplasia. *Prenat Diagn.* 2014;34(13):1326–1331.
25. Victoria T, Epelman M, Bebbington M, et al. Low-dose fetal CT for evaluation of severe congenital skeletal anomalies: preliminary experience. *Pediatr Radiol.* 2012;42(suppl 1):S142–S149.
26. Cassart M, Massez A, Cos T, et al. Contribution of three-dimensional computed tomography in the assessment of fetal skeletal dysplasia. *Ultrasound Obstet Gynecol.* 2007;29:537–543.
27. Miyazaki O, Nishimura G, Sago H, et al. Prenatal diagnosis of fetal skeletal dysplasia with 3D CT. *Pediatr Radiol.* 2012;42:842–852.
28. Victoria T, Epelman M, Coleman BG, et al. Low-dose fetal CT in the prenatal evaluation of skeletal dysplasias and other severe skeletal abnormalities. *AJR.* 2013;200:989–1000.
29. McCollough CH, Schueler BA, Atwell TD, et al. Radiation exposure andregnancy: when should we be concerned? *Radiographics.* 2007;27:909–917; discussion 17–18.
30. Wagner LK, Hayman LA. Pregnancy and women radiologists. *Radiology.* 1982;145:559–562.
31. Victoria T, Zhu X, Lachman R, et al. What is new in prenatal skeletal dysplasias? *AJR.* 2018;210:1022–1033.
32. Superti-Furga A. Achondrogenesis type 1B. *J Med Genet.* 1996;33:957–961.
33. Trujillo-Tiebas MJ, Fenollar-Cortes M, Lorda-Sanchez I, et al. Prenatal diagnosis of skeletal dysplasia due to FGFR3 gene mutations: a 9-year experience: prenatal diagnosis in FGFR3 gene. *J Assist Reprod Genet.* 2009;26:455–460.
34. Manikkam SA, Chetcuti K, Howell KB, et al. Temporal lobe malformations in chondroplasi: expanding the brain imaging pheotype associated with FGR3-related skeletal dysplasias. *AJNR.* 2018;39:380–384.
35. Chitty LS, Griffin DR, Meaney C, et al. New aids for the non-invasive prenatal diagnosis of achondroplasia: dysmorphic features, charts of fetal size and molecular confirmation using cell-free fetal DNA in maternal plasma. *Ultrasound Obstet Gynecol.* 2011;37(3):283–289.
36. Lachman RS, Taybi H. *Taybi and Lachman's Radiology of Syndromes, Metabolic Disorders, and Skeletal Dysplasias.* 5th ed. Philadelphia, PA: Mosby Elsevier; 2007.
37. Modaff P, Horton VK, Pauli RM. Errors in the prenatal diagnosis of children with achondroplasia. *Prenat Diagn.* 1996;16:525–530.
38. Spranger JW, Brill PW, Poznanski AK. *Bone Dysplasias: An Atlas of Genetic Disorders of Skeletal Development.* 2nd ed. Oxford; New York: Oxford University Press; 2002.
39. Bevan WP, Hall JG, Bamshad M, et al. Arthrogryposis multiplex congenita (amyoplasia): an orthopaedic perspective. *J Pediatr Orthop.* 2007;27:594–600.
40. Rink BD. Arthrogryposis: a review and approach to prenatal diagnosis. *Obstet Gynecol Surv.* 2011;66:369–377.
41. Hall JG. Genetic aspects of arthrogryposis. *Clin Orthop Relat Res.* 1985;194:44–53.
42. Robson CD, Barnewolt CE. MR imaging of fetal head and neck anomalies. *Neuroimag Clin N Am.* 2004;14:273–291, viii.
43. Fjortoft MI, Sevely A, Boetto S, et al. Prenatal diagnosis of craniosynostosis: value of MR imaging. *Neuroradiology.* 2007;49:515–521.
44. Irving MD, Chitty LS, Mansour S, et al. Chondrodysplasia punctata: a clinical diagnostic and radiological review. *Clin Dysmorphol.* 2008;17:229–241.
45. Kaufmann HJ, Mahboubi S, Spackman TJ, et al. [Tracheal stenosis as a complication of chondrodysplasia punctata]. *Ann Radiol.* 1976;19:203–209.
46. Zwijnenburg PJ, Deurloo KL, Waterham HR, et al. Second trimester prenatal diagnosis of rhizomelic chondrodysplasia punctata type 1 on ultrasound findings. *Prenat Diagn.* 2010;30:162–164.
47. Ulla M, Aiello H, Cobos MP, et al. Prenatal diagnosis of skeletal dysplasias: contribution of three-dimensional computed tomography. *Fetal Diagn Ther.* 2011;29:238–247.
48. Whyte MP. Hypophosphatasia and the role of alkaline phosphatase in skeletal mineralization. *Endocr Rev.* 1994;15(4):439–461.
49. Whyte MP, Essmyer K, Geimer M, et al. Homozygosity for TNSALP mutation 1348c>T (Arg433Cys) causes infantile hypophosphatasia manifesting transient disease correction and variably lethal outcome in a kindred of black ancestry. *J Pediatr.* 2006;148(6):753–758.

50. Mornet E. Hypophosphatasia: the mutations in the tissue-nonspecific alkaline phosphatase gene. *Hum Mutat.* 2000;15(4):309–315.

51. Khandwala HM, Mumm S, Whyte MP. Low serum alkaline phosphatase activity and pathologic fracture: case report and brief review of hypophosphatasia diagnosed in adulthood. *Endocr Pract.* 2006;12(6):676–681.

52. Vseticka J, Gattnarova Z, Marik I, et al. Ultrasound diagnosis of severe mesomelic dysplasia in two fetuses, associated with increased neck translucency and tetralogy of Fallot in one and cystic hygroma in the other. *Am J Med Genet A.* 2010;152A:815–818.

53. Thomas NS, Maloney V, Bass P, et al. SHOX mutations in a family and a fetus with Langer mesomelic dwarfism. *Am J Med Genet A.* 2004;128A:179–184.

54. Niyibizi C, Wang S, Mi Z, et al. Gene therapy approaches for osteogenesis imperfecta. *Gene Ther.* 2004;11:408–416.

55. Sillence DO, Senn A, Danks DM. Genetic heterogeneity in osteogenesis imperfecta. *J Med Genet.* 1979;16:101–116.

56. Basel D, Steiner RD. Osteogenesis imperfecta: recent findings shed new light on this once well-understood condition. *Genet Med.* 2009;11:375–385.

57. Elcioglu NH, Hall CM. Diagnostic dilemmas in the short rib-polydactyly syndrome group. *Am J Med Genet.* 2002;111:392–400.

58. Keppler-Noreuil KM, Adam MP, Welch J, et al. Clinical insights gained from eight new cases and review of reported cases with Jeune syndrome (asphyxiating thoracic dystrophy). *Am J Med Genet A.* 2011;155A:1021–1032.

59. den Hollander NS, Robben SG, Hoogeboom AJ, et al. Early prenatal sonographic diagnosis and follow-up of Jeune syndrome. *Ultrasound Obstet Gynecol.* 2001;18:378–383.

60. Rahmani R, Sterling CL, Bedford HM. Prenatal diagnosis of Jeune-like syndromes with two-dimensional and three-dimensional sonography. *J Clin Ultrasound.* 2012;40:222–226.

61. McInerney-Leo AM, Schmidts M, Cortés CR, et al. Short-rib polydactyly and Jeune syndromes are caused by mutations in WDR60. *Am J Hum Genet.* 2013;93(3):515–523.

62. Warman ML, Cormier-Daire V, Hall C, et al. Nosology and classification of genetic skeletal disorders: 2010 revision. *Am J Med Genet A.* 2011;155A:943–968.

63. Vasilj O, Miškoviæ B. Diagnosis and counseling of thanatophoric dysplasia with four-dimensional ultrasound. *J Matern Fetal Neonatal Med.* 2012;25(12):2786–2788.

64. Giancotti A, Castori M, Spagnuolo A, et al. Early ultrasound suspect of thanatophoric dysplasia followed by first trimester molecular diagnosis. *Am J Med Genet A.* 2011;155A(7):1756–1758.

65. Foldynova-Trantirkova S, Wilcox WR, Krejci P. Sixteen years and counting: the current understanding of fibroblast growth factor receptor 3 (FGFR3) signaling in skeletal dysplasias. *Hum Mutat.* 2012;33:29–41.

66. Toriello HV. Thrombocytopenia-absent radius syndrome. *Semin Thromb Hemost.* 2011;37:707–712.

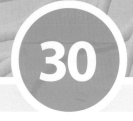

30 Chromosomal and Genetic Syndromes[1]

Stephanie L. Santoro • Robert J. Hopkin • Teresa Chapman • Beth M. Kline-Fath

Advances in prenatal imaging using ultrasound (US) and magnetic resonance imaging (MRI) have enabled earlier and more accurate identification of developmental features that point to various chromosomal abnormalities and syndromes. Because of the high perinatal death rate and childhood disability rates associated with these abnormalities, prenatal testing by cell-free DNA, chorionic villous sampling, amniocentesis, or cordocentesis may be legitimately pursued. The body of identified genes attributed causally to a wide array of developmental anomalies and syndromes continues to expand, enabling families and physicians to make steadily more informed decisions about pregnancy management and future family planning.

In this chapter, the pathogenesis, imaging characteristics, and management issues are described for several common and/or well-described conditions, including the most important chromosomal anomalies, heritable and sporadic syndromes, craniofacial abnormalities, and nongenetic associations leading to multisystem anomalies.

OVERVIEW OF GENETIC/ CHROMOSOMAL TESTING

Over the past few years, there has been a great deal of change in genetic testing options. This adds to the power of genetic diagnosis in identifying specific causes for malformations or in determining whether a fetus is affected by a condition for which there is a known risk. Because of the degree of change in options, a brief review of current testing is provided.

Screening for chromosomal abnormalities has been the standard approach to prenatal testing. It can be performed through multiple methods. In addition to maternal serum screening, often combined with US, laboratory techniques that allow for isolation of cell-free fetal DNA from maternal serum are now widely available. Cell-free fetal DNA can be used to detect abnormal chromosome ratios.[1] This testing is considered by the National Society of Genetic Counselors (NSGC) to be a form of screening and not diagnostic at this time.[2] There are significant false-positive and false-negative reports. This is due primarily to the relatively low risk for the specific abnormalities being screened.

Abnormal screens should be followed by diagnostic testing. This can be performed via amniocentesis or chorionic villus

sampling (CVS), followed by karyotyping (chromosome analysis), microarray, and/or fluorescence in situ hybridization (FISH). These tests have different strengths and limitations, which vary depending on the diagnosis in question and the specific clinical situation. The sensitivity of karyotyping to detect chromosomal anomalies differs depending on laboratory technique and banding resolution. In general, karyotyping can detect chromosomal abnormalities that are larger and may not allow for visualization of specific breakpoints. Karyotyping produces a karyogram, a visualization of the arrangement of chromosomes; as such, it can detect differences in positioning of chromosomal material such as translocations, or inversions including balanced rearrangements. Using single-nucleotide polymorphism (SNP) probes, a microarray analyzes the chromosome complement at higher resolution and can detect microdeletion and microduplication syndromes with much greater sensitivity than standard chromosome analysis. The microarray analysis includes a ratio comparing copy number. As such, it does not show the overall arrangement of the chromosomes and cannot detect translocation or inversions. FISH is specific to locations of interest and can detect deletion or duplication. FISH has utility for its rapid turnaround time, but may be followed up with subsequent testing depending on the chromosomal anomaly in question. For partial deletions or duplications, FISH studies will not determine the size of the abnormality, while microarray will give an accurate assessment of size as well as location.

Molecular Testing

In instances in which a single-gene syndrome, rather than a chromosomal anomaly, is suspected, testing of specific gene(s) may be considered. Depending on the syndrome suspected, there may be a single gene or multiple genes identified to cause that syndrome. In some instances, single-gene testing may be of greatest diagnostic yield. However, often, a panel of genes associated with a given syndrome may be of greater yield (e.g., for suspected Noonan syndrome that has been found to be related to changes in >20 genes). Gene panels involve sequencing multiple genes simultaneously and may provide more genetic information with a shorter turnaround time than testing singles genes one at a time. As the field of genetics advances, gene panels change frequently as new genes are discovered. In addition to gene panels for specific syndromes, there are many gene panels for specific clinical features that are available through clinical genetic laboratories, such as a brain malformation panel or ciliopathy gene panel. The size and scope of panels is also variable and may range from 5 to 10 genes to more than 3,000. Some gene panels may include coverage of copy number variants (deletions and duplications) within the genes that are analyzed. The ability to detect a genetic variant in a gene and the completeness of the coverage may also differ among panels and clinical laboratories. Due to the increasing complexity of ordering genetic testing, it is likely best practice to involve a geneticist or genetic counselor in decisions regarding choice of gene panels.

---

[1]Editors' note: An overwhelming number of genetic and nongenetic associations can be encountered in the fetus. Determining which entities to include in this chapter was difficult, but the synopsis is a review of disorders that may be imaged more commonly in a perinatal practice. The section is separated into chromosomal, genetic, craniosynostosis syndromes, and nongenetic associations. The review of each of these disorders focuses on the most common organ systems affected but cannot include every anomaly cited in the literature. For tables or lists of all abnormalities possible in the syndromes discussed below and for others not reviewed, dedicated genetic texts or internet resources, especially OMIM (Online Mendelian Inheritance in Man www.omim.org) or Genereviews (http://www.ncbi.nlm.nih.gov/books/NBK1116/), may be helpful.

Broad-Based Testing

Beyond testing of chromosome complement and for variants in selected genes, broader testing is clinically available, such as whole exome sequencing (WES). Rather than analyzing specific genes of interest, WES studies approximately 20,000 genes, accounting for 2% of all human genetic material.[3] WES targets the exons, which are the protein-coding regions of the human genome. Exons are captured, sequenced using massively parallel sequencing, and analyzed for sequence variants using tools and algorithms. The process of WES includes a detailed consenting process for carrier status, secondary findings, and can take months to receive a result. A geneticist or genetic counselor should be included from initial discussions if a prenatal WES is considered. In the future, additional testing, such as whole genome sequencing, is likely to become more widely available on a clinical basis.

Overall Considerations

Before offering a genetic test, many factors weigh into the decision of which is the best test to offer. Geneticists weigh aspects of the diagnosis in question—such as how likely is the suspected diagnosis (based on prevalence, how well a patient's phenotype fits, and if it follows any inheritance patterns in the family), how important is it to exclude other conditions (in terms of diagnostic, prognostic, and treatment options), and how will the diagnosis impact the expectant parents (in terms of pregnancy decision-making, emotional state). Geneticists and genetic counselors also consider details such as clinical status, insurance coverage, difference in cost between tests, lab availability, and turnaround time when selecting a test.

CHROMOSOMAL ANOMALIES

Any individual pregnant woman's background risk of having a baby affected by a chromosomal abnormality is influenced by her age (the higher the age of the mother, the higher the risk), the gestational age (GA) (the earlier the gestation, the higher the risk), and a history of having had a previous fetus or infant with a chromosomal defect. Specifically, the risk for trisomies in women who have had a prior fetus or child with a trisomy is 0.75% higher than the risk would be otherwise.[4] Maternal age positively correlates with various chromosomal abnormalities, including trisomies 13, 18, and 21, XXX and XXY, but not with 45,X.[5] Further noninvasive tests can contribute to the calculation of a risk for a trisomy or chromosomal defect. First-trimester tests performed at 11 to 14 weeks include nuchal translucency (NT) screening and maternal serum biochemistry assessment of human chorionic gonadotropin (hCG) and pregnancy-associated plasma protein A (PAPP-A). In the second trimester, a fetal anatomy screening US typically between 18 and 22 weeks and cell-free DNA and/or maternal serum biochemistry assessment at 15 to 20 weeks known as the quad or tetra screen includes measurements of alpha-fetoprotein (AFP), hCG, estriol, and inhibin-A. Any time a screening test is performed, the background risk, based on maternal age, GA, and prior history of a trisomy, is factored into a complex calculation that includes all variables measured, and this product becomes the updated background risk for the pregnancy.

Trisomy 21

Down syndrome (DS) is also known as trisomy 21, as it is caused by the presence of additional genetic material from chromosome 21. DS is the most common autosomal trisomy and is also the most common genetic cause of developmental delay. There is an increased risk of trisomy 21 with increasing maternal age (Table 30.1). DS is associated with a number of congenital anomalies and medical issues.[6]

Incidence: The incidence of DS is approximately 1.3 in 1,000 live births, with a similar prevalence across ethnicities.[7]

Pathogenesis/Etiology: The additional chromosomal material can be identified as an entire additional copy of chromosome 21,

TABLE 30.1 Risk for Trisomy 21 Based on Maternal Age	
MATERNAL AGE (yrs)	ODDS (1 in_)
20	1,176
21	1,160
22	1,136
23	1,114
24	1,087
25	1,040
26	990
27	928
28	855
29	760
30	690
31	597
32	508
33	421
34	342
35	274
36	216
37	168
38	129
39	98
40	74
41	56
42	42
43	31
44	23

Data from Snijders RJ, Sundberg K, Holzgreve W, et al. Maternal age- and gestation-specific risk for trisomy 21. *Ultrasound Obstet Gynecol*. 1999;13(3):167–170.

which is known as full trisomy 21 and is present in 90% to 95% of individuals with DS. An unbalanced Robertsonian translocation has been noted in 3% to 4% of individuals, wherein a portion of chromosome 21 translocates to another acrocentric chromosome, usually to chromosome 14, or from mosaicism for chromosome 21 in 1% of cases.[8] In a Robertsonian translocation, all the genes on each chromosome are included since the p arms of the acrocentric chromosomes contain only repeat elements. Translocations of part of the q arm are also possible but are much less common. The additional chromosomal material is due to either nondisjunction, in the case of full trisomy, or from random inheritance of a derivative chromosome in the case of an unbalanced translocation. A known relationship between increasing maternal age and prevalence of DS is theorized to be due to prolonged time in meiotic arrest and increased likelihood of meiotic nondisjunction during egg formation.[9] In the subset of cases attributable to translocation, however, the age of the mother does not seem to be relevant.

Diagnosis: Diagnosis typically cannot be made from US or MRI findings or first-trimester screening alone. Measurement of the NT, combined with the maternal age and maternal serum markers, including hCG and PAPP-A, can increase the detection of chromosomal defects substantially.[10] New laboratory techniques have allowed for isolation of cell-free fetal DNA from maternal serum and for detection of increased ratios of the presence of chromosome 21 suggestive of DS.[1] This testing is considered by the NSGC to be a form of screening and not diagnostic at this time.[2] Further diagnostic testing via chromosome analysis, not microarray, of amniocentesis or CVS should be offered. Chromosome analysis is the gold standard as it provides diagnosis and distinguishes among types of trisomy 21 (free, translocation, or mosaic). If the diagnosis of DS is made by chromosome analysis, parents should be offered referral to a geneticist to discuss outcomes and options.

Imaging: First-trimester US between 11 and 14 weeks for measurement of the fetal NT, when combined with maternal serum biochemical evaluation, can detect 90% of trisomy 21 cases with a false-positive rate of 5%.[10] At the same time that the NT is measured, the nasal bone should be evaluated. Either an absent or short nasal bone is an important imaging feature associated with trisomy 21 and other chromosomal defects. At the 11- to 14-week scan, the absence of the nasal bone may be seen in as high as 70%

of fetuses affected by trisomy 21 (Fig. 30.1A). In contrast, a normal nasal bone is visualized in 97.3% to 99.5% of chromosomally normal fetuses.[11] As with measurement of the NT, assessment of the fetal nasal bone is technically difficult, and the UK Fetal Medicine Foundation has established standards for this technique. A midline sagittal view of the fetal profile is captured, and the image is magnified such that only the fetal head and thorax fill the screen. The angle between the US transducer and the midline of the face should be about 45°. The observer should look for three echogenic lines, representing the skin of the nose, the nasal bone, and the nasal tip (Fig. 30.1B).

The fetal anatomic assessment by US in the second trimester serves to identify both minor and major defects (Table 30.2 and Fig. 30.2). Minor defects include increased nuchal fold thickness, echogenic bowel, echogenic intracardiac focus, mild hydronephrosis, short humerus, and short femur (Fig. 30.3). Major defects include cardiac anomalies (most commonly endocardial cushion defects), duodenal atresia, cervical lymphatic malformation, and hydrops. The risk for a chromosomal abnormality increases with the number of defects identified.[12]

A second-trimester US examination to screen for abnormal fetal anomalies may show few or extensive systems affected by trisomy 21. The "genetic sonogram" refers to evaluation for anatomic abnormalities, or markers, seen in the second-trimester fetal anatomic assessment. Detection of even minor markers increases the risk of an abnormal karyotype (Table 30.3). A meta-analysis of 48 studies summarizing prenatal US from 14 to 24 weeks GA found that the combined negative likelihood ratio of all markers, including short femur, but not short humerus, was 0.13, implying that if a systematic US examination excludes all markers, there is a 7.7-fold reduction in risk.[13]

Skull and facial imaging should evaluate for acrobrachycephaly, mild ventriculomegaly, nasal bone hypoplasia, and nuchal thickening. Nasal bone length should be compared to standard measurements (see Table 25 in Appendix A1) and although controversial hypoplasia can be diagnosed when less than 2.5 or 10th percentile or less than 0.7 multiples of the mean (MoM) or via an abnormal ratio of biparietal distance to nasal bone. A recent study suggested that the best screening performance is achieved when utilizing percentiles adjusted for maternal ethnicity and when combined with other aneuploidy markers.[14] Cardiac defects might include ventricular septal defect, atrioventricular canal defect, tetralogy of Fallot, or the finding of an echogenic intracardiac focus. Intra-abdominal abnormalities to consider

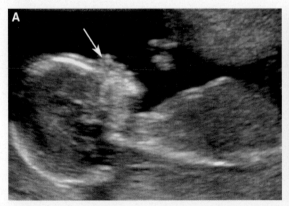
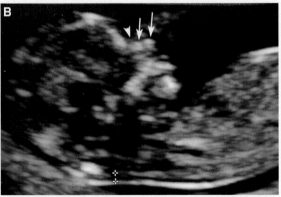

FIGURE 30.1: Absent and normal nasal bone. **A:** First-trimester fetal US showing the absence of a nasal bone (*arrow* indicates nasal soft tissue) in a fetus at gestational age 16 weeks with trisomy 21. **B:** First-trimester US in a different fetus at gestational age 13 weeks showing the expected echogenicity of the skin (*arrowhead*) and nasal bone and tip (*arrows*).

TABLE 30.2	Common Features of Major Trisomies		
	TRISOMY 21	**TRISOMY 18**	**TRISOMY 13**
Major	Cardiac defects, duodenal atresia, cystic hygroma, hydrops	Cardiac defects, spina bifida, cerebellar dysgenesis, micrognathia, diaphragmatic hernia, omphalocele, clenched hands/wrists, radial aplasia, clubfeet, cystic hygroma	Cardiac defects, central nervous system abnormalities, facial anomalies, cleft lip/palate, urogenital anomalies/echogenic kidneys, omphalocele, polydactyly, rocker-bottom feet, cystic hygroma
Minor	Nuchal thickening, hyperechoic bowel, EIF, shortened limbs, pyelectasis, mild ventriculomegaly, widened pelvic angle, shortened frontal lobe, clinodactyly, widened sandal gap, hypoplastic or absent nasal bone	Choroid cysts, brachycephaly, shortened limbs, IUGR, single umbilical artery	EIF, mild ventriculomegaly, pyelectasis, IUGR, single umbilical artery

EIF, echogenic intracardiac focus; *IUGR*, intrauterine growth retardation.
Reprinted with permission from Nyberg DA, Souter VL. Chromosomal abnormalities. In: Nyberg DA, McGahan JP, Pretorius DH, et al., eds. *Diagnostic Imaging of Fetal Anomalies*. Philadelphia, PA: Lippincott Williams & Wilkins; 2003:861–906.

are duodenal atresia, echogenic bowel, and pyelectasis. Duodenal atresia would be inferred by duodenal bulb distension proximal to the atretic segment. This pathology results in the "double-bubble" sign (Fig. 30.4A), reflecting the fluid-filled stomach adjacent to the distended duodenal bulb. In a study of prenatally diagnosed cases of double bubble, approximately 10% were found to have trisomy 21, suggesting that noninvasive screening may be helpful when present.[15] Trisomy 21 may also affect musculoskeletal development and manifest with short humerus and femur, clinodactyly, hypoplasia of the fifth digit middle phalanx, and sandal-foot deformity (Fig. 30.4B). Transient myeloproliferative disorders (transient leukemia) can manifest with heterogeneous hepatosplenomegaly and hydrops.

Fetal MRI is not commonly required for the diagnosis of trisomy 21, given the number of identifiable abnormalities evident sonographically and the biochemical and genetic testing available for diagnosis. There is no published literature showing improved diagnosis of trisomy 21 by fetal MRI. However, brain abnormalities, including mild ventriculomegaly (Fig. 30.5), are common indications for fetal MRI. When imaging a fetus for ventriculomegaly, it is important to focus not only on the fetal brain, but on the entire fetal body to exclude other associated anomalies. In the presence of DS, mild ventriculomegaly is often present without associated central nervous system (CNS) anomalies.

Gastrointestinal (GI) anomalies, such as Hirschsprung disease or anal atresia, may also be detected on second- or third-trimester MRI.

Differential Diagnosis: In the first trimester, an abnormally thick NT (>3.0 mm) can offer useful information, even with a normal chromosomal evaluation, as a thick NT is also associated with other developmental anomalies, including cardiac defects, diaphragmatic hernia, abdominal wall defects, and renal abnormalities. The NT is also useful in multiple gestation pregnancies, where maternal serum evaluation is not applicable. Discordant NT measurements in a dichorionic pregnancy would be concerning for genetic abnormalities and in a monochorionic pregnancy would be concerning for twin-to-twin transfusion.[16]

In the second trimester, multisystem developmental anomalies may be identified, and taken separately, each of these developmental anomalies has its own set of differential considerations. Thickening of the nuchal soft tissues could indicate a cervical lymphatic malformation, which may be present in isolation or as part of other trisomies (13 and 18), Turner syndrome (TS), microdeletion syndromes (13q-, 18p-), and triploidy. Nonimmune hydrops fetalis, characterized by generalized skin edema, ascites, and pericardial and pleural effusions, is a nonspecific condition resulting from a wide variety of maternal, placental, and fetal disorders.[17]

Echogenic bowel is also a nonspecific finding and is most often seen in normal fetuses. However, in addition to its increased frequency among fetuses with aneuploidy, and particularly trisomy 21, it is also associated with bowel atresia, congenital infection, and, uncommonly, with meconium ileus secondary to cystic fibrosis. Further, an increased risk of intrauterine growth retardation (IUGR), fetal demise, and placenta-related complications has been associated with echogenic bowel.[18]

Duodenal atresia, manifested by the "double-bubble" sign and polyhydramnios (see Fig. 30.4A), may not be apparent until well into the second trimester, after 20 weeks' GA. It is important to keep in mind that this sign may be seen in the normal fetus, and it is not specific for trisomy 21. Approximately 40% of prenatally detected duodenal atresia cases are not associated with a genetic defect.[19] In up to one-third of these cases, the fetus will be affected by trisomy 21. Other conditions leading to distension of the descending duodenum would include nonsyndromic duodenal

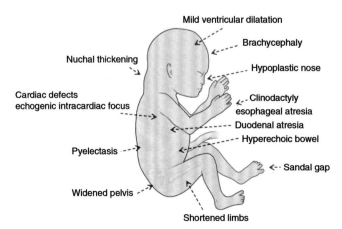

Mild ventricular dilatation
Brachycephaly
Nuchal thickening
Hypoplastic nose
Cardiac defects echogenic intracardiac focus
Clinodactyly esophageal atresia
Duodenal atresia
Hyperechoic bowel
Pyelectasis
Sandal gap
Widened pelvis
Shortened limbs

FIGURE 30.2: Common features of trisomy 21.

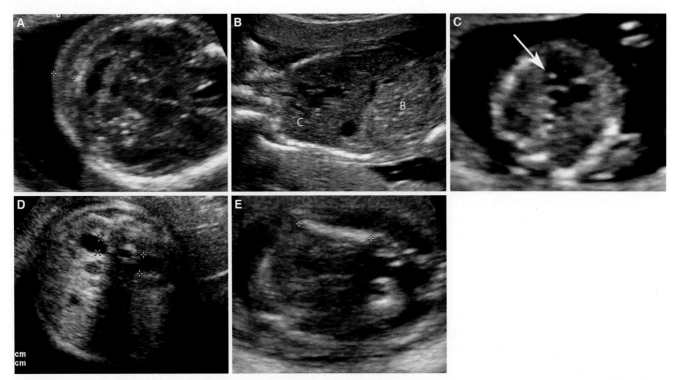

FIGURE 30.3: Minor defects detected by US in trisomy 21. **A:** Thickened nuchal fold, measuring greater than 5 mm, is marked by *calipers* in this fetus at 17 weeks' gestational age (GA). **B:** Echogenic bowel is recognized by its brightness similar to that of bone, as seen in a different fetus at 18 weeks' GA. *C,* chest; *B,* bowel. **C:** Echogenic intracardiac focus is present in the left ventricle (*arrow*) of the same fetus in **B**. **D:** Mild hydronephrosis in fetus at 24 weeks is noted with bilaterally dilated renal pelves, as determined by measuring the anteroposterior renal pelvis diameter. **E:** Short long bones (<5th percentile; femur length is 21 mm = 16 and 2/7 weeks ± 1.38 weeks) present in the same fetus as in **A**.

TABLE 30.3 Pooled Estimates of Detection Rate (DR), False-Positive Rate (FPR), and Positive and Negative Likelihood Ratios (LR1 and LR2) of Sonographic Markers for Trisomy 21 and Estimated Likelihood Ratio (LR) of Individual Isolated Markers

MARKER	DR (95% CI) (%)	FPR (95% CI) (%)	LR1 (95% CI) (%)	LR2 (95% CI) (%)	LR ISOLATED MARKER[a]
Intracardiac echogenic focus	24.4 (20.9–28.2)	3.9 (3.4–4.5)	5.83 (5.02–6.77)	0.80 (0.75–0.86)	0.95
Ventriculomegaly	7.5 (4.2–12.9)	0.2 (0.1–0.4)	27.52 (13.61–55.68)	0.94 (0.91–0.98)	3.81
Increased nuchal fold	26.0 (20.3–32.9)	1.0 (0.5–1.9)	23.30 (14.35–37.83)	0.80 (0.74–0.85)	3.79
Echogenic bowel	16.7 (13.4–20.7)	1.1 (0.8–1.5)	11.44 (9.05–14.47)	0.90 (0.86–0.94)	1.65
Mild hydronephrosis	13.9 (11.2–17.2)	1.7 (1.4–2.0)	7.63 (6.11–9.51)	0.92 (0.89–0.96)	1.08
Short humerus	30.3 (17.1–47.9)	4.6 (2.8–7.4)	4.81 (3.49–6.62)	0.74 (0.63–0.88)	0.78
Short femur	27.7 (19.3–38.1)	6.4 (4.7–8.8)	3.72 (2.79–4.97)	0.80 (0.73–0.88)	0.61
Absent or hypoplastic NB	59.8 (48.9–69.9)	2.8 (1.9–4.0)	23.27 (14.23–38.06)	0.46 (0.36–0.58)	6.58

[a]Derived by multiplying the positive LR for the given marker by the negative LR of each of all other markers.
NB, nasal bone.
From Agathokleous M, Chaveeva P, Poon LC, et al. Meta-analysis of second-trimester markers for trisomy 21. *Ultrasound Obstet Gynecol.* 2013;41(3):247–261. Copyright © 2012 ISUOG. Adapted by permission of John Wiley & Sons, Inc.

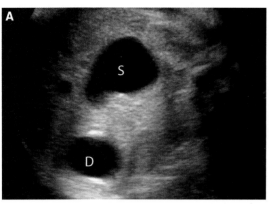
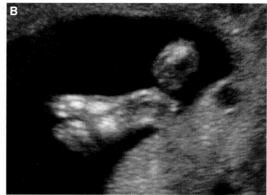

FIGURE 30.4: Additional anomalies in fetus affected by trisomy 21. **A:** Duodenal atresia is evident by a fluid-distended stomach *(S)* and proximal duodenum *(D)* in this 30-week-GA fetus. Polyhydramnios was also was also present (not shown here). **B:** Sandal-foot deformity in a 20-week-GA fetus can omit with trisomy 21. There is a gap between the first and second toes. Considerations for a gap between the second and third toes include syndactyly, ectrodactyly spectrum, and amniotic band syndrome.

atresia, pyloric atresia, extrinsic compression by a mass or by annular pancreas (a diagnosis further supported by the presence of echogenic bands around the descending duodenum), midgut volvulus secondary to malrotation, diaphragmatic hernia, or colonic duplication.[20]

Pelvocaliectasis is currently diagnosed when the anterior-to-posterior renal pelvis diameter measures ≥ 4 mm when less than 28 weeks' gestation or when ≥ 7 mm when greater than 28 weeks' gestation.[21] Although this finding has been shown to be associated with aneuploidy (and specifically, trisomy 21), the abnormality is commonly seen on screening US. The main etiological considerations include an obstructive lesion, such as ureteropelvic junction, and vesicoureteral reflux. The anomaly may be isolated or may be seen as part of a number of multisystemic syndromes.

Short long bones (femur and humerus) and other limb reduction anomalies are seen in many syndromes. Trisomy 21 should be considered if the measured-to-expected femur length ratio is less than 0.91. It would then be relevant to measure the humerus,

which is confirmed abnormal if the measured-to-expected humerus length ratio is less than 0.90.[22] Primary differential considerations include constitutional shortening of the limbs or the femurs, the latter being more common in Hispanic and Asian populations,[22] and skeletal dysplasias with either rhizomelic or micromelic shortening.

Prognosis: The prognosis for infants and children with trisomy 21 varies greatly and depends on the combination of the congenital malformations. Approximately 75% of fetuses known to have trisomy 21 will spontaneously abort or are stillborn.[23] The median age at death of individuals with DS has risen significantly in the United States, from 25 years in the early 1980s to 60 years today (http://www.ndss.org). Congenital heart disease (CHD) and respiratory infections are the most frequently reported medical cause of death.[24] Trisomy 21 is the most common genetic cause of intellectual disability, and affected individuals have intelligent quotients typically ranging from 40 to 70.[25] By 40 years of age, approximately 22% to 25% of individuals with DS develop Alzheimer dementia.[26] With the current life expectancy, approximately 70% will develop dementia in their lifetime.[27]

Management: With early prenatal diagnosis, education regarding trisomy 21 should be offered to the family to help them evaluate options and identify needed resources. Decisions regarding pregnancy termination or planning for delivery and care may be influenced by detailed imaging to identify malformations that require immediate postnatal attention or impact long-term prognosis. Following delivery, the infant should have a complete physical examination, chromosome analysis, and evaluation by a geneticist shortly after delivery. Common issues immediately after birth can include hypotonia and feeding difficulties.[6] GI anomalies (duodenal atresia, imperforate anus, Hirschsprung disease, celiac disease, and pancreas abnormalities) are seen in up to 12% of patients with DS.[6] CHD is also common, affecting up to 50% of children with DS. The CHD can range from AV canal defects (40% to 60%) to tetralogy of Fallot to atrial septal defect or ventricular septal defect.[6] For this reason, echocardiography should be performed in the first month of life or sooner if symptomatic. Pulmonary hypoplasia is common in patients with DS and can result in respiratory difficulty.[6] Blood abnormalities commonly seen include transient myeloproliferative disorder or

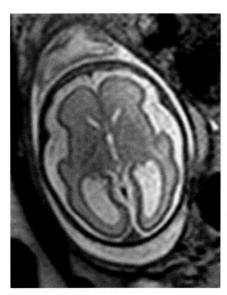

FIGURE 30.5: Axial T2 MRI of a 24-week fetus with mild ventriculomegaly measuring 12 mm at atrium but no other associated central nervous system abnormalities.

hyperviscosity syndrome, but thrombocytopenia, polycythemia, and leukemias are also possible; therefore, a screening complete blood count at the time of birth is necessary.[28] Hypothyroidism is common and is diagnosed through newborn screen.[6] Referral to appropriate specialty services should be made in the first few months after birth.[6]

Recurrence Risk: Genetic counseling should be offered to all parents of a child with DS for review of their specific recurrence risks based on the chromosomal pathogenesis. If a translocation is present (3% to 4% of cases), parents should be offered chromosome analysis to determine whether one of them is a carrier of a balanced translocation. If the translocation is de novo and neither parent has a balanced translocation, then there is no increased risk of recurrence. If the mother carries a balanced translocation, then the risk for future pregnancies is about 10% to 15%, whereas if the father carries the balanced translocation, the risk is about 3% to 5%.[8] Rarely, the translocation involves both of the chromosomes 21. In this circumstance, the carrier parent of the 21/21 translocation would have a 100% risk of recurrence. There is not an increased rate of trisomy 21 in second-degree relatives.[29]

Trisomy 18

Trisomy 18 is the second most common autosomal trisomy in live-born infants. It was described by Edwards in 1960 and is also known as Edwards syndrome. It is associated with multiple congenital anomalies, including cardiac defects, neural tube defects, congenital diaphragmatic hernia, omphalocele, cervical lymphatic malformation, limb anomalies, as well as profound developmental delay and short life expectancy.

Incidence: Trisomy 18 affects 1 in 3,000 live births.[30]

Pathogenesis/Etiology: Trisomy 18 is caused by additional genetic material from chromosome 18. Eighty percent to 85% of cases are the result of a full trisomy, 5% are due to unbalanced translocation, and 10% are mosaic. The additional chromosomal material is due to either nondisjunction in the case of full trisomy or from random inheritance of a derivative chromosome in the case of an unbalanced translocation. Trisomy 18 from a translocation is always partial trisomy since chromosome 18 is not an acrocentric chromosome and some genes will be lost at the break point. The phenotype is often different for partial trisomy 18 due to a translocation than for classical trisomy 18 secondary to nondisjunction. Trisomies 18 and 21 differ, in that the majority of meiotic errors in trisomy 18 occur in meiosis II, while trisomy 21 is typically due to meiosis I errors.[31]

Diagnosis: First-trimester screening shows low PAPP-A and low hCG. The second-trimester serum screening shows low estriol and AFP.[32] Maternal serum–derived cell-free fetal DNA testing can also detect most cases of trisomy 18, with a sensitivity and specificity similar to that found in trisomy 21. The suspected diagnosis should be confirmed with chromosome analysis on CVS or amniocentesis, regardless of the screening method used.

Imaging: Concern for aneuploidy may arise in the first trimester if the NT is thickened. Approximately 75% of cases can be detected by screening when taking into account maternal age and NT. This increases to about 96% if abnormal nasal bone, tricuspid valve, and ductus venosus flow are present.[33]

In the second trimester, suspicion for trisomy 18 is typically due to multiple anomalies seen on US.[34,35] Sonographic markers seen with trisomy 18 are summarized in Table 30.2 and Figure 30.6 and include a strawberry-shaped cranium (narrow frontal diameter and wide occipitoparietal diameter), choroid plexus cysts, clenched hands with overlapping fingers, a small omphalocele, single umbilical artery, shortened limbs, and cavovarus/clubfoot, and rocker-bottom foot deformities (Fig. 30.7). Major abnormalities include early-onset growth restriction (IUGR), cardiac defects, cervical lymphatic malformation, radial aplasia, spina bifida, esophageal atresia, and cerebellar anomalies (Fig. 30.8).

IUGR is seen in 51% of fetuses with trisomy 18 before 24 weeks' and in 89% of fetuses after 24 weeks' gestation.[35] CHD is seen in 73% to 90% of fetuses and can include atrioventricular canal defect, tetralogy of Fallot, and left heart disease.[36] Cervical lymphatic malformations can be evident by both US and fetal MRI and may range in appearance from mere nuchal thickening to a large cystic neck mass.

Neural tube defects suspected on US may be better seen by fetal MRI. Fetal karyotyping is recommended after the diagnosis of spina bifida, as approximately 17% of prenatally diagnosed cases of spina bifida are later recognized as having aneuploidy, including trisomy 18, trisomy 13, triploidy, and translocation.[37]

A mild marker for trisomies 18 and 21 are choroid plexus cysts. These are visualized commonly in the second trimester by US and bear no implication on prognosis when the karyotype is normal. The finding, when isolated, can be considered a transient, benign observation. A meta-analysis by Yoder et al.[38] reports a likelihood ratio of 13.8 (confidence interval [CI], 7.7 to 25.0) for trisomy 18 and 1.87 (CI, 0.78 to 4.46) for trisomy 21. In this study, including 1,346 fetuses with isolated choroid plexus cysts, 7 had trisomy 18, and 5 had trisomy 21. Two important variables that further increase the risk of trisomy 18 are a size greater than 10 mm and advanced maternal age.[39]

Brain malformations that are recognized in fetuses affected by trisomy 18 may include cerebellar hypoplasia, cerebellar vermian hypoplasia, agenesis of the corpus callosum, and holoprosencephaly. These disorders can be recognized by US, but fetal MRI is ideal for further evaluation of the cerebellar vermis and hemispheres (Fig 30.8). The degree of incomplete fusion of the hemispheres in holoprosencephaly is also readily detected by fetal MRI.

Facial abnormalities that may be found in trisomy 18 fetuses include cleft lip, cleft palate, ocular abnormalities (particularly in

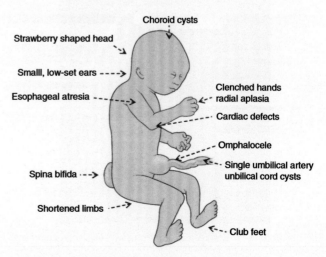

FIGURE 30.6: Common features of trisomy 18.

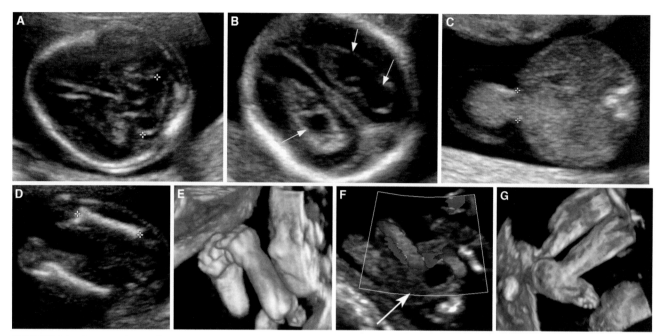

FIGURE 30.7: Sonographic markers of trisomy 18. **A:** A strawberry-shaped calvarium in a 19-week-gestaional age fetus. **B:** Choroid plexus cysts are noted as well-demarcated anechoic spaces within the bulk (*arrows*) of the echogenic choroid. **C:** Small omphaloceles are additional features of this disorder. **D:** Bilateral femurs and remaining long bones are abnormally short (<5th percentile; femur length of 22 mm = 16 and 4/7 weeks = ±1.38 weeks). **E:** Clenched hands may be observed by two-dimensional US and easily seen with three-dimensional US. **F:** A single umbilical artery in isolation is usually of no clinical significance but, with other malformations, contributes to the likelihood of a chromosomal anomaly. *Arrow* indicates the expected location of a nonvisualized umbilical artery. **G:** Foot abnormalities include rocker-bottom foot, as seen in a different 23-week fetus on three-dimensional US.

the context of severe midline brain anomalies), and micrognathia. Cleft defects, ocular anomalies, and micrognathia are well seen by US. However, brain anomalies not detected by US may accompany these facial anomalies and could be elucidated by the adjunctive use of MRI.

Intrathoracic and abdominal malformations, including diaphragmatic hernia and omphalocele, are typically recognized in the second trimester. Fetal MRI can clarify location of intrathoracic and intra-abdominal structures and assess compromise of pulmonary development by calculation of fetal lung volumes. Skeletal anomalies can be evaluated in real time with US, and it is uncommon that fetal MRI is required for clarification of clubfoot and rocker-bottom deformities or radial ray anomalies. When performing MRI for other reasons, however, it is important to attempt to visualize the extremities, and thick-slab T2 images and cine sequences can allow for a global assessment of skeletal position and movement.

Differential Diagnosis: First-trimester findings of increased nuchal thickness and early IUGR may be seen with other major chromosomal abnormalities. It has been reported that the risk for aneuploidy is substantially increased (odds ratio of 9.04) when the crown-rump length is shortened by 14 mm or more from that expected for the menstrual age.[40]

There are a number of prenatally detected anatomic features of trisomy 18 that each independently has other differential considerations. A single umbilical artery is a frequent association of congenital anomalies and chromosomal abnormalities.[41] Over 50% of fetuses with trisomy 18 have a single umbilical artery. Other entities with a high incidence of single umbilical artery include trisomy 13, Turner syndrome, and triploidy.

CNS abnormalities may be seen in trisomy 18, and there is wide overlap with other syndromes and disease processes in this category. Cerebellar hemispheric and vermian hypoplasia may also be seen with various chromosomal abnormalities, including trisomy 13, and may be seen in the context of other more complex hindbrain malformations such as Dandy–Walker malformations, rhombencephalosynapsis, and Joubert syndrome. Holoprosencephaly has a high association with chromosomal anomalies, most often trisomy 13, but is also seen with trisomy 18, triploidy, and many chromosomal deletions (see Table 15.1-5 in Chapter 15.1). Congenital diaphragmatic hernia (CDH) and omphalocele are each observed in a wide number of fetuses affected by chromosomal abnormalities. CDH is most often associated with trisomies 18, 13, and 21 and Turner syndrome.[42] Omphalocele carries an even higher risk of aneuploidy than does CDH, particularly if the omphalocele contains the liver. Trisomies 18 and 13 are reported most often, followed by trisomy 21, Turner syndrome, and triploidy. A syndrome that often presents with an omphalocele is Beckwith–Wiedemann.

Prognosis: Trisomy 18 is highly lethal in utero. A recent meta-analysis showed that only 48% of fetuses with trisomy 18 are live born, and of these, 39% survive beyond 48 hours and 11% beyond 1 month.[43] Therefore, trisomy 18 is not uniformly lethal. Interestingly, females with trisomy 18 are more likely to be born alive and survive longer than males with trisomy 18.[44] Although US abnormalities are present in the majority of cases, the findings are not predictive of outcome.[43]

A review of outcomes of patients with trisomy 18 has shown that the average survival is 7 to 14 days. For infants discharged home, median survival is 1 to 2 months for males and 9 to 10

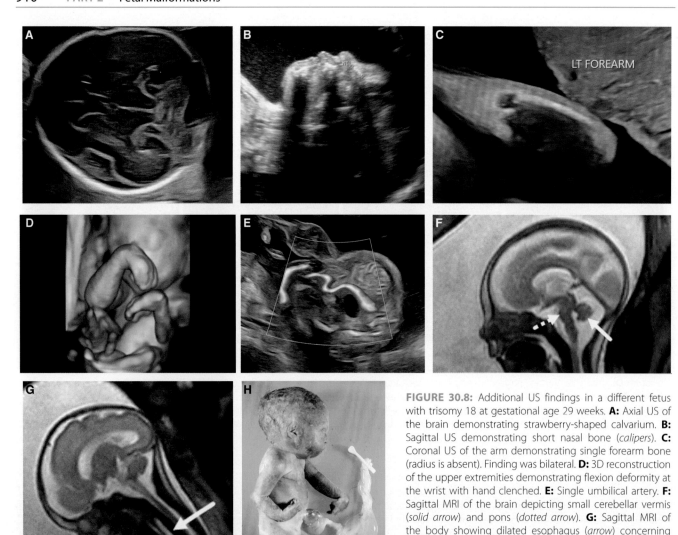

FIGURE 30.8: Additional US findings in a different fetus with trisomy 18 at gestational age 29 weeks. **A:** Axial US of the brain demonstrating strawberry-shaped calvarium. **B:** Sagittal US demonstrating short nasal bone (*calipers*). **C:** Coronal US of the arm demonstrating single forearm bone (radius is absent). Finding was bilateral. **D:** 3D reconstruction of the upper extremities demonstrating flexion deformity at the wrist with hand clenched. **E:** Single umbilical artery. **F:** Sagittal MRI of the brain depicting small cerebellar vermis (*solid arrow*) and pons (*dotted arrow*). **G:** Sagittal MRI of the body showing dilated esophagus (*arrow*) concerning for tracheoesophageal fistula. There was polyhydramnios present. **H:** A postmortem photograph of a different fetus with trisomy 18 showing multiple anomalies, including flexed hands and wrists, clubfeet, brachycephaly, omphalocele, and umbilical cord pseudocyst. (Courtesy of Raj Kapur, Pathology Department, Seattle Children's Hospital, Washington, DC.)

months for females.[45] Five percent to 10% of infants with trisomy 18 survive up to 1 year.[44] The most common causes of death include apnea, cardiopulmonary arrest, CHD, and pneumonia.[45] Of patients who survive beyond 1 year of age, major medical problems include scoliosis, hearing loss, and Wilms tumor.[46] Developmental delays are severe to profound. Patients with trisomy 18 may require significant inpatient hospital care.[47]

Management: If not obtained prenatally, chromosome analysis should be performed to confirm the diagnosis. If the pregnancy is not terminated electively, infants who survive to delivery can have multiple complications. A complete physical examination should evaluate for growth restriction, abnormal head shape, and an abnormal thorax due to a short sternum and narrow transverse chest diameter. Other typical findings include hypertonia, hypoplastic toenails, micrognathia, and low-arch dermal ridges.[30] Because of the high likelihood of CHD, echocardiography should be performed after birth.[46] Very few infants with trisomy 18 are able to feed orally, so nasogastric or gastrostomy tube feedings is often necessary.

Recurrence Risk: Families should receive genetic counseling when a diagnosis is made or suspected. The recurrence risk for full trisomy 18 is 1% or maternal age–associated risk or whichever is greater. The recurrence risk for parents with a balanced translocation may be as high as 50%.[45]

Trisomy 13

Trisomy 13 is the third most common autosomal aneuploidy in live-born infants. It was described by Patau in 1960 and is also known as Patau syndrome. It is associated with multiple congenital anomalies, including cardiac defects, CNS and facial anomalies, urogenital defects, omphalocele, cervical lymphatic malformation, and limb anomalies, as well as profound developmental delay and short life expectancy.[45]

Incidence: Trisomy 13 affects 1 in 5,000 live births.[45]

Pathogenesis/Etiology: Trisomy 13 is caused by additional genetic material from chromosome 13. Eighty percent of cases are the result of a full trisomy, and 20% are due to unbalanced translocation or mosaicism. The additional chromosomal material is due to either nondisjunction usually during maternal meiosis I in the case of full trisomy, or random inheritance of a derivative chromosome in the presence of an unbalanced translocation.[48] Both Robertsonian and non-Robertsonian translocations are associated with trisomy 13. Non-Robertsonian translocations are more likely to be associated with long-term survival. The phenotype of trisomy 13 with Robertsonian translocation is similar to that associated with nondisjunction.

Diagnosis: The standard tetra biochemistry serum screening does not detect fetuses with trisomy 13; however, screening for PAPP-A in the first trimester can identify trisomy 13.[49] Maternal serum cell-free fetal DNA testing can detect trisomy 13, but is not as sensitive for chromosome 13 as for chromosome 18 or 21. This may lead to false-negative results. Amniocentesis or CVS should be offered to confirm an abnormal screen or in case of high suspicion based on the pattern of malformations identified. FISH may be performed to obtain a more rapid diagnosis.

Imaging: Abnormal US findings are a common cause for suspicion of the diagnosis of trisomy 13. In the first trimester, the only discernible abnormality might be a thickened NT.[50] Approximately 75% of cases can be detected by screening when taking into account maternal age and NT. This increases to about 96% if abnormal nasal bone, tricuspid valve, and ductus venosus flow are present.[33]

There are minor and major markers that should be excluded on the second-trimester fetal anatomy US (summarized in Table 30.2 and Fig. 30.9). The more subtle sonographic abnormalities that might raise suspicion for trisomy 13 include low-set ears, cleft lip or palate, mild ventriculomegaly, polydactyly, echogenic intracardiac focus, small omphalocele, single umbilical artery, and cavovarus deformity (Fig. 30.10A–D).[51] Severe abnormalities include holoprosencephaly, cardiac defects, and renal anomalies (Fig. 30.10E, F). The most common US finding is holoprosencephaly and can be seen as early as 12 weeks of gestation.[50] Cardiac defects are often seen (in 80% to 100% of cases), and lesions include atrioventricular septal defect, hypoplastic left ventricle, or double outlet right ventricle.[51]

Fetal MRI may clarify findings of the fetal brain, specifically features of holoprosencephaly. Delineation of anatomic structures using MRI may be required for further evaluation of congenital diaphragmatic hernia, omphalocele, and renal and genitourinary abnormalities.

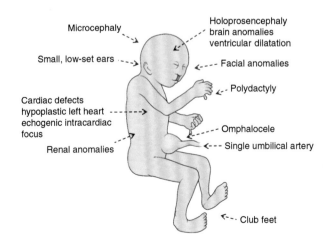

FIGURE 30.9: Common features of trisomy 13.

Differential Diagnosis: The observation of multisystem anomalies strongly supports a chromosomal abnormality or a severe manifestation of a syndrome. Many of the abnormalities overlap with trisomies 21 and 18, which would be differential consideration. Additional considerations could include Smith–Lemli–Opitz syndrome and Meckel–Gruber syndrome.

Prognosis: Trisomy 13 is highly lethal in utero. In a study evaluating the timing of miscarriage in fetuses with trisomy 13, it has been noted that the mean gestation is approximately 80 days and that only 5 of 62 fetuses carried beyond 100 days will survive beyond gestation.[52] This suggests that there are specific times during development when fetuses with trisomy 13 are more likely to die. Median postnatal survival is 7 to 10 days, and only 5% to 10% of infants with trisomy 13 survive for 1 year.[44] Those who live beyond the perinatal period have severe developmental disabilities, feeding difficulties, apnea, poor growth, seizures, and hypertension, thus receiving significant inpatient hospital care.[4,46,47] A case report of a female with trisomy 13 at age 12 years has been described.

Management: Once diagnosed, implications exist for both the fetus and the mother. Mothers of infants with trisomy 13 have an increased risk of developing severe preeclampsia.[53] This is theorized to be due to an increase in soluble fms-like tyrosine kinase (sFlt-1), an antiangiogenic protein whose gene is on chromosome 13. The protein can be released from the placenta into the maternal circulation and lead to endothelial dysfunction that may result in hypertension, proteinuria, and edema.[54]

Infants who survive to delivery should have chromosomal confirmation if not performed prenatally. Complete physical examination may show scalp defects, microcephaly, microphthalmia, cleft lip and palate, omphalocele, genital abnormalities, and polydactyly. Supportive care may be necessary for feeding difficulties and seizures.

Recurrence Risk: The recurrence risk for full trisomy 13 is 1% or the maternal age–associated risk or whichever is greater. The recurrence risk for parents with a balanced translocation is highly variable. The risk is estimated to be 20% for spontaneous abortion.[55] Recurrence risk for trisomy 13 can range from less than 1% for cases that involve mosaicism to 100% for rare cases of a parental balanced 13–13 Robertsonian translocation.

Triploidy and Tetraploidy

Triploidy and tetraploidy are two forms of polyploidy syndromes. Unlike the aneuploidy syndromes described with a single extra chromosome, the polyploidy syndromes consist of entire additional sets of genetic material. A haploid cell has 23 chromosomes; therefore, a triploid cell has 69 chromosomes and a tetraploid cell 92 chromosomes.

Incidence: Polyploidies can occur in up to 1% to 2% of conceptions, but are only seen in 1 in 10,000 live births.[56]

Pathogenesis/Etiology: In triploidy, the additional set of chromosomal material is due to failure of division in meiosis I or II in the spermatocyte (diandry) or oocyte (digyny), or, alternatively, the additional chromosomal material may arise from double fertilization of a normal ovum (dispermy). The source is most often paternal (75%), with the most common karyotype being 69 XXY (60%), and less frequent 69 XXX (37%) or 69 XXX (3%).[56] There is no association between triploidy and advanced maternal

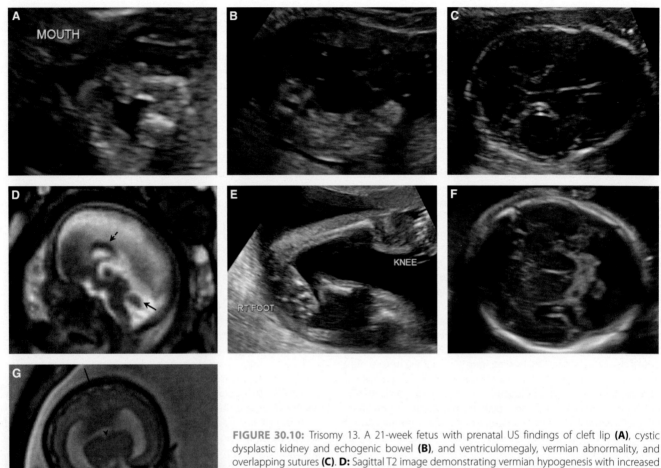

FIGURE 30.10: Trisomy 13. A 21-week fetus with prenatal US findings of cleft lip **(A)**, cystic dysplastic kidney and echogenic bowel **(B)**, and ventriculomegaly, vermian abnormality, and overlapping sutures **(C)**. **D:** Sagittal T2 image demonstrating vermian hypogenesis with increased tegmentovermian angle (*solid arrow*) and thickened corpus callosum (*dotted arrow*). **E:** US demonstrating clubfoot deformity. **F:** US of a fetus at 31-week gestation demonstrating fused thalami and lack of hemispheric separation consistent with holoprosencephaly. **G:** Coronal MRI of the same fetus in **F** confirming fusion of the thalami (*arrowhead*) and hemispheres (*solid arrow*). The ears are prominent and low in position (*dashed arrows*).

age, but there have been associations made between triploidy and delayed fertilization, for example, in the presence of prolonged menstrual cycles or with oral contraceptive discontinuation.[57]

Triploid fetuses can have variable features that range from nearly normal-appearing to multiple anomalies (Fig. 30.11). Interestingly, the underlying meiotic error has been associated with the features of the fetus.[58] In one type, typically due to diandry (paternal origin or dispermy), the fetus is well developed, but the placenta is large and cystic. The second type usually of digyny (maternal origin of diploid oocyte) is associated with a growth-restricted fetus having a relatively large head, but a small and noncystic placenta.

Diagnosis: An increased AFP level on quad screen may suggest triploidy. A low PAPP-A can also be seen with triploidy.[59] It is possible to diagnose fetal tetraploidy from amniocentesis or CVS, although it is important to consider false-positive results on CVS due to confined placental mosaicism and placental artifact.[60] Maternal serum cell-free fetal DNA testing does not detect triploidy or tetraploidy. Chromosome analysis should be offered to confirm the suspected diagnosis based on screening or imaging studies.

Imaging: Triploidy can be suggested by transvaginal US between 12 and 16 by the presence of molar changes in the placenta or a

cluster of unusual findings.[61] These include asymmetric growth restriction with abdominal circumference lagging 2 weeks behind head circumference, oligohydramnios, abnormal posterior fossa or enlarged fourth ventricle, and absent gallbladder[61] (Fig. 30.12).

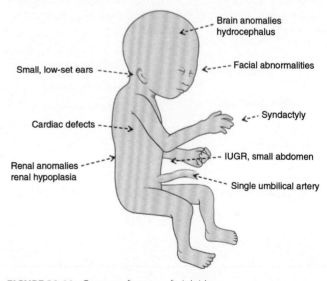

FIGURE 30.11: Common features of triploidy.

Other features that can be seen on US include hydrocephalus, micrognathia, microphthalmia, omphalocele, neural tube defects, cardiac and renal abnormalities, hypoplastic lungs, clenched hands, and 3–4 digital syndactyly.[61,62]

Tetraploidy is even more rare than triploidy. Less than 30 fetuses with tetraploidy have been reported to date. Tetraploid fetuses can also have variable features, including growth retardation, limb anomalies, abnormal positioning, low-set ears, increased nuchal thickness, and internal abnormalities.[63]

Differential Diagnosis: The differential diagnosis may include IUGR-related causes or other aneuploidy. A complete molar pregnancy (complete mole or hydatidiform mole) should also be considered. A complete mole occurs when a single sperm or two sperm fertilize an egg that has lost its DNA. If two sperm fertilize the egg, a diploid karyotype of either 46,XX or 46,XY could be seen. If a single sperm fertilizes such an egg, mitosis leads to replication of its genetic material, the genotype is diploid (46,XX or 46,YY is not seen). The result is gestational trophoblastic disease, wherein a mass of trophoblastic tissue with dilated chorionic villi, grossly appearing as a cluster of grapes, grows within the uterus.[64]

Prognosis: Most triploid fetuses miscarry. Triploidy is one of the most common diagnoses seen in first-trimester products of conception.[65] For each triploid born alive, approximately 1,200 are miscarried. There are no known triploidy survivals beyond 10.5 months.[66] There are no known tetraploidy survivals beyond 2 years.[64]

Management: Triploid diagnosis has implications for the mother as there is increased risk of vaginal bleeding and severe preeclampsia. The large placenta can also cause postpartum hemorrhage.[67] Maternal risks and fetal prognosis should be discussed. Elective termination should be offered, if early in gestation before time of legal termination. Cesarean section is indicated only to assist in delivery for maternal health.

In all cases of triploidy and tetraploidy, chromosome analysis should be performed to confirm the diagnosis. Supportive comfort care is recommended as both typically present with multiple complications. Infants with triploidy who survive to delivery often have growth restriction, macrocephaly, colobomas, cleft palate, micrognathia, and hypotonicity. Infants with

tetraploidy have growth restriction, developmental delay, and dysmorphic features, such as microcephaly, a prominent narrow forehead, microphthalmia or anophthalmia, and cleft palate.[63] It is important to keep in mind that examination findings can be subtle, so the diagnosis can be unsuspected for both disorders.

Recurrence Risk: The cause of triploidy and tetraploidy is unclear. Parents with a fetus with triploidy or tetraploidy are thought to be at slightly increased risk for chromosomal abnormalities, not solely triploidy or tetraploidy.[63]

Turner Syndrome

Turner syndrome (TS), also known as XO syndrome and monosomy X owing to loss of the second sex chromosome, is the most common sex chromosomal abnormality.[68] The syndrome was first described in 1938 by Henry Turner.

Incidence: TS is present in 1 in 2,500 female live births.[68] However, it is highly lethal in utero.[69] There is no relationship between increasing maternal age and prevalence of TS.[70]

Pathogenesis/Etiology: The loss of chromosomal material is variable and can be seen as an entirely lost chromosome, full 45X, in 50% of individuals, a structural abnormality of one X chromosome in 10% to 20%, or a mosaicism in 30% to 40%.[70] A common structural abnormality is the formation of an isochromosome, wherein one arm of the chromosome is duplicated and the other portion of the arm is lost. The lost sex chromosome can be due to either nondisjunction in the case of full 45X or from random inheritance of a derivative chromosome, as in the case of a structural chromosomal abnormality.

The severity of clinical phenotype cannot be predicted by type of karyotype, but the phenotype may differ depending on parental origin of remaining X chromosome.[71] In some infants with TS, the disease may not become apparent until later in life when a female presents with short stature and primary amenorrhea.[69] Mosaicism is quite common in TS. In cases with mosaicism, the unaffected cells may contain a Y chromosome.

Diagnosis: Serum screening findings include reduced AFP, reduced estriol, and elevated β-hCG.[72] Detection of abnormal X

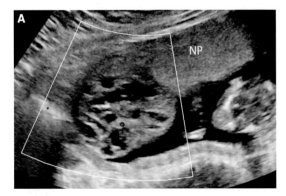
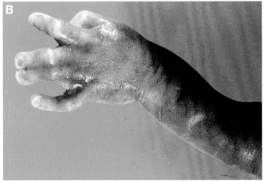

FIGURE 30.12: Cystic placental changes in triploidy. **A:** US of a twin pregnancy at 17 weeks' gestational age showing the normal placenta (*NP*) of a healthy twin adjacent to an abnormally cystic placenta of the twin affected by triploidy. **B:** A pathological photograph showing characteristic syndactyly of the third and fourth fingers. (Courtesy of Joe Siebert, Pathology Department, Seattle Children's Hospital, Washington, DC.)

chromosome ratios in cell-free fetal DNA is available as a clinical screening test. Amniocentesis or CVS should be offered.

Imaging: Multiple anomalies may be present on US (Fig. 30.13), though biochemical markers and chromosome analysis are more accurate at diagnosis. MRI typically is not necessary to aid in diagnosis. Approximately 75% of cases can be detected by screening US when taking into account NT, which increases to about 96% if abnormal nasal bone, tricuspid valve, and ductus venosus flow are present.[33]

TS results in lymphangiectasia and lymphatic malformations, manifesting in early pregnancy by fetal hydrops and large, septated cervical anechoic masses. The first-trimester manifestation of TS is typically an increased NT. A large yolk sac greater than 6 mm has also been reported.[73] Fetal hydrops may develop in either the first or the second trimester and is evident by pronounced skin thickening, pleural effusions, and ascites (Fig. 30.14A, B). Additional systems affected include the heart, kidneys, and the skeletal system.

A full anatomy assessment in the second trimester may reveal left heart congenital anomalies, such as coarctation or hypoplastic left heart syndrome. These cardiac lesions are the most common prenatal finding, whereas bifid aortic valve followed by mitral valve disease is the most common postnatally.[74] Findings

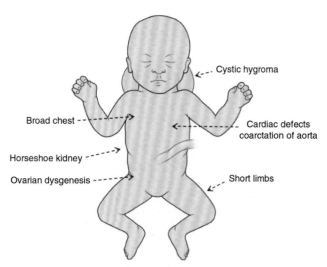

FIGURE 30.13: Common features of Turner syndrome (45X).

of coarctation on grayscale and Doppler imaging are poststenotic dilatation distal to the level of narrowing in the descending thoracic aorta and an abrupt velocity increase at the site of stenosis. Renal abnormalities in affected fetuses are usually not evident

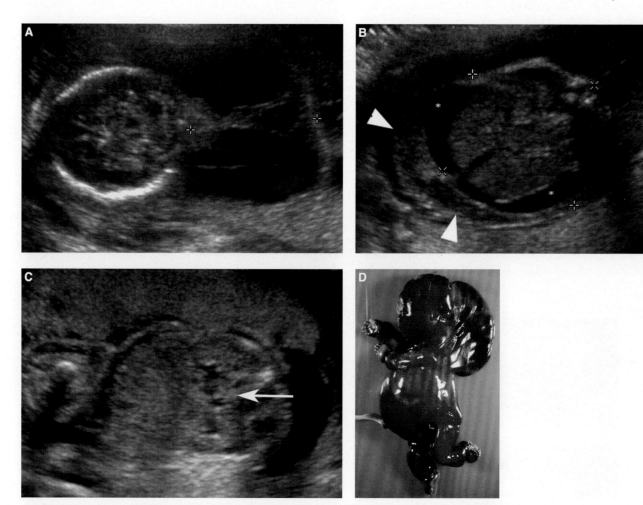

FIGURE 30.14: Turner syndrome in a 17-week fetus. **A:** A complex predominantly anechoic structure containing multiple septations along the posterior subcutaneous tissues of the neck (*calipers demarcating*), consistent with a lymphatic malformation. **B:** Fetal hydrops was also observed, with ascites (*asterisks*) and extensive skin thickening (*arrowheads*). **C:** The kidneys of this fetus are fused across the midline consistent with horseshoe kidney (*arrow*). **D:** A postmortem photograph of another fetus with Turner syndrome showing a large nuchal lymphatic malformation.

until the second trimester. Malformations of the urinary system are present in 30% to 40% of patients with TS, with collecting system anomalies most common, followed by horseshoe kidneys (Fig. 30.14C), malrotation, and ectopia.[75]

Short stature is a common clinical feature of TS, and the earliest prenatal manifestation of this is IUGR and short femur. Other skeletal abnormalities manifest postnatally and may include hip dislocation in infancy, scoliosis, and kyphosis. Short neck, broad chest, cubitus valgus, genu valgum, and short fourth metacarpals are also seen in TS.[76] Edema of the hands and feet in female fetuses is also potentially suggestive of TS. This may be seen both prenatally and postnatally.

Differential Diagnosis: In the first trimester of a monosomy X fetus, a thick NT reflects the development of a lymphatic malformation. The differential diagnosis for a thick NT is extensive and includes aneuploidy and multiple syndromes (Table 30.4). Observed chromosomal syndromes other than TS include trisomy 13, trisomy 18, trisomy 21, and triploidy with mosaicism. In one series, the most frequently observed abnormality in nonseptated cervical lymphatic malformation was trisomy 21 and that in septated malformations was TS.[77]

Prognosis: A small minority of conceptions with TS will survive to delivery. Girls with mosaicism for TS may have cells with all or a portion of the Y chromosome and are at risk for gonadoblastoma.[78] Intelligence is typically normal, but girls with TS may have learning disabilities.[69] Infants with TS may have a wide variety of clinical manifestations, but some are clinically normal at birth. The prognosis is generally good for those with only mild manifestations on prenatal imaging.

Management: The presence of a cervical lymphatic malformation, particularly in the setting of an abnormal karyotype, merits offering the option of termination of pregnancy due to the high risk of fetal loss. The newborn infant should have a complete physical examination with confirmed chromosome analysis. The typical phenotype includes short stature and a webbed appearance of the neck soft tissues, attributable to regression of the lymphatic malformation. Common issues immediately after birth include small for gestational age, lymphedema, and feeding difficulty due to inefficient sucking and swallowing.[69]

Increasing recognition of silent CHD leading to shorter life span has led to an increased referral to pediatric cardiologist with echocardiography and cardiac MRI as needed. Cardiac lesions, such as coarctation, most commonly require intervention. Renal anomalies may require renal US with routine follow-up to ensure continued normal renal function and to evaluate for complications, such as recurrent urinary tract infection and nephrolithiasis. Evaluation for congenital hip dysplasia is indicated.[69]

TABLE 30.4	**Differential Diagnosis for Abnormally Thick Nuchal Translucency (≥3 mm)[a]**		
CHROMOSOMAL ANOMALIES	**SKELETAL ABNORMALITIES**	**OTHER SYNDROMES AND SEQUENCES**	**OTHER CAUSES**
Trisomies: • Trisomy 21 (Down syndrome) • Trisomy 18 (Edwards syndrome) • Trisomy 13 (Patau syndrome) • Other trisomies (9, 10, 22)	Limb deletions syndromes: • Fanconi anemia • Holt–Oram syndrome • Roberts syndrome • Cornelia de Lange syndrome • Smith–Lemli–Opitz syndrome • Ectrodactyly–ectodermal dysplasia–clefting (EEC) syndrome • Thrombocytopenia-absent radius (TAR) syndrome • Orofaciodigital syndrome type IV	Noonan syndrome CHARGE syndrome Limb-body-wall complex Caudal regression syndrome Arthrogryposis Congenital adrenal hyperplasia Congenital high airway obstruction syndrome	Congenital cardiac disease. Chance of CHD increases exponentially with increasing NT: 0.6%–5% with NT between 2.5 and 3.5 mm; 64% with NT > 8.5 mm
Turner syndrome (XO syndrome) Triploidy Tetraploidy Deletion syndromes: • DiGeorge syndrome (22q11.2) • Deletion 5p (Cri-du-chat syndrome) • Deletion 11q (Jacobsen syndrome)	Skeletal dysplasias: • Achondrogenesis • Achondroplasia • Camptomelic dysplasia • Ellis–van Creveld syndrome • Jeune thoracic dystrophy • Thanatophoric dysplasia • Spondylothoracic dysplasia • Diastrophic dysplasia • Spondyloepiphyseal dysplasia congenita (SEDC) Split-hand/foot malformation Spinal muscular atrophy	Fryns syndrome Cerebrofrontofacial syndrome Multiple pterygium syndrome	

[a]Over 100 chromosomal aberrations and syndromes have been described in association with a thickened NT, and this table only includes the more commonly seen entities. CHD, congenital heart disease; NT, nuchal translucency.

Long-term management of TS includes hormone treatment, especially growth hormone for short stature and estrogen for feminization and bone health. Close monitoring for other medical complications such as cardiovascular and autoimmune disease are warranted.[69–75]

Recurrence Risk: The recurrence risk for TS is very low as inheritance is sporadic. However, when women with TS conceive, amniocentesis should be offered as there is up to 30% risk of chromosomal or congenital abnormalities.[78]

GENETIC SYNDROMES

Beckwith–Wiedemann Syndrome

Beckwith–Wiedemann syndrome (BWS) is one in a group of syndromes known as the overgrowth syndrome.[79] Affected individuals may have asymmetric growth of the body, including hemihypertrophy of solid organs, and patients with BWS have an increased risk of Wilms tumor, hepatoblastoma, neuroblastoma, rhabdomyosarcoma, and adrenocortical carcinoma.[79]

Incidence: BWS affects 1 in 13,700 live births.[79] BWS is more common in women who have undergone in vitro fertilization (IVF) treatment. It is seen in 1 in 4,000 deliveries that have used assisted reproductive technology.

Pathogenesis/Etiology: Abnormal imprinting on chromosome 11p15.5 is the underlying genetic cause of this syndrome.[80] Imprinting refers to the phenomenon whereby addition of methyl groups to the genetic material from one parent determines its expression. In general, children of parents with impaired fertility who are conceived by assisted reproductive technology may have an increased risk for all imprinting disorders.[80]

Most individuals with BWS are reported to have normal chromosome studies or karyotypes, and approximately 85% of individuals with BWS have no family history.[81] Up to 20% of BWS is due to paternal uniparental disomy. In this scenario, both copies of 11p15.5 come from the father, and the maternal copy is lost. The parental origin of chromosomal material on routine chromosome analysis is not discernible; therefore, this genetic abnormality is undetectable on karyotype. Methylation studies for the critical region on chromosome 11 are the most sensitive initial study. A minority of cases are due to mutation in the *CDKN1C* gene. This accounts for up to 15% of cases but is the most common cause of cases with apparent autosomal dominant inheritance.[82] Only 1% to 2% of cases have a recognizable cytogenetic abnormality, with duplication, inversion, or deletion as the cause.[79]

Diagnosis: Consideration of chromosome analysis and/or molecular genetic testing should be based on US findings (e.g., omphalocele, macrosomia, macroglossia). Molecular studies for BWS are clinically available, but must be specifically requested (Table 30.5). In cases with a known genetic mechanism in the family, testing could be performed on an amniocentesis sample. Without a known genetic mechanism, testing may be negative, but this does not exclude BWS due to the complex genetics of this syndrome; consultation with a geneticist may aid in testing.[83] Regardless, diagnostic testing should be offered to evaluate for chromosomal abnormalities by amniocentesis or CVS.

Imaging: In a recent large study, the prenatal detection rate for BWS has been cited at approximately 64%, with mean age at diagnosis of 19 to 20 weeks.[84] Abdominal wall defects are

TABLE 30.5 Summary of Molecular Genetic Testing Used in Beckwith–Wiedemann Syndrome

CAUSE OF BWS BY MOLECULAR MECHANISM	TEST METHOD	MUTATIONS/ALTERATIONS DETECTED	PROPORTION OF BWS ALTERATIONS DETECTED[1]
Loss of methylation at IC2 on the maternal chromosome	Methylation analysis	Methylation abnormalities at IC2 on the maternal chromosome	50%
Gain of methylation at IC1 on the maternal chromosome		Methylation abnormalities at IC1 on the maternal chromosome	5%
Mutation of the maternal *CDKN1C* allele	Sequence analysis	*CDKN1C* mutations	5% in persons with no family history of BWS ~40% in persons with a positive family history of BWS
Paternal uniparental disomy of 11p15.5	UPD analysis	11p15.5 paternal uniparental disomy	20%
Duplication, inversion, or translocation of 11p15.5	Cytogenetic analysis (karyotype) FISH	Cytogenetic duplication, inversion, or translocation Primarily used to clarify the relative positions of a chromosome 11 inversion or translocation and to confirm duplication of chromosome 11	1%
Submicroscopic genomic alteration within chromosome 11p15.5	Microdeletion/ microduplication analysis	Genomic alterations involving IC1 and/or IC2	Not yet accurately determined

UPD, uniparental disomy; *FISH,* fluorescence in situ hybridization.

common in BWS.[81] The diagnosis may be suspected as early as 12 weeks' GA if an omphalocele is observed. Between 10% and 43% of fetuses with apparently isolated omphalocele have BWS.[85] An exclusively bowel containing small omphalocele is the most common finding and routinely identified early in gestation with 100% accuracy.[86]

Second-trimester fetal anatomic US may detect the classic features of BWS, including global macrosomia, macroglossia, omphalocele, enlargement and echogenicity of the kidneys, and polyhydramnios (Fig. 30.15A). Beckwith–Wiedemann should always be considered when macrosomia and an omphalocele are both observed either via US or MRI (Fig. 30.15B, C). However, the development of macrosomia, macroglossia, visceromegaly, and retrognathia are not usually seen until later gestation, typically the late second trimester or third trimester.[86] Routine US may also detect placentomegaly, with placental abnormalities suggesting a partial mole or mesenchymal dysplasia.[87] A higher level focused US can reveal cardiomyopathy with cardiomegaly.

Additional occasional findings that standard US screening is unlikely to detect include cryptorchidism, hypospadias, embryonal tumors, pancreas enlargement, and renal cystic dysplasia. Although fetal MRI is not generally indicated to make this diagnosis, more detailed evaluation of the anatomy by MRI may be pursued for suboptimal imaging by US. On MRI, renal or adrenal enlargement, a suspected neoplasm, and more subtle findings of BWS might be discernible (Fig. 30.15D).[88] Not only will MRI allow for evaluation of the extent of newly recognized fetal tumors in fetuses with BWS, but the technique has been shown to be useful in the distinction of adrenal cystic changes from neuroblastoma.[89]

Differential Diagnosis: Other causes of macrosomia include incorrect dates, maternal diabetes, genetic anomalies, and chromosomal defects (Table 30.6). Genetic syndromes, including Perlman

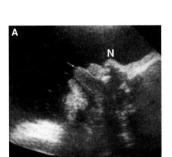
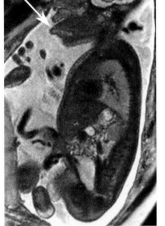
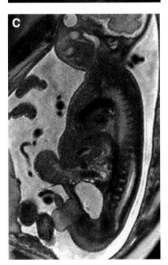
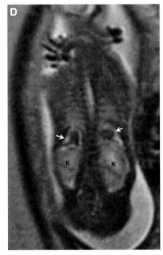

FIGURE 30.15: Beckwith–Wiedemann syndrome (BWS) US and MRI in three separate fetuses. **A:** Third-trimester sagittal view of the face showing macroglossia (*arrow*). *N*, nose. **B:** Sagittal T2 MRI in a 30-week fetus with enlargement of the tongue (*arrow*) persistently protruding beyond the lips. **C:** Sagittal T2 image of same fetus demonstrating a small omphalocele containing loops of bowel. (Courtesy of Dr. Chris Cassady, Houston, TX.) **D:** Coronal T2 image of a third fetus with BWS. Fetus has enlarged adrenal glands (*arrow*) and kidneys (*K*) bilaterally.

TABLE 30.6	Differential Diagnosis of Fetal Overgrowth	
	GENE INVOLVED	**INHERITANCE PATTERN**
Incorrect GA	NA	NA
Maternal diabetes	NA	NA
Genetic		
Sotos syndrome	*NSD1*	Sporadic/AD
Weaver syndrome	*NSD1*	Sporadic/AD
Beckwith–Wiedemann syndrome	Imprinted gene on 11p15	85% sporadic/ 15% AD
Simpson–Golabi–Behmel syndrome	*GPC3*	X-linked
Bannayan–Riley–Ruvalcaba syndrome	*PTEN*	AD
Costello (other RASopathies)	*HRAS*	AD
PIK3CA overgrowth	*PIK3CA-ART*	sporadic
Chromosome		
Trisomy 4p16.3	NA	NA
Trisomy 5p	NA	NA
Trisomy 12p	NA	NA
Pallister–Killian syndrome (mosaic tetrasomy 12p)	NA	NA
Trisomy 15q25	NA	NA
Deletion (monosomy) 22q13	NA	NA
Mosaic trisomy 8	NA	NA

AD, autosomal dominant; *NA,* not applicable.

(small mouth, small upturned nose, bilateral renal enlargement, macrosomia, renal hamartomas, hydronephrosis, hydroureter, developmental delay, and cryptorchidism), Sotos (prenatal and postnatal overgrowth, developmental delay, macrocephaly, dolichocephaly, a prominent forehead, large hands and feet, advanced bone age, prominent jaw, and variable psychomotor developmental delay), Weaver (prenatal overgrowth, developmental delay, macrocephaly, and camptodactyly), and Simpson–Golabi–Behmel (prenatal and postnatal overgrowth, macrocephaly, congenital diaphragmatic hernia, coarse facies, palatal abnormalities, congenital heart defects, generalized hypotonia, and ventriculomegaly).[87] Chromosomal abnormalities associated with fetal overgrowth, as noted in Table 30.6, include mosaic tetrasomy 12p, also known as Pallister–Killian syndrome, which is characterized by normal growth or overgrowth, congenital diaphragmatic hernia, heart disease, and postaxial polydactyly.[90]

Confirmation of gestational dates and evaluation for maternal diabetes should be done first. Next, a detailed US should be performed to evaluate for renal and cardiac anomalies. BWS is rarely associated with cardiac anomalies, but other overgrowth syndromes (e.g., Simpson–Golabi–Behmel syndrome) have a high incidence of cardiac defects (up to 50%).[80]

Prognosis: The reported perinatal mortality rate in BWS from prematurity, macroglossia, and cardiomyopathy is as high as 20%.[91] Patients with BWS have a higher risk of developing tumors in their first decade of life, after which the risk approaches the baseline risk of the general population. The most frequently observed tumors in BWS are Wilms tumor and hepatoblastoma, which comprise 43% and 12% of reported cancers, respectively.[92] Less common tumors include adrenocortical carcinoma, neuroblastoma, and rhabdomyosarcoma, as well as other benign or malignant neoplasms.[93] Intelligence and development are often normal.[94]

Management: The degree of macrosomia may influence the mode of delivery. An antenatal diagnosis can prepare the neonatology team for management of airway obstruction in the presence of macroglossia and for the severe hypoglycemia that can affect these patients.[91] Conservative postnatal surveillance for intra-abdominal tumors is performed with renal US examinations every 3 months until the age of 8 years; liver US examinations every 3 months until the age of 4 years; and measurements of serum AFP levels every 6 weeks until the age of 4 years.[92] AFP is normally very high in neonates, and it is not until 6 to 8 months of age that the AFP in a normal patient decreases to adult levels. AFP levels in BWS patients are less abnormal than previously expected; however, an increase in the AFP level in these patients, even if the levels remain relatively low, could indicate the growth of a hepatoblastoma.[92]

Recurrence Risk: Identification of the underlying genetic mechanism causing BWS permits better estimation of recurrence risk. In families with suspected autosomal dominant inheritance (15%), the recurrence risk is up to 50%, but in other forms of inheritance (e.g., methylation abnormalities), the recurrence risk would be expected to be very low.[95]

Holt–Oram Syndrome

Holt–Oram syndrome (HOS), also known as Heart and Hand syndrome, was first described in 1960 as a disease affecting cardiac

and skeletal development.[96] The syndrome is characterized by asymmetric abnormalities of the limbs (usually the left upper extremity) and cardiac defects (most commonly secundum atrial septal defects).

Incidence: HOS affects approximately 1 in 100,000 live births.[97]

Pathogenesis/Etiology: HOS is caused by mutations in the T-box transcription factor 5 (*TBX5*) gene at 12q24.1.[98,99] Point mutations and other sequence variants account for more than 70% of cases, while deletions and duplications are seen in less than 1%.[99] Interestingly, the sal-like 4 (Drosophila) *SALL4* gene at 20q13 has also been associated with a phenotype clinically indistinguishable from HOS and accounts for a small portion of the identified mutations, but mutations in this syndrome may be associated with additional congenital anomalies, especially renal, tympanic, and ocular.[100]

Diagnosis: There is no recognized serum screening abnormality that would alert the clinician to a diagnosis of HOS prenatally. If HOS is suspected, amniocentesis could be offered, though genetic testing is not required for diagnosis and could be falsely negative. Karyotype alone would not be expected to detect the vast majority of molecular genetic causes of HOS; *TBX5* gene testing would be required.

Imaging: The only first-trimester abnormality that may be evident with this syndrome is an abnormal NT. The diagnosis is typically made in the mid-to-late second trimester by US, although the findings may be overlooked depending on the ability to view the extremities carefully. Three-dimensional (3D) US offers significant detail of the bones and soft tissues of the fetus, enabling the diagnosis to be made more accurately in the second trimester.[101] It has been suggested that the ideal time to sonographically evaluate the upper extremity is between 13 and 16 weeks of gestation when the amniotic fluid volume enables free movement of the fetus, thereby permitting rotation of the forearm such that the radius and ulna can be viewed in a single plane. Outside this gestational period, hypoplasia of the ulna or radius can be more easily missed.[101]

HOS may present in a highly variable way, with limb anomalies identified from the shoulder through the hand, as summarized in Table 30.7 (Fig. 30.16).[102] Deformity of the sternum has also been described.[103]

Cardiac defects affect approximately 85% of fetuses with this disorder. The most common cardiac defect is an ostium secundum ASD.[96] The cardiac abnormalities span a spectrum from normal cardiac development to combined severe ASD, ventricular septal defect, and pulmonic stenosis.[104] Other reported cardiac anomalies include Ebstein anomaly, mitral valve prolapse, transposition of the great vessels, tetralogy of Fallot, and anomalous pulmonary venous return.[103]

Differential Diagnosis: Numerous conditions may lead to an abnormal NT (see Table 30.4). Other conditions that manifest with limb anomalies include the VACTERL/VATER association, thrombocytopenia-absent radius syndrome, Goldenhar syndrome, trisomy 13, and trisomy 18. Rare conditions such as Fanconi syndrome, Nager syndrome, Townes–Brocks syndrome, and Roberts syndrome should be considered in the differential diagnosis, but additional findings, such as micrognathia or in

TABLE 30.7	Extremity Findings That May Be Seen in Holt–Oram Syndrome
Shoulder	Clavicle hypoplasia Deformity of scapula Deformed head of humerus Accessory bones at shoulder joint
Forearm	Synostosis of radius and ulna Partial or complete radial hypoplasia
Carpus	Deformed carpal bones Supernumerary carpal bones
Thumb and digits	Hypoplastic thenar eminences Triphalangia Absent thumbs Clinodactyly of thumb Syndactyly Absent first metacarpal Short middle phalanx of fifth digit Clinodactyly of fifth digit
Whole limb	Phocomelia

utero growth restriction, microcephaly, and radial ray deficiencies, would be apparent. Poorly controlled diabetes may also lead to overlapping findings, including heart disease and radial malformations.

Prognosis: This syndrome is not associated with an increased rate of fetal demise. The prognosis will depend on the severity of cardiac disease.

Management: When an infant with suspected HOS is born, complete physical examination should be performed. Postnatal diagnostic criteria include (1) upper limb malformation involving carpal bone, (2) personal or family history of congenital heart malformation, and (3) personal history of cardiac conduction disease.[76] Exclusion criteria for HOS include other specific congenital anomalies such as ulnar ray anomalies only; lower limb anomalies; the presence of renal, vertebral, craniofacial, or anal anomalies; or abnormalities in auditory or visual systems.[76] Because of the varied clinical presentations, hand x-rays should be taken to evaluate for carpal bone anomalies.[102] If an infant meets the clinical diagnosis of HOS, *TBX5* gene testing should be sent. Cardiology consultation, electrocardiography, and echocardiography should be performed in view of the high incidence of cardiac disease.[99]

Recurrence Risk: The recurrence risk depends on the underlying genetic mechanism. If one parent carries the same mutation, the recurrence risk would be expected to be up to 50%; if neither parent carries the mutation, the syndrome is isolated with a very low recurrence risk.

Meckel–Gruber Syndrome

Meckel-Gruber syndrome (MGS) is also referred to as dysencephalia splanchnocystica and is invariably lethal.[105] The syndrome was first described by Meckel in 1822 and later by Gruber in 1934[106] and is most frequently characterized by an occipital encephalocele in 80% of cases, nephromegaly with microcystic dysplasia, and postaxial polydactyly.[106,107]

Incidence: The incidence of MGS ranges from 1 in 13,250 to 1 in 140,000 live births worldwide, with a predilection for the Finnish population (up to 1 in 9,000).[97,108]

Pathogenesis/Etiology: MGS is inherited autosomal recessive and has some variability to its expression, even among affected siblings.[106] The disease is secondary to a ciliary dysfunction and is categorized with other primary ciliopathies such as Bardet–Biedl and Joubert syndromes.

MGS demonstrates locus heterogeneity. There are a number of genes associated with MGS, including *TMEM216*, *TMEM67*, *CEP290*, *RPGRIP1L*, *CC2D2A*, *B9D1*, *B9D2*, and *MKS1*, which are located on a number of different chromosomes.[109,110] Regardless of the specific gene change, the result in embryogenesis is dysfunction of primary cilia.[111] The diagnosis is made clinically, though there is controversy over the specific criteria that should be used.[97,112]

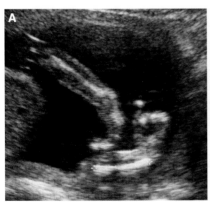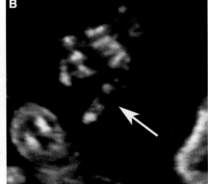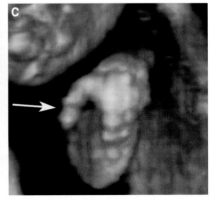

FIGURE 30.16: Radial deficiencies and suspected Holt–Oram syndrome. **A:** US of the left upper extremity in a 17-week-GA fetus showing a single forearm bone and radial angulation of the wrist. **B, C:** In a different fetus evaluated at 20-week-GA with suspected Holt–Oram syndrome, there is absence of the thumb and pollicization of the index finger (*arrows*) of the right hand seen by 2D (**B**) and 3D (**C**) US. Findings were symmetric. Anatomic assessment was also notable for a two-vessel cord and an atrial septal defect.

Diagnosis: There is no recognized serum screening abnormality that would alert the clinician to a diagnosis of MGS prenatally. In instances when MGS is suspected, genetic testing through a gene panel could be considered from a sample obtained via amniocentesis or CVS.

Imaging: The diagnosis may be made as early as the first trimester at 10 to 11 weeks, with visualization of the posterior encephalocele and polydactyly.[112,113] Anomalies of the CNS may be detected by screening US and further evaluated with fetal MRI.

Malformations of the brain and face, in addition to an occipital encephalocele noted in 80% of cases, might include a Dandy–Walker malformation (approximately one-third of cases), cerebellar hypoplasia, ventriculomegaly, microcephaly, brainstem dysplasia, cleft palate, and micrognathia (Fig. 30.17A, B).[106,112]

Renal disease may be evident sonographically by abnormal renal enlargement, microcystic changes, heterogeneous corticomedullary differentiation, and large hypoechoic medullary regions. When present, hyperechogenicity of affected kidneys is appreciable as early as 17 weeks' gestational age, when the renal cortex appears brighter than that of the fetal liver and spleen. Nephromegaly and abnormally increased T2 signal are appreciable on fetal MRI (Fig. 30.17C). The renal disease may manifest with oligohydramnios, although the amniotic fluid volume may remain normal. In the setting of oligohydramnios, fetal MRI is particularly helpful, given the limitations of evaluation by US without sufficient amniotic fluid.[114] Hepatic fibrosis may also be evident on necropsy, although this is not discernible on prenatal imaging.

Other features that could be detected prenatally include sloping forehead and bowing of the long bones of extremities. Cleft lip and palate, micrognathia, microphthalmia, and genital ambiguity are also reported.

Differential Diagnosis: Other syndromes that manifest with both brain and renal anomalies and polydactyly include trisomy 13, Joubert syndrome, oral-facial-digital syndromes types I and II, short rib polydactyly syndrome, and Smith-Lemli-Opitz syndrome. Another closely related ciliopathy to MGS is Joubert syndrome, a nonlethal condition characterized by vermian hypoplasia, thick horizontal superior cerebellar peduncles, and a deep interpeduncular cistern, creating a molar tooth sign.[115] Distinguishing the two syndromes from one another is important, given the fatality of MGS.[116]

The primary differential for cystic renal disease in the absence of other associated anomalies is autosomal recessive and autosomal dominant polycystic kidney disease. The increased renal echogenicity seen with MGS can be similar in other renal conditions that have innumerable microscopic cysts, tubular dilatation, or parenchymal dysplasia. Other syndromes to consider in the differential diagnosis of large and echogenic kidneys include Bardet–Biedl (also features ventriculomegaly and polydactyly), Ivermark II, and Jarcho–Levin syndromes (also features platyspondyly and spondylocostal dysplasia).[117]

Prognosis: This syndrome is lethal, and infants who survive gestation die within a few days after birth.[97,105]

Management: Families should receive genetic counseling if the diagnosis is suspected. Amniocentesis should be offered to exclude a chromosomal abnormality, though MGS has complex genetics and cannot be diagnosed by karyotype alone. Termination can be offered in the United States if diagnosis is made early. If an infant with suspected MGS is carried to delivery, supportive comfort care should be suggested at the time of birth. An autopsy should be performed, and genetic testing be done to provide counseling for future pregnancies.

Recurrence Risk: As MGS is autosomal recessive, the recurrence risk is 25%.[97]

Cornelia de Lange Syndrome

Cornelia de Lange syndrome (CdLS) is also known as Brachmann de Lange syndrome, as Brachmann first described it in the early 1900s, and later, de Lange contributed to the description. The features of this syndrome (summarized in Table 30.8) include prenatal and postnatal growth restriction, limb anomalies,

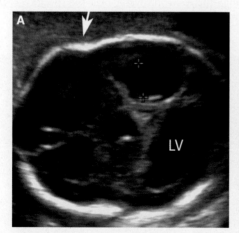 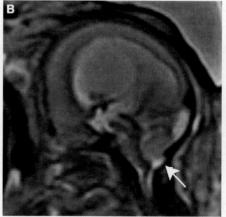 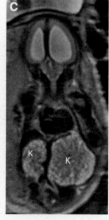

FIGURE 30.17: Meckel–Gruber syndrome in a 23-week-GA fetus. **A:** Axial US through the brain showing abnormally dilated ventricles (*LV*, lateral ventricle and calipers), as well as abnormal shape of the skull, with a buckled appearance in the region of the coronal suture (*arrow*), possibly related to hydrocephalus or to an abnormal suture. **B:** Subsequent fetal T2 MRI in sagittal plane showing aqueductal stenosis (*asterisk* marks the tectum, dorsal to the expected aqueduct), kinked deformity of the brainstem, and a small occipital cephalocele (*arrow*). **C:** Coronal T2 MRI shows marked enlargement and abnormal widespread cystic change of the bilateral renal parenchyma (denoted by *K*).

TABLE 30.8	Features of Cornelia de Lange Syndrome and Their Respective Frequencies	
		FREQUENCY (%)
Growth failure		>95
Intellectual disability		>95
Limb abnormalities		>95
Hirsutism		>80
Micrognathia		80
High and arched palate with clefts		30
Mandibular spurs		42
Seizures		25
GI abnormalities		1–4
Sensorineural hearing loss		>80
Ptosis or other ocular problems		50
Cryptorchidism		73
Congenital heart disease		25

GI, gastrointestinal.

distinctive facial features, cardiac defects, and congenital diaphragmatic hernia.[119] The facial features include hypertrophy and fusion of the eyebrows, arhed eyebrows, long eyelashes, small upturned nose, and microcephaly.[120]

Incidence: Estimates of the incidence of CdLS vary from 1 in 10,000 to 1 in 100,000.[119,120]

Pathogenesis/Etiology: Several genes are known to cause CdLS.[121,122] The gene responsible determines the inheritance pattern; *NIPBL*, *RAD21*, and *SMC3* are inherited in an autosomal dominant manner, while *SMC1A* and *HDAC8* show X-linked inheritance. Both point mutations and deletions/duplications are known to cause CdLS.

Diagnosis: A helpful adjunct to first- and second-trimester imaging may be measurement of PAPP-A, which is abnormally low in this syndrome.[123] Diagnostic testing with amniocentesis or CVS can be offered to families in which a diagnosis of CdLS is suspected, but typically, karyotype does not demonstrate abnormality. Further, even if the genes known to cause CdLS are tested through a gene panel, a negative result does not exclude the diagnosis of CdLS. Amniocentesis can evaluate for other chromosomal anomalies in the differential diagnosis.

Imaging: US is the primary mode of detection, with fetal MRI less helpful given the anatomic areas affected. The syndrome may be among many suspected as early as the first trimester on the basis of sonographic detection of a thickened NT and generalized skin edema (Fig. 30.18A, B). The diagnosis of CdLS can be suspected on the basis of US features of limb reduction defects, cardiac defects, and IUGR, although the in utero growth restriction is not usually recognized until 20 to 25 gestational weeks (Fig. 30.18C, D). Growth retardation typically occurs prenatally and is symmetric.[124] If moderate-to-severe fetal growth restriction and limb anomalies are noted, especially of the upper extremities, there should be a high suspicion for CdLS.[125]

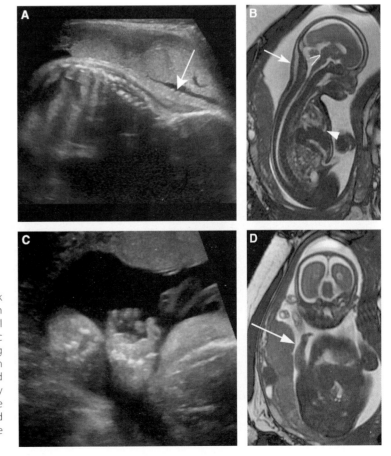

FIGURE 30.18: Cornelia de Lange syndrome in a 29-week fetus. **A:** Progressive hydrops had been monitored, with worsening pleural effusions, a small pericardial effusion, minimal ascites, diffuse skin thickening (*arrow*), and increasing amniotic fluid index. **B:** Sagittal SSFP T2 MRI showing skin thickening (*arrow*), pericardial effusion (*arrowhead*), and cerebellar vermian hypoplasia, with an increased tegmentovermian angle (marked by *white lines*). **C:** US of the extremities was notable for abnormally short right upper extremity containing a single forearm bone and an abnormal number of digits. The left hand was in a fixed flexed position (not shown here). **D:** Coronal MRI depicting the abnormal shortened right upper extremity (*arrow*).

Head and facial abnormalities that may be detected prenatally include brachycephaly, microcephaly, micrognathia, short broad nose with anteverted nares, fusion of eyebrows, low-set ears, hypertrichosis, and long eyelashes (Fig. 30.19A, B).[126] A mandibular spur, located below the mandible as a triangular bony structure, can also be seen in this syndrome.[125] Recognition of the facial features seen in CdLS is enhanced by 3D US in the second and third trimesters.

The limb malformations, if present, are quite variable, although most commonly affect the ulnar aspect of the upper extremities and also include syndactyly, micromelia, contractures at the elbows, oligodactyly, and short first metacarpal (Fig. 30.18C, D). Lower extremities are less likely to show abnormalities.

Cardiac abnormalities frequently identified are atrial and ventricular septal defects, but there have also been descriptions of hypoplastic left ventricle and coarctation of the aorta.[127] Genitourinary tract anomalies include polycystic kidneys, renal ectopia, pyelectasis, cryptorchidism, and ambiguous genitalia.[128] Bilateral diaphragmatic hernia is a rarer finding, but confirmation with fetal MRI can be helpful (Fig. 30.19C).

Interestingly, despite the number of systems that are maldeveloped in this syndrome, prenatal diagnosis can be elusive, with one report showing nearly 70% of postnatally diagnosed cases of de Lange syndrome missed by routine prenatal imaging.[129] The disease should be suspected with the observations of IUGR, ulnar deficiencies of the upper extremities, and cardiac defects and/or congenital diaphragmatic hernia.[119]

Differential Diagnosis: CdLS overlaps with a number of other syndromes. Abnormal NT and limb anomalies may be seen with Apert syndrome, chromosomal abnormalities, multiple pterygium syndrome, Roberts and Smith-Lemli-Opitz syndromes. The facial appearance in CdLS is similar to that seen in Roberts syndrome, but the limb anomalies will distinguish the two. Short radial ray may be observed in Fanconi anemia, thombocytopenia absent radius and Holt Oram syndrome.

Prognosis: Developmental delay is nearly universal (up to 95%), but varies in severity. Mean IQ is 53 but can range from below 30 to 100.[130] Behavioral problems are also seen and include autistic features and self-mutilating behaviors. Life expectancy can

be normal, as patients with CdLS have been reported to live into their 60s. The causes of death are varied but can include aspiration pneumonia, apnea, heart disease, intestinal obstruction, and postsurgical complications.[131]

Management: Prenatal surveillance of the IUGR is routine. Genetic evaluation should be sought shortly after birth to discuss diagnosis and options for testing. Postnatal difficulties are numerous and require multidisciplinary attention. Children affected by this syndrome have severe developmental delay and behavioral difficulties, failure to thrive, feeding difficulties, swallowing difficulties, and postnatal growth restriction. Early intervention should be initiated to optimize psychomotor development and communication skills.

After an infant with suspected CdLS is born, complete physical examination should be performed. Common issues after birth include gastroesophageal reflux disease and feeding difficulties, which may require gastrostomy tube or supplemental formula. Gastrointestinal evaluation should be completed and include upper gastrointestinal series, endoscopy, and, possibly, pH probe.[119] Growth parameters should be plotted on CdLS-specific growth charts.[132] With increased risk of cardiac defects, echocardiography should be performed. Upper extremity radiographs should be considered to evaluate any upper extremity anomalies.[119] Ophthalmology evaluation including dilated examination and evaluation for blocked tear ducts should be performed.[133] Renal US should be obtained to evaluate for renal anomalies, physical examination for cryptorchidism, and hearing tests to exclude hearing loss.[119]

Recurrence Risk: With a negative family history, recurrence risk is estimated at 1.5% because of the potential for germline mosaicism. With family history of CdLS, recurrence risk is based on genetic transmission, but may be as high as 50%.[121]

Smith–Lemli–Opitz Syndrome

Smith-Lemli-Opitz syndrome (SLOS) was first recognized in 1964 as a constellation of clinical findings, including microcephaly, broad alveolar ridge, severe feeding disorder, hypospadias, and global developmental delay.[134]

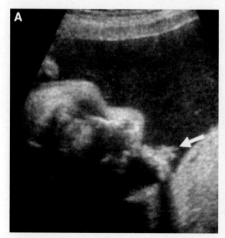
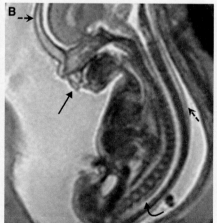
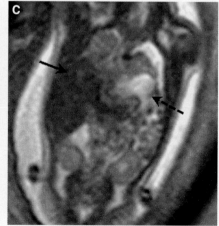

FIGURE 30.19: Cornelia de Lange syndrome. **A:** Axial view of the orbits showing the characteristic long eyelashes (*arrow*) seen in this syndrome. **B:** Fetal MRI at 23 weeks. Sagittal T2 MRI demonstrates prominent philtrum (*arrow*), diffuse soft-tissue edema (*dashed arrows*), and low conus (*curved arrow*). **C:** Coronal MRI in the same fetus showing bilateral congenital diaphragmatic hernia with liver in the right chest (*arrow*) and stomach in the left (*dashed arrow*).

Incidence: Incidence is 1 in 20,000 to 1 in 40,000 live births.[135]

Pathogenesis/Etiology: This syndrome arises from a genetic abnormality causing absent or deficient levels of 7-dehydrocholesterol reductase (DHCR7), an enzyme required in the cholesterol formation pathway.[135] The resulting overproduction of 7-dehydrocholesterol (a cholesterol precursor) is thought to affect several systems during fetal development, and the phenotypic manifestations cover a spectrum from mild developmental delay and syndactyly to lethality.[136] The wide variability of malformations is reflected in a scoring system (Table 30.9) used by Bialer et al.[137] to analyze phenotypic correlations between individuals and siblings. The study assigned a numeric value of 0, 1, or 2 to the relative severity of various anomalies across all systems. This

---

TABLE 30.9 Features Seen in Smith–Lemli–Opitz Syndrome in a Scoring System to Evaluate Phenotypic Correlations between Individuals and Siblings

ORGAN	SCORE	CRITERIA
Brain	1	Seizures; qualitative MR abnormality
	2	Major CNS malformations; gyral abnormalities
Oral	1	Bifid uvula or submucous cleft
	2	Cleft hard palate or median cleft lip
Skeletal	0	Non–Y-shaped minimal toe syndactyly;
	1	Y-shaped 2/3 toe syndactyly; club foot; upper or lower polydactyly; other syndactyly
Eye	2	Cataract; frank microphthalmia
Heart	0	Functional defects
	1	Single-chamber or vessel defect
	2	Complex cardiac malformation
Kidney	0	Functional defect
	1	Simple cystic kidney disease
	2	Renal agenesis; cystic disease
Liver	0	Induced hepatic abnormality
	1	Simple structural abnormality
	2	Progressive liver disease
Lung	0	Functional pulmonary disease
	1	Abnormal lobation; hypoplasia
	2	Pulmonary cysts; other major malformations
Bowel	0	Functional GI disease
	1	Pyloric stenosis
	2	Hirschsprung disease
Genitalia	1	Simple hypospadias
	2	Ambiguous for female genitalia in 46,XY; Genital malformation in 46,XX

CNS, central nervous system; GI, gastrointestinal; MR, magnetic resonance.
From Bialer MG, Penchaszadeh VB, Kahn E, et al. Female external genitalia and mullerian duct derivatives in a 46,XY infant with the Smith-Lemli-Opitz syndrome. Am J Med Genet. 1987;28(3):723–731. Copyright © 1987 Wiley-Liss, Inc. Adapted by permission of John Wiley & Sons, Inc.

---

evaluation determined that males with complete feminization, tending to have polydactyly and cleft palate, are among the more severely affected patients. Other findings in SLOS include cleft palate and cardiac defects.[138]

Diagnosis: Mutations in *DHCR7* are detected by sequence analysis in 96% of SLOS cases.[139] Elevated levels of 7-dehydrocholesterol in the amniotic fluid, as well as absence of unconjugated estriol, confirms the diagnosis.[140] However, up to 10% of affected patients may have estriol and cholesterol levels in the normal range.[141]

Prenatal diagnostic testing options for ambiguous genitalia include multiple molecular tests and amniotic fluid hormone concentrations. In the absence of other fetal anomalies or growth retardation on US, prenatal karyotype with testing for the sex-determining region Y (*SRY*) gene on the Y chromosome is the most useful test when ambiguous genitalia is suspected.

Imaging: US findings that may raise suspicion for SLOS include growth restriction, limb anomalies, holoprosencephaly, and cardiac defects. The primary features present in SLOS include microcephaly, limb malformations, and genital abnormalities, and variable features include brain malformations, cardiac defects, renal anomalies, and late-onset IUGR. Syndactyly of the second and third toes is clinically present in 97% of cases.[141]

The prenatal detection of this disorder might be seen in the late first trimester by recognition of a thick NT.[142] Abnormalities of the limbs, such as polydactyly, might be apparent as early as 12 weeks'. At this stage, karyotyping is helpful to rule out chromosomal causes.

Second-trimester US and fetal MRI may show findings that range from normal to multisystem anomalies. The most frequent detectable trait prenatally is IUGR.[136,143] Previously described brain anomalies in SLOS fetuses include ventriculomegaly, agenesis of the corpus callosum, cerebellar hypoplasia, and holoprosencephaly, which may be better elucidated on fetal MRI (Fig. 30.20A, B). Facial abnormalities that may be detected prenatally include hypertelorism, micrognathia, and cleft palate (Fig. 30.20C).

Limb abnormalities may involve the upper or lower extremities. Postaxial polydactyly of the hands, clenched hands, and valgus deformity of the feet are additional findings described in this syndrome (Fig. 30.20D). Soft-tissue syndactyly of the second and third toes is the most common anomaly of the skeletal system (Fig. 30.20E). Renal abnormalities seen in SLOS include hypoplasia, hydronephrosis, or cystic change.[143] Although the fetal genitalia can usually be assessed by 20 weeks', the prenatal recognition of ambiguous genitalia is difficult, with studies showing prenatal identification in only approximately 25% of postnatal diagnosed cases.[144] Fetal MRI may be helpful in genitalia evaluation.

Differential Diagnosis: The differential considerations for a thickened NT are extensive (see Table 30.4). In the presence of postaxial polydactyly and genital anomalies, two main categories of syndromes should be considered in the differential of SLOS. Polydactyly syndromes include Meckel Gruber, Joubert and orofacial digital syndrome, trisomy 13, Ellis–van Creveld syndrome, and short rib polydactyly syndrome. Many of these syndromes have associated limb anomalies, but they do not include the 2–3 syndactyly classically associated with SLOS. Syndromes manifesting with genital abnormalities include Carpenter syndrome, which also shares abnormal head shape and polydactyly in common with SLOS, congenital adrenal hyperplasia, Cornelia de-Lange, Opitz G/BBB syndrome (hypertelorism, defects of larynx, males

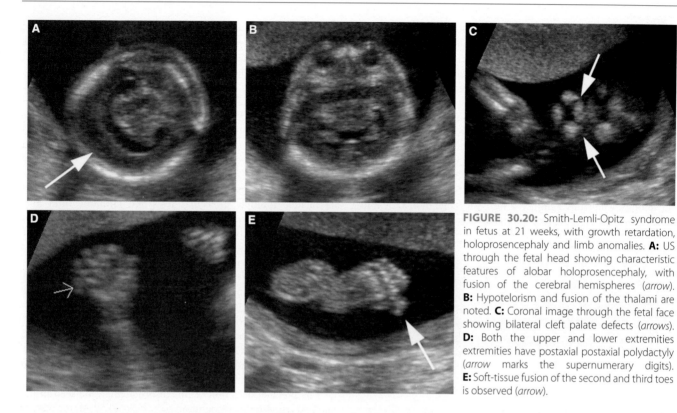

FIGURE 30.20: Smith-Lemli-Opitz syndrome in fetus at 21 weeks, with growth retardation, holoprosencephaly and limb anomalies. **A:** US through the fetal head showing characteristic features of alobar holoprosencephaly, with fusion of the cerebral hemispheres (*arrow*). **B:** Hypotelorism and fusion of the thalami are noted. **C:** Coronal image through the fetal face showing bilateral cleft palate defects (*arrows*). **D:** Both the upper and lower extremities extremities have postaxial postaxial polydactyly (*arrow* marks the supernumerary digits). **E:** Soft-tissue fusion of the second and third toes is observed (*arrow*).

with genital anomalies), and the MURCS association (Müllerian duct aplasia, renal aplasia, cervicothoracic somite dysplasia).

Prognosis: The severity of disease depends on the amount of DHCR7 activity. Two types of SLOS have been described: type I and type II. Type II is associated with absent DHCR7 activity altogether, whereas in type I, some amount of activity is present. In type II, neonatal death occurs. In less severe cases (type I), the children exhibit growth retardation, intellectual disability, behavior abnormalities, and failure to thrive. Life expectancy depends on the degree of internal malformations and the amount of supportive care during childhood and adulthood.[136]

Management: Infants with suspicion for SLOS should have complete physical examination. During the newborn period, feeding difficulty is the most likely complication, and gastrostomy is frequently required. Airway management may be necessary.

Other medical issues include GI problems (pyloric stenosis, gastroesophageal reflux, Hirschsprung disease, or constipation), recurrent acute otitis media, and eye problems (cataracts, ptosis, or strabismus). Ophthalmology evaluation should be obtained to evaluate for associated eye findings, as up to 20% of patients with SLOS have congenital cataracts.[145] Hearing screening should be completed to evaluate for conductive or sensorineural hearing loss.

CNS malformations are seen in SLOS (including Dandy–Walker malformation, holoprosencephaly); therefore, postnatal brain MRI is often helpful for accurate diagnosis.[146] Renal malformations (hypoplastic or cystic kidneys) have been reported, and renal US is typically performed.[147]

Cholesterol supplementation has been reported to result in improved growth, reduced photosensitivity, and increased nerve conduction velocity.[148,149] However, improvement in cognitive outcomes has not been documented. Cholesterol

supplementation in young patients can be given with dried or pasteurized egg yolk and has minimal side effects.[150] Patients with SLOS may require stress-dosed steroid treatment during acute illness.[151]

Developmental delay ranges from near-normal intelligence to severe cognitive disability, but is generally severe. Long-term issues include failure to thrive, risk of behavioral problems, and psychiatric disorders.[152]

Recurrence Risk: Gene testing may provide information to allow for prenatal testing in future at-risk pregnancies.[153] SLOS demonstrates autosomal recessive inheritance; thus, recurrence risk is 25%.[139]

Klippel–Trenaunay Syndrome

Klippel–Trenaunay syndrome (KTS) is characterized by asymmetric limb or trunk enlargement coupled with deep and superficial lymphatic malformations, venous malformations, and cutaneous hemangiomata of the affected limb or body part. The entity was first described by Klippel and Trenaunay in 1900 as a syndrome with cutaneous hemangiomas, asymmetric limb overgrowth, and varicosities, and later in 1907, Weber contributed the observation of occasional arteriovenous malformations in affected individuals.[154] The first prenatal recognition of this syndrome was described in 1988 as limb hypertrophy and numerous subcutaneous cysts.[155]

Incidence: The incidence of KTS is less than 1 in 10,000.[154]

Pathogenesis/Etiology: The genetic basis for KTS is thought to be a somatic mutation, resulting in vascular malformations. Inheritance is sporadic with all cases thought to involve mosaicism.[154] Multiple candidate genes have been identified, but currently, no clinical genetic testing is available. Diagnosis is clinical and is documented with two of the following three criteria: (1) capillary malformation, (2) venous malformation or atypical varicose veins, and (3) hypertrophy of the soft tissues and/or bone.[156] Most patients (63%) have all three clinical criteria.[157]

Diagnosis: There is no recognized serum screening abnormality that would alert the clinician to a diagnosis of KTS prenatally.

Imaging: The diagnosis may be made as early as middle second trimester, based on marked enlargement of the soft tissues of the involved limb or body part (Fig. 30.21A). The soft-tissue abnormalities may appear as mass-like tumors. US may be insufficient to completely evaluate the extent of abnormalities, in which case fetal MRI may offer additional information (Fig. 30.21B, C).[158] Evaluation of the brain may be important, especially in the presence of ventriculomegaly, given association with overgrowth in the brain, in particular hemimegalencephaly.[159]

The vascular malformations may enlarge rapidly, leading to life-threatening complications, including high-output cardiac failure and platelet trapping with a consumptive coagulopathy.[155] Overgrowth of the long bones in the affected limb will be apparent by prenatal US. Occasionally, the syndrome can affect the face and manifest with asymmetric facial hypertrophy. Intrapelvic and intra-abdominal involvement is also possible, evidenced by either distinct masses or visceromegaly. There has also been description of a case diagnosed by hemihypertrophy and subcutaneous cysts coupled with ascites and an abnormal maternal serum panel, and it is theorized that the ascites was secondary to cardiac failure or lymphatic abnormalities.[160]

Differential Diagnosis: Other syndromes that might present prenatally with lymphatic malformations, lymphedema, and limb hypertrophy include Beckwith–Wiedemann, disseminated hemangiomatosis syndrome, Maffucci syndrome, Bannayan–Riley–Ruvalcaba syndrome, Proteus syndrome, Russell–Silver syndrome, and Turner syndrome. Soft-tissue masses in the sacrococcygeal region should prompt consideration of a sacrococcygeal teratoma in the differential diagnosis, and fetal MRI would be advantageous for evaluating the intrapelvic extent of disease in this situation.

Prognosis: Prognosis of KTS depends on the location, size, and type of malformations seen. In severe fetal cases, hydrops may develop, and this is likely to lead to in utero demise. Routine monitoring for signs of cardiac failure is important, and if detected, delivery should be promptly performed in a medical setting where intensive neonatal care is available. Intelligence is normal. Life expectancy can be in the normal range.[157]

Management: Fetal congestive heart failure associated with KTS has been observed, so close monitoring during the pregnancy is warranted.[155] An infant with suspected KTS should have a screening complete blood count after birth to evaluate for thrombocytopenia that can develop from platelet consumption in the hemangioma.[154] Because some of the diagnoses in the differential have associated cardiac defects and the risk of heart failure, echocardiography is typically performed.

Depending on the severity of the hemangioma and hypertrophy, limb amputations in the neonatal period have been required.[158] In those infants who are stable postnatal, the disorder is treated symptomatically. Options for therapy include observation only, compressive stockings, anticoagulation, steroid therapy, laser ablation, sclerotherapy, and surgical resection.[158]

Recurrence Risk: Recurrence risk is expected to be very low owing to sporadic nature, though some reports of familial recurrence suggest the possibility of higher recurrence risk.[154]

Roberts Syndrome

Roberts syndrome (RBS), also called pseuduothalidomide syndrome or SC syndrome, was first described in 1919 as a combination of cleft lip, cleft palate, and maldevelopment of all four extremities. Numerous cases have since been described, sharing the primary features of IUGR, severe shortening of the limbs, cleft lip and palate, hypertelorism, microcephaly, and micrognathia.[161]

Incidence: RBS is rare; around 150 cases have been reported.[162]

Pathogenesis/Etiology: RBS is an autosomal recessive inherited disorder.[161] Clinical variability is even seen among affected individuals in families.[162] There is one gene known to cause RBS

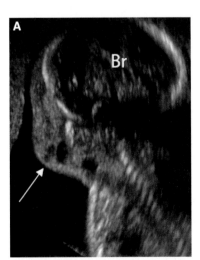
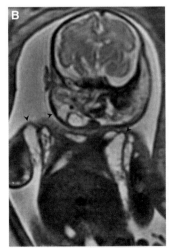
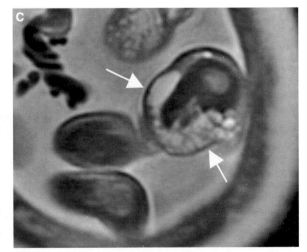

FIGURE 30.21: Klippel–Trenaunay syndrome. **A:** Sagittal US of the fetal head and neck at 17 weeks' showing abnormal subcutaneous soft-tissue thickening (*arrow; Br*, brain) containing cystic spaces. **B:** Coronal T2 MRI showing the extent of the superficial soft-tissue abnormality (*arrowheads*), involving the bilateral neck and chest. **C:** Extension along an upper extremity (marked by *arrows*) was also observed.

(*ESCO2*), and diagnosis is based on genetic testing.[163] A mutation in the *ESCO2* gene has been found in all patients with RBS. A negative result from amniocentesis nearly excludes RBS.[163]

Diagnosis: Karyotyping will show premature centromere separation of some chromosomes, and therefore, if a genetic workup is time sensitive, a search for these chromosomal abnormalities can provide information about the diagnosis.[163] Similar, but distinct, metaphase abnormalities can be seen in other syndromes (aneuploidies and Cornelia de-Lange).[164] Typically, if these findings are not seen, the diagnosis of RBS is unlikely but not definitively excluded.

Imaging: Fetuses with growth delay and limb anomalies on US may be suspected to have RBS. This disorder may be recognized as early as 12 weeks, on the basis of limb shortening, cervical lymphatic malformation, and polyhydramnios (Fig. 30.22). The degree of limb reduction in the upper and lower extremities is variable, and the bones may be absent or hypoplastic. Tetraphocomelia is classically observed. Flexion contractures are typically seen. Oligo syndactyly and syndactyly are also common features, which are more readily detected by 3D US than by 2D US.[165]

Additional less common findings in RBS are numerous: cryptorchidism, CNS malformations, cardiac lesions, renal anomalies, abnormal genitalia, and cervical lymphatic malformations.[161] Confusing findings on US may be elaborated with MRI, although there is no published case of a prenatal diagnosis of RBS by fetal MRI.

Differential Diagnosis: Other syndromes that can cause these severe limb abnormalities include amniotic band syndrome, Fanconi anemia (in utero growth restriction, microcephaly, and radial ray deficiencies), Holt Oram, autosomal recessive tetra-amelia associated with *WNT3* gene, thalidomide embryopathy, Nager syndrome, orofacial digital syndrome, and thrombocytopenia absent radius. Table 30.10 lists the recognized disorders that manifest with limb reduction abnormalities.[166]

Prognosis: The prognosis is poor. Rates of pregnancy loss and postnatal mortality are high.[162] Affected children who survive generally die after a few years, owing to associated malformations.

Management: An infant born with features of RBS should receive genetic counseling and confirmatory gene testing. A complete physical examination and extremity radiographs are typically performed to evaluate for limb reduction malformations. Prostheses

may be indicated.[167] In the neonatal period, feeding is often an issue, especially if cleft lip or palate is present.[168] In addition, echocardiography and cardiology evaluation are recommended because of the association with congenital heart defects.[161] Renal US is performed to evaluate for renal cysts.[167] Ophthalmology evaluation should be completed as corneal clouding and visual impairment are often seen.[161] Intellectual disability is nearly universal. However, patients with mild disease can have had normal intelligence and survive into adulthood.[169]

Recurrence Risk: Recurrence risk in future pregnancies is 25%.[154]

Noonan Syndrome

Noonan syndrome (NS) is similar to Turner syndrome (TS), but with a normal karyotype. The syndrome is characterized by postnatal short stature, identified in 50% to 70% of cases; a broad and webbed neck; and anterior chest wall deformity due to superior pectus carinatum and inferior pectus excavatum.[170] Characteristic facies are low-set and posteriorly rotated ears, hypertelorism, epicanthic folds, and thick eyelids. Coagulation defects, lymphatic dysplasias, renal anomalies, and ocular abnormalities are also associations.[171,172]

Incidence: The incidence of NS is estimated to be between 1 in 1,000 and 1 in 2,500 live births.[171]

Pathogenesis/Etiology: NS is inherited autosomal dominant, but with a normal karyotype. The genetic basis of NS is complex with numerous genes identified.[173] All of the genes identified are in the RAS pathway (group of proteins in human cells), which lead to RAS overactivation, turning on genes responsible for cell growth, proliferation, and survival. A *PTPN11* gene mutation is found in approximately 50% of patients.[174]

Diagnosis: When this syndrome is suspected, an NS gene panel could be considered. A positive result would have prognostic implications, but a negative result would not exclude NS.

Imaging: There is a 21% positive detection rate for NS utilizing prenatal US, whether there is only one or more abnormalities detected.[175] Molecular positive NS is more likely to have cardiac defects, followed by lymphatic malformation and then increased NT.[175]

Therefore, the diagnosis may be considered in the late first trimester based on a thickened NT. The primary prenatal feature is cervical lymphatic malformation, particularly in the

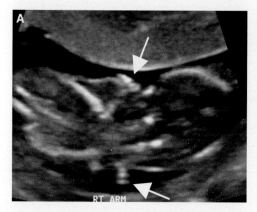
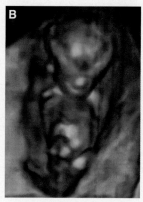

FIGURE 30.22: Tetraphocomelia in a 14-week fetus, raising suspicion for Roberts syndrome. **A:** 2D coronal US showing the absence of the bilateral arms and forearms, with discernible bilateral hands (*arrows*) arising directly from the shoulder regions. **B:** 3D US showing four diminutive limbs.

TABLE 30.10   Expected Limb Reduction Anomalies in Recognized Chromosomal and Syndromic Conditions

DIAGNOSIS	MALFORMATIONS
Trisomy 18	Hypoplasia of phalanges and/or short hallux
Poland anomaly	Hypoplasia of hands; hypoplasia of entire arm
Ectrodactyly–ectodermal dysplasia–clefting (EEC)	Ectrodactyly of hands and/or feet
Thrombocytopenia-absent radius (TAR) syndrome	Bilateral absence of the radius, mild shortening and bending of the ulna
Smith–Lemli–Opitz syndrome	Terminal transverse limb deficiencies
Oral-facial-digital syndrome	Asymmetric shortening of digits
Townes–Brocks	Hypoplasia of the thumb and of the third toe
Moebius	Terminal transverse limb deficiencies
Du Pan	Bilateral absence of the fibula, short metacarpals
Hypoglossia/hypodactyly	Absence of digits
Cornelia de Lange	Oligodactyly
Fanconi anemia	Hypoplasia of the thumb
Roberts	Phocomelia
Holt–Oram	Radial hypoplasia
VACTERL association	Hypoplasia of the thumb and/or radius
Oculo-auriculo-vertebral defect spectrum	Bilateral or unilateral hypoplasia of fingers
Amniotic bands	Terminal transverse limb deficiencies

Adapted from Stoll C, Alembik Y, Dott B, et al. Associated malformations in patients with limb reduction deficiencies. *Eur J Med Genet*. 2010;53(5):286–290. Copyright © 2010 Elsevier Masson SAS. With permission.

lateral aspects of the neck. In the presence of a normal karyotype and cervical lymphatic lesion, NS should be suspected. In a minority of cases, the lymphatic abnormalities will lead to overt development of fetal hydrops, which portends a poor prognosis (Fig. 30.23A).

Whereas IUGR is a feature of TS, prenatal growth restriction is not a feature of NS. Body length is usually normal in affected infants, and subsequently, short stature becomes apparent later in 50% to 70% of children.[170]

Cardiac defects are seen in 50% to 80% of individuals with this syndrome. While left heart lesions are more common in TS, right heart lesions, especially pulmonic stenosis and septal defects, are typically seen in NS (Fig. 30.23B). Pulmonary valve stenosis should raise suspicion for NS. Other types of cardiac diseases that might be prenatally diagnosed include AV canal defect, pulmonary artery stenosis, and tetralogy of Fallot.[176]

Additional findings that may be seen with NS include hypertelorism; low-set ears; cryptorchidism; micropenis; renal anomalies, including solitary kidney and collecting system anomalies; and scoliosis secondary to hemivertebrae.[170,177]

These features can be typically detected by prenatal US. There is no published description of fetal MRI offering further advantage in the prenatal diagnosis of NS, but when imaging in a fetus with multiple anomalies, soft tissue edema, and known normal karyotype, NS should be high on the differential (Fig. 30.23C).

Differential Diagnosis: There are several rare syndromes caused by mutations in RAS pathway genes. These include LEOPARD, Costello, and cardiofaciocutaneous syndromes. As with many of the syndromes and genetic abnormalities discussed in this chapter (see Table 30.4), the NT is abnormal in fetuses affected by NS. Cervical lymphatic malformations may be seen with a number of genetic abnormalities and have a high association with other major congenital anomalies.[178] This finding, combined with detection of cardiac defects, might also be seen with DiGeorge syndrome, Pallister–Killian syndrome, trisomy 10, trisomy 13, trisomy 18, trisomy 21, and TS.

Prognosis: Survival through gestation and in the first year of life typically depends on the severity of cardiac disease. Twenty percent to 30% of NS patients are affected by hypertrophic cardiomyopathy. The leading genetic cause of infantile hypertrophic cardiomyopathy is NS.[176] The combination of hypertrophic cardiomyopathy and NS carries a significant mortality, 22% at 1 year.[179]

Interestingly, some cases of NS are mild and may not be diagnosed until adulthood when the affected person has an affected child. Diagnosis of an affected fetus or neonate should prompt evaluation of family members.

Management: Prenatally, fetuses should be routinely assessed by US to monitor for the development of diffuse lymphedema,

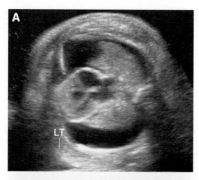

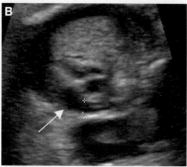

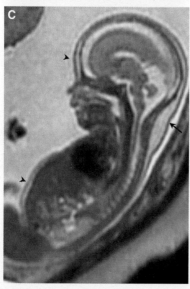

FIGURE 30.23: Noonan syndrome. **A, B:** Fetus at 35 weeks. **A:** Axial US of the chest showing large bilateral anechoic pleural effusions (*Lt,* left). **B:** Focused image of the right ventricular outflow tract showing the pulmonary artery (marked by *calipers*) and poststenotic dilatation (*arrow*). Pulmonic stenosis and evidence of hydrops portend a poor prognosis. **C:** Fetus at 23 weeks with significant nuchal soft-tissue thickening (*arrow*) and diffuse soft-tissue edema (*arrowheads*). Atrioventricular canal was also present.

which places the fetus at risk for intrauterine death. Children born with this syndrome can develop peripheral edema, and like children affected by TS, the neck appears webbed owing to regression of the lymphatic malformations.

Feeding difficulties are common in the newborn period but are typically self-limited.[180] Newborns should have screening echocardiography, renal US, and an ophthalmology examination.[177] Growth parameters should be plotted on NS-specific growth charts.[180] Approximately 80% of affected males will

have cryptorchidism.[177] Management of scoliosis secondary to vertebral segmentation anomalies may require orthopedic intervention.

Approximately 25% of children with NS have some degree of intellectual disability, but it is often mild.[181] Early referral for intervention should be obtained to limit developmental delay. Individuals with NS have a genetic predisposition to leukemia and certain solid tumors, including neuroblastoma and embryonal rhabdomyosarcoma.[182] In addition, a variety of coagulation defects have been seen in patients with NS; thus, laboratory tests to evaluate for coagulation defects should be performed.[177]

Recurrence Risk: Recurrence risk is up to 50% if the parents are found to carry a mutation.[173]

Velocardiofacial Syndrome (DiGeorge Syndrome)

Velocardiofacial syndrome (VCFS), also referred to as DiGeorge syndrome, is characterized by palate anomalies, characteristic facial features, and developmental delay. Conotruncal heart defects, such as tetralogy of Fallot, interrupted aorta, ventricular septal defects, and truncus arteriosus, are seen in up to 74% of patients.[183] Immune problems are less common but may be severe.[183] Other features include hypocalcemia, seizures, hearing loss, feeding difficulty, renal anomalies, and growth hormone deficiency.[183] Marked variability is seen both within and among families with VCFS.[184]

Incidence: Incidence estimates range from 1 in 4,000 to 1 in 6,395 live births.[183]

Pathogenesis/Etiology: The syndrome arises from a deletion on chromosome 22q11.2.[184] Ninety percent of cases are due to new mutations, but the remaining 10% are autosomal dominant.

Diagnosis: FISH specific for VCFS can detect the submicroscopic deletion on chromosome 22.[185] The deletion can also be identified on microarray. Microarray will also detect smaller or atypical deletions in this region. Karyotype from amniocentesis alone would not be expected to detect the deletion associated with most cases of VCFS.

Imaging: In a recent review of fetuses diagnosed with VCFS, cardiac disease is cited as the most common finding, present in 95% of cases (Fig. 30.24).[186] Amniocentesis should be offered for all pregnancies with a conotruncal heart defect since 10% to 20% will have abnormal FISH for VCFS. VCFS should also be considered in cases of right aortic arch without intracardiac anomalies, as approximately 10% or more have been shown to present with these findings.[187]

Extracardiac abnormalities are also present in 90% of cases and, when associated with cardiac disease, may warrant microarray testing for VCFS. The extracardiac anomalies that are found include CNS (38%), polyhydramnios (30%), small thymus (26%), facial (21%), genitourinary (17%), skeletal (19%), gastrointestinal (14%), and pulmonary (7%). Of note, cleft lip and cleft palate was only detected in 10% of cases.[186] 3D US may assist further in the diagnosis by demonstrating hypotelorism, small low-set ears with abnormal helices, downturned oral commissures, small mouth and jaw, and a straight facial profile (Fig. 30.25).[188]

Severe CNS malformations have also been described in fetuses affected by 22q11.2 microdeletion syndromes and include polymicrogyria, posterior encephalocele, myelomeningocele, and

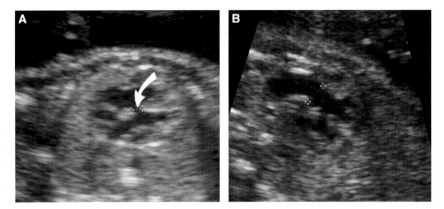

FIGURE 30.24: Velocardiofacial syndrome. **A:** A transverse view of the heart showing a ventricular septal defect (*arrow*) measuring 3 mm. **B:** A single great vessel (marked by *calipers*) arises from the heart. Single umbilical artery was also present. Fluorescent in situ hybridization analysis revealed a 22q deletion.

holoprosencephaly.[188] Fetal MRI would be ideal for evaluating brain and facial anomalies.

Differential Diagnosis: Other syndromes to consider in the differential diagnosis include CHARGE, diabetic embryopathy, Smith-Lemli-Opitz syndrome, Alagille syndrome, VATER, or Goldenhar.

Prognosis: The heart defects associated with deletion 22q11.2 are generally repairable, but feeding problems are very common, and cognitive impairment is essentially universal. Mental health problems, especially schizophrenia, may be seen in up to 30% of affected adults and adolescents. Combination of heart disease, kidney disease, and/or other malformations may complicate management. Severe T-cell deficiency with congenital heart has a mortality rate of approximately 65% to 70%.[183]

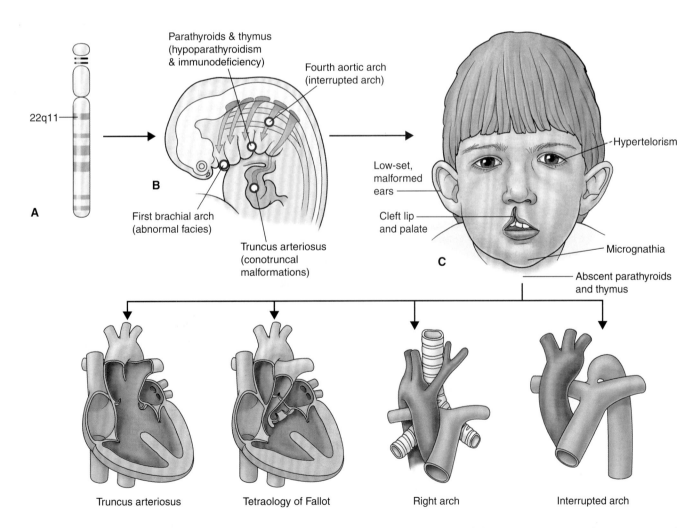

FIGURE 30.25: Characteristic features of velocardiofacial syndrome. (Adapted from Sze RW, Yutzey KE. The molecular genetic revolution in congenital heart disease. *AJR Am J Roentgenol.* 2001;176:575–581. Copyright © 2001 American Roentgen Ray Society.)

Management: Infants with suspicion for VCFS or DiGeorge syndrome should receive a number of evaluations at the time of birth. A complete physical examination should be performed. Feeding evaluation may be necessary as many infants have difficulty with suck and swallow (30%) and often require nasogastric tube feedings or gastrostomy tube.[189] Serum-ionized calcium level should be checked as hypocalcemia is common and is most severe in neonatal period. A lymphocyte count screens for immune defects; an abnormal value should prompt further testing and referral to an immunologist or hematologist. Ophthalmology evaluation is performed on the basis of the wide variety of eye findings associated with VCFS, including cataracts, colobomas, ptosis, and small optic nerves.[185] Hearing loss has been reported and should be screened.

Postnatal imaging is important to evaluate the extent of anomalies. Renal anomalies are seen in approximately 20% of affected patients and are evaluated with renal US. Radiography is performed to evaluate for vertebral anomalies.[190] Echocardiography and referral to a cardiologist should be obtained.[183] CNS malformations include reduced cerebellar volume, polymicrogyria, cystic white matter lesions, and pituitary gland defects. MRI could be considered, especially with seizure activity.[191]

Many long-term issues are present in VCFS. Developmental delays, behavioral problems, and psychiatric disorders are nearly universal, but have varying significance. Delays can range from mild, isolated language delay to significant global delay.[192] Speech assessment by age 1 year is recommended in view of the high incidence of velopalatine insufficiency and speech disorders, even without clefts.[193]

Recurrence Risk: Since 90% of cases are due to new mutations, recurrence risks are generally low. However, if a parent is affected, recurrence risk is 50%. Because of the variability in presentation, a mildly affected parent could have the 22q11.2 deletion and have gone undiagnosed.[193]

CHARGE Syndrome

CHARGE syndrome is a rare set of associations consisting of *c*olobomas, *h*eart defects, choanal *a*tresia, *r*etarded growth and development, *g*enital abnormalities, and *e*ar anomalies.[194] Please see chapter 21 for further review of ear anomalies.

Incidence: The incidence of CHARGE syndrome is from 1 in 8,500 to 1 in 10,000 live births.[194]

Pathogenesis/Etiology: The majority of CHARGE cases are sporadic because of new mutations. Rare recurrence has been attributed to germline mosaicism in a parent.[195] The chromodomain helicase DNA-binding protein 7 (*CHD7*) is the only gene known to be associated with CHARGE syndrome. An abnormality in *CHD7* is seen in 65% to 70% of patients, but is not necessary for diagnosis.[195] Truncating mutations (those that induce a premature translational "stop" signal) may cause haploinsufficiency of *CHD7* in some cases. Missense mutations (resulting in a single-nucleotide change rendering its encoded protein nonfunctional) seem to be related to a less severe, less specific phenotype.[196] There is one patient with CHARGE phenotype and an abnormality in the *SEMA3E* gene.[197]

Diagnosis: An amniocentesis with gene testing for *CHD7* could be offered and has been described in confirming a prenatally suspected case of CHARGE syndrome.[198] Karyotype from amniocentesis is expected to be normal.

Imaging: Postnatal diagnosis is based on clinical findings and temporal bone imaging.[194,199] Colobomas, which are seen in 80% to 90% of patients with CHARGE syndrome, can be unilateral or bilateral and can involve the iris, retina-choroid, or disc (Fig. 30.26A, B). Heart defects are variable but common in 75% to 85% of cases. Choanal atresia or stenosis can be unilateral or bilateral in 50% to 60% of patients (Fig. 30.26C, D). Growth deficiency is noted in 70% to 80%.[200] Genital anomalies seen in CHARGE include cryptorchidism or hypogonadotropic hypogonadism.[201] Ear abnormalities, seen in greater than 90% of affected individuals, include abnormal outer ears, malformed ossicles, cochlear defects, or abnormal semicircular canals (Fig. 30.26E, F).[202] Other features of CHARGE syndrome include cranial nerve dysfunction, orofacial clefts, and tracheoesophageal fistula.[195]

Prenatal suspicion for CHARGE syndrome could be raised owing to abnormal prenatal US and MRI findings. Sanlaville et al.[203] summarize a series of 10 fetuses affected by a *CDH7* gene mutation. The most commonly seen findings included bilateral and asymmetric external ear abnormalities manifesting as low-set, posteriorly rotated, and triangular or square-shaped auricle, semicircular canal hypoplasia or agenesis, and arhinencephaly. Seven of 10 fetuses also had a coloboma, always affecting the retina or choroid segment. Nine of 10 fetuses had a congenital heart defect, usually complex lesions and often involving the conotruncal region with septal defects. Six of the fetuses had choanal atresia. Less common findings included polyhydramnios, microphthalmia, and cleft lip and/or palate.

On the basis of their observation that four of six major criteria of CHARGE (coloboma, choanal atresia and/or cleft lip/palate, heart defect, arhinencephaly, semicircular canal agenesis, and external ear anomalies) were sufficient for the diagnosis of CHARGE, it has been proposed that the presence of four of these major findings are necessary for the prenatal diagnosis of CHARGE syndrome. Major and minor diagnostic criteria are summarized in Tables 30.11 and 30.12.

2D and 3D US can readily evaluate the pinna; however, sonographic evaluation of the temporal bone is limited. Identification of the fetal cochlea caudal to the temporal lobes can be obtained in approximately 50% of cases in the second trimester by using the fetal anterior fontanelle and coronal plane insonation.[204] The semicircular canals may be identified by second-trimester US as well, although with limited resolution. Fetal MRI has been shown to distinguish the cochlea from the semicircular canals, and it also permits the identification of the external auditory canals, with improved resolution as gestational age advances.[205] The fetal ear anomalies seen in CHARGE syndrome may be found by prenatal MRI, but it is important to keep in mind that evaluation of the cochlea, semicircular canals, and vestibule in the fetus by T2 MRI is usually not possible until later in gestation. Of note, the vestibule is more readily discernible than the cochlea and the ossicles earlier in gestation. Fetal MRI can also define subtle anomalies like coloboma (see Fig. 30.26B), absence of the olfactory tracts after 30 weeks' (Fig. 30.26D), choanal atresia (see Fig. 30.26C), cleft palate, or genital anomalies.[205]

Differential Diagnosis: The differential diagnosis includes mosaic trisomy 9, diabetic embryopathy, Carpenter syndrome, velocardiofacial syndrome, VACTERL association, Kabuki syndrome, and Joubert syndrome. These could be differentiated on the basis

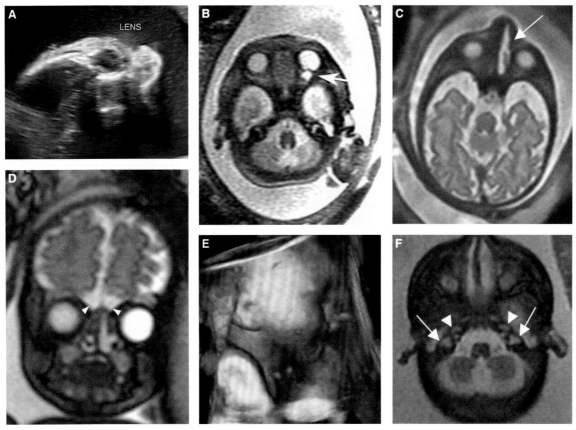

FIGURE 30.26: CHARGE syndrome. **A:** Axial US demonstrating globe with eccentric posterior cyst protrusion consistent with coloboma. **B:** Axial T2 MRI in a 33-week fetus showing a small well-demarcated T2-hyperintense structure posterior to the globe (*arrow*), consistent with a small coloboma. **C, D:** Axial SSFSE **(C)** and coronal T2 MRI SSFP **(D)** demonstrating fluid-distended nasal cavity (*arrow*), proven to represent choanal atresia. On the coronal imaging, there is also absence of the olfactory bulbs (*arrowheads*). **E, F:** Fetus at 31 weeks GA. **E:** 3D US demonstrating malformed ear. **F:** Axial SSFP demonstrating misshapen ears and dysplasia of the lateral semicircular canals (*arrows*), which should be distinct from the vestibule at this gestational age (*arrowheads* mark the cochlea).

TABLE 30.11	Major Diagnostic Characteristics of CHARGE Syndrome	
CHARACTERISTICS	**MANIFESTATIONS**	**FREQUENCY**
Ocular coloboma	Coloboma of the iris, retina, choroid, disc; microphthalmos	80%–90%
Choanal atresia or stenosis	Unilateral/bilateral: bony or membranous atresia/stenosis	50%–60%
Cranial nerve dysfunction or anomaly	I: hyposmia or anosmia VII: facial palsy (unilateral or bilateral) VIII: hypoplasia of auditory nerve IX/X: swallowing problems with aspiration	Frequent >40% Frequent 70%–90%
Characteristic CHARGE syndrome ear	Outer ear: short, wide ear with little or no lobe, "snipped off" helix, prominent antihelix that is often discontinuous with tragus, triangular concha, decreased cartilage; often protruding and usually asymmetric Middle ear: ossicular malformations Mondini defect of the cochlea Temporal bone abnormalities; absent or hypoplastic semicircular canals	80%–100%

Data from Sanlaville D, Etchevers HC, Gonzales M, et al. Phenotypic spectrum of CHARGE syndrome in fetuses with CHD7 truncating mutations correlates with expression during human development. *J Med Genet.* 2006;43:211–217.

TABLE 30.12   Minor Diagnostic Characteristics of CHARGE Syndrome

CHARACTERISTICS	MANIFESTATIONS	FREQUENCY
Genital hypoplasia	Males: micropenis, cryptorchidism Females: hypoplastic labia	50%–60%
	Males and females: delayed puberty secondary to hypogonadotropic hypogonadism	Frequent
Developmental delay	Delayed milestones, hypotonia	≤100%
Cardiovascular malformation	Including conotruncal defects (e.g., tetralogy of Fallot), AV canal defects, and aortic arch anomalies	75%–85%
Growth deficiency	Short stature, usually postnatal with or without growth hormone deficiency	70%–80%
Orofacial cleft	Cleft lip and/or palate	15%–20%
Tracheoesophageal (TE) fistula	TE defects of all types	15%–20%
Distinctive facial features	Square face with broad prominent forehead, prominent nasal bridge and columella, flat midface	

AV, atrioventricular.
Data from Sanlaville D, Etchevers HC, Gonzales M, et al. Phenotypic spectrum of CHARGE syndrome in fetuses with CHD7 truncating mutations correlates with expression during human development. *J Med Genet*. 2006;43:211–217.

of physical findings, but some may be subtle and might not be identified until the child is born.

Prognosis: Survival depends on the severity of an individual's phenotype. Cyanotic heart disease, tracheoesophageal fistula, and bilateral choanal atresia have the lowest survival.[206] It is highly recommended that affected infants be delivered at a tertiary care center. Observed IQs tend to be below average, and cognitive impairments may be partially explained by sensory deficits and by dysfunction in integrating regions of the brain.[202]

Management: An infant born with suspected CHARGE syndrome should have a full physical examination. In the newborn period, associated medical conditions can be life-threatening.[206] Airway management typically requires tracheostomy and surgical correction of choanal atresia.[207] Feeding difficulties are common, and evaluation by a speech pathologist should be performed. Need for gastrostomy is not uncommon.[208] Echocardiography as well as cardiology consultation, renal US, and hearing screening should be included in management shortly after birth.

Long-term needs include hearing and vision evaluations, assessment for hypogonadism as puberty onset can be delayed, and consideration of airway anomalies if anesthesia is required.[206]

Recurrence Risk: If parents are unaffected, risk is approximately 1% to 2% due to germline mosaicism.[209]

CRANIOSYNOSTOSIS

There are a number of craniosynostosis syndromes; however, only the most common types are described. Apert, Pfeiffer, and Crouzon syndromes are related syndromes as all are characterized by craniosynostosis resulting from abnormalities of fibroblast growth factor receptor (*FGFR*) genes.[210] In addition to the *FGFR* genes, there are many additional genes that can cause either syndromic or nonsyndromic craniosynostosis. Whereas the skull

base develops from enchondral ossification, the calvarial ossification occurs within membrane-derived mesodermal tissue. The gradually apposing calvarial ossification centers meet at fibrous sutures. Complete, solid fusion of these sutures in a normal individual does not occur until well into adulthood, with the exception of the metopic and mendosal suture, which typically fuse within the first year of life.

Clinically, the most important growth occurs along the sagittal and coronal sutures. The growth of the cranium is perpendicular to the suture, so that the skull increases in width through the sagittal suture and in anteroposterior diameter through the coronal sutures.[210] Premature fusion of the sutures leads to abnormal head shape, as summarized in Table 30.13 (Fig. 30.27).

Characteristic facial features include hypertelorism, downslanting palpebral fissures, proptosis, midface hypoplasia, small beaked nose, and prognathism. Other common features include high arch or cleft palate abnormalities, hearing loss, visual problems, and choanal stenosis or atresia. Developmental delay is also common.[211]

In this section, global features of the main craniosynostosis syndromes are provided, followed by more specific details about the clinical features, genetics, imaging, and management of Apert, Pfeiffer, Crouzon, and Antley–Bixler syndromes.

Incidence: The incidence of craniosynostosis is approximately 1 in 2,000 live births. Interestingly, advanced paternal age has been shown to be associated with de novo mutations in Apert, Pfeiffer, and Crouzon syndromes.[212]

Pathogenesis/Etiology: The specific genetics of each syndrome will be discussed separately.

Diagnosis: Genetic testing for all three of the *FGFR* genes, as well as larger craniosynostosis gene panels, is clinically available. Karyotype from amniocentesis would be expected to be normal.

TABLE 30.13 Summary of Resulting Head Shapes with Various Calvarial Suture Synostoses and the Syndromes Featuring Each

FUSED SUTURE	HEAD SHAPE	DESCRIPTION OF CONDITION	SYNDROME
Sagittal	Scaphocephaly	Long, narrow skull	Crouzon, Philadelphia type
Coronal, bilateral	Acrobrachycephaly	Broad, short skull	Apert, Crouzon, Pfeiffer, Saethre–Chotzen, Muenke, Antley–Bixler
Unilateral lambdoid or unilateral coronal	Plagiocephaly	Asymmetric, trapezoid	
Metopic	Trigonocephaly	Keel forehead	Baller–Gerold
All sutures	Oxycephaly Kleeblattschädel	Cloverleaf skull	Carpenter, Pfeiffer

Adapted from Flores-Sarnat L. New insights into craniosynostosis. *Semin Pediatr Neurol.* 2002;9(4):274–291. Copyright © 2009 Elsevier. With permission.

First-trimester diagnosis may be made with CVS and genetic analysis in patients with a known family history.

Imaging: It is possible to detect the presence of craniosynostosis prenatally by US. The biparietal diameter measures the transverse plane where the skull is widest. The occipitofrontal diameter represents the anterior to posterior direction with the measurement obtained from outer skull to outer skull. The cephalic index is the ratio of the biparietal to occipitofrontal diameters, calculated as a percentage. Eighty percent is the normal intrauterine cephalic index (Fig. 30.28A). Brachycephaly, correctly known as acrobrachycephaly, is diagnosed if the cephalic index is more than 85% (Fig. 30.28B). Scaphocephaly, also previously called dolichocephaly, is defined if the index is less than 75% (Fig. 30.28C). Head measurements may be correlated with abdominal circumference or femur length. The normal head/abdominal circumference (HC/AC) is 1.07% to 1.26%. An abnormal ratio should raise suspicion of a cranial anomaly.[213]

Fetal MRI may also show findings that suggest craniosynostosis.[214] Abnormal skull shape is readily apparent. Bone thickening and slight temporal indentations suggest bilateral coronal synostosis (Fig. 30.29A), whereas an indentation in the midline with scaphocephaly is suggestive of sagittal synostosis (Fig. 30.30A).

In general, prenatal diagnosis of craniosynostosis is very challenging and often missed particularly in early gestation.[214] The diagnosis of syndromic synostosis relies mainly on cranial deformity and associated abnormalities, in particular, limb malformations.

Differential Diagnosis: Differentiating between Apert, Crouzon, and Pfeiffer is based on characteristic features (see Tables 30.13 and 30.14). However, accurate diagnosis is often difficult prenatally and may be dependent on postnatal clinical findings and genetic testing.[211] The differential diagnosis includes other craniosynostosis syndromes (Muenke syndrome, Saethre–Chotzen syndrome, Antley–Bixler syndrome, Carpenter syndrome, or Baller–Gerold syndrome) or isolated, nonsyndromic craniosynostosis. Muenke syndrome has variable findings that may include unilateral coronal synostosis or megalencephaly without craniosynostosis.[215] Saethre–Chotzen syndrome is typically diagnosed via characteristic ear findings.[216] Baller–Gerold

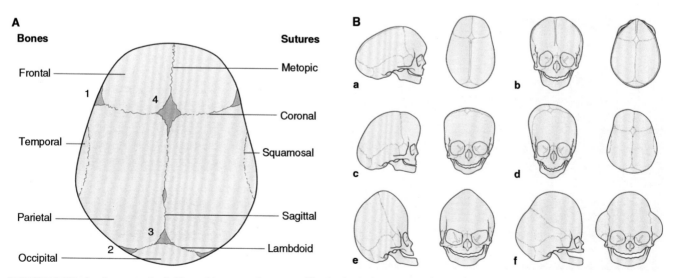

FIGURE 30.27: Craniosynostosis. **A:** Normal bones and sutures of fetal calvaria *(top view)* and anterolateral *(1)*, posterolateral *(2)*, posterior *(3)*, and anterior *(4)* fontanelles. **B:** Forms of craniosynostosis resulting from premature closure of the sagittal suture *(a)*, metopic suture *(b)*, coronal sutures *(c)*, unilateral coronal suture *(d)*, coronal and sagittal sutures *(e)*, and cloverleaf skull deformity with fusion of all sutures *(f)*.

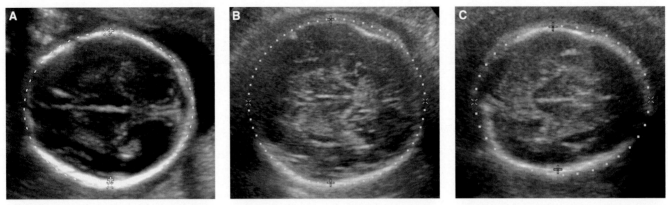

FIGURE 30.28: Assessment of the skull shape by US. **A:** The cephalic index is the ratio of the biparietal diameter to the occipitofrontal diameter, and this is typically near 80% (19 weeks' GA). **B:** An abnormally high index is diagnostic of acrobrachycephaly (19 weeks' GA). **C:** An abnormally low index is diagnostic of scaphocephaly (27 weeks' GA) + calipers represent biparietal and X calipers represent occipitofrontal diameters.

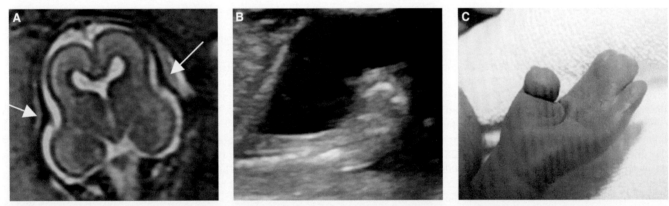

FIGURE 30.29: Apert syndrome diagnosed prenatally in a 21-week fetus. **A:** Coronal T2 MRI through the fetal head showing abnormal indentations (*arrows*) in the bilateral frontotemporal regions, indicating early coronal synostosis. **B:** US of the right hand showing abnormal clenching of the hand and fingers, with indistinct digits indicating complete syndactyly, called the "mitten" hand deformity. **C:** Photograph of hand of a newborn infant with Apert syndrome showing syndactyly deformity.

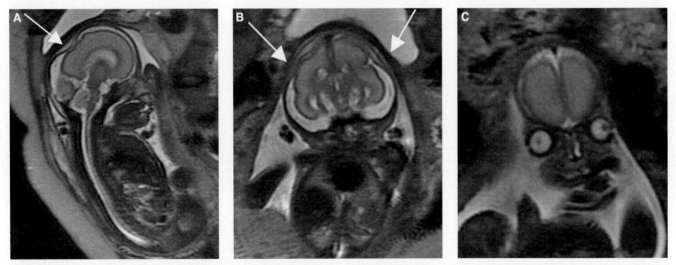

FIGURE 30.30: Pfeiffer syndrome diagnosed prenatally in a 27-week fetus. Sagittal **(A)** and coronal **(B)** T2 SSFSE MRI through the fetal head showing abnormal concave contours of the skull in the midline (*arrow in* **A**) at the vertex and along the frontotemporal regions (*arrows in* **B**), creating a cloverleaf-shaped skull. Midface hypoplasia is also appreciable. **C:** Coronal SSFSE T2 image through the fetal face demonstrating hypertelorism. No polydactyly or syndactyly was appreciable.

TABLE 30.14 Classic Extremity Abnormalities Commonly Observed in Each Craniosynostosis Syndromes

CRANIOSYNOSTOSIS SYNDROME	EXTREMITY ANOMALY
Apert	Mitten syndactyly
Pfeiffer	Broad toes and thumbs
Antley–Bixler	Arachnodactyly
Crouzon	Normal extremities

syndrome typically has radial ray defects. Carpenter syndrome has preaxial polydactyly of the feet.[210]

Isolated craniosynostosis will present without other extremity or craniofacial anomalies, other than hypertelorism or hypotelorism due to abnormal skull shape. There are a number of other syndromes that can present with craniosynostosis as a minor feature. Evaluation by a geneticist is warranted.

Prognosis: The prognosis varies with each syndrome and depends on the associated features. Pfeiffer syndrome has a higher morbidity and mortality than the other syndromes owing to the severity of airway abnormalities, including midface hypoplasia, nasopharyngeal stenosis, and tracheal anomalies.[217] Obstruction to the airway can cause failure to thrive, suboptimal neurological development, and developmental delay.

Management: An infant with syndromic craniosynostosis often has breathing problems in the first few months of life.[211] Respiratory issues are typically due to upper airway obstruction as a result of midface hypoplasia or choanal atresia/stenosis. Tracheostomy is often needed. Feeding difficulties are also common and can result in failure to thrive, if not addressed.[210] Management of syndromic craniosynostosis involves care at a multidisciplinary craniofacial clinic. Head imaging with computed tomography (CT) using 3D surface reconstructions of the face and skull is typically obtained in preparation for possible surgical management. MRI of the brain may be added to evaluate for hydrocephalus.[218] Craniosynostosis typically requires serial surgical procedures. Earlier surgical treatment, including craniotomy and fronto-orbital advancement, can reduce the risk of complications such as hydrocephalus and cognitive impairment. Ophthalmology evaluation and treatment may be necessary, especially if proptosis is present, as this can lead to exposure keratopathy.[219] Spinal radiographs are performed to evaluate for vertebral anomalies.[220]

Recurrence Risk: Inheritance of the *FGFR* gene is autosomal dominant; therefore, recurrence risk is 50% for affected individuals.[221]

Apert Syndrome

Apert syndrome, also known as acrocephalosyndactyly, was first described in the early 20th century and is one of the most severe craniosynostosis syndromes.[218,219] Patients with this disorder have a short anterior to posterior skull diameter owing to bilateral

coronal synostosis, a high forehead, a flat occiput, shallow orbits, hypertelorism, a flat face, midface hypoplasia, and a small nose.[210] Apert syndrome classically presents with fused fingers or toes and soft-tissue or bony syndactyly in hands or feet. Occasionally, rhizomelic shortening or elbow ankylosis can be seen. During infancy, there is a large midline calvarial defect replacing the sagittal and metopic suture. This defect gradually closes by the age of 3 to 4 years.[222] Other features of Apert syndrome include fused cervical vertebrae, hydrocephalus, and cardiac and gastrointestinal abnormalities.[223]

Incidence: The incidence of Apert is approximately 1 in 100,000.[224]

Pathogenesis/Etiology: Apert syndrome results from *FGFR2* mutations, which map to chromosome 10q25–q16 and apparently arise exclusively from the paternally derived chromosome. The disorder has been associated with older paternal age.[223] Two specific mutations, p.Ser252Trp and p.Pro253Arg, are most common.

Diagnosis: Targeted testing for the two mutations, p.Ser252Trp and p.Pro253Arg, can be performed, though typically sequencing of the *FGFR2* gene is done based on similar costs and turnaround time with greater information gained.[225]

Imaging: Prenatal recognition of Apert syndrome is difficult because the characteristic features of craniosynostosis do not usually present until the third trimester. Affected fetuses are usually identified by US between gestational weeks 20 and 27 when there is notation of either a brain abnormality, an abnormal skull shape, or syndactyly.[226] Both US and MRI may show the abnormal head shape (see Fig. 30.29A). The most common brain abnormality is ventriculomegaly, which may be assessed by MRI. Overexpansion and overconvolution of the temporal lobe, a common association with the *FGFR2* gene, is evident antenatally and may be more conspicuous earlier in gestation when the normal brain is still smooth, preceding the onset of craniosynostosis (Fig. 30.31A–B).[227] Corpus callosum agenesis/dysgenesis may also be detected. In all, 100% of patient have inner ear anomalies, with the most common being a common cavity formation of the lateral semicircular canal and vestibule, which also may be detected via MRI (Fig. 30.31C).[228]

3D US, MRI, and 3D printing can illustrate the craniofacial abnormalities more readily than 2D US.[229] This technique may not only decisively influence diagnosis, it may assist the parents in understanding the anomalies when being counseled.[226] US is ideal for evaluating the feet and hands, which are characteristically affected by bilateral syndactyly. A clenched "mitten" type appearance of the hand is typical and reflects near-complete syndactyly (Figs. 30.29B, C, 30.31D). The feet may appear small and unusually arched. Other associated abnormalities such as congenital cardiac lesions may be directly visualized on prenatal sonography.

Prognosis and Management: Neonates may require management of their airway. Surgery, such as craniofacial expansion or ventricular shunting, is often performed in early childhood to reduce intracranial pressure, as it has been shown to diminish the incidence of developmental delay. Affected individuals are at risk for developmental delay, although the degree of developmental delay is variable.[211] Management of a patient with Apert

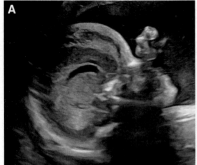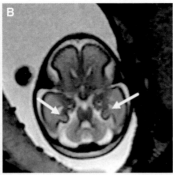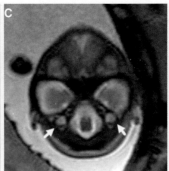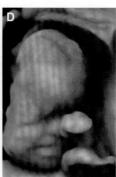

FIGURE 30.31: Apert syndrome in a 26-week fetus. **A:** Sagittal US demonstrating frontal bossing and midface hypoplasia. **B:** Axial MRI demonstrating oversulcation of the medial temporal lobes (*arrows*). **C:** Axial T2 image demonstrating common cavity of the lateral semicircular canals with vestibule (*arrows*) bilaterally. **D:** 3D US reformat demonstrating mitten hand deformities.

syndrome should include management of hydrocephalus, screening echocardiography for cardiac defects, and imaging to evaluate for intestinal malrotation or esophageal atresia.

Pfeiffer Syndrome

Pfeiffer syndrome, also called Pfeiffer-type acrocephalosyndactyly, was initially described in 1964 and is characterized by acrobrachycephaly, hypertelorism, depressed nasal bridge, broad-appearing and medially deviated thumb and great toe, as well as partial syndactyly in the hands and feet.[230] Pfeiffer syndrome can be subdivided into three types, with all having extremity findings but varying on other features. Pfeiffer syndrome type I typically has normal cognition, characteristic moderate-to-severe midface hypoplasia, hearing loss, and hydrocephalus. Type I is less common and less severe than types II and III. Pfeiffer syndrome types II and III commonly present with developmental delay, characteristic extreme proptosis, choanal and palatal abnormalities, hydrocephalus, and seizures.[231] Proptosis is often so severe that patients are unable to close their eyelids.[230] Visceral anomalies, including cardiac and genitourinary anomalies, also occur. Type II is more likely to include a broad thumb and great toe than type III. Skull shape is also a distinguishing feature in Pfeiffer syndrome types II and III. Type II typically has a cloverleaf skull shape, while type III presents with an oxycephalic skull shape, which is a conical shape secondary to coronal and lambdoid synostosis.[232]

Incidence: The incidence of Pfeiffer syndrome is approximately 1 to 1.6 in 100,000.[224] Nearly all cases of Pfeiffer syndrome result from de novo mutation.[212]

Pathogenesis/Etiology: Regardless of subtype, nearly all mutations in Pfeiffer syndrome are related to the *FGFR2* gene, which map at chromosome 10q25–q26. However, it should be noted that 5% of mutations in Pfeiffer syndrome type I are associated with the *FGFR1* gene, which map at chromosome 8p11.22–p1.[233] Approximately 80% of mutations are in exons 8 and 10.

Diagnosis: In a stepwise gene analysis for this suspected disorder, exons 8 and 10 can be sequenced first, followed by other exons if negative.[233] Alternatively, gene sequencing with copy number variant analysis could analyze both concurrently.

Imaging: In a recent review, the most common prenatal US finding in Pfeiffer syndrome is a skull shape abnormality, present in almost three-fourths of cases (Fig. 30.30).[234] Other US abnormalities include malformations of the nose in 50%, proptosis and hypertelorism in 45%, and frontal bossing in 22%. Thumb anomalies are noted in 33% and toe in 40%.[234] The lack of detection of craniosynostosis prenatally does not exclude Pfeiffer syndrome.

Sonographic findings of Pfeiffer syndrome type I in the second trimester include acrobrachycephaly, hypertelorism, a small nose, syndactyly, a broad thumb, and large toes.[235] MRI may also show these findings, as well as better detailing abnormal brain development.[214,232] Although US is superior for evaluation of the bones, MRI may improve assessment of the hands in certain cases using a thick-slab imaging technique that provides detail about the surface of the extremities. This has been shown to be useful in demonstrating the broad thumb of a fetus affected by Pfeiffer syndrome type II, thereby differentiating it from a fetus affected by the other craniosynostoses.[232]

Prognosis and Management: Prognosis depends on the severity of associated anomalies and primarily on the severity of the CNS compromise. Type I is compatible with life, and the individual is expected to have normal intelligence. Postnatal evaluation includes management of the craniosynostosis and surgical correction of the extremity anomalies. Types II and III usually result in early death.

Crouzon Syndrome

Crouzon syndrome, also known as craniofacial dysostosis, was initially described in 1912. This craniosynostosis syndrome does not have clinically apparent abnormalities of the hands and feet, although radiographs may show shortening of metacarpals and phalanges. Facial features that are more distinct in Crouzon syndrome include significant proptosis, external strabismus, and mandibular prognathism.[231] Progressive hydrocephalus occurs in approximately 30% of individuals affected by Crouzon syndrome. Development and cognition are typically normal in Crouzon syndrome.[236]

Incidence: Crouzon syndrome is the most common autosomal dominant craniosynostosis and occurs in 1 in 25,000 live births.[224]

Pathogenesis/Etiology: The most common gene known to be associated with Crouzon syndrome is the *FGFR2*, which maps to chromosome 10q25–q26.[210] A variant of this syndrome is Crouzon syndrome with acanthosis nigricans, which is associated with the *FGFR3* gene.[220]

Diagnosis: Gene sequencing can be approached as in Pfeiffer syndrome with sequencing exons 8 and 10 first, then sequencing others if negative or with concurrent full sequencing. If a young child presents with acanthosis nigricans or other characteristic findings including choanal atresia, hydrocephalus, or skeletal abnormalities that overlap with achondroplasia, testing for the most common mutation in the *FGFR3* gene could be considered.[237]

Imaging: Imaging does not play a diagnostic role until the second or third trimester.[238] Both second and third trimester US and MRI are capable of demonstrating the abnormal skull shape and striking ocular features of Crouzon syndrome. However, these findings may be apparent only late in pregnancy and may escape diagnosis.

Prognosis and Management: The severe proptosis frequently associated with Crouzon syndrome leads to exposure conjunctivitis and keratitis. Visual abnormalities include poor acuity and nystagmus. Scaphocephaly and acrobrachycephaly are the most common calvarial manifestations that are approached surgically with cranial osteotomies and orbitofacial advancement. Conductive hearing loss is also a prominent feature and will require postnatal management. Crouzon syndrome individuals uncommonly have intracranial hypertension or hydrocephalus. There are no associated extremity malformations. Development and cognition are typically normal.[220]

Antley–Bixler Syndrome

Antley–Bixler syndrome, also known as trapezoidocephaly or multiple synostosis syndrome, involves premature closure of the coronal and lambdoidal sutures, resulting in brachycephaly with frontal bossing.[239] Characteristic facial features include proptosis, downslanting palpebral fissures, depressed nasal bridge, and low-set and protruding ears. Choanal stenosis and atresia are frequent. Limb defects include radiohumeral synostosis, ulnar and femoral bowing, slender hands and feet, contractures, fractures, and advanced bone age. Other congenital abnormalities include cardiac defects, renal anomalies, and genital abnormalities. Renal anomalies that can be associated include ectopic kidney, duplication, horseshoe kidney, hypoplasia, or hydronephrosis. Congenital adrenal hyperplasia may be seen.[239]

Incidence: The incidence is unknown because of diagnostic controversies in the reporting of *FGFR*-related craniosynostosis as Antley–Bixler syndrome. More than 60 cases have been reported.

Pathogenesis/Etiology: The underlying etiology is a defect in sterol biosynthesis caused by mutation in a gene for cytochrome P450 reductase. The only gene known to be associated with Antley–Bixler syndrome is the cytochrome P450 oxidoreductase (*POR*).

Diagnosis: Diagnosis is based on clinical findings, but gene sequencing of the *POR* gene is available to confirm the diagnosis.[240] Amniocentesis with cytochrome P450 reductase (*POR*) gene sequencing can be offered, though not required for diagnosis and not routinely performed. During pregnancy, some mothers of fetuses with Antley–Bixler syndrome will have abnormal virilization that does not require intervention and resolves after delivery. Low maternal serum unconjugated estriol or lack of increase in urinary unconjugated estriol may be noted. If fetal craniosynostosis is identified and there is low unconjugated estriol, Antley–Bixler syndrome is the most likely diagnosis. There are reports of abnormal sterol profiles, particularly dimethylated and trimethylated sterols, in the amniotic fluid, although the finding is not specific for this syndrome.[241] Some infants are not diagnosed until the newborn screen is abnormal for 21-hydroxylase deficiency.[240]

Imaging: US findings of brachycephaly with frontal bossing and limb anomalies, especially radiohumeral synostosis, ulnar and femoral bowing, contractures, and fractures, may be evident with 2D US. Dedicated fetal echocardiography is recommended to assess for congenital cardiac lesions. 3D US will increase the ability to detect characteristic facial features, such as depressed nasal bridge and low-set ears. Renal and genital abnormalities as well as choanal atresia/stenosis may be more readily detected by prenatal MRI than US if sonography is limited owing to maternal factors, fetal positioning, or oligohydramnios. Prenatally discernible features of congenital adrenal hyperplasia, including adrenal gland enlargement and ambiguous genitalia, may be seen.[242]

Differential Diagnosis: The differential diagnosis includes other craniosynostosis syndromes, including Pfeiffer syndrome, thanatophoric dysplasia, and Shprintzen–Goldberg syndrome. Shprintzen–Goldberg syndrome lacks the characteristic facial features and ambiguous genitalia seen in Antley–Bixler syndrome.[243]

Prognosis and Management: Prognosis is guarded. Respiratory complications, typically due to choanal stenosis and atresia, can result in early death, but if respiratory issues are addressed, outcomes can be reasonably good. Interventions that have been utilized include endotracheal intubation, nasal stents, tracheotomy, and tracheostomy. Evaluation by an endocrinologist and assessment of adrenal axis should be performed even without ambiguous genitalia.[240] Identification of ambiguous genitalia requires a multidisciplinary team working with the family, ideally prenatally.[144] Imaging with CT or MRI should be done to describe location and extent of craniosynostosis, the presence of choanal stenosis, and the evaluation of orbital depth, to assist with surgical planning. Radiographs of long bone should be performed to evaluate for fractures, bowing, synostoses or joint contractures.[244] Congenital heart defects, such as transposition of the great vessels, atrioventricular septal defects, patent foramen ovale, and hypoplastic right atrium, should be excluded by screening echocardiography. Gastrointestinal malformations are rare, but screening for malrotation and imperforate anus should be considered.[239] Hydrocortisone replacement therapy is often needed for cortisol deficiency with stress-dose steroids.[240] Joint contractures are common, requiring physical therapy referral.[244]

Recurrence Risk: Inheritance is autosomal recessive; thus, recurrence risk is 25%.

SYNDROMES CHARACTERIZED BY MANDIBULAR ANOMALIES

Please see Mandible/Micrognathia in Chapter 20.

NONHERITABLE SYNDROMES AND ASSOCIATIONS

The following section includes multisystemic disorders arising from sporadic mutations or nongenetic processes.

VATER/VACTERL Association

The VATER association refers to a nonrandom association of the following anomalies: *v*ertebral defects, *a*nal atresia, *t*racheo-esophageal fistula with *e*sophageal atresia, and *r*enal dysplasia. The association, originally described in 1973, was later expanded to include *c*ardiac anomalies and *l*imb anomalies in the VACTER*L* association. The entity is not considered syndromic, as there is no known common underlying etiology. Of the cardiac defects in patients with VACTERL, the most common type is ventricular septal defect.[245] The most common type of renal anomaly is renal agenesis, and the most common limb defects are reduction deformities and polydactyly. Three of the core findings are required to make the diagnosis of VATER.[245]

Incidence: The incidence ranges from 1 in 10,000 to 1 in 40,000.[246]

Pathogenesis/Etiology: It is postulated that the grouping of disorders arises from abnormal mesodermal organization before 35 weeks' gestational age.[247] Interestingly, nearly all cases are sporadic, and no established gene has been found, although one patient with features was found to have a mutation in the Homeobox protein Hox-D13 (*HOXD13*) gene.[248] There are a few reports of families with inherited VACTERL features.[249] There is also a published report of both dichorionic, diamniotic twin fetuses affected by the VATER association. However, this twin pregnancy was conceived with intracytoplasmic sperm injection (ICSI) and embryo transfer, and the incidence of anomalies in pregnancies arising from ICSI is higher than seen with spontaneous conceptions.[250]

Diagnosis/Imaging: Prenatal imaging can detect anomalies that may lead to suspicion of the VACTERL association (Fig. 30.32). Diagnosis of VACTERL by US has been described as early as 17 weeks.[251] The most commonly recognized findings include radial ray anomalies, vertebral anomalies, and renal agenesis. Other less commonly identified findings include absent stomach, ventricular septal defect, hydronephrosis, and lower extremity reduction defects. The minority of diagnosed cases exhibit more than three of the classic findings.[252] In many cases, there are anomalies that are not detected, such as anal atresia, with prenatal US imaging.[253] Utilization of MRI, although not cited in the literature, may help in detection of anomalies that are not as easy to detect as on US.

Esophageal atresia may be difficult to diagnose by US, inferred either by an absent stomach or by polyhydramnios, and fluid may still be present in the stomach owing to an esophageal fistula. The diagnosis of esophageal atresia can be made by MRI, which may show fluid distension of the hypopharynx and upper esophagus, and absence of the intrathoracic esophagus (Fig. 30.32E).[254] MRI may be useful for further evaluation of the abdomen, elucidating details of renal development, and allowing for problem-solving in cases of urogenital sinus formation and obstructive renal lesions, which may be confusing due to cyst formation. Spine and limb anomalies may also be discernible. Normal appearance of the fetal brain is typical. Though VATER with hydrocephalus can be a genetically distinct condition, in the presence of significant brain abnormalities, other diagnosis must be considered.

Secondary findings of VACTERL include single umbilical artery, abnormal fetal respirations, and IUGR.[251]

Differential Diagnosis: Findings present determine the differential diagnosis, but could include CHARGE syndrome, diabetic embryopathy, mandibulofacial dysostosis with microcephaly, and Townes–Brocks syndrome, which share features including anorectal malformation, ear anomalies, vertebral anomalies, renal hypoplasia or dysplasia, cardiac anomalies, and limb anomalies. Fanconi anemia, chromosomal abnormalities, or MURCS association, which includes Müllerian hypoplasia/aplasia, renal agenesis, and cervicothoracic somite dysplasia, may be considered. There is also a genetically distinct condition referred to as VATER with hydrocephaly that has overlapping features but may be X linked, and with hydrocephaly as a feature, is often associated with intellectual disability.

Prognosis: Neonatal survival is high with the VACTERL association; however, affected infants may require considerable medical and surgical attention.[251]

Management: An infant born with features of VACTERL should have full physical examination and imaging to identify all anomalies. Examination should focus on detecting malformations that could exclude or verify diagnoses. Screening should include spine and extremity radiographs, echocardiography, and renal US. If there is difficulty or hypoxia with feeding, airway and esophageal evaluation should be performed to exclude tracheoesophageal fistula. Postnatal management of patients with VACTERL/VATER association focuses on surgical correction of the specific congenital anomalies. Long-term medical management is aimed at addressing the sequela of congenital malformations. If optimal surgical correction is achievable, the prognosis can be relatively positive. However, some patients will continue to be affected by their congenital malformations throughout life. Importantly, patients with VACTERL association do not tend to have neurocognitive impairment.

Recurrence Risk: VACTERL association is typically sporadic.

Amniotic Band Syndrome

Amniotic band syndrome (ABS) refers to fetal anomalies resulting from fibrous bands adhering to and entrapping fetal parts, leading potentially to structural deformity and even amputation. The anomalies may involve multiple locations, including limbs, trunk, and craniofacial regions.[255] Other synonyms for this disorder include constriction band syndrome, amniotic band disruption complex, amniotic deformity, adhesion and mutilation (ADAM) complex, amniotic adhesion malformation syndrome, and limb and body wall defect complex.[256]

Incidence: Depending on how ABS is defined, incidence ranges from 1 in 1,200 to 1 in 15,000 live births.[272]

Pathogenesis/Etiology: Numerous theories for the underlying mechanism of ABS exist. Common considerations include a disruption in embryogenesis due to primary rupture of amnion early in gestation or a vascular disruption event.[256,257] Most cases

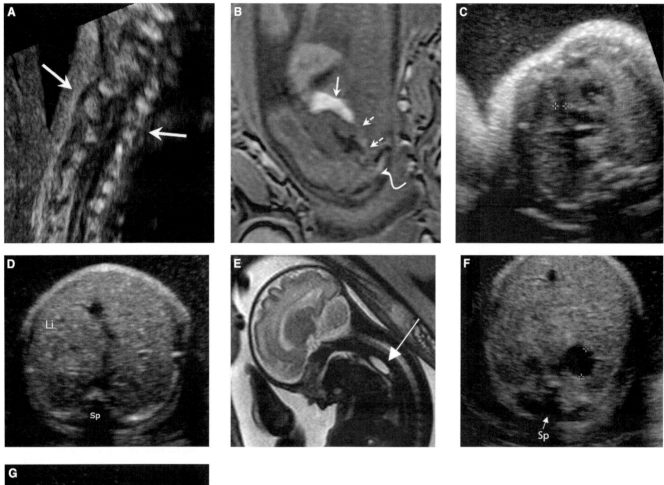

FIGURE 30.32: VACTERL association in multiple fetuses. **A: V**ertebral defects. Coronal US demonstrating curvature of the spine and multiple segmentation errors (*arrows*). **B: A**nal atresia. Sagittal T1 MRI demonstrating dilated meconium (*solid arrow*) proximal to diminutive meconium in rectosigmoid (*dotted arrows*), and complete absence in the rectum (*curved arrow*) in fetus at 28 weeks GA. **C: C**ardiac. US showing a ventricular septal defect. **D: T**racheoesophageal fistula. Survey demonstrates an abnormally high amniotic fluid index (30 mm) and absence of the stomach (*Li*, liver; *Sp*, spine). **E: E**sophageal atresia. Sagittal T2 MRI depicting a fluid-distended esophageal pouch above the atresia, which was noted transiently during imaging. (Courtesy of Dr. Chris Cassady, Houston, TX.) **F: R**enal anomalies. Axial view at the level of the kidneys shows abnormally dilated renal pelvis with an anteroposterior diameter of 15 mm on the right (calipers). *Sp*, spine. **G: L**imb defects. Polydactyly was observed in the left hand.

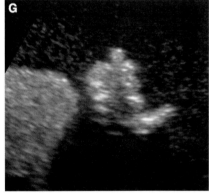

of ABS are sporadic. However, a higher risk has been noted in pregnancies preceded by uterine procedures or with twin gestations.[257] No genes have been found to predispose to ABS.

Diagnosis: Amniocentesis is not necessary in situations in which diagnosis of ABS is clear. If diagnosis is unclear owing to the appearance of associated anomalies, amniocentesis should be offered.

Imaging: Amniotic bands can be identified by both 2D US and MRI with a similar sensitivity, although the two modalities used in conjunction may aid the diagnosis in a small percentage of cases. The bands usually appear as thin, wispy strands that are freely floating within the amniotic fluid (Fig. 30.33A). In approximately one-third of focal or regional cases, an amniotic band will be identified in close approximation to the involved fetal part (Fig. 30.33B).

3D US has been shown to solidify the diagnosis by visualizing the physical relationship of a band with the affected fetal part.[258]

Limb involvement is appreciable as focal constriction of the soft tissues, possibly with edema distal to the site of constriction (Fig. 30.33C). This edema appears as hypoechoic subcutaneous skin thickening on US and as fluid signal thickening the subcutaneous space on MRI (Fig. 30.33D, E). On MRI, steady-state free process (SSFP) or heavy T2 images can improve visualization of the amniotic bands (Fig. 30.33F). Real-time imaging by US or cine imaging with MRI may show synchronous movement of separate fetal parts bound by a single band. Circumferential involvement by a band or bands may cause constriction of growth and deformity of the chest, abdomen, and skull or may also cause amputation of a limb.[258]

Involvement of the umbilical cord by amniotic bands is also a potential complication of this disorder. The bands may envelop

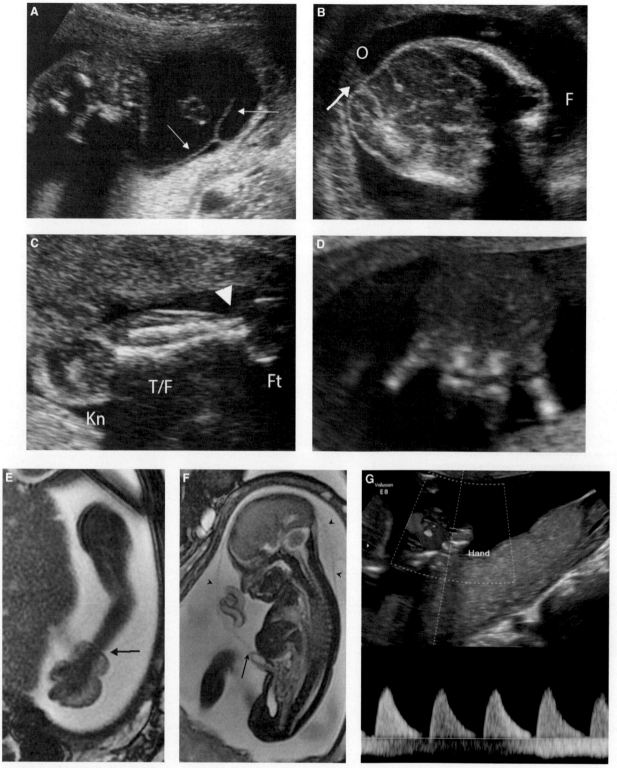

FIGURE 30.33: Amniotic band syndrome. **A–C:** A 19-week-GA fetus. **A:** Images through the lower left quadrant of the amniotic cavity showing abnormal septations, consistent with amniotic bands (*arrows*). **B:** Axial US through the fetal head showing apparent herniation of the occipital lobes through the posterior skull, consistent with encephalocele caused by amniotic bands next to defect, *arrow* (*O*, occiput; *F*, face). **C:** The left lower extremity is abnormal, with constriction of the soft tissues around the ankle (*arrowhead*), and swelling of the subcutaneous tissues in the foot, distal to the constriction (*Kn*, knee; *T/F*, tibia/fibula; *Ft*, foot). **D, E:** A 23-week GA fetus. **D:** There is amputation of the distal second and third digits. **E:** Sagittal SSFP MRI through the hand demonstrates constriction (*arrow*) from the band and distal T2 hyperintense swelling. **F:** SSFP imaging best depicting bands on this sagittal image of a fetus in which the band is identified as a thin membrane attaching to the umbilical cord (*arrow*), deforming abdominal wall, and encircling fetus (*arrowheads*). **G:** A 18-week GA fetus with bands encircling umbilical cord. Spectral Doppler of the tangled compromised cord demonstrates loss of diastolic flow in the umbilical artery and slightly pulsatile umbilical vein.

several loops of cord or may constrict a focal segment, leading to congestion of flow. Doppler spectral wave analysis may show pulsatility of the umbilical vein, absent end-diastolic flow in the umbilical artery, and elevation of the middle cerebral artery peak systolic velocity (Fig. 30.33G).[258]

Differential Diagnosis: The differential diagnosis is based on the findings and could include lymphatic or vascular malformations in the setting of focal limb soft-tissue swelling. More severe limb involvement with distortion of normal bone development may raise the question of limb reduction defects in other syndromes, such as Fanconi anemia or Adams–Oliver syndrome. Constriction and deformity of the skull may mimic a craniosynostosis.

Prognosis: The long-term outcome depends on the location and severity of deformations.

Management: In an infant with features of ABS, umbilical cord involvement may necessitate intrauterine lysis or early delivery if fetal compromise develops.[259] After birth, care is focused on management of deformities present, many requiring surgical therapy.[255] Reconstructive surgery for craniofacial clefts, anophthalmia, and encephalocele may be required.

Recurrence Risk: Most cases of ABS are sporadic with low recurrence.[255] A small number of families have reported recurrent pregnancies with amniotic bands.

Arthrogryposis Multiplex Congenita

Arthrogryposis multiplex congenita (AMC) describes two or more joint contractures in many different states, all resulting in diminished fetal movement. Other nomenclature utilized for this disorder includes multiple congenital contractures and fetal akinesia deformation sequence. Arthrogryposis was first described in 1841.[260] There is a debate on the use of the phrase "multiple congenital contractures" versus the term "arthrogryposis." Although both names may be used interchangeably, it should be emphasized that the term "arthrogryposis" is a descriptive rather than a definitive diagnosis.

Incidence: The incidence is approximately 1 in 2,000 to 5,000 live births.[261,262] Lethal forms are noted between 1 in 6985 to 25,250 depending on etiology and population.[262]

Pathogenesis/Etiology: Embryonic onset of immobility results in abnormal limb development, fixed joints, and pterygium formation. Prevention of fetal movement lasting for more than 3 weeks after 10 to 12 weeks will result in fixed joints.[263] The time of onset and length of immobility determines the severity of the contractures.[264]

The causes for AMC are both extrinsic and intrinsic to the fetus. Table 30.15 summarizes some of the disorders leading to AMC. AMC can be part of a clinical finding in over 400 disorders, of which more than 50% have a genetic origin.[265] These disorders may be inherited autosomal dominant, autosomal recessive, X-linked, via mitochondrial abnormalities, chromosomal or as a single-gene disorders.[262] The primary disorders in the fetus that result in AMC are extensive and involve major organs: brain, spinal cord, peripheral nerves, muscles, bones tendons, and/or joints. The pathology may also be secondary or extrinsic to the fetus, such as related to intrauterine crowding in the presence of

TABLE 30.15 Major Pathways and Associated Disorder Associated with Development of Arthrogryposis

EXTRINSIC	INTRINSIC (FETAL)	UNKNOWN
Uterine anomalies	Central nervous system disorder	Amyoplasia
Uterine tumors	Peripheral neuropathies	
Multifetal pregnancies	Neuromuscular junction abnormality	
Maternal illness	Myopathies	
Maternal exposures	Bone abnormalities Dermopathies Connective tissue/ ligament disorder Metabolic disturbance Genetic disorders	

uterine anomalies/tumors and multiple gestations or acquired from maternal disorders such as diabetes mellitus, myasthenia gravis, and toxic effect from drugs or infection.[260] However, in many cases, the etiology of arthrogryposis is unknown.

In general, one-third of cases with arthrogryposis will have isolated limb abnormalities and normal intelligence, one-third will have additional systems affected but generally normal neurological outcome, and one-third will have significant neurodevelopmental delay.[262] Overall, intrinsic causes of AMC will result in worse outcome than those due to extrinsic etiologies. Extrinsic causes from crowding tend to result in deformity with good outcome; however, acquired extrinsic disorders are more disruptive with a variable outcome. Intrinsic fetal etiologies usually result in malformations, which may be difficult to treat and have higher risk for lethality.[262]

AMC refers to categorized types of arthrogryposis, some associated with a genetic defect. The most commonly seen form of AMC is a sporadic, symmetric disorder known as *amyoplasia*.[266] This type of AMC represents approximately one-third of cases and is of unknown etiology but is characterized by symmetric replacement of extremity muscles by fat and connective tissue. Affected patients have normal cognitive function. Characteristically, affected patients have internal rotation of the shoulders with hands pronated and elbows extended. The knees are straight but feet equinovarus. Facial features include round face, high forehead, frontal bossing, and nevus flammeus over middle of forehead. The disorder is also associated with midline hemangiomas, gastroschisis, intestinal atresia, shortened digits, and monozygotic twins.[262]

Another subtype of AMC is called *distal arthrogryposis*, which is transmitted autosomal dominant but can have variable expression. In this disorder, there is characteristic involvement of distal joints with talipes equinovarus, calcaneovalgus, vertical talus, and metatarsus varus. The upper limbs can also be affected and may show ulnar deviation, camptodactyly, hypoplastic, or absent flexed overriding fingers. The large joints are spared. Intelligence is normal. A number of distal arthrogryposis syndromes have been described.[267] Multiple genes, including *TPM2*, *TNN12*, *TNNT3*, *MYH3*, and *MYBPC1*, have been found responsible for

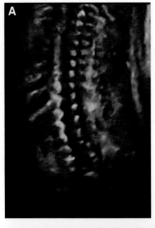
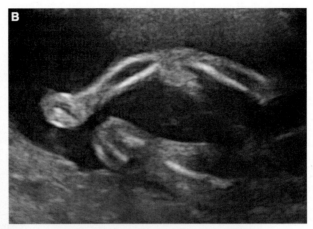
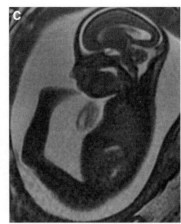
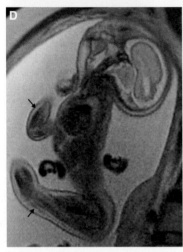
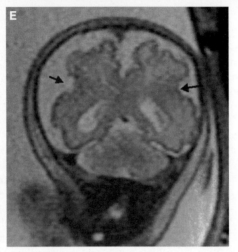

FIGURE 30.34: Arthrogryposis. **A–C:** Fetus at 22 weeks. **A:** Fixed curvature of the spine on 3D US. **B:** Unusual fixed positioning of the lower extremities with persistent hyperextension and rotation at the knee. **C:** Sagittal SSFP MRI showing similar findings. **D, E:** Fetus at 27 weeks. **D:** Sagittal SSFSE T2 MRI demonstrating fixed flexion deformities at the elbow and knee. The subcutaneous fat (*arrows*) is prominent, and the muscles (*dark signal*) are thin. **E:** Coronal SSFSE T2 MRI of the brain demonstrating irregular nodular cortex in Sylvian fissures (*arrows*), consistent with polymicrogyria. Patient expired with postmortem diagnosis of arthrogryposis, Pena–Shokeir phenotype.

the distal arthrogryposis syndromes and are available for clinical testing. The testing, however, is not required for diagnosis and may be falsely negative because of the number of subtypes and locus heterogeneity.[268,269]

Another subtype of AMC, *multiple pterygium syndrome*, is a group of autosomal dominant, recessive, or X-linked inherited syndromes that manifests with multiple contractures associated with webbing ("pterygia") of the joints, micrognathia, low-set ears, cardiac abnormalities, lung hypoplasia, cystic hygroma, and hydrops.[260] As opposed to the above-described entities, abnormal neurological function is common in this group of disorders.

Also worthy of mention is *Pena–Shokeir syndrome*,[270,271] which is a recessive disorder characterized by generalized contractures with short limbs, growth retardation, pulmonary hypoplasia, and craniofacial abnormalities. The pathophysiology in this disorder may reflect a primary motor neuropathy with a paucity of anterior horn cells in the spinal cord, although it has also been postulated that the phenotype results from fetal akinesia.

Diagnosis: A detailed history is essential, including family history of contractures, stillbirth, maternal illnesses, and exposures. Families of infants with arthrogryposis should be evaluated by a geneticist to assist with diagnosis of the underlying mechanism for the features seen, to discuss potential for genetic testing, and to receive counseling on recurrence risk.

Amniocentesis should be offered to exclude chromosomal abnormalities. Microarray will be much more sensitive and specific for this than standard chromosome analysis. There are

also panels focused on arthrogryposis, but given the extreme heterogeneity WES or whole genome sequence may be more likely to identify a specific diagnosis. This would, however, also be associated with increased numbers of variants of unclear significance.

Imaging: Previous studies have suggested low prenatal detection of AMC, being around 25%.[263] Prenatal detection is difficult, given the variability in presentation, different times of appearance, range of severity, and presence of other fetal or maternal anomalies.

First-trimester US may detect no more than 10% of cases.[265] The most common manifestations noted in the first trimester include increased NT, lymphatic malformations, or major anomaly with limb positioning deformities.[262] The remaining cases identified prenatal are usually detected in the second trimester.[265] Arthrogryposis should be suspected when decreased or lack of fetal movement is observed along with an abnormal fetal position. These observations should prompt a careful inspection of the joints, muscle mass, bone mineralization and fractures, jaw shape and swallowing, spine, and thoracic circumference (Fig. 30.34A–C). Features seen by prenatal imaging are summarized in Table 30.16. However, any major structural defect with joint anomaly and polyhydramnios should prompt careful evaluation for AMC, which includes assessment for absence or atypical fetal movements. Fetal MRI is extremely helpful in identifying CNS malformations; for example, polymicrogyria can be present in some types (Fig. 30.34D, E). Fetal MRI has also been utilized

TABLE 30.16	List of Features of Arthrogryposis Seen by Prenatal Imaging
First trimester/Other	Increased nuchal thickness
	Lymphatic malformation
	Hydrops
	Fetal akinesia
	Short umbilical cord
	Single umbilical artery
	Growth restriction
	Polyhydramnios
	Oligohydramnios
Musculoskeletal	Abnormal fetal position
	Fixed flexion/extension abnormalities
	Feet and hand deformities
	Scoliosis
	Hypomineralization of long bones
	Multiple fractures
	Low muscle mass
Central Nervous System	Ventriculomegaly
	Corpus callosum abnormalities
	Cerebellar abnormalities
	Brainstem abnormalities
	Delayed sulcation/gyration
	Lissencephaly/Polymicrogyria
	Cystic basal ganglia lesions
	Microcephaly
Craniofacial	Beak-like nose
	Cleft lip and palate
	Micrognathia/Retrognathia
	Microtia
Cardiac	Cardiomegaly
	Pericardial effusion
Thorax	Narrow chest
	Pleural effusion
	Pulmonary hypoplasia
	Thin ribs
	Congenital diaphragmatic hernia
Genitourinary and Gastrointestinal	Absent stomach bubble
	Gastroschisis
	Hydronephrosis

From Niles KM, Blaser S, Shannon P, et al. Fetal arthrogryposis multiplex congenital/fetal akinesia deformation sequence-Aetiology, diagnosis and management. *Prenat Diagn*. 2019;39(9):720–731. Copyright © 2019 John Wiley & Sons, Ltd. Adapted by permission of John Wiley & Sons, Inc.

to assess for pulmonary hypoplasia, decreased muscle mass, and facial anomalies.[272]

Differential Diagnosis: Arthrogryposis is not a diagnosis; it is a physical finding that simply refers to contractures of multiple joints, regardless of etiology. Therefore, any condition that may lead to multiple congenital contractures can be included in the differential.

Prognosis: Short- and long-term prognosis depends on the extent of abnormalities and number of systems impacted. Some patients with AMC may require intubation. Those patients with

AMC who require ventilator support have much worse long-term outcomes.[262]

Management: If there is interruption of the pregnancy or loss prenatal and/at birth, an autopsy and/or postmortem imaging should be offered. Pregnancies with AMC are more likely to require cesarean section due to atypical presentation, labor failure, and gracile bones that predispose the infant to fractures. An infant with AMC should have a complete physical examination with attention to joints. Characteristic features include rigidity of joints from contractures, dislocations, absence of normal skin creases, increase in subcutaneous fat, deep skin dimples, and decreased muscle mass.[273]

Respiratory distress may be seen in patients with AMC shortly after birth owing to pulmonary hypoplasia. Feeding issues may also occur. Management of joint abnormalities includes physical therapy, which should be initiated in the newborn period to maintain and develop joint mobility.[273] It is important to exclude CNS abnormalities; therefore, MRI of the brain and spine is recommended.[273] Renal dysfunction and cholestasis can be associated with some subtypes of the distal arthrogryposis syndromes and should be screened with US and biochemical testing.[274]

Long-term management issues focus on joint disorders, including potential for knee contractures. There is an increased incidence of hip dislocation and scoliosis. A study of teens and adults with AMC showed that they had limited shoulder motion and elbow deformities, but no other significant handicaps. Half of the study group walked independently, and most had normal intelligence.[274] A more recent study found that severe disability is seen in most adults with congenital arthrogryposis.[275] Historically, complex cases of arthrogryposis did not survive and were not included in studies; thus, there is a great deal of uncertainty about long-term functional outcomes for most forms of arthrogryposis.

Recurrence Risk: Recurrence risk varies according to the underlying cause and inheritance pattern. Distal arthrogryposis syndromes have a 50% recurrence risk, while amyoplasia is sporadic and has a low recurrence risk. In cases in which no etiology has been identified for AMC, there is a 3% to 5% recurrence risk, which increases to 7% in cases with CNS abnormality.[276]

REFERENCES

1. Canick JA, Kloza EM, Lambert-Messerlian GM, et al. DNA sequencing of maternal plasma to identify Down syndrome and other trisomies in multiple gestations. *Prenat Diagn*. 2012;32:730–734.
2. Devers PL, Cronister A, Ormond KE, et al. Noninvasive prenatal testing/noninvasive prenatal diagnosis: the position of the National Society of Genetic Counselors. *J Genet Couns*. 2013;22(3):291–295.
3. Bamshad MJ, Ng SB, Bigham AW, et al. Exome sequencing as a tool for Mendelian disease gene discovery. *Nat Rev Genet*. 2011;12(11):745–755. doi:10.1038/nrg3031.
4. Snijders RJ, Sundberg K, Holzgreve W, et al. Maternal age- and gestation-specific risk for trisomy 21. *Ultrasound Obstet Gynecol*. 1999;13:167–170.
5. Munné S, Sultan KM, Weier HU, et al. Assessment of numeric abnormalities of X, Y, 18, and 16 chromosomes in preimplantation human embryos before transfer. *Am J Obstet Gynecol*. 1995;172:1191–1199.
6. Bull MJ. Health supervision for children with Down syndrome. *Pediatrics*. 2011;128:393–406.
7. de Graaf G, Buckley F, Skotko BG. Estimates of the live births, natural losses, and elective terminations with Down syndrome in the United States. *Am J Med Genet A*. 2015;167(4):756–767. doi:10.1002/ajmg.a.37001.
8. Antonarakis SE. Parental origin of the extra chromosome in trisomy 21 as indicated by analysis of DNA polymorphisms: Down Syndrome Collaborative Group. *N Engl J Med*. 1991;324:872–876.
9. Huether CA, Ivanovich J, Goodwin BS, et al. Maternal age specific risk rate estimates for Down syndrome among live births in whites and other races from Ohio and metropolitan Atlanta, 1970–1989. *J Med Genet*. 1998;35:482–490.

10. Cicero S, Bindra R, Rembouskos G, et al. Integrated ultrasound and biochemical screening for trisomy 21 using fetal nuchal translucency, absent fetal nasal bone, free beta-hCG and PAPP-A at 11 to 14 weeks. *Prenat Diagn.* 2003;23:306–310.

11. Vintzileos A, Walters C, Yeo L. Absent nasal bone in the prenatal detection of fetuses with trisomy 21 in a high-risk population. *Obstet Gynecol.* 2003;101:905–908.

12. Canick J. Prenatal screening for trisomy 21: recent advances and guidelines. *Clin Chem Lab Med.* 2012;50:1003–1008.

13. Agathokleous M, Chaveeva P, Poon LC, et al. Meta-analysis of second-trimester markers for trisomy 21. *Ultrasound Obstet Gynecol.* 2013;41:247–261.

14. Papasozomenou P, Athanasiadis AP, Zafrakas M, et al. Screening performance of different methods defining fetal nasal gone hypoplasia as a single and combined marker for the detection of trisomy 21 in the second trimester. *J Matern Fetal Neonatal Med.* 2016;29(20):3368–3373.

15. Huang LY, Zhen L, Pan M, et al. Application of noninvasive prenatal testing in pregnancies with fetal double bubble sign: Is it feasible? *Prenat Diagn.* 2018;38:402–405.

16. Nicolaides KH, Heath V, Cicero S. Increased fetal nuchal translucency at 11–14 weeks. *Prenat Diagn.* 2002;22:308–315.

17. Holzgreve W, Curry CJ, Golbus MS, et al. Investigation of nonimmune hydrops fetalis. *Am J Obstet Gynecol.* 1984;150:805–812.

18. Sepulveda W, Reid R, Nicolaidis P, et al. Second-trimester echogenic bowel and intraamniotic bleeding: association between fetal bowel echogenicity and amniotic fluid spectrophotometry at 410 nm. *Am J Obstet Gynecol.* 1996;174:839–842.

19. Choudhry MS, Rahman N, Boyd P, et al. Duodenal atresia: associated anomalies, prenatal diagnosis and outcome. *Pediatr Surg Int.* 2009;25:727–730.

20. Dankovcik R, Jirasek JE, Kucera E, et al. Prenatal diagnosis of annular pancreas: reliability of the double bubble sign with periduodenal hyperechogenic band. *Fetal Diagn Ther.* 2008;24:483–490.

21. Nguyen HT, Benson CB, Bromley B, et al. Multidisciplinary consensus on the classification of prenatal and postnatal urinary tract dilation (UTD classification system). *J Pediatr Urol.* 2014;10:982–999.

22. Kovac CM, Brown JA, Apodaca CC, et al. Maternal ethnicity and variation of fetal femur length calculations when screening for Down syndrome. *J Ultrasound Med.* 2002;21:719–722.

23. Ranweiler R. Assessment and care of the newborn with Down syndrome. *Adv Neonatal Care.* 2009;9:17–24; quiz 25–16.

24. Yang Q, Rasmussen SA, Friedman JM. Mortality associated with Down's syndrome in the USA from 1983 to 1997: a population-based study. *Lancet.* 2002;359:1019–1025.

25. Roberts JE, Price J, Malkin C. Language and communication development in Down syndrome. *Ment Retard Dev Disabil Res Rev.* 2007;13:26–35.

26. Holland AJ, Hon J, Huppert FA, et al. Incidence and course of dementia in people with Down's syndrome: findings from a population-based study. *J Intellect Disabil Res.* 2000;44(pt 2):138–146.

27. Hartley D, Blumenthal T, Carrillo M, et al. Down syndrome and Alzheimer's disease: common pathways, common goals. *Alzheimers Dement.* 2015;11(6):700–709. doi:10.1016/j.jalz.2014.10.007.

28. Henry E, Walker D, Wiedmeier SE, et al. Hematological abnormalities during the first week of life among neonates with Down syndrome: data from a multihospital healthcare system. *Am J Med Genet A.* 2007;143:42–50.

29. Eunpu DL, McDonald DM, Zackai EH. Trisomy 21: rate in second-degree relatives. *Am J Med Genet.* 1986;25:361–363.

30. Lin HY, Lin SP, Chen YJ, et al. Clinical characteristics and survival of trisomy 18 in a medical center in Taipei, 1988–2004. *Am J Med Genet A.* 2006;140:945–951.

31. Eggermann T, Nöthen MM, Eiben B, et al. Trisomy of human chromosome 18: molecular studies on parental origin and cell stage of nondisjunction. *Hum Genet.* 1996;97:218–223.

32. Palomaki GE, Neveux LM, Knight GJ, et al. Maternal serum-integrated screening for trisomy 18 using both first- and second-trimester markers. *Prenat Diagn.* 2003;23:243–247.

33. Wagner P, Sonek J, Hoopmann M, et al. First trimester screening for trisomies 18 and 13, triploidy and Turner syndrome by detailed early anomaly scan. *Ultra Obstet Gynecol.* 2016;48:446–451.

34. Nyberg DA, Kramer D, Resta RG, et al. Prenatal sonographic findings of trisomy 18: review of 47 cases. *J Ultrasound Med.* 1993;12:103–113.

35. Hill LM. The sonographic detection of trisomies 13, 18, and 21. *Clin Obstet Gynecol.* 1996;39:831–850.

36. Moyano D, Huggon IC, Allan LD. Fetal echocardiography in trisomy 18. *Arch Dis Child.* 2005;90:F520–F522.

37. Babcook CJ, Goldstein RB, Filly RA. Prenatally detected fetal myelomeningocele: is karyotype analysis warranted? *Radiology.* 1995;194:491–494.

38. Yoder PR, Sabbagha RE, Gross SJ, et al. The second-trimester fetus with isolated choroid plexus cysts: a meta-analysis of risk of trisomies 18 and 21. *Obstet Gynecol.* 1999;93:869–872.

39. Snijders RJ, Shawa L, Nicolaides KH. Fetal choroid plexus cysts and trisomy 18: assessment of risk based on ultrasound findings and maternal age. *Prenat Diagn.* 1994;14:1119–1127.

40. Bahado-Singh RO, Lynch L, Deren O, et al. First-trimester growth restriction and fetal aneuploidy: the effect of type of aneuploidy and gestational age. *Am J Obstet Gynecol.* 1997;176:976–980.

41. Byrne J, Blanc WA. Malformations and chromosome anomalies in spontaneously aborted fetuses with single umbilical artery. *Am J Obstet Gynecol.* 1985;151:340–342.

42. Benjamin DR, Juul S, Siebert JR. Congenital posterolateral diaphragmatic hernia: associated malformations. *J Pediatr Surg.* 1988;23:899–903.

43. Russo FM, Pozzi E, Verderio M, et al. Parental counseling in trisomy 18: novel insights in prenatal features and postnatal survival. *Am J Med Genet A.* 2016;170A(2):329–336.

44. Rasmussen SA, Wong LY, Yang Q, et al. Population-based analyses of mortality in trisomy 13 and trisomy 18. *Pediatrics.* 2003;111:777–784.

45. Baty BJ, Blackburn BL, Carey JC. Natural history of trisomy 18 and trisomy 13, I: growth, physical assessment, medical histories, survival, and recurrence risk. *Am J Med Genet.* 1994;49:175–188.

46. Carey JC. Health supervision and anticipatory guidance for children with genetic disorders (including specific recommendations for trisomy 21, trisomy 18, and neurofibromatosis I). *Pediatr Clin North Am.* 1992;39:25–53.

47. Nelson KE, Hexem KR, Feudtner C. Inpatient hospital care of children with trisomy 13 and trisomy 18 in the United States. *Pediatrics.* 2012;129(5):869–876. doi:10.1542/peds.2011-2139.

48. Hassold T, Jacobs PA, Leppert M, et al. Cytogenetic and molecular studies of trisomy 13. *J Med Genet.* 1987;24:725–732.

49. Brizot ML, Snijders RJ, Bersinger NA, et al. Maternal serum pregnancy-associated plasma protein A and fetal nuchal translucency thickness for the prediction of fetal trisomies in early pregnancy. *Obstet Gynecol.* 1994;84:918–922.

50. Lehman CD, Nyberg DA, Winter TC III, et al. Trisomy 13 syndrome: prenatal US findings in a review of 33 cases. *Radiology.* 1995;194:217–222.

51. Wladimiroff JW, Bhaggoe WR, Kristelijn M, et al. Sonographically determined anomalies and outcome in 170 chromosomally abnormal fetuses. *Prenat Diagn.* 1995;15:431–438.

52. Jacobs PA, Hassold TJ, Henry A, et al. Trisomy 13 ascertained in a survey of spontaneous abortions. *J Med Genet.* 1987;24:721–724.

53. Tuohy JF, James DK. Pre-eclampsia and trisomy 13. *Br J Obstet Gynaecol.* 1992;99:891–894.

54. Bdolah Y, Palomaki GE, Yaron Y, et al. Circulating angiogenic proteins in trisomy 13. *Am J Obstet Gynecol.* 2006;194:239–245.

55. Schreinemachers DM, Cross PK, Hook EB. Rates of trisomies 21, 18, 13 and other chromosome abnormalities in about 20 000 prenatal studies compared with estimated rates in live births. *Hum Genet.* 1982;61:318–324.

56. Hassold T, Chen N, Funkhouser J, et al. A cytogenetic study of 1000 spontaneous abortions. *Ann Hum Genet.* 1980;44:151–178.

57. Rochon L, Vekemans MJ. Triploidy arising from a first meiotic non-disjunction in a mother carrying a reciprocal translocation. *J Med Genet.* 1990;27(11):724–726.

58. McFadden DE, Kalousek DK. Two different phenotypes of fetuses with chromosomal triploidy: correlation with parental origin of the extra haploid set. *Am J Med Genet.* 1991;38:535–538.

59. de Graaf IM, van Bezouw SM, Jakobs ME, et al. First-trimester non-invasive prenatal diagnosis of triploidy. *Prenat Diagn.* 1999;19:175–177.

60. Schluth C, Doray B, Girard-Lemaire F, et al. Prenatal diagnosis of a true fetal tetraploidy in direct and cultured chorionic villi. *Genet Couns.* 2004;15:429–436.

61. Zalel Y, Shapiro I, Weissmann-Brenner A, et al. Prenatal sonographic features of triploidy at 12–16 weeks. *Prenat Diagn.* 2016;36:65–55.

62. Pircon RA, Porto M, Towers CV, et al. Ultrasound findings in pregnancies complicated by fetal triploidy. *J Ultrasound Med.* 1989;8:507–511.

63. Stefanova I, Jenderny J, Kaminsky E, et al. Mosaic and complete tetraploidy in live-born infants: two new patients and review of the literature. *Clin Dysmorphol.* 2010;19:123–127.

64. Di Cintio E, Parazzini F, Rosa C, et al. The epidemiology of gestational trophoblastic disease. *Gen Diagn Pathol.* 1997;143:103–108.

65. Lindor NM, Ney JA, Gaffey TA, et al. A genetic review of complete and partial hydatidiform moles and nonmolar triploidy. *Mayo Clin Proc.* 1992;67:791–799.

66. Sherard J, Bean C, Bove B, et al. Long survival in a 69,XXY triploid male. *Am J Med Genet.* 1986;25:307–312.

67. Jauniaux E. Partial moles: from postnatal to prenatal diagnosis. *Placenta.* 1999;20:379–388.

68. Gravholt CH, Juul S, Naeraa RW, et al. Prenatal and postnatal prevalence of Turner's syndrome: a registry study. *BMJ.* 1996;312:16–21.

69. Frias JL, Davenport ML. Health supervision for children with Turner syndrome. *Pediatrics.* 2003;111:692–702.

70. Jacobs P, Dalton P, James R, et al. Turner syndrome: a cytogenetic and molecular study. *Ann Hum Genet.* 1997;61:471–483.

71. Sagi L, Zuckerman-Levin N, Gawlik A, et al. Clinical significance of the parental origin of the X chromosome in turner syndrome. *J Clin Endocrinol Metab.* 2007;92:846–852.

72. Ruiz C, Lamm F, Hart PS. Turner syndrome and multiple-marker screening. *Clin Chem.* 1999;45:2259–2261.

73. Gersak K, Veble A, Mulla ZD, et al. Association between increased yolk sac diameter and abnormal karyotypes. *J Perinat Med.* 2012;40:251–254.

74. Carvalho AB, Guerra Junior G, Baptista MT, et al. Cardiovascular and renal anomalies in Turner syndrome. *Rev Assoc Med Bras.* 2010;56:655–659.

75. Bondy CA. Care of girls and women with Turner syndrome: a guideline of the Turner Syndrome Study Group. *J Clin Endocrinol Metab.* 2007;92:10–25.

76. McDermott DA, Bressan MC, He J, et al. TBX5 genetic testing validates strict clinical criteria for Holt-Oram syndrome. *Pediatr Res.* 2005;58:981–986.

77. Gedikbasi A, Oztarhan K, Aslan G, et al. Multidisciplinary approach in cystic hygroma: prenatal diagnosis, outcome, and postnatal follow up. *Pediatr Int.* 2009;51:670–677.

78. Bianco B, Lipay MV, Melaragno MI, et al. Detection of hidden Y mosaicism in Turner's syndrome: importance in the prevention of gonadoblastoma. *J Pediatr Endocrinol Metab.* 2006;19:1113–1117.

79. Baujat G, Rio M, Rossignol S, et al. Clinical and molecular overlap in overgrowth syndromes. *Am J Med Genet C Semin Med Genet.* 2005;137C:4–11.

80. Cytrynbaum CS, Smith AC, Rubin T, et al. Advances in overgrowth syndromes: clinical classification to molecular delineation in Sotos syndrome and Beckwith-Wiedemann syndrome. *Curr Opin Pediatr.* 2005;17:740–746.

81. Reish O, Lerer I, Amiel A, et al. Wiedemann-Beckwith syndrome: further prenatal characterization of the condition. *Am J Med Genet.* 2002;107:209–213.

82. Shuman C, Beckwith JB, Smith AC, et al. Beckwith-Wiedemann syndrome. In: Pagon RA, Adam MP, Bird TD, et al., eds. *GeneReviews*™ [Internet]. Seattle, WA: University of Washington; 2000. Available from http://www.ncbi.nlm.nih.gov/books/NBK1394/. Updated December 14, 2010.

83. Eggermann T, Brioude F, Russo S, et al. Prenatal molecular testing for Beckwith–Wiedemann and Silver–Russell syndromes: a challenge for molecular analysis and genetic counseling. *Eur J Hum Genet.* 2016;24(6):784–793. doi:10.1038/ejhg.2015.224.

84. Barisic I, Boban L, Akhmedzhanova D, et al. Beckwith Wiedemann syndrome: A population based study on prevalence, prenatal diagnosis, associated anomalies and survival in Europe. *Eur J Med Genet.* 2018;61:499–507.

85. Porter A, Benson CB, Hawley P, et al. Outcome of fetuses with a prenatal ultrasound diagnosis of isolated omphalocele. *Prenat Diagn.* 2009;29:668–673.

86. Shieh HF, Estroff JA, Barnewolt CE, et al. Prenatal imaging throughout gestation in Beckwith-Wiedemann syndrome. *Prenat Diagn.* 2109;39:792–795.

87. Elliott M, Bayly R, Cole T, et al. Clinical features and natural history of Beckwith-Wiedemann syndrome: presentation of 74 new cases. *Clin Genet.* 1994;46:168–174.

88. Storm DW, Hirselj DA, Rink B, et al. The prenatal diagnosis of Beckwith-Wiedemann syndrome using ultrasound and magnetic resonance imaging. *Urology.* 2011;77:208–210.

89. Gocmen R, Basaran C, Karcaaltincaba M, et al. Bilateral hemorrhagic adrenal cysts in an incomplete form of Beckwith-Wiedemann syndrome: MRI and prenatal US findings. *Abdom Imaging.* 2005;30:786–789.

90. Vora N, Bianchi DW. Genetic considerations in the prenatal diagnosis of overgrowth syndromes. *Prenat Diagn.* 2009;29:923–929.

91. Williams DH, Gauthier DW, Maizels M. Prenatal diagnosis of Beckwith-Wiedemann syndrome. *Prenat Diagn.* 2005;25:879–884.

92. Zarate YA, Mena R, Martin LJ, et al. Experience with hemihyperplasia and Beckwith-Wiedemann syndrome surveillance protocol. *Am J Med Genet Part A.* 2009;149A:1691–1697.

93. Lapunzina P. Risk of tumorigenesis in overgrowth syndromes: a comprehensive review. *Am J Med Genet C Semin Med Genet.* 2005;137C:53–71.

94. Slavotinek A, Gaunt L, Donnai D. Paternally inherited duplications of 11p15.5 and Beckwith-Wiedemann syndrome. *J Med Genet.* 1997;34:819–826.

95. Sparago A, Cerrato F, Vernucci M, et al. Microdeletions in the human H19 DMR result in loss of IGF2 imprinting and Beckwith-Wiedemann syndrome. *Nat Genet.* 2004;36:958–960.

96. Majeed SM, Khan A, ul Haq M, et al. Holt-Oram syndrome. J Pak Med Assoc. 1991;41:139–140.

97. Salonen R, Norio R. The Meckel syndrome in Finland: epidemiologic and genetic aspects. *Am J Med Genet.* 1984;18:691–698.

98. Terrett JA, Newbury-Ecob R, Smith NM, et al. A translocation at 12q2 refines the interval containing the Holt-Oram syndrome 1 gene. *Am J Hum Genet.* 1996;59:1337–1341.

99. Basson CT, Bachinsky DR, Lin RC, et al. Mutations in human TBX5 [corrected] cause limb and cardiac malformation in Holt-Oram syndrome. *Nat Genet.* 1997;15:30–35.

100. Borozdin W, Wright MJ, Hennekam RC, et al. Novel mutations in the gene SALL4 provide further evidence for acro-renal-ocular and Okihiro syndromes being allelic entities, and extend the phenotypic spectrum. *J Med Genet.* 2004;41:e102.

101. Sunagawa S, Kikuchi A, Sano Y, et al. Prenatal diagnosis of Holt-Oram syndrome: role of 3-D ultrasonography. *Congenit Anom.* 2009;49:38–41.

102. Poznanski AK, Gall JC Jr, Stern AM. Skeletal manifestations of the Holt-Oram syndrome. *Radiology.* 1970;94:45–53.

103. Tongsong T, Chanprapaph P. Prenatal sonographic diagnosis of Holt-Oram syndrome. *J Clin Ultrasound.* 2000;28:98–100.

104. Hurst JA, Hall CM, Baraitser M. The Holt-Oram syndrome. *J Med Genet.* 1991;28:406–410.

105. Hartill V, Szymanska K, Sharif SM, et al. Meckel-Gruber syndrome: an update on diagnosis, clinical management, and research advances. *Front Pediatr.* 2017;5:244. doi:10.3389/fped.2017.00244.

106. Ickowicz V, Eurin D, Maugey-Laulom B, et al. Meckel-Gruber syndrome: sonography and pathology. *Ultrasound Obstet Gynecol.* 2006;27:296–300.

107. Eckmann-Scholz C, Jonat W, Zerres K, et al. Earliest ultrasound findings and description of splicing mutations in Meckel-Gruber syndrome. *Arch Gynecol Obstet.* 2012;286:917–921.

108. Auber B, Burfeind P, Herold S, et al. A disease causing deletion of 29 base pairs in intron 15 in the MKS1 gene is highly associated with the campomelic variant of the Meckel-Gruber syndrome. *Clin Genet.* 2007;72:454–459.

109. Valente EM, Logan CV, Mougou-Zerelli S, et al. Mutations in TMEM216 perturb ciliogenesis and cause Joubert, Meckel and related syndromes. *Nat Genet.* 2010;42:619–625.

110. Tallila J, Jakkula E, Peltonen L, et al. Identification of CC2D2A as a Meckel syndrome gene adds an important piece to the ciliopathy puzzle. *Am J Hum Genet.* 2008;82:1361–1367.

111. Kyttala M, Tallila J, Salonen R, et al. MKS1, encoding a component of the flagellar apparatus basal body proteome, is mutated in Meckel syndrome. *Nat Genet.* 2006;38:155–157.

112. Wright C, Healicon R, English C, et al. Meckel syndrome: what are the minimum diagnostic criteria? *J Med Genet.* 1994;31:482–485.

113. Celentano C, Prefumo F, Liberati M, et al. Prenatal diagnosis of Meckel-Gruber syndrome in a pregnancy obtained with ICSI. *J Assist Reprod Genet.* 2006;23:281–283.

114. Liu SS, Cheong ML, She BQ, et al. First-trimester ultrasound diagnosis of Meckel-Gruber syndrome. *Acta Obstet Gynecol Scand.* 2006;85:757–759.

115. Hosny IA, Elghawabi HS. Ultrafast MRI of the fetus: an increasingly important tool in prenatal diagnosis of congenital anomalies. *Magn Reson Imaging.* 2010;28:1431–1439.

116. Maria BL, Quisling RG, Rosainz LC, et al. Molar tooth sign in Joubert syndrome: clinical, radiologic, and pathologic significance. *J Child Neurol.* 1999;14:368–376.

117. Mougou-Zerelli S, Thomas S, Szenker E, et al. CC2D2A mutations in Meckel and Joubert syndromes indicate a genotype-phenotype correlation. *Hum Mutat.* 2009;30:1574–1582.

118. Chaumoitre K, Brun M, Cassart M, et al. Differential diagnosis of fetal hyperechogenic cystic kidneys unrelated to renal tract anomalies: a multicenter study. *Ultrasound Obstet Gynecol.* 2006;28:911–917.

119. Kline AD, Krantz ID, Sommer A, et al. Cornelia de Lange syndrome: clinical review, diagnostic and scoring systems, and anticipatory guidance. *Am J Med Genet A.* 2007;143A:1287–1296.

120. Jackson L, Kline AD, Barr MA, et al. de Lange syndrome: a clinical review of 310 individuals. *Am J Med Genet.* 1993;47:940–946.

121. Borck G, Redon R, Sanlaville D, et al. NIPBL mutations and genetic heterogeneity in Cornelia de Lange syndrome. *J Med Genet.* 2004;41:e128.

122. Deardorff MA, Kaur M, Yaeger D, et al. Mutations in cohesin complex members SMC3 and SMC1A cause a mild variant of cornelia de Lange syndrome with predominant mental retardation. *Am J Hum Genet.* 2007;80:485–494.

123. Arbuzova S, Nikolenko M, Krantz D, et al. Low first-trimester pregnancy-associated plasma protein-A and Cornelia de Lange syndrome. *Prenat Diagn.* 2003;23:864.

124. Bruner JP, Hsia YE. Prenatal findings in Brachmann-de Lange syndrome. *Obstet Gynecol.* 1990;76:966–968.

125. Thellier E, Levaillant M, Roume J, et al. Cornelia de Lange syndrome: specific features for prenatal diagnosis. *Ultra Obstet Gynecol.* 2017;49:668–670.

126. Spaggiari E, Vuillard E, Khung-Savatovsky S, et al. Ultrasound detection of eyelashes: a clue for prenatal diagnosis of Cornelia de Lange syndrome. *Ultrasound Obstet Gynecol.* 2013;41:341–342.

127. Ranzini AC, Day-Salvatore D, Farren-Chavez D, et al. Prenatal diagnosis of de Lange syndrome. *J Ultrasound Med.* 1997,16.755–758.

128. Charles AK, Porter HJ, Sams V, et al. Nephrogenic rests and renal abnormalities in Brachmann-de Lange syndrome. *Pediatr Pathol Lab Med.* 1997;17:209–219.

129. Barisic I, Tokic V, Loane M, et al. Descriptive epidemiology of Cornelia de Lange syndrome in Europe. *Am J Med Genet A.* 2008;146A:51–59.

130. Kline AD, Stanley C, Belevich J, et al. Developmental data on individuals with the Brachmann-de Lange syndrome. *Am J Med Genet.* 1993;47:1053–1058.

131. Beck B, Fenger K. Mortality, pathological findings and causes of death in the de Lange syndrome. *Acta Paediatr.* 1985;74:765–769.

132. Kline AD, Barr M, Jackson LG. Growth manifestations in the Brachmann-de Lange syndrome. *Am J Med Genet.* 1993;47:1042–1049.

133. Levin AV, Seidman DJ, Nelson LB, et al. Ophthalmologic findings in the Cornelia de Lange syndrome. *J Pediatr Ophthalmol Strabismus.* 1990;27:94–102.

134. Kelley RI, Hennekam RC. The Smith-Lemli-Opitz syndrome. *J Med Genet.* 2000;37:321–335.

135. Tint GS, Irons M, Elias ER, et al. Defective cholesterol biosynthesis associated with the Smith-Lemli-Opitz syndrome. *N Engl J Med.* 1994;330:107–113.

136. Porter FD. Smith-Lemli-Opitz syndrome: pathogenesis, diagnosis and management. *Eur J Hum Genet.* 2008;16:535–541.

137. Bialer MG, Penchaszadeh VB, Kahn E, et al. Female external genitalia and Müllerian duct derivatives in a 46,XY infant with the Smith-Lemli-Opitz syndrome. *Am J Med Genet.* 1987;28:723–731.

138. Lin AE, Ardinger HH, Ardinger RH Jr, et al. Cardiovascular malformations in Smith-Lemli-Opitz syndrome. *Am J Med Genet.* 1997;68:270–278.

139. Witsch-Baumgartner M, Loffler J, Utermann G. Mutations in the human DHCR7 gene. *Hum Mutat.* 2001;17:172–182.

140. Bradley LA, Palomaki GE, Knight GJ, et al. Levels of unconjugated estriol and other maternal serum markers in pregnancies with Smith-Lemli-Opitz (RSH) syndrome fetuses. *Am J Med Genet.* 1999;82:355–358.

141. Cunniff C, Kratz LE, Moser A, et al. Clinical and biochemical spectrum of patients with RSH/Smith-Lemli-Opitz syndrome and abnormal cholesterol metabolism. *Am J Med Genet.* 1997;68:263–269.

142. Hyett JA, Clayton PT, Moscoso G, et al. Increased first trimester nuchal translucency as a prenatal manifestation of Smith-Lemli-Opitz syndrome. *Am J Med Genet.* 1995;58:374–376.

143. Goldenberg A, Wolf C, Chevy F, et al. Antenatal manifestations of Smith-Lemli-Opitz (RSH) syndrome: a retrospective survey of 30 cases. *Am J Med Genet A.* 2004;124A:423–426.

144. Moshiri M, Chapman T, Fechner PY, et al. Evaluation and management of disorders of sex development: multidisciplinary approach to a complex diagnosis. *Radiographics*. 2012;32:1599–1618.

145. Finley SC, Finley WH, Monsky DB. Cataracts in a girl with features of the Smith-Lemli-Opitz syndrome. *J Pediatr*. 1969;75:706–707.

146. Caruso PA, Poussaint TY, Tzika AA, et al. MRI and 1H MRS findings in Smith-Lemli-Opitz syndrome. *Neuroradiology*. 2004;46:3–14.

147. Thompson E, Baraitser M. An autosomal recessive mental retardation syndrome with hepatic fibrosis and renal cysts. *Am J Med Genet*. 1986;24:151–158.

148. Starck L, Lovgren-Sandblom A, Bjorkhem I. Cholesterol treatment forever? The first Scandinavian trial of cholesterol supplementation in the cholesterol-synthesis defect Smith-Lemli-Opitz syndrome. *J Intern Med*. 2002;252:314–321.

149. Azurdia RM, Anstey AV, Rhodes LE. Cholesterol supplementation objectively reduces photosensitivity in the Smith-Lemli-Opitz syndrome. *Br J Dermatol*. 2001;144:143–145.

150. Nwokoro NA, Mulvihill JJ. Cholesterol and bile acid replacement therapy in children and adults with Smith-Lemli-Opitz (SLO/RSH) syndrome. *Am J Med Genet*. 1997;68:315–321.

151. Chemaitilly W, Goldenberg A, Baujat G, et al. Adrenal insufficiency and abnormal genitalia in a 46XX female with Smith-Lemli-Opitz syndrome. *Horm Res*. 2003;59:254–256.

152. Tierney E, Nwokoro NA, Porter FD, et al. Behavior phenotype in the RSH/Smith-Lemli-Opitz syndrome. *Am J Med Genet*. 2001;98:191–200.

153. Abuelo DN, Tint GS, Kelley R, et al. Prenatal detection of the cholesterol biosynthetic defect in the Smith-Lemli-Opitz syndrome by the analysis of amniotic fluid sterols. *Am J Med Genet*. 1995;56:281–285.

154. Berry SA, Peterson C, Mize W, et al. Klippel-Trenaunay syndrome. *Am J Med Genet*. 1998;79:319–326.

155. Zoppi MA, Ibba RM, Floris M, et al. Prenatal sonographic diagnosis of Klippel-Trenaunay-Weber syndrome with cardiac failure. *J Clin Ultrasound*. 2001;29:422–426.

156. Aelvoet GE, Jorens PG, Roelen LM. Genetic aspects of the Klippel-Trenaunay syndrome. *Br J Dermatol*. 1992;126:603–607.

157. Samuel M, Spitz L. Klippel-Trenaunay syndrome: clinical features, complications and management in children. *Br J Surg*. 1995;82:757–761.

158. Peng HH, Wang TH, Chao AS, et al. Klippel-Trenaunay-Weber syndrome involving fetal thigh: prenatal presentations and outcomes. *Prenat Diagn*. 2006;26:825–830.

159. Calvo-Garcia MA, Kline-fath BM, Adams DM, et al. Imaging evaluation of fetal vascular anomalies. *Pediatr Radiol*. 2015;45(8):1218–1229.

160. Chen CP, Lin SP, Chang TY, et al. Prenatal sonographic findings of Klippel-Trenaunay-Weber syndrome. *J Clin Ultrasound*. 2007;35:409–412.

161. Van Den Berg DJ, Francke U. Roberts syndrome: a review of 100 cases and a new rating system for severity. *Am J Med Genet*. 1993;47:1104–1123.

162. Maheshwari A, Kumar P, Dutta S, et al. Roberts-SC phocomelia syndrome. *Indian J Pediatr*. 2001;68:557–559.

163. Shule B, Oviedo A, Johnston K, et al. Inactivating mutations in ESCO2 cause SC phocomelia and Roberts syndrome: no phenotype-genotype correlation. *Am J Hum Genet*. 2005;77:1117–1128.

164. Kaur H, DeScipio C, McCallum J, et al. Precocious sister chromatid separation (PSCS) in Cornelia de Lange syndrome. *Am J Med Genet A*. 2005;138:27–31.

165. Rios LT, Araujo Junior E, Caetano AC, et al. Prenatal Diagnosis of EEC syndrome with "lobster claw" anomaly by 3D ultrasound. *J Clin Imaging Sci*. 2012;2:40.

166. Stoll C, Alembik Y, Dott B, et al. Associated malformations in patients with limb reduction deficiencies. *Eur J Med Genet*. 2010;53:286–290.

167. Holden KR, Jabs EW, Sponseller PD. Roberts/pseudothalidomide syndrome and normal intelligence: approaches to diagnosis and management. *Dev Med Child Neurol*. 1992;34:534–539.

168. Karabulut AB, Aydin H, Erer M, et al. Roberts syndrome from the plastic surgeon's viewpoint. *Plast Reconstr Surg*. 2001;108:1443–1445.

169. Goh ES, Li C, Horsburgh S, et al. The Roberts syndrome/SC phocomelia spectrum—a case report of an adult with review of the literature. *Am J Med Genet A*. 2010;152A:472–478.

170. Chacko E, Graber E, Regelmann MO, et al. Update on turner and Noonan syndromes. *Endocrinol Metab Clin North Am*. 2012;41:713–734.

171. van der Burgt I. Noonan syndrome. *Orphanet J Rare Dis*. 2007;2:4.

172. Burch M, Sharland M, Shinebourne E, et al. Cardiologic abnormalities in Noonan syndrome: phenotypic diagnosis and echocardiographic assessment of 118 patients. *J Am Coll Cardiol*. 1993;22:1189–1192.

173. Jongmans M, Otten B, Noordam K. Genetics and variation in phenotype in Noonan syndrome. *Horm Res*. 2004;62(suppl 3):56–59.

174. Beneteau C, Cave H, Moncla A, et al. SOS1 and PTPN11 mutations in five cases of Noonan syndrome with multiple giant cell lesions. *Eur J Hum Genet*. 2009;17:1216–1221.

175. Hakami F, Dillon MW, Lebo M, et al. Retrospective study of prenatal ultrasound findings in newborns with a Noonan spectrum disorder. *Prenat Diagn*. 2016;36:418–423.

176. Marino B, Digilio MC, Toscano A, et al. Congenital heart diseases in children with Noonan syndrome: an expanded cardiac spectrum with high prevalence of atrioventricular canal. *J Pediatr*. 1999;135:703–706.

177. Romano AA, Allanson JE, Dahlgren J, et al. Noonan syndrome: clinical features, diagnosis, and management guidelines. *Pediatrics*. 2010;126:746–759.

178. Descamps P, Jourdain O, Paillet C, et al. Etiology, prognosis and management of nuchal cystic hygroma: 25 new cases and literature review. *Eur J Obstet Gynecol Reprod Biol*. 1997;71:3–10.

179. Wilkinson JD, Lowe AM, Salbert BA, et al. Outcomes in children with Noonan syndrome and hypertrophic cardiomyopathy: a study from the Pediatric Cardiomyopathy Registry. *Am Heart J*. 2012;164:442–448.

180. Otten BJ, Noordam C. Growth in Noonan syndrome. *Horm Res*. 2009;72(suppl 2):31–35.

181. van der Burgt I, Thoonen G, Roosenboom N, et al. Patterns of cognitive functioning in school-aged children with Noonan syndrome associated with variability in phenotypic expression. *J Pediatr*. 1999;135:707–713.

182. Jongmans MC, van der Burgt I, Hoogerbrugge PM, et al. Cancer risk in patients with Noonan syndrome carrying a PTPN11 mutation. *Eur J Hum Genet*. 2011;19:870–874.

183. Shprintzen RJ, Higgins AM, Antshel K, et al. Velo-cardio-facial syndrome. *Curr Opin Pediatr*. 2005;17:725–730.

184. Yamagishi H, Srivastava D. Unraveling the genetic and developmental mysteries of 22q11 deletion syndrome. *Trends Mol Med*. 2003;9:383–389.

185. Emanuel BS, McDonald-McGinn D, Saitta SC, et al. The 22q11.2 deletion syndrome. *Adv Pediatr*. 2001;48:39–73.

186. Schindewolf E, Khaled N, Johnson MP, et al. Expanding the fetal phenotype: prenatal sonographic findings and perinatal outcomes in a cohort of patients with a confirmed 22q11.2 deletion syndrome. *Am J Med Genet*. 2018;176A:1735–1741.

187. Perolo A, De Roberis V, Cataneo I, et al. Risk of 22q11.2 deletion in fetuses with right aortic arch with and without intracardiac anomalies. *Ultrasound Obstet Gyncol*. 2016;48:200–205.

188. Basgul A, Kavak ZN, Kotiloglu E, et al. Antenatal diagnosis of velocardiofacial syndrome by 3D ultrasonography. *J Perinat Med*. 2006;34:177–178.

189. Eicher PS, McDonald-Mcginn DM, Fox CA, et al. Dysphagia in children with a 22q11.2 deletion: unusual pattern found on modified barium swallow. *J Pediatr*. 2000;137:158–164.

190. Ming JE, McDonald-McGinn DM, Megerian TE, et al. Skeletal anomalies and deformities in patients with deletions of 22q11. *Am J Med Genet*. 1997;72:210–215.

191. Kates WR, Burnette CP, Bessette BA, et al. Frontal and caudate alterations in velocardiofacial syndrome (deletion at chromosome 22q11.2). *J Child Neurol*. 2004;19:337–342.

192. McDonald-McGinn DM, Tonnesen MK, Laufer-Cahana A, et al. Phenotype of the 22q11.2 deletion in individuals identified through an affected relative: cast a wide FISHing net! *Genet Med*. 2001;3:23–29.

193. Bassett AS, Chow EW, Husted J, et al. Clinical features of 78 adults with 22q11 deletion syndrome. *Am J Med Genet A*. 2005;138:307–313.

194. Issekutz KA, Graham JM Jr, Prasad C, et al. An epidemiological analysis of CHARGE syndrome: preliminary results from a Canadian study. *Am J Med Genet A*. 2005;133A:309–317.

195. Bergman JE, Janssen N, Hoefsloot LH, et al. CHD7 mutations and CHARGE syndrome: the clinical implications of an expanding phenotype. *J Med Genet*. 2011;48:334–342.

196. Pampal A. CHARGE: an association or a syndrome? *Int J Pediatr Otorhinolaryngol*. 2010;74:719–722.

197. Martin DM, Sheldon S, Gorski JL. CHARGE association with choanal atresia and inner ear hypoplasia in a child with a de novo chromosome translocation t(2;7)(p14;q21.11). *Am J Med Genet*. 2001;99(2):115–119.

198. Colin E, Bonneau D, Boussion F, et al. Prenatal diagnosis of CHARGE syndrome by identification of a novel CHD7 mutation in a previously unaffected family. *Prenat Diagn*. 2012;32:692–694.

199. Amiel J, Attiee-Bitach T, Marianowski R, et al. Temporal bone anomaly proposed as a major criteria for diagnosis of CHARGE syndrome. *Am J Med Genet*. 2001;99:124–127.

200. Davenport SL, Hefner MA, Mitchell JA. The spectrum of clinical features in CHARGE syndrome. *Clin Genet*. 1986;29:298–310.

201. Ragan DC, Casale AJ, Rink RC, et al. Genitourinary anomalies in the CHARGE association. *J Urol*. 1999;161:622–625.

202. Davenport SL, Hefner MA, Thelin JW. CHARGE syndrome, part I: external ear anomalies. *Int J Pediatr Otorhinolaryngol*. 1986;12:137–143.

203. Sanlaville D, Etchevers HC, Gonzales M, et al. Phenotypic spectrum of CHARGE syndrome in fetuses with CHD7 truncating mutations correlates with expression during human development. *J Med Genet*. 2006;43:211–217.

204. Leibovitz Z, Egenburg S, Arad A, et al. Sonography of the fetal cochlea in the early second trimester of pregnancy. *J Ultrasound Med*. 2013;32:53–59.

205. Moreira NC, Teixeira J, Raininko R, et al. The ear in fetal MRI: what can we really see? *Neuroradiology*. 2011;53:1001–1008.

206. Blake KD, Davenport SL, Hall BD, et al. CHARGE association: an update and review for the primary pediatrician. *Clin Pediatr*. 1998;37:159–173.

207. Roger G, Morisseau-Durand MP, Van Den Abbeele T, et al. The CHARGE association: the role of tracheotomy. *Arch Otolaryngol Head Neck Surg*. 1999;125:33–38.

208. Dobbelsteyn C, Marche DM, Blake K, et al. Early oral sensory experiences and feeding development in children with CHARGE syndrome: a report of five cases. *Dysphagia*. 2005;20:89–100.

209. Jongmans MC, Hoefsloot LH, van der Donk KP, et al. Familial CHARGE syndrome and the CHD7 gene: a recurrent missense mutation, intrafamilial recurrence and variability. *Am J Med Genet A*. 2008;146A:43–50.

210. Flores-Sarnat L. New insights into craniosynostosis. *Semin Pediatr Neurol*. 2002;9:274–291.

211. Passos-Bueno MR, Serti Eacute AE, Jehee FS, et al. Genetics of craniosynostosis: genes, syndromes, mutations and genotype-phenotype correlations. *Front Oral Biol*. 2008;12:107–143.

212. Glaser RL, Jiang W, Boyadjiev SA, et al. Paternal origin of FGFR2 mutations in sporadic cases of Crouzon syndrome and Pfeiffer syndrome. *Am J Hum Genet.* 2000;66:768–777.
213. Miller C, Losken HW, Towbin R, et al. Ultrasound diagnosis of craniosynostosis. *Cleft Palate Craniofac J.* 2002;39:73–80.
214. Fjortoft MI, Sevely A, Boetto S, et al. Prenatal diagnosis of craniosynostosis: value of MR imaging. *Neuroradiology.* 2007;49:515–521.
215. Muenke M, Gripp KW, McDonald-McGinn DM, et al. A unique point mutation in the fibroblast growth factor receptor 3 gene (FGFR3) defines a new craniosynostosis syndrome. *Am J Hum Genet.* 1997;60:555–564.
216. Gebb J, Demasio K, Dar P. Prenatal sonographic diagnosis of familial Saethre-Chotzen syndrome. *J Ultrasound Med.* 2011;30:420–422.
217. Greig AV, Wagner J, Warren SM, et al. Pfeiffer syndrome: analysis of a clinical series and development of a classification system. *J Craniofac Surg.* 2013;24:204–215.
218. Renier D, Lajeunie E, Arnaud E, et al. Management of craniosynostoses. *Childs Nerv Syst.* 2000;16:645–658.
219. Wong GB, Kakulis EG, Mulliken JB. Analysis of fronto-orbital advancement for Apert, Crouzon, Pfeiffer, and Saethre-Chotzen syndromes. *Plast Reconstr Surg.* 2000;105:2314–2323.
220. Schweitzer DN, Graham JM Jr, Lachman RS, et al. Subtle radiographic findings of achondroplasia in patients with Crouzon syndrome with acanthosis nigricans due to an Ala391Glu substitution in FGFR3. *Am J Med Genet.* 2001;98:75–91.
221. Ferreira JC, Carter SM, Bernstein PS, et al. Second-trimester molecular prenatal diagnosis of sporadic Apert syndrome following suspicious ultrasound findings. *Ultrasound Obstet Gynecol.* 1999;14:426–430.
222. Kanauchi Y, Muragaki Y, Ogino T, et al. FGFR2 mutation in a patient with Apert syndrome associated with humeroradial synostosis. *Congenit Anom.* 2003;43:302–305.
223. Lajeunie E, Cameron R, El Ghouzzi V, et al. Clinical variability in patients with Apert's syndrome. *J Neurosurg.* 1999;90:443–447.
224. Wilkie AO, Byren JC, Hurst JA, et al. Prevalence and complications of single-gene and chromosomal disorders in craniosynostosis. *Pediatrics.* 2010;126:e391–e400.
225. Moloney DM, Slaney SF, Oldridge M, et al. Exclusive paternal origin of new mutations in Apert syndrome. *Nat Genet.* 1996;13:48–53.
226. Mahieu-Caputo D, Sonigo P, Amiel J, et al. Prenatal diagnosis of sporadic Apert syndrome: a sequential diagnostic approach combining three-dimensional computed tomography and molecular biology. *Fetal Diagn Ther.* 2001;16:10–12.
227. Stark Z, McGillivray G, Sampson A, et al. Apert syndrome: temporal lobe abnormalities on fetal brain imaging. *Prenat Diagn.* 2015;35:179–182.
228. Ketwaroo PD, Robson CD, Estroff JA. Prenatal imaging of craniosynostosis syndromes. *Semin Ultrasound CT MR.* 2015;36:453–464.
229. Werner H, Castro P, Daltro P, et al. Prenatal diagnosis of Apert syndrome using ultrasound, magnetic resonance imaging and three dimensional virtual/physical models: three case series and literature review. *Childs Nerv Syst.* 2018;34:1563–1571.
230. Cohen MM Jr. Pfeiffer syndrome update, clinical subtypes, and guidelines for differential diagnosis. *Am J Med Genet.* 1993;45:300–307.
231. Stoler JM, Rosen H, Desai U, et al. Cleft palate in Pfeiffer syndrome. *J Craniofac Surg.* 2009;20:1375–1377.
232. Itoh S, Nojima M, Yoshida K. Usefulness of magnetic resonance imaging for accurate diagnosis of Pfeiffer syndrome type II in utero. *Fetal Diagn Ther.* 2006;21:168–171.
233. Cornejo-Roldan LR, Roessler E, Muenke M. Analysis of the mutational spectrum of the FGFR2 gene in Pfeiffer syndrome. *Hum Genet.* 1999;104:425–431.
234. Giancotti A, D'Ambrosio V, Marchionni E, et al. Pfeiffer syndrome: literature review of prenatal sonographic findings and genetic diagnosis. *J Matern Fetal Neonatal Med.* 2017;30(18):2225–2231.
235. Medina M, Cortes E, Eguiluz I, et al. Three-dimensional features of Pfeiffer syndrome. *Int J Gynaecol Obstet.* 2009;105:266–267.
236. Dodge HW Jr, Wood MW, Kennedy RL. Craniofacial dysostosis: Crouzon's disease. *Pediatrics.* 1959;23:98–106.
237. Reardon W, Winter RM, Rutland P, et al. Mutations in the fibroblast growth factor receptor 2 gene cause Crouzon syndrome. *Nat Genet.* 1994;8:98–103.
238. Gollin YG, Abuhamad AZ, Inati MN, et al. Sonographic appearance of craniofacial dysostosis (Crouzon syndrome) in the second trimester. *J Ultrasound Med.* 1993;12:625–628.
239. McGlaughlin KL, Witherow H, Dunaway DJ, et al. Spectrum of Antley-Bixler syndrome. *J Craniofac Surg.* 2010;21:1560–1564.
240. Huang N, Pandey AV, Agrawal V, et al. Diversity and function of mutations in p450 oxidoreductase in patients with Antley-Bixler syndrome and disordered steroidogenesis. *Am J Hum Genet.* 2005;76:729–749.
241. Shackleton C, Marcos J, Arlt W, et al. Prenatal diagnosis of P450 oxidoreductase deficiency (ORD): a disorder causing low pregnancy estriol, maternal and fetal virilization, and the Antley-Bixler syndrome phenotype. *Am J Med Genet A.* 2004;129A:105–112.
242. New MI, Abraham M, Yuen T, et al. An update on prenatal diagnosis and treatment of congenital adrenal hyperplasia. *Semin Reprod Med.* 2012;30:396–399.
243. Robinson PN, Neumann LM, Demuth S, et al. Shprintzen-Goldberg syndrome: fourteen new patients and a clinical analysis. *Am J Med Genet A.* 2005;135:251–262.
244. Rumball KM, Pang E, Letts RM. Musculoskeletal manifestations of the Antley-Bixler syndrome. *J Pediatr Orthop B.* 1999;8:139–143.
245. Khoury MJ, Cordero JF, Greenberg F, et al. A population study of the VACTERL association: evidence for its etiologic heterogeneity. *Pediatrics.* 1983;71:815–820.
246. Solomon BD. VACTERL/VATER association. *Orphanet J Rare Dis.* 2011;6:56.
247. Weaver DD, Mapstone CL, Yu PL. The VATER association: analysis of 46 patients. *Am J Dis Child.* 1986;140:225–229.
248. Garcia-Barcelo MM, Wong KK, Lui VC, et al. Identification of a HOXD13 mutation in a VACTERL patient. *Am J Med Genet A.* 2008;146A:3181–3185.
249. Solomon BD, Pineda-Alvarez DE, Raam MS, et al. Analysis of component findings in 79 patients diagnosed with VACTERL association. *Am J Med Genet A.* 2010;152A:2236–2244.
250. Sunagawa S, Kikuchi A, Yoshida S, et al. Dichorionic twin fetuses with VACTERL association. *J Obstet Gynaecol Res.* 2007;33:570–573.
251. Miller OF, Kolon TF. Prenatal diagnosis of VACTERL association. *J Urol.* 2001;166:2389–2391.
252. Tongsong T, Wanapirak C, Piyamongkol W, et al. Prenatal sonographic diagnosis of VATER association. *J Clin Ultrasound.* 1999;27:378–384.
253. Debost-Legrand A, Goumy C, Laurichesse-Delmas H, et al. Prenatal diagnosis of the VACTERL association using routine ultrasound examination. *Birth Defects Res A Clin Mol Teratol.* 2015;103(10):880–886. doi: 10.1002/bdra.23346.
254. Langer JC, Hussain H, Khan A, et al. Prenatal diagnosis of esophageal atresia using sonography and magnetic resonance imaging. *J Pediatr Surg.* 2001;36:804–807.
255. Seeds JW, Cefalo RC, Herbert WN. Amniotic band syndrome. *Am J Obstet Gynecol.* 1982;144:243–248.
256. Orioli IM, Ribeiro MG, Castilla EE. Clinical and epidemiological studies of amniotic deformity, adhesion, and mutilation (ADAM) sequence in a South American (ECLAMC) population. *Am J Med Genet A.* 2003;118A:135–145.
257. Barzilay E, Harel Q, Haas J, et al. Prenatal diagnosis of amniotic band syndrome-risk factors and ultrasonic signs. *J Matern Fetal Neonatal Med.* 2015;28(3):281–283.
258. Neuman J, Calvo-Garcia MA, Kline-Fath BM, et al. Prenatal imaging of amniotic band sequence: utility and role of fetal MRI as an adjunct to prenatal US. *Pediatr Radiol.* 2012;42:544–551.
259. Kanayama MD, Gaffey TA, Ogburn PL Jr. Constriction of the umbilical cord by an amniotic band, with fetal compromise illustrated by reverse diastolic flow in the umbilical artery: a case report. *J Reprod Med.* 1995;40:71–73.
260. Kalampokas E, Kalampokas T, Sofoudis C, et al. Diagnosing arthrogryposis multiplex congenita: a review. *ISRN Obstet Gynecol.* 2012;2012:264918.
261. Lowry Rb, Sibbald B, Bedard T, et al. Prevalence of multiple congenital contractures including arthrogryposis multiplex congenital in Alberta, Canada and a strategy for classification and coding. *Birth Defects Res A Clin Mol Teratol.* 2010;88:1057–1061.
262. Niles KM, Blaser S, Shannon P, et al. Fetal arthrogryposis multiplex congenita/fetal akinesia deformation sequence (FADS)—Aetiology, diagnosis, and management. *Prenat Diagn.* 2019;39(9):720–731.
263. Filges I, Tercanli S, Hall JG. Fetal arthrogryposis: Challenges and perspectives for prenatal detection and management. *Am J Med Genet.* 2019;181C:327–336.
264. Hall JG. Arthrogryposis (multiple congenital contractures): diagnostic approach to etiology, classification, genetics and general principles. *Eur J Med Genet.* 2014;57:464–472.
265. Witters I, Moerman P, Fryns JP. Fetal akinesia deformation sequence: a study of 30 consecutive in utero diagnoses. *Am J Med Genet.* 2002;113(1):23–38.
266. Bevan WP, Hall JG, Bamshad M, et al. Arthrogryposis multiplex congenita (amyoplasia): an orthopaedic perspective. *J Pediatr Orthop.* 2007;27:594–600.
267. Beals RK. The distal arthrogryposes: a new classification of peripheral contractures. *Clin Orthop Relat Res.* 2005;(435):203–210.
268. Zhao N, Jiang M, Han W, et al. A novel mutation in TNNT3 associated with Sheldon-Hall syndrome in a Chinese family with vertical talus. *Eur J Med Genet.* 2011;54:351–353.
269. Toydemir RM, Rutherford A, Whitby FG, et al. Mutations in embryonic myosin heavy chain (MYH3) cause Freeman-Sheldon syndrome and Sheldon-Hall syndrome. *Nat Genet.* 2006;38:561–565.
270. Pena SDJ, Shokeir MHK. Syndrome of camptodactyly, multiple ankyloses facial anomalies and pulmonary hypoplasia: a lethal condition. *J Pediatr.* 1974;85:373–375.
271. Moerman P, Fryns JP, Goddeeris P, et al. Multiple ankyloses, facial anomalies, and pulmonary hypoplasia associated with severe antenatal spinal muscular atrophy. *J Pediatr.* 1983;103:238–241.
272. Nemec SF, Hoftberger R, Nemec U, et al. Fetal akinesia and associated abnormalities on prenatal MRI. *Prenat Diagn.* 2011;31(5):484–490.
273. Hageman G, Ippel EP, Beemer FA, et al. The diagnostic management of newborns with congenital contractures: a nosologic study of 75 cases. *Am J Med Genet.* 1988;30:883–904.
274. Carlson WO, Speck GJ, Vicari V, et al. Arthrogryposis multiplex congenita: a long-term follow-up study. *Clin Orthop Relat Res.* 1985;(194):115–123.
275. Dai S, Dieterich K, Jaeger M, et al. Disability in adults with arthrogryposis is severe, partly invisible, and varies by genotype. *Neurology.* 2018;90(18):e1596–e1604.
276. Rink BD. Arthrogryposis: a review and approach to prenatal diagnosis. *Obstet Gynecol Surv.* 2011;66(6):369–377.

31 Congenital Infections

Cristiano D. Jodicke • Paul Singh • Dev Maulik

Fetal infections account for 2% to 3% of all congenital anomalies.[1] Infections acquired during pregnancy may be associated with significant maternal–fetal morbidity and mortality. Pregnant women are commonly exposed to young children who may be a potential source of infectious disease. Maternal infections may be transmitted to the fetus, leading to poor perinatal and neonatal outcomes. Congenital infections pose many difficult issues for physicians and parents because of the obscure short-term and potential long-term sequelae that may adversely affect a variety of organ systems. Over the past few decades the prevention, detection, and treatment of congenital infections have improved dramatically. Despite being more common in underdeveloped countries, perinatal infections remain a concern worldwide. Thus, a sound knowledge of congenital infections is important for the clinician involved in maternal–child health. It is estimated that congenital infections account for nearly 20% of fetal and neonatal diseases.

Several organisms, such as cytomegalovirus (CMV), parvovirus, herpes simplex virus (HSV), human immunodeficiency virus (HIV), *Toxoplasma gondii*, varicella zoster virus (VZV), rubella, and *Treponema pallidum* are known to cause fetal infections. Less commonly considered pathogens include enteroviruses, *Listeria monocytogenes*, *Plasmodium*, and *Mycobacterium tuberculosis*. Efforts such as universal immunizations, preconceptional screening, and good hygienic practices have been instrumental in the reduction in incidence of these diseases.

Concern about exposure to infectious agents during pregnancy should prompt the workup of both the mother and fetus. Sonographic findings may assist in fetal prognostication, aid in patient counseling, and influence perinatal management. Apart from ultrasound (US), other commonly employed methods for prenatal diagnosis of congenital infection include magnetic resonance imaging (MRI) and amniotic fluid and fetal blood sampling.

Improvement in US technology has enhanced our understanding of fetal diagnosis and management. However, US is not a sensitive test for fetal infection and a normal targeted sonogram cannot reliably predict a favorable outcome. Although most affected fetuses appear sonographically normal, serial imaging may reveal evolving findings. Crino[2] reported that the initial screening US may not demonstrate any abnormalities; however, the fetus may show signs of undetected clinical infection only during the latter part of pregnancy. Various sonographic abnormalities have been associated with congenital infections, such as ascites, hydrops, ventriculomegaly, intracranial calcifications, hydrocephaly, microcephaly, cardiac anomalies, hepatosplenomegaly, echogenic bowel, and placentomegaly. Multiple organ systems are affected in approximately 50% of cases. Different intrauterine infections may have similar sonographic findings, but certain patterns of images in high-risk patients may lead to a specific diagnosis. Thus, practitioners should understand the limitations of US for the detection of congenital infection.

Since the central nervous system (CNS) is often affected by infectious exposures, fetal MRI may be utilized as an adjunct to US to provide further definition of brain injury. MRI is not emphasized in this chapter, but findings with regard to CNS infection can be found in Chapter 17.1 (Supratentorial Anomalies). Sometimes, MRI may also be helpful in evaluation of the gastrointestinal (GI) tract and hydropic fetus when the etiology of abnormality is unknown. Discussion of US and MRI in the evaluation of the GI tract and nonimmune hydrops can be found in Chapters 26.1 and 28.2, respectively.

This chapter reviews the agents most commonly associated with congenital infection and their respective US findings. In addition, a discussion about pathogenesis and other maternal–fetal diagnostic modalities and management is provided.

VIRAL INFECTIONS

Cytomegalovirus

Definition and Incidence: CMV occurs in 0.2% to 2.2% of all live births and is the most common cause of intrauterine infection and the leading infectious cause of sensorineural hearing loss and mental retardation.[3–5]

Pathogenesis: CMV is the largest known member of the human herpes virus family. These viruses are large, enveloped, DNA viruses sharing the biologic properties of latency and reactivation. Endogenous latent virus reactivation may occur regularly. Although CMV is found throughout all geographic locations, it is more widespread in developing countries and in areas of lower socioeconomic conditions. The seroprevalence increases with age and is due to many other factors such as poor hygiene, underdeveloped infrastructure, and high-risk sexual behavior.[6] Transmission of CMV occurs from person to person and requires intimate contact with infected excretions, such as saliva, urine, breast milk, or other body fluids.[7,8]

Vertical transmission can occur through the placenta from maternal–fetal hematogenous exchange. In addition, fetal infection can also occur as a result of exposure to infected cervical secretions and blood during delivery. The risk for transmission of the virus to the fetus is higher in primary-infected mothers than in those with reactivated disease. Although primary CMV infections are reported in 1% to 4% of seronegative women during pregnancy, the risk of viral transmission to the fetus is 30% to 40%.[5] Pregnant women who experience recurrent or reactivated CMV infection are much less likely to transmit infection to their fetus. While reactivation of CMV infection during pregnancy is reported to occur in 10% to 30% of seropositive women, the risk of transmitting the virus is only 1% to 3%.

The overall risk of congenital infection is highest when maternal CMV occurs during the third trimester; however, the probability of severe fetal injury is greatest when fetal infection takes place during the first trimester. During early pregnancy, CMV infection may cause disturbances during early brain development. CMV infections acquired during delivery or via breast milk have no effect on future, neurodevelopmental outcome in full-term infants. In contrast, in premature infants (<32 weeks), sepsis-like symptoms have been reported after exposure to contaminated secretions.[6]

Diagnosis: During diagnosis, two important steps must be followed. Initially, maternal infection must be investigated, and differentiation should be made between maternal primary and secondary infection based on serologic testing. Next, after maternal infection has been demonstrated, congenital infection should be investigated using both noninvasive (US examination) and invasive (amniocentesis) prenatal testing.

The best method for the diagnosis of asymptomatic maternal primary infection is seroconversion; however, this is clinically problematic due to the lack of universal screening. The detection of immunoglobulin (Ig) M antibodies in maternal sera can be helpful, but interpretation is somewhat complicated. Although CMV-IgM antibodies occur in all primary infections, they may also be detected after reactivation or reinfection and remain present for months. Hence, finding CMV-IgM antibodies in a single serum sample is not definitive for the diagnosis of a primary CMV infection and may indicate either remote primary infection acquired before pregnancy or recurrent disease.[5,9]

Apart from seroconversion, the combination of anti-CMV-IgM and low-avidity anti-CMV-IgG testing is the best way to diagnose a primary maternal infection. Antibody avidity is an indirect measure of the tightness of antibody binding to its target antigen and increases during the first months after a primary infection. The IgG avidity assay can be a useful tool to assist in distinguishing primary infection from past or recurrent infection as well as to determine when the primary infection occurred. An avidity index less than 30% strongly suggests a primary infection of less than 12 weeks.[10,11]

The clinical spectrum of congenital CMV infection is wide, ranging from a complete lack of symptoms to severe disease with multiorgan involvement and postnatal complications. The most sensitive and specific test for diagnosing congenital CMV infection is the identification of CMV in amniotic fluid using virus culture or CMV-DNA analysis by polymerase chain reaction (PCR). CMV-DNA and CMV-IgM antibody activity may also be demonstrable in cord blood. Amniocentesis is generally the procedure of choice because it is safer and has a higher diagnostic sensitivity compared to cordocentesis. The amniotic fluid should be sampled after the 21st week of pregnancy and at least 5 to 6 weeks after the estimated onset of infection.[6]

Approximately 5% to 15% of infants who develop congenital CMV infection as a result of primary maternal infection are symptomatic at birth. The most common clinical manifestations of severe neonatal infection are hepatosplenomegaly, intracranial calcifications, jaundice, growth restriction, microcephaly, chorioretinitis, hearing loss, thrombocytopenia, hyperbilirubinemia, and hepatitis.[6] Approximately 30% of severely infected infants die, and 80% of survivors have major morbidity. Among the 85% to 90% of infants with congenital CMV infection who are asymptomatic at birth, 10% to 15% subsequently develop hearing loss, chorioretinitis, or dental defects within the first 2 years of life.[12,13]

Ultrasound: US evaluation is invaluable in providing information about the condition of the fetus. The presence of characteristic US findings has a high predictive value for fetal infection and also may have prognostic significance. Because routine maternal CMV screening is not recommended, congenital CMV infection is underdiagnosed, and detection during pregnancy is often noted when suspicious sonographic abnormalities are found during routine screening examinations.

The main sonographic findings suggestive of congenital CMV infection are echogenic bowel (Fig. 31.1), ventriculomegaly (Fig. 31.2), microcephaly, periventricular calcifications (Fig. 31.3), fetal hydrops, intrauterine growth restriction (IUGR), placentomegaly (Fig. 31.4), and oligohydramnios. Less common findings include supraventricular tachycardia, meconium peritonitis, renal dysplasia, ascites, and pleural effusions.

Ventriculomegaly is frequently diagnosed during fetal life and has multiple etiologies, including CMV infection. Around 5% of all cases of ventriculomegaly are caused by fetal infection. de Vries et al.[14] found periventricular calcifications associated with mild-to-moderate ventriculomegaly in 10 out of 11 children with symptomatic congenital CMV infection. Malinger et al. demonstrated similar findings in five of eight affected fetuses with congenital CMV. In addition, fetuses with ventriculomegaly were identified at a more advanced gestational age (28.6 weeks) and had other associated sonographic findings than in those without ventriculomegaly.[15]

Microcephaly is associated with a poor prognosis in cases of congenital CMV, usually due to mental retardation. Noyola et al.[16] reported that microcephaly is the most specific predictor for mental retardation (100%; 95% CI, 84.5–100) and major motor disability (92.3%; 95% CI, 74.8–90) in children with symptomatic congenital CMV infection. Of note, microcephaly may not be apparent during the second-trimester US examination and generally is not an isolated finding. More common associated findings

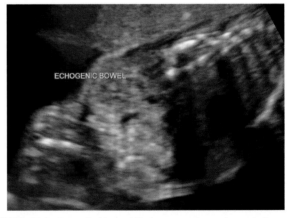

FIGURE 31.1: Sagittal-oblique US demonstrating echogenic bowel at 26 gestational weeks in a fetus with known congenital cytomegalovirus.

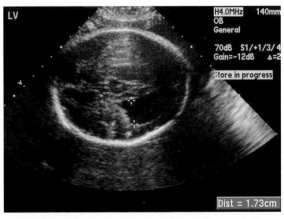

FIGURE 31.2: Axial US showing ventriculomegaly in a patient with known congenital cytomegalovirus at 27 weeks' gestation.

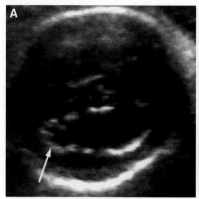
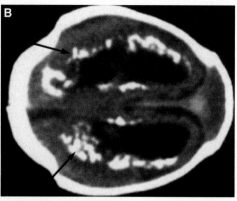

FIGURE 31.3: Cytomegalovirus. A: Transverse US of fetal brain shows ventricular dilatation and periventricular echogenic nodules (arrow). B: Computed tomography scan (oriented to correspond with ultrasound image) after birth confirms hydrocephalus and marked periventricular calcifications (arrows). (Courtesy of Luis Izquierdo, MD, Miami, FL.)

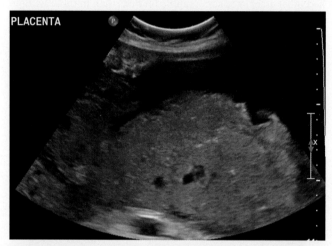

FIGURE 31.4: Thickened placenta in a pregnancy diagnosed with congenital cytomegalovirus at 30 weeks' gestation.

include intracranial calcifications, increased echogenicity of the lining of the ventricles, and ventriculomegaly.

Ventriculitis, which manifests as an increased echogenicity surrounding the lateral ventricles, is an US finding that may be present in CMV infection, although it also may be a normal variant. As with ventriculomegaly, it will rarely be an isolated US finding. Periventricular pseudocysts and intraventricular synechiae (IVS) have also been described in association with CMV infection.

Brain calcifications are considered a strong and common US marker of intrauterine infections. It is not an exclusive US finding in CMV infection and has been described in fetuses with other infections such as congenital toxoplasmosis, rubella, HSV, and varicella. The calcifications do not usually have an acoustic shadowing, and although they may be found in any portion of the brain, they have particular predilection for the periventricular zone.

Congenital CMV infection during the late first or early second trimester may interfere with neuronal proliferation and migration, and result in abnormal cortical development, including lissencephaly and schizencephaly. Microcephaly, ventriculomegaly, callosal dysgenesis, and abnormally developed sulci and gyration are the most common initial US findings in fetuses with congenital CMV infection and malformations of cortical development. A detailed US, including dedicated neurosonography, and perinatal MRI are indicated when the abovementioned intracranial US findings are detected during the initial routine screening examination.

Hyperechogenic bowel and ventriculomegaly are the most common abnormal US findings in CMV infection, although they may also be seen in uninfected fetuses. Guerra et al.[17] reported the following sonographic abnormalities in 23 cases of CMV-infected fetuses/infants: hyperechogenic bowel ($n = 7$), cerebral ventriculomegaly ($n = 7$), IUGR ($n = 3$), hydronephrosis ($n = 1$), hydrops ($n = 1$), cerebral periventricular echogenicity ($n = 1$), and the association of two or more fetal abnormalities (hyperechogenic bowel and cerebral ventriculomegaly, $n = 3$).

Hepatomegaly and hepatic calcifications may be also found in cases of fetal infection. Hydrops and ascites have been documented and may be related to hepatic dysfunction and portal hypertension from liver congestion. Supraventricular tachycardia and pericardial effusion have also been reported in association with CMV infection. During a 6-year study period, Gonce et al.[18] diagnosed 19 fetuses with CMV infection. The main sonographic findings were the following: brain abnormalities ($n = 14$), fetal hydrops ($n = 4$), hyperechogenic bowel ($n = 4$), pericardial effusion ($n = 1$), cardiomegaly ($n = 1$), oligohydramnios ($n = 4$), and placentomegaly ($n = 2$).

Although US is a valuable tool in evaluating a fetus with CMV infection, its limitations should be discussed when counseling patients. Guerra et al.[17] studied the effectiveness of US in the antenatal detection of symptomatic congenital CMV infection. Six hundred and fifty US examinations of fetuses from mothers with primary CMV infection were correlated to fetal or neonatal outcome. US abnormalities were found in 51 of 600 mothers with primary infection (8.5%) and 23 of 154 congenitally infected fetuses (14.9%). They concluded that US abnormalities predict symptomatic congenital infection in only a third of cases. Liesnard et al.[9] reported characteristic sonographic findings in 9 of 55 infected fetuses (16.4%), but the majority of infected newborns were asymptomatic. Another issue is that abnormal sonographic findings may be only detected for the first time during the third trimester after a normal US examination earlier in the pregnancy. Although repeat US examination during the third-trimester scan may lead to a more accurate diagnosis and help with counseling, pregnancy termination would not be an option due to advanced gestational age.

Management: The best prevention for congenital CMV infection is primary prevention with personal hygiene practices, such as handwashing and avoiding intimate contact with salivary secretions and urine from young children. Vaccination for CMV is currently under investigation and is not available for clinical use yet.

Although there are several methods for the prenatal diagnosis of congenital CMV infection, there is no effective treatment to offer once a diagnosis has been made. The use of CMV-specific hyperimmune globulin for treatment was evaluated by Nigro et al.[19] in 157 pregnant women with primary CMV infection. Forty-five women who had a primary infection longer than 6 weeks and congenital infection confirmed by amniocentesis were enrolled. Thirty-one of these women received intravenous treatment with CMV-specific hyperimmune globulin (200 U per kg of maternal body weight), and only one had an infant with clinical CMV disease at birth. In comparison, of the 14 women who declined treatment, 7 had infants who were symptomatic at delivery (adjusted odds ratio [OR], 0.02, $P < 0.001$). The maternal administration of valaciclovir and ganciclovir to treat intrauterine CMV infection has also been reported.[20,21] Although these studies were not randomized, they are promising and offer a possible treatment option for congenital CMV infection.

Intrauterine therapy with CMV hyperimmunoglobulin has also been attempted. Negishi et al.[22] was the first to report intraperitoneal CMV hyperimmunoglobulin administration in a fetus at 28 and 29 weeks of pregnancy. Since then, other investigators have reported the use of intraperitoneal CMV hyperimmunoglobulin as a possible treatment alternative for congenital CMV.[23–25] In addition, both the intraumbilical and intra-amniotic fluid administration of CMV-specific hyperimmune globulin has been performed.[26]

Parvovirus

Definition and Incidence: Human parvovirus B19 is a small single-stranded DNA virus from the Parvoviridae family that is responsible for erythema infectiosum, also known as fifth disease, and is a common childhood illness. It is a worldwide infection that affects individuals from infancy through adulthood. Infection can occur at any age but most commonly affects children from 6 to 10 years of age. The prevalence of parvovirus IgG antibodies steadily rises throughout life. In children aged from 1 to 5 years and from 6 to 19 years, the prevalence of IgG antibodies is 2% to 15% and 15% to 60%, respectively. In the geriatric population, the prevalence is more than 85%.[27,28]

More than half of reproductive-age women have developed immunity to parvovirus B19. About 35% to 45% of women of childbearing age, however, do not have protective IgG antibodies against parvovirus. During pregnancy, the risk of acquiring parvovirus infection is low. The incidence of acute infection in pregnancy is approximately 1% to 2% during endemic periods.[29] Women at increased risk include mothers of preschool and school-age children, workers at day-care centers, and school teachers. Vertical transmission occurs in about 30% to 50% of mothers infected with parvovirus during pregnancy.[30] Congenital infection can cause severe fetal consequences, such as anemia, nonimmune hydrops fetalis (NIHF), and fetal death. The risk of adverse fetal outcome is increased if maternal infection occurs during the first two trimesters of pregnancy; however, fetal infection can still occur during the third trimester.[31–33] It is highly unlikely that fetal infection will occur if the mother has IgG antibodies, since prior infection with parvovirus B19 confers lifelong immunity.[34]

Pathogenesis: The risk of fetal complications depends upon the gestational age at the time of maternal infection. The incidence of fetal morbidity and mortality decreases with gestational age. The highest risk for fetal loss happens when maternal infection develops during the 9th through the 16th weeks of pregnancy.[35,36] The risk of vertical transmission is maximal at the time IgM

antibodies appear. This coincides with maternal peak viral load, which occurs generally 7 days after maternal inoculation.[37]

The virus is spread by respiratory droplets, hand-to-mouth contact, and by blood products containing factor XIII and IX concentrates.[31–33,38,39] Outbreaks usually occur during the spring every 4 to 5 years and may last up to 6 months. Viremia occurs 4 to 14 days after exposure and may last up to 20 days. Serum and respiratory secretions become positive for parvovirus DNA 5 to 10 days after intranasal inoculation. Symptoms such as erythema infectiosum, mild fever, arthralgias, and headaches start approximately 10 to 14 days after infection; however, many people remain asymptomatic. By the time erythema infectiosum develops, the person is usually no longer infectious.

The fetal liver, the main site of erythrocyte production, is the virus's main target of infection.[31] The fetus is more vulnerable during the second trimester when the liver is the main source of hematopoietic activity, and the half-life of red blood cells is short. Parvovirus is a potent inhibitor of hematopoiesis because it infects erythroid precursor cells such as erythroblasts and megakaryocytes. Resultant severe anemia may occur, leading to congestive heart failure and the development of hydrops fetalis. Parvovirus may infect fetal cardiac myocytes and hepatocytes, resulting in myocarditis and impaired hepatic function, respectively.[40] Subsequent development of fetal high-output cardiac failure, generalized edema, and death may occur.[40] Thus, the development of hydrops may not correlate with the severity of fetal anemia. Placental trophoblastic cells also express the P antigen, the main cellular receptor for the virus, and are thus susceptible to infection by parvovirus. Poor fetal outcomes have been associated with placental villous trophoblast apoptosis in patients with congenital infection.[41] Such observations suggest that parvovirus infection may be associated with placental insufficiency. Stillbirth in nonhydropic fetuses may result from placental damage and occurs in 0.9% to 23% of pregnancies with documented maternal infection.[42,43]

Diagnosis: Serologic examination of maternal blood is the initial and most useful diagnostic tool for parvovirus. Specific IgM and IgG testing should be performed as soon as possible once maternal infection is suspected during pregnancy.[44] IgM antibodies become detectable in maternal serum within 7 to 10 days after infection, sharply peak at 10 to 14 days, and can persist in the circulation for 3 to 4 months or longer.[45] IgG antibodies will rise considerably more slowly and reach a plateau at 4 weeks after infection. Of note, after a recent contact, there will be a serologic window of 7 days, during which both IgG and IgM remain undetectable.[44] Women who are IgG-positive and IgM-negative can be reassured that there is no evidence of recent infection. Patients with IgG- and IgM-negative–specific antibody should be considered susceptible, and further serological testing should be carried out 4 weeks after the last contact or if signs of the disease develop.[35] IgM-positive patients, irrespective of IgG status, should receive serial fetal evaluation to rule out congenital infection.

Since most infected pregnancies have a favorable outcome, invasive prenatal diagnostic testing should only be used if there are definitive signs of fetal anemia or hydrops fetalis.[35] US must be used for diagnosis and surveillance. Fetal infection may be identified by using PCR of parvovirus viral DNA in amniotic fluid or fetal cord blood. Amniocentesis is the preferred method of choice due to less complications and increased availability. Serologic examination of fetal blood samples is highly unreliable since the IgG and IgM response to parvovirus is not produced during intrauterine life. Detection of parvovirus using specific IgM in fetal blood has a sensitivity of 29% compared to almost 100% for PCR.[35,44,46]

Ultrasound: As soon as a recent parvovirus maternal infection is suspected during pregnancy, US examination should be performed to exclude the presence of fetal anemia and hydrops. The virus infects the liver, which is the main site of erythrocyte production in the fetus, leading to anemia, most often occurring during the second trimester. Increased cardiac output and decreased viscosity of fetal blood caused by anemia are responsible for the changes in fetal blood during congenital infection. An increase in the middle cerebral artery peak systolic velocity (MCA-PSV) (Fig. 31.5) is a very sensitive measure to identify fetal anemia caused by parvovirus infection.[47] Weekly measurements of MCA-PSV are recommended after maternal infection is documented. Timing of intrauterine transfusion (IUT) for treatment of fetal anemia and prevention of fetal hydrops can be based on these MCA-PSV measurements. The infection causes anemia and possible myocarditis, leading to high-output cardiac failure and subsequent development of generalized edema. Fetal hydrops, an accumulation of excess fluid in at least two body

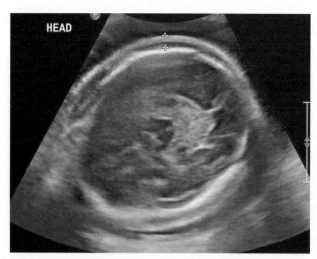

FIGURE 31.7: Axial US of the fetal head showing scalp edema in a pregnancy exposed to parvovirus and positive immunoglobulin IgM titers.

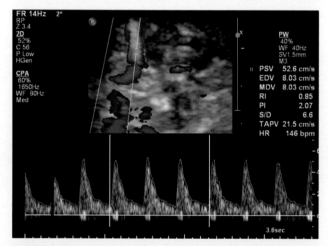

FIGURE 31.5: Duplex Doppler of the middle cerebral artery at 24 gestational weeks demonstrating increased peak systolic velocity in a fetus exposed to parvovirus.

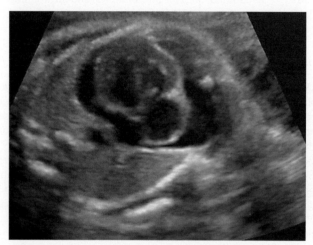

FIGURE 31.8: Cross-sectional US of the fetal chest demonstrating marked pericardial effusion in a pregnancy with confirmed parvovirus infection by amniotic fluid polymerase chain reaction.

compartments of the fetus, can be easily seen with US. The median interval between maternal parvovirus infection and diagnosis of hydrops fetalis is about 3 weeks, but may vary between 1 and 20 weeks.[48] The ultrasonographic findings include fetal ascites, skin edema, pericardial effusion, pleural effusions, and placental edema (Figs. 31.6 to 31.11). Enlargement and thickening of the fetal heart also may be documented during the examination. Fetal structural anomalies associated with parvovirus are uncommon; however, US findings such as hydrocephalus, hyperechogenic bowel, meconium peritonitis, fetal liver calcifications, cleft lip and palate, and increased fetal nuchal translucency have been reported.[48–52]

Management: Maternal infection with parvovirus is self-limited and is treated symptomatically. Acute red cell aplasia may rarely occur and requires serial measurements of hemoglobin and possible blood transfusions to prevent maternal complications due to severe anemia. The confirmation of fetal infection is not required for suspected maternal infection.

If serologic evidence suggests possible maternal infection, weekly measurements of fetal MCA-PSV and US assessment for

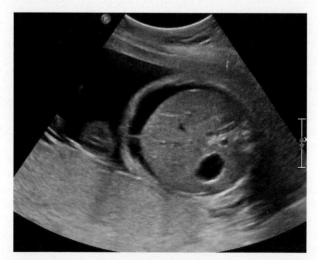

FIGURE 31.6: Cross-sectional US of the abdomen showing marked ascites in a fetus with congenital parvovirus.

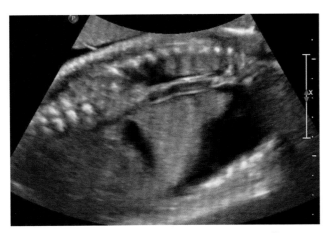

FIGURE 31.9: Sagittal US of chest demonstrating pleural effusion at 20 gestational weeks in a fetus with congenital parvovirus.

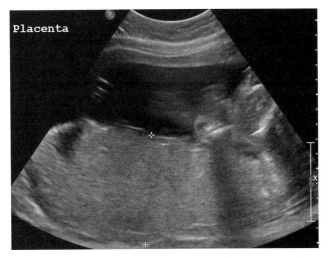

FIGURE 31.10: Placentomegaly demonstrated by ultrasound in a pregnancy complicated by fetal parvovirus infection.

hydrops should be performed. The MCA-PSV may diagnose significant fetal anemia with a sensitivity of as high as 100%.[53] In parvovirus infection, the MCA-PSV was reported to have a sensitivity of 94.1% for the diagnosis of fetal anemia.[47] Percutaneous umbilical blood sampling (PUBS) should be considered once the MCA-PSV reaches 1.5 multiples of the median (MOM) for gestational age. If fetal anemia is confirmed, fetal blood transfusion is indicated. IUT with packed red blood cells for cases of severe fetal anemia has been shown to reduce perinatal morbidity and mortality. Fetal survival may be as high as 60% to 80% when IUT is attempted, compared to only 15% to 30% with hydrops and no intervention. Fairley et al.[54] compared outcomes of expectant management with IUT in cases of maternal parvovirus infection, and found a greater than seven-fold reduction in fetal death with the use of IUT.

In addition, a targeted fetal US and echocardiography should be performed, especially in cases complicated by hydrops fetalis. Delivery is recommended at 34 gestational weeks in pregnancies affected with hydrops fetalis. An attempt to correct fetal anemia should be considered before delivery to improve neonatal outcome.

Prognosis: The long-term prognosis for children who received IUT for congenital parvovirus infection is controversial. Some studies have shown that children who underwent a successful IUT have good neurodevelopmental outcomes.[36,55] Miller et al.[36] described seven cases of fetal hydrops, two of which received IUT. They were unable to find any long-term developmental problems in the patients who received fetal blood transfusion. Similarly, Dembinski et al.[55] followed up on 20 children with parvovirus infection treated with IUT and found no evidence of developmental delay. On the other hand, de Jong et al.[44] described an increased risk of both neurodevelopmental delay and cerebral palsy in children treated with IUTs for congenital parvovirus infection. Parvovirus DNA has been detected within white matter multinucleated, reactive microglial cells, suggesting that the virus itself may play a direct role in perivascular changes and white matter damage.[56] Alternatively, severe fetal anemia and hydrops may cause hypoxic-ischemic cerebral injury, thereby, contributing to the increased rate of neurodevelopmental complications. Lindenburg et al.[57] demonstrated similar findings of developmental delay and cerebral palsy in neonates that underwent IUT for severe fetal anemia. However, for a number of reasons, these fetuses are likely to be delivered prematurely, which is itself a significant risk factor for pediatric developmental disorders.

Rubella Virus

Definition and Incidence: Rubella, also known as German measles and "third" disease, is caused by a lipid-enveloped, single-stranded RNA togavirus.[58] Congenital rubella syndrome (CRS) was one of the earliest described vertically transmitted infections in the newborn infant.[59] The last major epidemic of rubella in the United States occurred between 1964 and 1965, during which time 20,000 cases of infants were born with CRS. Cases of infection during pregnancy have been significantly reduced following vaccine development in 1969. From 1995 to 2000, an average of five cases of CRS has been reported annually in the United States. Newborns affected by CRS are most commonly born in countries where routine rubella vaccination programs are not used.

Pathogenesis: Rubella is an airborne transmitted infection spread by small respiratory droplets which become infectious

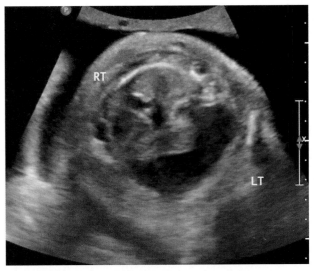

FIGURE 31.11: Cross-sectional US of the chest in a fetus with congenital parvovirus showing bilateral pleural effusions, more prominent in the left hemithorax. The fetal heart is displaced to the right side of the chest.

7 days prior to the appearance of the initial symptoms. Vertical transmission is hypothesized to occur 5 to 7 days following maternal inoculation.[60] The clinical features of rubella are a rash, fever, arthralgias, and lymphadenopathy. The rash generally manifests initially on the face and then gradually migrates toward the trunk and then to the lower extremities.[60] Generally, self-limited complications such as encephalitis, thrombocytopenia, neuritis, conjunctivitis, and orchitis have rarely been reported to occur as a result of rubella.[60–62] Importantly, encephalitis from rubella infection has been associated with a 50% mortality. Subclinical infection can occur in up to 50% of patients; however, in these patients, fetal anomalies as a result of congenital infection rarely occur. Reinfection with rubella after prior documented infection or immunization is extremely rare during pregnancy.[63,64] Antibody titers lower than 1/64 have been associated with reinfection.[65] The risk of vertical transmission depends upon gestational age and is 90%, 25%, and 95% during the first, second, and third trimesters, respectively. During the first trimester, CRS is extremely rare if the maternal rash occurs within the first 2 gestational weeks. If the rash appears during the third gestational week, the infection rate is 31%, and nearly 100% afterwards.[66] Congenital heart defects and deafness most commonly occur in infected fetuses during the first trimester, but are rare afterwards.

Diagnosis: Serological analysis is based on the detection of IgG, IgM, and also on IgG avidity antibodies.[60,67] The enzyme-linked immunosorbent assays (ELISA), hemagglutination inhibition (HI) test, and the immunofluorescent antibody assay (IFA) are the most common methods of antibody detection.[59,60,67–69] Acute rubella infection is characterized by the appearance of rubella IgM about 5 days after the onset of the maternal rash and persists for 6 weeks.[70] The presence of IgM antibodies does not always correspond to an acute infection. A false-positive IgM for rubella can result in patients with parvovirus, mononucleosis, or a positive rheumatoid factor.[71] In addition, IgM antibodies may persist for 1 year or more in a chronic rubella carrier. Thus, in order to properly establish a timeline of infection, it is important to measure the rubella IgG avidity. A high IgG avidity indicates chronic carrier status, while a lower IgG avidity indicates a more recent infection. The evaluation of IgG, IgM, or the RNA virus in the saliva instead of in the blood has been proposed to diagnose rubella.[72–75] Ramsay et al.[75] found a sensitivity of 98% and a specificity of 100% for IgG, and a specificity of 99% for IgM detected in the saliva.

Amniotic fluid sampling for fetal diagnosis of CRS should be performed 6 to 8 weeks after maternal infection to avoid false-negative results. Samples of amniotic fluid may be sent for viral cultures; however, this method lacks sensitivity and final results may take up to 6 weeks. PCR technology may be used to diagnose CRS, having the advantage of increased detection rates and faster result times.[69] The diagnosis of CRS via chorionic villus sampling has been described.[76]

Ultrasound: US has an important role in the prenatal diagnosis of CRS. Migliucci et al.[77] performed a retrospective study on 175 women referred for rubella infection. Sonographic findings of IUGR, polyhydramnios, cardiomegaly, atrial septal defect, hepatosplenomegaly, ascites, echogenic bowel, and placentomegaly were detected. Ugurbas et al.[78] reported an association between microphthalmos and CRS. Ventricular septal defect and pulmonary stenosis have also been reported in cases of CRS.[79] Exencephaly was diagnosed in one case.[80]

Management: Maternal rubella is a self-limited disease requiring only symptomatological care. Severe complications of rubella infection such as encephalitis, thrombocytopenia, neuritis, conjunctivitis, and orchitis should be aggressively managed. Termination of pregnancy may be offered in cases of maternal infection. The maternal administration of immune globulin in large doses (20 mL in adults) in cases of susceptible women exposed to rubella during gestation has been proposed.[67] This treatment, however, has not produced encouraging results because it does not seem to prevent fetal infection. Post exposure prophylaxis for rubella in early pregnancy is not recommended due to unproven clinical efficacy. The rubella vaccine is contraindicated during pregnancy; therefore, susceptible women should be immunized postpartum.

Prognosis: Up to two-thirds of children with congenital rubella may be asymptomatic at birth, but they will develop sequelae within the first 5 years of life.[74] Classic findings associated with neonatal rubella are low birth weight with a cluster of abnormalities, including cataracts, sensorineural deafness, and cardiac defects such as patent ductus arteriosus, pulmonary artery stenosis, and coarctation of aorta. Less common neonatal heart defects that have been reported are aortic stenosis and Ebstein anomaly.[81–84] Purpura (blueberry muffin spots), microphthalmia, corneal opacity, glaucoma, hepatosplenomegaly, thrombocytopenia, and radiolucent bone lesions may also be found.[85] Late manifestations of congenital rubella include hearing loss, pancreatic insufficiency, and behavioral disorders.[74,85] Diagnosis is made by serum detection of rubella IgM before 3 months of age or persistent IgG between 6 and 12 months of age.

Herpes Simplex Virus

Definition and Incidence: Genital HSV type 1 (HSV-1) or HSV type 2 (HSV-2) is a common infection in United States, affecting 16.2% or 1 in 6 people between the ages of 14 and 49 years.[86] Approximately 25% to 65% of pregnant patients in the United States have genital infection with HSV. The frequency of neonatal HSV infection in the United States varies according to the patient population, with the rate of infection ranging from 1 case per 12,500 to 1 case per 1,700 live births. Whitley et al.[87] analyzed the data from 30 U.S. health plans and showed a rate of 60 cases per 100,000 live births. This incidence is higher than that of congenital syphilis, toxoplasmosis, and congenital rubella.

Pathogenesis: HSV belongs to the family of double-stranded DNA viruses known as Alphaherpesvirinae, a subfamily of the Herpesviridae. HSV type 1 (HSV-1) and type 2 (HSV-2) are differentiated on the basis of the glycoproteins within the lipid envelope. Glycoproteins G1 and G2 are associated with HSV-1 and HSV-2, respectively. The hallmark of herpes infection is the ability to infect epithelial mucosal cells where replication occurs. The virus, then, gains access to sensory neurons and stays latent in the sensory ganglia for years, followed by reactivation.

HSV is transmitted from person to person through direct contact. HSV-1 is usually acquired orally, but may also be sexually transmitted. HSV-2 is primarily a sexually transmitted infection. Most neonatal infections result from exposure to HSV in the genital tract during delivery, although both viruses may also be transmitted vertically during pregnancy. Traditionally, HSV-1 was typically associated with orofacial lesions, while HSV-2 was felt to cause genital herpes. Although HSV-2 still predominates as the major etiology for genital herpes, an increasing proportion has been ascribed to HSV-1 recently, especially in younger women. According to the Centers for Disease Control and Prevention (CDC), the rate of HSV-2 seroprevalence in the United States has remained stable since the mid-1990s at 16.2%.[86]

The three categories of genital herpes infections are primary, nonprimary, and recurrent. A primary HSV infection is a newly acquired infection in the absence of preexisting antibodies to either HSV-1 or HSV-2. Primary symptomatic genital herpes have an incubation of a period of 2 to 20 days and cause ulceration of the external genitalia and cervix as well as blistering lesions on the internal thigh, buttocks, and perineal skin. Primary HSV infections can also be associated with a number of systemic symptoms such as fever, malaise, and headache.

Nonprimary episode infection refers to newly acquired antibodies to HSV-1 or 2 in the presence of preexisting antibodies to the other type. Nonprimary infections tend to be less severe than do primary HSV infections and to have less systemic symptoms and quicker recovery times. HSV-2 antibodies are highly protective against new HSV-1 infection; thus, nonprimary HSV-1 infections are much less common.

Recurrent genital HSV infections refer to the reactivation of a latent genital HSV. The HSV type obtained from the lesion matches the HSV type obtained from the serum. Recurrent infections are typically less severe, unilateral, and have fewer lesions than do either primary or nonprimary infections.[88] As in nonprimary HSV, recurrent genital HSV infections are more common with HSV-2 as opposed to HSV-1. Asymptomatic viral shedding may occur during phases in between clinical outbreaks of genital herpes, where HSV reactivates within the sensory neurons of the genital mucosa. Most sexual transmission of HSV occurs during periods of asymptomatic viral shedding because patients are unaware that they are infectious.[89] Most cases of genital HSV infection in women occur without signs or symptoms of disease and are associated with cervical viral shedding.

Diagnosis: There are a variety of methodologies for the diagnosis of HSV infection, including viral culture, PCR, direct fluorescent antibodies, Tzanck smears, and serologic identification of IgG and IgM. Pregnant women who present with symptoms suggestive of genital herpes should undergo both type-specific assay and viral identification testing. Routine antepartum screening in asymptomatic patients is not recommended.

Ultrasound: Since intrauterine HSV infection is very uncommon, limited experience exists regarding the sonographic prenatal diagnosis. Various fetal malformations have been associated with congenital herpes, including microcephaly, cerebral atrophy, hydranencephaly, intracranial calcifications, ventriculomegaly, microphthalmia, chorioretinitis, cataracts, congenital herpetic keratitis, congenital heart disease, hepatic calcifications, nonimmune hydrops, bullous skin lesions and scars, lower limb hypoplasia, and abnormal digits. Fetal cerebral malformation, echogenic bowel (Fig. 31.12), and skin lesions seem to be more common US findings in fetuses with congenital herpes. Brain lesions are considered as secondary to the cytotoxic virus effects, or subsequent ischemia caused by vascular occlusion of cerebral vessels. Lanouette et al.[90] reported a 14-fold increase in alpha-fetoprotein (AFP) noted during second-trimester screening in a patient with multiple fetal congenital anomalies. At 19 weeks' gestation, the patient underwent an amniocentesis and cordocentesis with results consistent with HSV infection.

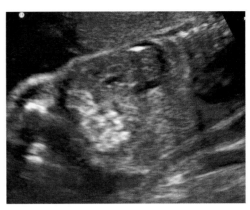

FIGURE 31.12: Sagittal-oblique US demonstrating echogenic bowel at 26 gestational weeks in a fetus with congenital herpes simplex virus.

Jayaram and Wake[91] reported a case with confirmed maternal HSV-2 infection in which a screening US at 20 weeks did not show any abnormalities. During the third trimester, the patient was admitted with reduced fetal movements. An US examination then noted absent corpus callosum and gross ventriculomegaly associated with absent end-diastolic flow of umbilical artery Doppler. Interestingly, an irregular heart rate with fluctuating baseline between 60 and 160 beats per minute was also documented.

In a case report by Diguet et al.,[92] during a screening US at 23 weeks of gestation, IUGR, absence of limb movements, thickened skin, hyperechogenic bowel, placental micronodular alterations, moderate pericardial effusion, and a reverse flow of the ductus venosus were noted. Because of a previous clinical episode of HSV at the beginning of pregnancy, amniocentesis was performed, revealing a positive PCR for HSV-1. On follow up sonographic examination at 27 weeks of gestation, oligohydramnios associated with fetal abdominal and lower limb skin irregular thickness, esophageal hyperechogenicity, and persistence of IUGR were found. The pregnancy was terminated, and fetal examination revealed extensive skin ulceration on the trunk and limbs, splenomegaly, and cardiomegaly.

Duin et al.[93] reported a case in a patient with confirmed HSV in which a normal US at 20 weeks' gestation with symmetric fetal growth was obtained; however, during a third-trimester examination, marked cerebral ventriculomegaly, third ventricle enlargement, frontal thinning of the cerebral cortex, and microcephaly were noted. A follow-up US demonstrated a slight dissolution of the cortical mantle. Severe parenchymal destruction, particularly in the temporal and parietal lobes, was confirmed by a prenatal MRI. The occipital cerebral cortex was also globally thinned with microgyria. Postmortem examination confirmed the prenatal diagnosis of hydranencephaly. This report suggests that fetal MRI may provide significant additional information in assessing the extensiveness of the fetal HSV infection. Interestingly, fetal malformation caused by congenital herpes infection may be only evident during the late part of pregnancy despite an initial normal screening US. Thus, third-trimester US evaluation for an anatomy follow-up and biometry should be considered in pregnancies with known herpes virus infection.

Management: Although considerable effort is made for the viral identification of genital HSV, treatment regimens do not vary by virus type. During a primary outbreak in pregnancy, oral antibiotic therapy is indicated to reduce the duration and severity of symptoms. Viral shedding is also decreased with proper therapy. No data indicates that maternal treatment reduces the risk of neonatal herpes. Acyclovir is not teratogenic and may be administered either orally in pregnant women with a first episode of genital herpes or intravenously in pregnant women with severe genital or disseminated herpetic disease.

Transabdominal invasive procedures, such as chorionic villus sampling, amniocentesis, and percutaneous umbilical sampling, may be performed even when genital lesions are present. Transcervical procedures should not be performed during the presence of active lesions.

Prognosis: Neonatal HSV infection is defined as infection in a newborn within 28 days of birth. There are three categories of neonatal infections: cutaneous disease, CNS disease, and disseminated disease. Cutaneous disease is an HSV disease localized to the skin, eye, and/or mouth. Although cutaneous disease has a low mortality, it may progress to CNS or disseminated disease. CNS disease manifests with neurological symptoms as well as positive CSF PCR findings and carries a mortality of approximately 15%. Disseminated disease has the worst prognosis with the highest fatality rate. Involvement of multiple organs (e.g., hepatitis, pneumonitis, or disseminated intravascular coagulation) is common and has a mortality rate of 31% and 85%, with and without therapy, respectively.

Human Immunodeficiency Virus

Definition and Incidence: Acquired immune deficiency syndrome (AIDS) is a severe immunological disorder caused by the HIV RNA retrovirus, resulting in a defect in cell-mediated immune response leading to an increased susceptibility to opportunistic infections. Despite aggressive efforts by the health community to reduce vertical transmission, HIV remains a significant perinatal risk globally. Almost 33.3 million people worldwide are infected, with 88% of infected infants born to mothers who did not receive any antiretroviral (ARV) treatment.[94,95] In the United States, approximately 21% of patients with HIV are unaware of their infection[96]; so the CDC recommends routine preconceptional HIV testing for all women.[97]

Pathogenesis: HIV attaches to the CD4 molecule on T lymphocytes via the external glycoprotein (gp120) and the transmembrane protein (gp41) located on the HIV envelope.[98] Following release into the cell cytoplasm, the viral RNA is reverse transcribed into DNA by the virus' own reverse transcriptase enzyme. After host-cell synthesis of HIV viral proteins, they are transported in close proximity to the cell membrane for assembly and egress. Destruction of the host's immune system ensues as CD4 T cells are consumed by the HIV virus. HIV is transmitted primarily by exposure to contaminated body fluids, especially blood and semen. During pregnancy, HIV may be transmitted to the fetus either transplacentally, at the time of vaginal delivery, or through breast milk.

Diagnosis: The ELISA performed on a blood sample or the rapid HIV test performed on blood or oral mucosa is the screening test of choice. Any positive HIV screening test should be followed by a confirmatory Western blot assay. Patients with a positive confirmatory testing result are considered to be infected with HIV and should be referred for consultation to an HIV specialist.

A thorough laboratory evaluation, including CD4+ T-cell count and plasma HIV RNA PCR is recommended.

Ultrasound: HIV infection has not been associated with any specific fetal anomalies. Joao et al.[99] followed up 995 HIV-infected pregnant patients undergoing antiretroviral therapy (ART). No significant increase in the rate of congenital anomalies was found compared to the overall population. In addition, they found that the prevalence of congenital anomalies was not affected by the timing of ART exposure during pregnancy.[99] However, the increasing complexity of ARV regimens used antenatally for HIV treatment may result in potential drug-related adverse events such as low birth weight and preterm birth.[100-103] Late IUGR has been demonstrated in HIV-infected pregnant women.[104] Similarly, in a prospective cohort study, Aaron et al.[105] found an increase in small for gestational age (SGA) births in HIV patients compared to an HIV-negative population. Therefore, it is suggested to follow up HIV patients with serial growth ultrasounds. US has been used to investigate abnormal placental implantation in HIV-positive women. Savvidou et al. investigated the effect of maternal HIV infection on the degree of placental invasion through pulsatility index measurements of the uterine arteries during the first trimester. No significant differences, however, were found in placental perfusion of HIV patients compared to non-HIV patients.[106]

Management: All women should be tested immediately upon diagnosis of pregnancy. Repeat testing should be done during the third trimester for patients at high risk of acquiring HIV antenatally. Instrumentation and invasive procedures, such as fetal scalp electrodes, forceps, vacuum suction devices, amniocentesis, cordocentesis, and chorionic villus sampling, may increase the risk of vertical transmission and should be avoided. Davies et al.[107] reviewed the risk of fetal infection with amniocentesis in women with HIV. They concluded that in HIV-positive women noninvasive screening tools, such as maternal serum and fetal US screening, be preferentially performed prior to the consideration of amniocentesis.[107] Furthermore, artificial rupture of membranes should be avoided in the absence of obstetrical indications.

Plasma viral load prior to delivery is the strongest predictor of vertical transmission and also will determine the mode of delivery. The American College of Obstetricians and Gynecologists (ACOG) recommend a scheduled cesarean delivery at 38 weeks of gestation for HIV-infected women with viral loads >1,000 copies per mL regardless of the ART regimen.[108] The combination of ART antenatally and intrapartum Zidovudine (AZT) has led to a significant decrease in the rate of vertical transmission of HIV. Prior to vaginal delivery, patients should receive a 2 mg per kg intravenous loading dose of AZT over 1 hour, followed by 1 mg per kg of intravenous AZT until cord clamp.[109] For HIV patients undergoing cesarean delivery, AZT should begin 3 hours before the surgery. Aside from AZT, all other ART drugs should be continued intrapartum.[109] Lastly, antibiotic prophylaxis for *Pneumocystis* and *Mycobacterium avium* complex may be required according to the CD4 count.

Prognosis: Pregnant patients affected with HIV should be counseled that in the absence of ART, the risk of vertical transmission is approximately 25%. With AZT, the risk is reduced to 5% to 8%. When care includes both AZT and scheduled cesarean delivery, the risk is decreased to 2% or less. A similar risk is seen among women with viral loads of less than 1,000 copies per mL despite the mode of delivery. Neonatal administration of ART has been shown to decrease the rate of seroconversion in the newborn of an HIV-infected mother.[110]

Varicella Zoster Virus

Definition and Incidence: Varicella infection, also known as chickenpox, is uncommon during pregnancy, although an important cause of maternal and fetal complications. An incidence of 1.6 to 4.6 per 1,000 has been reported among individuals between 15 and 45 years of age in the United States.[111,112] Approximately 90% of adults born in the United States and Europe are immune to VZV. The introduction of universal varicella vaccination has reduced the rate of VZV transmission in some countries.

Serious fetal complications have been associated with varicella acquired during pregnancy. Congenital varicella syndrome (CVS) is more common with maternal infection during the first half of pregnancy and may lead to multiple fetal anomalies. Since the first description of CVS in 1947 by Laforet et al.,[113] several other cases have been reported. Primary VZV during pregnancy may result in congenital infection 25% of the time.[114] Fetal outcomes depend on the time when the infection occurs. If maternal infection takes place during the first 20 weeks of gestation, the incidence of CVS is approximately 1% to 2%. The risk for spontaneous abortion is also increased during this period.[115]

Pathogenesis: VZV is a DNA virus of the herpes family and is highly contagious. The primary infection, also referred to as chickenpox, is self-limited. It is transmitted from person to person by direct contact, via respiratory droplets or secretions, or via aerosolization of vesicular fluid from skin lesions. The virus enters the host through the upper respiratory tract.[116] The incubation period usually lasts between 14 and 16 days but can vary from as few as 10 or as many as 21 days after contact.[115] Initially, nonspecific prodromal symptoms, such as fever, chills, headache, malaise, and sore throat, occur, followed by pruritus and a maculopapular rash that becomes vesicular. The rash will crust over in approximately 5 days. The period of contagiousness is 1 to 2 days before the onset of the rash and continues until all lesions are crusted.

Intrauterine infection occurs via transplacental transmission following maternal viremia. The vertical transmission rate increases with advancing gestation age. In a large prospective study, Enders et al.[117] demonstrated that IgM was detected in 5%, 10%, and 25% of infants at birth, following maternal varicella infection during the first, second, and third trimester, respectively. The type of fetal infection depends on the gestational age when the disease takes place. Infection during the first half of pregnancy may be complicated by CVS, while maternal disease around the time of delivery results in neonatal varicella.[118,119]

Diagnosis: The diagnosis of varicella generally is based on its classic clinical manifestations, and laboratory testing is unnecessary. Cases in which clinical manifestations are ambiguous but infection is suspected, culture, fluorescent antigen staining, or PCR testing for VZV DNA can be performed on vesicular fluid or scrapings from the lesions. Serologic tests are generally not of use for diagnosis, because specific antibodies only become detectable after the rash has occurred. At present, there are no reliable prenatal markers to predict fetal disease or severity. Serial US examinations of the fetus may be useful since some anomalies are not detected sonographically during the first examination.[120] PCR testing has been used to detect VZV infection in amniotic fluid with a high sensitivity and specificity.[121,122] Amniocentesis should

not be performed until 1 month after maternal infection to avoid false-negative results.[120,123] VZV cultures from amniotic fluid have a poor sensitivity.[124] Disruptions in the fetal skin may cause an elevation of AFP in maternal blood and amniotic fluid as well as an increase in acetylcholinesterase within the amniotic fluid.[120]

Ultrasound: Targeted US is recommended for all patients with documented infection to identify fetal anomalies associated with congenital varicella. Possible findings include IUGR, microcephaly, ventriculomegaly, cerebellar dysplasia, polyhydramnios, oligohydramnios, hydrops, and calcifications in the liver (Fig. 31.13), abdomen, and lungs.[120,125,126] Limb anomalies, including hypoplasia and contractures, are commonly found in cases of congenital varicella. Free-floating echogenic material and spicular echo reflections surrounding the skin may be indicative of cutaneous lesions.[126] Fetal ocular defects such as cataracts and microphthalmia may be visualized, as well. Interestingly, during a second-trimester US in a patient with documented varicella infection, a case of congenital pulmonary airway malformation (CPAM) was documented.[127] Multiple bilateral, diffuse hyperechogenic lesions in the lungs as well as multiple sonolucent areas in the liver were the only other noted abnormal images. Of note, sonographic findings associated with varicella fetopathy are nonspecific and may be associated with several other congenital infections, creating a difficulty in obtaining a clear diagnosis.

Fetal MRI may be a valuable adjunct to prenatal US. Verstraelen et al.[126] reported a case of congenital varicella infection in which additional information was obtained using MRI. During a routine prenatal US at 26 weeks' gestation, diminished gross fetal body movements, left lower limb hypoplasia with club foot deformity, right-kidney pyelectasis, echogenic bowels, and multiple calcifications in the liver and thorax were visualized. CNS lesions including cerebellar hypoplasia, pachygyria, and incomplete opercularization of the Sylvian fissure were missed by US, but were clearly demonstrated by MRI at 32 weeks. Prenatal MRI may, therefore, contribute to initial sonographic findings which may help enhance patient counseling.[126]

Management: Among adults who do not recall having varicella, the majority of patients are actually immune.[128] A history of varicella or two-dose vaccination is sufficient to reassure a pregnant patient that she is not susceptible to varicella infection. If maternal

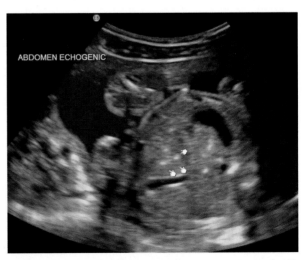

FIGURE 31.13: Liver calcifications seen on cross-sectional US of abdomen in a fetus with suspected congenital varicella syndrome.

serology is negative, secondary prevention during pregnancy must be considered. Susceptible pregnant seronegative women exposed to varicella should be offered varicella zoster immunoglobulin (VZIG) to limit maternal disease. Although optimum protection is obtained when the dose is administered within 96 hours of exposure, some experts suggest that VZIG may be administered with benefit up to 10 days after exposure.[129] VZIG should not be given once active disease has begun.[116] The recommended dose of VZIG is 125 units per 10 kg of body weight, up to a maximum of 625 units. Intravenous immune globulin (IVIG) can be substituted if necessary at a dose of 400 mg per kg if VZIG is not available. If VZIG is not administered within 4 to 10 days of exposure, antiviral therapy may be considered for postexposure prophylaxis; however, some authorities question its safety or efficacy compared to VZIG.

Even though VZIG has been shown to reduce the incidence of symptomatic disease in pregnant women, it does not influence the risk of development of CVS. Since serial US may lack sensitivity or specificity as a diagnostic tool for fetal varicella syndrome (FVS), invasive prenatal diagnosis to confirm congenital infection should be considered. Although there is no validated *in utero* treatment for FVS, a negative amniocentesis result can reassure parents that their child has no risk of FVS or of any long-term impairment.

Prognosis: Maternal infection during the second trimester and early third trimester most often does not result in CVS and is associated with a good prognosis.[130–133] Generally, neonates born with CVS have poor outcomes. Isolated cases of more favorable scenarios have been reported.[134,135] Neonatal death usually occurs from intractable gastroesophageal reflux, severe recurrent aspiration pneumonia, or respiratory failure. Structural anomalies are usually not seen with neonatal varicella syndrome. Before VZIG was available, the mortality rate from neonatal varicella syndrome was 31%.[136] Since the introduction of VZIG, the mortality rate has dropped to 7%.[118]

Zika Virus

Definition and Incidence: Zika virus is a single-stranded neurotropic and neurotoxic RNA Flavivirus, similar to dengue virus, that may cause severe fetal brain malformations during pregnancy, a period of rapid and critical CNS development. Transmission is typically from the bite of an infected mosquito, although mother-to-child, sexual, and blood donation transmissions can occur. Although maternal symptoms are uncommon and rarely severe, the consequences of congenital infections are devastating.

Diagnosis and Management: Prevention is the mainstay of infection control as there is currently no vaccine or therapy available. The CDC recommends that pregnant women should not travel to areas with a Zika outbreak.

Pregnant women with Zika symptoms and with possible Zika exposure should be tested for Zika virus infection. Pregnant women with no Zika symptoms but who have ongoing Zika exposure (e.g., live in or frequently travel to an area with risk of Zika) should be offered Zika testing. The CDC recommends women and men diagnosed with Zika or who have possible exposure to Zika through sex or travel to wait at least 3 months before trying to conceive.

Ultrasound: About 2 in 20 (10%) babies of women with confirmed Zika virus infection during pregnancy in US states and about 1 in 20 (5%) in US territories had Zika-associated birth defects. Congenital Zika virus infection causes a spectrum of adverse birth outcomes, including severe birth defects of the CNS.

In congenital Zika virus syndrome (CZS), the most frequent ultrasonographic findings are calcifications in the cortical white matter, ventriculomegaly, enlargement of the cisterna magna and the extra-axial subarachnoid space, corpus callosum abnormalities, and reduced brain volume (microcephaly). This infection can also result in a decrease in the brainstem and cerebellum. Placentomegaly, arthrogryposis, and eye abnormalities also have been associated with Zika virus infection.

Fetal growth restriction is generally a common finding associated with congenital Zika virus infection. For pregnant women with confirmed or possible Zika virus infection, serial fetal ultrasounds (every 3–4 weeks) should be considered to assess fetal anatomy, particularly fetal neuroanatomy, and to monitor growth closely.

Other Viral Infections

Congenital viral infection with Coxsackie B1 and B5 during the first trimester has been associated with fetal myocarditis resulting in severe heart failure.[79(pp762–763)] Intrauterine infection with enterovirus has been postulated as a possible cause of future development of type 1 diabetes during adolescence.[137]

PARASITIC INFECTIONS

Toxoplasmosis

Definition and Incidence: Toxoplasmosis is a parasitic infection caused by *Toxoplasma gondii*. It is estimated that 400 to 4,000 cases occur in the United States each year.[138–140] Furthermore, recent data suggests that congenital toxoplasmosis occurs in approximately 1 in 10,000 live births.[139] Treatment has been shown to decrease fetal infection rate, thus underscoring the importance of prenatal diagnosis.

Pathogenesis: *T. gondii* undergoes a complex life cycle comprised of three stages known as the tachyzoite, bradyzoite, and sporozoite phases. The tachyzoite phase represents the acute stage of infection where the protozoan invades and replicates within host cells. The bradyzoite phase represents the latent stage of infection where the protozoan exists as a tissue cyst. During the sporozoite phase, the protozoan exists as an environmentally resistant cyst. It is the tachyzoite form of the organism that is responsible for congenital infection. Members of the family Felidae are the definitive reservoir of *T. gondii*, while humans are temporary hosts only. During acute infections, cats excrete *T. gondii* oocysts in their feces, and humans are then infected by fecal–oral contact. Other routes of transmission to humans include ingestion of raw or inadequately cooked infected meat or unwashed fruits or vegetables and exposure to contaminated soil from gardening.[141] Sporozoites penetrate the human host's GI mucosa and are released in the tachyzoite phase into the systemic circulation. A woman can then transmit the infection to her fetus transplacentally. The incubation period may range from 10 to 23 days after ingestion of undercooked meat, and from 5 to 20 days after ingestion of oocysts from cat feces.[142]

Maternal infection with *T. gondii* prior to conception rarely results in congenital infection.[143] The prevalence of maternal infection is 0.4%, and out of those patients, 40% will develop congenital toxoplasmosis. The risk of congenital infection is directly related to the fetal gestational age. While acute maternal infection occurs between 10% and 25% of the time during the first trimester, it will occur between 60% and 90% of the time during the third trimester.[144,145] The severity of congenital toxoplasmosis, however, is inversely related to fetal gestational age, with the most devastating fetal infections occurring during the first half of pregnancy. Significant fetal morbidity and mortality decreases from 75% during the first trimester to almost 0% toward the end of the pregnancy.[79(p763)]

Diagnosis: In adults, the severity of *T. gondii* infection is correlated with the immune status of the host.[142] Generally, for immunocompetent adults, toxoplasmosis infections result in mild symptoms of lymphadenopathy, fever, fatigue, and malaise that are self-limited and resolve in weeks to months without any specific treatments. In contrast, however, patients who are immunocompromised as a result of AIDS, organ transplants, malignancies, or chronic steroid administration demonstrate severe neurological manifestations such as meningoencephalitis.

The most common method of diagnosis for acute toxoplasmosis is maternal serum antibody detection; however, individual variation in titers may confound the serologic results. Also, IgM antibodies have been reported to persist for up to 18 months post infection.[146] A negative IgM with a positive IgG result indicates chronic infection. A positive IgM result, on the other hand, may indicate more recent infection or a false-positive reaction. Commercially available test kits for *Toxoplasma* IgG and IgM antibodies have significant variation in sensitivities and specificities.[147] In response to this problem, the U.S. Food and Drug Administration (FDA) in 1997 issued a guide for the interpretation of toxoplasmosis serologic results.[148] Determining when *T. gondii* infection occurred in a pregnant woman is important since infection before conception poses little risk for transmission to the fetus. IgG avidity testing measures the strength with which IgG binds to *T. gondii* and may help determine when the infection occurred. High IgG avidity indicates that the infection occurred at least 5 months ago, while low IgG avidity reflects a more recent infection.[149] Women with positive serum IgM antibodies should undergo IgG avidity testing by an experienced toxoplasmosis reference laboratory.[149]

After maternal infection is confirmed, congenital toxoplasmosis must be investigated. The identification of *T. gondii* intrauterine infection by amniocentesis using PCR testing has been found to have both high sensitivities and specificities.[150] Foulon et al.[151] reported that a combination of PCR and mouse inoculation of amniotic fluid may improve sensitivities even further. Given the advances in PCR testing of amniotic fluid as well as the risk associated with cordocentesis, amniocentesis is the procedure of choice for the diagnosis of congenital toxoplasmosis infection.

Ultrasound: US findings of congenital toxoplasmosis include hydrocephalus, intracranial calcifications, fetal growth restriction, ascites (Fig. 31.14), and hepatosplenomegaly. In a case series published by Hohlfeld et al.,[152] 32 of 89 fetuses with proven congenital toxoplasmosis developed sonographic signs of infection. Ventriculomegaly was found in 25 fetuses, while intracranial calcifications (Fig. 31.15) were found in only 6 fetuses.[152] Furthermore, a number of false negatives were found, with postnatal brain examinations revealing multiple areas of brain necrosis and abscesses in normally reported prenatal studies.[152] With the improvement of US resolution, the advent of neurosonography, and the addition of fetal MRI, recent studies have been able to better

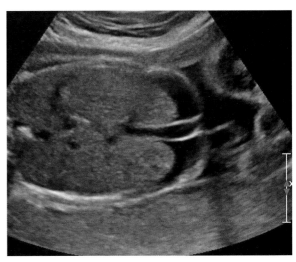

FIGURE 31.14: Cross-sectional US of the abdomen at the level of the cord insertion demonstrating ascites in a fetus with congenital toxoplasmosis.

delineate fetal neurological signs of congenital toxoplasmosis. Malinger et al.[153] in a recent review of eight patients with congenital toxoplasmosis described ventriculomegaly ($n = 7$) and multiple echogenic nodular foci consistent with calcifications in the brain parenchyma ($n = 7$), in the periventricular zone ($n = 3$), and in the caudothalamic zone 9 ($n = 3$). Good correlation has been demonstrated between US and fetal MRI for diagnosing brain abnormalities in fetal toxoplasmosis.[154,155] Interestingly, while US signs of fetal toxoplasmosis are not identified during the routine second-trimester US examination, they may be more commonly detected during the third trimester. It has been speculated that this occurs because of the prolonged time for the fetal insult to develop.[156] Unlike in CMV infection where intracranial echogenic nodules occur most often in the periventricular zone,[157] in toxoplasmosis they may be found dispersed in multiple areas of the fetal brain. Furthermore, periventricular cysts and microcephaly which are characteristic of CMV infections are not common in fetal toxoplasmosis.[153,158] Other non-CNS US findings such as thickened placenta with hypoechoic areas, liver echogenicities (Fig. 31.16), and hepatomegaly may be visualized, but are not specific for fetal toxoplasmosis.[153]

Management: Since the prevalence of congenital toxoplasmosis is so rare, routine screening during pregnancy for acute toxoplasmosis is not advocated by the ACOG [159] and the Royal College of Obstetrics and Gynecology.[160] Routine screening may not be cost effective, but, more importantly, may result in equivocal or false-positive values, leading to unnecessary treatment and fetal interventions. Interestingly, other countries such as Austria and France have implemented screening programs for toxoplasmosis, demonstrating a decline in the incidence of congenital infection.[161,162] It is difficult to determine whether the proportion of the decline is directly attributable to the program or to the overall general decline in European toxoplasmosis rate.

Treatment for toxoplasmosis infection is available and should be instituted as soon as maternal infection is confirmed. Spiramycin should be started at a maximum dose of 3 g per day in all pregnant women found to have serologic evidence of toxoplasmosis. In the United States, however, spiramycin is not available, but it may be obtained from Europe with special approval from

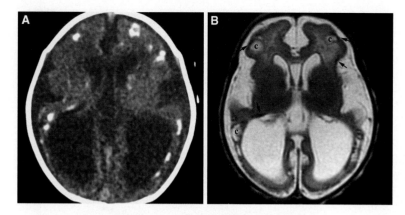

FIGURE 31.15: Congenital toxoplasmosis. **A:** Axial noncontrast computed tomography in a newborn shows extensive parenchymal calcifications that are predominantly cortical and subcortical in location. Also note moderate ventriculomegaly. Hydrocephalus is more common in toxoplasmosis than in cytomegalovirus (CMV) infection. **B:** Axial T2 MRI shows multiple foci of T2 hypointensity corresponding to CT-confirmed calcification *(black arrows)*. Also note the subcortical cysts *(c)*. Ventriculomegaly is moderate. (Reprinted with permission from Hedlund G, Bale JF, Barkovich AJ. Infections of the developing and mature nervous system. In: Barkovich AJ, Raybaud C, eds. *Pediatric Neuroimaging*. 5th ed. Philadelphia, PA: Wolters Kluwer Health/ Lippincott Williams & Wilkins; 2012:954–1050.)

the FDA. Spiramycin is a macrolide antibiotic that itself does not cross the placenta, but is thought to prevent passage of toxoplasmosis to the fetus.[79(p165)] A combination of pyrimethamine and sulfadiazine has been recommended when congenital infection is confirmed by amniocentesis.[163] Both drugs, however, are contraindicated during the first trimester due to their teratogenicity. Pyrimethamine is a folic acid antagonist, thus increasing the risk of neural tube defects if used early in pregnancy. Also, pyrimethamine has been associated with fetal heart and kidney malformations as well as maternal and fetal bone marrow suppression.[164] Sulfadiazine has been associated with an increased incidence of oral clefting. Thus, spiramycin is generally prescribed initially and changed to a pyrimethamine and sulfonamide combination if fetal infection is diagnosed after 15 weeks.[165]

In 2000, the CDC published primary prevention recommendations for pregnant women to avoid toxoplasmosis infection. These guidelines centered around patient and provider education as well as on specific hygienic and dietary precautions.[162] Foulon et al.[166] examined the impact of primary prevention on the incidence of toxoplasmosis in pregnancy. Periconceptional education and antenatal education are fundamental in the prevention of maternal and fetal infections. It has been demonstrated that pregnant women who received education sessions were associated with a 63% decrease in toxoplasmosis seroconversion rates compared to women who did not.[166]

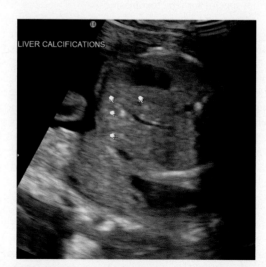

FIGURE 31.16: Axial cross-sectional US of multiple nonshadowing hepatic calcifications at 28 weeks' gestation.

Prognosis: The likelihood of long-term sequelae as a result of congenital toxoplasmosis decreases as gestational age increases. Toxoplasmosis acquired during the first trimester may result in a spontaneous abortion, while infection incurred during third trimester may be asymptomatic. Although the classic neonatal triad of chorioretinitis, intracranial calcifications, and hydrocephalus is suggestive of congenital toxoplasmosis, up to 90% of neonates affected with congenital toxoplasmosis do not demonstrate obvious signs on routine examination.[152,167] Other findings often seen in congenital toxoplasmosis include lymphadenopathy, hepatosplenomegaly, mental retardation, seizures, encephalitis, malaise, arthralgia, low-grade fever, and occipital and cervical lymphadenopathy. Indeed, disease sequelae may only become apparent when visual impairment, mental and cognitive abnormalities of variable severity, seizures, or learning disabilities present after several months or years.

Other Parasitic Infections

Apart from congenital toxoplasmosis, other sources of congenital parasitic infections include malaria, schistosomiasis, and trypanosomiasis. Malaria infection during pregnancy can have a huge impact on both the mother and the fetus, leading to still birth, premature delivery, or fetal growth restriction. Fetal anemia and splenomegaly have also been described in cases of congenital malaria.[168] Considering the poor outcomes associated with congenital malaria,[169,170] fetal US surveillance in endemic areas to detect and treat cases during pregnancy needs to be actively implemented.

Schistosomiasis mansoni has also been demonstrated to cause placental insufficiency, leading to fetal growth restriction.[171] *Trypanosoma cruzi* can cause congenital Chagas disease. Fetal organs, including the heart, brain, and integumentary and GI systems, may be affected, leading to hepatosplenomegaly, anemia, jaundice, and encephalitis.

BACTERIAL INFECTIONS

Syphilis

Definition and Incidence: Syphilis is a sexually transmitted disease caused by the bacterium *Treponema pallidum*. According to the World Health Organization (WHO), 12 million people are infected with syphilis each year.[172] In the United States, the rate of syphilis among women was 1.1 cases per 100,000 women in 2010, while the rate of congenital syphilis was 8.7 cases per 100,000 live births.[173] In 2008, the WHO reported that approximately

1.9 million pregnant women had active syphilis.[174] The importance of accurate prenatal diagnosis of syphilis was emphasized by Hawkes et al.[175] in a recent meta-analysis, who stated that approximately 70% of pregnant women infected with syphilis will have an adverse pregnancy outcome. Both the ACOG and the American Academy of Pediatrics recommend screening for syphilis at the first prenatal visit and again at 32 to 36 weeks, in high-risk women. Furthermore, the CDC recommends screening at delivery.[176]

Pathogenesis: Syphilis is horizontally transmitted via vaginal, anal, or oral sex. Approximately 3 weeks after infection, a round, small, and painless syphilitic chancre may appear on the vulva, vagina, cervix, anus, or rectum indicating primary infection. This lesion may last for 3 to 6 weeks and often goes unrecognized by the host. Eventually, *Treponema spirochetes* disseminate systemically, resulting in the cutaneous and mucosal manifestations of secondary infection, lasting for up to a year. During this time, the disease can be especially contagious. After primary or secondary syphilis, the infection may enter a latent phase, causing no symptoms to the host. This phase of the disease is divided into early and late depending on the duration of the infection. Initial infection occurring within the previous 12 months and beyond 12 months is characterized as early latent and late latent syphilis respectively. Importantly, during the latent phase, transmission to the fetus may still occur.[177] In approximately one-third of the people who go untreated, tertiary syphilis may develop. Skin, bone, or liver gumma, CNS abnormalities, and cardiovascular disorders are associated with tertiary syphilis. During this stage, individuals are not considered infectious.[178]

Diagnosis: The most specific test for the diagnosis of syphilis when an active chancre or condyloma latum is present is dark field microscopy. In the absence of active lesions, serologic testing for syphilis is performed. Serologic testing includes nontreponemal tests (NTTs) and treponemal tests (TTs). Generally, NTTs are used for screening and monitoring therapy, while TTs are for diagnostic confirmation. The Venereal Disease Research Laboratory (VDRL) test and the rapid plasma reagin (RPR) test are the most commonly used NTTs. Since NTTs detect antibodies to cardiolipin, a compound commonly found in human tissue, false-positive reactions can occur. TTs detect an interaction between serum immunoglobulins and surface antigens of *T. pallidum*. They include the fluorescent treponemal antibody absorption (FTA-ABS) test, the treponemal-specific, microhemagglutination assay for *T. pallidium* (MHA-TP), and *T. pallidum* particle agglutination test (TP-PA). Although far less common than in NTTs, false-positive reactions may still occur in diseases such as Lyme disease and leptospirosis.[177] Unlike NTTs which may become negative, TTs usually remain positive for life.

Ultrasound: In the presence of maternal syphilis, US findings of fetal hydrops, hepatosplenomegaly (Fig. 31.17), polyhydramnios, and thick placenta strongly suggest congenital syphilis. Other sonographic features include intrahepatic calcifications, ascites, hyperechogenic bowel, and even fetal death. Amniotic fluid dark field testing or PCR may be performed for confirmatory diagnosis. Hematologic sampling for fetal IgM anti-treponemal antibodies has been reported.[179] The degree of fetal hepatomegaly in pregnancies with syphilis has been correlated with amniotic fluid infection.[180] Dilatation of fetal bowel segments has been reported in case of congenital syphilis.[181] Hill and Maloney[182] reported

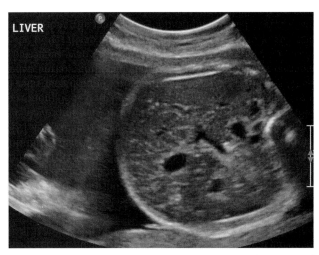

FIGURE 31.17: Axial US of the abdomen demonstrating hepatomegaly in a fetus with congenital syphilis.

fetal GI tract obstruction involving the stomach and small bowel in a case of congenital syphilis. Treponemal involvement of the intestine causing syphilitic enterocolitis has been described previously in stillbirths.[183] Wendel and Gilstrap[184] reported an association between hyperechogenicity of the vasculature in the basal ganglia and congenital syphilis. It has been demonstrated that congenital infection can result in placental villitis and obliterative arteritis, thereby resulting in placentomegaly and increased placental vascular resistance.[182] Lucas et al.[185] showed that mean systolic/diastolic (S/D) ratios of both the uterine and umbilical arteries were significantly increased in pregnancies affected by syphilis. Interestingly, in a case described by Schulman et al.[186] where decreased fetal movement was the initial complaint, fetal cardiac failure followed by bradycardia was noted. The pathological examination revealed acute syphilitic funisitis. Using 3D US, Araujo et al.[187] demonstrated oligodactyly and twisting of the toes in a case of congenital syphilis.

Management: Treatment of maternal infection is effective for both the prevention and the treatment of congenital syphilis. Penicillin G, parenterally administered, is the recommended treatment. In a randomized controlled trial performed by Radcliffe et al.,[188] penicillin G was found to be the most effective treatment for syphilis. The appropriate penicillin regimen varies according to the stage of infection.[189] A single dose of 2.4 million units of benzathine penicillin G is recommended for the treatment of primary syphilis, secondary syphilis, and early latent syphilis.[189] In cases of late latent syphilis or latent syphilis of unknown duration, the same dosage should be given and repeated twice at weekly intervals.[189] Because penicillin G does not cross the blood–brain barrier, aqueous crystalline penicillin G of 3 to 4 million units parenterally every 4 hours for 10 to 14 days is the treatment of choice for neurosyphilis.[189] Pregnant women who have a history of a penicillin allergy should be desensitized and treated. The titer of NTT antibodies reflects disease activity, with a four-fold decrease suggesting adequate therapy and a four-fold increase indicating active disease.

Prognosis: Congenital syphilis is classified as either early congenital syphilis (ECS) or late congenital syphilis (LCS). ECS appears in the first 2 years of life, while LCS appears afterwards. Both ECS and LCS affect a variety of organ systems. Findings of

ECS include hepatomegaly, splenomegaly, anemia, thrombocytopenia, leukopenia, macular–papular lesions over the hands and feet, ulceration of the nasal mucosa and cartilage (saddle nose deformity), periostitis, osteochondritis, nephrosis, neurosyphilis, and ocular malformations. Findings of LCS include peg-shaped, notched central incisors (Hutchinson teeth); multicuspid first molars (mulberry molars); interstitial keratitis; palsy of cranial nerve 8; rhinitis; impaired maxillary growth; saddle nose deformity; mental retardation; hydrocephalus; seizure disorders; periostitis of the skull, tibia (saber shin), and the clavicle (Higouménakis sign); and symmetric, tender joints (Clutton joints). The prognosis of congenital syphilis is dependent upon a number of factors, including the gestational age when vertical transmission occurred, stage of maternal syphilis, maternal treatment, and immunological response of the fetus.[190]

Other Bacterial Infections

Other bacteria that may cause congenital infections include *Listeria, Chlamydia, Mycoplasma, Mycobacterium,* and *Coxiella.* Q fever infection in pregnancy, caused by *Coxiella burnetii,* is associated with various maternal and neonatal adverse outcomes, including IUGR, stillbirth, preterm delivery, and oligohydramnios.[191,192] Shinar et al.[192] described two pregnancies complicated by Q fever that resulted in placental infection and abruption remote from term.

Although congenital tuberculosis is rare, a perinatal mortality of nearly 50% has been reported.[193] Clinical presentation of tuberculosis during pregnancy and infancy is often nonspecific, making recognition difficult. Tuberculosis has been associated with increased antenatal admission, premature delivery, IUGR, and maternal–fetal mortality.[194–196] Abramowsky et al.[197] described two cases of placental involvement with *Mycobacterium tuberculosis* causing acute villitis and Intervillositis. Principal neonatal sites of involvement include the liver and lungs; however, the bones, kidneys, spleen, GI tract, skin, and lymph nodes may also be affected. Generally, the diagnosis of congenital infection only occurs during the early neonatal period when clinical manifestations present. Common nonspecific clinical symptoms such as fever, respiratory distress, and hepatosplenomegaly most commonly appear within 2 to 3 weeks of delivery.[198] A high index of suspicion by health professionals is paramount in order to detect and manage tuberculosis in pregnancy and the early newborn period.

Listeria monocytogenes infection is a rare complication of pregnancy.[199] Intrauterine infection by *L. monocytogenes* has been associated with preterm delivery, meconium-stained amniotic fluid, hydrocephalus, chorioamnionitis, stillbirth, and neonatal death.[200,201] Prompt treatment with antibiotics is paramount in improving maternal and neonatal outcome.[202]

Mycoplasma and ureaplasma have been associated with chorioamnionitis, preterm delivery, and pregnancy loss.[203,204] Intrauterine infection with ureaplasma has also been associated with congenital pneumonia.[205]

Intra-amniotic Sludge

Intra-amniotic sludge is represented by the sonographic appearance of free-floating hyperechoic matter close to the internal cervical os (Fig. 31.18). It has been associated with an increased risk of preterm delivery and other adverse pregnancy outcomes. The precise nature of this material is unclear; however, it has been attributed to bleeding, meconium, vernix, and intrauterine infection.[206–209] For a more comprehensive review, refer to Chapters 7 and 10.

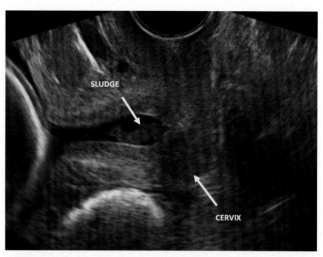

FIGURE 31.18: Transvaginal US demonstrating intra-amniotic sludge associated with cervical funneling at 24 gestational weeks.

SUMMARY

In summary, the global impact of congenital infections is significant. Although sonography by itself is not a sensitive test for fetal infection, the utilization of US technology assisted by fetal MRI along with other markers for congenital infection may influence clinical management, assist in prognostication, and aid in patient counseling. Indeed, particular findings such as an elevated MCA-PSV in the setting of congenital parvovirus may indicate the need for *in utero* fetal treatment. As diagnostic fetal imaging continues to advance, sonography will remain an invaluable tool for clinicians involved in the prenatal diagnosis of congenital infections.

REFERENCES

1. Stegmann BJ, Carey JC. TORCH infections: toxoplasmosis, other (syphilis, varicella-zoster, parvovirus B19), rubella, cytomegalovirus (CMV), and herpes infections. *Curr Womens Health Rep.* 2002;2(4):253–258.
2. Crino JP. Ultrasound and fetal diagnosis of perinatal infection. *Clin Obstet Gynecol.* 1999;42(1):71–80.
3. Pultoo A, Jankee H, Meetoo G, et al. Detection of cytomegalovirus in urine of hearing-impaired and mentally retarded children by PCR and cell culture. *J Commun Dis.* 2000;32(2):101–108.
4. Stagno S, Pass RF, Cloud G, et al. Primary cytomegalovirus infection in pregnancy: incidence, transmission to fetus, and clinical outcome. *JAMA.* 1986;256(14):1904–1908.
5. Yinon Y, Farine D, Yudin MH. Screening, diagnosis, and management of cytomegalovirus infection in pregnancy. *Obstet Gynecol Surv.* 2010;65(11):736–743.
6. Malm G, Engman ML. Congenital cytomegalovirus infections. *Semin Fetal Neonatal Med.* 2007;12(3):154–159.
7. Hanshaw JB. Cytomegalovirus infections. *Pediatr Rev.* 1995;16(2):43–48.
8. Stagno S, Pass RF, Dworsky ME, et al. Maternal cytomegalovirus infection and perinatal transmission. *Clin Obstet Gynecol.* 1982;25(3):563–576.
9. Liesnard C, Donner C, Brancart F, et al. Prenatal diagnosis of congenital cytomegalovirus infection: prospective study of 237 pregnancies at risk. *Obstet Gynecol.* 2000;95(6, pt 1):881–888.
10. Adler SP, Nigro G, Pereira L. Recent advances in the prevention and treatment of congenital cytomegalovirus infections. *Semin Perinatol.* 2007;31(1):10–18.
11. Grangeot-Keros L, Mayaux MJ, Lebon P, et al. Value of cytomegalovirus (CMV) IgG avidity index for the diagnosis of primary CMV infection in pregnant women. *J Infect Dis.* 1997;175(4):944–946.
12. Boppana SB, Pass RF, Britt WJ, et al. Symptomatic congenital cytomegalovirus infection: neonatal morbidity and mortality. *Pediatr Infect Dis J.* 1992;11(2):93–99.
13. Jones CA. Congenital cytomegalovirus infection. *Curr Probl Pediatr Adolesc Health Care.* 2003;33(3):70–93.
14. de Vries LS, Gunardi H, Barth PG, et al. The spectrum of cranial ultrasound and magnetic resonance imaging abnormalities in congenital cytomegalovirus infection. *Neuropediatrics.* 2004;35(2):113–119.
15. Malinger G, Lev D, Lerman-Sagie T. Imaging of fetal cytomegalovirus infection. *Fetal Diagn Ther.* 2011;29(2):117–126.

16. Noyola DE, Demmler GJ, Nelson CT, et al. Early predictors of neurodevelopmental outcome in symptomatic congenital cytomegalovirus infection. *J Pediatr.* 2001;138(3):325–331.

17. Guerra B, Simonazzi G, Puccetti C, et al. Ultrasound prediction of symptomatic congenital cytomegalovirus infection. *Am J Obstet Gynecol.* 2008;198(4):380.e1–380.e7.

18. Goncé A, Marcos MA, Borrell A, et al. Maternal IgM antibody status in confirmed fetal cytomegalovirus infection detected by sonographic signs. *Prenat Diagn.* 2012;32(9):817–821.

19. Nigro G, Adler SP, La Torre R, et al. Passive immunization during pregnancy for congenital cytomegalovirus infection. *N Engl J Med.* 2005;353(13):1350–1362.

20. Jacquemard F, Yamamoto M, Costa JM, et al. Maternal administration of valaciclovir in symptomatic intrauterine cytomegalovirus infection. *BJOG.* 2007;114(9):1113–1121.

21. Puliyanda DP, Silverman NS, Lehman D, et al. Successful use of oral ganciclovir for the treatment of intrauterine cytomegalovirus infection in a renal allograft recipient. *Transpl Infect Dis.* 2005;7(2):71–74.

22. Negishi H, Yamada H, Hirayama E, et al. Intraperitoneal administration of cytomegalovirus hyperimmunoglobulin to the cytomegalovirus-infected fetus. *J Perinatol.* 1998;18(6, pt 1):466–469.

23. Sato A, Hirano H, Miura H, et al. Intrauterine therapy with cytomegalovirus hyperimmunoglobulin for a fetus congenitally infected with cytomegalovirus. *J Obstet Gynaecol Res.* 2007;33(5):718–721.

24. Japanese Congenital Cytomegalovirus Infection Immunoglobulin Fetal Therapy Study Group. A trial of immunoglobulin fetal therapy for symptomatic congenital cytomegalovirus infection. *J Reprod Immunol.* 2012;95(1–2):73–79.

25. Matsuda H, Kawakami Y, Furuya K, et al. Intrauterine therapy for a cytomegalovirus-infected symptomatic fetus. *BJOG.* 2004;111(7):756–757.

26. Buxmann H, Stackelberg OM, Schlößer RL, et al. Use of cytomegalovirus hyperimmunoglobulin for prevention of congenital cytomegalovirus disease: a retrospective analysis. *J Perinat Med.* 2012;40(4):439–446.

27. Brown T, Anand A, Ritchie LD, et al. Intrauterine parvovirus infection associated with hydrops fetalis. *Lancet.* 1984;2(8410):1033–1034.

28. Heegaard ED, Brown KE. Human parvovirus B19. *Clin Microbiol Rev.* 2002;15(3):485–505.

29. Dembinski J, Eis-Hübinger AM, Maar J, et al. Long term follow up of serostatus after maternofetal parvovirus B19 infection. *Arch Dis Child.* 2003;88(3):219–221.

30. Chisaka H, Morita E, Yaegashi N, et al. Parvovirus B19 and the pathogenesis of anaemia. *Rev Med Virol.* 2003;13(6):347–359.

31. Nyman M, Tolfvenstam T, Petersson K, et al. Detection of human parvovirus B19 infection in first-trimester fetal loss. *Obstet Gynecol.* 2002;99(5, pt 1):795–798.

32. Wattre P, Dewilde A, Subtil D, et al. A clinical and epidemiological study of human parvovirus B19 infection in fetal hydrops using PCR Southern blot hybridization and chemiluminescence detection. *J Med Virol.* 1998;54(2):140–144.

33. Yaegashi N, Okamura K, Yajima A, et al. The frequency of human parvovirus B19 infection in nonimmune hydrops fetalis. *J Perinat Med.* 1994;22(2):159–163.

34. Rodis JF. Parvovirus infection. *Clin Obstet Gynecol.* 1999;42(1):107–120.

35. Enders M, Weidner A, Zoellner I, et al. Fetal morbidity and mortality after acute human parvovirus B19 infection in pregnancy: prospective evaluation of 1018 cases. *Prenat Diagn.* 2004;24(7):513–518.

36. Miller E, Fairley CK, Cohen BJ, et al. Immediate and long term outcome of human parvovirus B19 infection in pregnancy. *BJOG.* 1998;105(2):174–178.

37. DeHann T, Oepkes D, Beersma MFC. Aetiology, diagnosis and treatment of hydrops foetalis. *Curr Pediatr Rev.* 2005;1:63–72.

38. Jordan J, Tiangco B, Kiss J, et al. Human parvovirus B19: prevalence of viral DNA in volunteer blood donors and clinical outcomes of transfusion recipients. *Vox Sang.* 1998;75(2):97–102.

39. Torok T. Human parvovirus B19. In: Remington JS, Klein JO, eds. *Infectious Disease of the Fetus and Newborn Infant.* 4th ed. Philadelphia, PA: Saunders; 1995:668–702.

40. Rouger P, Gane P, Salmon C. Tissue distribution of H, Lewis and P antigens as shown by a panel of 18 monoclonal antibodies. *Rev Fr Transfus Immunohematol.* 1987;30(5):699–708.

41. Jordan JA, Butchko AR. Apoptotic activity in villous trophoblast cells during B19 infection correlates with clinical outcome: assessment by the caspase-related M30 Cytodeath antibody. *Placenta.* 2002;23(7):547–553.

42. Prospective study of human parvovirus (B19) infection in pregnancy. Public Health Laboratory Service Working Party on fifth disease. *BMJ.* 1990;300(6733):1166–1170.

43. Koch WC, Harger JH, Barnstein B, et al. Serologic and virologic evidence for frequent intrauterine transmission of human parvovirus B19 with a primary maternal infection during pregnancy. *Pediatr Infect Dis J.* 1998;17(6):489–494.

44. de Jong EP, de Haan TR, Kroes AC, et al. Parvovirus B19 infection in pregnancy. *J Clin Virol.* 2006;36(1):1–7.

45. Anderson MJ, Higgins PG, Davis LR, et al. Experimental parvoviral infection in humans. *J Infect Dis.* 1985;152(2):257–265.

46. Beersma MF, Claas EC, Sopaheluakan T, et al. Parvovirus B19 viral loads in relation to VP1 and VP2 antibody responses in diagnostic blood samples. *J Clin Virol.* 2005;34(1):71–75.

47. Cosmi E, Mari G, Delle Chiaie L, et al. Noninvasive diagnosis by Doppler ultrasonography of fetal anemia resulting from parvovirus infection. *Am J Obstet Gynecol.* 2002;187(5):1290–1293.

48. Ergaz Z, Ornoy A. Parvovirus B19 in pregnancy. *Reprod Toxicol.* 2006;21(4):421–435.

49. Markenson G, Correia LA, Cohn G, et al. Parvoviral infection associated with increased nuchal translucency: a case report. *J Perinatol.* 2000;20(2):129–131.

50. Simchen MJ, Toi A, Bona M, et al. Fetal hepatic calcifications: prenatal diagnosis and outcome. *Am J Obstet Gynecol.* 2002;187(6):1617–1622.

51. Yaron Y, Hassan S, Geva E, et al. Evaluation of fetal echogenic bowel in the second trimester. *Fetal Diagn Ther.* 1999;14(3):176–180.

52. Zerbini M, Gentilomi GA, Gallinella G, et al. Intra-uterine parvovirus B19 infection and meconium peritonitis. *Prenat Diagn.* 1998;18(6):599–606.

53. Mari G, Deter RL, Carpenter RL, et al.; for the Collaborative Group for Doppler Assessment of the Blood Velocity in Anemic Fetuses. Noninvasive diagnosis by Doppler ultrasonography of fetal anemia due to maternal red-cell alloimmunization. *N Engl J Med.* 2000;342(1):9–14.

54. Fairley CK, Smoleniec JS, Caul OE, et al. Observational study of effect of intrauterine transfusions on outcome of fetal hydrops after parvovirus B19 infection. *Lancet.* 1995;346(8986):1335–1337.

55. Dembinski J, Haverkamp F, Maara H, et al. Neurodevelopmental outcome after intrauterine red cell transfusion for parvovirus B19-induced fetal hydrops. *BJOG.* 2002;109(11):1232–1234.

56. Isumi H, Nunoue T, Nishida A, et al. Fetal brain infection with human parvovirus B19. *Pediatr Neurol.* 1999;21(3):661–663.

57. Lindenburg IT, Smits-Wintjens VE, van Klink JM, et al.; The LOTUS study Group. Long-term neurodevelopmental outcome after intrauterine transfusion for hemolytic disease of the fetus/newborn. *Am J Obstet Gynecol.* 2012;206(2):141.e1–141.e8.

58. Weisse ME. The fourth disease, 1900–2000. *Lancet.* 2001;357(9252):299–301.

59. Zimmerman L, Reef S. Congenital rubella syndrome. In: Roush SW, Baldy LM, Hall MAK, ed. *VPD Surveillance Manual.* 3rd ed. Washington, DC: Centers for Disease Control and Prevention; 2002.

60. Centers for Disease Control and Prevention. Rubella. In: Atkinson W, Hamborsky J, Wolfe S, et al., eds. *Epidemiology and Prevention of Vaccine-Preventable Disease.* 12th ed. Second printing. Washington, DC: Public Health Foundation, 2012.

61. Ciofi Degli Atti ML, Salmaso S, Bella A, et al. Pediatric sentinel surveillance of vaccine-preventable diseases in Italy. *Pediatr Infect Dis J.* 2002;21(8):763–768.

62. Gabutti G, Rota MC, Salmaso S, et al. Epidemiology of measles, mumps and rubella in Italy. *Epidemiol Infect.* 2002;129(3):543–550.

63. Best JM, Bantavala J. Rubella. In: Pattison JR, ed. *Principles and Practice of Clinical Virology.* 4th ed. New York: John Wiley & Sons; 2000:387–418.

64. Horstmann DM, Liebhaber H, Kohorn EI. Post-partum vaccination of rubella-susceptible women. *Lancet.* 1970;2(7681):1003–1006.

65. Miron D, On A. Congenital rubella syndrome after maternal immunization [in Hebrew]. *Harefuah.* 1992;122(5):291–293.

66. Enders G, Nickerl-Pacher U, Miller E, et al. Outcome of confirmed periconceptional maternal rubella. *Lancet.* 1988;1(8600):1445–1447.

67. Remington J. *Infectious Diseases of the Fetus and Newborn Infant.* 5th ed. Philadelphia, PA: WB Saunders; 2001.

68. Best JM, Tipples G, Al-Khusaiby SM, et al. Interpretation of rubella serology in pregnancy—pitfalls and problems. *BMJ.* 2002;325(7356):147–148.

69. Bosma TJ, Corbett KM, O'Shea S, et al. PCR for detection of rubella virus RNA in clinical samples. *J Clin Microbiol.* 1995;33(5):1075–1079.

70. Hudson P, Morgan-Capner P. Evaluation of 15 commercial enzyme immunoassays for the detection of rubella-specific IgM. *J Clin Virol.* 1996;5(1):21–26.

71. Almeida JD, Griffith AH. Viral infections and rheumatic factor. *Lancet.* 1980;2(8208–8209):1361–1362.

72. Akingbade D, Cohen BJ, Brown DW. Detection of low-avidity immunoglobulin G in oral fluid samples: new approach for rubella diagnosis and surveillance. *Clin Diagn Lab Immunol.* 2003;10(1):189–190.

73. Ben Salah A, Zaâtour A, Pomery L, et al. Validation of a modified commercial assay for the detection of rubella-specific IgG in oral fluid for use in population studies. *J Virol Methods.* 2003;114(2):151–158.

74. World Health Organization. *Report of a Meeting on Preventing Congenital Rubella Syndrome: Immunization Strategies, Surveillance Needs.* Geneva: World Health Organization; 2000:12–14.

75. Ramsay ME, Brugha R, Brown DW, et al. Salivary diagnosis of rubella: a study of notified cases in the United Kingdom, 1991–4. *Epidemiol Infect.* 1998;120(3):315–319.

76. Terry GM, Ho-Terry L, Warren RC, et al. First trimester prenatal diagnosis of congenital rubella: a laboratory investigation. *Br Med J (Clin Res Ed).* 1986;292(6525):930–933.

77. Migliucci A, Di Fraja D, Sarno L, et al. Prenatal diagnosis of congenital rubella infection and ultrasonography: a preliminary study. *Minerva Ginecol.* 2011;63(6):485–489.

78. Ugurbas SH, Zilelioglu G, Günalp I, et al. Microphthalmos: clinical and ultrasonographic findings. *Ann Ophthalmol (Skokie).* 2007;39(2):112–122.

79. Boyle MK, Pretorius DH. Fetal infections. In: Nyberg DA, McGahan JP, Pretorius DH, et al., eds. *Diagnostic Imaging of Fetal Anomalies.* Philadelphia, PA: Lippincott Williams & Wilkins; 2003:756.

80. Andrade J. Congenital Rubella syndrome and fetal exencephaly: a case report. *Ultrasound Obstet Gynecol.* 2000;16(suppl S1):72.

81. Ferreira SM, Ferreira AG Jr, Furlan IM, et al. Semilunar valvar stenosis associated with congenital Rubella syndrome. *Braz J Infect Dis.* 1998;2(5):256–259.

82. Moore JW, Mullins CE. Severe subaortic stenosis associated with congenital rubella syndrome: palliation by percutaneous transcatheter device occlusion of a patent ductus arteriosus. *Pediatr Cardiol.* 1986;7(4):221–223.

83. Varghese PJ, Izukawa T, Rowe RD. Supravalvular aortic stenosis as part of rubella syndrome, with discussion of pathogenesis. *Br Heart J.* 1969;31(1):59–62.

84. Wui ET, Ling LH, Yang H. Severe aortic regurgitation: an exceptional cardiac manifestation of congenital rubella syndrome. *Int J Cardiol.* 2006;113(2):e46–e47.

85. Levy-Bruhl D, Six C, Parent I. Rubella control in France. *Euro Surveill.* 2004; 9(4):15–16.

86. Centers for Disease Control and Prevention. Seroprevalence of herpes simplex virus type 2 among persons aged 14–49 years: United States, 2005–2008. *MMWR Morb Mortal Wkly Rep.* 2010;59(15):456–459.

87. Whitley R, Davis EA, Suppapanya N. Incidence of neonatal herpes simplex virus infections in a managed-care population. *Sex Transm Dis.* 2007;34(9):704–708.

88. Mitty J. Epidemiology, clinical manifestations, and diagnosis of genital herpes simplex virus infection. *UpToDate.* 2011. http://www.uptodate.com/contents/epidemiology-clinical-manifestations-and-diagnosis-of-genital-herpes-simplex-virus-infection. Updated December 13, 2018.

89. Dickson N, van Roode T, Herbison P, et al. Risk of herpes simplex virus type 2 acquisition increases over early adulthood: evidence from a cohort study. *Sex Transm Infect.* 2007;83(2):87–90.

90. Lanouette JM, Duquette DA, Jacques SM, et al. Prenatal diagnosis of fetal herpes simplex infection. *Fetal Diagn Ther.* 1996;11(6):414–416.

91. Jayaram PM, Wake CR. A rare case of absent corpus callosum with severe ventriculomegaly due to congenital herpes simplex infection. *J Obstet Gynaecol.* 2010;30(3):316.

92. Diguet A, Patrier S, Eurin D, et al. Prenatal diagnosis of an exceptional intrauterine herpes simplex type 1 infection. *Prenat Diagn.* 2006;26(2):154–157.

93. Duin LK, Willekes C, Baldewijns MM, et al. Major brain lesions by intrauterine herpes simplex virus infection: MRI contribution. *Prenat Diagn.* 2007;27(1):81–84.

94. World Health Organization. Global summary of the AIDS epidemic: 2009. http://data.unaids.org/pub/report/2009/jc1700_epi_update_2009_en.pdf. Accessed February 26, 2020.

95. World Health Organization. Towards universal access: scaling up priority HIV/AIDS interventions in the health sector. *Progress Rep.* 2010:97. http://whqlibdoc.who.int/publications/2010/9789241500395_eng.pdf. Accessed February 26, 2020.

96. Branson BM, Handsfield HH, Lampe MA, et al.; Centers for Disease Control and Prevention. Revised recommendations for HIV testing of adults, adolescents, and pregnant women in health-care settings. *MMWR Recomm Rep.* 2006;55:1–17.

97. Center, N.H.A.C.C., Compendium of State HIV Testing Laws. 2011. www.hivlawandpolicy.org/…/compendium-state-hiv-testing-laws-quick-reference-guide-clinicians-national-hivaids.

98. Ray N, Doms RW. HIV-1 coreceptors and their inhibitors. *Curr Top Microbiol Immunol.* 2006;303:97–120.

99. Joao EC, Calvet GA, Krauss MR, et al. Maternal antiretroviral use during pregnancy and infant congenital anomalies: the NISDI perinatal study. *J Acquir Immune Defic Syndr.* 2010;53(2):176–185.

100. Cotter AM, Garcia AG, Duthely ML, et al. Is antiretroviral therapy during pregnancy associated with an increased risk of preterm delivery, low birth weight, or stillbirth? *J Infect Dis.* 2006;193(9):1195–1201.

101. Kourtis AP, Schmid CH, Jamieson DJ, et al. Use of antiretroviral therapy in pregnant HIV-infected women and the risk of premature delivery: a meta-analysis. *AIDS.* 2007;21(5):607–615.

102. Szyld EG, Warley EM, Freimanis L, et al. Maternal antiretroviral drugs during pregnancy and infant low birth weight and preterm birth. *AIDS.* 2006;20(18):2345–2353.

103. Tuomala RE, Watts DH, Li D, et al. Improved obstetric outcomes and few maternal toxicities are associated with antiretroviral therapy, including highly active antiretroviral therapy during pregnancy. *J Acquir Immune Defic Syndr.* 2005;38(4):449–473.

104. Palaii N. Late intrauterine growth restriction in HIV pregnant women in developed countries. *Ultrasound Obstet Gynecol.* 2009;34(S1):151.

105. Aaron E, Bonacquisti A, Mathew L, et al. Small-for-gestational-age births in pregnant women with HIV, due to severity of HIV disease, not antiretroviral therapy. *Infect Dis Obstet Gynecol.* 2012;2012:135030.

106. Savvidou MD, Samuel MI, Akolekar R, et al. First trimester maternal uterine artery Doppler examination in HIV-positive women. *HIV Med.* 2011;12(10):632–636.

107. Davies G, Wilson RD, Désilets V, et al. Amniocentesis and women with hepatitis B, hepatitis C, or human immunodeficiency virus. *J Obstet Gynaecol Can.* 2003;25(2):145–148, 149–152.

108. Opinion AC, Scheduled cesarean delivery and the prevention of vertical transmission of HIV infection. *Int J Gynaecol Obstet.* 2001;73:279–281.

109. Davis JA, Yawetz S. Management of HIV in the pregnant woman. *Clin Obstet Gynecol.* 2012;55(2):531–540.

110. Department of Health and Human Services, P.o.A.G.f.A.a.A., Guidelines for the Use of Antiretroviral Agents in Pediatric HIV Infection, 2011:1–268. http://aidsinfo.nih.gov/contentfiles/PediatricGuidelines003005.pdf.

111. Enders G, Miller E. Varicella and herpes zoster in pregnancy and the newborn. In: Arvin AM, Gershon AA, eds. *Varicella-Zoster Virus Virology and Clinical Management.* Cambridge: Cambridge University Press; 2000:317–347.

112. Lamont RF, Sobel JD, Carrington D, et al. Varicella-zoster virus (chickenpox) infection in pregnancy. *BJOG.* 2011;118(10):1155–1162.

113. Laforet EG, Lynch CL Jr. Multiple congenital defects following maternal varicella; report of a case. *N Engl J Med.* 1947;236(15):534–537.

114. Paryani SG, Arvin AM. Intrauterine infection with varicella-zoster virus after maternal varicella. *N Engl J Med.* 1986;314(24):1542–1546.

115. Smith CK, Arvin AM. Varicella in the fetus and newborn. *Semin Fetal Neonatal Med.* 2009;14(4):209–217.

116. Gardella C, Brown ZA. Managing varicella zoster infection in pregnancy. *Cleve Clin J Med.* 2007;74(4):290–296.

117. Enders G, Miller E, Cradock-Watson J, et al. Consequences of varicella and herpes zoster in pregnancy: prospective study of 1739 cases. *Lancet.* 1994;343(8912):1548–1551.

118. Miller E, Cradock-Watson JE, Ridehalgh MK. Outcome in newborn babies given anti-varicella-zoster immunoglobulin after perinatal maternal infection with varicella-zoster virus. *Lancet.* 1989;2(8659):371–373.

119. Sauerbrei A, Wutzler P. Neonatal varicella. *J Perinatol.* 2001;21(8):545–549.

120. Mandelbrot L. Fetal varicella: diagnosis, management, and outcome. *Prenat Diagn.* 2012;32(6):511–518.

121. Leung J, Harpaz R, Baughman AL, et al. Evaluation of laboratory methods for diagnosis of varicella. *Clin Infect Dis.* 2010;51(1):23–32.

122. Mendelson E, Aboudy Y, Smetana Z, et al. Laboratory assessment and diagnosis of congenital viral infections: rubella, cytomegalovirus (CMV), varicella-zoster virus (VZV), herpes simplex virus (HSV), parvovirus B19 and human immunodeficiency virus (HIV). *Reprod Toxicol.* 2006;21(4):350–382.

123. Koren G. Congenital varicella syndrome in the third trimester. *Lancet.* 2005;366(9497):1591–1592.

124. Mouly F, Mirlesse V, Méritet JF, et al. Prenatal diagnosis of fetal varicella-zoster virus infection with polymerase chain reaction of amniotic fluid in 107 cases. *Am J Obstet Gynecol.* 1997;177(4):894–898.

125. Tan M, Koren G. Chickenpox in pregnancy: revisited. *Reprod Toxicol.* 2006;21(4):410–420.

126. Verstraelen H, Vanzieleghem B, Defoort P, et al. Prenatal ultrasound and magnetic resonance imaging in fetal varicella syndrome: correlation with pathology findings. *Prenat Diagn.* 2003;23:705–709.

127. Fernández-Aguilar S, Noël JC, Donner C, et al. Congenital pulmonary airway malformation and congenital varicella infection—a possible association. *Ultrasound Obstet Gynecol.* 2005;26(6):680–682.

128. Watson B, Civen R, Reynolds M, et al. Validity of self-reported varicella disease history in pregnant women attending prenatal clinics. *Public Health Rep.* 2007;122(4):499–506.

129. Salisbury D, Ramsay M, Noakes K. *Immunisation Against Infectious Disease: The Green Book.* 3rd ed. London: The Department of Health; 2006:421–442.

130. Balducci J, Rodis JF, Rosengren S, et al. Pregnancy outcome following first-trimester varicella infection. *Obstet Gynecol.* 1992;79:5–6.

131. Siegel M. Congenital malformations following chickenpox, measles, mumps and hepatitis. *JAMA.* 1973;226:1521–1524.

132. Darfour P, de Bievre P, Vinatier N, et al. Varicella and pregnancy. *Eur J Obstet Gynecol Reprod Biol.* 1996;66:119–123.

133. Michie CA, Acolet D, Charlton R, et al. Varicella-zoster contracted in the second trimester of pregnancy. *Pediatr Infect Dis J.* 1992;11:1050–1053.

134. Kotchmar GS Jr, Grose C, Brunell PA. Complete spectrum of the varicella congenital defects syndrome in 5-year-old child. *Pediatr Infect Dis.* 1984;3(2):142–145.

135. Schulze A, Dietzsch HJ. The natural history of varicella embryopathy: a 25-year follow-up. *J Pediatr.* 2000;137(6):871–874.

136. Meyers JD. Congenital varicella in term infants: risk reconsidered. *J Infect Dis.* 1974;129(2):215–217.

137. Elfving M, Svensson J, Oikarinen S, et al. Maternal enterovirus infection during pregnancy as a risk factor in offspring diagnosed with type 1 diabetes between 15 and 30 years of age. *Exp Diabetes Res.* 2008;2008:271958.

138. Alford CA Jr, Stagno S, Reynolds DW. Congenital toxoplasmosis: clinical, laboratory, and therapeutic considerations, with special reference to subclinical disease. *Bull N Y Acad Med.* 1974;50(2):160–181.

139. Guerina NG, Hsu HW, Meissner HC, et al. Neonatal serologic screening and early treatment for congenital *Toxoplasma gondii* infection. The New England Regional Toxoplasma Working Group. *N Engl J Med.* 1994;330(26):1858–1863.

140. Kimball AC, Kean BH, Fuchs F. Congenital toxoplasmosis: a prospective study of 4,048 obstetric patients. *Am J Obstet Gynecol.* 1971;111(2):211–218.

141. Dubey JP. Toxoplasmosis. *J Am Vet Med Assoc.* 1994;205(11):1593–1598.

142. Jones JL, Lopez A, Wilson M, et al. Congenital toxoplasmosis: a review. *Obstet Gynecol Surv.* 2001;56(5):296–305.

143. Vogel N, Kirisits M, Michael E, et al. Congenital toxoplasmosis transmitted from an immunologically competent mother infected before conception. *Clin Infect Dis.* 1996;23(5):1055–1060.

144. Dunn D, Wallon M, Peyron F, et al. Mother-to-child transmission of toxoplasmosis: risk estimates for clinical counselling. *Lancet.* 1999;353(9167):1829–1833.

145. Foulon W, Villena I, Stray-Pedersen B, et al. Treatment of toxoplasmosis during pregnancy: a multicenter study of impact on fetal transmission and children's sequelae at age 1 year. *Am J Obstet Gynecol.* 1999;180(2, pt 1):410–415.

146. Montoya JG. Laboratory diagnosis of *Toxoplasma gondii* infection and toxoplasmosis. *J Infect Dis.* 2002;185(suppl 1):S73–S82.

147. Wilson M, Remington JS, Clavet C, et al. Evaluation of six commercial kits for detection of human immunoglobulin M antibodies to *Toxoplasma gondii*. The FDA Toxoplasmosis Ad Hoc Working Group. *J Clin Microbiol.* 1997;35(12):3112–3115.

148. Dhakal R, Gajurel K, Pomares C, Talucod J, Press CJ, Montoya JG. Significance of a Positive Toxoplasma Immunoglobulin M Test Result in the United States. *J Clin Microbiol.* 2015;53(11):3601–3605.

149. Montoya JG, Liesenfeld O, Kinney S, et al. VIDAS test for avidity of *Toxoplasma*-specific immunoglobulin G for confirmatory testing of pregnant women. *J Clin Microbiol*. 2002;40(7):2504–2508.

150. Hohlfeld P, Daffos F, Costa JM, et al. Prenatal diagnosis of congenital toxoplasmosis with a polymerase-chain-reaction test on amniotic fluid. *N Engl J Med*. 1994;331(11):695–699.

151. Foulon W, Pinon JM, Stray-Pedersen B, et al. Prenatal diagnosis of congenital toxoplasmosis: a multicenter evaluation of different diagnostic parameters. *Am J Obstet Gynecol*. 1999;181(4):843–847.

152. Hohlfeld P, MacAleese J, Capella-Pavlovski M, et al. Fetal toxoplasmosis: ultrasonographic signs. *Ultrasound Obstet Gynecol*. 1991;1(4):241–244.

153. Malinger G, Werner H, Rodriguez Leonel JC, et al. Prenatal brain imaging in congenital toxoplasmosis. *Prenat Diagn*. 2011;31(9):881–886.

154. Cuillier F, Avignon MS. Case of the week #168. TheFetus.net. 2006-02-27.

155. Garel C. MRI of the fetal brain. In: *Normal Development and Cerebral Pathologies*. Berlin: Springer; 2004.

156. Gay-Andrieu F, Marty P, Pialat J, et al. Fetal toxoplasmosis and negative amniocentesis: necessity of an ultrasound follow-up. *Prenat Diagn*. 2003;23(7):558–560.

157. Becker LE. Infections of the developing brain. *AJNR*. 1992;13(2):537–549.

158. Baron J, Youngblood L, Siewers CMF, et al. The incidence of cytomegalovirus, herpes simplex, rubella, and toxoplasma antibodies in microcephalic, mentally retarded, and normocephalic children. *Pediatrics*. 1969;44(6):932–939.

159. ACOG Practice Bulletin. Perinatal viral and parasitic infections. Number 20, September 2000. (Replaces educational bulletin number 177, February 1993.) American College of Obstetrics and Gynecologists.

160. Newton LH, Hall SM. Survey of local policies for prevention of congenital toxoplasmosis. *Commun Dis Rep CDR Rev*. 1994;4(10):R121–R124.

161. Aspock H, Pollak A. Prevention of prenatal toxoplasmosis by serological screening of pregnant women in Austria. *Scand J Infect Dis Suppl*. 1992;84:32–37.

162. Lopez A, Dietz VJ, Wilson M, et al. Preventing congenital toxoplasmosis. *MMWR Recomm Rep*. 2000;49(RR-2):59–68.

163. Dorangeon PH, Marx-Chemla C, Quereux C, et al. The risks of pyrimethamine-sulfadoxine combination in the prenatal treatment of toxoplasmosis. *J Gynecol Obstet Biol Reprod (Paris)*. 1992;21(5):549–556.

164. Remington J. Toxoplasmosis. In: Remington JS, Klein J, eds. *Infectious Diseases of the Fetus and Newborn Infant*. 5th ed. Philadelphia, PA: WB Saunders; 2001:205–346.

165. Gilbert R, Gras L. Effect of timing and type of treatment on the risk of mother to child transmission of *Toxoplasma gondii*. *BJOG*. 2003;110(2):112–120.

166. Foulon W, Naessens A, Lauwers S, et al. Impact of primary prevention on the incidence of toxoplasmosis during pregnancy. *Obstet Gynecol*. 1988;72(3, pt 1):363–366.

167. Wilson CB, Remington JS, Stagno S, et al. Development of adverse sequelae in children born with subclinical congenital *Toxoplasma* infection. *Pediatrics*. 1980;66(5):767–774.

168. Chigozie JU. Impact of placental *Plasmodium falciparum* malaria on pregnancy and perinatal outcome in Sub-Saharan Africa. *Yale J Biol Med*. 2007;80(3):95–103.

169. Desai M, ter Kuile FO, Nosten F, et al. Epidemiology and burden of malaria in pregnancy. *Lancet Infect Dis*. 2007;7(2):93–104.

170. Poespoprodjo JR, Fobia W, Kenangalem E, et al. Vivax malaria: a major cause of morbidity in early infancy. *Clin Infect Dis*. 2009;48(12):1704–1712.

171. Bittencourt AL, Cardoso de Almeida MA, Iunes MA, et al. Placental involvement in schistosomiasis mansoni: report of four cases. *Am J Trop Med Hyg*. 1980;29(4):571–575.

172. World Health Organization. The global elimination of congenital syphilis: rationale and strategy for action. 2007. http://www.who.int/reproductivehealth/publications/rtis/9789241595858/en/. Accessed February 26, 2020.

173. Centers for Disease Control and Prevention. Sexually transmitted diseases surveillance. 2010. http://www.cdc.gov/STD/stats10/default.htm. Accessed February 26, 2020.

174. World Health Organization. Methods for surveillance and monitoring of congenital syphilis elimination within existing systems. 2011. https://www.who.int/reproductivehealth/publications/rtis/9789241503020/en/. Accessed February 26, 2020.

175. Hawkes S, Matin N, Broutet N, et al. Effectiveness of interventions to improve screening for syphilis in pregnancy: a systematic review and meta-analysis. *Lancet Infect Dis*. 2011;11(9):684–691.

176. Centers for Disease Control and Prevention. Syphilis. CDC Fact Sheet. 2012.

177. Ingall D. Syphilis. In: Remington JS, Klein JO, eds. *Infectious Diseases of the Fetus and Newborn Infant*. 5th ed. Philadelphia, PA: WB Saunders; 2001:643–681.

178. Kent ME, Romanelli F. Reexamining syphilis: an update on epidemiology, clinical manifestations, and management. *Ann Pharmacother*. 2008;42(2):226–236.

179. Hallak M, Peipert JF, Ludomirsky A, et al. Nonimmune hydrops fetalis and fetal congenital syphilis: a case report. *J Reprod Med*. 1992;37(2):173–176.

180. Nathan L, Twickler DM, Peters MT, et al. Fetal syphilis: correlation of sonographic findings and rabbit infectivity testing of amniotic fluid. *J Ultrasound Med*. 1993;12(2):97–101.

181. Satin AJ, Twickler DM, Wendel GD Jr. Congenital syphilis associated with dilation of fetal small bowel: a case report. *J Ultrasound Med*. 1992;11(1):49–52.

182. Hill LM, Maloney JB. An unusual constellation of sonographic findings associated with congenital syphilis. *Obstet Gynecol*. 1991;78(5, pt 2):895–897.

183. D'Aunoy R, Pearson B. Intestinal lesions in congenital syphilis. *Arch Pathol*. 1939;27:239–248.

184. Wendel G, Gilstrap LC. Syphilis during pregnancy. In: Gilstrap LC, Faro S, eds. *Infections in Pregnancy*. New York, NY: Alan R. Liss; 1990:115–125.

185. Lucas MJ, Theriot SK, Wendel GD Jr. Doppler systolic-diastolic ratios in pregnancies complicated by syphilis. *Obstet Gynecol*. 1991;77(2):217–222.

186. Schulman H, Miller JN, Dolisi F. The pathophysiology of acute syphilitic funisitis. *Ultrasound Obstet Gynecol*. 1991;1:353–356.

187. Araujo Júnior E, Martins Santana EF, Rolo LC, et al. Prenatal diagnosis of congenital syphilis using two- and three-dimensional ultrasonography: case report. *Case Rep Infect Dis*. 2012;2012:478436.

188. Radcliffe M, Meyer M, Roditi D, et al. Single-dose benzathine penicillin in infants at risk of congenital syphilis—results of a randomised study. *S Afr Med J*. 1997;87(1):62–65.

189. Workowski K. Sexually transmitted diseases treatment guidelines. *MMWR Morb Mortal Wkly Rep*. 2010;59(RR-12):1–113.

190. Saloojee H. The prevention and management of congenital syphilis: an overview and recommendations. *Bull World Health Organ*. 2004;82(6):424–430.

191. Jover-Diaz F, Robert-Gates J, Andreu-Gimenez L, et al. Q fever during pregnancy: an emerging cause of prematurity and abortion. *Infect Dis Obstet Gynecol*. 2001;9(1):47–49.

192. Shinar S, Skornick-Rapaport A, Rimon E. Placental abruption remote from term associated with Q fever infection. *Obstet Gynecol*. 2012;120(2, pt 2):503–505.

193. Peker E, Bozdogan E, Dogan M. A rare tuberculosis form: congenital tuberculosis. *Tuberk Toraks*. 2010;58(1):93–96.

194. Carter EJ, Mates S. Tuberculosis during pregnancy: the Rhode Island experience, 1987 to 1991. *Chest*. 1994;106(5):1466–1470.

195. Hamadeh MA, Glassroth J. Tuberculosis and pregnancy. *Chest*. 1992;101(4):1114–1120.

196. Llewelyn M, Cropley I, Wilkinson RJ, et al. Tuberculosis diagnosed during pregnancy: a prospective study from London. *Thorax*. 2000;55(2):129–132.

197. Abramowsky CR, Gutman J, Hilinski JA. *Mycobacterium tuberculosis* infection of the placenta: a study of the early (innate) inflammatory response in two cases. *Pediatr Dev Pathol*. 2012;15(2):132–136.

198. Peng W, Yang J, Liu E. Analysis of 170 cases of congenital TB reported in the literature between 1946 and 2009. *Pediatr Pulmonol*. 2011;46(12):1215–1224.

199. Rivera-Alsina ME, Saldana LR, Kohl S, et al. Listeria monocytogenes: an important pathogen in premature labor and intrauterine fetal sepsis. *J Reprod Med*. 1983;28(3):212–214.

200. Cheng BR, Kuo DM, Hsieh TT. Perinatal listeriosis: a case report. *Chang Gung Med J*. 1990;13(2):152–156.

201. Valkenburg MH, Essed GG, Potters HV. Perinatal listeriosis underdiagnosed as a cause of pre-term labour? *Eur J Obstet Gynecol Reprod Biol*. 1988;27(4):283–288.

202. Nolla-Salas J, Bosch J, Gasser I, et al. Perinatal listeriosis: a population-based multicenter study in Barcelona, Spain (1990–1996). *Am J Perinatol*. 1998;15(8):461–467.

203. Cassell G. Mycoplasmal infections. In: Remington JS, Klein JO, eds. *Infectious Diseases of the Fetus and Newborn Infant*. 5th ed. Philadelphia, PA: WB Saunders; 2001:733–767.

204. Cassell GH, Waites KB, Watson HL, et al. Ureaplasma urealyticum intrauterine infection: role in prematurity and disease in newborns. *Clin Microbiol Rev*. 1993;6(1):69–87.

205. Cassell GH, Davis RO, Waites KB, et al. Isolation of *Mycoplasma hominis* and *Ureaplasma urealyticum* from amniotic fluid at 16–20 weeks of gestation: potential effect on outcome of pregnancy. *Sex Transm Dis*. 1983;10(4 suppl):294–302.

206. Benacerraf BR, Gatter MA, Ginsburgh F. Ultrasound diagnosis of meconium-stained amniotic fluid. *Am J Obstet Gynecol*. 1984;149(5):570–572.

207. DeVore GR, Platt LD. Ultrasound appearance of particulate matter in amniotic cavity: vernix or meconium? *J Clin Ultrasound*. 1986;14(3):229–230.

208. Romero R, Kusanovic JP, Espinoza J, et al. What is amniotic fluid "sludge"? *Ultrasound Obstet Gynecol*. 2007;30(5):793–798.

209. Sherer DM, Abramowicz JS, Smith SA, et al. Sonographically homogeneous echogenic amniotic fluid in detecting meconium-stained amniotic fluid. *Obstet Gynecol*. 1991;78(5, pt 1):819–822.

32 Fetal Surgeries and Interventions

Alireza A. Shamshirsaz • Amy R. Mehollin-Ray • Ahmed A. Nassr • Michael A. Belfort

INTRODUCTION

In the United States, congenital birth defects and malformations occur in 3% of children.[1] Modern prenatal imaging techniques, particularly the invention and improvement of ultrasound technology, have allowed for earlier detection and the characterization of congenital anomalies. Innovative therapies have been developed to intervene *in utero* to change the course of fetal disease. This chapter provides a brief overview of the history of fetal surgery, ethical considerations, basics of imaging in interventional procedures, types of surgeries currently in use, and future directions of the field.

HISTORY

Experimental fetal surgery in animal models began in the 1920s, and evolved into the well-known lamb model developed by Barcroft in the 1940s.[1] These models were developed to mimic human pathologies and then studied with the employment of various therapeutic approaches including the use of safe and effective medications. This research also encouraged the development of criteria for biological plausibility and the rationale for selected fetal interventions, all essential to the eventual achievement of ethical human fetal surgery.

In 1963, Sir William Liley completed the first successful human fetal intervention procedure when he performed an intraperitoneal blood transfusion for hydrops fetalis in New Zealand.[2] The first open fetal surgery was performed in 1981 by Dr. Michael Harrison and his team at University of California-San Francisco (UCSF), treating urinary obstruction with a vesicostomy. With growing widespread access to ultrasound technology, other fetal conditions were diagnosed prenatally and evaluated for potential benefit of surgical intervention *in utero* in the 1980s, including obstructive uropathy, hydrocephalus, congenital cystic adenomatoid malformation (CCAM)/congenital pulmonary airway malformation (CPAM), and congenital diaphragmatic hernia (CDH).[3]

As the field of fetal intervention grew, a meeting was convened in 1982 gathering physicians involved in fetal treatment and procedures. This pioneering group agreed to a set of guiding actions including (1) peer-reviewed publication of work, (2) confining intervention to well-understood and lethal diseases, and (3) strict adherence to ethical guidelines.[4] The importance of shared case material in a fetal-treatment registry was emphasized to ensure rapid, evidence-based evolution of the field. Harrison published the decided upon principles for the guidance of practitioners performing fetal surgery based on the abovementioned propositions.[4] Rapid advancement of imaging technology and prenatal diagnosis allowed for the progressive development of fetal surgeries in the subsequent decades following the principles laid out at the first meeting of the International Fetal Medicine and Surgery Society (IFMSS).

Techniques for fetal surgery evolved from "open surgery" on the fetus via a hysterotomy, to less invasive techniques or "closed surgery," performed using a needle or through a trochar(s) inserted through the uterine wall. Digital optics and miniaturized instruments gave birth to the field of fetoscopic intervention, allowing direct visualization and surgery for fetal anomalies inside the uterine cavity.

ETHICAL CONSIDERATIONS

The ethics of fetal surgery have been intertwined with the evolution of the field. If, when, and how to intervene are the central questions in every potential case. Final decisions regarding invasive fetal therapy must abide by the following criteria[5]:

I. The proposed intervention has a high probability of being life-saving, or of preventing serious and irreversible disease, injury, or disability for the fetus and future child.
II. The intervention poses a low mortality risk and a low, or manageable, risk of serious disease, injury, or disability to the fetus and future child.
III. Maternal mortality or morbidity risk is very low or manageable.

As in traditional ethics discussions, the autonomy of the pregnant woman is paramount in decision making about interventions that subject her to risk for the potential benefit of the fetus.

Concern for fetal pain has also been an ethical consideration in the development of the field of fetal intervention. Although there is minimal evidence for the presence, or nature, of the perception of fetal pain, nociceptive sensory pathways and electroencephalographic (EEG) activity are present at 18 to 20 weeks.[6] To address this concern, however, analgesia is routinely administered beyond this gestational age during procedures that have the potential to elicit fetal pain. Intraoperatively, a combination of medications is given to suppress the fetal bradycardic response to stress, to decrease fetal movement, and to provide analgesia for potential fetal pain control. A common anesthetic combination consists of atropine, vecuronium, and fentanyl adjusted for estimated fetal weight (20 µg/kg, 0.2 mg/kg, and 15 µg/kg, respectively, dosed every 45 minutes) intravenously or intramuscularly via a 22-gauge needle under ultrasound guidance.

IMAGING PRINCIPLES FOR FETAL INTERVENTIONAL AND SURGICAL PROCEDURES

A clear understanding of basic ultrasound principles is important for the successful training of interventionists on needle orientation in various interventional procedures. Simulation models are great tools for initial training on needle orientation. Curved ultrasound transducers are commonly used to guide fetal interventional procedures. Linear transducers may be used for specific procedures, but, in general, most fetal interventions are performed using a curvilinear transducer.

After initial training on various available simulation models, amniocentesis procedures are a good opportunity to improve the operator's needle orientation skills. While simple invasive procedures can be usually completed by a single operator holding the ultrasound probe and inserting the needle, more complex procedures usually require two operators. The main reason for having a separate operator for ultrasound guidance in complex interventional procedures is to enable the surgeon to perform fine adjustments using two hands, where one hand supports and directs the needle at its interface with the patient's skin, and the other hand is used to advance (and also direct) the needle.

Steps of the Procedure

Careful Ultrasound Evaluation

Planning for any fetal interventional procedure or surgery is of utmost importance. Careful ultrasound evaluation should be performed in the operating (or procedure) room to determine the best access to the target (fetal or placental part). Location of the placenta and presence of uterine windows free of the placenta should be noted. Attention should be paid to the entire track through the maternal abdominal wall to the uterine target. In some circumstances, especially when extreme angulation of the transducer (and/or significant pressure) is required to image the target, pressure on the abdominal wall can compress maternal bowel loops against the uterus or adnexa. This may result in a false impression of uninterrupted tissue, and the needle can inadvertently be advanced through a trapped and compressed loop of bowel. After careful selection of the line of access, color Doppler should be applied to ensure absence of major uterine vascularity. This is particularly important when the area of access is located laterally as uterine or adnexal blood vessels could be accidently injured during the procedure.

Thorough examination of the placental location is critical, especially in open fetal surgical procedures. In fetoscopic procedures, transplacental access should be avoided as it is likely to cause significant bleeding, which can impair the fetoscopic visualization. In ultrasound-guided needle procedures, transplacental access should be avoided as much as possible because of the risk of puncturing surface fetal vessels. However, in certain circumstances, transplacental access is unavoidable and an informed and individualized decision has to be made.

Preparation

All invasive fetal interventional procedures are best performed in the operating room with standard sterile precautions. The ultrasound control panel should be covered by a transparent sterile cover with adhesive at the top to adhere to the panel. This allows one operator to control the ultrasound buttons. The transducer is placed in a sterile cover with sterile gel inside.

OPEN FETAL SURGERY

Open fetal surgery utilizes a hysterotomy to access the fetus and requires a uterine incision that has to be closed upon conclusion of the intervention. This technique is employed in limited circumstances to treat congenital disease that cannot be fully addressed by a minimally invasive approach. In some cases, a less invasive fetoscopic approach may have been attempted initially, but then because of inability to complete the procedure, conversion to an open surgery is required. Compared with a minimally invasive approach, open fetal surgery carries an increased risk of maternal complications such as preterm labor, rupture of the membranes, chorioamniotic separation, dehiscence of the uterine scar, and risk of placenta accreta in subsequent pregnancies because of the need for repeated cesarean deliveries. All fetal

surgeries carry additional complications such as those related to tocolytic and neuroprotective medications and these include respiratory and cardiac depression as well as pulmonary edema. Fetal surgery, in general, also carries increased risks to the fetus, such as fetal bradycardia or rarely death during the procedure, and risks associated with prematurity in the event of preterm delivery. In all cases of open fetal surgery, delivery by cesarean section is required in both the concurrent and subsequent pregnancies to avoid the risk of uterine rupture. It is recommended for women to space pregnancies by at least 2 years after open fetal surgery.

Open Spina Bifida Repair

Neural tube defects (NTDs) occurred frequently before standardized folic acid supplementation, and now occur in approximately 3.5 of 10,000 live births per year.[7] A NTD is due to failure of closure of the neural tube during embryogenesis (24 to 28 days after conception), and occurs in a range of severity from anencephaly (primarily affecting the brain), to encephalocele (affecting the brain and skull), to spina bifida (primarily affecting the spine with secondary brain complications such as hindbrain herniation). Myelomeningocele (MMC), the most severe form of spina bifida, can be associated with significant lifelong disability including paralysis, hydrocephalus, loss of bowel and bladder control, and cognitive, neurobehavioral, and learning disabilities (Fig. 32.1). In the event of progressive hydrocephalus after birth, many babies with MMC need a ventriculoperitoneal shunt, which has significant lifelong healthcare implications.[8]

The "two-hit hypothesis" provides an explanation for the neurological sequelae from MMC and is explained as follows: the "first hit" occurs at the time of embryogenesis from failure of closure of the spinal canal, while the "second hit" is progressive and is the result of ongoing exposure of the neural tissue to direct trauma and toxic agents in the amniotic fluid.[8] Secondary to MMC, ventriculomegaly occurs in more than 50% of fetuses by 24 weeks of gestation, and almost all will have ventriculomegaly at term.[9] Traditional treatment of ventriculomegaly postnatally with a ventriculoperitoneal shunt is associated with a significant amount of morbidity. The shunt failure rate after 2 years is almost 50%, and these children can require multiple shunt revisions, and have other complications including shunt infection and/or intraventricular hemorrhage.[10] The "two-hit hypothesis" theory generated the hypothesis that fetal MMC repair would prevent the

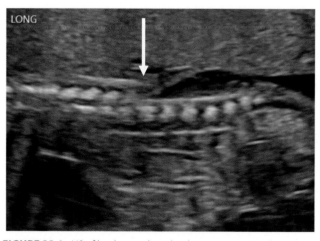

FIGURE 32.1: US of lumbosacral myeloschisis starting at L1 (*arrow*).

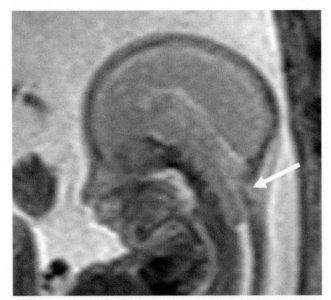

FIGURE 32.2: Preoperative sagittal T2 MRI showing hindbrain herniation into the cervical spinal canal (*arrow*).

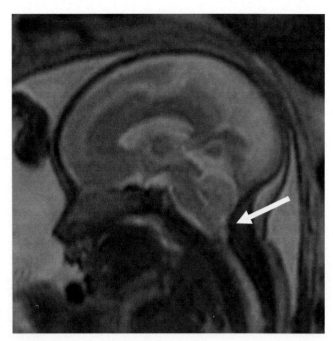

FIGURE 32.3: Postoperative sagittal T2 MRI of the same fetus showing improvement in posterior fossa (*arrow*) and increase in extra-axial cerebrospinal fluid.

"second hit" and improve morbidity. Initial fetoscopic attempts at *in utero* repair[11,12] were disappointing and led to the subsequent development of the open hysterotomy approach by Bruner et al.[13] Following initial enthusiasm for this type of repair, a randomized controlled trial was designed and funded by the National Institutes of Health.

The Management of Myelomeningocele Study (MOMS) trial was the first multicenter randomized controlled trial to comprehensively evaluate the obstetric, fetal, and neonatal effects of open fetal surgery for MMC[14] (Figs. 32.2 and 32.3). This study demonstrated a decrease in the need for postnatal shunting from 82% to 40% in the fetal surgery cohort (relative risk [RR] 0.48, 0.36 to 0.64), with concomitant significant improvements in mental and motor function and ambulation at 30 months of age ($P = 0.007$). However, the study also found higher rates of maternal and neonatal complications including uterine dehiscence and preterm birth.[14] More recent data have suggested a high rate of uterine rupture (10%) and fetal death (50%) when this occurs.[15] These complications are potentially addressed by more minimally invasive techniques. Different minimally invasive techniques have been described, including either a direct percutaneous fetoscopic approach or a technique that employs a laparotomy with uterine exteriorization. Both approaches use gas insufflation with carbon dioxide to improve visualization. The latter approach has been performed using two or three ports with encouraging results.[16]

The open MMC repair procedure follows the general outline of open surgery.

Treatment Approach
1. Keep mother and fetus warm intraoperatively (maternal temperature as close to 37°C as possible).
2. Monitor fetal cardiac function frequently.
3. Infuse warmed saline with antibiotics into the amniotic cavity to prevent placental abruption.
4. Use a no-touch technique when handling the neural placode.
5. Complete, water-tight coverage of the defect is the primary goal.
6. Perform vertical relaxing skin incisions lateral to the defect to aid in midline skin coverage if necessary.
7. Utilize magnesium sulfate bolus and infusion prior to case completion.

Congenital Pulmonary Airway Malformation

Congenital lung malformations (CLMs) occur in 1 in 30,000 pregnancies, and they can vary widely in character.[17] Congenital cystic adenomatoid malformation now typically referred to as congenital pulmonary airway malformation (CPAM) is one form of CLM (Figs. 32.4 and 32.5) and can be classified as either large cyst or small cyst in terms of type.[18]

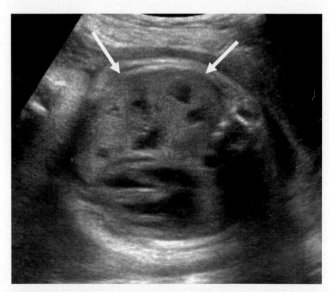

FIGURE 32.4: Axial US in a 25-week fetus with large left-sided multicystic lung lesion (*arrows*).

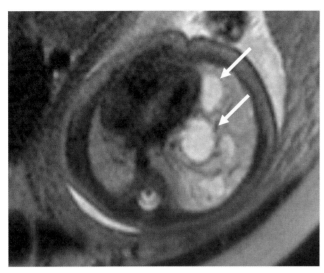

FIGURE 32.5: Axial T2 MRI shows a predominantly cystic lesion with macrocysts (*arrows*), compatible with large-cyst CPAM.

Complications from CPAM can arise prenatally if the lesion becomes large enough to shift thoracic structures, causing hydrops secondary to venocaval compression. Treatment with steroids without further intervention is successful in up to 78% of cases, despite the lack of an understanding of the mechanism.[19] A standard regimen consists of two doses of 12 mg intramuscular betamethasone 24 hours apart at approximately mid-gestation.[20]

For lesions with dominant cysts, thoracoamniotic shunting (detailed in a further section) can decompress the mass and improve cardiac compression–driven hydrops. In cases where the fetus is not yet viable (i.e., >24 weeks) and where there has not been adequate response to steroids (especially in fetuses with microcystic lesions), open fetal surgery might be an option in specific centers with such experience. Cases are selected up to 32 weeks on the basis of evidence of hydrops and cardiac dysfunction secondary to mass effect, but this indication is now quite rare since the advent of steroid treatment.[20] After 32 weeks, fetuses nonresponsive to steroids are offered *ex utero* intrapartum treatment (EXIT) to resection.

Treatment Approach for Open Surgery
1. If symptomatic polyhydramnios occurs, perform amnioreduction.
2. If open surgery is indicated, the following steps are recommended:
   A. Position the fetus for exteriorization of the affected side, including the arm and posterior chest.
   B. Keep mother and fetus warm intraoperatively.
   C. Monitor fetal cardiac function frequently, especially following exteriorization of the mass and during its removal because of the significant fluid shifts and cardiac stress.

Treatment Approach for EXIT to Resection
1. Prepare two operating rooms (one for the EXIT and one for the subsequent neonatal mass resection after umbilical cord clamping).
2. Upon exposure of the fetus, gain intravenous (IV) access and intubate the neonate without providing ventilation.
3. Perform posterolateral thoracotomy on the affected side.

4. Ventilate the neonate. This is because, in some cases, there is a "ball valve effect" that traps the ventilated gas inside the lung, leading to progressive expansion and intrathoracic pressure that can deviate the mediastinum and cause cardiac decompensation (much like a tension pneumothorax); if ventilation is tolerated, disconnect from placental circulation and transfer to second operating room for mass resection.
5. If ventilation is not tolerated, perform mass resection on placental circulation.

Sacrococcygeal Teratoma

Teratomas are the most common fetal solid tumor, the majority of which occur in the sacrococcygeal region (Fig. 32.6). The incidence is approximately 1 in 27,000 pregnancies. Half of prenatally diagnosed sacrococcygeal teratomas (SCTs) do not require any fetal treatment; however, severe complications can occur with large or highly vascular tumors.[21] High cardiac output failure, mass effect, arteriovenous fistula, and fetal demise can result, and, therefore, close prenatal monitoring of tumor size, fetal growth rate, and fetal cardiac function is required.[22] Treatment of babies with SCT at high risk of mortality with fetal surgery prior to 28 weeks' gestation is reasonable under appropriate circumstances; after 28 weeks, steroid administration and delivery, if necessary, is the preferred first-line therapy given the excellent neonatal outcomes now expected in level IV neonatal intensive care units (NICUs).[21]

Fetal interventions focus on decreasing the vascularity of SCTs and reducing cardiac failure from arteriovenous fistula. Both minimally invasive interventions (utilizing laser or radiofrequency ablation [RFA]) and open techniques have been used.[23,24] Only fetuses identified with cardiac dysfunction prior to development of hydrops are considered candidates for open fetal surgery (Figs. 32.7 and 32.8). Data are few and the published studies have yielded conflicting outcomes. Treatment is thus best individualized.

The Texas Children's Fetal Center Treatment Approach for open surgery is as follows:

1. Create hysterotomy wide enough to accommodate exteriorization of the lesion.
2. Debulk exterior portion of tumor only, focusing on minimizing debulking time.
3. Close remaining tumor with complete skin coverage.

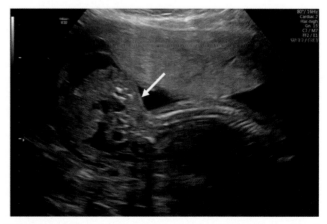

FIGURE 32.6: Sagittal US of a 20-week fetus with large predominantly external sacrococcygeal teratoma (*arrow*) containing both cystic and solid components.

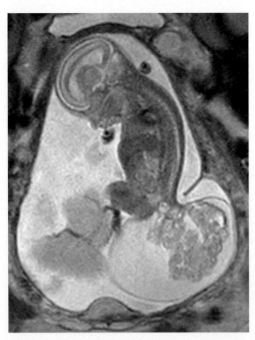

FIGURE 32.7: Sagittal T2 MRI of the same fetus in 32.6, again demonstrating large complex sacrococcygeal teratoma.

CLOSED FETAL SURGERY

The maternal morbidity associated with open fetal surgery from the hysterotomy has provoked some centers to develop a minimally invasive technique with "closed" or endoscopic fetal surgery techniques. These procedures involve two separate approaches: percutaneously without need for laparotomy and via laparotomy used to exteriorize the uterus. Both approaches

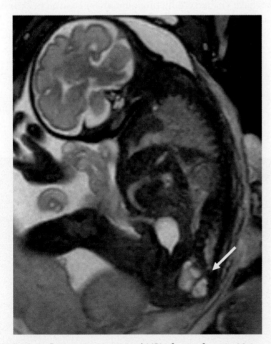

FIGURE 32.8: Postoperative sagittal MRI of same fetus in 32.6 and 32.7, 8 weeks after surgery, with small residual teratoma in the lower pelvis (*arrow*).

employ trocars or ports inserted through the uterine wall to access the uterine cavity under ultrasound guidance. The exteriorized uterus approach allows direct uterine access in cases of complete anterior placenta and direct fetal manipulation through the uterine wall to aid in positioning, and also allows anchoring of the membranes to the uterine wall prior to placement of the ports. Both the percutaneous and exteriorized uterus approaches employ a low-pressure CO_2 *in utero* environment to further improve visualization, and have been used to treat spina bifida and amniotic bands.[16,25] Flexible plastic ports or rigid metal cannulas are used to access the uterine cavity, through which fetoscopes and other instruments can be inserted.

Fetoscopic Procedures

All fetoscopic procedures utilize a fetoscope: an endoscopic instrument introduced into the amniotic cavity to provide direct intrauterine visual feedback on a monitor. Additional instruments, including microscissors and graspers, and even a laser fiber such as that used in treating twin-to-twin transfusion syndrome (TTTS), can be deployed alongside the fetoscope. The combination of fetoscopic and ultrasound visualization are frequently used (i.e., during endotracheal balloon placement in fetoscopic endoluminal tracheal occlusion [FETO]) providing a unique capacity to see both inside and outside of the target region.

Laser Photocoagulation

The most frequently utilized fetal intervention is laser photocoagulation with which TTTS, a condition affecting 9% to 15% of monochorionic diamniotic pregnancies, can be treated. TTTS is the result of vascular placental connections (both surface and deep) between the twins that for some unknown reason become unbalanced, resulting in unidirectional blood flow from the so-called donor twin to the so-called recipient twin. This imbalance can progress to cause cardiovascular stress in both babies (most commonly in the recipient twin who experiences increased preload, subsequent right ventricular hypertrophy, hypertension, and, ultimately, cardiomyopathy, and hydrops).

There are four types of vascular anastomoses: arteriovenous (AV), venoarterial (VA), arterioarterial (AA), and venovenous (VV). AV and VA connections are unidirectional, while AA and VV connections allow for bidirectional flow. The pathophysiology of TTTS is presumed to be from predominant AV anastomoses, with AA connections providing protection from this condition. Unbalanced VV connections carry the highest complication rate.

Diagnosis of TTTS is made by identifying a polyhydramnios/oligohydramnios sequence in monochorionic, diamniotic pregnancies. The Quintero staging system defines the initial step in this sequence as a deepest vertical pocket (DVP) of 8 cm or more in the recipient amniotic sac and 2 cm or less in the donor sac (Figs. 32.9 to 32.11).[26] Ultrasound imaging with Doppler is used to further classify progression of TTTS. European definitions of TTTS divide staging further by gestational age, requiring a DVP of 10 cm or more in the recipient sac if the pregnancy is more than 20 weeks.[27]

Ideally, TTTS should be rapidly identified and considered for fetal intervention. This is often not the case, and advanced cases of TTTS are frequently referred for urgent management.

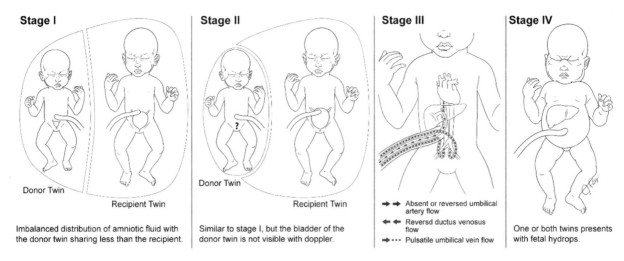

FIGURE 32.9: Stages of twin-to-twin transfusion syndrome. Courtesy of Texas Children's Hospital, with permission.

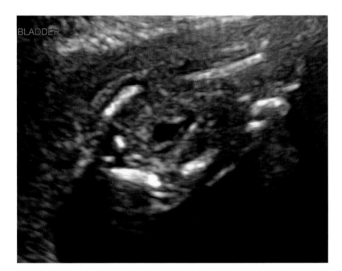

FIGURE 32.10: Axial US in a donor twin with small bladder and severe oligohydramnios.

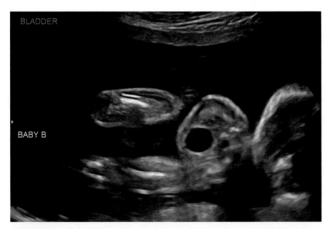

FIGURE 32.11: Axial US in a recipient twin with polyhydramnios and full bladder.

Treatment options include expectant management, repeated amnioreduction, septostomy of the inter-twin dividing membrane, laser ablation, selective twin reduction, or termination of pregnancy. Randomized controlled trials have shown that treatment of stage 1 to 4 TTTS with laser ablation, as compared to amnioreduction, improves 28-day and 6-month survival ($P = 0.009$, $P = 0.002$), and reduces neurological complications at 6 months ($P = 0.003$).[28] Laser therapy is generally accepted now as standard of care for patients with Quintero stage 2 to 4 TTTS.

Treatment of stage 1 TTTS is currently controversial. In cases of stage 1 TTTS with rapidly progressive polyhydramnios, preterm contractions, progressive cervical shortening, or significant maternal discomfort, laser therapy is indicated.[29] However, a study by the North American Fetal Therapy Network (NAFTNet) found that while a few cases stabilized with expectant management, the majority advanced within 1 to 2 weeks or had fetal demise.[30] While this study showed improved outcomes with fetal intervention in stage 1, further evidence is being collected to definitely answer this question (ClinicalTrials.gov NCT 01220011). Currently, treatment with expectant management and close ultrasound monitoring is recommended.

Laser therapy in the treatment of TTTS consists of photocoagulation of vascular anastomoses on the placental surface.[31] Several techniques for coagulation have been used. Initially, all anastomoses were ablated along the "membranous equator," or the placental midline separating the donor and recipient twins. Improvements to this technique have resulted in the practice of identifying the "vascular equator," and then focusing on selective laser coagulation of the placental vessels (SLCPVs) with an attempt to coagulate the artery before the vein in AV connections.[32] The latest improvement in laser therapy technique involves "solomonization," initially pioneered by Chalouhi et al., which involves connecting the sites of coagulation of the individual anastomoses from placental-edge to placental-edge along the "vascular equator." Solomonization decreases the risk of recurrent TTTS and twin anemia polycythemia sequence (TAPS).[33–35]

Laser photocoagulation can be challenging in cases of complete anterior placenta. Techniques to ameliorate this challenge include laparotomy and exteriorization of the uterus, the use of curved fetoscopes, the use of intracannula laser, and laparoscopy-assisted fetoscopic entry through the posterior uterus.[36-38]

Selected "pearls" regarding laser ablation:

1. Avoid creating septostomy by entering the uterus away from the donor.
2. To visualize hidden anastomoses, use a 70° scope.
3. "Solomonize" the vascular equator by marking each anastomosis and connecting markings from one edge of the placenta to the other.
4. In cases of anterior placenta, use a curved fetoscope.
5. In cases of anterior placenta without a window, the uterus can be accessed posteriorly with laparoscopic assistance.

Fetoscopic Endoluminal Tracheal Occlusion

This intervention is utilized in cases of CDH, a condition occurring in 1 in 5,000 to 10,000 live births.[39] CDH is a condition involving failure of proper embryogenesis of a portion of the diaphragm, allowing herniation of abdominal organs into the thoracic space. In many cases, this thoracic compression can result in significant pulmonary hypoplasia. The majority of cases develop on the left, although right-sided and bilateral cases also occur (13% and 2%, respectively).[40] From 26% to 58% of fetuses have associated abnormalities (neurological, cardiac, gastrointestinal, renal), and sometimes there is an accompanying genetic syndrome.[41] Isolated, severe cases of left- and right-sided CDH have a 24.1% and 0% survival rates without treatment, respectively, and are therefore considered candidates for fetal intervention.[42,43]

Diagnosis of CDH by ultrasound imaging demonstrates abdominal organs in the chest cavity (e.g., stomach, intestine, or liver). This herniation can progress to cause mediastinal shift and esophageal or cardiac compression and dysfunction. Esophageal compression can lead to polyhydramnios. Parameters used in diagnostic imaging on ultrasound and magnetic resonance imaging (MRI) include the lung-to-head ratio (LHR) (Fig. 32.12), observed-to-expected LHR, and observed-to-expected total lung volume (TLV).[44] The latter measurement is calculated using planimetry and a semiautomatic hand-tracing tool to outline lung volume in three planes.[45] CDH can be classified as mild, moderate, or severe based on these measurements and on liver involvement.

In indicated cases, the fetal treatment of CDH is by FETO with the goal of reducing pulmonary hypoplasia (Fig. 32.13). The procedure involves placement of a latex balloon (Fig. 32.14) into the fetal trachea to prevent intrapulmonary fluid from escaping, with subsequent removal in 4 to 6 weeks depending on fetal lung response (Fig. 32.15). The proposed mechanism for this treatment is that increased airway and alveolar pressure from the collected fluid allows normalization of pulmonary proliferation and pulmonary vascular development.[46] FETO is currently being evaluated with a randomized controlled trial (TOTAL [Tracheal Occlusion to Accelerate Lung Growth] trial—http://www.totaltrial.eu/). Data analysis of the TOTAL

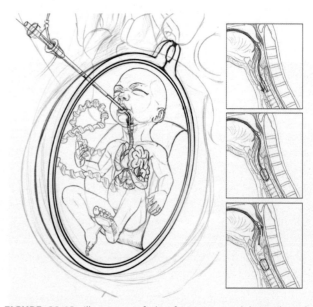

FIGURE 32.13: Illustration of the fetoscopic endoluminal tracheal occlusion procedure. Courtesy of Texas Children's Hospital, with permission.

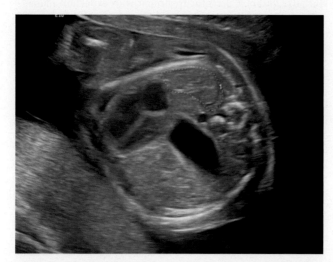

FIGURE 32.12: Axial US in a fetus with a left-sided congenital diaphragmatic hernia, with right lung area being measured by tracing method for calculation of lung-head ratio.

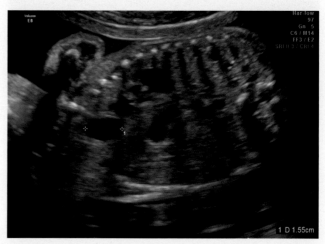

FIGURE 32.14: Coronal US showing the tracheal balloon (*calipers*) within the intrathoracic trachea.

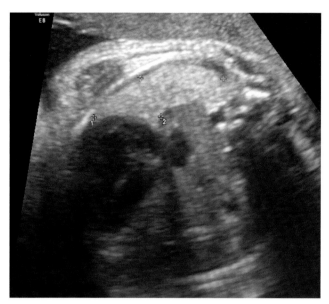

FIGURE 32.15: Axial US in a fetus with left CDH demonstrating increased size and echogenicity of the right lung (*measurements*) 4 weeks following fetoscopic endoluminal tracheal occlusion procedure.

trial registry shows increased likelihood of survival with FETO from 24.1% up to 49.1% in cases of severe left-sided CDH and from 0% up to 35.5% in cases of severe right-sided CDH ($P < 0.001$).[42,43] Although preliminary data is promising, FETO treatment should only be offered under a research protocol at a tertiary care fetal center.

Particular caution must be taken when utilizing the FETO intervention, as the endotracheal balloon must be removed prior to delivery. Failure to do this can be fatal due to persistent tracheal occlusion at birth. This requires an available fetal surgery team in close proximity to the fetal center in the event of unexpected preterm delivery so that balloon removal or EXIT delivery can be timely performed.

The following techniques for FETO are possible with an adequate lateral window in either anterior or posterior placentation.

Treatment Approach for Balloon Placement and Removal:

1. Preload the curved scope with the balloon.
2. Position the fetus face up, ideally in the upper half of the uterus.
3. Administer fetal anesthesia as described in the first section of this chapter.
4. Identify the complete fetal profile in a sagittal plane with sonographic imaging.
5. Access the fetal trachea.
6. Identify both vocal cords and the carina for optimal balloon positioning.
7. Use the same technique for balloon retrieval.

Amniotic Band Syndrome

Amniotic band syndrome (ABS) is a rare, sporadic condition occurring when fibrous amniotic bands entrap fetal parts (usually digits or limbs). These bands can interrupt fetal blood supply, resulting in constriction and eventual amputation. This syndrome occurs in 1 in 3,000 to 15,000 live births.[47] Severe cases can lead to major deformities of the body, head, abdominal wall, or even fetal death with strangulation of the umbilical cord.[48] The etiology of

ABS is not well understood. Possible pathophysiologies include early spontaneous or iatrogenic rupture of membranes and congenital abnormalities of the amnion.[49]

Diagnosis of ABS is made via ultrasound imaging, usually by asymmetry of cranial, facial, thoracic, abdominal wall, spinal, or limb defects. Other congenital diagnoses should be excluded, including developmental facial clefts, anencephaly, encephalocele, MMC, omphalocele, and limb–body wall anomaly.

Treatment of ABS using fetoscopy to preserve limb structure and function, and to prevent fetal death in cases of umbilical cord strangulation, has been described. Interventions utilize fetoscopy and laser ablation to release constrictive amniotic bands and are successful in preserving function in 50% of cases.[47]

Case selection for intervention is controversial. Husler et al. presented a classification system for amniotic bands, but this cannot be applied universally due to a failure of the classification to include cord strangulation. Fetoscopic band release should be reserved for cases in which the benefit of functional preservation clearly outweighs the risk of precipitating preterm birth, fetal loss, and preterm premature rupture of membranes (Figs. 32.16 and 32.17).[47] This is particularly relevant in cases of cord strangulation which can result in *in utero* demise.

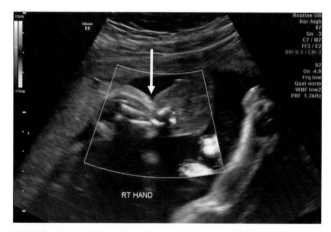

FIGURE 32.16: Color Doppler US of an amniotic band (*arrow*) constricting the right fetal hand with marked distal edema but preserved blood flow.

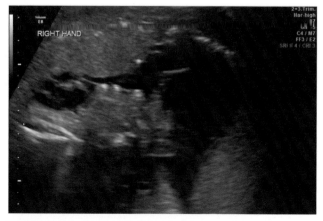

FIGURE 32.17: US of the right hand of the same fetus in figure 32.16 after fetoscopic release of the amniotic band.

Treatment Approach

1. Direct percutaneous fetoscopic approach
2. In cases of complete anterior placenta or inadequate visualization, a low-pressure CO_2 uterine environment can be utilized for amniotic band release.

Vasa Previa

Vasa previa (Figs. 32.18 and 32.19) is a condition involving exposed placental vessels from either velamentous cord insertion (type I) or bilobed/succenturiate placenta (type II).[50] Prenatal diagnosis is crucial in this pathology, and treatment with planned cesarean section at 35 to 36 weeks is necessary to prevent lethal hemorrhage from the fetus.[51,52] Fetal intervention has been suggested in selected cases in an attempt to resolve the condition prenatally and eliminate need for cesarean delivery.

In order to diagnose vasa previa, it is necessary to entertain a high sense of vigilance, especially when the placentation appears bilobed or succenturiate. Close monitoring with ultrasound is recommended, including serial assessment of cervical length from 28 to 32 weeks. This is helpful in determining optimal management, and to rule out a funic presentation. Vasa previa is identified on two-dimensional ultrasound by an echolucent area adjacent to the placental edge coursing over the internal cervical os. Color and spectral Doppler are helpful in confirming the diagnosis.

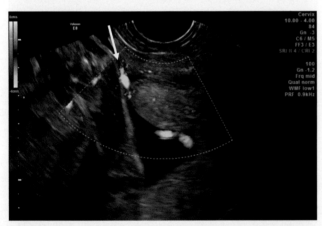

FIGURE 32.18: Sagittal color Doppler US demonstrating velamentous cord insertion and vasa previa (*arrow*).

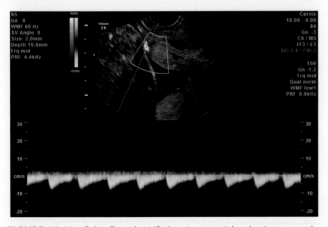

FIGURE 32.19: Color Doppler US showing arterial pulsations over the internal os region.

Laser photocoagulation has been used sparingly to successfully treat type II vasa previa.[53,54] Treatment should occur at tertiary centers with expertise, and is ideally undertaken in the third trimester.

Chorioangioma

Chorioangiomas are vascular tumors of the placenta, the majority of which are benign and asymptomatic. Some of these vascular tumors may be associated with poor perinatal outcome (especially those larger than 4 cm) by acting as arteriovenous shunts resulting in high cardiac output failure and fetal hydrops (Fig. 32.20).[55] In fetuses at risk for cardiac failure, fetoscopic laser ablation can be performed to interrupt the blood supply of the tumor.[56]

The diagnosis of chorioangiomas can be challenging. Sonographically, they appear as solid, circumscribed masses growing on the fetal surface of the placenta near the umbilical cord insertion. The differential diagnosis includes placental teratomas, mesenchymal metaplasia, and preplacental bleeding. Maternal serum alpha fetoprotein can be an early diagnostic indicator if elevated. Careful monitoring of fetuses with placental chorioangiomas is recommended, including serial growth ultrasounds, amniotic fluid assessment, Doppler studies, and fetal echocardiogram(s) to identify complications such as fetal anemia, polyhydramnios, hydrops, and growth restriction.

In those rare cases that require therapy, management options range from supportive treatment (therapeutic amnioreduction, intrauterine transfusion) to definitive therapy (fetoscopic vs. interstitial ablation). Currently, none of these approaches is preferable and therapy is applied on a case-by-case basis.

SURGERY BY GUIDED ULTRASOUND

Fetal procedures that do not use fetoscopic visualization and that are guided by real-time ultrasound imaging include needle-based or shunt-placement interventions.

Lower Urinary Tract Obstruction

Fetal urinary tract obstruction is caused by a range of conditions that obstruct the fetal urinary bladder neck, most commonly by posterior urethral valves (PUVs) in males. Other potential diagnoses include anterior urethral valves, urethral stenosis, urethral atresia, and obstructive ureterocele.[57] These conditions can progress to lower urinary tract obstruction (LUTO), occurring in approximately 2.2 of 10,000 live births.[58] Complete urethral obstruction carries a high risk of perinatal mortality due to the development of severe pulmonary hypoplasia and renal failure.

The initial diagnosis of LUTO often occurs at the time of fetal anatomy imaging around 18 to 20 weeks of gestation. The diagnostic signs on sonography include megacystis (enlarged urinary bladder), "keyhole" sign (dilation of proximal urethra), bilateral hydroureter and hydronephrosis, and oligohydramnios (Figs. 32.21 and 32.22). Further ultrasound imaging focusing on renal morphology and function is conducted if any of the abovementioned are detected. If LUTO has been prolonged or is severe, the kidneys may show renal cortical cysts, hyperechogenicity, or the absence of corticomedullary differentiation indicating dysplastic change.[59] Further imaging with MRI can better define the ureters, urachus, and bladder especially in patients with oligohydramnios. A multidisciplinary approach to manage LUTO is recommended, including fetal echocardiography,

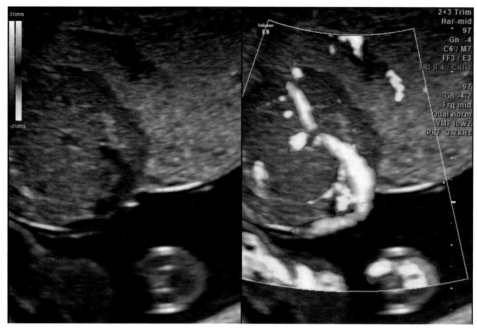

FIGURE 32.20: Side by side axial grayscale and color Doppler US of a 7-cm solid mass on fetal surface of the placenta just below cord insertion and supplied by the two main vessels to the lower half of the placenta.

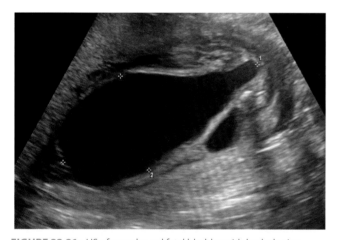

FIGURE 32.21: US of an enlarged fetal bladder with keyhole sign.

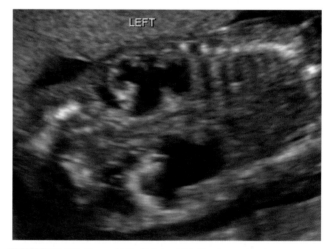

FIGURE 32.22: Coronal US of bilateral fetal hydronephrosis.

genetic consultation with amniocentesis or cordocentesis, and consultation with pediatric nephrologists and urologists. Cases of isolated LUTO can benefit from fetal intervention.

Selection of appropriate cases of LUTO for fetal intervention is imperative. Fetal urinary biochemistry is utilized in analyzing renal function via vesicocentesis after 18 weeks' gestation (Table 32.1).[60] Repeated fetal urinary studies are used to identify cases with favorable renal parameters, that is, chemistry and imaging studies demonstrating the potential for regaining renal function.[60,61]

Vesicoamniotic shunting (VAS) utilizes a double pigtail catheter inserted simultaneously into the fetal bladder and the amniotic space to allow for bladder decompression (Figs. 32.23 and 32.24).[62] VAS improves the likelihood of perinatal survival; however, neonatal survival and benefits to long-term renal function are unclear.[63] Other interventions include repeated vesicocentesis and fetal cystoscopy with mechanical or laser fulguration for treatment of PUV.[64] Currently, the success of the

latter procedure is limited by the precision of technical instruments and the risk of fetal fistula from tissue destruction from laser energy. Therefore, this intervention is limited to use under fetal therapy board oversight or institutional review board (IRB) protocol.[65]

TABLE 32.1 Normal Levels of Fetal Urinary Biochemistry (after 18 Weeks)

PARAMETER	NORMAL VALUE
Sodium	<100 mmol/L
Chloride	<90 mmol/L
Calcium	<8 mg/L
Osmolarity	<200 mOsm/L
Beta-2 microglobulin	<6 mg/L

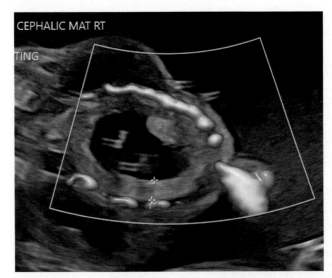

FIGURE 32.23: Color Doppler US demonstrating decompressed thick-wall fetal bladder (*calipers*) after insertion of vesicoamniotic shunt (Rocket shunt).

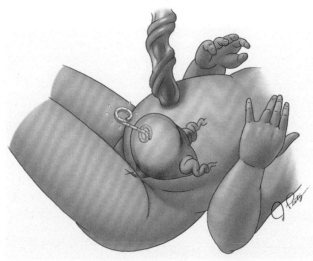

FIGURE 32.24: Illustration showing the correct placement of vesicoamniotic shunt (Harrison shunt). Courtesy of Texas Children's Hospital, with permission.

Treatment Approach

1. Sufficient amnioinfusion is necessary for deployment of the amniotic end of the shunt.
2. The "Rocket" or Kings College shunt is preferred to the Harrison shunt for increased likelihood of remaining in place after deployment.[62]
3. Shunt placement in the lower fetal bladder is preferred for adequate drainage.
4. The trocar should initially be directed into the amniotic fluid pocket and then redirected into the fetal bladder (to avoid deployment of the proximal end of the shunt into the uterine wall).
5. Fetoscopy can be utilized in difficult cases to ensure correct shunt placement.

Thoracoamniotic Shunt

Shunt interventions in the thoracic cavity are used for fetal pleural effusions or fluid-filled space-occupying chest lesions. Effusions and lung lesions can compress thoracic structures causing mediastinal shift and eventual pulmonary hypoplasia or hydrops in severe cases.[66] Pulmonary hypoplasia significantly increases the risk of morbidity and mortality postnatally.[67] Fetuses that develop cardiac dysfunction and/or hydrops may benefit from fetal intervention.

The majority of primary fetal pleural effusions are caused by abnormal lymphatic development and inadequate drainage (Fig. 32.25). Secondary pleural effusions are most often due to chromosomal or structural fetal defects.[68] Evaluation of fetuses with pleural effusion(s) involves a detailed diagnostic workup including ultrasound/MRI evaluation of structural abnormalities, genetic consultation and amniocentesis for genetic studies, infectious testing for TORCH (Toxoplasmosis, Other [Syphilis, Parvovirus B19, Varicella, Zika], Rubella, CMV, Herpes and HIV) infections, maternal blood-type and antibody test, and the Kleihauer–Betke test.[68] Fetal echocardiography is also recommended to evaluate structure and function of the affected fetal heart. Diagnoses related to significant structural abnormalities or lethal chromosomal disorders are contraindications for fetal surgery.

Common space-occupying lesions include congenital pulmonary airway malformations (CPAMs) and bronchopulmonary sequestration.[69] CPAMs with a large macrocystic component are most appropriate for fetal percutaneous intervention. CPAM volume ratio (CVR) is an ultrasound measurement developed to predict fetal prognosis and risk of hydrops.

$$CVR = (length \times height \times width \times 0.52)/head\ circumference$$

Cases of CVR greater than 1.6 cm are associated with 80% risk of developing hydrops, and are therefore candidates for fetal intervention. Cases with CVR less than 1.2 cm are followed up by ultrasound imaging weekly, and cases with CVR between 1.2 and 1.6 cm are followed up biweekly.

For both pleural effusions and fetal lung masses, cases with developing cardiac dysfunction are evaluated for fetal intervention. The primary therapeutic procedure for both conditions involves decompression with thoracoamniotic shunting by placement of in-dwelling, double-pigtail catheters (Fig. 32.26).

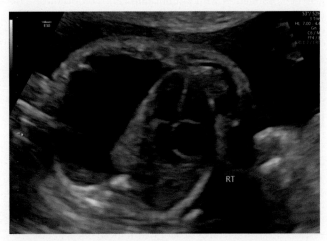

FIGURE 32.25: Axial US of a large left fetal hydrothorax.

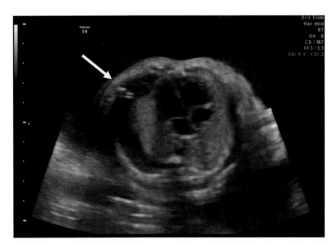

FIGURE 32.26: Axial US of the same fetus in 32.25 after insertion of a thoracoamniotic shunt (*Rocket shunt, arrow*).

For fetuses with a CPAM that is precipitating hydrops, shunting is associated with improved survival.[70] However, shunting may not be beneficial in fetuses with hydrops without concurrent cardiac dysfunction.[71] In rare cases, nonviable (i.e., <24 weeks gestational age) fetuses with hydrops and cardiac dysfunction secondary to CPAM may benefit from open surgery and resection of the mass. In addition, cases of bronchopulmonary sequestration have been successfully treated with percutaneous interstitial laser ablation of the supplying blood vessel.[72]

Fetuses with pleural effusions causing hydrops or preterm labor/shortened cervix secondary to polyhydramnios are also considered for fetal intervention. Other criteria occasionally used include (1) isolated effusion occupying more than 50% of the chest and (2) mediastinal shift and rapid increase of pleural effusion size.[68]

Treatment Approach for Pleural Effusion

1. Attempt initial thoracentesis with sampling of pleural fluid for biochemical and genetic testing as appropriate, and evaluate the response in terms of reexpansion of the lungs.
2. If the effusion rapidly reaccumulates, shunt placement is thought to be beneficial.
3. Placement of a double pig-tail catheter(s) (Harrison or Rocket) under real-time ultrasound guidance.

Selective Termination in Monochorionic Gestation

Complications of monochorionic twin pregnancies may in some cases, such as in TTTS, selective fetal growth restriction (sFGR), twin reversed arterial perfusion (TRAP) sequence, or twin anemia polycythemia sequence (TAPS), necessitate the selective termination of one fetus to protect the healthy fetus. In these cases, the traditional method of intrafetal injection used for selective termination poses a lethal risk to the cotwin due to vascular connections across the shared placenta. Identification of the chorionicity of the twins is crucial in consideration of selective feticide.

Techniques for selective termination include monopolar diathermy, laser, radiofrequency ablation (RFA), or microwave energy.[73] A 14- to 18-gauge needle is introduced by ultrasound guidance into the fetal abdomen adjacent to the umbilical cord insertion and used to occlude vessels using some form of coagulating energy (Figs. 32.27 and 32.28).[74] In cases of termination at later gestation where RFA and laser energy may be insufficient

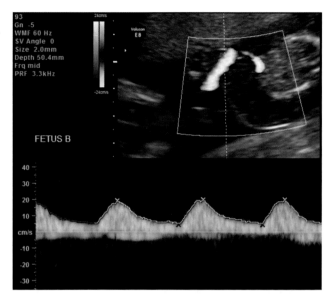

FIGURE 32.27: Color Doppler of an acardiac twin demonstrating reversed arterial perfusion.

to have effect in large vessels, bipolar diathermy forceps (2.4 to 3 mm) can be used to occlude and then coagulate the umbilical cord.[75] Laser photocoagulation of placental anastomoses, followed by intracardiac potassium chloride (KCl) has been described as a treatment approach with survival of the healthy fetus.[76]

Treatment Considerations

1. In monochorionic twins with TRAP sequence, early intervention after 12 weeks using intrafetal laser has improved outcomes compared to expectant management.[77]
2. Monochorionic, monoamniotic twins with TRAP sequence or significant fetal anomalies should be treated with both umbilical cord occlusion and cord transection.

Cardiac Intervention

Fetal cardiac intervention (FCI) has been used to treat several congenital cardiac conditions including severe aortic stenosis, restrictive foramen ovale in hypoplastic left heart syndrome (HLHS), and severe pulmonary stenosis with intact septum (Fig. 32.29).[78,79] Valvuloplasty in cases of stenosis and stent placement in cases of occlusion are the treatments of choice; however,

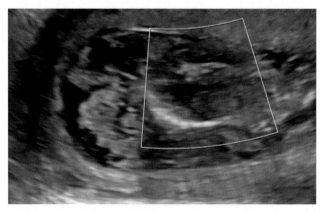

FIGURE 32.28: Color Doppler of an acardiac twin with no detectable blood flow after radiofrequency ablation procedure.

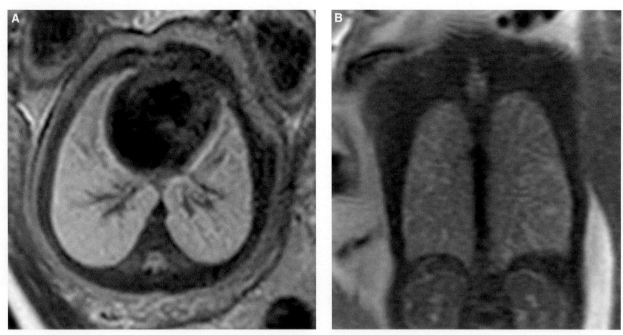

FIGURE 32.29: A/B: Axial and coronal T2 MRI shows nutmeg lung in a fetus with hypoplastic left heart syndrome and intact interatrial septum.

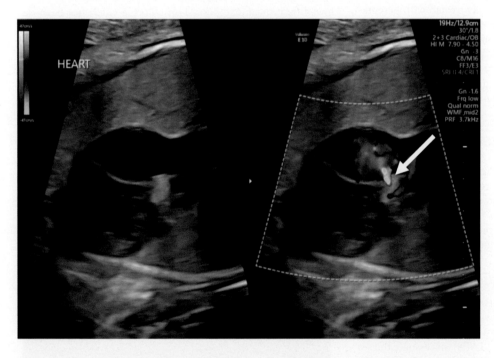

FIGURE 32.30: Axial side by side grayscale and color Doppler US in the same fetus as in figure 32.29 following atrial septostomy with interatrial stent placement. Color Doppler shows jet of blood through the stent (*arrow*).

FCI currently presents significant risks of morbidity and mortality to the fetus. There are uncertain long-term risks and benefits to the child, and no benefit in neurodevelopmental outcomes in cases of HLHS has been identified.[80] The primary goal of FCI is prevention of single ventricle physiology (such as in HLHS) which is associated with poor prognosis. Therefore, timing of the intervention is essential. Early identification and close monitoring of these conditions in order to recognize progressive ventricular dysfunction are essential so that, if indicated, fetal intervention may be offered in an attempt to prevent postnatal single-ventricle physiology (Fig. 32.30).

The primary congenital cardiac condition treated with FCI is severe aortic stenosis, often first recognized only in the second trimester of pregnancy. Aortic balloon valvuloplasty is used to prevent HLHS and is successful in 43% of surviving neonates.[81] Valvuloplasty is only indicated in critical stenosis as a bridge to biventricular repair postnatally.

Treatment Approach for Aortic Stenosis

1. Administration of fetal anesthesia
2. A 17- to 19-gauge needle is directed into the fetal heart under continuous ultrasound guidance.

3. The needle is aligned with the left ventricular outflow tract, the trocar is removed, and a guide wire with the preloaded balloon is advanced.
4. The balloon is positioned and confirmed with ultrasound to be across the valve.
5. The balloon is inflated, resulting in immediate valve dilation.
6. The balloon is deflated and removed along with the needle.

Pericardial effusion is an expected complication of any FCI, often with accompanying bradycardia. The effusion should be aspirated, and medications for fetal resuscitation should be available for use.

FUTURE DIRECTIONS

Fetal surgery has evolved rapidly in recent decades and continues to progress with the advent of improved imaging, diagnostic techniques and instrumentation technologies. Minimally invasive techniques are preferred to open fetal surgery in order to prevent the maternal morbidity associated with hysterotomy in the current and any future pregnancy.

A treatment approach involving CO_2 introduction to the uterus with only two 12-French ports, pioneered by Texas Children's Hospital, has been demonstrated to be of use in the treatment of some select congenital conditions without the need for open surgery. These conditions include NTDs, amniotic band release, and entrapment of a fetal limb by a previously placed shunt for pleural effusion drainage. Despite the theoretical concern for fetal acidosis (which has not materialized as data becomes increasingly available), this exteriorized uterus, two-port technique, is associated with a decreased risk of rupture of membranes and chorioamniotic separation because of an ability to anchor the fetal membranes to the uterus.[16,82]

Looking toward the future, there is some enthusiasm for expansion of fetoscopic treatment to the management of additional congenital diagnoses, such as gastroschisis. If early identification of gastroschisis becomes possible, closure of the abdominal wall defect may prevent some of the associated morbidity and mortality seen in this condition.

The goal of fetal surgery is to improve outcomes in otherwise lethal conditions, or in situations where significant and permanent progression of nonlethal prenatal disease may occur. This should be undertaken in an evidence-based, risk-reduced, and well supervised manner for both mother and child. As technology and data improve, so too will the outcomes of, and indications for, fetal intervention.

REFERENCES

1. Rosenkrantz JG, Simon RC, Carlisle JH. Fetal surgery in the pig with a review of other mammalian fetal technics. *J Pediatr Surg.* 1968;3(3):392–397.
2. Liley AW. *Intrauterine Transfusion of Foetus in Haemolytic Disease. Rhesus Haemolytic Disease.* Berlin, Germany: Springer; 1963:121–125.
3. Jancelewicz T, Harrison MR. A history of fetal surgery. *Clin Perinatol.* 2009;36(2):227–236.
4. Harrison MR, Filly RA, Golbus MS, et al. *Fetal Treatment.* Waltham, MA: Mass Medical Soc; 1982.
5. Moaddab A, Nassr AA, Belfort MA, et al. Ethical issues in fetal therapy. *Best Pract Res Clin Obstet Gynaecol.* 2017;43:58–67.
6. Myers LB, Cohen D, Galinkin J, et al. Anaesthesia for fetal surgery. *Pediatr Anesth.* 2002;12(7):569–578.
7. Centers for Disease Control and Prevention. National center on birth defects and developmental disabilities. CDC "Learn the signs Act early": child care providers materials pre-testing results. 2009.
8. Meuli M, Meuli-Simmen C, Hutchins GM, et al. The spinal cord lesion in human fetuses with myelomeningocele: implications for fetal surgery. *J Pediatr Surg.* 1997;32(3):448–452.
9. Babcook C, Goldstein RB, Barth RA, et al. Prevalence of ventriculomegaly in association with myelomeningocele: correlation with gestational age and severity of posterior fossa deformity. *Radiology.* 1994;190(3):703–707.
10. Drake J, Kestle J, Tuli S. CSF shunts 50 years on: past, present and future. *Childs Nerv Syst.* 2000;16(10–11):800–804.
11. Bruner JP, Tulipan NE, Richards WO. Endoscopic coverage of fetal open myelomeningocele in utero. *Am J Obstet Gynecol.* 1997;176(1):256–257.
12. Von Koch CS, Peacock WJ, Danielpour M, et al. In utero repair of myelomeningocele: experimental pathophysiology, initial clinical experience, and outcomes. *Arch Surg.* 2003;138(8):872–878.
13. Bruner JP, Tulipan NB, Richards WO, et al. In utero repair of myelomeningocele: a comparison of endoscopy and hysterotomy. *Fetal Diagn Ther.* 2000;15(2):83–88.
14. Adzick NS, Thom EA, Spong CY, et al. A randomized trial of prenatal versus postnatal repair of myelomeningocele. *N Engl J Med.* 2011;364(11):993–1004.
15. Goodnight WH, Bahtiyar O, Bennett KA, et al. Subsequent pregnancy outcomes after open maternal-fetal surgery for myelomeningocele. *Am J Obstet Gynecol.* 2019;220:494.e1–494.e7.
16. Belfort MA, Whitehead WE, Shamshirsaz AA, et al. Fetoscopic open neural tube defect repair: development and refinement of a two-port, carbon dioxide insufflation technique. *Obstet Gynecol.* 2017;129(4):734–743.
17. Bolde S, Pudale S, Pandit G, et al. Congenital pulmonary airway malformation: a report of two cases. *World J Clin Cases.* 2015;3(5):470.
18. Stocker JT, Madewell JE, Drake RM. Congenital cystic adenomatoid malformation of the lung: classification and morphologic spectrum. *Hum Pathol.* 1977;8(2):155–171.
19. Curran PF, Jelin EB, Rand L, et al. Prenatal steroids for microcystic congenital cystic adenomatoid malformations. *J Pediatr Surg.* 2010;45(1):145–150.
20. Cass DL, Olutoye OO, Cassady CI, et al. Prenatal diagnosis and outcome of fetal lung masses. *J Pediatr Surg.* 2011;46(2):292–298.
21. Peiró JL, Sbragia L, Scorletti F, et al. Management of fetal teratomas. *Pediatr Surg Int.* 2016;32(7):635–647.
22. Bond SJ, Harrison MR, Schmidt KG, et al. Death due to high-output cardiac failure in fetal sacrococcygeal teratoma. *J Pediatr Surg.* 1990;25(12):1287–1291.
23. Van Mieghem T, Al-Ibrahim A, Deprest J, et al. Minimally invasive therapy for fetal sacrococcygeal teratoma: case series and systematic review of the literature. *Ultrasound Obstet Gynecol.* 2014;43(6):611–619.
24. Hedrick HL, Flake AW, Crombleholme TM, et al. Sacrococcygeal teratoma: prenatal assessment, fetal intervention, and outcome. *J Pediatr Surg.* 2004;39(3):430–438.
25. Belfort MA, Whitehead WE, Ball R, et al. Fetoscopic amniotic band release in a case of chorioamniotic separation: an innovative new technique. *Am J Perinatol Rep.* 2016;6(02):e222–e225.
26. Quintero RA, Morales WJ, Allen MH, et al. Staging of twin-twin transfusion syndrome. *J Perinatol.* 1999;19(8):550.
27. Simpson LL, Society for Maternal-Fetal Medicine. Twin-twin transfusion syndrome. *Am J Obstet Gynecol.* 2013;208(1):3–18.
28. Senat M-V, Deprest J, Boulvain M, et al. Endoscopic laser surgery versus serial amnioreduction for severe twin-to-twin transfusion syndrome. *N Engl J Med.* 2004;351(2):136–144.
29. Johnson A. Diagnosis and management of twin-twin transfusion syndrome. *Clin Obstet Gynecol.* 2015;58(3):611–631.
30. Emery SP, Hasley SK, Catov JM, et al. North American Fetal Therapy Network: intervention vs expectant management for stage I twin-twin transfusion syndrome. *Am J Obstet Gynecol.* 2016;215(3):346.e1–346.e7.
31. De JL, Cruikshank DP, Keye JW. Fetoscopic neodymium: YAG laser occlusion of placental vessels in severe twin-twin transfusion syndrome. *Obstet Gynecol.* 1990;75(6):1046–1053.
32. Ville Y, Hyett J, Hecher K, et al. Preliminary experience with endoscopic laser surgery for severe twin–twin transfusion syndrome. *N Engl J Med.* 1995;332(4):224–227.
33. Chalouhi G, Essaoui M, Stirnemann J, et al. Laser therapy for twin-to-twin transfusion syndrome (TTTS). *Prenat Diagn.* 2011;31(7):637–646.
34. Ruano R, Rodo C, Peiro J, et al. Fetoscopic laser ablation of placental anastomoses in twin–twin transfusion syndrome using "Solomon technique." *Ultrasound Obstet Gynecol.* 2013;42(4):434–439.
35. Slaghekke F, Lopriore E, Lewi L, et al. Fetoscopic laser coagulation of the vascular equator versus selective coagulation for twin-to-twin transfusion syndrome: an open-label randomised controlled trial. *Lancet.* 2014;383(9935):2144–2151.
36. Shamshirsaz AA, Javadian P, Ruano R, et al. Comparison between laparoscopically assisted and standard fetoscopic laser ablation in patients with anterior and posterior placentation in twin-twin transfusion syndrome: a single center study. *Prenat Diagn.* 2015;35(4):376–381.
37. Papanna R, Johnson A, Ivey R, et al. Laparoscopy-assisted fetoscopy for laser surgery in twin–twin transfusion syndrome with anterior placentation. *Ultrasound Obstet Gynecol.* 2010;35(1):65–70.
38. Middeldorp JM, Lopriore E, Sueters M, et al. Laparoscopically guided uterine entry for fetoscopy in twin-to-twin transfusion syndrome with completely anterior placenta: a novel technique. *Fetal Diagn Ther.* 2007;22(6):409–415.
39. Torfs CP, Curry CJ, Bateson TF, et al. A population-based study of congenital diaphragmatic hernia. *Teratology.* 1992;46(6):555–565.

40. Deprest J, Jani J, Van Schoubroeck D, et al. Current consequences of prenatal diagnosis of congenital diaphragmatic hernia. *J Pediatr Surg.* 2006;41(2):423–430.

41. Holder A, Klaassens M, Tibboel D, et al. Genetic factors in congenital diaphragmatic hernia. *Am J Hum Genet.* 2007;80(5):825–845.

42. Jani J, Keller RL, Benachi A, et al. Prenatal prediction of survival in isolated left-sided diaphragmatic hernia. *Ultrasound Obstet Gynecol.* 2006;27(1):18–22.

43. Jani J, Nicolaides KH, Gratacos E, et al. Severe diaphragmatic hernia treated by fetal endoscopic tracheal occlusion. *Ultrasound Obstet Gynecol.* 2009;34(3):304–310.

44. Ruano R, Lazar D, Cass D, et al. Fetal lung volume and quantification of liver herniation by magnetic resonance imaging in isolated congenital diaphragmatic hernia. *Ultrasound Obstet Gynecol.* 2014;43(6):662–669.

45. Rypens F, Metens T, Rocourt N, et al. Fetal lung volume: estimation at MR imaging—initial results. *Radiology.* 2001;219(1):236–241.

46. Deprest J, Gratacos E, Nicolaides K. Fetoscopic tracheal occlusion (FETO) for severe congenital diaphragmatic hernia: evolution of a technique and preliminary results. *Ultrasound Obstet Gynecol.* 2004;24(2):121–126.

47. Javadian P, Shamshirsaz A, Haeri S, et al. Perinatal outcome after fetoscopic release of amniotic bands: a single-center experience and review of the literature. *Ultrasound Obstet Gynecol.* 2013;42(4):449–455.

48. Garza A, Cordero JF, Mulinare J. Epidemiology of the early amnion rupture spectrum of defects. *Am J Dis Child.* 1988;142(5):541–544.

49. Sentilhes L, Verspyck E, Eurin D, et al. Favourable outcome of a tight constriction band secondary to amniotic band syndrome. *Prenat Diagn.* 2004;24(3):198–201.

50. Catanzarite V, Maida C, Thomas W, et al. Prenatal sonographic diagnosis of vasa previa: ultrasound findings and obstetric outcome in ten cases. *Ultrasound Obstet Gynecol.* 2001;18(2):109–115.

51. Oyelese Y, Catanzarite V, Prefumo F, et al. Vasa previa: the impact of prenatal diagnosis on outcomes. *Obstet Gynecol.* 2004;103(5):937–942.

52. Vintzileos AM, Ananth CV, Smulian JC. Using ultrasound in the clinical management of placental implantation abnormalities. *Am J Obstet Gynecol.* 2015;213(4):S70–S77.

53. Chmait RH, Chavira E, Kontopoulos EV, et al. Third trimester fetoscopic laser ablation of type II vasa previa. *J Maternal Fetal Neonatal Med.* 2010;23(5):459–462.

54. Quintero RA, Kontopoulos EV, Bornick PW, Allen MH. In utero laser treatment of type II vasa previa. *J Maternal Fetal Neonatal Med.* 2007;20(12):847–851.

55. Amer HZM, Heller DS. Chorangioma and related vascular lesions of the placenta—a review. *Fetal Pediatr Pathol.* 2010;29(4):199–206.

56. Hosseinzadeh P, Shamshirsaz AA, Javadian P, et al. Prenatal therapy of large placental chorioangiomas: case report and review of the literature. *Am J Perinatol Rep.* 2015;5(02):e196–e202.

57. Pinette MG, Blackstone J, Wax JR, et al. Enlarged fetal bladder: differential diagnosis and outcomes. *J Clin Ultrasound.* 2003;31(6):328–334.

58. Anumba DO, Scott JE, Plant ND, et al. Diagnosis and outcome of fetal lower urinary tract obstruction in the northern region of England. *Prenat Diagn.* 2005;25(1):7–13.

59. Morris RK, Malin GL, Quinlan-Jones E, et al. Percutaneous vesicoamniotic shunting versus conservative management for fetal lower urinary tract obstruction (PLUTO): a randomised trial. *Lancet.* 2013;382(9903):1496–1506.

60. Nassr AA, Koh CK, Shamshirsaz AA, et al. Are ultrasound renal aspects associated with urinary biochemistry in fetuses with lower urinary tract obstruction? *Prenat Diagn.* 2016;36(13):1206–1210.

61. Ruano R, Sananes N, Wilson C, et al. Fetal lower urinary tract obstruction: proposal for standardized multidisciplinary prenatal management based on disease severity. *Ultrasound Obstet Gynecol.* 2016;48(4):476–482.

62. Morris R, Khan K, Kilby M. Vesicoamniotic shunting for fetal lower urinary tract obstruction: an overview. *Arch Dis Child Fetal Neonatal Ed.* 2007;92(3):F166–F168.

63. Nassr AA, Shazly SA, Abdelmagied AM, et al. Effectiveness of vesicoamniotic shunt in fetuses with congenital lower urinary tract obstruction: an updated systematic review and meta-analysis. *Ultrasound Obstet Gynecol.* 2017;49(6):696–703.

64. Ruano R, Sananes N, Sangi-Haghpeykar H, et al. Fetal intervention for severe lower urinary tract obstruction: a multicenter case–control study comparing fetal cystoscopy with vesicoamniotic shunting. *Ultrasound Obstet Gynecol.* 2015;45(4):452–458.

65. Sananes N, Favre R, Koh C, et al. Urological fistulas after fetal cystoscopic laser ablation of posterior urethral valves: surgical technical aspects. *Ultrasound Obstet Gynecol.* 2015;45(2):183–189.

66. Wilson RD, Baxter JK, Johnson MP, et al. Thoracoamniotic shunts: fetal treatment of pleural effusions and congenital cystic adenomatoid malformations. *Fetal Diagn Ther.* 2004;19(5):413.

67. Laberge J, Flageole H, Pugash D, et al. Outcome of the prenatally diagnosed congenital cystic adenomatoid lung malformation: a Canadian experience. *Fetal Diagn Ther.* 2001;16(3):178–186.

68. Yinon Y, Kelly E, Ryan G. Fetal pleural effusions. *Best Pract Res Clin Obstet Gynaecol.* 2008;22(1):77–96.

69. Khalek N, Johnson MP, eds. *Management of Prenatally Diagnosed Lung Lesions. Seminars in Pediatric Surgery.* Philadelphia, PA: Elsevier; 2013.

70. Knox E, Kilby M, Martin W, et al. In-utero pulmonary drainage in the management of primary hydrothorax and congenital cystic lung lesion: a systematic review. *Ultrasound Obstet Gynecol.* 2006;28(5):726–734.

71. Cass DL, Olutoye OO, Ayres NA, et al. Defining hydrops and indications for open fetal surgery for fetuses with lung masses and vascular tumors. *J Pediatr Surg.* 2012;47(1):40–45.

72. Ruano R, da Silva MM, Salustiano EM, et al. Percutaneous laser ablation under ultrasound guidance for fetal hyperechogenic microcystic lung lesions with hydrops: a single center cohort and a literature review. *Prenat Diagn.* 2012;32(12):1127–1132.

73. Stephenson CD, Temming LA, Pollack R, et al. Microwave ablation for twin-reversed arterial perfusion sequence: a novel application of technology. *Fetal Diagn Ther.* 2015;38(1):35–40.

74. Bebbington M. Selective reduction in multiple gestations. *Best Pract Res Clin Obstet Gynaecol.* 2014;28(2):239–247.

75. Bebbington M, Danzer E, Moldenhauer J, et al. Radiofrequency ablation vs bipolar umbilical cord coagulation in the management of complicated monochorionic pregnancies. *Ultrasound Obstet Gynecol.* 2012;40(3):319–324.

76. Bebbington M. Selective reduction in complex monochorionic gestations. *Am J Perinatol.* 2014;31(suppl 1):S51–S58.

77. Berg C, Holst D, Mallmann M, et al. Early vs late intervention in twin reversed arterial perfusion sequence. *Ultrasound Obstet Gynecol.* 2014;43(1):60–64.

78. Marshall AC, van der Velde ME, Tworetzky W, et al. Creation of an atrial septal defect in utero for fetuses with hypoplastic left heart syndrome and intact or highly restrictive atrial septum. *Circulation.* 2004;110(3):253–258.

79. Tulzer G, Arzt W, Franklin RC, et al. Fetal pulmonary valvuloplasty for critical pulmonary stenosis or atresia with intact septum. *Lancet.* 2002;360(9345):1567–1568.

80. Laraja K, Sadhwani A, Tworetzky W, et al. Neurodevelopmental outcome in children after fetal cardiac intervention for aortic stenosis with evolving hypoplastic left heart syndrome. *J Pediatr.* 2017;184:130.e4–136.e4.

81. McElhinney DB, Marshall AC, Wilkins-Haug LE, et al. Anatomic predictors of technical success and postnatal biventricular outcome after in utero aortic valvuloplasty for aortic stenosis with evolving hypoplastic left heart syndrome. *Am Heart Assoc.* 2008;120:1482–1490.

82. Belfort M, Shamshirsaz A, Whitehead W, et al. Unusual pleuroamniotic shunt complication managed using a two-port in-CO2 fetoscopic technique: technical and ethical considerations. *Ultrasound Obstet Gynecol.* 2016;47(1):123–124.

FIRST-TRIMESTER VALUES

TABLE 1	Combined Data Comparing Menstrual Age with Mean Gestational Sac Diameter, Crown–Rump Length, and HCG Levels				
MENSTRUAL AGE (d)	MENSTRUAL AGE (wk)	GESTATIONAL SAC SIZE (mm)	CROWN–RUMP LENGTH (mm)	HCG LEVEL (FIRST IRP), MEAN (U/L)	HCG LEVEL (FIRST IRP), RANGE (U/L)
30	4.3	—	—	—	—
31	4.4	—	—	—	—
32	4.6	3	—	1,710	(1,050–2,800)
33	4.7	4	—	2,320	(140–3,760)
34	4.9	5	—	3,100	(1,940–4,980)
35	5	5.5	—	4,090	(2,580–6,330)
36	5.1	6	—	5,340	(3,400–8,450)
37	5.3	7	—	6,880	(4,420–10,810)
38	5.4	8	—	8,770	(5,680–13,660)
39	5.6	9	—	11,040	(7,220–17,050)
40	5.7	10	0.2	13,730	(9,050–21,040)
41	5.9	11	0.3	15,300	(10,140–23,340)
42	6	12	0.4	16,870	(11,230–25,640)
43	6.1	13	0.4	30,480	(13,750–30,880)
44	6.3	14	0.5	24,560	(16,650–36,750)
45	6.4	15	0.6	29,110	(19,910–43,220)
46	6.6	16	0.7	34,100	(25,530–50,210)
47	6.7	17	0.8	39,460	(27,470–57,640)
48	6.9	18	0.9	45,120	(31,700–65,380)
49	7	19	1.0	50,970	(36,130–73,280)
50	7.1	20	1.0	56,900	(40,700–81,150)
51	7.3	21	1.1	62,760	(45,300–88,790)
52	7.4	22	1.2	68,390	(49,810–95,990)
53	7.6	23	1.3	73,640	(54,120–102,540)
54	7.7	24	1.4	78,350	(58,100–108,230)
55	7.9	25	1.5	82,370	(61,640–112,870)
56	8	26	1.6	85,560	(64,600–116,310)
57	8.1	26.5	1.7	—	—
58	8.3	27	1.8	—	—
59	8.4	28	1.9	—	—
60	8.6	29	2.0	—	—
61	8.7	30	2.1	—	—
62	8.9	31	2.2	—	—
63	9	32	2.3	—	—
64	9.1	33	2.4	—	—
65	9.3	34	2.5	—	—
66	9.4	35	2.6	—	—
67	9.6	36	2.8	—	—
68	9.7	37	2.9	—	—
69	9.9	38	3.0	—	—
70	10	39	3.1	—	—
71	10.1	40	3.2	—	—
72	10.3	41	3.4	—	—
73	10.4	42	3.5	—	—
74	10.6	43	3.7	—	—
75	10.7	44	3.8	—	—
76	10.9	45	4.0	—	—
77	11	46	4.1	—	—
78	11.1	47	4.2	—	—
79	11.3	48	4.4	—	—
80	11.4	49	4.6	—	—
81	11.6	50	4.8	—	—
82	11.7	51	5.0	—	—
83	11.9	52	5.2	—	—
84	12	53	5.4	—	—

HCG, human chorionic gonadotropin; IRP, international reference preparation.
Reproduced with permission from Nyberg DA, Hill LM, Bohm-Velez M. *Transvaginal Ultrasound.* St Louis, MO: Mosby-Year Book; 1992; Hadlock FP, Shah YP, Kanon DJ, et al. Crown-rump length: reevaluation of relation to menstrual age (5–18 weeks) with high-resolution real-time US. *Radiology.* 1992;182:501; and Robinson HP. "Gestational sac" volumes as determined by sonar in the first trimester of pregnancy. *BJOG.* 1975;82:100; and data from Daya S, Woods S. Transvaginal ultrasound scanning in early pregnancy and correlation with human chorionic gonadotropin levels. *J Clin Ultrasound.* 1991;19:139.

TABLE 2	Predicted Menstrual Age from Crown–Rump Length Measurements		
CROWN–RUMP LENGTH (mm)	MENSTRUAL AGE (wk)	CROWN–RUMP LENGTH (mm)	MENSTRUAL AGE (wk)
0.2	5.7	4.2	11.1
0.3	5.9	4.4	11.3
0.4	6.0	4.6	11.4
0.4	6.1	4.8	11.6
0.5	6.3	5.0	11.7
0.6	6.4	5.2	11.9
0.7	6.6	5.4	12.0
0.8	6.7	5.5	12.1
0.9	6.9	5.6	12.2
1.0	7.0	5.7	12.3
1.0	7.1	5.8	12.3
1.1	7.3	5.9	12.4
1.2	7.4	6.0	12.5
1.3	7.6	6.1	12.6
1.4	7.7	6.2	12.6
1.5	7.9	6.3	12.7
1.6	8.0	6.4	12.8
1.7	8.1	6.5	12.8
1.8	8.3	6.6	12.9
1.9	8.4	6.7	13.0
2.0	8.6	6.8	13.1
2.1	8.7	6.9	13.1
2.2	8.9	7.0	13.2
2.3	9.0	7.1	13.3
2.4	9.1	7.2	13.4
2.5	9.3	7.3	13.4
2.6	9.4	7.4	13.5
2.8	9.6	7.5	13.6
2.9	9.7	7.6	13.7
3.0	9.9	7.7	13.8
3.1	10.0	7.8	13.8
3.2	10.1	7.9	13.9
3.4	10.3	8.0	14.0
3.5	10.4	8.1	14.1
3.7	10.6	8.2	14.2
3.8	10.7	8.3	14.2
4.0	10.9	8.4	14.3
4.1	11.0	—	—

Reproduced with permission from Hadlock FP, Shah YP, Kanon DJ, et al. Fetal crown-rump length: reevaluation of relation to menstrual age (5–18 weeks) with high-resolution real-time US. *Radiology*. 1992;182:501–505.

TABLE 3   Reference Values for Crown–Rump Length Compared with Gestational Sac Size

GESTATIONAL SAC (mm)[a]	CROWN–RUMP LENGTH (mm)[b] PERCENTILES		
	5TH	50TH	95TH
10	0	4	8
11	0	5	9
12	0	5	10
13	1	5	10
14	1	6	11
15	1	7	12
16	1	7	13
17	2	8	14
18	2	8	15
19	2	9	15
20	3	10	16
21	3	10	17
22	4	11	18
23	4	12	19
24	5	12	20
25	5	13	21
26	6	14	22
27	6	15	24
28	7	16	25
29	7	17	26
30	8	18	27
31	9	18	28
32	9	19	29
33	10	20	31
34	11	21	32
35	12	22	33
36	12	23	34
37	13	25	36
38	14	26	37
39	15	27	38
40	16	28	40
41	17	29	41
42	18	30	43
43	19	31	44
44	20	33	46
45	21	34	47
46	22	35	49
47	23	37	50
48	24	38	52
49	25	39	54
50	26	41	55

[a]Standard deviation = 0.9185 + 0.1599 × gestational sac size.
[b]Crown–rump length = 0.012 × gestational sac size^2 + 0.9708 + 0.192 × gestational sac size.
Adapted from Grisolia G, Milano V, Pilu G, et al. Biometry of early pregnancy with transvaginal sonography. *Ultrasound Obstet Gynecol.* 1993;3:403–411.

AMNIOTIC FLUID INDEX

TABLE 4A	Amniotic Fluid Index in Normal Pregnancy (cm)				
GESTATIONAL AGE (wk)	5TH PERCENTILE	10TH PERCENTILE	50TH PERCENTILE	90TH PERCENTILE	95TH PERCENTILE
18	4.6	5.1	6.8	9.7	11.1
19	5.1	5.6	7.4	10.4	12
20	5.5	6.1	8	11.3	12.9
21	5.9	6.6	8.7	12.2	13.9
22	6.3	7.1	9.3	13.2	14.9
23	6.7	7.5	10	14.2	15.9
24	7	7.9	10.7	15.2	16.9
25	7.3	8.2	11.4	16.1	17.8
26	7.5	8.4	12	17	18.7
27	7.6	8.6	12.6	17.8	19.4
28	7.6	8.6	13	18.4	19.9
29	7.6	8.6	13.4	18.8	20.4
30	7.5	8.5	13.6	18.9	20.6
31	7.3	8.4	13.6	18.9	20.6
32	7.1	8.1	13.6	18.7	20.4
33	6.8	7.8	13.3	18.2	20
34	6.4	7.4	12.9	17.7	19.4
35	6	7	12.4	16.9	18.7
36	5.6	6.5	11.8	16.2	17.9
37	5.1	6	11.1	15.3	16.9
38	4.7	5.5	10.3	14.4	15.9
39	4.2	5	9.4	13.7	14.9
40	3.7	4.5	8.6	12.9	13.9
41	3.3	4	7.8	12.3	12.9

AFI, amniotic fluid index.
Data from Magann EF, Sanderson M, Martin JN, et al. The amniotic fluid index, single deepest pocket, and two-diameter pocket in normal human pregnancy. *Am J Obstet Gynecol*. 2000;182(6):1581–1588.

TABLE 4B	Maximum Vertical Pocket in Normal Pregnancy (cm)				
GESTATIONAL AGE (wk)	5TH PERCENTILE	10TH PERCENTILE	50TH PERCENTILE	90TH PERCENTILE	95TH PERCENTILE
18	2.7	2.9	4.1	5.9	6.4
19	2.8	3.1	4.3	6.1	6.6
20	2.9	3.2	4.4	6.2	6.7
21	2.9	3.3	4.5	6.3	6.8
22	3	3.3	4.6	6.3	6.8
23	3	3.4	4.6	6.3	6.8
24	3.1	3.4	4.7	6.3	6.8
25	3	3.3	4.7	6.3	6.8
26	3	3.3	4.8	6.4	6.8
27	3	3.3	4.8	6.4	6.9
28	3	3.3	4.8	6.4	6.9
29	2.9	3.3	4.8	6.4	6.9
30	2.9	3.3	4.8	6.4	6.9
31	2.9	3.2	4.8	6.5	7
32	2.9	3.2	4.8	6.6	7.1
33	2.9	3.2	4.82	6.6	7.2
34	2.8	3.2	4.8	6.6	7.2
35	2.8	3.1	4.7	6.6	7.2
36	2.7	3.1	4.7	6.6	7.1
37	2.6	2.9	4.5	6.5	7
38	2.4	2.8	4.4	6.3	6.8
39	2.3	2.7	4.2	6.1	6.6
40	2.1	2.5	3.9	5.8	6.2
41	1.9	2.2	3.7	5.4	5.7

SDP - deepest pocket, maximal vertical pocket.
Data from Magann EF, Sanderson M, Martin JN, et al. The amniotic fluid index, single deepest pocket, and two-diameter pocket in normal human pregnancy. *Am J Obstet Gynecol*. 2000;182(6):1581–1588..

BASIC ULTRASOUND BIOMETRY

| | TABLE 5 | Predicted Fetal Measurements at Specific Gestation Age (GA) | | |

GA (wk)	BIPARIETAL DIAMETER (cm)[a]	HEAD CIRCUMFERENCE (cm)[b]	FEMUR LENGTH (cm)[c]	ABDOMINAL CIRCUMFERENCE (cm)[d]
12	1.7	6.8	0.7	4.6
13	2.1	8.2	1.1	6.0
14	2.5	9.7	1.4	7.3
15	2.9	11.1	1.7	8.6
16	3.2	12.4	2.1	9.9
17	3.6	13.8	2.4	11.2
18	3.9	15.1	2.7	12.5
19	4.3	16.4	3.0	13.7
20	4.6	17.7	3.3	15.0
21	5.0	18.9	3.6	16.2
22	5.3	20.1	3.8	17.4
23	5.6	21.3	4.1	18.5
24	5.9	22.4	4.4	19.7
25	6.2	23.5	4.6	20.8
26	6.5	24.6	4.9	21.9
27	6.8	25.6	5.1	23.0
28	7.1	26.6	5.4	24.0
29	7.3	27.5	5.6	25.1
30	7.6	28.4	5.8	26.1
31	7.8	29.3	6.1	27.1
32	8.0	30.1	6.3	28.1
33	8.3	30.8	6.5	29.1
34	8.5	31.5	6.7	30.0
35	8.7	32.2	6.9	30.9
36	8.8	32.8	7.1	31.8
37	9.0	33.3	7.2	32.7
38	9.2	33.8	7.4	33.6
39	9.3	34.2	7.6	34.4
40	9.4	34.6	7.7	35.3

[a]Biparietal diameter $= -3.08 + 0.41 \times GA - 0.000061 \times GA^2$ (standard deviation, 3 mm).
[b]Head circumference $= -11.48 + 1.56 \times GA - 0.0002548 \times GA^2$ (standard deviation, 1 cm).
[c]Femur length $= -3.91 + 0.427 \times GA - 0.0034 \times GA^2$ (standard deviation, 3 mm).
[d]Abdominal circumference $= -13.3 + 1.61 \times GA - 0.00998 \times GA^2$ (standard deviation, 1.34 cm).
GA, gestational age.
Data from Hadlock FP, Deter RL, Harrist RB, et al. Estimating fetal age: computer assisted analysis of multiple fetal growth parameters. *Radiology*. 1984;152:497–501..

TABLE 6	Reference Values for Abdominal Circumference				
	ABDOMINAL CIRCUMFERENCE (cm)				
	PERCENTILES				
MENSTRUAL AGE (wk)	**3RD**	**10TH**	**50TH**	**90TH**	**97TH**
14.0	6.4	6.7	7.3	7.9	8.3
15.0	7.5	7.9	8.6	9.3	9.7
16.0	8.6	9.1	9.9	10.7	11.2
17.0	9.7	10.3	11.2	12.1	12.7
18.0	10.9	11.5	12.5	13.5	14.1
19.0	11.9	12.6	13.7	14.8	15.5
20.0	13.1	13.8	15.0	16.3	17.0
21.0	14.1	14.9	16.2	17.6	18.3
22.0	15.1	16.0	17.4	18.8	19.7
23.0	16.1	17.0	18.5	20.0	20.9
24.0	17.1	18.1	19.7	21.3	22.3
25.0	18.1	19.1	20.8	22.5	23.5
26.0	19.1	20.1	21.9	23.7	24.8
27.0	20.0	21.1	23.0	24.9	26.0
28.0	20.9	22.0	24.0	26.0	27.1
29.0	21.8	23.0	25.1	27.2	28.4
30.0	22.7	23.9	26.1	28.3	29.5
31.0	23.6	24.9	27.1	29.4	30.6
32.0	24.5	25.8	28.1	30.4	31.8
33.0	25.3	26.7	29.1	31.5	32.9
34.0	26.1	27.5	30.0	32.5	33.9
35.0	26.9	28.3	30.9	33.5	34.9
36.0	27.7	29.2	31.8	34.4	35.9
37.0	28.5	30.0	32.7	35.4	37.0
38.0	29.2	30.8	33.6	36.4	38.0
39.0	29.9	31.6	34.4	37.3	38.9
40.0	30.7	32.4	35.3	38.2	39.9

Adapted from Hadlock FP, Deter RL, Harrist RB, et al. Estimating fetal age: computer-assisted analysis of multiple fetal growth parameters. *Radiology*. 1984;152:497–501.

TABLE 7	Reference Values for Head Circumference				
	HEAD CIRCUMFERENCE (cm)				
	PERCENTILES				
MENSTRUAL AGE (wk)	3RD	10TH	50TH	90TH	97TH
14.0	8.8	9.1	9.7	10.3	10.6
15.0	10.0	10.4	11.0	11.6	12.0
16.0	11.3	11.7	12.4	13.1	13.5
17.0	12.6	13.0	13.8	14.6	15.0
18.0	13.7	14.2	15.1	16.0	16.5
19.0	14.9	15.5	16.4	17.4	17.9
20.0	16.1	16.7	17.7	18.7	19.3
21.0	17.2	17.8	18.9	20.0	20.6
22.0	18.3	18.9	20.1	21.3	21.9
23.0	19.4	20.1	21.3	22.5	23.2
24.0	20.4	21.1	22.4	23.7	24.3
25.0	21.4	22.2	23.5	24.9	25.6
26.0	22.4	23.2	24.6	26.0	26.8
27.0	23.3	24.1	25.6	27.0	27.9
28.0	24.2	25.1	26.6	28.1	29.0
29.0	25.0	25.9	27.5	29.1	30.0
30.0	25.8	26.8	28.4	30.0	31.0
31.0	26.7	27.6	29.3	31.0	31.9
32.0	27.4	28.4	30.1	31.8	32.8
33.0	28.0	29.0	30.8	32.6	33.6
34.0	28.7	29.7	31.5	33.3	34.3
35.0	29.3	30.4	32.2	34.1	35.1
36.0	29.9	30.9	32.8	34.7	35.8
37.0	30.3	31.4	33.3	35.2	36.3
38.0	30.8	31.9	33.8	35.8	36.8
39.0	31.1	32.2	34.2	36.2	37.3
40.0	31.5	32.6	34.6	36.6	37.7

Adapted from Hadlock FP, Deter RL, Harrist RB, et al. Estimating fetal age: computer-assisted analysis of multiple fetal growth parameters. *Radiology*. 1984;152:497–501.

TABLE 8	Reference Values for Femur Length				
	FEMUR LENGTH (cm)				
	PERCENTILES				
MENSTRUAL AGE (wk)	**3RD**	**10TH**	**50TH**	**90TH**	**97TH**
14.0	1.2	1.3	1.4	1.5	1.6
15.0	1.5	1.6	1.7	1.9	1.9
16.0	1.7	1.8	2.0	2.2	2.3
17.0	2.1	2.2	2.4	2.6	2.7
18.0	2.3	2.5	2.7	2.9	3.1
19.0	2.6	2.7	3.0	3.3	3.4
20.0	2.8	3.0	3.3	3.6	3.8
21.0	3.0	3.2	3.5	3.8	4.0
22.0	3.3	3.5	3.8	4.1	4.3
23.0	3.5	3.7	4.1	4.5	4.7
24.0	3.8	4.0	4.4	4.8	5.0
25.0	4.0	4.2	4.6	5.0	5.2
26.0	4.2	4.5	4.9	5.3	5.6
27.0	4.4	4.6	5.1	5.6	5.8
28.0	4.6	4.9	5.4	5.9	6.2
29.0	4.8	5.1	5.6	6.1	6.4
30.0	5.0	5.3	5.8	6.3	6.6
31.0	5.2	5.5	6.0	6.5	6.8
32.0	5.3	5.6	6.2	6.8	7.1
33.0	5.5	5.8	6.4	7.0	7.3
34.0	5.7	6.0	6.6	7.2	7.5
35.0	5.9	6.2	6.8	7.4	7.8
36.0	6.0	6.4	7.0	7.6	8.0
37.0	6.2	6.6	7.2	7.9	8.2
38.0	6.4	6.7	7.4	8.1	8.4
39.0	6.5	6.8	7.5	8.2	8.6
40.0	6.6	7.0	7.7	8.4	8.8

Adapted from Hadlock FP, Deter RL, Harrist RB, et al. Estimating fetal age: computer-assisted analysis of multiple fetal growth parameters. *Radiology.* 1984;152:497–501.

	HC/AC[a]			AC/FL[b]			BPD/FL[c]		
GA (wk)	**5TH**	**50TH**	**95TH**	**5TH**	**50TH**	**95TH**	**5TH**	**50TH**	**95TH**
14	1.13	1.23	1.34	4.93	5.51	6.16	1.75	1.92	2.11
15	1.12	1.22	1.33	4.73	5.29	5.92	1.66	1.82	2.00
16	1.11	1.21	1.32	4.57	5.11	5.71	1.58	1.74	1.91
17	1.10	1.20	1.31	4.43	4.95	5.54	1.52	1.67	1.83
18	1.09	1.19	1.30	4.32	4.83	5.40	1.47	1.61	1.77
19	1.08	1.18	1.29	4.23	4.73	5.29	1.42	1.56	1.71
20	1.07	1.17	1.28	4.16	4.65	5.20	1.39	1.52	1.67
21	1.06	1.17	1.27	4.11	4.59	5.13	1.36	1.49	1.64
22	1.05	1.16	1.26	4.07	4.55	5.08	1.34	1.47	1.61
23	1.04	1.15	1.25	4.04	4.52	5.05	1.32	1.45	1.59
24	1.03	1.14	1.24	4.03	4.50	5.03	1.30	1.43	1.57
25	1.02	1.13	1.23	4.02	4.50	5.03	1.29	1.42	1.56
26	1.01	1.12	1.22	4.03	4.50	5.03	1.29	1.41	1.55
27	1.00	1.11	1.21	4.04	4.51	5.04	1.28	1.41	1.54
28	0.99	1.10	1.20	4.05	4.53	5.06	1.28	1.40	1.54
29	0.98	1.09	1.19	4.07	4.55	5.09	1.28	1.40	1.54
30	0.97	1.08	1.18	4.10	4.58	5.12	1.27	1.40	1.53
31	0.96	1.07	1.17	4.12	4.61	5.15	1.27	1.40	1.53
32	0.95	1.06	1.16	4.15	4.64	5.18	1.27	1.39	1.53
33	0.94	1.05	1.16	4.17	4.67	5.22	1.27	1.39	1.52
34	0.94	1.04	1.15	4.20	4.69	5.24	1.26	1.38	1.52
35	0.93	1.03	1.14	4.21	4.71	5.27	1.25	1.37	1.51
36	0.92	1.02	1.13	4.23	4.73	5.28	1.24	1.36	1.50
37	0.91	1.01	1.12	4.23	4.73	5.29	1.23	1.35	1.48
38	0.90	1.00	1.11	4.23	4.73	5.29	1.21	1.33	1.46
39	0.89	0.99	1.10	4.22	4.71	5.27	1.19	1.30	1.43
40	0.88	0.98	1.09	4.19	4.69	5.24	1.16	1.28	1.40

TABLE 9   Normal Biometric Ratios of HC/AC, AC/FL, and BPD/FL

[a] HC/AC = $0.3668952 - 0.0096 \times GA$ (SD = 0.064) (modified formula to fit published tabular data).
[b] Log (AC/FL) = $1.3260806 - 0.0693157 \times GA + 0.0023154 \times GA^2 - 0.0000248 \times GA^3$ (SD = 0.02942).
[c] Log (BPD/FL) = $1.0205449 - 0.0865895 \times GA + 0.0028771 \times GA^2 - 0.0000321 \times GA^3$ (SD = 0.02458).
AC, abdominal circumference; BPD, biparietal diameter; GA, gestational age; FL, femur length; HC, head circumference.
Reproduced with permission from Snijders RJM, Nicolaides KH. Fetal biometry at 14–40 weeks' gestation. *Ultrasound Obstet Gynecol.* 1994;4:34–38.

TABLE 10	Fetal Weight Percentiles by Gestational Age				
	FETAL WEIGHT PERCENTILES (g)				
GA (wk)	3RD	10TH	50TH	90TH	97TH
10	26	29	35	41	44
11	34	37	45	53	56
12	43	48	58	68	73
13	54	61	73	85	92
14	69	77	93	109	117
15	87	97	117	137	147
16	109	121	146	171	183
17	135	150	181	212	227
18	166	185	223	261	280
19	204	227	273	319	342
20	247	275	331	387	415
21	298	331	399	467	500
22	357	397	478	559	599
23	424	472	568	664	712
24	500	556	670	784	840
25	586	652	785	918	984
26	681	758	913	1,068	1,145
27	787	876	1,055	1,234	1,323
28	903	1,005	1,210	1,415	1,517
29	1,029	1,145	1,379	1,613	1,729
30	1,163	1,294	1,559	1,824	1,955
31	1,306	1,454	1,751	2,048	2,196
32	1,457	1,621	1,953	2,285	2,449
33	1,613	1,795	2,162	2,529	2,711
34	1,773	1,973	2,377	2,781	2,981
35	1,936	2,154	2,595	3,036	3,254
36	2,098	2,335	2,813	3,291	3,528
37	2,259	2,514	3,028	3,542	3,797
38	2,414	2,687	3,236	3,785	4,058
39	2,563	2,852	3,435	4,018	4,307
40	2,700	3,004	3,619	4,234	4,538
41	2,825	3,144	3,787	4,430	4,749
42	2,935	3,266	3,934	4,602	4,933

Ln (Wt) = 0.578 + 0.332 MA − 0.00354 × MA^2; standard deviation = 12.7% of predicted weight.
Ln, natural log; MA, menstrual age; Wt, weight.
Reproduced with permission from Hadlock FP, Harrist RB, Marinez-Poyer J. In utero analysis of fetal growth: a sonographic weight standard. *Radiology.* 1991;181: 129–133, extrapolated to 42 weeks from 40 weeks.

TABLE 11	Fitted Percentiles for Fractional Arm Volume							
MENSTRUAL AGE (wk)		**FRACTIONAL ARM VOLUME (mL)**						
	n	**5TH**	**10TH**	**25TH**	**50TH**	**75TH**	**90TH**	**95TH**	**1 SD**
18–18.9	16	1.3	1.4	1.6	1.9	2.2	2.6	2.8	1.27
19–19.9	12	1.5	1.7	1.9	2.3	2.7	3.1	3.4	1.27
20–20.9	11	1.9	2.1	2.4	2.9	3.3	3.8	4.2	1.26
21–21.9	17	2.3	2.5	2.9	3.4	4.0	4.6	5.0	1.26
22–22.9	15	2.7	2.9	3.4	3.9	4.6	5.3	5.8	1.26
23–23.9	12	3.4	3.7	4.3	5.0	5.8	6.7	7.3	1.26
24–24.9	10	3.8	4.1	4.8	5.5	6.4	7.4	8.0	1.25
25–25.9	14	4.6	5.0	5.7	6.7	7.8	8.9	9.6	1.25
26–26.9	13	5.4	5.9	6.7	7.8	9.1	10.4	11.3	1.25
27–27.9	12	6.3	6.8	7.8	9.0	10.5	12.0	13.0	1.25
28–28.9	14	7.2	7.8	8.9	10.3	11.9	13.6	14.7	1.24
29–29.9	11	8.2	8.9	10.1	11.7	13.6	15.5	16.8	1.24
30–30.9	14	9.5	10.3	11.7	13.6	15.7	17.9	19.3	1.24
31–31.9	13	10.8	11.7	13.4	15.4	17.8	20.3	22.0	1.24
32–32.9	15	12.5	13.5	15.4	17.8	20.5	23.3	25.2	1.24
33–33.9	14	14.3	15.4	17.5	20.2	23.3	26.5	28.6	1.24
34–34.9	9	15.3	16.5	18.8	21.6	24.9	28.3	30.6	1.23
35–35.9	13	17.3	18.7	21.2	24.4	28.1	32.0	34.5	1.23
36–36.9	13	19.7	21.3	24.1	27.7	31.9	36.2	39.1	1.23
37–37.9	15	22.0	23.7	26.9	30.9	35.6	40.3	43.5	1.23
38–38.9	45	25.0	27.0	30.6	35.1	40.3	45.7	49.2	1.23
39–39.9	49	26.9	28.9	32.8	37.6	43.2	48.9	52.7	1.23
40–40.9	9	29.4	31.6	35.8	41.1	47.1	53.3	57.4	1.23
41–41.9	13	33.6	36.1	40.8	46.8	53.7	60.7	65.3	1.22
42–42.9	8	35.0	37.7	42.6	48.8	55.9	63.2	68.0	1.22

SD, standard deviation.
Reproduced with permission from Lee W, Balasubramaniam M, Deter RL, et al. Fractional limb volume—a soft tissue parameter of fetal body composition: validation, technical considerations and normal ranges during pregnancy. *Ultrasound Obstet Gynecol.* 2009;33:427–440.

TABLE 12	Fitted Percentiles for Fractional Thigh Volume							
MENSTRUAL AGE (wk)		FRACTIONAL THIGH VOLUME (mL)						
	n	5TH	10TH	25TH	50TH	75TH	90TH	95TH	1 SD
18–18.9	16	2.4	2.6	2.9	3.4	3.9	4.4	4.7	1.23
19–19.9	12	2.9	3.2	3.6	4.1	4.7	5.4	5.8	1.23
20–20.9	11	3.7	4.0	4.6	5.3	6.1	6.9	7.4	1.23
21–21.9	17	4.5	4.9	5.6	6.4	7.4	8.4	9.1	1.23
22–22.9	15	5.3	5.7	6.5	7.5	8.6	9.8	10.6	1.24
23–23.9	12	6.9	7.4	8.4	9.7	11.2	12.8	13.8	1.24
24–24.9	10	7.6	8.2	9.4	10.8	12.5	14.2	15.4	1.24
25–25.9	14	9.3	10.1	11.5	13.3	15.3	17.5	18.9	1.24
26–26.9	13	11.1	12.0	13.7	15.8	18.3	20.8	22.5	1.24
27–27.9	12	13.0	14.0	16.0	18.5	21.3	24.3	26.3	1.24
28–28.9	14	14.9	16.1	18.3	21.2	24.5	27.9	30.2	1.24
29–29.9	11	17.2	18.6	21.2	24.5	28.4	32.3	35.0	1.24
30–30.9	14	20.1	21.8	24.8	28.7	33.2	37.9	41.0	1.24
31–31.9	13	23.1	25.0	28.6	33.1	38.3	43.7	47.2	1.24
32–32.9	15	26.9	29.2	33.3	38.5	44.6	50.9	55.1	1.24
33–33.9	14	31.0	33.5	38.3	44.3	51.4	58.7	63.5	1.24
34–34.9	9	33.3	36.1	41.2	47.8	55.4	63.2	68.4	1.24
35–35.9	13	38.0	41.2	47.0	54.5	63.2	72.2	78.2	1.25
36–36.9	13	43.6	47.2	54.0	62.6	72.6	83.0	89.9	1.25
37–37.9	15	49.1	53.1	60.8	70.5	81.8	93.5	101.3	1.25
38–38.9	45	56.2	61.0	69.7	80.9	93.9	107.4	116.4	1.25
39–39.9	49	60.6	65.7	75.1	87.2	101.3	115.9	125.6	1.25
40 40.9	9	66.6	72.2	82.6	95.9	111.4	127.5	138.2	1.25
41–41.9	13	76.7	83.2	95.2	110.7	128.6	147.2	159.6	1.25
42–42.9	8	80.2	87.0	99.6	115.8	134.5	154.0	167.0	1.25

SD, standard deviation.
Reproduced with permission from Lee W, Balasubramaniam M, Deter RL, et al. Fractional limb volume—a soft tissue parameter of fetal body composition: validation, technical considerations and normal ranges during pregnancy. *Ultrasound Obstet Gynecol*. 2009;33:427–440.

ULTRASOUND EXTREMITY MEASUREMENTS

TABLE 13A	Ultrasound Reference Values for Humeral Length (mm)					

WEEKS OF GESTATION	n	PER CENTILES					SD
		3RD	10TH	50TH	90TH	97TH	
12	8	3.7	4.8	7.1	9.5	10.6	1.8
13	18	7.2	8.3	10.7	13.1	14.2	1.9
14	18	10.5	11.7	14.1	16.5	17.7	1.9
15	14	13.7	14.8	17.3	19.8	21.0	2.0
16	15	16.7	17.9	20.4	23.0	24.2	2.0
17	22	19.6	20.8	23.4	26.0	27.2	2.0
18	18	22.3	23.6	26.2	28.9	30.1	2.1
19	22	24.9	26.2	28.9	31.6	32.9	2.1
20	21	27.4	28.7	31.5	34.2	35.5	2.2
21	22	29.8	31.2	34.0	36.8	38.1	2.2
22	20	32.1	33.5	36.3	39.2	40.5	2.2
23	2.2.	34.3	35.7	35.6	41.5	419	2.3
24	24	36.4	37.8	40.7	43.7	45.1	2.3
25	20	38.4	39.8	42.8	45.8	47.2	2.4
26	19	40.3	41.7	44.8	47.9	49.3	2.4
27	24	421	43.6	46.7	44.8	51.3	2.4
28	20	43.9	45.3	48.5	51.7	53.2	2.5
29	21	45.5	47.0	50.2	53.5	55.0	2.5
30	19	47.1	48.6	51.9	55.2	56.7	2.6
31	26	48.6	50.2	53.5	56.8	58.4	2.6
32	25	50.0	51.6	55.0	58.4	59.9	2.6
33	23	51.4	53.0	56.4	59.8	61.5	2.7
34	20	52.7	54.3	57.8	61.3	62.9	2.7
35	20	53.9	55.6	59.1	62.6	64.3	2.8
36	24	55.1	56.8	60.3	63.9	65.6	2.8
37	19	56.2	57.9	61.5	65.1	66.8	2.8
38	20	57.2	58.9	62.6	66.3	68.0	2.9
39	14	58.2	60.0	63.7	67.4	69.2	2.9
40	13	59.1	60.9	64.7	66.5	70.3	3.0
41	25	60.0	61.8	65.6	69.5	71.3	3.0
42	17	60.8	62.6	66.5	70.4	72.2	3.0
Total	613						

SD, standard deviation.

Reproduced with permission from Chitty LS, Altman DG BJOG. *An International Journal of Obstetrics and Gynaecology* 2002;109:919–929.

TABLE 13B Ultrasound Reference Values for Radius Length (mm)

WEEKS OF GESTATION	n	PERCENTILES					SD
		3RD	10TH	50TH	90TH	97TH	
12	6	2.2	3.3	5.5	7.8	8.8	1.7
13	8	4.8	5.9	8.2	10.5	11.6	1.8
14	16	7.6	8.7	11.0	13.4	14.5	1.8
15	11	10.3	11.5	13.9	16.3	17.4	1.9
16	12	13.0	14.2	16.7	19.1	20.3	1.9
17	16	15.6	16.8	19.3	21.9	23.1	2.0
18	15	18.1	19.3	21.9	24.5	25.7	2.0
19	24	20.4	21.7	24.4	27.0	28.3	2.1
20	22	22.7	23.9	26.7	29.4	30.7	2.1
21	21	24.8	26.1	28.9	31.6	32.9	2.2
22	19	26.8	28.1	30.9	33.8	35.1	2.2
23	21	28.6	30.0	32.9	35.8	37.1	2.3
24	20	30.4	31.8	34.7	37.7	39.1	2.3
25	22	32.0	33.5	36.5	39.5	40.9	2.4
26	20	33.6	35.0	38.1	41.2	42.6	2.4
27	24	35.1	36.5	39.7	42.8	44.3	2.4
28	21	36.5	38.0	41.2	44.3	45.8	2.5
29	21	37.8	39.3	42.6	45.8	47.3	2.5
30	19	39.0	40.6	43.9	47.2	48.7	2.6
31	26	40.2	41.8	45.1	48.5	50.1	2.6
32	25	41.3	42.9	46.4	49.8	51.4	2.7
33	23	42.4	44.0*	47.5	51.0	52.6	2.7
34	19	43.4	45.0	48.6	52.1	53.8	2.8
35	22	44.3	46.0	49.6	53.2	54.9	2.8
36	22	45.2	46.9	50.6	54.3	56.0	2.9
37	18	46.1	47.8	51.6	55.3	57.0	2.9
38	18	46.9	48.7	52.5	56.2	58.0	3.0
39	11	47.7	49.5	53.3	57.2	59.0	3.0
40	14	48.4	50.3	54.2	58.1	59.9	3.0
41	21	49.1	51.0	55.0	58.9	60.8	3.1
42	15	49.8	51.7	55.7	59.7	61.6	3.1
Total	572						

SD, standard deviation.

Reproduced with permission from Chitty LS, Altman DG BJOG. *An International Journal of Obstetrics and Gynaecology* 2002;109:919–929.

| TABLE 13C | | Ultrasound Reference Values for Ulna Length (mm) | | | | | |

WEEKS OF GESTATION	n	PERCENTILES					SD
		3RD	10TH	50TH	90TH	97TH	
12	6	3.9	5.0	7.3	9.6	10.7	1.8
13	13	6.2	7.3	9.6	12.0	13.1	1.8
14	15	8.8	9.9	12.4	14.8	15.9	1.9
15	12	11.6	12.8	15.3	17.8	18.9	1.9
16	11	14.5	15.7	18.2	20.8	22.0	2.0
17	18	17.3	18.6	21.2	23.8	25.0	2.0
18	16	20.1	21.4	24.0	26.7	28.0	2.1
19	24	22.8	24.0	26.8	29.5	30.8	2.1
20	22	25.3	26.6	29.4	32.2	33.5	2.2
21	20	27.8	29.1	32.0	34.8	36.2	2.2
22	20	30.1	31.4	34.4	37.3	38.7	2.3
23	21	32.3	33.7	36.6	39.6	41.0	2.3
24	21	34.3	35.8	38.8	41.9	43.3	2.4
25	22	36.3	37.8	40.9	44.0	45.5	2.4
26	20	38.2	39.7	42.8	46.0	47.5	2.5
27	24	39.9	41.5	44.7	47.9	49.5	2.5
28	20	41.6	43.2	46.5	49.8	51.3	2.6
29	21	43.2	44.8	48.2	51.5	53.1	2.6
30	20	44.7	46.3	49.8	53.2	54.8	2.7
31	27	46.2	47.8	51.3	54.8	56.4	2.7
32	25	47.5	49.2	52.7	56.3	58.0	2.8
33	23	48.8	50.5	54.1	57.7	59.4	2.8
34	17	50.0	51.8	55.4	59.1	60.8	2.9
35	21	51.2	53.0	56.7	60.4	62.2	2.9
36	20	52.3	54.1	57.9	61.7	63.5	3.0
37	19	53.4	55.2	59.1	62.9	64.7	3.0

SD, standard deviation.

Reproduced with permission from Chitty LS, Altman DG BJOG. *An International Journal of Obstetrics and Gynaecology* 2002;109:919–929.

TABLE 13D	Ultrasound Reference Values for Femoral Length (mm)					
WEEKS OF GESTATION	*n*	**PERCENTILES**				
		3RD	**10TH**	**50TH**	**90TH**	**97TH**	**SD**
12	10	4.4	5.5	7.7	10.0	11.1	1.8
13	18	7.5	8.6	10.9	13.3	14.4	1.8
14	18	10.6	11.7	14.1	16.5	17.6	1.9
15	15	13.6	14.7	17.2	19.7	20.8	1.9
16	20	16.5	17.7	20.3	22.8	24.0	2.0
17	23	19.4	20.7	23.3	25.9	27.2	2.1
18	20	22.3	23.6	26.3	29.0	30.2	2.1
19	25	25.1	26.4	29.2	32.0	33.3	2.2
20	22	27.9	29.2	32.1	34.9	36.3	2.2
21	23	30.6	32.0	34.9	37.8	39.2	2.3
22	22	33.2	34.6	37.6	40.6	42.0	2.3
23	22	35.8	37.2	40.3	43.4	44.8	2.4
24	25	38.3	39.8	42.9	46.1	47.6	2.5
25	22	40.8	42.3	45.5	48.7	50.2	2.5
26	22	43.1	44.7	48.0	51.3	52.8	2.6
27	24	45.4	47.0	50.4	53.8	55.3	2.6
28	20	47.6	49.3	52.7	56.2	57.8	2.7
29	22	49.8	51.4	55.0	58.5	60.1	2.8
30	21	51.8	53.5	57.1	60.7	62.4	2.8
31	27	53.8	55.5	59.2	62.9	64.6	2.9
32	26	55.7	57.4	61.2	64.9	66.7	2.9
33	23	57.5	59.3	63.1	66.9	68.7	3.0
34	20	59.2	61.0	64.9	68.8	70.6	3.0
35	22	60.8	62.6	66.6	70.6	72.4	3.1
36	25	62.3	64.2	68.2	72.3	74.1	3.2
37	19	63.7	65.6	69.7	73.8	75.8	3.2
38	21	64.9	66.9	71.1	75.3	77.3	3.3
39	14	66.1	68.1	72.4	76.7	78.7	3.3
40	15	67.2	69.2	73.6	77.9	79.9	3.4
41	26	68.1	70.2	74.6	79.0	81.1	3.5
42	17	69.0	71.1	75.6	80.1	82.2	3.5
Total	649						

SD, standard deviation.

Reproduced with permission from Chitty LS, Altman DG BJOG. *An International Journal of Obstetrics and Gynaecology* 2002;109:919–929.

TABLE 13E	Ultrasound Reference Values for Tibial Length (mm)

WEEKS OF GESTATION	n	PERCENTILES					SD
		3RD	**10TH**	**50TH**	**90TH**	**97TH**	
12	7	4.4	5.4	7.6	9.8	10.5	1.7
13	9	5.8	6.9	9.2	11.4	12.5	1.8
14	14	8.0	9.1	11.4	13.7	14.8	1.8
15	11	10.6	11.7	14.1	16.4	17.6	1.9
16	16	13.3	14.5	16.9	19.4	20.5	1.9
17	20	16.2	17.4	19.9	22.4	23.5	2.0
18	15	19.0	20.2	22.8	23.4	26.6	2.0
19	22	21.8	23.1	25.7	28.3	29.6	2.1
20	20	24.5	25.8	28.5	31.2	32.5	2.1
21	21	27.2	28.5	31.2	34.0	35.3	2.2
22	16	29.7	31.0	33.8	36.7	38.0	2.2
23	19	32.1	33.5	36.4	39.2	40.6	2.3
24	22	34.4	35.8	38.8	41.7	43.1	2.3
25	21	36.6	38.0	41.0	44.1	45.5	2.4
26	20	38.7	40.1	43.2	46.3	47.8	2.4
27	21	40.7	42.2	45.3	48.5	49.9	2.5
28	17	42.6	44.1	47.3	50.5	52.0	2.5
29	21	44.4	45.9	49.2	52.5	54.0	2.6
30	17	46.1	47.7	51.0	54.3	55.9	2.6
31	23	47.7	49.3	52.7	56.1	57.7	2.7
32	21	49.3	50.9	54.4	57.8	59.5	2.7
33	21	50.8	52.4	55.9	59.5	61.1	2.8
34	19	52.2	53.9	57.5	61.0	62.7	2.8
35	19	53.5	55.2	58.9	62.6	64.3	2.9
36	20	54.8	56.6	60.3	64.0	65.7	2.9
37	14	56.0	57.8	61.6	65.4	67.2	3.0
38	18	57.2	59.0	62.9	66.7	68.5	3.0
39	11	58.3	60.2	64.1	68.0	69.8	3.1
40	12	59.4	61.3	65.2	69.2	71.1	3.1
41	22	60.4	62.3	66.4	70.4	72.3	3.2
42	16	61.4	63.3	67.4	71.6	73.5	3.2
Total	544						

SD, standard deviation.

Reproduced with permission from Chitty LS, Altman DG BJOG. *An International Journal of Obstetrics and Gynaecology* 2002;109:919–929.

| TABLE 13F | Ultrasound Reference Values for Fibular Length (mm) | | | | | |

WEEKS OF GESTATION	n	PERCENTILES					SD
		3RD	10TH	50TH	90TH	97TH	
12	5	3.6	4.6	6.8	9.0	10.0	1.7
13	5	5.2	6.2	8.5	10.7	11.8	1.7
14	11	7.4	8.5	10.8	13.1	14.2	1.8
15	10	10.0	11.1	13.5	15.9	17.0	1.9
16	15	12.8	14.0	16.4	18.8	20.0	1.9
17	19	15.6	16.8	19.3	21.8	23.0	2.0
18	14	18.4	19.7	22.2	24.8	26.0	2.0
19	21	21.2	22.4	25.1	27.7	29.0	2.1
20	19	23.9	25.1	27.9	30.6	31.8	2.1
21	21	26.4	27.7	30.5	33.3	34.6	2.2
22	17	28.9	30.2	33.1	35.9	37.3	2.2
23	19	31.2	32.6	35.5	38.5	39.8	2.3
24	24	33.5	34.9	37.9	40.9	42.3	2.3
25	19	35.6	37.0	40.1	43.2	44.6	2.4
26	21	37.6	39.1	42.2	45.4	46.8	2.4
27	21	39.6	41.1	44.3	47.5	49.0	2.5
28	17	41.4	42.9	46.2	49.5	51.0	2.6
29	21	43.1	44.7	48.0	51.4	52.9	2.6
30	20	44.8	46.4	49.8	53.2	54.8	2.7
31	23	46.4	48.0	51.5	54.9	56.6	2.7
32	21	47.9	49.5	53.1	56.6	58.3	2.8
33	20	49.3	51.0	54.6	58.2	59.9	2.8
34	20	50.7	52.4	56.1	59.7	61.5	2.9
35	20	52.0	53.7	57.5	61.2	63.0	2.9
36	20	53.2	55.0	58.8	62.6	64.4	3.0
37	14	54.4	56.2	60.1	64.0	65.8	3.0
38	18	55.5	57.4	61.3	65.3	67.1	3.1
39	10	56.6	58.5	62.5	66.5	68.4	3.1
40	12	57.6	59.5	63.6	67.7	69.6	3.2
41	22	58.6	60.5	64.7	68.9	70.8	3.3
42	16	59.5	61.5	65.8	70.0	72.0	3.3
Total	535						

SD, standard deviation.

Reproduced with permission from Chitty LS, Altman DG BJOG. *An International Journal of Obstetrics and Gynaecology* 2002;109:919–929.

TABLE 14 Prenatal Multipliers for Prediction of Bone Length at Birth

GA (wk)	MULTIPLIER
12	10.00
13	7.28
14	5.53
15	4.33
16	3.65
17	3.14
18	2.84
19	2.54
20	2.30
21	2.11
22	1.97
23	1.82
24	1.71
25	1.62
26	1.54
27	1.47
28	1.41
29	1.35
30	1.31
31	1.26
32	1.21
33	1.18
34	1.15
35	1.12
36	1.09
37	1.07
38	1.05
39	1.03
40	1.01
41	1.01
42	1.00

GA, gestational age.
Adapted with permission from Paley J, Gelman A, Paley D, et al. The prenatal multiplier method for prediction of limb length discrepancy. *Prenat Diagn.* 2005: 25(6):435–438.

TABLE 15 Ultrasound Reference for Foot Length (mm)

WEEKS OF GESTATION	n	3RD	10TH	50TH	90TH	97TH	SD
12	3	5.9	6.8	8.9	10.9	11.8	1.6
13	3	8.5	9.6	11.7	13.9	14.9	1.7
14	7	11.3	12.3	14.6	16.9	18.0	1.8
15	7	14.0	15.2	17.6	20.0	21.2	1.9
16	12	16.8	18.0	20.6	23.2	24.4	2.0
17	16	19.6	20.9	23.6	26.3	27.6	2.1
18	11	22.4	23.7	26.6	29.5	30.8	2.2
19	16	25.2	26.6	29.6	32.6	34.0	2.3
20	15	28.0	29.5	32.6	35.8	37.2	2.5
21	21	30.8	32.3	35.6	38.9	40.4	2.6
22	18	33.5	35.1	38.6	42.0	43.6	2.7
23	18	36.2	37.9	41.5	45.0	46.7	2.8
24	22	38.9	40.7	44.4	48.0	49.8	2.9
25	17	41.5	43.3	47.2	51.0	52.8	3.0
26	20	44.1	46.0	50.0	53.9	55.8	3.1
27	22	46.6	48.6	52.7	56.8	58.7	3.2
28	20	49.1	51.1	55.3	59.6	61.6	3.3
29	20	51.4	53.5	57.9	62.3	64.3	3.4
30	18	53.7	55.8	60.4	64.9	67.0	3.5
31	24	55.9	58.1	62.8	67.4	69.6	3.6
32	22	58.0	60.3	65.1	69.9	72.1	3.8
33	19	60.0	62.3	67.3	72.2	74.5	3.9
34	11	61.9	64.3	69.4	74.5	76.8	4.0
35	15	63.7	66.1	71.4	76.6	79.0	4.1
36	16	65.4	67.9	73.3	78.6	81.1	4.2
37	11	66.9	69.5	75.0	80.5	83.1	4.3
38	12	68.4	71.0	76.7	82.3	85.0	4.4
39	6	69.7	72.4	78.2	84.0	86.7	4.5
40	10	70.9	73.7	79.6	85.5	88.3	4.6
41	10	71.9	74.8	80.8	86.9	89.7	4.7
42	8	72.8	75.7	81.9	88.1	91.0	4.8
Total	450						

SD, standard deviation.
Reproduced with permission from Chitty LS, Altman DG BJOG. *An International Journal of Obstetrics and Gynaecology* 2002;109:919–929.

TABLE 16	Ultrasound Scapular Length (±2 SD) Compared with Gestational Age		

GA (wk)	SCAPULAR LENGTH (mm)		
	−2 SD	MEAN	+2 SD
14	10	10	10
15	11	11	11
16	12	12	12
17	13	13	13
18	14	14	14
19	14	15	15
20	15	16	16
21	16	17	17
22	17	18	18
23	18	19	19
24	19	20	20
25	20	21	21
26	21	22	22
27	22	23	23
28	23	23	24
29	24	24	25
30	25	25	26
31	26	26	27
32	27	27	28
33	28	28	29
34	29	29	30
35	30	30	31
36	31	31	32
37	32	32	32
38	33	33	33
39	34	34	34
40	35	35	35
41	35	36	36
42	36	37	37

GA, gestational age; SD, standard deviation.
Data from Sherer DM, Plessinger MA, Allen TA. Fetal scapular length in the ultrasonographic assessment of gestational age. *J Ultrasound Med.* 1994;13:523–528.

TABLE 17	Ultrasound Reference Values for Clavicle Length (mm)		

GA (wk)	YARKONI[a]		
	PERCENTILES		
	5TH	50TH	95TH
12	—	—	—
13	—	—	—
14	—	—	—
15	11	16	21
16	12	17	22
17	13	18	23
18	14	19	24
19	15	20	25
20	16	21	26
21	17	22	27
22	18	23	28
23	19	24	29
24	20	25	30
25	21	26	31
26	22	27	32
27	23	28	33
28	24	29	34
29	25	30	35
30	26	31	36
31	27	32	37
32	28	33	38
33	29	34	39
34	30	35	40
35	31	36	41
36	32	37	42
37	33	38	43
38	34	39	44
39	35	40	45
40	36	41	46

Used modified formula to fit tabular data. Clavicle = $1.118303 + 0.988639 \times GA$ (SD = 2.920).
[a] Reproduced with permission from Yarkoni S, Schmidt W, Jeanty P, et al. Clavicular measurement: a new biometric parameter for fetal evaluation. *J Ultrasound Med.* 1985;4:467–470.
GA, gestational age; SD, standard deviation.

TABLE 18	Ultrasound Reference Values for Rib Length		

GA (wk)	RIB LENGTH (mm)		
	PERCENTILES		
	5TH	50TH	95TH
14	1.4	2.3	3.1
15	1.6	2.5	3.3
16	1.8	2.7	3.5
17	2.0	2.9	3.7
18	2.2	3.1	3.9
19	2.5	3.3	4.1
20	2.7	3.5	4.3
21	2.9	3.7	4.5
22	3.1	3.9	4.7
23	3.3	4.1	4.9
24	3.5	4.3	5.1
25	3.7	4.5	5.3
26	3.9	4.7	5.5
27	4.1	4.9	5.7
28	4.3	5.1	5.9
29	4.5	5.3	6.1
30	4.7	5.5	6.3
31	4.9	5.7	6.5
32	5.1	5.9	6.7
33	5.3	6.1	6.9
34	5.5	6.3	7.1
35	5.7	6.5	7.3
36	5.9	6.7	7.5
37	6.1	6.9	7.8
38	6.3	7.1	8.0
39	6.5	7.3	8.2
40	6.7	7.5	8.4

Rib length = $-0.5834 + 0.203 \times GA$ (SD = 0.5).
GA, gestational age.
Adapted from Abuhamad AZ, Sedule-Murphy SJ, Kolm P, et al. Prenatal ultrasonographic fetal rib length measurement: correlation with gestational age. *Ultrasound Obstet Gynecol.* 1996;7:193–196.

BRAIN AND FACE MEASUREMENTS

TABLE 19	Ultrasound Transcerebellar Diameter Measurements	
GA (wk)	MEAN (cm)	SD (cm)
15	1.46	0.14
16	1.61	0.1
17	1.71	0.1
18	1.83	0.12
19	1.94	0.11
20	2.03	0.12
21	2.14	0.13
22	2.28	0.18
23	2.43	0.16
24	2.59	0.17
25	2.76	0.16
26	2.91	0.18
27	3.08	0.17
28	3.25	0.18
29	3.41	0.21
30	3.6	0.22
31	3.78	0.24
32	3.92	0.24
33	4.14	0.26
34	4.29	0.27
35	4.47	0.3
36	4.66	0.34
37	4.8	0.32
38	4.98	0.33

GA, gestational age; SD, standard deviation.
Adapted from Chaves MR, Ananth CV, Smulian JC, et al. Fetal transcerebellar diameter nomogram in singleton gestations with special emphasis in the third trimester: a comparison with previously published nomograms. *Am J Obstet Gynecol.* 2003;189:1021.

TABLE 20 **Ultrasound Reference Intervals for the Cerebellar Vermis, Basilar Pons, and the Brain Stem**

| | VERMIS | | | | | | | | |
| | SAGITTAL CC (mm) | | | SAGITTAL AP (mm) | | | SAGITTAL SURFACE AREA (cm²) | | |
GA (wk)	5%	50%	95%	5%	50%	95%	5%	50%	95%
18–19	8.4	9.2	11.3	7.8	8.8	10.6	0.61	0.65	0.80
20–21	10.0	12.2	14.0	8.3	10.0	13.2	0.80	1.06	1.34
22–23	11.3	13.4	15.1	11.2	12.6	15.5	1.07	1.25	1.56
24–25	14.6	15.7	17.3	13.3	14.7	16.9	1.32	1.63	1.87
26–27	15.6	17.3	18.6	13.7	16.2	18.7	1.9	2.20	2.50
28–29	16.4	18.5	22.2	16.1	18.6	20.6	1.73	2.48	2.97
30–31	19.1	20.3	22.8	16.5	19.1	22.8	2.59	3.12	3.52
32–33	19.6	22.3	23.5	18.3	20.2	22.4	2.84	3.27	3.90
34–35	20.6	22.1	25.4	18.6	22.0	23.6	3.12	3.81	4.38
36–37	22.0	24.7	27.1	20.5	24.7	26.0	3.71	4.00	4.78
38–39	24.3	26.5	28.2	18.8	22.7	25.8	4.30	4.64	5.02

| | PONS | | | | | | | | | | BRAIN STEM | | |
| | SAGITTAL CC (mm) | | | SAGITTAL AP (mm) | | | SAGITTAL SURFACE AREA (cm²) | | | | SAGITTAL SURFACE AREA (cm²) | | |
GA (wk)	5%	50%	95%	5%	50%	95%	5%	50%	95%	GA (wk)	5%	50%	95%
18–19	4.5	5.5	6.8	3.4	4.2	4.7	0.13	0.22	0.28	18–19	1.08	1.26	1.66
20–21	4.8	6.7	8.4	4.3	5.2	6.7	0.22	0.30	0.39	20–21	1.51	1.75	1.98
22–23	5.8	7.1	9.3	3.6	5.2	6.5	0.30	0.40	0.56	22–23	1.66	2.14	2.57
24–25	7.4	8.6	10.9	5.4	6.3	8.0	0.41	0.48	0.54	24–25	1.89	2.34	2.92
26–27	6.4	9.1	10.9	4.7	5.9	7.7	0.40	0.69	0.86	26–27	2.62	3.09	3.61
28–29	9.3	10.1	14.1	5.8	7.6	9.5	0.50	0.69	0.78	28–29	2.85	3.74	4.40
30–31	10.0	12.3	13.9	6.7	7.9	9.9	0.62	0.83	0.98	30–31	3.15	4.00	4.58
32–33	11.2	13.1	15.7	7.9	8.9	10.5	0.75	0.99	1.23	32–33	3.59	4.36	5.08
34–35	11.5	13.5	15.1	7.6	8.6	10.3	0.92	1.11	1.37	34–35	3.59	4.72	5.56
36–37	12.1	13.7	14.4	6.8	8.9	10.1	1.00	1.28	1.35	36–37	5.04	5.26	5.59
38–39	12.5	13.4	14.0	9.3	9.4	10.1	1.20	1.51	1.67	38–39	4.76	5.02	5.57

AP, anteroposterior; CC, craniocaudal; GA, gestational age.
Reproduced from Ginath S, Lerman-Sagie T, Haratz Krajden K, et al. The fetal vermis, pons and brainstem: normal longitudinal development as shown by dedicated neurosonography. *J Matern Fetal Neonatal Med.* 2013;26:757–762, with permission.

TABLE 21   **MRI Measurements of the Fetal Brain**

FRONTO-OCCIPITAL DIAMETER (FOD)

Maximum Distance between Frontal and Occipital Lobes (Sagittal)

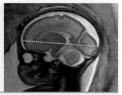

GA	COUNT	MEAN	SD	MIN	MAX	MEDIAN	10TH (%)	90TH (%)
16	21	35.05	1.62	32.17	37.90	34.95	32.90	37.51
17	19	38.23	1.72	35.97	42.21	38.20	36.35	41.64
18	22	43.54	2.17	38.64	47.80	43.65	41.14	46.43
19	21	47.04	2.11	42.20	50.51	46.89	44.20	49.50
20	33	51.09	2.47	47.11	56.42	50.95	48.16	55.04
21	22	56.75	2.52	50.70	61.00	56.50	53.81	60.60
22	23	59.24	2.74	54.30	64.70	58.70	56.00	63.50
23	20	64.54	1.76	61.67	69.10	64.37	62.42	66.80
24	23	66.71	1.92	63.81	71.40	66.46	64.67	68.50
25	24	68.94	2.54	64.30	73.00	69.86	64.42	72.15
26	20	75.27	2.89	70.40	81.60	75.39	70.83	78.56
27	16	77.65	3.06	72.68	84.00	77.87	73.49	82.30
28	20	79.99	3.90	72.00	88.05	79.95	75.23	85.14
29	17	83.94	3.03	78.50	88.00	84.20	79.07	87.95
30	16	87.60	3.37	81.00	94.20	87.23	83.00	92.60
31	14	91.80	4.36	82.00	100.00	92.65	87.05	97.10
32	17	92.99	1.87	89.00	96.41	92.91	90.40	95.19
33	19	93.91	4.29	86.20	101.89	94.90	87.20	99.19
34	15	99.92	4.15	90.00	106.64	100.70	92.30	105.00
35	18	101.12	5.15	91.80	110.58	100.92	93.17	108.90
36	16	102.10	4.04	93.60	108.00	103.60	97.10	107.00
37+	14	104.78	4.23	98.30	111.15	104.49	100.00	111.00

CORPUS CALLOSUM LENGTH (ANTERIOR TO POSTERIOR)

Between Genu and Splenium (Midline Sagittal)

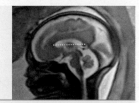

GA	COUNT	MEAN	SD	MIN	MAX	MEDIAN	10TH (%)	90TH (%)
16	21	7.37	0.83	5.32	8.65	7.24	6.31	8.44
17	19	9.41	1.03	7.59	12.23	9.36	8.33	10.61
18	21	13.20	2.18	10.14	17.70	13.05	10.61	16.40
19	19	16.01	2.18	12.47	19.90	15.49	12.53	19.40
20	31	19.50	1.28	17.24	22.50	19.81	17.74	20.60
21	19	22.77	1.43	20.50	26.70	22.75	21.10	24.60
22	23	23.66	1.92	20.31	27.90	23.49	21.75	26.60
23	20	27.24	1.84	23.50	30.20	27.42	24.61	29.75
24	22	27.80	1.46	24.64	30.90	27.82	26.35	29.50
25	22	29.64	2.33	27.00	35.00	29.19	27.19	34.27
26	18	31.72	2.28	26.47	35.40	31.58	29.08	35.00
27	17	32.05	2.37	25.79	35.00	31.93	29.36	35.00
28	18	34.32	1.87	31.03	37.00	34.41	31.34	36.89
29	17	36.03	2.10	32.43	41.50	36.50	33.00	37.72
30	16	36.37	1.54	32.00	38.75	36.85	34.38	38.00
31	14	37.61	2.73	33.90	42.00	36.75	34.30	41.70
32	18	38.13	2.58	32.30	44.10	38.08	35.38	41.26
33	18	39.76	2.20	37.15	44.22	38.92	37.43	43.42
34	14	41.20	2.77	36.80	47.95	40.85	37.60	44.10
35	18	41.38	2.60	37.62	45.98	41.13	37.90	45.79
36	16	41.97	3.14	35.10	48.00	40.95	39.35	47.80
37+	14	44.60	2.38	40.80	48.21	45.14	40.90	47.00

TABLE 21   MRI Measurements of the Fetal Brain (*continued*)

CEREBRAL BIPARIETAL DIAMETER

Maximum Transverse Diameter of Brain at Level of Sylvian Fissure and Third Ventricle (Coronal)

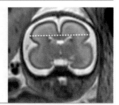

GA	COUNT	MEAN	SD	MIN	MAX	MEDIAN	10TH (%)	90TH (%)
16	21	29.10	1.30	26.27	31.63	29.19	27.69	30.94
17	19	31.17	1.11	29.32	33.46	30.83	29.74	32.76
18	22	34.05	1.96	31.27	40.00	33.99	31.88	35.65
19	20	36.13	1.86	33.30	39.31	35.98	34.28	38.84
20	33	38.52	1.88	34.63	43.00	38.47	36.00	41.01
21	21	41.84	2.64	37.20	47.70	41.47	38.20	45.20
22	23	44.25	1.74	41.20	48.50	43.80	42.45	47.00
23	20	47.52	0.99	45.00	49.20	47.59	46.11	48.81
24	23	49.15	1.50	47.00	53.20	48.97	47.40	50.75
25	24	51.10	3.89	42.50	61.60	51.38	45.80	54.30
26	20	54.99	2.61	49.54	59.80	54.60	52.25	58.85
27	17	58.69	3.56	53.90	67.40	57.80	53.98	66.50
28	19	60.95	2.18	58.00	65.69	60.47	58.00	65.02
29	18	64.86	2.49	58.25	68.90	65.23	62.00	68.14
30	16	66.76	2.25	62.00	71.10	66.58	64.23	69.70
31	14	70.03	3.25	65.59	75.10	70.25	66.00	75.05
32	17	73.31	2.55	70.10	79.70	72.54	70.28	77.90
33	19	74.63	2.24	71.40	79.40	74.78	71.40	78.40
34	15	79.93	4.09	71.80	86.50	80.88	74.00	85.19
35	19	80.05	3.47	74.80	86.00	80.00	75.00	85.64
36	16	82.66	4.25	75.90	90.20	81.30	77.00	90.10
37+	14	83.30	5.73	74.20	96.00	83.55	75.00	89.97

BONE BIPARIETAL DIAMETER

Maximum Transverse Diameter Outside to Inside Skull at Level of Sylvian Fissure and Third Ventricle (Coronal)

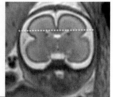

GA	COUNT	MEAN	SD	MIN	MAX	MEDIAN	10TH (%)	90TH (%)
16	21	33.63	1.92	30.56	37.72	33.95	31.71	35.92
17	19	35.79	1.58	32.90	39.32	35.38	34.14	38.58
18	22	39.29	2.36	35.01	45.00	38.86	36.39	42.65
19	20	42.51	1.92	39.31	46.02	42.18	39.86	45.63
20	33	45.98	2.23	40.25	49.62	46.29	43.00	49.30
21	22	50.35	2.77	45.70	56.30	50.25	47.00	53.80
22	23	52.17	3.68	42.60	59.40	53.14	48.50	54.46
23	20	56.73	2.31	53.30	62.90	56.41	54.10	60.52
24	23	57.68	2.37	54.42	63.30	57.56	54.72	60.12
25	24	60.80	4.17	52.40	70.60	61.36	55.40	65.11
26	20	64.73	3.77	57.10	71.60	65.61	60.07	69.14
27	16	67.19	3.01	61.40	72.00	67.00	63.63	71.76
28	18	69.74	3.32	64.80	76.90	68.86	66.25	75.05
29	18	73.10	3.32	63.92	78.90	73.60	69.20	76.93
30	16	75.03	2.84	70.00	80.20	75.03	70.00	79.70
31	14	78.77	3.61	72.10	86.10	78.33	74.00	85.00
32	17	81.86	4.14	76.00	93.40	80.82	76.50	85.40
33	19	82.96	2.56	78.02	87.20	83.64	78.45	86.80
34	14	85.98	3.86	78.20	91.89	87.25	80.00	89.48
35	19	86.43	4.48	78.20	93.50	86.05	79.93	93.00
36	16	90.20	6.77	75.50	103.30	88.60	84.80	100.70
37+	14	90.48	6.94	76.00	102.00	92.10	79.00	98.30

(*continued*)

TABLE 21	MRI Measurements of the Fetal Brain (*continued*)

VERMIS CRANIOCAUDAL

Maximum Craniocaudal Dimension of Vermis, Parallel to Long Axis of Brainstem (Midline Sagittal)

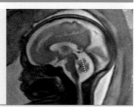

GA	COUNT	MEAN	SD	MIN	MAX	MEDIAN	10TH (%)	90TH (%)
16	21	4.83	0.49	3.94	5.89	4.83	4.22	5.55
17	19	5.76	0.52	4.67	6.52	5.61	5.16	6.52
18	22	6.68	0.57	5.40	7.89	6.57	6.08	7.66
19	19	7.10	0.84	5.30	8.40	7.13	5.90	8.14
20	33	8.39	1.04	5.80	11.10	8.14	7.40	9.70
21	21	9.25	1.44	6.10	11.30	9.40	7.30	10.80
22	23	10.33	0.93	7.90	11.65	10.33	8.90	11.35
23	19	11.50	1.22	8.10	13.06	11.65	10.00	13.06
24	22	12.16	0.73	10.30	13.34	12.24	11.50	13.01
25	24	12.58	1.03	10.30	14.34	12.57	11.50	13.84
26	20	13.45	1.13	11.60	15.70	13.44	12.06	15.10
27	17	14.95	0.87	13.32	17.00	15.00	13.90	15.84
28	20	15.36	1.28	12.00	17.22	15.62	13.40	16.62
29	17	16.13	1.28	14.50	19.83	15.97	14.60	18.00
30	16	16.81	1.48	14.00	19.80	16.87	15.00	18.79
31	14	17.52	0.86	16.10	19.00	17.40	16.40	18.77
32	18	18.67	1.14	16.40	21.20	18.88	16.80	19.78
33	19	19.13	1.20	16.40	20.82	19.48	17.00	20.73
34	14	20.00	1.26	16.00	21.33	20.20	19.01	21.20
35	17	20.07	1.23	17.00	21.80	20.50	17.60	21.40
36	16	21.94	3.06	17.00	29.70	21.73	17.21	27.20
37+	14	22.50	1.86	19.90	27.00	22.19	20.00	24.80

VERMIS ANTERIOR TO POSTERIOR

Maximum Anterior to Posterior Diameter of Vermis Perpendicular to Craniocaudal Measure (Midline Sagittal)

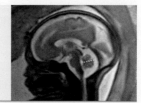

GA	COUNT	MEAN	SD	MIN	MAX	MEDIAN	10TH (%)	90TH (%)
16	21	3.53	0.34	2.88	4.19	3.52	3.16	3.94
17	19	4.15	0.29	3.52	4.75	4.12	3.73	4.55
18	22	4.85	0.36	4.20	5.58	4.89	4.34	5.31
19	19	5.37	0.58	4.10	6.11	5.58	4.38	5.89
20	33	6.07	0.59	4.50	6.90	6.07	5.30	6.87
21	20	6.63	0.74	5.10	7.90	6.86	5.56	7.54
22	22	7.22	0.43	6.59	8.30	7.23	6.59	7.70
23	17	7.75	0.58	6.50	8.59	7.73	7.00	8.50
24	22	8.20	0.50	7.41	9.38	8.20	7.50	8.90
25	24	9.17	1.02	7.90	12.50	8.93	8.20	10.70
26	20	9.59	1.00	7.70	11.30	9.60	7.97	10.80
27	17	10.20	1.04	8.49	12.20	10.14	9.02	11.80
28	20	10.70	1.18	8.64	14.00	10.48	9.44	12.31
29	17	11.54	0.90	9.70	13.08	11.72	10.10	12.60
30	16	11.65	0.80	10.48	13.00	11.65	10.48	12.93
31	14	12.48	1.29	10.09	15.00	12.55	10.56	14.00
32	18	12.61	1.11	10.80	14.60	12.34	11.00	14.60
33	19	14.00	1.12	11.60	15.80	14.11	12.58	15.41
34	13	14.68	0.88	12.22	15.80	15.00	13.70	15.38
35	16	14.82	0.93	13.00	16.90	14.65	13.70	16.06
36	16	15.98	1.37	13.26	18.40	16.05	13.42	18.20
37+	14	17.00	2.15	13.80	21.40	16.45	14.40	21.20

TABLE 21   MRI Measurements of the Fetal Brain (*continued*)

TRANSVERSE CEREBELLAR DIAMETER

Maximum Transverse Diameter of Cerebellum (Axial or Coronal)

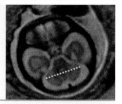

GA	COUNT	MEAN	SD	MIN	MAX	MEDIAN	10TH (%)	90TH (%)
16	21	14.72	0.75	13.10	16.47	14.54	13.94	15.64
17	19	15.84	0.71	14.86	17.27	15.66	15.09	17.00
18	22	16.96	1.22	12.70	19.60	17.15	15.99	18.00
19	20	17.83	1.13	15.70	19.57	18.03	15.95	19.22
20	32	19.56	1.26	17.30	22.80	19.48	18.20	21.20
21	20	20.61	1.27	18.00	22.70	20.82	18.70	22.17
22	23	22.29	1.50	19.60	25.00	22.30	20.30	24.31
23	20	24.79	1.26	22.00	27.22	24.75	23.05	26.45
24	22	25.27	1.64	22.02	29.30	25.17	23.50	27.35
25	24	27.62	2.22	22.80	33.40	27.33	25.00	29.90
26	19	28.50	1.32	25.70	30.85	28.51	26.40	30.30
27	16	30.61	1.62	27.60	34.00	30.48	27.80	32.88
28	20	33.03	1.43	30.00	36.47	32.92	31.22	34.77
29	18	35.18	1.53	32.20	37.40	35.36	32.90	36.99
30	16	36.20	2.25	32.00	40.08	36.28	33.00	39.81
31	14	38.71	1.98	35.00	42.20	38.84	36.00	41.00
32	17	40.80	2.30	35.50	44.50	41.20	37.09	43.62
33	18	41.58	1.90	37.70	45.03	41.77	38.50	44.10
34	15	44.60	3.34	38.40	49.80	43.70	41.00	49.80
35	19	45.70	2.11	40.60	49.40	45.90	43.00	49.00
36	16	48.37	3.51	41.10	53.70	48.73	43.00	52.80
37+	14	49.68	3.39	43.90	56.00	49.06	46.40	55.00

PONS ANTERIOR TO POSTERIOR

Maximum Anterior to Posterior Diameter of Pons (Midline Sagittal)

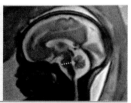

GA	COUNT	MEAN	SD	MIN	MAX	MEDIAN	10TH (%)	90TH (%)
16	21	4.95	0.37	4.08	5.86	4.88	4.58	5.24
17	19	5.37	0.24	5.01	5.89	5.31	5.06	5.86
18	21	6.06	0.50	4.90	7.03	6.09	5.47	6.67
19	18	6.23	0.65	5.00	7.73	6.18	5.50	7.34
20	33	6.59	0.59	5.10	7.93	6.59	5.90	7.37
21	19	6.99	0.73	5.60	8.57	7.00	6.10	8.10
22	20	7.07	0.71	6.00	8.39	7.09	6.05	8.01
23	19	7.98	0.65	7.00	9.62	7.90	7.00	9.32
24	22	8.18	0.71	7.13	9.65	7.97	7.34	9.32
25	24	8.50	0.76	7.40	10.10	8.40	7.60	9.78
26	19	9.09	0.62	7.40	10.10	8.96	8.40	9.97
27	16	9.36	1.05	7.10	11.50	9.48	7.50	10.90
28	20	10.28	1.00	7.20	12.00	10.46	9.20	11.36
29	17	11.00	0.76	9.70	12.70	10.98	9.83	12.01
30	15	11.50	0.66	10.76	13.10	11.25	10.90	12.56
31	14	11.99	0.70	10.20	13.12	12.24	11.00	12.58
32	18	12.30	1.19	9.20	14.90	12.47	11.20	13.70
33	19	12.48	1.14	9.70	15.00	12.54	10.90	14.10
34	14	12.85	0.82	10.90	14.19	13.05	11.70	14.10
35	17	13.38	0.67	11.90	14.80	13.40	12.50	14.20
36	16	13.60	1.58	10.90	16.40	13.92	11.00	15.50
37+	14	13.74	1.36	10.30	15.50	13.67	11.90	15.20

(continued)

TABLE 21	MRI Measurements of the Fetal Brain (*continued*)

PONS CRANIOCAUDAL

Maximum Craniocaudal Dimension of Pons (Midline Sagittal)

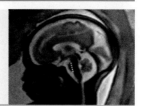

GA	COUNT	MEAN	SD	MIN	MAX	MEDIAN	10TH (%)	90TH (%)
16	21	4.89	0.58	4.01	5.98	5.01	4.14	5.47
17	19	5.38	0.69	4.17	6.55	5.24	4.35	6.38
18	20	5.98	0.63	4.60	7.08	6.03	5.18	6.83
19	16	5.98	0.67	4.60	7.11	6.09	5.20	7.00
20	30	6.55	0.76	4.90	7.89	6.57	5.45	7.53
21	17	6.79	1.27	4.70	9.40	6.99	4.70	8.40
22	23	7.17	1.01	5.10	9.50	7.18	5.90	8.40
23	19	8.12	1.08	5.70	9.83	8.00	6.70	9.62
24	19	8.42	0.76	6.40	9.38	8.60	7.00	9.38
25	23	8.82	1.60	6.30	13.70	8.90	6.80	10.20
26	19	9.15	2.31	4.60	13.60	9.37	5.40	12.10
27	16	10.14	1.40	8.50	14.30	9.89	8.60	12.30
28	20	10.53	0.75	9.14	11.93	10.45	9.58	11.75
29	17	11.15	0.75	9.60	12.80	11.06	9.90	12.00
30	15	11.49	1.12	9.60	14.10	11.27	10.10	13.40
31	13	12.27	1.05	10.00	13.80	12.40	10.79	13.60
32	18	12.31	0.94	10.00	13.80	12.49	10.61	13.65
33	19	12.65	1.17	9.80	13.88	13.01	10.00	13.80
34	14	13.03	1.16	11.00	15.90	12.96	11.60	14.34
35	16	13.12	0.89	11.30	14.70	12.89	11.90	14.20
36	16	13.60	1.98	8.90	16.70	13.75	10.20	16.20
37+	14	14.42	1.30	10.80	15.90	14.50	13.26	15.90

INDICES AND VENTRICLES

	CRANIOCEREBRAL	CORPUS CALLOSUM/BRAIN	THIRD VENTRICLE			FOURTH VENTRICLE		
	Bone BPD–Cerebral BPD/Bone BPD	Length Corpus Callosum/FOD	Maximum Transverse Diameter (Coronal)			Maximum Anterior to Posterior (Midline Sagittal)		
GA	INDEX	INDEX	COUNT	MEAN	SD	COUNT	MEAN	SD
16	13.48	21.02	21	1.84	0.44	21	2.54	0.61
17	12.92	24.62	19	1.85	0.44	19	2.78	0.40
18	13.34	30.33	22	1.97	0.55	22	3.01	0.75
19	15.01	34.04	17	1.93	0.42	20	2.49	0.54
20	16.23	38.17	32	1.74	0.46	33	2.55	0.73
21	16.88	40.12	21	1.97	0.47	20	2.72	0.57
22	15.19	39.95	22	1.81	0.47	23	2.78	0.60
23	16.24	42.21	20	1.93	0.43	19	2.84	0.58
24	14.80	41.67	23	1.93	0.50	22	2.91	0.53
25	15.96	42.99	24	1.87	0.37	24	3.03	0.74
26	15.04	42.15	20	1.93	0.43	19	3.22	0.71
27	12.64	41.27	17	2.09	0.52	17	3.04	0.82
28	12.60	42.91	20	2.04	0.39	20	3.72	0.63
29	11.26	42.92	17	2.05	0.43	17	3.53	0.80
30	11.02	41.52	16	2.00	0.70	16	3.45	0.64
31	11.10	40.97	14	2.14	0.70	14	3.29	0.70
32	10.45	41.00	18	1.99	0.57	18	3.90	0.75
33	10.04	42.34	19	2.64	0.51	19	4.14	0.56
34	7.04	41.23	15	2.44	0.56	14	3.70	0.81
35	7.38	40.92	19	2.33	0.68	17	3.89	0.96
36	8.36	41.11	16	2.42	0.70	16	4.26	0.68
37+	7.93	42.56	14	2.31	0.83	14	4.43	0.93
Total			426	2.06	0.53	424	3.28	0.68

TABLE 21   MRI Measurements of the Fetal Brain (*continued*)

INDEX AND SPACES

	INTERHEMISPHERIC (IHD)	CISTERNA MAGNA AP	CISTERNA MAGNA CC
	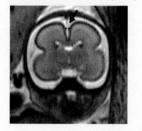	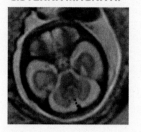	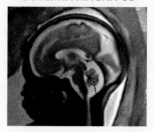

	IHD/Cerebral BPD	Width of IH Space at the level of the BPD (Coronal)			Diameter Posterior Cerebellum to Skull (Axial)			Inferior Vermis to Inferior Skull (Sagittal)		
GA	INDEX	COUNT	MEAN	SD	COUNT	MEAN	SD	COUNT	MEAN	SD
16	8.17	21	2.38	0.65	21	4.33	1.38	21	4.07	0.87
17	8.28	19	2.58	0.58	19	5.75	1.41	19	4.72	0.85
18	7.45	22	2.54	0.50	22	5.59	1.63	19	5.05	1.21
19	7.57	21	2.73	0.45	20	5.88	1.93	13	5.31	1.04
20	6.41	33	2.47	0.78	32	5.74	1.56	23	5.71	1.28
21	6.47	22	2.71	0.76	21	5.25	1.52	7	5.30	1.27
22	5.63	22	2.49	0.75	23	5.72	1.15	11	6.10	1.17
23	5.30	20	2.52	0.71	20	5.41	1.25	10	6.24	0.74
24	4.95	22	2.43	0.52	22	5.52	1.71	17	6.60	1.25
25	4.59	24	2.35	0.67	24	5.67	1.38	14	6.18	1.19
26	4.76	20	2.62	0.78	20	5.42	1.79	8	6.46	1.6
27	3.92	17	2.30	0.53	17	6.02	1.10	10	6.06	1.01
28	4.27	20	2.60	0.55	20	6.74	2.10	18	7.03	1.98
29	3.77	18	2.45	0.64	17	6.89	2.05	13	7.52	1.32
30	3.52	16	2.35	0.62	15	6.03	1.75	11	6.81	1.24
31	3.32	14	2.33	0.71	13	6.25	2.02	11	6.82	1.18
32	3.34	18	2.45	0.55	18	6.28	2.09	12	7.01	1.12
33	3.40	19	2.54	0.51	19	6.67	2.04	11	7.77	1.46
34	3.27	15	2.62	0.54	14	6.19	1.50	9	7.20	1.32
35	3.33	19	2.67	0.64	18	5.54	2.14	12	7.49	1.15
36	2.66	16	2.20	0.73	15	5.07	1.97	7	7.07	1.17
37+	2.98	14	2.49	0.80	14	5.73	1.67	10	7.30	1.82
Total		432	2.49	0.64	424	5.80	1.69	286	6.36	1.24

AP, anteroposterior; BPD, biparietal diameter; CC, craniocaudal; FOD, fronto-occipital diameter; GA, gestational age; IHD, interhemispheric distance; SD, standard deviation.

Measurements from normal imaging fetuses, small lung lesions, abdominal pathology. Studies measured by Egloff A, Bulas D and Kline-Fath, BM. Special thanks to Thomas Fath and Paul Horn for charting and statistical analysis.

TABLE 22A	Ultrasound Reference Values for Binocular Diameter, Interocular Diameter, and Ocular Diameter by Gestational Age											

	IOD (mm)			OD (mm)			TAL (mm)			BOD (mm)		
GA	95%	50%	5%	95%	50%	5%	95%	50%	5%	95%	50%	5%
14	12.2	8.9	5.5	8.2	5.9	3.7	6.8	5.5	4.4	27.9	23.5	19.1
15	12.6	9.2	5.9	8.5	6.2	3.9	7.1	5.8	4.7	28.8	24.4	20.0
16	13.1	9.7	6.3	8.8	6.6	4.3	7.7	6.2	5.0	30.1	25.7	21.3
17	13.6	10.2	6.9	9.3	7.0	4.8	8.3	6.8	5.5	31.6	27.2	22.9
18	14.2	10.9	7.5	9.8	7.5	5.3	9.1	7.4	6.0	33.4	29.0	24.6
19	14.7	11.3	8.0	10.2	7.9	5.7	9.7	7.9	6.4	34.7	30.3	25.9
20	15.5	12.1	8.7	10.8	8.5	6.3	10.7	8.7	7.0	36.8	32.4	28.0
21	16.0	12.6	9.2	11.2	8.9	6.7	11.4	9.2	7.5	38.2	33.8	29.4
22	16.4	13.0	9.7	11.6	9.3	7.0	12.0	9.7	7.8	39.4	35.0	30.7
23	17.0	13.6	10.2	12.0	9.7	7.5	12.7	10.3	8.3	40.9	36.5	32.2
24	17.6	14.3	10.9	12.6	10.3	8.0	13.5	11.0	8.9	42.8	38.4	34.0
25	18.1	14.8	11.4	13.0	10.7	8.4	14.2	11.5	9.3	44.2	39.8	35.4
26	18.8	15.4	12.0	13.5	11.2	9.0	15.0	12.1	9.8	45.9	41.5	37.2
27	19.3	15.9	12.5	13.9	11.6	9.4	15.5	12.6	10.2	47.3	42.9	38.6
28	19.7	16.4	13.0	14.3	12.0	9.7	16.1	13.0	10.5	48.6	44.2	39.8
29	20.2	16.9	13.5	14.7	12.4	10.1	16.6	13.4	10.9	50.0	45.6	41.2
30	20.8	17.5	14.1	15.2	12.9	10.6	17.2	13.9	11.3	51.7	47.3	42.9
31	21.4	18.0	14.7	15.6	13.3	11.1	17.7	14.3	11.6	53.2	48.8	44.5
32	22.0	18.6	15.3	16.1	13.8	11.6	18.1	14.7	11.9	54.9	50.5	46.1
33	22.5	19.2	15.8	16.5	14.3	12.0	18.5	14.9	12.1	56.4	52.0	47.6
34	23.2	19.8	16.4	17.0	14.8	12.5	18.8	15.2	12.3	58.1	53.7	49.3
35	23.4	20.0	16.6	17.2	15.0	12.7	18.9	15.3	12.4	58.7	54.3	49.9
36	24.2	20.8	17.4	17.9	15.6	13.3	19.1	15.5	12.5	60.9	56.5	52.1
37	24.7	21.3	17.9	18.3	16.0	13.7	19.2	15.5	12.6	62.2	57.8	53.4
38	25.3	21.9	18.5	18.8	16.5	14.2	19.2	15.5	12.5	63.9	59.5	55.1
39	25.7	22.4	19.0	19.1	16.9	14.6	19.2	15.5	12.5	65.2	60.8	56.4
40	26.2	22.8	19.5	19.5	17.3	15.0	19.1	15.4	12.4	66.6	62.2	57.8
41	26.9	23.5	20.1	20.1	17.8	15.5	18.9	15.2	12.2	68.5	64.1	59.6

Mean (50th centile) and 90% reference interval for measurements of the BOD, TAL, OD, and IOD of the fetal or bit calculated for individual values of gestational age from 14 to 41 gestational weeks.
BOD, binocular distance; IOD, intraocular distance; OD, ocular diameter; TAL, total axial length.
From Feldman N, Melcer Y, Levinsohn-Tavor O, et al. Prenatal ultrasound charts of orbital total axial length measurement (TAL): a valuable data for correct fetal eye malformation assessment. *Prenat Diagn*. 2015;35:558–563.

TABLE 22B — Ultrasound Reference Values for Diameter of Fetal Lens (mm)

GA (wk)	MEAN	PERCENTILES		
		10TH	50TH	90TH
15	2.5 ± 0.3	2.1	2.5	2.9
16	2.7 ± 0.2	2.5	2.8	3.0
17	3.1 ± 0.2	2.8	3.1	3.4
18	3.2 ± 0.2	3.0	3.2	3.5
19	3.7 ± 0.2	3.3	3.7	4.1
20	3.8 ± 0.3	3.4	3.8	4.1
21	3.9 ± 0.3	3.6	3.9	4.2
22	4.0 ± 0.2	3.7	4.0	4.2
23	4.0 ± 0.3	3.5	4.1	4.4
24	4.1 ± 0.3	3.8	4.2	4.4
25	4.2 ± 0.2	4.0	4.3	4.5
26	4.3 ± 0.2	4.0	4.4	4.6
27	4.5 ± 0.2	4.1	4.5	4.8
28	4.6 ± 0.3	4.3	4.6	5.0
29	4.7 ± 0.3	4.3	4.6	5.0
30	4.7 ± 0.3	4.3	4.7	5.0
31	4.8 ± 0.3	4.4	4.8	5.2
32	4.9 ± 0.2	4.5	5.0	5.3
33	5.1 ± 0.3	4.8	5.1	5.4
34	5.2 ± 0.2	4.9	5.1	5.5
35	5.3 ± 0.3	5.0	5.2	5.7
36	5.3 ± 0.2	5.0	5.4	5.7
37	5.4 ± 0.3	4.9	5.5	5.8
38	5.6 ± 0.4	5.0	5.7	6.1
39	5.7 ± 0.3	5.2	5.7	6.1
40	5.8 ± 0.3	5.3	5.8	6.2

GA, gestational age.
From Sukonpan K, Phupong V. A biometric study of the fetal orbit and lens in normal pregnancies. *J Clin Ultrasound.* 2009;37:69–74.

TABLE 22C — Ultrasound Reference Values for Circumference of Fetal Lens (mm)

GA	MEAN	PERCENTILES		
		10TH	50TH	90TH
15	8.5 ± 0.7	7.8	8.3	9.8
16	9.1 ± 0.6	8.4	9.0	9.9
17	10.4 ± 0.8	9.7	10.2	11.8
18	10.9 ± 0.8	10.2	10.7	11.9
19	12.3 ± 0.9	11.1	11.9	13.6
20	13.0 ± 0.7	12.0	12.9	14.0
21	13.3 ± 0.8	12.2	13.2	14.5
22	13.4 ± 0.7	12.5	13.5	14.7
23	13.6 ± 0.7	12.7	13.7	14.8
24	14.2 ± 0.6	13.6	14.2	15.3
25	14.4 ± 0.6	13.6	14.3	15.4
26	14.6 ± 0.5	13.9	14.6	15.5
27	15.2 ± 0.6	14.4	15.2	15.9
28	15.6 ± 0.7	14.9	15.6	16.5
29	15.9 ± 0.7	14.9	15.9	16.8
30	16.2 ± 0.7	15.5	1601	17.3
31	16.6 ± 0.6	15.7	16.6	17.4
32	16.9 ± 0.5	16.3	16.9	17.9
33	17.3 ± 0.5	16.6	17.3	18.0
34	17.6 ± 0.5	16.9	17.7	12.1
35	18.2 ± 0.6	17.6	18.1	19.1
36	18.4 ± 0.6	17.7	18.3	19.4
37	18.8 ± 0.6	18.2	18.8	19.5
38	19.1 ± 0.5	18.4	18.9	20.0
39	19.3 ± 0.6	18.4	19.3	20.0
40	19.6 ± 0.6	18.9	19.4	20.6

From Sukonpan K, Phupong V. A biometric study of the fetal orbit and lens in normal pregnancies. *J Clin Ultrasound.* 2009;37:69–74.

TABLE 22D Ultrasound Reference Values for Surface Area of Fetal Lens (mm²)

GA	MEAN	PERCENTILES		
		10TH	50TH	90TH
15	5.8 ± 0.9	5.1	5.3	7.1
16	6.7 ± 1.0	6.0	6.2	8.0
17	8.5 ± 1.0	7.7	8.1	10.8
18	9.6 ± 1.3	8.0	9.0	11.0
19	11.8 ± 1.8	10.0	11.0	14.0
20	13.4 ± 1.4	11.7	13.0	15.0
21	13.9 ± 1.6	12.0	14.0	16.5
22	14.2 ± 1.3	13.0	14.0	16.7
23	14.7 ± 1.5	13.0	15.0	16.8
24	15.9 ± 1.3	14.7	16.0	18.0
25	16.4 ± 1.1	15.0	16.0	18.0
26	16.8 ± 1.1	15.3	17.0	18.0
27	18.0 ± 1.2	16.3	18.0	19.7
28	19.2 ± 1.5	18.0	19.0	21.0
29	19.9 ± 1.5	18.0	20.0	22.0
30	20.7 ± 1.4	19.0	20.1	23.2
31	21.6 ± 1.2	19.6	22.0	23.0
32	22.8 ± 1.4	21.0	23.0	25.0
33	23.5 ± 1.2	22.0	24.0	25.0
34	24.2 ± 1.3	23.0	24.1	26.0
35	26.0 ± 1.5	24.0	25.5	28.7
36	26.4 ± 1.9	24.0	26.0	29.7
37	27.6 ± 2.0	26.0	27.0	29.7
38	28.5 ± 1.7	26.3	28.0	31.4
39	29.1 ± 1.6	26.3	29.5	31.5
40	29.8 ± 2.1	27.3	29.7	33.0

From Sukonpan K, Phupong V. A biometric study of the fetal orbit and lens in normal pregnancies. *J Clin Ultrasound*. 2009;37:69–74.

TABLE 22E Ultrasound Reference Ranges for Fetal Optic Tract Diameter (in mm)

GA	PERCENTILE				
	3RD	5TH	50TH	95TH	97TH
21	1.6	1.7	2.0	2.3	2.3
22	1.7	1.8	2.1	2.4	2.4
23	1.8	1.9	2.2	2.5	2.5
24	1.9	2.0	2.3	2.6	2.6
25	2.0	2.1	2.4	2.6	2.7
26	2.1	2.2	2.5	2.7	2.8
27	2.2	2.3	2.5	2.8	2.9
28	2.3	2.4	2.6	2.9	3.0
29	2.4	2.4	2.7	3.0	3.1
30	2.5	2.5	2.8	3.1	3.2
31	2.6	2.6	2.9	3.2	3.3
32	2.7	2.7	3.0	3.3	3.3
33	2.8	2.8	3.1	3.4	3.4
34	2.9	2.9	3.2	3.5	3.5
35	2.9	3.0	3.3	3.6	3.6
36	3.0	3.1	3.4	3.7	3.7

GA in weeks. Reproduced from Bault JP, Salomon LJ, Guibaud L, et al. Role of three-dimensional ultrasound measurement of the optic tract in fetuses with agenesis of the septum pellucidum. Ultrasound Obstet Gynecol. 2011;37(5):570–575. Copyright © International Society of Ultrasound in Obstetrics and Gynecology. With permission of John Wiley & Sons Ltd.

		BINOCULAR				INTEROCULAR				OCULAR			
TABLE 23A		**MRI Reference Values for Binocular Diameter, Interocular Diameter, and Ocular Diameter by Gestational Age (mm)**											
GA	**#**	**MEAN**	**SD**	**MIN**	**MAX**	**MEAN**	**SD**	**MIN**	**MAX**	**MEAN**	**SD**	**MIN**	**MAX**
16	8	24.39	1.46	21.90	27.08	9.10	0.99	7.84	10.70	6.14	0.76	4.96	7.15
17	8	26.85	1.62	23.86	29.43	10.56	1.27	9.22	12.87	7.39	0.53	6.85	8.28
18	7	28.23	1.09	26.25	29.48	10.74	0.50	9.79	11.27	7.84	0.39	7.41	8.40
19	8	30.29	1.05	28.18	31.68	12.39	1.43	10.20	15.40	8.05	0.41	7.29	8.62
20	21	31.85	2.00	27.90	35.84	12.49	1.46	10.33	15.83	8.69	0.75	7.30	10.74
21	24	33.43	2.56	29.42	38.30	14.29	1.31	12.50	17.57	9.21	1.03	6.14	10.95
22	21	36.19	1.41	32.80	38.67	14.51	1.64	11.51	17.66	9.96	0.64	8.05	10.80
23	18	37.70	2.29	33.86	41.67	15.25	1.21	13.58	17.58	10.49	0.86	9.37	11.88
24	17	38.58	1.39	36.31	41.16	15.55	1.51	11.51	17.14	10.98	0.51	9.79	11.65
25	16	40.75	1.49	38.60	44.10	15.63	1.52	14.06	19.74	11.65	0.68	10.24	13.42
26	18	42.27	2.28	38.10	46.07	17.08	1.59	14.55	20.32	11.97	0.53	10.66	12.95
27	12	44.04	2.40	39.33	47.02	17.28	1.50	15.21	21.06	12.54	0.66	11.35	13.94
28	19	45.65	1.87	41.80	49.77	18.37	1.41	15.72	20.65	13.01	0.50	12.22	13.90
29	15	46.28	1.72	43.30	48.43	18.50	1.44	15.03	20.25	13.35	0.90	12.20	15.15
30	9	46.56	2.15	42.40	48.94	18.58	0.73	17.30	19.64	13.61	0.63	12.55	14.83
31	10	48.06	2.87	44.30	55.37	18.75	2.08	15.65	22.30	13.76	0.81	12.30	14.82
32	12	49.55	1.45	47.21	51.78	19.31	1.76	15.95	22.30	14.76	0.70	13.70	16.22
33	15	49.80	1.74	46.40	53.40	19.89	1.44	16.98	23.14	14.89	0.75	13.25	16.08
34	10	52.19	2.11	48.75	55.39	20.52	1.27	17.81	21.84	15.55	0.90	14.06	16.90
35	9	52.46	1.84	50.00	55.10	20.86	2.07	17.71	24.60	15.58	0.55	15.05	17.00
36	3	54.14	0.33	53.67	54.38	22.13	0.40	21.58	22.52	15.75	0.35	15.26	16.02
37+	4	56.48	1.85	53.79	59.00	23.53	1.96	21.37	26.65	16.00	0.60	15.00	16.60

Biometry from Ashley Robinson and Beth Kline-Fath.

TABLE 23B	MRI Reference Values for Binocular Diameter, Interocular Diameter, Ocular Diameter, and Volume by Gestational Age

	BOD		IOD		OD		VOLUME	
GA (wk)	MEAN (mm)	SD	MEAN (mm)	SD	MEAN (mm)	SD	MEAN (mL)	SD
19	29.51	—	13.00	—	9.36	—	0.32	—
20	31.34	1.77	13.02	0.03	9.76	0.64	0.34	0.06
21	32.28	1.33	13.84	1.28	10.17	0.38	0.39	0.05
22	35.77	1.88	14.03	0.98	11.56	0.48	0.56	0.06
23	36.08	1.39	15.43	0.84	11.72	0.92	0.54	0.08
24	37.52	0.65	16.00	1.15	12.18	0.53	0.67	0.07
25	42.88	—	17.22	—	13.37	—	0.80	—
26	42.08	1.09	16.60	0.77	13.81	0.52	0.98	0.10
27	42.97	1.40	17.13	0.83	13.79	0.68	1.02	0.16
28	45.27	1.36	17.73	0.63	14.77	0.63	1.20	0.09
29	46.19	1.48	17.69	0.96	15.07	0.50	1.36	0.19
30	46.65	1.12	17.58	0.54	15.40	0.62	1.38	0.10
31	47.37	1.46	18.44	1.56	15.76	0.96	1.38	0.09
32	48.31	2.95	18.80	2.18	15.58	0.46	1.47	0.09
33	50.75	2.32	18.84	2.03	17.05	0.67	1.78	0.12
34	51.54	2.26	20.10	0.18	16.64	0.81	1.80	0.12
35	53.61	1.95	20.33	1.02	17.37	0.70	2.07	0.23
36	53.17	1.14	20.50	1.29	17.18	0.39	2.05	0.07
37	52.80	1.28	19.61	1.23	17.66	0.45	2.12	0.14
38	55.47	0.18	21.51	0.69	18.22	1.00	2.15	0.23

Mean and standard deviation (SD) per gestational age (GA) week for normative binocular distance (BOD), interocular distance (IOD), ocular diameter (OD), and volume at each GA.
MRI, magnetic resonance imaging.
From Velasco-Annis C, Gholipour A, Afacan O, et al. Normative biometrics for fetal ocular growth using volumetric MRI reconstruction. *Prenat Diagn*. 2015:35:400–408.

TABLE 24	Ultrasound Reference Values for Mandible Length

	MANDIBLE LENGTH (mm)		
	PERCENTILES		
GA (wk)	5TH	50TH	95TH
15	11	14	18
16	13	17	20
17	15	19	22
18	17	21	24
19	19	23	26
20	21	25	28
21	23	26	30
22	25	28	32
23	27	30	33
24	28	32	35
25	30	33	37
26	31	35	38
27	33	36	40
28	34	38	41
29	36	39	43
30	37	41	44
31	39	42	45
32	40	43	47
33	41	45	48
34	42	46	49
35	43	47	50
36	44	48	51
37	45	49	52
38	46	50	53
39	47	51	54

Mandible length (mm) $= -20.41 + 2.97 \times GA - 0.027 \times GA^2$ (SD $= 2.077$).
GA, gestational age; MA, menstrual age.
Reproduced with permission from Otto C, Platt LD. The fetal mandible measurement: an objective determination of fetal jaw size. *Ultrasound Obstet Gynecol*. 1991;1:12–17.

TABLE 25	Ultrasound Reference Values for Length of Nasal Bone

	LENGTH OF NASAL BONE (mm)		
GA (wk)	−2 SD	MEAN	+2 SD
14	3.3	4.2	5.0
16	3.1	5.2	7.3
18	5.0	6.3	7.6
20	5.7	7.6	9.5
22	6.0	8.2	10.4
24	6.8	9.4	12.0
26	7.2	9.7	12.3
28	7.8	10.7	13.6
30	8.3	11.3	14.4
32	8.0	11.6	15.2
34	7.5	12.3	17.0

GA, gestational age.
Reproduced with permission from Guis F, Ville Y, Vincent Y, et al. Ultrasound evaluation of the length of the fetal nasal bones throughout gestation. *Ultrasound Obstet Gynecol*. 1995;5:304–307.

NECK AND CHEST MEASUREMENTS

		THYROID CIRCUMFERENCE BY PERCENTILE (cm)				
GESTATIONAL AGE (wk)	NUMBER OF PATIENTS	5TH	10TH	50TH	90TH	95TH
16	5	1.3	1.7	2.3	2.8	3.0
17	5	1.4	1.8	2.3	2.9	3.1
18	14	1.5	1.8	2.4	3.0	3.2
19	10	1.7	1.8	2.5	3.1	3.3
20	25	1.8	1.9	2.5	3.2	3.4
21	13	1.9	2.0	2.6	3.3	3.5
22	11	2.1	2.1	2.8	3.4	3.6
23	4	2.2	2.2	2.9	3.6	3.8
24	11	2.3	2.3	3.0	3.7	3.9
25	11	2.5	2.4	3.1	3.9	4.1
26	15	2.6	2.5	3.3	4.0	4.3
27	7	2.7	2.7	3.4	4.2	4.4
28	10	2.9	2.8	3.6	4.4	4.6
29	9	3.0	3.0	3.8	4.6	4.8
30	6	3.1	3.1	4.0	4.8	5.0
31	5	3.3	3.3	4.2	5.0	5.2
32	9	3.4	3.5	4.4	5.2	5.5
33	11	3.5	3.7	4.6	5.5	5.7
34	1	3.7	3.9	4.8	5.7	6.0
35	7	3.8	4.1	5.0	6.0	6.2
36	7	3.9	4.3	5.3	6.2	6.5
37	4	4.1	4.6	5.5	6.5	6.8

TABLE 26 Ultrasound Thyroid Circumference Based on Gestational Age

Reproduced from Ranzini AC, Ananth CV, Smulian JC, et al. Ultrasonography of the fetal thyroid: nomograms based on biparietal diameter and gestational age. *J Ultrasound Med.* 2001;20(6):613–617, with permission from the American Institute for Ultrasound in Medicine.

TABLE 27	Ultrasound Percentile Reference Values for Thoracic Circumference (cm)									
		PREDICTIVE PERCENTILES								
GA (wk)	*n*	**2.5TH**	**5TH**	**10TH**	**25TH**	**50TH**	**75TH**	**90TH**	**95TH**	**97.5TH**
16	6	5.9	6.4	7.0	8.0	9.1	10.3	11.3	11.9	12.4
17	22	6.8	7.3	7.9	8.9	10.0	11.2	12.2	12.8	13.3
18	31	7.7	8.2	8.8	9.8	11.0	12.1	13.1	13.7	14.2
19	21	8.6	9.1	9.7	10.7	11.9	13.0	14.0	14.6	15.1
20	20	9.5	10.0	10.6	11.7	12.8	13.9	15.0	15.5	16.0
21	30	10.4	11.0	11.6	12.6	13.7	14.8	15.8	16.4	16.9
22	18	11.3	11.9	12.5	13.5	14.6	15.7	16.7	17.3	17.8
23	21	12.2	12.8	13.4	14.4	15.5	16.6	17.6	18.2	18.8
24	27	13.2	13.7	14.3	15.3	16.4	17.5	18.5	19.1	19.7
25	20	14.1	14.6	15.2	16.2	17.3	18.4	19.4	20.0	20.6
26	25	15.0	15.5	16.1	17.1	18.2	19.3	20.3	21.0	21.5
27	24	15.9	16.4	17.0	18.0	19.1	20.2	21.3	21.9	22.4
28	24	16.8	17.3	17.9	18.9	20.0	21.2	22.2	22.8	23.3
29	24	17.7	18.2	18.8	19.8	21.0	22.1	23.1	23.7	24.2
30	27	18.6	19.1	19.7	20.7	21.9	23.0	24.0	24.6	25.1
31	24	19.5	20.0	20.6	21.6	22.8	23.9	24.9	25.5	26.0
32	28	20.4	20.9	21.5	22.6	23.7	24.8	25.8	26.4	26.9
33	27	21.3	21.8	22.5	23.5	24.6	25.7	26.7	27.3	27.8
34	25	22.2	22.8	23.4	24.4	25.5	26.6	27.6	28.2	28.7
35	20	23.1	23.7	24.3	25.3	26.4	27.5	28.5	29.1	29.6
36	23	24.0	24.6	25.2	26.2	27.3	28.4	29.4	30.0	30.6
37	22	24.9	25.5	26.1	27.1	28.2	29.3	30.3	30.9	31.5
38	21	25.9	26.4	27.0	28.0	29.1	30.2	31.2	31.9	32.4
39	7	26.8	27.3	27.9	28.9	30.0	31.1	32.2	32.8	33.3
40	6	27.7	28.2	28.8	29.8	30.9	32.1	33.1	33.7	34.2

GA, gestational age.
Reproduced with permission from Chitkara U, Rosenberg J, Chervenak FA, et al. Prenatal sonographic assessment of the fetal thorax: normal values. *Am J Obstet Gynecol*. 1987;156:1069–1074.

TABLE 28	3D Ultrasound Reference Values for Lung Volumes									
		RIGHT LUNG VOLUME (cm^3)			LEFT LUNG VOLUME (cm^3)			TOTAL LUNG VOLUME (cm^3)		
GA (wk)	n	10%	50%	90%	10%	50%	90%	10%	50%	90%
20	8	4.31	5.37	6.75	3.60	4.66	6.05	8.03	9.95	12.45
21	7	5.21	6.49	8.17	4.44	5.58	7.03	9.67	12.09	15.20
22	8	6.23	7.77	9.68	5.21	6.69	8.58	11.59	14.66	18.28
23	9	7.61	9.39	11.59	6.36	8.08	10.18	14.39	17.70	22.07
24	10	8.94	11.25	14.15	7.61	9.68	12.30	16.83	21.22	26.88
25	8	10.80	13.46	16.61	8.85	11.47	14.73	20.28	25.24	31.68
26	7	12.81	15.96	20.09	10.28	13.60	17.12	23.66	29.70	37.52
27	9	14.88	18.54	22.87	12.55	15.80	20.09	27.92	34.56	43.50
28	8	17.12	21.54	27.11	14.15	18.36	23.34	31.97	39.74	50.17
29	9	20.09	24.53	30.88	16.61	20.70	26.58	36.37	45.13	56.19
30	7	21.98	27.66	34.47	18.73	23.34	29.96	40.73	50.63	63.99
31	8	24.78	30.57	38.86	19.69	25.79	32.46	44.76	56.12	71.33
32	7	27.39	33.78	42.95	21.98	28.22	35.87	49.47	61.50	76.90
33	10	29.67	36.60	45.60	24.29	30.27	38.09	53.27	66.70	83.40
34	9	32.14	39.25	49.90	24.78	32.46	41.68	57.84	71.62	92.03
35	7	33.45	41.68	52.46	27.39	34.12	43.38	60.74	76.22	96.01
36	7	35.87	43.82	54.60	27.66	35.87	46.53	64.55	80.47	101.85
37	8	36.97	46.06	57.97	29.37	37.34	46.99	66.76	84.35	106.62

3D, three-dimensional; GA, gestational age.
Reproduced with permission from Ruano R, Joubin L, Aubry MC, et al. A nomogram of fetal lung volumes estimated by 3-dimentional ultrasonography using the rotational technique (virtual organ computer-aided analysis). *J Ultrasound Med.* 2006;25:701–709.

TABLE 29	3D Ultrasound Values for Right Lung Volume

		LUNG VOLUME (cm³)							
		PERCENTILES							
EFW (g)	*n*	2.5TH	5TH	10TH	50TH	90TH	95TH	97.5TH	SD
200	23	0.48	0.92	1.42	3.99	6.56	7.07	7.50	1.566
300	27	1.42	1.97	2.60	5.85	9.10	9.74	10.28	1.980
400	28	2.35	3.02	3.78	7.71	11.63	12.41	13.07	2.393
500	17	3.28	4.07	4.97	9.57	14.17	15.08	15.86	2.806
600	20	4.22	5.12	6.15	11.43	16.71	17.74	18.64	3.219
700	16	5.15	6.17	7.33	13.29	19.25	20.41	21.43	3.633
800	13	6.09	7.22	8.51	15.15	21.78	23.08	24.21	4.046
900	15	7.02	8.27	9.70	17.01	24.32	25.75	27.00	4.459
1,000	16	7.96	9.32	10.88	18.87	26.86	28.42	29.78	4.872
1,100	11	8.89	10.37	12.06	20.73	29.40	31.09	32.57	5.286
1,200	10	9.82	11.42	13.24	22.59	31.94	33.76	35.36	5.699
1,300	9	10.76	12.47	14.42	24.45	34.47	36.43	38.14	6.112
1,400	12	11.69	13.52	15.61	26.31	37.01	39.10	40.93	6.525
1,500	13	12.63	14.57	16.79	28.17	39.55	41.77	43.71	6.939
1,600	8	13.56	15.62	17.97	30.03	42.09	44.44	46.50	7.352
1,700	8	14.50	16.67	19.15	31.89	44.62	47.11	49.28	7.765
1,800	14	15.43	17.72	20.34	33.75	47.16	49.78	52.07	8.179
1,900	6	16.36	18.77	21.52	35.61	49.70	52.45	54.86	8.592
2,000	7	17.30	19.82	22.70	37.47	52.24	55.12	57.64	9.005
2,100	5	18.23	20.87	23.88	39.33	54.78	57.79	60.43	9.418
2,200	6	19.17	21.92	25.07	41.19	57.31	60.46	63.21	9.832
2,300	4	20.10	22.97	26.25	43.05	59.85	63.13	66.00	10.249
2,400	5	21.04	24.02	27.43	44.91	62.39	65.80	68.78	10.658

3D, three-dimensional; EFW, estimated fetal weight; SD, standard deviation.
Reproduced with permission from Gerards FA, Engels MAJ, Twisk JWR, et al. Normal fetal lung volume measured with three-dimensional ultrasound. *Ultrasound Obstet Gynecol*. 2006;27:134–144.

TABLE 30	3D Ultrasound Reference Values for the Left Lung Volume

LUNG VOLUME (cm³)

PERCENTILES

EFW (g)	n	2.5TH	5TH	10TH	50TH	90TH	95TH	97.5TH	SD
200	23	0.41	0.77	1.18	3.30	5.42	5.84	6.19	1.291
300	27	1.19	1.63	2.14	4.73	7.32	7.82	8.27	1.582
400	28	1.98	2.50	3.10	6.15	9.20	9.80	10.32	1.862
500	17	2.77	3.37	4.06	7.57	11.08	11.78	12.37	2.143
600	20	3.55	4.23	5.00	9.00	12.99	13.76	14.45	2.434
700	16	4.34	5.10	5.97	10.42	14.87	15.74	16.50	2.714
800	13	5.12	5.96	6.92	11.84	16.76	17.72	18.56	3.000
900	15	5.91	6.83	7.88	13.27	18.66	19.70	20.63	3.286
1,000	16	6.70	7.70	8.84	14.69	20.54	21.68	22.68	3.566
1,100	11	7.48	8.56	9.79	16.11	22.43	23.66	24.74	3.852
1,200	10	8.27	9.43	10.75	17.54	24.33	25.64	26.81	4.138
1,300	9	9.05	10.29	11.71	18.96	26.21	27.63	28.87	4.423
1,400	12	9.84	11.16	12.67	20.38	28.09	29.61	30.92	4.704
1,500	13	10.63	12.03	13.63	21.81	29.99	31.59	32.99	4.990
1,600	8	11.41	12.89	14.58	23.23	31.88	33.57	35.05	5.275
1,700	8	12.20	13.76	15.54	24.65	33.76	35.55	37.10	5.556
1,800	14	12.98	14.62	16.49	26.08	35.67	37.53	39.18	5.847
1,900	6	13.77	15.49	17.45	27.50	37.55	39.51	41.23	6.128
2,000	7	14.57	16.36	18.41	28.92	39.43	41.49	43.27	6.408
2,100	5	15.34	17.22	19.36	30.35	41.34	43.47	45.36	6.699
2,200	6	16.14	18.09	20.32	31.77	43.22	45.45	47.40	6.980
2,300	4	16.93	18.96	21.28	33.19	45.10	47.43	49.45	7.260
2,400	5	17.70	19.81	22.23	34.61	46.99	49.41	51.52	7.551

3D, three-dimensional; EFW, estimated fetal weight; SD, standard deviation.
Reproduced with permission from Gerards FA, Engels MA, Twisk JW, et al. Normal fetal lung volume measured with three-dimensional ultrasound. *Ultrasound Obstet Gynecol.* 2006;27:134–144.

TABLE 31 MRI Reference Values for Lung Volumes

GA (wk)	n	FLV RANGE (mL)	MEAN FLV (mL)	MEDIAN FLV (mL)	SD	SKEWNESS	95% CI
21.0–25.0	13	16–48	26.15	24	9.15	1.18	13.00–47.55
26.0–27.5	29	23–66	38.83	37	10.12	0.57	22.33–63.27
28.0–30.0	34	29–89	52.97	53	14.20	0.59	29.73–88.00
31.0–31.5	26	35–101	65.04	64	15.91	0.18	37.71–105.53
32.0	32	38–109	70.22	67.5	18.16	0.41	40.30–114.62
32.5–33.0	34	47–110	72.29	69	17.18	0.69	44.38–111.73
33.5–35.0	30	52–129	80.73	77.50	24.32	0.73	43.34–138.38
35.5–38.0	16	38–150	88.63	77.50	31.77	0.42	39.45–175.58

CI, confidence interval; FLV, fetal lung volume; MRI, magnetic resonance imaging; SD, standard deviation.
Reproduced with permission from Rypens F, Metens T, Rocourt N, et al. Fetal lung volume: estimation at MR Imaging—initial results. *Radiology.* 2001;219:236–241.

TABLE 32 MRI Reference Values for Fetal TLV from 18 to 38 weeks Gestation

GA (wk)	NUMBER OF PATIENTS	TOTAL FETAL LUNG VOLUME VALUES (mL)						
		MEAN	SD	MEDIAN	MINIMUM	MAXIMUM	LOWER QUARTILE	UPPER QUARTILE
18	13	11.1	2.2	10.9	6.7	13.7	9.7	13.2
19	27	12.4	2.5	12.5	7.2	17.1	10.9	13.7
20	32	15.5	3.9	15.4	6.8	25.6	12.6	18.3
21	43	17.4	5.0	17.0	7.8	29.8	14.1	19.6
22	52	20.4	4.9	20.0	8.3	32.3	18.0	23.8
23	56	24.1	6.1	24.3	11.0	45.5	19.7	27.5
24	45	28.8	7.6	26.7	15.0	58.4	24.0	32.0
25	47	31.6	7.2	31.0	15.6	46.2	26.3	37.4
26	31	34.8	6.7	36.5	22.5	44.2	29.0	40.3
27	33	40.3	10.2	40.6	21.3	58.5	32.2	46.1
28	40	48.8	15.8	46.5	22.6	81.6	36.8	58.1
29	31	54.2	13.8	57.3	23.5	81.6	43.7	62.8
30	37	63.3	14.0	60.6	33.4	92.9	56.7	72.2
31	35	66.2	19.1	66.1	25.2	114.3	54.9	78.1
32	33	74.3	22.0	71.8	46.7	142.7	56.5	86.3
33	30	75.2	24.1	71.6	31.8	126.6	59.9	83.3
34	26	93.8	27.2	94.7	36.6	141.8	72.5	115.9
35	27	93.6	27.0	94.3	49.9	159.5	68.2	109.5
36	16	86.9	27.6	74.4	54.4	151.2	71.4	102.8
37	9	85.5	20.9	80.6	53.4	121.7	72.7	99.8
38	2	98.8	3.9	98.8	96.0	10.16	96.0	101.6

MRI, magnetic resonance imaging; SD, standard deviation; TLV, total lung volume; GA, gestational age.
Reproduced with permission from Meyers ML, Garcia JR, Blough KL, et al. Fetal lung volumes by MRI: normal weekly values from 18 through 38 weeks' gestation. *Am J Roentgenol.* 2018;211:432–438; Rypens F, Metens T, Rocourt N, et al. Fetal lung volume: estimation at MR imaging—initial results. *Radiology.* 2001;219:236–241.

ABDOMINAL MEASUREMENTS

TABLE 33	Ultrasound Reference Values for Renal Length (mm)						
		PERCENTILES					
GA (wk)	*n*	**3RD**	**10TH**	**50TH**	**90TH**	**97TH**	**SD**[a]
14	3	7.5	8.0	9.3	10.8	11.6	0.12
15	3	8.8	9.5	11.0	12.8	13.7	0.12
16	2	10.2	11.0	12.7	14.8	15.8	0.12
17	12	11.6	12.5	14.5	16.8	18.1	0.12
18	10	13.1	14.1	16.3	18.9	20.3	0.12
19	15	14.6	15.6	18.2	21.1	22.6	0.12
20	15	16.1	17.2	20.0	23.2	24.9	0.12
21	15	17.5	18.8	21.8	25.4	27.2	0.12
22	14	19.0	20.4	23.6	27.4	29.4	0.12
23	16	20.4	21.9	25.4	29.5	31.6	0.12
24	17	21.8	23.4	27.1	31.5	33.8	0.12
25	18	23.1	24.8	28.8	33.4	35.8	0.12
26	20	24.4	26.2	30.4	35.3	37.8	0.12
27	24	25.6	27.5	31.9	37.1	39.7	0.12
28	18	26.8	28.7	33.4	38.7	41.5	0.12
29	19	27.9	29.9	34.7	40.3	43.2	0.12
30	19	28.9	31.0	36.0	41.8	44.8	0.12
31	23	29.9	32.1	37.2	43.2	46.3	0.12
32	23	30.8	33.0	38.3	44.5	47.7	0.12
33	22	31.6	33.9	39.4	45.7	49.0	0.12
34	19	32.4	34.7	40.3	46.8	50.2	0.12
35	20	33.1	35.4	41.1	47.8	51.2	0.12
36	23	33.7	36.1	41.9	48.7	52.2	0.12
37	14	34.2	36.7	42.6	49.4	53.0	0.12
38	17	34.7	37.2	43.2	50.1	53.8	0.12
39	13	35.1	37.6	43.7	50.7	54.4	0.12
40	14	35.4	38.0	44.1	51.2	54.9	0.12
41	26	35.7	38.3	44.5	51.6	55.4	0.12
42	17	36.0	38.6	44.8	52.0	55.7	0.12

[a]Denotes standard deviation of log of measurement (constant).
GA, gestational age; SD, standard deviation.
Reproduced with permission from Chitty LS, Altman DG. Charts of fetal size: kidney and renal pelvis measurements. *Prenat Diagn*. 2003;23:891–897.

TABLE 34	MRI Reference Values for Mean Renal Length				
GA (wk)	MEAN KIDNEY LENGTH (mm)	STANDARD DEVIATION (mm)	95% CONFIDENCE INTERVAL, LOWER LIMIT (mm)	95% CONFIDENCE INTERVAL, UPPER LIMIT (mm)	NUMBER OF INVESTIGATED CASES
16	13.54	—	—	—	1
17	18.56	—	—	—	1
18	16.55	1.66	11.19	21.47	4
19	17.29	2.06	12.52	22.79	5
20	19.50	1.47	13.86	24.11	12
21	20.29	1.80	15.19	25.43	14
22	20.86	1.60	16.53	26.76	12
23	22.22	2.13	17.86	28.08	15
24	24.11	1.13	19.19	29.41	14
25	25.13	3.35	20.53	30.74	12
26	26.20	2.55	21.86	32.07	12
27	29.41	1.72	23.19	33.40	12
28	30.68	2.83	24.52	34.73	18
29	31.64	3.51	25.85	36.06	12
30	31.19	1.45	27.17	37.39	6
31	33.91	3.54	28.50	38.72	13
32	35.34	2.35	29.83	40.05	14
33	37.31	2.47	31.15	41.39	8
34	35.78	3.49	32.47	42.72	10
35	38.23	3.91	33.80	44.06	10
36	41.19	3.06	35.12	45.39	5
37	42.52	0.89	36.44	46.73	3
38	42.55	4.01	37.76	48.07	2
39	43.09	2.43	39.08	49.41	3

GA, gestational age
From Witzani L, Brugger PC, Hörmann M. Normal renal development investigated with fetal MRI. *Eur J Radiol*. 2006;57:294–302.

TABLE 35	MRI Reference Values for Adrenal Length and Thickness Based on Gestational Age				
	LENGTH (mm)		THICKNESS (mm)		
GA GROUP (wk)	MEAN (SD)	RANGE	MEAN (SD)	RANGE	
18–22	8.2 (1.50)	5.5–14.2	1.8 (0.29)	1.2–3.1	
23–26	8.9 (1.48)	6.1–12.4	1.8 (0.30)	1.0–2.7	
27–30	10.0 (1.74)	6.0–15.1	1.9 (0.40)	1.0–3.6	
31–34	9.6 (1.14)	8.1–12.6	2.0 (0.37)	1.3–2.9	
35–37	11.0 (1.87)	8.7–14.0	2.4 (0.57)	1.7–3.1	

GA, gestational age; MRI, magnetic resonance imaging; SD, standard deviation.
Reproduced from Smitthimedhin A, Rubio EI, Blask AR et al Normal size of the fetal adrenal gland on prenatal MRI. *Pediatr Radiol*. 2020. Pediatr Radiol 2020. [Epub ahead of print]

TABLE 36A		Ultrasound Reference Values for Fetal Penile Length		
95%	**5%**	**MEAN (cm)**	*n*	**GA (wk)**
1.32	0.40	0.86	8	22
1.40	0.48	0.94	5	23
1.47	0.56	1.02	6	24
1.55	0.64	1.09	5	25
1.62	0.71	1.17	6	26
1.70	0.79	1.25	6	27
1.78	0.87	1.32	6	28
1.85	0.95	1.40	6	29
1.93	1.02	1.47	8	30
2.00	1.10	1.55	7	31
2.08	1.17	1.63	8	32
2.16	1.25	1.70	7	33
2.24	1.33	1.78	6	34
2.31	1.40	1.86	10	35
2.39	1.48	1.93	6	36

GA, gestational age
Reference values for fetal penile measurement.
Danon D, Ben-Shitrit G, Bardin R, et al. Reference values for fetal penile length and width from 22 to 36 gestational weeks. *Prenat Diagn*. 2012;32:829–832.

TABLE 36B		Ultrasound Reference Values for Fetal Penile Width		
95%	**5%**	**MEAN (cm)**	*n*	**GA (wk)**
0.82	0.38	0.60	8	22
0.86	0.43	0.65	5	23
0.91	0.47	0.69	6	24
0.95	0.51	0.73	5	25
0.99	0.56	0.78	6	26
1.04	0.60	0.82	6	27
1.08	0.65	0.86	6	28
1.12	0.69	0.91	6	29
1.17	0.73	0.95	8	30
1.21	0.78	0.99	7	31
1.25	0.82	1.04	8	32
1.30	0.86	1.08	7	33
1.34	0.90	1.12	6	34
1.38	0.95	1.17	10	35
1.43	0.99	1.21	6	36

GA, gestational age.
Reference values for fetal penile measurement.
Danon D, Ben-Shitrit G, Bardin R, et al. Reference values for fetal penile length and width from 22 to 36 weeks gestational weeks. *Prenat Diagn*. 2012;32:829–832.

TABLE 37	Normal Ultrasound Colon Diameters		
	COLON DIAMETERS (mm)		
GA (wk)	**−2 SD**	**MEAN**	**+2 SD**
22	2	4	6
24	3	5	7
26	4	6	9
28	4	7	10
30	5	8	11
32	6	9	12
34	7	10	13
36	8	12	16
38	9	14	18
40	10	16	20

SD, standard deviation; GA, gestational age.
Data adapted from Harris RD, Nyberg DA, Mack LA, et al. Anorectal atresia: prenatal sonographic diagnosis. *AJR Am J Roentgenol*. 1987;149:395–400.

DOPPLER ULTRASOUND

TABLE 38	Doppler Ultrasound Intervals for Mean Uterine Artery Pulsatility Index		

	PERCENTILES		
GA (wk)	5TH	50TH	95TH
11	1.18	1.79	2.7
12	1.11	1.68	2.53
13	1.05	1.58	2.38
14	0.99	1.49	2.24
15	0.94	1.41	2.11
16	0.89	1.33	1.99
17	0.85	1.27	1.88
18	0.81	1.2	1.79
19	0.78	1.15	1.7
20	0.74	1.1	1.61
21	0.71	1.05	1.54
22	0.69	1	1.47
23	0.66	0.96	1.41
24	0.64	0.93	1.35
25	0.62	0.89	1.3
26	0.6	0.86	1.25
27	0.58	0.84	1.21
28	0.56	0.81	1.17
29	0.55	0.79	1.13
30	0.54	0.77	1.1
31	0.52	0.75	1.06
32	0.51	0.73	1.04
33	0.5	0.71	1.01
34	0.5	0.7	0.99
35	0.49	0.69	0.97
36	0.48	0.68	0.95
37	0.48	0.67	0.94
38	0.47	0.66	0.92
39	0.47	0.65	0.91
40	0.47	0.65	0.9
41	0.47	0.65	0.89

GA, gestational age.
Reproduced with permission from Gómez O, Figueras F, Fernández S, et al. Reference ranges for uterine artery mean pulsatility index at 11–41 weeks of gestation. *Ultrasound Obstet Gynecol.* 2008;32(2):128–132.

TABLE 39	Doppler Ultrasound Values for Umbilical Artery S/D Ratio							
	PERCENTILES							
GA (wk)	**2.5TH**	**5TH**	**10TH**	**25TH**	**50TH**	**75TH**	**90TH**	**95TH**	**97.5TH**
19	2.73	2.93	3.19	3.67	4.28	5	5.75	6.26	6.73
20	2.63	2.83	3.07	3.53	4.11	4.8	5.51	5.99	6.43
21	2.51	2.7	2.93	3.36	3.91	4.55	5.22	5.67	6.09
22	2.43	2.6	2.83	3.24	3.77	4.38	5.03	5.45	5.85
23	2.34	2.51	2.72	3.11	3.62	4.21	4.82	5.22	5.61
24	2.25	2.41	2.62	2.99	3.48	4.04	4.63	5.02	5.38
25	2.17	2.33	2.52	2.88	3.35	3.89	4.45	4.83	5.18
26	2.09	2.24	2.43	2.78	3.23	3.75	4.3	4.66	5
27	2.02	2.17	2.35	2.69	3.12	3.63	4.15	4.5	4.83
28	1.95	2.09	2.27	2.6	3.02	3.51	4.02	4.36	4.67
29	1.89	2.03	2.2	2.52	2.92	3.4	3.89	4.22	4.53
30	1.83	1.96	2.13	2.44	2.83	3.3	3.78	4.1	4.4
31	1.77	1.9	2.06	2.36	2.75	3.2	3.67	3.98	4.27
32	1.71	1.84	2	2.29	2.67	3.11	3.57	3.87	4.16
33	1.66	1.79	1.94	2.23	2.6	3.03	3.48	3.77	4.06
34	1.61	1.73	1.88	2.16	2.53	2.95	3.39	3.68	3.96
35	1.57	1.68	1.83	2.11	2.46	2.87	3.3	3.59	3.86
36	1.52	1.64	1.78	2.05	2.4	2.8	3.23	3.51	3.78
37	1.48	1.59	1.73	2	2.34	2.74	3.15	3.43	3.69
38	1.44	1.55	1.69	1.95	2.28	2.67	3.08	3.36	3.62
39	1.4	1.51	1.64	1.9	2.23	2.61	3.02	3.29	3.54
40	1.36	1.47	1.6	1.85	2.18	2.56	2.96	3.22	3.48
41	1.33	1.43	1.56	1.81	2.13	2.5	2.9	3.16	3.41

GA, gestational age; S/D, systolic-to-atrial.
Reproduced from Acharya G, Wilsgaard T, Berntsen GK, et al. Reference ranges for serial measurements of umbilical artery Doppler indices in the second half of pregnancy. *Am J Obstet Gynecol.* 2005;192(3):937–944.

TABLE 40	Doppler Ultrasound Values for Umbilical Artery Pulsatility Index							
	PERCENTILES							
GA (wk)	**2.5TH**	**5TH**	**10TH**	**25TH**	**50TH**	**75TH**	**90TH**	**95TH**	**97.5TH**
19	0.97	1.02	1.08	1.18	1.3	1.44	1.57	1.66	1.74
20	0.94	0.99	1.04	1.14	1.27	1.4	1.54	1.62	1.7
21	0.9	0.95	1	1.1	1.22	1.36	1.49	1.58	1.65
22	0.87	0.92	0.97	1.07	1.19	1.32	1.46	1.54	1.62
23	0.84	0.89	0.94	1.04	1.15	1.29	1.42	1.5	1.58
24	0.81	0.86	0.91	1	1.12	1.25	1.38	1.47	1.55
25	0.78	0.83	0.88	0.97	1.09	1.22	1.35	1.44	1.51
26	0.76	0.8	0.85	0.94	1.06	1.19	1.32	1.41	1.48
27	0.73	0.77	0.82	0.92	1.03	1.16	1.29	1.38	1.45
28	0.71	0.75	0.8	0.89	1	1.13	1.26	1.35	1.43
29	0.68	0.72	0.77	0.86	0.98	1.1	1.23	1.32	1.4
30	0.66	0.7	0.75	0.84	0.95	1.08	1.21	1.29	1.37
31	0.64	0.68	0.73	0.82	0.93	1.05	1.18	1.27	1.35
32	0.62	0.66	0.7	0.79	0.9	1.03	1.16	1.25	1.32
33	0.6	0.64	0.68	0.77	0.88	1.01	1.14	1.22	1.3
34	0.58	0.62	0.66	0.75	0.86	0.99	1.12	1.2	1.28
35	0.56	0.6	0.64	0.73	0.84	0.97	1.09	1.18	1.26
36	0.54	0.58	0.63	0.71	0.82	0.95	1.07	1.16	1.24
37	0.53	0.56	0.61	0.69	0.8	0.93	1.05	1.14	1.22
38	0.51	0.55	0.59	0.68	0.78	0.91	1.04	1.12	1.2
39	0.49	0.53	0.57	0.66	0.76	0.89	1.02	1.1	1.18
40	0.48	0.51	0.56	0.64	0.75	0.87	1	1.09	1.17
41	0.47	0.5	0.54	0.63	0.73	0.85	0.98	1.07	1.15

GA, gestational age.
Reproduced from Acharya G, Wilsgaard T, Berntsen GK, et al. Reference ranges for serial measurements of umbilical artery Doppler indices in the second half of pregnancy. *Am J Obstet Gynecol.* 2005;192:937–944.

TABLE 41	Doppler Ultrasound Values for Umbilical Artery Resistance Index								
	PERCENTILES								
GA (wk)	**2.5TH**	**5TH**	**10TH**	**25TH**	**50TH**	**75TH**	**90TH**	**95TH**	**97.5TH**
19	0.64	0.66	0.68	0.72	0.77	0.81	0.85	0.88	0.9
20	0.63	0.65	0.67	0.71	0.75	0.8	0.84	0.87	0.89
21	0.62	0.64	0.66	0.7	0.74	0.79	0.83	0.85	0.88
22	0.6	0.62	0.65	0.68	0.73	0.78	0.82	0.84	0.87
23	0.59	0.61	0.63	0.67	0.72	0.76	0.81	0.83	0.86
24	0.58	0.6	0.62	0.66	0.71	0.75	0.8	0.82	0.85
25	0.56	0.58	0.61	0.65	0.69	0.74	0.79	0.81	0.84
26	0.55	0.57	0.59	0.64	0.68	0.73	0.78	0.8	0.83
27	0.54	0.56	0.58	0.62	0.67	0.72	0.77	0.79	0.82
28	0.53	0.55	0.57	0.61	0.66	0.71	0.76	0.78	0.81
29	0.51	0.53	0.56	0.6	0.65	0.7	0.75	0.77	0.8
30	0.5	0.52	0.54	0.59	0.64	0.69	0.74	0.76	0.79
31	0.49	0.51	0.53	0.58	0.63	0.68	0.73	0.76	0.78
32	0.47	0.5	0.52	0.56	0.61	0.67	0.72	0.75	0.77
33	0.46	0.48	0.51	0.55	0.6	0.66	0.71	0.74	0.77
34	0.45	0.47	0.5	0.54	0.59	0.65	0.7	0.73	0.76
35	0.44	0.46	0.48	0.53	0.58	0.64	0.69	0.72	0.75
36	0.42	0.45	0.47	0.52	0.57	0.63	0.68	0.71	0.74
37	0.41	0.43	0.46	0.51	0.56	0.62	0.67	0.7	0.73
38	0.4	0.42	0.45	0.5	0.55	0.61	0.66	0.7	0.73
39	0.39	0.41	0.44	0.48	0.54	0.6	0.65	0.69	0.72
40	0.38	0.4	0.43	0.47	0.53	0.59	0.65	0.68	0.71
41	0.36	0.39	0.41	0.46	0.52	0.58	0.64	0.67	0.7

GA, gestational age.
Reproduced with permission from Acharya G, Wilsgaard T, Berntsen GK, et al. Reference ranges for serial measurements of umbilical artery Doppler indices in the second half of pregnancy. *Am J Obstet Gynecol*. 2005;192:937–944.

TABLE 42	Doppler Ultrasound Values for Peak Systolic Velocity of the Middle Cerebral Artery				
	PSV MCA (cm/s)				
	MULTIPLES OF THE MEDIAN				
GA (wk)	**1**	**1.3**	**1.5**	**1.7**	**2**
15	20	26	30	34	40
16	21	27	32	36	42
17	22	29	33	37	44
18	23	30	35	39	46
19	24	31	36	41	48
20	25	33	38	43	50
21	26	34	39	44	52
22	28	36	42	48	56
23	29	38	44	49	58
24	30	39	45	51	60
25	32	42	48	54	64
26	33	43	50	56	66
27	35	46	53	60	70
28	37	48	56	63	74
29	38	49	57	65	76
30	40	52	60	68	80
31	42	55	63	71	84
32	44	57	66	75	88
33	46	60	69	78	92
34	48	62	72	82	96
35	50	65	75	85	100
36	53	69	80	90	106
37	55	72	83	94	110
38	58	75	87	99	116
39	61	79	92	104	122
40	63	82	95	107	126

Peak systolic velocity (cm/s) = $e^{(2.31 + 0.046 \times GA)}$.

GA, gestational age; PSV, peak systolic velocity; MCA, middle cerebral artery.
Reproduced with permission from Mari G, Deter RL, Carpenter RL, et al. Noninvasive diagnosis by Doppler ultrasonography of fetal anemia due to maternal red-cell alloimmunization. Collaborative Group for Doppler Assessment of the Blood Velocity in Anemic Fetuses. *N Engl J Med*. 2000;342:9–14.

TABLE 43	Doppler Ultrasound Middle Cerebral Artery Pulsatility Index				
	MCA PI				
	PERCENTILES				
GA (wk)	**5TH**	**10TH**	**50TH**	**90TH**	**95TH**
21	1.18	1.26	1.6	2.04	2.19
22	1.25	1.33	1.69	0.15	2.30
23	1.32	1.41	1.78	2.25	2.41
24	1.38	1.47	1.86	2.36	2.52
25	1.44	1.54	1.94	2.45	2.62
26	1.50	1.6	2.01	2.53	2.71
27	1.55	1.65	2.06	2.60	2.78
28	1.58	1.69	2.11	2.66	2.84
29	1.61	1.71	2.15	2.70	2.88
30	1.62	1.73	2.16	2.72	2.90
31	1.62	1.73	2.16	2.71	2.90
32	1.61	1.71	2.14	2.69	2.87
33	1.58	1.68	2.10	2.64	2.82
34	1.53	1.63	2.04	2.57	2.74
35	1.47	1.56	1.96	2.47	2.64
36	1.39	1.48	1.86	2.36	2.52
37	1.30	1.39	1.75	2.22	2.38
38	1.20	1.29	1.63	2.07	2.22
39	1.1	1.18	1.49	1.91	2.05

GA, gestational age; MCA, middle cerebral artery; PI, pulsatility index.
Reproduced with permission from Ebbing C, Rasmussen S, Kiserud T. Middle cerebral artery blood flow velocities and pulsatility index and the cerebroplacental pulsatility ratio: longitudinal reference ranges and terms for serial measurements. *Ultrasound Obstet Gynecol*. 2007;30:287–296.

| TABLE 44 | Doppler Ultrasound Pulsatility Index in the Umbilical and Middle Cerebral Arteries and Cerebroplacental Doppler Ratio |

		UA		MCA		CPR	
GA (wk)	n	MEAN	SD	MEAN	SD	MEAN	SD
20	25	1.31	0.26	1.76	0.24	1.37	0.40
21	15	1.27	0.18	1.79	0.20	1.44	0.25
22	9	1.28	0.17	1.87	0.33	1.48	0.29
23	11	1.12	0.12	1.65	0.16	1.49	0.23
24	21	1.21	0.14	1.85	0.21	1.53	0.22
25	13	1.13	0.16	2.03	0.41	1.83	0.48
26	14	1.11	0.13	2.09	0.43	1.92	0.55
27	17	1.07	0.17	2.18	0.68	2.12	0.61
28	17	1.05	0.13	2.21	0.41	2.13	0.52
29	17	1.11	0.19	2.02	0.31	1.86	0.43
30	12	1.04	0.23	2.34	0.33	2.34	0.55
31	19	0.99	0.13	2.21	0.31	2.29	0.34
32	10	0.93	0.19	1.81	0.19	2.03	0.48
33	17	0.92	0.17	1.90	0.38	2.10	0.40
34	21	0.89	0.13	1.79	0.27	2.10	0.45
35	13	0.91	0.11	1.81	0.31	2.01	0.34
36	19	0.93	0.18	1.80	0.27	2.01	0.46
37	6	0.95	0.24	2.06	0.68	2.25	0.66
38	11	0.89	0.16	1.66	0.30	1.90	0.41
39	8	1.01	0.17	1.64	0.26	1.64	0.29
40	11	0.75	0.16	1.29	0.21	1.80	0.44

CPR, cerebroplacental Doppler ratio; UA, umbilical artery; MCA, middle cerebral artery; GA, gestational age; SD, standard deviation.
Reproduced with permission from Baschat AA, Gembruch U. The cerebroplacental Doppler ratio revisited. *Ultrasound Obstet Gynecol.* 2003;21:124–127.

| TABLE 45 | Doppler Ultrasound Ranges for the Systolic-to-Atrial Ratio of the Ductus Venosus |

	PERCENTILES		
GA (wk)	5TH	MEAN	95TH
14	3.583	4.497	5.78
15	3.153	4.047	5.304
16	2.767	3.641	4.871
17	2.44	3.295	4.497
18	2.171	3.007	4.182
19	1.955	2.771	3.919
20	1.785	2.582	3.703
21	1.654	2.432	3.526
22	1.557	2.315	3.381
23	1.486	2.225	3.264
24	1.437	2.157	3.169
25	1.406	2.107	3.092
26	1.389	2.07	3.028
27	1.382	2.044	2.974
28	1.383	2.025	2.929
29	1.39	2.013	2.889
30	1.401	2.005	2.854
31	1.415	1.999	2.821
32	1.431	1.996	2.791
33	1.449	1.994	2.762
34	1.467	1.993	2.734
35	1.486	1.993	2.706
36	1.505	1.993	2.678
37	1.524	1.992	2.651
38	1.543	1.992	2.624
39	1.563	1.992	2.597
40	1.582	1.992	2.57
41	1.601	1.992	2.542

GA, gestational age.
Modified from Bahlmann F, Wellek S, Reinhardt I, et al. Reference values of ductus venosus flow velocities and calculated waveform indices. *Prenat Diagn.* 2000;20:623–634.

TABLE 46	Doppler Ultrasound Ranges for the Pulsatility Index for Veins (PIV) of the Ductus Venosus								
	PERCENTILES								
GA (wk)	**2.5TH**	**5TH**	**10TH**	**25TH**	**50TH**	**75TH**	**90TH**	**95TH**	**97.5TH**
21	0.27	0.32	0.38	0.47	0.57	0.68	0.77	0.83	0.88
22	0.28	0.32	0.38	0.47	0.57	0.68	0.77	0.83	0.88
23	0.28	0.32	0.38	0.47	0.57	0.68	0.77	0.83	0.88
24	0.27	0.32	0.38	0.47	0.57	0.68	0.77	0.83	0.88
25	0.27	0.32	0.37	0.47	0.57	0.67	0.77	0.83	0.88
26	0.27	0.31	0.37	0.46	0.57	0.67	0.77	0.82	0.87
27	0.26	0.31	0.36	0.46	0.56	0.67	0.76	0.82	0.87
28	0.26	0.31	0.36	0.45	0.56	0.66	0.76	0.81	0.86
29	0.25	0.30	0.35	0.45	0.55	0.65	0.75	0.81	0.86
30	0.25	0.29	0.35	0.44	0.54	0.65	0.74	0.80	0.85
31	0.24	0.28	0.34	0.43	0.53	0.64	0.73	0.79	0.84
32	0.23	0.28	0.33	0.42	0.53	0.63	0.73	0.78	0.83
33	0.22	0.27	0.32	0.41	0.52	0.62	0.72	0.77	0.82
34	0.21	0.26	0.31	0.40	0.51	0.61	0.71	0.76	0.81
35	0.20	0.25	0.30	0.39	0.50	0.60	0.70	0.75	0.80
36	0.19	0.24	0.29	0.38	0.49	0.59	0.69	0.74	0.79
37	0.18	0.23	0.28	0.37	0.48	0.58	0.67	0.73	0.78
38	0.17	0.22	0.27	0.36	0.46	0.57	0.66	0.72	0.77
39	0.16	0.21	0.26	0.35	0.45	0.56	0.65	0.71	0.76

GA, gestational age; PIA, pulsatility index for veins.
Modified from Kessler J, Rasmussen S, Hanson M, et al. Longitudinal reference ranges for ductus venosus flow velocities and waveform indices. *Ultrasound Obstet Gynecol.* 2006;28:890–898.

ANEUPLOIDY TABLES

TABLE 47	Comparison of Likelihood Ratios for Sonographic Markers of Fetal Aneuploidy		
SONOGRAPHIC MARKER	**NYBERG ET AL.[a]** LIKELIHOOD RATIOS (95% CI)	**BROMLEY ET AL.[b]** LIKELIHOOD RATIOS	**SMITH-BINDMAN ET AL.[c]** LIKELIHOOD RATIOS (95% CI)
Nuchal thickening	11.0 (5.5–22.0)	12	17 (8–38)
Hyperechoic bowel	6.7 (2.7–16.8)	—	6.1 (3–12.6)
Short humerus	5.1 (1.6–16.5)	6	7.5 (4.7–12)
Short femur	1.5 (0.8–2.8)	1	2.7 (1.2–6)
Echogenic intracardiac focus	1.8 (1.0–3.0)	1.2	2.8 (1.5–5.5)
Pyelectasis	1.5 (0.6–3.6)	1.3	1.9 (0.7–5.1)
Normal ultrasound	0.36	0.2	—

CI, confidence interval.

[a]Reproduced with permission from Nyberg DA, Souter VL, El-Bastawissi A, et al. Isolated sonographic markers for detection of fetal Down syndrome in the second trimester of pregnancy. *J Ultrasound Med*. 2001;20:1053–1063.

[b]Reproduced with permission from Bromley B, Lieberman E, Shipp T, et al. The genetic sonogram: a method of risk assessment for Down syndrome in the mid-trimester. *J Ultrasound Med*. 2002;21:1087–1096.

[c]Reproduced with permission from Smith-Bindman R, Hosmer W, Feldstein VA, et al. Second-trimester ultrasound to detect fetuses with Down syndrome: a meta-analysis. *JAMA*. 2001;285:1044–1055.

| TABLE 48 | Maternal Age–Specific Odds (1:___) of Fetal Down Syndrome during the Second Trimester Based on Sonographic Markers of Fetal Aneuploidy | | | | | | | |

MATERNAL AGE (wk)	PREULTRASOUND ODDS (1:__)	NORMAL ULTRASOUND (1:__) LR 0.36	NUCHAL THICKNESS (1:__) LR 11.0	HYPERECHOIC BOWEL (1:__) LR 6.7	SHORT FEMUR LENGTH (1:__) LR 1.5	SHORT HUMERUS LENGTH (1:__) LR 5.1	ECHOGENIC INTRACARDIAC FOCUS (1:__) LR 1.8	RENAL PELVIS (1:__) LR 1.5
20	1,176	3,265	108	176	784	231	654	784
21	1,160	3,220	106	174	774	228	645	774
22	1,136	3,154	104	170	758	224	632	758
23	1,114	3,093	102	167	743	219	619	743
24	1,087	3,018	100	163	725	214	604	725
25	1,040	2,887	95	156	694	205	578	694
26	990	2,748	91	149	660	195	550	660
27	928	2,576	85	139	619	183	516	619
28	855	2,373	79	128	570	168	475	570
29	760	2,109	70	114	507	150	423	507
30	690	1,915	64	104	460	136	384	460
31	597	1,657	55	90	398	118	332	398
32	508	1,409	47	77	339	100	283	339
33	421	1,168	39	64	281	83	234	281
34	342	948	32	52	228	68	190	228
35	274	759	26	42	183	55	153	183
36	216	598	21	33	144	43	120	144
37	168	465	16	26	112	34	94	112
38	129	357	13	20	86	26	72	86
39	98	270	10	15	66	20	55	66
40	74	204	8	12	50	15	42	50
41	56	154	6	9	38	12	32	38
42	42	115	5	7	28	9	24	28
43	31	84	4	5	21	7	18	21
44	23	62	3	4	16	5	13	16

Assuming LRs of Nyberg et al. in Table 58.
Odds ratio (O) based on formula O (Down syndrome) = O (maternal age)/LR + 1 − 1/LR.
LR, likelihood ratio.
Reproduced with permission from Nyberg DA, Souter VL, El-Bastawissi A, et al. Isolated sonographic markers for detection of fetal Down syndrome in the second trimester of pregnancy. *J Ultrasound Med.* 2001;20:1053–1063.

Note: Page numbers followed by *f* denote figures; those followed by *t* denote tables.

CCS0420